PART ONE Basic Concepts of Pathophysiology

UNIT 1 The Cell
1. Cellular Biology, 1
2. Genes and Genetic Diseases, 38
3. Epigenetics and Disease, 62
4. Altered Cellular and Tissue Biology, 72
5. Fluids and Electrolytes, Acids and Bases, 112

UNIT 2 Mechanisms of Self-Defence
6. Innate Immunity: Inflammation and Wound Healing, 133
7. Adaptive Immunity, 157
8. Infection and Defects in Mechanisms of Defence, 176
9. Stress and Disease, 215

UNIT 3 Cellular Proliferation: Cancer
10. Biology of Cancer, 233
11. Cancer Epidemiology, 266
12. Cancer in Children and Adolescents, 294

PART TWO Body Systems and Diseases

UNIT 4 The Neurological System
13. Structure and Function of the Neurological System, 299
14. Pain, Temperature, Sleep, and Sensory Function, 328
15. Alterations in Cognitive Systems, Cerebral Hemodynamics, and Motor Function, 351
16. Disorders of the Central and Peripheral Nervous Systems and Neuromuscular Junction, 382
17. Developmental Alterations of Neurological Function, 411

UNIT 5 The Endocrine System
18. Mechanisms of Hormonal Regulation, 426
19. Alterations of Hormonal Regulation, 447

UNIT 6 The Hematological System
20. Structure and Function of the Hematological System, 477
21. Alterations of Hematological Function, 500
22. Developmental Alterations of Hematological Function, 537

UNIT 7 The Cardiovascular and Lymphatic Systems
23. Structure and Function of the Cardiovascular and Lymphatic Systems, 551
24. Alterations of Cardiovascular Function, 579
25. Developmental Alterations of Cardiovascular Function, 637

UNIT 8 The Pulmonary System
26. Structure and Function of the Pulmonary System, 653
27. Alterations of Pulmonary Function, 669
28. Developmental Alterations of Pulmonary Function, 701

UNIT 9 The Renal and Urological Systems
29. Structure and Function of the Renal and Urological Systems, 713
30. Alterations of Renal and Urinary Tract Function, 730
31. Developmental Alterations of Renal and Urinary Tract Function, 756

UNIT 10 The Reproductive Systems
32. Structure and Function of the Reproductive Systems, 763
33. Alterations of the Female Reproductive System, 785
34. Alterations of the Male Reproductive System, 832

UNIT 11 The Digestive System
35. Structure and Function of the Digestive System, 861
36. Alterations of Digestive Function, 882
37. Developmental Alterations of Digestive Function, 927

UNIT 12 The Musculoskeletal and Integumentary Systems
38. Structure and Function of the Musculoskeletal System, 942
39. Alterations of Musculoskeletal Function, 964
40. Developmental Alterations of Musculoskeletal Function, 1007
41. Structure, Function, and Disorders of the Integument, 1021
42. Developmental Alterations of the Integument, 1053

Appendix, 1064
Index, 1081

HEALTH PROMOTION BOXES

Gene Therapy, 58
Low-Level Lead Exposure Harms Children: A Renewed Call for Primary Prevention, 87
Low-Risk Alcohol Drinking Guidelines, 91
Cannabis and Canada's Youth, 92
Hyponatremia and Older Persons, 120
Potassium Intake: Hypertension and Stroke, 122
Tuberculosis and the Indigenous Population in Canada, 178
Risk of HIV Transmission Associated With Sexual Practices, 196
Glucocorticoids, Insulin, Inflammation, and Obesity, 221
Psychosocial Stress and Progression to Coronary Heart Disease, 222
Stress and the Gut–Brain Axis, 223
Acute Emotional Stress and Adverse Heart Effects, 228
Partner's Survival and Spouse's Hospitalizations and/or Death, 228
World Health Organization Cancer Prevention Strategies, 272
Magnetic Fields and Development of Pediatric Cancer, 297
Bone Marrow Transplantation: Improving Outcomes for Canadian Children and Adolescent Cancer Patients, 298
Neuroplasticity, 304
Reducing Risk Factors Associated With Alzheimer's Disease, 365
Tourette Syndrome, 371
Prevention of Stroke in Women, 395
West Nile Virus, 402
Prevention of Fetal Alcohol Spectrum Disorders, 412
Growth Hormone Supplementation in Aging, 432
Vitamin D, 438
Type 1 Diabetes Mellitus, 462
Type 2 Diabetes Mellitus, 464
Sticky Platelets, 492
B-type Natriuretic Peptide and Heart Failure, 575

Hypertension, 585
Obesity and Hypertension, 586
Recommendations for Managing Cholesterol, 596
Women and Microvascular Angina, 599
Canadian Heart Failure Statistics, 617
Sepsis Prevention: Central Line–Associated Bloodstream Infection, 629
The Surviving Sepsis Guidelines, 630
Endocarditis Risk, 641
Asthma, 682
Tips to Keep Lungs Healthy, 685
Ventilator-Associated Pneumonia, 689
Facts on Tobacco Use, 695
Lung Cancer, 697
Urinary Tract Infection and Antibiotic Resistance, 738
Nutrition and Premenstrual Syndrome, 793
Nonsurgical Management of Vaginal Prolapse, 799
Screening With the Papanicolaou Test and With the Human Papillomavirus DNA Test, 803
Cervical Cancer Primary Prevention, 805
Breast Cancer Screening Mammography, 816
Clostridium difficile and Diarrhea, 885
Promotion of Physical Activity in Canadian Schools, 902
Tendon and Ligament Repair, 961
Managing Tendinopathy, 971
The Management of Postmenopausal Osteoporosis, 977
Calcium, Vitamin D, and Bone Health, 979
Musculoskeletal Molecular Imaging, 988
Psoriasis and Comorbidities, 1031
Melanoma in People With Darkly Pigmented Skin, 1041

Huether and McCance's
Understanding Pathophysiology

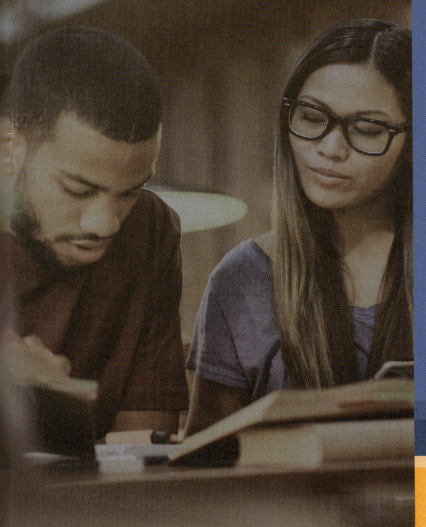

A tailored education experience —

Sherpath book-organized collections

Sherpath is the digital teaching and learning technology designed specifically for healthcare education.

Sherpath book-organized collections offer:

Objective-based, digital lessons, mapped chapter-by-chapter to the textbook, that make it easy to find applicable digital assignment content.

Adaptive quizzing with personalized questions that correlate directly to textbook content.

Teaching materials that align to the text and are organized by chapter for quick and easy access to invaluable class activities and resources.

Elsevier ebooks that provide convenient access to textbook content, even offline.

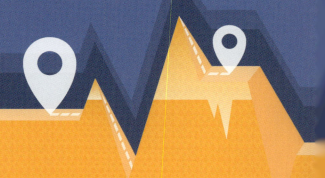

**VISIT
myevolve.us/sherpath**
today to learn more!

21-CS-0280 TM/AF 6/21

Second Canadian Edition

Huether and McCance's Understanding Pathophysiology

Kelly Power-Kean, MHS, NP, RN
Centre for Nursing Studies
Memorial University
St. John's, Newfoundland

Stephanie Zettel, BN, BSc (Hon.), MN
Associate Professor
School of Nursing and Midwifery
Faculty of Health, Community, and Education
Mount Royal University
Calgary, Alberta

Mohamed Toufic El-Hussein, RN, PhD, NP
Professor, School of Nursing and Midwifery
Faculty of Health, Community & Education
Mount Royal University;
Adjunct Associate Professor
Faculty of Nursing, University of Calgary
Acute Care Nurse Practitioner
Medical Cardiology, Coronary Care Unit - Rockyview General Hospital
Calgary, Alberta

U.S. AUTHORS

Sue E. Huether, MS, PhD
Professor Emerita
College of Nursing
University of Utah
Salt Lake City, Utah

Kathryn L. McCance, MS, PhD
Professor Emerita
College of Nursing
University of Utah
Salt Lake City, Utah

U.S. Section Editor

Valentina L. Brashers, MD, FACP, FNAP
Professor Emerita
University of Virginia
Charlottesville, Virginia

ELSEVIER

HUETHER AND McCANCE'S UNDERSTANDING PATHOPHYSIOLOGY, SECOND CANADIAN EDITION

ISBN: 978-0-323-77884-8

Copyright © 2023 Elsevier, Inc. All rights reserved.
Previous edition copyrighted 2018 by Elsevier Canada, a division of Reed Elsevier Canada, Ltd.

Adapted from *Understanding Pathophysiology*, Seventh Edition, by Sue E. Huether and Kathryn L. McCance. Copyright © 2020 by Elsevier, Inc. ISBN 978-0-323-63908-8 (softcover). Previous editions copyrighted 2012, 2008, 2004, 2000 and 1996.

All rights reserved. No part of this publication may be reproduced or transmitted in any form or by any means, electronic or mechanical, including photocopying, recording, or any information storage and retrieval system, without permission in writing from the publisher. Reproducing passages from this book without such written permission is an infringement of copyright law.

Requests for permission to make copies of any part of the work should be mailed to: College Licensing Officer, access ©, 1 Yonge Street, Suite 1900, Toronto, ON M5E 1E5. Fax: (416) 868-1621. All other inquiries should be directed to the publisher, www.elsevier.com/permissions.

Every reasonable effort has been made to acquire permission for copyrighted material used in this text and to acknowledge all such indebtedness accurately. Any errors and omissions called to the publisher's attention will be corrected in future printings.

The book and the individual contributions contained in it are protected under copyright by the Publisher (other than as may be noted herein).

Notice

Practitioners and researchers must always rely on their own experience and knowledge in evaluating and using any information, methods, compounds, or experiments described herein. Because of rapid advances in the medical sciences, in particular, independent verification of diagnoses and drug dosages should be made. To the fullest extent of the law, no responsibility is assumed by Elsevier, authors, editors, or contributors for any injury and/or damage to persons or property as a matter of products liability, negligence or otherwise, or from any use or operation of any methods, products, instructions, or ideas contained in the material herein.

Library of Congress Control Number: 2021947466

Managing Director, Global ERC: Kevonne Holloway
Senior Content Strategist (Acquisitions, Canada): Roberta A. Spinosa-Millman
Director, Content Development: Laurie Gower
Content Development Specialist: Martina van de Velde
Publishing Services Manager: Shereen Jameel
Senior Project Manager: Manikandan Chandrasekaran
Cover Design and Design Direction: Margaret Reid

Working together to grow libraries in developing countries

www.elsevier.com • www.bookaid.org

REVIEWERS

Christina McMillan Boyles, RN, MScN
Assistant Professor
School of Nursing
Laurentian University
Sudbury, Ontario

Sheri Fox-McPhee, RN, MN, NP
Program Coordinator/Instructor
Faculty of Health
University College of the North
Flin Flon, Manitoba

Joanne Jones, RN, MSN, CCNE
Associate Teaching Professor
School of Nursing
Thompson Rivers University
Kamloops, British Columbia

Terri Kean, RN, MN, NP, PhD(c), CDE
Assistant Professor/Nurse Practitioner
Faculty of Nursing
University of Prince Edward Island
Charlottetown, Prince Edward Island

Anne-Marie Kowatsch, MSc
Instructor
Baccalaureate Nursing Program
Red River College
Winnipeg, Manitoba

Jana Lok, RN, MN, PhD, ENC(C)
Assistant Professor, Teaching Stream
Bloomberg Faculty of Nursing
University of Toronto
Toronto, Ontario

Dr. Harminder Mathur, PID, DGO, MBBS
Instructor, Health Sciences
Department of Health Care
Stenberg College
Surrey, British Columbia

Allison McFadden-Squire, RN, MEd, BScN
Curriculum Lead
Practical Nurse Program
NorQuest College
Edmonton, Alberta

Jennifer Perry, RN(EC), NP-PHC, PhD
Professor
School of Baccalaureate Nursing
St. Lawrence College
Kingston, Ontario

Janet Purvis, RN, MN, PhD(c), CCHN(c)
Assistant Professor
Faculty of Nursing
St. Francis Xavier University
Antigonish, Nova Scotia

Kara Sealock, RN, MEd, EdD, CNCC(C), CCNE
Senior Instructor
Faculty of Nursing
University of Calgary
Calgary, Alberta

Karen Sutton, RN, MN, CNCC(C)
Professor
Program Coordinator, RN Critical Care Nursing
School of Health & Community Services
Durham College
Oshawa, Ontario

Claudette Taylor, PhD, NP
Associate Professor
Faculty of Nursing
Cape Breton University
Sydney, Nova Scotia

CONTRIBUTORS

The editors would like to acknowledge the following contributors, whose work is the foundation on which the Second Canadian Edition is based:

Barbara J. Boss, RN, PHD, CFNP, CANP
Retired Professor of Nursing
University of Mississippi Medical Center
Jackson, Mississippi

Valentina L. Brashers, MD, FACP, FNAP
Professor Emerita
University of Virginia
Charlottesville, Virginia

Lois E. Brenneman, MSN, FNP
Adjunct Faculty
Fairleigh Dickinson University
Florham Park, New Jersey

Russell J. Butterfield, MD, PhD
Assistant Professor
Neurology and Pediatrics
University of Utah
Salt Lake City, Utah

Sara J. Fidanza, MS, RN, CNS-BC, CPNP-BC
Digestive Health Institute
Children's Hospital Colorado
Clinical Faculty
University of Colorado College of Nursing
Aurora, Colorado

Diane P. Genereux, PhD
Assistant Professor
Department of Biology
Westfield State
Westfield, Massachusetts

Lynn B. Jorde, PhD
H. A. and Edna Benning Presidential Professor and Chair
Department of Human Genetics
University of Utah School of Medicine
Salt Lake City, Utah

Lauri A. Linder, PhD, APRN, CPON
Assistant Professor
College of Nursing
University of Utah
Salt Lake City, Utah
Clinical Nurse Specialist
Cancer Transplant Center
Primary Children's Hospital
Salt Lake City, Utah

Sue Ann McCann, MSN, RN
Programmatic Nurse Specialist
Nursing
Clinical Research Coordinator
Dermatology
University of Pittsburgh Medical Center
Pittsburgh, Pennsylvania

Noreen Heer Nicol, PhD, RN, FNP, NEA-BC
Associate Professor
College of Nursing
University of Colorado
Denver, Colorado

Jennifer Peterson, PhD, RN, CCNS
Sue and Bill Gross School of Nursing
University of California, Irvine
Irvine, California

Nancy Pike, PhD, RN, CPNP-AC, FAAN
Associate Professor
UCLA School of Nursing
Pediatric Nurse Practitioner
Cardiothoracic Surgery
Children's Hospital Los Angeles
Los Angeles, California

Geri C. Reeves, PhD, APRN, FNP-BC
Assistant Professor
School of Nursing
Vanderbilt University
Nashville, Tennessee

Patricia Ring, RN, MSN, PNP, BC
Retired
Renal/Voiding Improvement Program
Children's Hospital of Wisconsin
Milwaukee, Wisconsin

George W. Rodway, PhD, APRN
Associate Clinical Professor
UC Davis School of Nursing
Sacramento, California

Neal S. Rote, PhD
Academic Vice-Chair and Director of Research
Department of Obstetrics and Gynecology
University Hospitals Case Medical Center
Case Western Reserve University School of Medicine
Cleveland, Ohio

Sharon Sables-Baus, PhD, MPA, RN, PCNS-BC, CPPS, FAAN
Associate Professor
University of Colorado
College of Nursing and School of Medicine
Department of Pediatrics
Aurora, Colorado

Benjamin A. Smallheer, PhD
Assistant Professor
School of Nursing
Duke University, Durham
North Carolina
Acute Care Nurse Practitioner
Critical Care Medicine
Duke Raleigh Hospital
Raleigh, North Carolina

Lorey K. Takahashi, PhD
Professor of Psychology
Department of Psychology
University of Hawaii at Manoa
Honolulu, Hawaii

PREFACE

We have updated the Second Canadian Edition of *Huether and McCance's Understanding Pathophysiology* with consideration of the rapid advances in molecular and cellular biology. We rewrote and reorganized many sections to provide a foundation for better understanding of the mechanisms of disease. We have also integrated concepts from the basic sciences, including genetics, epigenetics, gene–environment interaction, immunity, and inflammation throughout the text. The nature of these revisions will assist students with the translation of the concepts and processes of pathophysiology into clinical practice and promote lifelong learning.

Some of the more specific changes we have made include a new discussion of comorbidities/multimorbidities in relevant chapters. We also pared down and balanced the amount of content focused on children with more focus on the older person. In addition, the titles of the chapters focusing on children reflect a more developmental aspect of the pathophysiology of disease. Similarly, "Geriatric Considerations" in relevant chapters redirect the focus to the special population of older persons.

We introduced new case studies that are associated with the main "alterations" chapter of each unit. These case studies pull together the content of the unit and reinforce application of that knowledge. They also allow students to develop their critical reasoning and clinical judgement skills as they apply them to actual nursing practice. The latter addition is timely, as it prepares the students for the new generation NCLEX, scheduled to be launched in April 2023.

Based on feedback from instructors and students, we have revised the chapters with the aim of reducing the complexity of the reading level to be more appropriate for undergraduate students. The Flesch-Kincaid Grade Level readability score guided this writing process, and we simplified language and explanations as much as possible. We also requested the input of undergraduate nursing students by having them review various revised chapters for readability and clarity.

We updated all references (with the exception of seminal research) to include citations published in the last 5 years. Furthermore, we have added an Appendix of Common Laboratory Values to this edition, which can be found at the end of the book. We have also highlighted a special emphasis on COVID-19, threading some its effects on different body systems throughout relevant chapters.

Other updates include Canadian statistics, based on data from Health Canada, the Canadian Institute for Health Information, and other relevant governmental organizations. Furthermore, we updated and explored Indigenous perspectives in relation to the epidemiology of pathophysiological conditions in Canada. Lastly, we are thankful for the feedback from Canadian reviewers and addressed their comments with a critical appreciation of relevant issues and application in current nursing practice.

Although the primary focus of the text is pathophysiology, we include discussions of the following interconnected topics to highlight their importance for clinical practice:
- A lifespan approach that includes special sections on aging and separate chapters on developmental aspects of pathophysiology
- Epidemiology and incidence rates showing regional and worldwide differences that reflect the importance of environmental and lifestyle factors on disease initiation and progression
- Sex differences that affect epidemiology and pathophysiology
- Molecular biology—mechanisms of normal cell function and how their alteration leads to disease
- Clinical manifestations, summaries of treatment, and health promotion/risk reduction

The authors and contributors of the text recognize and acknowledge the diverse histories of the First Peoples of the lands now referred to as Canada. It is recognized that individual communities identify themselves in various ways; within this text, the term Indigenous will be used to refer to all First Nations, Inuit, and Métis people within Canada.

This Second Canadian Edition also recognizes that language concerning sex, gender, and identity are fluid and continually evolving. The language and terminology presented in this text endeavours to be inclusive of all peoples and reflects what is, to the best of our knowledge, current at the time of publication.

ORGANIZATION AND CONTENT

The book has two parts: Part One, Basic Concepts of Pathophysiology, and Part Two, Body Systems and Diseases.

Part One: Basic Concepts of Pathophysiology

Part One introduces basic principles and processes that are important for a contemporary understanding of the pathophysiology of common diseases. The concepts include descriptions of cellular communication; forms of cell injury; genes and genetic disease; epigenetics; fluid and electrolytes and acid and base balance; immunity and inflammation; mechanisms of infection; stress, coping, and illness; and tumour biology. Chapter 3, *Epigenetics and Disease*, explains the way heritable changes in gene expression—*phenotype* without a change in *genotype*—are influenced by several factors, including age, environment and lifestyle, and disease state.

Part Two: Body Systems and Diseases

Part Two presents the pathophysiology of the most common alterations according to body system. To promote readability and comprehension, we use a logical sequence and uniform approach in presenting the content of the units and chapters. Each unit focuses on a specific organ system and contains chapters related to anatomy and physiology, the pathophysiology of the most common diseases, and common developmental concerns. The anatomy and physiology content serves as a review to enhance the learner's understanding of the structural and functional changes inherent in pathophysiology. A brief summary of normal aging effects at the end of these review chapters helps to reinforce how pathophysiology changes throughout the lifespan. The general organization of each disease or disorder discussion includes an introductory paragraph on relevant risk factors and epidemiology, a significant focus on pathophysiology and clinical manifestations, and then a brief review of evaluation and treatment.

Other significant topics for Part Two in the Second Canadian Edition include new and updated information on the following topics, with a focus on how COVID-19 may lead to alterations in the relevant systems:
- Mechanisms of pain transmission, pain syndromes, and categories of sleep disorders (Chapter 14)
- Alterations in levels of consciousness, seizure disorders, and delirium. Pathogenesis of degenerative brain diseases, the dementias, movement disorders, traumatic brain and spinal cord injury, stroke syndromes, headache, and infections and structural malformations of the central nervous system (Chapters 15, 16, 17)
- The pathogenesis of type 2 diabetes mellitus (Chapter 19)
- Platelet function and coagulation; anemias, alterations of leukocyte function and myeloid and lymphoid tumours (Chapters 20 and 21)

- Extensive chapter revisions of developmental alterations of hematological function (Chapter 22)
- Extensive chapter revisions on structure and function of the cardiovascular and lymphatic systems (Chapter 23)
- Mechanisms of atherosclerosis, hypertension, coronary artery disease, heart failure, and shock (Chapter 24)
- Pediatric valvular disorders, heart failure, hypertension, obesity, and heart disease (Chapter 25)
- Pathophysiology of acute lung injury, asthma, pneumonia, lung cancer, respiratory distress in the newborn, and cystic fibrosis (Chapters 27 and 28)
- Mechanisms of kidney stone formation, immune processes of glomerulonephritis, and acute and chronic kidney injury (Chapters 30 and 31)
- Female and male reproductive disorders, female and male reproductive cancers, breast diseases and mechanisms of breast cancer, prostate cancer, male breast cancer, and sexually transmitted infections (Chapters 33 and 34)
- Gastroesophageal reflux, nonalcoholic liver disease, inflammatory bowel disease, viral hepatitis, obesity, gluten-sensitive enteropathy, and necrotizing enterocolitis (Chapters 36 and 37)
- Bone cells, bone remodelling, joint and tendon diseases, osteoporosis, rheumatoid arthritis, and osteoarthritis (Chapters 38 and 39)
- Congenital and acquired musculoskeletal disorders, and muscular dystrophies in children (Chapter 40)
- Psoriasis, discoid lupus erythematosus, and atopic dermatitis (Chapters 41 and 42)
- Cancer of the various organ systems was updated for all chapters.

FEATURES TO PROMOTE LEARNING

A number of features are incorporated into this text that guide and support learning and understanding, including:

- *Learning Objectives* begin each chapter to help students focus on the key information that follows.
- *Chapter Outlines* including page numbers for easy reference
- *Key Terms* set in blue boldface in text and listed, with page numbers, at the beginning of each chapter
- *Quick Check* questions strategically placed throughout each chapter to help readers prepare for and confirm their understanding of the material; answers are included on the textbook's Evolve website
- *Health Promotion* boxes with a strategic focus on evidence-informed health promotion and current health practices
- *Risk Factors* boxes for selected diseases
- Special boxes for *Pediatric Considerations* and *Geriatric Considerations* that highlight discussions of lifespan alterations
- *Case Studies* appear at the end of the "Alterations" chapters to help students apply and synthesize concepts learned for each body system, through the addition of Critical Thinking and Clinical Judgement questions. (Suggested answers to these case study questions are included on the book's Evolve website.)
- *Comorbidities* boxes appear in selected chapters to help students link pathophysiology to pharmacology for these topics.
- End-of-chapter *Did You Understand?* summaries that condense the major concepts of each chapter into an easy-to-review list format; printable versions of these are available on the textbook's Evolve website.

ART PROGRAM

All of the figures and photographs have been carefully reviewed, and some have been revised or updated. This edition features approximately 950 images. The figures are designed to help students visually understand sometimes difficult and complex material. Hundreds of high-quality photographs show clinical manifestations, pathological specimens, and clinical imaging techniques. Micrographs show normal and abnormal cellular structure. The combination of illustrations, algorithms, photographs, and use of colour for tables and boxes allows a more precise understanding of essential information.

TEACHING/LEARNING PACKAGE

For Students

The free electronic **Student Resources** on Evolve include Next-Generation NCLEX (NGN)-Style Case Studies, review questions and answers, numerous animations, answers to the Quick Check questions in the book, answers to the Case Study questions in the book, printable key points, and bonus case studies with questions and answers. A comprehensive *Glossary* of pathophysiological conditions for the textbook of more than 600 terms helps students with the often-difficult terminology related to pathophysiology; this is available both on Evolve and in the electronic version of the textbook. These electronic resources enhance learning options for students. Go to https://evolve.elsevier.com/Canada/Huether/pathophysiology.

A new **Study Guide** includes many different question types, aiming to help the broad spectrum of student learners. Question types include the following:

Match the Definitions
Choose the Correct Words
Complete These Sentences
Categorize These Clinical Examples
Describe the Differences
Explain the Pictures
Order the Steps
Teach These People about Pathophysiology
Plus many more…

In addition, the Study Guide features new *Concept-Based Critical Thinking Exercises* focused on 10 pathophysiological concepts that are common to understanding pathophysiological processes in the body. These exercises feature 10 patient scenarios accompanied by critical thinking questions that use formats common to the National Council Licensure Examination's (NCLEX-RN) Next Generation Project. Answers to all questions, as well as answers and rationales for the Critical Thinking Exercises, are found in the back of the **Study Guide** for easy reference for students.

For Instructors

The electronic **Instructor Resources** on Evolve are available free to instructors with qualified adoptions of the textbook and include: Next-Generation NCLEX (NGN)-Style Case Studies, TEACH Lesson Plans with case studies to assist with clinical application; a Test Bank of more than 1 200 items; PowerPoint Presentations for each chapter, with integrated images, audience response questions, and case studies; and an Image Collection of approximately 950 key figures from the text. All of these teaching resources are also available to instructors on the book's Evolve website. Additionally, the Evolve Learning System provides a comprehensive suite of course communication and organization tools that allow you to upload your class calendar and syllabus, post scores and announcements, and more. Go to https://evolve.elsevier.com/Canada/Huether/pathophysiology

The most exciting part of the learning support package is **Pathophysiology Online**, a complete set of online modules that provide thoroughly developed lessons on the most important and difficult topics in pathophysiology supplemented with illustrations, animations, interactive activities, interactive algorithms, self-assessment reviews, and exams. Instructors can use it to enhance traditional classroom lecture courses or for distance and online-only courses. Students can use it as a self-guided study tool.

NEXT GENERATION NCLEX (NGN)

The National Council for the State Boards of Nursing (NCSBN), is a not-for-profit organization whose members include nursing regulatory bodies. In empowering and supporting nursing regulators in their mandate to protect the public, the NCSBN is involved in the development of nursing licensure examinations, such as the NCLEX-RN. In Canada, the NCLEX-RN was introduced in 2015 and is as of the writing of this text, the recognized licensure exam required for practising RNs in Canada.

The NCLEX-RN as of 2023 will be changing to ensure that its item types adequately measure clinical judgement, critical thinking, and problem-solving skills on a consistent basis. The NCSBN will also be incorporating into the examination, what they call the Clinical Judgement Measurement Model (CJMM), which is a framework the NCSBN has created to measure a novice nurse's ability to apply clinical judgement in practice.

These changes to the examination come as a result of findings indicating that novice nurses have a much higher than desirable error rate with patients (errors causing patient harm) and upon NCSBN's investigation, discovering that the overwhelming majority of these errors were caused by failures of clinical judgement.

Clinical judgement has been a foundation underlying nursing education for decades, based on the work of a number of nursing theorists. The theory of clinical judgement that most closely aligns to what NCSBN is basing their CJMM is the work by Christine A. Tanner.

The new version of the NCLEX-RN is identified loosely as the "Next-Generation NCLEX" or "NGN" and will feature:
- Six key skills in the CJMM: recognizing cues, analyzing cues, prioritizing hypotheses, generating solutions, taking actions, and evaluating outcomes.
- Approved item types as of March 2021: multiple response, extended drag and drop, cloze (drop-down), enhanced hot-spot (highlighting), matrix/grid, bowtie, and trend. More question types may be added.
- All new item types are accompanied by mini-case studies with comprehensive patient information—some of it relevant to the question, and some of it not.
- Case information may present a single, unchanging moment in time (a "single episode" case study) or multiple moments in time as a patient's condition changes (an "unfolding" case study).
- Single-episode case studies may be accompanied by 1 to 6 questions; unfolding case studies are accompanied by 6 questions.

For more information (and detail) regarding the NCLEX-RN and changes coming to the exam, visit the NCSBNs website: https://www.ncsbn.org/11447.htm and https://ncsbn.org/Building_a_Method_for_Writing_Clinical_Judgment_It.pdf.

For further NCLEX-RN examination preparation resources, see *Elsevier's Canadian Comprehensive Review for the NCLEX-RN Examination*, Second Edition, ISBN 9780323709385.

Prior to preparing for any nursing licensure examination, please refer to your provincial or territorial nursing regulatory body to determine which licensure examination is required in order for you to practice in your chosen jurisdiction.

ACKNOWLEDGEMENTS

This book would not be possible without the knowledge and expertise of the contributors to the previous US editions. Their reviews and synthesis of the evidence and clear and concise presentation of information are strengths of this text and facilitated the adaptation of this information for the Canadian context.

The reviewers for this edition provided excellent recommendations for focus of content and revisions, based on the Canadian context, with thoughtful consideration of Indigenous perspectives on health, wellness, and disease. We appreciate their insightful work.

We are thankful to Martina van de Velde, our Content Development Specialist, for overseeing this wonderful project, providing insights regarding formatting, and suggesting content to maintain a streamlined manuscript that flows seamlessly from one section to another. We are also thankful to Roberta A. Spinosa-Millman, Senior Content Strategist, for recruiting such a great team! Collaborating with one another on this project has been a great learning experience, and one that would not have been possible without Roberta having brought us all together.

We have respected the contributions from U.S. authors, Sue E. Huether and Kathryn L. McCance, in this Second Canadian Edition and recognize the innovation and clarity that these authors bring to pathophysiology.

Lastly, we would like to thank our families for their undying support. They are what makes this work possible!

Kelly Power-Kean
Stephanie Zettel
Mohamed Toufic El-Hussein

INTRODUCTION TO PATHOPHYSIOLOGY

The word root *"patho"* is derived from the Greek word *pathos*, which means suffering. The Greek word root *"logos"* means discourse or, more simply, system of formal study, and *"physio"* refers to functions of an organism. Altogether, pathophysiology is the study of the underlying changes in body physiology (molecular, cellular, and organ systems) that result from disease or injury. Important, however, is the inextricable component of suffering and the psychological, spiritual, social, cultural, and economic implications of disease.

The science of pathophysiology seeks to provide an understanding of the mechanisms of disease and to explain how and why alterations in body structure and function lead to the signs and symptoms of disease. Understanding pathophysiology guides health care providers in the planning, selection, and evaluation of therapies and treatments.

Knowledge of human anatomy and physiology and the interrelationship among the various cells and organ systems of the body is an essential foundation for the study of pathophysiology. Review of this subject matter enhances comprehension of pathophysiological events and processes. Understanding pathophysiology also entails the utilization of principles, concepts, and basic knowledge from other fields of study including pathology, genetics, epigenetics, immunology, and epidemiology. A number of terms are used to focus the discussion of pathophysiology; they may be used interchangeably at times, but that does not necessarily indicate that they have the same meaning. Those terms are reviewed here for the purpose of clarification.

Pathology is the investigation of structural alterations in cells, tissues, and organs, which can help identify the cause of a particular disease. Pathology differs from **pathogenesis**, which is the pattern of tissue changes associated with the *development* of disease. **Etiology** refers to the study of the *cause* of disease. Diseases may be caused by infection, heredity, gene–environment interactions, alterations in immunity, malignancy, malnutrition, degeneration, or trauma. Diseases that have no identifiable cause are termed **idiopathic**. Diseases that occur as a result of medical treatment are termed **iatrogenic** (e.g., some antibiotics can injure the kidney and cause kidney failure). Diseases that are acquired as a consequence of being in a hospital environment are called **health care–associated diseases**. An infection that develops as a result of a person's immune system being depressed after receiving cancer treatment during a hospital stay would be defined as a health care–associated infection.

Diagnosis is the naming or identification of a disease. A diagnosis is made from an evaluation of the evidence accumulated from the presenting signs and symptoms, health and medical history, physical examination, laboratory tests, and imaging. A **prognosis** is the expected outcome of a disease. **Acute disease** is the sudden appearance of signs and symptoms that last only a short time. **Chronic disease** develops more slowly, and the signs and symptoms last for a long time, perhaps for a lifetime. Chronic diseases may have a pattern of remission and exacerbation. **Remissions** are periods when symptoms disappear or diminish significantly. **Exacerbations** are periods when the symptoms become worse or more severe. A **complication** is the onset of a disease in a person who is already coping with another existing disease (e.g., a person who has undergone surgery to remove a diseased appendix may develop the complication of a wound infection or pneumonia). **Sequelae** are unwanted outcomes of having a disease or are the result of trauma, such as paralysis resulting from a stroke or severe scarring resulting from a burn.

Clinical manifestations are the signs and symptoms or *evidence* of disease. **Signs** are objective alterations that can be observed or measured by another person, measures of bodily functions such as pulse rate, blood pressure, body temperature, or white blood cell count. Some signs are **local**, such as redness or swelling, and other signs are **systemic**, such as fever. **Symptoms** are subjective experiences reported by the person with disease, such as pain, nausea, or shortness of breath; and they vary from person to person. The **prodromal period** of a disease is the time during which a person experiences vague symptoms such as fatigue or loss of appetite before the onset of specific signs and symptoms. The term **insidious symptoms** describes vague or nonspecific feelings and an awareness that there is a change within the body. Some diseases have a **latent period**, a time during which no symptoms are readily apparent in the affected person, but the disease is nevertheless present in the body; an example is the incubation phase of an infection or the early growth phase of a tumour. A **syndrome** is a group of symptoms that occur together and may be caused by several interrelated problems or a specific disease; severe acute respiratory syndrome (SARS), for example, presents with a set of symptoms that include headache, fever, body aches, an overall feeling of discomfort, and sometimes dry cough and difficulty breathing. A **disorder** is an abnormality of function; this term also can refer to an illness or a particular problem such as a bleeding disorder.

Epidemiology is the study of tracking patterns or disease occurrence and transmission among populations and by geographical areas. **Incidence** of a disease is the number of new cases occurring in a specific time period. **Prevalence** of a disease is the number of existing cases within a population during a specific time period.

Risk factors, also known as **predisposing factors**, increase the probability that disease will occur, but these factors are not the *cause* of disease. Risk factors include heredity, age, gender, race, environment, and lifestyle. A **precipitating factor** is a condition or event that *does* cause a pathological event or disorder. For example, asthma is precipitated by exposure to an allergen, or angina (pain) is precipitated by exertion.

Pathophysiology is an exciting field of study that is ever-changing as new discoveries are made. Understanding pathophysiology empowers health care providers with the knowledge of how and why disease develops and informs their decision making to ensure optimal health care outcomes. Embedded in the study of pathophysiology is understanding that suffering is a personal, individual experience and a major component of disease.

CONTENTS

PART ONE Basic Concepts of Pathophysiology

UNIT 1 The Cell

1 Cellular Biology, 1
Stephanie Zettel, with originating chapter contributions by Kathryn L. McCance
- Prokaryotes and Eukaryotes, 2
- Cellular Functions, 2
- Structure and Function of Cellular Components, 3
  - *Nucleus,* 3
  - *Cytoplasmic Organelles,* 3
  - *Plasma Membranes,* 3
  - *Cellular Receptors,* 10
- Cell-to-Cell Adhesions, 11
  - *Extracellular Matrix,* 11
  - *Specialized Cell Junctions,* 12
- Cellular Communication and Signal Transduction, 14
- Cellular Metabolism, 15
  - *Role of Adenosine Triphosphate,* 15
  - *Food and Production of Cellular Energy,* 16
  - *Oxidative Phosphorylation,* 17
- Membrane Transport: Cellular Intake and Output, 18
  - *Electrolytes as Solutes,* 19
  - *Transport by Vesicle Formation,* 22
  - *Movement of Electrical Impulses: Membrane Potentials,* 24
- Cellular Reproduction: The Cell Cycle, 25
  - *Phases of Mitosis and Cytokinesis,* 26
  - *Rates of Cellular Division,* 26
  - *Growth Factors,* 27
- Tissues, 27
  - *Tissue Formation,* 28
  - *Types of Tissues,* 28

2 Genes and Genetic Diseases, 38
Stephanie Zettel, with originating chapter contributions by Lynn B. Jorde
- DNA, RNA, and Proteins: Heredity at the Molecular Level, 39
  - *Definitions,* 39
  - *From Genes to Proteins,* 40
- Chromosomes, 41
  - *Chromosome Aberrations and Associated Diseases,* 43
- Elements of Formal Genetics, 49
  - *Phenotype and Genotype,* 49
  - *Dominance and Recessiveness,* 50
- Transmission of Genetic Diseases, 50
  - *Autosomal Dominant Inheritance,* 50
  - *Autosomal Recessive Inheritance,* 53
  - *X-Linked Inheritance,* 54
- Linkage Analysis and Gene Mapping, 56
  - *Classic Pedigree Analysis,* 56
  - *Complete Human Gene Map: Prospects and Benefits,* 56
- Multifactorial Inheritance, 58

3 Epigenetics and Disease, 62
Stephanie Zettel, with originating chapter contributions by Diane P. Genereux
- Epigenetic Mechanisms, 62
  - *DNA Methylation,* 63
  - *Histone Modifications,* 64
  - *RNA-Based Mechanisms,* 64
- Epigenetics and Human Development, 64
- Genomic Imprinting, 64
  - *Prader-Willi and Angelman Syndromes,* 65
  - *Beckwith-Wiedemann Syndrome,* 65
  - *Russell-Silver Syndrome,* 66
- Inheritance of Epigenetic States, 66
  - *Epigenetics and Nutrition,* 66
  - *Epigenetics and Maternal Care,* 66
- Epigenetics and Ethanol Exposure During Gestation 67
  - *Epigenetics and Mental Illness,* 67
  - *Epigenetic Disease in the Context of Genetic Abnormalities,* 67
  - *Twin Studies Provide Insights on Epigenetic Modification,* 68
  - *Molecular Approaches to Understand Epigenetic Disease,* 68
- Epigenetics and Cancer, 68
  - *DNA Methylation and Cancer,* 68
  - *microRNAs and Cancer,* 68
  - *Epigenetic Screening for Cancer,* 68
  - *Emerging Strategies for the Treatment of Epigenetic Disease,* 69
  - *DNA Demethylating Agents,* 69
  - *Histone Deacetylase Inhibitors,* 69
  - *microRNA Coding,* 70
- Future Directions, 70

4 Altered Cellular and Tissue Biology, 72
Stephanie Zettel, with originating chapter contributions by Kathryn L. McCance and Lois E. Brenneman
- Cellular Adaptation, 73
  - *Atrophy,* 73
  - *Hypertrophy,* 74
  - *Hyperplasia,* 76
  - *Dysplasia: Not a True Adaptive Change,* 76
  - *Metaplasia,* 77
- Cellular Injury, 77
  - *General Mechanisms of Cellular Injury,* 78
  - *Unintentional and Intentional Injuries,* 92
  - *Infectious Injury,* 95
  - *Immunological and Inflammatory Injury,* 95
- Manifestations of Cellular Injury: Accumulations, 95
  - *Water,* 95
  - *Lipids and Carbohydrates,* 95
  - *Glycogen,* 97
  - *Proteins,* 97
  - *Pigments,* 97
  - *Calcium,* 99

Urate, 100
Systemic Manifestations, 100
Cellular Death, 100
Necrosis, 101
Apoptosis, 103
Autophagy, 105
Aging and Altered Cellular and Tissue Biology, 106
Normal Lifespan, Life Expectancy, and Quality-Adjusted Life Year, 107
Degenerative Extracellular Changes, 107
Cellular Aging, 107
Tissue and Systemic Aging, 108
Frailty, 108
Somatic Death, 108

5 **Fluids and Electrolytes, Acids and Bases,** 112
Stephanie Zettel, with originating chapter contributions by Lois E. Brenneman and Sue E. Huether
Distribution of Body Fluids and Electrolytes, 113
Water Movement Between Plasma and Interstitial Fluid, 114
Water Movement Between ICF and ECF, 114
Alterations in Water Movement, 114
Edema, 114
Sodium, Chloride, and Water Balance, 116
Alterations in Sodium, Chloride, and Water Balance, 118
Isotonic Alterations, 118
Hypertonic Alterations, 118
Hypotonic Alterations, 120
Alterations in Potassium and Other Electrolytes, 121
Potassium, 121
Other Electrolytes—Calcium, Phosphate, and Magnesium, 124
Acid–Base Balance, 124
Hydrogen Ion and pH, 124
Buffer Systems, 124
Acid–Base Imbalances, 126
PEDIATRIC CONSIDERATIONS: Distribution of Body Fluids, 130
GERIATRIC CONSIDERATIONS: Distribution of Body Fluids, 130

UNIT 2 Mechanisms of Self-Defence

6 **Innate Immunity: Inflammation and Wound Healing,** 133
Stephanie Zettel, with originating chapter contributions by Valentina L. Brashers and Lois E. Brenneman
Human Defence Mechanisms, 134
First Line of Defence: Physical and Biochemical Barriers and the Human Microbiome, 134
Second Line of Defence: Inflammation, 137
Plasma Protein Systems and Inflammation, 138
Cellular Components of Inflammation, 141
Acute and Chronic Inflammation, 149
Local Manifestations of Acute Inflammation, 149
Systemic Manifestations of Acute Inflammation, 149
Chronic Inflammation, 150
Wound Healing, 151
Phase I: Inflammation, 152
Phase II: Proliferation and New Tissue Formation, 152
Phase III: Remodelling and Maturation, 153
Dysfunctional Wound Healing, 153
PEDIATRIC CONSIDERATIONS: Age-Related Factors Affecting Innate Immunity in the Newborn Child, 154
GERIATRIC CONSIDERATIONS: Age-Related Factors Affecting Innate Immunity in Older Persons, 154

7 **Adaptive Immunity,** 157
Stephanie Zettel, with originating chapter contributions by Valentina L. Brashers and Kathryn L. McCance
Third Line of Defence: Adaptive Immunity, 158
Antigens and Immunogens, 159
Antibodies, 161
Classes of Immunoglobulins, 161
Antigen–Antibody Binding, 162
Function of Antibodies, 162
Immune Response: Collaboration of B Cells and T Cells, 164
Generation of Clonal Diversity, 164
Development of B Lymphocytes, 164
Clonal Selection, 167
Cell-Mediated Immunity, 172
T-Lymphocyte Function, 172
PEDIATRIC CONSIDERATIONS: Age-Related Factors Affecting Mechanisms of Self-Defence in the Newborn Child, 174
GERIATRIC CONSIDERATIONS: Age-Related Factors Affecting Mechanisms of Self-Defence in Older Persons, 174

8 **Infection and Defects in Mechanisms of Defence,** 176
Stephanie Zettel, with originating chapter contributions by Valentina L. Brashers and Sue E. Huether
Infection, 177
Microorganisms and Humans: A Dynamic Relationship, 177
Countermeasures Against Infectious Microorganisms, 188
Deficiencies in Immunity, 191
Initial Clinical Presentation, 191
Primary (Congenital) Immune Deficiencies, 191
Secondary (Acquired) Immune Deficiencies, 194
Evaluation and Care of Those With Immune Deficiency, 194
Replacement Therapies for Immune Deficiencies, 194
AIDS, 195
Hypersensitivity: Allergy, Autoimmunity, and Alloimmunity, 199
Mechanisms of Hypersensitivity, 200
Antigenic Targets of Hypersensitivity Reactions, 208

9 **Stress and Disease,** 215
Stephanie Zettel, with originating chapter contributions by Lorey K. Takahashi and Kathryn L. McCance
Historical Background and General Concepts, 216

Stress Overview: Allostasis, Multiple Mediators, and Systems, 218
The Stress Response, 219
Regulation of the Hypothalamic–Pituitary–Adrenal System, 219
Neuroendocrine Regulation: Autonomic Nervous System, 220
Histamine and Other Hormones, 224
Role of the Immune System, 224
Stress, Personality, Coping, and Illness, 227
Coping, 229
GERIATRIC CONSIDERATIONS: Aging and the Stress–Age Syndrome, 230

UNIT 3 Cellular Proliferation: Cancer

10 Biology of Cancer, 233
Stephanie Zettel, with originating chapter contributions by Kathryn L. McCance and Neal S. Rote

Cancer Terminology and Characteristics, 234
Tumour Classification and Nomenclature, 234
The Biology of Cancer Cells, 235
Sustained Proliferative Signalling, 239
Evading Growth Suppressors, 242
Genomic Instability, 244
Enabling Replicative Immortality, 246
Inducing Angiogenesis, 246
Reprogramming Energy Metabolism, 247
Resisting Apoptotic Cell Death, 248
Tumour-Promoting Inflammation, 249
Evading Immune Destruction, 251
Activating Invasion and Metastasis, 252
Clinical Manifestations of Cancer, 255
Paraneoplastic Syndromes, 255
Pain, 255
Fatigue, 255
Cachexia, 255
Anemia, 258
Leukopenia and Thrombocytopenia, 258
Infection, 258
Gastrointestinal Tract, 258
Hair and Skin, 258
Diagnosis, Characterization, and Treatment of Cancer, 259
Diagnosis and Staging, 259
Classification of Tumours: Classic Histology and Modern Genetics, 261
Treatment, 261

11 Cancer Epidemiology, 266
Stephanie Zettel, with originating chapter contributions by Kathryn L. McCance and Lois E. Brenneman

Genetics, Epigenetics, and Tissue, 266
Incidence and Mortality Trends, 272
In Utero and Early Life Conditions, 272
Environmental and Lifestyle Factors, 274
Tobacco Use, 274
Diet, 276
Nutrition, Obesity, Alcohol Consumption, and Physical Activity: Impacts on Cancer, 276
Ionizing Radiation, 282
Ultraviolet Radiation, 285
Electromagnetic Radiation, 287
Infection, and Sexual and Reproductive Behaviour, 288
Other Viruses and Microorganisms, 288
Air Pollution, 289
Chemical and Occupational Hazards as Carcinogens, 289

12 Cancer in Children and Adolescents, 294
Stephanie Zettel, with originating chapter contributions by Lauri A. Linder

Incidence, Etiology, and Types of Childhood Cancer, 294
Etiology, 295
Genetic and Genomic Factors, 295
Environmental Factors, 296
Prognosis, 297

PART TWO Body Systems and Diseases

UNIT 4 The Neurological System

13 Structure and Function of the Neurological System, 299
Kelly Power-Kean, with originating chapter contributions by Sue E. Huether

Overview and Organization of the Nervous System, 300
Cells of the Nervous System, 301
The Neuron, 301
Neuroglia and Schwann Cells, 302
Nerve Injury and Regeneration, 302
The Nerve Impulse, 304
Synapses, 304
Neurotransmitters, 304
The Central Nervous System, 305
The Brain, 305
The Spinal Cord, 311
Motor Pathways, 311
Sensory Pathways, 312
Protective Structures of the Central Nervous System, 313
Blood Supply of the Central Nervous System, 316
The Peripheral Nervous System, 318
The Autonomic Nervous System, 319
Anatomy of the Sympathetic Nervous System, 319
Anatomy of the Parasympathetic Nervous System, 322
Neurotransmitters and Neuroreceptors, 322
Functions of the Autonomic Nervous System, 322
GERIATRIC CONSIDERATIONS: Aging and the Nervous System, 326

14 Pain, Temperature, Sleep, and Sensory Function, 328
Kelly Power-Kean, with originating chapter contributions by George W. Rodway and Sue E. Huether

Pain, 329
Theories of Pain, 329
Neuroanatomy of Pain, 330
Pain Modulation, 331
Clinical Descriptions of Pain, 333

Temperature Regulation, 334
  Control of Body Temperature, 335
  Temperature Regulation in Infants and Older Persons, 336
  Pathogenesis of Fever, 336
  Benefits of Fever, 337
  Disorders of Temperature Regulation, 337
Sleep, 338
  Sleep Disorders, 339
The Special Senses, 340
  Vision, 340
  Hearing, 344
  Olfaction and Taste, 347
Somatosensory Function, 347
  Touch, 347
  Proprioception, 347
GERIATRIC CONSIDERATIONS: Aging and Changes in Vision, 348
GERIATRIC CONSIDERATIONS: Aging and Changes in Hearing, 348
GERIATRIC CONSIDERATIONS: Aging and Changes in Olfaction and Taste, 348

15 Alterations in Cognitive Systems, Cerebral Hemodynamics, and Motor Function, 351
Kelly Power-Kean, with originating chapter contributions by Barbara J. Boss and Sue E. Huether
Alterations in Cognitive Systems, 352
  Alterations in Arousal, 352
  Alterations in Awareness, 358
  Data-Processing Deficits, 360
  Seizure Disorders, 365
  Types of Seizure, 366
Alterations in Cerebral Hemodynamics, 367
  Increased Intracranial Pressure, 367
  Cerebral Edema, 368
  Hydrocephalus, 369
Alterations in Neuromotor Function, 369
  Alterations in Muscle Tone, 369
  Alterations in Muscle Movement, 371
  Upper and Lower Motor Neuron Syndromes, 374
  Motor Neuron Diseases, 376
  Amyotrophic Lateral Sclerosis, 377
Alterations in Complex Motor Performance, 378
  Disorders of Posture (Stance), 378
  Disorders of Gait, 378
  Disorders of Expression, 378
Extrapyramidal Motor Syndromes, 378
CASE STUDY: Seizure, 379

16 Disorders of the Central and Peripheral Nervous Systems and Neuromuscular Junction, 382
Kelly Power-Kean, with originating chapter contributions by Barbara J. Boss and Sue E. Huether
Central Nervous System Disorders, 383
  Traumatic Brain and Spinal Cord Injury, 383
  Degenerative Disorders of the Spine, 391
  Cerebrovascular Disorders, 394
  Primary Headache Syndrome, 398
  Infection and Inflammation of the Central Nervous System, 400
  Demyelinating Disorders, 402
Peripheral Nervous System and Neuromuscular Junction Disorders, 403
  Peripheral Nervous System Disorders, 404
  Neuromuscular Junction Disorders, 404
Tumours of the Central Nervous System, 405
  Brain Tumours, 405
  Spinal Cord Tumours, 408

17 Developmental Alterations of Neurological Function, 411
Kelly Power-Kean, with originating chapter contributions by Russell J. Butterfield and Sue E. Huether
Development of the Nervous System in Children, 412
Structural Malformations, 413
  Defects of Neural Tube Closure, 413
  Craniostenosis, 414
  Malformations of Brain Development, 415
Alterations in Function: Encephalopathies, 416
  Static Encephalopathies, 416
  Inherited Metabolic Disorders of the Central Nervous System, 417
  Acute Encephalopathies, 419
  Infections of the Central Nervous System, 420
Cerebrovascular Disease in Children, 420
  Perinatal Stroke, 420
  Childhood Stroke, 420
  Epilepsy and Seizure Disorders in Children, 420
Childhood Tumours, 421
  Brain Tumours, 421
  Embryonal Tumours, 422

UNIT 5 The Endocrine System

18 Mechanisms of Hormonal Regulation, 426
Kelly Power-Kean, with originating chapter contributions by Valentina L. Brashers and Sue E. Huether
Mechanisms of Hormonal Regulation, 427
  Regulation of Hormone Release, 428
  Hormone Transport, 428
  Mechanisms of Hormone Action, 429
Structure and Function of the Endocrine Glands, 431
  Hypothalamic–Pituitary System, 431
  Pineal Gland, 436
  Thyroid and Parathyroid Glands, 436
  Endocrine Pancreas, 438
  Adrenal Glands, 439
GERIATRIC CONSIDERATIONS: Aging and Its Effects on Specific Endocrine Glands, 444

19 Alterations of Hormonal Regulation, 447
Kelly Power-Kean, with originating chapter contributions by Valentina L. Brashers and Sue E. Huether
Mechanisms of Hormonal Alterations, 448
Alterations of the Hypothalamic–Pituitary System, 449
  Diseases of the Posterior Pituitary, 449
  Diseases of the Anterior Pituitary, 450

Alterations of Thyroid Function, 453
  Thyrotoxicosis/Hyperthyroidism, 453
  Hypothyroidism, 455
  Thyroid Carcinoma, 457
Alterations of Parathyroid Function, 457
  Hyperparathyroidism, 457
  Hypoparathyroidism, 458
Dysfunction of the Endocrine Pancreas: Diabetes Mellitus, 458
  Types of Diabetes Mellitus, 460
  Acute Complications of Diabetes Mellitus, 465
  Chronic Complications of Diabetes Mellitus, 466
Alterations of Adrenal Function, 470
  Disorders of the Adrenal Cortex, 470
  Tumours of the Adrenal Medulla, 473
CASE STUDY: Type 2 Diabetes Mellitus, 474

UNIT 6 The Hematological System

20 Structure and Function of the Hematological System, 477
Kelly Power-Kean, with originating chapter contributions by Sue E. Huether

Components of the Hematological System, 478
  Composition of Blood, 478
  Lymphoid Organs, 482
  The Mononuclear Phagocyte System, 484
Development of Blood Cells, 485
  Hematopoiesis, 485
  Development of Erythrocytes, 487
  Development of Leukocytes, 490
  Development of Platelets, 491
Mechanisms of Hemostasis, 491
  Function of Platelets and Blood Vessels, 491
  Function of Clotting Factors, 494
  Retraction and Lysis of Blood Clots, 495
PEDIATRIC CONSIDERATIONS: Hematological Value Changes, 497
GERIATRIC CONSIDERATIONS: Hematological Value Changes, 498

21 Alterations of Hematological Function, 500
Kelly Power-Kean, with originating chapter contributions by Kathryn L. McCance

Alterations of Erythrocyte Function, 501
  Classification of Anemias, 501
  Macrocytic-Normochromic Anemias, 503
  Microcytic-Hypochromic Anemias, 505
  Normocytic-Normochromic Anemias, 507
Myeloproliferative Red Blood Cell Disorders, 507
  Polycythemia Vera, 508
  Iron Overload, 509
Alterations of Leukocyte Function, 510
  Quantitative Alterations of Leukocytes, 510
Alterations of Lymphoid Function, 518
  Lymphadenopathy, 518
  Malignant Lymphomas, 518
Alterations of Splenic Function, 524
Hemorrhagic Disorders and Alterations of Platelets and Coagulation, 526
  Disorders of Platelets, 526
  Alterations of Platelet Function, 529
  Disorders of Coagulation, 529
CASE STUDY: Iron Deficiency Anemia, 534

22 Developmental Alterations of Hematological Function, 537
Kelly Power-Kean, with originating chapter contributions by Laura A. Linder and Kathryn L. McCance

Disorders of Erythrocytes, 537
  Acquired Disorders, 538
  Inherited Disorders, 540
Disorders of Coagulation and Platelets, 545
  Inherited Hemorrhagic Disease, 545
  Antibody-Mediated Hemorrhagic Disease, 546
Neoplastic Disorders, 547
  Leukemia, 547
  Lymphomas, 548

UNIT 7 The Cardiovascular and Lymphatic Systems

23 Structure and Function of the Cardiovascular and Lymphatic Systems, 551
Mohamed Toufic El-Hussein, with originating chapter contributions by Kathryn L. McCance

The Circulatory System, 552
The Heart, 552
  Structures That Direct Circulation Through the Heart, 553
  Structures That Support Cardiac Metabolism: The Coronary Vessels, 555
  Structures That Control Heart Action, 556
  Factors Affecting Cardiac Output, 563
The Systemic Circulation, 566
  Structure of Blood Vessels, 566
  Factors Affecting Blood Flow, 568
  Regulation of Blood Pressure, 571
  Regulation of the Coronary Circulation, 575
The Lymphatic System, 575

24 Alterations of Cardiovascular Function, 579
Mohamed Toufic El-Hussein, with originating chapter contributions by Valentina L. Brashers

Diseases of the Veins, 580
  Varicose Veins and Chronic Venous Insufficiency, 580
  Thrombus Formation in Veins, 580
  Superior Vena Cava Syndrome, 581
Diseases of the Arteries, 581
  Hypertension, 581
  Orthostatic (Postural) Hypotension, 588
  Aneurysm, 589
  Thrombus Formation, 590
  Embolism, 590
  Peripheral Vascular Disease, 590
  Atherosclerosis, 591
  Peripheral Artery Disease, 592
  Coronary Artery Disease, Myocardial Ischemia, and Acute Coronary Syndromes, 595
Disorders of the Heart Wall, 606
  Disorders of the Pericardium, 606

Pericardial Effusion, 607
Disorders of the Myocardium: The Cardiomyopathies, 608
Disorders of the Endocardium, 609
Cardiac Complications in AIDS, 616
Manifestations of Heart Disease, 616
    Heart Failure, 616
    Dysrhythmias, 620
Shock, 621
    Impairment of Cellular Metabolism, 621
    Impairment of Oxygen Use, 621
    Clinical Manifestations of Shock, 625
    Treatment for Shock, 625
    Types of Shock, 625
    Multiple Organ Dysfunction Syndrome, 630
COMORBIDITIES: Cardiovascular Comorbidities, 633
GERIATRIC CONSIDERATIONS: Aging and Cardiovascular Function, 634
CASE STUDY: Coronary Artery Disease, 634

25 Developmental Alterations of Cardiovascular Function, 637
Mohamed Toufic El-Hussein, with originating chapter contributions by Nancy Pike and Jennifer Peterson
Congenital Heart Disease, 637
    Obstructive Defects, 639
    Defects With Increased Pulmonary Blood Flow, 641
    Defects With Decreased Pulmonary Blood Flow, 643
    Mixing Defects, 644
    Heart Failure, 646
Acquired Cardiovascular Disorders, 647
    Kawasaki Disease, 648
    Systemic Hypertension, 649

UNIT 8   The Pulmonary System

26 Structure and Function of the Pulmonary System, 653
Mohamed Toufic El-Hussein, with originating chapter contributions by Valentina L. Brashers
Structures of the Pulmonary System, 654
    Conducting Airways, 654
    Gas-Exchange Airways, 655
    Pulmonary and Bronchial Circulation, 655
    Control of the Pulmonary Circulation, 656
    Chest Wall and Pleura, 657
Function of the Pulmonary System, 657
    Ventilation, 658
    Neurochemical Control of Ventilation, 659
    Mechanics of Breathing, 660
    Gas Transport, 662
GERIATRIC CONSIDERATIONS: Aging and the Pulmonary System, 666

27 Alterations of Pulmonary Function, 669
Mohamed Toufic El-Hussein, with originating chapter contributions by Valentina L. Brashers and Sue E. Huether
Clinical Manifestations of Pulmonary Alterations, 670
    Signs and Symptoms of Pulmonary Disease, 670
    Conditions Caused by Pulmonary Disease or Injury, 672
Disorders of the Chest Wall and Pleura, 673
    Chest Wall Restriction, 673
    Pleural Abnormalities, 674
Pulmonary Disorders, 675
    Restrictive Lung Diseases, 675
    Obstructive Lung Diseases, 682
    Respiratory Tract Infections, 688
    Pulmonary Vascular Disease, 691
    Malignancies of the Respiratory Tract, 693
COMORBIDITIES: The Negative Impact of Comorbidities on the Disease Course of COVID-19, 697
COMORBIDITIES: Chronic Obstructive Pulmonary Disease Comorbidities, 698
GERIATRIC CONSIDERATIONS: Chronic Obstructive Pulmonary Disease in Older Persons, 699
CASE STUDY: Chronic Obstructive Pulmonary Disease, 699

28 Developmental Alterations of Pulmonary Function, 701
Mohamed Toufic El-Hussein, with originating chapter contributions by Valentina L. Brashers
Disorders of the Upper Airways, 702
    Infections of the Upper Airways, 702
    Aspiration of Foreign Bodies, 703
    Obstructive Sleep Apnea Syndrome, 704
Disorders of the Lower Airways, 704
    Respiratory Distress Syndrome of the Newborn, 704
    Bronchopulmonary Dysplasia, 705
    Respiratory Tract Infections, 706
    Aspiration Pneumonitis, 708
    Asthma, 709
    Acute Lung Injury/Acute Respiratory Distress Syndrome, 710
    Cystic Fibrosis, 710
Sudden Unexpected Infant Death, 711

UNIT 9   The Renal and Urological Systems

29 Structure and Function of the Renal and Urological Systems, 713
Mohamed Toufic El-Hussein, with originating chapter contributions by Sue E. Huether
Structures of the Renal System, 714
    Structures of the Kidney, 714
Urinary Structures, 718
    Ureters, 718
Renal Blood Flow, 719
    Autoregulation of Intrarenal Blood Flow, 719
    Neural Regulation of Renal Blood Flow, 720
    Hormones and Other Factors Regulating Renal Blood Flow, 720
Kidney Function, 720
    Nephron Function, 720
    Hormones and Nephron Function, 724
    Aldosterone, 725

　　　　Natriuretic Peptides, 725
　　　　Renal Hormones, 725
　　　Tests of Renal Function, 726
　　　　Renal Clearance, 726
　　　　Plasma Creatinine Concentration, 726
　　　　Blood Urea Nitrogen, 726
　　　PEDIATRIC CONSIDERATIONS: Pediatrics and Renal Function, 728
　　　GERIATRIC CONSIDERATIONS: Aging and Renal Function, 728

30 **Alterations of Renal and Urinary Tract Function,** 730
　Mohamed Toufic El-Hussein, with originating chapter contributions by Sue E. Huether
　　　Urinary Tract Obstruction, 731
　　　　Upper Urinary Tract Obstruction, 731
　　　　Lower Urinary Tract Obstruction, 733
　　　　Tumours, 736
　　　Urinary Tract Infection, 736
　　　　Causes of Urinary Tract Infection, 737
　　　　Types of Urinary Tract Infection, 737
　　　Glomerular Disorders, 739
　　　　Glomerulonephritis, 739
　　　　Nephrotic and Nephritic Syndromes, 742
　　　Acute Kidney Injury, 744
　　　　Classification of Kidney Dysfunction, 744
　　　　Classification of Acute Kidney Injury, 744
　　　　COVID-19-Associated Acute Kidney Injury, 747
　　　Chronic Kidney Disease, 748
　　　　Creatinine and Urea Clearance, 750
　　　　Fluid and Electrolyte Balance, 750
　　　　Calcium, Phosphate, and Bone, 751
　　　　Protein, Carbohydrate, and Fat Metabolism, 751
　　　　Cardiovascular System, 751
　　　　Pulmonary System, 752
　　　　Hematological System, 752
　　　　Immune System, 752
　　　　Neurological System, 752
　　　　Gastro-intestinal System, 752
　　　　Endocrine and Reproductive Systems, 752
　　　　Integumentary System, 752
　　　COMORBIDITIES: Comorbidities Relating to End-Stage Kidney Disease, 753
　　　GERIATRIC CONSIDERATIONS: Aging and Chronic Kidney Disease, 753
　　　CASE STUDY: Urinary Tract Infection, 754

31 **Developmental Alterations of Renal and Urinary Tract Function,** 756
　Mohamed Toufic El-Hussein, with originating chapter contributions by Patricia Ring and Sue E. Huether
　　　Structural Abnormalities, 757
　　　　Hypospadias, 757
　　　　Epispadias and Exstrophy of the Bladder, 757
　　　　Bladder Outlet Obstruction, 758
　　　　Ureteropelvic Junction Obstruction, 758
　　　　Hypoplastic or Dysplastic Kidneys, 758
　　　　Polycystic Kidney Disease, 758
　　　　Renal Agenesis, 758
　　　Glomerular Disorders, 758
　　　　Glomerulonephritis, 758
　　　　Immunoglobulin A Nephropathy, 759
　　　　Nephrotic Syndrome, 759
　　　　Hemolytic Uremic Syndrome, 759
　　　Nephroblastoma, 760
　　　Bladder Disorders, 760
　　　　Urinary Tract Infections, 760
　　　　Vesicoureteral Reflux, 761
　　　Urinary Incontinence, 761
　　　　Types of Incontinence, 761

UNIT 10　The Reproductive Systems

32 **Structure and Function of the Reproductive Systems,** 763
　Kelly Power-Kean, with originating chapter contributions by George W. Rodway and Sue E. Huether
　　　Development of the Reproductive Systems, 764
　　　　Sexual Differentiation in Utero, 765
　　　　Puberty and Reproductive Maturation, 767
　　　The Female Reproductive System, 767
　　　　External Genitalia, 767
　　　　Internal Genitalia, 768
　　　　Female Sex Hormones, 772
　　　　Menstrual Cycle, 772
　　　Structure and Function of the Breast, 775
　　　　Female Breast, 775
　　　　Male Breast, 777
　　　The Male Reproductive System, 777
　　　　External Genitalia, 777
　　　　Internal Genitalia, 779
　　　　Spermatogenesis, 780
　　　　Male Sex and Reproductive Hormones, 780
　　　Aging and Reproductive Function, 781
　　　　Aging and the Female Reproductive System, 781
　　　　Aging and the Male Reproductive System, 782

33 **Alterations of the Female Reproductive System,** 785
　Kelly Power-Kean, with originating chapter contributions by Kathryn L. McCance
　　　Abnormalities of the Female Reproductive Tract, 786
　　　Alterations of Sexual Maturation, 786
　　　　Delayed or Absent Puberty, 787
　　　　Precocious Puberty, 787
　　　Disorders of the Female Reproductive System, 787
　　　　Hormonal and Menstrual Alterations, 788
　　　　Infection and Inflammation, 793
　　　　Pelvic Organ Prolapse, 797
　　　　Benign Growths and Proliferative Conditions, 798
　　　　Cancer, 802
　　　　Sexual Dysfunction, 811
　　　　Impaired Fertility, 811
　　　Disorders of the Female Breast, 812
　　　　Galactorrhea, 812
　　　　Benign Breast Disease and Conditions, 813
　　　　Breast Cancer, 814
　　　CASE STUDY: Breast Cancer, 829

34 Alterations of the Male Reproductive System, 832
Kelly Power-Kean, with originating chapter contributions by George W. Rodway
- Alterations of Sexual Maturation, 833
  - *Delayed or Absent Puberty, 833*
  - *Precocious Puberty, 833*
- Disorders of the Male Reproductive System, 833
  - *Disorders of the Urethra, 833*
  - *Disorders of the Penis, 833*
  - *Disorders of the Scrotum, Testis, and Epididymis, 836*
  - *Disorders of the Prostate Gland, 840*
  - *Sexual Dysfunction, 852*
- Disorders of the Male Breast, 855
  - *Gynecomastia, 855*
  - *Carcinoma, 855*
- Sexually Transmitted Infections, 856
- CASE STUDY: Benign Prostatic Hyperplasia, 859

UNIT 11 The Digestive System

35 Structure and Function of the Digestive System, 861
Mohamed Toufic El-Hussein, with originating chapter contributions by Sue E. Huether
- The Gastro-intestinal Tract, 862
  - *Mouth and Esophagus, 862*
  - *Stomach, 864*
  - *Large Intestine, 871*
  - *Intestinal Microbiome, 873*
  - *Splanchnic Blood Flow, 873*
- Accessory Organs of Digestion, 873
  - *Liver, 874*
  - *Gallbladder, 877*
  - *Exocrine Pancreas, 877*
- **GERIATRIC CONSIDERATIONS:** Aging and the Gastro-intestinal System, 880

36 Alterations of Digestive Function, 882
Mohamed Toufic El-Hussein, with originating chapter contributions by Sue E. Huether
- Disorders of the Gastro-intestinal Tract, 883
  - *Clinical Manifestations of Gastro-intestinal Dysfunction, 883*
  - *Disorders of Motility, 887*
  - *Gastritis, 892*
  - *Peptic Ulcer Disease, 893*
  - *Malabsorption Syndromes, 897*
  - *Inflammatory Bowel Disease, 898*
  - *Diverticular Disease of the Colon, 900*
  - *Appendicitis, 901*
  - *Mesenteric Vascular Insufficiency, 901*
  - *Disorders of Nutrition, 902*
- Disorders of the Accessory Organs of Digestion, 905
  - *Common Complications of Liver Disorders, 906*
  - *Disorders of the Liver, 910*
  - *Disorders of the Gallbladder, 914*
  - *Disorders of the Pancreas, 915*
  - *Digestive Symptoms and Intestinal Inflammation in COVID-19 Patients, 917*
- Cancer of the Digestive System, 917
  - *Cancer of the Gastro-intestinal Tract, 917*
  - *Cancer of the Accessory Organs of Digestion, 921*
- COMORBIDITIES: Comorbidities Related to Digestive Function, 924
- **GERIATRIC CONSIDERATIONS:** Age-Related Gastric Changes, 926
- CASE STUDY, 927

37 Developmental Alterations of Digestive Function, 927
Mohamed Toufic El-Hussein, with originating chapter contributions by Sharon Sables-Baus and Sara J. Fidanza
- Disorders of the Gastro-intestinal Tract, 928
  - *Congenital Impairment of Motility, 928*
  - *Acquired Impairment of Motility, 931*
  - *Impairment of Digestion, Absorption, and Nutrition, 932*
  - *Diarrhea, 936*
- Disorders of the Liver, 937
  - *Disorders of Biliary Metabolism and Transport, 937*
  - *Inflammatory Disorders, 938*
  - *Portal Hypertension, 939*
  - *Metabolic Disorders, 939*
- Gastro-intestinal Malignancies in Children, 939
  - *Hepatoblastoma, 940*
  - *Pancreatic Tumours, 940*

UNIT 12 The Musculoskeletal and Integumentary Systems

38 Structure and Function of the Musculoskeletal System, 942
Stephanie Zettel, with originating chapter contributions by Geri C. Reeves
- Structure and Function of Bones, 943
  - *Elements of Bone Tissue, 943*
  - *Types of Bone Tissue, 947*
  - *Characteristics of Bone, 948*
  - *Maintenance of Bone Integrity, 949*
- Structure and Function of Joints, 950
  - *Fibrous Joints, 950*
  - *Cartilaginous Joints, 950*
  - *Synovial Joints, 953*
- Structure and Function of Skeletal Muscles, 953
  - *Whole Muscle, 953*
  - *Components of Muscle Function, 958*
  - *Tendons and Ligaments, 961*
- Aging and the Musculoskeletal System, 961
  - *Aging of Bones, 961*
  - *Aging of Joints, 962*
  - *Aging of Muscles, 962*

39 Alterations of Musculoskeletal Function, 964
Stephanie Zettel, with originating chapter contributions by Benjamin A. Smallheer
- Musculoskeletal Injuries, 965
  - *Skeletal Trauma, 965*
  - *Support Structures, 968*
- Disorders of Bones, 973
  - *Metabolic Bone Diseases, 974*
  - *Infectious Bone Disease: Osteomyelitis, 981*

Disorders of Joints, 982
  Osteoarthritis, 982
  Classic Inflammatory Joint Disease, 985
Disorders of Skeletal Muscle, 994
  Secondary Muscular Dysfunction, 994
  Fibromyalgia, 994
  Chronic Fatigue Syndrome, 996
  Muscle Membrane Abnormalities, 996
  Metabolic Muscle Diseases, 996
  Inflammatory Muscle Diseases: Myositis, 997
  Toxic Myopathies, 999
Musculoskeletal Tumours, 1000
  Bone Tumours, 1000
  Muscle Tumours, 1004
CASE STUDY: Fractures from a Fall, 1004

40 Developmental Alterations of Musculoskeletal Function, 1007
Stephanie Zettel, with originating chapter contributions by Kathryn L. McCance

Congenital Defects, 1008
  Clubfoot, 1008
  Developmental Dysplasia of the Hip, 1008
  Osteogenesis Imperfecta, 1009
Bone Infection, 1010
  Osteomyelitis, 1010
  Septic Arthritis, 1010
Juvenile Idiopathic Arthritis, 1012
Osteochondroses, 1012
  Legg-Calvé-Perthes Disease, 1013
  Osgood-Schlatter Disease, 1014
Scoliosis, 1014
Muscular Dystrophy, 1015
  Duchenne Muscular Dystrophy, 1015
  Becker Muscular Dystrophy, 1016
  Facioscapulohumeral Muscular Dystrophy, 1017
  Myotonic Muscular Dystrophy, 1017
Musculoskeletal Tumours, 1017
  Benign Bone Tumours, 1017
  Malignant Bone Tumours, 1018
Nonaccidental Trauma, 1019
  Fractures in Nonaccidental Trauma, 1019

41 Structure, Function, and Disorders of the Integument, 1021
Stephanie Zettel, with originating chapter contributions by Sue Ann McCann and Sue E. Huether

Structure and Function of the Skin, 1022
  Layers of the Skin, 1022
  Clinical Manifestations of Skin Dysfunction, 1024
Disorders of the Skin, 1029
  Inflammatory Disorders, 1029
  Papulosquamous Disorders, 1030
  Vesiculobullous Diseases, 1033
  Infections, 1034
  Vascular Disorders, 1038
  Benign Tumours, 1039
  Skin Cancer, 1039
  Burns, 1042
  Cold Injury, 1046
Disorders of the Hair, 1047
  Alopecia, 1047
  Hirsutism, 1049
Disorders of the Nail, 1049
  Paronychia, 1049
  Onychomycosis, 1049
GERIATRIC CONSIDERATIONS: Aging and Changes in Skin Integrity, 1049

42 Developmental Alterations of the Integument, 1053
Stephanie Zettel, with originating chapter contributions by Noreen Heer Nicol and Sue E. Huether

Acne Vulgaris, 1053
Dermatitis, 1054
  Atopic Dermatitis, 1054
  Diaper Dermatitis, 1055
Infections of the Skin, 1055
  Bacterial Infections, 1055
  Fungal Infections, 1056
  Viral Infections, 1057
Insect Bites and Parasites, 1060
  Scabies, 1060
  Pediculosis (Lice Infestation), 1060
  Fleas, 1060
  Bedbugs, 1061
Cutaneous Hemangiomas and Vascular Malformations, 1061
  Cutaneous Hemangiomas, 1061
  Cutaneous Vascular Malformations, 1061
Other Skin Disorders, 1062
  Miliaria, 1062
  Erythema Toxicum Neonatorum, 1062

Appendix, 1064
Index, 1081

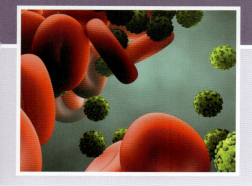

1

Cellular Biology

Stephanie Zettel, with originating chapter contributions by Kathryn L. McCance

Additional resources are available online at http://evolve.elsevier.com/Canada/Huether/pathophysiology

CHAPTER OUTLINE

Prokaryotes and Eukaryotes, 2
Cellular Functions, 2
Structure and Function of Cellular Components, 3
  Nucleus, 3
  Cytoplasmic Organelles, 3
  Plasma Membranes, 3
  Cellular Receptors, 10
Cell-To-Cell Adhesions, 11
  Extracellular Matrix, 11
  Specialized Cell Junctions, 12
Cellular Communication and Signal Transduction, 14
Cellular Metabolism, 15
  Role of Adenosine Triphosphate, 15
  Food and Production of Cellular Energy, 16
  Oxidative Phosphorylation, 17
Membrane Transport: Cellular Intake and Output, 18
  Electrolytes as Solutes, 19
  Transport by Vesicle Formation, 22
  Movement of Electrical Impulses: Membrane Potentials, 24
Cellular Reproduction: The Cell Cycle, 25
  Phases of Mitosis and Cytokinesis, 26
  Rates of Cellular Division, 26
  Growth Factors, 27
Tissues, 27
  Tissue Formation, 28
  Types of Tissues, 28

LEARNING OBJECTIVES

1. Compare and contrast prokaryotes and eukaryotes.
2. Identify the eight specialized functions of a cell.
3. Discuss the functions of the principal cytoplasmic organelles.
4. Discuss the plasma membrane, addressing both structural and functional aspects.
5. Discuss the importance of the amphipathic properties of the membrane lipid layer.
6. Discuss the importance of plasma membrane proteins.
7. Discuss the functions of cell membrane receptors and principal types of ligands.
8. Discuss the importance and structure of the extracellular matrix.
9. Describe methods and processes of cellular communication and types of signalling.
10. Describe the process of energy generation and utilization by the cell to support cellular function.
11. Describe the role of ATP in the cell.
12. Describe the processes of passive transport, diffusion, hydrostatic pressure, and osmosis.
13. Define mediated active and passive transport, endocytosis, and exocytosis, and give examples of each.
14. Discuss the electrochemical changes in the plasma membrane that result in an action potential.
15. Describe cellular reproduction within the four phases of the cell cycle and the four stages of the M phase.
16. Describe the three ways that cells adhere to each other to form tissues and organs.
17. Name the four basic tissue types.

KEY TERMS

Absolute refractory period, 25
Action potential, 24
Active transport, 18
Amphipathic, 4
Anabolism, 15
Anaphase, 26
Anion, 19
Antiport, 19
Arrested (resting) (G_0) state, 27
Autocrine signalling, 14
Basal lamina, 11
Basement membrane, 11
Binding site, 10
Catabolism, 15
Cation, 19
Caveolae, 22
Cell adhesion molecule (CAM), 8
Cell cortex, 9
Cell cycle, 25
Cell junction, 12
Cell polarity, 3
Cell-to-cell adhesion, 11
Cellular metabolism, 15
Cellular receptor, 10
Centromere, 26
Channel, 18
Chemical synapse, 14
Chromatid, 26
Chromatin, 26
Citric acid cycle (Krebs cycle, tricarboxylic acid cycle), 17
Clathrin, 22
Coated vesicle, 22
Collagen, 11
Concentration gradient, 20
Connective tissue, 11
Connexon, 14
Contact-dependent signalling, 14
Cytokinesis, 25
Cytoplasm, 3
Cytoplasmic matrix, 3
Cytosol, 3
Daughter cell, 26
Depolarization, 24

Desmosome, 13
Differentiation, 3
Diffusion, 20
Digestion, 16
Effective osmolality, 21
Elastin, 12
Electrolyte, 19
Electron-transport chain, 17
Endocytosis, 22
Endosome, 22
Equatorial plate (metaphase plate), 26
ER stress, 9
Eukaryote, 2
Exocytosis, 22
Extracellular matrix (ECM), 11
Fibroblast, 11
Fibronectin, 12
Filtration, 20
G_0 phase, 25
G_1 phase, 25
G_2 phase, 25
Gap junction, 14
Gating, 14
Glycocalyx, 10
Glycolipid, 4
Glycolysis, 17
Glycoprotein, 4
Growth factor (cytokine), 27
Histones, 3
Homeostasis, 14
Hormonal signalling, 14
Hyperpolarized state, 25
Hypopolarized state, 25
Interphase, 25
Ions, 8
Junctional complex, 14
Ligand, 10
Lipid bilayer, 8
M phase, 25
Macromolecule, 11
Mediated transport, 18
Meiosis, 25
Membrane lipid raft (MLR), 6
Membrane transport protein, 18
Metabolic pathway, 15
Metaphase, 26
Mitosis, 25
Neurohormonal signalling, 14
Neurotransmitter, 14
Nuclear envelope, 3
Nuclear pores, 3
Nucleolus 3
Nucleus, 3
Oncotic pressure (colloid osmotic pressure), 21
Organelle, 3
Osmolality, 20
Osmolarity, 21
Osmosis, 21
Osmotic pressure, 21
Oxidation, 17
Oxidative phosphorylation, 17
Paracrine signalling, 14
Passive transport, 18
Phagocytosis, 22
Phospholipid, 6
Phospholipid bilayer, 3
Pinocytosis, 22
Plasma membrane (plasmalemma), 3
Plasma membrane receptor, 10
Platelet-derived growth factor (PDGF), 27
Polarity, 19
Polypeptide, 6
Post-translational modification (PTM), 6
Prokaryote, 2
Prophase, 26
Protein, 6
Proteolytic, 9
Receptor protein, 14
Receptor-mediated endocytosis (ligand internalization), 22
Relative refractory period, 25
Repolarization, 25
Resting membrane potential, 22
Retinoblastoma (Rb) protein, 27
S phase, 25
Signalling cell, 14
Signal transduction pathway, 14
Solute, 18
Spindle fibre, 26
Stem cell, 28
Stroma, 27
Substrate, 15
Substrate phosphorylation (anaerobic glycolysis), 17
Symport, 19
Target cell, 14
Telophase, 26
Terminally differentiated, 28
Threshold potential, 24
Tight junction, 13
Tonicity, 21
Transfer reaction, 17
Transmembrane protein, 8
Transporter, 18
Unfolded-protein response (UPR), 9
Uniport, 19
Valence, 19

It is important to understand the structure of cells in order to understand mechanisms of disease, because cells communicate with each other and work together within an entire system. Messages are transmitted, received, interpreted, and used by the cell in a variety of ways, and streamlined conversation between, among, and within cells maintains cellular function and specialization. When cells resemble each other and work more effectively together, they are well-differentiated and work to promote the integrity of the entire organism. For example, prokaryotic and eukaryotic cells are organized differently, and this accounts for the difference in their response to pharmacotherapy. Anti-infectives, such as penicillin, are only effective against bacteria, whereas pharmacotherapy against eukaryotic cells results in more severe adverse effects, because they are more closely related to human cells When cells become less differentiated (as a result of injury or mutation) or less like the surrounding cells, the conversation breaks down, and cells either adapt (sometimes altering function) or become vulnerable to isolation, injury, or diseases such as cancer.

PROKARYOTES AND EUKARYOTES

Living cells generally are divided into eukaryotes and prokaryotes. The cells of higher animals and plants are eukaryotes, as are the single-celled organisms, fungi, protozoa, and most algae. Prokaryotes include cyanobacteria (blue-green algae), bacteria, and rickettsiae.

Eukaryotes (*eu* = good; *karyon* = nucleus; also spelled *eucaryotes*) are larger and have more extensive intracellular anatomy and organization than prokaryotes. Eukaryotic cells also have a characteristic set of membrane-bound intracellular compartments, called *organelles*, that includes a well-defined nucleus. **Prokaryotes**, on the other hand, contain no organelles, and their nuclear material is not encased by a nuclear membrane. There is no distinct nucleus.

Prokaryotic and eukaryotic cells differ in chemical composition and biochemical activity. The *nuclei* of prokaryotic cells carry genetic information in a single circular chromosome, and they lack a class of proteins called *histones*, which in eukaryotic cells bind with deoxyribonucleic acid (DNA) and are involved in the supercoiling of DNA. Eukaryotic cells have several or many chromosomes. Protein production, or synthesis, in the two classes of cells also differs because of major structural differences in ribonucleic acid (RNA)–protein complexes. Other distinctions include differences in mechanisms of transport across the outer cellular membrane and in enzyme content.

CELLULAR FUNCTIONS

QUICK CHECK 1.1
1. Why is the process of differentiation essential to specialization? Give an example.
2. Describe at least two cellular functions.

Cells become specialized through the process of **differentiation**, or maturation, so that some cells eventually perform one kind of function and other cells perform other functions. Cells with a highly developed function, such as movement, often lack some other property, such as hormone production, which is more highly developed in other cells.

All cells share essentially eight common functions, which are listed below:

1. *Movement.* Muscle cells can generate forces that produce motion. Muscles that are attached to bones produce limb movements. Muscles that enclose hollow tubes or cavities also move or empty contents when they contract (e.g., the colon).
2. *Conductivity.* Conductivity is the chief function of nerve cells. A stimulus creates an electrical potential across the cell membrane that is then propagated to other cells and cellular components.
3. *Metabolic absorption.* All cells can take in and use nutrients and other substances from their surroundings.
4. *Secretion.* Certain cells, such as mucous gland cells, can synthesize new substances from substances they absorb and then secrete the new substances to serve as needed elsewhere.
5. *Excretion.* All cells can create waste products resulting from the metabolic breakdown of nutrients. Membrane-bound sacs (lysosomes) within cells contain enzymes that break down, or digest, large molecules, turning them into waste products that are released from the cell.
6. *Respiration.* Cells absorb oxygen, which is used to transform nutrients into energy in the form of adenosine triphosphate (ATP). Cellular respiration, or oxidation, occurs in organelles called *mitochondria*.
7. *Reproduction.* Tissue growth occurs as cells enlarge and reproduce. Even without growth, tissue maintenance requires that new cells be produced to replace cells that are lost normally through cellular death. Not all cells are capable of continuous division (see Chapter 4).
8. *Communication.* Communication is vital for cells to survive as a society of cells. Appropriate communication allows the maintenance of a dynamic steady state.

STRUCTURE AND FUNCTION OF CELLULAR COMPONENTS

Figure 1.1A shows a "typical" eukaryotic cell, which consists of three components: an outer membrane called the **plasma membrane, or plasmalemma**; a fluid "filling" called **cytoplasm** (Figure 1.1B); and the "organs" of the cell—the membrane-bound intracellular **organelles**, among them the nucleus.

Nucleus

The **nucleus**, which is surrounded by the cytoplasm and generally is located in the centre of the cell, is the largest membrane-bound organelle. Two pliable membranes compose the **nuclear envelope** (Figure 1.2A). The nuclear envelope has **nuclear pores**, which allow chemical messages to exit and enter the nucleus (Figure 1.2B). The outer membrane is continuous with membranes of the endoplasmic reticulum (see Figure 1.1). The nucleus contains the **nucleolus** (a small, dense structure composed largely of RNA), most of the cellular DNA, and the DNA-binding proteins (i.e., the histones) that regulate its activity. The DNA "chain" in eukaryotic cells is so long that it is easily broken. **Histones** are proteins that are essential for cell division in eukaryotes. They bind to DNA and cause DNA to fold into chromosomes (Figure 1.2C), thus decreasing the risk of breaks in the DNA chain.

The primary functions of the nucleus are cell division and control of genetic information. Other functions include the replication and repair of DNA and the transcription of the information stored in DNA. Genetic information is transcribed into RNA, which can be processed into various forms of RNA (such as messenger, transport, and ribosomal RNAs) and introduced into the cytoplasm, where it directs cellular activities. Most of the processing of RNA occurs in the nucleolus. (The roles of DNA and RNA in protein synthesis are discussed in Chapter 2.)

Cytoplasmic Organelles

Cytoplasm is an aqueous solution (also called the **cytosol**) that fills the **cytoplasmic matrix**—the space between the nuclear envelope and the plasma membrane. The cytosol represents about half the volume of a eukaryotic cell. It contains thousands of enzymes involved in intermediate metabolism and is *crowded* with ribosomes making proteins (see Figure 1.1B).[1] The organelles suspended in the cytoplasm have their own biological membranes, because they simultaneously carry out essential cellular functions requiring different biochemical environments. Many of these functions are directed by coded messages carried from the nucleus by RNA. The functions include protein and hormone synthesis and transport, the maintenance of cellular structure and motility, cellular metabolism, as well as the processing and elimination of waste (including cellular debris and foreign proteins or antigens). The cytosol is a storage unit for fat, carbohydrates, and secretory vesicles. Table 1.1 lists the principal cytoplasmic organelles.

Plasma Membranes

Every cell is contained within a membrane with gates, channels, and pumps. Membranes surround the cell or enclose an intracellular organelle and are important to normal physiological function because they control the composition of the space, or compartment, they enclose. Membranes can allow or exclude various molecules and, because of selective transport systems, they can move molecules in or out of the space (Figure 1.3). By controlling the movement of substances from one compartment to another, membranes exert a powerful influence on metabolic pathways. Directional transport is facilitated by the distribution of charge within a cell, as well as differences in the structure of one aspect of the cell when compared with another. **Cell polarity**, the direction of cellular transport, maintains normal cell and tissue structure for numerous functions (e.g., movement of nutrients in and out of the cell) and becomes altered with diseases (Figure 1.4). The plasma membrane also has an important role in cell-to-cell recognition. Other functions of the plasma membrane include cellular mobility and the maintenance of cellular shape (Table 1.2).

Membrane Composition

The basic structure of cell membranes is the **phospholipid bilayer**, which is composed of two layers of lipid molecules, one layer with a phospholipid head attached to two fatty acid chains. Proteins also span the bilayer to form channels and receptors that alter processes inside the cell. (Figure 1.5). The phospholipid bilayer is a complex structure where lipids and proteins are not uniformly distributed but can separate into discrete units called *microdomains*, differing in their protein and lipid compositions[2] and different membranes have varying percentages of lipids and proteins. For instance, intracellular membranes

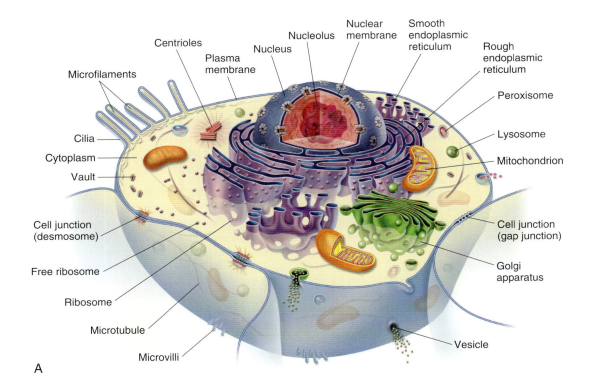

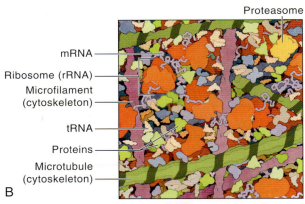

FIGURE 1.1 Typical Components of a Eukaryotic Cell and Structure of the Cytoplasm. A, Artist's interpretation of cell structure. Note the many mitochondria known as the "power plants of the cell." **B,** Colour-enhanced electron micrograph of a cell. The cell is crowded. Note, too, the innumerable dots bordering the endoplasmic reticulum. These are ribosomes, the cell's "protein factories." *mRNA*, Messenger RNA; *tRNA*, transfer RNA. ([B] from Patton, K. T. [2019]. *Anatomy & physiology* [10th ed.]. Elsevier.)

may have a higher percentage of proteins than plasma membranes, most likely because most enzymatic activity occurs within organelles. The cell membrane exists in different physical states called *phases*: solid gel phase, fluid liquid-crystalline phase, and liquid-ordered phase (Figure 1.5B). These phases, which are determined by physical bonds between larger proteins in the bilayer, are dynamic and can change under physiological factors such as temperature and pressure fluctuations. Carbohydrates can be associated with plasma membranes when they are chemically combined with lipids (**glycolipids**), and with proteins (**glycoproteins**) (see Figure 1.5).

The outer surface of the plasma membrane in many types of cells, especially endothelial cells and adipocytes, is not smooth but dimpled with flask-shaped invaginations known as caveolae ("tiny caves"). Caveolae serve as a storage site for many receptors, provide a route for transport into the cell, and act as the initiator for relaying signals from several extracellular chemical messengers into the cell's interior.

Lipids. Each lipid molecule is said to be polar, or **amphipathic**, which means that one part is hydrophobic (uncharged, or "water hating") and another part is hydrophilic (charged, or "water loving") (Figure 1.6). The membrane spontaneously organizes itself into two layers because of these two incompatible solubilities. The bilayer serves as a barrier to the diffusion of water and hydrophilic substances, while allowing lipid-soluble molecules, such as oxygen (O_2) and carbon dioxide (CO_2), to diffuse through the membrane readily. The structure of

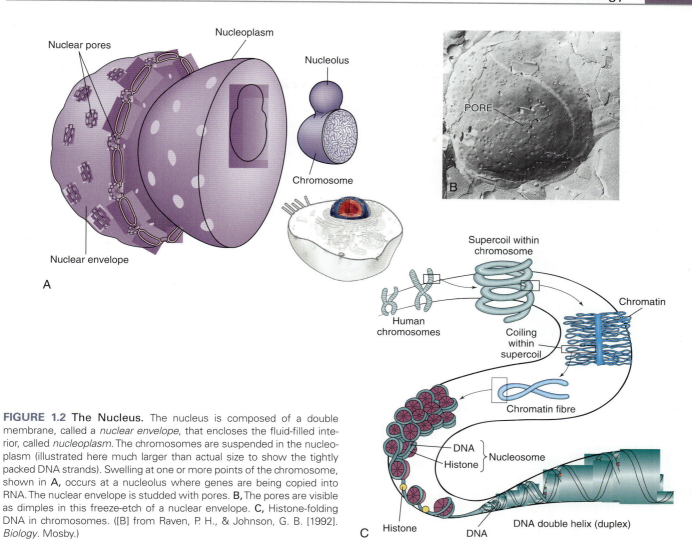

FIGURE 1.2 The Nucleus. The nucleus is composed of a double membrane, called a *nuclear envelope*, that encloses the fluid-filled interior, called *nucleoplasm*. The chromosomes are suspended in the nucleoplasm (illustrated here much larger than actual size to show the tightly packed DNA strands). Swelling at one or more points of the chromosome, shown in **A**, occurs at a nucleolus where genes are being copied into RNA. The nuclear envelope is studded with pores. **B,** The pores are visible as dimples in this freeze-etch of a nuclear envelope. **C,** Histone-folding DNA in chromosomes. ([B] from Raven, P. H., & Johnson, G. B. [1992]. *Biology*. Mosby.)

TABLE 1.1	Principal Cytoplasmic Organelles
Organelle	**Characteristics and Description**
Ribosomes	RNA-protein complexes (nucleoproteins) synthesized in nucleolus and secreted into cytoplasm. They provide sites for cellular protein synthesis.
Endoplasmic reticulum	Network of tubular channels (cisternae) that extend throughout outer nuclear membrane. It specializes in synthesis and transport of protein and lipid components of most organelles.
Golgi complex	Network of smooth membranes and vesicles located near nucleus. It is responsible for processing and packaging proteins onto secretory vesicles that break away from the complex and migrate to various intracellular and extracellular destinations, including the plasma membrane. Best-known vesicles are those that have coats largely made of the protein *clathrin*. Proteins in the complex bind to the cytoskeleton, generating tension that helps organelle function and keep the complex's stretched shape intact.
Lysosomes	Saclike structures that originate from the Golgi complex and contain enzymes for digesting most cellular substances to their basic form, such as amino acids, fatty acids, and carbohydrates (sugars). Cellular injury leads to release of lysosomal enzymes that cause cellular self-destruction.
Peroxisomes	Structures similar to lysosomes, but contain several oxidative enzymes (e.g., catalase, urate oxidase) that produce or use hydrogen peroxide; reactions detoxify various wastes.
Mitochondria	Structures that contain metabolic machinery needed for cellular energy metabolism. Enzymes of respiratory chain (electron-transport chain), found in the inner membrane of mitochondria, generate most of a cell's ATP (oxidative phosphorylation). They have a role in osmotic regulation, pH control, calcium homeostasis, and cell signalling.
Cytoskeleton	"Bone and muscle" of a cell. It is composed of a network of protein filaments, including microtubules and actin filaments (microfilaments); it forms cell extensions (microvilli, cilia, flagella).
Caveolae	Tiny indentations (caves) that can capture extracellular material and shuttle it inside the cell or across the cell.
Vaults	Cytoplasmic ribonucleoproteins shaped like octagonal barrels. They are thought to act as "trucks," shuttling molecules from the nucleus to elsewhere in the cell.

ATP, Adenosine triphosphate.

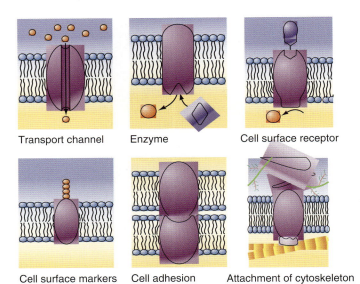

FIGURE 1.3 Functions of Plasma Membrane Proteins. The plasma membrane proteins illustrated here show a variety of functions performed by the different types of plasma membranes. (From Raven, P. H., & Johnson, G. B. [1995]. *Understanding biology* [3rd ed.]. William C. Brown Communications.)

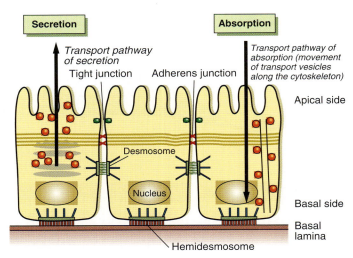

FIGURE 1.4 Cell Polarity of Epithelial Cells. Schematic of cell polarity (cell direction) of epithelial cells. Shown are the directions of the basal side and the apical side. Organelles and cytoskeleton are also arranged directionally to enable, for example, intestinal cell secretion and absorption. (Adapted from *Life science web textbook*, The University of Tokyo.)

TABLE 1.2	Plasma Membrane Functions
Cellular Mechanism	**Membrane Functions**
Structure	Usually thicker than membranes of intracellular organelles
	Containment of cellular organelles
	Maintenance of relationship with cytoskeleton, endoplasmic reticulum, and other organelles
	Maintenance of fluid and electrolyte balance
	Outer surfaces of plasma membranes in many cells are not smooth but are dimpled with cavelike indentations called *caveolae*; they are also studded with cilia or even smaller cylindrical projections called *microvilli*; both are capable of movement
Protection	Barrier to toxic molecules and macromolecules (proteins, nucleic acids, polysaccharides)
	Barrier to foreign organisms and cells
Activation of cell	Hormones (regulation of cellular activity)
	Mitogens (cellular division; see Chapter 2)
	Antigens (antibody synthesis; see Chapter 6)
	Growth factors (proliferation and differentiation; see Chapter 10)
Storage	Storage site for many receptors
Transport	Diffusion and exchange diffusion
	Endocytosis (pinocytosis, phagocytosis)
	Exocytosis (secretion)
	Active transport
Cell-to-cell interaction	Communication and attachment at junctional complexes
	Symbiotic nutritive relationships
	Release of enzymes and antibodies to extracellular environment
	Relationships with extracellular matrix

Modified from King, D. W., Fenoglio, C. M., & Lefkowitch, J. H. (1983). *General pathology: Principles and dynamics*. Lea & Febiger.

the cell membrane also makes it more difficult for water-soluble medications and ionized medications to enter the cell.

The most abundant lipids in the cell membrane are phospholipids. **Phospholipids** have a phosphate-containing hydrophilic head connected to a hydrophobic tail. Phospholipids and glycolipids (lipids bound to carbohydrates) form self-sealing lipid bilayers. Lipids and associated proteins act as "molecular glue" for the structural integrity of the membrane and form **membrane lipid rafts (MLRs)**. MLRs appear to be structurally and functionally distinct regions of the plasma membrane[3,4] and consist of numerous microdomains that form a network of various lipid–lipid, protein–protein, and protein–lipid interactions (Figures 1.5B and 1.7). Lipid rafts have several functions that include (1) cellular polarity and the corresponding communication of cellular signals; (2) platforms for extracellular matrix (ECM) adhesion and cellular structure through cell adhesion molecules (CAMs); (3) signalling across the membrane, which can alter the structure of the cytosol and regulate cell growth, movement, and other functions; and (4) entry of viruses, bacteria, toxins, and nanoparticles.[3]

Proteins. A **protein** is made from a chain of amino acids known as **polypeptides**. There are 20 types of amino acids in proteins, and each type of protein has a unique sequence of amino acids. A protein is synthesized through the translation of RNA (see Chapter 2). A protein might then undergo a series of **post-translational modifications (PTMs)** that further impact and diversify protein function in the cell. These PTMs can alter the activity and functions of proteins and have become very important in understanding the nature of disease. For instance, researchers have known for decades that pathogens can interfere with the host's PTMs.[5]

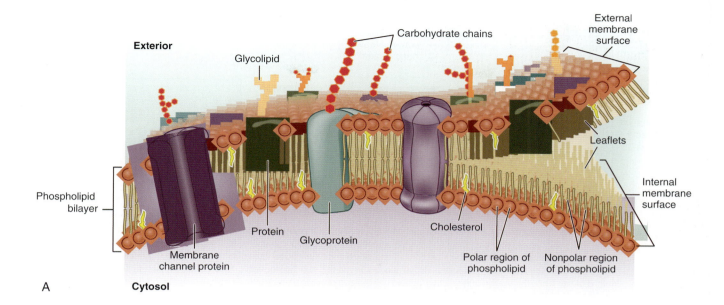
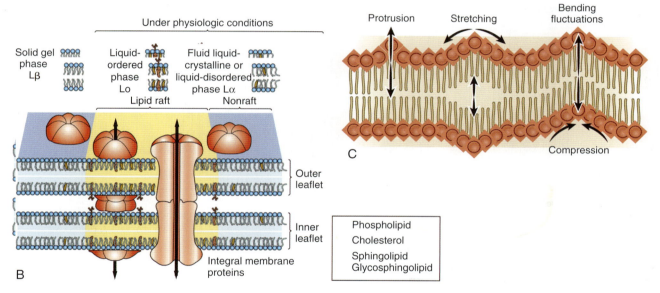

FIGURE 1.5 Lipid Bilayer Membranes. A, Lipids and proteins are not evenly distributed but can isolate into microdomains, differing in their protein and lipid composition. **B,** An example of a microdomain is lipid rafts (*yellow*). Rafts are dynamic domain structures composed of cholesterol, sphingolipids, and membrane proteins important in different cellular processes. Various models exist to clarify the functions of domains. The three major phases of lipid bilayer organization include a solid gel phase (e.g., with low temperatures), a liquid-ordered phase (high temperatures), and a fluid liquid-crystalline (or liquid-disordered) phase. Some membrane-associated proteins are integrated into the lipid bilayer; other proteins are loosely attached to the outer and inner surfaces of the membrane. Transmembrane proteins protrude through the entire outer and inner surfaces of the membrane, and they can be attracted to microdomains through specific interactions with lipids. Interaction of the membrane proteins with distinct lipids depends on the hydrophobic thickness of the membrane, the lateral pressures of the membrane (mechanical force may shift protein channels from an open to closed state), the polarity or electrical charges at the lipid-protein interface, and the presence on the protein side of amino acid side chains. Protein-lipid interactions can be critical for correct insertion, folding, and orientation of membrane proteins. For example, diseases related to lipids that interfere with protein folding are becoming more prevalent. **C,** The cell membrane is not static but is always moving. Observed for the first time from measurements taken at the National Institute of Standards and Technology (NIST) and France's Institut Laue-Langevin (ILL). (Adapted from Bagatolli, L. A., Ipsen, J. H., Simonsen, A. C., et al. [2010]. *Progress in Lipid Research, 49*[4], 378–389; Contreras, F. X., Ernst, A. M., Wieland, F., et al. [2011]. *Cold Spring Harbor Perspectives in Biology, 3*[6], a004705; Cooper, G. M. [2000]. *The cell—a molecular approach* [2nd ed.]. Sunderland (MA): Sinauer Associates; Defamie, N., & Mesnil, M. [2012]. *Biochimica et Biophysica Acta, 1818*[8], 1866–1869; Woodka, A. C., Butler, P. D., Porcar, L. et al. [2012]. *Physical Review Letters, 109*[5], 058102.)

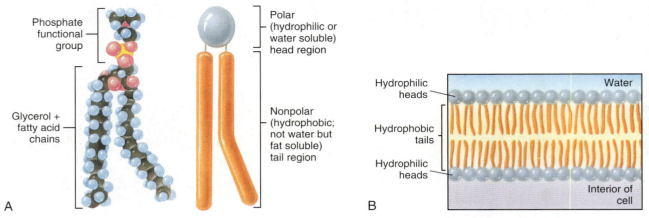

FIGURE 1.6 Structure of a Phospholipid Molecule. A, Each phospholipid molecule consists of a phosphate functional group and two fatty acid chains attached to a glycerol molecule. **B,** The fatty acid chains and glycerol form nonpolar, hydrophobic "tails," and the phosphate functional group forms the polar, hydrophilic "head" of the phospholipid molecule. When placed in water, the hydrophobic tails of the molecule face inward, away from the water, and the hydrophilic head faces outward, toward the water. (From Raven, P. H., & Johnson, G. B. [1995]. *Understanding biology* [3rd ed.]. W.C. Brown Communications.)

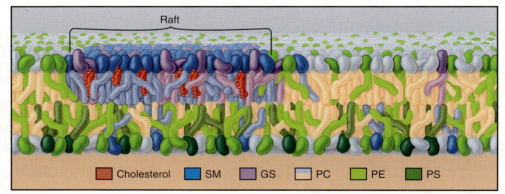

FIGURE 1.7 Lipid Rafts. The plasma membrane is composed of many lipids, including sphingomyelin (*SM*) and cholesterol, shown here as a small raft in the external leaflet. *GS,* Glycosphingolipid; *PC,* phosphatidylcholine; *PE,* phosphatidylethanolamine; *PS,* phosphatidylserine. (From Pollard, T. D., & Ernshaw, W. C. [2004]. *Cell biology.* Saunders/Elsevier.)

Membrane proteins associate with the lipid bilayer in different ways (Figure 1.8), including (1) **transmembrane proteins** that extend across the bilayer and are exposed to an aqueous environment on both sides of the membrane (Figure 1.8A); (2) proteins located almost entirely in the cytosol and are associated with the cytosolic half of the lipid bilayer by an α helix exposed on the surface of the protein (Figure 1.8B); (3) proteins that exist outside the bilayer, on one side or the other, and are attached to the membrane by one or more covalently (or chemically-bonded) attached lipid groups (Figure 1.8C); and (4) proteins bound indirectly to one or the other bilayer membrane face, held in place by their interactions with other proteins (Figure 1.8D).[1]

Proteins exist in densely folded molecular configurations rather than straight chains; so most hydrophilic (water soluble) units are at the surface of the molecule, and most hydrophobic (water insoluble) units are inside. Membrane proteins, like other proteins, are synthesized by the ribosome and then make their way in a process called *trafficking*, to different membrane locations of a cell.[6] Trafficking places unique demands on membrane proteins for folding, translocation, and stability.[6] Thus, much research is now being done to understand misfolded proteins and how they can result in disease (Box 1.1).

Although membrane structure is determined by the **lipid bilayer**, membrane functions are determined largely by proteins. Proteins act as (1) recognition and binding units (receptors) for substances moving into and out of the cell; (2) pores or transport channels for various electrically charged particles, called **ions** or *electrolytes,* and specific carriers for amino acids and monosaccharides; (3) specific enzymes that drive active pumps to promote concentration of certain ions, particularly potassium (K^+), within the cell while keeping concentrations of other ions (e.g., sodium, Na^+) less than concentrations found in the extracellular environment; (4) cell surface markers, such as glycoproteins (proteins attached to carbohydrates), that identify a cell to its neighbour; (5) **cell adhesion molecules (CAMs),** or proteins that allow cells to hook together and form attachments of the cytoskeleton for maintaining cellular shape; and (6) catalysts of chemical reactions (e.g., conversion of lactose to glucose; see Figure 1.3). Membrane proteins are key components of energy transduction, converting chemical energy into electrical energy, or electrical energy into either mechanical energy or synthesis of ATP.[6] ATP enzymes affect the shape of biological membranes, particularly mitochondrial membranes, and this relationship impacts aging and disease.[7-9]

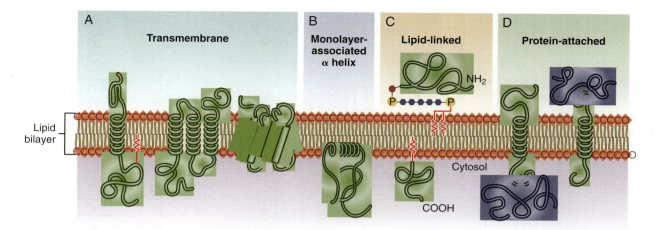

FIGURE 1.8 Proteins Attach to the Plasma Membrane in Different Ways. **A,** Transmembrane proteins extend through the membrane as a single α helix, as multiple α helices, or as a rolled-up barrel-like sheet called a β barrel. **B,** Some membrane proteins are anchored to the cytosolic side of the lipid bilayer by an amphipathic α helix. **C,** Some proteins are linked on either side of the membrane by a covalently attached lipid molecule. **D,** Proteins are attached by weak noncovalent interactions with other membrane proteins. *COOH,* Carboxyl group; *NH₂,* amino group; *P,* protein. ([D] adapted from Alberts, B. [2014]. *Essential cell biology* [4th ed.]. Garland.)

BOX 1.1 Endoplasmic Reticulum, Protein Folding, and ER Stress

Protein folding in the endoplasmic reticulum (ER) is critical for its function. Proteins perform vital functions in every cell and must fold into complex three-dimensional structures to do so (see Figure). The ER is the primary site for protein folding in the cell. Most secreted proteins *fold* and are modified in an error-free manner, but ER or cell stress, mutations, or random (stochastic) errors during protein synthesis can decrease or alter the rate of folding. Pathophysiological processes, such as viral infections, environmental toxins, and mutant protein expression, can disrupt the sensitive ER environment. Natural processes also can perturb the environment, such as the large protein-synthesizing load placed on the ER. These perturbations cause the accumulation of immature and abnormal proteins in cells, leading to **ER stress**. Fortunately, the ER is loaded with protective ways to help folding; for example, protein *chaperones* facilitate folding and prevent the formation of malformed proteins. Misfolded proteins that are not repaired in the ER have been observed in some diseases and can initiate apoptosis or cell death. The ER can actually mediate intracellular signalling pathways in response to the accumulation of unfolded or misfolded proteins, and these pathways are known as the **unfolded-protein response (UPR)**. Interestingly, investigators are studying UPR-associated inflammation and how the UPR is coupled to inflammation in health and disease.[a] Specific diseases include Alzheimer's disease, Parkinson's disease, prion disease (such as Creutzfeldt-Jacob disease, where a particular protein can cause irregular protein folding in the brain), amyotrophic lateral sclerosis, and diabetes mellitus. ER stress might also accelerate age-related dysfunction.[b]

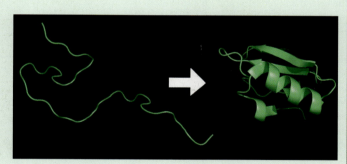

Protein Folding. Each protein exists as an unfolded polypeptide (*left*) or a random coil after the process of translation from a sequence of mRNA to a linear string of amino acids. From amino acids interacting with each other they produce a three-dimensional structure called the folded protein (*right*) that is its native state.

[a] Grootjans, J., Kaser, A., Kaufman, R. J., et al. (2016). The unfolded protein response in immunity and inflammation. *Nature Reviews Immunology, 16*(8), 469–484. https://doi.org/10.1038/nri.2016.62.

[b] Salminen, A., Kaarniranta, K., & Kaupinnin, A. (2020). ER stress activates immunosuppressive network: implications for aging and Alzheimer's disease. *Journal of Molecular Medicine, 98,* 633–650. https://doi.org/10.1007/s00109-020-01904-z.

Data from Brodsky, J., & Skach, W. R. (2011). *Curr Opin Cell Biol, 23,* 464–475; Jäger, R., Bertrand, M. J. M., Gorman, A. M., et al. (2012). *Biol Cell, 104*(5), 259–270; Ron, D., & Walter, P. (2007). *Nat Rev Mol Cell Biol, 8,* 519–529.

In animal cells, the plasma membrane is stabilized by a meshwork of proteins attached to the underside of the membrane called the **cell cortex**. Similarly, human red blood cells have a cell cortex that maintains their flattened biconcave shape (and thus, their corresponding function of oxygen transport).[1]

Protein regulation in a cell: protein homeostasis. The cellular protein pool is in a state of constant flux. The number of copies of a protein in a cell depends on how quickly it is made and how long it survives or is broken down. This adaptable system of protein homeostasis is defined by the "proteostasis" network that comprises ribosomes (makers); chaperones (helpers); and two protein breakdown systems or **proteolytic** systems—*lysosomes* and the *ubiquitin–proteasome system (UPS)*. These systems regulate protein homeostasis under a large variety of conditions, which include variations in nutrient supply, the

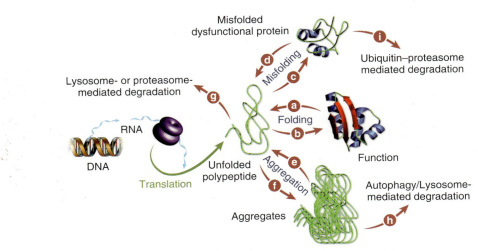

FIGURE 1.9 **Protein Homeostasis System and Outcomes.** A main role of the protein homeostasis network (*proteostasis*) is to minimize protein misfolding and protein aggregation. The network includes ribosome-mediated protein synthesis, chaperone- (folding helpers in the endoplasmic reticulum) and enzyme-mediated folding, breakdown systems of lysosome- and proteasome-mediated protein degradation, and vesicular trafficking. The network integrates biological pathways that balance folding, trafficking, and protein degradation depicted by arrows *a*, *b*, *c*, *d*, *e*, *f*, *g*, *h*, and *i*. (Adapted from Lindquist, S. L., & Kelly, J. W. [2011]. *Cold Spring Harbor Perspectives in Biology, 3*[12], a004507.)

existence of oxidative stress or free radicals, cellular differentiation, changes in temperature, and the presence of heavy metal ions and other sources of stress.[10] Malfunction or failure of the proteostasis network is associated with human disease[11] (Figure 1.9).

Carbohydrates. The short chains of sugars or carbohydrates (oligosaccharides) contained within the plasma membrane are generally bound to membrane proteins (glycoproteins) and lipids (glycolipids). Long polysaccharide chains attached to membrane proteins are called *proteoglycans*. All of the carbohydrate on the glycoproteins, proteoglycans, and glycolipids is located on the outside of the plasma membrane, and the carbohydrate coating is called the **glycocalyx**. The glycocalyx helps protect the cell from mechanical damage.[1] Additionally, the layer of carbohydrate gives the cell a slimy surface that assists the mobility of other cells, like leukocytes, to squeeze through the narrow spaces.[1] Other functions of carbohydrate in the cell include specific cell–cell recognition and adhesion. Intercellular recognition is an important function of membrane oligosaccharides; for example, the transmembrane proteins called *lectins*, which bind to a particular oligosaccharide, recognize neutrophils at the site of bacterial infection. This recognition allows the neutrophil to adhere to the blood vessel wall and migrate from the blood into the infected tissue to help eliminate the invading bacteria.[1]

Cellular Receptors

Cellular receptors are protein molecules on the plasma membrane, in the cytoplasm, or in the nucleus that can recognize and bind with specific smaller molecules called **ligands** (from the Latin *ligare*, "to bind") (Figure 1.10). The region of a protein that associates with a ligand is called its **binding site**. Hormones, for example, are ligands. Recognition and binding depend on the chemical configuration of the receptor and its smaller ligand, which must fit together somewhat like pieces of a jigsaw puzzle (see Chapter 18). Binding selectively to a protein receptor with high affinity to a ligand depends on formation of weak, noncovalent interactions—hydrogen bonds, electrostatic attractions, and Van der Waals attractions—and favourable hydrophobic forces.[1] Numerous receptors are found in most cells, and ligand binding to receptors activates or inhibits the receptor's associated signalling or biochemical pathway.

Plasma membrane receptors protrude from or are exposed at the external surface of the membrane and are important for cellular uptake of ligands (see Figure 1.10). The ligands that bind with membrane receptors include hormones, neurotransmitters, antigens, complement components, lipoproteins, infectious agents, medications, and metabolites. Many new discoveries concerning the specific interactions of cellular receptors with their respective ligands have provided a basis for understanding disease.

Although the chemical nature of ligands and their receptors differs, receptors are classified based on their location and function. Cellular type determines overall cellular function, but plasma membrane receptors determine which ligands a cell will bind with and how the cell will respond to the binding. Specific processes also control intracellular mechanisms.

Receptors for different medications are found on the plasma membrane, in the cytoplasm, and in the nucleus. Membrane receptors have been found for certain anaesthetics, opiates, endorphins, enkephalins, antibiotics, cancer chemotherapeutic agents, digitalis, and other medications. Membrane receptors for endorphins, which are opiatelike peptides isolated from the pituitary gland, are found in large quantities in pain pathways of the nervous system (see Chapters 13 and 14). The endorphins (or medications such as morphine) change the cell's permeability to ions when bound to a receptor, as well as increasing the concentration of molecules that regulate intracellular protein synthesis, and initiating molecular events that modulate pain perception.

Receptors for infectious microorganisms, or antigen receptors, bind bacteria, viruses, and parasites to the cell membrane. Similarly, antigen receptors on white blood cells (e.g., lymphocytes, monocytes, macrophages, granulocytes) recognize and bind with antigenic

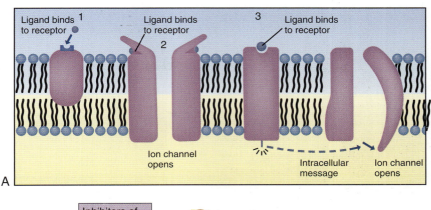

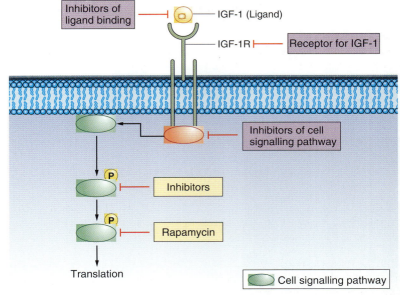

FIGURE 1.10 Cellular Receptors. **A**, 1, Plasma membrane receptor for a ligand (here, a hormone molecule) on the surface of an integral protein. A neurotransmitter can exert its effect on a postsynaptic cell by means of two fundamentally different types of receptor proteins: 2, channel-linked receptors, and 3, non–channel-linked receptors. Channel-linked receptors are also known as *ligand-gated channels*. **B**, Example of ligand-receptor interaction. Insulinlike growth factor 1 (*IGF-1*) is a ligand and binds to the insulinlike growth factor 1 receptor (*IGF-1R*). With binding at the cell membrane the intracellular signalling pathway is activated, causing translation of new proteins (*P*) to act as intracellular communicators. This pathway is important for cancer growth. Researchers are developing pharmacological strategies to reduce signalling at and downstream of the IGF-1R, hoping this will lead to compounds useful in cancer treatment.

microorganisms and activate the immune and inflammatory responses (see Chapter 6).

CELL-TO-CELL ADHESIONS

Plasma membranes not only serve as the outer boundaries of all cells but also allow groups of cells to be held together robustly, in **cell-to-cell adhesions**, to form tissues and organs. Once arranged, cells are linked by three different means: (1) CAMs in the cell's plasma membrane, (2) the ECM, and (3) specialized cell junctions.

Extracellular Matrix

The **extracellular matrix (ECM)** is secreted by the **fibroblasts** and includes the **basement membrane** (or **basal lamina**). The matrix and the cells within it are known collectively as **connective tissue** because they interconnect cells to form tissues and organs. Cells adhere to one another through this ECM, which is an intricate meshwork of fibrous proteins embedded in a watery, gel-like substance composed of complex carbohydrates (Figure 1.11). The matrix is similar to glue; however, it also provides a pathway for diffusion of nutrients, wastes, and other water-soluble substances between the blood and tissue cells. Moreover, the matrix helps regulate the function of the cells within it. Common examples of such functions include cellular growth and differentiation.

There are three groups of **macromolecules** within the matrix: (1) fibrous structural proteins, including collagen and elastin; (2) adhesive glycoproteins, such as fibronectin; and (3) proteoglycans and hyaluronic acid.

- **Collagen** forms cablelike fibres or sheets that provide tensile strength or resistance to longitudinal stress. In osteoarthritis, for

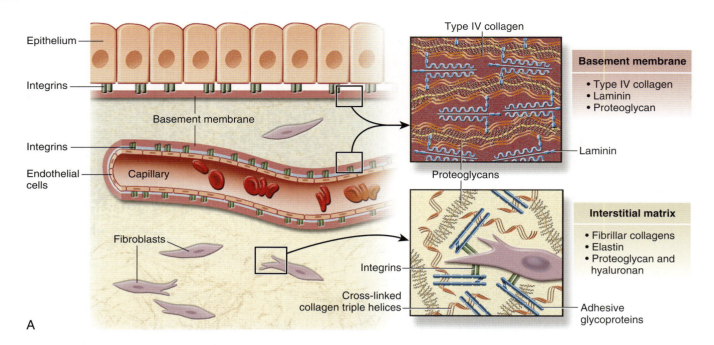

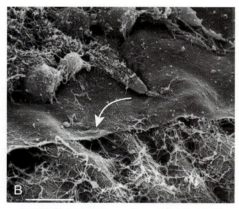

FIGURE 1.11 Extracellular Matrix. A, Tissues are not just cells but also extracellular space. The extracellular space is an intricate network of macromolecules called the extracellular matrix (*ECM*). The macromolecules that constitute the ECM are secreted locally (by mostly fibroblasts) and assembled into a meshwork in close association with the surface of the cell that produced them. Two main classes of macromolecules include proteoglycans, which are bound to polysaccharide chains called glycosaminoglycans, and fibrous proteins (e.g., collagen, elastin, fibronectin, and laminin), which have structural and adhesive properties. Together the proteoglycan molecules form a gel-like ground substance in which the fibrous proteins are embedded. The gel permits rapid diffusion of nutrients, metabolites, and hormones between the blood and the tissue cells. Matrix proteins modulate cell-matrix interactions, including normal tissue remodelling (which can become abnormal, e.g., with chronic inflammation). Disruptions of this balance result in serious diseases such as arthritis, tumour growth, and other pathological conditions. **B,** Scanning electron micrograph of a chick embryo where a portion of the epithelium has been removed, exposing the curtainlike ECM *(white arrow)*. ([A] adapted from Kumar, V., Abbas, A. K., & Aster, J. C. [Eds.]. [2015]. *Robbins and Cotran pathologic basis of disease* [9th ed.]. Saunders; [B] from Gartner, L. P., & Hiatt, J. L. [2006]. *Color textbook of histology* [3rd ed.]. Saunders/Elsevier.)

example, collagen breakdown destroys the fibrils that give cartilage its tensile strength.
- **Elastin** is a rubberlike protein fibre most abundant in tissues that must be capable of stretching and recoiling. For instance, the lungs have an abundance of elastin, which is responsible for the passive recoil of the lungs on expiration.
- **Fibronectin**, a large glycoprotein, promotes cell adhesion and cell anchorage. Some cancer cells actually have less fibronectin, and this allows cancer cells to travel, or metastasize, to other parts of the body.

Human connective tissue can be hard and dense, like bone; flexible, like tendons or the dermis of the skin; resilient and shock absorbing, like cartilage; or soft and transparent, similar to the jellylike substance that fills the eye.

Specialized Cell Junctions

Specialized **cell junctions** are unique membrane regions where cells come into direct physical contact with other cells of the same tissue, and they are classified by their function: (1) some hold cells together

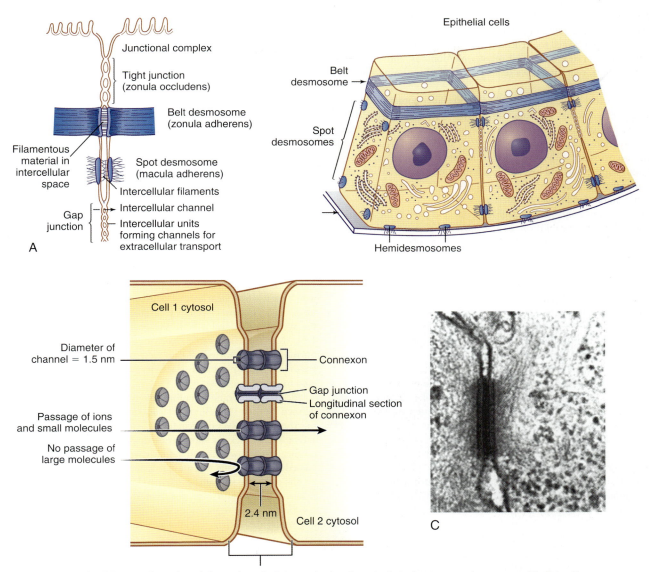

FIGURE 1.12 Junctional Complex. A, Schematic drawing of a belt desmosome between epithelial cells. This junction, also called the *zonula adherens*, encircles each of the interacting cells. The spot desmosomes and hemidesmosomes, like the belt desmosomes, are adhering junctions. This tight junction is an impermeable junction that holds cells together but seals them in such a way that molecules cannot leak between them. The gap junction, as a communicating junction, mediates the passage of small molecules from one interacting cell to the other. **B,** Connexons. The connexin gap junction proteins (i.e., they span the cell membrane) have four transmembrane domains and they play a vital role in maintaining cell and tissue function and homeostasis. Cells connected by gap junctions are considered ionically (electrically) and metabolically coupled. Gap junctions coordinate the activities of adjacent cells; for example, they are important for synchronizing contractions of heart muscle cells through ionic coupling and for permitting action potentials to spread rapidly from cell to cell in neural tissues. The reason gap junctions occur in tissues that are not electrically active is unknown. Although most gap junctions are associated with junctional complexes, they sometimes exist as independent structures. **C,** Electron micrograph of desmosomes. ([A and C] from Raven, P. H., & Johnson, G. B. [1992]. *Biology*. Mosby; [B] adapted from Gartner, L. P., & Hiatt, J. L. [2006]. *Color textbook of histology* [3rd ed.]. Saunders Elsevier; Sherwood, L. [2013]. *Learning* [8th ed.]. Brooks/Cole CENGAGE.)

and form a tight seal (*tight junctions*); (2) some provide strong mechanical attachments (*adherens junctions*, **desmosomes**, *hemidesmosomes*); (3) some provide a special type of chemical communication (e.g., *gap junctions*, which involve the movement of ions and small water-soluble molecules and cause an electrical wave); and (4) some maintain polarity across the apical and basal aspects of individual epithelial cells (*tight junctions*) (Figure 1.12). Overall, cell junctions protect the integrity of the epithelium through mechanical attachment and provide communication of the cells with each other while maintaining cell polarity.

Tight junctions are barriers to diffusion, prevent the movement of substances through transport proteins in the plasma membrane, and prevent the leakage of small molecules between the plasma membranes of adjacent cells. Gap junctions are clusters of communicating tunnels or *connexons* that allow small ions and molecules to pass directly from the inside of one cell to the inside of another. Connexons extend outward from each of the adjacent plasma membranes, and are composed of small protein molecules (called *connexins*) spanning the cell membrane. (Figure 1.12C).

Multiple factors regulate gap junction intercellular communication, including voltage across the junction, intracellular pH, intracellular Ca^{++} concentration, and protein phosphorylation. The most abundant human connexin is connexin 43 (Cx43).[12] A shorter cancer-free survival rate is correlated with a loss of Cx43 in colorectal tumours.[13] Cx43 is a tumour suppressor, and loss of the gap junctions provided by Cx43 contributes further to colorectal cancer. This makes Cx43 an important prognostic marker and target for therapy.[13]

The junctional complex is a highly permeable part of the plasma membrane. This permeability is controlled by a process called gating, where increased levels of cytoplasmic calcium from injured cells cause decreased permeability at the junctional complex. Gating enables uninjured cells to protect themselves from injured neighbouring cells.

CELLULAR COMMUNICATION AND SIGNAL TRANSDUCTION

Cells need to communicate with each other for four main reasons: (1) maintenance of a stable internal environment, or homeostasis; (2) regulation of growth and division; (3) development and organization of cells into tissues; and (4) coordination of their functions. Cells communicate by using hundreds of different signal molecules. Insulin is just one example (Figure 1.10B). Similarly, cells communicate with each other in three main ways: (1) they display plasma membrane–bound signalling molecules (receptors) that affect the cell itself and other cells in direct physical contact (Figure 1.13A); (2) they affect receptor proteins *inside* the target cell, and the signal molecule has to enter the cell to bind to them (Figure 1.13B); and (3) they form protein channels (gap junctions) that directly coordinate the activities of adjacent cells (Figure 1.13C). Alterations in cellular communication affect disease onset and progression. For instance, if a cell cannot perform gap junctional intercellular communication, normal growth control and cell differentiation is not possible, and cancerous tumours can develop (see Chapter 10). Chemical signals from cells involve both local and distance communication. Primary modes of intercellular signalling are contact-dependent, paracrine (hormones working on nearby cells), autocrine (hormones from the cell target the same cell), neurohormonal (e.g., renin-angiotensin-aldosterone and the sympathetic nervous system), and neurotransmitter (e.g., norepinephrine, acetylcholine) (Figure 1.14).

Contact-dependent signalling requires cells to be in close membrane–membrane contact. In paracrine signalling, cells secrete local chemical mediators that are quickly taken up, destroyed, or immobilized. Paracrine signalling usually involves different cell types; however, cells also can produce signals to which they alone respond, called autocrine signalling (see Figure 1.14). For example, cancer cells use this form of signalling to stimulate their survival and proliferation. The mediators act only on nearby cells. Hormonal signalling involves specialized endocrine cells that secrete chemicals called *hormones*; hormones are released by one set of cells and travel through the bloodstream to produce a response in other sets of cells (see Chapter 18). In neurohormonal signalling, hormones are released into the blood by neurosecretory neurons. Like endocrine cells, neurosecretory neurons release bloodborne chemical messengers, whereas ordinary neurons secrete short-range neurotransmitters into a small discrete space (i.e., synapse). Neurons communicate directly with the cells they innervate by releasing chemicals or neurotransmitters at specialized junctions called chemical synapses; the neurotransmitter diffuses across the synaptic cleft and acts on the postsynaptic target cell (see Figure 1.14). Many of these same signalling molecules are receptors used in hormonal, neurohormonal, and paracrine signalling. Important differences lie in the speed and selectivity with which the signals are delivered to their targets.[1]

Plasma membrane receptors belong to one of three classes that are defined by their signalling (transduction) mechanism. Table 1.3 summarizes these classes of receptors. Cells respond to external stimuli by activating a variety of signal transduction pathways, which are communication pathways, or signalling cascades (Figure 1.15C). Signals are passed between cells when a particular type of molecule is produced by one cell—the signalling cell—and received by another—the target cell—by means of a receptor protein that recognizes and responds specifically to the signal molecule (Figure 1.15A,B). In turn, the signalling molecules activate a pathway of intracellular protein kinases that results in various responses, such as growth and reproduction, death, survival, or differentiation (Figure 1.15D). If deprived of appropriate signals, most cells undergo a form of cell suicide known as *programmed cell death*, or *apoptosis* (see Chapter 4).

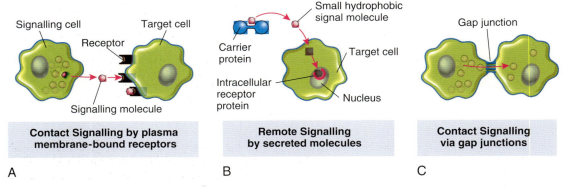

FIGURE 1.13 Cellular Communication. Three primary ways cells communicate with one another. ([B] adapted from Alberts, B., Johnson, A., Lewis, J., et al. [2008]. *Molecular biology of the cell* [5th ed.]. Garland Publishers.)

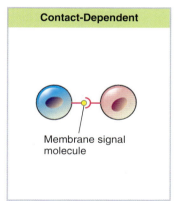
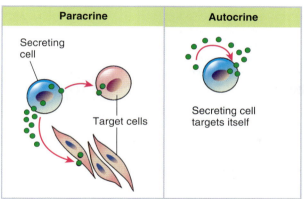
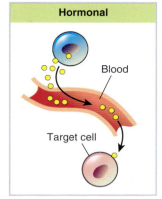
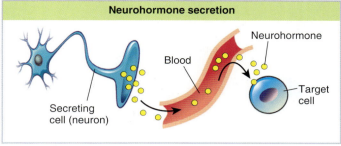
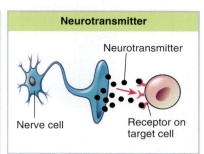

FIGURE 1.14 Primary Modes of Chemical Signalling. Five forms of signalling mediated by secreted molecules. Hormones, paracrines, neurotransmitters, and neurohormones are all intercellular messengers that accomplish communication between cells. Autocrines bind to receptors on the same cell. Not all neurotransmitters act in the strictly synaptic mode shown; some act in a contact-dependent mode as local chemical mediators that influence multiple target cells in the area.

TABLE 1.3 Classes of Plasma Membrane Receptors

Type of Receptor	Description
Ion channel coupled	Involve rapid synaptic signalling between electrically excitable cells; also called *transmitter-gated* ion channels. Channels open and close briefly in response to neurotransmitters, changing ion permeability of plasma membrane of postsynaptic cell.
Enzyme coupled	Once activated by ligands, function directly as enzymes or associate with enzymes.
G-protein coupled	Indirectly activate or inactivate plasma membrane enzyme or ion channel; interaction mediated by *GTP-binding regulatory protein (G-protein)*. May also interact with inositol phospholipids, which are significant in cell signalling, and with molecules involved in *inositol-phospholipid transduction pathway*.

GTP, Guanosine-5′-triphosphate.

CELLULAR METABOLISM

Cellular metabolism is the sum of chemical reactions involved in the maintenance of cellular function. **Anabolism** is the energy-using process of metabolism (*ana* = upward) by which cellular structures are made, whereas the energy-releasing process is known as **catabolism** (*kata* = downward) by which cellular structures are broken down. Metabolism provides the cell with the energy it needs to produce cellular structures.

Dietary proteins, fats, and starches (i.e., carbohydrates) are hydrolyzed in the intestinal tract into amino acids, fatty acids, and glucose, respectively. They are then absorbed, circulated, and incorporated into the cell, where they may be used for various vital cellular processes, including the production of ATP. ATP production is one example of a series of reactions called a **metabolic pathway** where biochemical reactions by protein catalysts or enzymes result in further **substrates** for chemical reactions in the chain. Furthermore, each enzyme has a high affinity for a particular **substrate**, a specific substance converted to a product of the reaction.

Role of Adenosine Triphosphate

ATP is the basic unit of intracellular energy (or fuel) used by all cells, and it is this fuel or energy that drives all biological reactions necessary for cells to function. Cellular function depends on the cell's ability to extract and use the chemical energy in organic molecules. For example, when 1 mol of glucose metabolically breaks down into carbon dioxide and water under the influence of oxygen, 686 kcal of chemical energy are released. The chemical energy lost by one molecule is then transferred to the chemical structure of another molecule by an energy-carrying or energy-transferring molecule, such as ATP.

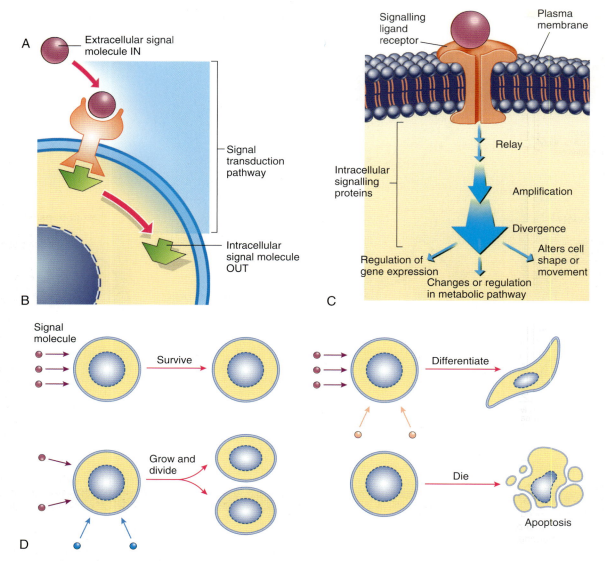

FIGURE 1.15 Schematic of a Signal Transduction Pathway. Like a telephone receiver that converts an electrical signal into a sound signal, a cell converts an extracellular signal, A, into an intracellular signal, B. C, An extracellular signal molecule (ligand) bonds to a receptor protein located on the plasma membrane, where it is transduced into an intracellular signal. This process initiates a signalling cascade that relays the signal into the cell interior, amplifying and distributing it during transit. Amplification is often achieved by stimulating enzymes. Steps in the cascade can be modulated by other events in the cell. D, Different cell behaviours rely on multiple extracellular signals.

The energy stored in ATP can be used in various energy-requiring reactions and is generally converted to adenosine diphosphate (ADP) and inorganic phosphate (Pi) in the process. When ATP is converted to ADP, the release of energy is about 7 kcal/mol of ATP. The cell uses ATP for various process such as muscle contraction and active transport of molecules across cellular membranes. ATP not only stores energy but also *transfers* it from one molecule to another. For example, energy stored by carbohydrate, lipid, and protein is catabolized and transferred to ATP. Recent literature suggests that ATP has a role outside cells as well. (Box 1.2).

Food and Production of Cellular Energy

Catabolism (or breakdown) of the proteins, lipids, and polysaccharides found in food can be divided into the following three phases (Figure 1.16):

Phase 1: **Digestion**. Large molecules are broken down into smaller subunits: proteins into amino acids, polysaccharides into simple sugars

> **BOX 1.2   Role of Adenosine Triphosphate Outside Cells**
>
> ATP is a messenger outside cells as well, and its role in inflammation has been well-documented in the pathogenesis of systemic inflammatory response syndrome (SIRS). ATP stimulates the production of proinflammatory cytokines. The removal of extracellular ATP has promise in treating inflammatory disorders such as SIRS.
>
> From Cauwels, A., Rogge, E., Vandendriessche, B, Shiva, S., & Brouckaert, P. (2014). Extracellular ATP drives systemic inflammation, tissue damage and mortality. *Cell Death & Disease,* 5, e1102. doi:10.1038/cddis.2014.70.

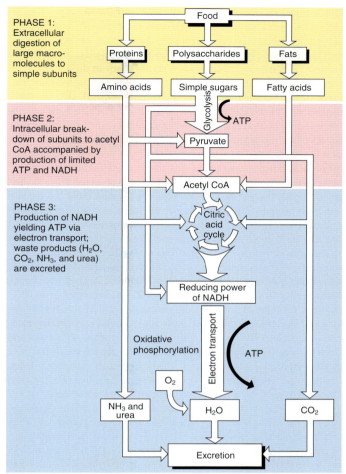

FIGURE 1.16 Three Phases of Catabolism, Which Lead from Food to Waste Products. These reactions produce adenosine triphosphate *(ATP)*, which is used to power other processes in the cell. CO_2, Carbon dioxide; *CoA*, coenzyme A; H_2O, water; *NADH*, reduced nicotinamide adenine dinucleotide; NH_3, ammonia; O_2, oxygen.

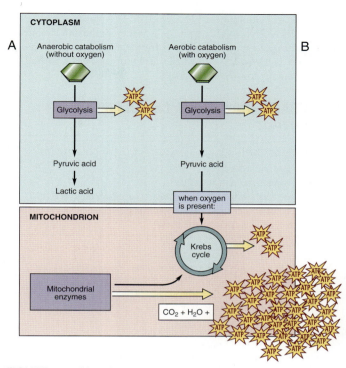

FIGURE 1.17 Glycolysis. Sugars are important for fuel or energy and they are oxidized in small steps to carbon dioxide (CO_2) and water (H_2O). Glycolysis is the process for oxidizing sugars or glucose. Breakdown of glucose. **A,** Anaerobic catabolism, to lactic acid and little adenosine triphosphate *(ATP)*. **B,** Aerobic catabolism, to carbon dioxide, water, and lots of ATP. (From Herlihy, B. [2018]. *The human body in health and illness* [6th ed.]. Elsevier.)

(i.e., monosaccharides), and fats into fatty acids and glycerol. These processes occur outside the cell and are activated by enzymes.

Phase 2: **Glycolysis** and **oxidation**. The most important part of phase 2 is glycolysis, the splitting of glucose. Glycolysis produces two molecules of ATP per glucose molecule through oxidation, or the removal and transfer of a pair of electrons. The total process is called *oxidative cellular metabolism* and involves 10 biochemical reactions (Figure 1.17).

Phase 3: **Citric acid cycle (Krebs cycle, tricarboxylic acid cycle)**. Most of the ATP is generated during this final phase, which begins with the citric acid cycle and ends with oxidative phosphorylation. About two thirds of the total oxidation of carbon compounds in most cells is accomplished during this phase. The major end products are CO_2 and two dinucleotides—reduced nicotinamide adenine dinucleotide (NADH) and the reduced form of flavin adenine dinucleotide ($FADH_2$)—both of which transfer their electrons into the electron-transport chain and create ATP.

Oxidative Phosphorylation

Oxidative phosphorylation occurs in the mitochondria and is the mechanism by which the energy produced from carbohydrates, fats, and proteins is transferred to ATP. During the breakdown (catabolism) of foods, many reactions involve the removal of electrons from various intermediates. These reactions generally require a coenzyme (a nonprotein carrier molecule), such as nicotinamide adenine dinucleotide (NAD), to transfer the electrons and thus are called **transfer reactions**.

Molecules of NAD and flavin adenine dinucleotide (FAD) transfer electrons they have gained from the oxidation of substrates to molecular oxygen. The electrons from reduced NAD and FAD (NADH and $FADH_2$, respectively) are transferred to the **electron-transport chain** on the inner surfaces of the mitochondria with the release of hydrogen ions. Some carrier molecules are brightly coloured, iron-containing proteins known as *cytochromes* that accept a pair of electrons. These electrons eventually combine with molecular oxygen.

If oxygen is not available to the electron-transport chain, ATP will not be formed by the mitochondria. Instead, an anaerobic (without oxygen) metabolic pathway synthesizes ATP. This process, called **substrate phosphorylation or anaerobic glycolysis**, is linked to the breakdown (glycolysis) of carbohydrate (see Figure 1.17). Because glycolysis occurs in the cytoplasm of the cell, it provides energy for cells that lack mitochondria. The reactions in anaerobic glycolysis involve the conversion of glucose to pyruvic acid (pyruvate) with the simultaneous production of ATP. With the glycolysis of one molecule of glucose, two ATP molecules and two molecules of pyruvate are liberated. If oxygen is present, the two molecules of pyruvate move into the mitochondria, where they enter the citric acid cycle (Figure 1.18).

If oxygen is absent, pyruvate is converted to lactic acid, which is released into the extracellular fluid. The conversion of pyruvic acid to lactic acid is reversible; therefore, once oxygen is restored, lactic acid is quickly converted back to either pyruvic acid or glucose. The anaerobic generation of ATP from glucose through glycolysis is not as efficient as the aerobic generation process (2 molecules ATP via glycolysis versus 36 molecules ATP via oxidative phosphorylation in the mitochondria). Adding an oxygen-requiring stage to the catabolic process (phase 3; see Figure 1.16) provides cells with a much more powerful method for extracting energy from food molecules.

MEMBRANE TRANSPORT: CELLULAR INTAKE AND OUTPUT

> ✓ **QUICK CHECK 1.2**
> 1. What does glycolysis produce?
> 2. Define *membrane transport proteins*.
> 3. What are the differences between passive and active transport?
> 4. Why do water and small, electrically charged molecules move easily through pores in the plasma membrane?

Cell survival and growth depend on the constant exchange of molecules with their environment. Cells continually import nutrients, fluids, and chemical messengers from the extracellular environment and expel metabolites, or the products of metabolism, and end products of lysosomal digestion. Cells also must regulate ions in their cytosol and organelles. Simple diffusion across the lipid bilayer of the plasma membrane occurs for such important molecules as O_2 and CO_2. However, the majority of molecular transfer depends on specialized **membrane transport proteins** that span the lipid bilayer and provide private conduits for select molecules.[1] Membrane transport proteins occur in many forms and are present in all cell membranes.[1] Transport by membrane transport proteins is sometimes called **mediated transport**. Most of these transport proteins allow selective passage (e.g., Na^+ but not K^+ or K^+ but not Na^+). Each type of cell membrane has its own transport proteins that determine which solute can pass into and out of the cell or organelle.[1] The two main classes of membrane transport proteins are *transporters* and *channels*. These transport proteins differ in the type of **solute**—small particles of dissolved substances—they transport. A **transporter** is specific, allowing only those ions that fit the unique binding sites on the protein (Figure 1.19A). A transporter undergoes conformational changes to enable membrane transport. A **channel**, when open, forms a pore across the lipid bilayer that allows ions and selective polar organic molecules to diffuse across the membrane (Figure 1.19B). Transport by a channel depends on the size and electrical charge of the molecule. Some channels are controlled by a gate mechanism that determines which solute can move into it. Ion channels are responsible for the electrical excitability of nerve and muscle cells and play a critical role in the membrane potential.

The mechanisms of membrane transport depend on the characteristics of the substance to be transported. In **passive transport**, water and small, electrically uncharged molecules move easily through pores in the plasma membrane's lipid bilayer (Figure 1.19). This process can occur naturally through any semipermeable barrier. Molecules will easily flow "downhill" from a region of higher concentration to a region of lower concentration; this movement is called *passive* because it does not require expenditure of energy or a driving force and is driven by osmosis, hydrostatic pressure, and/or diffusion.

Other molecules may be too large to pass through pores or are ligands bound to receptors on the cell's plasma membrane. Some of these molecules move into and out of the cell by **active transport**, which requires the cell's expenditure of metabolic energy (Figure 1.20). Unlike passive transport, active transport involves living membranes that have to drive the flow "uphill" by coupling it to an energy source. Movement of a solute against its concentration gradient occurs by special types of transporters called *pumps* (see Figure 1.20). These

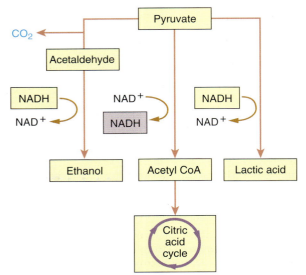

FIGURE 1.18 What Happens to Pyruvate, the Product of Glycolysis? In the presence of oxygen, pyruvate is oxidized to acetyl coenzyme A (*Acetyl CoA*) and enters the citric acid cycle. In the absence of oxygen, pyruvate instead is reduced, accepting the electrons extracted during glycolysis and carried by reduced nicotinamide adenine dinucleotide (*NADH*). When pyruvate is reduced directly, as it is in muscles, the product is lactic acid. When carbon dioxide (*CO2*) is first removed from pyruvate and the remainder is reduced, as it is in yeasts, the resulting product is ethanol. *NAD+*, Oxidized nicotinamide adenine dinucleotide.

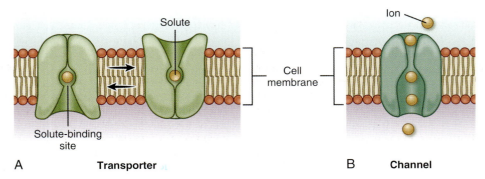

FIGURE 1.19 Inorganic Ions and Small, Polar Organic Molecules Can Cross a Cell Membrane Through Either a Transporter or a Channel. (Adapted from Alberts, B. [2014]. *Essential cell biology* [4th ed.]. Garland.)

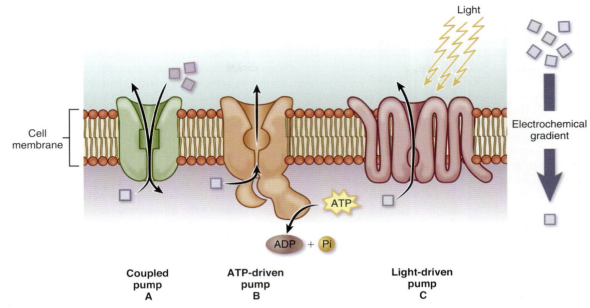

FIGURE 1.20 Pumps Carry Out Active Transport in Three Ways. A, *Coupled pumps* link the uphill transport of one solute to the downhill transport of another solute. B, *ATP-driven pumps* drive uphill transport from hydrolysis of ATP. C, *Light-driven pumps* are mostly found in bacteria and use energy from sunlight to drive uphill transport. *ADP,* Adenosine diphosphate; *ATP,* adenosine triphosphate; *Pi,* inorganic phosphate. (Adapted from Alberts, B. [2014]. *Essential cell biology* [4th ed.]. Garland.)

transporter pumps must harness an energy source to power the transport process. This energy can come from ATP hydrolysis, a transmembrane ion gradient, or sunlight (see Figure 1.20). A common energy source present in all cell membranes is the Na^+–K^+-dependent adenosine triphosphatase (ATPase) pump (see Figure 1.25). It continuously regulates the cell's volume by controlling leaks through pores or protein channels and maintaining the ionic concentration gradients needed for cellular excitation and membrane conductivity. Large molecules (macromolecules), along with fluids, are transported by endocytosis (taking in) and exocytosis (expelling). Receptor-macromolecule complexes enter the cell by means of receptor-mediated endocytosis.

Mediated transport systems can move solute molecules singly or two at a time. Two molecules can be moved simultaneously in one direction (a process called **symport**; e.g., sodium-glucose in the digestive tract) or in opposite directions (called **antiport**; e.g., the sodium–potassium pump in all cells), or a single molecule can be moved in one direction (called **uniport**; e.g., glucose) (Figure 1.21).

Electrolytes as Solutes

Body fluids are composed of **electrolytes**, which are electrically charged and form ions when dissolved in solution, as well as non-electrolytes, such as glucose, urea, and creatinine, which do not have a charge. Electrolytes account for approximately 95% of the solute molecules in body water. Electrolytes exhibit **polarity** by orienting themselves toward the positive or negative pole. Ions with a positive charge are known as **cations** and migrate toward the negative pole, or *cathode* when an electrical current is passed through the electrolyte solution. Similarly, **anions** carry a negative charge and migrate toward the positive pole, or *anode*, in the presence of electrical current. Anions and cations are located in both the intracellular fluid (ICF) and the extracellular fluid (ECF) compartments, although their concentration depends on their location. (Fluid and electrolyte balance between body compartments is discussed in Chapter 5.) For

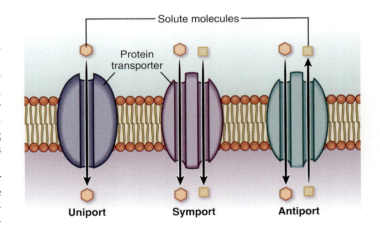

FIGURE 1.21 Mediated Transport. The illustration shows simultaneous movement of a single solute molecule in one direction *(uniport)*, of two different solute molecules in one direction *(symport)*, and of two different solute molecules in opposite directions *(antiport)*.

example, sodium (Na^+) is the predominant extracellular cation, and potassium (K^+) is the principal intracellular cation. The difference in ICF and ECF concentrations of these ions is important for the transmission of electrical impulses across the plasma membranes of nerve and muscle cells.

Electrolytes are measured in milliequivalents per litre (mEq/L) or millimoles per litre (mmol/L). The term *milliequivalent* indicates the chemical-combining activity of an ion, which depends on the electrical charge, or **valence**, of its ions. In abbreviations, valence is indicated by the number of plus or minus signs. One milliequivalent of any cation can combine chemically with 1 mEq of any anion: one monovalent anion will combine with one monovalent cation. Divalent ions (i.e., with 2 charges) combine more strongly than monovalent ions. To maintain electrochemical balance, one divalent ion will combine with two monovalent ions (e.g., $Ca^{++} + 2Cl^- \rightleftharpoons CaCl_2$).

Passive Transport: Diffusion, Filtration, and Osmosis

Diffusion. **Diffusion** is the movement of a solute molecule from an area of greater solute concentration to an area of lesser solute concentration. This difference in concentration is known as a **concentration gradient**. If the concentration of particles is greater on one side of a permeable membrane than on the other side, the particles diffuse spontaneously from the area of greater concentration to the area of lesser concentration until equilibrium is reached. When there is a higher concentration on one side of the membrane, the rate of diffusion is greater.

The *diffusion rate* is also influenced by differences of electrical potential across the membrane. For example, because the pores in the lipid bilayer are often lined with Ca^{++}, other cations (e.g., Na^+ and K^+) diffuse slowly because they are repelled by positive charges in the pores.

Similarly, the rate of diffusion of a substance depends on its size (or diffusion coefficient) and its lipid solubility (Figure 1.22). Usually, smaller molecules that are more fat-soluble are more hydrophobic and nonpolar, and they will more readily diffuse across the lipid bilayer. Nonpolar molecules include oxygen, carbon dioxide, and steroid hormones (e.g., androgens and estrogens), and common lipophilic ("lipid-loving") molecules are fatty acids and steroids. As such, these particles diffuse rapidly across the cell membrane. On the other hand, water-soluble substances, such as glucose and inorganic ions, diffuse very slowly, as do ions and other polar molecules.

Water, however, readily diffuses through biological membranes because water molecules are small and uncharged. The dipolar structure of water also allows it to rapidly cross the regions of the bilayer containing the lipid head groups that constitute the two outer regions of the lipid bilayer.

Filtration: hydrostatic pressure. **Filtration** is the movement of water and solutes through a membrane because of a greater *hydrostatic pressure*, or mechanical force of water, on one side of the membrane than on the other side. (Figure 1.23A). In the vascular system, hydrostatic pressure is the blood pressure generated in vessels when the heart contracts. Blood reaching the capillary bed has a hydrostatic pressure of 25 to 30 mm Hg, which is sufficient force to push water across the thin capillary membranes into the interstitial space. The hydrostatic pressure of water moving out of the capillaries is partially balanced by osmotic forces that tend to pull water back into the capillaries (Figure 1.23B). The water that is not osmotically attracted back into the capillaries moves into the lymph system (see the discussion of Starling forces in Chapter 5).

Osmosis. **Osmosis** is the movement of water "down" a concentration gradient—that is, across a semipermeable membrane from a region of higher water concentration to one of lower water concentration. For osmosis to occur, (1) the membrane must be more permeable to water than to solutes, and (2) the concentration of solutes on one side of the membrane must be greater than that on the other side so that water moves more easily. Osmosis is directly related to both hydrostatic pressure and solute concentration but is independent of particle size or weight. For example, particles of the plasma protein albumin are small but are more concentrated in body fluids than the larger and heavier particles of globulin. Therefore, albumin exerts a greater osmotic force than does globulin.

Osmolality controls the distribution and movement of water between body compartments. The terms *osmolality* and *osmolarity* are often used interchangeably in reference to osmotic activity, but they define different measurements. **Osmolality** measures the number of milliosmoles per kilogram (mOsm/kg) of water, or the concentration of molecules per *weight* of water. **Osmolarity** measures the number of milliosmoles per litre of solution, or the concentration of molecules per *volume* of solution.

In solutions that contain only ions such as sodium and chloride the difference between the two measurements is negligible. When

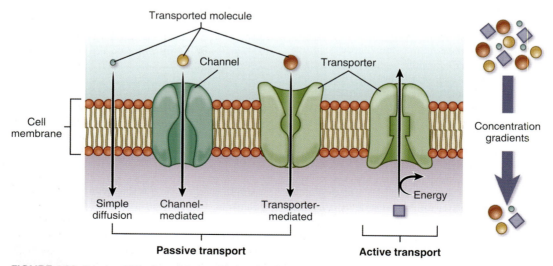

FIGURE 1.22 Passive Diffusion of Solute Molecules Across the Plasma Membrane. Oxygen, nitrogen, water, urea, glycerol, and carbon dioxide can diffuse readily down the concentration gradient. Macromolecules are too large to diffuse through pores in the plasma membrane. Ions may be repelled if the pores contain substances with identical charges. If the pores are lined with cations, for example, other cations will have difficulty diffusing because the positive charges will repel one another. Diffusion can still occur, but it occurs more slowly.

CHAPTER 1 Cellular Biology

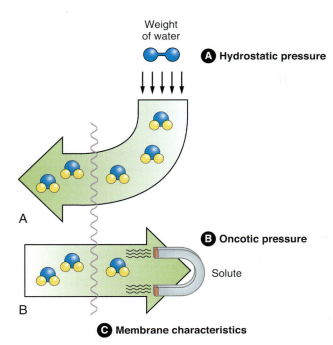

FIGURE 1.23 Hydrostatic Pressure and Oncotic Pressure in Plasma. **A,** Hydrostatic pressure in plasma. **B,** Oncotic pressure exerted by proteins in the plasma usually tends to *pull* water into the circulatory system. The proteins are too big to cross the semipermeable membrane and have a negative charge. **C,** Individuals with low protein levels (e.g., starvation) are unable to maintain a normal oncotic pressure; therefore, water is not reabsorbed into the circulation and, instead, causes body edema.

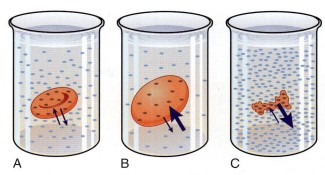

FIGURE 1.24 Tonicity. Tonicity is important, especially for red blood cell function. **A,** Isotonic solution. **B,** Hypotonic solution. **C,** Hypertonic solution. (From Waugh, A., & Grant, A. [2012]. *Ross and Wilson anatomy and physiology in health and illness* [12th ed.]. Churchill Livingstone.)

considering all the different solutes in plasma (e.g., proteins, glucose, lipids), however, the difference between osmolality and osmolarity becomes more significant. Osmolarity tends to be less than osmolality because solute content is considered part of the solution volume. On the other hand, the osmolality of a solution is a measure of weight, and the solvent weight is separate from that of the solutes. Though the distinction between the two measurements is negligible, because of the relatively large proportion of solutes dissolved in plasma compared with the amount of water (or solvent), osmolality is the preferred modality for human clinical assessment.

The normal osmolality of body fluids is 280 to 294 mOsm/kg. The osmolalities of intracellular and extracellular fluids tend to equilibrate, providing a measure of body fluid concentration hydration status. Hydration is also affected by hydrostatic pressure because the movement of water by osmosis (or **osmotic pressure**) can be opposed by an equal amount of hydrostatic pressure. Factors that determine osmotic pressure are the type and thickness of the plasma membrane, the size of the molecules, the concentration of molecules or the concentration gradient, and the solubility of molecules within the membrane.

Effective osmolality is sustained osmotic activity and depends on the concentration of solutes remaining on one side of a permeable membrane. If the solutes penetrate the membrane and equilibrate with the solution on the other side of the membrane, the osmotic effect will be diminished or lost.

Plasma proteins influence osmolality because they have a negative charge (see Figure 1.23B). When the fluid in one compartment contains small, diffusible ions, such as Na^+ and chloride (Cl^-), together with large, nondiffusible, charged particles, such as plasma proteins, the body tends to maintain an electrical equilibrium, and the nondiffusible protein molecules create asymmetry in the distribution of small ions. The protein-containing compartment maintains a state of electroneutrality, but the osmolality is higher because they are heavier than the smaller ions dissolved in solution. The overall osmotic effect of colloids (large molecules that are either soluble or insoluble and are suspended in solution), such as plasma proteins, is called **oncotic pressure or colloid osmotic pressure**.

Tonicity describes the effective osmolality of a solution. (The terms *osmolality* and *tonicity* may be used interchangeably.) Solutions have relative degrees of tonicity. An isotonic solution (or isosmotic solution) has the same osmolality or concentration of particles (285 mOsm) as the ICF or ECF. A hypotonic solution has a lower concentration and is thus more dilute than body fluids (Figure 1.24). A hypertonic solution has a concentration of more than 285 to 294 mOsm/kg. The concept of tonicity is important when correcting water and solute imbalances by administering different types of replacement solutions (see Figure 1.24) (see Chapter 5).

Active Transport of Na^+ and K^+

The active transport system for Na^+ and K^+ is found in virtually all mammalian cells. The Na^+–K^+-antiport system (i.e., Na^+ moving out of the cell and K^+ moving into the cell) uses the direct energy of ATP to transport these cations. The transporter protein is ATPase, which requires Na^+, K^+, and magnesium (Mg^{++}) ions. The concentration of ATPase in plasma membranes is directly related to Na^+–K^+-transport activity. Approximately 60 to 70% of the ATP synthesized by cells, especially muscle and nerve cells, is used to maintain the Na^+–K^+-transport system. Excitable tissues have a high concentration of Na^+–K^+ ATPase, as do other tissues that transport significant amounts of Na^+. For every hydrolyzed ATP molecule, three molecules of Na^+ are transported out of the cell, and only two molecules of K^+ move into the cell. The process leads to an electrical potential with the inside of the cell becoming more negative than the outside. The ATPase induces the transporter protein to undergo several conformational changes, causing Na^+ and K^+ to move short distances (Figure 1.25). The conformational change lowers the affinity of Na^+ and K^+ for the ATPase transporter, resulting in the release of the cations after transport.

Table 1.4 summarizes the major mechanisms of transport through pores and protein transporters in the plasma membranes. Many disease states involve the loss of these membrane transport systems.

Endocytosis and Exocytosis

The active transport mechanisms by which the cells move large proteins, polynucleotides, or polysaccharides (macromolecules) across the plasma membrane are very different from those that control small solute and ion transport. Transport of macromolecules involves the sequential formation and fusion of membrane-bound vesicles.

In **endocytosis**, a section of the plasma membrane enfolds substances from outside the cell, and separates from the plasma membrane, forming a vesicle that moves into the cell (Figure 1.26A). There are two types of endocytosis, based on the size of the vesicle formed. **Pinocytosis** (cell drinking) involves the ingestion of fluids, bits of the plasma membrane, and solute molecules through formation of small vesicles; and **phagocytosis** (cell eating) involves the ingestion of large particles, such as bacteria, through formation of large vesicles (vacuoles).

Because most cells continually ingest fluid and solutes by pinocytosis, the terms *pinocytosis* and *endocytosis* often are used interchangeably. In pinocytosis, the vesicle fuses with a lysosome, and lysosomal enzymes digest the vesicle's contents for use by the cell. Vesicles that bud from membranes have a particular protein coat formed by the protein **clathrin** on their cytosolic surface and are called **coated vesicles**, which allow the cell to designate which metabolic pathway is most suitable for the contents of the vesicle. Pinocytosis occurs mainly by the clathrin-coated pits and vesicles (Figure 1.27). After the coated pits pinch off from the plasma membrane, they quickly shed their coats and fuse with an **endosome**. This membrane-bound vesicle's main function is to sort its contents and determine whether they will be broken down by lysosomes or whether they are destined to be recycled by the plasma membrane. In phagocytosis, the large molecular substances are engulfed by the plasma membrane and enter the cell so that they can be isolated and destroyed by lysosomal enzymes (see Chapter 6). Substances that are not degraded by lysosomes are isolated in residual bodies and released by exocytosis. Both pinocytosis and phagocytosis require metabolic energy and often involve binding of the substance with plasma membrane receptors before membrane invagination and fusion with lysosomes in the cell. New data are revealing that endocytosis has an even larger and more important role than previously known (Box 1.3).

In eukaryotic cells, secretion of macromolecules almost always occurs by exocytosis (Figure 1.26). **Exocytosis** has two main functions: (1) replacement of portions of the plasma membrane that have been removed by endocytosis and (2) release of molecules synthesized by the cells into the ECM.

Receptor-Mediated Endocytosis

The internalization process, called **receptor-mediated endocytosis (ligand internalization)**, is rapid and enables the cell to ingest large amounts of receptor-macromolecule complexes in clathrin-coated vesicles without ingesting large volumes of extracellular fluid (see Figure 1.27). The cellular uptake of cholesterol, for example, depends on receptor-mediated endocytosis. Many essential metabolites (e.g., vitamin B_{12} and iron) and the influenza virus also depend on receptor-mediated endocytosis.

Caveolae

The outer surface of the plasma membrane is dimpled with tiny flask-shaped pits called **caveolae**. Caveolae are thought to form from membrane microdomains or lipid rafts. Caveolae are cholesterol- and glycosphingolipid-rich microdomains where the protein *caveolin* is thought to be involved in several processes, including clathrin-independent endocytosis, cellular cholesterol regulation and transport, and cellular communication. Many proteins, including a variety of receptors, cluster in these tiny chambers.

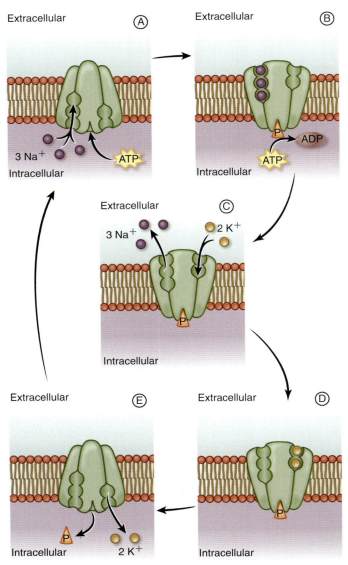

FIGURE 1.25 Active Transport and the Sodium–Potassium Pump. *A,* Three sodium (Na^+) ions bind to sodium-binding sites on the carrier's inner face. *B,* At the same time, an energy-containing adenosine triphosphate *(ATP)* molecule produced by the cell's mitochondria binds to the carrier. The ATP dissociates, transferring its stored energy to the carrier. *C* and *D,* The carrier then changes shape, releases the three Na^+ ions to the outside of the cell, and attracts two potassium (K^+) ions to its potassium-binding sites. *E,* The carrier then returns to its original shape, releasing the two K^+ ions and the remnant of the ATP molecule to the inside of the cell. The carrier is now ready for another pumping cycle. *ADP,* Adenosine diphosphate; *P,* protein.

Transport by Vesicle Formation

> ✓ **QUICK CHECK 1.3**
> 1. Identify examples of molecules transported in one direction (symport) and opposite directions (antiport).
> 2. If oxygen is no longer available to make ATP, what happens to the transport of Na^+?
> 3. Describe the differences between pinocytosis, phagocytosis, and receptor-mediated endocytosis.

TABLE 1.4 Major Transport Systems in Mammalian Cells

Substance Transported	Mechanism of Transport[a]	Tissues
Carbohydrates		
Glucose	Passive: protein channel	Most tissues
	Active: symport with Na+	
Fructose	Active: symport with Na+	Small intestines and renal tubular cells
	Passive	Intestines and liver
Amino Acids		
Amino acid specific transporters	Coupled channels	Intestines, kidney, and liver
All amino acids except proline	Active: symport with Na+	Liver
Specific amino acids	Active: group translocation	Small intestine
	Passive	
Other Organic Molecules		
Cholic acid, deoxycholic acid, and taurocholic acid	Active: symport with Na+	Intestines
Organic anions (e.g., malate, α-ketoglutarate, glutamate)	Antiport with counter–organic anion	Mitochondria of liver cells
ATP–ADP	Antiport transport of nucleotides; can be active	Mitochondria of liver cells
Inorganic Ions		
Na+	Passive	Distal renal tubular cells
Na+/H+	Active antiport, proton pump	Proximal renal tubular cells and small intestines
Na+/K+	Active: ATP driven, protein channel	Plasma membrane of most cells
Ca++	Active: ATP driven, antiport with Na+	All cells, antiporter in red blood cells
H+/K+	Active	Parietal cells of gastric cells secreting H+
HCO3 (perhaps other anions)	Mediated: antiport (anion transporter–band 3 protein)	Erythrocytes and many other cells
Water	Osmosis passive	All tissues

[a]The known transport systems are listed here; others have been proposed. Most transport systems have been studied in only a few tissues and their sites of activity may be more limited than indicated.

ADP, Adenosine diphosphate; *ATP*, adenosine triphosphate, *Ca++*, calcium; *Cl-*, chloride; *H+*, hydrogen; *HCO3-*, bicarbonate; *K+*, potassium; *Na+*, sodium.

Data from Alberts, B., Bray, D., Hopkin, K., et al. (2014). *Essential cell biology* (4th ed.). Garland Publishing; Alberts, B., Johnson, A., Lewis, J., et al. (2001). *Molecular biology of the cell* (4th ed.). Wiley; Devlin, T. M. (Ed.). (1992). *Textbook of biochemistry: with clinical correlations* (3rd ed.). Wiley; Raven, P. H., & Johnson, G. B. (1995). *Understanding biology* (3rd ed.). Brown.

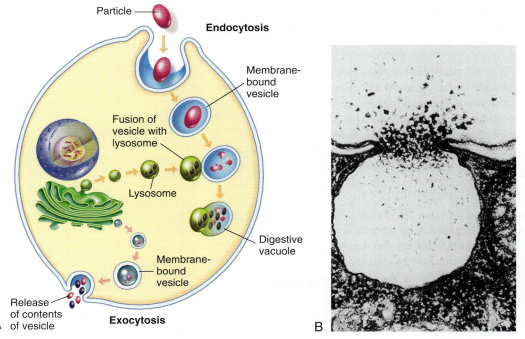

FIGURE 1.26 Endocytosis and Exocytosis. **A,** Endocytosis and fusion with lysosome and exocytosis. **B,** Electron micrograph of exocytosis. ([B] from Raven, P. H., & Johnson, G. B. [1999]. *Biology* [5th ed.]. McGraw-Hill.)

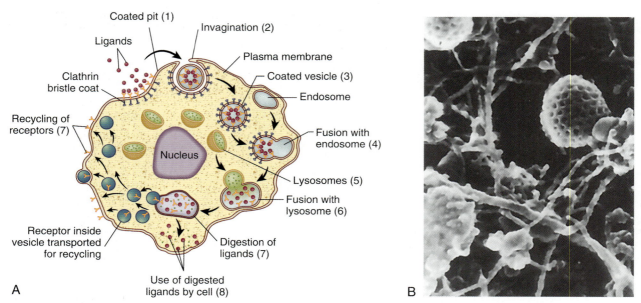

FIGURE 1.27 Ligand Internalization by Means of Receptor-Mediated Endocytosis. **A,** The ligand attaches to its surface receptor (through the clathrin coat) and, through receptor-mediated endocytosis, enters the cell. The ingested material fuses with a lysosome and is processed by hydrolytic lysosomal enzymes. Processed molecules can then be transferred to other cellular components. **B,** Electron micrograph of a coated pit showing different sizes of filaments of the cytoskeleton (×82 000) receptor-mediated endocytosis with coated pit and vesicle. ([B] from Erlandsen, S. L., & Magney, J. E. [1992]. *Color atlas of histology.* Mosby.)

BOX 1.3 The New Endocytic Matrix

An explosion of new data is disclosing a much more involved role for endocytosis than just a simple way to internalize nutrients and membrane-associated molecules. These new data show that endocytosis appears to control signalling and has a major role in determining the net output of biochemical pathways. Endocytosis modulates the presence of receptors and their ligands, as well as effectors both at the plasma membrane or at intermediate stations of the endocytic route. The overall processes and anatomy of these new functions are sometimes called the *endocytic matrix*. All of these functions ultimately have a large impact on almost every cellular process, including the nucleus.

From Sigismund, S., & Scita, G. (2018). The "endocytic matrix reloaded" and its impact on the plasticity of migratory strategies. *Current Opinion in Cell Biology, 54,* 9–17. doi:10.1016/j.ceb.2018.02.006.

Caveolae are also important sites for signal transduction, where extracellular chemical messages or *signals* are communicated to the cell's interior for execution. For example, plasma membrane estrogen receptors can localize in caveolae, and facilitate several intracellular biological actions.[14] This new understanding has the potential for developing effective therapies to treat complications of pregnancy such as preeclampsia.[15]

Movement of Electrical Impulses: Membrane Potentials

All body cells are electrically polarized, with the inside of the cell more negatively charged than the outside. The difference in electrical charge, or voltage, is known as the **resting membrane potential** and is about −70 to −85 mV. The difference in voltage across the plasma membrane results from the differences in ionic composition of ICF and ECF. Sodium ions are more concentrated in the ECF, and potassium ions are more concentrated in the ICF. The concentration difference is maintained by the active transport of Na^+ and K^+ (the sodium–potassium pump), which transports sodium outward and potassium inward (Figure 1.28). Because the resting plasma membrane is more permeable to K^+ than to Na^+, K^+ diffuses easily from the ICF to the ECF. Because both Na^+ and K^+ are cations, the net result is an excess of anions inside the cell, resulting in the negative resting membrane potential.

Nerve and muscle cells are excitable and can change their resting membrane potential in response to electrochemical stimuli. Changes in resting membrane potential convey messages from cell to cell. When a nerve or muscle cell receives a stimulus that exceeds the membrane threshold value, a rapid change occurs in the resting membrane potential, known as the **action potential**. The action potential carries signals along the nerve or muscle cell and propagates information along a particular electrical pathway. Nerve impulses are described in Chapter 13. When a resting cell is stimulated through voltage-regulated channels, the cell membranes become more permeable to sodium. Sodium moves into the cell and the membrane potential moves from a negative value (in millivolts) to zero. This movement is known as **depolarization**. The depolarized cell is more positively charged, and its polarity is neutralized.

To generate an action potential and depolarization of the cell, the **threshold potential** must be reached. Generally, this occurs when the cell has depolarized by 15 to 20 mV. When the threshold is reached, the cell will continue to depolarize with no further stimulation. The sodium gates open, and sodium rushes into the cell. The membrane potential is now zero and then becomes positive

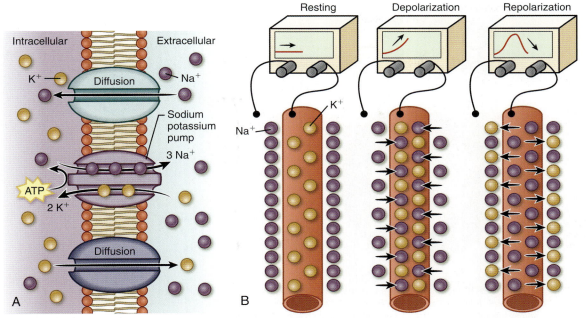

FIGURE 1.28 Sodium–Potassium Pump and Propagation of an Action Potential. **A,** Concentration difference of sodium (Na+) and potassium (K+) intracellularly and extracellularly. The direction of active transport by the sodium–potassium pump is also shown (black arrows). **B,** The left diagram represents the polarized state of a neuronal membrane when at rest. The middle and right diagrams represent changes in sodium and potassium membrane permeabilities with depolarization and repolarization. *ATP,* Adenosine triphosphate.

(depolarization). The rapid reversal in polarity results in the action potential.

During **repolarization**, the negative polarity of the resting membrane potential is re-established. As the voltage-gated sodium channels begin to close, voltage-gated potassium channels open. Membrane permeability to sodium decreases and potassium permeability increases. Potassium ions leave the cell. As the sodium gates close and potassium leaves the cell, the membrane potential of the cell becomes more negative. The Na+–K+ pump then finishes this journey to the negative resting membrane potential by actively pumping potassium back into the cell and sodium out of the cell.

During most of the action potential, the plasma membrane cannot respond to an additional stimulus. This time is known as the **absolute refractory period** and is related to changes in permeability to sodium. During the latter phase of the action potential, when permeability to potassium increases, a stronger-than-normal stimulus can evoke an action potential; this time is known as the **relative refractory period**.

When the membrane potential is more negative than normal, there is more charge across the cell membrane, and the cell is in a **hyperpolarized state**. The cell is less excitable, and a stronger-than-normal stimulus is required to reach the threshold potential and generate an action potential. Similarly, when the membrane potential is more positive than normal, there is less charge across the cell membrane, and the cell is in a **hypopolarized state**. The cell is more excitable, and a weaker-than-normal stimulus is required to reach the threshold potential. Changes in the intracellular and extracellular concentrations of ions or a change in membrane permeability can cause these alterations in membrane excitability.

CELLULAR REPRODUCTION: THE CELL CYCLE

Cellular reproduction is necessary for the maintenance of life and is categorized as either meiosis or mitosis (with cytokinesis), depending on the types of cells that are involved. Reproduction of *gametes* (sperm and egg cells) occurs through a process called **meiosis**, described in Chapter 2. On the other hand, the reproduction, or division, of other body cells (*somatic cells*) involves two sequential phases—**mitosis**, or nuclear division, and **cytokinesis**, or cytoplasmic division. Before a cell can divide, however, it must double its mass and duplicate all its contents. **Interphase** is the stage when the cell grows and prepares for actual cell division. The alternation between mitosis and interphase in all tissues is known as the **cell cycle**. As cells die, more cells receive the signal to enter the cell cycle and divide.

The four designated phases of the cell cycle (Figure 1.29) are (1) the **S phase** (S = synthesis), in which DNA is synthesized in the cell nucleus; (2) the **G2 phase** (G = gap), in which RNA and protein synthesis occurs, namely, the period between the completion of DNA synthesis and the next phase (M); (3) the **M phase** (M = mitosis), which includes both nuclear and cytoplasmic division; and (4) the **G1 phase**, which is the period between the M phase and the start of DNA synthesis. When cells are in the **G0 phase**, they are neither dividing nor preparing to divide. Rather, they are continuing on with their regular function as part of the tissue or organ to which they belong. Understanding the cell cycle is important when considering the effectiveness of antineoplastic medications and the growth of cancer cells. This will be covered in Chapter 10.

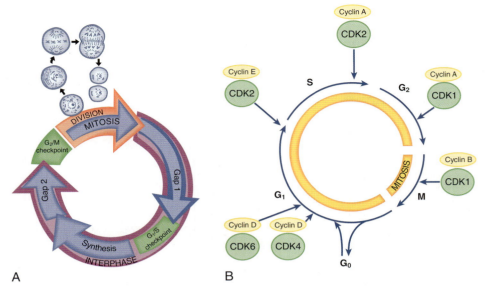

FIGURE 1.29 Interphase and the Phases of Mitosis. **A,** The G_1/S checkpoint is to "check" for cell size, nutrients, growth factors, and DNA damage. See text for resting phases. The G_2/M checkpoint checks for cell size and DNA replication. **B,** The orderly progression through the phases of the cell cycle is regulated by *cyclins* (so called because levels rise and fall) and cyclin-dependent protein kinases *(CDKs)* and their inhibitors. When cyclins are complexed with CDKs, cell cycle events are triggered.

Phases of Mitosis and Cytokinesis

Interphase (the G_1, S, and G_2 phases) is the longest phase of the cell cycle. During interphase, the **chromatin** (the substance that gives the nucleus its granular appearance) consists of very long, slender rods jumbled together in the nucleus. Late in interphase, strands of chromatin begin to coil, causing shortening and thickening.

The M phase of the cell cycle, mitosis and cytokinesis, begins with **prophase**, the first appearance of chromosomes. As the phase proceeds, each chromosome is seen as two identical halves called **chromatids**, which lie together and are attached by a spindle site called a **centromere**. (The two chromatids of each chromosome, which are genetically identical, are sometimes called *sister chromatids*.) The nuclear membrane, which surrounds the nucleus, disappears. **Spindle fibres** are microtubules formed in the cytoplasm. They radiate from two centrioles located at opposite poles of the cell and pull the chromosomes to opposite sides of the cell. This is the beginning of **metaphase**. Next, the centromeres become aligned in the middle of the spindle, which is called the **equatorial plate (or metaphase plate)** of the cell. In this stage, chromosomes are easiest to observe microscopically because they are highly condensed and arranged in a relatively organized fashion.

Anaphase begins when the centromeres split, and the sister chromatids are pulled apart. The spindle fibres shorten, causing the sister chromatids to be pulled apart from the centromere toward opposite sides of the cell. When the sister chromatids are separated, each is considered to be a chromosome. The cell has 92 chromosomes during this stage. By the end of anaphase, there are 46 chromosomes lying at each side of the cell. Barring mitotic errors, each of the two groups of 46 chromosomes is identical to the original 46 chromosomes present at the start of the cell cycle.

During **telophase**, the final stage, a new nuclear membrane is formed around each group of 46 chromosomes, the spindle fibres disappear, and the chromosomes begin to uncoil. Cytokinesis causes the cytoplasm to divide into almost equal parts during this phase. At the end of telophase, two identical diploid cells, called **daughter cells**, have been formed from the original cell.

Rates of Cellular Division

Although the complete cell cycle lasts 12 to 24 hours, about 1 hour is required for the four stages of mitosis and cytokinesis. All types of cells undergo mitosis during formation of the embryo, but many adult cells—such as nerve cells, lens cells of the eye, and muscle cells—lose their ability to replicate and divide. The cells of other tissues, particularly epithelial cells (e.g., cells of the intestine, lung, or skin), divide continuously and rapidly, completing the entire cell cycle in less than 10 hours.

The difference between cells that divide slowly and cells that divide rapidly is the length of time spent in the G_1 phase of the cell cycle. Once the S phase begins, however, progression through mitosis takes a relatively constant amount of time.

The mechanisms that control cell division depend on the integrity of genetic, epigenetic (heritable changes in genome function that occur without alterations in the DNA sequence; see Chapter 3), and protein growth factors. Protein growth factors govern the proliferation of different cell types. Individual cells are focused on survival of the entire organism. When a need arises for new cells, as in repair of injured cells, previously nondividing cells must be triggered rapidly to re-enter the cell cycle. With continual wear and tear, the cell birth rate and the cell death rate must be kept in balance.

Growth Factors

Growth factors, also called cytokines, are peptides (protein fractions) that transmit signals within and between cells. They have a major role in the regulation of tissue growth and development (Table 1.5). Having nutrients is not enough for a cell to proliferate; it must also receive stimulatory chemical signals (growth factors) from other cells, usually its neighbours or the surrounding supporting tissue called stroma. These signals act to overcome intracellular braking mechanisms that tend to restrain cell growth and block progress through the cell cycle (Figure 1.30).

An example of a brake that regulates cell proliferation is the retinoblastoma (Rb) protein, first identified through studies of a rare childhood eye tumour called *retinoblastoma*, in which the Rb protein is missing or defective. The Rb protein is abundant in the nucleus of all vertebrate cells. It binds to gene regulatory proteins, preventing them from stimulating the transcription of genes required for cell proliferation (see Figure 1.30). Extracellular signals, such as growth factors, activate intracellular signalling pathways that inactivate the Rb protein, leading to cell proliferation.

Different types of cells require different growth factors; for example, platelet-derived growth factor (PDGF) stimulates the production of connective tissue cells. Table 1.5 summarizes the most significant growth factors. Some growth factors also regulate other cellular processes, such as cellular differentiation. In addition to growth factors that stimulate cellular processes, there are factors that inhibit these processes. Cells that are starved of growth factors come to a halt after mitosis and enter the arrested (resting) G0 state of the cell cycle.[1]

TISSUES

> **QUICK CHECK 1.4**
> 1. What is the cell cycle?
> 2. Describe the five types of intracellular communication.
> 3. Why is the extracellular matrix important for tissue cells?

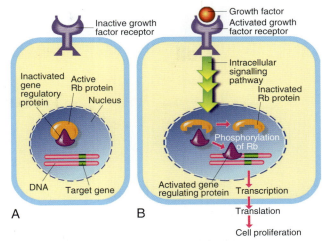

FIGURE 1.30 How Growth Factors Stimulate Cell Proliferation. A, Resting cell. With the absence of growth factors, the retinoblastoma (Rb) protein is not phosphorylated; thus, it holds the gene regulatory proteins in an inactive state. The gene regulatory proteins are required to stimulate the transcription of genes needed for cell proliferation. **B**, Proliferating cell. Growth factors bind to the cell surface receptors and activate intracellular signalling pathways, leading to activation of intracellular proteins. These intracellular proteins phosphorylate and thereby inactivate the Rb protein. The gene regulatory proteins are now free to activate the transcription of genes, leading to cell proliferation. *DNA*, Deoxyribonucleic acid.

TABLE 1.5	Examples of Growth Factors and Their Actions
Growth Factor	**Physiological Actions**
Platelet-derived growth factor (PDGF)	Stimulates proliferation of connective tissue cells and neuroglial cells
Epidermal growth factor (EGF)	Stimulates proliferation of epidermal cells and other cell types
Insulinlike growth factor 1 (IGF-1)	Collaborates with PDGF and EGF; stimulates proliferation of fat cells and connective tissue cells
Vascular endothelial growth factor (VEGF)	Mediates functions of endothelial cells; proliferation, migration, invasion, survival, and permeability
Insulinlike growth factor 2 (IGF-2)	Collaborates with PDGF and EGF; stimulates or inhibits response of most cells to other growth factors; regulates differentiation of some cell types (e.g., cartilage)
Transforming growth factor-beta (TGF-β; multiple subtypes)	Stimulates or inhibits response of most cells to other growth factors; regulates differentiation of some cell types (e.g., cartilage)
Fibroblast growth factor (FGF; multiple subtypes)	Stimulates proliferation of fibroblasts, endothelial cells, myoblasts, and other multiple subtypes
Interleukin-2 (IL-2)	Stimulates proliferation of T lymphocytes
Nerve growth factor (NGF)	Promotes axon growth and survival of sympathetic and some sensory and central nervous system neurons
Hematopoietic cell growth factors (IL-3, GM-CSF, G-CSF, erythropoietin)	Promote proliferation of blood cells

G-CSF, Granulocyte colony-stimulating factor; *GM-CSF*, granulocyte-macrophage colony-stimulating factor.

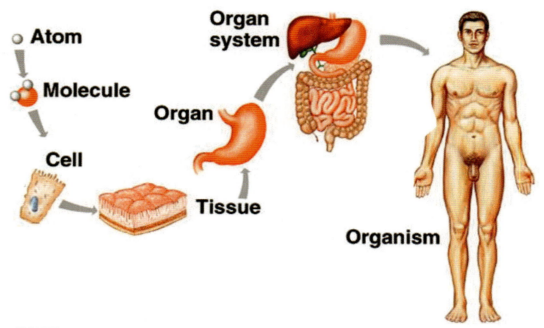

FIGURE 1.31 Cells, Tissues, Organs, and Organ Systems. The smallest level of organization shown in this diagram is the cell. Cells working together make up a tissue, which in turn is part of an organ. Organs working together form the different organ systems that make up a whole organism.

Cells of one or more types are organized into tissues, and different types of tissues compose organs. Finally, organs are integrated to perform complex functions as tracts or systems (Figure 1.31).

Tissue Formation

To form tissues, cells must exhibit intercellular recognition and communication, adhesion, and memory. Specialized cells sense their environment through signals, such as growth factors, from other cells. This type of communication ensures that new cells are produced only when and where they are required. Different cell types have different adhesion molecules in their plasma membranes and stick selectively to other cells of the same type. They can also adhere to ECM components and increase the strength of the ECM and the strength of the cytoskeleton. Cells have memory because of specialized patterns of gene expression from signals during embryonic development. Memory allows cells to autonomously preserve their distinctive character and pass it on to their progeny.[1]

Fully specialized or **terminally differentiated** cells that are lost are regenerated from proliferating *precursor cells*. These precursor cells have been derived from a smaller number of stem cells.[1] **Stem cells** are cells with the potential to develop into many different cell types during early development and growth. In many tissues, stem cells serve as an internal repair and maintenance system, and they are capable of dividing indefinitely. These cells can maintain themselves over very long periods of time and can generate all the differentiated cell types of the tissue. This stem cell–driven tissue renewal is very evident in the epithelial lining of the intestine, stomach, blood cells, and skin, which is continuously exposed to environmental factors. When a stem cell divides, each daughter cell has a choice: it can remain as a stem cell or it can follow a pathway that results in terminal differentiation (Figure 1.32).

Types of Tissues

The four basic types of tissues are nerve, epithelial, connective, and muscle tissues. The structure and function of these four types underlie the structure and function of each organ system. Neural tissue is composed of highly specialized cells called *neurons*, which receive and transmit electrical impulses rapidly across junctions called *synapses* (see Figure 13.1). Different types of neurons have special characteristics that depend on their distribution and function within the nervous system. Epithelial, connective, and muscle tissues are summarized in Tables 1.6, 1.7, and 1.8, respectively.

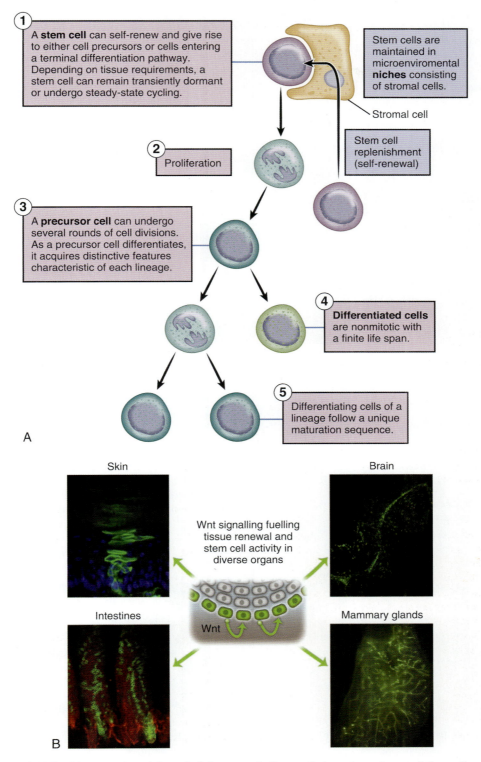

FIGURE 1.32 Properties of Stem Cell Systems. A, Stem cells have three characteristics: self-renewal, proliferation, and differentiation into mature cells. Stem cells are housed in niches consisting of stromal cells that provide factors for their maintenance. Stem cells of the embryo can give rise to cell precursors that generate all the tissues of the body. This property defines stem cells as multipotent. Stem cells are difficult to identify anatomically. Their identification is based on specific cell surface markers (cell surface antigens recognized by specific monoclonal antibodies) and on the lineage they generate following transplantation. **B,** Wnt signalling fuels tissue renewal. ([A] from Kierszenbaum, A. [2012]. *Histology and cell biology: An introduction to pathology* [3rd ed.]. Elsevier. [B] from Clevers, H., Loh, K. M., & Nusse, R. [2014]. *Science, 346*[6205], 54.)

TABLE 1.6 Characteristics of Epithelial Tissues

Simple Squamous Epithelium
Structure

Single layer of cells

Location and Function

Lining of blood vessels leads to diffusion and filtration

Lining of pulmonary alveoli (air sacs) leads to separation of blood from fluids in tissues

Bowman's capsule (kidney), where it filters substances from blood, forming urine

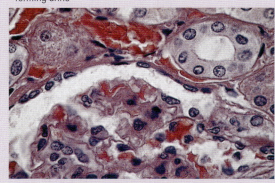

Simple Squamous Epithelial Cell. Photomicrograph of simple squamous epithelial cell in parietal wall of Bowman's capsule in kidney. (From Erlandsen, S. L., & Magney, J. E. [1992]. *Color atlas of histology*. Mosby.)

Stratified Squamous Epithelium
Structure

Two or more layers, depending on location, with cells closest to basement membrane tending to be cuboidal

Location and Function

Epidermis of skin and linings of mouth, pharynx, esophagus, and anus provide protection and secretion

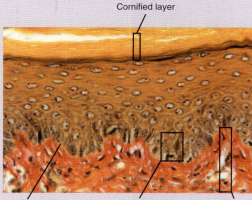

Cornified Stratified Squamous Epithelium. Diagram of stratified squamous epithelium of skin. (Copyright Ed Reschke. Used with permission.)

Transitional Epithelium
Structure

Vary in shape from cuboidal to squamous, depending on whether basal cells of bladder are columnar or are composed of many layers; when bladder is full and stretched, the cells flatten and stretch like squamous cells

Location and Function

Linings of urinary bladder and other hollow structures stretch, allowing expansion of the hollow organs

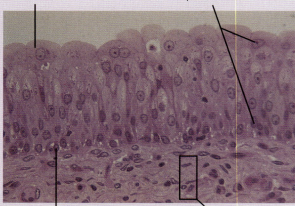

Stratified Squamous Transitional Epithelium. Photomicrograph of stratified squamous transitional epithelium of urinary bladder. (Copyright Ed Reschke. Used with permission.)

Simple Cuboidal Epithelium
Structure

Simple cuboidal cells; rarely stratified (layered)

Location and Function

Glands (e.g., thyroid, sweat, salivary) and parts of the kidney tubules and outer covering of ovary secrete fluids

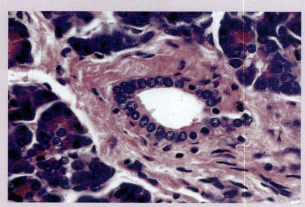

Simple Cuboidal Epithelium. Photomicrograph of simple cuboidal epithelium of pancreatic duct. (From Erlandsen, S. L., & Magney, J. E. [1992]. *Color atlas of histology*. Mosby.)

(Continued)

TABLE 1.6 Characteristics of Epithelial Tissues—cont'd

Simple Columnar Epithelium
Structure

Large amounts of cytoplasm and cellular organelles

Location and Function

Ducts of many glands and lining of digestive tract allow secretion and absorption from stomach to anus

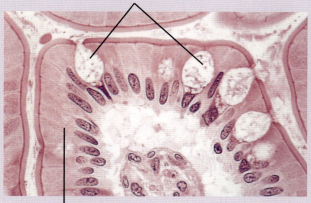

Simple Columnar Epithelium. Photomicrograph of simple columnar epithelium. (Copyright Ed Reschke. Used with permission.)

Ciliated Simple Columnar Epithelium
Structure

Same as simple columnar epithelium but ciliated

Location and Function

Linings of bronchi of lungs, nasal cavity, and oviducts allow secretion, absorption, and propulsion of fluids and particles

Stratified Columnar Epithelium
Structure

Small and rounded basement membrane (columnar cells do not touch basement membrane)

Location and Function

Linings of epiglottis, part of pharynx, anus, and male urethra provide protection

Pseudostratified Ciliated Columnar Epithelium
Structure

All cells in contact with basement membrane
Nuclei found at different levels within cell, giving stratified appearance
Free surface often ciliated

Location and Function

Linings of large ducts of some glands (parotid, salivary), male urethra, respiratory passages, and eustachian tubes of ears transport substances

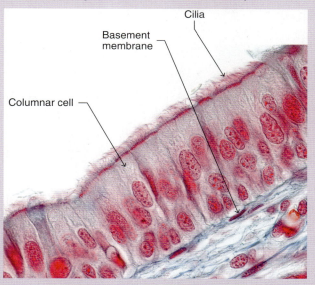

Pseudostratified Ciliated Columnar Epithelium. Photomicrograph of pseudostratified ciliated columnar epithelium of trachea. (iStockphoto/Jose Luis Calvo Martin & Jose Enrique Garcia-Mauriño)

TABLE 1.7 Connective Tissues

Loose or Areolar Tissue
Structure
Unorganized; spaces between fibres
Most fibres collagenous, some elastic and reticular
Includes many types of cells (fibroblasts and macrophages most common) and large amount of intercellular fluid

Location and Function
Attaches skin to underlying tissue; holds organs in place by filling spaces between them; supports blood vessels
Intercellular fluid transports nutrients and waste products
Fluid accumulation causes swelling (edema)

Loose Areolar Connective Tissue. (Copyright Ed Reschke. Used with permission.)

Dense Irregular Tissue
Structure
Dense, compact, and areolar tissue, with fewer cells and greater number of closely woven collagenous fibres than in loose tissue

Location and Function
Dermis layer of skin; acts as protective barrier

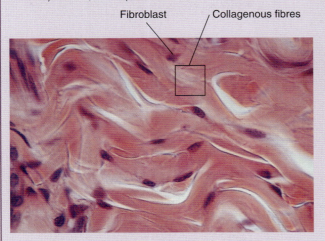

Dense, Irregular Connective Tissue. (Copyright Ed Reschke. Used with permission.)

Dense, Regular (White Fibrous) Tissue
Structure
Collagenous fibres and some elastic fibres, tightly packed into parallel bundles, with only fibroblast cells

Location and Function
Forms strong tendons of muscle, ligaments of joints, some fibrous membranes, and fascia that surrounds organs and muscles

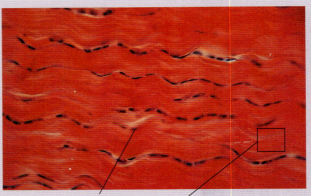

Dense, Regular (White Fibrous) Connective Tissue. (Copyright Ed Reschke. Used with permission.)

Elastic Tissue
Structure
Elastic fibres, some collagenous fibres, fibroblasts

Location and Function
Lends strength and elasticity to walls of arteries, trachea, vocal cords, and other structures

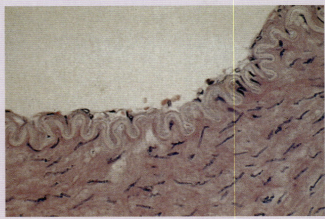

Elastic Connective Tissue. (From Erlandsen, S. L., & Magney, J. E. [1992]. *Color atlas of histology.* Mosby.)

(Continued)

TABLE 1.7 Connective Tissues—cont'd

Adipose Tissue
Structure

Fat cells dispersed in loose tissues; each cell containing a large droplet of fat flattens nucleus and forces cytoplasm into a ring around cell's periphery

Location and Function

Stores fat, which provides padding and protection

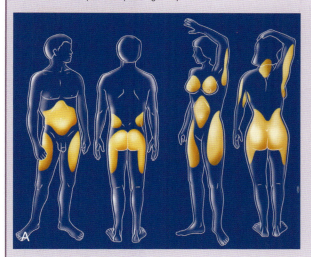

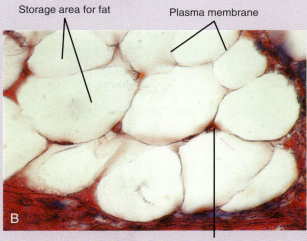

Adipose Tissue. **A**, Fat storage areas—distribution of fat in male and female bodies. **B**, Photomicrograph of adipose tissue. ([A] modified from Patton, K. T. [2019]. *Anatomy & physiology* [10th ed.]. Elsevier; [B] copyright Ed Reschke. Used with permission.)

Cartilage (Hyaline, Elastic, Fibrous)
Structure

Collagenous fibres embedded in a firm matrix (chondrin); no blood supply

Location and Function

Gives form, support, and flexibility to joints, trachea, nose, ear, vertebral disks, embryonic skeleton, and many internal structures

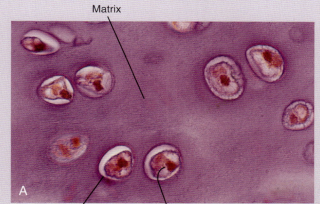

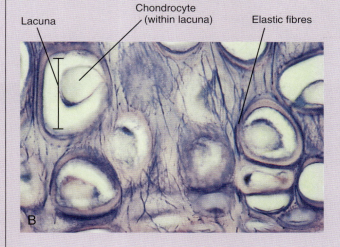

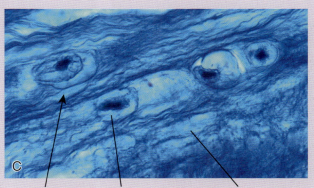

Cartilage. **A**, Hyaline cartilage. **B**, Elastic cartilage. **C**, Fibrous cartilage. ([A, B, and C] copyright Ed Reschke. Used with permission.)

(Continued)

TABLE 1.7 Connective Tissues —cont'd

Bone
Structure

Rigid connective tissue consisting of cells, fibres, ground substances, and minerals

Location and Function

Lends skeleton rigidity and strength

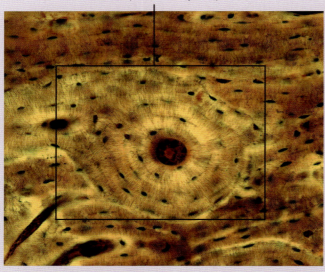

Bone. (Steve Gschmeissner/Science Source.)

Special Connective Tissues
Plasma

Structure

Fluid

Location and Function

Serves as matrix for blood cells

Macrophages in Tissue, Reticuloendothelial, or Macrophage System

Structure

Scattered macrophages (phagocytes) called Kupffer cells (in liver), alveolar macrophages (in lungs), microglia (in central nervous system)

Location and Function

Facilitate inflammatory response and carry out phagocytosis in loose connective, lymphatic, digestive, medullary (bone marrow), splenic, adrenal, and pituitary tissues

TABLE 1.8 Muscle Tissues

Skeletal (Striated) Muscle
Structure Characteristics of Cells

Long, cylindrical cells that extend throughout length of muscles
Striated myofibrils (proteins)
Many nuclei on periphery

Location and Function

Attached to bones directly or by tendons and provide voluntary movement of skeleton and maintenance of posture

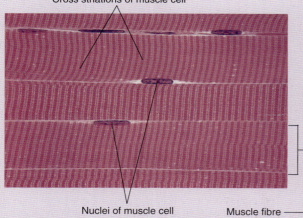

Skeletal (Striated) Muscle. (From Thibodeau, G. A., & Patton, K. T. [2007]. *Anatomy & physiology* [6th ed.]. Mosby.)

Cardiac Muscle
Structure Characteristics of Cells

Branching networks throughout muscle tissue
Striated myofibrils

Location and Function

Cells attached end-to-end at intercalated disks with tissue forming walls of heart (myocardium) to provide involuntary pumping action of heart

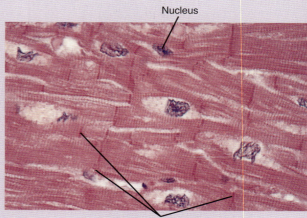

Cardiac muscle. (Copyright Ed Reschke. Used with permission.)

(Continued)

TABLE 1.8 Muscle Tissues—cont'd

Smooth (Visceral) Muscle
Structure Characteristics of Cells

Long spindles that taper to a point
Absence of striated myofibrils

Location and Function

Walls of hollow internal structures, such as digestive tract and blood vessels (viscera), provide voluntary and involuntary contractions that move substances through hollow structures

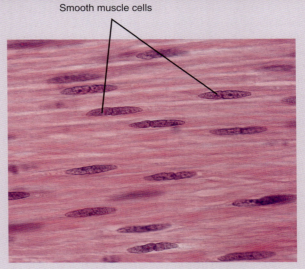

Smooth (visceral) muscle. (iStockphoto/Jose Luis Calvo Martin & Jose Enrique Garcia-Mauriño)

DID YOU UNDERSTAND?

Cellular Functions
1. Cells become specialized through the process of differentiation or maturation.
2. The eight specialized cellular functions are movement, conductivity, metabolic absorption, secretion, excretion, respiration, reproduction, and communication.

Structure and Function of Cellular Components
1. The eukaryotic cell consists of three general components: the plasma membrane, the cytoplasm, and the intracellular organelles.
2. The nucleus is the largest membrane-bound organelle and is found usually in the cell's centre. The chief functions of the nucleus are cell division and control of genetic information.
3. Cytoplasm is an aqueous solution (cytosol) that fills the cytoplasmic matrix—the space between the nuclear envelope and the plasma membrane.
4. The endoplasmic reticulum is a network of tubular channels (cisternae) that extend throughout the outer nuclear membrane. It specializes in the synthesis and transport of protein and lipid components of most of the organelles.
5. The Golgi complex is a network of smooth membranes and vesicles located near the nucleus. The Golgi complex is responsible for processing and packaging proteins into secretory vesicles that break away from the Golgi complex and migrate to a variety of intracellular and extracellular destinations, including the plasma membrane.
6. Lysosomes are saclike structures that originate from the Golgi complex and contain digestive enzymes. These enzymes are responsible for digesting most cellular substances to their basic form, such as amino acids, fatty acids, and carbohydrates (sugars).
7. Cellular injury leads to a release of the lysosomal enzymes, causing cellular self-digestion.
8. Mitochondria contain the metabolic machinery necessary for cellular energy metabolism. The enzymes of the respiratory chain (electron-transport chain), found in the inner membrane of the mitochondria, generate most of the cell's ATP.
9. The cytoskeleton is the "bone and muscle" of the cell. The internal skeleton is composed of a network of protein filaments, including microtubules and actin filaments (microfilaments).
10. The plasma membrane encloses the cell and, by controlling the movement of substances across it, exerts a powerful influence on metabolic pathways.
11. Proteins are the major workhorses of the cell. Membrane proteins, like other proteins, are synthesized by the ribosome and then make their way, called *trafficking*, to different locations in the cell. Trafficking places unique demands on membrane proteins for folding, translocation, and stability. Misfolded proteins are emerging as an important cause of disease.
12. Protein regulation in a cell is called *protein homeostasis* and is defined by the proteostasis network. This network is composed of ribosomes (makers), chaperones (helpers), and protein breakdown or proteolytic systems. Malfunction of these systems is associated with disease.
13. Carbohydrates contained within the plasma membrane are generally bound to membrane proteins (glycoproteins) and lipids (glycolipids).
14. Protein receptors (recognition units) on the plasma membrane enable the cell to interact with other cells and with extracellular substances.
15. Membrane functions are determined largely by proteins. These functions include recognition by protein receptors and transport of substances into and out of the cell.

Cell-to-Cell Adhesions
1. Cell-to-cell adhesions are formed on plasma membranes, thereby allowing the formation of tissues and organs. Cells are held together by three different means: (a) the extracellular matrix, (b) cell adhesion molecules in the cell's plasma membrane, and (c) specialized cell junctions.
2. The extracellular matrix includes three groups of macromolecules: (a) fibrous structural proteins (e.g., collagen and elastin), (b) adhesive glycoproteins, and (c) proteoglycans and hyaluronic acid. The matrix helps regulate cell growth, movement, and differentiation.
3. The basement membrane is a tough layer of extracellular matrix underlying the epithelium of many organs; it is also called the *basal lamina*.
4. Cell junctions can be classified as symmetrical and asymmetrical. Symmetrical junctions include tight junctions, the belt desmosome, desmosomes, and gap junctions. An asymmetrical junction is the hemidesmosome.

Cellular Communication and Signal Transduction
1. Cells communicate in three main ways: (a) they form protein channels (gap junctions); (b) they display receptors that affect intracellular processes or other cells in direct physical contact; and (c) they use receptor proteins *inside* the target cell.
2. Primary modes of intercellular signalling include contact-dependent, paracrine, hormonal, neurohormonal, and neurotransmitter.
3. Signal transduction involves signals or instructions from extracellular chemical messengers that are conveyed to the cell's interior for execution. If deprived of appropriate signals, cells undergo a form of cell suicide known as programmed cell death, or apoptosis.

Cellular Metabolism
1. The chemical tasks of maintaining essential cellular functions are referred to as *cellular metabolism*. Anabolism is the energy-using process of metabolism, whereas catabolism is the energy-releasing process.
2. Adenosine triphosphate (ATP) functions as an energy-transferring molecule. It is fuel for cell survival. Energy is stored by molecules of carbohydrate, lipid, and protein, which, when catabolized, transfers energy to ATP.
3. Oxidative phosphorylation occurs in the mitochondria and is the mechanism by which the energy produced from carbohydrates, fats, and proteins is transferred to ATP.

Membrane Transport: Cellular Intake and Output
1. Cell survival and growth depends on the constant exchange of molecules with their environment. The two main classes of membrane transport proteins are transporters and channels. The majority of molecular transfer depends on specialized membrane transport proteins.
2. Water and small, electrically uncharged molecules move through pores in the plasma membrane's lipid bilayer in the process called *passive transport*.
3. Passive transport does not require the expenditure of energy; rather, it is driven by the physical effect of osmosis, hydrostatic pressure, and diffusion.
4. Larger molecules and molecular complexes are moved into the cell by active transport, which requires the cell to expend energy (by means of ATP).
5. The largest molecules (macromolecules) and fluids are transported by the processes of endocytosis (ingestion) and exocytosis (expulsion). Endocytosis, or vesicle formation, is when the substance to be transported is engulfed by a segment of the plasma membrane, forming a vesicle that moves into the cell.
6. Pinocytosis is a type of endocytosis in which fluids and solute molecules are ingested through formation of small vesicles.
7. Phagocytosis is a type of endocytosis in which large particles, such as bacteria, are ingested through formation of large vesicles, called *vacuoles*.
8. In receptor-mediated endocytosis, the plasma membrane receptors are clustered in specialized areas called *coated pits*.
9. Endocytosis occurs when coated pits invaginate, internalizing ligand-receptor complexes in coated vesicles.
10. Inside the cell, lysosomal enzymes process and digest material ingested by endocytosis.
11. Two types of solutes exist in body fluids: electrolytes and nonelectrolytes. Electrolytes are electrically charged and dissociate into constituent ions when placed in solution. Nonelectrolytes do not dissociate when placed in solution.
12. Diffusion is the passive movement of a solute from an area of higher solute concentration to an area of lower solute concentration.
13. Filtration is the measurement of water and solutes through a membrane because of a greater mechanical pressure.
14. Hydrostatic pressure is the mechanical force of water pushing against cellular membranes.
15. Osmosis is the movement of water across a semipermeable membrane from a region of lower solute concentration to a region of higher solute concentration.
16. The amount of hydrostatic pressure required to oppose the osmotic movement of water is called the *osmotic pressure* of the solution.
17. The overall osmotic effect of colloids, such as plasma proteins, is called the *oncotic pressure*, or *colloid osmotic pressure*.
18. All body cells are electrically polarized, with the inside of the cell more negatively charged than the outside. The difference in voltage across the plasma membrane is the resting membrane potential.
19. When an excitable (nerve or muscle) cell receives an electrochemical stimulus, cations enter the cell and cause a rapid change in the resting membrane potential, known as the *action potential*. The action potential "moves" along the cell's plasma membrane and is transmitted to an adjacent cell. This is how electrochemical signals convey information from cell to cell.

Cellular Reproduction: The Cell Cycle
1. Cellular reproduction in body tissues involves mitosis (nuclear division) and cytokinesis (cytoplasmic division).
2. Only mature cells are capable of division. Maturation occurs during a stage of cellular life called *interphase* (the growth phase).
3. The cell cycle is the reproductive process that begins after interphase in all tissues with cellular turnover. There are four phases of the cell cycle: (a) the S phase, during which DNA synthesis takes place in the cell nucleus; (b) the G_2 phase, the period between the completion of DNA synthesis and the next phase (M); (c) the M phase, which involves both nuclear (mitotic) and cytoplasmic (cytokinetic) division; and (d) the G_1 phase (growth phase), after which the cycle begins again.

4. The M phase (mitosis) involves four stages: prophase, metaphase, anaphase, and telophase.
5. The mechanisms that control cellular division depend on the integrity of genetic, epigenetic, and protein growth factors.

Tissues

1. Cells of one or more types are organized into tissues, and different types of tissues compose organs. Organs are organized to function as tracts or systems.
2. Three key factors that maintain the cellular organization of tissues are (a) recognition and cell communication, (b) selective cell-to-cell adhesion, and (c) memory.
3. Tissue cells are linked at cell junctions, which are specialized regions on their plasma membranes. Cell junctions attach adjacent cells and allow small molecules to pass between them.
4. The four basic types of tissues are epithelial, muscle, nerve, and connective tissues.
5. Neural tissue is composed of highly specialized cells called *neurons* that receive and transmit electrical impulses rapidly across junctions called *synapses*.
6. Epithelial tissue covers most internal and external surfaces of the body. The functions of epithelial tissue include protection, absorption, secretion, and excretion.
7. Connective tissue binds various tissues and organs together, supporting them in their locations and serving as storage sites for excess nutrients.
8. Muscle tissue is composed of long, thin, highly contractile cells or fibres called *myocytes*. Muscle tissue that is attached to bones enables voluntary movement. Muscle tissue in internal organs enables involuntary movement, such as the heartbeat.

2

Genes and Genetic Diseases

Stephanie Zettel, with originating chapter contributions by Lynn B. Jorde

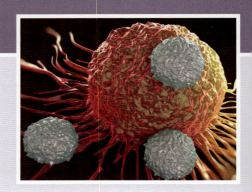

Additional resources are available online at http://evolve.elsevier.com/Canada/Huether/pathophysiology

CHAPTER OUTLINE

DNA, RNA, and Proteins: Heredity at the Molecular Level, 39
    Definitions, 39
    From Genes to Proteins, 40
Chromosomes, 41
    Chromosome Aberrations and Associated Diseases, 43
Elements of Formal Genetics, 49
    Phenotype and Genotype, 49
    Dominance and Recessiveness, 50

Transmission of Genetic Diseases, 50
    Autosomal Dominant Inheritance, 50
    Autosomal Recessive Inheritance, 53
    X-Linked Inheritance, 54
Linkage Analysis and Gene Mapping, 56
    Classic Pedigree Analysis, 56
    Complete Human Gene Map: Prospects and Benefits, 56
Multifactorial Inheritance, 58

LEARNING OBJECTIVES

1. Describe the structure and function of DNA, compared to RNA.
2. Discuss the processes of DNA mutation.
3. Define the processes of transcription, gene splicing, and translation.
4. Describe the differences between somatic cells, gametes, autosomes, and sex chromosomes.
5. Describe the normal karyotype.
6. Discuss the differences between euploid and aneuploid cells.
7. Identify the different mechanisms of mutation and discuss the effect of these mutations on survival.
8. Identify the major chromosomal abnormalities.
9. Differentiate between genotype and phenotype and give examples of each.
10. Differentiate between autosomal dominant, autosomal recessive, and X-linked recessive inheritance modes.
11. Discuss the concept of pedigrees and how they are useful.
12. Define the terms *penetrance* and *expressivity* and give examples of each.
13. Describe sex-limited and sex-linked traits and give an example of each.
14. Discuss the process and significance of gene mapping.
15. Discuss the concept of multifactorial inheritance.

KEY TERMS

Adenine, 39
Allele, 49
Amino acid, 39
Aneuploid cell, 43
Anticodon, 41
Autosome, 41
Barr body, 54
Base pair substitution, 40
Carrier, 50
Carrier detection test, 54
Chromosomal mosaic, 43
Chromosomal theory of inheritance, 50
Chromosome, 39
Chromosome band, 42
Chromosome breakage, 47
Clastogen, 47
Codominance, 50
Codon, 39
Complementary base pairing, 40
Consanguinity, 54
CpG islands, 52
Cri du chat syndrome, 47
Crossover, 56
Cytokinesis, 41
Cytosine, 39
Delayed age of onset, 51
Deletion, 47
Deoxyribonucleic acid (DNA), 39
Diploid cell, 41
DNA methylation, 52
DNA polymerase, 40
Dominant, 50
Dosage compensation, 54
Double-helix model, 39
Down syndrome, 43
Duplication, 47
Dystrophin, 55
Empirical risk, 59
Epigenetic, 52
Euploid cell, 43
Exon, 41
Expressivity, 52
Fragile site, 48
Frameshift mutation, 40
Gamete, 41
Gene, 39
Genomic imprinting, 52
Genotype, 49
Germline mosaicism, 51
Guanine, 39
Haploid cell, 41
Hemizygous, 54
Heterozygote, 50
Heterozygous, 49
Homologous, 41
Homozygote, 50
Homozygous, 49
Inbreeding, 54
Intron, 41
Inversion, 48
Karyotype (karyogram), 42
Klinefelter's syndrome, 46
Linkage, 56
Linkage analysis, 56
Locus, 49
Meiosis, 41
Messenger RNA (mRNA), 40
Metaphase spread, 41
Methylation, 52
Missense, 40
Mitosis, 41
Mode of inheritance, 50
Monosomy, 43
Multifactorial inheritance, 58
Mutagen, 40
Mutation, 40
Mutational hot spot, 40
Nondisjunction, 43
Nonsense, 40
Nucleotide, 39
Obligate carrier, 52

CHAPTER 2 Genes and Genetic Diseases

Partial trisomy, 43	Principle of segregation, 50	RNA polymerase, 40	Thymine, 39
Pedigree, 50	Proband, 50	Robertsonian translocation, 48	Transcription, 40
Penetrance, 51	Promoter site, 40	Sex-influenced trait, 56	Transfer RNA
Phenotype, 49	Purine, 39	Sex-limited trait, 56	(tRNA), 41
Polygenic trait, 58	Pyrimidine, 39	Sex linked (inheritance), 54	Translation, 41
Polymorphic (polymorphism), 49	Recessive, 50	Silent mutation, 40	Translocation, 48
Polypeptide, 39	Reciprocal translocation, 48	Somatic cell, 41	Triploidy, 43
Polyploid cell, 43	Recombination, 56	Spontaneous mutation, 40	Trisomy, 43
Position effect, 48	Recurrence risk, 51	Template, 40	Tumour-suppressor
Principle of independent assortment, 50	Ribonucleic acid (RNA), 40	Termination sequence, 41	gene, 52
	Ribosomal RNA (rRNA), 41	Tetraploidy, 43	Turner's syndrome, 46
	Ribosome, 41	Threshold of liability, 58	X inactivation, 54

Genetics is the study of biological inheritance; the cell nucleus is composed of chromatin and plays an integral role in ensuring that certain cellular traits are reproduced in daughter cells. Chromatin gives the nucleus a granular appearance in nondividing cells and, just before the cell divides, the chromatin condenses to form discrete, dark-staining organelles, which are called **chromosomes**. (Cell division is discussed in Chapter 1.) Gregor Mendel determined that chromosomes contained **genes**, the basic units of inheritance, by studying how traits are passed on from the parents to the progeny cells in pea plants. This understanding can also be applied to human cells (Figure 2.1).

The primary constituent of chromatin is **deoxyribonucleic acid (DNA)**. Genes are composed of sequences of DNA. By serving as the blueprints of proteins in the body, genes ultimately influence all aspects of body structure and function. Humans have approximately 20 000 protein-coding genes and an additional 9 000 to 10 000 genes that encode various types of RNA (see the following section) that are not translated into proteins. An error in one of these genes often leads to a recognizable genetic disease (e.g., hypertension, coronary artery disease, diabetes, and cancer).

Great progress is being made both in understanding the diagnosis of genetic diseases and their genetic mechanisms. This new understanding has paved the way for innovative "gene therapy", where normal genes can be used to correct genetic diseases.

DNA, RNA, AND PROTEINS: HEREDITY AT THE MOLECULAR LEVEL

> ✓ **QUICK CHECK 2.1**
> 1. What is the major composition of DNA?
> 2. Define the terms *mutation, autosomes,* and *sex chromosomes*.
> 3. What is the significance of mRNA?
> 4. What is the significance of chromosomal translocation?

Definitions
Composition and Structure of DNA
Genes are composed of DNA, which has three basic components: the five-carbon monosaccharide deoxyribose; a phosphate molecule; and four types of nitrogenous bases. Two of the bases, **cytosine** and **thymine**, are single carbon-nitrogen rings called **pyrimidines**. The other two bases, **adenine** and **guanine**, are double carbon-nitrogen rings called **purines**. The four bases are commonly represented by their first letters: A (adenine), C (cytosine), T (thymine), and G (guanine).

The **double-helix model** postulated by Watson and Crick proposes a structure for h DNA, where DNA appears like a twisted ladder with chemical bonds as its rungs (Figure 2.2). The two sides of the ladder consist of deoxyribose and phosphate molecules, which are united by strong phosphodiester bonds. Nitrogenous bases extend from each side of the ladder and are joined by a weak hydrogen bond to form the rungs of the ladder; adenine pairs with thymine, and guanine pairs with cytosine. Each DNA subunit—consisting of one deoxyribose molecule, one phosphate group, and one base—is called a **nucleotide**.

DNA as the Genetic Code
DNA directs the synthesis of all the body's proteins. Proteins are composed of one or more **polypeptides** (intermediate protein compounds), which in turn, consist of sequences of **amino acids**. The body contains 20 different types of amino acids and each is determined by a certain sequence of 3 nitrogenous bases that is known as a **codon**. Because there are 64 (4×4×4) possible codons but only 20 amino acids, there are many cases in which several codons can code for the same amino acid. DNA is in all living organisms and uses the same codes to make protein. Mitochondria, however, have their own DNA and code for different proteins that are involved with cellular respiration and metabolism.

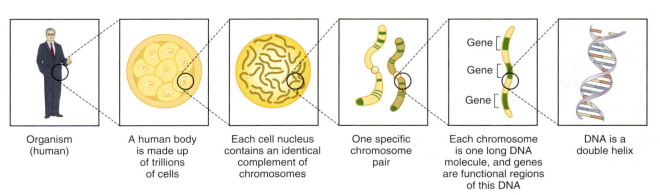

Organism (human) — A human body is made up of trillions of cells — Each cell nucleus contains an identical complement of chromosomes — One specific chromosome pair — Each chromosome is one long DNA molecule, and genes are functional regions of this DNA — DNA is a double helix

FIGURE 2.1 Successive Enlargements from a Human to the Genetic Material.

key to accurate replication. The unpaired base attracts a free nucleotide only if the nucleotide has the proper complementary base. When replication is complete, a new double-stranded molecule identical to the original is formed. The single strand is said to be a **template**, or molecule on which a complementary molecule is built.

Several different proteins are involved in DNA replication. The most important of these proteins is an enzyme known as **DNA polymerase**. This enzyme travels along the single DNA strand, adding the correct nucleotides to the free end of the new strand and checking to ensure that its base is actually complementary to the template base. This mechanism of DNA proofreading substantially enhances the accuracy of DNA replication.

Mutation

A **mutation** is any inherited alteration of genetic material. One type of mutation is the **base pair substitution**, in which one base pair replaces another. This replacement *can* result in a change in the amino acid sequence. However, because of the redundancy of the genetic code, many of these mutations do not change the amino acid sequence. Such mutations are called **silent mutations** and have no effect on the final product. Base pair substitutions altering amino acids consist of two basic types: **missense** mutations, which produce a change in a single amino acid; and **nonsense** mutations, which produce one of the three stop codons (UAA, UAG, or UGA) in the messenger RNA (mRNA) (Figure 2.4). Missense mutations (Figure 2.4A) produce a single amino acid change, whereas nonsense mutations (Figure 2.4B) produce a premature stop codon in the mRNA and terminate translation of the polypeptide.

The **frameshift mutation** involves the insertion or deletion of one or more base pairs of the DNA molecule. As Figure 2.5 shows, these mutations change the entire "reading frame" of the DNA sequence because the deletion or insertion is not a multiple of three base pairs (the number of base pairs in a codon). Consequently, frameshift mutations can greatly alter the amino acid sequence. When multiples of 3 bases are inserted or deleted, these mutations are *in frame* and result in less severe disease consequences than frameshift mutations.

Agents known as **mutagens** increase the frequency of mutations by directly altering DNA. Examples include radiation and chemicals such as nitrogen mustard, vinyl chloride, alkylating agents, formaldehyde, and sodium nitrite.

Mutations are rare events. The rate of **spontaneous mutations** (those occurring in the absence of exposure to known mutagens) in humans is about 1.1×10^{-8} per gene per generation,[1] but varies from one gene to another. Some DNA sequences have particularly high mutation rates and are known as **mutational hot spots** (Box 2.1).[2]

From Genes to Proteins

DNA is formed and replicated in the cell nucleus, but protein synthesis takes place in the cytoplasm. The DNA code is transported from the nucleus to the cytoplasm, and subsequent protein is formed through the processes of transcription and translation, which are mediated by **ribonucleic acid (RNA)**. RNA is chemically similar to DNA with a few notable differences: the sugar molecule is ribose rather than deoxyribose; uracil, though similar in structure and still able to bind with adenine, replaces thymine as one of the four nitrogenous bases; and RNA exists as a single strand.

Transcription

Transcription involves the synthesis of **messenger RNA (mRNA)** from a DNA template. The process begins when **RNA polymerase** binds to a **promoter site**, a sequence of DNA that specifies the beginning of a gene. RNA polymerase then separates a portion of the DNA,

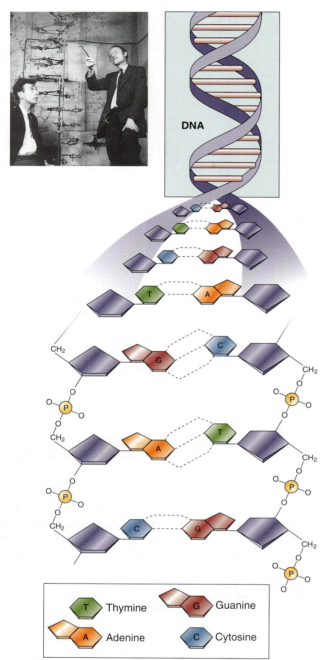

FIGURE 2.2 Watson–Crick Model of the DNA Molecule. The DNA structure illustrated here is based on that published by James Watson *(photograph, left)* and Francis Crick *(photograph, right)* in 1953. Note that each side of the DNA molecule consists of alternating sugar and phosphate groups. Each sugar group is bonded to the opposing sugar group by a pair of nitrogenous bases (adenine-thymine or cytosine-guanine). The sequence of these pairs constitutes a genetic code that determines the structure and function of a cell. (Illustration from Herlihy, B. [2015]. *The human body in health and illness* [5th ed.]. Saunders. Photo from Barrington Brown/Science Source.)

Replication of DNA

DNA replication consists of breaking the weak hydrogen bonds between the bases, leaving a single strand with an unpaired base (Figure 2.3). The consistent pairing of adenine with thymine and of guanine with cytosine, known as **complementary base pairing**, is the

CHAPTER 2 Genes and Genetic Diseases

exposing unattached DNA bases. One DNA strand then provides the template for the sequence of mRNA nucleotides, and the sequence of bases in the mRNA is complementary to the template strand (with the exception of uracil instead of thymine). The mRNA sequence is identical to that of the other DNA strand. Transcription continues until the RNA polymerase reaches a **termination sequence** which consists of codons that signal the end of transcription. At this point, the RNA polymerase detaches from the DNA, and the transcribed mRNA moves out of the nucleus and into the cytoplasm (Figures 2.6 and 2.7).

Gene Splicing

In eukaryotes, many RNA sequences are removed by nuclear enzymes, and the remaining sequences are spliced together to form the functional mRNA that migrates to the cytoplasm. The excised sequences are called **introns** (intervening sequences), and the sequences that are left to code for proteins are called **exons**.

Translation

In **translation**, mRNA directs the synthesis of a polypeptide (see Figure 2.7), interacting with **transfer RNA (tRNA)**, a cloverleaf-shaped strand of about 80 nucleotides. The tRNA molecule has a site on the cloverleaf "stem" where an amino acid attaches. A site at the opposite end of the centre "leaflet" attracts a three-nucleotide sequence called the **anticodon**. This complementary base pairing specifies the sequence of amino acids through tRNA.

The site of actual protein synthesis is in the **ribosome**, which consists of approximately equal parts of protein and **ribosomal RNA (rRNA)**. During translation, the ribosome initiates translation of the mRNA by binding both tRNA and mRNA to enable base pairing between tRNA and mRNA. The ribosome then moves along the mRNA sequence, processing each codon and translating an amino acid by way of this interaction of mRNA and tRNA.

The ribosome also provides an enzyme that catalyzes the formation of covalent peptide bonds between the adjacent amino acids, resulting in a growing polypeptide. When the ribosome arrives at a termination signal on the mRNA sequence, translation and polypeptide formation stop; the mRNA, ribosome, and polypeptide separate from one another; and the polypeptide is released into the cytoplasm to perform its required function.

CHROMOSOMES

Human cells can be categorized into **gametes** (sperm and egg cells) and **somatic cells**, which include all cells other than gametes. Each somatic cell nucleus has 46 chromosomes in 23 pairs (Figure 2.8). These are **diploid cells** because the individual's father and mother each donate one chromosome per pair. New somatic cells are formed through **mitosis** and **cytokinesis**. Gametes are **haploid cells** because they have only 1 member of each chromosome pair, for a total of 23 chromosomes. Haploid cells are formed from diploid cells by **meiosis** (Figure 2.9).

In 22 of the 23 chromosome pairs, the 2 members of each pair are virtually identical in microscopic appearance and are **homologous** (Figure 2.10B). These 22 chromosome pairs are homologous in both males and females and are termed **autosomes**. The remaining pair of chromosomes, the sex chromosomes, consists of two homologous X chromosomes in females and a nonhomologous pair, X and Y, in males.

Figure 2.10A illustrates a **metaphase spread**, which is a photograph of the chromosomes as they appear in the nucleus of a somatic cell during metaphase. (Chromosomes are easiest to visualize during

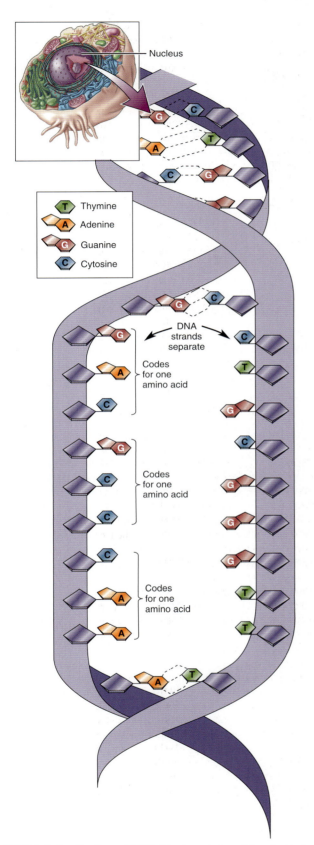

FIGURE 2.3 Replication of DNA. The two chains of the double helix separate and each chain serves as the template for a new complementary chain. (From Herlihy, B. [2015]. *The human body in health and illness* [5th ed.]. Saunders.)

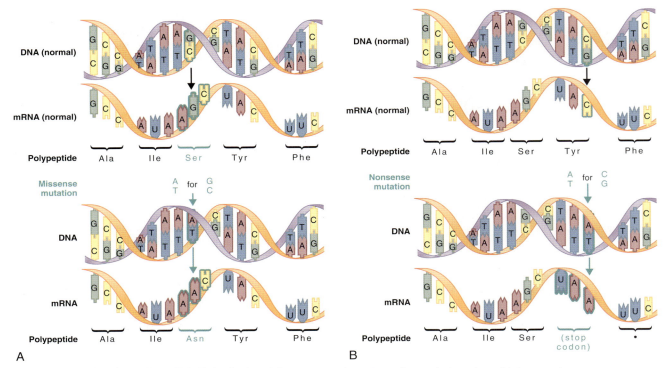

FIGURE 2.4 Base Pair Substitution. Missense mutations, **A**, produce a single amino acid change, whereas nonsense mutations, **B**, produce a stop codon in the messenger RNA *(mRNA)*. Stop codons terminate translation of the polypeptide. *Ala*, Alanine; *Asn*, asparagine; *Ile*, isoleucine; *Phe*, phenylalanine; *Ser*, serine; *Tyr*, tyrosine. (From Roach, J. C., Glusman, G., Smit, A. F., et al. [2010]. Analysis of genetic inheritance in a family quartet by whole-genome sequencing. *Science, 328*[5978], 636–639. doi:10.1126/science.1186802.)

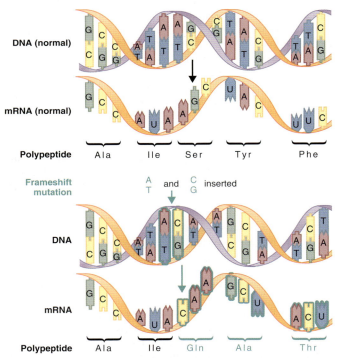

FIGURE 2.5 Frameshift Mutations. Frameshift mutations result from the addition or deletion of a number of bases that is not a multiple of 3. This mutation alters all of the codons downstream from the site of insertion or deletion. *Ala*, Alanine; *Asn*, asparagine; *Gln*, glutamine; *Ile*, isoleucine; *mRNA*, messenger RNA; *Phe*, phenylalanine; *Ser*, serine; *Tyr*, tyrosine. (From Jorde, L. B., Carey, J. C., & Bamshad, M. J. [2010]. *Medical genetics* [4th ed.]. Mosby.)

BOX 2.1 Mutational Hot Spots and Antibiotic Resistance

Zhang and colleagues investigated mechanisms of antibiotic resistance (clofazimine [Lamprene]) in *Mycobacterium tuberculosis* and discovered two nucleotide sequences that accounted for more than 50% of the mutations resulting in resistance to clofazimine. The authors also discovered two new genes responsible for resistant organisms and suggested that this research will assist in more rapidly identifying those who are resistant to this antibiotic and enable the discovery of more effective treatments.

From Zhang, S., Chen, J., Cui, P., et al. (2015). *Journal of Antimicrobial Chemotherapy, 70*(9), 2507–2510. doi:10.1093/jac/dkv150.

---

this stage of mitosis.) In Figure 2.10A, the chromosomes are arranged according to size, with the homologous chromosomes in their pairs. The 22 autosomes are numbered according to length, with chromosome 1 being the longest and chromosome 22 the shortest. A karyotype, or karyogram, is an ordered display of chromosomes. Chromosomal length varies from person to person, so it is not always possible to distinguish each chromosome by its length. The position of the centromere (region of DNA responsible for movement of the replicated chromosomes into the two daughter cells during mitosis and meiosis) also is used to classify chromosomes (see Figures 2.10B and 2.11).

The chromosomes in Figure 2.10 were stained with Giemsa stain, resulting in distinctive chromosome bands. These bands form various patterns in different chromosomes that distinguish each from the others. Such banding techniques allow for the numbering of chromosomes and the study of individual variations. Missing or duplicated portions of chromosomes can result in serious diseases and are also readily

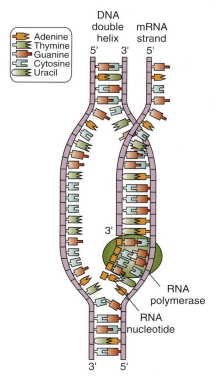

FIGURE 2.6 General Scheme of RNA Transcription. In transcription of messenger RNA *(mRNA)*, a DNA molecule "unzips" in the region of the gene to be transcribed. RNA nucleotides already present in the nucleus temporarily attach themselves to exposed DNA bases along one strand of the unzipped DNA molecule according to the principle of complementary pairing. As the RNA nucleotides attach to the exposed DNA, they bind to each other and form a chainlike RNA strand called an *mRNA molecule*. Notice that the new mRNA strand is an exact copy of the base sequence on the opposite side of the DNA molecule. As in all metabolic processes, the formation of mRNA is controlled by an enzyme—in this case, the enzyme is called *RNA polymerase*. (From Ignatavicius, D. D., & Workman, L. D. [2010]. *Medical-surgical nursing* [6th ed.]. Saunders.)

identified. Moreover, to facilitate the identification and diagnosis of chromosomal traits, each chromosome can be given its own colour.

Chromosome Aberrations and Associated Diseases

Chromosome abnormalities are the leading known cause of intellectual disability and miscarriage, with chromosome aberrations occurring in at least 1 in 12 conceptions. Most of these fetuses do not survive to term, and about 50% of all recovered aborted fetuses from the first trimester have major chromosome aberrations.[3] Chromosomal abnormalities are present in about 1 in 150 live births.

Polyploidy

Cells with a multiple of the normal number of chromosomes are **euploid cells** (Greek *eu*=good or true). When a euploid cell has more than the diploid number of chromosomes, it is said to be a **polyploid cell**. Several types of body tissues, including some liver, bronchial, and epithelial tissues, are normally polyploid. A zygote that has three copies of each chromosome, rather than the usual two, has a form of polyploidy called **triploidy**. Nearly all triploid fetuses are spontaneously aborted or stillborn. The prevalence of triploidy among live births is approximately 1 in 10 000. **Tetraploidy**, a condition in which euploid cells have 92 chromosomes, has been found primarily in early aborted fetuses, although some affected infants have been born alive. Triploidy and tetraploidy are relatively common conditions, accounting for approximately 10% of all known miscarriages, and fetuses generally do not survive to term.[4]

Aneuploidy

A cell that does not contain a multiple of 23 chromosomes is an **aneuploid cell**. A cell containing three copies of one chromosome is said to be trisomic (a condition termed **trisomy**) and is aneuploid. **Monosomy**, the presence of only one copy of a given chromosome in a diploid cell, is the other common form of aneuploidy. Among the autosomes, monosomy of any chromosome is lethal, but newborns with trisomy of chromosomes 13, 18, 21, or X can survive. *Loss of chromosome material generally has more serious consequences than duplication of chromosome material.*

Sex chromosomes are often aneuploid with less serious consequences than those of autosomes. This is because very little genetic material—only about 40 genes—is located on the Y chromosome. Similarly, inactivation of extra X chromosomes largely diminishes their effect. A zygote bearing *no* X chromosome, however, will not survive.

Aneuploidy is usually the result of **nondisjunction**, an error in which homologous chromosomes or sister chromatids fail to separate normally during meiosis or mitosis (Figure 2.12). Nondisjunction produces some gametes that have two copies of a given chromosome and others that have no copies of the chromosome. When such gametes unite with normal haploid gametes, the resulting zygote is monosomic or trisomic for that chromosome. Occasionally, a cell can be monosomic or trisomic for more than one chromosome.

Autosomal aneuploidy. Trisomy can occur for any chromosome, but fetuses with trisomies of chromosomes (other than 13, 18, 21, or X) do not survive to term. Trisomy 16, for example, is the most common trisomy among aborted fetuses, but it is not seen in live births.[5]

Partial trisomy, in which only an extra portion of a chromosome is present in each cell, can also occur. Trisomies may occur in only some cells of the body, and individuals who are affected are **chromosomal mosaics**, meaning that the body has two or more different cell lines, each of which has a different karyotype. Mosaics are often formed by early mitotic nondisjunction occurring in one embryonic cell but not in others.

The best-known example of aneuploidy in an autosome is trisomy of chromosome 21, which causes **Down syndrome** (named after J. Langdon Down, who first described the syndrome in 1866). Down syndrome is seen in approximately 1 in 800 live births (from https://cdss.ca/resources/general-information); its principal features are shown and outlined in Figure 2.13 and Table 2.1.

The risk of having a child with Down syndrome increases greatly with maternal age. As Figure 2.14 demonstrates, women younger than 30 years have a risk ranging from about 1 in 1 000 births to 1 in 2 000 births. The risk begins to rise substantially after 35 years of age and reaches 3 to 5% for women older than 45 years. This dramatic increase in risk is caused by the age of maternal egg cells, which are held in an arrested state of prophase I from the time they are formed in the female embryo until they are shed in ovulation: an egg cell formed by a 45-year-old woman is essentially 45 years old. This long, suspended state may allow defects to accumulate in the cellular proteins responsible for meiosis and nondisjunction of the chromosome. Therefore, the risk of Down syndrome increases with maternal age.[6]

Sex chromosome aneuploidy. Among live births, about 1 in 500 males and 1 in 900 females have a form of sex chromosome aneuploidy.[7]

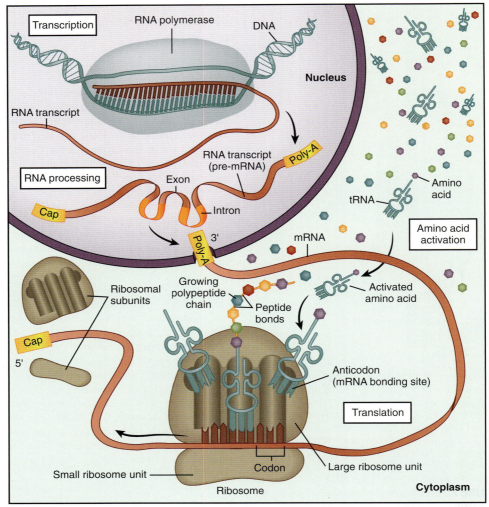

FIGURE 2.7 Protein Synthesis. The site of transcription is the nucleus and the site of translation is the cytoplasm. See the text for details. *mRNA*, Messenger RNA; *tRNA*, transfer RNA.

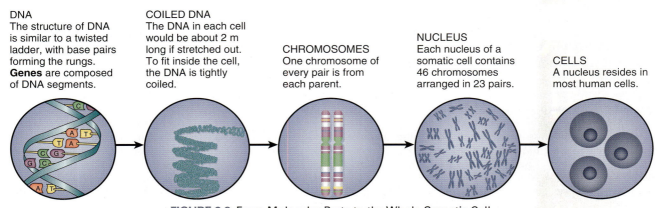

FIGURE 2.8 From Molecular Parts to the Whole Somatic Cell.

One of the most common sex chromosome aneuploidies, affecting about 1 in 1000 newborn females, is trisomy X. Instead of two X chromosomes, these females have three X chromosomes in each cell. Most of these females have no overt physical abnormalities, although sterility, menstrual irregularity, or intellectual disability is sometimes seen. Some females have four X chromosomes, and they are more often intellectually disabled. Those with five or more X chromosomes generally are more severely intellectually disabled and have various physical defects.

A condition that leads to somewhat more serious problems is the presence of a single X chromosome and no homologous X or Y chromosome, and the individual has a total of 45 chromosomes.

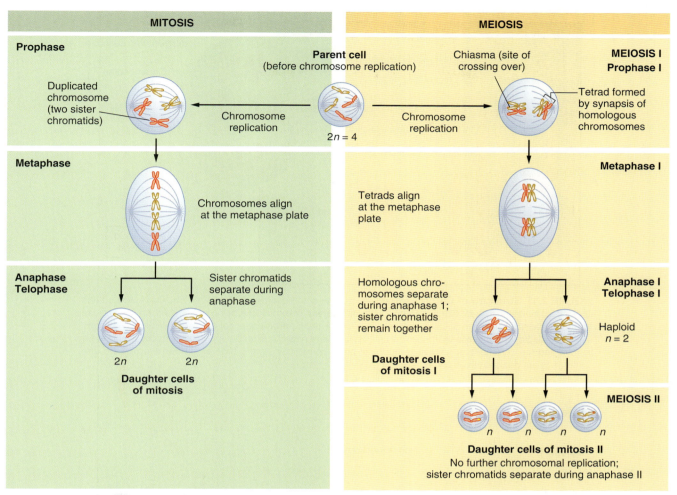

FIGURE 2.9 Phases of Meiosis and Comparison to Mitosis. (From Jorde, L. B., Carey, J. C., & Bamshad, M. J. [2010]. *Medical genetics* [4th ed.]. Mosby.)

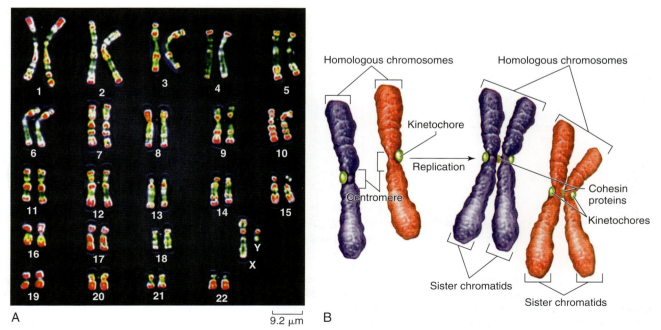

FIGURE 2.10 Karyotype of Chromosomes. A, Human karyotype. B, Homologous chromosomes and sister chromatids. (From Raven, P. H., Johnson, G., Mason, K., et al. [2008]. *Biology* [8th ed.]. McGraw-Hill.)

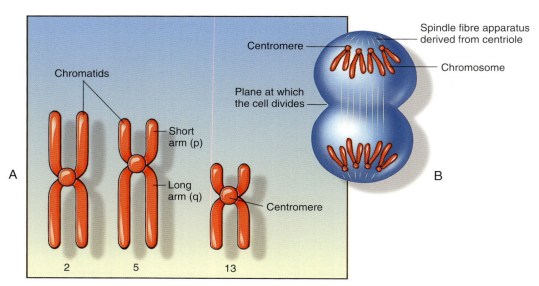

FIGURE 2.11 Structure of Chromosomes. A, Human chromosomes 2, 5, and 13. Each is replicated and consists of two chromatids. Chromosome 2 is a metacentric chromosome because the centromere is close to the middle; chromosome 5 is submetacentric because the centromere is set off from the middle; chromosome 13 is acrocentric because the centromere is at or very near the end. **B,** During mitosis, the centromere divides and the chromosomes move to opposite poles of the cell. At the time of centromere division, the chromatids are designated as chromosomes.

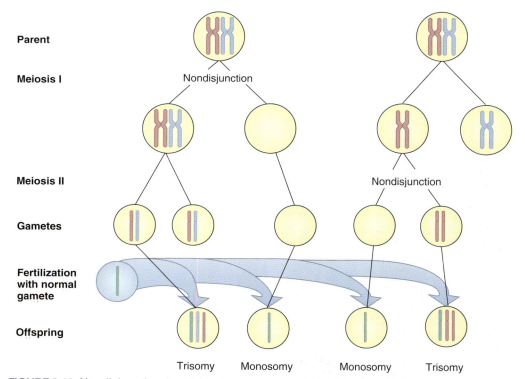

FIGURE 2.12 Nondisjunction. Nondisjunction causes aneuploidy when chromosomes or sister chromatids fail to divide properly. (From Jorde, L. B., Carey, J. C., & Bamshad, M. J. [2010]. *Medical genetics* [4th ed.]. Mosby.)

The karyotype is usually designated as 45,X and results in a set of symptoms known as **Turner's syndrome** (Figure 2.15; see Table 2.1). Individuals with at least two X chromosomes and one Y chromosome in each cell (47,XXY karyotype) have **Klinefelter's syndrome** (Figure 2.16; see Table 2.1).

Abnormalities of Chromosome Structure

In addition to the loss or gain of whole chromosomes, parts of chromosomes can be lost or duplicated as gametes are formed, and the arrangement of genes on chromosomes can change. Unlike aneuploidy and polyploidy, these changes sometimes have no serious consequences for an individual's health. Some of them can even remain entirely unnoticed, especially when very small pieces of chromosomes are involved. Nevertheless, abnormalities of chromosome structure can also produce serious disease in individuals or their offspring.

During meiosis and mitosis, chromosomes usually maintain their structural integrity, but **chromosome breakage** occasionally occurs. Mechanisms exist to "heal" these breaks and usually repair them perfectly with no damage to the daughter cell. However, some breaks remain or heal in a way that alters the chromosome's structure. The risk of chromosome breakage increases with exposure to harmful agents called **clastogens** (e.g., ionizing radiation, viral infections, and some types of chemicals).

Deletions. Broken chromosomes and lost DNA cause **deletions** (Figure 2.17). Usually, a gamete with a deletion unites with a normal gamete to form a zygote. The zygote thus has one chromosome with the normal complement of genes and one with some missing genes. Serious consequences can result with this loss, even though one normal chromosome is present. One common example is **cri du chat syndrome**. The term literally means "cry of the cat" and describes the characteristic cry of the affected child. Other symptoms include low birth weight, severe intellectual disability, microcephaly (smaller than normal head size), and heart defects. This disease is caused by a deletion of part of the short arm of chromosome 5.

Duplications. A deficiency of genetic material is more harmful than an excess, so **duplications** usually have less serious consequences

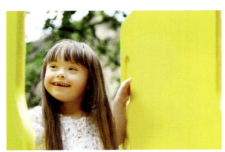

FIGURE 2.13 Child With Down Syndrome. (iStockphoto/DenKuvaiev)

TABLE 2.1	Characteristics of Various Chromosome Disorders
Disease/Disorder	**Features**
Down Syndrome	
Trisomy of Chromosome 21	
IQ	It usually ranges from 20 to 70 (intellectual disability).
Male/female findings	Virtually all males are sterile; some females can reproduce.
Face	Distinctive features include low nasal bridge, epicanthal folds, protruding tongue, low-set ears.
Musculoskeletal system	Features include poor muscle tone (hypotonia) and short stature.
Systemic disorders	Features include congenital heart disease (one third to one half of cases), reduced ability to fight respiratory tract infections, and increased susceptibility to leukemia—overall reduced survival rate; by age 40 years usually develop symptoms similar to those of Alzheimer's disease.
Mortality	About 75% of fetuses with Down syndrome abort spontaneously or are stillborn; 20% of infants die before age 10 years; those who live beyond 10 years have life expectancy of about 60 years.
Causative factors	97% of cases are caused by nondisjunction during formation of one parent's gametes or during early embryonic development; 3% result from translocations; in 95% of cases, nondisjunction occurs when mother's egg cell is formed; the remainder involve paternal nondisjunction; 1% are mosaics—these have a large number of normal cells, and effects of trisomic cells are attenuated and symptoms are generally less severe.
Turner's Syndrome	
(45,X) Monosomy of X Chromosome	
IQ	Individuals with this syndrome are not considered to be intellectually disabled, although the syndrome is associated with some impairment of spatial and mathematical reasoning ability.
Male/female findings	It is found only in females.
Musculoskeletal system	Short stature is common; other features are characteristic webbing of neck, widely spaced nipples, and reduced carrying angle at elbow.
Systemic disorders	Features include coarctation (narrowing) of aorta, edema of feet in newborns; females are usually sterile and have gonadal streaks rather than ovaries; streaks are sometimes susceptible to cancer.
Mortality	About 15–20% of spontaneous abortions with chromosome abnormalities have this karyotype, most common single-chromosome aberration; highly lethal during gestation, only about 0.5% of these conceptions survive to term.
Causative factors	75% of cases inherit X chromosome from mother, thus caused by meiotic error in father; frequency is low compared with other sex chromosome aneuploidies (1:5000 newborn females); 50% have simple monosomy of X chromosome; the remainder have more complex abnormalities; combinations of 45,X cells with XX or XY cells common.
Klinefelter's Syndrome	
(47,XXY) XXY Condition	
IQ	A moderate degree of mental impairment may be present.
Male/female findings	Individuals have a male appearance but are usually sterile; 50% develop female-like breasts (gynecomastia); occurs in 1:1000 male births.
Voice	Voice is somewhat high pitched.
Systemic disorders	Features include sparse body hair, sterility, and small testicles.
Causative factors	50% of cases are the result of nondisjunction of X chromosomes in mother, and frequency rises with increasing maternal age; also involves XXY and XXXY karyotypes with degree of physical and mental impairment increasing with each added X chromosome; mosaicism fairly common with most prevalent combination of XXY and XY cells.

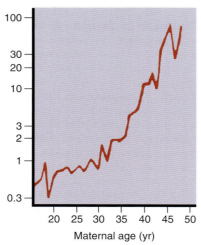

FIGURE 2.14 Down Syndrome Increases With Maternal Age. Rate is per 1 000 live births related to maternal age.

than deletions. For example, a deletion of a region of chromosome 5 causes cri du chat syndrome, but a duplication of the same region causes intellectual disability with less serious physical defects.

Inversions. An **inversion** occurs when two breaks take place on a chromosome, followed by the reinsertion of the missing fragment at its original site but in inverted order. Therefore, a chromosome symbolized as ABCDEFG might become ABEDCFG after an inversion.

Unlike deletions and duplications, no loss or gain of genetic material occurs. Inversions are "balanced" alterations of chromosome structure, and they often have no apparent physical effect. Some genes, however, are influenced by neighbouring genes and this **position effect** can change a gene's expression, sometimes resulting in physical defects. Inversions can also cause serious problems in the offspring of individuals carrying the inversion because the inversion can lead to duplications and deletions in the chromosomes as it is transmitted to the offspring.

Translocations. The interchange of genetic material between nonhomologous chromosomes is called **translocation**. A **reciprocal translocation** occurs when breaks take place in two different chromosomes and the material is exchanged (Figure 2.18A). As with inversions, the carrier of a reciprocal translocation is usually normal, but their offspring can have duplications and deletions.

A second and clinically more important type of translocation is **Robertsonian translocation**. In this disorder, the long arms of two nonhomologous chromosomes fuse at the centromere, forming a single chromosome. Robertsonian translocations are confined to chromosomes 13, 14, 15, 21, and 22 because the short arms of these chromosomes are very small and contain no essential genetic material. The short arms are usually lost during subsequent cell divisions. Because the carriers of Robertsonian translocations lose no important genetic material, they are unaffected, although they have only 45 chromosomes in each cell. Their offspring, however, may have serious monosomies or trisomies. For example, a common Robertsonian translocation involves the fusion of the long arms of chromosomes 21 and 14. An offspring who inherits a gamete carrying the fused chromosome can receive an extra copy of the long arm of chromosome 21 and develop Down syndrome. Robertsonian translocations are responsible for approximately 3% to 5% of Down syndrome cases. Parents who carry a Robertsonian translocation involving chromosome 21 have an increased risk of producing multiple offspring with Down syndrome.

Fragile sites. **Fragile sites** are chromosomal regions that are susceptible to gaps or breaks that often occur during the stress of

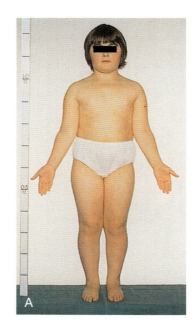

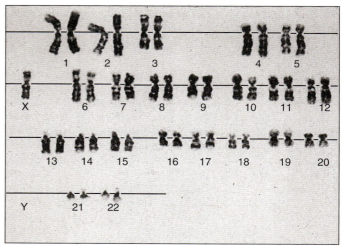

FIGURE 2.15 Turner's Syndrome. A, A sex chromosome is missing, and the person's chromosomes are 45,X. Characteristic signs are short stature, female genitalia, webbed neck, shieldlike chest with underdeveloped breasts and widely spaced nipples, and imperfectly developed ovaries. **B,** As this karyotype shows, Turner's syndrome results from monosomy of sex chromosomes (genotype XO). (From Patton, K. T., & Thibodeau, G. A. [2013]. *Anatomy & physiology* [8th ed.]. Mosby. Courtesy Nancy S. Wexler, PhD., Columbia University.)

replication. Although most of these fragile sites do not appear to be related to disease, these sites are often rearranged in disorders such as cancer. One fragile site, located on the long arm of the X chromosome, is associated with *fragile X syndrome*. The most important feature of this syndrome is intellectual disability. With a relatively high population prevalence (affecting approximately 1 in 4 000 males and 1 in 8 000 females), fragile X syndrome is the second most common genetic cause of intellectual disability (after Down syndrome).

In fragile X syndrome, females who inherit the mutation do not necessarily express the disease condition, but they can pass it on to descendants who do express it. Ordinarily, a male who inherits a

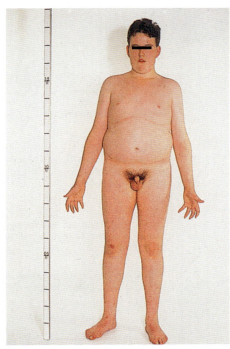

FIGURE 2.16 Klinefelter's Syndrome. This young man exhibits many characteristics of Klinefelter's syndrome: small testes, some development of the breasts, sparse body hair, and long limbs. This syndrome results from the presence of two or more X chromosomes with one Y chromosome (e.g., genotypes XXY or XXXY). (From Patton, K. T. [2019]. *Anatomy & physiology* [10th ed.]. Elsevier. Courtesy Nancy S. Wexler, PhD., Columbia University.)

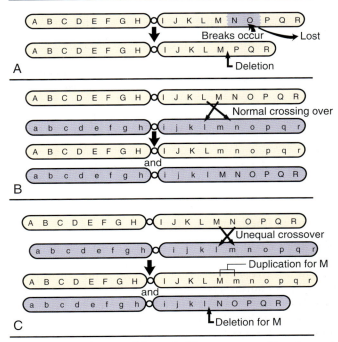

FIGURE 2.17 Abnormalities of Chromosome Structure. A, Deletion occurs when a chromosome segment is lost. **B,** Normal crossing over. **C,** The generation of duplication and deletion through unequal crossing over.

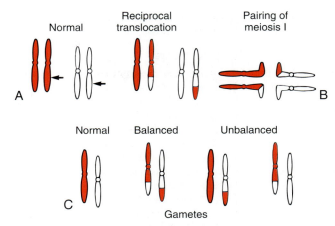

FIGURE 2.18 Normal and Abnormal Chromosome Translocation. A, Normal chromosomes and reciprocal translocation. **B,** Pairing at meiosis I. **C,** Consequences of translocation in gametes; unbalanced gametes result in zygotes that are partially trisomic and partially monosomic and consequently develop abnormally.

disease gene on the X chromosome expresses the condition because he has only one X chromosome. About one third of carrier females are affected, although less severely than males. Interestingly, unaffected males with the defect have been shown to have more than about 50 repeated DNA sequences near the beginning of the fragile X gene. These repeating CGG trinucleotide sequences cause fragile X syndrome when the number of copies exceeds 200,[8] and the number of these repeats can increase from generation to generation. More than 20 other genetic diseases, including Huntington's disease and myotonic dystrophy, also are caused by this mechanism.[9]

ELEMENTS OF FORMAL GENETICS

Traits caused by single genes are called *Mendelian traits* (after Gregor Mendel). Each gene occupies a position, or **locus**, on a chromosome. The genes at a particular locus can have different forms (i.e., they can be composed of different nucleotide sequences) called **alleles**. A locus that has two or more alleles that each occur with an appreciable frequency in a population is said to be **polymorphic** (or a **polymorphism**).

Because humans are diploid organisms, each chromosome is represented twice, with one member of the chromosome pair contributed by the father and one by the mother. At a given locus, an individual has one allele whose origin is paternal and one whose origin is maternal. When the two alleles are identical, the individual is **homozygous** at that locus. When the alleles are not identical, the individual is **heterozygous** at that locus.

Phenotype and Genotype

The composition of genes at a given locus is known as the **genotype**. The outward appearance of an individual, which is the result of both genotype and environment, is the **phenotype**. For example, an infant who is born with an inability to metabolize the amino acid phenylalanine has the single-gene disorder known as phenylketonuria (PKU) and thus has the PKU genotype. If the condition is left untreated, abnormal metabolites of phenylalanine will begin to accumulate in the infant's brain, and irreversible intellectual disability will occur. Intellectual disability is one aspect of the PKU phenotype. By imposing dietary restrictions to exclude food that contains phenylalanine, however, intellectual disability can be prevented. Foods high in phenylalanine include proteins found in milk, dairy products, meat, fish, chicken, eggs, beans, and nuts. Although the child still has the PKU genotype, a modification of the environment (in this case, the child's diet) produces an outwardly normal phenotype.

Dominance and Recessiveness

In many loci, the effects of one allele mask those of another when the two are found together in a **heterozygote**. The allele whose effects are observable is said to be **dominant**. The allele whose effects are hidden is said to be **recessive** (from the Latin root for "hiding"). Traditionally, for loci having two alleles, the dominant allele is denoted by an uppercase letter and the recessive allele is denoted by a lowercase letter. When one allele is dominant over another, the heterozygote genotype *Aa* has the same phenotype as the dominant homozygote *AA*. For the recessive allele to be expressed, the genotype must exist in the **homozygote** form, *aa*. When the heterozygote is distinguishable from both homozygotes, the locus is said to exhibit **codominance**.

A **carrier** is an individual who has a disease gene but is phenotypically normal. Many genes for a recessive disease occur in heterozygotes who carry one copy of the gene but do not express the disease. When recessive genes are lethal in the homozygous state, they are eliminated from the population when they occur in homozygotes. By "hiding" in carriers, however, recessive genes for diseases are passed on to the next generation.

TRANSMISSION OF GENETIC DISEASES

> ✓ **QUICK CHECK 2.2**
> 1. Why is the influence of environment significant to phenotype?
> 2. Describe the differences between a dominant and a recessive allele.
> 3. Why are the concepts of variable expressivity, incomplete penetrance, and delayed age of onset so important in relation to genetic diseases?
> 4. What is the recurrence risk for autosomal dominant inheritance and recessive inheritance?

The pattern in which a genetic disease is inherited through generations is termed the **mode of inheritance**. Knowing the mode of inheritance can reveal much about the disease-causing gene itself and allow for more reliable genetic counselling.

Mendel systematically studied modes of inheritance and formulated two basic laws of inheritance. His **principle of segregation** states that homologous genes separate from one another during reproduction and that each reproductive cell carries only one copy of a homologous gene. Mendel's second law, the **principle of independent assortment**, states that the hereditary transmission of one gene does not affect the transmission of another. Mendel discovered these laws in the mid-nineteenth century by performing breeding experiments with garden peas, even though he had no knowledge of chromosomes. Early twentieth-century geneticists found that chromosomal behaviour essentially corresponds to Mendel's laws, which now form the basis for the **chromosomal theory of inheritance**.

The known single-gene diseases can be classified into four major modes of inheritance: autosomal dominant, autosomal recessive, X-linked dominant, and X-linked recessive. The first two types involve genes known to occur on the 22 pairs of autosomes. The last two types occur on the X chromosome. Very few disease-causing genes occur on the Y chromosome.

The **pedigree** chart summarizes family relationships and shows which members of a family are affected by a genetic disease (Figure 2.19). Generally, the pedigree begins with one individual in the family, the **proband**. This individual is usually the first person in the family diagnosed or seen in a clinic.

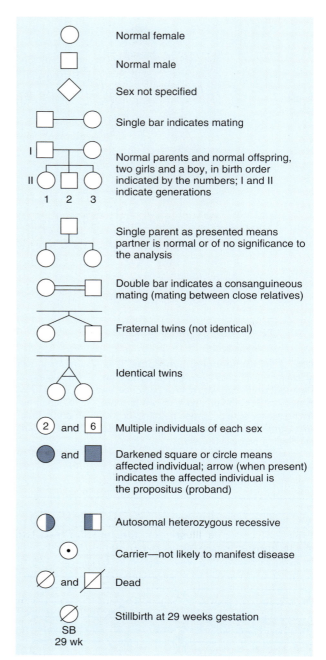

FIGURE 2.19 Symbols Commonly Used in Pedigrees. (From Jorde, L. B., Carey, J. C., & Bamshad, M. J. [2010]. *Medical genetics* [4th ed.]. Mosby.)

Autosomal Dominant Inheritance
Characteristics of Pedigrees

Diseases caused by autosomal dominant genes are rare, with the most common occurring in fewer than 1 in 500 individuals. Therefore, it is uncommon for two individuals who are both affected by the same autosomal dominant disease to produce offspring together. Figure 2.20A illustrates this unusual pattern. Affected offspring are usually produced by the union of a normal parent with an affected heterozygous parent. The Punnett square in Figure 2.20B illustrates this mating. The affected parent can pass either a disease-causing allele or a normal allele to the next generation. On average, half the children will be heterozygous and will express the disease, and half will be normal.

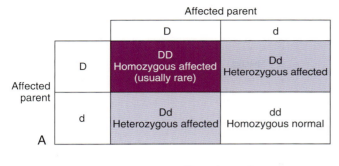

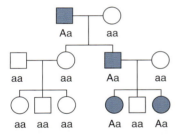

FIGURE 2.20 Punnett Square and Autosomal Dominant Traits. **A,** Punnett square for the mating of two individuals with an autosomal dominant gene. Here both parents are affected by the trait. **B,** Punnett square for the mating of a normal individual with a carrier for an autosomal dominant gene.

FIGURE 2.21 Pedigree Illustrating the Inheritance Pattern of Postaxial Polydactyly, an Autosomal Dominant Disorder. Affected individuals are represented by shading. (From Jorde, L. B., Carey, J. C., & Bamshad, M. J. [2010]. *Medical genetics* [4th ed.]. Mosby.)

The pedigree in Figure 2.21 shows the transmission of an autosomal dominant allele. Several important characteristics of this pedigree support the conclusion that the trait is caused by an autosomal dominant gene:
- The two sexes exhibit the trait in approximately equal proportions; males and females are equally likely to transmit the trait to their offspring.
- No generations are skipped. If an individual has the trait, one parent must also have it. If neither parent has the trait, none of the children have it (with the exception of new mutations, as discussed later).
- Affected heterozygous individuals transmit the trait to approximately half their children, and because gamete transmission is subject to chance fluctuations, all or none of the children of an affected parent may have the trait. As large numbers of matings of this type are studied, the proportion of affected children closely approaches one half. Skipped generations are not seen in classic autosomal dominant pedigrees.

Recurrence Risks

Parents at risk of producing children with a genetic disease nearly always ask the question, "What is the *chance* that our child will have this disease?" The probability that an individual will develop a genetic disease is termed the **recurrence risk**. When one parent is affected by an autosomal dominant disease (and is a heterozygote) and the other is unaffected, the recurrence risk for each child is one half.

An important principle is that each birth is an independent event, much like a coin toss. Thus, even though parents may have already had a child with the disease, their recurrence risk remains one half. Even if they have produced several children, all affected (or all unaffected) by the disease, the law of independence dictates the probability their next child will have the disease is still one half. Parents' misunderstanding of this principle is a common problem encountered in genetic counselling.

If a child is born with an autosomal dominant disease, and there is no history of the disease in the family, the child is probably the product of a new mutation: the gene transmitted by one of the parents has undergone a mutation from a normal to a disease-causing allele. The alleles at this locus in most of the parent's other germ cells are still normal. In this situation, the recurrence risk for the parent's subsequent offspring is not greater than that of the general population, but the offspring of the affected child will have a recurrence risk of one half.

Occasionally, two or more offspring have symptoms of an autosomal dominant disease when there is no family history of the disease. It is unlikely that this disease would be a result of multiple mutations in the same family because mutation is a rare event. The mechanism most likely responsible is termed **germline mosaicism**, where a mutation likely occurred that affected all or part of a germline during the embryonic development of one of the parents. Only the germline cells were involved, and few or none of the somatic cells of the embryo were affected. Thus, the parent carries the mutation in his or her germline but does not actually express the disease. As a result, the unaffected parent can transmit the mutation to multiple offspring. This phenomenon, although relatively rare, can have significant effects on recurrence risks.[10]

Delayed Age of Onset

One of the best-known autosomal dominant diseases is Huntington's disease, a neurological disorder whose main features are progressive dementia and increasingly uncontrollable limb movements (chorea; discussed further in Chapter 15). A key feature of this disease is its **delayed age of onset**: symptoms usually are not seen until 40 years of age or later. Thus, those who develop the disease often have borne children before they are aware they have the disease-causing mutation. If the disease was present at birth, nearly all affected persons would die before reaching reproductive age and the occurrence of the disease-causing allele in the population would be much lower. An individual whose parent has the disease has a 50% chance of developing it during middle age. He or she is thus confronted with a torturous question: Should I have children, knowing that there is a 50–50 chance that I may have this disease-causing gene and will pass it to half of my children? A DNA test can now be used to determine whether an individual has inherited the trinucleotide repeat mutation that causes Huntington's disease.

Penetrance and Expressivity

The **penetrance** of a trait is the percentage of individuals with a specific genotype who also exhibit the expected phenotype. Incomplete penetrance means individuals who have the disease-causing genotype may not exhibit the disease phenotype at all, even though the genotype and the associated disease may be transmitted to the next generation. A pedigree illustrating the transmission of an autosomal dominant mutation with incomplete penetrance is provided in Figure 2.22. Retinoblastoma, the most common malignant eye tumour affecting children, typically

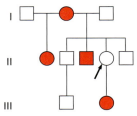

FIGURE 2.22 Pedigree for Retinoblastoma Showing Incomplete Penetrance. Female with *black arrow* in line II must be heterozygous, but she does not express the trait.

exhibits incomplete penetrance. About 10% of the individuals who are **obligate carriers** of the disease-causing mutation (i.e., those who have an affected parent and affected children and therefore must themselves carry the mutation) do not have the disease. The penetrance of the disease-causing genotype is then said to be 90%.

The gene responsible for retinoblastoma is a **tumour-suppressor gene**: the normal function of its protein product is to regulate the cell cycle so cells do not divide uncontrollably. When the protein is altered because of a genetic mutation, its tumour-suppressing capacity is lost and a tumour can form[11] (see Chapters 10 and 17).

Expressivity is the extent of variation in phenotype associated with a particular genotype. If the expressivity of a disease is variable, penetrance may be complete but the severity of the disease can vary greatly. A good example of variable expressivity in an autosomal dominant disease is neurofibromatosis type 1, or von Recklinghausen disease. As in retinoblastoma, the mutations that cause neurofibromatosis type 1 occur in a tumour-suppressor gene.[12] The expression of this disease varies from a few harmless café-au-lait (light brown) spots on the skin to numerous neurofibromas, scoliosis, seizures, gliomas, neuromas, malignant peripheral nerve sheath tumours, hypertension, and learning disorders (Figure 2.23).

Several factors cause variable expressivity. Genes at other loci sometimes modify the expression of a disease-causing gene. Environmental factors also can influence expression of a disease-causing gene. Finally, different mutations at a locus can cause variation in severity. For example, a mutation that alters only one amino acid of the factor VIII gene usually produces a mild form of hemophilia A, whereas a "stop" codon (premature termination of translation) usually produces a more severe form of this blood coagulation disorder.

Epigenetics and Genomic Imprinting

Although this chapter focuses on DNA sequence variation and its consequence for disease, there is increasing evidence that the same DNA sequence can produce dramatically different phenotypes because of chemical modifications to the DNA once it is formed, altering the *expression* of genes (these modifications are collectively termed **epigenetic**, Chapter 3). An important example of such a modification is **DNA methylation**, the attachment of a methyl group to a cytosine base followed by a guanine base in the DNA sequence (Figure 2.24). These sequences, which are common near many genes, are termed **CpG islands**. When the CpG islands located near a gene become heavily methylated, the gene is less likely to be transcribed into mRNA. In other words, the gene becomes transcriptionally inactive. Identical (monozygotic) twins can accumulate different methylation patterns in the DNA sequences of their somatic cells as they age, causing increasing numbers of phenotypic differences.[13] Intriguingly, twins with more differences in their lifestyles (e.g., smoking versus nonsmoking) accumulated larger numbers of differences in their **methylation** patterns. The twins, despite having identical DNA sequences, become more and

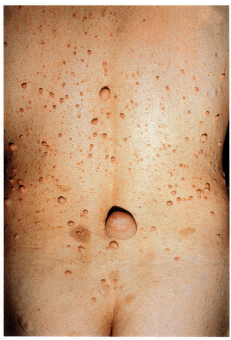

FIGURE 2.23 Neurofibromatosis. Tumours. The most common types are either sessile or pedunculated. Early tumours are soft, dome-shaped papules or nodules that have a distinctive violaceous hue. Most are benign. (From Habif, T. P., Campbell, J. L. Jr, Chapman, M. S., et al. [2005]. *Skin disease: Diagnosis and treatment* [2nd ed.]. Elsevier.)

more different as a result of epigenetic changes, which in turn affect the expression of genes (see Figure 3.5).

Epigenetic alteration of gene activity can have important disease consequences. For example, a major cause of one form of inherited colon cancer (termed *hereditary nonpolyposis colorectal cancer [HNPCC]*) is the methylation of a gene whose protein product repairs damaged DNA. When this gene becomes inactive, damaged DNA accumulates, eventually resulting in colon tumours. Epigenetic changes are also discussed in Chapters 3, 10, and 11.

Approximately 100 human genes are thought to be methylated differently, depending on which parent transmits the gene. This epigenetic modification, characterized by methylation and other changes, is termed **genomic imprinting**. For each of these genes, one of the parents *imprints* the gene (inactivates it) when it is transmitted to the offspring. An example is the insulin-like growth factor 2 (*IGF-2*) gene on chromosome 11, which is transmitted by both parents, but the copy inherited from the mother is normally methylated and inactivated (imprinted). Thus, only one copy of *IGF-2* is active in normal individuals. However, the maternal imprint is occasionally lost, resulting in two active copies of *IGF-2*. Having two active copies of *IGF-2* causes excess fetal growth and contributes to a condition known as *Beckwith-Wiedemann syndrome*.

A second example of genomic imprinting is a deletion of part of the long arm of chromosome 15 (15q11–q13), which, when inherited from the father, causes the offspring to manifest a disease known as *Prader-Willi syndrome* (short stature, obesity, hypogonadism). When the same deletion is inherited from the mother, the offspring develop *Angelman syndrome* (intellectual disability, seizures, ataxic gait). The two different phenotypes reflect the fact that different genes are normally active in the maternally and paternally transmitted copies of this region of chromosome 15.

CHAPTER 2 Genes and Genetic Diseases

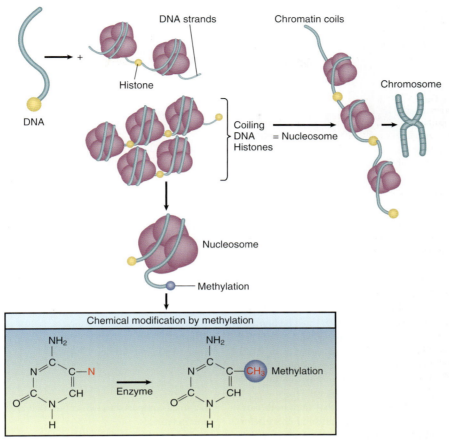

FIGURE 2.24 Epigenetic Modifications. Because DNA is a long molecule, it needs packaging to fit in the tiny nucleus. Packaging involves *coiling* of the DNA in a "left-handed" spiral around spools, made of four pairs of proteins individually known as histones and collectively termed the *histone octamer*. The entire spool is called a *nucleosome* (see also Figure 1.2). Nucleosomes are organized into chromatin, the repeating building blocks of a chromosome. Histone modifications are correlated with methylation, are reversible, and occur at multiple sites. Methylation occurs at the 5 position of cytosine and provides a "footprint" or signature as a unique epigenetic alteration *(red)*. When genes are expressed, chromatin is open or active; however, when chromatin is condensed because of methylation and histone modification, genes are inactivated.

Autosomal Recessive Inheritance
Characteristics of Pedigrees

Like autosomal dominant diseases, diseases caused by autosomal recessive genes are rare in populations, although there can be numerous carriers. The most common lethal recessive disease in White children, cystic fibrosis, occurs in about 1 in 2500 births. Approximately 1 in 25 White people carries a copy of a mutation that causes cystic fibrosis (see Chapter 28). Carriers are phenotypically unaffected. Some autosomal recessive diseases are characterized by delayed age of onset, incomplete penetrance, and variable expressivity.

Figure 2.25 shows a pedigree for cystic fibrosis. The gene responsible for cystic fibrosis encodes a chloride ion channel in some epithelial cells. Defective transport of chloride ions leads to a salt imbalance that results in secretions of abnormally thick, dehydrated mucus. Some digestive organs, particularly the pancreas, become obstructed, causing malnutrition, and the lungs become clogged with mucus, making them highly susceptible to bacterial infections. Death from lung disease or heart failure occurs before 40 years of age in about half of persons with cystic fibrosis.

Important criteria for discerning autosomal recessive inheritance include:

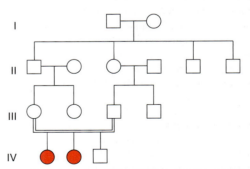

FIGURE 2.25 Pedigree for Cystic Fibrosis. Cystic fibrosis is an autosomal recessive disorder. The double bar denotes a consanguineous mating. Because cystic fibrosis is relatively common in European populations, most cases do not involve consanguinity.

- Males and females are affected in equal proportions.
- Consanguinity (marriage between related individuals) is sometimes present, especially for rare recessive diseases.
- The disease may be seen in siblings of affected individuals but usually not in their parents.
- On average, one fourth of the offspring of carrier parents will be affected.

	D	d
D	DD Homozygous normal	Dd Heterozygous carrier
d	Dd Heterozygous carrier	dd Homozygous affected

FIGURE 2.26 Punnett Square for the Mating of Heterozygous Carriers Typical of Most Cases of Recessive Disease.

Recurrence Risks

In most cases of recessive disease, both of the parents of affected individuals are heterozygous carriers. On average, one fourth of their offspring will be normal homozygotes, half will be phenotypically normal carrier heterozygotes, and one fourth will be homozygotes with the disease (Figure 2.26). Thus, the recurrence risk for the offspring of carrier parents is 25%. However, in any given family, there are chance fluctuations.

If two parents have a recessive disease, they each must be homozygous for the disease. Therefore, all their children also must be affected. Homozygous genes for the disease distinguish recessive from dominant inheritance because two parents both affected by a dominant gene are nearly always both heterozygotes, resulting in only one fourth of their children being unaffected (i.e., having the recessive trait).

Because carrier parents usually are unaware that they both carry the same recessive allele, they often produce an affected child before becoming aware of their condition. Carrier detection tests can identify heterozygotes by analyzing the DNA sequence to reveal a mutation. Some recessive diseases for which carrier detection tests are routinely used include phenylketonuria, sickle cell disease, cystic fibrosis, Tay-Sachs disease, hemochromatosis, and galactosemia.

Consanguinity

Consanguinity and inbreeding are related concepts. Consanguinity refers to the mating of two related individuals, and the offspring of such matings are said to be *inbred*. Consanguinity is sometimes an important characteristic of pedigrees for recessive diseases because relatives share a certain proportion of genes received from a common ancestor. The proportion of shared genes depends on the closeness of their biological relationship. Consanguineous matings produce a significant increase in recessive disorders and are seen most often in pedigrees for rare recessive disorders.

X-Linked Inheritance

Some genetic conditions are caused by mutations in genes located on the sex chromosomes, and this mode of inheritance is termed sex linked. Only a few diseases are known to be inherited as X-linked dominant or Y chromosome traits. Only the more common X-linked recessive diseases are discussed here.

Because females receive two X chromosomes, one from the father and one from the mother, they can be homozygous for a disease allele at a given locus, homozygous for the normal allele at the locus, or heterozygous. Males, having only one X chromosome, are hemizygous for genes on this chromosome. If a male inherits a recessive disease gene on the X chromosome, he will be affected by the disease since the Y chromosome does not carry a normal allele to counteract the effects of the disease gene. More males are affected by X-linked recessive diseases than females because a single X-linked recessive gene will cause disease

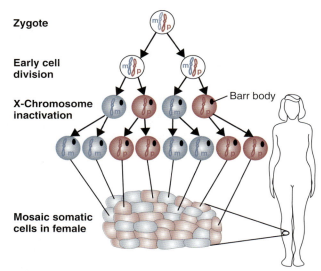

FIGURE 2.27 The X-Inactivation Process. The maternal *(m)* and paternal *(p)* X chromosomes are both active in the zygote and in early embryonic cells. X inactivation then takes place, resulting in cells having either an active paternal X or an active maternal X. Females are thus X chromosome mosaics, as shown in the tissue sample at the bottom of the figure. (From Jorde, L. B., Carey, J. C., & Bamshad, M. J. [2010]. *Medical genetics* [4th ed.]. Mosby.)

in a male compared to two copies that are required for disease expression in females.

X Inactivation

In the late 1950s, Mary Lyon proposed that one X chromosome in the somatic cells of females is permanently inactivated, a process termed X inactivation.[14,15] This proposal, the *Lyon hypothesis*, explains why most gene products coded by the X chromosome are present in equal amounts in males and females, even though males have only one X chromosome and females have two X chromosomes. This phenomenon is called dosage compensation. The inactivated X chromosomes are observable in many interphase cells as highly condensed intranuclear chromatin bodies, termed **Barr bodies** (after Barr and Bertram, who discovered them in the late 1940s). Normal females have one Barr body in each somatic cell, whereas normal males have no Barr bodies.

X inactivation occurs very early in embryonic development—approximately 7 to 14 days after fertilization. In each somatic cell, one of the two X chromosomes is inactivated. In some cells, the inactivated X chromosome is the one contributed by the father; in other cells, it is the one contributed by the mother. Once the X chromosome has been inactivated in a cell, all the descendants of that cell have the same inactivated chromosome (Figure 2.27).

Some individuals do not have the normal number of X chromosomes in their somatic cells. For example, males with Klinefelter's syndrome typically have two X chromosomes and one Y chromosome. These males do have one Barr body in each cell. Females whose cell nuclei have three X chromosomes have two Barr bodies in each cell, and females whose cell nuclei have four X chromosomes have three Barr bodies in each cell. Females with Turner's syndrome have only one X chromosome and no Barr bodies. Thus, the number of Barr bodies is always one less than the number of X chromosomes in the cell. All but one X chromosome are always inactivated.

Persons with abnormal numbers of X chromosomes, such as those with Turner's syndrome or Klinefelter's syndrome, are not physically normal. This situation presents a puzzle because they presumably have only one active X chromosome, the same as individuals with normal numbers of chromosomes. The difference in the number of X chromosomes is probably because the distal tips of the short and long arms of the X chromosome, as well as several other regions on the chromosome arm, are not inactivated. X inactivation in these cases is *incomplete*.

The DNA of an inactivated X chromosome is heavily methylated. Inactive X chromosomes can also be partially reactivated in vitro by administering 5-azacytidine, a demethylating agent.

Sex Determination

The process of sexual differentiation, in which the embryonic gonads become either testes or ovaries, begins during the sixth week of gestation. A key principle of mammalian sex determination is that one copy of the Y chromosome is sufficient to initiate the process of gonadal differentiation that produces a male fetus. The number of X chromosomes does not alter this process. For example, an individual with two X chromosomes and one Y chromosome in each cell is still phenotypically a male. Thus, the Y chromosome contains a gene that begins the process of male gonadal development.

This gene, termed *SRY* (for "sex-determining region on the Y"), has been located on the short arm of the Y chromosome[7] (Figure 2.28), which pairs with the distal tip of the short arm of the X chromosome during meiosis and exchanges genetic material with it (crossover), just as autosomes do. The DNA sequences of these regions on the X and Y chromosomes are highly similar, whereas the rest of the X and Y chromosomes do not exchange material and are not similar in DNA sequence.

Other genes that contribute to male differentiation are located on other chromosomes, and *SRY* triggers the action of these genes. The *SRY* protein product is very similar to other proteins known to regulate gene expression.

Occasionally, the crossover between X and Y occurs closer to the centromere than it should, placing the *SRY* gene on the X chromosome after crossover. This variation can result in offspring with an apparently normal XX karyotype but a male phenotype. Such XX males are seen in about 1 in 20 000 live births and resemble males with Klinefelter's syndrome. Conversely, it is possible to inherit a Y chromosome that has lost the *SRY* gene (the result of either a crossover error or a deletion of the gene). This situation produces an XY female. Such females have gonadal streaks rather than ovaries and have poorly developed secondary sex characteristics.

Characteristics of Pedigrees

X-linked pedigrees show distinctive modes of inheritance. The most striking characteristic is that females seldom are affected. To express an X-linked recessive trait fully, a female must be homozygous such that either both her parents are affected, or her father is affected and her mother is a carrier. These matings are rare.

Four important principles of X-linked recessive inheritance are:
1. The trait is seen much more often in males than in females.
2. Because a father can give a son only a Y chromosome, the trait is never transmitted from father to son.
3. The gene can be transmitted through a series of carrier females, causing the appearance of one or more "skipped generations."
4. The gene is passed from an affected father to all his daughters, who, as phenotypically normal carriers, transmit it to approximately half their sons, who then become affected.

A relatively common X-linked recessive disorder is Duchenne muscular dystrophy (DMD), which affects approximately 1 in 3 500 males. As its name suggests, this disorder is characterized by progressive muscle degeneration. Affected individuals usually are unable to walk by age 10 or 12 years. The disease affects the heart and respiratory muscles, and death caused by respiratory or cardiac failure usually occurs before 20 years of age. Identification of the disease-causing gene (on the short arm of the X chromosome) has greatly increased our understanding of the disorder.[16] The *DMD* gene is the largest gene ever found in humans, spanning more than 2 million DNA bases. It encodes a previously undiscovered muscle protein, termed **dystrophin**. Extensive study of dystrophin indicates that it plays an essential role in maintaining the structural integrity of muscle cells; it may also help to regulate the activity of membrane proteins. When dystrophin is absent, as in DMD, the cell cannot survive, and muscle deterioration ensues. Most cases of DMD are caused by frameshift deletions of portions of the *DMD* gene and with corresponding alterations of the amino acids encoded by the DNA following the deletion.

Recurrence Risks

The most common mating type involving X-linked recessive genes is the combination of a carrier female and a normal male (Figure 2.29A). On average, the carrier mother will transmit the disease-causing allele to half her sons (who are affected) and half her daughters (who are carriers).

The other common mating type is an affected father and a normal mother (Figure 2.29B). In this situation, all the sons will be normal because the father can transmit only his Y chromosome to them. Because all the daughters must receive the father's X chromosome, they will all be heterozygous carriers. None of the children in this situation will be affected.

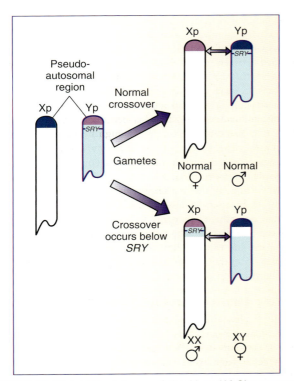

FIGURE 2.28 Distal Short Arms of the X and Y Chromosomes Exchange Material During Meiosis in the Male. The region of the Y chromosome in which this crossover occurs is called the *pseudoautosomal region*. The *SRY* gene, which triggers the process leading to male gonadal differentiation, is located just outside the pseudoautosomal region. Occasionally, the crossover occurs on the centromeric side of the *SRY* gene, causing it to lie on an X chromosome instead of a Y chromosome. An offspring receiving this X chromosome will be an XX male, and an offspring receiving the Y chromosome will be an XY female.

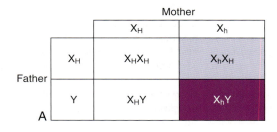

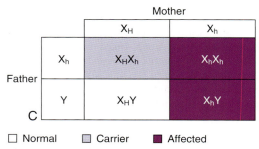

☐ Normal   ☐ Carrier   ■ Affected

FIGURE 2.29 Punnett Square and X-linked Recessive Traits. A, Punnett square for the mating of a normal male ($X_H Y$) and a female carrier of an X-linked recessive gene ($X_H X_h$). **B,** Punnett square for the mating of a normal female ($X_H X_H$) with a male affected by an X-linked recessive disease ($X_h Y$). **C,** Punnett square for the mating of a female who carries an X-linked recessive gene ($X_H X_h$) with a male who is affected with the disease caused by the gene ($X_h Y$).

The final mating pattern, less common than the other two, involves an affected father and a carrier mother (Figure 2.29C). With this pattern, on average, half the daughters will be heterozygous carriers, and half will be homozygous for the disease allele (and be affected by the condition). Half the sons will be normal, and half will be affected. Some X-linked recessive diseases, such as DMD, are fatal or incapacitating before the affected individual reaches reproductive age, and affected fathers are rare.

Sex-Limited and Sex-Influenced Traits

A **sex-limited trait** can occur in only one sex, often because of anatomical differences. Inherited uterine and testicular defects are two obvious examples. A **sex-influenced trait** occurs much more often in one sex than the other. For example, male-pattern baldness occurs in both males and females but is much more common in males. Autosomal dominant breast cancer, which is much more commonly expressed in females than males, is another example of a sex-influenced trait.

LINKAGE ANALYSIS AND GENE MAPPING

Locating genes on specific regions of chromosomes has been one of the most important goals of human genetics. The location and identification of a gene can tell much about the function of the gene, the interaction of the gene with other genes, and the likelihood that certain individuals will develop a genetic disease.

Classic Pedigree Analysis

Genes located close together on the same chromosome tend to be transmitted together to the offspring. Mendel's principle of independent assortment holds true for most pairs of genes but not those that occupy the same region of a chromosome. Such loci demonstrate **linkage**.

During the first meiotic stage, the arms of homologous chromosome pairs intertwine and sometimes exchange portions of their DNA (Figure 2.30) in a process known as **crossover**. During crossover, new combinations of alleles can be formed. For example, two loci on a chromosome have alleles A_1 and A_2 and alleles B_1 and B_2. Alleles A_1 and B_1 are located together on one member of a chromosome pair, and alleles A_2 and B_2 are located on the other member. The genotype of this individual is denoted as $A_1 B_1 / A_2 B_2$.

As Figure 2.30A, shows, the allele pairs $A_1 B_1$ and $A_2 B_2$ would be transmitted together when no crossover occurs. However, when crossover occurs (Figure 2.30B), all four possible pairs of alleles can be transmitted to the offspring: $A_1 B_1$, $A_2 B_1$, $A_1 B_2$, and $A_2 B_2$. The process of forming such new arrangements of alleles is called **recombination**. Crossover does not necessarily lead to recombination, however, because double crossover between two loci can result in no actual recombination of the alleles at the loci (Figure 2.30C).

Once a close linkage has been established between a disease-gene locus and a "marker" locus (a DNA sequence that varies among individuals) and once the alleles of the two loci that are inherited together within a family have been determined, reliable predictions can be made as to whether a member of a family will develop the disease. This type of analysis is called **linkage analysis**. For example, linkage has been established between several DNA polymorphisms and each of the two major genes that can cause autosomal dominant breast cancer (about 5% of breast cancer cases are caused by these autosomal dominant genes). Determining this kind of linkage means that it is possible for offspring of an individual with autosomal dominant breast cancer to know whether they also carry the gene and can pass it on to their own children. In most cases, specific disease-causing mutations can be identified, allowing direct detection and diagnosis. For some genetic diseases, prophylactic treatment is available if the condition can be diagnosed in time. An example of this is *hemochromatosis*, a recessive genetic disease in which excess iron is absorbed, causing degeneration of the heart, liver, brain, and other vital organs. Individuals at risk of developing the disease can be determined by testing for a mutation in the hemochromatosis gene and through clinical tests. Preventive therapy (periodic phlebotomy) can then be initiated to deplete iron stores and ensure a normal lifespan.

Complete Human Gene Map: Prospects and Benefits

The major goals of the Human Genome Project were to find the locations of all human genes (the "gene map") and to determine the entire human DNA sequence. These goals have now been accomplished, and the genes responsible for more than 4000 Mendelian conditions have been identified (Figure 2.31).[3,17,18] The project has greatly increased our understanding of the mechanisms that underlie many diseases, such as retinoblastoma, cystic fibrosis, neurofibromatosis, and Huntington's disease. The project also has led to more accurate diagnosis of these conditions and, in some cases, more effective treatment.

DNA sequencing is now much less expensive and more efficient. Consequently, many thousands of individuals have now been

CHAPTER 2 Genes and Genetic Diseases

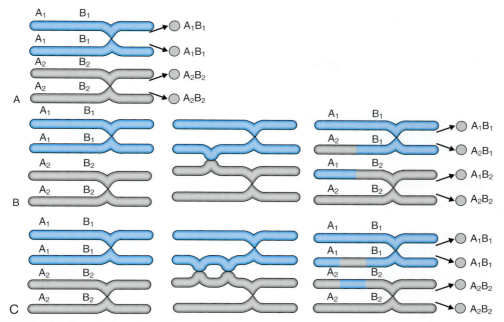

FIGURE 2.30 Genetic Results of Crossing Over. **A**, No crossing over. **B**, Crossing over with recombination. **C**, Double crossing over, resulting in no recombination.

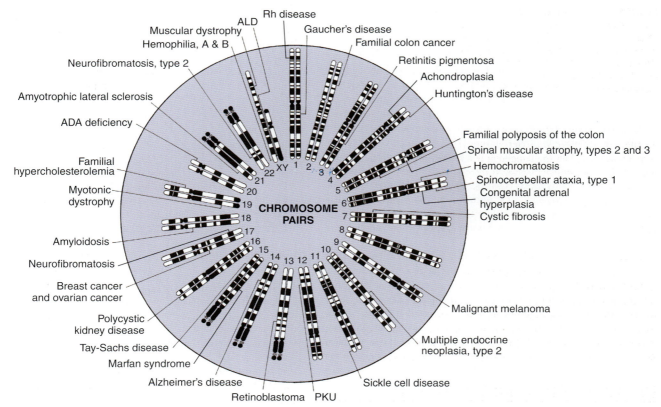

FIGURE 2.31 Example of Diseases: A Gene Map. *ADA*, Adenosine deaminase; *ALD*, adrenoleukodystrophy; *PKU*, phenylketonuria.

completely sequenced, leading in some cases to the identification of disease-causing genes (see *Health Promotion: Gene Therapy*).[19]

HEALTH PROMOTION: GENE THERAPY

Thousands of subjects are currently enrolled in more than 1000 gene therapy protocols. Most of these protocols involve the genetic alteration of cells to combat various types of cancer. Others involve the treatment of inherited diseases, such as β-thalassemia, hemophilia B, severe combined immunodeficiency, and retinitis pigmentosa.

MULTIFACTORIAL INHERITANCE

✓ QUICK CHECK 2.3
1. Define linkage analysis; cite an example.
2. Why is "threshold of liability" an important consideration in multifactorial inheritance?
3. Describe the concept of multifactorial inheritance and include two examples.

Not all traits are produced by single genes; some traits result from several genes acting together. These are called **polygenic traits**. When environmental factors also influence the expression of the trait (as is usually the case), the term **multifactorial inheritance** is used. Many multifactorial and polygenic traits tend to follow a normal distribution in populations. Figure 2.32 shows how three loci acting together can cause grain colour in wheat to vary in a gradual way from white to red, exemplifying multifactorial inheritance. If both alleles at each of the three loci are white alleles, the colour is pure white. If most alleles are white but a few are red, the colour is somewhat darker; if all are red, the colour is dark red.

Other examples of multifactorial traits include height and IQ. Although both height and IQ are determined in part by genes, they are also influenced by the environment. For example, the average height of many human populations has increased by 5 to 10 cm in the past 100 years because of improvements in nutrition and health care. Also, IQ scores can be improved by exposing individuals (especially children) to enriched learning environments. Thus, both genes and environment contribute to variation in these traits.

A number of diseases do not follow a normal distribution. Instead, they appear to be either present in or absent from an individual but do not follow the patterns expected of single-gene diseases. Many of them are probably polygenic or multifactorial, but a certain **threshold of liability** must be crossed before the disease is expressed. Below the threshold, the individual appears normal; above it, the individual is affected by the disease (Figure 2.33).

A good example of such a threshold trait is pyloric stenosis, a disorder characterized by a narrowing or obstruction of the pylorus, the area between the stomach and small intestine. Chronic vomiting, constipation, weight loss, and electrolyte imbalance can result from the condition, but the condition is easily corrected by surgery. The prevalence of pyloric stenosis is about 3 in 1000 live births in White people. This disorder is much more common in males than females, affecting 1 in 200 males and 1 in 1000 females. The apparent reason for this difference is that the threshold of liability is much lower in males than females, as shown in Figure 2.33. Thus, fewer defective alleles are required to generate the disorder in males. This situation also means the offspring of affected females are more likely to have pyloric stenosis because affected females carry more disease-causing alleles than most affected males.

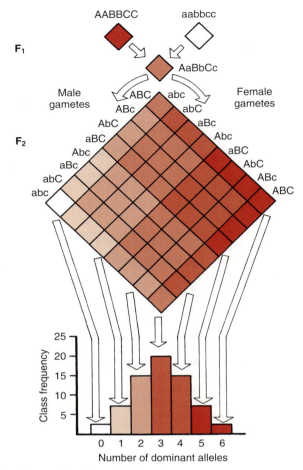

FIGURE 2.32 Multifactorial Inheritance. Analysis of mode of inheritance for grain colour in wheat. The trait is controlled by three independently assorted gene loci.

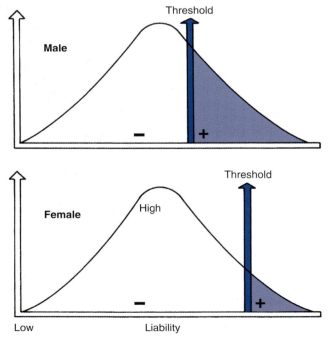

FIGURE 2.33 Threshold of Liability for Pyloric Stenosis in Males and Females.

A number of other common diseases are thought to correspond to a threshold model. They include cleft lip and cleft palate, neural tube defects (anencephaly, spina bifida), clubfoot (talipes), and some forms of congenital heart disease.

Although recurrence risks can be given with confidence for single-gene diseases (e.g., 50% for autosomal dominants, 25% for autosomal recessives), attributing a recurrence risk is considerably more difficult for multifactorial diseases: the number of genes contributing to the disease is not known, the precise allelic constitution of the biological parents is not known, and the extent of environmental effects can vary from one population to another. Empirical risks (i.e., those based on direct observation) are helpful to explain the inheritance of a multifactorial disease or trait and can be determined by examining large samples of biological families where one child has developed the disease/condition. The siblings of each child are then surveyed to calculate the percentage who also develop the disease/condition.

Another difficulty is distinguishing polygenic or multifactorial diseases from single-gene diseases having incomplete penetrance or variable expressivity. Large data sets and good epidemiological data often are necessary to make the distinction. Box 2.2 lists criteria commonly used to define multifactorial diseases.

The genetics of common disorders such as hypertension, heart disease, and diabetes is complex and often confusing. Nevertheless, the public health impact of these diseases, together with the evidence for hereditary factors in their etiology, demands further study in genetics. Hundreds of genes contributing to susceptibility for these diseases have been discovered, and the next decade will undoubtedly witness substantial advancements in our understanding of these disorders.

BOX 2.2 Criteria Used to Define Multifactorial Diseases

1. The recurrence risk becomes higher if more than one family member is affected. For example, the recurrence risk for neural tube defects in a British family increases to 10% if two siblings have been born with the disease. By contrast, the recurrence risk for single-gene diseases remains the same regardless of the number of siblings affected.
2. If the expression of the disease is more severe, the recurrence risk is higher. This finding is consistent with the liability model; a more severe expression indicates that the individual is at the extreme end of the liability distribution. Relatives of the affected individual are thus at a higher risk of inheriting disease genes. Cleft lip or cleft palate is a condition in which relatives are at a higher risk of inheriting disease genes.
3. Relatives of probands of the less commonly affected are more likely to develop the disease. As with pyloric stenosis, development of the disease occurs because an affected individual of the less susceptible sex is usually at a more extreme position on the liability distribution.
4. Generally, if the population frequency of the disease is f, the risk for offspring and siblings of probands is approximately $\sqrt{f}$. The same principle does not usually hold true for single-gene traits.
5. The recurrence risk for the disease decreases rapidly in more remotely related relatives. Although the recurrence risk for single-gene diseases decreases by 50% with each degree of relationship (e.g., an autosomal dominant disease has a 50% recurrence risk for siblings, 25% for uncle-nephew relationship, 12.5% for first cousins), the risk for multifactorial inheritance decreases much more quickly.

DID YOU UNDERSTAND?

DNA, RNA, and Proteins: Heredity at the Molecular Level

1. Genes, the basic units of inheritance, are composed of deoxyribonucleic acid (DNA) and are located on chromosomes.
2. DNA is composed of deoxyribose, a phosphate molecule, and four types of nitrogenous bases. The physical structure of DNA is a double helix.
3. The DNA bases code for amino acids, which in turn make up proteins. The amino acids are specified by triplet codons of nitrogenous bases.
4. DNA replication is based on complementary base pairing, in which a single strand of DNA serves as the template for attracting bases that form a new strand of DNA.
5. DNA polymerase is the primary enzyme involved in replication. It adds bases to the new DNA strand and performs "proofreading" functions.
6. A mutation is an inherited alteration of genetic material (i.e., DNA).
7. Substances that cause mutations are called *mutagens*.
8. Transcription and translation, the two basic processes in which proteins are specified by DNA, both involve ribonucleic acid (RNA). RNA is chemically similar to DNA, but it is single stranded, has a ribose sugar molecule, and has uracil rather than thymine as one of its four nitrogenous bases.
9. Transcription is the process by which DNA specifies a sequence of messenger RNA (mRNA).
10. Much of the RNA sequence is spliced from the mRNA before the mRNA leaves the nucleus. The excised sequences are called *introns*, and those that remain to code for proteins are called *exons*.
11. Translation is the process by which RNA directs the synthesis of polypeptides. This process takes place in the ribosomes, which consist of proteins and ribosomal RNA (rRNA).
12. During translation, mRNA interacts with transfer RNA (tRNA), a molecule that has an attachment site for a specific amino acid.

Chromosomes

1. Human cells consist of diploid somatic cells (body cells) and haploid gametes (sperm and egg cells).
2. Humans have 23 pairs of chromosomes. Twenty-two of these pairs are autosomes. The remaining pair consists of the sex chromosomes. Females have two homologous X chromosomes as their sex chromosomes; males have an X and a Y chromosome.
3. A karyotype is an ordered display of chromosomes arranged according to length and the location of the centromere.
4. Various types of stains can be used to make chromosome bands more visible.
5. About 1 in 150 live births has a major diagnosable chromosome abnormality. Chromosome abnormalities are the leading known cause of intellectual disability and miscarriage.
6. Polyploidy is a condition in which a euploid cell has some multiple of the normal number of chromosomes. Humans have been observed to have triploidy (three copies of each chromosome) and tetraploidy (four copies of each chromosome); both conditions are lethal.
7. Somatic cells that do not have a multiple of 23 chromosomes are aneuploid. Aneuploidy is usually the result of nondisjunction.

8. Trisomy is a type of aneuploidy in which one chromosome is present in three copies in somatic cells. A partial trisomy is one in which only part of a chromosome is present in three copies.
9. Monosomy is a type of aneuploidy in which one chromosome is present in only one copy in somatic cells.
10. In general, monosomies cause more severe physical defects than do trisomies, illustrating the principle that the loss of chromosome material has more severe consequences than the duplication of chromosome material.
11. Down syndrome, a trisomy of chromosome 21, is the best-known disease caused by a chromosome aberration. It affects 1 in 800 live births and is much more likely to occur in the offspring of women older than 35 years.
12. Most aneuploidies of the sex chromosomes have less severe consequences than those of the autosomes.
13. The most commonly observed sex chromosome aneuploidies involve alterations in the number of X chromosomes, namely the 47,XXX karyotype, 45,X karyotype (Turner's syndrome), and 47,XXY karyotype (Klinefelter's syndrome).
14. Abnormalities of chromosome structure include deletions, duplications, inversions, and translocations.

Elements of Formal Genetics

1. Mendelian traits are caused by single genes, each of which occupies a position, or locus, on a chromosome.
2. Alleles are different forms of genes located at the same locus on a chromosome.
3. At any given locus in a somatic cell, an individual has two genes, one from each parent. An individual may be homozygous or heterozygous at a locus.
4. An individual's genotype is their genetic makeup, and the phenotype reflects the interaction of genotype and environment.
5. In a heterozygote, a dominant gene's effects mask those of a recessive gene. The recessive gene is expressed only when it is present in two copies.

Transmission of Genetic Diseases

1. Genetic diseases caused by single genes usually follow autosomal dominant, autosomal recessive, or X-linked recessive modes of inheritance.
2. Pedigree charts are important tools in the analysis of modes of inheritance.
3. Skipped generations are not seen in classic autosomal dominant pedigrees.
4. Recurrence risks specify the probability that future offspring will inherit a genetic disease. For single-gene diseases, recurrence risks remain the same for each offspring, regardless of the number of affected or unaffected offspring.
5. The recurrence risk for autosomal dominant diseases is usually 50%.
6. Germline mosaicism can alter recurrence risks for genetic diseases because unaffected parents can produce multiple affected offspring. This situation occurs because the germline of one parent is affected by a mutation but the parent's somatic cells are unaffected.
7. Males and females are equally likely to exhibit autosomal dominant diseases and to pass them on to their offspring.
8. Many genetic diseases have a delayed age of onset.
9. A gene that is not always expressed phenotypically is said to have incomplete penetrance.
10. Variable expressivity is a characteristic of many genetic diseases.
11. Genomic imprinting, which is associated with methylation, results in differing expression of a disease gene, depending on which parent transmitted the gene.
12. Epigenetics involves changes, such as the methylation of DNA bases that do not alter the DNA sequence but can alter the expression of genes.
13. Most commonly, biological parents of children with autosomal recessive diseases are both heterozygous carriers of the disease gene.
14. The recurrence risk for autosomal recessive diseases is 25%.
15. Males and females are equally likely to be affected by autosomal recessive diseases.
16. Consanguinity is sometimes present in families with autosomal recessive diseases, and it becomes more prevalent with rarer recessive diseases.
17. Carrier detection tests for an increasing number of autosomal recessive diseases are available.
18. In each normal female somatic cell, one of the two X chromosomes is inactivated early in embryogenesis.
19. X inactivation is random, fixed, and incomplete (i.e., only part of the chromosome is actually inactivated). It may involve methylation.
20. Gender is determined embryonically by the presence of the *SRY* gene on the Y chromosome. Embryos that have a Y chromosome (and thus the *SRY* gene) become males, whereas those lacking the Y chromosome become females. When the Y chromosome lacks the *SRY* gene, an XY female can be produced. Similarly, an X chromosome that contains the *SRY* gene can produce an XX male.
21. X-linked genes are those that are located on the X chromosome. Nearly all known X-linked diseases are caused by X-linked recessive genes.
22. Males are hemizygous for genes on the X chromosome.
23. X-linked recessive diseases are seen much more often in males than in females because males need only one copy of the gene to express the disease.
24. Biological fathers cannot pass X-linked genes to their sons.
25. Skipped generations often are seen in X-linked recessive disease pedigrees because the gene can be transmitted through carrier females.
26. Recurrence risks for X-linked recessive diseases depend on the carrier and affected status of the mother and father.
27. A sex-limited trait is one that occurs only in one sex (gender).
28. A sex-influenced trait is one that occurs more often in one sex than the other.

Linkage Analysis and Gene Mapping

1. During meiosis I, crossover occurs and can cause recombinations of alleles located on the same chromosome.
2. The frequency of recombinations can be used to infer the map distance between loci on the same chromosome.
3. A marker locus, when closely linked to a disease-gene locus, can be used to predict whether an individual will develop a genetic disease.
4. The major goals of the Human Genome Project were to find the locations of all human genes (the "gene map") and to determine the entire human DNA sequence. These goals have now been accomplished, and the genes responsible for more than 4000 Mendelian conditions have been identified.

Multifactorial Inheritance

1. Traits that result from the combined effects of several loci are polygenic. When environmental factors also influence the expression of the trait, the term *multifactorial inheritance* is used.
2. Many multifactorial traits have a threshold of liability. Once the threshold of liability has been crossed, the disease may be expressed.
3. Empirical risks, based on direct observation of large numbers of families, are used to estimate recurrence risks for multifactorial diseases.
4. Recurrence risks for multifactorial diseases become higher if more than one biological family member is affected or if the expression of the disease in the proband is more severe.
5. Recurrence risks for multifactorial diseases decrease rapidly for more remote relatives.

3

Epigenetics and Disease

Stephanie Zettel, with originating chapter contributions by Diane P. Genereux

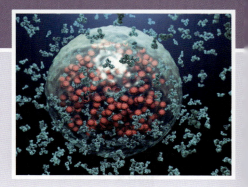

Additional resources are available online at http://evolve.elsevier.com/Canada/Huether/pathophysiology

CHAPTER OUTLINE

Epigenetic Mechanisms, 62
   DNA Methylation, 63
   Histone Modifications, 64
   RNA-Based Mechanisms, 64
Epigenetics and Human Development, 64
Genomic Imprinting, 64
   Prader-Willi and Angelman Syndromes, 65
   Beckwith-Wiedemann Syndrome, 65
   Russell-Silver Syndrome, 66
Inheritance of Epigenetic States, 66
   Epigenetics and Nutrition, 66
   Epigenetics and Maternal Care, 66
Epigenetics and Ethanol Exposure During Gestation 67
   Epigenetics and Mental Illness, 67

Epigenetic Disease in the Context of Genetic Abnormalities, 67
   Twin Studies Provide Insights on Epigenetic Modification, 68
   Molecular Approaches to Understand Epigenetic Disease, 68
Epigenetics and Cancer, 68
   DNA Methylation and Cancer, 68
   microRNAs and Cancer, 68
   Epigenetic Screening for Cancer, 68
   Emerging Strategies for the Treatment of Epigenetic Disease, 69
   DNA Demethylating Agents, 69
   Histone Deacetylase Inhibitors, 69
   microRNA Coding, 70
Future Directions, 70

LEARNING OBJECTIVES

1. Identify the three major types of epigenetic modifications.
2. Describe how epigenetics affect embryogenesis.
3. Discuss how epigenetic changes affect disease risk.
4. Identify ways in which epigenetic changes can be reversed.
5. Describe the process of imprinting and how this can affect disease.

KEY TERMS

5-Azacytidine, 69
Angelman syndrome, 65
Beckwith-Wiedemann syndrome, 65
Biallelic, 64
DNA methylation, 63
Embryonic stem cell, 64
Epigenetics, 62
Facioscapulohumeral muscular dystrophy (FHMD), 68
Fragile X, 67
Histone, 64
Histone modification, 64
Housekeeping genes, 64
Imprinted, 64
Locus, 63
microRNA (miRNA), 64
Monoallelic, 64
Noncoding RNA (ncRNA), 64
Prader-Willi syndrome, 65
Russell-Silver syndrome, 66

Epigenetic ("upon genetic") modification is an important contributor to human diversity. It involves a change in phenotype or gene expression that occurs without a DNA mutation or changes in the nucleotide sequence. Epigenetics is the study of mechanisms that can turn genes "on" (i.e., increase their expression) and "off" (i.e., stop them from being expressed). Epigenetic mechanisms include chemical modifications to DNA (where methyl groups are added to the DNA structure) and associated histones, as well as the production of small RNA molecules. Gene regulation by epigenetic processes can occur with transcription or translation. Epigenetic modification plays a fundamental role in human development, particularly with the differentiation of embryonic stem cells into specific cell types, and the inactivation of one of the two X chromosomes in each cell of a genetic female. Some genes are actually *imprinted*, where the expression of a gene depends on whether it is inherited from the mother or the father.

EPIGENETIC MECHANISMS

> ✓ **QUICK CHECK 3.1**
> 1. Define *epigenetics*.
> 2. What are the three types of epigenetic mechanisms?
> 3. Compare and contrast the molecular and phenotypic features of Prader-Willi and Angelman syndromes.

A variety of diseases can result from abnormal epigenetic states. For instance, metabolic disease can occur when there is irregular expression

CHAPTER 3 Epigenetics and Disease

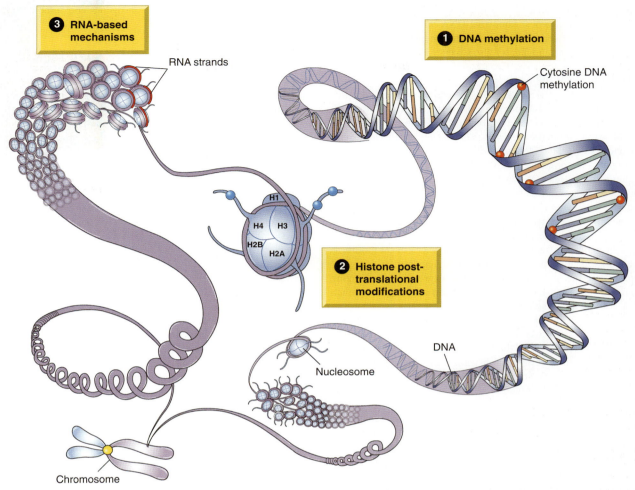

FIGURE 3.1 Three Types of Epigenetic Mechanisms. Investigators are studying three epigenetic mechanisms: (1) DNA methylation, (2) histone modifications, and (3) RNA-based mechanisms. See text for discussion. *H*, Histone.

of both copies of a locus (i.e., a specific, fixed position of a gene on a chromosome) that is typically imprinted. Environmental stressors can also greatly increase the risk for the expression of these epigenetic modifications and are strongly associated with some cancers. Research into how abnormal epigenetic states can result in disease is currently a focus of both preventive efforts and pharmaceutical intervention. Common epigenetic mechanisms include DNA methylation, histone modifications, and RNA-based mechanisms (Figure 3.1).

DNA Methylation

DNA methylation (see Figure 3.1) occurs through the attachment of a methyl group (CH_3) to a cytosine. Substantial DNA methylation essentially "insulates" the DNA and silences the genes by blocking access to the DNA by the transcription factors. Histones are the structural proteins that support the DNA, and DNA methylation often occurs with histone modification (or *hypoacetylation*, the removal of an acetyl group from the histone protein which results in a change in structure of the protein) (see "Histone Modifications"). Together, DNA methylation and histone hypoacetylation can disrupt transcription of the gene and the production of the encoded protein. A guanine base generally follows methylated cytosines (sometimes known as cytosines in "CpG dinucleotides"). In human embryonic stem cells, methylation can also occur at cytosines in sequence with other nucleotide bases (see Figure 2.24).

DNA methylation plays a prominent role in both human health and disease. For example, in each cell of a normal human female, methylation silences one of the two X chromosomes, and the other X chromosome is transcriptionally active and not methylated. Epigenetic inactivation of one X chromosome, either that inherited from the mother or that from the father, in each human female takes place during early embryonic development. The determination of which chromosome is to be silenced occurs both randomly and independently in each cell, and the silent state of that chromosome is inherited by all subsequent copies of that chromosome. If a woman's two X chromosomes carry different alleles at a given position on the chromosome (or locus), random X inactivation can lead to *somatic mosaicism*, where active alleles in two different cells can result in two very different traits. Striking examples include the patchy coloration of calico cats, as well as *anhidrotic ectodermal dysplasia* in humans, characterized by abnormal development of ectodermal tissues such as the skin, hair, teeth and sweat glands. Affected females have patchy presence and absence of sweat glands with one X chromosome bearing a normal allele and one X chromosome with a mutant allele at the same locus. As a result of this somatic mosaicism, females typically tend to have less severe phenotypes than males for a variety of X-linked disorders, including colour blindness and fragile X syndrome.

DNA methylation can also lead to misregulation of tumour-suppressor genes and oncogenes. Abnormal DNA methylation states are a common feature of several human cancers, including those of the colon[1-3] (see Figures 3.1 and 3.6; see also Chapter 10).

Histone Modifications

Histone modifications (see Figure 3.1) whereby histones, the proteins that support DNA and organizes it in the nucleus of the cell, are changed include histone acetylation (or the addition of an acetyl group) and deacetylation (or the deletion of an acetyl group) to the end of a histone protein. Like DNA methylation, these changes can alter the expression state of chromatin. *Chromatin* is also known as DNA that is bound to histones. When the DNA of the human genome is wound around histones, it is in a compressed state, and at any given time, various regions of chromatin are typically in one of two forms: (1) *euchromatin*, an open state where most or all nearby genes are transcriptionally active; and (2) *heterochromatin*, a closed state where most or all nearby genes are transcriptionally inactive. Chemical modification of histones in a region of DNA can either upregulate (i.e., increase) or downregulate (i.e., decrease) nearby gene expression by changing the interaction between DNA and histones and affecting how much DNA is accessible to transcription factors.

Chromatin structure plays a critical role in determining the developmental potential of a given cell lineage and can undergo dramatic changes during development of the organism. For example, chromatin states differ substantially between embryonic stem cells and terminally differentiated cells. The fraction of DNA that is in the heterochromatic state increases as cells differentiate. Similarly, there is a reduction in the number of active genes as cells progress from pluripotent stem cells to terminally differentiated cells that take on the structure and function of a given tissue. Histone modification is critical for normal development, but mutations in genes that encode histone-modifying proteins have been implicated in conditions such as congenital heart disease.[4]

Sperm cells, in contrast, express *protamines* rather than histones. These are evolutionarily derived from histones,[5] and enable sperm DNA to wind into an even more compact state than histone-bound DNA in somatic cells. This tight compaction has an evolutionary advantage because it improves the hydrodynamic features of the sperm head and facilitates its movement toward the egg.

RNA-Based Mechanisms

RNA-based mechanisms such as noncoding RNAs (ncRNAs) (see Figure 3.1) play an important role in regulating a wide variety of cellular processes, including RNA splicing and DNA replication. These ncRNAs are similar to "sponges" because they can "sop up" complementary RNAs and inhibit their function (see, e.g., http://www.ncbi.nlm.nih.gov/pmc/articles/PMC2957044/). Hairpin-shaped microRNAs (miRNAs), which are encoded by DNA sequences of approximately 22 nucleotides and exist typically within the introns (a segment of a DNA molecule that does not code for proteins) of genes or in noncoding DNA located between genes (see Chapter 2) are particularly important to gene regulation. In contrast to DNA methylation and histone modification, both of which principally affect gene expression at the level of transcription to RNA, miRNAs affect the translation of messenger RNAs (mRNAs) encoded at other loci. miRNAs may bind to regions of mRNA where there are complementary base pairs, and miRNAs can actually be both specific enough (and not bind to *all* of the mRNAs in a cell) and general enough to regulate a large number of different mRNA sequences. miRNAs also directly modulate translation by impairing ribosomal function. They regulate diverse signalling pathways such as those that stimulate cancer development and progression, which are called *oncomirs*. miRNAs have been linked to carcinogenesis because they alter the activity of oncogenes and tumour-suppressor genes (see Chapter 10).

EPIGENETICS AND HUMAN DEVELOPMENT

Each of the cells in the very early embryo has the potential to give rise to a somatic cell of any type. These embryonic stem cells are therefore said to be totipotent ("possessing all powers"). A key process in early development then is the epigenetic modification of specific DNA nucleotide sequences within these embryonic stem cells. These modifications ultimately lead to the gene-expression profiles that characterize the various differentiated somatic cell types, and ensure that specific genes are expressed only in the cells and tissue types where their gene products typically function (e.g., factor VIII expression primarily in hepatocytes, or dopamine receptor expression in neurons).

All of the cells in a given individual contain almost exactly the same genetic information. It is the epigenetic modification that enables them to achieve the diverse functions of differentiated somatic cells. A small percentage of genes, termed housekeeping genes, are necessary for the function and maintenance of all cells. These genes escape epigenetic silencing and remain transcriptionally active in all (or nearly all) cells. Housekeeping genes include encoding histones, DNA and RNA polymerases, and ribosomal RNA genes.

How can embryonic stem cells maintain their ability to differentiate into many cell types? Fertilization actually triggers a global *loss* of DNA methylation at most loci in both the oocyte-contributed and the sperm-contributed genomes, and methylation is not directly copied by the DNA replication process. As embryonic cell division proceeds in the absence of DNA methyltransferases, cell division continues, eventually yielding cells that have nearly all of their loci in unmethylated, transcriptionally active states. Around the time of implantation in the uterus, the DNA methyltransferases become active again, and allow for differentiation of the cells into organ systems characteristic of the fetus.

GENOMIC IMPRINTING

A baby inherits two copies of each autosomal gene: one from its mother and one from its father. For a large subset of these genes, expression is biallelic, meaning that both the maternally and the paternally inherited copies contribute to offspring phenotype. For another, smaller subset of these genes, expression is monoallelic,[6] and the maternal copy is randomly chosen for inactivation in some somatic cells where the paternal copy is randomly chosen for inactivation in other somatic cells. For a third and smaller subset of autosomes (about 1%) either the maternal copy or the paternal copy is imprinted, meaning that either the copy inherited through the sperm or the copy inherited through the egg is inactivated and remains in this inactive state in all of the somatic cells of the individual.

The subset of genes that are subject to imprinting is much greater for loci involved with organismal growth. The *genetic conflict hypothesis*[6] is a potential explanation for this pattern. There are differences in how the mother and the father genes are expressed in the offspring. The mother uses relatively fewer resources than the father to secure the survival of their child because she needs to secure her own survival in order to be able to have more children. As a result, imprinting of maternally inherited genes tends to reduce offspring size, and imprinting of paternally inherited genes tends to increase offspring size. When the disease is as a result of imprinting, the phenotypes (or observable characteristics) of affected individuals are critically dependent on whether the mutation is inherited from the mother or from the father. Some examples of such imprinting disorders are below.

Prader-Willi and Angelman Syndromes

Prader-Willi syndrome is associated with a deletion of about 4 million base pairs on the long arm of chromosome 15 when the deletion is inherited from the father. Features include short stature, hypotonia (decreased muscle tone), small hands and feet, obesity, mild to moderate intellectual disability, and hypogonadism[7] (Figure 3.2A). Those affected by Prader-Willi syndrome are constantly hungry and are at risk for developing type 2 diabetes. On the other hand, the same 4-Mb deletion, when inherited from the mother, causes Angelman syndrome and is characterized by severe intellectual disability, seizures, and an ataxic gait (Figure 3.2B).[8] Children with Angelman syndrome are generally happy with an increased interest in water. These diseases each occur in about 1 of every 15 000 live births, and chromosome deletions are responsible for about 70% of cases of both diseases. The other 25 to 30% of cases occur when a child either has two copies of chromosome 15 from the mother with none from the father (e.g., Prader-Willi syndrome), or two copies of chromosome 15 from the father with none from the mother (e.g., Angelman syndrome). The deletions that cause Prader-Willi and Angelman syndromes are indistinguishable at the DNA sequence level and affect the same group of genes.

The 4-Mb deletion (the *critical region*) contains several genes that are normally transcribed only on the copy of chromosome 15 that is inherited from the father,[9] and these genes are transcriptionally inactive (or imprinted) on the copy of chromosome 15 inherited from the mother. Similarly, other genes in this region are only transcriptionally active on the chromosome inherited from the mother. Several genes in this region are normally active on only one chromosome copy (Figure 3.3). If the single active copy of one of these genes is lost because of a chromosome deletion, then no gene product is produced, resulting in disease.

Beckwith-Wiedemann Syndrome

Beckwith-Wiedemann syndrome is an overgrowth condition with a predisposition toward cancer and is usually identifiable at birth because of the presence of large size for gestational age, neonatal hypoglycemia, a large tongue, creases on the earlobe, and omphalocele (an abdominal wall defect where the intestines, liver, and other organs remain outside of the abdomen in a separate sac because they have not returned to the abdominal cavity during the sixth week of intrauterine development).[10] Children with Beckwith-Wiedemann syndrome have an increased risk of developing Wilms tumour (which starts in the kidneys) or hepatoblastoma (a form of liver cancer). Both of these tumours can be treated effectively if they are detected early, and screening at regular intervals is an important part of management. Some children with Beckwith-Wiedemann syndrome also develop asymmetrical overgrowth of a limb or one side of the face or trunk (hemihyperplasia).

About 20 to 30% of Beckwith-Wiedemann syndrome cases can be caused by the inheritance of two copies of chromosome 11 from the father and no copy of the chromosome from the mother. Several genes on the short arm of chromosome 11 are imprinted on either the paternally or the maternally transmitted chromosome. These genes are found in two separate regions of the chromosome, depending on the degree of DNA methylation. In the first differentially methylated region (DMR1), the gene that encodes insulin-like growth factor 2 *(IGF-2)* is inactive on the maternally transmitted chromosome but active on the

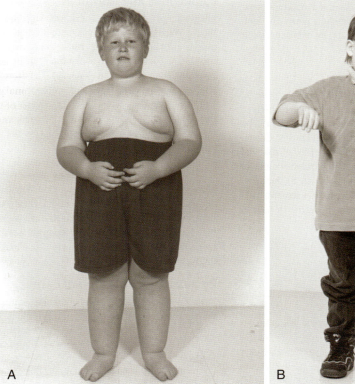
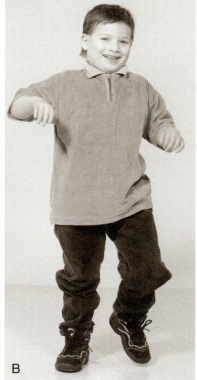

FIGURE 3.2 Prader-Willi and Angelman Syndromes. **A,** A child with Prader-Willi syndrome (truncal obesity, small hands and feet, inverted V-shaped upper lip). **B,** A child with Angelman syndrome (characteristic posture, ataxic gait, bouts of uncontrolled laughter). (From Jorde, L. B., Carey, J. C., & Bamshad, M. J. [2010]. *Medical genetics* [4th ed.]. Mosby.)

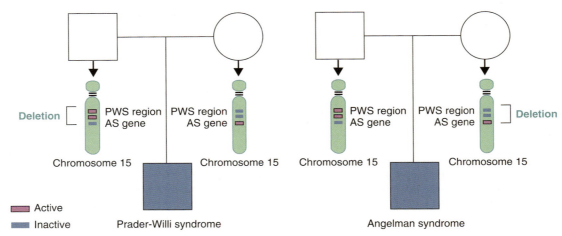

FIGURE 3.3 Prader-Willi Syndrome Pedigrees. These pedigrees illustrate the inheritance patterns of Prader-Willi syndrome *(PWS)*, which can be caused by a deletion of about 4 million base pairs (Mb) of chromosome 15q when inherited from the father. In contrast, Angelman syndrome *(AS)* can be caused by the same deletion but only when it is inherited from the mother. The reason for this difference is that different genes in this region are normally imprinted (inactivated) in the copies of 15q transmitted by the mother and the father. (From Jorde, L. B., Carey, J. C., & Bamshad, M. J. [2010]. *Medical genetics* [4th ed.]. Mosby.)

paternally transmitted chromosome. Thus, a normal individual has only one active copy of *IGF-2*. When two copies of the paternal chromosome are inherited, or there is loss of imprinting on the maternal copy of *IGF-2*, an active *IGF-2* gene is present in double dose. These changes produce increased levels of IGF-2 during fetal development and contribute to the overgrowth features of Beckwith-Wiedemann syndrome. Note that, in contrast to Prader-Willi and Angelman syndromes, which are generally the result of a missing gene product, Beckwith-Wiedemann syndrome is caused, in part, by overexpression of a gene product.

Russell-Silver Syndrome

Russell-Silver syndrome is characterized by delayed growth, proportionate short stature, leg length discrepancy, and a small, triangular face. About one third of Russell-Silver syndrome cases are caused by imprinting abnormalities of chromosome 11p15.5 that lead to downregulation of *IGF-2* and diminished growth. Another 10% of cases of Russell-Silver syndrome are caused by an inheritance of two copies of the maternal gene with none from the father. In contrast to the extra copies of active *IGF-2* (and overgrowth) in Beckwith-Wiedemann syndrome, downregulation of *IGF-2* causes the diminished growth seen in Russell-Silver syndrome.

INHERITANCE OF EPIGENETIC STATES

> **✓ QUICK CHECK 3.2**
> 1. Evaluate the statement: "Epigenetic information is highly dynamic in early development."
> 2. How does the epigenetic regulation of imprinted genes compare with that of the rest of the genome?
> 3. Compare and contrast the molecular mechanisms leading to fragile X syndrome and to FSHD.
> 4. Why are pairs of identical twins especially useful in the study of epigenetic phenomena?

Imprinting occurs not only with genetic modification in utero but also during childhood and adolescence, and these epigenetic changes can be transmitted across generations.[11] The following discussion includes some examples that further explain how the environment can impact genetic expression through epigenetics.

Epigenetics and Nutrition

Many people in the Netherlands suffered from starvation during World War II because of a Nazi blockade that occurred in 1943. Dutch individuals who suffered nutritional deprivation in utero during this 1943 blockade were more likely to develop obesity and diabetes as adults than those who had not. Furthermore, the impact of these changes was passed on to future generations—the offspring of these children were also found to be significantly smaller when compared to the rest of the Dutch population. These data are supported with other studies where there was increased risk of cardiovascular and metabolic disease when individuals were subject to starvation conditions in utero.[12]

The *IGF-2* gene is a possible explanation for the relationships between nutritional deprivation and disease risk across generations and is a possible target of epigenetic modifications due to nutritional deprivation. Exposure to chemicals such as bisphenol A (a component in some plastics) in utero and through lactation also seems to lead to epigenetic modifications similar to those that arise through nutritional deprivation in early life.[13]

Epigenetics and Maternal Care

Parenting style can also affect epigenetic states, and this information can be transmitted from one generation to the next. For example, mice and other rodents can exhibit two alternate styles of nursing behaviour: (1) frequent arched-back nursing with a high level of licking and grooming behaviour, and (2) an alternate style with infrequent arched-back nursing and much reduced licking and grooming behaviour. Pups of mothers that engaged in frequent arched-backed nursing were found to have significantly lower methylation levels of DNA and higher transcription activity of a glucocorticoid receptor–encoding locus. Most of the products of these genes influence hypothalamic-pituitary-adrenal function.[14] These findings suggest that alteration to methylation states of DNA could help explain the finding that exposure to stress early in life can modulate behaviour in adulthood. These findings also suggest that epigenetic processes can tell us about the environment, and that the certain epigenetic modifications can modulate behaviour later in life.

EPIGENETICS AND ETHANOL EXPOSURE DURING GESTATION

The impact of ethanol exposure in utero on skeletal and neural development was first reported in 1973[15] and led to broad awareness of fetal alcohol spectrum disorder. At first, researchers found alcohol exposure in utero can affect the DNA methylation states of various genomic elements, but without specific emphasis on loci directly relevant to skeletal and neural development.[10] More recently, treating cultured neural stem cells with ethanol impaired their ability to differentiate to functional neurons, and this impairment seems to be correlated with abnormal methylation of DNA at loci that are active in normal neuronal tissue.[16] Ethanol exposure in utero most likely modulates fetal expression of the DNA methyltransferases.[17]

Epigenetics and Mental Illness

Epigenetics also plays a role in psychiatric illness, resulting in many different phenotypes.[11] Schizophrenia, major depressive disorder, and bipolar disorder are just a few examples of how epigenetic influences can alter the course of an illness. These disorders are associated with alternating remissions and relapses, and the epigenetic changes that occur demonstrate how genetic activity is altered by the interactions of the organism with its environment. These epigenetic influences are reversible and can change over time. Further research in this area is considering how the environment impacts the expression of psychiatric conditions and the possibility of understanding the effect of environmental stimuli on the course of the illness with the intention to better treat and support individuals with these conditions.

Epigenetic Disease in the Context of Genetic Abnormalities

In some diseases, both genetic and epigenetic factors contribute to the origin of abnormal phenotypes. For example, several abnormal phenotypes can arise in individuals with mutations at the **fragile X** locus *FMR1* (Figure 3.4A). Some of these phenotypes occur in individuals who have both epigenetic and genetic changes. For example,

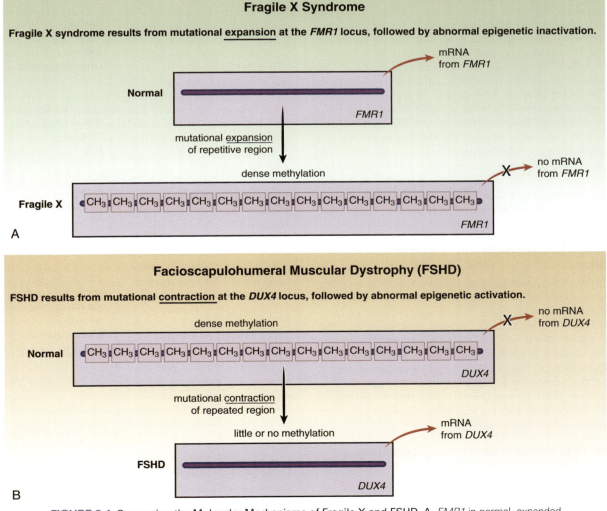

FIGURE 3.4 Comparing the Molecular Mechanisms of Fragile X and FSHD. **A**, *FMR1* in normal, expanded permutation, and full-mutation states. **B**, *DUX4* in normal and contracted states. *FSHD*, Facioscapulohumeral muscular dystrophy; *mRNA*, messenger RNA.

the most common genetic abnormality at *FMR1* involves expansion in the number of cytosine-guanine (CG) dinucleotide repeats in the gene promoter. Females who have CG repeats that exceed what is normal at this locus (about 35) are at risk for fragile X–associated primary ovarian insufficiency, characterized by an elevated risk for early menopause.[18] Moreover, males with similar moderate expansions of this base sequence are at risk for fragile X tremor ataxia syndrome (FXTAS), characterized by a late-onset intention tremor.[19] Both of these conditions seem to arise through accumulation of excess levels of *FMR1* mRNAs in nuclear inclusion bodies.[18,20] Individuals with 200 repeats are at risk for fragile X syndrome, characterized by reduced IQ and a set of behavioural abnormalities. Remarkably, although possession of a large CG repeat in the *FMR1* promoter dramatically increases the probability that an individual will have fragile X syndrome, the disease can be present in males who have the large repeat but be absent in their brothers who have inherited an allele of very similar size.[21] This difference can be explained, at least in part, by the observation that acquisition of methylation-based silencing at *FMR1* is random. The presence of a large sequence of repeats increases the probability of the abnormal methylation and consequent gene silencing but does not guarantee it. This dense methylation at *FMR1* might be affected by diet or the environment in individuals with the full-mutation allele.

In yet another example, the disease phenotype of **facioscapulohumeral muscular dystrophy (FSHD)** (Figure 3.4B) arises through loss of normal methylation rather than a gain of abnormal methylation. Symptoms of the disease include adverse impacts on skeletal musculature. Though lifespan is not typically reduced by the disease, wheelchair use becomes necessary late in life for a subset of individuals. The primary genetic event in FSHD is deletion of a nucleotide repeat in the *DUX4* gene (see Figure 3.4B). In normal individuals, the *D4Z4* gene promoter has between 11 and 150 copies, but those individuals with FSHD have only 1 to 10 such repeats. In healthy individuals with a normal-sized allele, the *D4Z4* promoter typically is highly methylated. In individuals with reduced copy-counts, the normally dense methylation is lost (see Figure 3.4B).[22] The disease allele typically also has fewer repressive histone marks than the normal allele.[23] Together, fragile X syndrome and FSHD highlight that both abnormal gain and abnormal loss of epigenetic modifications can result in disease.

Twin Studies Provide Insights on Epigenetic Modification

Identical (monozygotic) twin pairs, whose DNA sequences are essentially the same, offer a unique opportunity to isolate and examine the impacts of epigenetic modifications. As twins age, they exhibit increasingly substantial differences in methylation patterns of the DNA sequences of their somatic cells, and these changes are often reflected in increasing numbers of phenotypic differences. Twins with significant lifestyle differences (e.g., smoking versus nonsmoking) tend to accumulate larger numbers of differences in their methylation patterns. These results, along with findings generated in animal studies, suggest that changes in epigenetic patterns may be an important part of the aging process.[24]

Molecular Approaches to Understand Epigenetic Disease

Conventional sequencing approaches are not sufficient to reveal epigenetic differences between normal individuals and those who have epigenetic modifications associated with disease because epigenetic information is not encoded by DNA but rather by chemical modifications to these molecules. To collect information on DNA methylation states of individual nucleotides, DNA is typically subjected to bisulfite conversion before sequencing. Bisulfite treatment does not alter most nucleotides, including methylated cytosines, but deaminates unmethylated cytosines to uracil.[25] Uracil base pairs with adenine, not guanine; thus, methylated and unmethylated cytosines can be distinguished in resulting sequence data, so long as the genetic sequence is known. Similarly, antibodies specific for histones (with various modifications) are useful for understanding the extent of histone modifications in epigenetic disease.[26]

EPIGENETICS AND CANCER

QUICK CHECK 3.3
1. Evaluate the statement: "Cancer is, in many cases, an epigenetic disease."
2. Describe the role of miRNAs in cancer.
3. Describe a potential strategy for the treatment of epigenetic disease.
4. Describe some of the challenges of developing pharmaceutical approaches to remedy abnormal epigenetic states.

DNA Methylation and Cancer

Some of the most extensive evidence for the role of epigenetic modification in human disease comes from studies of cancer (Figure 3.5).[27,28] Tumour cells typically exhibit genome-wide hypomethylation (decreased methylation), which can increase the activity of oncogenes (see Chapter 10). Hypomethylation increases as tumours progress from benign neoplasms to malignancy. In addition, the promoter regions of tumour-suppressor genes are often hypermethylated, which decreases their rate of transcription and their ability to inhibit tumour formation. For example, hypermethylation of the promoter region of the *RB1* gene is often seen in retinoblastoma;[29] hypermethylation of the *BRCA1* gene is seen in some cases of inherited breast cancer (Chapter 33).[30]

A major cause of one form of inherited colon cancer (hereditary nonpolyposis colorectal cancer [HNPCC]) is the methylation of the promoter region of a gene, *MLH1*, whose protein product repairs damaged DNA. When *MLH1* becomes inactive, DNA damage accumulates, eventually resulting in colon tumours.[31,32] Abnormal methylation of tumour-suppressor genes also is common in the progression of Barrett esophagus, a condition in which the lining of the esophagus is replaced by cells that have features associated with the lower intestinal tract, and to adenocarcinoma possibly through upregulation of one of the enzymes that adds methyl groups to DNA.[33]

microRNAs and Cancer

Hypermethylation also occurs in miRNA genes, which encode small (22 base pair) RNA molecules that bind to the ends of mRNAs, degrading them and preventing their translation. More than 1 000 miRNA sequences have been identified in humans, and hypermethylation of specific subgroups of miRNAs is associated with tumourigenesis. When miRNA genes are methylated, their mRNA targets are overexpressed, and this overexpression has been associated with metastasis.[27]

Epigenetic Screening for Cancer

The common finding of epigenetic alteration in cancerous tissue raises the possibility that epigenetic screening approaches could complement

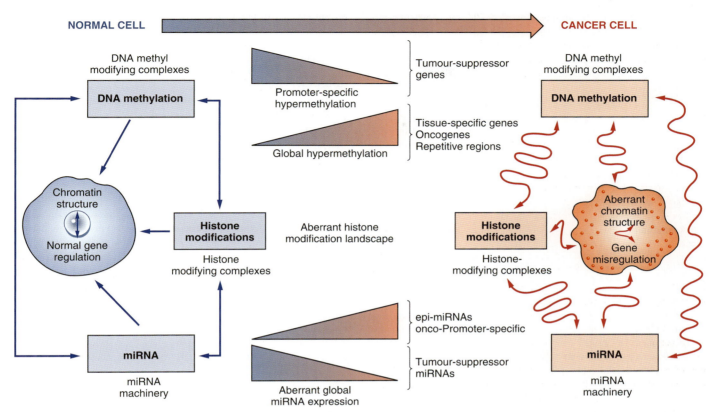

FIGURE 3.5 Global Epigenomic Alterations and Cancer. Oncogenesis often occurs through a combination of genetic mutations and epigenetic change. In cancer cells, the promoters of tumour-suppressor genes typically become hypermethylated, leading, in combination with histone modifications, to abnormal gene silencing. Because tumour-suppressor genes typically help to control cell division, their silencing can result in tumour progression. Global hypomethylation leads to chromosomal instability and fragility and increases the risk of additional genetic mutations. As well, these modifications create abnormal messenger RNA and microRNA (miRNA) expression, which leads to activation of oncogenes and silencing of tumour-suppressor genes. (Reprinted with permission from Sandoval, J., & Esteller, M., Cancer epigenomics: beyond genomics. *Current Opinion in Genetics & Development, 22*(1), 50–55.)

or even replace existing early-detection methods. In some cases, epigenetic screening could be done using bodily fluids, such as urine or sputum, eliminating the need for the more invasive, costly, and risky strategies currently in place. Monitoring for misregulation of miRNAs has shown promise as a tool for early diagnosis of cancers of the colon,[34] breast,[35] and prostate.[36] Other epigenetics-based screening approaches have shown promise for detection of cancers of the bladder,[37] lung,[38] and prostate.[39]

Emerging Strategies for the Treatment of Epigenetic Disease

Epigenetic modifications are potentially reversible: DNA can be demethylated, histones can be modified to change the transcriptional state of nearby DNA, and miRNA-encoding loci can be upregulated or downregulated. This possibility raises the prospect for treating epigenetic disease with pharmaceutical agents that directly reverse the changes associated with the disease phenotype. In recent years, interventions involving all three types of epigenetic modulators (DNA methylation, histone modification, and miRNAs) have shown considerable promise for the treatment of disease.

DNA Demethylating Agents

5-Azacytidine has been used as a therapeutic drug in the treatment of leukemia and myelodysplastic syndrome (5-azacytosine, the active component of 5-azacytidine, is shown in Figure 3.6).[40] A cytosine analogue, 5-azacytidine, is incorporated into DNA opposite its complementary nucleotide, guanine. 5-Azacytidine differs from cytosine in that it has a nitrogen, rather than a carbon, in the fifth position of its cytidine ring. As a result, the DNA methyltransferases cannot add methyl groups to 5-azacytidine, and DNA that contains 5-azacytidine declines in its methylation density over successive rounds of DNA replication.[41] Administration of 5-azacytidine is associated with various adverse effects, including digestive disturbance, but it has shown promise in the treatment of diseases such as pancreatic cancer[42] and myelodysplastic syndromes.[43,44]

Histone Deacetylase Inhibitors

The activity of the histone deacetylases (HDACs) increases chromatin compaction, decreasing transcriptional activity (Figure 3.7). In many cases, excessive activity of HDACs results in transcriptional inactivation of tumour-suppressor genes, leading ultimately to the development of tumours. Treatment with HDAC inhibitors, either alone or in combination with other medications, has shown promise in the treatment of cancers of the breast[45] and prostate,[46] but only very limited success in the treatment of pancreatic cancer.[47]

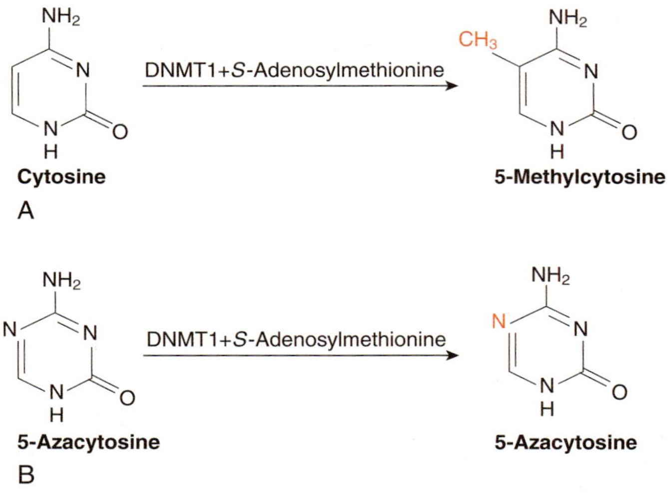

microRNA Coding

A major challenge in developing medications that modify epigenetic alterations is to target only the genes responsible for a specific cancer. Therapeutic approaches that use miRNA offer a potential solution to this problem because treatment can be targeted to individual loci using sequence characteristics of relevant RNA molecules.

FUTURE DIRECTIONS

Robust experimental observations are clarifying the roles of epigenetic states in determining cell fates and disease phenotypes. The well-documented involvement of epigenetic abnormalities in carcinogenesis and the mounting evidence for these epigenetic changes in other common diseases (discussed in other chapters) will likely provide possibilities for reversing the epigenetic abnormalities and possibly preventing their establishment in utero.

FIGURE 3.6 **5-Azacytosine as Demethylating Agent. A,** Unmethylated cytosines in DNA are typically subject to the addition of methyl groups by DNMT1, a DNA methyltransferase, using methyl groups supplied by the methyl donor S-adenosylmethionine. **B,** In 5-azacytosine, the 5' carbon of cytosine is replaced with a nitrogen. This chemical difference is sufficient both to block the addition of a methyl group and to confer irreversible binding to DNMT1. Incorporation of 5-azacytosine into DNA is therefore sufficient to drive passive loss of methylation from replicating DNA, and thus to reactivate hypermethylated loci. 5-Azacytosine, bound to a sugar, can be integrated into DNA, and has been administered with some success in treating epigenetic diseases that arise through hypermethylation of individual loci.

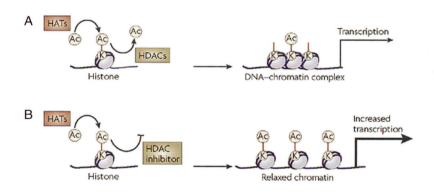

FIGURE 3.7 Effect of HDAC Inhibitors on Chromatin Remodelling and Transcription. **A,** Levels of histone acetylation at specific lysine (K) residues are determined by concurrent reactions of acetylation (Ac) and deacetylation, which are mediated by histone acetyltransferases (HATs) and histone deacetylases (HDACs). This histone acetylation is vital for establishing the conformational structure of DNA–chromatin complexes, and, subsequently, transcriptional gene expression. **B,** By blocking the deacetylation reaction, HDAC inhibitors change the equilibrium of histone acetylation levels, leading to increased acetylation, chromatin modification to relax conformation, and transcription upregulation. (Reprinted with permission from Kazantsev, A., G., & Thompson, L., M. (2008). Therapeutic application of histone deacetylase inhibitors for central nervous system disorders. Nature Reviews Drug Discovery, 7(10), 854–868.)

DID YOU UNDERSTAND?

Epigenetic Mechanisms

1. Investigators are studying three major types of epigenetic mechanisms: (a) DNA methylation, which results from attachment of a methyl group to a cytosine; in the somatic cells, all or nearly all methylation occurs at cytosines that are followed by guanines ("CpG dinucleotides"); (b) histone modifications, through the addition of various chemical groups, including methyl and acetyl; and (c) noncoding RNAs (ncRNAs) or microRNAs (miRNAs), short nucleotides derived from introns of protein coding genes or transcribed as independent genes from regions of the genome whose functions, if any, remain poorly understood. miRNAs regulate diverse signalling pathways.
2. DNA methylation is, at present, the best-studied epigenetic process. When a gene becomes heavily methylated, the DNA is less likely to be transcribed into mRNA.
3. Methylation, along with histone hypoacetylation and condensation of chromatin, inhibits the binding of proteins that promote transcription, such that the gene becomes transcriptionally inactive.
4. Environmental factors, such as diet and exposure to certain chemicals, may cause epigenetic modification.
5. The heritable transmission to future generations of epigenetic modifications is called *transgenerational inheritance*.

Epigenetics and Human Development

1. Epigenetic modification alters gene expression without changes to DNA sequence.
2. Housekeeping genes are necessary for the function and maintenance of all cells, and they escape epigenetic silencing, remaining transcriptionally active in all (or nearly all) cells.
3. Fertilization triggers loss of DNA methylation and suppression of DNA methyltransferases (enzymes that add methyl groups to DNA), yielding cells that have nearly all of their loci in unmethylated and transcriptionally active states.
4. Implantation in the uterus activates the DNA methyltransferases and allows for cell-lineage–specific marks required for the development of organ systems.

Genomic Imprinting

1. Gregor Mendel's experiments with garden peas demonstrated that the phenotype is the same whether a given allele is inherited from the mother or the father. This principle, which has long been part of the central dogma of genetics, does not always hold. For some human genes, a given gene is transcriptionally active on only one copy of a chromosome (e.g., the copy inherited from the father). On the other copy of the chromosome (the one inherited from the mother) the gene is transcriptionally inactive. This process of gene silencing, in which genes are silenced depending on which parent transmits them, is known as *imprinting*; the transcriptionally silenced genes are said to be "imprinted."
2. When an allele is imprinted, it typically has heavy methylation. By contrast, the nonimprinted allele is typically not methylated.
3. A well-known disease example of imprinting is associated with a deletion of about 4 million base pairs (Mb) of the long arm of chromosome 15. When this deletion is inherited from the father, the child manifests Prader-Willi syndrome.
4. The same 4-Mb deletion, when inherited from the mother, causes Angelman syndrome.
5. Another well-known example of imprinting is Beckwith-Wiedemann syndrome, an overgrowth condition accompanied by an increased predisposition to cancer.
6. Whereas upregulation, or extra copies, of active *IGF-2* causes overgrowth in Beckwith-Wiedemann syndrome, downregulation of *IGF-2* causes the diminished growth seen in Russell-Silver syndrome.

Inheritance of Epigenetic States

1. Events encountered in utero, in childhood, and in adolescence can result in specific epigenetic changes that yield a wide range of phenotypic abnormalities, including metabolic syndromes.
2. Fetal alcohol spectrum disorder, which results from ethanol exposure in utero, may be mediated by the repressive impact of ethanol on the DNA methyltransferases.
3. Both abnormal gain of methylation, as in the case of fragile X syndrome, and abnormal loss of methylation, as in the case of facioscapulohumeral muscular dystrophy, can produce disease phenotypes.
4. As twins age, they demonstrate increasing differences in methylation patterns of their DNA sequences, causing increasing numbers of phenotypic differences.
5. In studies of twins with significant lifestyle differences (e.g., smoking versus nonsmoking) large numbers of differences in their methylation patterns are observed to accrue over time.

Epigenetics and Cancer

1. The best evidence for epigenetic effects on human disease risk comes from studies of cancer.
2. Methylation densities decline as tumours progress, which can increase the activity of oncogenes, causing tumours to progress from benign neoplasms to malignancy. Additionally, the promoter regions of tumour-suppressor genes are often hypermethylated. These elevated methylation levels decrease their rate of transcription at these critical genes, thus reducing the ability to inhibit tumour formation.
3. Hypermethylation also is seen in miRNA genes and is associated with tumourigenesis.
4. Unlike DNA sequence mutations, epigenetic modifications can be reversed through pharmaceutical intervention. For example, 5-azacytidine, a demethylating agent, has been used as a therapeutic drug in the treatment of leukemia and myelodysplastic syndrome.

Future Directions

1. Robust experimental observations are defining the roles of epigenetic states in shaping cell fates.
2. The well-documented involvement of epigenetic abnormalities in carcinogenesis and the mounting evidence for these epigenetic changes in other common diseases (discussed throughout the text) will likely elucidate new therapies with the possibilities of reversing the epigenetic abnormalities.

4

Altered Cellular and Tissue Biology

Stephanie Zettel, with originating chapter contributions by Kathryn L. McCance and Lois E. Brenneman

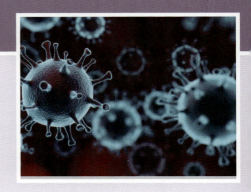

Additional resources are available online at http://evolve.elsevier.com/Canada/Huether/pathophysiology

CHAPTER OUTLINE

Cellular Adaptation, 73
- Atrophy, 73
- Hypertrophy, 74
- Hyperplasia, 76
- Dysplasia: Not a True Adaptive Change, 76
- Metaplasia, 77

Cellular Injury, 77
- General Mechanisms of Cellular Injury, 78
- Unintentional and Intentional Injuries, 92
- Infectious Injury, 95
- Immunological and Inflammatory Injury, 95

Manifestations of Cellular Injury: Accumulations, 95
- Water, 95
- Lipids and Carbohydrates, 95
- Glycogen, 97
- Proteins, 97

Pigments, 97
Calcium, 99
Urate, 100
Systemic Manifestations, 100

Cellular Death, 100
- Necrosis, 101
- Apoptosis, 103
- Autophagy, 105

Aging and Altered Cellular and Tissue Biology, 106
- Normal Lifespan, Life Expectancy, and Quality-Adjusted Life Year, 107
- Degenerative Extracellular Changes, 107
- Cellular Aging, 107
- Tissue and Systemic Aging, 108
- Frailty, 108

Somatic Death, 108
CASE STUDY, 109

LEARNING OBJECTIVES

1. Describe the cellular adaptations made in each of the following processes: atrophy, hypertrophy, hyperplasia, dysplasia, and metaplasia.
2. Discuss causative factors of each of the above cellular adaptations.
3. Identify the most common cause of cellular injury.
4. Describe the mechanism of cellular injury that can occur because of: hypoxia, free radicals, and reactive oxygen species.
5. Describe cellular injury caused by physical trauma such as blunt force trauma, abrasions, lacerations, and gunshots.
6. Describe cellular injury caused by infection and inflammation.
7. Describe the major mechanism of tissue damage caused by chemical injury.
8. Discuss the importance of alcoholism.
9. Discuss unintentional vs. intentional injuries.
10. Discuss the manifestations of cellular injury, including hydropic changes, protein, lipid and carbohydrate alterations, pigment changes, and electrolyte changes.
11. Discuss the manifestations of cellular death, including the four major types of necrosis, and give examples of the tissue types affected by each type of necrosis.
12. Discuss apoptosis.
13. Discuss the cellular mechanisms of normal degenerative changes of aging.
14. Discuss the types of tissue necrosis.
15. Identify the clinical manifestations of somatic death.

KEY TERMS

Adaptation, 73
Aging, 106
Algor mortis, 108
Anoxia, 79
Anthropogenic, 92
Apoptosis, 101
Asphyxial injuries, 92
Atrophy, 73
Autolysis, 101

Autophagic vacuole, 74
Autophagy, 105
Bilirubin, 99
Carbon monoxide (CO), 87
Carboxyhemoglobin, 88
Caseous necrosis, 102
Caspase, 105
Cellular accumulations (infiltrations), 95

Cellular swelling, 95
Chemical asphyxiant, 94
Choking asphyxiation, 92
Coagulative necrosis, 102
Compensatory hyperplasia, 76
Cyanide, 94
Cytochrome, 98
Disuse atrophy, 74
Drowning, 94

Dry-lung drowning, 94
Dysplasia (atypical hyperplasia), 76
Dystrophic calcification, 99
Electrophile, 84
ER stress, 104
Ethanol, 88
Fat-free mass (FFM), 108
Fatty change (steatosis), 96

CHAPTER 4 Altered Cellular and Tissue Biology

Fatty necrosis, 102
Fetal alcohol spectrum disorder, 91
Frailty, 108
Free radical, 81
Gangrenous necrosis, 102
Gas gangrene, 103
Hanging strangulation, 94
Hemoprotein, 98
Hemosiderin, 98
Hemosiderosis, 99
Hormonal hyperplasia, 76
Hydrogen sulphide, 94
Hyperplasia, 76
Hypertrophy, 74
Hypoxia, 78
Hypoxia-inducible transcription factor (HIF), 79
Infarct, 102
Irreversible injury, 77
Ischemia, 79
Ischemia-reperfusion injury, 81
Karyolysis, 101
Karyorrhexis, 101
Lead (Pb), 86
Life expectancy, 107
Lifespan, 106
Ligature strangulation, 94
Lipid peroxidation, 82
Lipofuscin, 74
Liquefactive necrosis, 102
Livor mortis, 108
Manual strangulation, 94
Maximal lifespan, 107
Melanin, 97
Mesenchymal (tissue from embryonic mesoderm) cell, 77
Metaplasia, 77
Metastatic calcification, 100
Mitochondrial DNA (mtDNA), 108
Necrosis, 101
Nucleophile, 84
Oncosis (vacuolar degeneration), 95
Oxidative stress, 81
Pathological atrophy, 73
Pathological hyperplasia, 76
Physiological atrophy, 73
Postmortem autolysis, 109
Postmortem change, 108
Programmed necrosis (necroptosis), 101
Proteasome, 74
Protein adduct, 84
Psammoma bodies, 100
Pyknosis, 101
Quality-adjusted life year (QALY), 107
Reperfusion injury, 81
Reversible injury, 77
Rigor mortis, 109
Sarcopenia, 108
Somatic death, 108
Strangulation, 92
Suffocation, 92
Toxicophore, 84
Ubiquitin, 74
Ubiquitin–proteasome pathway, 74
Urate, 100
Vacuolation, 80
Xenobiotic, 83

Diseases are generally *multifactorial* in nature. Injury to cells and their surrounding environment, called the *extracellular matrix* (ECM), leads to tissue and organ injury. A narrow range of structure and functions, including metabolism and specialization, restricts the normal cell; however, it can *adapt* to physiological demands or stress to maintain a steady state called *homeostasis*. When one organ system is damaged, multiple organ systems adapt to maintain this homeostasis through the process of *allostasis*. **Adaptation** is a reversible structural or functional response both to normal or physiological conditions and to adverse or pathological conditions. For example, the uterus adapts to pregnancy—a normal physiological state—by enlarging. Enlargement occurs because of an increase in the size and number of uterine cells. Adverse conditions such as high blood pressure (hypertension) stimulate myocardial cells to enlarge to accommodate the increased work of pumping. Like most of the body's adaptive mechanisms, however, cellular adaptations to adverse conditions are usually only temporarily successful. Severe or long-term stressors overwhelm adaptive processes, and cellular injury or death is the result. Adaptation, injury, neoplasia, accumulations, aging, and death are all mechanisms that alter cellular and tissue biology. (Neoplasia is discussed in Chapters 10 and 11.)

Knowledge of the structural and functional reactions of cells and tissues to injurious agents, including genetic defects, is vital to understanding disease processes. Any factor that disrupts cellular structures or deprives the cell of oxygen and nutrients required for survival can cause cellular injury. Injury may be reversible (*sublethal*) or irreversible (*lethal*) and is classified broadly as chemical, hypoxic (lack of sufficient oxygen), free radical, intentional, unintentional, immunological, infection, and inflammatory. Cellular injuries from various causes have different clinical and pathophysiological manifestations. Stresses from metabolic derangements may be associated with intracellular *accumulations* and include carbohydrates, proteins, and lipids. Sites of cellular death can cause accumulations of calcium resulting in *pathological calcification*. Examination of cells with particular staining patterns can actually confirm structural changes that lead to cellular death. The two main types of cellular death are *necrosis* and *apoptosis*, and nutrient deprivation can initiate *autophagy* that results in cellular death. This chapter includes a discussion of pathways of cellular death.

Cellular aging causes structural and functional changes that eventually may lead to cellular death or a decreased capacity to recover from injury. There is still much to learn about the aging process, and distinguishing between pathological changes and physiological changes that occur with aging is often difficult. Aging clearly causes alterations in cellular structure and function, yet *senescence*, growing old, is both inevitable and normal.

CELLULAR ADAPTATION

Cells adapt to their environment to escape and protect themselves from injury. An adapted cell is neither normal nor injured; its condition lies somewhere between these two states. Adaptations are reversible changes in cell size, number, phenotype, metabolic activity, or functions of cells.[1] Adaptive responses have limits, however, and additional cell stresses can affect essential cell function leading to *cellular injury*. Cellular adaptations also can be a common and central part of many disease states. In the early stages of a successful adaptive response, cells may have enhanced function, making it hard to distinguish between a pathological response and an extreme adaptation to an excessive functional demand. The most significant adaptive changes in cells include atrophy (decrease in cell size), hypertrophy (increase in cell size), hyperplasia (increase in cell number), and metaplasia (reversible replacement of one mature cell type by another less mature cell type or a change in the phenotype). Dysplasia (deranged cellular growth) is not a true cellular adaptation but rather an atypical hyperplasia. These changes are in Figure 4.1.

Atrophy

Atrophy is a decrease or shrinkage in cellular size. If atrophy occurs in a sufficient number of an organ's cells, the entire organ shrinks or becomes atrophic. Atrophy can affect any organ, but it is most common in skeletal muscle, the heart, secondary sex organs, and the brain. Atrophy is *physiological* or *pathological*. **Physiological atrophy** occurs with early development. For example, the thymus gland undergoes physiological atrophy during childhood. **Pathological atrophy** occurs because of decreases in workload, pressure, use, blood supply, nutrition, hormonal stimulation, and nervous system stimulation (Figure 4.2).

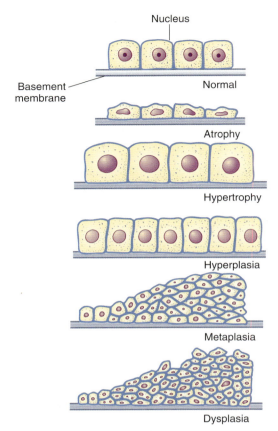

FIGURE 4.1 Adaptive and Dysplastic Alterations in Simple Cuboidal Epithelial cells.

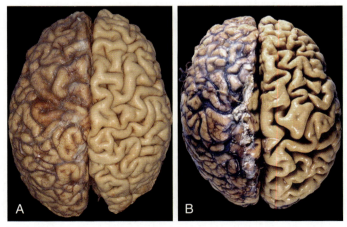

FIGURE 4.2 Atrophy. A, Normal brain of a young adult. B, Atrophy of the brain in an 82-year-old male with atherosclerotic cerebrovascular disease, resulting in reduced blood supply. Note that loss of brain substance narrows the gyri and widens the sulci. The meninges have been stripped from the right half of each specimen to reveal the surface of the brain. (From Kumar, V., Abbas, A. K., & Aster, J. C. [Eds.]. [2021]. *Robbins and Cotran pathologic basis of disease* [10th ed.]. Elsevier.)

Individuals immobilized in bed for a prolonged period of time exhibit a type of skeletal muscle atrophy called **disuse atrophy**. Aging causes brain cells to become atrophic and endocrine-dependent organs, such as the gonads, to shrink as hormonal stimulation decreases. Whether atrophy results from normal physiological conditions or by pathological conditions, atrophic cells exhibit the same basic changes.

The atrophic muscle cell contains less endoplasmic reticulum (ER) and fewer mitochondria and myofilaments (part of the muscle fibre that controls contraction) than found in the normal cell. There is an immediate reduction of oxygen consumption and amino acid uptake in muscular atrophy caused by nerve loss. The mechanisms of atrophy include decreased protein synthesis, increased protein catabolism, or both. *Ribosome biogenesis*, or the synthesis of ribosomes, may also play a role. Growth and division of the cell depend on ribosome function and its ability to convert mRNA into protein. Ribosome biogenesis is a tightly regulated process involving upwards of 200 different proteins that relies on a number of factors in both the external and internal environment of the cell.[2] The primary pathway of protein catabolism is the **ubiquitin–proteasome pathway**, and catabolism involves **proteasomes** (protein-degrading complexes). Proteins degraded in this pathway are first conjugated to **ubiquitin** (another small protein) and then degraded by proteasomes. An increase in proteasome activity is characteristic of atrophic muscle changes. Deregulation of this pathway often leads to abnormal cell growth and is associated with cancer and other diseases (see Chapters 3 and 10).

Atrophy resulting from chronic malnutrition is often accompanied by a "self-eating" process called *autophagy* that creates **autophagic vacuoles**. These vacuoles are membrane-bound vesicles within the cell that contain cellular debris and hydrolytic enzymes, which function to break down substances to the simplest units of fat, carbohydrate, or protein. The levels of hydrolytic enzymes rise rapidly in atrophy. The enzymes are isolated in autophagic vacuoles to prevent uncontrolled cellular destruction. Thus, the vacuoles form as needed in order to protect uninjured organelles from the injured organelles and are eventually engulfed and destroyed by lysosomes. Certain contents of the autophagic vacuole may resist destruction by lysosomal enzymes and persist in membrane-bound residual bodies. An example of granules that can persist and resist breakdown is granules containing **lipofuscin**, the yellow-brown age pigment. Lipofuscin accumulates primarily in liver cells, myocardial cells, and atrophic cells.

Hypertrophy

Hypertrophy is a compensatory increase in the size of cells in response to mechanical stimuli (also called *mechanical load* or *stress*, such as from repetitive stretching, chronic pressure, or volume overload) and consequently increases the size of the affected organ (Figures 4.3 and 4.4). The cells of the heart and kidneys are particularly prone to enlargement. Hypertrophy, as an adaptive response (muscular enlargement), occurs in the striated muscle cells of both the heart and skeletal muscles. Dilation of the cardiac chambers initially causes cardiac enlargement, which triggers an increased synthesis of cardiac muscle proteins, allowing muscle fibres to do more work. The increased accumulation of protein in the cellular components (plasma membrane, ER, myofilaments, mitochondria) accounts for the increase in cellular size, *not* an increase in cellular fluid. Yet, individual protein pools may expand or shrink.[3] Cardiac hypertrophy involves changes in signaling and transcription factor pathways resulting in increased protein synthesis, and this leads to left ventricular hypertrophy (LVH). Emerging evidence suggests that the ubiquitin–proteasome system (UPS) not only attends to damaged, misfolded, or mutant proteins by protein breakdown but also may attend to cell growth, eventually leading to LVH.[4] ECM remodeling and increased growth of adult myocytes characterizes cardiac hypertrophy over time. The myocytes progressively increase in size and reach a limit beyond which no further hypertrophy can occur (see Chapter 24).[5,6]

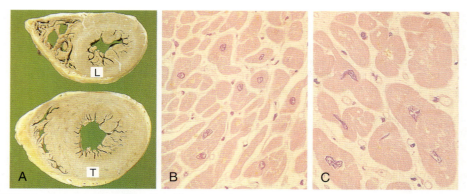

FIGURE 4.3 Hypertrophy of Cardiac Muscle in Response to Valve Disease. **A,** Transverse slices of a normal heart and a heart with hypertrophy of the left ventricle (*L,* normal thickness of left ventricular wall; *T,* thickened wall from heart in which severe narrowing of aortic valve caused resistance to systolic ventricular emptying). **B,** Histology of cardiac muscle from the normal heart. **C,** Histology of cardiac muscle from a hypertrophied heart. (From Stevens, A., & Lowe, J. [2000]. *Pathology: Illustrated review in color* [2nd ed.]. Mosby.)

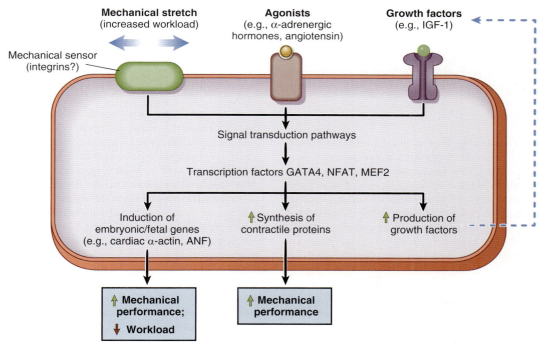

FIGURE 4.4 Mechanisms of Myocardial Hypertrophy. Mechanical sensors appear to be the main stimulators for physiological hypertrophy. Other stimuli possibly more important for pathological hypertrophy include agonists (initiators) and growth factors. These factors then signal transcription pathways whereby transcription factors then bind to DNA sequences, activating muscle proteins that are responsible for hypertrophy. These pathways include induction of embryonic/fetal genes, increased synthesis of contractile proteins, and production of growth factors. *ANF,* Atrial natriuretic factor; *GATA4,* a transcription factor that regulates genes with the DNA "GATA" sequence; *IGF-1,* insulinlike growth factor 1; *MEF2,* myocyte enhancer factor-2; *NFAT,* nuclear factor of activated T-cells. (Adapted from Kumar, V., Abbas, A. K., & Aster, J. C. [Eds.]. [2021]. *Robbins and Cotran pathologic basis of disease* [10th ed.]. Elsevier.)

As such, time may be the critical factor or determinant of the transition from physiological to pathological cardiac hypertrophy. Myocardial structure and function remain intact with *physical hypertrophy,* despite increased workload of the heart. Examples of physical hypertrophy include normal growth and development, moderate endurance exercise training, pregnancy, and the early phases of increased pressure and volume loading on the adult human heart. This physiological response is temporary. *Pathological hypertrophy* in the heart is associated with structural AND functional changes to the heart. Pathological hypertrophy is also secondary to hypertension, coronary heart disease, or problem valves, and is presumably a key risk factor for heart failure. Similarly, aging, strenuous exercise, and sustained workload or stress can lead to these same structural and functional manifestations. Increased interstitial fibrosis, cellular death, and abnormal cardiac function often are the results of this process (see Figure 4.3). Although the progression of pathological cardiac hypertrophy seems to be irreversible, emerging data from experimental studies and clinical observations indicate that it is possible to reverse this process in certain cases. Normalizing the increased wall stress can actually reverse the hypertrophy in a process termed *regression*.[7] For example, unloading of hemodynamic stress by a left ventricular assist device (used in individuals with heart failure for bridging to heart transplantation) induces regression of cardiac hypertrophy and improvement of left ventricular function in those with end-stage heart failure.[8] Regression of cardiac hypertrophy is accompanied by activation of unique sets of genes, including fetal-type genes and those involved in protein degradation.[9,10] Improvement in new blood vessel development (angiogenesis) in the hypertrophic heart can lead to regression of the hypertrophy and prevention of heart failure.[11,12] In mice, dietary supplementation of physiologically relevant levels of copper can reverse pathological cardiac hypertrophy.[12,13]

When a diseased kidney is removed, the remaining kidney adapts to the increased workload with an increase in both the size and the number of cells. The major contributing factor to this renal enlargement is hypertrophy. Another example of normal or physiological hypertrophy is the increased growth of the uterus and mammary glands in response to pregnancy.

Hyperplasia

Hyperplasia is an increase in the number of cells, resulting from an increased rate of cellular division. Hyperplasia, as a response to injury, occurs when the injury has been severe and prolonged enough to have caused cellular death. Loss of epithelial, liver, and kidney cells triggers deoxyribonucleic acid (DNA) synthesis and mitotic division. Increased cell growth is a multistep process involving the production of growth factors, which stimulate the remaining cells to synthesize new cell components and, ultimately, to divide. Hyperplasia and hypertrophy often occur together, and both take place if the cells can synthesize DNA.

Two types of normal, or physiological, hyperplasia are compensatory hyperplasia and hormonal hyperplasia. Compensatory hyperplasia is an adaptive mechanism that enables certain organs to regenerate. For example, removal of part of the liver leads to hyperplasia of the remaining liver cells (hepatocytes) to compensate for the loss. Even with removal of 70% of the liver, regeneration is complete in about 2 weeks. Several growth factors and cytokines (chemical messengers) are induced and play critical roles in liver regeneration.

Not all types of mature cells have the same capacity for compensatory hyperplastic growth. Nondividing tissues contain cells that can no longer (i.e., postnatally) go through the cell cycle and undergo mitotic division. These highly specialized cells, for example, neurons and skeletal muscle cells, never divide again once they have differentiated—that is, they are *terminally differentiated*.[14] In human cells, cell growth and cell division depend on signals from other cells; but cell growth, unlike cell division, does not depend on the cell-cycle control system.[14] Nerve cells and most muscle cells do most of their growing after they have terminally differentiated and permanently ceased dividing.[14] Significant compensatory hyperplasia occurs in epidermal and intestinal epithelia, hepatocytes, bone marrow cells, and fibroblasts; and some hyperplasia is noted in bone, cartilage, and smooth muscle cells. Another example of compensatory hyperplasia is the callus, or thickening, of the skin because of hyperplasia of epidermal cells in response to a mechanical stimulus.

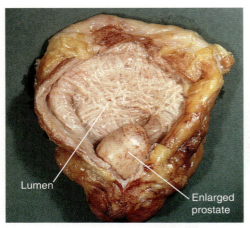

FIGURE 4.5 Hyperplasia of the Prostate with Secondary Thickening of the Obstructed Urinary Bladder (Bladder Cross-Section). The enlarged prostate is protruding into the lumen of the bladder, which appears trabeculated. These "trabeculae" result from hypertrophy and hyperplasia of smooth muscle cells that occur in response to increased intravesical pressure caused by urinary obstruction. (From Damjanov, I. [2012]. *Pathology for the health professions* [4th ed.]. Saunders.)

Hormonal hyperplasia occurs chiefly in estrogen-dependent organs, such as the uterus and breast. After ovulation, for example, estrogen stimulates the endometrium to grow and thicken in preparation for receiving the fertilized ovum. If pregnancy occurs, hormonal hyperplasia, as well as hypertrophy, enables the uterus to enlarge. (Hormone function is described in Chapters 19 and 33.)

Pathological hyperplasia is the abnormal proliferation of normal cells, usually in response to excessive hormonal stimulation or growth factors on target cells (Figure 4.5). The most common example is pathological hyperplasia of the endometrium (caused by an imbalance between estrogen and progesterone secretion, with oversecretion of estrogen) (see Chapter 33). Pathological endometrial hyperplasia, which causes excessive menstrual bleeding, is under the influence of regular growth-inhibition controls. If these controls fail, hyperplastic endometrial cells can undergo malignant transformation. Benign prostatic hyperplasia is another example of pathological hyperplasia and results from changes in hormone balance. In both of these examples, if the hormonal imbalance is corrected, hyperplasia regresses.[1]

Dysplasia: Not a True Adaptive Change

Dysplasia refers to abnormal changes in the size, shape, and organization of mature cells (Figure 4.6). Dysplasia is not a true adaptive process but is similar to hyperplasia and is atypical hyperplasia. Dysplastic changes often occur in epithelial tissue of the cervix and respiratory tract, where they are strongly associated with common neoplastic growths and are often adjacent to cancerous cells. Importantly, however, the term *dysplasia* does *not* indicate cancer and may not progress to cancer. Dysplasia can be mild, moderate, or severe; yet, because this classification scheme is somewhat subjective, it has prompted some to recommend the use of either "low grade" or "high grade" instead. If the inciting stimulus is removed, dysplastic changes often are reversible. (Dysplasia is discussed further in Chapter 10.)

CHAPTER 4 Altered Cellular and Tissue Biology

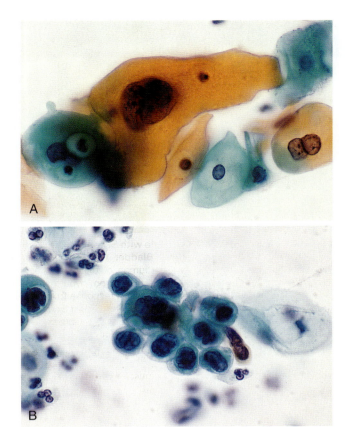

FIGURE 4.6 Dysplasia of the Uterine Cervix. **A,** Mild dysplasia. **B,** Severe dysplasia. (From Damjanov, I., & Linder, J. [1996]. *Anderson's pathology* [10th ed.]. Mosby.)

Metaplasia

Metaplasia is the reversible replacement of one mature cell type (epithelial or mesenchymal) by another, sometimes less differentiated, cell type. It develops (as an adaptive response better suited to withstand the adverse environment) from a reprogramming of stem cells that exist on most epithelia or of undifferentiated mesenchymal (tissue from embryonic mesoderm) cells present in connective tissue. These precursor cells mature along a new pathway because of signals generated by growth factors in the cell's environment. The best example of metaplasia is replacement of normal columnar ciliated epithelial cells of the bronchial (airway) lining by stratified squamous epithelial cells (Figure 4.7). The newly formed cells do not secrete mucus or have cilia and cause a loss of a vital protective mechanism. Bronchial metaplasia can be reversed if the inducing stimulus, usually cigarette smoking, is removed. With prolonged exposure to the inducing stimulus, however, dysplasia and cancerous transformation can occur.

CELLULAR INJURY

> ✓ **QUICK CHECK 4.1**
> 1. When does a cell become irreversibly injured? How would you know?
> 2. Describe the pathogenesis of hypoxic injury.
> 3. What are the mechanisms of ischemia-reperfusion injury?

Injury to cells and to the ECM leads to injury of tissues and organs, ultimately determining the structural patterns of disease. Loss of function comes from cell and ECM injury and cellular death. Cellular injury occurs if the cell is unable to maintain allostasis—a normal or adaptive steady state—in the face of injurious stimuli or stress. Injured cells may recover (reversible injury) or die (irreversible injury). Injurious stimuli include chemical agents, lack of sufficient oxygen (hypoxia), free radicals, infectious agents, physical and mechanical factors, immunological reactions, genetic factors, and nutritional imbalances. Table 4.1 and Figure 4.8 summarize the types of injuries and their responses.

The extent of cellular injury depends on the type, state (including level of cell differentiation and increased susceptibility to fully differentiated cells), and adaptive processes of the cell, as well as the type, severity, and duration of the harmful stimulus. Two individuals exposed to an identical stimulus may incur varying degrees of cellular

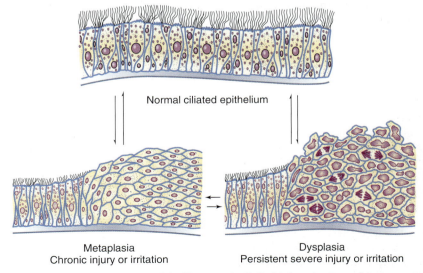

FIGURE 4.7 Reversible Changes in Cells Lining the Bronchi.

TABLE 4.1 Types of Progressive Cellular Injury and Responses

Type	Responses
Adaptation	Atrophy, hypertrophy, hyperplasia, metaplasia
Active cellular injury	Immediate response of "entire" cell
Reversible	Loss of ATP, cellular swelling, detachment of ribosomes, autophagy of lysosomes
Irreversible	"Point-of-no-return" structurally when severe vacuolization of mitochondria occurs and Ca^{++} moves into cell
Necrosis	Common type of cellular death with severe cell swelling and breakdown of organelles
Apoptosis, or programmed cellular death	Cellular self-destruction for elimination of unwanted cell populations
Autophagy	Eating of self, cytoplasmic vesicles engulf cytoplasm and organelles, recycling factory
Chronic cellular injury (subcellular alterations)	Persistent stimuli response may involve only specific organelles or cytoskeleton (e.g., phagocytosis of bacteria)
Accumulations or infiltrations	Water, pigments, lipids, glycogen, proteins
Pathological calcification	Dystrophic and metastatic calcification

ATP, Adenosine triphosphate; *Ca^{++}*, calcium.

TABLE 4.2 Common Mechanisms in Cellular Injury and Cellular Death

Mechanism	Comments
ATP depletion	Loss of mitochondrial ATP and decreased ATP synthesis; results include cellular swelling, decreased protein synthesis, decreased membrane transport, and lipogenesis, all changes that contribute to loss of integrity of plasma membrane
Reactive oxygen species (↑ROS)	Lack of oxygen is key in progression of cellular injury in ischemia (reduced blood supply); activated oxygen species (ROS, $O_2^{\bullet-}$, H_2O_2, $\bullet OH$) cause destruction of cell membranes and cell structure
Ca^{++} entry	Normally intracellular cytosolic calcium concentrations are very low; ischemia and certain chemicals cause an increase in cytosolic Ca^{++} concentrations; sustained levels of Ca^{++} continue to increase with damage to plasma membrane; Ca^{++} causes intracellular damage by activating a number of enzymes
Mitochondrial damage	Can be damaged by increases in cytosolic Ca^{++}, ROS; two outcomes of mitochondrial damage are loss of membrane potential, which causes depletion of ATP and eventual death or necrosis of cell, and activation of another type of cellular death (apoptosis)
Membrane damage	Early loss of selective membrane permeability found in all forms of cellular injury, lysosomal membrane damage with release of enzymes causing cellular digestion
Protein misfolding, DNA damage	Proteins may misfold, triggering *unfolded protein response* that activates corrective responses; if overwhelmed, response activates cell suicide program or apoptosis; DNA damage (genotoxic stress) also can activate apoptosis

ATP, Adenosine triphosphate; *Ca^{++}*, calcium.

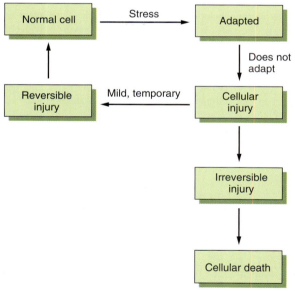

FIGURE 4.8 Stages of Cellular Adaptation, Injury, and Death. The normal cell responds to physiological and pathological stresses by adapting (atrophy, hypertrophy, hyperplasia, and metaplasia). Cellular injury occurs if the adaptive responses are exceeded or compromised by injurious agents, stress, and mutations. The injury is reversible if it is mild or transient, but if the stimulus persists, the cell suffers irreversible injury and eventually death.

General Mechanisms of Cellular Injury

The biochemical mechanisms involved with cellular injury and death are common to every cell, regardless of the injuring agent. These include adenosine triphosphate (ATP) depletion, mitochondrial damage, oxygen and oxygen-derived free radical membrane damage (depletion of ATP), protein folding defects, DNA damage defects, and calcium-level alterations (Table 4.2). Examples of common forms of cellular injury are (1) hypoxic injury, (2) free radicals and reactive oxygen species injury, and (3) chemical injury.

Hypoxic Injury

Hypoxia, or lack of sufficient oxygen within cells, is the single most common cause of cellular injury (Figure 4.9). Hypoxia can result from a reduced amount of oxygen in the air, loss of hemoglobin or decreased efficacy of hemoglobin, decreased production of red blood cells, diseases of the respiratory and cardiovascular systems, and poisoning of the oxidative enzymes (cytochromes) within the cells. Hypoxia plays a role in physiological processes including cell differentiation, angiogenesis, proliferation, erythropoiesis, and overall cell viability.[15] The main consumers of oxygen are mitochondria, and the production of reactive oxygen species (ROS) at the mitochondrial complex III mediates cellular responses to hypoxia.[15] ROS are also possible hypoxia signalling molecules.

injury. Modifying factors such as nutritional status can profoundly influence the extent of injury. The precise "point of no return" that leads to cellular death is a biochemical puzzle, but once changes to the nucleus occur and cell membranes are disrupted, the cell moves to irreversible injury and death.

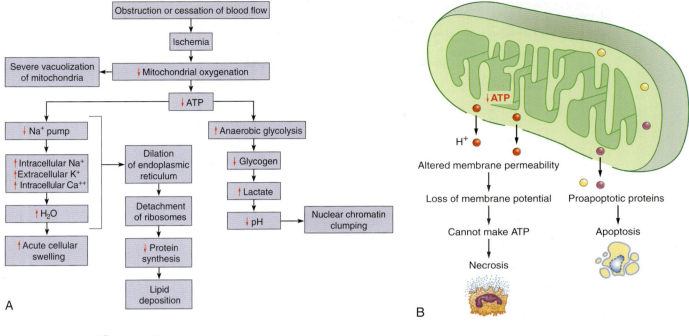
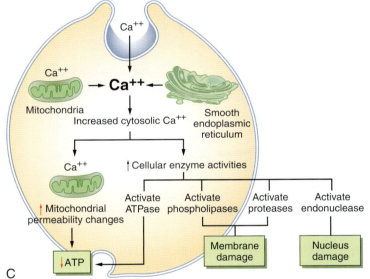

FIGURE 4.9 Hypoxic Injury Induced by Ischemia. A, Consequences of decreased oxygen delivery or ischemia with decreased adenosine triphosphate (ATP). The structural and physiological changes are reversible if oxygen (H_2O) is delivered quickly. Significant decreases in ATP result in cellular death, mostly by necrosis. B, Mitochondrial damage can result in changes in membrane permeability, loss of membrane potential, and decrease in ATP concentration. Between the outer and inner membranes of the mitochondria are proteins that can activate the cell's suicide pathways, called apoptosis. C, Calcium ions (Ca^{++}) are critical mediators of cellular injury. Ca^{++} are usually maintained at low concentrations in the cell's cytoplasm; thus, ischemia and certain toxins can initially cause an increase in the release of Ca^{++} from intracellular stores and later an increased movement (influx) across the plasma membrane. (Adapted from Kumar, V., Abbas, A. K., & Aster, J. C. [Eds.]. [2015]. *Robbins and Cotran pathologic basis of disease* [9th ed.]. Saunders.)

More commonly, hypoxia occurs with pathophysiological conditions such as inflammation, ischemia, and cancer. Hypoxia can induce inflammation, and inflamed lesions can become hypoxic (Figure 4.10).[16] Some cellular mechanisms involved in hypoxia and inflammation include activation of immune responses and oxygen-sensing compounds called *prolyl hydroxylases* (PHDs) and **hypoxia-inducible transcription factor (HIF)**. HIF is a family of transcription regulators that coordinate the expression of many genes in response to oxygen deprivation. Interestingly, mammalian development occurs in a hypoxic environment.[17] Hypoxia-induced signalling involves complicated cross-talk between hypoxia and inflammation, linking hypoxia and inflammation to inflammatory bowel disease, certain cancers, and infections.[16] Research is ongoing to understand the mechanisms of how tumours adapt to low oxygen levels by inducing angiogenesis, increasing glucose consumption, and promoting the metabolic state of glycolysis (see Chapter 10).[18]

The most common cause of hypoxia is **ischemia** (reduced blood supply). Common causes of ischemic injury include gradual narrowing of **arteries** (arteriosclerosis) or complete blockage by blood clots (thrombosis), or both. Progressive hypoxia caused by gradual arterial obstruction results in less severe outcomes than the acute **anoxia** (total lack of oxygen) caused by a sudden obstruction, as with an embolus (a blood clot or other blockage in the circulation). An acute obstruction in a coronary artery can cause myocardial cellular death (infarction) within minutes if the blood supply does not return, whereas the gradual onset of ischemia usually results in myocardial adaptation. Myocardial infarction and stroke, which are common causes of death in North America, generally result from atherosclerosis (a type of arteriosclerosis) and consequent ischemic injury. (Vascular obstruction is discussed in Chapter 24.)

Studies of the heart muscle have demonstrated cellular responses to hypoxic injury caused by ischemia. Within 1 minute after blood supply

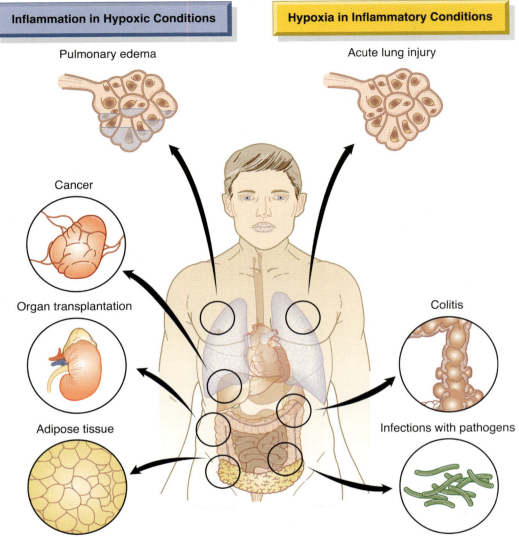

FIGURE 4.10 Hypoxia and Inflammation. Shown is a simplified drawing of clinical conditions characterized by tissue hypoxia that causes inflammatory changes *(left)* and inflammatory diseases that ultimately lead to hypoxia *(right)*. These diseases and conditions are discussed in more detail in their respective chapters. (From Eltzschig, H. K., & Carmeliet, P. [2011]. Hypoxia and inflammation. *The New England Journal of Medicine, 364,* 656–665. Reprinted with permission from Massachusetts Medical Society.)

to the myocardium stops, the heart becomes pale and has difficulty contracting normally. Within 3 to 5 minutes, the ischemic portion of the myocardium ceases to contract because of a rapid decrease in mitochondrial phosphorylation and consequent decreased ATP production. Lack of ATP leads to increased anaerobic metabolism, which generates ATP from glycogen when there is insufficient oxygen. When glycogen stores are depleted, even anaerobic metabolism ceases.

A reduction in ATP levels causes the plasma membrane's sodium–potassium (Na^+–K^+) pump and sodium–calcium exchange mechanism to fail, which leads to an intracellular accumulation of sodium and calcium and diffusion of potassium out of the cell. Sodium and water then can enter the cell freely, and cellular swelling, as well as early dilation of the ER, results. Dilation causes the ribosomes to detach from the rough ER, reducing protein synthesis. With continued hypoxia, the entire cell swells, with increased concentrations of sodium, water, and chloride and decreased concentrations of potassium. These disruptions are reversible if oxygen is restored. If oxygen is not restored, however, vacuolation (formation of vacuoles) occurs within the cytoplasm and swelling of lysosomes and marked mitochondrial swelling result from damage to the outer membrane. Continued hypoxic injury with accumulation of calcium subsequently activates multiple enzyme systems, resulting in membrane damage, cytoskeleton disruption, DNA and chromatin degradation, ATP depletion, and eventual cellular death (Figure 4.9C). Structurally, with plasma membrane damage, extracellular calcium readily moves into the cell and intracellular calcium stores escape. Increased intracellular calcium levels further activate cell enzymes (caspases) that promote cellular death by apoptosis. Persistent ischemia is associated with irreversible injury and necrosis. Irreversible injury is associated structurally with severe swelling of the mitochondria, severe damage to plasma membranes, and swelling of lysosomes. Overall, death due to ischemia is mainly by necrosis but apoptosis may also contribute through activation of cell enzymes (as above).[1]

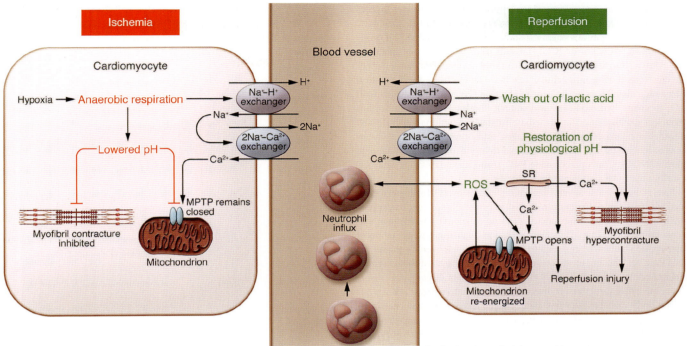

FIGURE 4.11 Reperfusion Injury. Without oxygen, or anoxia, the cells display hypoxic injury and become swollen. With reoxygenation, reperfusion injury increases because of the formation of reactive oxygen radicals that can cause cell necrosis. (Hausenly, D.J. & Yellon, D.M. [2013]. Myocardial-ischemia reperfusion injury: A neglected therapeutic target. *Journal of Clinical Investigation, 123*[1], 92–100.)

Restoration of blood flow and oxygen, however, can cause additional injury called **ischemia-reperfusion injury** (Figure 4.11). Ischemia-reperfusion injury is very important clinically because it is associated with tissue damage during myocardial and cerebral infarction. Several mechanisms for ischemia-reperfusion injury include:

- *Oxidative stress*—Reoxygenation causes the increased generation of ROS and nitrogen species.[1] These highly reactive oxygen intermediates (oxidative stress) include hydroxyl radical ($\cdot OH$), superoxide radical ($\cdot O_2^-$), and hydrogen peroxide (H_2O_2). The nitrogen species include nitric oxide (NO) generated by endothelial cells, macrophages, neurons, and other cells. These radicals can all cause further membrane damage and mitochondrial calcium overload. With **reperfusion injury**, neutrophils adhere more readily to the endothelium. Antioxidant treatment not only reverses neutrophil adhesion but also can reverse neutrophil-mediated heart injury. For example, one study of individuals undergoing elective percutaneous coronary intervention (PCI) showed that pretreatment with vitamin C was associated with less myocardial injury.[19] Similarly, the PREVEC Trial (prevention of reperfusion damage associated with percutaneous coronary angioplasty following acute myocardial infarction) seeks to evaluate whether vitamins C and E reduce infarct size in patients subjected to percutaneous coronary angioplasty after acute myocardial infarction.[20]
- *Increased intracellular calcium concentration*—Intracellular and mitochondrial calcium overload the cell during acute ischemia. Reperfusion causes even more calcium influx because of cell membrane damage and ROS-induced injury to the sarcoplasmic reticulum. The increased calcium increases mitochondrial permeability, eventually leading to depletion of ATP and further cellular injury.
- *Inflammation*—Ischemic injury increases inflammation because resident immune cells release danger signals (from cytokines) when cells die and this signalling initiates inflammation.
- *Complement activation*—The activation of complement may increase the tissue damage from reperfusion-ischemia injury.[1]

Free Radicals and Reactive Oxygen Species Injury: Oxidative Stress

An important mechanism of cellular injury is injury induced by free radicals, especially by ROS; this form of injury is **oxidative stress**. Oxidative stress occurs when *excess* ROS overwhelm endogenous antioxidant systems. A **free radical** is an electrically uncharged atom or group of atoms that has an unpaired electron. Having one unpaired electron makes the molecule unstable; the molecule becomes stabilized by either donating or accepting an electron from another molecule. When the attacked molecule loses its electron, it becomes a free radical. Therefore, it is capable of injurious chemical bond formation with proteins, lipids, and carbohydrates—key molecules in membranes and nucleic acids. Free radicals are difficult to control and initiate chain reactions. They are *highly* reactive because they have low chemical specificity, meaning that they can react with most molecules in their proximity. Oxidative stress can activate several intracellular signalling pathways because ROS can modulate enzymes and transcription factors. Oxidative stress is an important mechanism of cell damage in many conditions, including chemical and radiation injury, ischemia-reperfusion injury, cellular aging, and microbial killing by phagocytes, particularly neutrophils and macrophages.[1]

Free radicals develop within cells, first by the reduction–oxidation reactions (redox reactions) in normal metabolic processes such as respiration. Under normal physiological conditions, ROS serve as "redox messengers" in the regulation of intracellular signalling; however, excess ROS may produce irreversible damage to cellular components. All biological membranes contain redox systems, which also are important for cell defense (e.g., inflammation, iron uptake, growth and proliferation, and signal transduction). Second, absorption of extreme energy sources (e.g., ultraviolet light, radiation) produces free radicals. Third, enzymatic metabolism of exogenous chemicals or medications (e.g., CCl_3, a product of carbon tetrachloride [CCl_4]) results in the formation of free radicals. Fourth, transition metals (i.e., iron and copper) donate or accept free electrons during intracellular reactions and activate the formation of free radicals such as in the Fenton reaction (i.e., when they react with H_2O_2 to create hydroxyl ions and water). Finally, NO is an important colourless gas that is an intermediate in many reactions generated by endothelial cells, neurons, macrophages, and other cell types. NO can act as a free radical and can be converted to highly reactive peroxynitrite anion ($ONOO^-$), nitrogen dioxide (NO_2), and nitrate (NO_3^-). Table 4.3 describes the most significant free radicals.

Free radicals cause several damaging effects by (1) **lipid peroxidation**, which is the destruction of polyunsaturated lipids (the same process by which fats become rancid), leading to membrane damage and increased permeability; (2) protein alterations, causing fragmentation of polypeptide chains that can lead to loss and protein misfolding; and (3) DNA damage, causing mutations (Figure 4.12). Because of the increased understanding of free radicals, a growing number of diseases and disorders relate either directly or indirectly to these reactive species (Box 4.1).

The body can eliminate free radicals. The oxygen free radical, superoxide, may spontaneously decay into oxygen and hydrogen peroxide. Table 4.4 summarizes other methods that contribute to inactivation or termination of free radicals. The toxicity of certain medications and chemicals result from either conversion of these chemicals to free radicals or to the formation of oxygen-derived metabolites (see the following discussion).

Mitochondrial Effects
Mitochondria are key players in cellular injury and cellular death because they produce the life-sustaining energy of ATP. ROS and increases of cytosolic calcium ion (Ca^{++}) concentration can also damage mitochondria

TABLE 4.3 Free Radicals as Contributors to Oxidative Stress

Name	Formula	Characteristics
Hyperoxide/superoxide	$•O_2^-$	Highly unstable, signalling function, synaptic plasticity
Hydrogen peroxide	H_2O_2	Cell toxicity, signalling function, generation of other reactive oxygen species
Hydroxyl radical	$•OH$	Free radical, highly unstable, very reactive agent
Alkoxyl radical	$RO•$	Free radical, reaction product of lipids
Peroxyl radical	$ROO•$	Free radical, reaction product of lipids
Hypochlorite anion	OCl^-	Reactive oxygen species, reactive chlorine species, enzymatically generated by myeloperoxidase
Singlet oxygen	$^1O_2$	Induced/excited oxygen molecule, radical and nonradical form
Ozone	O_3	Environmental toxin
Nitric oxide	$•NO$	Environmental toxin, endogenous signal molecule
Peroxynitrite anion	$ONOO^-$	Highly reactive reaction intermediate of $•O_2$ and $•NO$
Nitrogen dioxide	$•NO_2$	Highly reactive radical, environmental toxin
Nitrogen oxides	NO_x	Environmental toxins, including NO and $•NO_2$, derived from the combustion process

From Oxidative stress and free radicals in COPD–implications and relevance for treatment. Domej W et al. International Journal of COPD 2014:9 1207–1224. Originally published by and used with permission from Dove Medical Press Ltd.

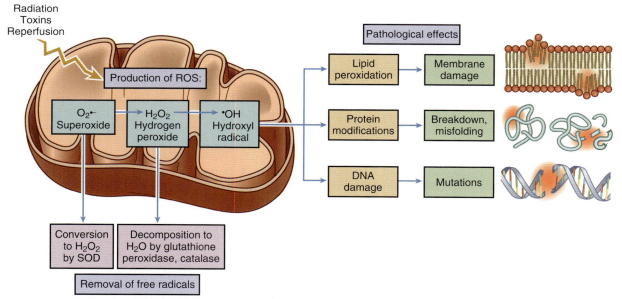

FIGURE 4.12 The Role of Reactive Oxygen Species in Cellular Injury. The production of reactive oxygen species (*ROS*) can be initiated by many cell stressors, such as radiation, toxins, and reperfusion of oxygen. Free radicals are removed by normal decay and enzymatic systems. ROS accumulate in cells because of insufficient removal or excess production leading to cellular injury, including lipid peroxidation, protein modifications, and DNA damage or mutations. *SOD*, Superoxide dismutase. (Adapted from Kumar, V., Abbas, A. K., & Aster, J. C. [Eds.]. [2021]. *Robbins and Cotran pathologic basis of disease* [10th ed.]. Elsevier.)

BOX 4.1 Diseases and Disorders Linked to Oxygen-Derived Free Radicals

Deterioration noted in aging
    Atherosclerosis
    Ischemic brain injury
    Alzheimer's disease
Neurotoxins
Cancer
Cardiac myopathy
Chronic granulomatous disease
Diabetes mellitus
    Eye disorders
        Macular degeneration
        Cataracts
Inflammatory disorders
Iron overload
Lung disorders
    Asbestosis
    Oxygen toxicity
    Emphysema
Nutritional deficiencies
Radiation injury
Reperfusion injury
Rheumatoid arthritis
Skin disorders
Toxic states
    Xenobiotics (CCl_4, paraquat, cigarette smoke, etc.)
    Metal irons (Ni, Cu, Fe, etc.)

BOX 4.2 Three Major Types and Consequences of Mitochondrial Damage

1. Damage to the mitochondria results in the formation of the *mitochondrial permeability transition pore*, a high-conductance channel or pore. The opening of this channel results in the loss of mitochondrial membrane potential, causing failure of oxidative phosphorylation, depletion of adenosine triphosphate, and damage to mitochondrial DNA, leading to necrosis of the cell.
2. Altered oxidative phosphorylation leads to the formation of reactive oxygen species that can damage cellular components.
3. Because mitochondria store several proteins between their membranes, increased permeability of the outer membrane may result in leakage of proapoptotic proteins and cause cellular death by apoptosis.

Data from Kumar, V., Abbas, A. K., & Aster, J. C. (Eds.). (2021). *Robbins and Cotran pathologic basis of disease* (10th ed.). Elsevier.

TABLE 4.4 Methods Contributing to Inactivation or Termination of Free Radicals

Method	Process
Antioxidants	Endogenous or exogenous; either blocks synthesis or inactivates (e.g., scavenges) free radicals; includes vitamin E, vitamin C, cysteine, glutathione, albumin, ceruloplasmin, transferrin, γ-lipoacid, others
Enzymes	Superoxide dismutase,[a] which converts superoxide to hydrogen peroxide (H_2O_2); catalase[a] (in peroxisomes) decomposes H_2O_2; glutathione peroxidase[a] decomposes hydroxyl radical (•OH) and H_2O_2

[a]These enzymes are important in modulating the cellular destructive effects of free radicals, also released in inflammation.

(see Figure 4.9). Box 4.2 summarizes the three major types of mitochondrial damage and their consequences. Currently, investigators are trying to identify the polypeptides (i.e., proteomes) directly involved in diseases associated with mitochondrial dysfunction. ROS not only damage proteins and mitochondria but also can promote damage in neighbouring cells. Furthermore, protein aggregates can increase mitochondrial damage and damaged mitochondria can induce even more protein damage. This happens with neuro-degeneration. An emerging area of research concerns mitochondrial DNA that escapes from autophagy, which may be a mechanism of tissue inflammation.[21]

Chemical or Toxic Injury

> **✓ QUICK CHECK 4.2**
> 1. Why are children more susceptible to the toxic effects of lead exposure?
> 2. Describe the sources of lead exposure.
> 3. Describe the mechanisms of cellular injury related to chronic alcoholism.
> 4. What are the sources of mercury exposure?

Mechanisms

Humans are constantly exposed to a variety of compounds termed **xenobiotics** (Greek *xenos*, "foreign"; *bios*, "life") that include toxic, mutagenic, and carcinogenic chemicals (Figure 4.13). Some of these chemicals are present in the human diet, for example, fungal

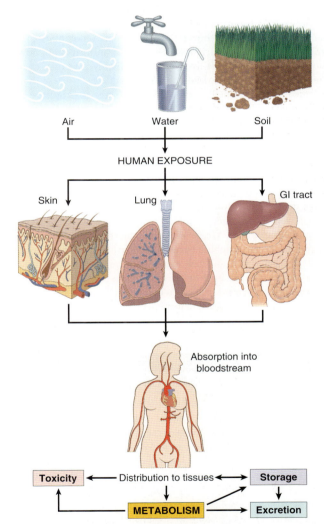

FIGURE 4.13 Human Exposure to Pollutants. Pollutants contained in air, water, and soil are absorbed through the lungs, gastro-intestinal (GI) tract, and skin. In the body, the pollutants may act at the site of absorption but are generally transported through the bloodstream to various organs where they can be stored or metabolized. Metabolism of xenobiotics may result in the formation of water-soluble compounds that are excreted, or a toxic metabolite may be created by activation of the agent. (From Kumar, V., Abbas, A. K., & Aster, J. C. [Eds.]. [2021]. *Robbins and Cotran pathologic basis of disease* [10th ed.]. Elsevier.)

mycotoxins such as aflatoxin B_1. Many xenobiotics are toxic to the liver (hepatotoxic). The liver is the initial site of contact for many ingested xenobiotics, medications, and alcohol, making this organ most susceptible to chemically induced injury. The toxicity of many chemicals results from absorption through the gastro-intestinal tract after oral ingestion. Certain dietary supplements (e.g., chaparral and ma-huang) are also potent hepatotoxins.[22] Other common routes of exposure for xenobiotics are absorption through the skin and inhalation. The severity of chemically induced liver injury varies from minor liver injury to acute liver failure, cirrhosis, and liver cancer.[23]

A systems biology approach to understanding the basis of cellular injury includes identification of toxicity pathways or altered cellular response pathways, which when disturbed can result in adverse health effects. Using this model of testing, investigators proposed screening and classifying compounds using a "cellular stress response pathway." Components or mechanisms of these pathways include oxidative stress, heat shock response, DNA damage response, hypoxia, ER stress (see Chapter 1), mental stress, inflammation, and osmotic stress.

The liver is the principal site for xenobiotic metabolism, called *biotransformation*, and converts the lipophilic xenobiotics to more hydrophilic forms for efficient excretion. Biotransformation, however, also can produce short-lived unstable highly reactive chemical intermediates that can lead to adverse effects.[24] These harmful intermediates, classified and catalogued, are **toxicophores**. The intermediates include electrophiles, nucleophiles, free radicals, and redox-active reactants. **Electrophiles** (electron lovers) are atoms or molecules attracted to electrons that will accept a pair of electrons to make a covalent bond. This process creates a partially or fully charged centre in electrophilic molecules.[24] A **nucleophile** is an atom or molecule that donates an electron pair to an electrophile to make a chemical bond. All chemical species with a free pair of electrons can act as nucleophiles. Nucleophiles are strongly attracted to positively charged regions in other chemicals and can be oxidized to free radicals and electrophiles.[24] In general, the majority of all *reactive* chemical species are electrophilic because the formation of nucleophiles is rare.[24] The generation of these excess reactive chemical species leads to molecular damage in liver cells. These reactive intermediates can interact with cellular macromolecules (such as proteins and DNA), can covalently bind to proteins and form **protein adducts** (chemical bound to protein) and DNA adducts, or can react directly with cell structures to cause cell damage.[25] Adduct formation can lead to adverse conditions including disruption in protein function, excess formation of fibrous connective tissue (fibrogenesis), and activation of immune responses.[24] The reactive metabolite target protein database contains the identity of proteins modified by xenobiotics.[26] The body has two major defense systems for counteracting these effects: (1) detoxification enzymes and their cofactors and (2) antioxidant systems. Phases of detoxification include phase I enzymes, such as cytochrome P-450 (CYP) oxidases, which are the most important oxidative reactions. Other phase I detoxification enzymes include those for reduction and hydrolysis. In phase II detoxification, conjugation enzymes, such as glutathione (GSH), detoxify reactive electrophiles and produce polar metabolites that cannot diffuse across membranes. Most conjugation enzymes are located in the cytosol. Phase III detoxification is often called the *efflux transporter system* because enzymes remove the parent medications, metabolites, and xenobiotics from cells. The liver has the highest supply of biotransformation enzymes of all organs and, therefore, has the key role in protection from chemical toxicity.[24] Figure 4.14 is a summary of chemically induced liver injury.

The consequence of self-propagating chain reactions of free radicals is lipid peroxidation. Free radicals react mainly with polyunsaturated fatty acids in membranes and can initiate lipid peroxidation. The breakdown of membrane lipids results in altered function of the mitochondria, ER, plasma membranes, and Golgi apparatus, and therefore has a role in acute liver cellular death (necrosis) and progression of liver injury (Figure 4.15).[24]

Chemical Agents, Including Medications

Numerous chemical agents cause cellular injury. Because chemical injury remains a constant problem in clinical settings, it is a major limitation to medication therapy. Over-the-counter and prescribed medications can cause cellular injury, sometimes leading to death. The leading cause of child poisoning is medications. The site of injury is frequently the liver, where many chemicals and medications are metabolized (see Figure 4.15). Long-term exposure to air pollutants, insecticides, and herbicides can also cause cellular injury (see *Health Promotion*: Air Pollution Reported as Largest Single Environmental Health Risk).

HEALTH PROMOTION

Air Pollution Reported as Largest Single Environmental Health Risk

The World Health Organization (WHO) reports that about 4.2 million people die every year from ambient air pollution, 3.8 million people die every year from exposure to household pollutions such as cookstoves, and 91% of the world's population lives in areas that exceed WHO guideline limits for pollution.[a,b] Air pollution is also a leading cause of heart, brain, and lung disease. Improved measurements and better technology have enabled scientists to better analyze the health risks associated with pollution. These findings confirm that air pollution is now the world's largest single environmental health risk and reducing air pollution could save millions of lives. New data show a stronger link between indoor and outdoor air pollution exposure and cardiovascular diseases (e.g., strokes and ischemic heart disease) as well as the link between air pollution and cancer. These data are in addition to the role of air pollution in the development of respiratory diseases, including infections and chronic obstructive pulmonary diseases. Statistics from 2017[c] indicate that most of the disease burden from air pollution (82%) stems from noncommunicable disease. Air pollution also accounted for 41% of global deaths related to chronic obstructive lung disease (COPD), 20% of global deaths related to type 2 diabetes, 19% of global deaths related to lung cancer, 16% of global deaths related to ischemic heart disease, and 11% of global deaths related to stroke.

[a] World Health Organization (WHO). (2019). *Ambient (outdoor) air pollution.* https://www.who.int/news-room/fact-sheets/detail/ambient-(outdoor)-air-quality-and-health.
[b] World Health Organization (WHO). (2019). *Household air pollution and health.* https://www.who.int/news-room/fact-sheets/detail/household-air-pollution-and-health.
[c] Health Effects Institute. (2019). *State of global air/2019: A special report on global exposure to air pollution and its disease burden.* https://www.stateofglobalair.org/sites/default/files/soga_2019_report.pdf.

WHO has suggested some recommendations for controlling air pollution in its *WHO Guideline for Indoor Air Quality: Household Fuel Combustion* (https://www.who.int/airpollution/guidelines/household-fuel-combustion/en/).

CHAPTER 4 Altered Cellular and Tissue Biology

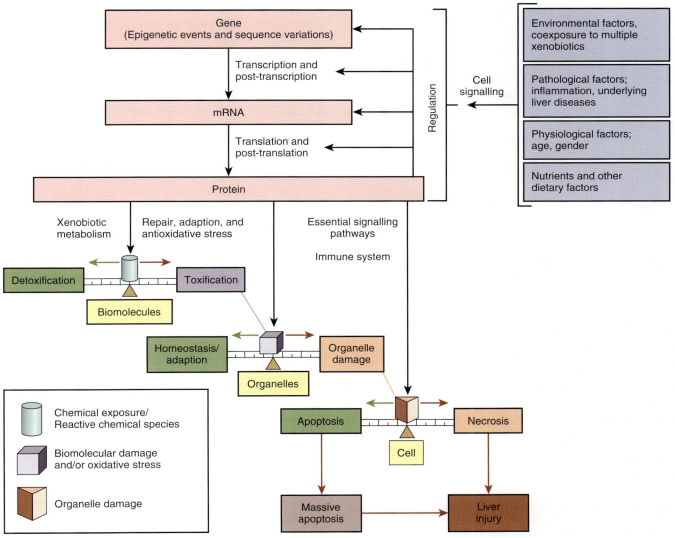

FIGURE 4.14 Chemical Liver Injury. Liver injury is a result of genetic, environmental, biological, and dietary factors. Certain chemicals can form toxic or chemically reactive metabolites. The risk of liver injury also can increase with increasing doses of a toxicant. Xenobiotic enzyme induction can lead to altered metabolism of chemicals, and medications can either inhibit or induce medication-metabolizing enzymes. These changes can lead to greater toxicity. The dose at the site of action is controlled by the Phase I to III xenobiotic metabolites, and metabolizing enzymes are encoded by numerous different genes. Therefore, the metabolism and toxicity outcomes can vary greatly among individuals. Additionally, all aspects of xenobiotic metabolism are regulated by certain transcription factors (cellular mediators of gene regulation). Overall, the extent of cell damage depends on the balance between reactive chemical species and protective responses aimed at decreasing oxidative stress, repairing macromolecular damage, or preserving cell health by inducing apoptosis or cellular death. Significant clinical outcomes of chemical-induced liver injury occur with necrosis and the immune response. Covalent binding of reactive metabolites to cellular proteins can produce new antigens (haptens) that initiate autoantibody production and T-cytotoxic cell responses. Necrosis, a form of cellular death, can result from extensive damage to the plasma membrane with altered ion transport, changes of membrane potential, cell swelling, and eventual dissolution. Altogether, the pathogenesis of chemically induced liver injury is determined by genetics, environmental factors, and other underlying pathological conditions. *Green arrows* are pathways leading to cell recovery; *red arrows* indicate pathways to cell damage or death; *black arrows* are pathways leading to chemically induced liver injury. *mRNA*, Messenger RNA. (Adapted from Gu, X., & Manautou, J.E. [2013]. Molecular mechanisms underlying chemical liver injury. *Expert Reviews in Molecular Medicine, 14*, e4.)

There are other ways to classify mechanisms by which medication actions, chemicals, and toxins produce injury. These include (1) direct damage, also called *on-target toxicity*; (2) exaggerated response at the target, including overdose; (3) biological activation to toxic metabolites, including free radicals; (4) hypersensitivity and related immunological reactions; and (5) rare toxicities.[27] These mechanisms are not mutually exclusive, and several may be operating concurrently.

Direct damage is when chemicals and medications injure cells by combining *directly* with critical molecular substances. For example, cyanide is highly toxic (i.e., poisonous) because it inhibits mitochondrial cytochrome oxidase and blocks electron transport. Many

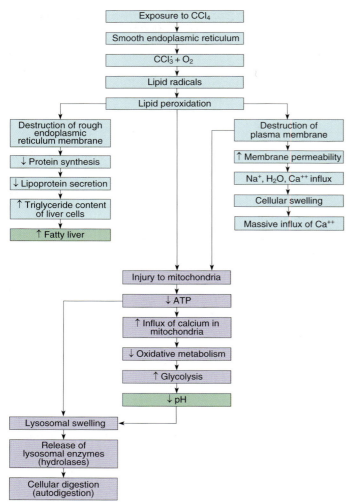

FIGURE 4.15 Chemical Injury of Liver Cells Induced by Carbon Tetrachloride Poisoning. *Light blue boxes* are mechanisms unique to chemical injury, *purple boxes* involve hypoxic injury, and *green boxes* are clinical manifestations. *ATP,* Adenosine triphosphate; Ca^{++}, calcium ion; CCl_4, carbon tetrachloride; CCl_3, trichloromethyl free radical; H_2O, water; Na^+, sodium; O_2, oxygen.

chemotherapeutic medications, known as antineoplastic agents, induce cell damage by direct cytotoxic effects. Examples of exaggerated pharmacological responses at the target include tumours caused by industrial chemicals and the birth defects attributed to thalidomide.[27] Similarly, another example includes common drugs of abuse (Table 4.5). Drug abuse can involve mind-altering substances beyond therapeutic or social norms (Table 4.6). Drug addiction and overdose are serious public health issues.

Most toxic chemicals are not biologically active in their parent (native) form but must be converted to reactive metabolites, which then act on target molecules. The cytochrome P-450 oxidase enzymes in the smooth ER of the liver and other organs usually perform this conversion. These toxic metabolites result in membrane damage and cellular injury mostly from formation of *free radicals* and subsequent membrane damage from lipid peroxidation (see Figure 4.15). For example, acetaminophen (Paracetamol) is converted to a toxic metabolite in the liver, causing cellular injury (Figure 4.16). Acetaminophen is one of the most common causes of poisoning worldwide.[28] Many investigators are studying hepatoprotective strategies.[29]

Hypersensitivity reactions are a common medication toxicity and range from mild skin rashes to immune-mediated organ failure.[27] One type of hypersensitivity reaction is the delayed-onset reaction, which occurs after multiple doses of a medication. Some protein medications and large polypeptide medications (e.g., insulin) can directly stimulate antibody production (see Chapter 8). Most medications, however, act as haptens and bind covalently to serum or cell-bound proteins. The binding makes the protein immunogenic, stimulating antidrug antibody production, T-cell responses against the medication, or both. For example, penicillin itself is not antigenic but its metabolic degradation products can become antigenic and cause an allergic reaction. Toxicities related to hypersensitivity reactions reflect individual genetic predispositions that affect medication or chemical metabolism, disposition, and immune responses.

Carbon monoxide, carbon tetrachloride, and social drugs, such as alcohol and marijuana, can significantly alter cellular function and injure cellular structures. Accidental or suicidal poisonings by chemical agents cause numerous deaths. The injurious effects on cells of some agents—lead, carbon monoxide, ethyl alcohol, mercury—are common.

Lead. Lead (Pb) is a heavy toxic metal that persists in older homes, the environment, and the workplace. Lead may be found in hazardous concentrations in food, water, and air, and it is one of the most common overexposures found in industry.[30] Despite efforts to reduce exposure through government regulation, exposure still persists for many people, and toxicity is still a primary hazard for children[31] (see *Health Promotion: Low-Level Lead Exposure Harms Children: A Renewed Call for Primary Prevention*). Although Pb was removed from paint in Europe in 1922 and regulations to reduce the amount of Pb in paint were created in Canada in 2002, many homes in Canada still contain leaded paint, and chipped and peeling leaded paint constitutes a major source of current childhood exposure.[32-35] The chipped paint can disintegrate at friction surfaces to form Pb dust.[35] Another source of contamination is Pb dust dispersed along roadways from previous leaded gasoline emissions.[35] When Pb was removed from gasoline, blood lead levels (BLLs) dropped significantly.[36-38] Previous emissions of leaded fuel created large dispersions of Pb dust in the environment. Particulate Pb (2 to 10 μm) does not degrade and persists in the environment, making it a notable source of human exposure.[39] Other airborne sources include smelters and piston-engine airplanes.[40] Drinking water exposed to Pb occurs from outdated fixtures, plumbing without corrosion control, and solders.[35] Well water may not be tested for Pb.[35] Although the average blood levels of Pb in children in Canada have dropped since the 1970s, there are at-risk populations with higher than average BLLs.[35] Children of lower social economic status or racial minority status are still at higher risk of Pb poisoning, and some regions in Canada have an increased prevalence of higher BLLs in children.[35] Common sources of Pb are included in Table 4.7.

Children are more susceptible to the effects of Pb than adults for several reasons, including:
(1) Children have increased hand-to-mouth behaviour and exposure from the ingestion of Pb dust
(2) The blood–brain barrier in children is immature during fetal development, contributing to greater Pb accumulation in the developing brain
(3) Infant absorption of Pb is greater than that in adults, and bone turnover (in adults the body burden of Pb is found in bone) in children from skeletal growth results in continuous leaching of Pb into blood, causing constant body exposure.[35,41] If nutrition is compromised, especially if dietary intake of iron and calcium is insufficient, children are more likely to have elevated BLLs.[35] Particularly worrisome is Pb exposure during pregnancy because the developing fetal nervous system is especially vulnerable; Pb exposure can result in lower IQ, learning disorders, hyperactivity, and attention problems.[31]

TABLE 4.5 Common Drugs of Abuse

Class	Molecular Target	Example
Opioid narcotics	Mu opioid receptor (agonist)	Heroin, hydromorphone (Dilaudid)
		Oxycodone (Percodan, Percocet, OxyContin)
		Methadone (Metadol)
		Meperidine (Demerol)
Sedative-hypnotics	$GABA_A$ receptor (agonist)	Barbiturates
		Ethanol
		Methaqualone (Quaalude)
		Glutethimide (Doriden)
		Etchlorvynol (Placidyl)
Psychomotor stimulants	Dopamine transporter (antagonist)	Cocaine
	Serotonin receptors (toxicity)	Amphetamines
		3,4-Methylenedioxymethamphetamine (MDMA, ecstasy)
Phencyclidinelike medications	NMDA glutamate receptor channel (antagonist)	Phencyclidine (PCP, angel dust)
		Ketamine
Cannabinoids	CB_1 cannabinoid receptors (agonist)	Marijuana
		Cannabis
		Hashish
Hallucinogens	Serotonin 5-HT_2 receptors (agonist)	Lysergic acid diethylamide (LSD)
		Mescaline
		Psilocybin

5-HT_2, 5-hydroxytryptamine; CB_1, cannabinoid receptor type 1; GABA, gamma-aminobutyric acid; NMDA, N-methyl-D-aspartate.
From Hyman, S.E. (2001). JAMA, 286, 2586; Oakes, S. A. (2021). Cell injury, cell death, and adaptations. In V. Kumar, A. K. Abbas, & J. C. Aster (Eds.), Robbins and Cotran pathologic basis of disease (10th ed., pp. 36–70). Elsevier.

HEALTH PROMOTION

Low-Level Lead Exposure Harms Children: A Renewed Call for Primary Prevention

Lead exposure is relatively low in Canada, and levels are often difficult to determine. Notable symptoms include headaches, irritability, abdominal pain, vomiting, anemia (general weakness, paleness), weight loss, poor attention span, noticeable learning difficulty, slowed speech development, and hyperactivity.

Low levels of lead exposure tend to create vague symptoms, and the cause often cannot be determined easily. Exposure to lead is mainly through oral ingestion or absorption by the skin. Because children tend to touch everything and put things into their mouths, they are at greater risk of exposure, although blood lead levels of Canadian children are generally low (at less than 0.483 μmol/L). Routine BLL testing may be necessary in communities with a history of soil contamination (from nearby industrial activity).

Further information on lead screening is available through Health Canada at https://www.canada.ca/en/health-canada/services/home-garden-safety/reduce-your-exposure-lead.html. *The Lead information package—Some commonly asked questions about lead and human health* is available at https://www.hc-sc.gc.ca/ewh-semt/contaminants/lead-plomb/asked_questions-questions_posees-eng.php.

The organ systems primarily affected by Pb ingestion include the nervous system, the hematopoietic system (tissues that produce blood cells), and the kidneys of the urological system. The neurological effect of Pb in exposed children is the driving factor for reducing Pb levels in the environment.[35] Elevated BLLs not only are linked to cognitive deficits but also are associated with behavioural changes including antisocial behaviour, acting out in school, and difficulty paying attention.[35] The cognitive and behavioural changes of Pb-exposed children persist after complete cessation of Pb exposure[35] (Figure 4.17). Studies in animals have led to the hypothesis that Pb targets the learning and memory processes by inhibiting the N-methyl-D-aspartate receptor (NMDAR), which is necessary for hippocampus-mediated learning and memory.[35,42] Similar changes also have been found in cultured neuron systems.[35] Inhibition of either voltage-gated calcium channels or NMDARs by Pb results in reduction of Ca^{++} entry into the cell, thereby disrupting the necessary Ca^{++} signalling for neurotransmission.[43,44] Pb induces cellular damage by increasing oxidative stress.[45] Pb toxicity involves the direct formation of ROS (singlet oxygen, hydrogen peroxides, hydroperoxides) and depletion of antioxidants.[45] Pb exposure leads to lowered levels of GSH, which is important for the metabolism of specific medications and other toxins. Therefore, low levels of Pb (and the blood levels of other metals) can increase the toxicity of GSH-metabolized substances.[45] Animal and human population studies indicate that low-level Pb exposure may also cause hypertension.[46] Pb interferes with the normal remodelling of cartilage and bone in children. Radiological studies show that "lead lines" are detectable in bone and are also seen as areas of hyperpigmentation in the gums. Pb inhibits several enzymes involved in hemoglobin synthesis and causes anemia (most obvious is a microcytic hypochromic anemia). Renal lesions can cause tubular dysfunction, resulting in glycosuria (glucose in the urine), aminoaciduria (amino acids in the urine), and hyperphosphaturia (excess phosphate in the urine). Gastro-intestinal symptoms are less severe and include nausea, loss of appetite, weight loss, and abdominal cramping.

Carbon monoxide. Gaseous substances can be classified according to their ability to asphyxiate (interrupt respiration) or irritate. Toxic asphyxiants, such as carbon monoxide, hydrogen cyanide, and hydrogen sulphide, directly interfere with cellular respiration.

Carbon monoxide (CO) is an odourless, colourless, nonirritating, and undetectable gas unless it is mixed with a visible or odorous

TABLE 4.6 Social or Street Drugs and Their Effects

Type of Drug	Description and Effects
Marijuana (pot)[a]	*Active substance:* Δ9-tetrahydrocannabinol (THC), found in resin of *Cannabis sativa* plant With smoking (e.g., "joints"), about 5–10% is absorbed through lungs; with heavy use the following adverse effects have been reported: alterations of sensory perception; cognitive and psychomotor impairment (e.g., inability to judge time, speed, distance); an increase in heart rate and blood pressure; an increase in susceptibility to laryngitis, pharyngitis, bronchitis; coughing and hoarseness; possible contribution to lung cancer (different dosages need study; it contains large number of carcinogens); based on data from animal studies, reproductive changes, including reduced fertility, decreased sperm motility, and decreased levels of circulatory testosterone; fetal abnormalities, including low birth weight; increased frequency of infectious illness, which is thought to be result of depressed cell-mediated and humoral immunity; beneficial effects include decreased nausea secondary to cancer chemotherapy and decreased pain in certain chronic conditions
Methamphetamine (meth)	An amine derivation of amphetamine ($C_{10}H_{15}N$) used as crystalline hydrochloride CNS stimulant; in large doses causes irritability, aggressive (violent) behaviour, anxiety, excitement, auditory hallucinations, and paranoia (delusions and psychosis); mood changes are common and abuser can swiftly change from friendly to hostile; paranoiac swings can result in suspiciousness, hyperactive behaviour, and dramatic mood swings Appeals to abusers because body's metabolism is increased and produces euphoria, alertness, and perception of increased energy Stages: • *Low intensity:* User is not psychologically addicted and uses methamphetamine by swallowing or snorting • *Binge and high intensity:* User has psychological addiction and smokes or injects to achieve a faster, stronger high • *Tweaking:* Most dangerous stage; user is continually under the influence, not sleeping for 3–15 days, extremely irritated, and paranoid
Cocaine and crack	Extracted from leaves of coca plant and sold as a water-soluble powder (cocaine hydrochloride) liberally diluted with talcum powder or other white powders; extraction of pure alkaloid from cocaine hydrochloride is "free-base" called *crack* because it "cracks" when heated Crack is more potent than cocaine; cocaine is widely used as an anaesthetic, usually in procedures involving oral cavity; it is a potent CNS stimulant, blocking reuptake of neurotransmitters norepinephrine, dopamine, and serotonin; also increases synthesis of norepinephrine and dopamine; dopamine induces sense of euphoria, and norepinephrine causes adrenergic potentiation, including hypertension, tachycardia, and vasoconstriction; cocaine can therefore cause severe coronary artery narrowing and ischemia; the reason cocaine increases thrombus formation is unclear; other cardiovascular effects include dysrhythmias, sudden death, dilated cardiomyopathy, rupture of descending aorta (i.e., secondary to hypertension); effects on fetus include premature labour, delayed fetal development, stillbirth, hyperirritability
Heroin	Opiate closely related to morphine, methadone, and codeine Highly addictive, and withdrawal causes intense fear ("I'll die without it"); sold "cut" with similar-looking white powder; dissolved in water it is often highly contaminated; feeling of tranquility and sedation lasts only a few hours and thus encourages repeated intravenous or subcutaneous injections; acts on the receptors enkephalins, endorphins, and dynorphins, which are widely distributed throughout body with high affinity to CNS; effects can include infectious complications, especially *Staphylococcus aureus*, granulomas of lung, septic embolism, and pulmonary edema—in addition, viral infections, including from HIV, from casual exchange of needles; sudden death is related to overdosage secondary to respiratory depression, decreased cardiac output, and severe pulmonary edema

[a]Marijuana became legalized in Canada on October 17, 2018 (https://www.justice.gc.ca/eng/cj-jp/cannabis/).
Data from Kumar, V., Abbas, A. K., & Aster, J. C. [Eds.]. [2021]. *Robbins and Cotran pathologic basis of disease* [10th ed.]. Elsevier; Nahas, G., Sutin, K., & Bennett, W. M. (2000). *New England Journal of Medicine, 343*(7), 514–515.
CNS, Central nervous system; *HIV*, human immunodeficiency virus.

pollutant. Interestingly, although CO is a chemical agent, it ultimately produces a hypoxic injury—namely, oxygen deprivation. As a systemic asphyxiant, CO causes death by inducing central nervous system (CNS) depression. Normally, oxygen molecules are carried to tissues bound to hemoglobin in red blood cells (see Chapter 27). Because CO's affinity for hemoglobin is 300 times greater than that of oxygen, CO quickly binds with the hemoglobin, preventing the oxygen molecules from binding to the hemoglobin. Minute amounts of CO can produce a significant percentage of **carboxyhemoglobin** (carbon monoxide bound with hemoglobin). With increasing levels of carboxyhemoglobin, hypoxia occurs insidiously, evoking widespread ischemic changes in the CNS. Symptoms related to CO poisoning include headache, giddiness, tinnitus (ringing in the ears), chest pain, confusion, nausea, weakness, and vomiting. However, people can die before experiencing any overt symptoms, as CNS depression causes most individuals to be unaware of their CO exposure, and they lapse into unconsciousness and die if not found quickly. Measuring carboxyhemoglobin levels in the blood confirms this diagnosis.

CO is an *air pollutant* found in combustion fumes produced by cars and trucks, small gasoline engines, stoves, gas ranges, gas refrigerators, heating systems, lanterns, burning charcoal or wood, and cigarette smoke. Chronic exposure can occur in people working in confined spaces, such as underground garages and tunnels. Fumes can accumulate in enclosed or semienclosed spaces, and poisoning from breathing CO can occur in humans and animals. Although all people and animals are at risk, those most susceptible to poisoning include unborn babies, infants, and people with chronic heart disease, respiratory problems, and anemia. For information on preventing CO poisoning from home appliances and on proper venting, see: http://www.healthycanadians.gc.ca.

Ethanol. Alcohol **(ethanol)** is the most abused drug in Canada. Heavy drinkers aged 12 and older (i.e., drinking more than five drinks on one occasion for males and more than four drinks on one occasion for females) accounted for about 19.1% of Canada's population in 2018.[47] A blood concentration of 17 mmol/L is the legal definition for drunk driving in Canada. This level of alcohol in an average person may be reached after consumption of three drinks (three 12-ounce bottles of beer, 15 ounces of wine, and 4 to 5 ounces of distilled liquor). The effects of alcohol vary by age, gender, and percentage of body fat; the rate of metabolism affects the blood alcohol level. Because alcohol is not only a psychoactive drug but also a food, it is part of the basic food supply in many societies.

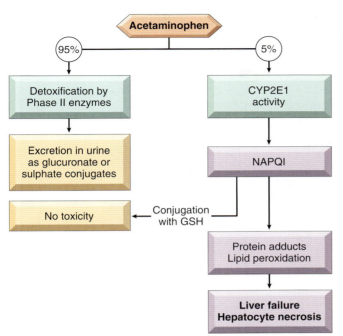

FIGURE 4.16 Acetaminophen Metabolism and Toxicity. *CYP2E1*, A cytochrome; *GSH*, glutathione; *NAPQI*, toxic by-product.

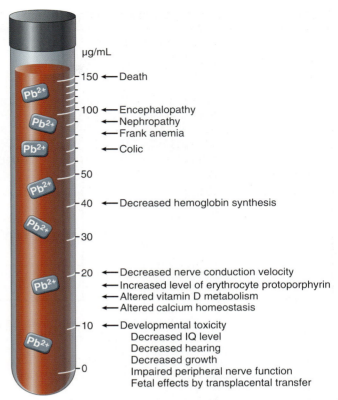

FIGURE 4.17 Lead Poisoning in Children Related to Blood Levels. (From Kumar, V., Abbas, A. K., & Aster, J. C. [Eds.]. [2021]. *Robbins and Cotran pathologic basis of disease* [10th ed.]. Elsevier.)

TABLE 4.7	Common Sources of Lead Exposure
Exposure	**Source**
Environmental	Lead paint, soil, or dust near roadways or lead-painted homes; plastic window blinds; plumbing materials (from pipes or solder); pottery glazes and ceramic ware; lead-core candle wicks; leaded gasoline; water (pipes)
Occupational	Lead mining and refining, plumbing and pipe fitting, auto repair, glass manufacturing, battery manufacturing and recycling, printing shop, construction work, plastic manufacturing, gas station attendant, firing-range attendant
Hobbies	Glazed pottery making, target shooting at firing ranges, lead soldering, preparing fishing sinkers, stained-glass making, painting, car or boat repair
Other	Gasoline sniffing, costume jewellery, cosmetics, contaminated herbal products

Data from Sanborn, M. D., Abelsohn, A., Campbell, M., et al. (2002). *Canadian Medical Association Journal, 166*(10), 1287–1292.

A large intake of alcohol has enormous effects on nutritional status. Liver and nutritional disorders are the most serious consequences of alcohol abuse. Major nutritional deficiencies include magnesium, vitamin B_6, thiamine, and phosphorus. Folic acid deficiency is a common problem in chronic alcoholic populations. Ethanol alters folic acid (folate) allostasis by decreasing intestinal absorption of folate, increasing liver retention of folate, and increasing the loss of folate through urinary and fecal excretion.[48] Folic acid deficiency becomes especially serious in pregnant women who consume alcohol and may contribute to fetal alcohol spectrum disorder.

Most of the alcohol in blood is metabolized to *acetaldehyde* in the liver by three enzyme systems: (1) alcohol dehydrogenase (ADH), (2) the microsomal ethanol-oxidizing system (MEOS; CYP2E1), and (3) catalase (Figure 4.18). The main metabolic pathway involves ADH, an enzyme located in the cytosol of hepatocytes. The MEOS depends on a specific cytochrome P-450 enzyme (CYP2E1) needed for cellular oxidation. Activation of CYP2E1 requires a high ethanol concentration and is thought to be important in the accelerated ethanol metabolism (i.e., tolerance) noted in persons with chronic alcoholism. Acetaldehyde has many toxic tissue effects and is responsible for some of the acute effects of alcohol and for development of head and neck cancer (HNC).[1] HNC risk may be influenced by alcohol-metabolizing genes (*ADH1B* and *ALDH2*) and oral hygiene.[49]

The major effects of acute alcoholism involve the CNS. After alcohol is ingested, it is absorbed, unaltered, in the stomach and small intestine. Fatty foods and milk slow absorption. Alcohol then is distributed to all tissues and fluids of the body in direct proportion to the blood concentration. Individuals differ in their capability to metabolize alcohol. Genetic differences in the metabolism of liver alcohol, including levels of aldehyde dehydrogenases, are present in everyone.[50] These genetic polymorphisms may account for ethnic and gender differences in ethanol metabolism. Persons with chronic alcoholism develop tolerance because of production of enzymes, leading to an increased rate of metabolism (e.g., CYP2E1).

Numerous studies have validated the so-called *J-* or *U-shaped* inverse association between alcohol and overall or cardiovascular mortality, such as from myocardial infarction and ischemic stroke.

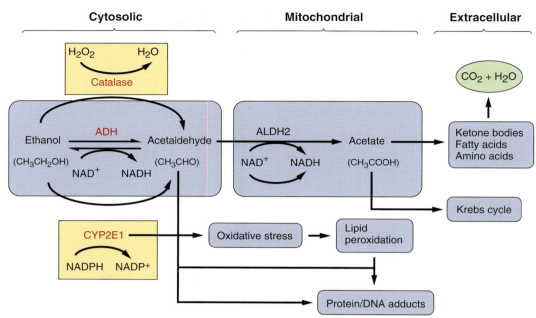

FIGURE 4.18 **Ethanol Metabolism Pathway.** Ethanol is metabolized into acetaldehyde through the cytosolic enzyme alcohol dehydrogenase *(ADH)*, the microsomal enzyme cytochrome P-450 2E1 *(CYP2E1)*, and the peroxisomal enzyme catalase. The ADH enzyme reaction is the main ethanol metabolic pathway involving an intermediate carrier of electrons, namely, nicotinamide adenine dinucleotide *(NAD⁺)*, which is reduced by two electrons to form *NADH*. Acetaldehyde is metabolized mainly by aldehyde dehydrogenase 2 *(ALDH2)* in the mitochondria to acetate and NADH before being cleared into the systemic circulation. CO_2, Carbon dioxide; H_2O_2, hydrogen peroxide; H_2O, water; $NADP^+$, oxidized form of nicotinamide adenine dinucleotide phosphate; *NADPH*, dihydronicotinamide-adenine dinucleotide phosphate. (Reprinted with permission from Zhang, Y., & Ren, J. [2011]. ALDH2 in alcoholic heart diseases: molecular mechanism and clinical implications. *Pharmacology & Therapeutics, 132*[1], 86–95. Elsevier.)

Light to moderate (nonbinge) drinkers tend to have lower mortality than nondrinkers, and heavy drinkers have higher mortality[51] (See *Health Promotion:* Low-Risk Alcohol Drinking Guidelines.) The suggested mechanisms for cardioprotection for light to moderate drinkers include:

1. An increase in levels of high-density lipoprotein–cholesterol (HDL-C)
2. A decrease in levels of low-density lipoprotein (LDL)
3. Prevention of clot formation
4. Reduction in platelet aggregation
5. A decrease in blood pressure
6. An increase in coronary vessel vasodilation
7. An increase in coronary blood flow
8. A decrease in coronary inflammation
9. A decrease in atherosclerosis
10. Limited ischemia–reperfusion injury (I/R injury)
11. A decrease in diabetic vessel pathology[52]

Similarly, the Canadian Heart and Stroke Association recommends no more than 15 drinks per week for men and 10 drinks per week for women (one 341-mL beer, 118 mL of wine, 44 mL of 80-proof spirits, or 29 mL of 100-proof spirits). Drinking more alcohol can increase the risks of alcoholism, high blood pressure, obesity, stroke, breast cancer, suicide, and accidents.[53] Individuals who do not consume alcohol should not be encouraged to start drinking.[54]

Acute alcoholism (drunkenness) affects the CNS. Alcohol intoxication causes CNS depression. Depending on the amount consumed, CNS depression is associated with sedation, drowsiness, loss of motor coordination, delirium, altered behaviour, and loss of consciousness. Toxic amounts (65 to 86 mmol/L) result in a lethal coma or respiratory arrest because of medullary centre depression.

Acute alcoholism may also induce reversible hepatic and gastric changes.[1] Chronic and binge drinking causes alcoholic liver disease (ALD), with a spectrum from hepatic steatosis (fatty change) to steatohepatitis (fatty change and inflammation) and cirrhosis (see Chapter 36). These alterations can eventually lead to hepatocellular carcinoma. Recent studies of ALD reveal a major role of mitochondria in its pathogenesis. Alcohol causes mitochondrial DNA damage, lipid accumulation, and oxidative stress. Acute alcoholism also contributes significantly to motor vehicle fatalities.

Chronic alcoholism causes structural alterations in practically all organs and tissues in the body because most tissues contain enzymes capable of ethanol oxidation or nonoxidative metabolism. The most significant activity, however, occurs in the liver. Alcohol is the leading cause of liver-related morbidity and mortality.[55] In general, hepatic changes initiated by acetaldehyde include inflammation, deposition of fat, enlargement of the liver, interruption of microtubular transport of proteins and their secretion, increase in intracellular water, depression of fatty acid oxidation in the mitochondria, increase in membrane rigidity, and acute liver cell necrosis (see Chapter 36). Specifically, chronic or binge alcohol consumption causes ALD with a spectrum ranging from simple fatty liver (steatosis), to steatohepatitis (fatty with inflammation), to cirrhosis (Figure 4.19) (see Chapter 36). Cirrhosis is associated with portal hypertension and an increased risk for hepatocellular carcinoma. Cellular damage increases with ROS and oxidative stress. Activation of proinflammatory cytokines from neutrophils and lymphocytes mediates liver damage.[56] Oxidative stress

HEALTH PROMOTION
Low-Risk Alcohol Drinking Guidelines

Canada's Low-Risk Alcohol Drinking Guidelines recommend no more than 10 drinks per week for women (15 drinks/week for men) with no more than 3 drinks at one time (4 drinks/one time for men). The annual national consumption of alcohol is 470 standard servings per person (or nine servings/week) for individuals 15 years and over. Risky alcohol consumption is common in underage drinkers (30% at least monthly in 2010) and peaks between 19 and 24 years, with more than 50% of males and 45% of females drinking more than the recommended levels monthly, or more often. The guidelines recommend not drinking when you are:

- operating a motor vehicle
- using machinery or tools
- pregnant or planning to be pregnant
- responsible for the safety of others
- taking medication or other drugs that interact with alcohol
- doing any kind of dangerous physical activity
- living with mental or physical health problems
- living with alcohol dependence
- making important decisions

The guidelines suggest the following safer drinking tips to prevent injury and illness:

- Set limits for yourself when you drink, and stick to them.
- Eat before and while you are drinking.
- Drink slowly: consume no more than two drinks in any 3 hours.
- Have one nonalcoholic drink for every drink of alcohol.
- Consider your age, body weight, and health problems that might suggest lower limits.
- Do not start to drink or increase your drinking for perceived health benefits.

From Canadian Centre on Substance Abuse (CCSA). (2018). *Drinking guidelines*. https://www.ccsa.ca/canadas-low-risk-alcohol-drinking-guidelines-brochure; Statistics Canada. (2012). *Table 183-0019: Volume of sales of alcoholic beverages in litres of absolute alcohol and per capita 15 years and over, fiscal years ended March 31, annual*. http://wwww5.statcan.gc.ca/cansim/a26?lang=eng&retrLang=eng&id=1830019&paSer=&pattern=&stByVal=2&p1=-1&p2=-1&tabMode=dataTable&csid=; Canadian Centre on Substance Abuse (CCSA). (2012). *Levels and Patterns of Alcohol Use in Canada. Alcohol Price Policy Series, Report 1 of 3*. http://www.ccsa.ca/Resource%20Library/CCSA-Patterns-Alcohol-Use-Policy-Canada-2012-en.pdf.

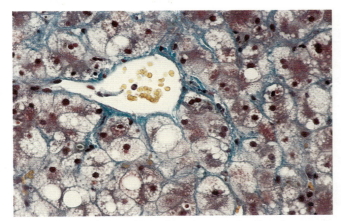

FIGURE 4.19 Alcoholic Hepatitis. Chicken-wire fibrosis extending between hepatocytes (Mallory trichrome stain). (From Damjanov, I., & Linder, J. [Eds.]. [1996]. *Anderson's pathology* [10th ed.]. Mosby.)

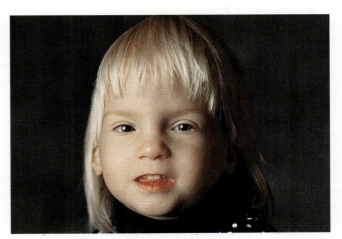

FIGURE 4.20 Fetal Alcohol Spectrum Disorder. When alcohol enters the fetal blood, the potential result can cause tragic congenital abnormalities, such as microcephaly ("small head"), low birth weight, and cardiovascular defects, as well as developmental disabilities, such as physical and intellectual disability, and even death. Note the small head, thinned upper lip, small eye openings (palpebral fissures), epicanthal folds, and receded upper jaw (retrognathia) typical of fetal alcohol spectrum disorder. (From Fortinash, K.M., & Holoday Worret, P.A. [2012]. *Psychiatric mental health nursing* [5th ed.]. Mosby.)

is associated with cell membrane phospholipid depletion, which alters the fluidity and function of cell membranes as well as intercellular transport. Chronic alcoholism affects several disorders, including injury to the myocardium (alcoholic cardiomyopathy); increased tendency to hypertension, acute gastritis, acute and chronic pancreatitis; and regressive changes in skeletal muscle. Chronic alcohol consumption is associated with an increased incidence of cancer of the oral cavity, liver, esophagus, and breast.

Ethanol also affects the onset of a variety of immune defects, including effects on the production of cytokines involved in inflammatory responses. Alcohol can induce epigenetic variations in the developmental pathways of many types of immune cells (e.g., granulocytes, macrophages, and T lymphocytes) that promote increased inflammation.[57] Alcohol increases the development of serious medical conditions related to immune system dysfunction, including acute respiratory distress syndrome (ARDS), as well as liver cancer and ALD.[57] Binge and chronic drinking increases susceptibility to many infectious microorganisms and can enhance the progression of human immunodeficiency virus (HIV) by affecting innate and adaptive immunity.[57]

The deleterious effects of prenatal alcohol exposure can cause mental deficiency and neurobehavioural disorders, as well as fetal alcohol syndrome. **Fetal alcohol spectrum disorder** includes delayed growth, facial anomalies, cognitive impairment, and ocular malformations (Figure 4.20). It is among the common causes of intellectual disability.[58] Evidence of epigenetic alterations has led to the hypothesis that alcohol effects on fetal development may be caused not only by maternal alcohol consumption but also by the father's exposure as well.[58] Epigenetic alterations may be carried through the male germline for generations.[59] Alcohol crosses the placenta, reaching the fetus, and blood levels of the fetus may reach equivalent levels to maternal levels in 1 to 2 hours.[60] Research has demonstrated an unimpeded bidirectional movement of alcohol between the fetus and the mother. The fetus may completely depend on maternal hepatic detoxification because the activity of ADH in the fetal liver is less than 10% of that in the adult liver.[60] Additionally, the amniotic fluid acts as a reservoir for alcohol, prolonging fetal exposure.[60] Some recent studies suggest that acetaldehyde can alter fetal development by disrupting differentiation and growth; DNA and protein synthesis; modification of carbohydrates, proteins, and fats; and flow of nutrients across the placenta; and neuro-circuitry dysfunction may be long-lasting.[58,60]

Mercury. Mercury is a global threat to human and environmental health. A recent report entitled *Global Mercury Assessment 2018* presents an overview.[61] This report provides the most recent information on worldwide atmospheric mercury emissions, releases to the aquatic environment, and the fate of mercury in the global environment. Human activities have increased total atmospheric mercury concentrations by about 450% above natural levels. The major sources of **anthropogenic** (i.e., relating to human activity) mercury emissions to air are artisanal and small-scale gold mining (ASGM) and coal burning. The next major sources are the production of ferrous and nonferrous metals, and cement production. Importantly, investigators report that emissions from industrial sectors have increased since 2010. Types of aquatic releases of mercury include industrial sites (power plants, factories), old mines, landfills, and waste disposal locations. ASGM is a significant producer of aquatic mercury release. More than 90% of mercury in marine animals is from anthropogenic emissions. Large amounts of inorganic mercury have accumulated in surface soils and in the oceans. Climate change, with thawing of enormous areas of frozen lands, may release even more long-stored mercury and organic matter into lakes, rivers, and oceans.

Dental amalgams, or "silver fillings," are made of two almost equal parts of liquid mercury and a powder containing silver, tin, copper, zinc, and other metals.[40] When amalgams are placed or removed, they can release a small amount of mercury vapour. Chewing can release a small amount of vapour, and people absorb the vapour by inhalation or ingestion.[40] Researchers are studying the effects of exposure to magnetic fields, such as from mobile phone use, and the release of mercury from amalgams.[62] Susceptibility to mercury toxicity varies in a dose-dependent fashion and, among individuals, based on multiple genes, not all of which have been identified.[63,64] Worldwide efforts are under way to phase down or eliminate the use of mercury dental amalgam.[64] Thimerosal, a mercury-containing preservative, was removed from all vaccines in 2001, with the exception of inactivated influenza vaccines.[65]

Unintentional and Intentional Injuries

> **QUICK CHECK 4.3**
> 1. Give examples of intentional and unintentional injury.
> 2. Describe unintentional injury as a form of injury in health care delivery in Canada.
> 3. What is the major mechanism of injury with drowning?

Unintentional and intentional injuries are an important health problem in Canada. Statistics on nonfatal injuries are harder to document accurately, but they can be a significant cause of morbidity and disability, and they can cost society billions of dollars annually. Examples include the opioid crisis and the effects of cannabis in youth (see *Health Promotion*: Cannabis and Canada's Youth). Table 4.8 describes and classifies these injuries further.

HEALTH PROMOTION
Cannabis and Canada's Youth

Cannabis, when used during adolescence, can cause devastating and permanent damage to the rapidly developing brain. Cannabis contains a chemical called delta-9-tetrahydrocannabinol (THC), which stimulates cannabinoid receptors in the brain. These receptors, in turn, modulate the secretion of gamma aminobutyric acid (GABA), which is an inhibitory neurotransmitter, and glutamate, which is an excitatory neurotransmitter. The frontal cortex of the brain, responsible for cognition and judgement, is particularly sensitive to THC, and the surrounding dopamine networks are also affected. Structural changes such as lower brain volumes, altered folding patterns, and thinning of the cortex are also evident on an MRI. In this age group, cannabis use can lead to increased tobacco use, mental illness (such as depression and anxiety), as well as impaired cognition and decreased performance in life.

In 2010, Canadian youth ranked first for cannabis use among 43 countries and regions across Europe and North America, with one-third of youth (regardless of gender) having tried cannabis at least once by age 15. Hospitalization of younger Canadians due to ingestion of cannabis is also increasing.

Although cannabis is now legal in Canada and has its therapeutic uses (e.g., relief of pain and nausea, sleep, and stimulation of appetite), there are still major systemic issues related to access and the need to safeguard today's youth from unintentional harm. The THC content in marijuana today is 2 to 4 times higher than it was 40 years ago, and cannabis can be both inhaled and ingested, depending on its form.

From Grant, N., Bélanger, R.E., & Canadian Paediatric Society Adolescent Health Committee. (2017). Position Statement: Cannabis and Canada's children and youth. *Paediatric & Child Health, 22*(2), 98–102. https://www.cps.ca/en/documents/position/cannabis-children-and-youth.

Asphyxial Injuries

Asphyxial injuries happen when cells fail to receive or use oxygen. Deprivation of oxygen may be partial (*hypoxia*) or total (*anoxia*). Asphyxial injuries comprise four general categories: suffocation, strangulation, chemical asphyxiants, and drowning.

Suffocation. Suffocation, or oxygen failing to reach the blood, can result from a lack of oxygen in the environment (entrapment in an enclosed space or filling of the environment with a suffocating gas) or blockage of the external airways. Classic examples of these types of asphyxial injuries are a child who is trapped in an abandoned refrigerator or a person who commits suicide by putting a plastic bag over their head. A reduction in the ambient oxygen level to 16% (normal is 21%) is immediately dangerous. If the level is below 5%, death can occur within a matter of minutes. The diagnosis of these types of asphyxial injuries depends on obtaining an accurate and thorough history because there will be no specific physical findings.

Diagnosis and treatment in **choking asphyxiation** (obstruction of the internal airways) depend on locating and removing the obstructing material. Injury or disease also may cause swelling of the soft tissues of the airway, leading to partial or complete obstruction and subsequent asphyxiation. Suffocation also may result from compression of the chest or abdomen (mechanical or compressional asphyxia), preventing normal respiratory movements. Usual signs and symptoms include florid facial congestion and petechiae (pinpoint hemorrhages) of the eyes and face.

Strangulation. Strangulation is the result of compression and closure of the blood vessels and air passages due to external pressure on

TABLE 4.8 Unintentional and Intentional Injuries

Type of Injury	Description
BLUNT-FORCE INJURIES 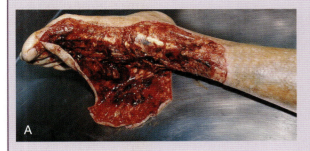	Mechanical injury to body resulting in tearing, shearing, or crushing; most common type of injury seen in health care settings; caused by blows or impacts; motor vehicle accidents and falls most common cause (see photo A) *Contusion* (*bruise*): Bleeding into skin or underlying tissues; initial colour will be red-purple, then blue-black, then yellow-brown or green (see Figure 4.24); duration of bruise depends on extent, location, and degree of vascularization; bruising of soft tissue may be confined to deeper structures; *hematoma* is collection of blood in soft tissue; *subdural hematoma* is blood between inner surface of dura mater and surface of brain; can result from blows, falls, or sudden acceleration/deceleration of head as occurs in *shaken baby syndrome*; *epidural hematoma* is collection of blood between inner surface of skull and dura; is most often associated with a skull fracture *Laceration:* Tear or rip resulting when tensile strength of skin or tissue is exceeded; is ragged and irregular with abraded edges; an extreme example is *avulsion*, where a wide area of tissue is pulled away; lacerations of internal organs are common in blunt-force injuries; lacerations of liver, spleen, kidneys, and bowel occur from blows to abdomen; thoracic aorta may be lacerated in sudden deceleration accidents; severe blows or impacts to chest may rupture heart with lacerations of atria or ventricles *Fracture:* Blunt-force blows or impacts can cause bone to break or shatter (see Chapter 39)
SHARP-FORCE INJURIES 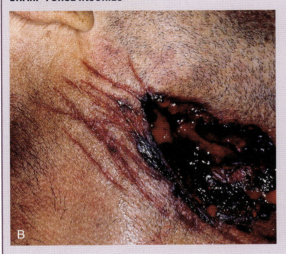	Sharp-force injuries are characterized by a relatively well-defined traumatic separation of tissues, occurring when a sharp-edged or pointed object comes into contact with the skin and underlying tissues. Three specific subtypes of sharp-force injuries exist, as follows: stab wounds, incised wounds, and chop wounds.[a] *Incised wound:* A wound that is *longer* than it is *deep*; wound can be straight or jagged with sharp, distinct edges without abrasion; usually produces significant external bleeding with little internal hemorrhage; these wounds are noted in sharp-force injury suicides; in addition to a deep, lethal cut, there will be superficial incisions in same area called *hesitation marks* (see photo B) *Stab wound:* A penetrating sharp-force injury that is *deeper* than it is *long;* if a sharp instrument is used, depths of wound are clean and distinct but can be abraded if object is inserted deeply and wider portion (e.g., hilt of a knife) impacts skin; depending on size and location of wound, external bleeding may be surprisingly small; after an initial spurt of blood, even if a major vessel or heart is struck, wound may be almost completely closed by tissue pressure, thus allowing only a trickle of visible blood despite copious internal bleeding *Puncture wound:* Instruments or objects with sharp points but without sharp edges produce puncture wounds; classic example is wound of foot after stepping on a nail; wounds are prone to infection, have abrasion of edges, and can be very deep *Chopping wound:* Heavy, edged instruments (axes, hatchets, propeller blades) produce wounds with a combination of sharp- and blunt-force characteristics
GUNSHOT WOUNDS 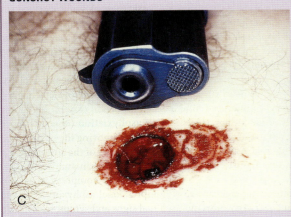	Gunshot wounds are either penetrating (bullet remains in body) or perforating (bullet exits body); bullet also can fragment; most important factors or appearances are whether it is an entrance or exit wound and range of fire *Entrance wound:* All wounds share some common features; overall appearance is most affected by range of fire *Contact range entrance wound:* Distinctive type of wound when gun is held so muzzle rests on or presses into skin surface; there is searing of edges of wound from flame and soot or smoke on edges of wound in addition to hole; hard contact wounds of head cause severe tearing and disruption of tissue (because of thin layer of skin and muscle overlying bone); wound is gaping and jagged, known as *blow back*; can produce a patterned abrasion that mirrors weapon used (see photo C)

(Continued)

Type of Injury	Description
	Intermediate (distance) range entrance wound: Surrounded by gunpowder tattooing or stippling; *tattooing* results from fragments of burning or unburned pieces of gunpowder exiting barrel and forcefully striking skin; *stippling* results when gunpowder abrades but does not penetrate skin (see photo D)
	Indeterminate range entrance wound: Occurs when flame, soot, or gunpowder does not reach skin surface but bullet does; *indeterminate* is used rather than *distant* because appearance may be same regardless of distance; for example, if an individual is shot at close range through multiple layers of clothing the wound may look the same as if the shooting occurred at a distance
	Exit wound: Has the same appearance regardless of range of fire; most important factors are speed of projectile and degree of deformation; size cannot be used to determine if hole is an exit or entrance wound; usually has clean edges that can often be re-approximated to cover defect; skin is one of toughest structures for a bullet to penetrate; thus it is not uncommon for a bullet to pass entirely through body but stop just beneath skin on "exit" side
	Wounding potential of bullets: Most damage done by a bullet is a result of amount of energy transferred to tissue impacted; speed of bullet has much greater effect than increased size; some bullets are designed to expand or fragment when striking an object, for example, *hollow-point* ammunition; lethality of a wound depends on what structures are damaged; wounds of brain may not be lethal; however, they are usually immediately incapacitating and lead to significant long-term disability; a person with a "lethal" injury (wound of heart or aorta) also may not be immediately incapacitated

*a*From Prahlow, J.A. (2016). *Forensic autopsy of sharp-force injuries.* http://emedicine.medscape.com/article/1680082-overview.

the neck. Strangulation causes cerebral hypoxia or anoxia secondary to the alteration or cessation of blood flow to and from the brain. It is important to remember that the amount of force needed to close the jugular veins (2 kg) or carotid arteries (5 kg) is significantly less than that required to crush the trachea (15 kg). It is the alteration of cerebral blood flow in most types of strangulation that causes injury or death—not the lack of airflow. With complete blockage of the carotid arteries, unconsciousness can occur within 10 to 15 seconds.

Hanging strangulations result from a noose around the neck, where the weight of the body causes constriction of the noose and compression of the neck. The body does not need to be completely suspended to produce severe injury or death. Depending on the type of ligature used, there usually is a distinct mark on the neck—an inverted V with the base of the V pointing toward the point of suspension. Internal injuries of the neck are actually quite rare in hangings, and only in judicial hangings, in which the body is weighted and dropped, is significant soft tissue or cervical spinal trauma seen. Petechiae of the eyes or face can happen, but they are rare.

In **ligature strangulation**, the mark on the neck is horizontal without the inverted V pattern seen in hangings. Petechiae may be more common because intermittent opening and closure of the blood vessels may occur from the victim's struggles. Internal injuries of the neck are rare.

Variable amounts of external trauma on the neck are found with contusions and abrasions in **manual strangulation** caused either by the assailant or by the victim clawing at his or her own neck in an attempt to remove the assailant's hands. Internal damage can be quite severe, with bruising of deep structures and even fractures of the hyoid bone and tracheal and cricoid cartilages. Petechiae are common.

Chemical asphyxiants. **Chemical asphyxiants** either prevent the delivery of oxygen to the tissues or block its use. Carbon monoxide is the most common chemical asphyxiant. **Cyanide** acts as an asphyxiant by combining with the ferric iron atom in cytochrome oxidase (an enzyme in the electron transport chain used to create ATP in mitochondria), thereby blocking the intracellular use of oxygen. A victim of cyanide poisoning will have the same cherry-red appearance as a carbon monoxide intoxication victim because cyanide blocks the use of circulating oxyhemoglobin. An odour of bitter almonds may also be present. (The ability to smell cyanide is a genetic trait that is absent in a significant portion of the general population.) **Hydrogen sulphide** (sewer gas) is a chemical asphyxiant in which victims of hydrogen cyanide poisoning may have brown-tinged blood in addition to the non-specific signs of asphyxiation.

Drowning. **Drowning** is an alteration of oxygen delivery to tissues resulting from the inhalation of fluid, usually water. In 2016, there were 408 drowning deaths in Canada.[66] Changes in blood electrolyte levels and volume from the absorption of fluid from the lungs may be an important factor in some drownings; however, the major mechanism of injury is hypoxemia (low blood oxygen levels). Even in freshwater drownings, where large amounts of water can pass through the alveolar-capillary interface, there is no evidence that increases in blood volume result in significant electrolyte disturbances or hemolysis, or that the amount of fluid loading is beyond the compensatory capabilities of the kidneys and heart. Airway obstruction is the more important pathological abnormality, underscored by the fact that in as many as 15% of drownings, little or no water enters the lungs because of vagal nerve–mediated laryngospasms. This phenomenon is **dry-lung drowning**.

No matter what mechanism is involved, cerebral hypoxia leads to unconsciousness in a matter of minutes. Whether this cerebral hypoxia progresses to death depends on a number of factors, including the age and the health of the individual. One of the most important factors is the temperature of the water. Irreversible injury develops much more rapidly in warm water than it does in cold water. Children have survived after submergence in very cold water for up to one hour. Complete submersion is not necessary for a person to drown. An incapacitated or helpless individual (e.g., epileptic, alcoholic, infant) may drown in water that is only a few centimetres deep.

It is important to remember that no specific or diagnostic findings *prove* that a person recovered from the water is actually a drowning victim. In cases where water has entered the lung, there may be large amounts of foam exiting the nose and mouth, although the same sign also exists in certain types of drug overdoses. A body recovered from water with signs of prolonged immersion could just as easily be a victim of some other type of injury with the immersion acting to obscure the actual cause of death. When working with a living victim recovered from water, it is essential to keep in mind that an underlying condition may have led to the person's becoming incapacitated and submerged—a condition that also may need to be treated or corrected while correcting hypoxemia and dealing with its complications.

Infectious Injury

The pathogenicity (virulence) of microorganisms lies in their ability to survive and proliferate in the human body, where they injure cells and tissues. The disease-producing potential of a microorganism depends on its ability to (1) invade and destroy cells, (2) produce toxins, and (3) produce damaging hypersensitivity reactions. (See Chapter 8 for a description of infection and infectious organisms.)

Immunological and Inflammatory Injury

Cellular membranes are injured by direct contact with cellular and chemical components of the immune and inflammatory responses, such as phagocytic cells (lymphocytes, macrophages) and substances such as histamine, antibodies, lymphokines, complement, and proteases (see Chapter 6). Complement is responsible for many of the membrane alterations that occur during immunological injury.

Membrane alterations are associated with a rapid leakage of K^+ out of the cell and a rapid influx of water. Antibodies can interfere with membrane function by binding with and occupying receptor molecules on the plasma membrane. Antibodies also can block or destroy cellular junctions, interfering with intercellular communication. Other mechanisms of cellular injury are genetic and epigenetic factors, nutritional imbalances, and physical agents. Table 4.9 summarizes these mechanisms.

MANIFESTATIONS OF CELLULAR INJURY: ACCUMULATIONS

> ✓ **QUICK CHECK 4.4**
> 1. Why is an increase in the concentration of intracellular calcium injurious?
> 2. Compare and contrast necrosis and apoptosis.
> 3. Why is apoptosis significant?
> 4. Define *autophagy*.

Intracellular accumulation of abnormal amounts of various substances and the resultant metabolic disturbances is an important manifestation of cellular injury. **Cellular accumulations**, also known as infiltrations, result not only from sublethal, sustained injury of cells but also from normal (but inefficient) cell function. Two categories of substances can produce accumulations: (1) *normal cellular substances* (such as excess water, proteins, lipids, and carbohydrates) and (2) *abnormal substances*, either endogenous (such as a product of abnormal metabolism or synthesis) or exogenous (such as infectious agents or a mineral). These products can accumulate transiently or permanently and can be toxic or harmless, depending on the substance. Four general mechanisms explain how accumulations abnormally accumulate inside the cell (Figure 4.21). Abnormal accumulations of these substances can occur in the cytoplasm (often in the lysosomes) or in the nucleus for a number of reasons:

(1) There is insufficient removal of the normal substance because of altered packaging and transport, such as what happens with fatty change in the liver, (e.g., *steatosis*).
(2) An abnormal substance, often the result of a mutated gene, accumulates because of defects in protein folding, transport, or abnormal degradation.
(3) There is inadequate metabolism of an endogenous substance (normal or abnormal), usually because of lack of a vital lysosomal enzyme, and these are called *storage diseases*.
(4) Harmful exogenous materials, such as heavy metals, mineral dusts, or microorganisms, accumulate because of inhalation, ingestion, or infection.

In all storage diseases, the cells attempt to digest, or catabolize, the "stored" substances. As a result, excessive amounts of metabolites (products of catabolism) accumulate in the cells and enter the ECM, where phagocytic cells called *macrophages* consume them (see Chapter 6). Some of these scavenger cells circulate throughout the body, whereas others remain fixed in certain tissues, such as the liver or spleen. As more and more macrophages and other phagocytes migrate to tissues that are producing excessive metabolites, the affected tissues begin to swell. This mechanism causes enlargement of the liver (hepatomegaly) or the spleen (splenomegaly) as a clinical manifestation of many storage diseases.

Water

Cellular swelling, the most common degenerative change, results from the shift of extracellular water into the cells. In hypoxic injury, movement of fluid and ions into the cell is associated with acute failure of metabolism and loss of ATP production. Normally, ATP and the enzyme involved in active transport, adenosine triphosphatase (ATPase), maintain the pump that transports sodium ions (Na^+) out of the cell. In metabolic failure caused by hypoxia, reduced levels of ATP and ATPase permit sodium to accumulate in the cell while potassium (K^+) diffuses outward. The increased intracellular sodium concentration increases osmotic pressure, drawing more water into the cell. The cisternae of the ER swell, rupture, and then unite to form large vacuoles that isolate the water from the cytoplasm, a process called *vacuolation*. Progressive vacuolation results in cytoplasmic swelling called **oncosis** (which has replaced the old term *hydropic [water] degeneration*) or vacuolar degeneration (Figure 4.22). If cellular swelling affects all the cells in an organ, the organ increases in weight and becomes distended and pale.

Cellular swelling is reversible and is sublethal. It is, in fact, an early manifestation of almost all types of cellular injury, including severe or lethal cellular injury. It is also associated with high fever, hypokalemia (abnormally low concentrations of potassium in the blood; see Chapter 5), and certain infections.

Lipids and Carbohydrates

Certain metabolic disorders result in the abnormal intracellular accumulation of carbohydrates and lipids. These substances may accumulate throughout the body but primarily favour the spleen, liver, and CNS. Accumulations in cells of the CNS can cause neurological dysfunction and severe intellectual disability. Lipids accumulate in Tay-Sachs disease, Niemann-Pick disease, and Gaucher's disease. The mucopolysaccharidoses, where carbohydrates are in excess, are progressive disorders that usually involve multiple organs, including the liver, spleen,

TABLE 4.9	Mechanisms of Cellular Injury	
Mechanism	**Characteristics**	**Examples**
Genetic Factors	Alter cell's nucleus and plasma membrane's structure, shape, receptors, or transport mechanisms	Sickle cell anemia, Huntington's disease, muscular dystrophy, abetalipoproteinemia, familial hypercholesterolemia
Epigenetic Factors	Induction of mitotically heritable alterations in gene expression without changing DNA	Gene silencing in cancer
Nutritional Imbalances	Pathophysiological cellular effects develop when nutrients are not consumed in diet and transported to body's cells *or* when excessive amounts of nutrients are consumed and transported	Protein deficiency, protein-calorie malnutrition, glucose deficiency, lipid deficiency (hypolipidemia), dyslipidemia (increased lipoproteins in blood causing deposits of fat in heart, liver, and muscle), vitamin deficiencies
Physical Agents		
Temperature extremes	*Hypothermic injury* results from chilling or freezing of cells, creating high intracellular sodium concentrations; abrupt drops in temperature lead to vasoconstriction and increased viscosity of blood, causing ischemic injury, infarction, and necrosis; reactive oxygen species are important in this process	Frostbite
	Hyperthermic injury is caused by excessive heat and varies in severity according to nature, intensity, and extent of heat	Burns, burn blisters, heat cramps usually from vigorous exercise with water and salt loss; heat exhaustion with salt and water loss causes heme contraction; heat stroke is life-threatening with a clinical rectal temperature of 41°C (106°F)
	Tissue injury caused by compressive waves of air or fluid impinging on body, followed by sudden wave of decreased pressure; changes may collapse thorax, rupture internal solid organs, and cause widespread hemorrhage: carbon dioxide and nitrogen that are normally dissolved in blood precipitate from solution and form small bubbles (gas emboli), causing hypoxic injury and pain	Blast injury (air or immersion), decompression sickness (caisson disease or "the bends"); recently reported in a few individuals with subdural hematomas after riding high-speed roller coasters
Ionizing radiation	Refers to any form of radiation that can remove orbital electrons from atoms; source is usually environment and medical use; damage is to DNA molecule, causing chromosomal aberrations, chromosomal instability, and damage to membranes and enzymes; also induces growth factors and extracellular matrix remodelling; uncertainty exists regarding effects of low levels of radiation	X-rays, γ-rays, and α- and β-particles cause skin redness, skin damage, chromosomal damage, cancer
Illumination	Fluorescent lighting and halogen lamps create harmful oxidative stresses; ultraviolet light has been linked to skin cancer	Eyestrain, obscured vision, cataracts, headaches, melanoma
Mechanical stresses	Injury is caused by physical impact or irritation; they may be overt or cumulative	Faulty occupational biomechanics, leading to overexertion disorders
Noise	Can be caused by acute loud noise or cumulative effects of various intensities, frequencies, and duration of noise; considered a public health threat	Hearing impairment or loss; tinnitus, temporary threshold shift, or loss can occur as a complication of critical illness, from mechanical trauma, ototoxic medications, infections, vascular disorders, and noise

heart, and blood vessels. T mucopolysaccharides accumulate in reticuloendothelial cells, endothelial cells, intimal smooth muscle cells, and fibroblasts throughout the body. In turn, these carbohydrate accumulations can cause clouding of the cornea, joint stiffness, and intellectual disability.

Although lipids sometimes accumulate in heart, muscle, and kidney cells, the most common site of intracellular lipid accumulation, or **fatty change (steatosis)**, is liver cells (Figure 4.23). Because hepatic metabolism and secretion of lipids are crucial to proper body function, imbalances and deficiencies in these processes lead to major pathological changes. In developed countries, the most common cause of fatty change in the liver is alcohol abuse (see Chapter 36). Other causes of fatty change include diabetes mellitus, protein malnutrition, toxins, anoxia, and obesity. As lipids fill the cells, vacuolation pushes the nucleus and other organelles aside. The liver's outward appearance is yellow and greasy.

Lipid accumulation in liver cells occurs after cellular injury instigates one or more of the following mechanisms:

1. Increased movement of free fatty acids into the liver (starvation, e.g., increases the metabolism of triglycerides in adipose tissue, releasing fatty acids that subsequently enter liver cells)
2. Failure of the metabolic process that converts fatty acids to phospholipids, resulting in the preferential conversion of fatty acids to triglycerides
3. Increased synthesis of triglycerides from fatty acids (increased levels of the enzyme α-glycerophosphatase can accelerate triglyceride synthesis)
4. Decreased synthesis of apoproteins (lipid-acceptor proteins)

CHAPTER 4 Altered Cellular and Tissue Biology

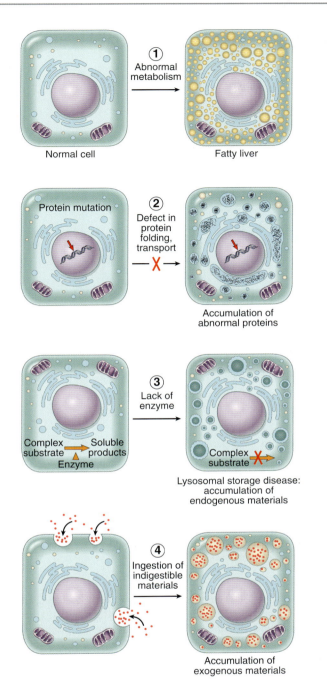

FIGURE 4.21 Mechanisms of Intracellular Accumulations. (From Kumar, V., Abbas, A. K., & Aster, J. C. [Eds.]. [2021]. *Robbins and Cotran pathologic basis of disease* [10th ed.]. Elsevier.)

5. Failure of lipids to bind with apoproteins and form lipoproteins
6. Failure of mechanisms that transport lipoproteins out of the cell
7. Direct damage to the ER by free radicals released by alcohol's toxic effects

Many pathological states show accumulation of cholesterol and cholesterol esters. These states include atherosclerosis, in which atherosclerotic plaques, smooth muscle cells, and macrophages within the intimal layer of the aorta and large arteries contain lipid-rich vacuoles of cholesterol and cholesterol esters. Other states include cholesterol-rich deposits in the gallbladder and Niemann-Pick disease (type C), which involve genetic mutations of an enzyme affecting cholesterol transport.

Glycogen

Glycogen storage is important as a readily available energy source in the cytoplasm of normal cells. Intracellular accumulations of glycogen occur in genetic disorders called *glycogen storage diseases* and in disorders of glucose and glycogen metabolism. As with water and lipid accumulation, glycogen accumulation results in excessive vacuolation of the cytoplasm. The most common cause of glycogen accumulation is the disorder of glucose metabolism (i.e., diabetes mellitus) (see Chapter 19).

Proteins

Proteins provide cellular structure and constitute most of the cell's dry weight. Ribosomes synthesize proteins in the cytoplasm from the essential amino acids lysine, threonine, leucine, isoleucine, methionine, tryptophan, valine, phenylalanine, and histidine. The accumulation of protein probably damages cells in two ways. Cellular organelle damage may occur when metabolites (enzymes produced when the cell attempts to digest some proteins) are released from lysosomes. Additionally, when excessive amounts of protein are present in the cytoplasm, they may push against cellular organelles, disrupting organelle function and intracellular communication.

Protein excess accumulates primarily in the epithelial cells of the renal convoluted tubules of the nephron unit and in the antibody-forming plasma cells (B lymphocytes) of the immune system. Several types of renal disorders cause excessive excretion of protein molecules in the urine (proteinuria). Normally, little or no protein is present in the urine, and its presence in significant amounts indicates cellular injury and altered cellular function.

Accumulations of protein in B lymphocytes can occur during active synthesis of antibodies during the immune response. These excess aggregates of protein are *Russell bodies* (see Chapter 6). Russell bodies are numerous in multiple myeloma (plasma cell tumour) (see Chapter 21).

Furthermore, mutations in protein can slow protein folding, resulting in the accumulation of partially folded intermediates. An example is α_1-antitrypsin deficiency, which can cause emphysema. Certain types of cellular injury are associated with the accumulation of cytoskeleton proteins. For example, the *neurofibrillary tangle* found in the brain in Alzheimer's disease contains these types of proteins.

Pigments

Pigment accumulations may be normal or abnormal, as well as endogenous (produced within the body) or exogenous (produced outside the body). Endogenous pigments come from amino acids, for example (e.g., tyrosine, tryptophan). They include melanin and the blood proteins porphyrins, hemoglobin, and hemosiderin. Lipid-rich pigments, such as lipofuscin (the aging pigment), give a yellow-brown colour to cells undergoing slow, regressive, and often atrophic changes. The most common exogenous pigment is carbon (coal dust), a pervasive air pollutant in urban areas. Inhaled carbon interacts with lung macrophages and travels by lymphatic vessels to regional lymph nodes. This accumulation blackens lung tissues and involved lymph nodes. Other exogenous pigments include mineral dusts containing silica and iron particles, lead, silver salts, and dyes for tattoos.

Melanin

Melanin accumulates in epithelial cells (keratinocytes) of the skin and retina. It is an extremely important pigment because it protects the skin

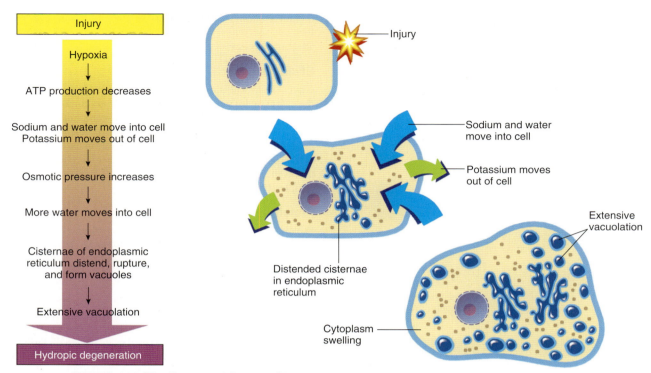

FIGURE 4.22 The Process of Oncosis (Formerly Referred to as "Hydropic Degeneration"). *ATP,* Adenosine triphosphate.

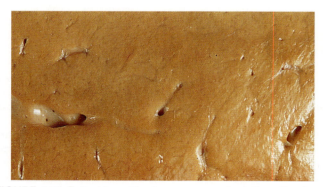

FIGURE 4.23 Fatty Liver. The liver appears yellow. (From Damjanov, I., & Linder, J. [2000]. *Pathology: A color atlas.* Mosby.)

against long exposure to sunlight and is an essential factor in the prevention of skin cancer (see Chapters 11 and 41). Ultraviolet light (e.g., sunlight) stimulates the synthesis of melanin, which probably absorbs ultraviolet rays during subsequent exposure. Melanin also may protect the skin by trapping the injurious free radicals produced by the action of ultraviolet light on skin.

Melanin is a brown-black pigment derived from the amino acid *tyrosine. Melanocytes* synthesize this pigment and *melanosomes*, membrane-bound cytoplasmic vesicles store it.

Melanin also accumulates in melanophores (melanin-containing pigment cells), macrophages, or other phagocytic cells in the dermis. Presumably, these cells acquire the melanin from nearby melanocytes or from pigment released from dying epidermal cells. This mechanism causes freckles. Melanin also occurs in the benign form of pigmented moles called *nevi* (see Chapter 41). Malignant melanoma is a cancerous skin tumour that contains melanin.

A decrease in melanin production occurs in the inherited disorder of melanin metabolism called *albinism*. Albinism is often diffuse, involving all the skin, the eyes, and the hair. Albinism also involves phenylalanine metabolism. In classic types, the person with albinism is unable to convert tyrosine to 3,4-dihydroxyphenylalanine (DOPA), an intermediate in melanin biosynthesis. Melanocytes are present in normal numbers, but they are unable to make melanin. Individuals with albinism are very sensitive to sunlight and quickly become sunburned. They are also at high risk for skin cancer.

Hemoproteins

Hemoproteins are among the most essential of the normal endogenous pigments. They include hemoglobin and the oxidative enzymes or **cytochromes**. A knowledge of iron uptake, metabolism, excretion, and storage is integral to an understanding of disorders involving these pigments (see Chapter 20). Excessive storage of iron can cause hemoprotein accumulations in cells, and this then transfers to the cells from the bloodstream. Iron enters the blood from three primary sources: (1) tissue stores, (2) the intestinal mucosa (mainly the stomach), and (3) macrophages that remove and destroy dead or defective red blood cells. The amount of iron in blood plasma depends also on the metabolism of the major iron transport protein, *transferrin*.

Iron is stored in tissue cells in two forms: as ferritin and, when increased levels of iron are present, as hemosiderin. **Hemosiderin** is a yellow-brown pigment derived from hemoglobin. With pathological states, excesses of iron cause hemosiderin to accumulate within cells, often in areas of bruising and hemorrhage and in the lungs and spleen after congestion caused by heart failure. With local hemorrhage, the skin first appears red-blue and then lysis of the escaped red blood cells occurs, causing transformation of hemoglobin to hemosiderin. The colour changes noted in bruising reflect this transformation (Figure 4.24).

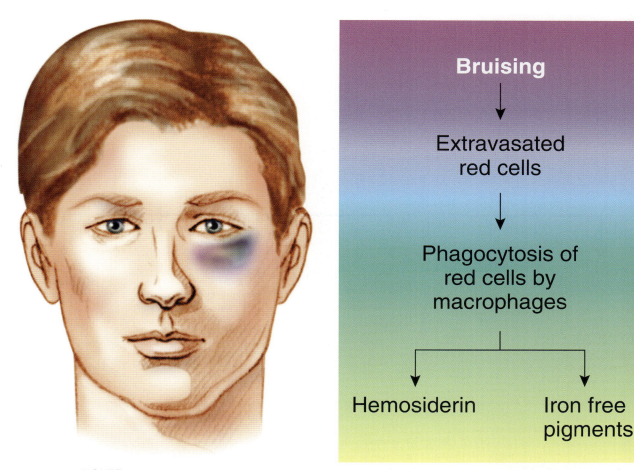

FIGURE 4.24 The Colour Changes in a "Black Eye" Highlight Hemoseridin Accumulation Post Trauma.

Hemosiderosis is a condition in which excess iron is stored as hemosiderin in the cells of many organs and tissues. This condition is common in individuals who have received repeated blood transfusions or prolonged parenteral administration of iron. Hemosiderosis is also associated with increased absorption of dietary iron, and conditions where iron storage and transport are impaired, as well as hemolytic anemia (when there is excessive breakdown of red blood cells). Excessive alcohol (e.g., wine) ingestion also can lead to hemosiderosis. Normally, an iron absorption process in the intestines prevents absorption of excessive dietary iron. Failure of this process can lead to total body iron accumulations in the range of 60 to 80 g, compared with normal iron stores of 4.5 to 5 g. Excessive accumulations of iron, such as occur in hemochromatosis (a genetic disorder of iron metabolism and the most severe example of iron overload), are associated with liver and pancreatic cell damage.

Bilirubin is a normal, yellow-to-green pigment of bile derived from the porphyrin structure of hemoglobin. Excess bilirubin within cells and tissues causes jaundice (icterus), or yellowing of the skin. Jaundice occurs when the bilirubin level exceeds 25 to 34 mmol/L of plasma, compared with the normal values of 6.8 to 17.1 mmol/L. Hyperbilirubinemia occurs with the following three circumstances: (1) mass destruction of red blood cells (erythrocytes), such as in hemolytic jaundice; (2) diseases affecting the metabolism and excretion of bilirubin in the liver; and (3) diseases that cause obstruction of the common bile duct, such as gallstones or pancreatic tumours. Certain medications (specifically chlorpromazine [Largactil] and other phenothiazine derivatives), estrogenic hormones, and halothane (Fluothane) (an anaesthetic) can cause the obstruction of normal bile flow through the liver.

Because unconjugated bilirubin is lipid soluble, it can injure the lipid components of the plasma membrane. Albumin, a plasma protein, provides significant protection by binding unconjugated bilirubin in plasma. Unconjugated bilirubin causes two cellular outcomes: uncoupling of oxidative phosphorylation and a loss of cellular proteins. These two changes could cause structural injury to the various membranes of the cell.

Calcium

Calcium salts accumulate in both injured and dead tissues (Figure 4.25). An important mechanism of cellular calcification is the influx of extracellular calcium in injured mitochondria. Another mechanism that causes calcium accumulation in alveoli (gas-exchange airways of the lungs), gastric epithelium, and renal tubules is the excretion of acid at these sites. This leads to the local production of hydroxyl ions. Hydroxyl ions then combine with calcium and precipitate out of solution as calcium hydroxide, $Ca(OH)_2$, and hydroxyapatite, $Ca_5(PO_4)_3OH$, a mixed salt. Damage occurs when calcium salts cluster and harden, interfering with normal cellular structure and function.

Pathological calcification can be dystrophic or metastatic. **Dystrophic calcification** occurs in dying and dead tissues in areas of necrosis (see also the types of necrosis: coagulative, liquefactive, caseous, and fatty). It is present in chronic tuberculosis of the lungs and lymph nodes, advanced atherosclerosis (narrowing of the arteries because of plaque

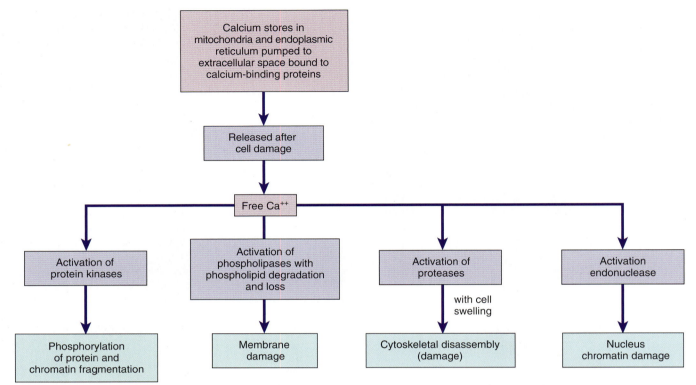

FIGURE 4.25 Free Cytosolic Calcium: A Destructive Agent. Adenosine triphosphate (ATP)–dependent calcium pumps normally remove calcium (Ca^{++}). Calcium is also bound to buffering proteins, such as calbindin or parvalbumin, in normal cells and is contained in the endoplasmic reticulum and the mitochondria. If there is abnormal permeability of calcium-ion channels, direct damage to membranes, or depletion of ATP (i.e., hypoxic injury), calcium increases in the cytosol. If calcium buffering or active transport of calcium from the cell does not occur, uncontrolled enzyme activation takes place, and this causes further damage. Uncontrolled entry of calcium into the cytosol is an important final common pathway in many causes of cellular death.

accumulation), and heart valve injury (Figure 4.26). Calcification of the heart valves interferes with their opening and closing and causes heart murmurs (see Chapter 24). Calcification of the coronary arteries predisposes them to severe narrowing and thrombosis, which can lead to myocardial infarction. Another site of dystrophic calcification is the centre of tumours. Over time, the centre is deprived of its oxygen supply, dies, and becomes calcified. The calcium salts appear as gritty, clumped granules that can become hard as stone. When several layers clump together, they resemble grains of sand and become **psammoma bodies**.

Metastatic calcification consists of mineral deposits that occur in undamaged normal tissues as the result of hypercalcemia (excess calcium in the blood; see Chapter 5). Conditions that cause hypercalcemia include hyperparathyroidism, toxic levels of vitamin D, hyperthyroidism, idiopathic hypercalcemia of infancy, Addison's disease (adrenocortical insufficiency), systemic sarcoidosis, milk-alkali syndrome, and the increased bone demineralization that results from bone tumours, leukemia, and disseminated cancers. Hypercalcemia also may occur in advanced renal failure with phosphate retention. As phosphate levels increase, the activity of the parathyroid gland increases, thus causing higher levels of circulating calcium.

Urate

In humans, uric acid (**urate**) is the major end product of purine catabolism because of the absence of the enzyme, urate oxidase. Serum urate concentration is, in general, stable: approximately 297.4 μmol/L in postpubertal males and 243.9 μmol/L in postpubertal females. Disturbances in maintaining serum urate levels result in hyperuricemia and the deposition of sodium urate crystals in the tissues, leading to painful disorders collectively called *gout*. These disorders include acute arthritis, chronic gouty arthritis, tophi (firm, nodular, subcutaneous deposits of urate crystals surrounded by fibrosis), and nephritis (inflammation of the nephron). Chronic hyperuricemia results in the deposition of urate in tissues, cellular injury, and inflammation. Because lysosomal enzymes do not degrade urate crystals, these crystals persist in dead cells.

Systemic Manifestations

Systemic manifestations of cellular injury include a general sense of fatigue and malaise, a loss of well-being, and altered appetite. Fever is often present because of biochemicals produced during the inflammatory response. Table 4.10 summarizes the most significant systemic manifestations of cellular injury.

CELLULAR DEATH

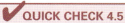 **QUICK CHECK 4.5**
1. Cellular aging is a complex process. What mechanisms are involved?
2. What are the body composition changes that occur with cellular aging?
3. Define *frailty* and possible endocrine–immune system involvement.

CHAPTER 4 Altered Cellular and Tissue Biology

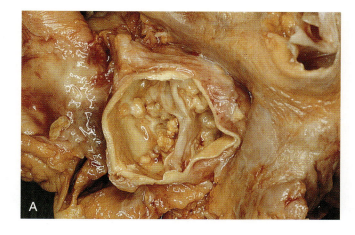

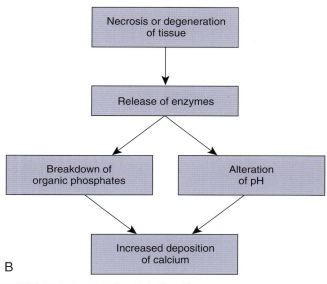

FIGURE 4.26 Aortic Valve Calcification. A, This calcified aortic valve is an example of dystrophic calcification. **B,** This algorithm shows the dystrophic mechanism of calcification. ([A] from Damjanov, I. [2012]. *Pathology for the health professions* [4th ed.]. Saunders.)

TABLE 4.10	Systemic Manifestations of Cellular Injury
Manifestation	**Cause**
Fever	Release of endogenous pyrogens (interleukin-1, tumour necrosis factor-alpha, prostaglandins) from bacteria or macrophages; acute inflammatory response
Increased heart rate	Increase in oxidative metabolic processes resulting from fever
Increase in leukocytes (leukocytosis)	Increase in total number of white blood cells because of infection; normal is 5 000–9 000/mm³ (increase is directly related to severity of infection)
Pain	Various mechanisms, such as release of bradykinins, obstruction, pressure
Presence of cellular enzymes	Release of enzymes from cells of tissue[a] in extracellular fluid
Lactate dehydrogenase (LDH) (LDH isoenzymes)	Release from red blood cells, liver, kidney, skeletal muscle
Creatine kinase (CK) (CK isoenzymes)	Release from skeletal muscle, brain, heart
Aspartate aminotransferase (AST/SGOT)	Release from heart, liver, skeletal muscle, kidney, pancreas
Alanine aminotransferase (ALT/SGPT)	Release from liver, kidney, heart
Alkaline phosphatase (ALP)	Release from liver, bone
Amylase	Release from pancreas
Aldolase	Release from skeletal muscle, heart

[a]The rapidity of enzyme transfer is a function of the weight of the enzyme and the concentration gradient across the cellular membrane. The specific metabolic and excretory rates of the enzymes determine how long levels of enzymes remain elevated.

In response to significant external stimuli, cellular injury becomes irreversible and cells die. Necrosis and apoptosis are two ways to classify cellular death. **Necrosis** is characterized by rapid loss of the plasma membrane structure, swelling of organelles, dysfunction of the mitochondria, and lack of typical features of apoptosis.[67] **Apoptosis** is known as a regulated or programmed cell process characterized by the "dropping off" of cellular fragments called *apoptotic bodies*. Many disorders involve too little or too much apoptosis, including neurodegenerative diseases, ischemic damage, autoimmune disorders, and cancers. Yet, apoptosis can have normal functions, and unlike necrosis, it is not always a pathological process. Necrosis is the main outcome in several common injuries including ischemia, toxin exposure, certain infections, and trauma. Necrosis may be *regulated* or *programmed* in a well-orchestrated way as a backup for apoptosis (apoptosis may progress to necrosis)[68]—hence the new term, **programmed necrosis**, or necroptosis. Necroptosis shares traits with both necrosis and apoptosis. Necroptosis is recognized in both normal physiological conditions and pathological conditions, including bone growth plate disorders, cellular death in fatty liver disease, acute pancreatitis, reperfusion injury, and certain neuro-degenerative disorders, such as Parkinson's disease.[1]

Historically, programmed cellular death only referred to apoptosis. Figure 4.27 illustrates the structural changes in cellular injury resulting in necrosis or apoptosis. Table 4.11 compares the unique features of necrosis and apoptosis. Other forms of cell loss include autophagy (self-eating).

Necrosis

Cellular death eventually leads to cellular dissolution, or necrosis. **Necrosis** is the sum of cellular changes after local cellular death and the process of cellular self-digestion, known as autodigestion or **autolysis** (see Figure 4.27). Cells die long before a light microscopy highlights any necrotic changes. The structural signs that indicate irreversible injury and progression to necrosis are dense clumping and progressive disruption both of genetic material and of plasma and organelle membranes. Because membrane integrity is lost, necrotic cell contents leak out and may cause the signalling of inflammation in surrounding tissue. In later stages of necrosis, disruption of most organelles occurs, and **karyolysis** (nuclear dissolution and lysis of chromatin from the action of hydrolytic enzymes) is under way. In some cells, the nucleus shrinks and becomes a small, dense mass of genetic material **(pyknosis)**. The pyknotic nucleus eventually dissolves (by karyolysis) through the action of hydrolytic lysosomal enzymes on DNA. **Karyorrhexis** means fragmentation of the nucleus into smaller particles, or "nuclear dust."

Although necrosis still refers to death induced by nonspecific trauma or injury (e.g., cell stress or the heat shock response), with the very recent identification of molecular mechanisms regulating the process

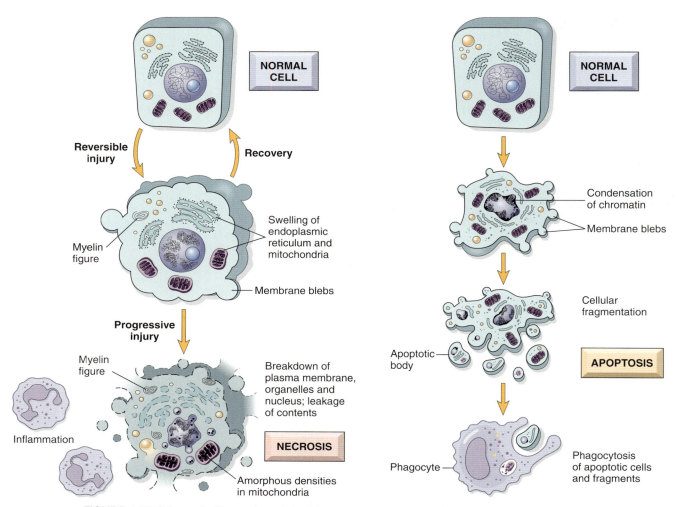

FIGURE 4.27 Schematic Illustration of the Morphological Changes in Cellular Injury Culminating in Necrosis or Apoptosis. Myelin figures come from degenerating cellular membranes and are noted within the cytoplasm or extracellularly. (From Oakes, S. A. [2021]. Cell injury, cell death, and adaptations. In V. Kumar, A. K. Abbas, & J. C. Aster [Eds.], *Robbins and Cotran pathologic basis of disease* [10th ed., pp. 33–70]. Elsevier.)

of necrosis, the study of necrosis has experienced a new twist. Cellular death by necrosis occurs in a seemingly disorganized and unregulated manner. Some molecular regulators governing programmed necrosis, however, communicate through a large network of signalling pathways.[69] Programmed necrosis is actually associated with pathological diseases and provides innate immune response to viral infection.[69]

Different types of necrosis tend to occur in different organs or tissues and sometimes can indicate the mechanism or cause of cellular injury. The four major types of necrosis are coagulative, liquefactive, caseous, and fatty. Another type, gangrenous necrosis, is *not* a distinctive type of cellular death but refers instead to larger areas of tissue death. A summary of these necroses follows:

1. **Coagulative necrosis**. It occurs primarily in the kidneys, heart, and adrenal glands; it commonly results from hypoxia caused by severe ischemia or hypoxia caused by chemical injury, especially ingestion of mercuric chloride. Coagulation is a result of protein denaturation, which causes the protein albumin to change from a gelatinous, transparent state to a firm, opaque state (Figure 4.28A). The area of coagulative necrosis is called an **infarct**.
2. **Liquefactive necrosis**. It commonly results from ischemic injury to neurons and glial cells in the brain (Figure 4.28B). Liquefactive necrosis readily affects dead brain tissue because brain cells are rich in digestive hydrolytic enzymes and lipids, and the brain contains little connective tissue. Cells initiate autodigestion by their own hydrolases, so the tissue becomes soft, liquefies, and segregates from healthy tissue, forming cysts. Bacterial infection, especially by *Staphylococci*, *Streptococci*, and *Escherichia coli*, causes this condition.
3. **Caseous necrosis**. It usually results from tuberculous pulmonary infection, especially by *Mycobacterium tuberculosis* (Figure 4.28C). It is a combination of coagulative and liquefactive necroses. The dead cells disintegrate, but the hydrolases do not completely remove all the debris. Tissues resemble clumped cheese in that they are soft and granular. A granulomatous inflammatory wall encloses areas of caseous necrosis.
4. **Fatty necrosis**. Fat necrosis is cellular dissolution caused by powerful enzymes, called *lipases* that occur in the breast, pancreas, and other abdominal structures (Figure 4.28D). Lipases break down triglycerides, releasing free fatty acids that then combine with calcium, magnesium, and sodium ions, creating soaps (saponification). The necrotic tissue appears opaque and chalk-white.
5. **Gangrenous necrosis**. Although it refers to death of tissue, this type of gangrene is not a specific pattern of cellular death. It results from severe hypoxic injury, which commonly occurs because of

CHAPTER 4 Altered Cellular and Tissue Biology

TABLE 4.11 Features of Necrosis and Apoptosis

Feature	Necrosis	Apoptosis
Cell size	Enlarged (swelling)	Reduced (shrinkage)
Nucleus	Pyknosis → karyorrhexis → karyolysis	Fragmentation into nucleosome-sized fragments
Plasma membrane	Disrupted	Intact; altered structure, especially orientation of lipids
Cellular contents	Enzymatic digestion; may leak out of cell	Intact; may be released in apoptotic bodies
Adjacent inflammation	Frequent	No
Physiological or pathological role	Invariably pathological (culmination of irreversible cellular injury)	Often physiological, means of eliminating unwanted cells; may be pathological after some forms of cellular injury, especially DNA damage

From Oakes, S. A. (2021). Cell injury, cell death, and adaptations. In V. Kumar, A. K. Abbas, & J. C. Aster (Eds.), *Robbins and Cotran pathologic basis of disease* (10th ed., pp. 33–70). Elsevier.

arteriosclerosis, or blockage, of major arteries, particularly those in the lower leg (Figure 4.29). With hypoxia and subsequent bacterial invasion, the tissues can undergo necrosis. *Dry gangrene* is usually the result of coagulative necrosis. The skin becomes very dry and shrinks, resulting in wrinkles, and its colour changes to dark brown or black. *Wet gangrene* develops when neutrophils invade the site, causing liquefactive necrosis. Wet gangrene also usually occurs in internal organs, causing the site to become cold, swollen, and black. A foul odour is present, and death is a possibility if systemic symptoms become severe.

6. **Gas gangrene.** This type of gangrene is the result of infection of injured tissue by one of many species of *Clostridium*. These anaerobic bacteria produce hydrolytic enzymes and toxins that destroy connective tissue and cellular membranes and cause bubbles of gas to form in muscle cells. Gas gangrene can be fatal if enzymes lyse the membranes of red blood cells, destroying their oxygen-carrying capacity. Shock is the main cause of death.

Apoptosis

Apoptosis ("dropping off") is an important distinct type of cellular death that differs from necrosis in several ways (see Figure 4.27 and Table 4.11). Apoptosis is an active process of cellular self-destruction called *programmed cellular death* and happens in both normal and pathological tissue changes. Cells need to die; otherwise, endless

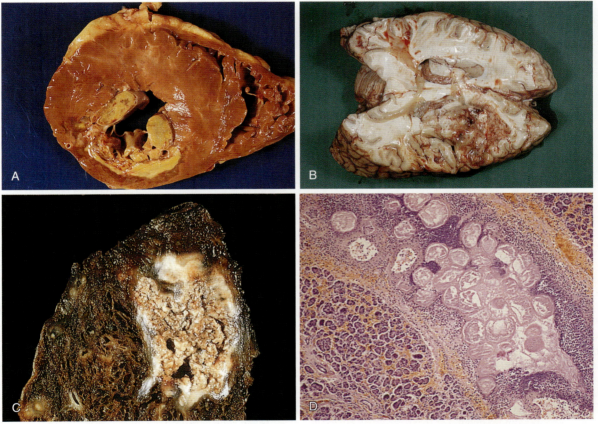

FIGURE 4.28 Types of Necrosis. **A,** Coagulative necrosis. A wedge-shaped kidney infarct (*yellow*). **B,** Liquefactive necrosis of the brain. The area of infarction softens because of liquefaction necrosis. **C,** Caseous necrosis. Tuberculosis of the lung, with a large area of caseous necrosis containing yellow-white and cheesy debris. **D,** Fat necrosis of pancreas. Interlobular adipocytes are necrotic; acute inflammatory cells surround these. ([A] from Kumar, V., Abbas, A. K., & Aster, J. C. [Eds.]. [2015]. *Robbins and Cotran pathologic basis of disease* [9th ed.]. Saunders. [B] from Damjanov, I. [2012]. *Pathology for the health professions* [4th ed.]. Saunders. [C] from Kumar, V., Abbas, A. K., & Aster, J. C. [Eds.]. [2021]. *Robbins and Cotran pathologic basis of disease* [10th ed.]. Elsevier. [D] from Damjanov, I., & Linder, J. [Eds.]. [1996]. *Anderson's pathology* [10th ed.]. Mosby.)

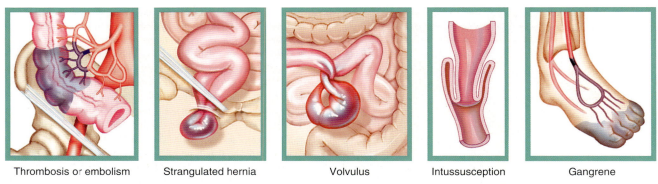

FIGURE 4.29 Gangrene, A Complication of Necrosis. In certain circumstances, necrotic tissue will be invaded by putrefactive organisms that are both saccharolytic and proteolytic. Foul-smelling gases are produced, and the tissue becomes green or black as a result of breakdown of hemoglobin. Obstruction of the blood supply to the bowel almost inevitably is followed by gangrene.

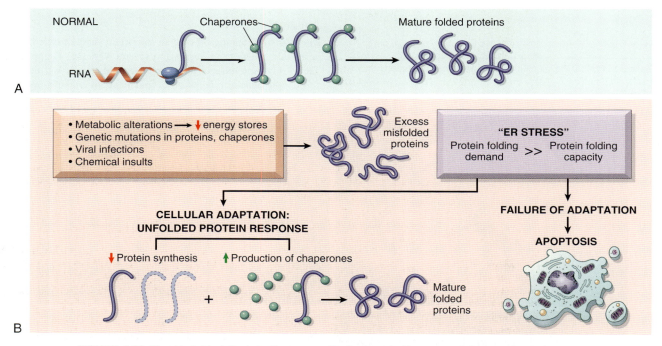

FIGURE 4.30 The Unfolded Protein Response, Endoplasmic Stress, and Apoptosis. A, In normal or healthy cells, chaperones help fold the newly made proteins and then either incorporate them into the cell or secrete them. **B,** Various stressors can cause endoplasmic reticulum *(ER)* stress whereby the cell is challenged to cope with the increased load of misfolded proteins. The accumulation of the protein load initiates the *unfolded protein response* in the ER; if restoration of the protein fails, the cell dies by apoptosis. An example of a disease caused by misfolding of proteins is Alzheimer's disease. (From Kumar, V., Abbas, A. K., & Aster, J. C. [Eds.]. [2021]. *Robbins and Cotran pathologic basis of disease* [10th ed.]. Elsevier.)

proliferation would lead to gigantic bodies. The average adult may create 10 billion new cells every day—and destroy the same number.[70] Death by apoptosis causes loss of cells in many pathological states, including:

- *Severe cellular injury.* When cellular injury exceeds repair mechanisms, the cell triggers apoptosis. *DNA damage* can result either directly or indirectly from production of free radicals.
- *Accumulation of misfolded proteins.* This state may result from genetic mutations or free radicals. Excessive accumulation of misfolded proteins in the ER leads to a condition known as **ER stress** (see Chapter 1). ER stress results in apoptotic cellular death. This mechanism explains several degenerative diseases of the CNS and other organs (Figure 4.30).
- *Infections (particularly viral).* Apoptosis results directly from the infection or indirectly from the host immune response. Cytotoxic T lymphocytes respond to viral infections by inducing apoptosis and, therefore, eliminating the infectious cells. This process can cause tissue damage, and it is the same for cellular death in tumours and rejection of tissue transplants.
- *Obstruction in tissue ducts.* In organs with duct obstruction, including the pancreas, kidney, and parotid gland, apoptosis causes pathological atrophy.

Dysregulated apoptosis is either excessive or insufficient apoptosis and contributes further to disease. For instance, a low rate of apoptosis can permit the survival of abnormal cells, for example, mutated cells that can increase cancer risk. Defective apoptosis may not eliminate lymphocytes

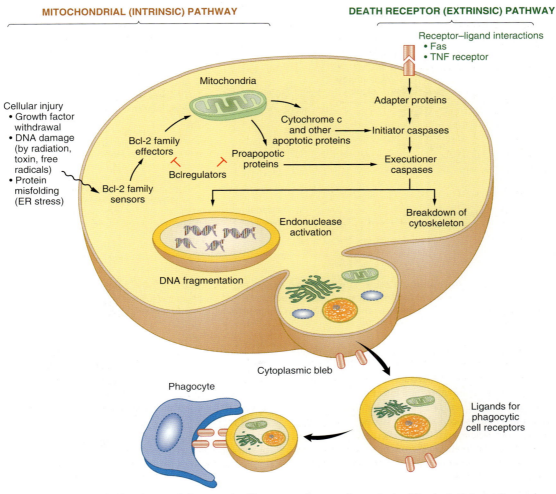

FIGURE 4.31 **Mechanisms of Apoptosis.** The two pathways of apoptosis differ in their induction and regulation, and both culminate in the activation of "executioner" caspases. The induction of apoptosis by the mitochondrial pathway involves the Bcl-2 family, which causes leakage of mitochondrial proteins. The regulators of the death receptor pathway involve the proteases, called *caspases*. *ER stress*, Endoplasmic reticulum stress; *TNF*, tumour necrosis factor. (Adapted from Kumar, V., Abbas, A. K., & Aster, J. C. [Eds.]. [2021]. *Robbins and Cotran pathologic basis of disease* [10th ed.]. Elsevier.)

that react against host tissue (self-antigens), leading to autoimmune disorders. Excessive apoptosis is known to occur in several neurodegenerative diseases, from ischemic injury (such as myocardial infarction and stroke), and from death of virus-infected cells (as seen in many viral infections).

Apoptosis depends on a tightly regulated cellular program for its initiation and execution.[70] This death program involves enzymes that divide other proteins—proteases (or **caspases**), which are activated by proteolytic activity in response to signals that induce apoptosis. The activated suicide caspases cleave and, thereby, activate other members of the family, resulting in an amplifying "suicide" cascade. The activated caspases then cleave other key proteins in the cell, killing the cell quickly and neatly. Two different pathways converge on caspase activation. These are the *mitochondrial (intrinsic) pathway* and the *death receptor (extrinsic) pathway* (Figure 4.31). Cells that die by apoptosis release chemical factors that recruit phagocytes that quickly engulf the remains of the dead cell, thus reducing chances of inflammation. With necrosis, cellular death is not tidy because cells that die from acute injury swell, burst, and spill their contents all over their neighbours, causing a likely damaging inflammatory response.

Autophagy

The Greek term **autophagy** means "eating of self." Autophagy, as a "recycling factory," is a self-destructive process and a survival mechanism. Autophagy involves the delivery of cytoplasmic contents to the lysosome for degradation. Box 4.3 contains the terms used to describe autophagy.

When cells are starved or nutrient deprived, the autophagic process institutes cannibalization and recycles the digested contents.[1,71] Autophagy can maintain cellular metabolism under starvation

BOX 4.3 The Major Forms of Autophagy

Macroautophagy, the most common term to refer to autophagy, involves the sequestration and transportation of parts (cargo) of the cytosol in an autophagic vacuole (autophagosome).

Microautophagy is the inward invagination of the lysosomal membrane for cargo delivery.

Chaperone-mediated autophagy is the chaperone-dependent proteins that direct cargo across the lysosomal membrane.

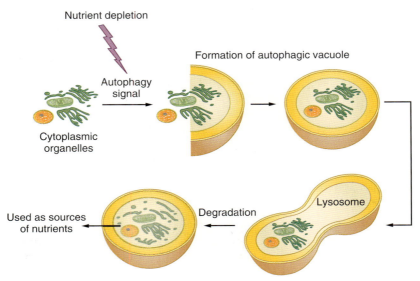

FIGURE 4.32 Autophagy. Cellular stresses, such as nutrient deprivation, activate autophagy genes that create vacuoles in which cellular organelles are sequestered and then degraded following fusion of the vesicles with lysosomes. The digested materials are recycled to provide nutrients for the cell.

conditions and remove damaged organelles under stress conditions, improving the survival of cells. With the central role of autophagy in cell allostasis, autophagy has been implicated in cancer, heart disease, neuro-degenerative diseases, inflammation, and infection.[72] Autophagy begins with a membrane, also known as a *phagophore* (although controversial) (Figure 4.32).[73] This cup-shaped, curved phagophore expands and engulfs intracellular cargo—organelles, ribosomes, proteins—forming a double membrane *autophagosome*. The cargo-laden autophagosome fuses with the lysosome, now called an *autophagolysosome*, which promotes the degradation of the autophagosome by lysosomal acid proteases. The phagophore membrane is highly curved along the rim of the open cup, suggesting that mechanisms responsible for its formation and growth may depend on membrane curvature–dependent events.[74] Lysosomal transporters export amino acids and other by-products of degradation out of the cytoplasm where they can be reused for the synthesis of macromolecules and for metabolism.[75,76] ATP is generated and cellular damage is reduced during autophagy that removes nonfunctional proteins and organelles.[71]

Autophagy has the potential for therapeutic use in many disease states. Autophagy is a critical garbage collecting and recycling process in healthy cells, and this process becomes less efficient and less discriminating as the cell ages. Consequently, harmful agents accumulate in cells, damaging cells and leading to aging: for example, failure to clear protein products in neurons of the CNS can cause dementia; failure to clear ROS-producing mitochondria can lead to nuclear DNA mutations and cancer. Thus, these processes may even partially define aging. Therefore, normal autophagy may potentially rejuvenate an organism and prevent cancer development as well as other degenerative diseases.[77] Autophagy may also be the last immune defense against infectious microorganisms that penetrate intracellularly.[78]

AGING AND ALTERED CELLULAR AND TISSUE BIOLOGY

The terms *aging* and *lifespan* are synonymous; however, they are not equivalent. Aging is usually a normal physiological process that is universal and inevitable, whereas lifespan is the time from birth to death and is useful to study the aging process.[79] Aging is associated with a gradual loss of homeostatic mechanisms with no known identifiable cause.[80] Aging is also a complex process with a focus on genetic, epigenetic, inflammatory, oxidative stress, and metabolic origins of aging. This includes the study of genetic signatures in humans with exceptional longevity, as well as the identification and recent discovery of epigenetic mechanisms that modulate gene expression. The roles of intrauterine environment and lifelong patterns of health help to explain aging even further. The effects of personality, behaviour, and social support, the influence of insulin/insulin-like growth factor 1 (IGF-1) signalling, and the contributions of cellular dysfunction and senescence to an inflammatory microenvironment can lead to chronic disease, frailty, and decreased lifespan. In summary, the factors that may be most important for aging include increased damage to the cell (or reduced capacity for repair) and reduced capacity to divide (or replicative senescence). Similarly, aging results in an increased likelihood of defective protein balance or allostasis as well.[1] A major challenge of aging research has been to separate the causes of cell and tissue aging from the vast changes that accompany it.[80] Public health issues related to healthy aging require understanding the nature of aging and the factors that predict healthy aging.

Aging is not a disease because it is "normal"; disease is usually "abnormal." Conceptually, this distinction seems clear until the concept of "injury" or "damage" comes into play; disease is typically the result of injury. *Chronological aging* is the time-dependent loss of structure and function that proceeds very slowly and in such small increments that it appears to be the result of the accumulation of small, imperceptible injuries—a gradual result of wear and tear. One of the hallmarks of aging is the accumulation of damaged macromolecules. DNA damage can lead to cellular dysfunction both directly and indirectly because of cellular responses to damage that can lead to altered gene expression.[81,82] Age-related changes to macromolecules for long-lived cells, such as neurons and myofibres, lead to gradual loss of structure and function.

Replicative aging or *senescence* is the accumulation of cellular damage in continuously dividing cells, for example, epithelia of the skin or gastro-intestinal tract. One mechanism of replicative senescence is the progressive shortening of telomeres—the repeated sequences of DNA at the ends of chromosomes. Replicative aging and chronological aging are particularly important for adult stem cells because they divide throughout life.[83] As mutations increase with age, cell fates include apoptosis, malignant transformation, cell-cycle arrest, or senescence.[84]

Genetic and environmental interventions have actually extended the lifespan of model organisms, such as the nematode worm *Caenorhabditis elegans* (*C. elegans*), the fruit fly *Drosophila melanogaster*, and mice.[85,86] Extending lifespan, however, is not equivalent to delaying aging![80] For example, treatment of an acute infection can prevent death but the fundamental *rate* of aging continues. Yet, investigators continue to study and try to isolate, manipulate, and reset so-called longevity genes to slow the rate of aging.

Recent advances in stem cell biology have begun to reveal the molecular mechanisms behind reprogramming events that occur during fertilization and when the nucleus of a mature somatic cell is transferred to an enucleated oocyte. Called *somatic cell nuclear transfer* (SCNT), this process gave rise to the first cloned mammal, Dolly the sheep, and led to the explosion of research in cloning.[80] SCNT is important in terms of demonstrating the ability of the oocyte cytoplasm to reprogram the donor nucleus. Induced pluripotent stem cells (iPSCs) are the result of such reprogramming events.[87] The major emphasis of reprogramming research is the reversal of the differentiated program and attainment of a pluripotent state (differentiated cells in all three germ layers of the embryo).[80,88]

Restoration of youthfulness to aged cells and tissues has created so-called rejuvenating interventions. Experiments to test whether cells and tissues from an old animal can be restored to a younger self include the approach called *heterochronic* (i.e., young-to-old or old-to-young) *transplantations* and *heterochronic parabiosis*, when the systemic circulations of two animals are joined. The systemic environment may become more youthful with restoration of protein components in the blood and tissues, especially chemokines and cytokines.[89] For example, investigators found a protein, GDF-11, may reverse age-associated cardiac hypertrophy when injected into old animals.[90]

Administration of the medication rapamycin (Sirolimus), an mTOR inhibitor, can extend the lifespan of mice.[91] These and future studies may not just change differentiation programs of cells and tissue but also possibly alter the aging clock. Observations in *C. elegans* suggest strongly that the causes of aging may be largely epigenetic.[80,92,93]

Normal Lifespan, Life Expectancy, and Quality-Adjusted Life Year

The maximal lifespan of humans is between 80 and 100 years and does not vary significantly among populations. Life expectancy is the *average* number of years of life remaining at a given age; however, it does not include quality of life. The quality-adjusted life year (QALY) is a measure of disease burden that includes quality and not just quantity of life lived. Statistics Canada reported in 2016 that the life expectancy at birth was 82.30 years (for both sexes).[94]

Degenerative Extracellular Changes

Extracellular factors that affect the aging process include the binding of collagen; the increase in the effects of free radicals on cells; the structural alterations of fascia, tendons, ligaments, bones, and joints; and the development of peripheral vascular disease, particularly arteriosclerosis (see Chapter 24).

Aging affects the ECM with increased cross-linking (e.g., aging collagen becomes more insoluble, chemically stable but rigid, resulting in decreased cell permeability), decreased synthesis, and increased degradation of collagen. The ECM determines the tissue's physical properties.[95] These changes, together with the disappearance of elastin and changes in proteoglycans and plasma proteins, cause disorders of the ground substance that result in dehydration and wrinkling of the skin (see Chapter 41).

Other age-related defects in the ECM include skeletal muscle alterations (e.g., atrophy, decreased tone, and loss of contractility), cataracts, diverticula, hernias, and rupture of intervertebral discs.

Free radicals of oxygen that result from oxidative cellular metabolism, *oxidative stress* (e.g., respiratory chain, phagocytosis, prostaglandin synthesis), damage tissues during the aging process. The oxygen radicals produced include superoxide radical, hydroxyl radical, and hydrogen peroxide. These oxygen products are extremely reactive and can damage nucleic acids, destroy polysaccharides, oxidize proteins, peroxidize unsaturated fatty acids, and kill and lyse cells. Oxidant effects on target cells can lead to malignant transformation, presumably through DNA damage. That progressive and cumulative damage from oxygen radicals may lead to harmful alterations in cellular function is consistent with those alterations of aging. The wear-and-tear theory of aging states that damages accumulate with time, decreasing the organism's ability to maintain a steady state. Because these oxygen-reactive species not only can permanently damage cells but also may lead to cellular death, there is new support for their role in the aging process.

Of much interest is the relationship between aging and the disappearance or alteration of extracellular substances important for vessel integrity. Aging causes lipid, calcium, and plasma proteins depositions in vessel walls. These depositions cause serious basement membrane thickening and alterations in smooth muscle functioning, resulting in arteriosclerosis (a progressive disease that causes such problems as stroke, myocardial infarction, renal disease, and peripheral vascular disease).

Cellular Aging

Cellular changes characteristic of aging include atrophy, decreased function, and loss of cells, possibly caused by apoptosis (Figure 4.33). Loss of cellular function from any of these causes initiates the

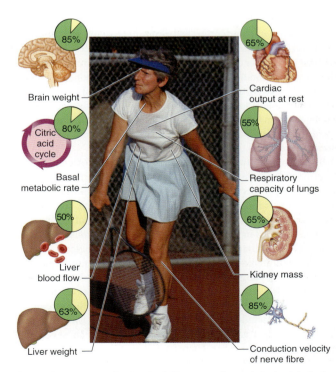

FIGURE 4.33 Some Biological Changes Associated with Aging. Insets show the proportion of remaining functions in the organs of a person in late adulthood compared with those of a 20-year-old.

compensatory mechanisms of hypertrophy and hyperplasia of the remaining cells, which can lead to metaplasia, dysplasia, and neoplasia. All of these changes can alter receptor placement and function, nutrient pathways, secretion of cellular products, and neuroendocrine control mechanisms. In the aged cell, DNA, RNA, cellular proteins, and membranes are most susceptible to injurious stimuli. DNA is particularly vulnerable to such injuries as breaks, deletions, and additions. Lack of DNA repair increases the cell's susceptibility to mutations that may be lethal or may promote the development of neoplasia (see Chapter 10).

Mitochondria are the organelles responsible for the generation of most of the energy used by eukaryotic cells. Mitochondrial DNA (mtDNA) encodes some of the proteins of the electron-transfer chain, the system necessary for the conversion of ADP to ATP. Mutations in mtDNA can deprive the cell of ATP, and mutations correlate with the aging process. Errors in replication or unrepaired damage could cause an accumulation of mutations.[96,97]

The most common age-related mtDNA mutation in humans is a large rearrangement called the *4977 deletion*, or *common deletion*, and is common in humans older than 40 years. It is a deletion that removes all or part of 7 of the 13 protein-encoding mtDNA genes and 5 of the 22 transfer RNA genes. Individual cells containing this deletion have a condition known as *heteroplasmy*. Heteroplasmy levels rise with aging. Cumulative damage of mtDNA results in the progression of such common diseases as diabetes, cancer, heart failure, and neuro-degenerative disorders.

Tissue and Systemic Aging

It is probably safe to say that every physiological process functions less efficiently with increasing age. The most characteristic tissue change with age is a progressive stiffness or rigidity that affects many systems, including the arterial, pulmonary, and musculoskeletal systems. A consequence of blood vessel and organ stiffness is a progressive increase in peripheral resistance to blood flow. The movement of intracellular and extracellular substances also decreases with age, as does the diffusion capacity of the lung. Blood flow through organs also decreases.

Changes in the endocrine and immune systems include thymus atrophy. Although this occurs at puberty, causing a decreased immune response to T-dependent antigens (foreign proteins), increased formation of autoantibodies and immune complexes (antibodies that are bound to antigens), and an overall decrease in the immunological tolerance for the host's own cells further diminish the effectiveness of the immune system later in life. In women the reproductive system loses ova, and in men spermatogenesis decreases. Responsiveness to hormones decreases in the breast and endometrium.

The stomach experiences decreases in the rate of emptying and secretion of hormones and hydrochloric acid. Muscular atrophy diminishes mobility by decreasing motor tone and contractility. Sarcopenia, loss of muscle mass and strength, can occur into old age. The skin of the aged individual is affected by atrophy and wrinkling of the epidermis and by alterations in the underlying dermis, fat, and muscle.

Total body changes include a decrease in height; a reduction in circumference of the neck, thighs, and arms; widening of the pelvis; and lengthening of the nose and ears. Several of these changes are the result of tissue atrophy and of decreased bone mass caused by osteoporosis and osteoarthritis. Some body composition changes include an increase in body weight, which begins in middle age (men gain until 50 years of age and women until 70 years), and an increase in fat mass followed by a decrease in stature, weight, fat-free mass, and body cell mass at older ages. Fat-free mass (FFM) includes all minerals, proteins, and water plus all other constituents except lipids. As the amount of fat increases, the percentage of total body water decreases. Increased body fat and centralized fat distribution (abdominal area) are associated with non–insulin-dependent diabetes and heart disease. Total body potassium concentration also decreases because of decreased cellular mass. An increased sodium–potassium ratio suggests that the decreased cellular mass correlates with an increased extracellular compartment.

Although some of these alterations are probably inherent in aging, others represent consequences of the process. Advanced age increases susceptibility to disease, and death occurs after an injury or insult because of diminished cellular, tissue, and organ function.

Frailty

Frailty is a common clinical syndrome in older persons, leaving a person vulnerable to falls, functional decline, disability, disease, and death. With an increasing aged population worldwide, efforts to promote independence and decrease frailty are challenging and needed. Sarcopenia and cachexia are a common consequence of aging and many acute and chronic illnesses.[98] Investigators are grappling with a common nomenclature to develop consensus for definitions of sarcopenia and cachexia. One proposal has been to define each condition simply as "muscle wasting disease," which can be applied in both acute and chronic settings.[98] An acceptable vocabulary and classification system is yet to be developed.

The determinants of sarcopenia include environmental and genetic factors.[99] Common themes of mechanisms for sarcopenia include: (1) decrease in the number of skeletal muscle fibres, mainly type II fibres; (2) decline in muscle protein synthesis with age; (3) decline in muscle fractions, such as myofibrillar and mitochondrial, with age; (4) reduction in protein turnover adversely affecting muscle function by inducing protein loss and protein accumulation; (5) loss of alpha motor neurons in the spinal column; (6) dysregulation of anabolic hormones; (7) cytokine productions and inflammation; (8) inadequate nutrition; and (9) sedentary history.[99,100] For research and clinical purposes, the criteria indicating compromised energetics include low grip strength, slowed walking speed, low physical activity, and unintentional weight loss.[101] The syndrome is complex and involves other alterations such as osteopenia, cognitive impairment, and anemia, as well as gender differences.

SOMATIC DEATH

Somatic death is death of the entire person. Unlike the changes that follow cellular death in a live body, postmortem change is diffuse and does not involve components of the inflammatory response. Within minutes after death, postmortem changes appear, eliminating any difficulty in determining that death has occurred. The most notable manifestations are complete cessation of respiration and circulation. The surface of the skin usually becomes pale and yellowish; however, the lifelike colour of the cheeks and lips may persist after death caused by carbon monoxide poisoning, drowning, or chloroform poisoning.[102]

Body temperature falls gradually immediately after death and then more rapidly (approximately 1°C/hr [33.8°F/hr]) until, after 24 hours, body temperature equals that of the environment.[103] After death caused by certain infective diseases, body temperature may continue to rise for a short time. Postmortem reduction of body temperature is called algor mortis.

Blood pressure within the retinal vessels decreases, causing muscle tension to decrease and the pupils to dilate. The face, nose, and chin become sharp or peaked-looking as blood and fluids drain from these areas.[104] Gravity causes blood to settle in the most dependent, or lowest, tissues, which develop a purple discolouration called livor mortis. Incisions made at this time usually fail to cause bleeding. The skin loses its elasticity and transparency.

Within 6 hours after death, acidic compounds accumulate within the muscles because of the breakdown of carbohydrates and the depletion of ATP. This increased acidity interferes with ATP-dependent detachment of myosin from actin (contractile proteins), and muscle stiffening, or **rigor mortis**, develops. The smaller muscles are usually affected first, particularly the muscles of the jaw. Within 12 to 14 hours, rigor mortis usually affects the entire body.

Signs of putrefaction are generally obvious about 24 to 48 hours after death. Rigor mortis gradually diminishes, and the body becomes flaccid at 36 to 62 hours. Putrefactive changes vary depending on the temperature of the environment. The most visible is greenish discoloration of the skin, particularly on the abdomen. The discoloration is thought to be related to the diffusion of hemolyzed blood into the tissues and the production of sulfhemoglobin, choleglobin, and other denatured hemoglobin derivatives.[103,104] Slippage or loosening of the skin from underlying tissues occurs at the same time. After this, swelling or bloating of the body and liquefactive changes occur, sometimes causing opening of the body cavities. At a microscopic level, putrefactive changes are associated with the release of enzymes and lytic dissolution called **postmortem autolysis**.

CASE STUDY

Mr. Harold, age 45 years, was involved in a motor vehicle collision (MVC). At the time of the accident, the road was slippery, and the outdoor temperature was −30°C. On impact, his arm was pinned between the door and the steering wheel, cutting off circulation to his arm. Initially his arm turned pale and he complained of tingling and burning while he was still in the vehicle.

It took 20 minutes for the ambulance to arrive and another 20 minutes for the paramedics to remove the door and release the pressure on his arm. While waiting for assistance, Mr. Harold's ring finger on his left hand turned white. His left hand was cool to touch, and he experienced 9/10 left arm pain. He then became lethargic and fatigued. The paramedics became concerned as Mr. Harold's ring finger then became cyanotic. At the hospital, Mr. Harold learned that his left ring finger would require amputation.

Critical Thinking and Clinical Judgement Questions

1. What issues and concerns did Mr. Harold experience?
2. What was the cause of his cellular injury?
3. How did his tissues adapt to the injury?
4. Is this an example of necrosis or apoptosis? Explain the nature of this type of cellular injury.
5. a) What is the pathogenesis for each of his clinical manifestations? b) What other manifestations might the nurse observe?
6. When blood flow was restored to Mr. Harold's arm, only one of his fingers required amputation. Explain the cellular basis of this reperfusion injury.
7. What medical and nursing treatment would the nurse expect Mr. Harold to require?
8. Compare and contrast impaired circulation to a limb versus insufficient circulation to the entire body.

DID YOU UNDERSTAND?

Cellular Adaptation

1. Cellular adaptation is a reversible, structural, or functional response both to normal or physiological conditions and to adverse or pathological conditions. Cells can adapt to physiological demands or stress to maintain a steady state called *allostasis*.
2. The most significant adaptive changes in cells include atrophy, hypertrophy, hyperplasia, and metaplasia.
3. Atrophy is a decrease in cellular size caused by aging, disuse, or reduced/absent blood supply, hormonal stimulation, or neural stimulation. The amounts of endoplasmic reticulum (ER), mitochondria, and microfilaments decrease. The mechanisms of atrophy probably include decreased protein synthesis, increased protein catabolism, or both. A new hypothesis called ribosome biogenesis involves the role of messenger RNA (mRNA) and protein translation.
4. Hypertrophy is an increase in the size of cells in response to mechanical stimuli and consequently increases the size of the affected organ. The amounts of protein in the plasma membrane, ER, microfilaments, and mitochondria increase. Hypertrophy is physiological or pathological.
5. Hyperplasia is an increase in the number of cells caused by an increased rate of cellular division. Hyperplasia is classified as physiological (compensatory and hormonal) and pathological.
6. Dysplasia, or *atypical hyperplasia*, is an abnormal change in the size, shape, and organization of mature tissue cells. It is atypical rather than a true adaptational change.
7. Metaplasia is the reversible replacement of one mature cell type by another, less mature, cell type.

Cellular Injury

1. Injury to cells and to the extracellular matrix (ECM) lead to injury of tissues and organs, ultimately determining the structural patterns of disease. Cellular injury occurs if the cell is unable to maintain allostasis—a normal or adaptive steady state—in the face of injurious stimuli or stress. Injured cells may recover (reversible injury) or die (irreversible injury).
2. Four biochemical themes are important to cellular injury: (a) adenosine triphosphate (ATP) depletion, resulting in mitochondrial damage; (b) accumulation of oxygen and oxygen-derived free radicals, causing membrane damage; (c) protein folding defects; and (d) increased intracellular calcium concentration and loss of calcium steady state.
3. Causes of injury include lack of oxygen (hypoxia), free radicals, caustic or toxic chemicals, infectious agents, inflammatory and immune responses, genetic factors, insufficient nutrients, or physical and mechanical trauma from many causes.
4. The sequence of events leading to cellular death is commonly decreased ATP production, failure of active transport mechanisms (the sodium–potassium pump), cellular swelling, detachment of ribosomes from the ER, cessation of protein synthesis, mitochondrial swelling as a result of calcium accumulation, vacuolation, leakage of digestive enzymes from lysosomes, autodigestion of intracellular structures, lysis of the plasma membrane, and death.
5. The initial insult in hypoxic injury is usually ischemia (the cessation of blood flow into vessels that supply the cell with oxygen and nutrients).

6. Free radicals cause cellular injury because they have an unpaired electron that makes the molecule unstable. To stabilize itself, the molecule either donates or accepts an electron from another molecule. Therefore, it forms injurious chemical bonds with proteins, lipids, and carbohydrates—key molecules in membranes and nucleic acids.
7. The damaging effects of free radicals, especially activated oxygen species such as superoxide radical ($\cdot O_2^-$), hydroxyl radical ($\cdot OH$), and hydrogen peroxide (H_2O_2), called oxidative stress, include (a) peroxidation of lipids, (b) alteration of ion pumps and transport mechanisms, (c) fragmentation of DNA, and (d) damage to mitochondria, releasing calcium into the cytosol.
8. Restoration of oxygen, however, can cause additional injury, called reperfusion injury. The mechanisms discussed for reperfusion injury include oxidative stress, increased intracellular calcium concentration, inflammation, and complement activation.
9. Injuries by blunt force are the result of the application of mechanical energy to the body, resulting in tearing, shearing, or crushing of tissues. The most common types of blunt-force injuries include motor vehicle accidents and falls.
10. A contusion is bleeding into the skin or underlying tissues from a blow. A collection of blood in soft tissues or an enclosed space is a *hematoma*.
11. An abrasion (scrape) results from removal of the superficial layers of the skin caused by friction between the skin and injuring object. Abrasions and contusions may have a patterned appearance that mirrors the shape and features of the injuring object.
12. A laceration is a tear or rip resulting when there is a loss of tensile strength in the skin or tissue.
13. An incised wound is a cut that is longer than it is deep. A stab wound is a penetrating sharp-force injury that is deeper than it is long.
14. Gunshot wounds may be either penetrating (bullet retained in the body) or perforating (bullet exits the body). The most important factors determining the appearance of a gunshot injury are whether it is an entrance or an exit wound and the range of fire.
15. Asphyxial injuries result from a failure of cells to receive or use oxygen. These injuries are in four general categories: suffocation, strangulation, chemical asphyxiants, and drowning.
16. Activation of inflammation and immunity, which occurs after cellular injury or infection, involves powerful biochemicals and proteins capable of damaging normal (uninjured and uninfected) cells.
17. Genetic disorders injure cells by altering the nucleus and the plasma membrane's structure, shape, receptors, or transport mechanisms.
18. Deprivation of essential nutrients (proteins, carbohydrates, lipids, vitamins) can cause cellular injury by altering cellular structure and function, particularly of transport mechanisms, chromosomes, the nucleus, and DNA.
19. Injurious physical agents include temperature extremes, changes in atmospheric pressure, ionizing radiation, illumination, mechanical stresses, and noise.

Manifestations of Cellular Injury: Accumulations

1. An important manifestation of cellular injury is the resultant metabolic disturbances of intracellular accumulation (infiltration) of abnormal amounts of various substances. Two categories of accumulations are (a) normal cellular substances (e.g., excess water, proteins, lipids, and carbohydrates) and (b) abnormal substances, either endogenous (e.g., a product of abnormal metabolism or synthesis) or exogenous (e.g., a virus).
2. Most accumulations result from four types of mechanisms, all abnormal: (a) an endogenous substance is produced in excess or at an increased rate; (b) an abnormal substance, often the result of a mutated gene, accumulates; (c) an endogenous substance is not effectively catabolized; and (d) a harmful exogenous substance accumulates because of inhalation, ingestion, or infection.
3. Accumulations harm cells by "crowding" the organelles and by causing excessive (and sometimes harmful) metabolites to accumulate during their catabolism. The metabolites enter the cytoplasm or the ECM.
4. Cellular swelling, the accumulation of excessive water in the cell, results from the failure of transport mechanisms and is a sign of many types of cellular injury. Oncosis is a type of cellular death resulting from cellular swelling.
5. Accumulations of organic substances—lipids, carbohydrates, glycogen, proteins, pigments—are caused by disorders in which (a) cellular uptake of the substance exceeds the cell's capacity to catabolize (digest) or use it or (b) cellular anabolism (synthesis) of the substance exceeds the cell's capacity to use or secrete it.
6. Dystrophic calcification (accumulation of calcium salts) is always a sign of pathological change because it occurs only in injured or dead cells. Metastatic calcification, however, can occur in uninjured cells in individuals with hypercalcemia.
7. Disturbances in urate metabolism can result in hyperuricemia and deposition of sodium urate crystals in tissue—leading to a painful disorder called gout.
8. Systemic manifestations of cellular injury include fever, leukocytosis, increased heart rate, pain, and serum elevations of enzymes in the plasma.

Cellular Death

1. Cellular death is necrosis and apoptosis. Necrosis consists of rapid loss of the plasma membrane structure, organelle swelling, mitochondrial dysfunction, and the lack of features of apoptosis. Apoptosis is regulated or programmed cellular death and is characterized by "dropping off" of cellular fragments, called apoptotic bodies. Necrosis is regulated or programmed under certain conditions; hence, the new term *programmed necrosis*, or necroptosis.
2. The four major types of necrosis are coagulative, liquefactive, caseous, and fatty. Different types of necrosis occur in different tissues.
3. Structural signs that indicate irreversible injury and progression to necrosis are the dense clumping and disruption of genetic material and the disruption of the plasma and organelle membranes.
4. Apoptosis, a distinct type of sublethal injury, is a process of selective cellular self-destruction that occurs in both normal and pathological tissue changes.
5. Death by apoptosis causes loss of cells in many pathological states, including (a) severe cellular injury, (b) accumulation of misfolded proteins, (c) infections, and (d) obstruction in tissue ducts.
6. Excessive accumulation of misfolded proteins in the ER leads to a condition known as *ER stress*. ER stress results in apoptotic cellular death, and this mechanism explains several degenerative diseases of the central nervous system and other organs.
7. Excessive or insufficient apoptosis is *dysregulated apoptosis*.
8. *Autophagy* means, "eating of self," and as a recycling factory it is a self-destructive process and a survival mechanism. The autophagic process institutes cannibalization and recycles the digested contents in starvation or nutrient-deprived states. Autophagy can maintain cellular metabolism under starvation conditions and remove damaged organelles under stress conditions, improving the survival of cells. Autophagy declines and becomes less efficient as the cell ages, thus contributing to the aging process.
9. Gangrenous necrosis, or gangrene, is tissue necrosis caused by hypoxia and the subsequent bacterial invasion.

Aging and Altered Cellular and Tissue Biology
1. It is difficult to determine the physiological (normal) from the pathological changes of aging. Current research is focusing on genetic, epigenetic, inflammatory, oxidative stress, and metabolic origins of aging.
2. Important factors in aging include increased damage to the cell, reduced capacity to divide, reduced ability to repair damaged DNA, and increased likelihood of defective protein balance or allostasis.
3. Frailty is a common clinical syndrome in older persons, leaving a person vulnerable to falls, functional decline, disability, disease, and death. Sarcopenia and cachexia are common consequences of aging.

Somatic Death
1. Somatic death is death of the entire person. Postmortem change is diffuse and does not involve components of the inflammatory response.
2. Manifestations of somatic death include cessation of respiration and circulation, gradual lowering of body temperature, dilation of the pupils, loss of elasticity and transparency in the skin, stiffening of the muscles (rigor mortis), and discoloration of the skin (livor mortis). Signs of putrefaction are obvious about 24 to 48 hours after death.

5

Fluids and Electrolytes, Acids and Bases

Stephanie Zettel, with originating chapter contributions by Lois E. Brenneman and Sue E. Huether

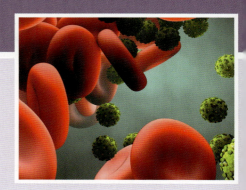

Additional resources are available online at http://evolve.elsevier.com/Canada/Huether/pathophysiology

CHAPTER OUTLINE

Distribution of Body Fluids and Electrolytes, 113
    Water Movement Between Plasma and Interstitial Fluid, 114
    Water Movement Between ICF and ECF, 114
Alterations in Water Movement, 114
    Edema, 114
Sodium, Chloride, and Water Balance, 116
Alterations in Sodium, Chloride, and Water Balance, 118
    Isotonic Alterations, 118
    Hypertonic Alterations, 118
    Hypotonic Alterations, 120

Alterations in Potassium and Other Electrolytes, 121
    Potassium, 121
    Other Electrolytes—Calcium, Phosphate, and Magnesium, 124
Acid–Base Balance, 124
    Hydrogen Ion and pH, 124
    Buffer Systems, 124
    Acid–Base Imbalances, 126
PEDIATRIC CONSIDERATIONS: Distribution of Body Fluids, 130
GERIATRIC CONSIDERATIONS: Distribution of Body Fluids, 130
CASE STUDY, 131

LEARNING OBJECTIVES

1. Discuss the two functional fluid compartments of the body.
2. Discuss the ways water moves between plasma and interstitial fluid.
3. Explain Starling forces.
4. Describe the causation, pathophysiological process, and clinical manifestations of edema.
5. Discuss the regulatory processes for sodium and water balance in the body, including the role of antidiuretic hormone, renin-angiotensin-aldosterone, and atrial natriuretic hormone.
6. Define hypotonic, isotonic, and hypertonic alterations in water balance and give an example of each.
7. Identify the basic causes and clinical manifestations of hypernatremia, hyponatremia, hyperchloremia, and hypochloremia.
8. Discuss the causes and clinical manifestations of water deficit.
9. Discuss the causes and clinical manifestations of water excess.
10. Discuss the clinical manifestations and treatments for the syndrome of inappropriate antidiuretic hormone (SIADH).
11. Discuss the distribution, function, and regulation of potassium in the body.
12. Identify the basic causes and clinical manifestations of hyperkalemia and hypokalemia.
13. Discuss the role of hydrogen ion concentration in cellular function and dysfunction.
14. Describe how the plasma buffering systems help prevent significant fluctuations in pH.
15. Explain how the lungs and the kidneys regulate acid–base balance.
16. Differentiate between respiratory and metabolic acid–base disorders by causes and mechanisms of compensation.

KEY TERMS

Acidemia, 126
Acidosis, 126
Aldosterone, 116
Alkalemia, 126
Alkalosis, 126
Angiotensin I, 116
Angiotensin II, 116
Anion gap, 127
Antidiuretic hormone (ADH), 116
Aquaporin, 114
Baroreceptor, 117
Buffer, 124
Buffering, 124
Capillary hydrostatic pressure (blood pressure), 114
Capillary (plasma) oncotic pressure, 114
Carbonic acid–bicarbonate buffer, 126
Chloride (Cl⁻), 117
Compensation, 126
Correction, 126
Dehydration, 119
Dilutional hyponatremia (water intoxication), 120
Edema, 114
Extracellular fluid (ECF), 113
Hypercapnia, 128
Hyperchloremia, 119
Hyperkalemia, 121
Hypernatremia, 118
Hypertonic fluid alterations, 118
Hypervolemic hypernatremia, 119
Hypervolemic hyponatremia, 120
Hypocapnia, 129
Hypochloremia, 120
Hypochloremic metabolic alkalosis, 128
Hypokalemia, 121
Hyponatremia, 120
Hypotonic fluid imbalance, 120
Hypovolemic hypernatremia, 119

CHAPTER 5 Fluids and Electrolytes, Acids and Bases

Hypovolemic hyponatremia, 119
Interstitial fluid, 113
Interstitial hydrostatic pressure, 114
Interstitial oncotic pressure, 114
Intracellular fluid (ICF), 113
Intravascular fluid, 113
Isotonic alteration, 118
Isotonic fluid excess, 118
Isotonic fluid loss, 118
Isovolemic hypernatremia, 118
Isovolemic hyponatremia, 120
Lymphedema, 116
Metabolic acidosis, 127
Metabolic alkalosis, 128
Natriuretic peptide, 116
Net filtration, 114
Net transendothelial flow theory, 114
Nonvolatile, 124
Nonvolatile acids, 124
Oncotic pressure, 114
Osmolality, 114
Osmoreceptor, 117
Potassium (K^+), 121
Potassium adaptation, 121
Renin, 116
Renin-angiotensin-aldosterone system, 116
Respiratory acidosis, 128
Respiratory alkalosis, 129
Sodium (Na^+), 116
Starling forces, 114
Total body water (TBW), 113
Urodilatin, 117
Volatile, 124
Volume-sensitive receptor, 117
Water balance, 117

The cells of the body live in a fluid environment with maintenance of electrolyte and acid–base concentrations within a narrow range. Changes in electrolyte concentration affect the electrical activity of nerve and muscle cells and cause shifts of fluid from one compartment to another. In turn, alterations in acid–base balance disrupt cellular functions. Fluid fluctuations also affect blood volume and cellular function. Disturbances in these functions are common and can be life-threatening. Understanding how alterations occur and how the body compensates or corrects the disturbance is important for comprehending many pathophysiological conditions.

DISTRIBUTION OF BODY FLUIDS AND ELECTROLYTES

Total body water (TBW) is the sum of fluids in all body compartments and is about 60% of body weight in adults (measured in kilograms) (Table 5.1). One litre of water weighs 1 kg. The rest of the body weight is fat and fat-free solids (most notably bone).

Body fluids distribute themselves among functional compartments, or spaces, and provide a transport medium for cellular and tissue function. **Intracellular fluid (ICF)** comprises all the fluid within cells, about two thirds of TBW. **Extracellular fluid (ECF)** is all the fluid outside the cells (about one third of TBW) and includes **interstitial fluid** (the space between cells and outside the blood vessels) and **intravascular fluid** (blood plasma) (Table 5.2). The total volume of body water for a 70-kg person is about 42 litres. Other ECF compartments include lymph and transcellular fluids, such as synovial, intestinal, and cerebrospinal fluid; sweat; urine; and pleural, peritoneal, pericardial, and intraocular fluids.

Electrolytes and other solutes distribute themselves throughout the intracellular and extracellular fluid (Table 5.3). Note that ECF contains a large amount of *sodium* and *chloride* and a small amount of *potassium*, whereas the opposite is true of ICF. The concentrations of *phosphates* and *magnesium* are greater in ICF, and the concentration of *calcium* is greater in ECF. These differences are important for the maintenance of electroneutrality between the extracellular and intracellular compartments, the transmission of electrical impulses, and the movement of water among body compartments (see Chapter 1).

Although the amount of fluid within the various compartments is relatively constant, solutes (e.g., salts) and water move between compartments to maintain their unique compositions. The percentage of TBW varies with the amount of body fat and age. Because fat is water repelling (hydrophobic), there is very little water in adipose (fat) cells. Individuals with more body fat have proportionately less TBW and tend to be more susceptible to dehydration.

TABLE 5.1 Total Body Water (%) in Relation to Body Weight

Body Build	Adult Male	Adult Female	Child (1–10 yr)	Infant (1 mo–1 yr)	Newborn (Up to 1 mo)
Normal	60	50	65	70	70–80
Lean	70	60	50–60	80	
Obese	50	42	50	60	

NOTE: Total body water is a percentage of body weight.
mo, Month; *yr*, year.

TABLE 5.2 Distribution of Body Water (70-kg Man)

Fluid Compartment	% of Body Weight	Volume (L)
Intracellular fluid (ICF)	40	28
Extracellular fluid (ECF)	20	14
Interstitial	15	11
Intravascular	5	3
Total body water (TBW)	60	42

TABLE 5.3 Representative Distribution of Electrolytes in Body Compartments

Electrolytes	ECF (mmol/L)	ICF (mmol/L)
Cations		
Sodium	142	12
Potassium	4.2	150
Calcium	2.5	0
Magnesium	1	12
TOTAL	149.7	174
Anions		
Bicarbonate	24	12
Chloride	103	4
Phosphate	2	100
Proteins	16	65
Other anions	8	6
TOTAL	153	187

ECF, Extracellular fluid; *ICF*, intracellular fluid.

TABLE 5.4 Normal Water Gains and Losses (70-kg Man)

	Daily Intake (mL)		Daily Output (mL)
Drinking	1400–1800	Urine	1400–1800
Water in food	700–1000	Stool	100
Water of oxidation	300–400	Skin	300–500
		Lungs	600–800
TOTAL	2400–3200	**TOTAL**	2400–3200

The distribution and the amount of TBW change with age (see the *Pediatric Considerations* and *Geriatric Considerations* boxes later in this chapter), and although daily fluid intake may fluctuate widely, the body regulates water volume within a relatively narrow range. Water obtained by drinking, water ingested in food, and water derived from oxidative metabolism are the primary sources of body water. Normally, the largest amounts of water are lost through renal excretion, with lesser amounts lost through the stool and vaporization from the skin and lungs (insensible water loss) (Table 5.4).

Water Movement Between Plasma and Interstitial Fluid

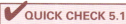

QUICK CHECK 5.1
1. What forces promote net filtration?
2. How do hormones regulate salt and water balance?
3. What are aquaporins?

The distribution of water and the movement of nutrients and waste products between the capillary and interstitial spaces occur as a result of changes in hydrostatic pressure (mechanical force pushing water outward) and osmotic or oncotic pressure (chemical force pulling water inward) at the arterial and venous ends of the capillary. Water, sodium, and glucose readily move across the capillary membrane. The plasma proteins (albumin, in particular) normally do not cross the capillary membrane and maintain effective **osmolality** by generating plasma **oncotic pressure**.

As plasma flows from the arterial to the venous end of the capillary, four forces determine fluid movement across the endothelium of the blood vessel. These four forces acting together are **net filtration** or **Starling forces**:

1. **Capillary hydrostatic pressure (blood pressure)** facilitates the outward movement of water from the capillary to the interstitial space.
2. **Capillary (plasma) oncotic pressure** osmotically attracts water from the interstitial space back into the capillary.
3. **Interstitial hydrostatic pressure** facilitates the inward movement of water from the interstitial space into the capillary.
4. **Interstitial oncotic pressure** osmotically attracts water from the capillary into the interstitial space.

The forces moving fluid back and forth across the capillary wall are:
Net filtration = (Forces favouring filtration)
  − (Forces opposing filtration)

Forces favouring filtration = Capillary hydrostatic pressure and interstitial oncotic pressure

Forces opposing filtration = Capillary oncotic pressure and interstitial hydrostatic pressure

The balance of the hydrostatic and osmotic/oncotic pressures between the capillary plasma and adjacent interstitium determines the net movement of fluid between these two compartments, and the **net transendothelial flow theory** explains how these forces change with blood flow through the capillary network.[1] At the arterial end of the capillary, autoregulatory mechanisms of the capillary endothelium ensure consistent blood flow that is capable of meeting metabolic demands over a wide range of blood pressures, and the hydrostatic pressure exceeds capillary oncotic pressure. This change in pressure favours the formation of filtrate through transendothelial flow (i.e., autoregulatory changes in blood flow at the level of the endothelium) from the capillary to the interstitial space. At the venous end of the capillary, capillary oncotic pressure exceeds capillary hydrostatic pressure. Rather than fluids being reabsorbed back into the capillary, the *net transendothelial flow theory* suggests that the filtrate is formed across the entire length of the capillary, and in a steady state, there is no reabsorption of fluid. Furthermore, the oncotic pressures are not strong enough to account for this fluid movement, and nearly all the filtrate returns to the venous circulation through lymph. Interstitial hydrostatic pressure promotes the movement of about 10% of the interstitial fluid along with small amounts of protein into the lymphatics, which then returns to the circulation. Because albumin does not normally cross the capillary membrane, interstitial oncotic pressure is normally minimal. Figure 5.1 illustrates net filtration.

Water Movement Between ICF and ECF

Water moves between ICF and ECF compartments primarily as a function of osmotic forces. Water moves freely by diffusion through the lipid bilayer cell membrane, as well as through **aquaporins**, a family of water channel proteins that provide permeability to water.[2] Sodium is responsible for the ECF osmotic balance, and potassium maintains the ICF osmotic balance. Active transport of ions out of the cell balances out the osmotic force of ICF proteins and other nondiffusible substances. Water crosses cell membranes freely, so the osmolality of TBW is normally at equilibrium. Normally ICF is not subject to rapid changes in osmolality, but when ECF osmolality changes, water moves from one compartment to another until re-establishment of osmotic equilibrium (see Isotonic Alterations).

ALTERATIONS IN WATER MOVEMENT

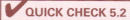

QUICK CHECK 5.2
1. How does an increase in capillary hydrostatic pressure cause edema?
2. How does a decrease in capillary oncotic pressure cause edema?

Edema

Edema is excessive accumulation of fluid within the interstitial spaces. Increased capillary hydrostatic pressure favours the movement of fluid from the capillaries or lymphatic channels into the tissues, as do decreased plasma oncotic pressure, increased capillary membrane permeability, and lymphatic channel obstruction[3] (Figure 5.2).

PATHOPHYSIOLOGY Capillary hydrostatic pressure increases because of venous obstruction or salt and water retention. Venous obstruction causes hydrostatic pressure to increase behind the obstruction, pushing fluid from the capillaries into the interstitial spaces. Thrombophlebitis (inflammation of veins), hepatic obstruction, tight clothing around the extremities, and prolonged standing are all common causes of venous obstruction. Heart failure, renal failure, and cirrhosis of the liver are

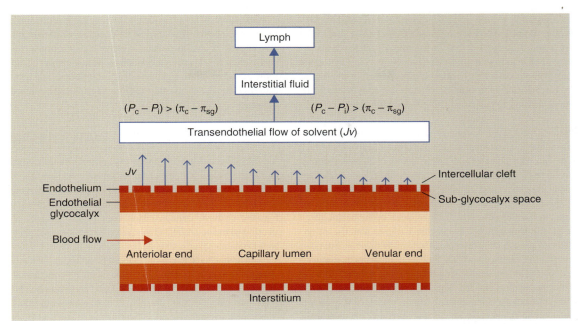

FIGURE 5.1 The Contemporary Model of Capillary Dynamics. The fluid that is filtered through the mesh-like glycocalyx and into the sub-glycocalyx space is nearly devoid of protein. Consequently, it is the glycocalyx layer that establishes the oncotic pressure gradient with the capillary plasma, rather than the interstitium, as originally proposed. This allows for more accurate definition of the true oncotic pressure gradient as $\pi_c - \pi_{sg}$ and to refine the equation that governs transendothelial solvent flow ($Jv = K[(P_c - P_i) - \sigma(\pi_c - \pi_{sg})]$). P_c, Hydrostatic capillary pressure; P_i, hydrostatic interstitial pressure; π_c, oncotic capillary pressure; π_{sg}, oncotic pressure of the subglycocalyx; Jv, transendothelial flow of solvent. (From Henderson, M., Gillon, S., & Al-Haddad, M. [2018]. Organization and composition of body fluids. *Physiology, 19*[10], 568–574, Figure 4. https://doi.org/10.1016/j.mpaic.2018.08.005.)

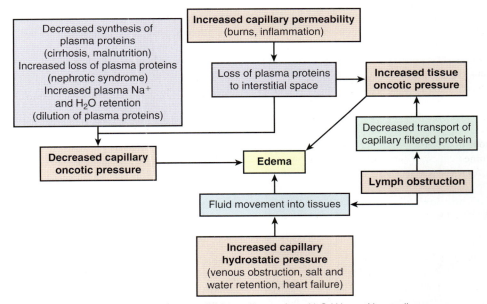

FIGURE 5.2 Mechanisms of Edema Formation. H_2O, Water; Na^+, sodium.

associated with excessive salt and water retention, which cause plasma volume overload, increased capillary hydrostatic pressure, and edema.

A loss or diminished production of albumin (e.g., from liver disease or protein malnutrition) contributes to decreased plasma oncotic pressure. This is because there are fewer particles in the plasma to attract the water to it. Plasma proteins are also lost in glomerular diseases of the kidney, serous drainage from open wounds, hemorrhage, burns, and cirrhosis of the liver. The decreased oncotic attraction of fluid within the capillary causes filtered capillary fluid to remain in the interstitial space, resulting in edema.

Capillaries become more permeable with inflammation and immune responses. Examples of events that trigger such responses include trauma (burns or crushing injuries), neoplastic disease, and allergic reactions. Proteins escape from the vascular space and produce edema through decreased capillary oncotic pressure and interstitial fluid protein accumulation.

The lymphatic system normally absorbs interstitial fluid and a small number of proteins. When lymphatic channels are blocked or surgically removed, proteins and fluid accumulate in the interstitial space, causing **lymphedema**.[4] For example, lymphedema of the arm or leg occurs after surgical removal of axillary or femoral lymph nodes, respectively, for treatment of carcinoma. Inflammation or tumours may cause lymphatic obstruction, leading to edema of the involved tissues.

CLINICAL MANIFESTATIONS *Localized edema* is usually limited to a site of trauma, as in a sprained finger. Another kind of localized edema occurs within particular organ systems and includes cerebral, pulmonary, and laryngeal edema; pleural effusion (fluid accumulation in the pleural space); pericardial effusion (fluid accumulation within the membrane around the heart); and ascites (accumulation of fluid in the peritoneal space). Edema of specific organs, such as the brain, lung, or larynx, can be life-threatening. *Generalized edema*, on the other hand, is the result of a more uniform distribution of fluid in interstitial spaces. Dependent edema, in which fluid accumulates in gravity-dependent areas of the body, might signal more generalized edema. Dependent edema appears in the feet and legs when standing and in the sacral area and buttocks when supine (lying on back). Assessing for dependent edema involves pressing on tissues overlying bony prominences. A pit left in the skin indicates edema (hence the term *pitting edema*) (Figure 5.3).

Edema usually is associated with weight gain, swelling and puffiness, tight-fitting clothes and shoes, limited movement of affected joints, and symptoms associated with the underlying pathological condition. Fluid accumulations increase the distance required for nutrients and waste products to move between capillaries and tissues. Blood flow may also be impaired. Therefore, wounds heal more slowly, and with prolonged edema, the risks of infection and pressure sores over bony prominences increase. Edematous fluid becomes trapped in a "third space" (i.e., the interstitial space, pleural space, pericardial space) as it accumulates and is unavailable for metabolic processes or perfusion. Dehydration is a common complication of this diversion of fluid. "Third spacing" occurs with severe burns, where large amounts of intravascular fluid are lost to the interstitial spaces, reducing plasma volume, and causing shock (see Chapter 24).

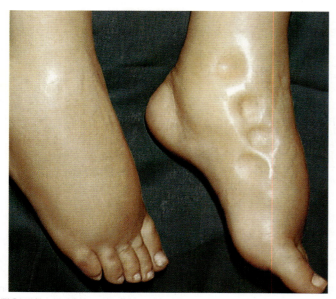

FIGURE 5.3 Pitting Edema. (From Bloom, A., & Ireland, J. [1992]. *Color atlas of diabetes* [2nd ed.]. Mosby.)

EVALUATION AND TREATMENT Specific conditions causing edema require diagnosis. The focus of treatment is on the underlying disorder, although it is also important to treat its symptoms. Supportive measures include elevating edematous limbs, using compression stockings, avoiding prolonged standing, restricting salt intake, and taking diuretics. Severe cases often require administration of intravenous (IV) albumin.

SODIUM, CHLORIDE, AND WATER BALANCE

The kidneys and hormones have a central role in maintaining sodium and water balance. Because water follows the osmotic gradients established by changes in salt concentration, sodium concentration and water balance are intimately related. The renal effects of aldosterone regulate sodium concentration (see Figure 18.18), whereas **antidiuretic hormone (ADH**; also known as *vasopressin*) primarily regulates water balance.

Sodium (Na^+) accounts for 90% of the ECF cations (positively charged ions) (see Table 5.3). Along with its constituent anions (negatively charged ions), chloride (Cl^-) and bicarbonate (HCO_3^-), sodium regulates extracellular osmotic forces. Consequently, sodium has a major role in water balance. Sodium is important in other functions, including maintenance of neuromuscular irritability for conduction of nerve impulses (in conjunction with potassium [K^+] and calcium [Ca^+]; see Figure 1.29), regulation of acid–base balance (using sodium bicarbonate [$NaCO_3$] and sodium phosphate [Na_3PO_4]), participation in cellular chemical reactions, and transport of substances across the cellular membrane.

The kidney, in conjunction with neural and hormonal mediators, maintains normal serum sodium concentration within a narrow range (136 to 145 mmol/L) primarily through renal tubular reabsorption. **Aldosterone** is a mineralocorticoid, synthesized and secreted from the adrenal cortex as a component of the **renin-angiotensin-aldosterone system**, and it mediates the hormonal regulation of sodium (and potassium) balance. Factors that influence aldosterone secretion include circulating blood volume, blood pressure, and plasma concentrations of sodium and potassium. When circulating blood volume or blood pressure decreases, sodium levels decrease, or potassium levels increase, the juxtaglomerular cells of the kidney release the hormone, **renin**. Renin stimulates the formation of **angiotensin I**, an inactive polypeptide, from its precursor from the liver, **angiotensinogen**. Angiotensin-converting enzyme (ACE) in pulmonary vessels then converts angiotensin I to **angiotensin II**, which stimulates both the secretion of aldosterone and ADH, and causes vasoconstriction. The aldosterone promotes renal sodium and water reabsorption with excretion of potassium, thus increasing blood volume (Figure 5.4; see also Figure 29.9). Vasoconstriction elevates the systemic blood pressure and restores renal perfusion (blood flow). This restoration inhibits the further release of renin.

Interestingly, the novel coronavirus, COVID-19, which is responsible for the recent global pandemic, uses ACE-2 (which is similar in origin to ACE) as an entry receptor in order to infect the host. Normal activation of the ACE-2 enzyme by angiotensin II results in angiotensin (1–7) and negatively regulates the renin-angiotensin-aldosterone system (RAS). ACE-2 has a protective function related to both the cardiovascular and renal systems, and this protective function is lost with COVID-19 infection. The impact of RAS extends beyond just the kidneys and affects all organs by altering the function of vascular endothelial cells (see https://www.rndsystems.com/resources/articles/ace-2-sars-receptor-identified).

Natriuretic peptides are hormones primarily produced by the myocardium. The atria produce atrial natriuretic hormone (or peptide)

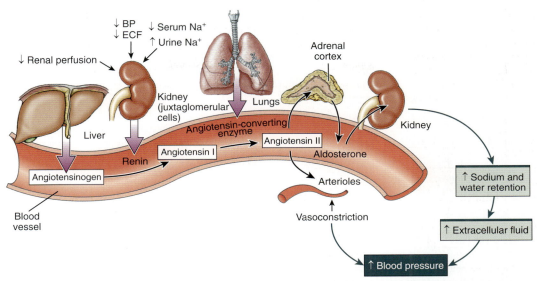

FIGURE 5.4 The Renin-Angiotensin-Aldosterone System. *BP*, Blood pressure; *ECF*, extracellular fluid; *Na+*, sodium. (Modified from Herlihy, B., & Maebius, N. [2011]. *The human body in health and disease* [4th ed.]. Philadelphia: Saunders. Borrowed from Lewis, S. L., Bucher, L., Heitkemper, M. M., et al. [2014]. *Medical-surgical nursing: Assessment and management of clinical problems* [9th ed.]. Mosby.)

(ANH or ANP), and the ventricles produce B-type natriuretic peptide (BNP). The kidney also synthesizes an ANP analogue called **urodilatin**, which is released by the distal convoluted tubule and collecting duct in response to increased mean arterial pressure. Cardiac endocrine cells release natriuretic peptides when there is an increase in transmural atrial pressure (increased volume), which may occur with heart failure, or similar to the cells in the nephron of the kidney, when there is an increase in mean arterial pressure[5] (Figure 5.5). ANPs are natural antagonists to the RAS. Natriuretic peptides cause vasodilation and increase sodium and water excretion, thus decreasing blood pressure.

Chloride (Cl^-) is the major anion in ECF and provides electroneutrality, particularly in relation to sodium. Chloride transport is generally passive and follows the active transport of sodium so that increases or decreases in chloride concentration are proportional to changes in sodium concentration. Chloride concentration tends to vary inversely with changes in the concentration of bicarbonate (HCO_3^-), the other major anion.

ADH regulates **water balance**. That is why an increase in plasma osmolality or a decrease in circulating blood volume (and blood pressure) triggers its release from the posterior pituitary gland (Figure 5.6). Increased plasma osmolality occurs with water deficit or sodium excess in relation to TBW. The increased osmolality stimulates hypothalamic **osmoreceptors**. In addition to causing thirst, these osmoreceptors signal the posterior pituitary gland to release ADH. Thirst stimulates water drinking, and ADH increases water reabsorption into the plasma from the distal tubules and collecting ducts of the kidney (see Chapter 29). The reabsorbed water results in decreased plasma osmolality, returning it toward normal, and urine concentration increases.

Similarly, with fluid loss (dehydration) from vomiting, diarrhea, or excessive sweating, a decrease in blood volume and blood pressure often occurs. **Volume-sensitive receptors** and **baroreceptors** (nerve endings that are sensitive to changes in volume and pressure) also stimulate the release of ADH from the pituitary gland and stimulate thirst. The volume receptors are located in the right and left atria and thoracic vessels; the aorta, pulmonary arteries, and carotid sinus all contain baroreceptors. ADH secretion also occurs when atrial pressure drops, as occurs with decreased blood volume and with the release of

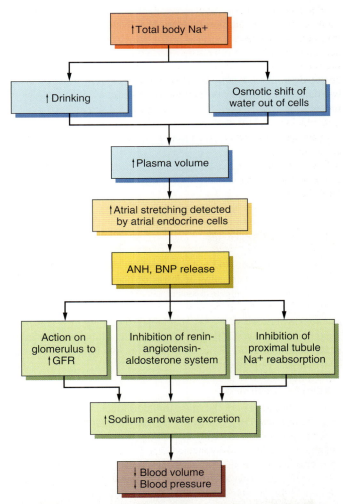

FIGURE 5.5 The Natriuretic Peptide System. *ANH*, Atrial natriuretic hormone; *BNP*, brain natriuretic peptide; *GFR*, glomerular filtration rate; *Na+*, sodium.

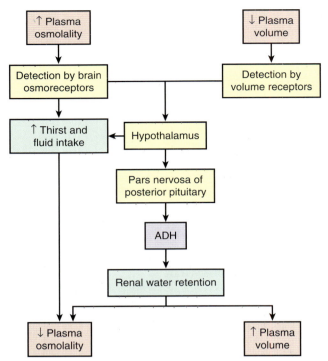

FIGURE 5.6 The Antidiuretic Hormone System. *ADH,* Antidiuretic hormone.

TABLE 5.5	Water and Solute Imbalances
Tonicity	**Mechanism**
Isotonic (iso-osmolar) imbalance Serum osmolality = 280–294 mOsm/kg	Gain or loss of ECF resulting in concentration equivalent to 0.9% sodium chloride solution (normal saline); no shrinking or swelling of cells
Hypertonic (hyperosmolar) imbalance Serum osmolality >294 mOsm/kg	Imbalances that result in ECF concentration >0.9% salt solution (i.e., water loss or solute gain); cells shrink in hypertonic fluid
Hypotonic (hypo-osmolar) imbalance Serum osmolality <280 mOsm/kg	Imbalance that results in ECF <0.9% salt solution (i.e., water gain or solute loss); cells swell in hypotonic fluid
Formula for calculating serum osmolality	(2 × [Na] + [Glu])/18 + BUN/2.8

BUN, Blood serum urea nitrogen level (mmol/L); *ECF,* extracellular fluid; *[Glu],* serum glucose concentration (mmol/L); *[Na],* serum sodium concentration (mmol/L).

angiotensin II (see Figure 29.9). The reabsorption of water mediated by ADH then promotes the restoration of plasma volume and blood pressure (see Figure 5.6).

ALTERATIONS IN SODIUM, CHLORIDE, AND WATER BALANCE

> **✓ QUICK CHECK 5.3**
> 1. What causes isotonic imbalance?
> 2. What are some causes of hypernatremia?
> 3. What is the most severe complication of hyponatremia?

Alterations in sodium and water balance are closely related. Sodium imbalances occur with gains or losses of body water. Water imbalances develop with gains or losses of salt. The tonicity of a fluid refers to the change in the concentration of solutes in relation to water: isotonic, hypertonic, or hypotonic (Table 5.5 and Figure 5.7; see also Figure 1.25). Changes in tonicity also alter the volume of water in the intracellular and extracellular compartments, resulting in isovolemia, hypervolemia, or hypovolemia.

Isotonic Alterations

Isotonic alterations are the most common kinds of alterations, and they occur when TBW changes accompany proportional changes in the concentrations of electrolytes (see Figure 5.7). **Isotonic fluid loss** causes dehydration and hypovolemia. For example, if an individual loses pure plasma or ECF, fluid volume is less but the concentration and type of electrolytes and the osmolality remain in the normal range (280 to 294 milliosmoles [mOsm]). Causes include hemorrhage, severe wound drainage, excessive diaphoresis (sweating), and inadequate fluid intake. There is loss of ECF volume with weight loss, dryness of skin and mucous membranes, decreased urine output, and symptoms of hypovolemia. Indicators of hypovolemia include a rapid heart rate, flattened neck veins, and normal or decreased blood pressure. In severe states, hypovolemic shock can occur (see Chapter 24). Isotonic fluids containing electrolytes and glucose are given orally, intravenously (i.e., 0.9% saline solution or 5% dextrose in 0.225% saline solution), or, in some cases, subcutaneously (hypodermoclysis).

Isotonic fluid excess causes hypervolemia. Common causes include excessive administration of IV fluids, hypersecretion of aldosterone, or the effects of medications such as cortisone (which causes renal reabsorption of sodium and water). As plasma volume expands, hypervolemia develops with weight gain. The diluting effect of excess plasma volume leads to decreased hematocrit and decreased plasma protein concentration. The neck veins may distend, and the blood pressure increases. Increased capillary hydrostatic pressure leads to edema formation. Ultimately, pulmonary edema and heart failure may develop. Diuretics are common treatment.

Hypertonic Alterations

Hypertonic fluid alterations develop when the osmolality of ECF is elevated above normal (greater than 294 mOsm). The most common causes are increased concentration of ECF sodium (hypernatremia) or deficit of ECF water, or both. In both instances, ECF hypertonicity attracts water from the intracellular space, causing ICF dehydration (see Figure 5.7).

Hypernatremia

PATHOPHYSIOLOGY Hypernatremia occurs when serum sodium levels exceed 145 mmol/L. Increased levels of serum sodium cause hypertonicity. Hypernatremia can be isovolemic, hypovolemic, or hypervolemic, depending on the accompanying ECF water volume.

Isovolemic hypernatremia is the most common type and occurs when there is a *loss of free water* with a near-normal body sodium concentration. Causes include inadequate water intake; excessive sweating (sweat is hypotonic), fever, or respiratory tract infections, which increase the respiratory rate and enhance water loss from the lungs; burns; vomiting; diarrhea; and central or nephrogenic diabetes

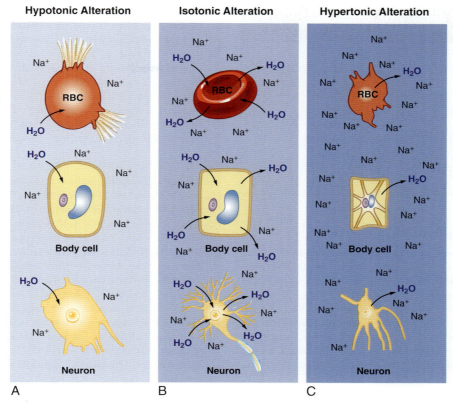

FIGURE 5.7 Effects of Alterations in Extracellular Sodium Concentration in Red Blood Cell, Body Cell, and Neuron. **A,** Decrease in extracellular fluid *(ECF)* sodium *(Na⁺)* concentration (hyponatremia) results in intracellular fluid osmotic attraction of water *(H₂O)* with swelling and potential bursting of cells. **B,** Isotonic alteration: Normal concentration of sodium in ECF and no change in shifts of fluid in or out of cells. **C,** Hypertonic alteration: An increase in ECF sodium concentration (hypernatremia) results in osmotic attraction of water out of cells with cell shrinkage. *RBC,* Red blood cell.

insipidus (lack of ADH or inadequate renal response to ADH). Infants with severe diarrhea are vulnerable and have increased risk because they cannot communicate thirst. Insufficient water intake occurs particularly in individuals who are comatose, confused, or immobilized, or who are receiving gastric feedings. **Dehydration** refers to water deficit but also is commonly used to indicate both sodium and water loss (isotonic or iso-osmolar dehydration).[6]

Hypovolemic hypernatremia occurs where there is loss of sodium accompanied by a relatively greater loss of body water. Causes include use of loop diuretics, osmotic diuresis (i.e., from hyperglycemia related to uncontrolled diabetes mellitus or use of mannitol), or failure of the kidneys to concentrate urine.

Hypervolemic hypernatremia is rare and occurs when there is increased TBW and a greater increase in total body sodium level, resulting in hypervolemia. Causes include infusion of hypertonic saline solutions (e.g., as sodium replacement for treatment of salt depletion, which can occur with renal impairment, heart failure, or gastro-intestinal losses); oversecretion of adrenocorticotropic hormone (ACTH) or aldosterone (e.g., Cushing's syndrome, adrenal hyperplasia); and near saltwater drowning.[7] High amounts of dietary sodium rarely cause hypernatremia in a healthy individual because the sodium is eliminated by the kidneys.

Because chloride follows sodium, **hyperchloremia** (elevation of serum chloride concentration greater than 106 mmol/L) often accompanies hypernatremia, as well as plasma bicarbonate deficits (such as in metabolic acidosis).[8] There are no specific symptoms or treatment for chloride excess.

CLINICAL MANIFESTATIONS When there is excessive sodium intake or decreased sodium loss in relation to water, water redistributes itself osmotically to the hypertonic extracellular space, resulting in hypervolemia and intracellular dehydration. Clinical manifestations include thirst, weight gain, bounding pulse, and increased blood pressure. Central nervous system signs are the most serious and result from alterations in membrane potentials and shrinking of brain cells (sodium cannot cross brain capillaries because of their tight endothelial junctions). Signs include muscle twitching and hyper-reflexia (hyperactive reflexes), confusion, coma, convulsions, and cerebral hemorrhage from stretching of veins. Signs and symptoms of intracellular and extracellular dehydration with volume depletion (Box 5.1) manifest hypernatremia with marked water deficit.

EVALUATION AND TREATMENT Serum sodium levels are greater than 145 mmol/L and urine specific gravity will be greater than 1.030. The history and physical examination provide information about underlying disorders and events. The treatment of hypernatremia and water deficit is oral fluids or isotonic salt-free fluid (5% dextrose in water) until the serum sodium level returns to normal. Administration of fluid is done slowly, in order to prevent cerebral edema. Monitoring serum sodium levels is important throughout treatment. Hypervolemia or hypovolemia requires treatment of the underlying clinical condition.

BOX 5.1 Signs and Symptoms of Dehydration

Increased serum sodium concentration	Soft eyeballs
Thirst	Sunken fontanels in infants
Headache	Prolonged capillary refill time
Weight loss	Tachycardia
Oliguria and concentrated urine	Weak pulses
Hard stools	Low blood pressure
Decreased skin turgor	Postural hypotension
Dry mucous membranes	Hypovolemic shock
Decreased sweating and tears	Confusion
Elevated temperature	Coma

Hypotonic Alterations

Hypotonic fluid imbalances occur when the osmolality of ECF is less than 280 mmol (see Figure 5.7). The most common causes are sodium deficit or water excess. Either leads to *intracellular overhydration* (cellular edema) and cell swelling. When there is a sodium deficit, the osmotic pressure of ECF decreases and water moves into the cell where the osmotic pressure is greater. The plasma volume then decreases, leading to symptoms of hypovolemia. With water excess, increases in both ICF and ECF volume occur, causing symptoms of hypervolemia and water intoxication with cerebral and pulmonary edema.

Hyponatremia
PATHOPHYSIOLOGY

1. **Hyponatremia** develops when the serum sodium concentration falls below 135 mmol/L. Hyponatremia occurs when there is loss of sodium, inadequate intake of sodium, or dilution of sodium by water excess.[9] Sodium depletion usually causes hypo-osmolality with movement of water into cells and rupture of cell membranes.
2. **Isovolemic hyponatremia** occurs when there is loss of sodium without a significant loss of water (pure sodium deficit). Causes can include syndrome of inappropriate antidiuretic hormone[10] (SIADH [see Chapter 19], which enhances water retention), hypothyroidism, pneumonia, and glucocorticoid deficiency. Inadequate intake of dietary sodium is rare but possible in individuals on low-sodium diets, particularly with use of diuretics.
3. **Hypervolemic hyponatremia** occurs when total body sodium level increases. The increased sodium leads to an increase in TBW and dilution of sodium in the extracellular space. Causes include heart failure, cirrhosis of the liver and nephrotic syndrome. Edema is present.
4. **Hypovolemic hyponatremia** occurs with a loss of TBW, but there is a greater loss of body sodium. There is decreased volume in the ECF. Causes include prolonged vomiting, severe diarrhea, inadequate secretion of aldosterone (e.g., adrenal insufficiency), and renal losses from diuretics.
5. **Dilutional hyponatremia** (water intoxication) occurs when there is intake of large amounts of free water or replacement of fluid loss with IV (5% dextrose in water), which dilutes sodium. Carbon dioxide and water are the products of glucose metabolism. As a result, IV infusion with 5% dextrose in water leaves a hypotonic solution and has an overall diluting effect. Excessive sweating stimulates thirst and intake of large amounts of free water (as can occur in endurance athletes), which dilutes sodium. Some individuals with psychogenic disorders develop water intoxication from compulsive water drinking. Other causes can include tap water enemas, near-freshwater drowning, and use of selective serotonin reuptake inhibitors (SSRIs). When the body is functioning normally, it is almost impossible to produce an excess of TBW because the kidneys play a key role in regulating water balance.
6. **Hypochloremia**, a low level of serum chloride (less than 98 mmol/L), usually occurs with hyponatremia or an elevated bicarbonate concentration, as in metabolic alkalosis. Sodium deficit related to restricted intake, use of diuretics, vomiting, or nasogastric suction usually accompanies chloride deficiency. Hypochloremia is also a characteristic of cystic fibrosis (see Chapter 28), and treatment of the underlying cause is required.

CLINICAL MANIFESTATIONS The serum sodium concentration will be less than 135 mmol/L. Sodium depletion usually causes hypo-osmolality with movement of water into cells. The hematocrit is low from the dilutional effect of water excess in dilutional hyponatremia. The high amount of intracellular solutes compared with the low amount of extracellular solutes because of the hyponatremia causes an intracellular osmotic shift of water, resulting in cell swelling. The most life-threatening consequence is cerebral edema and increased intracranial pressure. Neurological changes include lethargy, confusion, apprehension, seizures, and coma. A decrease in sodium concentration changes the cell's ability to depolarize and repolarize normally, altering the action potential in neurons and muscle (see Chapter 1). Muscle twitching, depressed reflexes, and weakness are common. Nausea and vomiting are more common with less severe hyponatremia (i.e., decreases between 120 and 130 mmol/L). Hypovolemic hyponatremia has signs of hypotension, tachycardia, and decreased urine output. Clinical manifestations of hypervolemic hyponatremia include weight gain, edema, ascites, and jugular vein distension. Hyponatremia is a major cause of morbidity and mortality in critical care units and in older persons (see *Health Promotion*: Hyponatremia and Older Persons).

HEALTH PROMOTION
Hyponatremia and Older Persons

Hyponatremia is the most common of the electrolyte disorders, and prevalence is highest among older hospitalized individuals. Isovolemic hyponatremia caused by SIADH is the most common cause and can occur with central nervous system injury, pulmonary disease, malignancies, nausea, pain, and aging changes. Other contributing factors include use of thiazide diuretics, proton pump inhibitors, age-related decrease in thirst with dehydration, and diminished urine concentrating ability. Hyponatremia contributes to cognitive deficits, gait disturbances, falls, fractures, long-term hospitalization, the need for long-term care, and death. Assessment of older persons for risk, implementation of preventive strategies, and early intervention is important.

SIADH, Syndrome of inappropriate antidiuretic hormone.
From Ayus, J. C., Negri, A. L., Kalantar-Zadeh, K., et al. (2012). *Nephrology Dialysis Transplantation, 27*(10), 3725–3731; Berl, T. (2013). *Clinical Journal of the American Society of Nephrology, 8*(3), 469–475; Cowen, L.E., Hodak, S.P., & Verbalis, J.G. (2013). *Endocrinology & Metabolism Clinics of North America, 42*(2), 349–370; Cumming, K., Hoyle, G.E., Hutchison, J.D., et al. (2014). *PLoS One, 9*(2), e88272; Mannesse, C.K., Vondeling, A.M., van Marum, R.J., et al. (2013). *Ageing Research Reviews, 12*(1), 165–173; Schrier, R.W., Sharma, S., & Shchekochikhin, D. (2013). *Nature Reviews: Nephrology, 9*(1), 37–50 (Erratum in [2013]. *Nature Reviews: Nephrology, 9*(3), 124).

EVALUATION AND TREATMENT The cause of hyponatremia must be determined and treatment planned accordingly. The treatment of hyponatremia consists of small amounts of IV hypertonic sodium chloride (i.e., 3% sodium chloride) given slowly (in order to prevent osmotic demyelination in the brain) when neurological manifestations are severe.[10] Most cases of dilutional hyponatremia require a restricted intake of water because body sodium levels may be normal or increased even though serum sodium levels are low. Arginine vasopressin (ADH) receptor antagonists (vaptans) are a class of medications used for the treatment of hypervolemic and euvolemic hyponatremia.[11] With each treatment, serum sodium levels must be monitored.[9]

ALTERATIONS IN POTASSIUM AND OTHER ELECTROLYTES

> ✓ **QUICK CHECK 5.4**
> 1. What role does potassium play in the body? What metabolic dysfunctions occur in potassium deficiency? In potassium excess?
> 2. Explain how a person can have normal total body potassium levels but still exhibit hypokalemia.
> 3. What is the most prominent electrocardiogram (ECG) change associated with hyperkalemia? With hypokalemia?

Potassium

Potassium (K^+) is the major intracellular electrolyte and is essential for normal cellular functions. Total body potassium content is about 4000 mmol, with most of it (98%) located in the cells. The ICF concentration of potassium is 150 to 160 mmol/L; the ECF potassium concentration is 3.5 to 5.0 mmol/L. A sodium–potassium adenosine-triphosphatase active transport system (Na^+–K^+ ATPase pump) maintains this difference in concentration (see Figure 1.26).

As the predominant ICF ion, potassium exerts a major influence on the regulation of ICF osmolality and fluid balance, as well as on intracellular electrical neutrality in relation to hydrogen (H^+) and sodium. Potassium is required for glycogen and glucose deposition in liver and skeletal muscle cells. It also maintains the resting membrane potential, as reflected in the transmission and conduction of nerve impulses (see Figure 1.29), the maintenance of normal cardiac rhythms, and the contraction of skeletal muscle and smooth muscle.

Dietary potassium moves rapidly into cells after ingestion. However, several factors influence the distribution of potassium between intracellular and extracellular fluids. Insulin, aldosterone, epinephrine, and alkalosis facilitate the shift of potassium into cells. Likewise, insulin deficiency, aldosterone deficiency, acidosis, cell lysis, and strenuous exercise facilitate the shift of potassium out of cells. Glucagon blocks entry of potassium into cells, and glucocorticoids promote potassium excretion. Potassium also will move out of cells along with water when there is increased ECF osmolality.

Although potassium exists in most body fluids, the kidney is the most efficient regulator of potassium balance. The renal glomerulus freely filters potassium, and the proximal tubule and loop of Henle reabsorb 90%. In the distal tubules, *principal cells* secrete potassium and *intercalated cells* reabsorb potassium. These cells determine the amount of potassium excreted from the body. The gut may also sense the amount of K^+ ingested and stimulate renal K^+ excretion, independent of aldosterone.[12]

The plasma concentration in the peritubular capillaries primarily determines the potassium concentration in the distal tubular cells. When plasma potassium concentration increases from increased dietary intake or shifts of potassium from ICF to ECF occur, there is potassium secretion into the urine by the distal tubules. Decreased levels of plasma potassium result in decreased distal tubular secretion, although approximately 5 to 15 mmol/day will continue to be lost. Changes in the rate of filtrate (urine) flow through the distal tubule also influence the concentration gradient for potassium secretion. When the urine flow rate is high, as with the use of diuretics, potassium concentration in the distal tubular urine is lower, leading to the secretion of potassium into the urine.

Changes in pH (hydrogen ion concentration) also affect potassium balance. During acute acidosis, hydrogen ions accumulate in the ICF and potassium shifts out of the cell to the ECF to maintain a balance of cations across the cell membrane. This response occurs in part because of a decrease in Na^+–K^+ ATPase pump activity. Decreased ICF potassium results in decreased secretion of potassium by the distal tubular cells, contributing to hyperkalemia. In acute alkalosis, intracellular fluid levels of hydrogen diminish and potassium shifts into the cell; in addition, the distal tubular cells increase their secretion of potassium, further contributing to hypokalemia.[13]

Besides conserving sodium, *aldosterone* also regulates potassium concentration. Elevated plasma potassium concentration causes the release of renin by renal juxtaglomerular cells and the adrenal secretion of aldosterone through the renin-angiotensin-aldosterone system. Aldosterone then stimulates the release of potassium into the urine by the distal renal tubules. Aldosterone also increases the secretion of potassium from sweat glands.

Insulin helps regulate plasma potassium levels by stimulating the Na^+–K^+ ATPase pump, thus promoting the movement of potassium into liver and muscle cells, particularly after eating. Insulin is also a treatment for hyperkalemia. Dangerously low levels of plasma potassium can result with insulin administration while potassium levels are depressed. Potassium balance is especially significant in the treatment of conditions requiring insulin administration, such as insulin-dependent diabetes mellitus.

Potassium adaptation is the ability of the body to adapt to increased levels of potassium intake over time. A sudden increase in potassium may be fatal, but if the increased intake of potassium is slow (up to 120 mmol/day), the kidney can increase the urinary excretion of potassium and maintain potassium balance.

Hypokalemia

PATHOPHYSIOLOGY Potassium deficiency, or **hypokalemia**, develops when the serum potassium concentration falls to less than 3.5 mmol/L. Plasma concentrations of potassium are a means to measure overall changes in potassium balance because cellular and total body stores are difficult to measure. Generally, lowered serum potassium level indicates loss of total body potassium. With potassium loss from ECF, the concentration gradient change favours movement of potassium from the cell to the ECF. This adjustment in potassium movement maintains the ICF/ECF concentration, but depletes the amount of total body potassium.

Factors contributing to the development of hypokalemia include reduced intake of potassium, increased entry of potassium into cells, and increased loss of body potassium. Dietary deficiency of potassium is more common in older persons with both low protein intake and inadequate intake of fruits and vegetables, as well as in individuals with alcoholism or anorexia nervosa (see *Health Promotion*: Potassium Intake: Hypertension and Stroke). Reduced potassium intake generally becomes a problem when combined with other causes of potassium depletion.

ECF hypokalemia can develop without losses of total body potassium. For example, potassium shifts from the ECF to the ICF in exchange for hydrogen to maintain plasma acid–base balance during respiratory or metabolic alkalosis. Insulin promotes cellular uptake of potassium, and insulin administration may cause an ECF potassium deficit.

Potassium shifts from the ICF to the ECF in conditions such as diabetic ketoacidosis, in which the increased hydrogen ion concentration in the ECF causes H^+ to shift into the cell in exchange for potassium. The plasma maintains a normal level of potassium, but the kidney

HEALTH PROMOTION
Potassium Intake: Hypertension and Stroke

Enriched dietary intake of potassium is associated with lower risk of hypertension and stroke. The Canadian diet often exceeds recommendations for sodium intake and has a deficiency in potassium intake. There is increased risk of high blood pressure, cardiovascular disease, and mortality when the plasma ratio of sodium concentration to potassium concentration is high. Potassium reduces the effects of high dietary salt with a decrease in blood pressure, stroke rates, and cardiovascular disease risk. Potassium affects blood pressure by various means, namely through the renal handling of sodium, endothelial cell function, decreased vascular resistance, and reduced oxidative stress.

A recent meta-analysis of potassium intake and risk of stroke[a] suggests an inverse relationship between potassium intake and risk of total, hemorrhagic, and ischemic stroke, with the lowest risk occurring at a potassium intake of around 90 mmol/day. The authors of the study further explain that the mechanisms by which potassium intake may affect stroke risk require further investigation, as blood pressure is only one factor. The benefit of potassium intake on reduced risk of stroke is particularly evident in decreasing blood pressure in the older female population.

[a] Vincetti, M., Fillipini, T., Crippa, A., des Sesmaisons, A., Wise, L. A., and Orsini, N. (2016). Meta-analysis of the potassium intake and the risk of stroke. *Journal of the American Heart Association, 5*(10). https://doi.org/10.1161/JAHA.116.004210.

continues to excrete potassium in the urine, causing a deficit in total body potassium. Insulin administration and IV rehydration must occur with potassium supplements in order to prevent severe, or even fatal, hypokalemia. Serum potassium measurements are important during therapy, as is the cautious administration of potassium in order to prevent hyperkalemia.

Gastro-intestinal and renal disorders are usually responsible for the loss of potassium from body stores. Diarrhea, intestinal drainage tubes or fistulae, and laxative abuse also result in hypokalemia. There is a loss of about 5 to 10 mmol of potassium and 100 to 150 mL of water in the stool each day. With diarrhea, fluid and electrolyte losses can be voluminous, with several litres of fluid and 100 to 200 mmol of potassium lost per day. Vomiting or continuous nasogastric suctioning is often associated with potassium depletion, partly because of the potassium lost from the gastric fluid but principally because of renal compensation for volume depletion and the metabolic alkalosis (elevated bicarbonate levels) that occurs from sodium, chloride, and hydrogen ion losses. The loss of fluid and sodium stimulates the secretion of aldosterone, which then causes renal losses of potassium.

Renal potassium losses occur with increased secretion of potassium by the distal tubule. Other explanations for urinary losses of potassium include the use of potassium-wasting diuretics, excessive aldosterone secretion, increased distal tubular flow rate, and low plasma magnesium concentration. When there is an increased flow of bicarbonate in the distal tubule, this electronegativity attracts potassium and contributes to further potassium loss in the urine.

Many diuretics inhibit the reabsorption of sodium chloride, causing the diuretic effect. The distal tubular flow rate then increases (because of more water and sodium in the filtrate) and promotes more potassium excretion (through the action of aldosterone). Primary hyperaldosteronism with excessive secretion of aldosterone from an adrenal adenoma (tumour) can also cause potassium wasting. Similarly, many kidney diseases reduce the ability to conserve sodium. The disordered sodium reabsorption produces a diuretic effect, and the increased distal tubule flow rate favours the secretion of potassium (again, due to aldosterone). Magnesium deficits increase renal potassium secretion and promote hypokalemia because magnesium blocks the channel that transports potassium out of the cell in the Na^+–K^+ ATPase pump. When there is a magnesium deficiency, there is a greater loss of potassium into the urine filtrate through these channels. Certain antibiotics (i.e., carbenicillin disodium [Geocillin] and amphotericin B [Fungizone]) also cause hypokalemia by increasing the rate of potassium excretion. Furthermore, rare hereditary defects in renal potassium transport (e.g., Bartter and Gitelman syndromes) can cause hypokalemia.

CLINICAL MANIFESTATIONS Mild losses of potassium usually have relatively few or no symptoms. Severe loss of potassium results in neuromuscular and cardiac manifestations. Neuromuscular excitability decreases because the cell is now *hyperpolarized*. As such, the resting membrane potential is more negative and requires a larger impulse in order to achieve an action potential. Resulting symptoms of hypokalemia include skeletal muscle weakness, smooth muscle atony, cardiac dysrhythmias, glucose intolerance, and impaired urinary concentrating ability.[14]

Symptoms also occur in relation to the *rate* of potassium depletion. Because the body can accommodate slow losses of potassium, the decrease in ECF concentration may allow potassium to shift from the intracellular space, restoring the potassium concentration gradient toward normal, with less severe neuromuscular changes. With acute and severe losses of potassium, changes in neuromuscular excitability are more profound. Skeletal muscle weakness occurs initially in the larger muscles of the legs and arms and ultimately affects the diaphragm and depresses ventilation. Paralysis and respiratory arrest can occur with severe losses. Signs of loss of smooth muscle tone include constipation, intestinal distension, anorexia, nausea, vomiting, and paralytic ileus (paralysis of the intestinal muscles).

The cardiac effects of hypokalemia correlate directly with changes in membrane excitability. As ECF potassium concentration decreases, the resting membrane potential becomes more negative (i.e., from -90 to $-100\,mV$ [hyperpolarization]). Because potassium contributes to the repolarization phase of the action potential, hypokalemia delays ventricular repolarization. Various dysrhythmias may occur, including sinus bradycardia, atrioventricular block, and paroxysmal atrial tachycardia. The characteristic changes in the electrocardiogram (ECG) reflect *delayed repolarization*. For example, the amplitude of the T wave decreases, the amplitude of the U wave increases, and the ST segment is depressed (Figure 5.8). In severe states of hypokalemia, P waves peak, the QT interval is prolonged, and T wave inversions are present. Hypokalemia enhances the therapeutic effect of digitalis and increases the risk of digitalis toxicity.

A wide range of metabolic dysfunctions may result from potassium deficiency (Table 5.6). Hypokalemia depresses insulin secretion and affects carbohydrate metabolism by altering hepatic and skeletal muscle glycogen synthesis. Renal function is impaired, with a decreased ability to concentrate urine. Polyuria (increased urine) and polydipsia (increased thirst) are associated with decreased responsiveness to ADH. Long-term potassium deficits lasting more than 1 month may damage renal tissue, with interstitial fibrosis and tubular atrophy.

EVALUATION AND TREATMENT The diagnosis of hypokalemia relates to the medical history and the identification of disorders associated with potassium loss or shifts of extracellular potassium to the intracellular space. Treatment involves an estimation of total body potassium losses and correction of acid–base imbalances. Prevention of further losses of potassium is key, and the individual should be encouraged to eat foods rich in potassium. The maximal rate of oral replacement is 40 to 80 mmol/day if renal function is normal. A maximal safe rate of IV replacement is 20 mmol/hr with a maximal

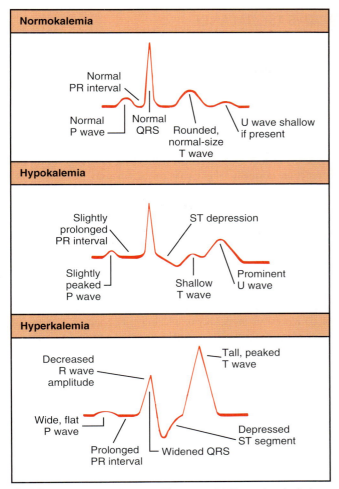

FIGURE 5.8 Electrocardiogram Changes with Potassium Imbalance.

concentration of 40 mmol/L. This is because potassium can be irritating to blood vessels. Monitoring of serum potassium values is important during treatment.

Hyperkalemia

PATHOPHYSIOLOGY Elevation of ECF potassium concentration greater than 5.0 mmol/L constitutes hyperkalemia.[15] Because of efficient renal excretion, increases in total body potassium level are relatively rare. The body handles acute increases in serum potassium level quickly through increased cellular uptake and renal excretion of body potassium excesses.

Causes of hyperkalemia include increased intake of potassium, a shift of potassium from cells to ECF, decreased renal excretion, or medications that decrease renal potassium excretion (i.e., ACE inhibitors, angiotensin receptor blockers, and aldosterone antagonists). The body generally tolerates slow, long-term increases in potassium intake through potassium adaptation when renal function is normal, and short-term sudden increases in potassium intake can actually exceed the capacity of the kidney to excrete it. Dietary excesses of potassium are uncommon, but accidental ingestion of potassium salt substitutes can cause toxicity. Use of stored whole blood and IV boluses of potassium penicillin G or replacement potassium can precipitate hyperkalemia, particularly with impaired renal function. Potassium moves from ICF to ECF with cell trauma (such as burns, massive crushing injuries, and surgeries) or a change in cell membrane permeability, acidosis, insulin deficiency, or cellular hypoxia. Potassium excretion continues with normal kidney function, and as cell repair begins, hypokalemia can develop without an adequate replacement of potassium.

In acidosis, ECF hydrogen ions shift into cells (according to the hydrogen ion gradient) in exchange for ICF potassium and sodium (in order to maintain electroneutrality). As such, hyperkalemia and acidosis often occur simultaneously. Because insulin promotes cellular entry of potassium, insulin deficits, which occur with such conditions as diabetic ketoacidosis, often accompany hyperkalemia. Hypoxia can also lead to hyperkalemia by diminishing the efficiency of cell membrane active transport, resulting in the escape of potassium to ECF. Digitalis overdose (toxicity) may cause hyperkalemia by inhibiting the Na^+-K^+ ATPase pump, and thus allowing potassium to remain outside the cell.

Decreased renal excretion of potassium commonly is associated with hyperkalemia. Renal failure that results in oliguria (urine output of 30 mL/hr or less) accompanies elevations of serum potassium level. The amount of potassium intake, the degree of acidosis and the rate of renal cell damage directly affect the severity of the hyperkalemia. Decreases in the secretion or renal effects of aldosterone also can cause decreases in the urinary excretion of potassium. For example, Addison's disease (a disease of adrenal cortical insufficiency) results in decreased production and secretion of aldosterone (and other steroids) and thus, contributes to hyperkalemia.

CLINICAL MANIFESTATIONS Symptoms vary with the severity of hyperkalemia. During mild attacks, increased neuromuscular irritability is evident as restlessness, intestinal cramping, and diarrhea. Severe hyperkalemia decreases the resting membrane potential (i.e., from −90 to −70 mV [hypopolarization]) and causes muscle weakness, loss of muscle tone, and paralysis. This happens because of the persistent depolarization and subsequent inactivation of sodium channels in the cell membrane. Cell membranes become less excitable, and this results in the muscle weakness or paralysis commonly seen with this condition. In mild states of hyperkalemia, there is more rapid repolarization, reflected in the ECG as narrow and taller T waves with a shortened QT interval. Severe hyperkalemia causes delayed cardiac conduction and prevents repolarization of the heart muscle. Severe hyperkalemia depresses the ST segment, prolongs the PR interval, and widens the QRS complex because of decreased conduction velocity from inactivated sodium channels (see Figure 5.8). Bradydysrhythmias and delayed conduction are common in hyperkalemia; severe hyperkalemia can even cause ventricular fibrillation or cardiac arrest.[16]

As with hypokalemia, changes in the ratio of intracellular to extracellular potassium concentration contribute to the symptoms of hyperkalemia (see Table 5.6). The neuromuscular effects of hyperkalemia relate to the increase in rate of repolarization and the presence of other contributing factors, such as acidosis and calcium balance. Acute elevations of extracellular potassium concentration affect neuromuscular irritability because of changes to the ratio of potassium in the ECF compared to the ICF. Similarly, changes in ECF calcium concentration can exert a similar effect on neuromuscular function, often overriding the effects of hyperkalemia because calcium is also a cation and affects the threshold potential (see Chapter 1).

EVALUATION AND TREATMENT Clinical investigations should include hyperkalemia when there is a history of renal disease, massive trauma, insulin deficiency, Addison's disease, use of potassium salt substitutes, or metabolic acidosis. There is a correlation between the acuity of the onset of symptoms and the underlying cause.

TABLE 5.6 Clinical Manifestations of Potassium Level Alterations

Organ System	Hypokalemia	Hyperkalemia
Cardiovascular	Dysrhythmias ECG changes (flattened T waves, U waves, ST depression, peaked P wave, prolonged QT interval) Cardiac arrest Weak, irregular pulse rate Postural hypotension	Dysrhythmias ECG changes (peaked T waves, prolonged PR interval, absent P wave with widened QRS complex) Bradycardia Heart block Cardiac arrest
Nervous	Lethargy Fatigue Confusion Paresthesias	Anxiety Tingling Numbness
Gastro-intestinal	Nausea and vomiting Decreased motility Distension Decreased bowel sounds Ileus	Nausea and vomiting Diarrhea Colicky pain
Kidney	Water loss Thirst Inability to concentrate urine Increased tubular production of ammonia and ammonium Kidney damage	Oliguria Kidney damage
Skeletal and smooth muscle	Weakness Flaccid paralysis Respiratory arrest Constipation Bladder dysfunction	Early: hyperactive muscles Late: weakness and flaccid paralysis

Management of hyperkalemia includes treating the contributing causes and correcting the potassium excess. When serum potassium levels are dangerously high, calcium gluconate is the recommended treatment to restore normal neuromuscular irritability and to stabilize the resting cardiac membrane potential by making the threshold potential less negative. Administration of glucose (which readily stimulates insulin secretion) or administration of both glucose and insulin for diabetic individuals facilitates cellular entry of potassium. Sodium bicarbonate corrects metabolic acidosis and lowers serum potassium concentration. Oral or rectal administration of cation exchange resins, which exchange sodium for potassium in the intestine, can be effective. Dialysis also effectively removes potassium when renal failure has occurred.

Other Electrolytes—Calcium, Phosphate, and Magnesium

Information for the other body electrolytes—calcium (Ca^{++}), phosphate (PO_4^{3+}), and magnesium (Mg^{++})—is in Table 5.7. Parathyroid hormone (PTH) and vitamin D are important for the regulation of these minerals[17] (see Chapter 18).

ACID–BASE BALANCE

QUICK CHECK 5.5
1. What is the difference between compensation and correction of acid–base disturbances?
2. What two chemicals change in metabolic acid–base disturbances?
3. How do alterations in carbon dioxide concentration influence acid–base status?

Regulation of acid–base balance is within a narrow range for the body to function normally. Slight changes in amounts of hydrogen and changes in pH can significantly alter biological processes in cells and tissues.[18] Hydrogen ions maintain membrane integrity and the speed of metabolic enzyme reactions. Most pathological conditions disturb acid–base balance, producing circumstances possibly more harmful than the disease process itself.

Hydrogen Ion and pH

The concentration of hydrogen ions in body fluids is approximately 0.000 000 1 mg/L (or 1×10^{-7} mg/L), is indicated as pH 7.0. The symbol *pH* represents the acidity or alkalinity of a solution. Changes of 1 unit in pH (e.g., from pH 7.0 to pH 6.0) reflect a tenfold change in the [H^+] ([H^+]=hydrogen ion concentration). A higher [H^+] indicates a more acidic solution and a lower pH. Likewise, a more alkaline or basic solution has a higher pH. In biological fluids, a pH of less than 7.4 is defined as acidic and a pH greater than 7.4 is defined as alkaline, or basic (Table 5.8).

Body acids are end products of protein, carbohydrate, and fat metabolism, and acids can release hydrogen ions. The body has mechanisms to balance the relative amounts of acids and bases to maintain normal pH. The lungs, kidneys, and bones are the major organs involved in regulating acid–base balance. The systems work together to regulate short- and long-term changes in acid–base status.

Body acids exist in two forms: **volatile** (eliminated as carbon dioxide [CO_2] gas) and **nonvolatile** (the kidney can eliminate these). The volatile acid is carbonic acid (H_2CO_3), a *weak acid* (i.e., it does not release its hydrogen easily). In the presence of the enzyme, carbonic anhydrase, it readily dissociates into CO_2 and water (H_2O). The lungs then eliminate the carbon dioxide through pulmonary ventilation.

Nonvolatile acids are sulphuric, phosphoric, and other organic acids. They are *strong acids* (readily release their hydrogens). The renal tubules secrete nonvolatile acids into the urine in amounts of about 60 to 100 mmol of hydrogen per day, or about 1 mmol per kilogram of body weight.

Buffer Systems

Buffering occurs in response to changes in acid–base status. **Buffers** can absorb excessive hydrogen ions (H^+) (acid) or hydroxyl ions (OH^-) (base) and prevent a significant change in pH. The buffer systems are located in both the ICF and the ECF compartments, and they function at different rates (Table 5.9). The most important plasma buffer systems are *carbonic acid–bicarbonate* and the protein *hemoglobin* (Figure 5.9). *Phosphate* and *protein* are the most important intracellular buffers and provide a first line of defence. Ammonia and phosphate can attach hydrogen ions and are important renal buffers.

TABLE 5.7 Alterations in Calcium, Phosphate, and Magnesium

Parameter	Calcium	Phosphate	Magnesium
Normal values	Serum: 2.1–2.6 mmol/L (total, adult), 1.9–2.6 mmol/L) total, less than 10 days), 1.05–1.30 mmol/L (ionized, adult); 99% in bone as hydroxyapatite; remainder in plasma and body cells with 50% bound to plasma proteins; 40% free or ionized; ionized form most important physiologically	Serum: 0.8–1.5 mmol/L (adult), 1.45–2.10 mmol/L in infants and young children; mainly in bone with some in ICF and ECF; exists as phospholipids, phosphate esters, and inorganic phosphate (ionized form)	Serum: 0.75–0.95 mmol/L (adult); 40–60% stored in bone, 33% bound to plasma proteins; primary intracellular divalent cation
Function	Needed for fundamental metabolic processes; major cation for structure of bone and teeth; enzymatic cofactor for blood clotting; required for hormone secretion and function of cell receptors; directly related to plasma membrane stability and permeability, transmission of nerve impulses, and contraction of muscles; parathyroid hormone, vitamin D_3, and calcitonin act together to control calcium absorption and excretion (see Chapter 18)	Intracellular and extracellular anion buffer in regulation of acid–base balance; provides energy for muscle contraction (as ATP); parathyroid hormone, vitamin D_3, and calcitonin act together to control phosphate absorption and excretion (see Chapter 18)	Cofactor in intracellular enzymatic reactions and causes neuromuscular excitability; often interacts with calcium and potassium in reactions at cellular level and has important role in smooth muscle contraction and relaxation; magnesium is absorbed in the intestine and eliminated by the kidney
Excess	**Hypercalcemia** (serum concentrations >2.6 mmol/L)	**Hyperphosphatemia** (serum concentrations >1.5 mmol/L)	**Hypermagnesemia** (serum concentrations >1.25 mmol/L)
Causes	Hyperparathyroidism; bone metastases with calcium resorption from breast, prostate, renal, and cervical cancer; sarcoidosis; excess vitamin D; many tumours that produce PTH	Acute or chronic renal failure with significant loss of glomerular filtration; treatment of metastatic tumours with chemotherapy that releases large amounts of phosphate into serum; long-term use of laxatives or enemas containing phosphates; hypoparathyroidism	Usually renal insufficiency or failure; also excessive intake of magnesium-containing antacids, adrenal insufficiency
Effects	Many nonspecific; fatigue, weakness, lethargy, anorexia, nausea, constipation; impaired renal function, kidney stones; dysrhythmias, bradycardia, cardiac arrest; bone pain, osteoporosis	Symptoms primarily related to low serum calcium levels (caused by high phosphate levels) similar to results of hypocalcemia; when prolonged, calcification of soft tissues in lungs, kidneys, joints	Skeletal smooth muscle contraction; excess nerve function; loss of deep tendon reflexes; nausea and vomiting; muscle weakness; hypotension; bradycardia; respiratory distress
Deficit	**Hypocalcemia** (serum calcium concentration <2.1 mmol/L)	**Hypophosphatemia** (serum phosphate concentration <0.4 mmol/L—critical value)	**Hypomagnesemia** (serum magnesium concentration <0.75 mmol/L)
Causes	Related to inadequate intestinal absorption, deposition of ionized calcium into bone or soft tissue, blood administration, or decreases in PTH and vitamin D; nutritional deficiencies occur with inadequate sources of dairy products or green leafy vegetables	Most commonly by intestinal malabsorption related to vitamin D deficiency, use of magnesium- and aluminum-containing antacids, long-term alcohol abuse, and malabsorption syndromes; respiratory alkalosis; increased renal excretion of phosphate associated with hyperparathyroidism	Malnutrition, malabsorption syndromes, alcoholism, urinary losses (renal tubular dysfunction, loop diuretics)
Effects	Increased neuromuscular excitability; tingling, muscle spasm (particularly in hands, feet, and facial muscles), intestinal cramping, hyperactive bowel sounds; severe cases show convulsions and tetany; prolonged QT interval, cardiac arrest	Conditions related to reduced capacity for oxygen transport by red blood cells and disturbed energy metabolism; leukocyte and platelet dysfunction; deranged nerve and muscle function; in severe cases, irritability, confusion, numbness, coma, convulsions; possibly respiratory failure (because of muscle weakness), cardiomyopathies, bone resorption (leading to rickets or osteomalacia)	Behavioural changes, irritability, increased reflexes, muscle cramps, ataxia, nystagmus, tetany, convulsions, tachycardia, hypotension

ATP, Adenosine triphosphate; *PTH*, parathyroid hormone.

Carbonic Acid–Bicarbonate Buffering

The carbonic acid–bicarbonate buffer pair *operates in both the lung and the kidney* and is a major extracellular buffer. The lungs are a second line of defence and can relatively quickly (within seconds to minutes) decrease the amount of carbonic acid by blowing off carbon dioxide. The kidneys are a third line of defence (hours to days) and can slowly reabsorb bicarbonate (a type of base) or regenerate new bicarbonate from carbon dioxide and water. The relationship between bicarbonate (HCO_3^-) and carbonic acid (H_2CO_3) is usually expressed as a ratio. Normal bicarbonate level is about 24 mmol/L, and normal carbonic acid level is about 1.2 mmol/L (when the partial pressure of carbon dioxide in arterial blood [$PaCO_2$] is 40 mm Hg), producing a 20:1 (24:1.2) ratio and the normal pH of 7.4 (Figure 5.10). These two systems are very effective together because the lungs can adjust acid concentration rapidly by ventilation, and bicarbonate is slowly reabsorbed or regenerated by the kidney tubules.

Compensation occurs with renal and respiratory adjustments to primary changes in pH. The respiratory system compensates for changes in pH by increasing or decreasing the concentration of carbon dioxide (carbonic acid) by changing ventilation. The renal system compensates by producing more acidic or more alkaline urine. The values for $PaCO_2$ and bicarbonate will vary from normal levels in an attempt to maintain a ratio of 20:1. Correction occurs when the values for both components of the buffer pair (carbonic acid and bicarbonate) return to normal levels.

Protein Buffering

Both intracellular and extracellular proteins have negative charges and can serve as buffers for hydrogen. Hemoglobin (Hb) is an excellent intracellular blood buffer because it can bind with hydrogen ions (H^+) (forming HHb) and carbon dioxide (forming $HHbCO_2$). Hemoglobin bound to hydrogen ion becomes a weak acid. Hemoglobin not saturated with oxygen (venous blood) is a better buffer than hemoglobin saturated with oxygen (arterial blood). Figure 5.9 depicts this pH control mechanism.

Renal Buffering

The distal tubule of the kidney regulates acid–base balance by secreting hydrogen into the urine and reabsorbing bicarbonate into the plasma. Dibasic phosphate (HPO_4^{2-}) and ammonia (NH_3) are two important renal buffers because they can attach hydrogen ions and be secreted into the urine. The renal buffering of hydrogen ions requires the use of carbon dioxide (CO_2) and water (H_2O) to form carbonic acid (H_2CO_3). The enzyme carbonic anhydrase catalyzes the reaction. The tubular cell then secretes the hydrogen in the carbonic acid, and phosphate and ammonia buffer the hydrogen in the lumen (i.e., forms $H_2PO_4^-$ and NH_4^+). The kidney reabsorbs the remaining bicarbonate. The end effect is the addition of new bicarbonate to the plasma, which further contributes to the alkalinity of the plasma because the hydrogen ions leave the body in the urine (Figure 5.11).

Acid–Base Imbalances

Pathophysiological changes in the concentration of hydrogen ions in the blood lead to acid–base imbalances.[19,20] In acidemia the pH of arterial blood is less than 7.4. A systemic increase in hydrogen ion concentration or a loss of base is termed acidosis. In alkalemia the pH of arterial blood is greater than 7.4. A systemic decrease in hydrogen ion concentration or an excess of base is termed alkalosis (Figure 5.12). Metabolic or respiratory processes may cause these changes. Figure 5.10 summarizes the relationship among pH, the partial pressure of carbon dioxide (respiratory regulation), and the concentration of bicarbonate (renal regulation) during alkalosis and acidosis. Acid–base imbalances are assessed using measurement of arterial blood gases, which includes the reporting of pH, $PaCO_2$, and HCO_3^-. The medical history and clinical symptoms are important in determining the cause of the disorder. Figure 5.13 summarizes the relationships among pH, $PaCO_2$, and bicarbonate during different acid–base alterations.

TABLE 5.8 pH of Body Fluids

Body Fluid	pH	Factors Affecting pH
Gastric juices	1.0–3.0	Hydrochloric acid production
Urine	5.0–6.0	Hydrogen ion excretion from waste products
Arterial blood	7.35–7.45	pH is slightly higher because there is less carbonic acid
Venous blood	7.37	pH is slightly lower because there is more carbonic acid
Cerebrospinal fluid	7.32	Decreased bicarbonate and higher carbon dioxide content decrease pH
Pancreatic fluid	7.8–8.0	Contains bicarbonate produced by exocrine cells
Bile	7.0–8.0	Contains bicarbonate
Small intestine fluid	6.5–7.5	Contains alkaline fluid from pancreas, liver, and gallbladder

TABLE 5.9 Buffer Systems

Buffer Pairs	Buffer System	Chemical Reaction	Rate
HCO_3^-/H_2CO_3	Bicarbonate	$H^+ + HCO_3^- \rightleftharpoons H_2O + CO_2$	Instantaneously
Hb^-/HHb	Hemoglobin	$HHb \rightleftharpoons H^+ + Hb^-$	Instantaneously
$HPO_4^{2-}/H_2PO_4^-$	Phosphate	$H_2PO_4^- + H^+ + HPO_4^{2-}$	Instantaneously
Pr^-/HPr	Plasma proteins	$HPr \rightleftharpoons H^+ + Pr^-$	Instantaneously

Organs	Physiological Mechanism		Rate
Lung ventilation	Regulates retention or elimination of CO_2 and therefore H_2CO_3 concentration		Minutes to hours
Ionic shifts	Exchange of intracellular potassium and sodium for hydrogen		2–4 hours
Kidney tubules	Bicarbonate reabsorption and regeneration, ammonia formation, phosphate buffering		Hours to days
Bone	Exchanges of calcium and phosphate and release of carbonate		Hours to days

CO_2, Carbon dioxide; H^+, hydrogen; Hb^-, hemoglobin; HCO_3^-, bicarbonate; H_2CO_3, carbonic acid; HHb, hydrogenated hemoglobin; H_2O, water; HPO_4^{2-}, dibasic phosphate; $H_2PO_4^-$, monobasic phosphate; HPr, hydrogenated protein; Pr^-, protein.

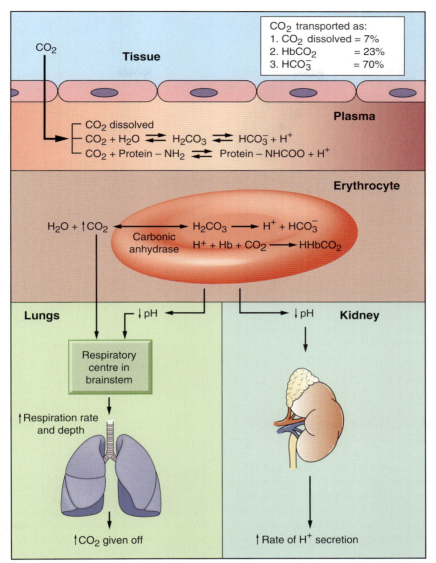

FIGURE 5.9 Integration of pH Control Mechanisms (Example for Acidosis). Carbon dioxide *(CO$_2$)* is produced in tissue cells and diffuses to plasma, where it is transported as dissolved CO$_2$, or it combines with water *(H$_2$O)* to form carbonic acid *(H$_2$CO$_3$)*, or it combines with protein from which hydrogen has been released. Most of the CO$_2$ diffuses into the red blood cells and combines with water to form H$_2$CO$_3$. The H$_2$CO$_3$ dissociates to form hydrogen ion *(H$^+$)* and bicarbonate *(HCO$_3^-$)*. Hydrogen combines with hemoglobin *(Hb)* that has released its oxygen to form HHb, which buffers the hydrogen and makes venous blood slightly more acidic than arterial blood. The increase in H$^+$ coupled with elevated CO$_2$ levels results in HhbCO$_2$ and an increase in the respiratory rate and secretion of H$^+$ by the kidneys. *HhbCO$_2$,* Carbaminohemoglobin; *NH$_2$,* amidogen; *NHCOO,* carbamate.

Metabolic Acidosis

In **metabolic acidosis**, the concentrations of non–carbonic acids increase or bicarbonate is lost from ECF or the kidney is unable to regenerate it (Table 5.10). Metabolic acidosis can occur either quickly, as in lactic acidosis caused by poor perfusion or hypoxemia, or slowly over an extended time, as in renal failure, diabetic ketoacidosis, or starvation (anion gap acidosis).[21] There is a decrease in the 20:1 ratio of HCO$_3^-$ to H$_2$CO$_3$.

The buffering systems normally compensate for excess acid and maintain arterial pH within normal range. When acidosis is severe, there is a depletion of buffers, and they cannot compensate; the ratio of the concentrations of bicarbonate to carbonic acid decreases to less than 20:1 (see Figure 5.10). An increase in the plasma concentration of chloride out of proportion of sodium causes hyperchloremic acidosis (nonanion gap acidosis). The specific type of acidosis can be determined by examining the serum **anion gap** (see Table 5.10).

Changes in the function of the neurological, respiratory, gastrointestinal, and cardiovascular systems occur with metabolic acidosis. Early symptoms include headache and lethargy, which progress to confusion and coma in severe acidosis. The respiratory system's efforts to compensate for the increase in metabolic acids result in what are termed *Kussmaul respirations* (a form of hyperventilation), which are deep and rapid. This response represents the body's attempt to increase pH by expelling carbon dioxide, which decreases carbonic acid concentration. Other symptoms include anorexia, nausea, vomiting, diarrhea, and abdominal discomfort. Death can result in the most severe and prolonged cases preceded by dysrhythmias and hypotension. Effective treatment is dependent on accurate diagnosis of the underlying condition.

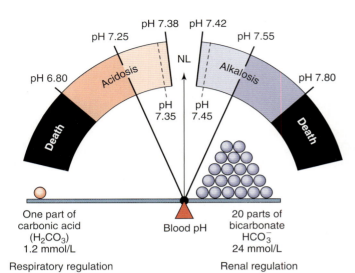

FIGURE 5.10 Ratio of Carbonic Acid and Bicarbonate Concentration in Maintaining pH Within Normal Limits. An increase in carbonic acid (H_2CO_3) or decrease in bicarbonate (HCO_3^-) concentration causes acidosis. A decrease in H_2CO_3 or increase in HCO_3^- concentration causes alkalosis. *NL,* Normal. (From Monahan, F. D. [2007]. *Medical-surgical nursing: health and illness perspectives* [8th ed.]. Mosby.)

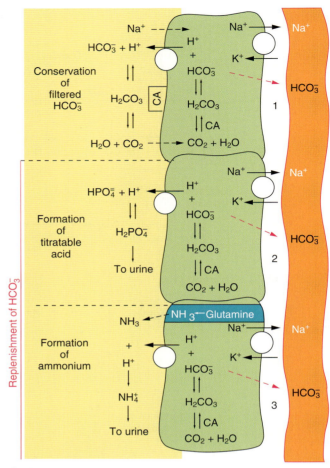

FIGURE 5.11 Renal Excretion of Acid. 1, Conservation of filtered bicarbonate. Filtered bicarbonate (HCO_3^-) combines with secreted hydrogen ion (H^+) in the presence of carbon anhydrase (*CA*) to form carbonic acid (H_2CO_3), which then dissociates to water (H_2O) and carbon dioxide (CO_2); both diffuse into the epithelial cell. The CO_2 and H_2O combine to form H_2CO_3 in the presence of CA, and the resulting bicarbonate ion (HCO_3^-) is reabsorbed into the capillary. **2, Formation of titratable acid.** Hydrogen ion is secreted and combines with dibasic phosphate (HPO_4^{2-}) to form monobasic phosphate ($H_2PO_4^-$). The secreted H^+ results from the dissociation of H_2CO_3, and the capillary reabsorbs the remaining HCO_3^-. **3, Formation of ammonium.** Ammonia (NH_3) is produced from glutamine in the epithelial cell and diffuses to the tubular lumen, where it combines with H^+ to form ammonium ion (NH_4^+). Once NH_4^+ has been formed, it cannot return to the epithelial cell (diffusional trapping), and the bicarbonate remaining in the epithelial cell is reabsorbed into the capillary. *K*+, Potassium; *NA*+, sodium.

Metabolic Alkalosis

When excessive loss of metabolic acids occurs, bicarbonate concentration increases, causing **metabolic alkalosis**[22] (see Figure 5.13). When acid loss results from vomiting, renal compensation is not very effective because loss of chloride (an anion) in hydrochloric acid (HCl) stimulates renal retention of bicarbonate (an anion). The result is **hypochloremic metabolic alkalosis**.[22] Hyperaldosteronism can also cause alkalosis because of sodium bicarbonate retention and loss of hydrogen and potassium. Diuretics may produce a mild alkalosis because they promote greater excretion of sodium, potassium, and chloride than of bicarbonate.

Some common signs and symptoms of metabolic alkalosis are weakness, muscle cramps, hyperactive reflexes, tetany, confusion, convulsions, and atrial tachycardia. Respirations may be shallow, and slow ventilation may manifest as the lungs attempt to compensate by increasing carbon dioxide retention. The manifestations vary with the cause and severity of the alkalosis. The symptoms of hyperactive reflexes and tetany occur because alkalosis increases binding of Ca^{++} to plasma proteins, thus decreasing ionized calcium concentration. The decreased ionized calcium concentration causes excitable cells to become hypopolarized, initiating an action potential more easily and causing muscle contraction.

Treatments should reflect the underlying cause of the condition. With hypochloremic alkalosis or contraction alkalosis with volume depletion, the first treatment for correction is sodium chloride solution because chloride replacement must occur before the kidney can excrete bicarbonate.

Respiratory Acidosis

Respiratory acidosis occurs when there is alveolar hypoventilation, resulting in an excess of carbon dioxide in the blood (**hypercapnia**). The arterial carbon dioxide tension (or pressure) ($PaCO_2$) is greater than 45 mm Hg and the pH is less than 7.35 (see Figure 5.13). A decrease in alveolar ventilation in relation to the metabolic production of carbon dioxide produces respiratory acidosis by an increase in the concentration of carbonic acid. Respiratory acidosis can be acute or chronic.[23] Common causes include depression of the respiratory centre (e.g., from medications or head injury), paralysis of the respiratory muscles, disorders of the chest wall (e.g., kyphoscoliosis or broken ribs), and disorders of the lung parenchyma (e.g., pneumonia, pulmonary edema, emphysema, asthma, bronchitis). Renal compensation occurs by elimination of hydrogen ion and retention of bicarbonate.

The signs and symptoms often include headache, blurred vision, breathlessness, restlessness, and apprehension followed by lethargy,

CHAPTER 5 Fluids and Electrolytes, Acids and Bases

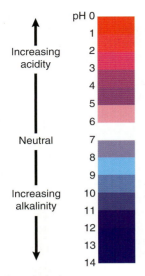

FIGURE 5.12 Acid–base Imbalances.

disorientation, muscle twitching, tremors, convulsions, and coma. Respiratory rate is rapid at first and gradually becomes depressed as the respiratory centre adapts to increasing levels of carbon dioxide. The skin may be warm and flushed because the elevated carbon dioxide concentration causes vasodilation. The restoration of adequate alveolar ventilation is necessary to remove the excess CO_2 (and decrease H_2CO_3).

Respiratory Alkalosis

Respiratory alkalosis occurs when there is alveolar hyperventilation (deep, rapid respirations). Excessive reduction in plasma carbon dioxide levels (**hypocapnia**) decreases carbonic acid concentration.[24,25] The $PaCO_2$ is less than 35 mm Hg and the pH is greater than normal (see Figure 5.13). Respiratory alkalosis can be chronic or acute. Hypoxemia (caused by pulmonary disease, heart failure, or high altitudes), hypermetabolic states (e.g., fever, anemia, thyrotoxicosis), early salicylate intoxication, hysteria, cirrhosis, and Gram-negative sepsis stimulate hyperventilation. Improper use of mechanical ventilators also can cause iatrogenic (treatment-related) respiratory alkalosis, and secondary alkalosis may develop because of hyperventilation stimulated by

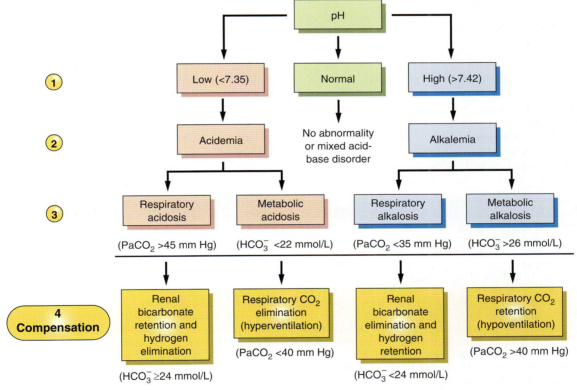

FIGURE 5.13 Primary and Compensatory Acid–base Changes. The interpretation of the cause of an acid–base imbalance uses a systematic approach. **1**, Is the pH low or high? **2**, If the pH is low (acidemia), is the cause respiratory (high $PaCO_2$) or metabolic (low HCO_3^-)? **3**, If the pH is high (alkalemia), is the cause respiratory (low $PaCO_2$) or metabolic (high HCO_3^-)? **4**, Is there compensation for the primary acid–base disorder? (a) HCO_3^- will be ≥ 24 mmol/L if there is renal compensation for a primary respiratory acidosis; (b) $PaCO_2$ will be <40 mm Hg if there is respiratory compensation of a primary metabolic acidosis; (c) HCO_3^- will be <24 mmol/L if there is renal compensation for primary respiratory alkalosis; (d) $PaCO_2$ will be >40 mm Hg if there is respiratory compensation for primary metabolic alkalosis. NOTE: Examine the pH first to determine whether there is acidemia or alkalemia. Then examine the changes in HCO_3^- and $PaCO_2$. **1**, HCO_3^- will be elevated when there is primary metabolic alkalosis or renal compensation for primary respiratory acidosis. **2**, HCO_3^- will be decreased when there is primary metabolic acidosis or renal compensation for primary respiratory alkalosis. **3**, $PaCO_2$ will be elevated when there is primary respiratory acidosis or respiratory compensation for primary metabolic alkalosis. **4**, A primary respiratory alkalosis or respiratory compensation for metabolic acidosis results in a decreased $PaCO_2$. HCO_3^-, Bicarbonate; $PaCO_2$, partial pressure of carbon dioxide in arterial blood.

TABLE 5.10 Causes of Metabolic Acidosis

Increased Non–Carbonic Acids (Elevated Anion Gap)[a]	Bicarbonate Loss or Hyperchloremic Acidosis (Normal Anion Gap)
Increased H+ load	Diarrhea
Ketoacidosis (e.g., diabetes mellitus, starvation)	Ureterosigmoidoscopy (due to bowel segments exposed to urine with chloride absorbed in excess of sodium in the small intestine)
Lactic acidosis (e.g., shock, hypoxemia)	Renal failure (loss of bicarbonate)
Ingestion (e.g., ammonium chloride, ethylene glycol, methanol, salicylates, paraldehyde)	Proximal renal tubular acidosis (loss of more renal sodium in relation to chloride)
Decreased renal H+ excretion	
Uremia	
Distal renal tubule acidosis	

[a]**Anion gap** refers to anions not usually measured in laboratory reports (e.g., sulphate, phosphate, and lactate). The anions usually measured are chloride (Cl−) and bicarbonate (HCO_3^-). When the sum of the concentrations of measured anions (e.g., chloride and bicarbonate) is subtracted from the sum of the concentrations of measured cations (e.g., sodium and potassium), there is a "gap" of approximately 10–12 mmol/L; this is the normal anion gap. An elevated anion gap provides clues to the cause of the acidosis (i.e., to the addition of endogenously or exogenously generated acids). In a normal anion gap acidosis, chloride accumulates to replace lost bicarbonate.

metabolic or respiratory acidosis. The kidneys compensate by decreasing hydrogen excretion and bicarbonate reabsorption.

Respiratory alkalosis stimulates the central and peripheral nervous systems, causing dizziness, confusion, tingling of extremities (paresthesias), convulsions, and coma. Cerebral vasoconstriction (due to reduced CO_2) reduces cerebral blood flow. Carpopedal spasm (spasm of muscles in the fingers and toes), tetany, and other symptoms of hypocalcemia (see Table 5.7) exist as the body strives to maintain electroneutrality by moving calcium into the ICF.

Arterial Blood Gas Analysis

Interpreting arterial blood gases (ABGs) is an essential component to understanding acid–base balance and the compensatory mechanisms involved with restoring (or attempting to restore) acid–base balance. The 6 *Easy Steps to ABG Analysis* is a useful resource for nurses to use for this process.[26] The six steps to ABG analysis are:

1. Is the pH normal?
2. Is the CO_2 normal?
3. Is the HCO_3^- normal?
4. Match the CO_2 or the HCO_3^- with the pH.
5. Does the CO_2 or the HCO_3^- go the opposite direction of the pH?
6. Are the partial pressure of oxygen in arterial blood (PaO_2) and the oxygen (O_2) saturation normal?

First, determine whether the pH is normal (7.35 to 7.45), acidic (less than 7.35), or alkaline (greater than 7.45). Then, look at the CO_2 level (normal is 35 to 45 mmol/L). Less than 35 mmol/L is alkalotic, whereas greater than 45 mmol/L is acidotic. Next, look at the HCO_3^- level (normal is 22 to 26 mmol/L). An HCO_3^- level that is less than 22 mmol/L is acidotic, and a level that is greater than 26 mmol/L is alkalotic. The next step is to match the CO_2 or the HCO_3^- level with the pH to determine the type of disorder—respiratory or metabolic. For example, an acidic CO_2 level of 50 mmol/L with a pH of 7.30 would indicate respiratory acidosis. To determine whether there is compensation, note whether the CO_2 level or the HCO_3^- level is in the opposite direction of the pH. For example, if the HCO_3^- is 27 mmol/L (alkalotic) and the pH is 7.30, that would indicate some compensation by the metabolic system (i.e., the kidneys; see Chapter 29) and other buffering systems in the body. The last step of the process is to look at PaO_2 and O_2 saturation. Low values of each are evidence of hypoxemia (see Chapter 27).

PEDIATRIC CONSIDERATIONS
Distribution of Body Fluids

Newborn Infants
At birth, TBW represents about 75 to 80% of body weight and decreases to about 67% during the first year of life. Physiological loss of body water amounting to 5% of body weight occurs as an infant adjusts to a new environment. Infants are particularly susceptible to significant changes in TBW because of a high metabolic rate and greater body surface area, as compared with adults. Consequently, they have a greater fluid intake and output in relation to their body size. Renal mechanisms of fluid and electrolyte conservation may not be mature enough to counter abnormal losses related to vomiting or diarrhea, thereby allowing dehydration to occur. Symptoms of dehydration include increased thirst, decreased urine output, decreased body weight, decreased skin elasticity, sunken fontanels, absent tears, dry mucous membranes, increased heart rate, and irritability.

Children and Adolescents
TBW slowly decreases to 60 to 65% of body weight. At adolescence, the percentage of TBW approaches adult levels and differences according to gender appear. Males have a greater percentage of body water because of increased muscle mass, and females have more body fat because of the influence of estrogen and thus less water.

GERIATRIC CONSIDERATIONS
Distribution of Body Fluids

The further decline in the percentage of TBW in older persons is in part the result of a decreased free fat mass and decreased muscle mass, as well as a reduced ability to regulate sodium and water balance. Kidneys are less efficient in producing either a concentrated or a diluted urine, and sodium-conserving responses are sluggish. Thirst perception also may decline, and loss of cognitive function can influence access to beverages. Healthy older persons can adequately maintain their hydration status. When disease is present, a decrease in TBW, dehydration, and hypernatremia can become life-threatening.

CASE STUDY

Fluids, Electrolytes, and Acid Base

Case #1

Conrad is a 28-year-old male who presents to the Emergency Department with severe fatigue and dehydration secondary to a four-day history of vomiting. During the interview, he describes attending a family reunion and states that perhaps he "ate something bad." Upon admission, his vital signs are temperature of 39°C, pulse 116, respirations deep and 24/min, and blood pressure 98/60 mm Hg. The nurse also notes the patient has dry mucous membranes and tenting of skin. The physician orders an IV of 0.45% normal saline with an arterial blood gas (ABG), serum electrolytes, blood urea nitrogen (BUN), creatinine, and glucose.

Conrad's lab results are:

ABG	Results
pH	7.46
$PaCO_2$	50 mm Hg
HCO_3^-	35 mmol/L
PaO_2	88 mm Hg (on room air)
Base excess	−3
Sodium (Na^+)	150 mmol/L
Potassium (K^+)	3.4 mmol/L
Chloride (Cl^-)	60 mmol/L
BUN	30 mmol/L
Creatinine	150 μmol/L
Glucose	4 mmol/L

Critical Thinking and Clinical Judgement Questions—Case 1

1. Is Conrad clinically dehydrated? b) How does the nurse know?
2. How would Conrad present differently if he were an infant (less than 1 year old)?
3. a) What is his acid–base imbalance? b) Why?
4. How might he be compensating for this acid–base imbalance?

Case #2

Henry is a 79-year-old man living in a long-term care facility. He has had multiple medical diagnoses, including heart failure (HF), chronic obstructive pulmonary disease (COPD), and a stroke. He is bedridden and receiving enteral tube feedings. He has chronic diarrhea from his tube feedings. He receives digoxin and furosemide (Lasix) to manage his heart failure.

Critical Thinking and Clinical Judgement Questions—Case 2

1. a) Does Henry have an ECF excess or deficit? b) Why?
2. a) What would be his most likely acid–base imbalance? b) Why?
3. Why is he at risk for hypernatremia?
4. Why is he at risk for hypokalemia?
5. Why is he at risk for hypercalcemia?
6. a) What are some other clinical manifestations the nurse would expect to see with each of these imbalances? b) Would the nurse see any edema (localized vs. generalized)?
7. What would the nurse anticipate for treatment of each imbalance?

DID YOU UNDERSTAND?

Distribution of Body Fluids and Electrolytes

1. The sum of all fluids is the total body water (TBW), which varies with age and amount of body fat.
2. Body fluids distribute themselves among functional compartments, classified as intracellular fluid (ICF) and extracellular fluid (ECF).
3. Water moves between ICF and ECF compartments principally by osmosis.
4. Water moves between plasma and interstitial fluid by osmosis (pulling of water) and hydrostatic pressure (pushing of water), which occur across the capillary membrane.
5. Movement across the capillary wall is *net filtration* and is according to Starling forces (the balance between hydrostatic and osmotic forces).

Alterations in Water Movement

1. Edema is a problem of fluid distribution that results in accumulation of fluid within the interstitial spaces.
2. The pathophysiological process that leads to edema involves an increase in forces favouring fluid filtration from the capillaries or lymphatic channels into the tissues (i.e., net transendothelial flow theory).
3. Causes of edema include arterial dilation, venous or lymphatic obstruction, increased vascular volume, loss of plasma proteins, or increased capillary permeability.
4. Edema is localized or generalized and has symptoms of weight gain, swelling and puffiness, tighter-fitting clothes and shoes, and limited movement of the affected area.

Sodium, Chloride, and Water Balance

1. There is an intimate relationship between the balance of sodium and water levels; chloride levels are generally proportional to changes in sodium levels.
2. The sensation of thirst and antidiuretic hormone (ADH) regulate water balance. An increase in plasma osmolality or a decrease in circulating blood volume triggers a release of ADH from the posterior pituitary.
3. Aldosterone regulates sodium balance and increases reabsorption of sodium from the urine into the blood by the distal tubules of the kidney.
4. Renin and angiotensin are hormones that promote secretion of aldosterone and thus, regulate sodium and water balance.
5. Natriuretic peptides decrease tubular reabsorption and promote urinary excretion of sodium.

Alterations in Sodium, Chloride, and Water Balance

1. Alterations in sodium and water balance are isotonic, hypertonic, or hypotonic.
2. Isotonic alterations occur when changes in TBW occur with proportional changes in electrolytes.
3. Hypertonic alterations develop when the osmolality of ECF is elevated above normal, usually because of an increased concentration of ECF sodium or a deficit of ECF water.
4. An acute increase in sodium level or a loss of water causes hypernatremia (sodium levels of more than 145 mmol/L)
5. Hypernatremia can be isovolemic, hypovolemic, or hypervolemic, depending on accompanying changes in the level of body water.

6. Hypovolemia and dehydration are common in hypernatremia with marked water deficit.
7. An excess of sodium or a deficit of plasma bicarbonate causes hyperchloremia.
8. Hypotonic alterations occur when the osmolality of ECF is less than normal.
9. Hyponatremia (serum sodium concentration less than 135 mmol/L) usually causes movement of water into cells.
10. Sodium loss, inadequate sodium intake, or dilution of the body's sodium level with excess water may cause hyponatremia.
11. Hyponatremia can be isovolemic, hypervolemic, hypovolemic, or dilutional, depending on accompanying changes in the amount of body water.
12. Hypochloremia usually is the result of hyponatremia or elevated bicarbonate concentrations.

Alterations in Potassium and Other Electrolytes

1. Potassium is the predominant ICF ion; it regulates ICF osmolality, maintains the resting membrane potential, and is required for deposition of glycogen in liver and skeletal muscle cells.
2. The kidney regulates potassium balance by aldosterone and insulin secretion, and by changes in pH.
3. Potassium adaptation allows the body to accommodate slowly to increased levels of potassium intake.
4. Hypokalemia (serum potassium concentration of less than 3.5 mmol/L) indicates loss of total body potassium, although ECF hypokalemia can develop without losses of total body potassium, and plasma potassium levels may be normal or elevated when there is a depletion of total body potassium.
5. Reduced potassium intake, a shift of potassium from ECF to ICF, increased aldosterone secretion, increased renal excretion, and alkalosis may cause hypokalemia.
6. Increased potassium intake, a shift of potassium from ICF to ECF, or decreased renal excretion can cause hyperkalemia.
7. Calcium is an ion necessary for bone and teeth formation, blood coagulation, hormone secretion and cell receptor function, and membrane stability.
8. Phosphate acts as a buffer in acid–base regulation and provides energy for muscle contraction.
9. The parathyroid hormone (PTH) rigidly controls calcium and phosphate concentrations, vitamin D, and calcitonin.
10. Inadequate intestinal absorption, deposition of calcium into bone or soft tissue, blood administration, or decreased PTH and vitamin D levels can contribute to hypocalcemia (serum calcium concentration less than 2.1 mmol/L).
11. A number of diseases, including hyperparathyroidism, bone metastases, sarcoidosis, and excess vitamin D cause hypercalcemia (serum calcium concentration greater than 2.6 mmol/L).
12. Intestinal malabsorption and increased renal excretion of phosphate are common causes of hypophosphatemia.
13. Hyperphosphatemia develops with acute or chronic renal failure when there is significant loss of glomerular filtration.
14. Magnesium is a major intracellular cation, and the main regulator of magnesium is PTH.
15. Magnesium functions in enzymatic reactions and often interacts with calcium at the cellular level.
16. Malabsorption syndromes can cause hypomagnesemia (serum magnesium concentration less than 0.75 mmol/L).
17. Hypermagnesemia (serum magnesium concentration greater than 1.25 mmol/L) is rare and usually results from renal insufficiency or failure.

Acid–Base Balance

1. Hydrogen ions, which maintain membrane integrity and the speed of enzymatic reactions, are within a narrow range if the body is to function normally.
2. Hydrogen ion concentration, [H^+], expressed as pH, represents the negative logarithm (i.e., 10^{-7}) of hydrogen ions in solution (i.e., 0.000 000 1 mg/L).
3. Different body fluids have different pH values; values less than 7.4 are acidic and values greater than 7.4 are alkaline, or basic.
4. The renal and respiratory systems, together with the body's buffer systems, are the principal regulators of acid–base balance.
5. Buffers are substances that can absorb excessive acid or base without a significant change in pH.
6. Buffers exist as acid–base pairs; the principal plasma buffers are carbonic acid (H_2CO_3), bicarbonate (HCO_3^-), protein (hemoglobin), and phosphate.
7. The lungs and kidneys act to compensate for primary changes in pH by increasing or decreasing ventilation and by producing more acidic or more alkaline urine.
8. Correction is a process different from compensation; correction occurs when the values for both components of the buffer pair return to normal as the primary disorder is treated or resolves.
9. Acid–base imbalances occur with changes in the concentration of hydrogen ions in the blood; an increase causes acidosis, and a decrease causes alkalosis.
10. An abnormal increase or decrease in bicarbonate concentration causes metabolic alkalosis or metabolic acidosis; changes in the rate of alveolar ventilation and removal of carbon dioxide produce respiratory acidosis or respiratory alkalosis.
11. Metabolic acidosis results from an increase in the levels of non–carbonic acids or the loss of bicarbonate from ECF.
12. Metabolic alkalosis occurs with an increase in bicarbonate concentration, often from loss of metabolic acids from conditions such as vomiting or gastro-intestinal suctioning or excessive bicarbonate intake, hyperaldosteronism, and diuretic therapy.
13. Respiratory acidosis occurs with decreased alveolar ventilation, which in turn causes hypercapnia (an increase in carbon dioxide concentration in the blood) and increased carbonic acid concentration.
14. Respiratory alkalosis occurs with alveolar hyperventilation and excessive reduction of carbon dioxide level, or hypocapnia with decreases in carbonic acid concentration.

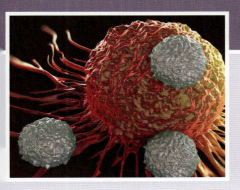

6

Innate Immunity: Inflammation and Wound Healing

Stephanie Zettel, with originating chapter contributions by Valentina L. Brashers and Lois E. Brenneman

Additional resources are available online at http://evolve.elsevier.com/Canada/Huether/pathophysiology

CHAPTER OUTLINE

Human Defence Mechanisms, 134
    First Line of Defence: Physical and Biochemical Barriers and the Human Microbiome, 134
    Second Line of Defence: Inflammation, 137
    Plasma Protein Systems and Inflammation, 138
    Cellular Components of Inflammation, 141

Acute and Chronic Inflammation, 149
    Local Manifestations of Acute Inflammation, 149
    Systemic Manifestations of Acute Inflammation, 149
    Chronic Inflammation, 150

Wound Healing, 151
    Phase I: Inflammation, 152
    Phase II: Proliferation and New Tissue Formation, 152
    Phase III: Remodelling and Maturation, 153
    Dysfunctional Wound Healing, 153

PEDIATRIC CONSIDERATIONS: Age-Related Factors Affecting Innate Immunity in the Newborn Child, 154
GERIATRIC CONSIDERATIONS: Age-Related Factors Affecting Innate Immunity in Older Persons, 154
CASE STUDY, 155

LEARNING OBJECTIVES

1. Identify innate immunity vs. adaptive immunity.
2. Describe the composition, function, and purpose of physical, mechanical, and biochemical barriers.
3. Discuss the importance of normal flora in relation to opportunistic infections.
4. Describe the process of inflammation.
5. Describe the steps of the acute inflammatory response.
6. Identify the three plasma protein systems that mediate the inflammatory response.
7. Discuss what the term *cascade* means.
8. Diagram the complement, clotting, and kinin systems, noting where they converge.
9. Describe two control mechanisms for the protein systems and explain how they provide a check and balance system for inflammation.
10. Discuss each of the cell types (granulocytes, platelets, lymphocytes, natural killer cells, and monocytes) involved in the inflammatory response, and explain their individual roles and relative importance to the process.
11. Discuss how phagocytosis can actually promote the inflammatory process.
12. Compare and contrast the roles of cellular products, particularly cytokines, in the inflammatory process.
13. Describe the process and sequence of phagocytosis.
14. Differentiate between local and systemic responses to acute inflammation based on clinical manifestations.
15. Identify the histological characteristics of chronic inflammation, focusing on the differences between resolution and repair.
16. Describe tissue healing by primary and secondary intention.
17. Describe the different types of dysfunctional wound healing that can occur during the reconstructive phase.

KEY TERMS

Abscess, 149
Acute inflammation, 149
Acute-phase reactant, 149
Adaptive (acquired) immunity, 134
α_1-Antitrypsin, 148
Alternative pathway, 140
Anaphylatoxin, 139
Angiogenesis, 152
Angiogenesis factor, 152
Antimicrobial peptide, 136
Basophil, 144

Blood clot, 140
Bradykinin, 140
C1 esterase inhibitor (C1 INH), 140
C1 INH deficiency, 140
Carboxypeptidase, 140
Cathelicidin, 136
Chemokine, 142
Chemotactic factor, 139
Chemotaxis, 145
Chronic inflammation, 150
Classical pathway, 140

Clotting (coagulation) system, 140
Collagen, 153
Collectin, 136
Common pathway, 140
Complement receptor, 142
Complement system, 139
Contact activation (intrinsic) pathway, 140
Contraction, 151
Contracture of scar tissue, 154
Cyst, 149

Cytokine, 142
Cytokine storm, 142
Damage-associated molecular pattern (DAMP), 141
Defensin, 136
Degranulation, 144
Dehiscence, 153
Dendritic cell, 146
Diapedesis, 146
Endogenous pyrogen, 149
Endothelial cell, 145
Eosinophil, 146

Eosinophil chemotactic factor of anaphylaxis (ECF-A), 145
Epithelialization, 151
Epithelioid cell, 150
Exudate, 149
Fc receptor, 148
Fever, 149
Fibrinolytic system, 140
Fibrinous exudate, 149
Fibroblast, 153
Giant cell, 150
Granulation tissue, 152
Granuloma, 150
Hageman factor (factor XII), 140
Hemorrhagic exudate, 149
Hereditary angioedema, 140
Hexose-monophosphate shunt, 148
Histaminase, 140
Histamine, 144
Hypertrophic scar, 153
Inflammasomes, 142
Inflammation, 137
Inflammatory phase, 152
Inflammatory response, 134
Innate immunity, 134
Interferon (IFN), 144
Interleukin (IL), 143
Interleukin-1 (IL-1), 143
Interleukin-6 (IL-6), 143
Interleukin-10 (IL-10), 144
Keloid, 153
Kinin system, 140
Lectin pathway, 140
Leukocytosis, 149
Leukotriene (slow-reacting substance of anaphylaxis [SRS-A]), 145
Lymphocyte 141
Lysozyme, 136
Macrophage, 146
Mannose-binding lectin (MBL), 136
Margination (pavementing), 146
Mast cell, 144
Matrix metalloproteinase (MMP), 152
Monocyte, 146
Myofibroblast, 153
Natural killer (NK) cell, 148
Neutrophil (polymorphonuclear neutrophil [PMN]), 146
Neutrophil chemotactic factor (NCF), 145
Nitric oxide (NO), 145
NOD-like receptors (NLRs), 142
Normal flora, 136
Normal microbiome, 136
Opportunistic microorganism, 137
Opsonin, 139
Opsonization, 148
Pathogen-associated molecular pattern (PAMP), 141
Pattern recognition receptor (PRR), 141
Phagocyte, 138
Phagocytosis, 146
Phagolysosome, 148
Phagosome, 148
Plasma protein system, 138
Plasmin, 140
Plasminogen, 140
Platelet, 146
Platelet-activating factor (PAF), 145
Primary intention, 151
Proliferation phase, 152
Prostacyclin (PGI_2), 145
Prostaglandin, 145
Purulent (suppurative) exudate, 149
Pyrogen, 149
Regeneration, 151
Repair, 151
Resolution, 151
Scar tissue, 151
Scavenger receptors, 142
Secondary intention, 152
Serous exudate, 149
T lymphocyte (T cell), 146
Tissue factor (extrinsic) pathway, 140
Tissue factor (TF; tissue thromboplastin), 140
Toll-like receptor (TLR), 141
Transforming growth factor, 144
Transforming growth factor-beta (TGF-β), 144
Tumour necrosis factor-alpha (TNF-α), 142
Wound contraction, 153

The human body is continually susceptible to a large variety of conditions that result in damage, such as sunlight, pollutants, agents that can cause physical trauma, and infectious agents (viruses, bacteria, fungi, parasites). Damage can also arise from within cells (cancer is an example). The damage may be at the level of a single cell, which the body can easily repair, or it may be at the level of multiple cells, tissues, or organs, which can result in disease and potentially the death of the individual. To protect us from these conditions, the body has developed a highly sophisticated, multilevel system of interactive defence mechanisms.

HUMAN DEFENCE MECHANISMS

QUICK CHECK 6.1
1. How do physical barriers contribute to defence mechanisms?
2. What are antimicrobial peptides?
3. What two types of defensins contribute to the biochemical barrier?
4. What is the normal microbiome? What is its role in defence?
5. What are opportunistic microorganisms?

The human body has developed several means of protecting itself from injury and infection. **Innate immunity**, also known as natural or native immunity, includes natural barriers (physical and biochemical) and inflammation. Physical and biochemical barriers form the first line of defence at the body's surfaces and are in place at birth to prevent damage by substances in the environment and thwart infection by pathogenic microorganisms. Surface barriers may also harbour a group of microorganisms known as the "normal flora" that can protect us from pathogens. If the injurious agent is able to break through these surface barriers, the second line of defence, the **inflammatory response**, is activated to protect the body from further injury, prevent infection of the injured tissue, and promote healing. The inflammatory response is a rapid activation of biochemical and cellular mechanisms that are relatively nonspecific, with initiation of similar responses, regardless of the type of tissue, against a wide variety of causes of tissue damage. The third line of defence, **adaptive (acquired) immunity** (also known as *specific immunity*), involves a relatively slower and more specific process and targets particular invading microorganisms for eradicating them. Adaptive immunity also involves "memory," which results in a more rapid response during future exposure to the same microorganism. Table 6.1 highlights the differences and compares the above three levels of defence mechanisms. The information presented in this chapter introduces the components and processes of innate immunity and sets the stage for Chapter 7, which presents an overview of adaptive immunity, and Chapter 8, which discusses processes of infection and alterations in immune defences. The *Pediatric* and *Geriatric Considerations* boxes at the end of the chapter explain innate immunity in the newborn and the changes in immunity associated with aging.

First Line of Defence: Physical and Biochemical Barriers and the Human Microbiome
Physical Barriers

The physical barriers that cover the external parts of the human body offer considerable protection from damage and infection. These barriers are composed of tightly associated epithelial cells of the skin and of the linings of the gastrointestinal, genitourinary, and respiratory tracts (Figure 6.1). When pathogens attempt to penetrate this physical barrier, mechanical processes in the body (such as coughing or sneezing, vomiting from the stomach, or flushing from the urinary tract by urine) remove them, along with dead epithelial (skin) cells, which continually replenish themselves. Epithelial cells of the upper respiratory tract also produce mucus and have hair-like cilia that trap and move pathogens upward. Coughing and

TABLE 6.1 Overview of Human Defences

Characteristics	Barriers	Innate Immunity	Adaptive (Acquired) Immunity
Level of defence	First line of defence against infection and tissue injury	Second line of defence; occurs as response to tissue injury or infection (inflammatory response)	Third line of defence; initiated when innate immune system signals cells of adaptive immunity
Timing of defence	Constant	Immediate response	Delay between primary exposure to antigen and maximal response; immediate against secondary exposure to antigen
Specificity	Broadly specific	Broadly specific	Response is very specific toward "antigen"
Cells	Epithelial cells Microbiome	Mast cells, granulocytes (neutrophils, eosinophils, basophils), monocytes/macrophages, natural killer (NK) cells, platelets, endothelial cells	T cells, B cells, macrophages, dendritic cells
Memory	No memory involved	No memory involved	Specific immunological memory by T and B cells
Active molecules	Defensins, cathelicidins, collectins, lactoferrin, bacterial toxins	Complement, clotting factors, kinins, cytokines	Antibodies, complement, cytokines
Protection	Protection includes anatomical barriers (i.e., skin and mucous membranes), cells and secretory molecules (e.g., lysozymes, low pH of stomach and urine), and ciliary activity	Protection includes vascular responses, cellular components (e.g., mast cells, neutrophils, macrophages), secretory molecules or cytokines, and activation of plasma protein systems	Protection includes activated T and B cells, cytokines, and antibodies

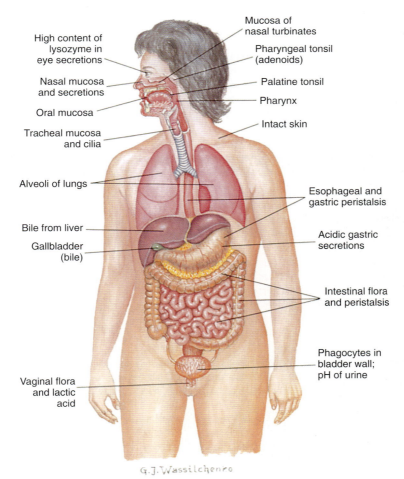

FIGURE 6.1 The Closed Barrier. The digestive, respiratory, and genitourinary tracts and skin form closed barriers between the internal organs and the environment. (From Grimes, D. E. [1991]. *Infectious diseases.* Mosby.)

sneezing then expel these pathogens. Additionally, the low temperature (such as on the skin) and the low pH (such as of the skin and stomach) generally inhibit microorganisms, most of which routinely require temperatures near 37°C (98.6°F) and pH near neutral for efficient growth.

Epithelial Cell–Derived Chemicals

Epithelial cells secrete an array of substances that protect against infection, including mucus, perspiration (or sweat), saliva, tears, and earwax. These can trap potential invaders and contain substances that will kill microorganisms. Perspiration, tears, and saliva contain an enzyme (lysozyme) that attacks the cell walls of Gram-positive bacteria. Sebaceous glands in the skin also secrete fatty acids and lactic acid that kill bacteria and fungi. These glandular secretions create an acidic (pH 3 to 5) and inhospitable environment for most bacteria.

Epithelial cell secretions also contain small-molecular-weight antimicrobial peptides that kill or inhibit the growth of disease-causing bacteria, fungi, and viruses.[1]

The cathelicidins are examples of such peptides, and only one of them is known to function in humans. Bacteria have cholesterol-free cell membranes into which cathelicidin can insert and disrupt the membrane, killing the bacteria. Epithelial cells of the skin, gut, urinary tract, and respiratory tract produce cathelicidin. Neutrophils, mast cells, and monocytes then store cathelicidin and release it during inflammation.

Human defensins are also examples of antimicrobial peptides. Defensin molecules exist as two different subtypes (alpha and beta), where the α-defensins often require activation by proteolytic enzymes, and the β-defensins require no enzymatic activation. The α-defensins work with neutrophils in killing bacteria. Paneth cells lining the small intestine also contain α-defensins, where they protect against a variety of disease-causing microorganisms. Epithelial cells lining the respiratory, urinary, and intestinal tracts, as well as in the skin, are rich in β-defensins. β-defensins may also help protect epithelial surfaces from infection with adenovirus (one of the causes of the common cold) and human immunodeficiency virus (HIV). Both classes of antimicrobial peptides can also activate cells of the next levels of defence: innate and acquired immunity.

The lung also produces and secretes a family of glycoproteins, collectins, which includes surfactant proteins A through D and mannose-binding lectin. Collectins react with carbohydrates on the surface of a wide array of pathogenic microorganisms and help macrophages (cells of the innate immune system) to recognize and kill the microorganism. Mannose-binding lectin (MBL) recognizes a sugar commonly found on the surface of microbes and is a powerful activator of a plasma protein system (complement), resulting in damage to bacteria or increased recognition by macrophages.

The Normal Microbiome

An array of microorganisms colonizes the body's surfaces and makes up the normal microbiome (previously known as normal flora) of the organism. Each colonizing combination of bacteria and fungi is unique to the particular location (i.e., skin and mucous membranes of the eyes, upper and lower gastro-intestinal [GI] tracts, upper respiratory tract, urethra, vagina) and individual[2] (Table 6.2). The microorganisms in the microbiome do not normally cause disease, and although their relationship with humans is *commensal* (to the benefit of one organism without affecting the other), the relationship may be more *mutualistic* (to the benefit of both organisms). For example, the lower gut is relatively sterile at birth but colonization with bacteria begins quickly, with the number, diversity, and concentration increasing progressively during the first year of life.

The normal microbiome benefits us in many ways; bacteria in the GI tract produce (1) enzymes that facilitate the digestion and utilization of many molecules in the human diet, such as fatty acids and large polysaccharides; (2) usable metabolites (e.g., vitamin K, B vitamins); and (3) antibacterial factors that prevent colonization by pathogenic microorganisms (see Chapter 8). For example, members of the normal microbiome in the colon produce chemicals (ammonia, phenols, indoles, and other toxic materials) and proteins *(bacteriocins)* that are toxic to more pathogenic microorganisms. They also compete with

TABLE 6.2 The Human Microbiome

Location	Microorganisms
Skin	Predominantly Gram-positive cocci and rods; *Staphylococcus epidermidis*, corynebacteria, mycobacteria, and streptococci are primary inhabitants; *Staphylococcus aureus* in some people; also yeasts (*Candida*, *Pityrosporum*) in some areas of skin
	Numerous transient microorganisms may become temporary residents
	In moist areas, Gram-negative bacteria
	Around sebaceous glands, *Propionibacterium* and *Brevibacterium*
	Mite *Demodex folliculorum* lives in hair follicles and sebaceous glands around face
Nose	Predominantly Gram-positive cocci and rods, especially *S. epidermidis*
	Some people are nasal carriers of pathogenic bacteria, including *S. aureus*, β-hemolytic streptococci, and *Corynebacterium diphtheria*
Mouth	Complex of bacteria that includes several species of streptococci, *Actinomyces*, lactobacilli, and *Haemophilus*
	Anaerobic bacteria and spirochetes colonize gingival crevices
Pharynx	Similar to flora in mouth plus staphylococci, *Neisseria*, and diphtheroids
	Some asymptomatic persons also harbour pathogens: pneumococcus, *Haemophilus influenzae*, *Neisseria meningitidis*, and *C. diphtheria*
Distal small intestine	Enterobacteria, streptococci, lactobacilli, anaerobic bacteria, and *C. albicans*
Colon	Bacteroides, lactobacilli, clostridia, *Salmonella*, *Shigella*, *Klebsiella*, *Proteus*, *Pseudomonas*, enterococci, and other streptococci, bacilli, and *Escherichia coli*
Distal urethra	Typical bacteria found on skin, especially *S. epidermidis* and diphtheroids; also lactobacilli and nonpathogenic streptococci
Vagina	Birth to 1 month: similar to adult
	1 month to puberty: *S. epidermidis*, diphtheroids, *E. coli*, and streptococci
	Puberty to menopause: *Lactobacillus acidophilus*, diphtheroids, staphylococci, streptococci, and variety of anaerobes
	Postmenopause: similar to prepubescence

Adapted from Bennett, J. E., Dolin, R., & Blaser, M. J. (Eds.). (2015). *Mandell, Douglas, and Bennett's principles and practice of infectious diseases* (8th ed.). Saunders.

pathogens for nutrients and block their attachment to the epithelium, which is an obligatory first step in the infectious process by most pathogens. Additionally, the normal microbiome of the gut helps train the adaptive immune system by inducing growth of gut-associated lymphoid tissue (where most cells of the adaptive immune system reside) and the development of both local and systemic adaptive immunity. GI bacteria also influence ongoing communication between the brain and GI tract *(brain–gut axis)* and play an important role in modulating cognitive function, behaviour, pain modulation, and stress responses.[3]

Prolonged treatment with broad-spectrum antibiotics can alter the normal microbiome, decreasing its protective activity, and lead to an overgrowth of pathogenic microorganisms. In the intestine, overgrowth of the yeast *Candida albicans* or the bacteria *Clostridium difficile* (a cause of pseudomembranous colitis, an infection of the colon) may occur. The bacterium *Lactobacillus* is also a major constituent of the normal GI and vaginal microbiome in healthy women[4] and produces a variety of chemicals (e.g., hydrogen peroxide, lactic acid, bacteriocins) that help prevent infections of the vagina and urinary tract by other bacteria and yeast. Prolonged antibiotic treatment can diminish colonization with *Lactobacillus* and increase the risk for urological or vaginal infections, such as vaginosis.

The physical integrity of the skin and mucosal epithelium, as well as other mechanisms that protect the microbiome from the immune and inflammatory systems (as described above) maintain its mutualistic relationship with the microbiome. Some members of the normal bacterial microbiome are opportunistic; **opportunistic microorganisms** can cause disease if there is a break in the individual's defences. The innate and adaptive immune systems normally control these microorganisms, and they can also contribute to our defences. For example, *Pseudomonas aeruginosa* is a member of the normal microbiome of the skin and produces a toxin that protects against infections with staphylococcal and other bacteria. However, severe burns compromise the integrity of the skin and may lead to life-threatening systemic infections with *Pseudomonas*.

Second Line of Defence: Inflammation

> ✓ **QUICK CHECK 6.2**
> 1. Why are innate immunity and inflammation described as "nonspecific"?
> 2. Describe how the five cardinal signs of inflammation are related to the process of inflammation.
> 3. Describe the basic steps in acute inflammation.
> 4. What are the benefits of inflammation?

Whereas the physical and biochemical barriers of the innate immune system are relatively static, **inflammation** is a systematic process that responds to cellular or tissue damage, whether the damaged tissue is septic or sterile. The response is a rapid initiation of an interactive system of humoral (or soluble in the blood) and cellular systems designed to limit the extent of tissue damage, destroy contaminating infectious microorganisms, initiate the adaptive immune response, and begin the healing process.

The inflammatory response has four particular characteristics: (1) it occurs in tissues with a blood supply (vascularized); (2) it is activated *rapidly* (within seconds) after damage occurs; (3) it depends on the activity of both *cellular and chemical components*; and (4) it is *nonspecific*, meaning that it takes place in approximately the same way, regardless of the type of stimulus or whether exposure to the same stimulus has occurred in the past.

Virtually any injury to vascularized tissues can activate the inflammatory response. This includes infection or tissue necrosis (e.g., ischemia, trauma, physical or chemical injury, foreign bodies, immune reactions).

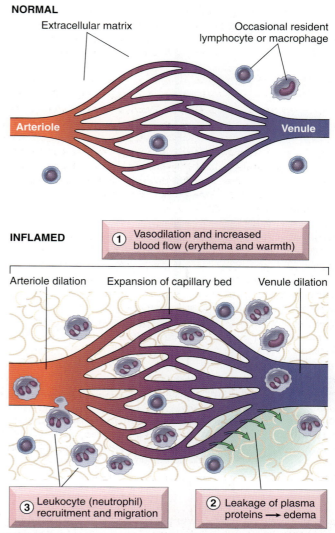

FIGURE 6.2 The Major Local Changes in the Process of Inflammation. Compared with normal circulation, inflammation is characterized by (1) dilation of the blood vessels and increased blood flow, leading to erythema and warmth; (2) increased vascular permeability with leakage of plasma from the vessels, leading to edema; and (3) movement of leukocytes from the vessels into the site of injury. (From Kumar, V., Abbas, A. K., Aster, J. C., et al. [Eds.]. [2010]. *Robbins and Cotran pathologic basis of disease* [8th ed.]. Saunders.)

In the first century, a Roman named Celsus described the classic or cardinal signs of acute inflammation as rubor (redness), calor (heat), tumour (swelling), and dolor (pain). *Functio laesa* (loss of function) is also a cardinal sign. Microscopic inflammatory changes occur within seconds in the microcirculation (arterioles, capillaries, and venules) near the site of an injury and include the following processes (Figure 6.2):

1. *Vasodilation* (increased size of the blood vessels), which causes slower blood velocity and increases blood flow to the injured site
2. *Increased vascular permeability* (the blood vessels become porous from contraction of endothelial cells) and leakage of fluid out of the vessel (exudation), causes swelling (edema) at the site of injury; as plasma moves outward, blood in the microcirculation becomes more viscous and flows more slowly, and the increased blood flow and increasing concentration of red blood cells at the site of inflammation cause locally increased redness (erythema) and warmth

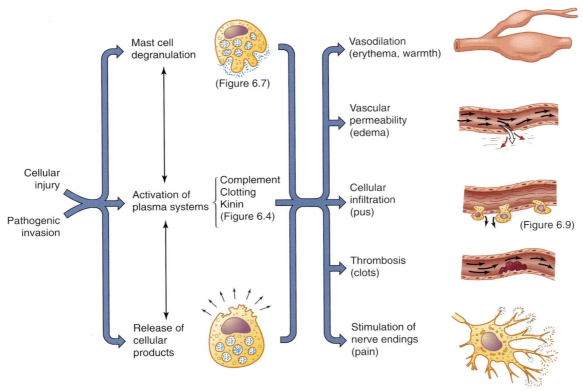

FIGURE 6.3 Acute Inflammatory Response. Inflammation is usually initiated by cellular injury and may be complicated by infection. Mast cell degranulation, the activation of three plasma systems, and the release of subcellular components from the damaged cells occur as a consequence. These systems are interdependent, so that induction of one (e.g., mast cell degranulation) can result in the induction of the other two. The result is the development of the characteristic microscopic and clinical hallmarks of inflammation. The figure numbers refer to additional figures in which more detailed information may be found on that portion of the response.

3. *White blood cell adherence* to the inner walls of vessels and their migration through enlarged junctions between the endothelial cells lining the vessels into the surrounding tissue

Each of the characteristic changes associated with inflammation is the direct result of the activation and interactions of a host of chemicals and cellular components found in the blood and tissues. The vascular changes deliver leukocytes (particularly neutrophils), plasma proteins, and other biochemical mediators to the site of injury, where they act in concert. Some of these chemical mediators activate pain fibres. The tissue injury, pain, and swelling contribute to loss of function. Figure 6.3 summarizes the process of acute inflammation. The lymphatic vessels drain the extravascular fluid to the lymph nodes and may also become secondarily inflamed: lymphangitis of the lymph vessels and lymphadenitis of the nodes, which become hyperplastic, enlarged, and frequently painful.

There are several benefits of inflammation, including:
- It prevents infection and further damage by invading microorganisms. The inflammatory exudate dilutes toxins produced by bacteria and released from dying cells. The activation of plasma protein systems (e.g., complement and clotting systems) helps contain and destroy bacteria. The influx of **phagocytes** (e.g., neutrophils, macrophages) destroys cellular debris and microorganisms.
- It limits and controls the inflammatory process. The influx of plasma protein systems (e.g., clotting system), plasma enzymes, and cells (e.g., eosinophils) prevents the inflammatory response from spreading to areas of healthy tissue.
- It interacts with components of the adaptive immune system to elicit a more specific response to contaminating pathogen(s) through the influx of macrophages and lymphocytes that destroy pathogens.
- It prepares the area of injury for healing and repair through removal of bacterial products, dead cells, and other products of inflammation (e.g., by way of channels through the epithelium or drainage by lymphatic vessels).

Fluid and debris that accumulate at an inflamed site are drained by lymphatic vessels. This process also facilitates the development of acquired immunity because microbial antigens in lymphatic fluid pass through the lymph nodes, where they encounter lymphocytes.

Plasma Protein Systems and Inflammation

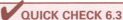 **QUICK CHECK 6.3**
1. What are the three most important products of the complement system?
2. How is the coagulation cascade activated? How is it related to the plasma kinin cascade?
3. What factors control the plasma protein systems of inflammation?

Three key **plasma protein systems** are essential to an effective inflammatory response: (1) the complement system, (2) the clotting system, and the (3) kinin system (Figure 6.4). Although each system has a unique role in inflammation, they have many similarities. Each

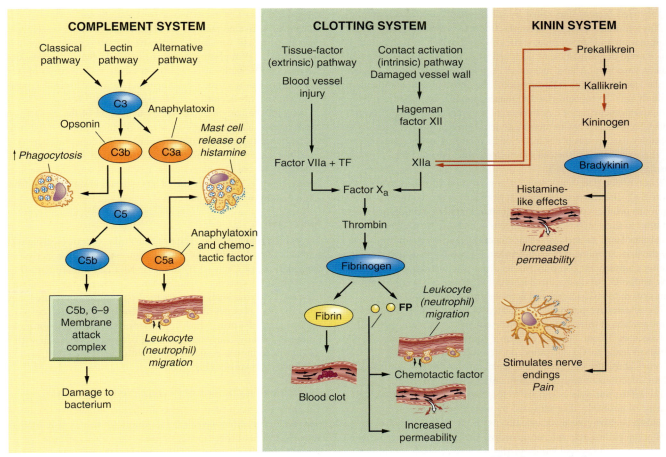

FIGURE 6.4 Plasma Protein Systems in Inflammation: Complement, Clotting, and Kinin Systems. Each plasma protein system consists of a family of proteins that are activated in sequence to create potent biological effects. The complement system can be activated by three mechanisms, each of which results in proteolytic activation of C3. The fragments of C3 activation, C3a and C3b, are major components of inflammation. C3a is a potent anaphylatoxin, which induces degranulation of mast cells. C3b can bind to the surface of cells, such as bacteria, and either serve as an opsonin for phagocytosis or proteolytically activate the next component of the complement cascade, C5. The smaller fragment of C5 activation is C5a, a powerful anaphylatoxin, and is also chemotactic for neutrophils, attracting them to the site of inflammation. The larger fragment, C5b, activates the components of the membrane attack complex (C5–C9), which damage the bacterial membrane and kill the bacteria. The clotting system can be activated by the tissue factor (extrinsic) pathway and the contact activation (intrinsic) pathway. All routes of clotting initiation lead to activation of factor X and thrombin. Thrombin is an enzyme that proteolytically activates fibrinogen to form fibrin and small fibrinopeptides (FPs). Fibrin polymerizes to form a clot, and the FPs are highly active as chemotactic factors and cause increased vascular permeability. The XIIa produced by the clotting system can also be activated by kallikrein of the kinin system *(red arrow)*. Prekallikrein is enzymatically converted to kininogen, which activates bradykinin. Bradykinin functions similarly to histamine and increases vascular permeability. Bradykinin can also stimulate nerve endings to cause pain. *FP,* Fibrinopeptide; *TF,* Tissue factor.

system consists of multiple proteins found in the blood, usually in inactive forms; several of these proteins are enzymes that circulate as proenzymes. Furthermore, each system contains a few proteins that can be activated early in inflammation. Activation of the first components results in sequential activation of other components of the system, leading to a biological function that helps protect the individual. This sequential activation or *cascade* of activations and the plasma protein systems are the complement cascade, the clotting cascade, or the kinin cascade. In some cases, activation of a particular protein in the system may require that it be enzymatically cut into two pieces of different size. Usually, the larger fragment continues the cascade by activating the next component, and the smaller fragment frequently has potent proinflammatory activities.

Complement System

The **complement system** consists of a large number of proteins (sometimes called *complement factors*) that together constitute about 10% of the total circulating serum protein. Activation of the complement system produces several factors that can destroy pathogens directly or can activate or increase the activity of many other components of the inflammatory and adaptive immune response. Factors produced during activation of the complement system are among the body's most potent defenders, particularly against bacterial infection.

The most important function of the complement cascade is activation of C3 and C5, which results in a variety of molecules that are (1) opsonins, (2) chemotactic factors, or (3) anaphylatoxins.[5] **Opsonins** coat the surface of bacteria and increase their susceptibility to being phagocytized (eaten) and killed by inflammatory cells, such as neutrophils and macrophages. **Chemotactic factors** diffuse from a site of inflammation and attract phagocytic cells to that site. **Anaphylatoxins** induce rapid degranulation of mast cells (i.e., release of histamine that induces vasodilation and increased capillary permeability), a major cellular component of inflammation. The most potent complement products are C3b (opsonin), C3a (anaphylatoxin), and C5a (anaphylatoxin, chemotactic factor). Activation of terminal complement components C5b through C9 (membrane attack complex, or MAC) results in a complex that creates pores in the outer membranes of cells or bacteria. The pores disrupt the cell's membrane and permit water to enter, causing the death of the cell.

Three major pathways control the activation of complement (see Figure 6.4). The **classical pathway** is primarily activated by *antibodies*, which are proteins of the acquired immune system. Antibodies must first bind to their targets, called *antigens*, which can be proteins or carbohydrates from bacteria or other infectious agents. Antibodies activate the first component of complement, C1, which leads to activation of other complement components, leading to activation of C3 and C5. Thus, antibodies of the acquired immune response can use the complement system to kill bacteria and activate inflammation.

The **alternative pathway** is activated by several substances found on the surface of infectious organisms such as bacteria and yeast. This pathway uses unique proteins to form a complex that activates C3. C3 activation leads to C5 activation and convergence with the classical pathway. Thus, the complement system can be directly activated by certain infectious organisms without antibody being present.

The **lectin pathway** is similar to the classical pathway but is independent of antibody. It is activated by several plasma proteins. These proteins recognize carbohydrate patterns found on the surface of a large number of pathogenic microorganisms, including bacteria, viruses, protozoa, and fungi, and binds to these polysaccharides. Binding of these polysaccharides then activates complement.[6] Thus, infectious agents that may not be able to activate the complement system directly by means of the alternative pathway are still susceptible to complement because of how certain plasma proteins bind to the carbohydrate patterns on their surfaces in the lectin pathway.

In summary, the complement cascade can be activated by at least three different means, and its products have four functions: (1) opsonization (C3b); (2) anaphylatoxic activity resulting in mast cell degranulation (C3a, C5a); (3) leukocyte chemotaxis (C5a); and (4) cell lysis (C5b–C9 [MAC]).

Clotting System

The **clotting (coagulation) system** is a group of plasma proteins that, when activated sequentially, form a blood clot. A **blood clot** is a meshwork of protein (fibrin) strands that contains platelets (the primary cellular initiator of clotting) and traps other cells, such as erythrocytes, phagocytes, and microorganisms. Clots have three basic functions: (1) they plug damaged vessels and stop bleeding, (2) they trap microorganisms and prevent their spread to adjacent tissues, and (3) they provide a framework for future repair and healing. Specific details and illustrations of the clotting system are presented in Chapter 20 (see also Figure 20.18), and only the relationship between clotting and inflammation is presented here.

The clotting system can be activated by many substances that are released during tissue injury and infection, including collagen, proteinases, kallikrein, and plasmin, as well as by bacterial products such as endotoxins. Like the complement cascade, different pathways that converge can activate the coagulation cascade and result in the formation of a clot (see Figure 6.4). **Tissue factor (TF)** (also called **tissue thromboplastin**) is released by damaged endothelial cells in blood vessels and activates the **extrinsic** (or **tissue factor**) **pathway**. TF then reacts with activated factor VII (VIIa). Damage to the vessel wall activates the **intrinsic** (or **contact activation**) **pathway** and **Hageman factor (factor XII)** in plasma contacts negatively charged subendothelial substances. The pathways converge at factor X. Activation of factor X begins a **common pathway** leading to activation of fibrin that polymerizes to form a fibrin clot.

As with the complement system, activation of the clotting system produces protein fragments known as fibrinopeptides (FPs) A and B that enhance the inflammatory response. Fibrinopeptides are released from fibrinogen when fibrin is produced. Both FPs (especially fibrinopeptide B) are chemotactic for neutrophils and increase vascular permeability by enhancing the effects of bradykinin (formed from the kinin system) on endothelial cells.

Kinin System

The third plasma protein system, the **kinin system** (see Figure 6.4), interacts closely with the coagulation system. The activation of Hageman factor (factor XII) to factor XIIa can initiate both the clotting and kinin systems. *Prekallikrein* is another name for factor XIIa because it enzymatically activates the first component of the kinin system. The final product of the kinin system is a small-molecular-weight molecule, **bradykinin**, which comes from a larger precursor molecule, kininogen. Bradykinin causes dilation of blood vessels, acts with prostaglandins to induce pain, causes smooth muscle cell contraction, and increases vascular permeability.

Control and Interaction of Plasma Protein Systems

The three plasma protein systems are highly interactive. Activation of one results in production of a large number of very potent, biologically active substances that further activate the other systems. Very tight regulation of these processes is essential for the following two reasons:

1. The inflammatory process is critical for an individual's survival, and efficient activation must be guaranteed, regardless of the cause of tissue injury. Furthermore, interaction among the plasma systems may result in activation of the entire inflammatory response, regardless of which system is activated initially.
2. The biochemical mediators generated during these processes are potent and potentially detrimental to the individual, and their action is limited to only injured or infected tissues.

Multiple mechanisms are available to either activate or inactivate (regulate) these plasma protein systems. For example, the plasma that enters the tissues during inflammation (edema) contains enzymes that destroy mediators of inflammation (e.g., **carboxypeptidase** inactivates C3a and C5a, kininases degrade kinins, and **histaminase** degrades histamine and kallikrein).

The formation of clots concurrently activates a **fibrinolytic system** which limits the size of the clot and removes the clot after bleeding has stopped. *Thrombin* of the clotting system activates **plasminogen** in the blood to form the enzyme **plasmin** which then degrades fibrin. However, plasmin can also activate both the complement cascade (through components C1, C3, and C5) and the kinin cascade (by activating factor XII and producing prekallikrein activator).

Other regulators of the inflammatory process include **C1 esterase inhibitor (C1 INH)** which inhibits complement activation, as well as clotting and kinin pathway components such as kallikrein and factor XIIa. Interestingly, a genetic defect in C1 INH (**C1 INH deficiency**) results in **hereditary angioedema**, which is a self-limiting edema of cutaneous and mucosal layers resulting from stress, illness, or a relatively minor or unapparent trauma. Characteristics of the disease include signs and symptoms from hyperactivation of all three plasma protein systems.

Many cells also have factors linked to the external surface of their cell membrane that protect them from inadvertent complement damage by preventing activation of C3 and inhibiting the MAC.

Cellular Components of Inflammation

> ✓ **QUICK CHECK 6.4**
> 1. What are pattern recognition receptors?
> 2. What are cytokines? How do cytokines promote inflammation?
> 3. What products do the mast cells release during inflammation, and what are their effects?
> 4. What two phagocytic cell types are involved in the acute inflammatory response? What is the role of each?
> 5. What are the five steps in the process of phagocytosis?

Inflammation is a process in vascular tissue, and the cellular components can be found in the blood or in tissue surrounding the blood vessels. The blood vessels are lined with endothelial cells, which actively maintain blood flow under normal conditions. During inflammation, the vascular endothelium becomes a principal coordinator of blood clotting and the passage of cells and fluid into the tissue. The tissues close to the vessels contain two types of cells involved with the inflammatory response: (1) mast cells, which are among the most important activators of inflammation, and (2) dendritic cells, which connect the innate and acquired immune responses. The blood contains a complex mixture of cells (Figure 6.5 and see also Chapter 20). Blood cells are erythrocytes (red blood cells), platelets, and leukocytes (white blood cells). Erythrocytes carry oxygen to the tissues, and platelets are small cell fragments involved in blood clotting. Leukocytes are granulocytes (containing many enzyme-filled cytoplasmic granules), monocytes, and lymphocytes. Granulocytes are the most common leukocytes and differ from each other according to the staining of their granules (e.g., basophils, eosinophils, and neutrophils). Monocytes are precursors of macrophages that are found in the tissue. Various forms of **lymphocytes** participate in the innate immune response (e.g., natural killer [NK] cells) and the acquired immune response (B and T cells).

Cells of both innate and acquired immune systems respond to molecules produced at a site of cellular damage that recruit these cells to that site to augment the protective response. These chemotactic molecules originate from destroyed or damaged cells, contaminating microbes, activation of the plasma protein systems, or secretions by other cells of the innate or acquired immune systems. Each cell has a set of cell surface receptors that specifically bind these molecules, resulting in activation of intracellular signalling pathways and activation of the cell itself. Activation may result in the cell gaining a function critical to the inflammatory response or the induction of the release of additional cellular products that increase inflammation, or both. Most of these inflammatory cells and protein systems, along with the substances they produce, act at the site of tissue injury to (1) confine the extent of damage; (2) kill microorganisms; (3) remove the cellular debris; and (4) activate healing, tissue regeneration (a process known as *resolution*), or repair.

Cellular Receptors

As will be discussed in Chapter 7, B and T lymphocytes of the adaptive immune system have evolved surface receptors (i.e., the T-cell antigen receptor, or TCR, and the B-cell antigen receptor, or BCR) that bind a large spectrum of antigens. Cells involved in innate immune responses have evolved a different set of receptors that recognize a much more limited array of specific molecules (or ligands). These receptors are

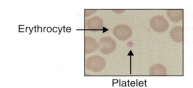
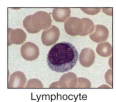
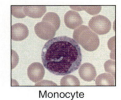
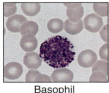
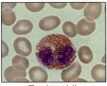
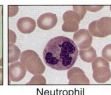

FIGURE 6.5 Cellular Components of the Blood. Cells in the blood are red blood cells (erythrocytes), cellular fragments (platelets), or white blood cells (leukocytes). Leukocytes consist of lymphocytes, monocytes, and granulocytes (neutrophils, eosinophils, basophils). (Erythrocyte plate from Goldman, L., & Schafer, A. I. [Eds.]. [2012]. *Goldman's Cecil medicine* [24th ed.]. Saunders; rest of plates from McPherson, R. A. [Ed.]. [2012]. *Henry's clinical diagnosis and management by laboratory methods* [22nd ed.]. Saunders.)

referred to as **pattern recognition receptors (PRRs)**. PRRs recognize two types of molecular *patterns*: (1) molecules that are expressed by infectious agents, either found on their surface or released as soluble molecules (**pathogen-associated molecular patterns**, or **PAMPs**); or (2) products of cellular damage (**damage-associated molecular patterns**, or **DAMPs**). This enables cells of the innate immune system to respond to both sterile (through DAMPs) and septic (through PAMPs and DAMPs) tissue damage. There are at least 100 different PRRs that, in turn, recognize more than 1 000 different molecules.

PRRs are generally present on cells in tissues near the body's surface (i.e., skin, respiratory tract, GI tract, genitourinary tract) where they monitor the environment for products of cellular damage and potentially infectious microorganisms. Classes of cellular PRRs primarily differ in the specificity of ligands they bind. PRRs can exist as cell surface receptors that bind extracellular ligands, in endosomes in contact with ingested microbes and other materials, in the cytosol where they bind intracellular materials resulting from cellular damage, or as secretions into the extracellular environment. MBL of the lectin pathway of complement activation is an example of a secreted PRR.

Toll-like receptors (TLRs) primarily recognize a large variety of PAMPs located on the microorganism's cell wall or surface (e.g., bacterial lipopolysaccharide [LPS], peptidoglycans, lipoproteins, yeast zymosan, viral coat proteins), other surface structures (e.g., bacterial flagellin), or microbial nucleic acid (e.g., bacterial DNA, viral double-stranded RNA).[7] There are currently 11 known TLRs in humans (Table 6.3). They present on the surface of many cells that have direct and early contact with potential pathogenic microorganisms, including mucosal epithelial cells, mast cells, neutrophils, macrophages, dendritic cells, and some subpopulations of lymphocytes. Similarly, TLRs

TABLE 6.3 Cellular Source and Microbial Target for Each Toll-Like Receptor

Receptor	Cellular Expression Pattern	PAMP Recognition
TLR1	Cell surface (ubiquitous): neutrophils, monocytes/macrophages, dendritic cells, T cells, B cells, natural killer (NK) cells	Fungal, bacterial, viral; forms heterodimer with TLR2 (see TLR2 recognition)
TLR2	Cell surface: neutrophils, monocytes/macrophages, dendritic cells	Fungal (yeast zymosan), bacterial (Gram-positive bacterial peptidoglycan, lipoproteins), viral (lipoproteins)
TLR3	Intracellular: monocytes/macrophages, dendritic cells, T cells, NK cells, epithelial cells	Double-stranded RNA produced by many viruses
TLR4	Cell surface: granulocytes, monocytes/macrophages, dendritic cells, T cells, B cells, epithelial cells	Bacterial (primarily Gram-negative bacterial LPS, lipoteichoic acids), viral (RSV F protein, hepatitis C)
TLR5	Cell surface: granulocytes, monocytes/macrophages, dendritic cells, NK cells, epithelial cells	Bacterial (flagellin); forms heterodimer with TLR4
TLR6	Cell surface: monocytes/macrophages, dendritic cells, B cells, NK cells	Fungal, bacterial, viral; forms heterodimer with TLR2 (see TLR2 recognition)
TLR7	Intracellular: monocytes/macrophages, dendritic cells, B cells	Natural ligand uncertain; may bind viral single-strand RNA
TLR8	Cell surface: monocytes/macrophages, dendritic cells, NK cells	Natural ligand uncertain; may bind fungal PAMPs or viral single-stranded RNA
TLR9	Intracellular: monocytes/macrophages, dendritic cells, B cells	Bacterial (unmethylated DNA [CpG dinucleotides])
TLR10	Cell surface: monocytes/macrophages, dendritic cells, B cells	Natural ligand uncertain; may form heterodimers with TLR2
TLR11	TLR11 gene does not code a full-length protein in humans	No known immune response

LPS, Lipopolysaccharide; *PAMP*, pathogen-associated molecular pattern; *RSV*, respiratory syncytial virus; *TLR*, toll-like receptor.

associate with pathways that produce two groups of transcription factors: (1) *NF-κB*, which controls synthesis and release of cytokines; and (2) *interferon regulatory factors* (*IRFs*), which control the production of antiviral type I interferons.[8]

Complement receptors are found on many cells of the innate and acquired immune responses (e.g., granulocytes, monocytes/macrophages, lymphocytes, mast cells, erythrocytes, platelets), as well as some epithelial cells. They recognize several fragments produced through activation of the complement system, particularly C3a, C5a, and C3b.

Scavenger receptors exist primarily on macrophages and facilitate recognition and phagocytosis of bacterial pathogens, as well as damaged cells and altered soluble lipoproteins associated with vascular damage (e.g., high-density lipoprotein [HDL], acetylated low-density lipoprotein [LDL], oxidized LDL).[9] Some scavenger receptors (e.g., SR-PSOX) recognize the cell membrane phospholipid phosphatidylserine (PS). Erythrocyte senescence and cellular apoptosis result in the externalization of this component of the cell membrane. As such, macrophages, through this receptor, can identify and remove old red blood cells and cells undergoing apoptosis.

NOD-like receptors (NLRs) are cytoplasmic receptors that recognize products of microbes and damaged cells. At least 22 NLRs exist in humans. NOD-1 and NOD-2 recognize fragments of peptidoglycans from intracellular bacteria and initiate production of proinflammatory mediators, such as tumour necrosis factor (TNF) and interleukin-6 (IL-6).[10] Other NLRs associate with intracellular multiprotein complexes called **inflammasomes**. Inflammasomes primarily bind cellular stress-related molecules, a type of DAMP, and control the production of the inflammatory cytokines interleukin-1β (IL-1β) and IL-18.[11]

Cellular Products

Intercellular communication and cooperation are necessary for an effective inflammatory (or adaptive immune) response. **Cytokines** constitute a large family of small-molecular-weight soluble intercellular-signalling molecules that come from cells, bind to specific cell membrane receptors, and regulate innate or adaptive immunity (Figure 6.6). Cytokines may be either *proinflammatory* or *anti-inflammatory* in nature, depending on whether they tend to induce or inhibit the inflammatory response. These molecules usually diffuse over short distances, but some effects occur over long distances, such as the systemic induction of fever by some inflammatory cytokines (i.e., endogenous pyrogens). Binding of cytokines to a target cell often induces synthesis of additional cellular products. For example, binding of the cytokine **tumour necrosis factor-alpha (TNF-α)** to a cell may result in synthesis and release of interleukin-1.

The novel COVID-19 coronavirus can actually produce a *cytokine storm syndrome* similar to that seen in sepsis in some individuals. A **cytokine storm** is an activation cascade of cytokine production that amplifies itself due to an unregulated host immune response to different triggers such as infections, malignancy, and other disorders. A cytokine storm is essentially a severe systemic inflammatory response to infections and drugs that leads to excessive activation of immune cells and the generation of proinflammatory cytokines.[12] The cytokine storm can lead to apoptosis of epithelial cells and endothelial cells, vascular leakage, acute respiratory dysfunction syndrome, and other syndromes affecting multiple organ systems (see Figure 7.12). Elevated cytokine levels are common with COVID-19 infection[13] and can often result in a poor prognosis. COVID-19 (or the SARS-CoV-2) selectively stimulates IL-6 and the subsequent exhaustion of lymphocytes. Research into the treatment for COVID-19 actually includes the production of monoclonal antibodies against IL-6 (i.e., tocilizumab).

There are many different types of cytokines, depending on where they come from and what they do.[14] The terms *lymphokines* and *monokines* refer respectively to cytokines secreted from lymphocytes or monocytes, although cytokines are secreted by many different types of cells. **Chemokines** are members of a special family of cytokines that are chemotactic and primarily attract leukocytes to sites of inflammation.[15] Many cell types produce chemokines, including macrophages, fibroblasts, and endothelial cells, in response to proinflammatory cytokines, such as TNF-α. There are currently more than 50 different human chemokines. Examples include those that primarily attract macrophages (e.g., monocyte/macrophage chemotactic proteins [MCP-1, MCP-2, and MCP-3]), macrophage inflammatory proteins (MIP-α and MIP-1β), or neutrophils (e.g., interleukin-8 [IL-8]).

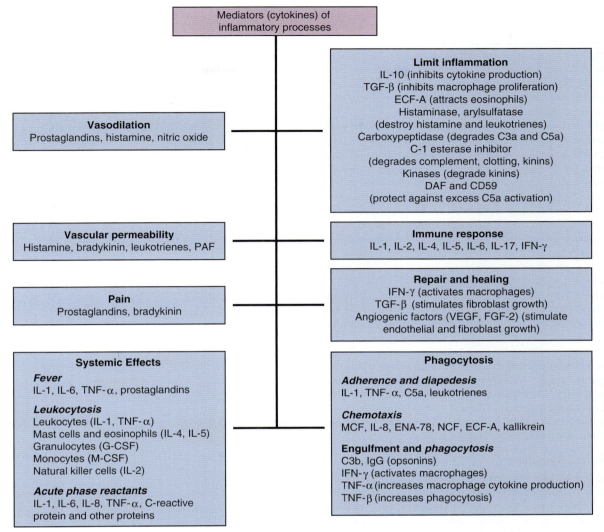

FIGURE 6.6 Principal Mediators of Inflammatory Processes. *C3b*, Large fragment produced from complement component C3; *C5a*, small fragment produced from complement component C5; *DAF*, decay accelerating factor; *ECF-A*, eosinophil chemotactic factor of anaphylaxis; *ENA-78*, epithelial neutrophil activating peptide-78; *FGF*, fibroblast growth factor; *G-CSF*, granulocyte colony-stimulating factor; *IFN*, interferon; *IgG*, immunoglobulin G (predominant class of antibody in the blood); *IL*, interleukin; *MCF*, monocyte chemotactic factor; *M-CSF*, macrophage colony-stimulating factor; *NCF*, neutrophil chemotactic factor; *PAF*, platelet-activating factor; *TGF*, T-cell growth factor; *TNF*, tumour necrosis factor; *VEGF*, vascular endothelial growth factor.

Macrophages and lymphocytes primarily produce **interleukins (ILs)** in response to stimulation of PRRs or by other cytokines.[16] There are more than 30 ILs, and their effects include:

- Alteration of adhesion molecule expression on many types of cells
- Attraction of leukocytes to a site of inflammation (chemotaxis)
- Induction of proliferation and maturation of leukocytes in the bone marrow
- General enhancement or suppression of inflammation
- Development of the acquired immune response

Two major proinflammatory ILs are interleukin-1 and interleukin-6, which cooperate closely with another cytokine, TNF-α. Macrophages mainly produce **interleukin-1 (IL-1)**, which has two forms, IL-1α and IL-1β.[17] IL-1 activates monocytes, other macrophages, and lymphocytes, thereby enhancing both innate and acquired immunity, and it acts as a growth factor for many cells. It has several effects on neutrophils, including (1) induction of proliferation (resulting in an increase in the number of circulating neutrophils), (2) attraction to an inflammatory site (chemotaxis), and (3) increased cellular respiration and lysosomal enzyme activity (both effects resulting in increased cellular killing of bacteria). IL-1 is an endogenous pyrogen (i.e., fever-causing cytokine) that reacts with receptors on cells of the hypothalamus and affects the body's thermostat, resulting in fever.

Macrophages, lymphocytes, and fibroblasts are the main producers of **interleukin-6 (IL-6)**. IL-6 directly induces hepatocytes (liver cells) to produce many of the proteins needed in inflammation (acute-phase reactants, discussed later in this chapter). IL-6 also stimulates growth and differentiation of blood cells in the bone marrow and the growth of fibroblasts (required for wound healing).

Although not classified as an interleukin, macrophages and other cells (e.g., mast cells) secrete TNF-α in response to stimulation of

TLRs. TNF-α induces a multitude of proinflammatory effects, particularly on the vascular endothelium and macrophages. When secreted in large amounts, TNF-α has systemic effects that include:
- Inducing fever by acting as an endogenous pyrogen
- Causing increased synthesis of inflammation-related serum proteins by the liver
- Causing muscle wasting (cachexia) and intravascular thrombosis in cases of severe infection and cancer

Very high levels of TNF-α can be lethal and are probably responsible for fatalities from shock caused by Gram-negative bacterial infections.

Some cytokines are anti-inflammatory and diminish the inflammatory response. The most important are interleukin-10 and transforming growth factor-beta. Lymphocytes primarily produce interleukin-10 (IL-10), which suppresses the growth of other lymphocytes and the production of proinflammatory cytokines by macrophages. This leads to downregulation of both inflammatory and acquired immune responses. Many cells in response to inflammation produce transforming growth factors, including transforming growth factor-beta (TGF-β). These growth factors induce cell division and differentiation of other cell types, such as immature blood cells.

Interferons (IFNs) are members of a family of cytokines that protect against viral infections and modulate the inflammatory response. (Mechanisms of viral infection are described in Chapter 8.) Virally infected cells produce and release type I interferons (primarily IFN-α, IFN-β) in response to viral double-stranded RNA and other viral PAMPs. These IFNs do not kill viruses directly but instead induce antiviral proteins and protection in neighbouring healthy cells. Lymphocytes primarily produce type II interferon (IFN-γ), which activates macrophages and results in increased capacity of the organism to kill infectious agents (including viruses and bacteria). Type II interferon also enhances the development of acquired immune responses against viruses.

Mast Cells and Basophils

The mast cell is probably the most important cellular activator of the inflammatory response. Mast cells are filled with granules and located in the loose connective tissues close to blood vessels near the body's outer surfaces (i.e., in the skin and lining of the GI and respiratory tracts). Basophils are found in the blood and probably function in the same way as tissue mast cells.[18] A great number of stimuli activate mast cells to release potent soluble inducers of inflammation. These inducers are released by (1) degranulation (the release of the contents of mast cell granules) and (2) *synthesis* (the new production and release of mediators in response to a stimulus) (Figure 6.7).

Degranulation. In response to a stimulus (and within seconds), mast cells release biochemical mediators in their granules, including histamine, chemotactic factors, and cytokines (e.g., TNF-α, IL-4), which exert their effects immediately. Histamine is a small-molecular-weight molecule with potent effects on many other cells, particularly those that control the circulation. Histamine is a *vasoactive amine*. Serotonin is another example of a vasoactive amine, produced as a result of inflammation, though it does not come from mast cells. These molecules cause temporary, rapid constriction of smooth muscle and dilation of the postcapillary venules, which results in increased blood flow into the microcirculation. Histamine also causes increased vascular permeability resulting from retraction of endothelial cells lining the capillaries and increased adherence of leukocytes to the endothelium. Histamine affects cells by binding to histamine H1 and H2 receptors on the target cell surface (Figure 6.8). Antihistamines are medications that block the binding of histamine to its receptors, resulting in decreased inflammation.

Binding of histamine to the *H1 receptor* is essentially proinflammatory; that is, it promotes inflammation. On the other hand, binding to

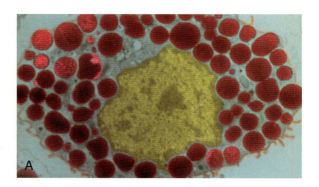

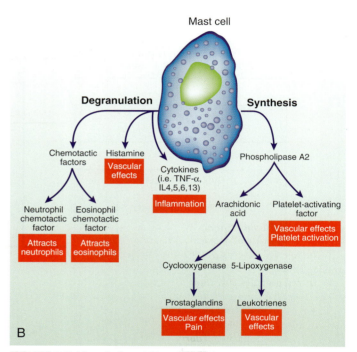

FIGURE 6.7 Mast Cell and Mast Cell Degranulation and Synthesis of Biological Mediators During Inflammation. A, Colourized photomicrograph of mast cell; dense red granules contain histamine and other biologically active substances. **B,** Mast cell degranulation *(left)* and synthesis *(right)*. Histamine and other biologically active substances are released immediately after stimulation of mast cells. Different pharmacological compounds block the synthesis or action of biological mediators during inflammation in specific ways: corticosteroids work by inhibiting phospholipases; nonsteroidal anti-inflammatory drugs inhibit cyclo-oxygenase from producing prostaglandins; and acetaminophen blocks a variant of cyclo-oxygenase (i.e., it has no anti-inflammatory effect). *IL,* Interleukin; *TNFα,* tumour necrosis factor-alpha. ([A] from Roitt, I. M., Broistoff, J., & Male, D. K. [1993]. *Immunology* [3rd ed.]. Mosby.)

the *H2 receptor* is generally anti-inflammatory because it results in suppression of leukocyte function. The H1 receptor is present on smooth muscle cells, especially those of the bronchi, and causes bronchial smooth muscle to contract (bronchoconstriction) when stimulated. Both types of receptors are distributed among many different cells and are often present on the same cells. They may also act in an antagonistic fashion. For example, stimulation of H1 receptors on neutrophils results in augmentation of neutrophil chemotaxis, whereas H2 receptor stimulation results in its inhibition. The H2 receptor is especially

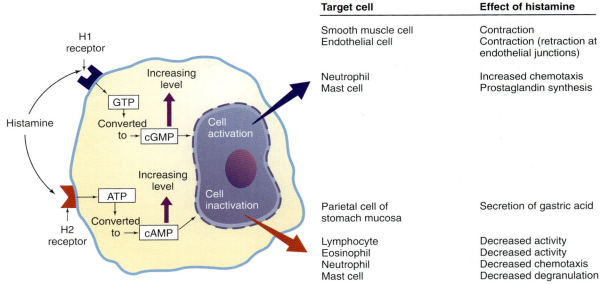

FIGURE 6.8 Effects of Histamine Through H1 and H2 Receptors. The effects depend on (1) the density and affinity of H1 or H2 receptors on the target cell and (2) the identity of the target cell. *ATP,* Adenosine triphosphate; *cAMP,* cyclic adenosine monophosphate; *cGMP,* cyclic guanosine monophosphate; *GTP,* guanosine triphosphate.

abundant on parietal cells of the stomach mucosa and induces the secretion of gastric acid as part of the normal physiology of the stomach. The role of histamine receptors and hypersensitivity is discussed in Chapter 8.

Mast cell granules also contain chemotactic factors, two of which are **neutrophil chemotactic factor (NCF)** and **eosinophil chemotactic factor of anaphylaxis (ECF-A)**. **Chemotaxis** is directional movement of cells along a chemical gradient created by a chemotactic factor. Neutrophils are predominant during the early stages of inflammation (and killing of bacteria). Eosinophils help regulate the inflammatory response. Both cells are discussed in more detail later in this chapter.

Synthesis of mediators. Activated mast cells initiate synthesis of other mediators of inflammation. These include leukotrienes, prostaglandins, and platelet-activating factor, which are produced from lipids (arachidonic acid) in the plasma membrane. **Leukotrienes (slow-reacting substances of anaphylaxis [SRS-A])** are sulphur-containing lipids produced by lipoxygenase that initiate histamine-like effects such as smooth muscle contraction and increased vascular permeability. Leukotrienes appear to be important in the later stages of the inflammatory response because they stimulate slower and more prolonged inflammatory responses than histamine.

Prostaglandins cause increased vascular permeability, neutrophil chemotaxis, and pain by direct effects on nerves. They are long-chain, unsaturated fatty acids produced by the action of the enzyme cyclooxygenase (COX) on arachidonic acid. Prostaglandins have different structures (e.g., E, D, A, F, and B) with numeral subscripts designating the number of double bonds. For example, prostaglandins E_1 and E_2 cause increased vascular permeability and smooth muscle contraction. COX also exists in two different forms. COX-1 is found in most tissues and has a general protective function, whereas COX-2 is associated with inflammation. Acetylsalicylic acid (Aspirin) and other nonsteroidal anti-inflammatory drugs (NSAIDs) inhibit both COX-1 and COX-2, but inhibition of COX-1 causes complications, such as GI toxicity. Selective COX-2 inhibitors are now available (e.g., Celebrex, or celecoxib).

Removal of a fatty acid from the plasma membrane phospholipids by phospholipase A_2 produces **platelet-activating factor (PAF)**. Although mast cells are a major source of PAF, neutrophils, monocytes, endothelial cells, and platelets can also produce PAF. The biological activity of PAF is virtually identical to that of leukotrienes: namely, PAF causes endothelial cell retraction to increase vascular permeability, leukocyte adhesion to endothelial cells, and platelet activation.

Endothelium

The lining of blood vessels consists of a layer of endothelial cells that adhere to an underlying matrix of connective tissue that contains a variety of proteins, including collagen, fibronectin, and laminins. **Endothelial cells** regulate circulating components of the inflammatory system and maintain normal blood flow by preventing spontaneous activation of platelets and members of the clotting system. Furthermore, **nitric oxide (NO)**, derived from its immediate precursor, arginine (an amino acid), is an important signalling molecule and can act as a second messenger, as well as an intercellular messenger in continually relaxing vascular smooth muscle (resulting in vasodilation) and suppressing the effects of low levels of cytokines. **Prostacyclin (PGI2)** comes from arachidonic acid; it both maintains blood flow and pressure and inhibits platelet activation. PGI_2 and NO are synergistic when it comes to regulating blood flow in that they work together to cause vasodilation more than either is able to do on its own. PGI_2 production varies a great deal and increases when there is a requirement for additional regulation of blood flow.

Damage to the endothelial cell lining of the vessel exposes the subendothelial connective tissue matrix, which is prothrombogenic and initiates platelet activation and formation of clots (the contact activation [intrinsic] clotting pathway). Proinflammatory mediators (e.g., histamine, prostacyclin, and many others) affect the endothelium, resulting in adherence of leukocytes to the vessel surface, invasion of leukocytes into the tissue, and movement of plasma from the vessel into the interstitium.

Platelets

Platelets are anucleate cytoplasmic fragments formed from *megakaryocytes*. They circulate in the bloodstream until vascular injury occurs, resulting in platelet activation by many products of tissue destruction and inflammation, including collagen, thrombin, and PAF. Activated platelets have many functions: (1) they interact with components of the coagulation cascade to stop bleeding; (2) they degranulate, releasing biochemical mediators such as serotonin, which has vascular effects similar to those of histamine; and (3) they synthesize thromboxane A_2 (TXA_2) from prostaglandin H_2. TXA_2 is a potent vasoconstrictor and inducer of platelet aggregation. Prolonged use of low-dose Aspirin (acetylsalicylic acid) preferentially suppresses production of TXA_2 without interfering with the production of anti-inflammatory PGI_2 by the endothelium. Platelets also release growth factors that promote wound healing. (Platelet function is described in detail in Chapter 20.)

Phagocytes

The primary role of most granulocytes (neutrophils, eosinophils, basophils) and monocytes/macrophages is **phagocytosis**—the process by which a cell ingests and disposes of damaged cells and foreign material, including microorganisms.

Neutrophils. The **neutrophil, or polymorphonuclear neutrophil (PMN)**, is a member of the granulocytic series of white blood cells. The staining pattern of its granules and the presence of its multilobed nucleus is characteristic of neutrophils. Neutrophils are the predominant phagocytes in the early inflammatory site, arriving within 6 to 12 hours after the initial injury. Several inflammatory mediators (e.g., some bacterial proteins, complement fragments C3a and C5a, and mast cell NCF) specifically and rapidly attract and activate neutrophils from the circulation.[19]

Because the neutrophil is a mature cell that is incapable of division and sensitive to acidic environments, it is short lived at the inflammatory site and becomes a component of the purulent exudate, or pus. Pus is removed from the body through the epithelium or drained from the infected site via the lymphatic system. (The lymphatic system is described in Chapter 23.) The primary roles of the neutrophil are removal of debris and dead cells in sterile lesions, such as burns, and destruction of bacteria in nonsterile lesions.

Eosinophils. Another population of granulocytes is the **eosinophil**. Although eosinophils are only mildly phagocytic, they have two specific functions: (1) they serve as the body's primary defence against parasites, and (2) they help regulate vascular mediators released from mast cells. The role of eosinophils in resistance to parasites occurs in collaboration with specific antibodies produced by the acquired immune system (discussed in Chapter 7).[20]

Regulation of mast cell–derived inflammatory mediators is critical to control inflammation. The acute inflammatory response is needed only in a circumscribed area and for a limited time. Therefore, control mechanisms are necessary to prevent biochemical mediators from evoking more inflammation than necessary. Mast cell eosinophil chemotactic factor of anaphylaxis (ECF-A) attracts eosinophils to the site of inflammation. Eosinophil lysosomal granules contain enzymes that degrade vasoactive molecules, thereby controlling the vascular effects of inflammation. For example, histaminase degrades histamine, and arylsulfatase B degrades leukotrienes.

Basophils. The basophil is the least prevalent granulocyte in the blood. It is very similar to mast cells in the content of its granules. In addition, it is an important source of the cytokine IL-4, which is a key regulator of the adaptive immune response. Although often associated with allergies and asthma, its primary role is yet unknown.

Monocytes and macrophages. **Monocytes** are the largest normal blood cells (14 to 20 μm in diameter). Monocytes are produced in the bone marrow, enter the circulation, and migrate to the inflammatory site where they develop into macrophages. Monocytes also appear to be the precursors of macrophages that are found in tissues (tissue macrophages) including Kupffer cells in the liver, alveolar macrophages in the lungs, and microglia in the brain. **Macrophages** are generally larger (20 to 40 μm) and are more active as phagocytes than their monocytic precursors. Macrophages, particularly those residing in the tissues, are often important cellular initiators of the inflammatory response.

Monocyte-derived macrophages from the circulation may appear at the inflammatory site as soon as 24 hours after the initial neutrophil infiltration, but usually arrive 3 to 7 days later. Neutrophils and monocytes/macrophages differ chiefly in the following ways:

- *Speed:* Neutrophils arrive at the injury site first, whereas macrophages move more sluggishly.
- *Active lifespan:* Macrophages survive and divide in the acidic inflammatory site, whereas neutrophils cannot.
- *Chemotactic factors:* Neutrophils and macrophages are not attracted by the same factors, such as macrophage chemotactic factor, which is released by neutrophils.
- *Enzymatic content of their lysosomes, or digestive vacuoles:* Neutrophils have a more active nicotinamide adenine dinucleotide phosphate (NADPH) oxidase and produce more hydrogen peroxide; macrophage phagolysosomes are more acidic, favouring the activity of acidic proteases and other enzymes.
- *Role in the immune response:* Macrophages, but not neutrophils, are involved in activation of the adaptive immune system.
- *Role in wound repair:* Macrophages are the primary cells that infiltrate tissue in wounds, remove cells and cellular debris, promote angiogenesis, and produce cytokines and growth factors that suppress further inflammation and initiate healing by promoting epithelial cell division, activating fibroblasts, and promoting synthesis of extracellular matrix and collagen.

The bactericidal activity of macrophages can increase markedly with the help of inflammatory cytokines produced by cells of the acquired immune system (subsets of T lymphocytes) or cells activated through TLRs. Macrophage activation results in two subpopulations of cells.[21] TLRs activate M1 macrophages at sites of inflammation and have greater bacterial killing capacity. whereas lymphocyte-produced cytokines activate M2 macrophages and have more of a healing and repair function.[22]

Several bacteria are resistant to killing by granulocytes and can even survive inside macrophages. Microorganisms, such as *Mycobacterium tuberculosis* (tuberculosis), *Mycobacterium leprae* (leprosy), *Salmonella typhi* (typhoid fever), *Brucella abortus* (brucellosis), and *Listeria monocytogenes* (listeriosis), can remain dormant or multiply inside the phagolysosomes of macrophages.

Dendritic cells. **Dendritic cells** provide one of the major links between the innate and acquired immune responses. They are the primary phagocytic cells located in the peripheral organs and skin, which encounter molecules released from infectious agents that undergo phagocytosis by means of the recognition of PRRs. Dendritic cells then migrate through the lymphatic vessels to lymphoid tissue, such as lymph nodes, and interact with **T lymphocytes (T cells)** to generate an acquired immune response.[23] Through the production of a family of cytokines, they guide development of a subset of T cells (T-helper cells) that coordinate the development of functional B and T cells (discussed in Chapter 7).

Phagocytosis. The two most important phagocytes are neutrophils and macrophages. Both cells are circulating in the blood and must first leave the circulation and migrate to the site of inflammation before initiating phagocytosis (Figure 6.9). Many products of inflammation affect expression of surface molecules involved in cell-to-cell

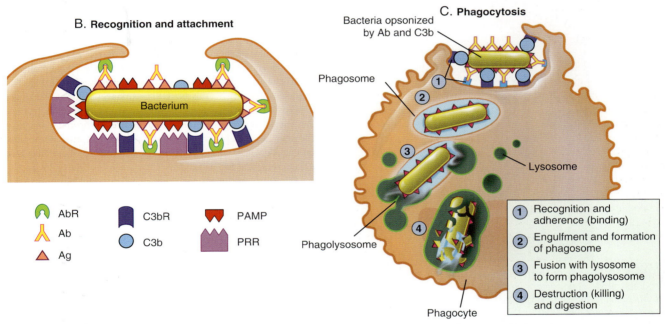

FIGURE 6.9 Process of Phagocytosis. The process that results in phagocytosis occurs via three interrelated steps: adherence and diapedesis, tissue invasion by chemotaxis, and phagocytosis. **A,** *Adherence, margination, diapedesis, and chemotaxis:* The primary phagocyte in the blood is the neutrophil, which usually moves freely within the vessel (1). At sites of inflammation, the neutrophil progressively develops increased adherence to the endothelium, leading to accumulation along the vessel wall (margination, or pavementing) (2). At sites of endothelial cell retraction, the neutrophil exits the blood by means of diapedesis (3). *Chemotaxis:* In the tissues, the neutrophil detects chemotactic factor gradients through surface receptors (1) and migrates toward higher concentrations of the factors (2). The high concentration of chemotactic factors at the site of inflammation immobilizes the neutrophil (3). **B,** *Specific receptors for recognition and attachment.* **C,** *Phagocytosis:* Opsonized microorganisms bind to the surface of a phagocyte through specific receptors (1). The phagocytic vacuole, or phagosome, ingests the microorganism (2). Lysosomes fuse with the phagosome, resulting in the formation of a phagolysosome (3). During this process, lysosomes expose the microorganism to various products, including a variety of enzymes and reactive oxygen species (e.g., hydrogen peroxide [H_2O_2], superoxide [O_2^-]). The microorganism is killed and digested (4). *Ab,* Antibody; *AbR,* antibody receptor; *Ag,* antigen; *C3b,* complement component C3b; *C3bR,* complement C3b receptor; *PAMP,* pathogen-associated molecular pattern; *PRR,* pattern recognition receptor.

adherence. Both leukocytes and endothelial cells begin expressing molecules (selectins and integrins) that increase adhesion, or stickiness, causing the leukocytes to adhere more avidly to the endothelial cells in the walls of the capillaries and venules in a process called **margination**, or **pavementing**. Leukocyte-endothelial interactions lead to **diapedesis**, or emigration of the cells through the junctions between the endothelial cells that have loosened in response to inflammatory mediators.[24]

Once inside the tissue, leukocytes undergo a process of directed migration (chemotaxis) by which chemotactic factors attract them

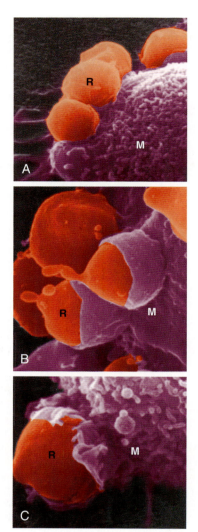

FIGURE 6.10 Phagocytosis of Red Blood Cell. This scanning electron micrograph shows the progressive steps in phagocytosis. **A,** Red blood cells *(R)* attach to the surface of a macrophage *(M).* **B,** Part of the macrophage *(M)* membrane starts to enclose the red blood cell *(R).* **C,** The red blood cells are almost totally engulfed by the macrophage. (Modified from King, D. W., Fenoglio, C. M., & Lefkowitch, J. H. [1983]. *General pathology: principles and dynamics.* Lea & Febiger.)

by acting as a glue to tighten the affinity of adherence between the phagocyte and the target cell. The most efficient opsonins are antibodies and C3b produced by the complement system. Antigens on the surface of bacteria initiate the production of antibodies that are highly specific to that particular microorganism. Certain bacterial and fungal polysaccharide coatings activate the alternative and lectin pathways of complement activation, which deposits C3b on the bacterial surface and increases phagocytosis. The surface of phagocytes contains a variety of specific receptors that will strongly bind to opsonins. These receptors include complement receptors that bind to C3b and **Fc receptors** that bind to the constant site on antibody molecules.

Small pseudopods that extend from the plasma membrane carry out *engulfment* (or endocytosis) and surround the adherent microorganism, forming an intracellular phagocytic vacuole, or **phagosome** (see Figures 6.9 and 6.10). After the formation of the phagosome, lysosomes converge, fuse with the phagosome, and discharge their contents, creating a **phagolysosome**. Destruction of the bacterium takes place within the phagolysosome through both oxygen-dependent and oxygen-independent mechanisms.

Oxygen-dependent killing mechanisms result from the production of toxic oxygen species. A burst of oxygen uptake by the phagocyte accompanies phagocytosis; this process is the *respiratory burst* and results from a shift in much of the cell's glucose metabolism to the **hexose-monophosphate shunt**, which produces NADPH. A membrane-associated enzyme, NADPH oxidase, uses NADPH to generate superoxide (O_2^-), hydrogen peroxide (H_2O_2), and other reactive oxygen species that can be highly damaging to bacteria. Hydrogen peroxide also can collaborate with the lysosomal enzyme *myeloperoxidase* and halide anions (chloride [Cl$^-$] and bromide [Br$^-$]) to form acids that kill bacteria and fungi.

Oxygen-independent mechanisms of microbial killing include (1) the acidic pH (3.5 to 4.0) of the phagolysosome, (2) cationic proteins that bind to and damage target cell membranes, (3) enzymatic attack of the microorganism's cell wall by lysozyme and other enzymes, and (4) inhibition of bacterial growth by lactoferrin binding of iron.

When a phagocyte dies at an inflammatory site, it frequently lyses (breaks open) and releases its cytoplasmic contents into the tissue. For example, contents of neutrophil primary granules (lysozyme, hydrolases, neutral proteases) and secondary granules (lysozyme, collagenase, gelatinase) can digest the connective tissue matrix, causing much of the tissue destruction associated with inflammation.[26] Natural inhibitors found in the blood, such as superoxide dismutase (breaks down O_2^-), catalase (breaks down H_2O_2), and the antiproteinases **α_1-antitrypsin** and α_2-macroglobulin (both produced by the liver), can minimize the destructive effects of many enzymes and reactive oxygen molecules released by dying phagocytes. An inherited deficiency of α_1-antitrypsin often leads to chronic lung damage and emphysema as a result of inflammation. (The pulmonary effects of α_1-antitrypsin deficiency are described in Chapter 27.)

Natural Killer Cells and Lymphocytes

The main function of **natural killer (NK) cells** is recognition and elimination of cells infected with viruses, although they also are somewhat effective at elimination of other abnormal cells, specifically cancer cells.[27] NK cells seem to be more efficient in this role when they encounter an infected cell within the circulatory system as opposed to within tissues. NK cells have inhibitory and activating receptors that allow differentiation between infected or tumour cells and normal cells. If the NK cell binds to a target cell through activating receptors, it produces several cytokines and toxic molecules that can kill the target.[28] NK cells and lymphocytes, which are the principal cells of the adaptive immune response, will be discussed in more detail in Chapter 7.

to the inflammatory site.[25] The primary chemotactic factors include many bacterial products, NCF produced by mast cells, the chemokine IL-8, complement fragments C3a and C5a, and products of the clotting and kinin systems. Red blood cells cannot repair themselves and undergo phagocytosis by macrophages at the end of their lifespan (Figure 6.10).

At the inflammatory site, the process of phagocytosis involves five steps: (1) recognition and adherence of the phagocyte to its target, (2) engulfment (ingestion or endocytosis), (3) formation of a phagosome, (4) fusion of the phagosome with lysosomal granules within the phagocyte, and (5) destruction of the target. Throughout the process, the membrane-bound vesicles isolate both the target and digestive enzymes. Isolation protects the actual phagocyte from both the harmful effects of the target microorganisms, as well as its own enzymes.

Most phagocytes can trap and engulf bacteria using PRRs, although the process is relatively slow. **Opsonization** greatly enhances adherence

ACUTE AND CHRONIC INFLAMMATION

> **QUICK CHECK 6.5**
> 1. Describe how acute inflammation differs from chronic inflammation. What characteristics do they share?
> 2. List the types of exudate produced in inflammation.

Inflammation can be acute and chronic. The acute inflammatory response is self-limiting; that is, it continues only until the threat to the host is eliminated. This usually takes 8 to 10 days from onset to healing. If the acute inflammatory response is inadequate, a chronic inflammation may develop and persist for weeks or months. Inflammation may progress to a granulomatous response that is designed to contain the cause of tissue damage so it no longer poses any harm to the individual with prolonged healing. Tuberculosis (TB) is one such example. A granuloma is formed most commonly in the lung as the infection is walled off from further potential damage, and caseous necrosis is the result. TB is a difficult infection to treat for this reason, and the spores can live in latent form for long periods of time, receiving the stimulus to divide when the host's immune defences are low. The characteristics of the early (i.e., acute) inflammatory response differ from those of the later (i.e., chronic) response, and each phase involves different biochemical mediators and cells that function together. Depending on the successful containment of tissue damage and infection, the acute and chronic phases may lead to healing with limited permanent tissue damage.

Local Manifestations of Acute Inflammation

The cells and plasma protein systems of the inflammatory response interact to produce all the characteristics of inflammation, whether local or systemic (discussed in the next section), as well as determine the duration of inflammation, either acute or chronic. All the local characteristics of **acute inflammation** (i.e., swelling, pain, heat, and redness [erythema]) result from vascular changes and the subsequent leakage of circulating components into the tissue.

The **exudate** of inflammation results from increased vascular permeability and varies in composition, depending on the stage of the inflammatory response and, to some extent, the injurious stimulus. In early or mild inflammation, the exudate may be watery (**serous exudate**) with very few plasma proteins or leukocytes, such as the fluid in a blister. In more severe or advanced inflammation, the exudate may be thick and clotted (**fibrinous exudate**), such as in the lungs of individuals with pneumonia. If a large number of leukocytes accumulate, as in persistent bacterial infections, the exudate consists of pus and is a **purulent (suppurative) exudate**. Purulent exudate is characteristic of walled-off lesions (**cysts** or **abscesses**). If bleeding occurs, the exudate is filled with erythrocytes and is a **hemorrhagic exudate**.

Systemic Manifestations of Acute Inflammation

The three primary systemic changes associated with the acute inflammatory response are (1) fever, (2) leukocytosis (a transient increase in the levels of circulating leukocytes), and (3) increased levels of circulating plasma proteins.

Fever

Fever is partially induced by specific cytokines (e.g., IL-1, released from neutrophils and macrophages). These cytokines are known as **endogenous pyrogens** to differentiate them from pathogen-produced *exogenous pyrogens*. **Pyrogens** act directly on the hypothalamus, the portion of the brain that controls the body's thermostat. (Mechanisms of temperature regulation and fever are discussed in Chapter 14.) A fever is often beneficial because some microorganisms (e.g., those that cause syphilis or gonococcal urethritis) are highly sensitive to small increases in body temperature. On the other hand, fever may have harmful adverse effects because it may enhance the host's susceptibility to the effects of endotoxins associated with Gram-negative bacterial infections (bacterial toxins are described in Chapter 8).

Leukocytosis

Leukocytosis is an increase in the number of circulating white blood cells (greater than $11\,000/mL^3$ in adults). During many infections, a *left shift* in the ratio of immature to mature neutrophils accompanies leukocytosis where more immature forms of neutrophils, such as band cells, metamyelocytes, and occasionally myelocytes, are present in relatively greater than normal proportions. (Chapter 20 contains a more complete discussion of the development and maturation of blood cells.) Production of immature leukocytes increases primarily from proliferation and release of granulocyte and monocyte precursors in the bone marrow.

Plasma Protein Synthesis

The synthesis of many plasma proteins, mostly products of the liver, increases during inflammation. These proteins, which can be either proinflammatory or anti-inflammatory in nature, are **acute-phase reactants** (Table 6.4). Acute-phase reactants reach maximal circulating levels within 10 to 40 hours after the start of inflammation. IL-1 is indirectly responsible for the synthesis of acute-phase reactants through the induction of IL-6, which directly stimulates liver cells to synthesize most of these proteins.

Common laboratory tests for inflammation measure levels of acute-phase reactants. For example, an increase in blood levels of acute-phase reactants, primarily fibrinogen, is associated with an increased adhesion among erythrocytes and a corresponding increase in the sedimentation rate. The erythrocyte sedimentation rate (ESR) is a measurement of the rate at which red blood cells sediment in a tube over a prescribed time span (usually an hour). Although increased erythrocyte sedimentation is a nonspecific reaction, it is a good indicator of an acute inflammatory response. Although the ESR has some utility in diagnosing inflammation, the C-reactive protein produced by the liver during acute inflammation is more commonly used as an indicator of inflammation in clinical practice.

TABLE 6.4 Circulating Levels of Acute-Phase Reactants During Inflammation

Function	Increased	Decreased
Coagulation components	Fibrinogen Prothrombin Factor VIII Plasminogen	None
Protease inhibitors	α_1-Antitrypsin α_1-Antichymotrypsin	Inter-α1-antitrypsin
Transport proteins	Haptoglobin Hemopexin Ceruloplasmin Ferritin	Transferrin
Complement components	C1s, C2, C3, C4, C5, C9, factor B, C1 inhibitor	Properdin
Miscellaneous proteins	α_1-Acid glycoprotein Fibronectin Serum amyloid A (SAA) C-reactive protein (CRP)	Albumin Prealbumin α_1-Lipoprotein β-Lipoprotein

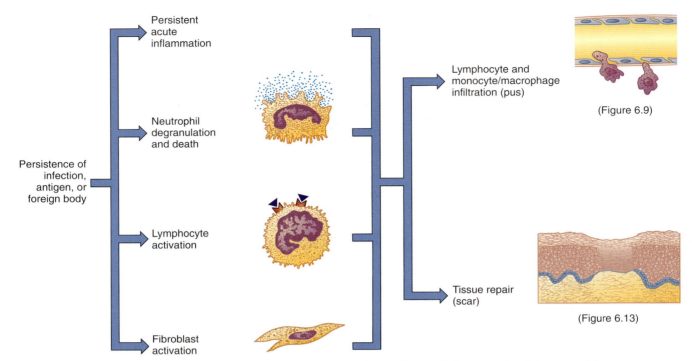

FIGURE 6.11 The Chronic Inflammatory Response. Inflammation usually becomes chronic because of the persistence of an infection, an antigen, or a foreign body in the wound. Chronic inflammation has many of the same processes of acute inflammation. In addition, large amounts of neutrophil degranulation and death, the activation of lymphocytes, and the concurrent activation of fibroblasts result in the release of mediators that induce the infiltration of more lymphocytes and monocytes/macrophages and the beginning of wound healing and tissue repair. For more detailed information on each portion of the response, see the figures referenced in this illustration.

Chronic Inflammation

Superficially, the difference between acute and chronic inflammation is duration; **chronic inflammation** lasts 2 weeks or longer, regardless of cause. Chronic inflammation is sometimes preceded by an unsuccessful acute inflammatory response (Figure 6.11). For example, if bacterial contamination or foreign objects (e.g., dirt, wood splinter, silica, and glass) persist in a wound, an acute response may last beyond 2 weeks. Pus formation, suppuration (purulent discharge), and incomplete wound healing are often present with this type of chronic inflammation.

Chronic inflammation can also occur as a distinct process without previous acute inflammation. Some microorganisms (e.g., mycobacteria that cause tuberculosis) have cell walls with a very high lipid and wax content, making them relatively insensitive to breakdown by phagocytes. Other microorganisms (e.g., those that cause leprosy, syphilis, and brucellosis) can survive within the macrophage and avoid removal by the acute inflammatory response. Furthermore, other microorganisms produce toxins that damage tissue and cause persistent inflammation, even after the organism is killed. Finally, chemicals, particulate matter, or physical irritants (e.g., inhaled dusts, wood splinters, and suture material) can cause a prolonged inflammatory response.

Chronic inflammation presents clinically with a dense infiltration of lymphocytes and macrophages. If macrophages are unable to protect the host from tissue damage, the body attempts to wall off and isolate the infected area, thus forming a **granuloma** (Figure 6.12). For example, infections caused by some bacteria (listeriosis, brucellosis, tuberculosis), fungi (histoplasmosis, coccidioidomycosis), and parasites (leishmaniasis, schistosomiasis, toxoplasmosis) can result in granuloma formation. TNF-α primarily drives granuloma formation.[29] Some macrophages differentiate into large **epithelioid cells**, which specialize

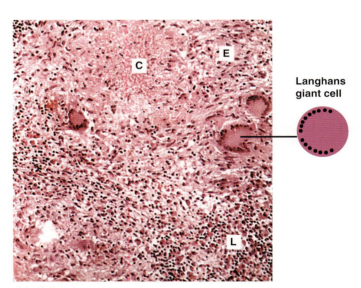

FIGURE 6.12 Tuberculous Granuloma. A central area of amorphous caseous necrosis (C) is surrounded by a zone of lymphocytes (L) and enlarged epithelioid cells (E). Activated macrophages frequently fuse to form multinucleated cells (Langhans giant cells). In tuberculoid granulomas the nuclei of the giant cells move to the cellular margins in a horseshoe-like formation.

in taking up debris and other small particles. Other macrophages fuse into multinucleated **giant cells**, which are active phagocytes that can engulf very large particles—larger than those that can be engulfed by a single macrophage. These two types of specialized cells form the centre of the granuloma, which is surrounded by a wall of lymphocytes. The granuloma itself is often encapsulated by fibrous deposits of collagen and may become cartilaginous or possibly calcified by deposits of calcium carbonate and calcium phosphate.

The classic granuloma associated with tuberculosis has a wall of epithelioid cells surrounding a cheese-like proteinaceous centre derived from dead and decaying tissue (caseous necrosis) and mycobacteria.[30] Decay of cells within the granuloma results in the release of acids and the enzymatic contents of lysosomes from dead phagocytes. In this inhospitable environment, the cellular debris breaks down into its basic constituents, and a clear fluid may remain (liquefactive necrosis). Eventually, this fluid diffuses out and leaves a hollow, thick-walled structure that has replaced normal tissue and reduced the function of the lung.

WOUND HEALING

QUICK CHECK 6.6
1. How does regeneration of tissue differ from repair of tissue?
2. What does it mean to heal by primary intention?
3. What is the role of fibroblasts in wound healing?
4. Describe various ways in which wound healing may be dysfunctional.

The conclusion of inflammation is healing and repair. The most favourable outcome is a return to normal structure and function if damage is minor, no complications occur, and destroyed tissues are capable of **regeneration** (replacement of damaged tissue with healthy tissue, such as what occurs in the epithelia of the skin and intestines, as well as in some organs, such as the liver) (Figure 6.13). This restoration is called **resolution** and may take up to 2 years. Local production of IL-10 appears to play a critical role in this process.[31] Resolution may not be possible if extensive damage is present, the tissue is not capable of regeneration, infection results in abscess or granuloma formation, or fibrin persists in the lesion. In those cases, repair takes place instead of resolution. **Repair** is the replacement of destroyed tissue with scar tissue. Collagen is the main component of **scar tissue** and fills in the lesion, restoring most of the tissue's strength. Unfortunately, collagen cannot carry out the physiological functions of destroyed tissue, resulting in loss of function.

Wound healing involves processes that (1) fill in, (2) seal, and (3) shrink the wound. These characteristics of healing vary in importance and duration among different types of wounds. A clean incision, such as a paper cut or a sutured surgical wound, heals primarily through the process of collagen synthesis. Because this type of wound has minimal tissue loss and close apposition of the wound edges, very little sealing (**epithelialization**) and shrinkage (**contraction**) occur. Wounds that heal under conditions of minimal tissue loss heal by **primary intention** (see Figure 6.13).

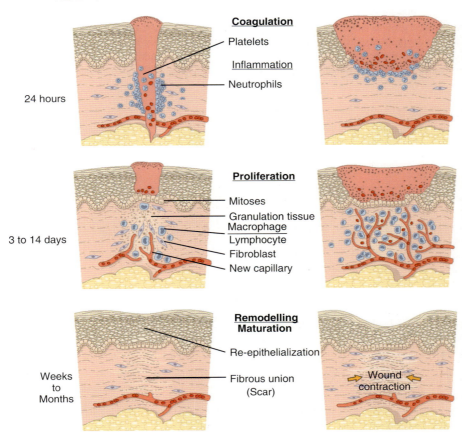

FIGURE 6.13 Wound Healing by Primary and Secondary Intention, and Phases of Wound Healing. Phases of wound healing (coagulation, inflammation, proliferation, remodelling, and maturation) and steps in wound healing by primary intention *(left)* and secondary intention *(right)*. Note large amounts of granulation tissue and wound contraction in healing by secondary intention. (From Roberts, J. R., & Custalow, C. B. [2013]. *Roberts and Hedges' clinical procedures in emergency medicine* [6th ed.]. Saunders.)

Other wounds do not heal as easily. Healing of an open wound, such as a stage IV pressure ulcer (decubitus ulcer), requires a great deal of tissue replacement, and epithelialization, scar formation, and contraction take longer. Healing occurs via secondary intention (see Figure 6.13). Similarly, healing by either primary or secondary intention may occur at different rates for different types of tissue injury.

Epidermal wounds that heal by secondary intention and unsutured internal lesions do not completely heal. At best, repaired tissue regains 80% of its original tensile strength. Only epithelial, hepatic (liver), and bone marrow cells are capable of the complete mitotic regeneration of the normal tissue known as *compensatory hyperplasia*. In fibrous connective tissue, such as joints and ligaments, normal healing results in replacement of the original tissue with new tissue that does not have exactly the same structure or function as that of the original. Some tissues heal without replacement of cells. For example, damage resulting from myocardial infarction heals with a scar composed of fibrous tissue rather than with cardiac muscle.

Wound healing occurs in three overlapping phases: (1) inflammation, (2) proliferation and new tissue formation, and (3) remodelling and maturation.

Phase I: Inflammation

The early phase of wound healing, the transition from acute inflammation to healing, begins almost immediately. The inflammatory phase includes coagulation or hemostasis and the infiltration of cells that participate in wound healing, including platelets, neutrophils, and macrophages (Figure 6.14). The fibrin mesh of the blood clot acts as a scaffold for cells that participate in healing. Platelets contribute to clot formation and, as they degranulate, release growth factors that initiate proliferation of undamaged cells. Neutrophils clear the wound of debris and bacteria. Macrophages take over as the primary phagocytic cell as inflammation progresses to wound healing and repair. Macrophages are essential to wound healing because they clear debris, release wound healing mediators and growth factors, recruit fibroblasts, and help promote formation of a new blood supply (angiogenesis) during the proliferative phase of wound healing.

Phase II: Proliferation and New Tissue Formation

The proliferative phase begins 3 to 4 days after the injury and continues for as long as 2 weeks. The fibrin that seals the wound is replaced by normal tissue or scar tissue during this phase. Macrophage invasion of the dissolving clot and recruitment and proliferation of fibroblasts (connective tissue cells), followed by fibroblast collagen synthesis, epithelialization, contraction of the wound, and cellular differentiation characterize the proliferation phase. Macrophages secrete a variety of biochemical mediators that promote healing, including:

- TGF-β, which stimulates fibroblasts entering the lesion to synthesize and secrete the collagen precursor procollagen.
- Angiogenesis factors, such as vascular endothelial growth factor (VEGF) and fibroblast growth factor-2 (FGF-2), which stimulate vascular endothelial cells to form capillary buds that grow into the lesion; decreased pH and decreased wound oxygen tension also promote angiogenesis.[32]
- Matrix metalloproteinases (MMPs), which degrade and remodel extracellular matrix proteins (e.g., collagen and fibrin) at the site of injury.[33]

Granulation tissue grows into the wound from surrounding healthy connective tissue and consists of invasive cells, new lymphatic vessels, and new capillaries derived from capillaries in the surrounding tissue, giving the granulation tissue a red, granular appearance. During this process, the healing wound must be protected. *Epithelialization* is the process by which epithelial cells grow into the wound from surrounding healthy tissue.[34] Epithelial cells migrate under the clot or scab using MMPs to unravel collagen. Migrating epithelial cells

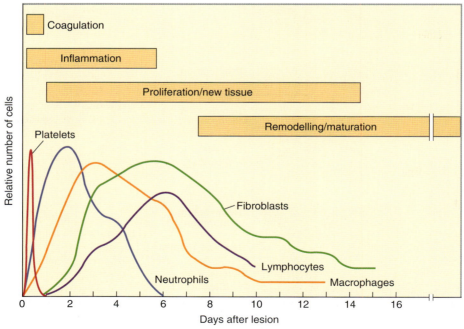

FIGURE 6.14 Time Course of Cells Infiltrating a Wound. Neutrophils and macrophages are the predominant cells that infiltrate a wound during inflammation. Lymphocytes appear later and peak at day 7. Fibroblasts are the predominant cells during the proliferative and remodelling phases of the healing process. (Adapted from Townsend, C. M., Beauchamp, D. R., Evers, B. M., et al. [Eds.]. [2012]. *Sabiston textbook of surgery* [19th ed.]. Elsevier.)

contact similar cells from all sides of the wound and seal it. The epithelial cells remain active, undergoing differentiation to give rise to the various epidermal layers (see Chapter 41). Epithelialization of a skin wound is faster if the wound is kept moist, preventing the fibrin clot from becoming a scab.

Fibroblasts are important cells during healing because they secrete collagen and other connective tissue proteins. Macrophage-derived TGF-β stimulate fibroblasts to proliferate, enter the lesion, and deposit connective tissue proteins in debrided areas about 6 days after the fibroblasts have entered the lesion. Collagen is the most abundant protein in the body.[35] It contains high concentrations of the amino acids glycine, proline, and lysine, many of which are further modified by enzymes in the fibroblasts. Modification of proline and lysine requires several cofactors that are absolutely necessary for proper collagen polymerization and function. These include iron, ascorbic acid (vitamin C), and molecular oxygen (O_2); absence of any of these results in impaired wound healing. As healing progresses, intermolecular covalent bonds cross-link collagen molecules to form collagen fibrils that undergo a further cross-linking to form collagen fibres. The complete process takes several months.

In granulation tissue, TGF-β induces some fibroblasts to transition into myofibroblasts, specialized cells responsible for wound contraction.[36] Myofibroblasts have features of both smooth muscle cells and fibroblasts. They appear microscopically similar to fibroblasts but differ in that their cytoplasm contains bundles of parallel fibres similar to those found in smooth muscle cells. Wound contraction occurs as extensions from the plasma membrane of myofibroblasts establish connections between neighbouring cells, contract their fibres, and exert tension on the neighbouring cells while anchoring themselves to the wound bed. Wound contraction is necessary for closure of all wounds, especially those that heal by secondary intention. Contraction is noticeable 6 to 12 days after injury.

Phase III: Remodelling and Maturation

Tissue remodelling and maturation begins several weeks after injury and is normally complete within 2 years. During this phase, there is continuation of cellular differentiation, scar formation, and scar remodelling. The fibroblast is the major cell of tissue remodelling with the deposition of collagen into an organized matrix. Tissue regeneration and wound contraction continue in the remodelling and maturation phase—a phase for recovering normal tissue structure that can persist for years. For wounds that heal by scarring, scar tissue contracts with the remodelling process and capillaries disappear, leaving the scar avascular. Within 2 to 3 weeks after maturation has begun, the scar tissue has gained about two thirds of its eventual maximal strength.

Dysfunctional Wound Healing

Dysfunctional wound healing and impaired epithelialization may occur during any phase of the healing process. The causes of dysfunctional wound healing include: (1) ischemia, (2) excessive bleeding, (3) obesity, (4) excessive fibrin deposition, (5) a predisposing disorder such as diabetes mellitus, (6) wound infection, (7) inadequate nutrients, (8) numerous medications, and (9) tobacco smoke.[37]

Oxygen-deprived (ischemic) tissue is susceptible to cellular death and infection, which prolongs inflammation and delays healing. *Ischemia* reduces energy production and impairs collagen synthesis and the tensile strength of regenerating connective tissue.

Healing is prolonged if there is *excessive bleeding*. Large clots increase the amount of space that granulation tissue must fill, and they serve as mechanical barriers to oxygen diffusion. Accumulated blood is an excellent culture medium for bacteria and promotes infection, thereby prolonging inflammation by increasing exudation and pus formation. Decreased blood volume also inhibits inflammation because of vessel constriction rather than the dilation required to deliver inflammatory cells, nutrients, and oxygen to the site of injury.

Obesity delays wound healing because of impaired leukocyte function and predisposition to infection, decreases in the number of growth factors, and increases in the levels of proinflammatory cytokines. Additionally, there is dysregulation in collagen synthesis and a decrease in angiogenesis.[38]

Excessive fibrin deposition is detrimental to healing. Fibrin released in response to injury must eventually be reabsorbed to prevent organization into fibrous adhesions. Adhesions formed in the pleural, pericardial, or abdominal cavities can bind organs together by fibrous bands and distort or strangulate the affected organ.

Persons with *diabetes* are at risk for prolonged wound healing. Wounds are often ischemic because of the potential for small-vessel diseases that impair the microcirculation and alter hemoglobin (e.g., increase glycosylation), which has an increased affinity for oxygen and thus, does not readily release oxygen in tissues. Consequences of hyperglycemia also include suppression of macrophages and increased risk for wound infection.

Infiltration of pathogens causes *wound infection*. Pathogens damage cells, stimulate the continued release of inflammatory mediators, consume nutrients, and delay wound healing.

Optimal *nutrition* is important during all phases of healing because metabolic needs increase. Leukocytes need glucose to produce the adenosine 5′-triphosphate (5′-adenosine triphosphate [ATP]) necessary for chemotaxis, phagocytosis, intercellular killing, and initiation of healing. When people with diabetes do not receive enough insulin (or do not use it effectively), wounds heal poorly. Hypoproteinemia impairs fibroblast proliferation and collagen synthesis. Prolonged lack of vitamins A and C results in poorly formed connective tissue and greatly impaired healing because they are cofactors required for collagen synthesis.[39] Other nutrients, including iron, zinc, manganese, and copper, are also cofactors for collagen synthesis. Malnutrition increases the risk for wound infection, delays healing, and reduces wound tensile strength.

Medications, including antineoplastic (anticancer) agents, NSAIDs, and steroids, delay wound healing. Antineoplastic agents slow cell division and inhibit angiogenesis. Although NSAIDs inhibit prostaglandin production and suppress acute inflammation and relieve pain, they also can delay wound healing, particularly bone formation, and may contribute to the formation of excessive scarring. Steroids prevent macrophages from migrating to the site of injury and inhibit release of collagenase and plasminogen activator. Steroids also inhibit fibroblast migration into the wound during the proliferative phase and delay epithelialization. Toxic agents in *tobacco smoke* (i.e., nicotine, carbon monoxide, and hydrogen cyanide) delay wound healing and increase the risk for wound infection.

Dysfunctional collagen synthesis may involve excessive production of collagen, leading to a hypertrophic scar or keloid.[40] A hypertrophic scar is raised but remains within the original boundaries of the wound and tends to regress over time (Figure 6.15A). A keloid is a raised scar that extends beyond the original boundaries of the wound, invades surrounding tissue, and is likely to recur after surgical removal (Figure 6.15B). There is a familial tendency to keloid formation, with a greater incidence in Black people than in White people.

Wound Disruption

A potential complication of wounds that are sutured closed is dehiscence, in which the wound pulls apart at the suture line. Dehiscence generally occurs 5 to 12 days after suturing, when collagen synthesis is at its peak. Wound infection occurs with approximately half of dehiscence occurrences, but they may also be the result of sutures breaking because of excessive strain. Obesity increases the risk for dehiscence because adipose tissue is difficult to suture. Wound dehiscence usually is heralded by increased serous drainage from the wound and a patient's perception that "something gave way." Wound dehiscence requires prompt surgical attention.

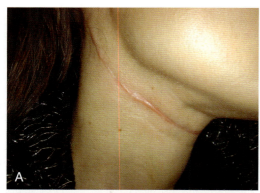

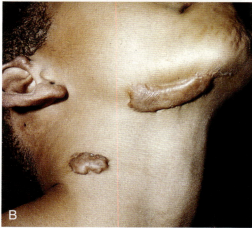

FIGURE 6.15 Hypertrophic Scar and Keloid Scar Formation. Hypertrophic scar (A) and keloid scar (B) caused by excessive synthesis of collagen at suture sites. ([A] from Flint, P. W., Haughey, B. H., Lund, V. J., et al. [2015]. *Cummings otolaryngology: head & neck surgery* [6th ed.]. Mosby; [B] from Damjanov, I., & Linder, J. [1996]. *Anderson's pathology* [10th ed.]. Mosby.)

Impaired Contraction

Wound contraction, although necessary for healing, may become excessive, resulting in a deformity or contracture of scar tissue. Burns of the skin are especially susceptible to contracture development, particularly at joints, resulting in loss of movement around the joints. Examples of internal contractures include duodenal strictures caused by dysfunctional healing of a peptic ulcer; esophageal strictures caused by chemical burns (such as lye ingestion); or abdominal adhesions caused by surgery, infection, or radiation. Contractures may occur in cirrhosis of the liver, constricting vascular flow and contributing to the development of portal hypertension and esophageal varices. Proper positioning, range-of-motion exercises, and surgery are among the physical means used to overcome excessive skin contractures. Surgery is one way to release internal contractures.

PEDIATRIC CONSIDERATIONS

Age-Related Factors Affecting Innate Immunity in the Newborn Child

- Newborn physiological immunity is acquired from the mother through the placenta and breast milk.
- Newborns have transiently depressed inflammatory responses.
- Neutrophils are incapable of chemotaxis, lacking fluidity in the plasma membrane.
- Complement levels are diminished, especially components of the alternative pathways (e.g., factor B), particularly in premature newborns.
- Monocyte/macrophage numbers are normal, but chemotaxis of monocytes is delayed.
- There is a tendency for infections associated with chemotactic defects, for example, cutaneous abscesses caused by staphylococci and cutaneous candidiasis.
- There are diminished oxidative and bacterial responses in those stressed by in utero infection or respiratory insufficiency.
- There is a tendency to develop severe overwhelming sepsis and meningitis when infected by bacteria against which no maternal antibodies are present.
- The establishment of the gut microbiome is facilitated by breast milk.
- Caesarean-delivered newborns have reduced gut microbial diversity.

GERIATRIC CONSIDERATIONS

Age-Related Factors Affecting Innate Immunity in Older Persons

- Older persons have normal numbers of cells of innate immunity, but the cells may have diminished function (e.g., decreased phagocytic activity and altered cytokine synthesis).
- The incidence of chronic inflammation is higher, possibly related to an increased production of proinflammatory mediators.
- Older persons are at risk for impaired healing and infection associated with chronic illness (e.g., diabetes mellitus, peripheral vascular disease, or cardiovascular disease) and decreased phagocytosis.
- The use of medications may interfere with healing (e.g., anti-inflammatory steroids).
- A loss of subcutaneous fat diminishes layers of protection against injury.
- Atrophied epidermis, including underlying capillaries, decreases perfusion and increases the risk of hypoxia in the wound bed.

CHAPTER 6 Innate Immunity: Inflammation and Wound Healing

CASE STUDY

John Doe is a 55-year-old man recently admitted to the hospital for an elective laparotomy (open abdominal surgery) to remove polyps in his large intestine. (The preliminary pathology report indicates that the polyps are benign.) John also has a medical history of type 2 diabetes. On the third postoperative day, the nurse notices the wound is dehisced, and there is purulent drainage coming from where the wound edges are no longer closely approximated. John's pain has also increased, and he is requiring more analgesic to relieve it. The physician is notified and orders the removal of some staples with packing of the wound and changing the dressing every shift.

Critical Thinking and Clinical Judgement Questions

1. What are some signs and symptoms that the wound is infected? What are some differences between a local infection versus a systemic infection?
2. What are some examples of breaks in the first line of defence? second line of defence?
3. How is this wound healing differently now? What is the difference between an acute surgical wound and a chronic wound?
4. What factors impact wound healing?

DID YOU UNDERSTAND?

Human Defence Mechanisms

1. The three lines of human defence from injury and infection are innate immunity (which includes natural barriers), inflammatory response, and adaptive (acquired) immunity.
2. Physical barriers are the first lines of defence that prevent damage to the individual and prevent invasion by pathogens; these include the skin and mucous membranes.
3. Antibacterial peptides (cathelicidins, defensins, collectins, and mannose-binding lectin) in mucous secretions, perspiration, saliva, tears, and other secretions provide a biochemical barrier against pathogenic microorganisms.
4. The skin and mucous membranes are colonized by commensal or mutualistic microorganisms that provide protection by releasing chemicals that facilitate immune responses, prevent colonization by pathogens, and facilitate digestion in the gastro-intestinal tract.
5. The second line of defence is the inflammatory response (inflammation), a rapid and nonspecific protective response to cellular injury from any cause. It can occur only in vascularized tissue.
6. The macroscopic hallmarks of inflammation are redness, swelling, heat, pain, and loss of function of the inflamed tissues.
7. The microscopic hallmarks of inflammation are vasodilation, increased capillary permeability, and an accumulation of fluid and cells at the inflammatory site.
8. Three key plasma protein systems mediate inflammation: the complement system, the clotting system, and the kinin system. The components of all three systems are a series of inactive proteins that are activated sequentially.
9. Antigen-antibody reactions (through the classical pathway) or by other products can activate complement, as well as bacterial polysaccharides (through the lectin pathway or the alternative pathway), resulting in the production of biologically active fragments that recruit phagocytes, activate mast cells, and destroy pathogens.
10. The most biologically potent products of the complement system are C3b (opsonin), C3a (anaphylatoxin), and C5a (anaphylatoxin, chemotactic factor).
11. The clotting system stops bleeding, localizes microorganisms, and provides a meshwork for repair and healing.
12. Bradykinin is the most important product of the kinin system and causes vascular permeability, smooth muscle contraction, and pain.
13. Control of inflammation regulates inflammatory cells and enzymes and localizes the inflammatory response to the area of injury or infection.
14. Carboxypeptidase, histaminase, and C1 esterase inhibitor are inactivating enzymes, and the fibrinolytic system and plasmin facilitate clot degradation after bleeding is stopped.
15. The inflammatory process involves many different types of cells, including mast cells, endothelial cells, platelets, phagocytes (neutrophils, eosinophils, monocytes/macrophages, dendritic cells), natural killer cells, and lymphocytes.
16. Most cells express plasma membrane pattern recognition receptors that recognize molecules produced by infectious microorganisms (pathogen-associated molecular patterns, or PAMPs), or products of cellular damage (damage-associated molecular patterns, or DAMPs). Many inflammatory cells express toll-like receptors and NOD-like receptors, recognize PAMPs and DAMPs, and promote release of cytokines and inflammatory mediators that eliminate damaged cells and protect against invasion by microbes.
17. The cells of the innate immune system secrete many biochemical mediators (cytokines) that are responsible for activating other cells and regulating the inflammatory response; these cytokines include chemokines, interleukins, interferons, and other molecules.
18. Chemokines induce chemotaxis of leukocytes, fibroblasts, and other cells to promote phagocytosis and wound healing.
19. Lymphocytes and macrophages primarily produce interleukins that promote or inhibit inflammation by activating growth and differentiation of leukocytes and lymphocytes.
20. The most important proinflammatory interleukins are interleukin-1 (IL-1), interleukin-6 (IL-6), and tumour necrosis factor-alpha. Interleukin-10 downregulates the inflammatory response.
21. Virally-infected cells produce interferons. Once released from infected cells, interferons can stimulate neighbouring healthy cells to produce substances that prevent viral infection.
22. The most important activator of the inflammatory response is the mast cell, which is located in connective tissue near capillaries and initiates inflammation by releasing biochemical mediators (histamine, chemotactic factors) from preformed cytoplasmic granules and synthesizing other mediators (prostaglandins, leukotrienes, and platelet-activating factor) in response to a stimulus. Basophils are in the blood and probably function in the same way as tissue mast cells.
23. Histamine is the major vasoactive amine released from mast cells. It causes dilation of capillaries and retraction of endothelial cells lining the capillaries, which increases vascular permeability.
24. The endothelial cells lining the circulatory system (vascular endothelium) normally regulate circulating components of the inflammatory system and maintain normal blood flow by preventing spontaneous activation of platelets and members of the clotting system.
25. Platelets interact with the coagulation cascade to stop bleeding and release a number of mediators that promote and control inflammation.

26. During inflammation, the endothelium expresses receptors that help leukocytes leave the vessel and retract to allow fluid to pass into the tissues.
27. The polymorphonuclear neutrophil, the predominant phagocytic cell in the early inflammatory response, exits the circulation by diapedesis through the retracted endothelial cell junctions and moves to the inflammatory site by chemotaxis.
28. Eosinophils release products that control the inflammatory response and are the principal cell that kills parasitic organisms.
29. The macrophage, the predominant phagocytic cell in the late inflammatory response, is highly phagocytic, is responsive to cytokines, and promotes wound healing.
30. Dendritic cells connect the innate and acquired immune systems by collecting antigens at the site of inflammation and transporting them to sites, such as the lymph nodes, where immunocompetent B and T cells reside and are transformed into functional cells.
31. Phagocytosis is a multistep cellular process for the elimination of pathogens and foreign debris. The steps are (a) recognition and attachment, (b) engulfment, (c) formation of a phagosome, (d) fusion of the phagosome with lysosomal granules within the phagocyte, and (e) destruction of the target. Phagocytic cells engulf microorganisms and enclose them in phagocytic vacuoles (phagolysosomes), within which toxic products (especially metabolites of oxygen) and degradative lysosomal enzymes kill and digest the microorganisms.
32. Opsonins, such as antibody and complement component C3b, coat microorganisms and make them more susceptible to phagocytosis by binding them more tightly to the phagocyte.

Acute and Chronic Inflammation

1. Acute inflammation is self-limiting and usually resolves within 8 to 10 days.
2. Local manifestations of inflammation are the result of the vascular changes associated with the inflammatory process, including vasodilation and increased capillary permeability. The symptoms include redness, heat, swelling, and pain.
3. The principal systemic effects of inflammation are fever and increases in levels of circulating leukocytes (leukocytosis) and plasma proteins (acute-phase reactants [i.e., IL-1 and IL-6]).
4. Chronic inflammation can be a continuation of acute inflammation that lasts 2 weeks or longer. It can also occur as a distinct process without much preceding acute inflammation.
5. Chronic inflammation is characterized by a dense infiltration of lymphocytes and macrophages. The body may wall off and isolate the infection to protect against tissue damage by formation of a granuloma.

Wound Healing

1. Resolution and regeneration refer to the return of tissue to nearly normal structure and function. Repair refers to healing by scar tissue formation.
2. Damaged tissue proceeds to resolution (restoration of the original tissue structure and function) if little tissue has been lost or if injured tissue is capable of regeneration. Wounds that heal under conditions of minimal tissue loss are said to heal by primary intention.
3. Tissues that sustained extensive damage or those incapable of regeneration heal by the process of repair, resulting in the formation of a scar. This process is *healing by secondary intention*.
4. Resolution and repair occur in two separate phases: the (1) reconstructive phase in which the wound begins to heal and the (2) maturation phase in which the healed wound undergoes remodelling.
5. Dysfunctional wound healing can be related to ischemia, excessive bleeding, obesity, excessive fibrin deposition, a predisposing disorder such as diabetes mellitus, wound infection, inadequate nutrients, numerous medications, and tobacco smoke.
6. Dehiscence is a disruption in which the wound pulls apart at the suture line.
7. A contracture of scar tissue is a deformity caused by the excessive shortening of collagen in scar tissue.

Pediatric Considerations: Age-Related Factors Affecting Innate Immunity in the Newborn Child

1. Newborns have transiently depressed inflammatory function, particularly neutrophil chemotaxis and alternative complement pathway activity.

Geriatric Considerations: Age-Related Factors Affecting Innate Immunity in Older Persons

1. Older persons are at risk for impaired wound healing, usually because of chronic illnesses.

7

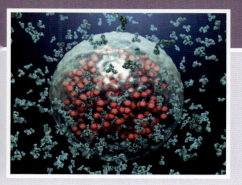

Adaptive Immunity

Stephanie Zettel, with originating chapter contributions by Valentina L. Brashers and Kathryn L. McCance

Additional resources are available online at http://evolve.elsevier.com/Canada/Huether/pathophysiology

CHAPTER OUTLINE

Third Line of Defence: Adaptive Immunity, 158
Antigens and Immunogens, 159
Antibodies, 161
    Classes of Immunoglobulins, 161
    Antigen–Antibody Binding, 162
    Function of Antibodies, 162
Immune Response: Collaboration of B Cells and T Cells, 164
    Generation of Clonal Diversity, 164
    Development of B Lymphocytes, 164
    Clonal Selection, 167

Cell-Mediated Immunity, 172
    T-Lymphocyte Function, 172
PEDIATRIC CONSIDERATIONS: Age-Related Factors Affecting Mechanisms of Self-Defence in the Newborn Child, 174
GERIATRIC CONSIDERATIONS: Age-Related Factors Affecting Mechanisms of Self-Defence in Older Persons, 174

LEARNING OBJECTIVES

1. Distinguish between natural and acquired immunity.
2. Define and describe humoral and cell-mediated immunity.
3. Describe the differences between active and passive immunity.
4. Define antigen and differentiate between the various types of antigens.
5. Describe the steps of antigen binding, presenting, and processing.
6. Define antibody, describing the molecular structure and function of an antibody.
7. Identify the classes of immunoglobulins.
8. Describe what is meant by direct and indirect effects of an antibody.
9. Define and describe the differences between secretory and systemic immune systems.
10. Discuss the roles of the various types of T lymphocytes and their development from stem cells.
11. Define and describe clonal diversity and clonal selection.
12. Describe what is meant by superantigens.
13. Differentiate between a primary and secondary immune response.
14. Discuss the alterations in immunity for infants and the elderly.

KEY TERMS

Active immunity (active acquired immunity), 158
Adaptive (acquired) immunity, 158
Agglutination, 162
Antibody, 161
Antibody-dependent cell-mediated cytotoxicity (ADCC), 173
Antigen, 158
Antigen-binding fragment (Fab), 161
Antigen-binding site (paratope), 162
Antigenic determinant (epitope), 162
Antigen processing, 168
Antigen-processing (antigen-presenting) cell (APC), 167
B cell antigen receptor (BCR), 164
B lymphocyte (B cell), 158
CD3, 166
CD4, 166
CD8, 166
Cellular immunity, 158
Central tolerance, 164
Class switch, 172
Clonal diversity, 158
Clonal selection, 158
Complementarity determining region (CDR), 161
Crystallizable fragment (Fc), 161
Dendritic cell, 167
Hapten, 159
Human leukocyte antigen (HLA), 167
Humoral immunity, 158
Immune response, 158
Immunity, 158
Immunocompetent, 164
Immunogen, 159
Immunoglobulin (Ig), 161
Lymphocyte, 158
Lymphoid stem cell, 164
Major histocompatibility complex (MHC), 167
Memory cell, 158
Natural killer (NK) cell, 172
Neutralization, 162
Passive immunity (passive acquired immunity), 158
Peripheral tolerance, 173
Plasma cell, 158
Precipitation, 162
Primary (central) lymphoid organ, 164
Primary immune response, 167
Secondary immune response, 167
Secondary lymphoid organ, 159
Secretory immunoglobulin, 164
Secretory (mucosal) immune system, 164
Somatic recombination, 164
Superantigen (SAG), 171
Systemic immune system, 164
T cell antigen receptor (TCR), 166
T lymphocyte (T cell), 158
T-cytotoxic cell (Tc cell), 158
Th1 cell, 170
Th2 cell, 170
Th17 cell, 170
T-helper cell (Th cell), 158
Titre, 167
T-regulatory cell (Treg cell), 158

157

The third line of defence in the human body is **adaptive (acquired) immunity**, often called the **immune response** or **immunity**, and consists of **lymphocytes** and serum proteins called *antibodies*. The adaptive immune response comes into play once there is both a break in the external barriers and activation of the processes of inflammation (innate immunity, see Chapter 6). Inflammation is the "first responder" that contains the initial injury and slows the spread of infection, whereas adaptive immunity slowly augments the initial defences against infection and provides long-term security against reinfection.

THIRD LINE OF DEFENCE: ADAPTIVE IMMUNITY

> ✓ **QUICK CHECK 7.1**
> 1. Define acquired immunity.
> 2. Distinguish between innate immunity and acquired immunity.
> 3. Distinguish between humoral immunity and cell-mediated immunity.
> 4. What are the differences among antigens, immunogens, and haptens?

Inflammation (or the innate immune response) and adaptive immunity differ in several key ways. First, activation of the components of inflammation occurs immediately after tissue damage. Adaptive immunity is *inducible*; in other words, the effectors of the immune response, lymphocytes and antibodies, do not pre-exist; it is the infection/damage that induces their production in response to a foreign antigen. This means adaptive immunity develops more slowly than inflammation, taking 7 to 14 days to respond. Second, the inflammatory response is similar in all tissues, regardless of differences in the cause of tissue damage or whether the inflammatory site is sterile or contaminated with infectious microorganisms. The adaptive immune response is exquisitely *specific*. The lymphocytes and antibodies induced in response to infection are extremely specific to the infecting microbe. Third, the residual mediators of inflammation must be removed quickly to limit damage to surrounding healthy tissue and allow healing. The effectors of the adaptive immune response are *long-lived* and systemic, providing long-term immunological protection (including immunological memory and memory response) against specific infections. Finally, the inflammatory response to both recurrent tissue damage and infection is identical. The immune response has *memory*. If reinfected with the same microbe, production of specific lymphocytes and specific antibodies occurs immediately, assuring permanent long-term protection against infection.

Despite the differences, the innate and adaptive immune systems are highly interactive and complementary. Many components of innate immunity are necessary for the development of the adaptive immune response. Conversely, products of the adaptive immune response activate components of innate immunity. Thus, both systems are essential for complete protection against infectious disease.

The basic mechanisms underlying the adaptive immune response will be discussed in this chapter. This chapter will focus on the key concepts and the most important, or well-studied, mediators of the immune response.

The adaptive immune response has its own vocabulary (Figure 7.1). **Antigens** are the molecular targets of antibodies and lymphocytes. Antigens are generally small molecules, usually within proteins, carbohydrates, or lipids, found on the surface of microbes or infected cells that are capable of stimulating an immune response because they are foreign to the body. In the fetus, well before being exposed to any infectious microorganisms, lymphocytes have undergone extensive differentiation. Some lymphoid stem cells enter the thymus and differentiate into **T lymphocytes (T cells**, *T* indicates thymus derived), whereas others enter specific regions of the bone marrow and differentiate into **B lymphocytes (B cells**, *B* indicates bone-marrow–derived). Each type of cell develops origin-specific cell surface proteins that identify them as T or B cells. Both B and T cells also develop cell surface antigen receptors. The receptors are remarkable because an individual lymphocyte is programmed to recognize only one specific antigen before having encountered that antigen. Before birth, each individual has a population of B and T cells capable of recognizing at least 10^8 different antigens. This generation of **clonal diversity** is the process by which B and T cells establish their diversity of antigen receptors (see Figure 7.1).

A second process, *clonal selection*, begins when an infection occurs. This process requires the cooperation among a variety of cells in the secondary lymphoid organs; an antigen needs to be *processed* by phagocytic cells, primarily dendritic cells, which also express the processed antigen on their surfaces and *present* the antigen to lymphocytes. This begins a symphony of cellular interactions, referred to as **clonal selection**, involving several subsets of B and T cells, intercellular adhesion through antigen receptors and specific intercellular adhesion molecules, the production and response to multiple cytokines, and eventual differentiation of immunocompetent B and T cells into highly specialized effector cells. B cells develop into **plasma cells** that become factories for the production of antibodies. T cells develop into several subsets that can identify and kill a target cell (**T-cytotoxic cells, Tc cells**), regulate the immune response by helping the clonal selection process (**T-helper cells, Th cells**), or suppress inappropriate immune responses (**T-regulatory cells, Treg cells**). Both B and T cells also differentiate into very long-lived **memory cells** that exist for decades or, in some cases, for the life of the individual. A second infection that occurs with the same microbe can rapidly activate memory cells.

Antibodies circulate in the blood and defend against extracellular microbes and microbial toxins. This response is the *humoral immune response*, or **humoral immunity**. Effector T cells circulate in the blood and tissues and defend against intracellular pathogens (e.g., viruses) and cancer cells. This response is the *cellular immune response*, or **cellular immunity** (also cell-mediated immunity).

The preceding overview describes **active immunity (active acquired immunity)**, which develops in response to antigens, and the individual develops antibodies to antigens. Antigens can be the result of exposure to an infection, or they can be administered in a vaccine. Vaccines can be live or attenuated forms of the pathogen (e.g., the influenza virus), or they can include bits of protein from the pathogen to which the individual develops antibodies. This is the case with the Pfizer and Moderna COVID-19 vaccines, which are mRNA vaccines. As such, these vaccines contain the genetic instructions for making the protein that is found on the surface of SARS-CoV-2. The vaccine then uses our cells to make this protein, which triggers an immune reaction to make antibodies and memory cells against it in case of future infection by the actual virus. The mRNA vaccine does not contain the virus and cannot cause actual infection.[1]

In certain clinical situations, preformed antibody or lymphocytes may be administered to an individual. This is **passive immunity (passive acquired immunity)**. Examples include individuals exposed to an infectious agent without having a pre-existing vaccine-induced immunity (e.g., hepatitis A virus or rabies virus) (Table 7.1). Other examples include the newborn receiving maternal antibodies via the placenta or through breast milk, Rh immunoglobulin injection to manage an Rh incompatibility between mom and baby, and an intravenous infusion of IgG to treat Guillain-Barré syndrome. Several forms

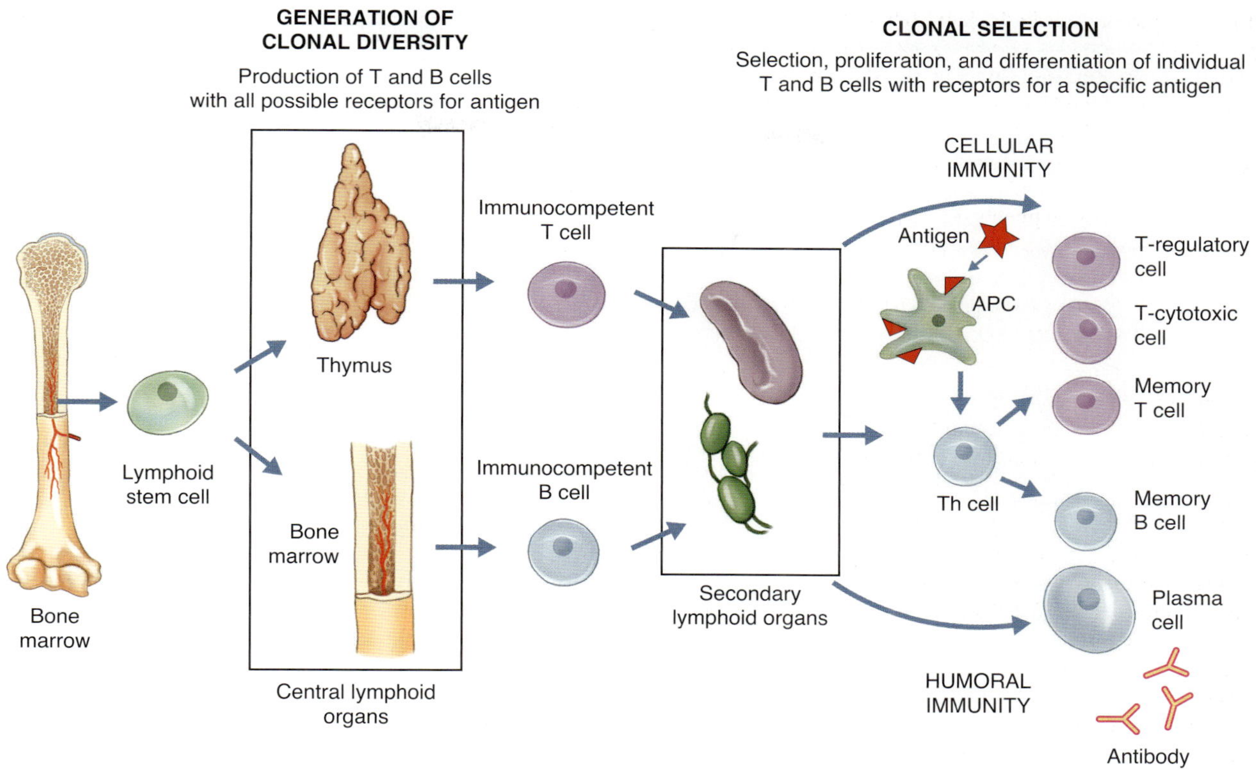

FIGURE 7.1 Overview of the Immune Response. The immune response exists in two phases: **1**, the *generation of clonal diversity* and **2**, *clonal selection*. During the generation of clonal diversity, lymphoid stem cells from the bone marrow migrate to the central lymphoid organs (the thymus or regions of the bone marrow), where they undergo a series of cellular division and differentiation stages resulting in either immunocompetent T cells from the thymus or immunocompetent B cells from the bone marrow. These cells are still naïve in that they have never encountered foreign antigen. These cells enter the blood and lymphatic vessels and migrate to the secondary lymphoid organs (e.g., lymph nodes, spleen) of the systemic immune system (Figure 7.2). Some take up residence in B-cell and T-cell–rich areas of those organs, and others re-enter the circulation. Approximately 60 to 70% of circulating lymphocytes are immunocompetent T cells, and 10 to 20% are immunocompetent B cells. A foreign antigen initiates the clonal selection phase. Antigen-presenting cells *(APCs)* usually process the antigen for presentation to T-helper cells *(Th cells)*. The intercellular cooperation among APCs, Th cells, and immunocompetent T and B cells results in a second stage of cellular proliferation and differentiation. Because the antigen has "selected" those T and B cells with compatible antigen receptors, only a small population of T and B cells undergo this process at one time. The result is an active cellular immunity or humoral immunity, or both. A population of effector T cells that can kill targets (T-cytotoxic cells) or regulate the immune response (T-regulatory cells) mediates cellular immunity, as well as a population of memory cells (memory T cells) that can respond more quickly to a second challenge with the same antigen. Similarly, a population of soluble proteins (antibodies) produced by plasma cells and by a population of memory B cells that can produce more antibody rapidly to a second challenge with the same antigen mediates humoral immunity.

of cancer have used passive immunization with specific T cells as treatment for the condition. Whereas active acquired immunity is long lived, passive immunity is only temporary because the donor's antibodies or T cells are eventually destroyed.

ANTIGENS AND IMMUNOGENS

Understanding the molecules against which an immune response is directed is integral to understanding the nature of the immune response itself. Although the terms *antigen* and *immunogen* are commonly used as synonyms, there are clinically important differences between the two. *Antigen* is commonly used to describe a molecule that can *bind with* antibodies or antigen receptors on B and T cells. A molecule that will *induce* an immune response is an **immunogen**. Thus, all immunogens are antigens but not all antigens are immunogens. For example, *immunogenicity* is frequently related to the size of the antigen. In general, large molecules (those greater than 10,000 daltons), such as proteins and polysaccharides, are most immunogenic. Many low-molecular-weight molecules can function as **haptens**; as such, they are too small to be immunogens by themselves but become immunogenic after combining with larger molecules that function as carriers for the hapten. For example, poison ivy contains an oily

TABLE 7.1 Antigens and Antibodies in Clinical Practice

Antigen Source	Protection: Combat Active Disease	Protection: Vaccination	Diagnosis (Determining "titre")	Therapy
Infectious agents	Neutralize or destroy pathogenic microorganisms (e.g., antibody response against viral infections)	Induce safe and protective immune response (e.g., recommended childhood vaccines)	Measure circulating antigen from infectious agent or antibody (e.g., diagnosis of hepatitis B infection)	Passive treatment with antibody to treat or prevent infection (e.g., administration of antibody against hepatitis A)
Cancers	Prevent tumour growth or spread (e.g., immune surveillance to prevent early cancers)	Prevent cancer growth or spread (e.g., vaccination with cancer antigens)	Measure circulating antigen (e.g., circulating PSA for diagnosis of prostate cancer)	Immunotherapy (e.g., treatment of cancer with antibodies against cancer antigens)
Environmental substances	Prevent entrance into body (e.g., secretory IgA limits systemic exposure to potential allergens)	No clear example	Measure circulating antigen or antibody (e.g., diagnosis of allergy by measuring circulating IgE)	Immunotherapy (e.g., administration of antigen for desensitization of individuals with severe allergies)
Self-antigens	Immune system tolerance to self-antigens, which can be altered by an infectious agent leading to autoimmune disease (see Chapter 8)	Some cases of vaccination alter tolerance to self-antigens, leading to autoimmune disease	Measure circulating antibody against self-antigen for diagnosis of autoimmune disease (see Chapter 8)	Oral administration of self-antigens to diminish production of autoimmune disease–associated autoantibodies

PSA, Prostate-specific antigen.

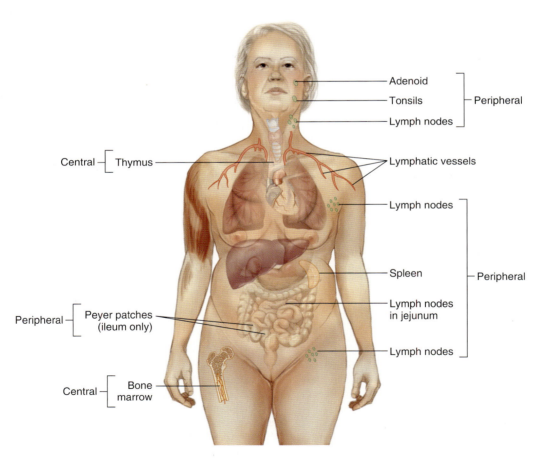

FIGURE 7.2 Lymphoid Tissues: Sites of B-Cell and T-Cell Differentiation. Immature lymphocytes migrate through central (primary) lymphoid tissues: the bone marrow (central lymphoid tissue for B lymphocytes) and the thymus (central lymphoid tissue for T lymphocytes). Mature lymphocytes later reside in the T- and B-lymphocyte–rich areas of the peripheral (secondary) lymphoid tissues.

sap called *urushiol* (molecular weight approximately 1,500 daltons), which is chemically altered upon contact with the skin, binds to large proteins in the skin, and becomes immunogenic, resulting in a T-cell response and onset of a classic poison ivy rash. Penicillin is another example of a hapten that can cause a delayed hypersensitivity response. Chapter 8 describes many similar conditions.

ANTIBODIES

> **QUICK CHECK 7.2**
> 1. What are the major functions of antibodies?
> 2. What is the difference between the secretory immune system and systemic immune system?

A basic understanding of antibodies and how they react with antigens provides a foundation for more complex topics, such as the B cell and T cell antigen receptors, the generation of clonal diversity, and intercellular collaborations during clonal selection, which are discussed later in this chapter. The terms **antibody** and **immunoglobulin (Ig)** are generally interchangeable: *immunoglobulin* is frequently used as a generic description of a general group of antibodies, whereas *antibody* commonly denotes one particular set of immunoglobulins known to have specificity for a particular antigen.

Classes of Immunoglobulins

There are five classes of immunoglobulins (IgG, IgA, IgM, IgE, and IgD), which have minor differences in structure and function (Figure 7.3). Both IgG and IgA have subclasses (Table 7.2).

IgG is the most abundant class of immunoglobulins, constituting 80 to 85% of the immunoglobulins in the blood and accounting for most of the protective activity against infections. During pregnancy, maternal IgG crosses the placenta and protects the newborn child during the first 6 months of life.

IgA is found in the blood and in bodily secretions as secretory IgA (subclass IgA2). Secretory IgA is a *dimer* consisting of two IgA2 molecules held together through a J chain and secretory piece. The secretory piece is attached to dimeric IgA during transportation through mucosal epithelial cells to protect against degradation by enzymes also found in secretions.

IgM is the largest immunoglobulin and usually exists as a pentamer (a molecule consisting of five identical smaller molecules) that has a J chain for stabilization. It is the first antibody produced during the initial, or primary, response to antigens. Synthesis of IgM usually begins early in neonatal life but increases as a response to infection in utero.

IgE is normally at low concentrations in the circulation. It has very specialized functions as a mediator of many common allergic responses (see Chapter 8) and in the defence against parasitic infections.[2]

IgD is also in low concentrations in the blood. Its primary function is as an antigen receptor on the surface of early B cells.

Molecular Structure

There are three parts to an antibody molecule (Figure 7.4). Two identical fragments have the ability to bind antigen and are termed **antigen-binding fragments (Fabs)**. The third fragment is termed the **crystallizable fragment (Fc)**. The Fab portions contain the recognition sites (receptors) for antigens and confer the molecule's specificity toward a particular antigen. The Fc portion is responsible for most of the biological functions of antibodies.[3]

An immunoglobulin molecule consists of four polypeptide chains: two identical light (L) chains and two identical heavy (H) chains. The different amino acid sequences in the heavy chains determine the class of antibody. The light and heavy chains are held together by noncovalent bonds and covalent disulphide linkages. A set of disulphide bridges between the heavy chains occurs in the hinge region and, in some instances, lends a degree of flexibility at that site.

Furthermore, each L and H chain has constant (C) and variable (V) regions. The constant regions have relatively stable amino acid sequences within a particular immunoglobulin class. Conversely, among different antibodies, the sequences of the variable regions have a large number of amino acid differences, and these variable regions are

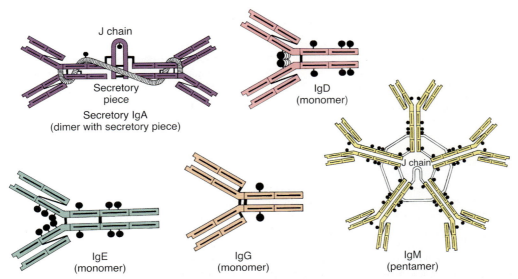

FIGURE 7.3 Structures of Different Immunoglobulins. Secretory IgA, IgD, IgE, IgG, and IgM. The black circles attached to each molecule represent carbohydrate residues.

TABLE 7.2 Properties of Immunoglobulins

Class	Adult Serum Levels (mcmol/L)	Present in Secretions	Complement Activation	Opsonin	Agglutinin	Mast Cell Activation	Placental Transfer
IgG	53–60	+	++	++	+	–	+++
	18–20	+	+	–	+	–	+
	6–6.8	+	+++	++	+	–	+++
	3.3	–	–	–	+	+	++
IgM	1.2–1.5	+	++++	–	++++	–	–
IgA	17.5–18.8	+	–	–	+	–	–
	3.1	+	–	–	+	–	–
	0.3	++++	–	–	+	–	–
IgD	3[a]	–	–	–	–	–	–
IgE	0.03[a]	+	–	–	–	+++	–

[a]Unit of measurement is mg/dL.

sIgA, Secretory immunoglobulin A; – indicates lack of activity; + to ++++ indicate relative activity or concentration.

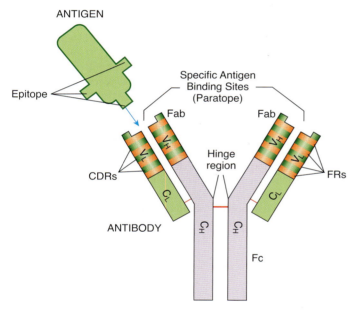

FIGURE 7.4 Antigen–Antibody Binding. *CDRs*, Complementarity determining regions; C_H, constant region heavy chain; C_L, constant region light chain; *Fab*, antigen-binding fragment; *Fc*, crystallizable fragment; *FRs*, framework regions; V_H, variable region heavy chain; V_L, variable region light chain; *red lines* are disulphide linkages.

called **complementarity determining regions (CDRs)**. They determine the specificity of an antibody for a particular antigen. The regions between CDRs are called *framework regions* (FRs), and they have more stable amino acid sequences (see Figure 7.4).

Antigen–Antibody Binding

Because antigens are relatively small, a large molecule (e.g., protein, polysaccharide, nucleic acid) usually contains multiple and diverse antigens. The precise area of the antigen that is recognized by an antibody is its **antigenic determinant**, or **epitope**. Similarly, the matching portion on the antibody is the **antigen-binding site**, or **paratope**. The antigen fits into the antigen-binding site of the antibody with the specificity of a key into a lock and noncovalent chemical interactions keep these bonds in place.

Function of Antibodies

The chief function of antibodies is to protect against infection. Antibodies do this either by *direct* mechanisms—through the action of antibody alone—or *indirect* mechanisms—requiring activation of other components of the innate immune response (Figure 7.5). Direct mechanisms by which antibodies can affect infectious agents or their toxic products include (1) **neutralization** (inactivating or blocking the binding of antigens to receptors), (2) **agglutination** (clumping insoluble particles that are in suspension), or (3) **precipitation** (making a soluble antigen into an insoluble precipitate). For example, many pathogens initiate infection by attaching to specific receptors on cells. Viruses that cause the common cold or the influenza virus must attach to specific receptors on respiratory tract epithelial cells. Some bacteria, such as *Neisseria gonorrhoeae* that causes gonorrhea, must attach to specific sites on urogenital epithelial cells. Antibodies may protect the host by covering sites on the microorganism that are needed for attachment, thereby preventing infection. Furthermore, vaccination with inactivated or attenuated (weakened) viruses, which are designed to induce neutralizing antibody production at the site of the entrance of the virus into the body, can prevent many viral infections. Vaccination against influenza using an inhaled vaccine particularly induces protective IgA in the respiratory tract.

Some bacteria secrete toxins that harm individuals. For example, specific bacterial toxins cause the symptoms of tetanus or diphtheria. Most toxins are proteins that bind to surface molecules on cells and damage those cells. Protective antibodies against the toxin (referred to as *antitoxins*) can bind to the toxins, prevent their interaction with host cells, and neutralize their biological effects (see Chapter 8).

Indirectly, through the Fc portion, antibodies activate components of the innate immune response, including complement and phagocytes (Figure 7.6). Antibody is an opsonin that facilitates phagocytosis of bacteria because phagocytic cells express receptors that bind the Fc portion of antibody. Simultaneous binding of the Fc regions of two adjacent antibodies bound to a microbe activates complement component C1 through the classical pathway. C1 activation then results in activation of the entire cascade.[4] IgM is the best complement-activating antibody, and IgG is the best opsonin. Cloning specific monoclonal antibodies for use in diagnostic tests and therapy is now a common procedure (Box 7.1).

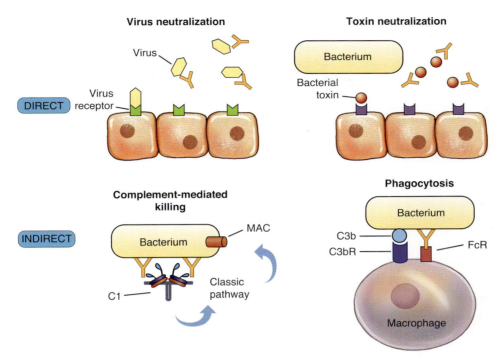

FIGURE 7.5 Direct and Indirect Functions of Antibodies. Protective activities of antibodies can be direct (through the action of antibodies alone) or indirect (requiring activation of other components of the innate immune response), usually through the crystallizable fragment (Fc) region. *Direct* means include neutralization of viruses or bacterial toxins before they bind to receptors on the surface of the host's cells. *Indirect* means include activation of the classical complement pathway through C1, resulting in formation of the membrane attack complex *(MAC)*, or increased phagocytosis of bacteria opsonized with antibody and complement components bound to appropriate surface receptors *(FcR* and *C3bR)*. *C3b,* Large fragment produced from complement component C3; *C3bR,* complement C3b receptor; *FcR,* crystallizable fragment receptor.

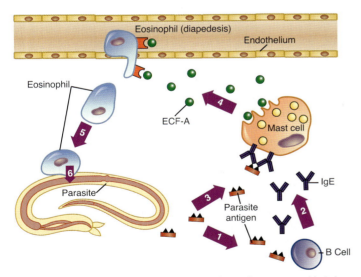

FIGURE 7.6 IgE Function. 1, Soluble antigens from a parasitic infection cause production of IgE antibody by B cells. **2,** Secreted IgE binds to IgE-specific receptors on the mast cell. **3,** Additional soluble parasite antigen cross-links the IgE on the mast cell surface, **4,** leading to mast cell degranulation and release of many proinflammatory products, including eosinophil chemotactic factor of anaphylaxis *(ECF-A)*. **5,** ECF-A attracts eosinophils from the circulation. **6,** The eosinophil attaches to the surface of the parasite and releases potent lysosomal enzymes that damage microorganisms.

BOX 7.1 Monoclonal Antibodies

Most humoral immune responses are polyclonal—that is, the responses involve a mixture of antibodies produced from multiple B cells. Most antigenic molecules have multiple antigenic determinants, each of which induces a different group of antibodies. Thus, a polyclonal response is a mixture of antibody classes, specificities, and function, some of which are more protective than others.

The cloning of one B cell in a laboratory setting results in a monoclonal antibody where the entire antibody is of the same class, specificity, and function. The advantages of monoclonal antibodies are that (1) the single antibody is of known antigenic specificity rather than a mixture of different antibodies; (2) monoclonal antibodies have a single, constant binding affinity; (3) dilution of the monoclonal antibodies in solution (or titre) is more specific because there is only one antibody in solution; and (4) purification of the antibody is easier. Thus, extremely specific and sensitive laboratory tests (e.g., home and laboratory pregnancy tests) and therapies (e.g., for certain infectious diseases or several experimental therapies for cancer) are now available because of the development of highly concentrated antibody with optimal function.

Immunoglobulin E

IgE is a special class of antibody that protects the individual from infection with large parasitic worms (helminths).[5] However, IgE is also the primary cause of common allergies (e.g., hay fever, dust, bee stings) when relatively innocuous environmental antigens (such as pollen, dust, and bee venom) promote its production. Chapter 8 further discusses the role of IgE in allergies.

Large multicellular parasites usually invade mucosal tissues. Many antigens from the parasites induce IgE, as well as other antibody classes. IgG, IgM, and IgA bind to the surface of parasites, activate complement, generate chemotactic factors for neutrophils and macrophages, and serve as opsonins for those phagocytic cells. This response, however, does not greatly damage parasites. The only inflammatory cell that can adequately damage a parasite is the eosinophil. This is because of the special contents of its granules which contain major basic protein, eosinophil cationic protein, eosinophil peroxidase, and eosinophil neurotoxin, each of which can damage infectious worms. IgE is effective for parasitic infections because it specifically initiates an inflammatory reaction that preferentially attracts eosinophils to the site of parasitic infection.

Mast cells in the tissues also have Fc receptors that bind IgE with high specificity and high affinity. IgE antibodies against antigens of the parasite rapidly bind to the mast cell surface. Soluble parasite molecules with multiple antigenic determinants diffuse to neighbouring mast cells and simultaneously bind to multiple IgE molecules. This reaction initiates a cascade of effects that can ultimately kill the parasite. The steps of the cascade are presented in Figure 7.6.

Secretory Immune System

Immunocompetent lymphocytes migrate among secondary lymphoid organs and tissues as part of the **systemic immune system**. Another, partially independent, immune system protects the external surfaces of the body through lacrimal and salivary glands and a network of lymphoid tissues residing in the breasts, bronchi, intestines, and genitourinary tract. This system is the **secretory (mucosal) immune system** (Figure 7.7). Plasma cells in those sites secrete antibodies in bodily secretions such as tears, sweat, saliva, mucus, and breast milk to prevent pathogenic microorganisms from both infecting and penetrating the body's surfaces to cause systemic disease.[6] Alternatively, the microorganisms may reside in the membranes without causing disease, be shed, and cause infection for other individuals. Thus, an individual may become a carrier for a particular infectious organism. For example, in the 1950s two vaccines were developed to prevent infection with poliovirus, which enters through the gastro-intestinal tract. The Sabin vaccine was an oral vaccine that contained an attenuated (i.e., inactivated so as to render relatively harmless) live virus. This route caused a transient, limited infection and induced effective systemic and secretory immunity that prevented both the disease and the establishment of a carrier state. The Salk vaccine, on the other hand, consisted of killed viruses administered by injection in the skin. It induced adequate systemic protection but did not generally prevent an intestinal carrier state. Thus, recipients of the Salk vaccine were protected from disease but could still shed the virus and infect others.

IgA is the dominant **secretory immunoglobulin**, although IgM and IgG also are present in secretions. The primary role of IgA is to prevent the attachment and invasion of pathogens through mucosal membranes, such as those of the gastro-intestinal, pulmonary, and genito-urinary tracts. Plasma cells of the mucosa produce dimeric IgA antibodies containing the J chain. Mucosal epithelium expresses a cell surface immunoglobulin receptor that binds and internalizes IgA. Secretory IgA (sIgA) is the IgA that is bound with the epithelial receptor (secretory piece).

The lymphoid tissues of the secretory immune system are connected. For example, many foreign antigens in a mother's gastro-intestinal tract (e.g., poliovirus) induce secretion of specific antibodies into the breast milk. Colostral antibodies (i.e., those found in the colostrum of breast milk) may protect the nursing newborn against infectious disease agents that enter through the gastro-intestinal tract. Although colostral antibodies provide the newborn with passive immunity against gastro-intestinal infections, they do not provide systemic immunity because transport across the newborn's gut into the bloodstream is discontinued after the first 24 hours of life. Maternal antibodies that pass across the placenta into the fetus before birth provide passive systemic immunity.

IMMUNE RESPONSE: COLLABORATION OF B CELLS AND T CELLS

Generation of Clonal Diversity

The immune response occurs in two phases: (1) generation of clonal diversity and (2) clonal selection (Table 7.3 and see Figure 7.1). *Clonal diversity* is the production of a large population of B cells and T cells before birth that have the capacity to recognize almost any foreign antigen found in the environment. This process mostly occurs in specialized lymphoid organs (the **primary [central] lymphoid organs**): the bone marrow for B cells, and the thymus for T cells.[7] The result is the differentiation of **lymphoid stem cells** into B and T cells with the ability to react against almost any antigen. B and T cells can collectively recognize more than 10^8 different antigenic determinants. The primary lymphoid organs release lymphocytes into the circulation as **immunocompetent** cells that have antigen-binding receptors that allow them to react with antigens and migrate to the circulation and other (secondary) lymphoid organs in the body.

Development of B Lymphocytes

Lymphocytes destined to become B cells circulate through the specialized regions of the bone marrow, where they are exposed to hormones and cytokines that induce proliferation and differentiation into mature (immunocompetent) B cells (see Figure 7.1). Lymphoid stem cells in the bone marrow interact with stromal cells (cells from the connective tissue) through a variety of intercellular adhesion molecules. As the stem cell begins to mature, it progressively develops a variety of necessary surface markers important for the further differentiation and proliferation of the B cell.[8] The next stage in development is formation of the B cell antigen receptor (BCR).

The **B cell antigen receptor (BCR)** is a complex of antibodies bound to the cell surface and other molecules involved in intracellular signalling (Figure 7.8). Its role is to recognize an antigen and communicate that information to the cell's nucleus. The BCRs in immunocompetent cells are membrane-associated IgM (mIgM) and IgD (mIgD) immunoglobulins that have identical specificities for antigens. The mIgM is a monomer rather than the pentamer primarily found in the blood.

As described previously, the variable regions of antibodies, as well as the BCR, contain CDR areas. The diversity of these CDRs is responsible for the variety of antigens that immunocompetent B cells can recognize.[9] The rearrangement of existing DNA during B-cell development in the primary lymphoid organs, a process known as **somatic recombination**, makes this enormous repertoire of specificities possible. Multiple loci in the DNA that encode for the variable regions of immunoglobulins recombine to generate receptors that can collectively recognize and bind to any possible antigen.[9] To create the variable region of a light chain, enzymes encoded by *recombination activating genes* (*RAG-1*, *RAG-2*) rearrange different regions. This cutting and splicing of DNA essentially enables the progeny of a single lymphocyte to synthesize immunoglobulins with identical variable regions. Each lymphocyte, however, has different variable regions because recombination of the DNA varies with each lymphocyte, making each cell unique and able to react with different antigens. The gene for the H chain undergoes similar rearrangement.

Somatic rearrangement of the variable regions will frequently result in a BCR that recognizes the individual's own antigens, which may

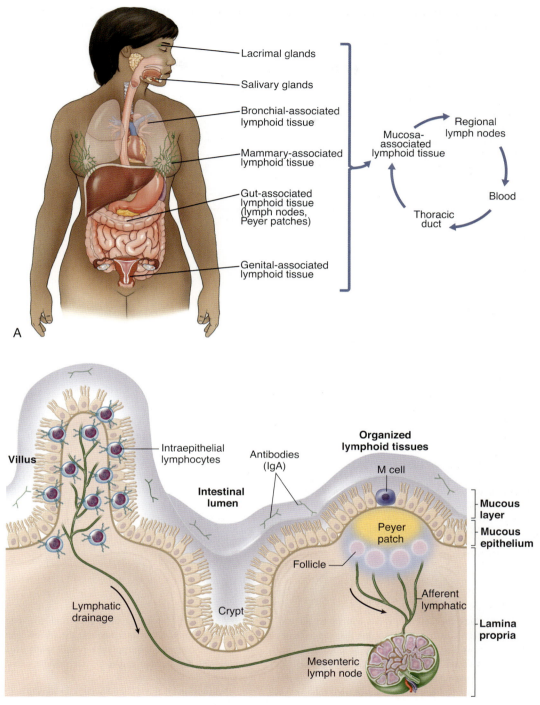

FIGURE 7.7 Secretory Immune System. A, Lymphocytes from the mucosal-associated lymphoid tissues circulate throughout the body in a pattern separate from other lymphocytes. For example, lymphocytes from the gut-associated lymphoid tissue circulate through the regional lymph nodes, the thoracic duct, and the blood and return to other mucosal-associated lymphoid tissues rather than to lymphoid tissue of the systemic immune system. **B,** Lymphoid tissue associated with mucous membranes is called *mucosa-associated lymphoid tissue* (MALT). *M cell,* Microfold cell.

TABLE 7.3 Generation of Clonal Diversity Versus Clonal Selection

	Generation of Clonal Diversity	Clonal Selection
Purpose?	To produce large numbers of T and B cells with maximum diversity of antigen receptors	To select, expand, and differentiate clones of T and B cells against specific antigens
When does it occur?	Primarily in fetus	Primarily after birth and throughout life
Where does it occur?	Central lymphoid organs: thymus for T cells, bone marrow for B cells	Peripheral lymphoid organs, including lymph nodes, spleen, and other lymphoid tissues
Is foreign antigen involved?	No	Yes, the antigen determines which clones of cells will be selected
What hormones or cytokines are involved?	Thymic hormones, IL-7, others	Many cytokines produced by Th cells and APCs
Final product?	Immunocompetent T and B cells that can react with the antigen, but have not seen the antigen, and migrate to secondary lymphoid organs	Plasma cells that produce antibodies, effector T cells that help (Th cells), kill targets (Tc cells), or regulate immune responses (Treg cells); memory B and T cells

APCs, Antigen-presenting cells; *IL-7*, interleukin-7; *Tc cells*, T-cytotoxic cells; *Th cells*, T-helper cells; *Treg cells*, T-regulatory cells.

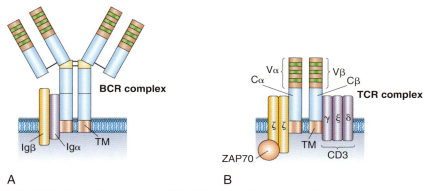

FIGURE 7.8 B Cell Antigen Receptor and T Cell Antigen Receptor. **A,** The antigen receptor on the surface of B cells (B cell antigen receptor *[BCR] complex*) is a monomeric (single) antibody with a structure similar to that of circulating antibody, with an additional transmembrane region *(TM)* that anchors the molecule to the cell surface. The active BCR complex contains molecules *(Igα and Igβ)* that are responsible for intracellular signalling after the receptor has bound antigen. **B,** The T-cell receptor *(TCR)* consists of an α- and a β-chain joined by a disulphide bond. Each chain consists of a constant region *(Cα and Cβ)* and a variable region *(Vα and Vβ)*. Each variable region contains complementarity determining regions and framework regions in a structure similar to that of an antibody.

result in an inadvertent attack on "self" antigens expressed on various tissues and organs, thereby causing autoimmune disease or hypersensitivities. The bone marrow destroys many of these "autoreactive" B cells, with upwards of 90% of developing B cells undergoing apoptosis. This process of **central tolerance** results in immunocompetent B cells that initiate a response against foreign antigens and are "tolerant" to *self-antigens*.

There is also a variety of important surface molecules that develop during B cell differentiation and are characteristic markers for B cells. These include CD21 (a complement receptor) and CD40 (adhesion molecule required for later interactions with T cells).

Development of T Lymphocytes

The process of T-cell proliferation and differentiation is similar to that for B cells (see Figure 7.1). The primary lymphoid organ for T-cell development is the thymus.[10] Lymphoid stem cells journey through the thymus, where, under influence of thymic hormones and the cytokine interleukin-7 (IL-7), they undergo cell division and simultaneously produce receptors (**T cell antigen receptors [TCRs]**) against the diversity of antigens the individual will encounter throughout life. They exit the thymus through the blood vessels and lymphatics as mature (immunocompetent) T cells with antigen-specific receptors on the cell surface and establish residence in secondary lymphoid organs.

Production of the TCR proceeds in a manner very similar to that described earlier for B cells. The most common TCR resembles an antibody Fab region and consists of two protein chains, α- and β-chains, each of which has a variable region and a constant region (see Figure 7.8). The variable regions also undergo somatic recombination. As with the BCR, a set of intracellular signalling molecules coassemble in the membrane with the TCR. The complex of these signalling molecules is called **CD3**.[11] Thus, all immunocompetent T cells can be identified by the presence of CD3 on the surface.

Differentiation of T cells in the thymus also results in expression of a variety of other important surface molecules. Initially, the developing cells express proteins called **CD4** and **CD8** concurrently. Th cells go on to express the CD4 surface protein, whereas Tc cells continue their development to express the CD8 surface protein. Approximately 60%

of immunocompetent T cells in the circulation express CD4 and 40% express CD8.

Central tolerance also occurs in the thymus, where destruction of more than 95% of developing T cells occurs. Like B cells, T cells can also become autoreactive.

Clonal Selection

Antigens initiate the second phase of the immune response, clonal selection. *Clonal selection* is the processing of antigen for a specific immune response. This process involves a complex interaction among cells in the secondary lymphoid organs (see Figure 7.1). *Processing* of most antigens is integral for the initiation of an effective immune response because they cannot react directly with most cells of the immune system. This process begins with *presentation* of the antigen to the immune cells in a specific manner. This is the job of antigen-processing (antigen-presenting) cells (APCs) (usually dendritic cells, macrophages, or similar cells). The interaction among APCs, subpopulations of T cells that facilitate immune responses (Th cells), and immunocompetent B or T cells results in differentiation of B cells into active antibody-producing cells (plasma cells) and T cells into effector cells, such as Tc cells. Both lines also develop into memory cells that respond even faster when that antigen enters the body again. Thus, activation of the immune system produces a long-lasting protection against specific antigens (see Figure 7.1). Defects in any aspect of cellular collaboration can lead to problems with cell-mediated immunity, humoral immunity, or both and, depending on the particular defect, potentially the individual's death from infection (see Chapter 8).

Primary and Secondary Immune Responses

The immune response to an antigen exists in two phases—the primary and secondary responses—and measuring concentrations of circulating antibodies over time differentiates each phase from the other (Figure 7.9). After a single initial exposure to most antigens, there is a latent period, or lag phase, during which clonal selection occurs. After approximately 5 to 7 days, detection of IgM antibody in the circulation is possible. This response is the primary immune response and occurs typically with initial production of IgM followed by production of IgG against the same antigen. The quantity of IgG may be about equal to or less than the amount of IgM. The titre is the amount of antibody in a serum sample, and a higher titre indicates more antibodies. If no further exposure to the antigen occurs, catabolism of the circulating antibody occurs, and measurable quantities fall. The individual's immune system, however, is now ready if there is a re-exposure to the antigen.

A second challenge by the same antigen results in the secondary immune response, where there is more rapid production of a larger amount of antibody than the primary response. The rapidity of the secondary immune response is the result of memory cells that require less further differentiation. IgM may be transiently produced in the secondary response, but IgG production increases considerably, making it the predominant antibody class. Natural infection (e.g., rubella) may even result in measurable levels of protective IgG for the life of the individual. Some vaccines (e.g., polio) also may produce extremely long-lived protection, although most vaccines require boosters at specified intervals.

Antigen Processing and Presentation

For most antigens, the first step in clonal selection is processing and presentation by APCs. *Exogenous antigens* (i.e., existing outside the cell) are usually expressed on large molecules found on microbes, which undergo phagocytosis and destruction by dendritic cells and macrophages. Other antigens, *endogenous antigens*, originate within a virally infected or cancerous cell.

Processing results in the release of small antigenic determinants, which are presented on the surface of APCs by specialized major histocompatibility complex (MHC) molecules. MHC molecules in humans are also called human leukocyte antigens (HLAs) (discussed in more detail in Chapter 8) and have a role in transplantation. MHC molecules are glycoproteins found on the surface of all human cells except red blood cells and exist in two general classes, class I and class II, based on their molecular structure, distribution among cell populations, and function in antigen presentation. MHC class I molecules have a large alpha (α) chain along with a smaller chain called β_2-microglobulin. MHC class II molecules have α- and β-chains that differ from the ones used for MHC class I. A large complex of different genetic loci within genes on human chromosome 6 encode the α- and β-chains of the MHC molecules (Figure 7.10). MHC genes are probably the most

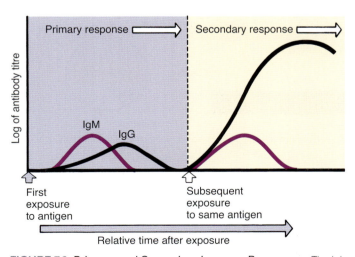

FIGURE 7.9 Primary and Secondary Immune Responses. The initial administration of antigen induces a primary response during which IgM is initially produced, followed by IgG. Another administration of the antigen induces the secondary response in which IgM is transiently produced and larger amounts of IgG are produced over a longer period of time.

Coded on Chromosome 6 HLA Molecules	
Class I MHC Molecules (HLA-A, HLA-B, HLA-C)	**Class II MHC Molecules** (HLA-DR, HLA-DP, HLA-DQ)
Expressed on all nucleated cells and platelets	Expressed only on antigen-presenting cells (APCs): Macrophages Dendritic cells B cells
Presents endogenous antigen	Presents exogenous antigen
Recruits CD8+ Tc-Cells	Recruits CD4+ Th-Cells

T cells recognize antigenic fragments complexed to HLA-encoded molecules as "non-self."

FIGURE 7.10 Antigen-Presenting Molecules. *HLA,* Human leukocyte antigen; *MHC,* major histocompatibility complex; *Tc cells,* T-cytotoxic cells; *Th cells,* T-helper cells.

polymorphic of any human genes; this means that no two individuals, except identical twins, will have a complete set of identical MHC molecules.

MHC class I molecules present endogenous antigens, which are primarily recognized by Tc cells. Because MHC class I molecules are expressed on *all* cells, except red blood cells, any change in that cell caused by viral infection or malignancy may result in presentation of foreign antigens to the immune system. On the other hand, MHC class II molecules present exogenous antigens (Figure 7.11). Th cells preferentially recognize antigens presented by MHC class II molecules to the immune system. Thus, antigen presentation to Tc cells is *MHC class I restricted* and presentation to Th cells is *MHC class II restricted*. A limited number of cells that have APC function, including macrophages and dendritic cells, and B cells can also coexpress both MHC class II molecules and MHC class I molecules.

Thus, the term **antigen processing** relates to the process by which enzymes cut up large exogenous and endogenous antigens into small antigenic fragments that link with the appropriate MHC molecules and are inserted into the membrane of the APC.[12] CD1, which is unrelated to the MHC, frequently presents lipid antigens to the immune system and is not discussed here.

Cellular Interactions in the Immune Response

The second step in clonal selection is a finely tuned set of intercellular collaborations that result in the production of effector cells (plasma cells, Th cells, Tc cells) and memory cells.[13] Each collaboration requires three complementary intracellular signalling events: (1) antigen-specific recognition through the TCR complex, (2) activation of intercellular adhesion molecules, and (3) the response to specific groups of cytokines. Without each signalling event, a protective immune response will not be produced. These signalling events are excessive in the cytokine storm typical of the body's response to COVID-19 infection and are the result of an abundance of cytotoxic CD8 T cells and Th17 T helper cells that further amplify this signal (see Figure 7.12).

T-helper lymphocytes. Regardless of whether an antigen primarily induces a cellular or humoral immune response, APCs usually must present antigens to Th cells. Th cells are the essential controllers of the adaptive immune response. The APC presents antigen which is both held by the polymorphic regions (α1 and β1) of the α- and β-chains of MHC class II molecules,[14] as well as the TCR on the Th cell (see Figure 7.8). More specifically, the strength of the intercellular antigen binding is increased by CD4 on the Th cell, which binds to a nonpolymorphic

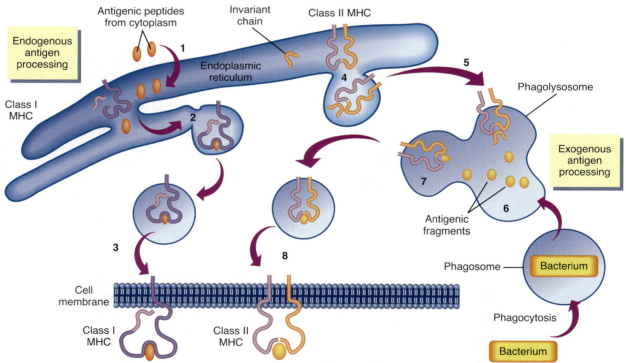

FIGURE 7.11 Antigen Processing. Initiation of most immune responses require antigen processing and presentation. Foreign antigens may be either endogenous (cytoplasmic protein) or exogenous (e.g., bacterium). Endogenous antigenic peptides are transported into the endoplasmic reticulum (ER) where **1,** the major histocompatibility complex *(MHC)* molecules are being assembled. **2,** In the ER, antigenic peptides bind to the α-chains of the MHC class I molecule and **3,** the complex is transported to the cell surface. **4,** The α- and β-chains of the MHC class II molecules are also being assembled in the ER, but the antigen-binding site is blocked by a small molecule (invariant chain) to prevent interactions with endogenous antigenic peptides. **5,** The MHC class II–invariant chain complex is transported to phagolysosomes, where **6,** exogenous antigenic fragments have been produced as a result of phagocytosis. In the phagolysosomes, **7,** the invariant chain is digested and replaced by exogenous antigenic peptides, **8,** after which the MHC class II–antigen complex is inserted into the cell membrane.

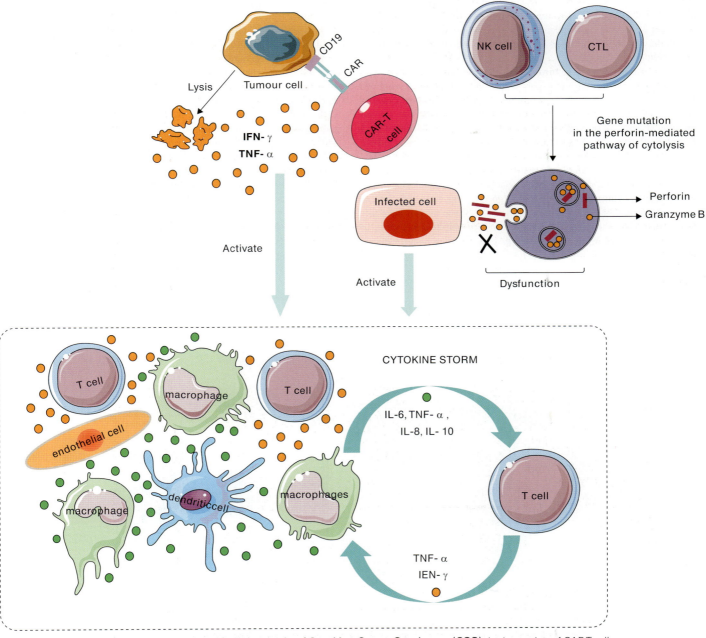

FIGURE 7.12 Proposed Pathogenesis of Cytokine Storm Syndrome (CSS). In the setting of CAR T-cell therapy, CAR T cells can recognize target cells (tumour cells) and induce the lysis of target cells, along with the activation of CAR T cells and T cell, causing a consecutive release of cytokines including IFN-γ or TNF-α. These cytokines trigger a cascade reaction by activation of innate immune cells including macrophages, dendritic cells, and endothelial cells with further cytokine releasing, which finally leads to a cytokine storm. In the setting of hemophagocytic lymphohistiocytosis, a cytokine syndrome where NK cells and cytotoxic T-cells are unable to kill their target cells effectively, mutations in perforin coding genes or genes essential for perforin transport will cause a failure of normal cytolytic function and inability to clear the antigenic stimulus, leading to the persistent activation of macrophages and T cells by the infected cells, accompanied by excessive secretion of proinflammatory cytokines, which finally leads to a cytokine storm. *CAR,* Chimeric antigen receptor; *CTL,* cytotoxic T lymphocytes; *IFN-γ,* interferon-gamma; *IL,* interleukin; *NK cell,* natural killer cell; *TNFα,* tumour necrosis factor-alpha. (From Gao, Y., Xu, G., Wang, B., & Liu, B. [2020]. Cytokine storm syndrome in coronavirus disease 2019: a narrative review. *Journal of Internal Medicine* [Figure 1]. https://onlinelibrary.wiley.com/doi/epdf/10.1111/joim.13144.)

region of the β2 region of the MHC class II molecule. The cytoplasmic portions of CD3 and CD4 interact to activate intracellular signalling pathways. A second costimulatory signal results from the interaction of a variety of adhesion molecules; the most critical is B7 on the APC and CD28 on the Th cell.

The third signal occurs through Th-cell cytokine receptors. The APC secretes IL-1 during the early stages of Th-cell differentiation. IL-1 then creates this signal by binding to the IL-1 receptor on the Th cell (Figure 7.13). The initial differentiation response by the Th cell includes the production of the cytokine IL-2 and upregulation of IL-2 receptors. IL-2 acts in an autocrine (self-stimulating) fashion to induce further maturation and proliferation of the Th cell. Without IL-2 production, the Th cell cannot efficiently mature into a functional helper cell.

At this point and depending on the predominant cytokines in the immediate environment, Th cells undergo differentiation into one of several subsets: Th1, Th2, Th17, or Treg cells.[15] These subsets have different functions: **Th1 cells** preferentially provide help in developing Tc cells (cell-mediated immunity); **Th2 cells** provide more help for developing B cells (humoral immunity); **Th17 cells** are lymphokine-secreting cells that activate macrophages; and **Treg cells** limit the immune response (Treg cells are discussed later in this chapter).[16] The Th subsets differ considerably in the spectrum of cytokines they produce. Additionally, Th1 and Th2 cells may suppress each other so that the immune response may favour either antibody formation, with suppression of a cell-mediated response, or the opposite. For example, antigens derived from viral or bacterial pathogens and those derived from cancer cells seem to induce a greater number of Th1 cells relative to Th2 cells, whereas antigens derived from multicellular parasites and allergens may result in production of more Th2 cells. Many antigens (e.g., tetanus vaccine), however, will produce excellent humoral and cell-mediated responses simultaneously. Th cells are necessary for development of most humoral and cellular immune responses. Moreover, the Th cell is the target of HIV, the human immunodeficiency virus, the virus that causes acquired immune deficiency syndrome (AIDS), and infection with this virus results in life-threatening conditions because Th cells are destroyed, resulting in genetic mutations (and cancer [see Chapter 10]), as well as deficient immune responses to pathogens and foreign antigens (see Chapter 8).

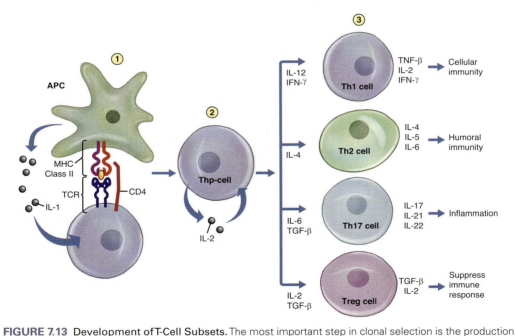

FIGURE 7.13 Development of T-Cell Subsets. The most important step in clonal selection is the production of populations of T-helper cells *(Th1, Th2, and Th17 cells)* and T-regulatory cells *(Treg cells)* that are necessary for the development of cellular and humoral immune responses. In this model, 1, antigen-presenting cells *(APC)* (probably multiple populations) may influence whether 2, a precursor Th cell *(Thp cell)* will differentiate into 3, a Th1, Th2, Th17, or Treg cell. Differentiation of the Thp cell is initiated by three signalling events. The interaction of the T-cell receptor *(TCR)* and CD4 with an antigen presented by major histocompatibility complex *(MHC)* class II molecules creates an antigen signal. Interactions between adhesion molecules also produce a set of costimulatory signals (not shown). The interactions of cytokines (particularly interleukin-1 *[IL-1]*) with appropriate cytokine receptors on the Thp cell produce a third signal. The Thp cell upregulates IL-2 production and expression of the IL-2 receptor, which acts in an autocrine fashion to accelerate Thp cell differentiation and proliferation. Commitment to a particular phenotype results from the relative concentrations of other cytokines. The production of IL-12 and interferon gamma *(IFN-γ)* by some populations of APCs favour differentiation into the Th1 cell phenotype; the production of IL-4 by a variety of cells favours differentiation into the Th2 cell phenotype; IL-6 and transforming growth factor-beta *(TGF-β)* facilitate differentiation into Th17 cells; and IL-2 and TGF-β induce differentiation into Treg cells. The production of cytokines that assist in the differentiation of T-cytotoxic cells, leading to cellular immunity characterizes the Th1 cell, whereas the Th2 cell produces cytokines that favour B-cell differentiation and humoral immunity. Th1 and Th2 cells affect each other through the production of inhibitory cytokines: IFN-γ will inhibit the development of Th2 cells, and IL-4 will inhibit the development of Th1 cells. Th17 cells produce cytokines that affect phagocytes and increase inflammation. Treg cells produce immunosuppressive cytokines that prevent the immune response from being excessive. *TNF-β*, Tumour necrosis factor-beta.

Superantigens. Several pathogenic microorganisms, particularly viruses and bacteria, manipulate the normal interaction between APCs and Th cells to the detriment of the individual and the benefit of the microbe through a group of microbial molecules called **superantigens (SAGs)** that bind to the portion of the TCR outside of its normal antigen-specific binding site, as well as to MHC class II molecules outside of their antigen-presentation sites (Figure 7.14). Some SAGs also react with CD28 on the Th cells and provide a costimulatory signal. Thus, SAGs are not processed by an APC to be presented to an immune cell. This binding, which is independent of antigen recognition, provides a signal for Th-cell activation, proliferation, and cytokine production. The normal antigen-specific recognition between Th cells and APCs results in activation of relatively few cells—only those cells with specific TCRs against that antigen, whereas SAGs activate a large population of Th cells, regardless of antigen specificity, and induce excessive production of cytokines, including IL-2, interferon gamma (IFN-γ), and tumour necrosis factor-alpha (TNF-α). The overproduction of inflammatory cytokines results in symptoms of a systemic inflammatory reaction, including fever, low blood pressure, and, potentially, fatal shock. Some examples of SAGs are the bacterial toxins produced by *Staphylococcus aureus* and *Streptococcus pyogenes* (SAGs that cause toxic shock syndrome and food poisoning).[17]

T-cytotoxic lymphocytes. The differentiation of immunocompetent T cells into effector Tc cells requires similar intercellular communications as described for Th cells, with some very important differences. Rather than interacting with an APC, the immunocompetent Tc cell recognizes antigen presented by MHC class I molecules on the surface of a virus-infected cell or cancerous cell (Figure 7.15). The Tc cell expresses CD8, rather than CD4. CD8 binds to the MHC class I molecule and, as with Th-cell differentiation, the proximity of the CD3 and CD8 cytoplasmic portions activates intercellular signalling pathways. Th1 cells produce cytokine signals, especially IL-2, and activate cytokine receptors on the Tc cells.

B-cell clonal selection. The production of an effective antibody response requires a further sequence of cellular interactions. The immunocompetent B cell is also an APC and expresses surface mIgM and mIgD BCRs (Figure 7.16). Unlike the TCR that can

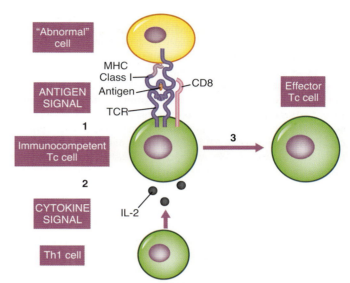

FIGURE 7.15 T-Cytotoxic Cell Clonal Selection. The immunocompetent T-cytotoxic cell *(Tc cell)* can react with the antigen but cannot yet kill target cells. During clonal selection, this cell reacts with the antigen presented by major histocompatibility complex *(MHC)* class I molecules on the surface of a virally infected or cancerous *abnormal* cell. **1,** The T cell antigen receptor *(TCR)* simultaneously recognizes the antigen–MHC class I complex, which binds to the antigen, and CD8, which binds to the MHC class I molecule. **2,** Cytokines provide a separate signal, particularly interleukin-2 *(IL-2)* from T-helper *(Th1)* cells. **3,** In response to these signals, the Tc cell develops into an effector Tc cell with the ability to kill abnormal cells.

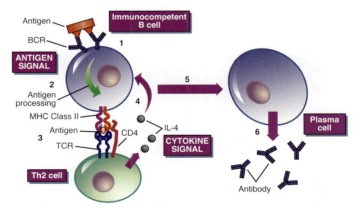

FIGURE 7.16 B-Cell Clonal Selection. Immunocompetent B cells undergo proliferation and differentiation into antibody-secreting plasma cells. **1,** Multiple signals are necessary. The B cell itself can directly bind a soluble antigen through the B cell antigen receptor *(BCR)* and act as an antigen-processing cell. The B cell internalizes the antigen (1), processes it **2,** and then presents it to the T cell antigen receptor *(TCR)* on a T-helper *(Th2)* cell **3,** by major histocompatibility complex *(MHC)* class II molecules **4.** Th2 cell cytokines (e.g., interleukin-4 *[IL-4]*) then react with the B cell **5.** The B cell differentiates into plasma cells that secrete the antibody **6.**

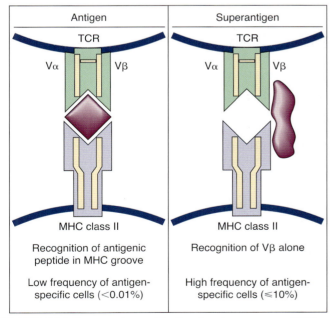

FIGURE 7.14 Superantigens. The T cell antigen receptor *(TCR)* and major histocompatibility complex *(MHC)* class II molecule are normally held together by a processed antigen. Superantigens, such as some bacterial exotoxins, bind directly to the variable region of the TCR-β-chain and the MHC class II molecule. Each superantigen activates sets of Vβ chains independently of the antigen specificity of the TCR. *Vα* and *Vβ*, Variable regions.

only *see* processed and presented antigens, the BCR can react with soluble antigens that have not been processed because they express antibodies with variable binding sites for antigens on their surfaces. B cells also express surface CD21, which is a receptor for opsonins produced by complement activation. Antigen binding through the BCR and CD21 activates the B cell, resulting in internalization, processing, and presentation of antigen fragments by MHC class II molecules.[18] A Th2 cell recognizes the antigen presented on the B cell surface through the TCR and CD4. Antigen and other intercellular adhesion molecules create intercellular bridges that induce the Th2 cell to secrete cytokines (particularly IL-4) that initiate B-cell proliferation and maturation into plasma cells.[19]

A major component of B cell maturation is **class switch**, the process that results in the change in antibody production from one class to another (e.g., IgM to IgG during the primary immune response). Before exposure to antigens and Th2 cells, the B cell produces IgM and IgD, which are used as cell membrane receptors. During the clonal selection process, a B cell proliferates and develops into antibody-secreting plasma cells, and each B cell has the option of becoming a secretor of IgM or changing the class of antibody to a secreted form of IgG, IgA, or IgE. Class switch occurs by another round of somatic recombination with the variable region of the antibody heavy chain combined with a different constant region of the heavy chain. Because the variable region is conserved and the light chain remains unchanged, the antigenic specificity of the antibody also remains unchanged. The particular constant region for each B cell during class switch appears to be, at least partially, under the control of specific Th2 cytokines. For example, IL-4 and IL-13 appear to preferentially stimulate switch to IgE secretion and transforming growth factor-beta (TGF-β) and IL-5 appear to play major roles in class switch to IgA secretion. Thus, during clonal selection, because the stimulating cytokine might differ, a B cell may produce a population of plasma cells that are capable of producing many different classes of antibodies against the same antigen.

Although most antigens require B cells to interact with Th cells, a few antigens can bypass the need for cellular interactions and can directly stimulate B-cell maturation and proliferation. These antigens are called *T-cell–independent antigens* (Figure 7.17). They are mostly bacterial products that are large and are likely to have repeating identical antigenic determinants that bind and cross-link several BCRs. The accumulated intracellular signal is adequate to induce differentiation into a plasma cell but is not adequate to induce a change in the class of antibody produced by the plasma cell. Therefore, T-cell–independent antigens usually induce relatively pure IgM primary and secondary immune responses.

Memory cells. During the clonal selection process, both B cells and T cells differentiate and proliferate into an extremely large population of long-lived memory cells.[20] Memory cells remain inactive until subsequent exposure to the same antigen. Upon re-exposure, these memory cells do not require much further differentiation and will therefore rapidly become new plasma cells or effector T cells without the previously described cellular interactions.

CELL-MEDIATED IMMUNITY

QUICK CHECK 7.3
1. What are antigen-presenting cells?
2. Describe B cell antigen receptors and T cell antigen receptors.
3. What is the role of T-helper cells?
4. Why are cytokines important to the immune response?
5. What is the difference between central tolerance and peripheral tolerance?

Although this chapter has already discussed the relatively straightforward function of antibodies, the function of effector T cells is more complex and involves the principles of intercellular recognition necessary for clonal selection.

T-Lymphocyte Function

The clonal selection process produces several subsets of effector T cells. This chapter has already discussed Th cells and T memory cells. Other effector T cells include Tc cells that attack and destroy cells expressing antigens from intracellular (endogenous) origins, Treg cells that limit (suppress) the immune response, and lymphokine-secreting T cells that secrete cytokines and activate other cells.

T-Cytotoxic Lymphocytes (Tc Cells)

Tc cells are responsible for the cell-mediated destruction of tumour cells or cells infected with viruses. In a fashion similar to intercellular recognition during the clonal selection process, the Tc cell must directly adhere to the target cell through antigen presented by MHC class I molecules and CD8 (Figure 7.18). Because of the broad cellular distribution of MHC class I molecules, Tc cells can recognize antigens on the surface of almost any type of cell that has been infected by a virus or has become cancerous. Unlike clonal selection, the roles of costimulatory signals through adhesion molecules and cytokines are of less importance here. Attachment to a target cell activates multiple killing mechanisms through which the Tc cell induces the target cell to undergo apoptosis.

Various other cells kill targets in a fashion similar to Tc cells. Prominent among these cells are natural killer cells. **Natural killer (NK) cells** are a special group of lymphoid cells that are similar to T cells but lack antigen-specific receptors. Instead, they express a

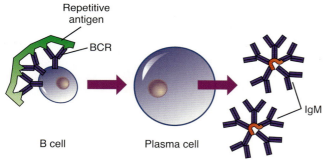

FIGURE 7.17 Activation of a B Cell by a T-Cell–Independent Antigen. Molecules containing repeating identical antigenic determinants may interact simultaneously with several receptors on the surface of the B cell and induce the proliferation and production of immunoglobulins. Because T-helper cells do not participate, class switch does not occur, and the resultant antibody response is IgM. *BCR,* B cell antigen receptor.

inactivation of the NK cell. As such, NK cells complement the effects of Tc cells. In some instances, a virus-infected or cancerous cell will "protect" itself by downregulating MHC class I molecule expression. Without surface MHC class I molecules, a cell becomes resistant to Tc-cell recognition and killing. NK cells primarily kill target cells that have suppressed the expression of MHC class I molecules.

NK cells, as well as some macrophages, can specifically kill targets through use of antibodies. For instance, NK cells express Fc receptors for IgG. If antigens on the infected or cancerous cell bind IgG, the NK cell can attach through Fc receptors and activate its normal killing mechanisms. This is referred to as **antibody-dependent cell-mediated cytotoxicity (ADCC)**.

Lymphokine-Secreting T Cells

Two subsets of Th cells amplify inflammation. Th1 cells, in addition to assisting Tc-cell clonal selection, secrete cytokines that activate M1 macrophages to increase phagocytic and microbial killing functions (described in Chapter 6). The most important cytokine for macrophage activation is IFN-γ. Th2 cells, in addition to assisting B-cell clonal selection, secrete cytokines (e.g., IL-4, IL-13) that activate M2 macrophages for healing and repair of damaged tissue (described in Chapter 6). Th17 cells secrete a set of cytokines (e.g., IL-17, IL-22, chemokines) that recruit phagocytic cells to a site of inflammation.[21] Th17-cell cytokines also may activate cells, particularly epithelial cells, to produce antimicrobial proteins in defence against certain bacterial and fungal pathogens.

T-Regulatory Lymphocytes

Treg cells are a diverse group of T cells that control the immune response, usually suppressing the response and maintaining tolerance against self-antigens.[22] This process of **peripheral tolerance**, in contrast to that of central tolerance (described earlier), occurs in the secondary lymphoid organs and other tissues. This population of Treg cells that differentiate from the Th-cell population expresses CD4 and binds to antigens presented by MHC class II molecules. Unlike other Th cells, however, Treg cells express consistently high levels of CD25 (the IL-2 receptor). TGF-β and IL-2 primarily control the differentiation of the Th precursor cell. Treg cells also produce very high levels of immunosuppressive cytokines TGF-β and IL-10, which generally decrease Th1 and Th2 activity by suppressing antigen recognition and Th-cell proliferation, are listed in the following *Pediatric Considerations* and *Geriatric Considerations* boxes contain age-related mechanisms of self-defence in the newborn child and in older persons respectively.

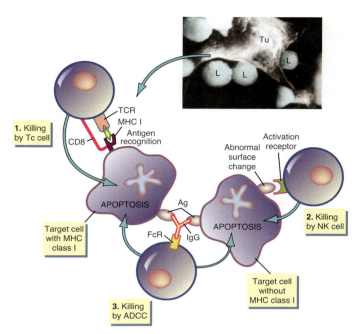

FIGURE 7.18 Cellular Killing Mechanisms. Several cells have the capacity to kill abnormal (e.g., virally infected, cancerous) target cells. **1,** T-cytotoxic cells *(Tc cells)* recognize an endogenous antigen presented by major histocompatibility complex *(MHC)* class I molecules. The Tc cell mobilizes multiple killing mechanisms that induce apoptosis of the target cell. **2,** Natural killer *(NK)* cells identify and kill target cells through receptors that recognize abnormal surface changes. NK cells specifically kill targets that do not express surface MHC class I molecules. **3,** Several cells, including macrophages and NK cells, can kill by antibody-dependent cell-mediated cytotoxicity *(ADCC)*. IgG antibodies bind to the foreign antigen *(Ag)* on the target cell, and cells involved in ADCC bind IgG through crystallizable fragment receptors *(FcR)* and initiate killing. The insert is a scanning electron microscopic view of Tc cells *(L)* attacking a much larger tumour cell *(Tu)*. (Insert from Abbas, A., & Lichtman, A. [2003]. *Cellular and molecular immunology* [5th ed.]. Saunders.)

variety of cell surface activation receptors (similar to pattern recognition receptors, see Chapter 6) that identify protein changes on the surface of cells infected with viruses or that have become cancerous. After attachment, the NK cell kills its target in a manner similar to that of Tc cells. NK cells also have receptors for MHC class I molecules. However, NK cells lack CD8, and binding to MHC class I molecules results in

PEDIATRIC CONSIDERATIONS
Age-Related Factors Affecting Mechanisms of Self-Defence in the Newborn Child

- The placenta transports maternal IgG antibodies into the fetal blood that protect the neonate for the first 6 months, after which the child is able to produce their own antibodies.
- Maternal antibodies provide protection within the newborn's circulation (see the figure in this box).
- Deficits in specific maternal transplacental antibody may lead to a tendency to develop severe, overwhelming sepsis and meningitis in the newborn.
- Normal human newborns are immunologically immature; they have deficient antibody production, phagocytic activity, and complement activity, especially components of alternative pathways (e.g., factor B).
- The newborn cannot produce all classes of antibody; the newborn produces IgM (develops in the last trimester) to in utero infections (e.g., cytomegalovirus, rubella virus, and *Toxoplasma gondii*), and only limited amounts of IgA; IgG production begins after birth and rises steadily throughout the first year of life.
- Neonates often have transiently depressed inflammatory function, particularly neutrophil chemotaxis and alternative complement pathway activity.
- The T-cell–independent immune response is adequate in the fetus and neonate, but the T-cell–dependent immune response develops slowly during the first 6 months of life.

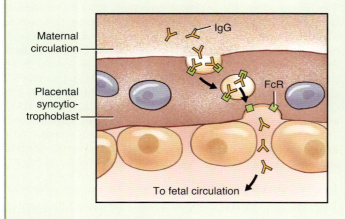
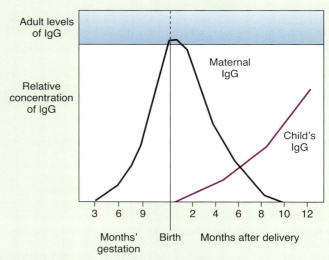

Antibody Levels in Umbilical Cord Blood and in Neonatal Circulation. Early in gestation, maternal IgG begins active transport across the placenta and enters the fetal circulation. At birth, the fetal circulation may contain nearly adult levels of IgG, which is almost exclusively from the maternal source. The fetal immune system has the capacity to produce IgM and small amounts of IgA before birth (not shown). After delivery, rapid destruction of maternal IgG occurs, and neonatal IgG production increases. *FcR*, Crystallizable fragment receptor.

GERIATRIC CONSIDERATIONS
Age-Related Factors Affecting Mechanisms of Self-Defence in Older Persons

- Immune function decreases with age; diminished T-cell function and reduced antibody responses to antigenic challenges occur with age.
- The thymus reaches maximum size at sexual maturity and then undergoes involution until it is a vestigial remnant by middle age; by 45 to 50 years of age, the thymus is only 15% of its maximum size.
- With age, there is a decrease in thymic hormone production and the organ's ability to mediate T-cell differentiation.
- T-cell function and antibody production are somewhat deficient in older persons. Older persons also tend to have increased levels of circulating autoantibodies (antibodies against self-antigens).
- Older persons are at risk for impaired wound healing, usually because of chronic illnesses.
- Older persons are less susceptible to the effect of vaccines.

DID YOU UNDERSTAND?

Third Line of Defence: Adaptive Immunity

1. Adaptive immunity is a state of protection, primarily against infectious agents, that differs from inflammation by being slower to develop, being more specific, and having memory that makes it much longer lived.
2. The cells of the innate system most often initiate the adaptive immune response. These cells process and present portions of invading pathogens (i.e., antigens) to lymphocytes in peripheral lymphoid tissue.

3. Two different types of lymphocytes—B cells and T cells—mediate the adaptive response. Each has distinct functions. B cells are responsible for humoral immunity and production of circulating antibodies (immunoglobulins), whereas T cells are responsible for cell-mediated immunity, in which they kill targeted cells directly or stimulate the activity of other leukocytes.
4. Adaptive immunity can be either active or passive, depending on whether immune response components originated in the host or came from a donor.
5. The humoral immune response consists of molecules (antibodies) produced by B cells.
6. The induction of an immune response, or clonal selection, begins when antigen enters the individual's body.

Antigens and Immunogens
1. Antigens are molecules that bind and react with components of the immune response, such as antibodies and antigen receptors on B and T cells. Most antigens can induce an immune response, and these antigens are called *immunogens*.
2. All immunogens are antigens but not all antigens are immunogens.
3. Large molecules, such as proteins, polysaccharides, and nucleic acids, are most immunogenic. Thus, molecular size is an important factor for antigen immunogenicity.
4. Haptens are antigens too small to be immunogens by themselves but become immunogenic after combining with larger molecules.

Antibodies
1. Antibodies are plasma glycoproteins that can be classified by chemical structure and biological activity as IgG, IgM, IgA, IgE, or IgD.
2. A typical antibody molecule has two identical heavy (H) chains and two identical light (L) chains, as well as two antigen-binding fragment portions (Fab) that bind antigen and a crystalline fragment portion (Fc) that interacts with complement or receptors on cells.
3. The antigenic determinant, or epitope, is the precise chemical structure with which an antibody or B cell or T cell antigen receptor reacts.
4. The protective effects of antibodies may be *direct* through the action of antibody alone or *indirect* requiring activation of other components of the innate immune response.
5. IgE is a special class of antibody produced against environmental antigens that are the primary cause of common allergies. It also protects the individual from infection caused by large parasitic worms (helminths).
6. The secretory immune system protects the external surfaces of the body by secreting antibodies in bodily secretions, such as tears, sweat, saliva, mucus, and breast milk. IgA is the dominant secretory immunoglobulin.

Immune Response: Collaboration of B Cells and T Cells
1. The generation of clonal diversity results in production of B and T cells with receptors against millions of antigens that possibly will be encountered in an individual's lifetime. This process occurs in the fetus in the primary lymphoid organs: the thymus for T cells and portions of the bone marrow for B cells.
2. The generation of clonal diversity concludes when immunocompetent T and B cells migrate from the primary lymphoid organs into the circulation and secondary lymphoid organs to await antigen.
3. Lymphoid stem cells interact with stromal cells through a variety of adhesion factors. As the stem cell matures, it develops a variety of surface markers or receptors, one of the earliest being interleukin-7 (IL-7) receptor. IL-7, produced by stromal cells, is critical for driving differentiation and proliferation of the B cell.
4. The role of the B cell antigen receptor (BCR) is to recognize an antigen and communicate that information to the cell's nucleus.
5. The variable regions of antibodies, as well as the BCR, contain complementarity determining regions (CDRs). The diversity of these CDRs is responsible for the variety of antigens recognized by immunocompetent B cells. The enormous repertoire of antibody specificities is made possible by rearrangement of existing DNA during B-cell development in the primary lymphoid organs, a process called *somatic recombination*.
6. Somatic rearrangement of the antibody variable regions will frequently result in a BCR that recognizes the individual's own antigens, which may result in attack on "self" antigens expressed on various tissue and organs. Many of these "autoreactive" B cells are eliminated in the bone marrow. Most of the developing B cells undergo apoptosis. This entire process is referred to as *central tolerance*.
7. The process of T-cell proliferation and differentiation is similar to that for B cells. The primary lymphoid organ for T-cell development is the thymus. Lymphoid stem cells travel through the thymus, where thymic hormones and the cytokine IL-7 promote lymphoid stem cell division and the production of receptors. They exit the thymus as mature immunocompetent T cells with antigen-specific receptors on the cell surface.
8. The T cell antigen receptor (TCR) proceeds in a manner similar to the BCR. Initially proteins called CD4 and CD8 are expressed on the developing cells. Eventually CD4 cells develop into T-helper cells (Th cells) and CD8 cells become T-cytotoxic cells (Tc cells). Other mature T cells include T-regulatory cells (Treg cells) and memory cells.
9. Most antigens must first interact with antigen-presenting cells (APCs) (e.g., macrophages). Dendritic cells present in the skin, mucosa, and lymphoid tissues also present antigens.
10. The response to antigens can be divided into two phases: primary immune response and secondary immune response. The primary immune response of humoral immunity is usually dominated by IgM, with lesser amounts of IgG. The secondary immune response has a more rapid production of a larger number of antibodies, predominantly IgG.
11. APCs process antigens and present them on the cell surface using molecules of the major histocompatibility complex (MHC). The particular MHC molecule (class I or class II) that presents the antigen determines which cell will respond to that antigen. Th cells require that the antigen be presented in a complex with MHC class II molecules. Tc cells require that the antigen be presented by MHC class I molecules.
12. Th cells consist of Th1 cells, which help Tc cells respond to antigens; Th2 cells, which help B cells develop into plasma cells; and Th17 cells, which help activate macrophages.
13. Tc cells bind to and kill cellular targets such as cells infected with viruses or cancer cells.
14. The T cell sees the presented antigen through the TCR and accessory molecules (CD4 or CD8). CD4 is found on Th cells and reacts specifically with MHC class II molecules. CD8 is found on Tc cells and reacts specifically with MHC class I molecules.
15. The natural killer (NK) cell has some characteristics of the Tc cells and is important for killing target cells in which viral infection or malignancy has resulted in the loss of cellular MHC molecules.
16. Self-antigens are antigens on an individual's own cells. The individual's immune system does not normally recognize self-antigens as immunogenic, and this condition is known as peripheral tolerance.

8

Infection and Defects in Mechanisms of Defence

Stephanie Zettel, with originating chapter contributions by Valentina L. Brashers and Sue E. Huether

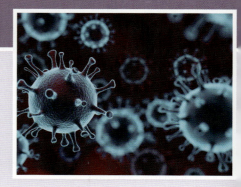

Additional resources are available online at http://evolve.elsevier.com/Canada/Huether/pathophysiology

CHAPTER OUTLINE

Infection, 177
  Microorganisms and Humans: A Dynamic Relationship, 177
  Countermeasures Against Infectious Microorganisms, 188
Deficiencies in Immunity, 191
  Initial Clinical Presentation, 191
  Primary (Congenital) Immune Deficiencies, 191
  Secondary (Acquired) Immune Deficiencies, 194
  Evaluation and Care of Those With Immune Deficiency, 194
  Replacement Therapies for Immune Deficiencies, 194
  AIDS, 195
Hypersensitivity: Allergy, Autoimmunity, and Alloimmunity, 199
  Mechanisms of Hypersensitivity, 200
  Antigenic Targets of Hypersensitivity Reactions, 208
CASE STUDY, 213

LEARNING OBJECTIVES

1. Describe the factors influencing infection by a pathogen.
2. Compare bacterial, viral, and fungal infections, including manifestations.
3. Explain how live, attenuated, and killed vaccines differ, as well as their relative risks and benefits.
4. Explain how bacterial resistance to antibiotics occurs.
5. Discuss the different congenital and acquired immune deficiencies.
6. Discuss the pathogenesis of acquired immune deficiency syndrome (AIDS).
7. Describe clinical symptoms that indicate potential human immunodeficiency virus (HIV) infection and its progression to AIDS.
8. Describe the treatment for AIDS.
9. Define the three stimuli of hypersensitivity: allergy, autoimmunity, and alloimmunity (also known as isoimmunity).
10. Describe and compare the four types of hypersensitivity reactions.
11. Describe how an individual becomes sensitized to an allergen in type I hypersensitivity reactions.
12. Describe the common clinical manifestations of allergy reactions and the underlying histological processes.
13. Differentiate between immediate and delayed hypersensitivities and give an example of each.
14. Define autoimmune disease and give an example.
15. Define alloimmune disease and give an example.
16. Discuss the different types of blood group antigens and the issues concerning blood type compatibility for blood transfusions.
17. Discuss the importance of the Rh antigen for women of childbearing age.
18. Discuss the significance of human leukocyte antigen (HLA, also known as major histocompatibility complex) in tissue or organ transplants.

KEY TERMS

ABO blood group, 210
Acquired immunodeficiency syndrome (AIDS), 195
Acute rejection, 212
Adenosine deaminase deficiency (ADA deficiency), 193
Agammaglobulinemia, 193
Allergen, 208
Allergy, 199
Allergic, 200
Alloimmune disease, 199
Alloimmunity, 199
Anaphylaxis, 200
Ankylosing spondylitis (AS), 208
Antibiotic resistance, 183
Antibody-dependent cell-mediated cytotoxicity (ADCC), 205
Antigenic drift, 185
Antigenic shift, 185
Antigenic variation, 185
Antitoxin, 182
Arthus reaction, 207
Atopic, 204
Attenuated virus, 190
Autoimmune disease, 199
Autoimmunity, 199
Bacteremia, 183
Bare lymphocyte syndrome, 193
β-Lactamase, 183
Biofilms, 179
Blood group antigen, 210
Bruton agammaglobulinemia, 193
C3 deficiency, 194
CCR5 antagonist, 197
Chronic granulomatous disease (CGD), 193
Chronic mucocutaneous candidiasis, 194
Chronic rejection, 212
Combined deficiencies, 192
Communicability, 178
Contact dermatitis, 208
Cryoglobulins, 207
Defects in innate immunity, 192
Delayed hypersensitivity reaction, 200
Delayed hypersensitivity skin test, 208
Dermatophyte, 185
Desensitization, 208
DiGeorge syndrome, 193
Dimorphic fungus (*pl.*, fungi), 185
Endotoxic shock, 183
Endotoxin (lipopolysaccharide [LPS]), 183
Erythema, 208

CHAPTER 8 Infection and Defects in Mechanisms of Defence

Exotoxin, 182
Graft-versus-host disease (GVHD), 194
Herd immunity, 190
Highly active antiretroviral therapy (HAART), 198
Histamine, 203
HIV fusion inhibitor, 197
HIV integrase, 196
HIV integrase inhibitor, 197
HIV protease, 196
HIV protease inhibitor, 197
Human immunodeficiency virus (HIV), 195
Human leukocyte antigen (HLA), 194
Hyperacute rejection, 212
Hypersensitivity, 199
Hypogammaglobulinemia, 193
Immediate hypersensitivity reaction, 200
Immune deficiency, 191
Immunogenicity, 190
Induration, 208
Infectious diseases, 177
Infectivity, 178
Influenza, 183
Isohemagglutinin, 211
Major histocompatibility complex (MHC), 193
Mannose-binding lectin (MBL) deficiency, 194
Mesenchymal stem cell (MSC), 194
Methicillin-resistant *Staphylococcus aureus* (MRSA), 183
Multiple-antibiotic resistance, 189
Mycosis (*pl.*, mycoses), 185
Parasitic microorganisms, 186
Passive immunotherapy, 191
Pathogenicity, 178
Phagocytic defects, 192
Portal of entry, 178
Predominantly antibody deficiency, 193
Primary (congenital) immune deficiency, 191
Raynaud phenomenon, 207
Reverse transcriptase, 196
Reverse transcriptase inhibitor, 197
Rh blood group, 211
Secondary (acquired) immune deficiency, 191
Selective IgA deficiency, 193
Sepsis, 183
Septicemia, 183
Serum sickness, 205
Severe combined immunodeficiency (SCID), 192
Severe congenital neutropenia, 193
Systemic lupus erythematosus (SLE), 209
Tissue-specific antigen, 204
Tolerance, 209
Toxigenicity, 178
Toxoid, 190
Tropism, 183
Type I hypersensitivity, 200
Type II hypersensitivity, 204
Type III hypersensitivity, 205
Type IV hypersensitivity, 207
Universal donor, 211
Universal recipient, 211
Urticaria (hives), 203
Vaccination, 190
Vaccine, 190
Virulence, 178
Wheal and flare reaction, 203
Wiskott-Aldrich syndrome (WAS), 193
X-linked SCID, 193
Zoonotic infection, 183

The defensive system of the body is a finely tuned network, but it is not perfect. Sometimes infectious agents can inhibit or escape defence mechanisms, or the system may break down, leading to inadequate protection or inappropriate activation. An inadequate response (commonly called an *immune deficiency*) may range from relatively mild defects to life-threatening severity. Inappropriate responses (hypersensitivity reactions) may be (1) exaggerated against noninfectious environmental substances (allergy); (2) misdirected against the body's own cells (autoimmunity); or (3) directed against beneficial foreign tissues, such as transfusions or transplants (alloimmunity). Several of these inappropriate responses can be serious or life-threatening. This chapter provides an overview of conditions under which human protective systems can fail.

INFECTION

> **QUICK CHECK 8.1**
> 1. How do antigenic changes in viral pathogens promote disease?
> 2. What are three mechanisms pathogens use to block the immune system?
> 3. What is the difference between an endotoxin and an exotoxin?
> 4. How do bacteria develop antibiotic resistance?

Efforts in the prevention and treatment of infectious disease have come a long way. In Canada, heart disease and malignancies greatly surpass infectious disease as major causes of death.[1] However, since the severe acute respiratory syndrome (SARS) epidemic that took place in 2003, and most recently, the novel coronavirus, COVID-19, in 2019–2021, the challenge of treating infectious diseases has become a key issue. Hospitals have implemented measures geared toward controlling health care–associated infections.[2] Most deaths related to infections occur in individuals whose protective systems are compromised (children, older persons, and those with chronic disease).

Infectious disease remains a significant threat to life in many parts of the world, including India, Africa, and Southeast Asia.[3] Sanitary living conditions, clean water, uncontaminated food, vaccinations, and antimicrobial medications have improved the health of many; but inefficient health care systems, endemic poverty, political unrest, and other factors have slowed progress in some regions. As a result of initiatives to prevent and treat infectious diseases, smallpox no longer exists (the last reported case was in 1975 in Somalia). Worldwide, the incidence of polio is down by more than 99%, with no cases in the Western hemisphere.[4] Although vaccines and antimicrobials have diminished the frequency of some infectious diseases such as measles, new diseases have emerged, such as West Nile virus, SARS, Middle East respiratory syndrome coronavirus (MERS-CoV), *Hantavirus*, and most recently, COVID-19. Some diseases have spread uncontrollably, such as Ebola virus disease into new regions of Africa, and the global pandemic of COVID-19, for which there is now an mRNA-based vaccine and an Adenovirus vector vaccine (AstraZeneca) (see Chapter 7). The resurgence of measles because of vaccine hesitancy (concerns related to side-effects of vaccines) poses an additional risk. As well, many multiple medication–resistant microorganisms continue to develop. All of these examples reflect the ongoing intense challenges in the struggle to prevent and control infectious diseases.

In Canada, First Nations people and the Inuit have higher rates of contagious disease, resulting in shorter life expectancies. Human immunodeficiency virus (HIV)/acquired immunodeficiency syndrome (AIDS), influenza, West Nile virus, and tuberculosis (TB) are just a few of the common conditions found in the Indigenous population[5] (see *Health Promotion:* Tuberculosis and the Indigenous Population in Canada).

Microorganisms and Humans: A Dynamic Relationship

In particular, the increase in antibiotic resistance places more importance on maintenance of an intact inflammatory and immune system. Individuals with immune deficiencies become easily infected with opportunistic microorganisms—those that normally would not cause disease but seize the opportunity provided by the person's decreased immune or inflammatory responses.

True pathogens have devised means to circumvent the normal controls provided by the innate and adaptive immune

HEALTH PROMOTION

Tuberculosis and the Indigenous Population in Canada

Indigenous people have one of the highest rates of tuberculosis (TB) in Canada. In 2017, the rate of active TB in Canada was 4.9 per 100 000 people, yet the rate of active TB among the Indigenous people in Canada was 21.4 per 100 000 population. The poor living conditions on many reserves partially explains the rate of TB incidence in the Indigenous population. For example, homes on reserves are often overcrowded and poorly ventilated. A lack of proper nutrition can further increase the risk for those with latent TB infection to progress to an active disease state. Many individuals in First Nations communities also have pre-existing comorbidities such as diabetes and HIV that further contribute to this risk. Moreover, many of these communities are remote and isolated, which results in decreased access to health care services.

In 2014, the federal government developed a framework for action to lower the incidence of TB in Canada. The key areas of focus for this framework are:

1. Optimizing and enhancing current efforts to prevent and control active TB disease
2. Facilitating the identification and treatment of latent TB infection for those at high risk for developing active TB disease
3. Championing collaborative action to address the underlying risk factors for TB

The report *Tuberculosis Prevention and Control in Canada: A Federal Framework for Action* presents the federal government's framework for action and associated initiatives in relation to addressing TB in Canada.

From Public Health Agency of Canada. (2014). *Tuberculosis Prevention and Control in Canada: A Federal Framework for Action.* http://www.phac-aspc.gc.ca/tbpc-latb/pubs/tpc-pct/assets/pdf/tpc-pcta-eng.pdf; Government of Canada. (2019). *Tuberculosis: Monitoring.* https://www.canada.ca/en/public-health/services/diseases/tuberculosis/surveillance.html.

TABLE 8.1 Classes of Microorganisms That Are Infectious to Humans

Class	Size	Site of Reproduction	Example
Virus	20–300 nm	Intracellular	Poliomyelitis
Chlamydiae	200–1 000 nm	Intracellular	Urethritis
Rickettsiae	300–1 200 nm	Intracellular	Rocky Mountain spotted fever
Mycoplasma	125–350 nm	Extracellular	Atypical pneumonia
Bacteria	0.8–15 mcg	Skin	Staphylococcal wound infection
		Mucous membranes	Cholera
		Extracellular	Streptococcal pneumonia
		Intracellular	Tuberculosis
Fungi	2–200 mcg	Skin	Tinea pedis (athlete's foot)
		Mucous membranes	Candidiasis (e.g., thrush)
		Extracellular	Sporotrichosis
		Intracellular	Histoplasmosis
Protozoa	1–50 mm	Mucosal	Giardiasis
		Extracellular	Sleeping sickness
Helminths	3 mm to 10 m	Intracellular	Trichinosis
		Extracellular	Filariasis

systems. Several factors influence the capacity of a pathogen to cause disease:

- **Communicability**: The ability to spread from one individual to others (e.g., measles and pertussis spread very easily; HIV is of lower communicability)
- **Infectivity**: The ability of the pathogen to invade and multiply in the host (e.g., herpes simplex virus can survive for long periods in a latent stage)
- **Virulence**: The capacity of a pathogen to cause severe disease (e.g., measles virus is of low virulence; rabies and Ebola viruses are highly virulent)
- **Pathogenicity**: The ability of an agent to produce disease—success depends on communicability, infectivity, extent of tissue damage, and virulence (e.g., HIV can kill T lymphocytes [T cells])
- **Portal of entry**: The route by which a pathogenic microorganism infects the host (e.g., direct contact, inhalation, ingestion, or bites of an animal or insect)
- **Toxigenicity**: The ability to produce soluble toxins or endotoxins, factors that greatly influence the pathogen's degree of virulence

The ability of pathogens to attach to cell surfaces increases their infectivity. Other features that influence their infectivity are the release of enzymes that dissolve protective barriers, a rapid rate of cell division, and their ability to escape the action of phagocytes, or resist the effect of low pH (as in *H. pylori* infection of the stomach). After penetrating protective barriers (invasion), pathogens then multiply and spread through the lymph and blood to tissues and organs, where they continue multiplying and cause disease. In humans the route of entry of many pathogenic microorganisms also becomes the site of shedding of new infectious agents to other individuals, completing a cycle of infection.

Microorganisms that range in size from 20 nm (poliovirus) to 10 m (tapeworm) can cause infectious disease. Table 8.1 summarizes the different classes and characteristics of pathogenic microorganisms. Table 8.2 summarizes some mechanisms of tissue damage caused by microorganisms. Chapters 6 and 7 describe the multiple layers of defence against infection. Furthermore, Table 8.3 contains examples of microorganisms that defeat our protective systems.

Bacterial Disease

Bacteria are prokaryotes in that they lack a discrete nucleus, and they are relatively small. They can be aerobic or anaerobic and motile or immotile. Spherical bacteria are *cocci*, rodlike forms are *bacilli*, and spiral forms are *spirochetes*. Gram stain differentiates the microorganisms as Gram-positive or Gram-negative bacteria. Table 8.4 lists examples of human diseases caused by specific bacteria. Figure 8.1 reviews the general structure of bacteria.

Bacterial survival and growth depend on the effectiveness of the body's defence mechanisms and on the bacterium's ability to resist these defences. Substantial information is available on the subject of bacterial pathogenesis. *Staphylococcus aureus* is a good example of how one species of bacteria has adapted to become a life-threatening pathogen.

S. aureus is a major cause of hospital-acquired (health care–associated) infections and is now spreading throughout communities. This microorganism is a common commensal inhabitant of normal skin and nasal passages (estimates indicate that from 30 to 80% of individuals may be nasal carriers) which derives some benefit (i.e., food and nourishment) from inhabiting the skin without harming the organism, and its main method of transmission is through direct skin-to-skin contact or contact with shared items or surfaces of contaminated individuals (e.g., towels, used bandages).[6]

TABLE 8.2 Examples of Microorganisms That Cause Tissue Damage

Pathogens That Directly Cause Tissue Damage

Produce Exotoxin

Streptococcus pyogenes	Tonsillitis, scarlet fever
Staphylococcus aureus	Boils, toxic shock syndrome, food poisoning
Corynebacterium diphtheria	Diphtheria
Clostridium tetani	Tetanus
Vibrio cholerae	Cholera

Produce Endotoxin

Escherichia coli	Gram-negative sepsis
Haemophilus influenzae	Meningitis, pneumonia
Salmonella typhi	Typhoid
Shigella	Bacillary dysentery
Pseudomonas aeruginosa	Wound infection
Yersinia pestis	Plague

Cause Direct Damage With Invasion

Variola	Smallpox
Varicella-zoster	Chickenpox, shingles
Hepatitis B virus	Hepatitis
Poliovirus	Poliomyelitis
Measles virus	Measles, subacute sclerosing panencephalitis
Influenza virus	Influenza
Herpes simplex virus	Cold sores

Pathogens That Indirectly Cause Tissue Damage

Produce Immune Complexes

Hepatitis B virus	Kidney disease
Streptococcus pyogenes	Glomerulonephritis
Treponema pallidum	Kidney damage in secondary syphilis
Most acute infections	Transient renal deposits

Cause Cell-Mediated Immunity

Mycobacterium tuberculosis	Tuberculosis
Mycobacterium leprae	Tuberculoid leprosy
Lymphocytic choriomeningitis virus	Aseptic meningitis
Borrelia burgdorferi	Lyme arthritis
Herpes simplex virus	Herpes stromal keratitis

Data modified from Janeway, C. A., Travers, P., Walport, M., et al. (2001). *Immunobiology: the system in health and disease* (5th ed.). Garland.

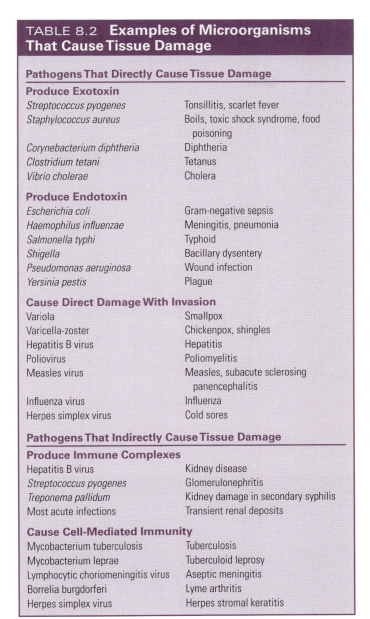

FIGURE 8.1 General Structure of Bacteria. A, The structure of the bacterial cell wall determines its staining characteristics with Gram stain. A Gram-positive bacterium has a thick layer of peptidoglycan *(left)*. A Gram-negative bacterium has a thick peptidoglycan layer and an outer membrane *(right)*. B, Example of a Gram-positive (darkly stained microorganisms, *arrow*) group A *Streptococcus*. This microorganism consists of cocci that frequently form chains. C, Example of a Gram-negative (pink microorganisms, *arrow*) *Neisseria meningitides* in cerebrospinal fluid. *Neisseria* form complexes of two cocci (diplococci). ([A] from Murray, P. R., Rosenthal, K. S., & Pfaller, M. A. [2013]. *Medical microbiology* [7th ed.]. Saunders; [B], [C] from Murray, P. R., Rosenthal, K. S., Kobayashi, G. S., et al. [2002]. *Medical microbiology* [4th ed.]. Mosby.)

S. aureus is one example of an opportunistic pathogen in that it is well-equipped to act as a life-threatening pathogen when the opportunity arises. Skin infections may occur at sites of trauma, such as cuts and abrasions, and at areas of the body covered by hair (e.g., back of neck, groin, buttock, armpit, beard area of men). Most infections are relatively mild and localized, appearing as red and swollen pustules on the skin, containing pus or other drainage. They can develop into abscesses, boils, carbuncles, cellulitis, or furunculosis. Invasive disease may originate from wound infections (e.g., trauma, surgical wounds, indwelling medical devices, prosthetic joints) and lead to fatal septicemia and abscesses in internal organs (e.g., lungs, kidney, bones, skeletal muscle, meninges, or heart) (Figure 8.2).

Microscopically, staphylococci are Gram-positive cocci that generally grow in grapelike clusters. However, this microorganism possesses a myriad of potential virulence factors that determine the severity, location, and clinical features of infection. It should be noted that individual strains of this opportunistic pathogen manifest only some of the entire array of virulence factors.

Microorganisms frequently exist as part of complex multicellular masses called *biofilms*. **Biofilms** consist of mixed species of microorganisms, including bacteria, fungi, and viruses. Growth of bacteria in biofilms offers survival advantage by protection from the host's responses and exposure to antibiotics. These structures are associated with otitis media; urinary tract infections secondary to indwelling catheters; foot ulcers in diabetic persons; infected burn wounds; vaginitis; osteomyelitis; pneumonia secondary to cystic fibrosis; and diseases of the oral cavity related to dental plaque, such as dental caries and periodontitis. *S. aureus* biofilms are associated

TABLE 8.3 Examples of Mechanisms Used by Pathogens to Resist the Immune System

Mechanisms	Effect on Immunity	Example of Specific Microorganisms
Destroy or Block Component of Immune System		
Produce toxins	Kills phagocyte or interferes with chemotaxis	*Staphylococcus*
	Prevents phagocytosis by inhibiting fusion between phagosome and lysosomal granules	*Streptococcus* *Mycobacterium tuberculosis*
Produce antioxidants (e.g., catalase, superoxide dismutase)	Prevents killing by oxygen-dependent mechanisms	*Mycobacterium* sp.
Produce protease to digest IgA	Promotes bacterial attachment	*Salmonella typhi* *Neisseria gonorrhoeae* (urinary tract infection), *Haemophilus influenzae*, and *Streptococcus pneumoniae* (pneumonia)
Produce surface molecules that mimic crystallizable fragment (Fc) receptors and bind antibodies	Prevents activation of complement system Prevents antibody functioning as opsonin	*Staphylococcus* Herpes simplex virus
Mimic Self-Antigens		
Produce surface antigens (e.g., M protein, red blood cell antigens) that are similar to self-antigens	Resembles individual's own tissue; in some individuals, antibodies can be formed against self-antigen, leading to hypersensitivity disease (e.g., antibody to M protein also reacts with cardiac tissue, causing rheumatic heart disease; antibody to red blood cell antigens can cause anemia)	Group A *Streptococcus* (M protein) *Mycoplasma pneumoniae* (red cell antigens)
Change Antigenic Profile		
Undergo mutation of antigens or activate genes that change surface molecules	Delays immune response because of failure to recognize new antigen	Influenza HIV Some parasites

TABLE 8.4 Examples of Common Bacterial Infections

Microorganism	Gram Stain	Respiratory Pathway	Intracellular or Extracellular
Respiratory Tract Infections			
Upper Respiratory Tract Infections			
Corynebacterium diphtheriae (diphtheria)	Gram +	Facultative anaerobic	Extracellular
Haemophilus influenzae	Gram −	Facultative anaerobic	Extracellular
Streptococcus pyogenes (group A)	Gram +	Facultative anaerobic	Extracellular
Otitis Media			
Haemophilus influenzae	Gram −	Facultative anaerobic	Extracellular
Streptococcus pneumoniae	Gram +	Facultative anaerobic	Extracellular
Lower Respiratory Tract Infections			
Bacillus anthracis (pulmonary anthrax)	Gram +	Facultative anaerobic	Extracellular
Bordetella pertussis (whooping cough)	Gram −	Aerobic	Extracellular
Chlamydia pneumonia	Not stainable	Aerobic	Obligate intracellular
Escherichia coli	Gram −	Facultative anaerobic	Extracellular
Haemophilus influenzae	Gram −	Facultative anaerobic	Extracellular
Legionella pneumophila	Gram −	Aerobic	Facultative intracellular
Mycobacterium tuberculosis	Gram + (weakly)	Aerobic	Extracellular
Mycoplasma pneumoniae	Not stainable	Aerobic	Extracellular
Neisseria meningitidis (develops into meningitis)	Gram −	Aerobic	Extracellular
Pseudomonas aeruginosa	Gram −	Aerobic	Extracellular
Streptococcus agalactiae (group B; develops into meningitis)	Gram +	Facultative anaerobic	Extracellular
Streptococcus pneumoniae	Gram +	Facultative anaerobic	Extracellular
Yersinia pestis (plague)	Gram −	Facultative anaerobic	Extracellular

(Continued)

TABLE 8.4 Examples of Common Bacterial Infections—cont'd

Microorganism	Gram Stain	Respiratory Pathway	Intracellular or Extracellular
Gastro-intestinal Infections			
Inflammatory Gastro-intestinal Infections			
Bacillus anthracis (gastro-intestinal anthrax)	Gram +	Facultative anaerobic	Extracellular
Clostridium difficile	Gram +	Anaerobic	Extracellular
Escherichia coli O157:H7	Gram −	Facultative anaerobic	Extracellular
Vibrio cholerae	Gram −	Facultative anaerobic	Extracellular
Invasive Gastro-intestinal Infections			
Brucella abortus (brucellosis, undulant fever, leading to sepsis, heart infection)	Gram −	Aerobic	Intracellular
Helicobacter pylori (gastritis and peptic ulcers)	Gram −	Microaerophilic	Extracellular
Listeria monocytogenes (leading to sepsis and meningitis)	Gram +	Aerobic	Intracellular
Salmonella typhi (typhoid fever)	Gram −	Anaerobic	Extracellular
Shigella sonnei	Gram −	Facultative anaerobic	Extracellular
Food Poisoning			
Bacillus cereus	Gram +	Facultative anaerobic	Extracellular
Clostridium botulinum	Gram +	Anaerobic	Extracellular
Clostridium perfringens	Gram +	Anaerobic	Extracellular
Staphylococcus aureus	Gram +	Facultative anaerobic	Extracellular
Sexually Transmitted Infections			
Chlamydia trachomatis (pelvic inflammatory disease)	Not stainable	Aerobic	Intracellular
Neisseria gonorrhoeae (urethritis)	Gram −	Aerobic	Facultative intracellular
Treponema pallidum (spirochete; syphilis)	Gram −	Aerobic	Extracellular
Skin and Wound Infections			
Bacillus anthracis (cutaneous anthrax)	Gram +	Facultative anaerobic	Extracellular
Borrelia burgdorferi (Lyme disease; spirochete)	Gram −	Aerobic	Extracellular
Clostridium tetani (tetanus)	Gram +	Anaerobic	Extracellular
Clostridium perfringens (gas gangrene)	Gram +	Anaerobic	Extracellular
Mycobacterium leprae (leprosy)	Gram + (weakly)	Aerobic	Extracellular
Pseudomonas aeruginosa	Gram −	Aerobic	Extracellular
Rickettsia prowazekii (rickettsia; typhus)	Gram −	Aerobic	Obligate intracellular
Staphylococcus aureus	Gram +	Facultative anaerobic	Extracellular
Streptococcus pyogenes (group A)	Gram +	Facultative anaerobic	Extracellular
Eye Infections			
Chlamydia trachomatis (conjunctivitis)	Not stainable	Aerobic	Obligate intracellular
Haemophilus aegyptius (pink eye)	Gram −	Facultative anaerobic	Extracellular
Zoonotic Infections			
Bacillus anthracis (anthrax)	Gram +	Facultative anaerobic	Extracellular
Brucella abortus (brucellosis, also called undulant fever)	Gram −	Aerobic	Intracellular
Borrelia burgdorferi (spirochete; Lyme disease)	Gram −	Aerobic	Extracellular
Listeria monocytogenes	Gram +	Aerobic	Intracellular
Rickettsia rickettsii (rickettsia; Rocky Mountain spotted fever)	Gram −	Aerobic	Obligate intracellular
Rickettsia prowazekii (rickettsia; typhus)	Gram −	Aerobic	Obligate intracellular
Yersinia pestis (plague)	Gram −	Facultative anaerobic	Extracellular
Health Care–Associated Infections			
Enterococcus faecalis	Gram +	Facultative anaerobic	Extracellular
Enterococcus faecium	Gram +	Facultative anaerobic	Extracellular
Escherichia coli (cystitis)	Gram −	Facultative anaerobic	Extracellular
Pseudomonas aeruginosa	Gram −	Obligate anaerobic	Extracellular
Staphylococcus aureus	Gram +	Facultative anaerobic	Extracellular
Staphylococcus epidermidis	Gram +	Facultative anaerobic	Extracellular

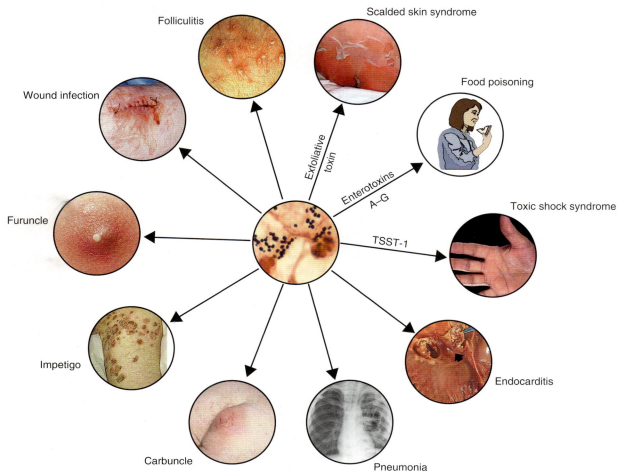

FIGURE 8.2 *Staphylococcus aureus* Infections. Different strains of Staphylococcus aureus (Gram-positive cocci in sputum from an individual with pneumonia [centre photograph]) cause a variety of infections. The particular infection may depend on the toxin produced: exfoliative toxin (scalded skin syndrome), enterotoxins A–G (food poisoning), or toxic shock syndrome toxin-1 (TSST-1). (Toxic shock syndrome, carbuncle, impetigo, and wound infection photos from Cohen, J., & Powderly, W. G. [2010]. *Infectious diseases* [3rd ed.]. Mosby; folliculitis photo from Goldman, L., & Ausiello, D. [2012]. *Cecil medicine* [24th ed.]. Saunders; centre photo and photos of food poisoning and endocarditis from Kumar, V., Abbas, A. K., & Aster, J. C. [Eds.] [2015]. *Robbins and Cotran pathologic basis of disease* [9th ed.]. Saunders; furuncle photo from Long, S. S., Pickering, L. K., & Prober, C. G. [2012]. *Principles and practice of pediatric infectious diseases* [4th ed.]. Saunders; scalded skin syndrome and pneumonia photos from Mandell, G., Bennett, J., & Dolin, R. [2010]. *Principles and practice of infectious diseases* [7th ed.]. Churchill Livingstone.)

with persistent nasopharyngeal colonization and colonization of implanted devices.[7]

A variety of surface proteins mediate adherence among microorganisms in biofilms and to connective tissue (laminin, fibrin, fibronectin) and endothelium. Attachment to collagen occurs in strains causing osteomyelitis and septic arthritis. The capsular polysaccharide mediates attachment to prosthetic devices and protects against phagocytosis. One surface protein, protein A, binds immunoglobulin G (IgG) by the crystallizable fragment (Fc) portion, resulting in the antigen-binding fragment (Fab) regions facing outward.

Thus, the bacteria appear coated with a self-protein, and, with the Fc bound directly to protein A, the IgG cannot activate complement or act as an opsonin.[8] Staphylococcal protein A and a protein called *staphylococcal binder of immunoglobulin* both bind and neutralize IgG. *Staphylococcus* also produces proteins that inhibit complement activity, including activation of C3 and C5, preventing production of C3b,

C3a, and C5a.[9] A coagulase that induces fibrin clotting on the bacterial surface also masks bacterial antigens under a surface of self-proteins.

Furthermore, some strains of *S. aureus* avoid innate immunity. They can produce inhibitors of antimicrobial peptides and avoid recognition by Toll-like receptors.[10] Even when engulfed by a phagocyte, *S. aureus* may resist intracellular oxidative killing by inactivating hydrogen peroxide and other reactive oxygen species. They also resist lysozyme by changing the chemistry of the cell wall.[11]

Many bacteria use toxins as virulence factors, including exotoxins and endotoxins. Some bacteria secrete exotoxins that are immunogenic, eliciting production of antibodies known as **antitoxins**. The most poisonous yet discovered is botulinum neurotoxin produced by *Clostridium botulinum*; less than 1 ng/kg is toxic to humans. Strains of *S. aureus* are capable of producing a wide array of secreted toxic molecules, or **exotoxins**. They include those that damage the cell membrane (α-toxin, which forms pores in membranes; hemolysin, which destroys erythrocytes; β-toxin, which is a sphingomyelinase; δ-toxin, a detergent-like toxin; and leukocidin, which lyses phagocytes). Other toxins include coagulase, which causes blood clots; staphylokinase, which breaks down clots; exfoliative toxins, which cause separation of the epidermis resulting in scalded skin syndrome; lipase, which degrades lipids on the skin surface and facilitates abscess formation; enterotoxins, which cause food poisoning; and superantigens (discussed in Chapter 7).[12] Each infectious strain of *S. aureus* may produce a few of these toxins so that strains differ in their capacities to cause particular diseases; thus, different strains may cause purulent dermal infections, food poisoning, or toxic shock syndrome.

Antibiotic resistance has become a major problem with *S. aureus*. For several decades pathogenic strains have commonly produced β-lactamase, an enzyme that destroys penicillin. More recently, staphylococci have developed resistance to broad-spectrum antibiotics, including methicillin-like antibiotics (methicillin-resistant *Staphylococcus aureus* [MRSA]), which were widely used to treat penicillin-resistant microorganisms.

S. aureus is an opportunistic pathogen because it has many virulence factors that neutralize important components of the innate and adaptive immune systems, destroy tissue, and resist the action of many common antibiotics. Vaccines are an option, but the task of vaccinating is sometimes difficult.[13]

Similarly, Gram-negative microbes produce an endotoxin (lipopolysaccharide [LPS]) that is a structural portion of the cell wall. Growth, lysis, or destruction of the bacteria, as well as treatment with antibiotics, may result in its release. Therefore, antibiotics cannot prevent the toxic effects of the endotoxin. Bacteria that produce endotoxins are called *pyrogenic bacteria* because they activate the inflammatory process and produce fever. The innermost part of the lipopolysaccharide, lipid A, consists of polysaccharide and fatty acids and is responsible for the substance's toxic effects.

Bacteremia occurs when bacteria are present in the blood. Gram-negative sepsis (sepsis or septicemia) occurs when bacteria are growing in the blood and release large amounts of endotoxin, which can cause endotoxic shock with up to 50% mortality.[14] Released endotoxin, as well as other bacterial products, reacts with pattern recognition receptors (PRRs) and induces the overproduction of proinflammatory cytokines, particularly tumour necrosis factor-alpha (TNF-α), interleukin-1 (IL-1), and interleukin-6 (IL-6).[15] Endotoxin also is a potent activator of the complement and clotting systems, leading to a degree of capillary permeability sufficient to permit escape of large volumes of plasma into surrounding tissue, contributing to hypotension and, in severe cases, cardiovascular shock (see Chapter 24). Activation of the coagulation cascade leads to the syndrome of disseminated (or diffuse) intravascular coagulation (see Chapter 21).

Viral Disease

Viral diseases are the most common afflictions of humans and range from the common cold (caused by many viruses) to the "cold sore" of herpes simplex virus to cancers to AIDS. Examples of human diseases caused by specific viruses are listed in Table 8.5. Viruses are very simple microorganisms consisting of nucleic acid protected from the environment by a layer or layers of proteins (capsid). The viral genome can be double-stranded DNA (dsDNA), single-stranded DNA (ssDNA), double-stranded RNA (dsRNA), or single-stranded RNA (ssRNA). A select group of viruses (e.g., HIV, herpesviruses, influenza virus) bud from the surface of an infected cell, retaining a portion of the cell's plasma membrane (envelope) as added protection. Viral replication depends totally on their ability to infect a permissive host cell—a cell that cannot resist viral invasion and replication. Thus, viruses are obligatory intracellular microbes. Transmission is usually from one infected individual to an uninfected individual by aerosols of respiratory tract fluids, contact with infected blood, sexual contact, or transmission from an animal reservoir (zoonotic infection) usually through a vector, such as mosquitoes.[16]

To understand the basic concepts of viral pathogenicity, it may be best to look closely at a single virus. Influenza is an ssRNA virus with a segmented genome (eight pieces of ssRNA). It is transmitted through aerosols or body fluids and is highly infectious. Symptoms begin 1 to 4 days after infection and may include chills, fever, sore throat, muscle aches, severe headaches, coughing, weakness, generalized discomfort, nausea, and vomiting and may lead to pneumonia. It can be fatal, particularly in young children and older persons.[17] The normal rate of infectivity is about 5 to 15%, with a mortality of about 0.1%, and in most cases, recovery occurs in 1 to 2 weeks. Yearly seasonal influenza outbreaks result in about 250 000 to 500 000 deaths worldwide.

The life cycle of every virus is completely intracellular and involves several steps, the first being *attachment* to a receptor on the target cell (Figure 8.3). The influenza virion expresses two surface proteins that are essential to virulence. The hemagglutinin (HA) protein is a glycoprotein that is necessary for entrance into cells by binding to glycan receptors on the surface of respiratory tract epithelium. The viral surface neuraminidase (NA) is an enzyme that is necessary for release of new virions from infected cells by cleaving cellular sialic acids (a common component of mammalian cell membranes). The specificity of this virus–receptor interaction (tropism) dictates the range of host cells that a particular virus will infect and, therefore, the clinical symptoms that reflect the alteration of the function of the infected cells. Other viruses also use specific receptors; for example, HIV attaches to CD4 on T-helper cells, Epstein-Barr virus (EBV, a cause of mononucleosis and Burkitt lymphoma) attaches to complement receptor 2 (CR2) on B lymphocytes (B cells), and rhinovirus (a group of viruses that cause the common cold) attaches to intracellular adhesion molecule-1 (ICAM-1) on respiratory tract epithelium. The SARS-CoV-2 virus responsible for the COVID-19 pandemic gains entry to the host via the ACE-2 receptor, which is expressed by the lungs, kidneys, and gastro-intestinal tract. The ACE-2 receptor serves a protective function and is a key regulator of angiotensin II. It is responsible for breaking down angiotensin II, and when the SARS-CoV-2 virus binds to it, more angiotensin II is available to injure tissues. Angiotensin II is a potent mediator of inflammation and the inhibition of the ACE-2 receptor allows the ACE to function unopposed increases the death of cells in the alveoli by reducing the production of surfactant, triggering inflammation, vasoconstriction, and acute respiratory distress syndrome.[18]

Attachment is followed by *penetration* (entrance into the cell by endocytosis or membrane fusion), *uncoating* (release of viral nucleic acid from the viral capsid by viral or host enzymes), *replication* (synthesis of messenger RNA [mRNA] and viral proteins), *assembly* (formation of new virions), and *release* (exit from the cell by lysis or budding). The influenza virus enters the respiratory tract epithelial cells by endocytosis. Low pH leads to intermembrane fusion between the endosome and viral envelop and uncoating.[19] The viral ssRNA is transported to the nucleus where transcription and replication occur using the viral RNA-dependent RNA polymerase.[20] Viral proteins assemble in the cytoplasm to form the matrix around the viral genome, and the virion buds from the cell surface. Infected cells usually die as a direct effect of the virus. The severity of clinical symptoms is usually secondary to the level of cytokines produced by the infected cells or in response to death of the cells.

The effects of a virus on the infected cell vary greatly. Some viruses, such as herpesviruses, will initiate a latency phase during which the

TABLE 8.5 Examples of Human Diseases Caused by Specific Viruses

Baltimore Classification	Family	Virus	Envelope	Main Route of Transmission	Disease
dsDNA	Adenoviruses	Adenovirus	No	Droplet contact	Acute febrile pharyngitis
	Herpesviruses	Herpes simplex type 1 (HSV-1)	Yes	Direct contact with saliva or lesions	Lesions in mouth, pharynx, conjunctivitis
		Herpes simplex type 2 (HSV-2)	Yes	Sexually, contact with lesions during birth	Sores on labia, meningitis in children
		Herpes simplex type 8 (HSV-8)	Yes	Sexually?, body fluids	Kaposi sarcoma
		Epstein-Barr virus (EBV)	Yes	Saliva	Mononucleosis, Burkitt lymphoma
		Cytomegalovirus (CMV)	Yes	Body fluids, mother's milk, transplacental	Mononucleosis, congenital infection
		Varicella-zoster virus (VZV)	Yes	Droplet contact	Chickenpox, shingles
ssDNA	Papovaviruses	Papillomavirus	No	Direct contact	Warts, cervical carcinoma
dsRNA	Reoviruses	Rotavirus	No	Fecal-oral	Severe diarrhea
ssRNA+	Picornaviruses	Coxsackievirus	No	Fecal-oral, droplet contact	Nonspecific febrile illness, conjunctivitis, meningitis
		Hepatitis A virus	No	Fecal-oral	Acute hepatitis
		Poliovirus	No	Fecal-oral	Poliomyelitis
		Rhinovirus	No	Droplet contact	Common cold
	Flaviviruses	Hepatitis C virus	Yes	Blood, sexually	Acute or chronic hepatitis, hepatocellular carcinoma
		Yellow fever virus	Yes	Mosquito vector	Yellow fever
		Dengue virus	Yes	Mosquito vector	Dengue fever
		West Nile virus	Yes	Mosquito vector	Meningitis, encephalitis
	Togaviruses	Rubella virus	Yes	Droplet contact, transplacental	Acute or congenital rubella
	Coronaviruses	SARS COVID-19	Yes	Droplets in aerosol or direct contact	Severe respiratory tract disease COVID-19 results in generalized endothelial dysfunction, resulting in a variety of circulatory and inflammatory conditions.[a]
ssRNA−	Caliciviruses	Norovirus	No	Fecal-oral	Gastroenteritis
	Orthomyxoviruses	Influenza virus	Yes	Droplet contact	Influenza
	Paramyxoviruses	Measles virus	Yes	Droplet contact	Measles
		Mumps virus	Yes	Droplet contact	Mumps
		Parainfluenza virus	Yes	Droplet contact	Croup, pneumonia, common cold
		Respiratory syncytial virus (RSV)	Yes	Droplet contact, hand-to-mouth	Pneumonia, influenza-like syndrome
	Rhabdoviruses	Rabies virus	Yes	Animal bite, droplet contact	Rabies
	Bunyaviruses	Hantavirus	Yes	Aerosolized animal fecal material	Viral hemorrhagic fever
	Filoviruses	Ebola virus	Yes	Direct contact with body fluids	Viral hemorrhagic fever
		Marburg virus	Yes	Direct contact with body fluids	Viral hemorrhagic fever
	Arenavirus	Lassa virus	Yes	Aerosolized animal fecal material	Viral hemorrhagic fever
ssRNA+ with RT	Retroviruses	HIV	Yes	Sexually, blood products	AIDS
dsDNA with RT	Hepadnaviruses	Hepatitis B virus	Yes	All body fluids	Acute or chronic hepatitis, hepatocellular carcinoma

[a]Varga, Z., Flammer, A. J., Steiger, P., et al. (2020). Endothelial cell infection and endotheliitis in COVID-19. *Lancet*, 395(10234), 1417–1418. https://doi.org/10.1016/S0140-6736(20)30937-5.

dsDNA, Double-stranded DNA; *dsRNA*, double-stranded RNA; *RT*, reverse transcriptase; *ssDNA*, single-stranded DNA; *ssRNA+*, positive-sense single-stranded RNA; *ssRNA−*, negative-sense single-stranded RNA.

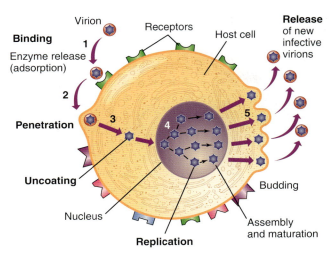

FIGURE 8.3 Stages of Viral Infection of a Host Cell. The virion (1) becomes attached to the cell's plasma membrane by absorption; (2) releases enzymes that weaken the membrane and allow it to penetrate the cell; (3) uncoats itself; (4) replicates; and (5) matures and escapes from the cell by budding from the plasma membrane. The infection then can spread to other host cells.

host cell transforms (i.e., herpes simplex viruses 1 and 2 establish latency in neurons). During this phase, the viral DNA integrates itself into the DNA of the host cell and becomes a permanent passenger in that cell and its progeny. In response to stimuli, such as stress, hormonal changes, or disease, the virus may exit latency and enter a productive cycle. Neurons release herpesviruses 1 and 2 and infect skin epithelium, where lesions in the skin are a result of the immune response against the infected epithelium.

Cytopathic effects caused by other viruses include:

- Cessation of DNA, RNA, and protein synthesis (e.g., herpesvirus)
- Disruption of lysosomal membranes, resulting in release of digestive lysosomal enzymes that can kill the cell (e.g., herpesvirus)
- Fusion of host cells, producing multinucleated giant cells (e.g., respiratory syncytial virus)
- Alteration of the antigenic properties, or identity, of the infected cell, causing the individual's immune system to attack the cell as if it were foreign (e.g., hepatitis B virus)
- Transformation of host cells into cancerous cells, resulting in uninhibited and unregulated growth (e.g., human papillomavirus)
- Promotion of secondary bacterial infection in tissues damaged by viruses
- Acute respiratory distress syndrome, vascular disease (leading to multiple organ failure), gastro-intestinal irritation, autoimmune disorders (e.g., SARS-CoV-2)

The principal method by which influenza virus eludes the immune system is by changing viral surface antigens, a process known as **antigenic variation**. Antibodies against the HA and NA antigens are responsible for protection against influenza infection. Infections are seasonal and protection gained from the previous year's infection does not totally protect against influenza in the following year because the HA and NA antigens undergo yearly change. Usually antigenic variation is relatively minor (**antigenic drift**) and results from mutations. Individuals frequently have partial protection resulting from the previous year's infection, which lessens the clinical effects of the disease. Two groups of influenza virus—influenza A and influenza B—infect humans, and the yearly vaccine against influenza is a trivalent mixture of inactivated proteins from two influenza A subtypes and one influenza B subtype. Influenza B almost exclusively infects humans and mutates at a much lower rate than influenza A. Influenza A has antigenically distinct subtypes based on HA (17 forms) and NA (10 forms) antigens. Currently, subtypes H1N1, H1N2, and H3N2 are the primary causes of influenza worldwide.

Influenza A periodically undergoes major antigenic changes (**antigenic shifts**) (Figure 8.4). Influenza A can infect birds and mammals, and shifts occur in animals coinfected by a human and an avian strain of influenza. The genome is segmented and the segments can undergo recombination, during which the human virus obtains a new HA or NA antigen. Without an antigenic shift, clinical influenza is usually epidemic (the number of new infections exceeds the number usually observed at other times of the year). When major antigenic changes occur, previous protection may not exist, resulting in a major pandemic (an epidemic that spreads over a large area, such as a continent or worldwide) and much more severe disease.

The SARS-CoV-2 virus responsible for COVID-19 has also undergone antigenic drift. There are now variants of the SARS-CoV-2 virus, most notably three main mutations to the virus, one of which was responsible for the global spread of the virus, and the other two variants that are more transmissible than existing strains.[21]

The concern with zoonotic influenza is that a lethal influenza virus that infects birds or other animals may suddenly develop the capacity to infect humans.[16] The World Health Organization (WHO) and the Public Health Agency of Canada (PHAC) (http://www.phac-aspc.gc.ca) closely monitor these and other novel infections, such as COVID-19. As of December 31, 2020, there were 87 247 114 global cases of COVID-19, with 1 815 893 confirmed, many of which were related to a second wave of infection.[22] Canada documented over 573 000 cases of COVID-19, with 15 472 deaths as of December 31, 2020.[23] In addition, the PHAC is currently monitoring human cases of several zoonotic influenza outbreaks, including swine influenza virus (H1N1), a pathogenic H5N1 avian influenza virus, and a new strain of avian influenza (H7N9).

Viral pathogens bypass many defence mechanisms by hiding within cells and away from normal inflammatory or immune responses. Some viruses spread from cell to cell through the bloodstream (e.g., influenza, rubella) and are highly sensitive to neutralizing antibodies that block viral spread and eventually cure the infection; these diseases are self-limiting. On the other hand, other viruses (e.g., measles, herpes) are inaccessible to antibodies after initial infection because they remain inside infected cells, spreading by direct cell-to-cell contact. Most viruses have developed additional defence mechanisms. For example, influenza virus produces NS1 protein (viral nonstructural protein-1) that blocks the antiviral effects of type I interferon.

Fungal Disease

Fungi are relatively large eukaryotic microorganisms with thick walls that have two basic structures: single-celled yeasts (spheres) or multicellular moulds (filaments or hyphae) (Figure 8.5). Some fungi can exist in either form and are called **dimorphic fungi**. The cell walls of fungi are rigid and multilayered and composed of polysaccharides different from the peptidoglycans of bacteria. The lack of peptidoglycans allows fungi to resist the action of bacterial cell wall inhibitors such as penicillin and cephalosporin. Moulds are aerobic, and yeasts are facultative anaerobes, which adapt to, but do not require, anaerobic conditions. They usually reproduce by simple division or budding.

Mycoses are diseases caused by fungi. Mycoses can be superficial, deep, or opportunistic. Superficial mycoses occur on or near skin or mucous membranes and usually produce mild and superficial disease. Fungi that invade the skin, hair, or nails are known as **dermatophytes**. The diseases they produce are called *tineas* (ringworm)—for example,

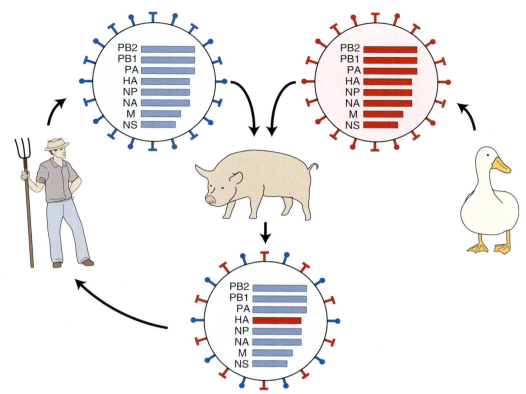

FIGURE 8.4 Antigenic Shifts in Influenza Virus. One theory proposes that antigenic shifts occur when a human influenza virus *(blue)* and an avian influenza virus *(red)* co-infect a species that is permissive for both. The eight single-stranded RNA strands are co-expressed in the same infected cell, resulting in mixing of the strands so that a hybrid virus can be produced. The hybrid virus indicated here contains all the genetic information of the original virus that infected humans but contains a new hemagglutinin *(HA)*-containing stand from the avian virus. This virus expresses a new HA antigen and will be less susceptible to residual immunity that normally provides partial protection against yearly influenza infections.

tinea capitis (scalp), tinea pedis (feet), and tinea cruris (groin). Chapter 41 discusses the various skin disorders caused by fungi.

Pathological fungi cause disease by adapting to the host environment. Fungi that colonize the skin can digest keratin. Other fungi can grow with wide temperature variations in lower oxygen environments. Still other fungi have the capacity to suppress host immune defences. Phagocytes and T cells are important in controlling fungi. Low white blood cell counts promote fungal infection, and infection control is particularly important for individuals who are immunosuppressed. Table 8.6 summarizes common pathological fungi.

Candida albicans is the most common cause of fungal infections in humans. It is an opportunistic yeast that is a commensal inhabitant in the normal microbiome of many healthy individuals, residing in the skin, gastro-intestinal tract, mouth (30 to 55% of healthy individuals), and vagina (20% of healthy women). *C. albicans* is normally under the control of local defence mechanisms, including members of the bacterial microbiome that produce antifungal agents. In healthy individuals, antibiotic therapy can diminish the microbiome (e.g., diminished levels of *Lactobacillus* in the gastro-intestinal or vaginal microbiome). *Candida* overgrowth may occur, resulting in localized infection such as vaginitis or oropharyngeal infection (thrush).

In immunocompromised individuals, particularly those with diminished levels of neutrophils (neutropenia), disseminated infection may occur. *Candida* is the most common fungal infection in people with cancer (particularly acute leukemia and other hematological cancers), transplantation (bone marrow and solid organ), and HIV/AIDS.

Invasive candidiasis also may be secondary to indwelling catheters, intravenous lines, or peritoneal dialysis, which provides direct entrance into the bloodstream.

Disseminated candidiasis may involve deep infections of several internal organs, including abscesses in the kidney, brain, liver, and heart, and is characterized by persistent or recurrent fever, Gram-negative shock-like symptoms (hypotension, tachycardia), and disseminated intravascular coagulation (DIC). The death rates of septic or disseminated candidiasis are in the range of 30 to 40%.

Parasitic Disease

Parasitic microorganisms establish a relationship in which the parasite benefits at the expense of the other species. Parasites range from unicellular protozoa to large worms. Parasitic worms (helminths) include intestinal and tissue nematodes (e.g., hookworm, roundworm), flukes (e.g., liver fluke, lung fluke), and tapeworms. A protozoan is a eukaryotic, unicellular microorganism with a nucleus and cytoplasm. Pathogenic protozoa include malaria (*Plasmodium*), amoebae (e.g., *Entamoeba histolytica*, which causes amoebic dysentery), and flagellates (e.g., *Giardia lamblia*, which causes diarrhea; *Trypanosoma*, which causes sleeping sickness). Although less common in Canada, parasites and protozoa are common causes of infections worldwide, with a significant effect on the mortality and morbidity of individuals in developing countries. Important parasites of humans are listed in Table 8.7.

Malaria is one of the most common infections worldwide. In 2018, the World Health Organization (WHO) estimated that there were

CHAPTER 8 Infection and Defects in Mechanisms of Defence

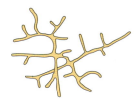

MOULDS
Filamentous fungi grow as multinucleate, branching hyphae, forming a mycelium (i.e., ringworm)

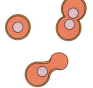

YEASTS
Yeasts grow as ovoid or spherical; single cells multiply by budding and division (i.e., *Histoplasma*)

A

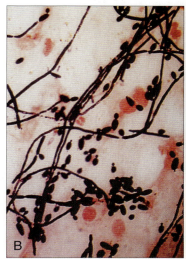
B

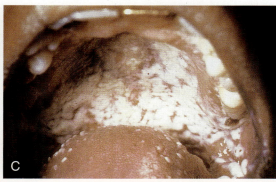
C

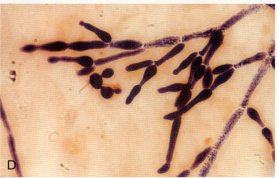
D

FIGURE 8.5 Morphology of Fungi. **A**, Fungi may be either mould or yeast forms, or dimorphic. **B**, Photograph showing *Candida albicans* with both the mycelial and the yeast forms. **C**, Oral infection with *C. albicans* (candidiasis, i.e., thrush). **D**, Gram stain of sputum showing that clinical isolates of *C. albicans* present as chains of elongated budding yeasts (×1000). ([A], [B] from Goering, R., Dockrell, H., Zuckerman, M., et al. [2013]. *Mims' medical microbiology* [5th ed.]. Saunders. [C] from McPherson, R., & Pincus, M. [2012]. *Henry's clinical diagnosis and management by laboratory methods* [22nd ed.]. Saunders; [D] courtesy Dr. Stephen Raffanti.)

TABLE 8.6 Common Pathogenic Fungi

Primary Site of Infection	Fungus	Disease (Primary)	Symptoms
Superficial (no tissue invasion, little inflammation)	*Malassezia furfur*	Tinea versicolour, seborrheic dermatitis, dandruff	Red rash on body
Cutaneous (no tissue invasion, inflammatory response)	Dermatophytes	Tinea pedis (athlete's foot)	Scaling, fissures, pruritus
	Trichophyton mentagrophytes	Tinea cruris (jock itch)	Rash, pruritus
	Trichophyton rubrum	Tinea corporis (ringworm)	Lesion, raised border, scaling
	Microsporum canis		
	Candida albicans	Cutaneous candidiasis	Lesions in most areas of skin, mucous membranes, thrush, vaginal infection
Subcutaneous (tissue invasion)	*Sporothrix schenckii*	Sporotrichosis	Ulcers or abscesses on skin and other organ systems
Systemic (dimorphic; causes disease in healthy individuals)	*Stachybotrys chartarum*, or "black mould"	Black mould disease	Rash, headaches, nausea, pain
	Coccidioides immitis	Coccidioidomycosis	Valley fever, flulike symptoms
	Histoplasma capsulatum	Histoplasmosis	Lung, flulike symptoms, disseminates to multiple organs, eye
	Blastomyces dermatitidis	Blastomycosis	Flulike symptoms, chest pains
Systemic (opportunistic)	*Aspergillus fumigatus*, *Aspergillus flavus*	Aspergillosis	Invasive to lungs and other organs
	Pneumocystis jiroveci	Pneumocystis pneumonia (PCP)	Pneumonia
	Cryptococcus neoformans	Cryptococcosis	Pneumonialike illness, skin lesions, disseminates to brain, meningitis
	C. albicans	Systemic candidiasis	Sepsis, endocarditis, meningitis

TABLE 8.7 Examples of Parasites That Are Important in Humans

Category	Subgroup	Species	Disease	Organs Affected/Symptoms
Protozoa	Ameboid	*Entamoeba histolytica*	Amebiasis	Dysentery, liver abscess
	Flagellate	*Giardia lamblia*	Giardiasis[a]	Diarrhea
		Trichomonas vaginalis	Trichomoniasis	Inflammation of reproductive organs
		Trypanosoma cruzi, T. brucei	Chagas disease: African sleeping sickness	Generalized, blood and lymph nodes, progressing to cardiac and central nervous system (CNS)
	Ciliate	*Balantidium coli*	Balantidiasis	Small intestines, invasion of colon, diarrhea
	Sporozoa (nonmotile)	*Cryptosporidium parvum, C. hominis*	Cryptosporidiosis[a]	Intestine, diarrhea
		Plasmodium spp.	Malaria	Blood, liver
		Toxoplasma gondii	Toxoplasmosis[a]	Intestine, eyes, blood, heart, liver
Helminths	Flukes (trematodes)	*Fasciola hepatica*	Fasciolosis	Liver destruction
		Schistosoma mansoni	Schistosomiasis	Blood, diarrhea, bladder, generalized symptoms
	Tapeworms (cestodes)	*Taenia solium*	Pork tapeworm	Encysts in muscle, brain, liver
	Roundworms (nematodes)	*Ascaris lumbricoides*	Ascariasis	Intestinal obstruction, bile duct obstruction
		Necator americanus (hookworm)	Hookworm disease	Intestinal parasite
		Trichinella spiralis	Trichinosis[a]	Intestine, diarrhea, muscle, CNS, death
		Wuchereria bancrofti	Filariasis, elephantiasis	Lymphatics
		Enterobius vermicularis (pinworm)	Pinworm infection	Intestines
		Onchocerca volvulus	Onchocerciasis	Blindness, dermatitis

[a]Most common in Canada and the United States.

228 million cases of malaria with an estimated 405 000 deaths; 94% were in Africa.[24] Malaria is caused by *Plasmodium falciparum*, a protozoan (unicellular) parasite.

Transmission of protozoan parasites occurs through vectors or ingestion. Vectors include the tsetse fly (*Trypanosoma cruzi*, which causes Chagas disease in South America; *Trypanosoma brucei*, which causes sleeping sickness in Africa) and sand fleas (leishmaniasis). Water and food can be contaminated with protozoal parasites (e.g., *E. histolytica, G. lamblia*). Transmission of *Plasmodium* is through the bite of an infected female *Anopheles* mosquito, where the parasite grows in the salivary gland.

The initial attachment to cells depends on the presence of the microorganism in the bloodstream or gastro-intestinal tract. Microorganisms in the bloodstream have surface proteins that allow them to attach to various receptors to infect macrophages, red blood cells, or organ cells such as the liver. For example, multiplication of *Plasmodium* occurs in erythrocytes and results in the release of additional parasites that infect other erythrocytes. Periodic (48 to 72 hours) lysis of the erythrocytes results in anemia and induction of cytokines (e.g., TNF-α, gamma interferon [IFN-γ], IL-1) that provoke fever, chills, sweating, headache, muscle pains, and vomiting. Severe symptoms include anemia, pulmonary edema, and other complications causing death. Neurological complications may result from infected red blood cells adhering to endothelium in capillaries of the brain.

Countermeasures Against Infectious Microorganisms

The body's innate and adaptive responses against microorganisms are numerous and involve an interaction between the immune and inflammatory systems. Pathogenic microorganisms, however, have developed means of circumventing the individual's protective defences. Therefore, prophylactic or interventive procedures are now available to either prevent the pathogen from initiating disease (vaccines, public health measures) or destroy the pathogen once the disease process has started (antimicrobials). Most vaccine development focuses on preventing the most severe and common infections (see Table 8.8). With the initial success of antibiotic therapy, vaccine development was not considered to be as important. The increase in antibiotic-resistant pathogens, however, has renewed the need for effective vaccines and a greater emphasis now is being placed on the development of new vaccines.

TABLE 8.8 Incidence of Vaccine-Preventable Disease (VPD) in Canada

ELIMINATION	LOW-LEVEL INCIDENCE	MODERATE-LEVEL INCIDENCE
(VPDs that have domestic and international programs to reduce their disease-specific incidence to zero)	(VPDs that generally have an annual incidence rate of less than one case per 100 000 population)	(VPDs that consistently have an annual incidence rate equal to or greater than one case per 100 000 population)
Measles	Tetanus	Pertussis
Rubella	Diphtheria	IPD (invasive pneumococcal disease)
CRS/CRI (congenital rubella syndrome/infection)	Invasive disease due to Hib (*Haemophilus influenzae* type b)	Varicella
Polio	IMD (invasive meningococcal disease)	
Mumps		

[a]As of December 31, 2017.
Data from Public Health Agency of Canada (PHAC). (2020). *Vaccine preventable disease surveillance report to December 31, 2017* (p. 5). https://www.canada.ca/content/dam/phac-aspc/documents/services/publications/vaccines-immunization/vaccine-preventable-disease-surveillance-report-december-31-2017/vaccine-preventable-disease-surveillance-report-eng.pdf.

Infection Control Measures

Although effective means of safeguarding populations from exposure to infectious disease are well-known, lack of implementation or breakdowns in application of these initiatives has led to the re-emergence of some infectious diseases, particularly in less developed countries. The following are some examples of environmental infection control measures:

- Hand hygiene
- Sanitary disposal of sewage, garbage, and animal waste
- Provision of water treatment and prevention of water contamination
- Maintenance of sanitation practices for the transport, preparation, and serving of food
- Control of insect vectors by draining standing water and implementation of mosquito eradication programs
- Support of research to develop safe agents for insecticide-resistant insect vectors

Antimicrobials

Since initiation of the widespread use of penicillin during World War II, antibiotics have significantly prevented the spread of infections. Antibiotics are natural products of fungi, bacteria, and related microorganisms that affect the growth of other microorganisms. Some antibacterial antibiotics are *bactericidal* (kill the microorganism), whereas others are *bacteriostatic* (inhibit growth until the microorganism is destroyed by the individual's own protective mechanisms). The mechanisms of action of most antibiotics include inhibition of the function or production of the cell wall or membrane; inhibition of protein synthesis; blockage of DNA replication; and interference with folic acid metabolism. See Table 8.9 for a list of mechanisms of action against a variety of pathogens. Because viruses use the enzymes of the host's cells, there has been far less success in developing antiviral antibiotics.

Antibiotic-resistant microorganisms arose as a result of the widespread use of antibiotics. Penicillin was very effective at treating infection in 1944, but by 1946, 14% of all *S. aureus* infections in a British hospital were penicillin resistant, producing β-lactamase, an enzyme that destroys penicillin. The same hospital reported an increase to 59% by 1950 and to greater than 89% in the 1990s.

More than 2 million individuals develop antibiotic-resistant infections yearly, resulting in more than 23 000 deaths. Antibiotic resistance to a single antibiotic has rapidly progressed to **multiple-antibiotic resistance**. The CDC released a lengthy report on the matter—*Antibiotic Resistance Threats in the United States, 2013*—in which 18 pathogens were sorted into "Urgent Threats," "Serious Threats," and "Concerning Threats."[25] The most urgent threats are *Clostridium difficile*, carbapenem (an "antibiotic of last resort" against penicillin-resistant organisms) resistant Enterobacteriaceae species (i.e., *Klebsiella* and *E. coli*), and medication-resistant *Neisseria gonorrhoeae*.

Similarly, the *Chief Public Health Officer's Report on the State of Public Health in Canada, 2013*, which focused specifically on infectious disease and its spread, addressed the following concerns: immunization and vaccine-preventable diseases (and how to improve programs across Canada), health care–associated infections (and some of the more common ones, such as *C. difficile*, MRSA, and vancomycin-resistant enterococci), antimicrobial resistance (including methods of spread and ways to minimize the impact on the population), the resurgence of TB (particularly in vulnerable populations), foodborne and waterborne infections, and sexually transmitted infections.[26]

Many other infections considered routine and easily treatable are now resistant to almost all currently available antibiotics, including MRSA and *Streptococcus pneumoniae*, which causes pneumonia, meningitis, and acute otitis media (middle ear infection), and which were once routinely susceptible to penicillin. Additionally, there are major increases in resistant *Salmonella typhi* (typhoid fever), *Shigella* (bloody diarrhea), *Acinetobacter* (pneumonia), *Campylobacter* (bloody diarrhea), *Enterococcus* (sepsis, wound infection, urinary tract infection), *Pseudomonas aeruginosa* (burn infection, sepsis), and *Mycobacterium tuberculosis* (tuberculosis).[27] Antibiotic-resistant fungi (e.g., fluconazole-resistant *C. albicans*) have evolved, and malarial parasites have recently developed broad medication resistance, including to chloroquine—the previous mainstay of the preventive and therapeutic arsenal of antimalarial medications.

Antibiotic resistance is usually a result of *genetic mutations* that can be transmitted directly to neighbouring microorganisms by plasmid exchange or incorporation of free DNA. Some microorganisms can *inactivate antibiotics*, penicillin resistance being the classic example. Other forms of resistance result from *modification of the target molecule*. Azidothymidine (AZT) is a family of antivirals that suppresses the enzymatic activity of reverse transcriptase, a viral-specific enzyme responsible for the replication of viral RNA and the production of a DNA copy. HIV frequently mutates and produces an AZT-resistant reverse transcriptase. Multidrug transporters in the microorganism's membrane mediate a third mechanism of resistance. These transporters affect the rate of intracellular accumulation of the antimicrobial by *preventing entrance* or, more commonly, by *increasing active efflux of the antibiotic*. Antibiotic-resistant strains of *M. tuberculosis* protect themselves from aminoglycosides and tetracycline by a multidrug pump that increases efflux.

Why have multiple-antibiotic–resistant microorganisms appeared? They have appeared for a number of reasons, including (1) lack of adherence in completing the therapeutic regimen with antibiotics allows the selective resurgence of microorganisms that are more relatively resistant to the antibiotic; (2) overuse of antibiotics can lead to the destruction of the normal microbiome, allowing the selective overgrowth of antibiotic-resistant strains or pathogens that had previously been controlled. There also is concern that overuse of antibiotics to promote growth in cattle results in ingestion of antibiotic-containing meat.[28]

TABLE 8.9 Chemicals or Antimicrobials Identified That Prevent Growth of or Destroy Microorganisms

Mechanism of Action	Agents
Inhibits synthesis of cell wall	Penicillins, cephalosporins, monobactams, carbapenems, vancomycin, bacitracin, cycloserine, fosfomycin
Inhibits cell membrane function	Amphotericin, ketoconazole, polymycin
Damages cytoplasmic membrane	Polymyxins, polyene antifungals, imidazoles
Alters metabolism of nucleic acid	Quinolones, rifampin, nitrofurans, nitroimidazoles
Inhibits protein synthesis	Aminoglycosides, tetracyclines, chloramphenicol, macrolides, clindamycin, spectinomycin
Inhibits folic acid synthesis (needed for protein synthesis)	Sulfonamides, trimethoprim
Alters energy metabolism	Trimethoprim, dapsone, isoniazid

Adapted from Adams, M. P., Urban, C. Q., Sutter, R. E., et al. (2020). *Pharmacology for nurses: a pathophysiological approach* (3rd Canadian Ed.). Pearson Canada Inc.

Active Immunization

Recovery from an infection generally results in the strongest resistance to a future infection with the same microbe. Vaccines are biological preparations of antigens that when administered, stimulate production of protective antibodies or cellular immunity against a specific pathogen without causing potentially life-threatening disease. The purpose of vaccination is to induce long-lasting protective immune responses under safe conditions. The primary immune response from vaccination is generally short lived; therefore, booster injections are used to push the immune response through multiple secondary responses that result in large numbers of memory cells and sustained protective levels of antibody or T cells, or both.

Mass vaccination programs have been tremendously successful and have led to major changes in the health of the world's population.[29] In the early 1950s an estimated 50 million cases of smallpox occurred each year, with about 15 million deaths. The WHO conducted an aggressive immunization campaign from 1967 to 1977 that resulted in the global eradication of smallpox by 1979. The Government of Canada publishes vaccine schedules at its website: https://www.canada.ca/en/public-health/services/provincial-territorial-immunization-information/provincial-territorial-routine-vaccination-programs-infants-children.html. Similarly, there is a global movement to develop a vaccine that is effective in preventing COVID-19. Many countries, including Canada, are collaborating in this aggressive immunization campaign effort.

Development of a successful vaccine is costly and depends on several factors. These include (1) identification of the protective immune response and (2) the appropriate antigen to induce that response. For example, individuals with ongoing HIV infection produce a great deal of antibody against several HIV antigens. However, for development of a successful vaccine, it is important to first understand which antibody, if any, will protect against an initial infection.

Once a good candidate antigen is identified, it must be developed into an effective, cost-efficient, stable, and safe vaccine. Most vaccines against viral infection (measles, mumps, rubella, varicella [chickenpox]) contain live viruses that are weakened (attenuated virus) so they continue to express appropriate antigens but establish only a limited and easily controlled infection. Limited replication of the virus appears to afford better long-term protection than using viral antigen. Current exceptions are the hepatitis B vaccine, which uses a recombinant viral protein, and the hepatitis A vaccine, which is an inactivated (killed) virus and normally should not cause an infection.

Even attenuated viruses can establish life-threatening infections in individuals whose immune systems are deficient or suppressed. The risk of infection by the vaccine strain of a virus is extremely small, but it may affect the choice of recommended vaccines. For example, the Sabin vaccine for polio was an attenuated virus that was administered orally. It provided systemic protection and induced a secretory immune response to prevent growth of the poliovirus in the intestinal tract. Being a live virus, the vaccine could cause polio in some children who had unsuspected immune deficiencies (about 1 case in 2.4 million doses). The Salk vaccine was a completely inactivated virus administered by injection. It induced protective systemic immunity but did not provide adequate secretory immunity. Therefore, even if the individual was protected from systemic infection by poliovirus, the virus could establish a limited infection in the individual's intestinal mucosa, be shed, and infect others. When polio was epidemic, the oral vaccine was preferred. However, the live attenuated vaccine itself caused about eight cases of paralytic polio per year in the United States in individuals with inadequate immune systems. As a result, the current recommendation of the CDC is vaccination with the killed virus. The Sabin vaccine, or trivalent vaccine, is also no longer recommended or available in Canada, because most cases of paralytic polio from 1980 to 1995 were associated with this vaccine.[30]

Some common bacterial vaccines are killed microorganisms or extracts of bacterial antigens. The vaccine against pneumococcal pneumonia consists of a mixture of capsular polysaccharides from 23 strains of *S. pneumoniae*. Of the more than 90 known strains of this microorganism, these 23 cause the most severe illnesses. However, the capsular vaccine is not very immunogenic in young children. A *conjugated* vaccine is available that contains capsular polysaccharides from 13 strains conjugated to carrier proteins to increase immunogenicity. A similar vaccine is available for *Haemophilus influenzae* type b (Hib).

Some bacterial pathogens are not invasive but colonize mucosal membranes or wounds and release potent exotoxins that act locally or systemically. Vaccination against systemic exotoxins (e.g., diphtheria, tetanus, pertussis) has been achieved using toxoids—purified exotoxins that have been chemically detoxified without loss of immunogenicity. Pertussis (whooping cough) vaccine has been changed from a killed whole-cell vaccine to cellular extract (acellular) vaccine that contains the pertussis toxoid and additional bacterial antigens. This change has dramatically reduced adverse effects (fever, local inflammatory reactions, and others) of vaccination.

With so many recommended vaccines, there has been an effort to combine vaccines to minimize the number of required injections. One of the first licensed vaccine mixtures was DPT, which now usually contains diphtheria (D) and tetanus (T) toxoids and acellular pertussis vaccine (aP). More recent mixtures include DTaP with inactivated poliovirus, either with Hib conjugate to tetanus toxoid or with hepatitis B antigen.

Common problems confronting vaccination programs include access to the programs in less developed countries or lack of adherence of the susceptible population even when vaccination programs are available. A certain percentage of the population will be genetically unresponsive or less responsive to a particular vaccine and therefore, will not produce a protective immune response. As many as 10% of the population may not respond adequately to the recommended series of injections. With most vaccines, the percentage of unresponsive individuals is low, and they will benefit from successful immunization of the rest of the population. Depending on the microorganism, a certain percentage of the population (usually about 85%) should be immunized to achieve protection of the total population. This form of immunity is referred to as herd immunity. Outbreaks of infection can occur if herd immunity does not exist. In 2017, 90.2% of children in Canada received the measles, mumps, and rubella (MMR) vaccine by the age of 2. This percentage is still lower than the suggested 95% for herd immunity against this virus, and there have been several recent outbreaks of both the mumps and measles in various regions across Canada.[31] In several European countries, as well as the United States, antivaccine groups have disrupted immunization programs. As a result, the incidence of pertussis (whooping cough) increased by 10 to 100 times in those countries compared with neighbouring countries that maintained a high incidence of immunization. Immunizations should be complete before children start school.

The reluctance to vaccinate has generally been based on potential vaccine dangers.[32] As with any medicine, complications can arise. In the case of vaccines, these complications include pain and redness at the injection site, fever, allergic reactions to vaccine ingredients, and infection associated with attenuated viruses in immune-deficient individuals. More severe dangers do exist, although they are extremely rare. More commonly the reluctance to vaccination is based on inadequate information.[33] A common fear relates to the presence of the preservative *thimerosal* in vaccines. Thimerosal is a mercury-containing compound that had been used as a preservative since the 1930s. Although no cases of mercury toxicity have been reported secondary to vaccination, thimerosal was removed from all vaccines in 2001, with the exception of some inactivated influenza vaccines. In 2003 groups in northern Nigeria claimed that the oral vaccine was unsafe and contained additional antifertility medications (estradiol), HIV, and cancer-causing agents.[34] The reasoning appeared to be secondary to mounting distrust of Western nations because of conflicts in the Middle East. The effect was suspension of polio immunization for almost 1 year in two Nigerian states and reduction of immunization in three other states. The incidence of polio rose dramatically, and more than 27 000 cases of paralysis resulted. The goal of the WHO is to eradicate polio worldwide by 2022. In 2019, the total global number of wild polio (naturally occurring) cases was 176, with the highest number of cases in Pakistan.[35]

Passive Immunotherapy

Passive immunotherapy is a form of countermeasure against pathogens in which the individual receives preformed antibodies. Passive immunotherapy with human immunoglobulin is an approved treatment for several infections, including hepatitis A and hepatitis B. Treatment of potential rabies infection after a bite also combines passive and active immunization. The rabies virus proliferates very slowly.[36] Individuals who have been bitten receive a onetime injection with human rabies immunoglobulin, or, more recently, with monoclonal antibody to slow further viral proliferation, followed by multiple injections with a killed viral vaccine to induce greater protective immunity. There is great potential for more specific therapy with monoclonal antibodies for other infectious diseases. Approval of a monoclonal antibody against respiratory syncytial virus (RSV) further enables treatment of the condition, and recently, an experimental monoclonal antibody preparation seems to have neutralized the Ebola virus. More importantly, there are currently many COVID-19 vaccine projects in progress that take advantage of various facets of the COVID-19 infection: triggering an immune response,[37] producing antibodies to neutralize the virus,[38] or the Imperial vaccine,[39] which uses synthetic RNA to mimic the virus and trains the immune system by synthesizing a protein that exists on the outside of the virus. Essentially, the body is fighting the coronavirus without actually developing COVID-19.

In the past, vaccines and therapeutic antibodies were developed only for the deadliest pathogens. With the increase in antibiotic-resistant microorganisms and novel pathogens such as the SARS-CoV-2 virus, the development and widespread use of new vaccines and antibodies against these microorganisms are paramount.[40]

DEFICIENCIES IN IMMUNITY

> **QUICK CHECK 8.2**
> 1. Why is the development of recurrent or unusual infections the clinical hallmark of immunodeficiency?
> 2. Compare and contrast the most common infections in individuals with defects in cell-mediated immune response and those with defects in humoral immune response.
> 3. What are the new treatments for HIV?

An **immune deficiency** (also called *immunodeficiency*) is the failure of the immune or inflammatory response to function normally, resulting in increased susceptibility to infections. Genetic defects are the cause of **primary (congenital) immune deficiency**, whereas other conditions such as cancer, infection, or normal physiological changes (such as aging) cause **secondary (acquired) immune deficiency**. Acquired forms of immune deficiency are far more common than the congenital forms.

Initial Clinical Presentation

The clinical hallmark of immune deficiency is a tendency to develop unusual or recurrent, severe infections. The most severe primary immune deficiencies develop in young children, 2 years old and younger. Preschool and school-age children normally may have 6 to 12 infections per year, and adults may have 2 to 4 infections per year. Most of these are not severe and are limited to viral infections of the upper respiratory tract, recurrent streptococcal pharyngitis, or mild otitis media (middle ear infection).

Potential immune deficiencies should be considered if the individual has experienced severe, documented bouts of pneumonia, otitis media, sinusitis (sinus infection), bronchitis, septicemia (blood infection), or meningitis or infections with rare opportunistic microorganisms (e.g., *Pneumocystis carinii*).[41] Infections are also generally recurrent with only short intervals of relative health, and multiple simultaneous infections are common. Individuals with immune deficiencies often have eight or more purulent ear infections, two or more serious sinus infections, and two or more pneumonias, recurrent abscesses, or persistent fungal infections (particularly thrush) within a year. Invasive fungal infections are rare in healthy individuals and strongly indicate a defective immune system. Recurrent internal infections, such as meningitis, osteomyelitis, or sepsis, are common. Prolonged antibiotic use is commonly ineffective by oral or injected routes and may necessitate intravenous administration. Children frequently present with failure to thrive because of chronic diarrhea and other chronic symptoms. Furthermore, some types of primary deficiency are the result of a familial history of immune deficiency.

Routine care of individuals with immune deficiencies must be tempered with the knowledge that the immune system may be totally ineffective. It is unsafe to administer conventional immunizing agents or blood products to many of these individuals because of the risk of causing an uncontrolled infection. Infection is a particular problem with the use of attenuated vaccines that contain live but weakened microorganisms (e.g., live polio vaccine; vaccines against measles, mumps, and rubella).

The type of recurrent infections may indicate the type of immune defect. For example, recurrent infections caused by certain viruses (e.g., varicella herpes, cytomegalovirus), fungi, and yeasts (e.g., *Candida*, *Histoplasma*), or atypical microorganisms (e.g., *P. carinii*) are the result of deficiencies in T-cell immune responses. Likewise, if the individual has documented, recurrent infections with microorganisms that require opsonization (e.g., encapsulated bacteria) or with viruses against which humoral immunity is normally effective (e.g., rubella), B-cell deficiencies and phagocyte deficiencies are likely the main cause. Some complement deficiencies resemble defects in antibody or phagocyte function, but others are associated with disseminated infections with bacteria of the genus *Neisseria* (*Neisseria meningitides* and *Neisseria gonorrhoeae*).

Primary (Congenital) Immune Deficiencies

Most primary immune deficiencies are the result of *single gene defects* (Table 8.10). Generally, the mutations are sporadic and not inherited: a family history exists in only about 25% of individuals. The sporadic mutations occur before birth, but the onset of symptoms may be early or later, depending on the particular syndrome. In some instances, symptoms of immune deficiency appear within the first 2 years of life. Other immune deficiencies are progressive, with the onset of symptoms appearing in the second or third decade of life.

TABLE 8.10 Examples of Primary Immune Deficiencies

Classification	Example	Immune Deficiency	Outcome
Combined Immune Deficiencies: Without Nonimmune Defects			
Defective development of both B cells and T cells	Severe combined immunodeficiencies (SCIDs)	Lack of both T and B cells, little or no antibody production or cellular immunity	Recurrent, life-threatening infections with variety of microorganisms
	X-linked SCID	Defective interleukin receptors needed for lymphocyte maturation	Recurrent, life-threatening infections with variety of microorganisms
Defects in cooperation among B cells, T cells, and antigen-presenting cells	Bare lymphocyte syndrome	No antigen presentation because of lack of major histocompatibility complex (MHC) class I or MHC class II molecules on cell surface	Recurrent, life-threatening infections with variety of microorganisms
Combined Immune Deficiencies: With Nonimmune Defects			
Defect in actin cytoskeleton	Wiskott-Aldrich syndrome	Decreased IgM antibody	Recurrent infections with encapsulated bacteria; thrombocytopenia; eczema
Defective development of T cells in central lymphoid organ (thymus)	DiGeorge syndrome	Lack of T cells	Recurrent, life-threatening fungal and viral infections; defective parathyroid gland; abnormal facial development
Predominantly Antibody Deficiencies			
Defect in class-switch to IgA	Selective IgA deficiency	Diminished or absent IgA	Asymptomatic or recurrent mild sinus, pulmonary, and gastro-intestinal infections
Defect in development of B cells in the bone marrow	Bruton agammaglobulinemia	Few B cells	Recurrent bacterial infections
Phagocytic Defects			
Defects in production of neutrophils	Severe congenital neutropenia	Lack of neutrophils	Recurrent, life-threatening bacterial infections
Defects in bacterial killing	Chronic granulomatous disease	Lack of production of oxygen products (e.g., hydrogen peroxide)	Recurrent infections with bacteria that are sensitive to killing by oxygen-dependent mechanisms
Defects in Innate Immunity			
Defect in development of cellular immunity against specific antigen	Chronic mucocutaneous candidiasis	Lack of T-cell response to *Candida*	Recurrent and disseminated infections with fungus *Candida albicans*
Complement Deficiencies			
Defective production of C3	C3 deficiency	Little or no C3 produced	Recurrent, life-threatening bacterial infections
Defective production of component of membrane attack complex	C6, C7, C8, or C9 deficiency	Little or no C6, C7, C8, or C9 produced	Recurrent disseminated infections with *Neisseria gonorrhoeae* or *Neisseria meningitides*
Defective production of component of lectin pathway	Mannose-binding lectin deficiency	Little or no activation of lectin pathway	Recurrent infections with bacteria and yeast with mannose-containing capsules

Individually, primary immune deficiencies are rare. On average, 1 in 1 200 Canadians suffer from the condition, and up to 70% are undiagnosed.[42] Many such conditions are subtle with minor deficiencies, but several result from major defects and lead to recurrent life-threatening infections. The distribution between genders is about even, although some specific diseases have a male or female predominance.

Primary immune deficiencies have recently been reclassified, based on the principal component of the immune or inflammatory system that is defective.[43] The major groups include (1) combined with or without nonimmune defects (where both B and T cells are deficient, although this group contains some diseases previously classified as T-cell defects), (2) predominantly antibody deficiencies, (3) immune dysregulation (defects in control of lymphocyte proliferation, T-regulatory cell defects), (4) **phagocytic defects** (inadequate numbers or function), (5) **defects in innate immunity**, and (6) complement defects. To provide a better understanding of the diversity and severity of primary immune deficiencies, a few select examples follow.

Combined Deficiencies

Combined deficiencies include the most life-threatening disorders and result from defects that directly affect the development of both T and B cells. However, the severity depends on the degree to which B and T cells are affected.[44] The most severe disorders are called **severe combined immunodeficiencies (SCIDs)**. Most individuals with SCIDs have few detectable lymphocytes in the circulation and secondary lymphoid organs (spleen, lymph nodes). The thymus is usually underdeveloped because of the absence of T cells. Immunoglobulin levels, especially IgM and IgA, are also absent or greatly reduced. Autosomal recessive enzymatic defects are the main cause of severe forms of SCID and result in the accumulation of toxic metabolites. Rapidly dividing cells, such as lymphocytes, are especially sensitive. For example, (ADA deficiency) results in the accumulation of toxic purines. X-linked SCID results from a common defect in most of the important IL receptors needed for lymphocyte maturation (e.g., IL-2, IL-4, IL-7).

Even if nearly adequate numbers of B and T cells are produced, their cooperation may be defective. The bare lymphocyte syndrome is an immune deficiency characterized by an inability of lymphocytes and macrophages to produce major histocompatibility complex (MHC) class I or class II molecules. Without MHC molecules, antigen presentation and intercellular cooperation cannot occur effectively. Children with this deficiency develop serious, life-threatening infections and usually die before the age of 5 years.

Some combined immune deficiencies result in depressed development of a small portion of the immune system. For example, an individual can be unable to produce a certain class of antibody, as in Wiskott-Aldrich syndrome (WAS, an X-linked recessive disorder), where IgM antibody production is greatly depressed. Antibody responses against antigens that elicit primarily an IgM response, such as polysaccharide antigens from bacterial cell walls (e.g., *P. aeruginosa*, *S. pneumoniae*, *H. influenzae*, and other microorganisms with polysaccharide outer capsules), are deficient.

Moreover, many combined immune deficiencies have other characteristic defects that are completely unrelated to the immune system but may be life-threatening on their own. These symptoms help in diagnosing and clarifying the pathophysiology of the condition. For example, WAS results from a mutation in the *WAS* gene that affects the actin cytoskeleton, which is important for platelet function. Thus, WAS has an associated major defect in platelet function and is classified as a combined deficiency with nonimmune defects. Clinical manifestations include bleeding secondary to thrombocytopenia (low platelet counts), eczema, and recurrent infections (e.g., otitis media, pneumonia, herpes simplex, cytomegalovirus).

DiGeorge syndrome (congenital thymic aplasia or hypoplasia and diminished parathyroid gland development) results from a lack or partial lack of the thymus, resulting in greatly decreased T-cell numbers and function. Defective development of the third and fourth pharyngeal pouches during embryonic development results in the thymic defects and the lack of the parathyroid gland (causing an inability to regulate calcium concentration). Low blood calcium levels cause the development of tetany or involuntary rigid muscular contraction. Abnormal development of facial features is common with DiGeorge syndrome because the same embryonic pouches control these facial movements; these include low-set ears, fish-shaped mouth, and other altered features (Figure 8.6). Other examples of combined immune deficiencies include defects in CD3 resulting in the loss of T cell antigen receptor intracellular signalling, defective somatic gene rearrangement of variable region genes or constant region genes, IL-2 receptor defects, and defects in DNA repair.

Predominantly Antibody Deficiencies

Predominantly antibody deficiencies result from defects in B-cell maturation or function and are the most common of immune deficiencies.[45] Pure B-cell deficiencies do not affect T-cell responses. People affected by this disorder have lower levels of circulating immunoglobulins (hypogammaglobulinemia) or occasionally, totally or nearly absent immunoglobulins (agammaglobulinemia).

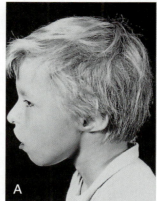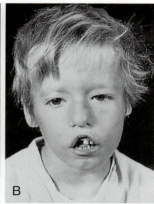

FIGURE 8.6 Facial Anomalies Sometimes Associated With DiGeorge Syndrome. Note the wide set eyes (B), as well as the low set ears, and shortened structure of the upper lip (A). (From Male, D., Brostoff, J., Roth, D., et al. [2013]. *Immunology* [8th ed.]. Mosby.)

Some defects may involve a particular *class* of antibody, such as selective IgA deficiency, in which only IgA is suppressed. This deficiency may result from a failure to class-switch to IgA and mature into IgA-producing plasma cells. Many individuals are asymptomatic, although others have a history of recurring sinus, pulmonary, and gastro-intestinal infections. Individuals with IgA deficiency often have chronic intestinal candidiasis (infection with *C. albicans*). Complications of IgA deficiency include severe allergic disease and autoimmune diseases. Secretory IgA normally may prevent the uptake of allergens from the environment; therefore, IgA deficiency may lead to a more intense challenge to the immune system by environmental antigens.

Blocked development of mature B cells in the bone marrow can result in Bruton agammaglobulinemia. With this condition, there are few or no circulating B cells, although T-cell number and function are normal, resulting in repeated bacterial infections, such as otitis media, streptococcal sore throat, and conjunctivitis, and more serious conditions, such as septicemia.

Other predominantly antibody deficiencies include severe reduction in particular classes or subclasses of antibody; defects in B-cell surface receptors, such as CD21 and CD40; and defects in class-switch, which may result in a *hyper-IgM syndrome*.

Phagocyte Defects

Phagocyte defects range from inadequate numbers of phagocytes (e.g., severe congenital neutropenia) to defects in phagocyte function that can result in recurrent infections with the same group of microorganisms (encapsulated bacteria) associated with antibody and complement deficiencies. Chronic granulomatous disease (CGD) is a severe defect in the myeloperoxidase–hydrogen peroxide system; a major means of bacterial destruction using the enzyme myeloperoxidase, halides (e.g., chloride ion), and hydrogen peroxide.[46] As a result of phagocytosis, neutrophils and other phagocytes switch much of their glucose metabolism to the hexose-monophosphate shunt. Conversion of molecular oxygen by nicotinamide adenine dinucleotide phosphate (NADPH) oxidase into by products of highly reactive oxygen derivatives, including hydrogen peroxide, occurs in this pathway. Mutations in NADPH oxidase result in deficient production of hydrogen peroxide and other oxygen products needed for phagocytic killing. In such cases, affected individuals have adequate myeloperoxidase and halide but lack the necessary hydrogen peroxide for neutralizing pathogens and foreign debris. A lack of hydrogen peroxide (and other highly reactive oxygen species) results in recurrent severe pneumonias; tumour-like granulomata in lungs, skin, and bones; and other infections with some opportunistic microorganisms, such as *S. aureus*, *Serratia marcescens*, and *Aspergillus* species. Other phagocytic deficiencies include defects in various leukocyte adhesion molecules, defects in the phagocytosis process or bacterial killing, and defects in cytokine receptors.

Defects in Innate Immunity

Some immune deficiencies are characterized by a defect in the capacity to produce an immune response against a particular antigen. In chronic mucocutaneous candidiasis, interaction between the Th17 lymphocytes and macrophages is ineffective related to a specific infectious agent, *C. albicans*. In this case, the macrophage cannot be activated, and individuals with this immune deficiency usually have mild to extremely severe recurrent *Candida* infections involving the mucous membranes and skin. Other defects in innate immunity include defects in Toll-like receptors and natural killer (NK) cells.

Complement Deficiencies

C3 deficiency is the most severe defect because of its central role in the complement cascade. Loss of C3b and C3a production and the inability to activate C5 result in recurrent life-threatening infections with encapsulated bacteria (e.g., *H. influenzae* and *S. pneumoniae*) at an early age. Increased infections with only one group of bacteria—those of the genus *Neisseria* (*N. meningitidis* or *N. gonorrhoeae*)—may exist with deficiencies of any of the terminal components of the complement cascade (C5, C6, C7, C8, or C9 deficiencies). *Neisseria* bacteria usually cause localized infections (meningitis or gonorrhea), but terminal pathway defects result in an 8 000-fold increased risk for systemic infections with atypical strains of these microorganisms.

Mannose-binding lectin (MBL) deficiency is the primary defect of the lectin pathway of complement activation. This defect, as well as defects in the alternative pathway, results in increased risk of infection with microorganisms that have polysaccharide capsules rich in mannose, particularly the yeast *Saccharomyces cerevisiae* and encapsulated bacteria such as *N. meningitidis* and *S. pneumoniae*. Other complement deficiencies include defects in components C1, C2, C4, C5, C1 inhibitor, factor B, factor D, properdin, complement control factors, MBL-associated serine protease, or complement receptors.

Secondary (Acquired) Immune Deficiencies

Secondary, or acquired, immune deficiencies are far more common than primary deficiencies. These deficiencies are complications of other physiological, psychological, or pathophysiological conditions. Box 8.1 summarizes some conditions that are associated with acquired immune deficiencies.

Although secondary deficiencies are common, many are not clinically relevant. In many cases, the degree of the immune deficiency is relatively minor and exists without any apparent increased susceptibility to infection. Alternatively, the immune system may be substantially suppressed, but only for a short time. This minimizes the incidence of clinically relevant infections. Some secondary immune deficiencies (e.g., AIDS or immunosuppression by cancer), however, are extremely severe and may result in recurrent life-threatening infections.

Evaluation and Care of Those With Immune Deficiency

A review of clinical characteristics can help select the appropriate tests. A basic screening test is a complete blood count (CBC) with a differential. The CBC provides information on the numbers of red blood cells, white blood cells, and platelets, and the differential indicates the quantities of lymphocytes, granulocytes, and monocytes in the blood. Quantitative determination of immunoglobulins (IgG, IgM, IgA) is a screening test for antibody production, and an assay for total complement (total hemolytic complement, CH_{50}) is useful if a complement defect is suspected. Table 8.11 describes further testing.

Replacement Therapies for Immune Deficiencies

Treatment of many immune deficiencies can involve replacing the missing component of the immune system. Administration of intravenous immune globulin (IVIg), antibody-rich fractions prepared from plasma pooled from large numbers of donors can help individuals with B-cell deficiencies that cause hypogammaglobulinemia or agammaglobulinemia.[47] This is because administration of IVIg replaces the individual's antibodies temporarily. Since these antibodies have a half-life of 3 to 4 weeks, individuals must be treated repeatedly to maintain a protective level of antibodies in the blood.

Replacement of stem cells through transplantation of bone marrow, umbilical cord cells, or other cell populations that are rich in stem cells can sometimes treat defects in lymphoid cell development in the primary lymphoid organs (e.g., SCID, WAS). Similarly, transplantation of fetal thymus tissue or thymic epithelial cells (the cells that produce thymic hormones) can treat thymic defects (e.g., DiGeorge syndrome, chronic mucocutaneous candidiasis). It is important to note that in most cases, improvement is only temporary.

Transfusions of glycerol frozen-packed erythrocytes can successfully treat enzymatic defects that cause SCID (e.g., ADA deficiency) because the donor erythrocytes contain the needed enzyme and can, at least temporarily, provide sufficient enzyme for normal lymphocyte function.

Blood and marrow stem cell transplants (see https://www.llscanada.org/sites/default/files/file_assets/f-73-14-7405621_AvrIWIiW_bloodmarrowstemcelltransplantation.pdf) containing hematopoietic stem cells are routinely used to treat SCID. However, as discussed later in this chapter, the donor and recipient should be matched as closely as possible for human leukocyte antigens (HLAs). Individuals with SCID are at risk for graft-versus-host disease (GVHD). GVHD occurs if T cells in a transplanted graft (e.g., transfused blood, bone marrow transplants) are mature and capable of cell-mediated immunity against the recipient's HLA. The primary targets for GVHD are the skin (e.g., rash, loss or increase of pigment, thickening of skin), liver (e.g., damage to bile duct, hepatomegaly), mouth (e.g., dry mouth, ulcers, infections), eyes (e.g., burning, irritation, dryness), and gastro-intestinal tract (e.g., severe diarrhea), and the disease may lead to death from infections. Removing mature T cells from tissue used to treat individuals with immune deficiencies can reduce the risk of acquiring GVHD.[48]

Injection of mesenchymal stem cells (MSCs) may also be useful in these individuals. Stem cells are relatively undifferentiated cells and come from a variety of sources (e.g., embryos, bone marrow, adult tissues). MSCs are present in all adult tissues. These particular stem cells undergo differentiation into other cell types and, more importantly, have potent immunosuppressive properties.[49] Several clinical trials have demonstrated complete suppression of GVHD in a large number of recipients of MSCs.[50]

Two girls with SCID related to an ADA deficiency successfully received the first therapeutic replacement of defective genes.[51] A retroviral vector carrying the normal gene for ADA[52] then infected bone marrow stem cells from these children, inserting the normal *ADA* gene into the individuals' genetic material. The children received these genetically altered stem cells via an IV transfusion, resulting in reconstitution of their immune systems. Other gene therapy trials have

BOX 8.1 Some Conditions Known to Be Associated With Acquired Immunodeficiencies

Normal Physiological Conditions
Pregnancy
Infancy
Aging

Psychological Stress
Emotional trauma
Eating disorders

Dietary Insufficiencies
Malnutrition caused by insufficient intake of large categories of nutrients, such as protein or calories
Insufficient intake of specific nutrients, such as vitamins, iron, or zinc

Infections
Congenital infections, such as rubella, cytomegalovirus, hepatitis B
Acquired infections, such as AIDS

Malignancies
Malignancies of lymphoid tissues, such as Hodgkin's disease, acute or chronic leukemia, or myeloma
Malignancies of nonlymphoid tissues, such as sarcomas and carcinomas

Physical Trauma
Burns

Medical Treatments
Stress caused by surgery
Anaesthesia
Immunosuppressive treatment with corticosteroids or antilymphocyte antibodies
Splenectomy
Cancer treatment with cytotoxic medications or ionizing radiation

Other Diseases or Genetic Syndromes
Diabetes
Alcoholic cirrhosis
Sickle cell disease
Systemic lupus erythematosus
Chromosome abnormalities, such as trisomy 21

TABLE 8.11 Laboratory Evaluation of Immune Deficiencies

Function Tested	Laboratory Test	Significance of Test
Tests of Humoral Immune Function		
Antibody production	Total immunoglobulin levels, including IgG, IgM, and IgA	Decrease or absence of total antibody production or of specific classes of antibody, which is associated with many B-cell and combined deficiencies
	Levels of isohemagglutinins	Production of specific IgM antibodies, which is decreased in some combined deficiencies; not useful with persons who are blood type AB and do not have naturally occurring isohemagglutinins
	Levels of antibodies against vaccines—especially diphtheria and tetanus toxoids	Production of specific IgG antibodies, which is decreased when B cells are deficient or class-switch is blocked
B-cell numbers	Numbers of lymphocytes with surface immunoglobulin	Production of circulating B cells, which is decreased in many severe B-cell or combined deficiencies
Antibody subclasses	Level-specific subclasses, particularly IgG1, IgG2, and IgG3	Decrease or absence of a particular subclass, which is characteristic of several immune deficiencies
Tests of Cellular Immune Function		
Delayed hypersensitivity skin test	Skin test reaction against previously encountered antigens, especially *Candida albicans* or tetanus toxoid	Defects in antigen-responsive T cells and skin test cellular interactions (e.g., lymphokine activity and macrophage function)
T-cell numbers	Numbers of T cells expressing characteristic membrane antigens (CD3 or CD11)	Defects in production of circulating T cells
T-cell proliferation in vitro	Proliferative response to nonspecific mitogens (e.g., phytohemagglutinin)	General T-cell defects in response to nonspecific stimulation (mitogens)
	Proliferative response to antigens (e.g., tetanus toxoid)	Defects in response of T cells to specific antigens
T-cell subpopulations	Quantify percentage of T cells with specific markers for total T cells (CD3), T-helper cells (CD4), T-cytotoxic cells (CD8)	Decrease in numbers of CD4 cells, which is related to AIDS progression

verified immune reconstitution in individuals with ADA deficiency, X-linked SCID, CGD, and WAS.[53] Some of the recipients, however, developed leukemia as a result of the gene therapy, and this raises questions concerning the use of retroviral vectors for the insertion of new genes.

AIDS

Acquired immunodeficiency syndrome (AIDS) is a secondary immune deficiency that develops in response to viral infection. The **human immunodeficiency virus (HIV)** infects and destroys the CD4-positive (CD4+) T-helper cells (Th cells), which are necessary for the development of both plasma cells and T-cytotoxic cells (Tc cells). Therefore, HIV suppresses the immune response against itself and secondarily creates a generalized immune deficiency by suppressing the development of immune responses against other pathogens and opportunistic microorganisms, leading to the development of AIDS. New developments in the management of HIV infection have made it more of a chronic illness when the condition is well managed (with immune modifiers and effective antiviral agents). Many people live with HIV infection for long periods without progressing to AIDS.

Despite major efforts by health care agencies around the world, the number of cases and deaths from HIV infection and AIDS (HIV/AIDS) remains a major health concern. The WHO estimated that at the end of 2019, 38 million people were living with HIV/AIDS worldwide, 67% of these people had access to antiretroviral therapy, and 7.1 million people did not even know they had HIV. Newly infected individuals with HIV reached 1.7 million, and 690 000 died of HIV-related causes.[54] Since 1980 it is estimated that more than 36 million individuals have died from AIDS worldwide. The majority of cases are in sub-Saharan Africa, where about 1 in 20 adults is living with HIV, but the epidemic is worldwide, and the number of new cases is increasing rapidly, particularly in Asia.

In Canada, the spread of HIV/AIDS remains somewhat stable. There were 2 561 cases of HIV in Canada reported in 2018 (an increase of 8.2% from 2017), and the disease is being diagnosed at a younger age.[55] The national diagnosis rate also increased to 6.9 per 100 000 population in 2018 from 6.5 per 100 000 population in 2017. Before the implementation of massive public health campaigns and the use of antiviral medications, the progression from HIV infection to AIDS and death was inevitable. With the advent of effective therapy to stabilize progression of the disease in the mid-1990s, HIV infection has become a chronic disease in Canada and the United States, with many fewer deaths.

Epidemiology of AIDS

HIV is a bloodborne pathogen with the following routes of transmission: (1) blood or blood products, (2) intravenous medication abuse, (3) both heterosexual and homosexual activity, and (4) maternal–child transmission before or during birth. Although the disease first gained attention in the United States related to sexual transmission between males, the most common route worldwide is through heterosexual activity (see *Health Promotion*: Risk of HIV Transmission Associated With Sexual Practices). Worldwide, women constitute more than half of those living with HIV/AIDS. In Canada, as in the rest of the world, the predominant means of transmission to women is through heterosexual contact. Hundreds of thousands of cases of HIV/AIDS have been reported in children who contracted the virus from their mothers across the placenta, through contact with infected blood during delivery, or through the milk during breastfeeding.

Pathogenesis of AIDS

HIV is a member of a family of viruses called *retroviruses*, which carry genetic information in the form of RNA rather than DNA (Figure 8.7). Retroviruses use a viral enzyme, **reverse transcriptase**, to convert RNA into dsDNA. **HIV integrase** then inserts the new DNA into the infected cell's genetic material, where it may remain dormant. If the cell enters the cell cycle and begins to divide, translation of the viral information may begin, resulting in the formation of new virions, lysis, and death of the infected cell, and shedding of infectious HIV particles. **HIV protease** is essential during this process as it packages proteins needed to form the viral internal structure (capsid). If, however, the cell remains relatively dormant, the viral genetic material may remain latent for years and is probably present for the life of the individual.

The primary surface receptor on HIV is the envelope protein gp120, which binds to the molecule CD4 on the surface of Th cells. The chemokine receptor, CCR5, is another essential co-receptor that must be present on target cells for HIV infection to occur. The decreasing number of $CD4^+$ Th cells is a key immunological finding in AIDS (Figure 8.8).

HEALTH PROMOTION

Risk of HIV Transmission Associated With Sexual Practices

Evolving evidence about the risk of sexual transmission of HIV supports the assertion that people living with HIV who are both consistently taking antiretroviral therapy (ART) and virally suppressed have effectively no risk of transmitting HIV to their sexual partners: "Undetectable equals untransmittable" (U = U).[a,b,c] A 2018 Canadian review of the literature concluded that the risk was "negligible", but only when there were no other sexually transmitted infections (STIs).[d] Even then, the results of numerous studies aligning the incidence of HIV infection with other STIs such as syphilis are inconclusive. Information on viral load (VL) testing history around the time of STI diagnosis informs the overall risk assessment for HIV sexual transmission risk. Other factors that affect the overall transmission risk include condom use, the presence of other (nonreportable) genital infections, and sexual practices.[e]

[a]Public Health Agency of Canada. (2017). *Statement on behalf of the Council of Chief Medical Officers of Health*. Ottawa: Government of Canada. Retrieved from https://www.canada.ca/en/public-health/news/2017/11/statement_on_behalfofthecouncilofchiefmedicalofficersofhealth.html.
[b]Centers for Disease Control and Prevention; National Center for HIV/AIDS, Viral Hepatitis, and TB Prevention. (2018). *Evidence of HIV treatment and viral suppression in preventing the sexual transmission of HIV*. https://www.cdc.gov/hiv/pdf/risk/art/cdc-hiv-art-viral-suppression.pdf.
[c]Pebody, R. (2020). Undetectable viral load transmission—information for people with HIV. *AIDSmap.com* (November). https://www.aidsmap.com/about-hiv/undetectable-viral-load-and-transmission-information-people-hiv#:~:text=Having%20an%20undetectable%20viral%20load%20does%20mean%20that%20there%20is,a%20sexual%20partner%20is%20zero.
[d]LeMessurier, J., Traversy, G., Varsaneux, O., et al. (2018). Risk of sexual transmission of human immunodeficiency virus with antiretroviral therapy, suppressed viral load and condom use: a systematic review. *Canadian Medical Association Journal, 190*(46), e1350–e1360. https://www.cmaj.ca/content/190/46/E1350.
[e]Public Health Ontario. (2019). *Evidence Brief: human immunodeficiency virus (HIV) sexual transmission risk with bacterial sexually transmitted infection (STI) co-infection*. https://www.publichealthontario.ca/-/media/documents/E/2019/eb-HIV-risk-bacterial-STI-co-infection.pdf?la=en.

Clinical Manifestations of AIDS

Depletion of $CD4^+$ Th cells has a profound effect on the immune system, causing a severely diminished response to a wide array of infectious pathogens and cancers (Box 8.2). At the time of diagnosis, the individual may present with one of several different conditions: (1) serologically negative (no detectable antibody), (2) serologically positive (positive for antibody against HIV proteins) but asymptomatic, (3) early stages of HIV disease, or (4) AIDS (Figure 8.9).

The presence of circulating antibody against the HIV protein p24 followed by more complex tests for antibodies against additional HIV proteins (e.g., Western blot analysis) or for HIV DNA (e.g., polymerase chain reaction) indicates infection by the virus, although many of these individuals are asymptomatic. Antibody appears rather rapidly after infection through blood products, usually within 4 to 7 weeks, although some individuals have been seronegative for longer periods. The period between infection and the appearance of antibody is referred to as the *window period*. Although a person does not have antibody against HIV, he or she may be cultivating the virus in blood and bodily fluids and be infectious to others.

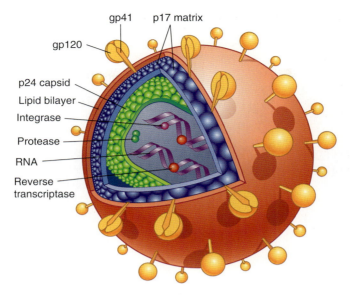
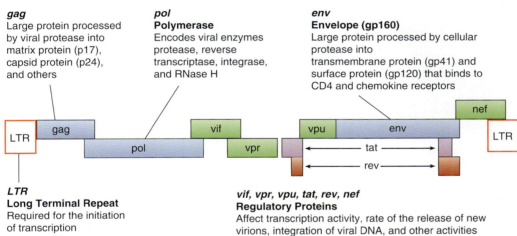

FIGURE 8.7 **The Structure and Genetic Map of HIV-1.** The human immunodeficiency virus type 1 (HIV-1) virion consists of a core of two identical strands of viral RNA molecules of viral enzymes (reverse transcriptase, protease, integrase) coated in a core capsid structure consisting primarily of the structural viral protein p24. The capsid is further encased in a matrix consisting primarily of viral protein p17. The outer surface is an envelope consisting of the plasma membrane of the cell from which the virus budded (lipid bilayer) and two viral glycoproteins: a transmembrane glycoprotein, gp41, and a noncovalently attached surface protein, gp120. The HIV-1 genome contains regions that encode the structural proteins *(gag)*, the viral enzymes *(pol)*, and the envelope proteins *(env)*. The genome of complex retroviruses, such as HIV-1, often contains a variety of small regions that regulate expression of the virus. (Modified from Kumar, V., Abbas, A. K., & Aster, J. C. [Eds.]. [2021]. *Robbins and Cotran pathologic basis of disease* [10th ed.]. Elsevier.)

Those with the early stages of HIV disease (early-stage disease) usually initially present with relatively mild and nonspecific symptoms resembling influenza, such as headaches, fever, or fatigue. These symptoms disappear after 1 to 6 weeks, and although individuals appear to be in clinical latency, the virus is actively proliferating in lymph nodes.

The currently accepted definition of AIDS relies on both laboratory tests and clinical symptoms. If the individual is positive for antibodies against HIV, it is the associated various clinical symptoms that enable the accurate diagnosis of AIDS (Figure 8.10; see also Box 8.2). The symptoms include atypical or opportunistic infections and cancers, as well as indications of debilitating chronic disease (e.g., wasting syndrome, recurrent fevers). Most commonly, new cases of AIDS are diagnosed initially by decreased CD4+ Th cell numbers. Individuals who are not HIV infected typically have 800 to 1 000 CD4+ Th cells per cubic millimetre of blood, with a range from 600 to 1 200/mm^3. A diagnosis of AIDS can be made if the CD4+ Th cell numbers decrease to less than 200/mm^3. Without treatment, the average time from infection to development of AIDS is just over 10 years. Some estimates are that approximately 99% of untreated HIV-infected individuals would eventually progress to AIDS.

Treatment and Prevention of HIV and AIDS

Approved HIV medications are classified by mechanism of action: (1) nucleoside and non-nucleoside inhibitors of reverse transcriptase (**reverse transcriptase inhibitors**), (2) inhibitors of the viral protease (**HIV protease inhibitors**), (3) inhibitors of the viral integrase (**HIV integrase inhibitors**), (4) inhibitors of viral entrance into the target cell (**HIV fusion inhibitors**), and a (5) **CCR5 antagonist** (inhibitor of viral attachment) (see Figure 8.8). Low dose aspirin has potential to

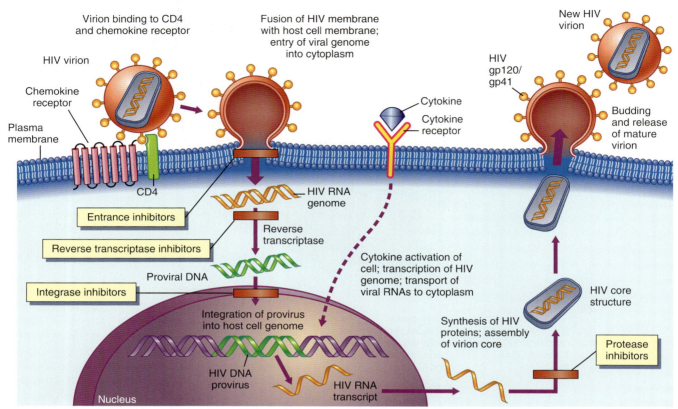

FIGURE 8.8 Life Cycle and Possible Sites of Therapeutic Intervention of HIV. The human immunodeficiency virus *(HIV)* virion consists of a core of two identical strands of viral RNA coated in a protein structure with viral proteins gp41 and gp120 on its surface (envelope). HIV infection begins when a virion binds to CD4 and chemokine co-receptors on a susceptible cell and follows the process described here. The provirus may remain latent in the cell's DNA until it is activated (e.g., by cytokines). The HIV life cycle is susceptible to blockage at several sites (see the text for further information), including entrance inhibitors, reverse transcriptase inhibitors, integrase inhibitors, and protease inhibitors. (Modified from Kumar, V., Abbas, A. K., & Aster, J. C. [Eds.]. [2021]. *Robbins and Cotran pathologic basis of disease* [10th ed.]. Elsevier.)

prevent the transmission of HIV by reducing the inflammation of cells in the female genitourinary tract, thus reducing the HIV target cells.[56] The current regimen for treatment of HIV infection is a combination of medications, termed **highly active antiretroviral therapy (HAART)**.[57] HAART protocols require a combination of synergist medications from different classes, and specific regimens (e.g., timing of medication administration, doses, medication combinations) are adapted on the basis of age of the individual, secondary clinical symptoms (renal or hepatic insufficiency), CD4+ Th cell levels, viral load, specific co-infections, pre-existing cardiac risk factors, past history of treatment failure, suspected medication resistance, and other parameters.[58] The clinical benefits of HAART are profound. The introduction of HAART has significantly reduced death from AIDS-related diseases. However, there are now resistant variants to these medications. Medication therapy for AIDS is not curative because HIV incorporates into the genetic material of the host, particularly CD4+ T memory cells, and may never be removed by antimicrobial therapy.[59] Therefore, medication administration to control the virus may have to continue for the lifetime of the individual. Additionally, HIV may persist in regions where the antiviral medications are not as effective, such as the central nervous system (CNS).

The chronic nature of HIV/AIDS resulting from successful HAART introduces additional concerns. Long-term toxicity of HAART medications increases the risk for cardiovascular disease, metabolic disorders, and organ failure. In many cases, treated individuals may always be immunocompromised and can even develop chronic immune activation, which is characterized by activation of monocytes and T cells, production of proinflammatory cytokines (e.g., IFN-γ, IL-6), and depletion of Th17 cells, thus decreasing the neutrophil and macrophage response to invading pathogens.[60] Chronic immune activation tends to exacerbate clinical disease in adults and neonates.[61]

Vaccine development should be the most effective means of preventing HIV infection and may be useful in treating pre-existing infection. Most of the common viral vaccines (e.g., rubella, mumps, influenza) induce protective antibodies that block the initial infection. Only one vaccine (rabies) is used after the infection has occurred. The rabies vaccine is successful because the rabies virus proliferates and spreads very slowly. However, the ability of an HIV vaccine to either successfully prevent or treat HIV infection is questionable for several reasons:[62] (1) the AIDS virus is genetically and antigenically *variable*, like the influenza virus, so that a vaccine created against one variant may not provide protection against another variant; (2) although individuals with HIV/AIDS have high levels of circulating antibodies against the virus, these *antibodies do not appear to be protective*. Therefore, even if a circulating antibody response can be induced by vaccination, that response might not be effective. A vaccine may have to induce both circulating and secretory (to prevent initial infection of the mucosal T cell) antibody and Tc cells.

BOX 8.2 AIDS-Defining Opportunistic Infections and Neoplasms Found in Individuals With HIV Infection

Infections

Protozoal and Helminthic Infections
Cryptosporidiosis or isosporiasis (enteritis)
Pneumocystosis (pneumonia or disseminated infection)
Toxoplasmosis (pneumonia or central nervous system [CNS] infection)

Fungal Infections
Candidiasis (esophageal, tracheal, or pulmonary)
Coccidioidomycosis (disseminated)
Cryptococcosis (CNS infection)
Histoplasmosis (disseminated)

Bacterial Infections
Mycobacteriosis ("atypical," e.g., *Mycobacterium avium-intracellulare*, disseminated or extrapulmonary
Mycobacterium tuberculosis, disseminated or extrapulmonary)
Nocardiosis (pneumonia, meningitis, disseminated)
Salmonella infections (septicemia, recurrent)

Viral Infections
Cytomegalovirus (pulmonary, intestinal, retinitis, or CNS)
Herpes simplex virus (localized or disseminated)
Progressive multifocal leukoencephalopathy
Varicella-zoster virus (localized or disseminated)

Neoplasms
Invasive cancer of the uterine cervix
Kaposi sarcoma
Non-Hodgkin's lymphomas (Burkitt, immunoblastic)
Primary lymphoma of brain

From Kumar, V., Abbas, A. K., & Aster, J. C. (Eds.). (2021). *Robbins and Cotran pathologic basis of disease* (10th ed.). Elsevier.

Pediatric AIDS and Central Nervous System Involvement

HIV can be transmitted from mother to child during pregnancy, at the time of delivery, or through breastfeeding. The risk of mother-to-child transmission has dropped precipitously since the use of antiretroviral medications in pregnant women. The clinical diagnosis of HIV infection in young children born of HIV-infected mothers is very often a difficult task because the presence of maternal antibodies may result in a misleading false-positive test for antibodies against HIV for as long as 18 months after birth. Testing for antibody against HIV can be performed recurrently from birth until 18 months; if the test results become negative and remain so after 12 months, the child can be considered uninfected.

The report *WHO Recommendations on the Diagnosis of HIV Infection in Infants and Children* suggests that in children younger than 18 months, testing for HIV or viral components should occur in two separate specimens, not including cord blood.[63] Testing involves detection of HIV nucleic acid or p24 antigen, or direct isolation of HIV in viral cultures.

HIV infection of babies is generally more aggressive than in adults; on average, an untreated child will die by his or her second birthday. Neurological involvement occurs more commonly in children than in adults and results from CNS involvement, rather than effects on peripheral portions of the nervous system. HIV encephalopathy occurs with varying degrees of severity and is a clinical component in the diagnosis of AIDS in children. Most HIV-infected newborns appear normal but may progressively develop signs of CNS involvement. These signs usually appear as failure to attain (or loss of) developmental milestones or loss of intellectual ability, verified by standard developmental scale or neuropsychological tests; acquired symmetrical motor deficits, seen in children older than age 1 month; impaired brain growth or acquired microcephaly, demonstrated by head circumference measurements; or brain atrophy, demonstrated by computed tomography (CT) or magnetic resonance imaging (MRI) (serial imaging is required in children younger than 2 years of age).

It may be difficult to completely differentiate the effect of HIV infection on the CNS from other risk factors, including prenatal medication exposure, prematurity, chronic illness, and a chaotic social atmosphere. The pathogenesis of HIV encephalopathy in children is poorly understood, but the presence of inflammatory mediators may be a contributing factor.

Because HIV infection in infants progresses very rapidly, treatment must begin at the diagnosis of infection. In older children the criteria for treatment are similar to those used in adults. A growing number of investigational protocols are available for treatment of children with HIV. In general, treatment is focused on the preservation and maintenance of the immune system, aggressive response to opportunistic infections, support and relief of symptomatic occurrences, and administration of HAART.

HYPERSENSITIVITY: ALLERGY, AUTOIMMUNITY, AND ALLOIMMUNITY

> ### ✓ QUICK CHECK 8.3
> 1. Distinguish among the four types of hypersensitivity mechanisms.
> 2. What is the mechanism of anaphylaxis?
> 3. What are some clinical examples of type IV hypersensitivity?

Allergy, autoimmunity, and alloimmunity are classified as *hypersensitivity reactions*. **Hypersensitivity** is an altered immunological response to an antigen that results in disease or damage to the individual. Allergy, autoimmunity, and alloimmunity (also termed *isoimmunity*) is most easily understood in relationship to the source of the antigen (e.g., environmental, tissue-specific/self-antigens, bacteria, and other foreign pathogens) against which the hypersensitivity response is directed (Table 8.12). For instance, **allergy** refers to a hypersensitivity to environmental antigens. These can include medicines, natural products (e.g., pollens, bee stings), infectious agents, and any other antigen that is not naturally found in the individual.

Autoimmunity is a disturbance in the immunological tolerance of self-antigens. The immune system normally does not strongly recognize the individual's own antigens. Healthy individuals of all ages, but particularly older persons, may produce low quantities of antibodies against their own antigens (*autoantibodies*) without developing overt autoimmune disease. Therefore, the presence of low quantities of autoantibodies does not necessarily indicate a disease state. Autoimmune diseases occur when the immune system reacts against self-antigens to such a degree that autoantibodies or autoreactive T cells damage the individual's tissues. Many clinical disorders are associated with autoimmunity and are generally referred to as **autoimmune diseases** (Table 8.13). Autoimmune diseases are more prevalent in women and the overall prevalence is rising.[64]

Alloimmune diseases occur when the immune system of one individual produces an immunological reaction against tissues of another individual. **Alloimmunity** can be observed during immunological reactions against transfusions, transplanted tissue, or the fetus during pregnancy.

How allergy, autoimmunity, or alloimmunity develops as the mechanism of hypersensitivity essentially remains a mystery. Because

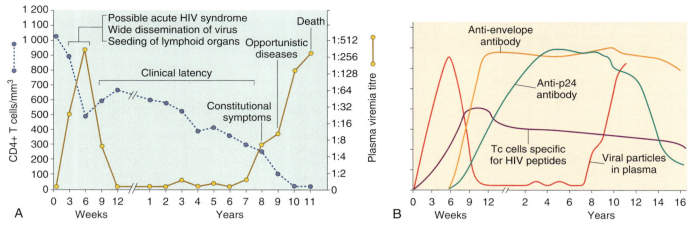

FIGURE 8.9 Typical Progression From HIV Infection to AIDS in Untreated Persons. A, Clinical progression begins within weeks after infection; the person may experience symptoms of acute human immunodeficiency virus (HIV) syndrome. During this early period, the virus progressively infects T cells and other cells and spreads to the lymphoid organs, with a sharp decrease in the number of circulating CD4+ Th cells. During a period of clinical latency, the virus replicates and T-cell destruction continues, although the person is generally asymptomatic. The individual may develop HIV-related disease (constitutional symptoms); a variety of symptoms of acute viral infection that do not involve opportunistic infections or malignancies. When the number of CD4+ Th cells is critically suppressed, the individual becomes susceptible to a variety of opportunistic infections and cancers with a diagnosis of acquired immunodeficiency syndrome (AIDS). The length of time for progression from HIV infection to AIDS may vary considerably from person to person. B, Laboratory tests are changing throughout infection. Antibody and Tc cell (T-cytotoxic cells [Tc cells]) levels change during the progression to AIDS. During the initial phase antibodies against HIV-1 are not yet detectable (window period), but viral products, including proteins and RNA, and infectious virus may be detectable in the blood a few weeks after infection. Most antibodies against HIV are not detectable in the early phase. During the latent phase of infection antibody levels against p24 and other viral proteins, as well as HIV-specific Tc cells, increase, and then remain constant until the development of AIDS. ([A] redrawn from Fauci, A. S., & Lane, H. C. [1997]. Human immunodeficiency virus disease: AIDS and related conditions. In: Fauci, A. S., Braunwald, E., Isselbacher, K. J., et al. [Eds.], *Harrison's principles of internal medicine* [14th ed.]. McGraw-Hill; [B] from Kumar, V., Abbas, A. K., & Aster, J. C. [Eds.]. [2021]. *Robbins and Cotran pathologic basis of disease* [10th ed.]. Elsevier.)

hypersensitivity reactions involve exaggerated immune responses, genetic, infectious, and possibly environmental factors contribute to the development of hypersensitivity reactions.

Mechanisms of Hypersensitivity

Hypersensitivity reactions are also characterized by the particular immune mechanism that results in the disease (Table 8.14). These mechanisms are apparent in most hypersensitivity reactions and exist as four distinct types: *type I* (IgE-mediated reactions), *type II* (tissue-specific reactions), *type III* (immune complex–mediated reactions), and *type IV* (cell-mediated reactions). This classification is artificial, and seldom is a particular disease associated with only a single mechanism. The four mechanisms are interrelated, and in most hypersensitivity reactions, several mechanisms can be functioning simultaneously or sequentially.

As with all immune responses, hypersensitivity reactions require sensitization against a particular antigen that results in a *primary immune response*. Disease symptoms appear after an adequate *secondary immune response* occurs. Hypersensitivity reactions are *immediate* or *delayed*, depending on the time required to elicit clinical symptoms after re-exposure to the antigen. Reactions that occur within minutes to a few hours after exposure to an antigen are termed **immediate hypersensitivity reactions**. **Delayed hypersensitivity reactions** may take several hours to appear and are at maximal severity days after re-exposure to the antigen. Generally, immediate reactions are caused by antibody, whereas delayed reactions are caused by cells (e.g., T cells, NK cells, macrophages).

The most rapid and severe immediate hypersensitivity reaction is **anaphylaxis**. Anaphylaxis occurs within minutes of re-exposure to the antigen and can be either systemic (generalized) or cutaneous (localized). Symptoms of systemic anaphylaxis include pruritus, erythema, vomiting, abdominal cramps, diarrhea, and breathing difficulties, and the most severe reactions may include contraction of bronchial smooth muscle, edema of the throat, and decreased blood pressure that can lead to shock and death.[65] Examples of systemic anaphylaxis are allergic reactions to bee stings, peanuts, shellfish, or eggs. Cutaneous anaphylaxis results in local symptoms, such as pain, swelling, and redness, which occur at the site of exposure to an antigen (e.g., a painful local reaction to an injected vaccine or medication).

Type I: IgE-Mediated Hypersensitivity Reactions

Antigen-specific IgE and the products of mast cells are the mediators of **type I hypersensitivity** reactions (Figure 8.11). Most common **allergic** reactions are type I reactions. In addition, as an allergic response, most type I reactions occur against environmental antigens. Because of this strong association, many health care providers use the term *allergy* to indicate only IgE-mediated reactions. However, IgE can contribute to some autoimmune and alloimmune diseases, and many common allergies (e.g., poison ivy) are not mediated by IgE.

IgE has a relatively short lifespan in the blood because it rapidly binds to Fc receptors on mast cells.[66] Unlike Fc receptors on phagocytes, which bind IgG that has previously reacted with an antigen, the Fc receptors on mast cells specifically bind IgE that has not previously

CHAPTER 8 Infection and Defects in Mechanisms of Defence

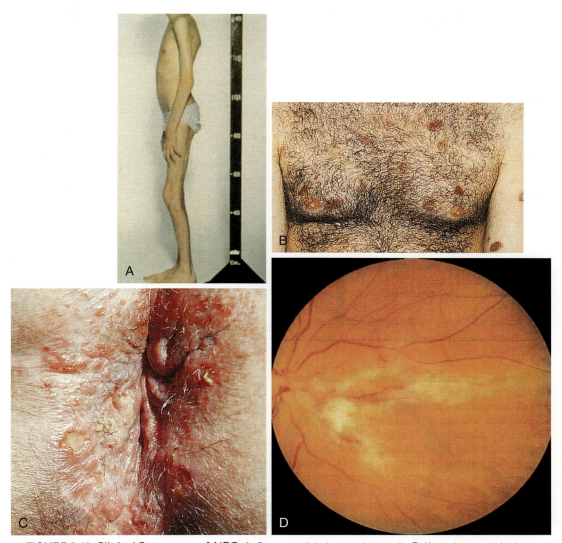

FIGURE 8.10 Clinical Symptoms of AIDS. **A**, Severe weight loss and anorexia. **B**, Kaposi sarcoma lesions. **C**, Perianal lesions of herpes simplex infection. **D**, Deterioration of vision from cytomegalovirus retinitis leading to areas of infection, which can lead to blindness. ([A], [D] from Taylor, P. K. [1995]. *Diagnostic picture tests in sexually transmitted diseases*. London: Mosby; [B], [C] from Morse, S. A., Holmes, K. K., & Balllard, R. C. [Eds.]. [2011]. *Atlas of sexually transmitted diseases and AIDS* [4th ed.]. Saunders.)

TABLE 8.12 Relative Incidence and Examples of Hypersensitivity Diseases

	MECHANISM			
	Type I (IgE Mediated)	Type II (Tissue Specific)	Type III (Immune Complex Mediated)	Type IV (Cell Mediated)
Allergy Target antigens: environmental antigens	++++ Hay fever	+ Hemolysis in medication allergies	+ Gluten (wheat) allergy	++ Poison ivy allergy
Autoimmunity Target antigens: self-antigens	+ May contribute to some type III reactions	++ Autoimmune thrombocytopenia	+++ Systemic lupus erythematosus	++ Hashimoto thyroiditis
Alloimmunity Target antigens: another person's antigens	+ May contribute to some type III reactions	++ Hemolytic disease of the newborn	+ Individuals who do not make their own IgA may have an anaphylactic response against IgA in human immune globulin	++ Graft rejection

[a]The frequency of each reaction is indicated in a range from rare (+) to very common (++++). An example of each reaction is given.

TABLE 8.13 Examples of Autoimmune Disorders

System Disease	Organ or Tissue	Probable Self-Antigen
Endocrine System		
Hyperthyroidism (Graves' disease)	Thyroid gland	Receptors for thyroid-stimulating hormone on plasma membrane of thyroid cells
Hashimoto's disease	Thyroid gland	Thyroid cell surface antigens, thyroglobulin
Insulin-dependent diabetes	Pancreas	Islet cells, insulin, insulin receptors on pancreatic cells
Addison's disease	Adrenal gland	Surface antigens on steroid-producing cells; microsomal antigens
Male infertility	Testis	Surface antigens on spermatozoa
Skin		
Pemphigus vulgaris	Skin	Intercellular substances in stratified squamous epithelium
Bullous pemphigoid	Skin	Basement membrane
Vitiligo	Skin	Surface antigens on melanocytes (melanin-producing cells)
Neuromuscular Tissue		
Multiple sclerosis	Neural tissue	Surface antigens of nerve cells
Myasthenia gravis	Neuromuscular junction	Acetylcholine receptors; striations of skeletal and cardiac muscle
Rheumatic fever	Heart	Cardiac tissue antigens that cross-react with group A streptococcal antigen
Cardiomyopathy	Heart	Cardiac muscle
Gastro-intestinal System		
Ulcerative colitis	Colon	Mucosal cells
Pernicious anemia	Stomach	Surface antigens of parietal cells; intrinsic factor
Primary biliary cirrhosis	Liver	Cells of bile duct
Chronic active hepatitis	Liver	Surface antigens of hepatocytes, nuclei, microsomes, smooth muscle
Eye		
Sjögren's syndrome	Lacrimal gland	Antigens of lacrimal gland, salivary gland, thyroid, and nuclei of cells
Connective Tissue		
Ankylosing spondylitis	Joints	Sacroiliac and spinal apophyseal joint
Rheumatoid arthritis	Joints	Collagen, IgG
Systemic lupus erythematosus	Multiple sites	Numerous antigens in nuclei, organelles, and extracellular matrix
Renal System		
Immune complex glomerulonephritis	Kidney	Numerous immune complexes
Goodpasture's syndrome	Kidney	Glomerular basement membrane
Hematological System		
Idiopathic neutropenia	Neutrophil	Surface antigens on polymorphonuclear neutrophils
Idiopathic lymphopenia	Lymphocytes	Surface antigens on lymphocytes
Autoimmune hemolytic anemia	Erythrocytes	Surface antigens on erythrocytes
Autoimmune thrombocytopenic purpura	Platelets	Surface antigens on platelets
Respiratory System		
Goodpasture's syndrome	Lung	Septal membrane of alveolus

TABLE 8.14 Immunological Mechanisms of Tissue Destruction

Type	Name	Rate of Development	Class of Antibody Involved	Principal Effector Cells Involved	Participation of Complement	Examples of Disorders
I	IgE-mediated reaction	Immediate	IgE	Mast cells	No	Seasonal allergic rhinitis, Asthma
II	Tissue-specific reaction	Immediate	IgG, IgM	Macrophages in tissues	Frequently	Autoimmune thrombocytopenic purpura, Graves' disease, autoimmune hemolytic anemia
III	Immune complex–mediated reaction	Immediate	IgG, IgM	Neutrophils	Yes	Systemic lupus erythematosus
IV	Cell-mediated reaction	Delayed	None	Lymphocytes, Macrophages	No	Contact sensitivity to poison ivy, metals (jewelry), and latex

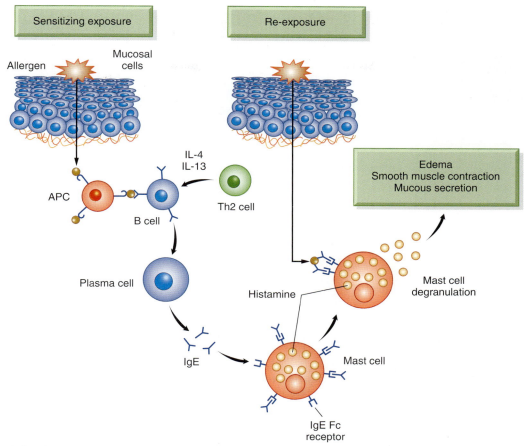

FIGURE 8.11 Mechanism of Type I, IgE-Mediated Reactions. First exposure to an allergen leads to antigen processing and presentation of antigen by an antigen-presenting cell (APC) to B cells, which is under the direction of T-helper 2 cells (Th2 cells). Th2 cells produce specific cytokines (e.g., interleukin-4 [IL-4], IL-13, and others) that favour maturation of the B cells into plasma cells that secrete IgE. The IgE is adsorbed to the surface of the mast cell by binding with IgE-specific crystallizable fragment (Fc) receptors. When an adequate amount of IgE is bound, the mast cell is sensitized. During re-exposure, the allergen cross-links the surface-bound IgE and causes degranulation of the mast cell. Contents of the mast cell granules, primarily histamine, induce local edema, smooth muscle contraction, mucous secretion, and other characteristics of an acute inflammatory reaction. (See Chapter 6 for more details on the role of mast cells in inflammation.)

interacted with antigen. After a large amount of IgE has bound to the mast cells, an individual is *sensitized*. Further exposure of a sensitized individual to the allergen results in degranulation of the mast cell and the release of mast cell products (see Chapter 6).

Mechanisms of IgE-mediated hypersensitivity. The most potent mediator of IgE-mediated hypersensitivity is **histamine**, which affects several key target cells. Acting through H1 receptors, histamine: (1) contracts bronchial smooth muscles (bronchial constriction), (2) increases vascular permeability (edema), and (3) causes vasodilation (increased blood flow) (see Chapter 6). The interaction of histamine with H2 receptors results in increased gastric acid secretion. Blocking histamine receptors with antihistamines can control some type I responses.

Clinical manifestations of IgE-mediated hypersensitivity. The clinical manifestations of type I reactions are attributable mostly to the biological effects of histamine. The tissues most commonly affected by type I responses contain large numbers of mast cells and are sensitive to the effects of histamine released from them. These tissues are found in the gastro-intestinal tract, the skin, and the respiratory tract (Figure 8.12 and Table 8.15).

Gastro-intestinal allergy develops as allergens such as food or medicines enter through the mouth. Symptoms include vomiting, diarrhea, or abdominal pain. Foods most often implicated in gastro-intestinal allergies are milk, chocolate, citrus fruits, eggs, wheat, nuts, peanut butter, and fish.[67] The most common food allergy in adults is shellfish, which may initiate an anaphylactic response and death.[68] When food is the source of an allergen, the active immunogen may be a result of how the food is processed during manufacture or broken down by digestive enzymes.[69] Sometimes the allergen is a medication, an additive, or a preservative in the food. For example, cows treated for mastitis with penicillin yield milk containing trace amounts of this antibiotic. Thus, hypersensitivity apparently caused by milk proteins may instead be the result of an allergy to penicillin.

Urticaria, or hives, is a dermal (skin) manifestation of allergic reactions (see Figure 8.12). The underlying mechanism is the localized release of histamine and increased vascular permeability, resulting in limited areas of edema. Urticaria is characterized by white fluid-filled blisters (wheals) surrounded by areas of redness (flares). This **wheal and flare reaction** is usually accompanied by pruritus. Immunological reactions do not cause all urticarial symptoms. Some urticarial

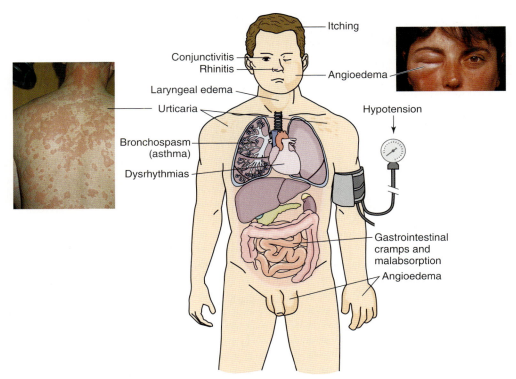

FIGURE 8.12 Type I, IgE-Mediated Hypersensitivity Reactions. Manifestations of allergic reactions as a result of type I hypersensitivity include pruritus, angioedema (swelling caused by exudation), edema of the larynx, urticaria (hives), bronchospasm (constriction of airways in the lungs), hypotension (low blood pressure), and dysrhythmias (irregular heartbeat) because of anaphylactic shock, and gastro-intestinal cramping caused by inflammation of the gastro-intestinal mucosa. Photographic inserts show a diffuse allergic-like eye and skin reaction on an individual. The skin lesions have raised edges and develop within minutes or hours, with resolution occurring after about 12 hours. (Inserts from Male, D., Brostoff, J., Roth, D., et al. [2013]. *Immunology* [8th ed.]. Mosby.)

symptoms, termed *nonimmunological urticaria*, result from exposure to cold temperatures, emotional stress, medications, systemic diseases, or malignancies (e.g., lymphomas).

Effects of allergens on the mucosa of the eyes, nose, and respiratory tract include conjunctivitis (inflammation of the membranes lining the eyelids) (see Figure 8.12), rhinitis (inflammation of the mucous membranes of the nose), and asthma (constriction of the bronchi). Vasodilation, hypersecretion of mucus, edema, and swelling of the respiratory mucosa contribute to the symptoms. The mucous membranes of the respiratory tract extend from the nose, mouth, and throat down to all lung tissues, and all become compromised during allergic reactions. The degree to which each is affected determines the symptoms of the disease; most anaphylactic reactions are type I hypersensitivities.

The central problem in allergic diseases of the lung is obstruction of the large and small airways (bronchi) of the lower respiratory tract by bronchospasm (constriction of smooth muscle in airway walls), edema, and thick secretions. This obstruction leads to ventilatory insufficiency, wheezing, and difficult or laboured breathing (see Chapter 27).

Certain individuals are genetically predisposed to develop allergies and are called **atopic**. In families in which one parent has an allergy, allergies develop in about 40% of the offspring. If both parents have allergies, the incidence may be as high as 80%. Atopic individuals tend to produce higher quantities of IgE and have more Fc receptors for IgE on their mast cells. The airways and the skin of atopic individuals have increased responsiveness to a wide variety of both specific and nonspecific stimuli.

Evaluation and treatment of IgE hypersensitivity. Allergic reactions can be life-threatening; therefore, it is essential that severely allergic individuals be informed of the specific allergen against which they are sensitized and instructed to avoid contact with that material. Several tests are available to evaluate allergic individuals. These include food challenges, skin tests with allergens, and laboratory tests for total IgE and allergen specific IgE.

Type II: Tissue-Specific Hypersensitivity Reactions

Type II hypersensitivities are generally reactions against a specific cell or tissue. Cells express a variety of antigens on their surfaces, some of which are called **tissue-specific antigens** because they are expressed on the plasma membranes of only certain cells. Platelets, for example, have groups of antigens that are found on no other cells of the body. The symptoms of many type II diseases are determined by which tissue or organ expresses the particular antigen. Environmental antigens (e.g., medications or their metabolites) may bind to the plasma membranes of specific cells (especially erythrocytes and platelets) and function as targets of type II reactions. The five general mechanisms by which type II hypersensitivity reactions can affect cells are shown in Figure 8.13. Each mechanism begins with antibody binding to tissue-specific antigens or antigens that have attached to particular tissues.

TABLE 8.15 Causes of Clinical Allergic Reactions

Typical Allergen	Mechanism of Hypersensitivity	Clinical Manifestation
Ingestants		
Foods	Type I	Gastro-intestinal allergy
Drugs	Types I, II, III	Urticaria, immediate medication reaction, hemolytic anemia, serum sickness
Inhalants		
Pollens, dust, moulds	Type I	Allergic rhinitis, bronchial asthma
Aspergillus fumigatus	Types I, III	Allergic bronchopulmonary aspergillosis
Thermophilic actinomycetes[a]	Types III, IV	Extrinsic allergic alveolitis
Injectants		
Drugs	Types I, II, III	Immediate medication reaction, hemolytic anemia, serum sickness
Bee venom	Type I	Anaphylaxis
Vaccines	Type III	Localized Arthus reaction
Serum	Types I, III	Anaphylaxis, serum sickness
Contactants		
Poison ivy, metals	Type IV	Contact dermatitis
Latex	Types I, IV	Contact dermatitis, anaphylaxis

[a]An order of fungi that grows best at high temperatures (between 45 and 80°C [113 and 176°F]).

Modified from Bellanti, J. A. (1985). *Immunology III.* Saunders.

The cell may be destroyed by antibodies and complement (Figure 8.13A). IgM or IgG reacts with an antigen on the surface of the cell, causing activation of the complement cascade through the classical pathway. Formation of the membrane attack complex (C5–9) damages the membrane and may result in lysis of the cell. For example, erythrocytes are destroyed by complement-mediated lysis in individuals with autoimmune hemolytic anemia (see Chapters 21 and 22) or as a result of an alloimmune reaction to mismatched transfused blood cells.

Antibody may cause cell destruction through phagocytosis by macrophages (Figure 8.13B). The antibody may additionally activate complement, resulting in the deposition of C3b on the cell surface. Receptors on the macrophage recognize and bind opsonins (e.g., antibody or C3b) and increase phagocytosis of the target cell. For example, antibodies against platelet-specific antigens or against red blood cell antigens of the Rh system cause their removal by phagocytosis in the spleen.

Tissue damage may be caused by toxic products produced by neutrophils (Figure 8.13C). Soluble antigens such as medications, molecules released from infectious agents, or molecules released from an individual's own cells may enter the circulation. In some instances, the antigens are deposited on the surface of tissues, where they bind antibody. The antibody may activate complement, resulting in the release of C3a and C5a, which are chemotactic for neutrophils, and the deposition of complement component C3b. Neutrophils are attracted, bind to the tissues through receptors for the Fc portion of antibody (Fc receptor) or for C3b, and release their granules onto the healthy tissue. The components of neutrophil granules, as well as the toxic oxygen products produced by these cells, will damage the tissue.

Antibody-dependent cell-mediated cytotoxicity (ADCC) *involves NK cells* (Figure 8.13D). The activation of ADCC involves the binding of IgG antibodies to antigens. The Fc portion of the antibody on the target cell is then recognized by Fc receptors on the NK cells, which release toxic substances that destroy the target cell. ADCC takes advantage of both innate and adaptive immunity because it uses the Fc portion of the antibody to activate NK cells, as well as monocytes, to mediate the cytotoxic effect. ADCC exists naturally with the response to the parasite, *Plasmodium* (in malaria), where ADCC causes lysis of red blood cells during acute infection,[70] and it has potential to treat conditions such as cancer and viral infection in the development of monoclonal antibodies.[71]

The last mechanism does not destroy the target cell but causes the cell to malfunction (Figure 8.13E). The antibody is usually directed against antigenic determinants associated with specific cell surface receptors. The antibody changes the function of the receptor by preventing interactions with their normal ligands, replacing the ligand and inappropriately stimulating the receptor, or destroying the receptor. For example, in the hyperthyroidism (excessive thyroid activity) of Graves' disease, the autoantibody binds to and activates receptors for thyroid-stimulating hormone (TSH) (a pituitary hormone that controls the production of the hormone thyroxine by the thyroid). In this way, the antibody stimulates the thyroid cells to produce thyroxine. Under normal conditions, the increasing levels of thyroxine in the blood would signal the pituitary to decrease TSH production, which would result in less stimulation of the TSH receptor in the thyroid and a concomitant decrease in thyroxine production. Increasing amounts of thyroxine in the blood have no effect on anti-TSH receptor antibodies, which continue to stimulate despite decreasing amounts of TSH (see Chapter 19).

Type III: Immune Complex–Mediated Hypersensitivity Reactions

Mechanisms of type III hypersensitivity. Most type III hypersensitivity disease reactions are caused by antigen–antibody (immune) complexes that are formed in the circulation and deposited later in vessel walls or other tissues (Figure 8.14). The primary difference between type II and type III mechanisms is that in type II hypersensitivity antibody binds to an antigen on the cell surface, whereas in type III, antibody binds to soluble antigen that is released into the blood or body fluids, and the complex is then deposited in the tissues. Type III reactions are not organ specific, and symptoms are mostly unrelated to the particular antigenic target of the antibody. The harmful effects of immune complex deposition are caused by complement activation, particularly through the generation of chemotactic factors for neutrophils. The neutrophils bind to antibody and C3b contained in the complexes and attempt to ingest the immune complexes. They are often unsuccessful because the complexes are bound to large areas of tissue. During the attempted phagocytosis, large quantities of lysosomal enzymes are released into the inflammatory site instead of into phagolysosomes. The attraction of neutrophils and the subsequent release of lysosomal enzymes cause most of the resulting tissue damage.

Immune complex disease. Two prototypic models of type III hypersensitivity help explain the variety of diseases in this category. Serum sickness is a model of systemic type III hypersensitivities, and the Arthus reaction is a model of localized or cutaneous reactions.

Serum sickness–type reactions are caused by the formation of immune complexes in the blood and their subsequent generalized deposition in target tissues. Typically affected tissues are the blood vessels, joints, and kidneys. Symptoms include fever, enlarged lymph

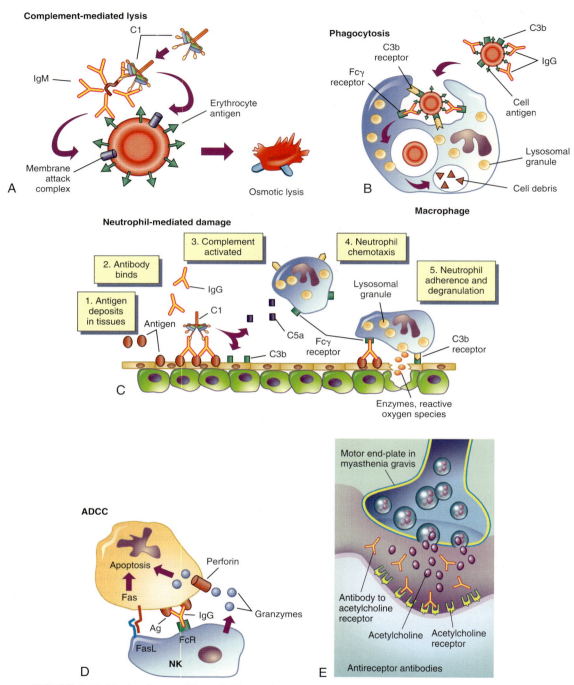

FIGURE 8.13 **Mechanisms of Type II, Tissue-Specific Hypersensitivity Reactions.** Antigens on the target cell bind with antibody and are destroyed or prevented from functioning by one of the following mechanisms: **A**, complement-mediated lysis (an erythrocyte target is illustrated here); **B**, clearance (phagocytosis) by macrophages in the tissue; **C**, neutrophil-mediated damage; **D**, antibody-dependent cell-mediated cytotoxicity *(ADCC)* (apoptosis of target cells is induced by natural killer *[NK]* cells by two mechanisms: by the release of granzymes and perforin, which is a molecule that creates pores in the plasma membrane, and enzymes [granzymes] that enter the target through the perforin pores; by the interactions of Fas ligand *[FasL;* a molecule similar to tumour necrosis factor-alpha] on the surface of NK cells with *Fas* [the receptor for FasL] on the surface of target cells); or **E**, modulation or blocking of the normal function of receptors by antireceptor antibody. This example of mechanism (E) depicts myasthenia gravis in which acetylcholine receptor antibodies block acetylcholine from attaching to its receptors on the motor endplates of skeletal muscle, thereby impairing neuromuscular transmission and causing muscle weakness. *Ag*, Antigen; *C1*, complement component C1; *C3b*, complement fragment produced from C3, which acts as an opsonin; *C5a*, complement fragment produced from C5, which acts as a chemotactic factor for neutrophils; *Fcγ receptor*, cellular receptor for the crystallizable fragment (Fc) portion of IgG; *FcR*, Fc receptor.

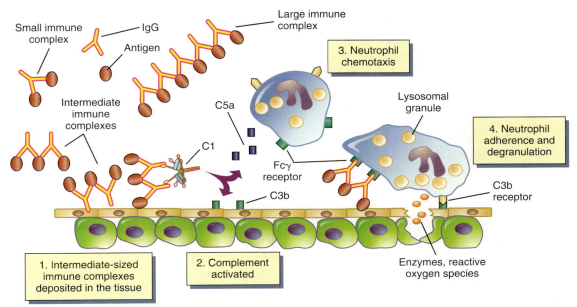

FIGURE 8.14 Mechanisms of Type III, Immune Complex–Mediated Hypersensitivity Reactions. Immune complexes form in the blood from circulating antigen and antibody. Both small and large immune complexes are removed successfully from the circulation and do not cause tissue damage. Intermediate-sized complexes are deposited in certain target tissues in which the circulation is slow or filtration of the blood occurs. The complexes activate the complement cascade through C1 and generate fragments including C5a and C3b. C5a is chemotactic for neutrophils, which migrate into the inflamed area and attach to the IgG and C3b in the immune complexes. The neutrophils attempt unsuccessfully to phagocytose the tissue and, in the process, release a variety of degradative enzymes that destroy the healthy tissues. *C1,* Complement component C1; *C3b,* complement fragment produced from C3, which acts as an opsonin; *C5a,* complement fragment produced from C5, which acts as a chemotactic factor for neutrophils; *Fcγ receptor,* cellular receptor for the crystallizable fragment (Fc) portion of IgG.

nodes, rash, and pain at sites of inflammation. Serum sickness was initially described as a complication of therapeutic administration of horse serum that contained antibody against tetanus toxin. Foreign serum is not administered to individuals today, although serum sickness reactions can be caused by the repeated intravenous administration of other antigens, such as medications, and the characteristics of serum sickness are observed in systemic type III autoimmune diseases.

A form of serum sickness is **Raynaud phenomenon**, a condition caused by the temperature-dependent deposition of immune complexes in the capillary beds of the peripheral circulation. Certain immune complexes precipitate at temperatures below normal body temperature, particularly in the tips of the fingers, toes, and nose, and are called **cryoglobulins**. The precipitates block the circulation and cause localized pallor and numbness, followed by cyanosis (a bluish tinge resulting from oxygen deprivation) and eventually gangrene if the circulation is not restored.

An **Arthus reaction** is caused by repeated local exposure to an antigen that reacts with preformed antibody and forms immune complexes in the walls of the local blood vessels. Symptoms of an Arthus reaction begin within 1 hour of exposure and peak 6 to 12 hours later. The lesions are characterized by a typical inflammatory reaction, with increased vascular permeability, an accumulation of neutrophils, edema, hemorrhage, clotting, and tissue damage.

Arthus reactions may be observed after injection, ingestion, or inhalation of allergens. Skin reactions can follow subcutaneous or intradermal inoculation with medications, fungal extracts, or antigens used in skin tests. Gastro-intestinal reactions, such as gluten-sensitive enteropathy (celiac disease), follow ingestion of an antigen, usually gluten from wheat products (see Chapter 37). Allergic alveolitis (farmer lung, pigeon breeder disease) is an Arthus-like acute hemorrhagic inflammation of the air sacs (alveoli) of the lungs resulting from inhalation of fungal antigens, usually particles from mouldy hay or pigeon feces (see Chapter 27).

Type IV: Cell-Mediated Hypersensitivity Reactions

Whereas types I, II, and III hypersensitivity reactions are mediated by antibody, **type IV hypersensitivity** reactions are mediated by T cells and do not involve antibody (Figure 8.15). Type IV mechanisms occur through either Tc cells or lymphokine-producing Th1 and Th17 cells. Tc cells attack and destroy cellular targets directly. Th1 and Th17 cells produce cytokines that recruit and activate phagocytic cells, especially macrophages. Destruction of the tissue is usually caused by direct killing by Tc cells or the release of soluble factors, such as lysosomal enzymes and toxic reactive oxygen species, from activated macrophages.

Clinical examples of type IV hypersensitivity reactions include graft rejection, the skin test for TB, and allergic reactions resulting from contact with such substances as poison ivy and metals. A type IV component also may be present in many autoimmune diseases. For example, T cells against type II collagen (a protein present in joint tissues) contribute to the destruction of joints in rheumatoid arthritis; T cells against a thyroid cell–surface antigen contribute to the destruction of the thyroid in autoimmune thyroiditis (Hashimoto's disease); and T cells against an antigen on the surface of pancreatic beta cells (the cell that normally produces insulin) are responsible for beta-cell destruction in insulin-dependent (type 1) diabetes mellitus.

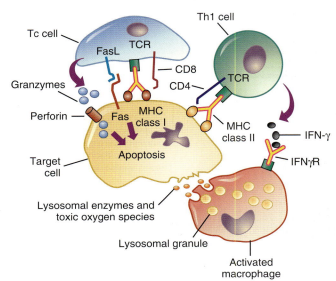

FIGURE 8.15 Mechanisms of Type IV, Cell-Mediated Hypersensitivity Reactions. Antigens from target cells stimulate T cells to differentiate into T-cytotoxic cells *(Tc cells)*, which have direct cytotoxic activity, and T-helper cells *(Th1 cells)* involved in delayed hypersensitivity. The Th1 cells produce lymphokines (especially interferon-γ *[IFN-γ]*) that activate the macrophage through specific receptors (e.g., IFN-γ receptor *[IFNγR]*). The macrophages can attach to targets and release enzymes and reactive oxygen species that are responsible for most of the tissue destruction. *FasL*, A molecule similar to tumour necrosis factor-alpha; *MHC*, major histocompatibility complex; *TCR*, T cell antigen receptor.

In 1891 Paul Ehrlich was the first to thoroughly describe a type IV hypersensitivity reaction in the skin, leading to the development of a diagnostic skin test for TB. The reaction follows an intradermal injection of tuberculin antigen into a suitably sensitized individual and is called a **delayed hypersensitivity skin test** because of its slow onset—24 to 72 hours to reach maximal intensity. The reaction site is infiltrated with T cells and macrophages, resulting in a clear hard centre (**induration**) and a reddish surrounding area (**erythema**).

Allergic type IV reactions are elicited by some environmental antigens that are haptens (Chapter 7) and become immunogenic after binding to larger (carrier) proteins in the individual. In allergic **contact dermatitis**, the carrier protein is in the skin. The best-known example is poison ivy (Figure 8.16). The antigen is a plant catechol, urushiol, which reacts with normal skin proteins and evokes a cell-mediated immune response. Skin reactions to industrial chemicals, cosmetics, detergents, clothing, food, metals, and topical medicines (such as penicillin) are elicited by the same mechanism. Contact dermatitis consists of lesions only at the site of contact with the allergen, such as a metal allergy to jewellery.

Antigenic Targets of Hypersensitivity Reactions

> ✓ **QUICK CHECK 8.4**
> 1. Why do certain medications become immunogenic to the host?
> 2. Why is systemic lupus erythematosus considered an autoimmune disease?
> 3. Define the different types of graft rejection.

Allergy

Allergens. Allergies are the most common hypersensitivity reactions. The majority of allergies are type I reactions that lead to annoying symptoms, including rhinitis, sneezing, and other relatively mild reactions. In some individuals, however, these reactions can be excessive and life-threatening (anaphylaxis). Antigens that cause allergic responses are called **allergens**. It is not known why some antigens are allergens and others are not. Typical allergens include pollens (e.g., ragweed), moulds and fungi (e.g., *Penicillium chrysogenum*), foods (e.g., milk, eggs, fish), animals (e.g., cat dander, dog dander), cigarette smoke, and components of house dust (e.g., fecal pellets of house mites). Often the allergen is contained within a particle that is too large to be phagocytosed or is surrounded by a protective nonallergenic coat. The actual allergen is released after enzymatic breakdown (e.g., by lysozyme in secretions) of the larger particle.

Allergic disease: bee sting allergy. Bee venoms contain a mixture of enzymes and other proteins that may serve as allergens and cause a type I hypersensitivity reaction. About 1% of children may have an anaphylactic reaction to bee venom.[72] Within minutes they may develop excessive swelling (edema) at the bee sting site, followed by generalized hives, pruritus, and swelling in areas distal from the sting (e.g., eyes, lips), and other systemic symptoms including flushing, sweating, dizziness, and headache. The most severe symptoms may include gastrointestinal (e.g., stomach cramps, vomiting), respiratory (e.g., tightness in the throat, wheezing, difficulty breathing), and vascular (e.g., low blood pressure, shock) reactions. Severe respiratory tract and vascular reactions may lead to death.

For an individual with known bee sting hypersensitivity, lifestyle changes include avoidance of stinging or biting insects. If a child has experienced a previous anaphylactic reaction, the chance of having another is about 60%. The primary life-threatening symptoms result from contraction of respiratory tract smooth muscle. Autonomic nervous system mediators, such as epinephrine, bind to specific receptors on smooth muscle and reverse the effects of histamine, resulting in muscle relaxation. Thus, most individuals with bee sting allergies carry self-injectable epinephrine. The administration of antihistamines has little effect because histamine has already bound H1 receptors and initiated severe bronchial smooth muscle contraction.

Clinical **desensitization** to allergens is possible with some individuals. The individual receives minute quantities of the allergen by injection in increasing doses over a prolonged period. The procedure may reduce the severity of the allergic reaction in the treated individual. However, this form of therapy may trigger systemic anaphylaxis, which can be severe and life-threatening. This approach works best for routine respiratory tract allergens and biting insect allergies (80 to 90% rate of desensitization over 5 years of treatment).[73] Food allergies are very difficult to suppress, but some promising trials are under way to evaluate desensitization by oral or sublingual administration of increasing amounts of allergen.

Autoimmunity

Autoimmune diseases originate from an initiating event in a genetically predisposed individual. Current models of factors related to autoimmune diseases include genetic factors, environmental factors, and random or stochastic changes.[74] Some autoimmune diseases can be familial and attributed to the presence of a very small number of susceptibility genes; affected family members may not all develop the same disease, but have different disorders characterized by a variety of hypersensitivity reactions, including autoimmune and allergic. For example, the HLA antigen B27 is a risk factor for developing **ankylosing spondylitis (AS)**, an autoimmune inflammatory disease of the spine; 95% of individuals diagnosed with AS express HLA-B27, whereas only 4 to 8% of the general population expresses this antigen.[75] Although most autoimmune diseases appear as isolated events without a positive family history, susceptibility for developing such diseases appears to be linked to a combination of multiple genes.

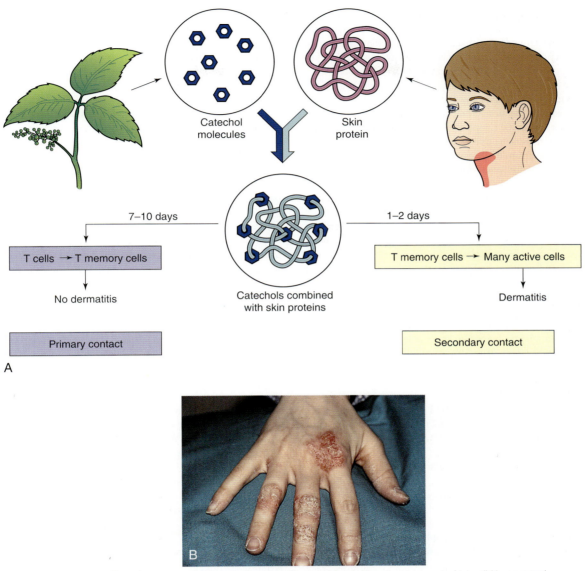

FIGURE 8.16 Development of Allergic Contact Dermatitis. **A,** The development of type IV hypersensitivity to poison ivy. The first (primary) contact with allergen sensitizes (produces reactive T cells) the individual but does not produce a rash (dermatitis). Secondary contact activates a type IV cell-mediated reaction that causes dermatitis. **B,** Contact dermatitis caused by a delayed hypersensitivity reaction leading to vesicles and scaling at the sites of contact. (From Damjanov, I., & Linder, J. [1996]. *Anderson's pathology* [10th ed.]. Mosby.)

Breakdown of tolerance. An individual is usually tolerant to his or her own antigens. **Tolerance** is a state of immunological control so that the individual does not make a detrimental immune response against his or her own cells and tissues. Autoimmune disease results from a breakdown of this tolerance.

The initiating event that breaks tolerance is unclear for most autoimmune diseases, as is why and how only certain tissues become involved.[74] Exploration of potential infectious initiators of autoimmune disease is ongoing,[76] with acute rheumatic fever being the most well-known. In a small number of individuals with group A streptococcal sore throats, the M proteins in the bacterial capsule mimic (*antigenic mimicry*) normal heart antigens and induce antibodies that also react with proteins in the heart valve, damaging the valve.[77] Thus acute rheumatic fever is a type II autoimmune hypersensitivity. Additionally, some streptococcal skin or throat infections release bacterial antigens into the blood that form circulating immune complexes. The complexes may deposit in the kidneys and initiate an immune complex–mediated glomerulonephritis (inflammation of the kidney).[78] Thus streptococcal antigens (an environmental antigen) may also cause a type III allergic hypersensitivity (poststreptococcal glomerulonephritis).

Autoimmune disease: systemic lupus erythematosus. **Systemic lupus erythematosus (SLE)** is the most common, complex, and serious of the autoimmune disorders. SLE is characterized by the production of a large variety of antibodies (autoantibodies) against self-antigens, including nucleic acids, erythrocytes, coagulation proteins, phospholipids, lymphocytes, platelets, and many other self-components. The most characteristic autoantibodies are against nucleic acids (e.g., ssDNA, dsDNA), histones, ribonucleoproteins, and other nuclear materials. Approximately 98% of persons with SLE have detectable antibodies against nuclear antigens. The blood normally contains many of these products of cellular turnover and breakdown so that autoantibodies react with the circulating antigen and form circulating immune complexes. The deposition of circulating DNA/anti-DNA complexes in the kidneys can cause severe kidney inflammation. Similar reactions can occur in the brain, heart, spleen, lung, gastro-intestinal tract, peritoneum, and skin. Thus, some of the symptoms of SLE result from a type III hypersensitivity reaction. Other symptoms, such as destruction of red blood cells (anemia), lymphocytes (lymphopenia), and other cells, may be type II hypersensitivity reactions.

SLE, like most autoimmune diseases, occurs more often in women (approximately a 9:1 predominance of females), especially in the 20- to 40-year-old age group.[79] Black individuals are affected more often than White individuals (about an eightfold increased risk). A genetic predisposition for the disease has been implicated based on increased incidence in twins and the existence of autoimmune disease in the families of individuals with SLE.

As with many autoimmune diseases, clinical manifestations of SLE may wax and wane; the individual may go through periods of remission and be relatively disease free until the onset of a *flare* (exacerbated disease activity). Symptoms include arthralgias or arthritis (90% of individuals), vasculitis and rash (70 to 80% of individuals), renal disease (40 to 50% of individuals), hematological abnormalities (50% of individuals, with anemia being the most common complication), and cardiovascular diseases (30 to 50% of individuals) (see "Discoid (Cutaneous) Lupus Erythematosus" in Chapter 41). Because the signs and symptoms affect nearly every body system and tend to vacillate, SLE is extremely difficult to diagnose. As a result, a list of 11 common clinical findings,[80] which has been modified slightly to increase sensitivity of the diagnosis,[81] is below. The serial or simultaneous presence of at least four of these findings indicates that the individual has SLE. The findings are:

1. Facial rash confined to the cheeks (malar rash) (see Figure 8.17).
2. Discoid rash (raised patches, scaling).
3. Photosensitivity (development of skin rash as a result of exposure to sunlight).
4. Oral or nasopharyngeal ulcers.
5. Nonerosive arthritis of at least two peripheral joints.
6. Serositis (inflammation of membranes of lung [pleurisy] or heart [pericarditis]).
7. Renal disorder (persistent proteinuria of greater than 0.5 g/day or greater than 3 by dipstick, or cellular casts).
8. Neurological disorders (seizures or psychosis in the absence of known causes).
9. Hematological disorders (hemolytic anemia, leukopenia, lymphopenia, or thrombocytopenia).
10. Immunological disorders (anti-dsDNA, anti–Smith [Sm] antigen, false-positive serological test for syphilis, or antiphospholipid antibodies [anticardiolipin antibody or lupus anticoagulant]).
11. Presence of antinuclear antibody (ANA).

Laboratory diagnosis is usually based on a positive ANA screening test; about 98% of individuals with SLE are positive, but a substantial number of false positives occur in healthy individuals and those with other diseases. Because SLE is a progressive and slowly developing disease, some laboratory tests, including the ANA, may be positive years before the onset of clinical symptoms.[76] Detection of a positive ANA is usually followed by one or more specific tests (e.g., antibodies against Sm, dsDNA) that are complicated by low sensitivity (only a portion of individuals with SLE will be positive, although the number of false positives is low).

There is no cure for SLE or most other autoimmune diseases. Fatalities resulting from SLE are usually related to infection, organ failure, or cardiovascular disease. The goals of treatment are to control symptoms and prevent further damage by suppressing the autoimmune response. Nonsteroidal anti-inflammatory drugs, such as acetylsalicylic acid (Aspirin), ibuprofen (Advil), or naproxen (Apo-Naproxen), reduce inflammation and relieve pain. Corticosteroids are often prescribed for more serious active disease. Immunosuppressive medications (e.g., methotrexate [Apo-Methotrexate], azathioprine [Nu-azathioprine], or cyclophosphamide [Procytox]) are used to treat severe symptoms involving internal organs. Antimalarial medications (e.g., hydroxychloroquine [Plaquenil]) are preferred treatments for individuals with stable disease.[76] Ultraviolet light may initiate flares, and protection from sun exposure is helpful. Prolonged use of certain medications can cause transient SLE-like symptoms, and the medication history is important for differential diagnosis.

Alloimmunity

Alloantigens. Genetic diversity is the norm in humans. Diversity also is observed among self-antigens, so that two individuals may have different antigens on their tissues and, therefore, make an immune response against each other's tissues. Some self-antigens, such as the ABO blood group, have limited diversity with very few different antigens being expressed in the population, whereas others, such as the HLA system, have tremendous diversity.

Alloimmune disease: transfusion reactions. Red blood cells (erythrocytes) express several important surface antigens, which are known collectively as the **blood group antigens** and can be targets of alloimmune reactions. More than 80 different red cell antigens are grouped into several dozen blood group systems. The most important of these, because they provoke the strongest humoral alloimmune response, are the ABO and Rh systems.

The **ABO blood group** consists of two major carbohydrate antigens, labelled A and B (Figure 8.18), that are expressed on virtually all cells. These are codominant, so both A and B can be simultaneously expressed, resulting in an individual having any one of four different blood types. The erythrocytes of blood type A express the type A carbohydrate antigen, those with blood type B express the B antigen, those with blood type AB express both A and B antigens on the same cell, and those of blood type O express neither the A nor the B antigen. A person with type A blood also has circulating antibodies to the B carbohydrate antigen. If this person receives blood from a type AB or B individual, a

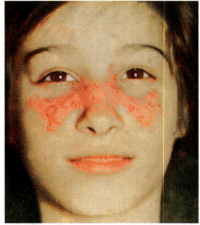

FIGURE 8.17 Butterfly Rash Manifestation of Systemic Lupus Erythematosus (SLE). (From Kliegman, R. M., Stanton, B. F., St. Geme III, J. W., et al. [Eds.], *Nelson handbook of pediatrics* [19th ed., Figure 152.1, A]. W. B. Saunders.)

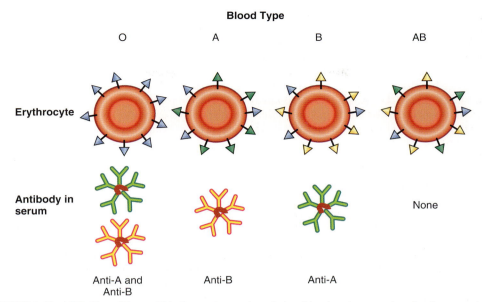

FIGURE 8.18 ABO Blood Types. This figure shows the relationship of antigens and antibodies associated with the ABO blood groups. The surfaces of erythrocytes of individuals with blood group O have a core carbohydrate that is present on cells of all ABO blood groups (H antigen). The sera of blood group O individuals contain IgM antibodies against both A and B carbohydrates. In individuals of the blood group A, some of the H antigens have been modified into A antigens. The sera of these individuals have IgM antibodies against the B antigen. In individuals with blood group B, some of the H antigens have been modified into B antigens. These individuals have IgM antibodies against the A antigen in their sera. In individuals of the blood group AB, some of the H antigens have been modified into both the A and B antigens. These individuals do not have antibodies to either A or B antigens.

severe transfusion reaction occurs, and the transfused erythrocytes are destroyed by agglutination or complement-mediated lysis. Similarly, a type B individual (whose blood contains anti-A antibodies) cannot receive blood from a type A or AB donor. Type O individuals, who have neither antigen but have both anti-A and anti-B antibodies, cannot accept blood from any of the other three types. These naturally occurring antibodies, called **isohemagglutinins**, are IgM immunoglobulins and are induced early in life against similar antigens expressed on naturally occurring bacteria in the intestinal tract.

Because individuals with type O blood lack both types of antigens, they are **universal donors**, meaning that anyone can accept their red blood cells. Similarly, type AB individuals are **universal recipients** because they lack both anti-A and anti-B antibodies and can receive transfusions with any ABO blood type. Only complete and careful ABO matching between donor and recipient can prevent harmful transfusion reactions.

The **Rh blood group** is a group of antigens expressed only on red blood cells. This blood group has the most diverse group of red cell antigens, consisting of at least 45 separate antigens, although only one is considered of major importance: the D antigen. Individuals who express the D antigen on their red cells are Rh-positive, whereas individuals who do not express the D antigen are Rh-negative. When discussing the gene for the Rh antigen, the letter *d* is used to indicate lack of D. Rh-positive individuals can have either a *DD* or *Dd* genotype, whereas Rh-negative individuals have the *dd* genotype. About 85% of North Americans are Rh-positive. Rh-negative individuals can make an IgG antibody to the D antigen (anti-D) if exposed to Rh-positive erythrocytes.

IgG anti-D alloantibody produced by Rh-negative mothers against erythrocytes of their Rh-positive fetuses produces a disease called *hemolytic disease of the newborn* (see Chapter 22). The mother's

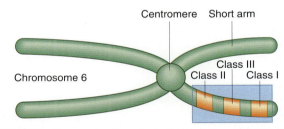

FIGURE 8.19 Human Leukocyte Antigens. The major histocompatibility complex is located on the short arm of chromosome 6 and contains genes that code for class I antigens, class II antigens, and class III proteins (i.e., complement proteins and cytokines). (From Peakman, M., & Vergani, D. [2009]. *Basic and clinical immunology* [2nd ed.]. Churchill Livingstone.)

antibody crosses the placenta and destroys the red blood cells of the fetus. The use of prophylactic anti-D immunoglobulin (i.e., WinRho) has greatly decreased the occurrence of this particular form of the disease. Administration of anti-D antibody within a few days of exposure to RhD-positive erythrocytes completely prevents sensitization against the D antigen. Control of hemolytic disease of the newborn related to the D antigen allows for greater understanding and exploration of alloantibodies against the other Rh antigens. In general, these alloantibodies are associated with a less severe hemolytic disease.

Alloimmune disease: transplant rejection. Chapter 7 discusses molecules of the MHC as antigen-presenting molecules. MHC molecules are also a major target of transplant rejection. *Human leukocyte antigen (HLA)* is another name for the human MHC molecule and the *HLA-A, HLA-B, HLA-C, HLA-DR, HLA-DQ,* and *HLA-DP* are other names for the different MHC loci (Figure 8.19). Additional genes for complement components (e.g., C4, factor B) also exist in the MHC region and they are class III loci. The class I (HLA-A, HLA-B, and HLA-C) and class II MHC loci (HLA-DR, HLA-DQ, and HLA-DP) are the most genetically diverse (polymorphic) of any human genetic loci. Within the human population, the number of possible different alleles (i.e., forms of the gene) expressed by each locus is astounding. For example, more than 300 different HLA-A molecules are expressed in the population. These numbers are based on the polymorphism of observed DNA sequences and may not reflect differences in function.

Clearly, not every allele is expressed in the same individual. Humans have two copies of each MHC locus (one inherited from each parent) that are codominant so that molecules encoded by each parent's genes are expressed on the surface of every cell, except erythrocytes. Within an individual, each locus will express only one allele. For example, each person will have at most two different HLA-A proteins (one from each parent). However, with the tremendous number of possible alleles that can be expressed throughout the population, it is unlikely that any two unrelated individuals will have the same MHC antigens.

The diversity of MHC molecules becomes clinically relevant during organ transplantation. The recipient of a transplant can mount an immune response against the foreign HLA antigens on the donor tissue, resulting in rejection. To minimize the chance of tissue rejection, the donor and recipient are often tissue-typed beforehand to identify differences in HLA antigens. Because of the large number of different alleles, it is highly unlikely that a perfect match can be found between someone who needs a transplant and a potential donor from the general population. The more similar two individuals are in their HLA tissue type, the more likely a transplant from one to the other will be successful. Clearly, the most successful transplants would be between identical twins because they are identical genetically.

The specific combination of alleles at the six major HLA loci on one chromosome (A, B, C, DR, DQ, and DP) is termed a *haplotype*. Everyone has two HLA haplotypes, one from the paternal chromosome 6 and another from the maternal chromosome (Figure 8.20). Each parent passes on one set of HLA antigens to each of his or her offspring, meaning that children usually share half their HLA antigens with each parent. Odds dictate that children will share one haplotype with half their siblings and either no haplotypes or both haplotypes with a quarter of their siblings. Thus, the chance of finding a match among siblings is much higher (25%) than the general population.

Transplant rejection may be classified as hyperacute, acute, or chronic, depending on the amount of time that elapses between transplantation and rejection. **Hyperacute rejection** is immediate and rare. When the circulation is re-established to the grafted area, the graft may immediately turn white (the so-called white graft) instead of a normal pink colour. Hyperacute rejection usually occurs because of pre-existing antibody (type II reaction) to HLA antigens on the vascular endothelial cells in the grafted tissue.

Acute rejection is a cell-mediated immune response that occurs within days to months after transplantation. This type of rejection occurs when the recipient develops an immune response against unmatched HLA antigens after transplantation. A biopsy of the rejected organ usually shows an infiltration of lymphocytes and macrophages characteristic of a type IV reaction.

Chronic rejection may occur after a period of months or years of normal function. It is characterized by slow, progressive organ failure. Chronic rejection usually results from a weak cell-mediated (type IV) reaction against minor histocompatibility antigens on the grafted tissue. However, antibodies against HLA and other antigens also may cause chronic rejection through activation of complement or ADCC with NK cells.

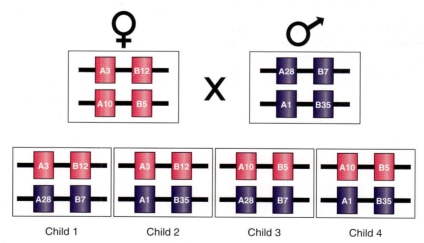

FIGURE 8.20 Inheritance of Human Leukocyte Antigens. Human leukocyte antigen (HLA) alleles are inherited in a codominant fashion; both maternal and paternal antigens are expressed. Specific HLA alleles are commonly given numbers to indicate different antigens. In this example, the mother has linked genes for HLA-A3 and HLA-B12 on one chromosome 6 and genes for HLA-A10 and HLA-B5 on the second chromosome 6. The father has HLA-A28 and HLA-B7 on one chromosome and HLA-A1 and HLA-B35 on the second chromosome. The children from this pairing may have one of four possible combinations of maternal and paternal HLA.

CHAPTER 8 Infection and Defects in Mechanisms of Defence

CASE STUDY

Edward, a 48-year-old unemployed auto mechanic, has come to the clinic complaining of a puffy, running nose and itchy, watery eyes that has been bothering him all day. He tells the nurse he has hay fever and this happens every spring. His history also includes myasthenia gravis and HIV. He has visible ptosis. He was diagnosed with HIV 6 years ago and believes he contracted the virus from a woman he met at a party and slept with twice.

Critical Thinking and Clinical Judgement Questions

1. a) How are viral infections different than bacterial infections in humans? Explain this difference in relation to MHC proteins and corresponding treatment. b) How is HIV different than other viruses?
2. a) How does Edward's HIV status put him at risk for opportunistic infections? b) What are some signs and symptoms of infection?
3. a) Is Edward a candidate for a vaccine? b) Explain active and passive immunity and how it relates to Edward. c) Why is there no vaccine for HIV?
4. a) What diagnostic tests would indicate if Edward's HIV was managed effectively and why? b) Why would he be given a combination of medications?
5. a) Explain the hypersensitivity reactions responsible for Edward's hay fever and myasthenia gravis. b) What other hypersensitivity reactions is Edward at risk for and why?
6. a) Edward recognizes that he is at greater risk of developing kidney failure related to his HIV. Why? b) Is he a candidate for a kidney transplant? Explain the risks associated with the various types of rejection and what needs to be done to minimize these risks.

DID YOU UNDERSTAND?

Infection

1. Infectious disease is a significant cause of morbidity and mortality worldwide.
2. Pathogens have unique characteristics that influence their ability to cause disease.
3. Bacteria injure cells by producing exotoxins or endotoxins. Exotoxins are enzymes that can damage the plasma membranes of host cells or can inactivate enzymes critical to protein synthesis, and endotoxins activate the inflammatory response and produce fever.
4. Septicemia is the proliferation of bacteria in the blood. Endotoxins released by bloodborne bacteria cause the release of vasoactive enzymes that increase the permeability of blood vessels. Leakage from vessels causes hypotension that can result in endotoxic shock.
5. Viruses enter host cells and use the metabolic processes of host cells to proliferate and cause disease.
6. Viruses that have invaded host cells may decrease protein synthesis, disrupt lysosomal membranes, form inclusion bodies where synthesis of viral nucleic acids is occurring, fuse with host cells to produce giant cells, alter antigenic properties of the host cell, transform host cells into cancerous cells, and promote bacterial infection.
7. Diseases caused by fungi are called *mycoses*, and they occur in two forms: yeasts (spheres) and multicellular moulds (filaments or hyphae).
8. Dermatophytes are fungi that infect skin, hair, and nails with diseases such as ringworm and athlete's foot.
9. Fungi release toxins and enzymes that are damaging to tissue. *Candida albicans* is the most common cause of fungal infections in humans.
10. Parasitic microorganisms range from unicellular protozoa to large worms. Although less common in Canada and the United States, parasites and protozoa are common causes of infection worldwide.
11. Parasitic and protozoal infections are rarely transmitted from human to human. Infection mainly spreads through vectors (e.g., by mosquito bites) or through contaminated water or food (i.e., malaria, Chagas disease, sleeping sickness, and leishmaniasis).
12. Infection control measures include implementation of clean food and water, management of sewage and waste, control of insects that transmit disease, vaccination, appropriate use of antimicrobials, and passive immunotherapy.

Deficiencies in Immunity

1. An immune deficiency is the failure of mechanisms of self-defence to function in their normal capacity.
2. Immunodeficiencies are either congenital (primary) or acquired (secondary). Congenital immunodeficiencies are caused by genetic defects that disrupt lymphocyte development, whereas acquired immunodeficiencies are secondary to disease or other physiological alterations.
3. The clinical hallmark of immunodeficiency is a propensity to unusual or recurrent severe infections. The type of infection usually reflects the immune system defect.
4. The most common infections in individuals with defects of cell-mediated immune response are fungal and viral, whereas infections in individuals with defects of the humoral immune response or complement function are primarily bacterial.
5. Severe combined immunodeficiency (SCID) is a total lack of T-cell function and a severe (either partial or total) lack of B-cell function.
6. Wiskott-Aldrich syndrome is caused by decreased production of IgM antibody.
7. DiGeorge syndrome (congenital thymic aplasia or hypoplasia) is characterized by complete or partial lack of the thymus (resulting in depressed T-cell immunity) and is frequently associated with diminished or absent parathyroid gland activity (resulting in hypocalcemia) and cardiac anomalies.
8. Antibody deficiencies result from defects in B-cell maturation or function, the lymphoid organs required for B-cell maturation (as in Bruton agammaglobulinemia), to deficiencies in a single class of immunoglobulins (e.g., selective IgA deficiency).
9. Phagocyte defects include inadequate numbers or alteration in function, such as inadequate adhesion to bacteria or ineffective killing.
10. Complement and mannose-binding lectin deficiencies also are rare causes of increased risk for infection.
11. Acquired immunodeficiencies are caused by superimposed conditions, such as malnutrition, medical therapies, physical trauma, psychological stress, or infections.
12. Immunodeficiency syndromes usually are treated by replacement therapy. Deficient antibody production is treated by replacement of missing immunoglobulins with commercial gamma-globulin preparations. Lymphocyte deficiencies are treated by the replacement of host lymphocytes with transplants of bone marrow, fetal liver, or fetal thymus from a donor. Gene therapy trials are ongoing.
13. AIDS is an acquired dysfunction of the immune system caused by a retrovirus (HIV) that infects and destroys CD4+ Th cells.

Hypersensitivity: Allergy, Autoimmunity, and Alloimmunity

1. Hypersensitivity is an immune response misdirected against the host's own tissues (autoimmunity) or directed against beneficial foreign tissues, such as transfusions or transplants (alloimmunity); or it can be exaggerated responses against environmental antigens (allergy).
2. Mechanisms of hypersensitivity are classified as type I (IgE-mediated reactions), type II (tissue-specific reactions), type III (immune complex–mediated reactions), and type IV (cell-mediated reactions).
3. Hypersensitivity reactions can be immediate (developing within seconds or hours) or delayed (developing within hours or days).
4. Anaphylaxis, the most rapid immediate hypersensitivity reaction, is an explosive reaction that occurs within minutes of re-exposure to the antigen and can lead to shock and death.
5. Type I (IgE-mediated) hypersensitivity reactions occur after antigen reacts with IgE on tissue mast cells, leading to mast cell degranulation and the release of histamine and other inflammatory substances.
6. Type II (tissue-specific) hypersensitivity reactions are caused by five possible mechanisms: complement-mediated lysis, phagocytosis by macrophages, neutrophil-mediated damage, antibody-dependent cell-mediated cytotoxicity, and modulation of cellular function.
7. Type III (immune complex–mediated) hypersensitivity reactions are caused by the formation of immune complexes that are deposited in target tissues, where they activate the complement cascade, generating chemotactic fragments that attract neutrophils into the inflammatory site.
8. Immune complex disease can be a systemic reaction, such as serum sickness (e.g., Raynaud phenomenon), or localized, such as the Arthus reaction.
9. Type IV (cell-mediated) hypersensitivity reactions are caused by specifically sensitized lymphocytes, which either kill target cells directly or release lymphokines that activate other cells, such as macrophages.
10. Allergens are antigens that cause allergic responses, usually a type I hypersensitivity response.
11. Autoimmune disease is loss of tolerance to self-antigens. There can be a genetic predisposition, and the diseases can be a type II or type III hypersensitivity reaction.
12. Alloimmunity is the immune system's reaction against antigens on the tissues of other members of the same species.
13. Alloimmune disorders include hemolytic disease of the newborn, in which the maternal immune system becomes sensitized against antigens expressed by the fetus; and transplant rejection and transfusion reactions, in which the immune system of the recipient of an organ transplant or blood transfusion reacts against foreign antigens on the donor's cells.

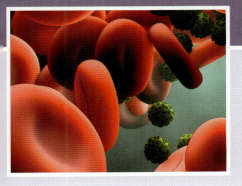

9

Stress and Disease

Stephanie Zettel, with originating chapter contributions by Lorey K. Takahashi and Kathryn L. McCance

Additional resources are available online at http://evolve.elsevier.com/Canada/Huether/pathophysiology.

CHAPTER OUTLINE

Historical Background and General Concepts, 216
  Stress Overview: Allostasis, Multiple Mediators, and Systems, 218
The Stress Response, 219
  Regulation of the Hypothalamic–Pituitary–Adrenal System, 219
  Neuroendocrine Regulation: Autonomic Nervous System, 220
  Histamine and Other Hormones, 224

Role of the Immune System, 224
Stress, Personality, Coping, and Illness, 227
  Coping, 229
GERIATRIC CONSIDERATIONS: Aging and the Stress–Age Syndrome, 232
CASE STUDY, 230

LEARNING OBJECTIVES

1. Describe the physiological basis of the general adaptation syndrome (GAS), as proposed by Selye.
2. Discuss the components of physiological stress and the stages of the GAS response.
3. Discuss the neuroendocrine stress response from initiation (by recognition of a stressor) through resolution (by exhaustion or adaptation).
4. List the effects of cortisol, epinephrine, and norepinephrine on the individual under stress.
5. Identify hormones, other than epinephrine and cortisol, affected by the physiological response to a stressor.
6. Describe the known mechanisms of interaction between the neuroendocrine and immune responses to stress.
7. Apply understanding of the stress response to a clinical or personal situation by describing the factors involved in the initiation of the response and manifestations observed or experienced.
8. Discuss the factors that mediate an individual's ability to cope with a stressor.
9. Describe the importance and functions of T helper 1 and T helper 2 cells and associated cytokines.

KEY TERMS

Adrenocorticotropic hormone (ACTH), 219
Alarm stage (in GAS), 216
Allostasis, 218
Allostatic overload, 218
Anticipatory response, 216
Coping, 229

Corticotropin-releasing hormone (CRH), 219
Cortisol, 219
Diseases of adaptation, 216
Exhaustion stage (in GAS), 216
General adaptation syndrome (GAS), 216
Homeostasis, 215

Hypothalamic–pituitary–adrenal (HPA) system, 219
Neuropeptide Y (NPY), 224
Peripheral (immune) CRH, 224
Physiological stress, 216
Psychoneuroimmunology (PNI), 216

Reactive response, 216
Resistance or adaptation stage (in GAS), 216
Stressor, 215
Stress response, 215
Th1 to Th2 shift, 220
White coat syndrome, 216

Stress is broadly defined as a perceived or anticipated threat that disrupts a person's well-being or **homeostasis**. Stress involves a complex interaction between the body and brain in the face of random and constant external and internal challenges called **stressors**.[1,2] A stressor may stem from psychological/emotional (fear, social rejection), physical (dramatic temperature changes, abuse), or physiological (infection, inflammation) stimuli that trigger the **stress response**.

Exposure to acute stress activates defensive neural, autonomic, and immune systems to facilitate adaptation and survival.[3–5] However, unremitting or toxic stress can have adverse effects because it promotes pathophysiology in the very systems that function to meet the challenges of acute stress. For example, acute stress can enhance the immune system to protect the individual, but prolonged stress may lead to immunosuppression that impairs the body's ability to fight diseases.[6]

Many events may be stressful and uncontrollable, such as loss of a family member, loss of a job, cancer diagnosis, physical abuse, social neglect, or financial hardships and can result in unhealthy coping strategies (e.g., smoking, drinking alcohol, drug abuse) and poor decisions, such as foregoing sleep, eating high-calorie comfort foods, and withdrawing from physical activity. Furthermore, continued engagement in these behavioural activities is linked to a number of serious illnesses, such as hypertension, depression, diabetes, and obesity (Figure 9.1).[4,7,8] There are positive benefits from good coping behaviour (e.g., mindfulness, yoga,

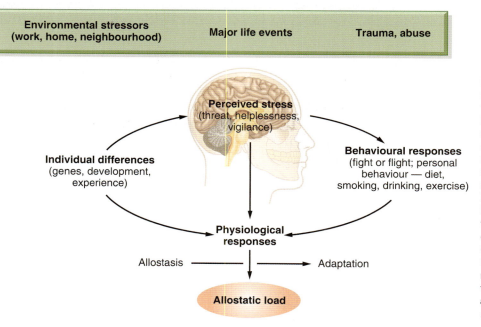

FIGURE 9.1 Physiological and Behavioural Stress Responses. Stress processes arise from bidirectional communication patterns between the brain and other physiological systems (autonomic, immune, neural, and endocrine). Importantly, these bidirectional mechanisms are protective, promoting short-term adaptation (allostasis). Chronic stress mechanisms, however, can lead to long-term dysregulation and promote behavioural responses and physiological responses that lead to stress-induced disorders/diseases (allostatic load), compromising health. (Reprinted with permission from McEwen, B. S. [2008]. Central effects of stress hormones in health and disease: understanding the protective and damaging effects of stress and stress mediators. *European Journal of Pharmacology, 583*[2–3], 174–185.)

exercise), and social support from others and health care providers also assists with maintaining a healthy behavioural and physiological profile.

HISTORICAL BACKGROUND AND GENERAL CONCEPTS

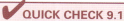

QUICK CHECK 9.1
1. How is stress related to unhealthy coping behaviours?
2. Briefly describe the three stages of the general adaptation syndrome.
3. Define *allostatic load* and *allostatic overload*.

Walter B. Cannon used the term *stress* in both a physiological and a psychological sense as early as 1914 and coined the term "fight-or-flight response" to describe the body's preparation to deal with threat.[9] He applied the engineering concepts of stress and strain in a physiological context and believed that emotional stimuli were also capable of causing stress. The physiological reactions to stress included increased heart rate and blood supply of oxygen and glucose to muscles and the brain, elevated respiration, dilation of pupils, and inhibition of gastric secretions.

In 1946, Hans Selye further popularized and advanced the concept of stress in terms of a chemical or physical change (i.e., physiological stress, in response either to the external environment or within the body itself): **physiological stress** involves (1) enlargement of the adrenal gland, (2) decreased lymphocyte levels in the blood from damage to lymphatic structures of the immune system, and (3) development of bleeding ulcers in the stomach and duodenal lining. Selye concluded that physiological stress can impair the ability of the organism to resist future stressors and described what is now known as the **general adaptation syndrome (GAS)**.[10]

GAS involves three successive stages: (1) the alarm stage, (2) the resistance or adaptation stage, and (3) the exhaustion stage. The **alarm stage** is the emergency reaction that prepares the body to fight or flee from threat. This stage involves the secretion of hormones and catecholamines to support physiological and metabolic activity (Figures 9.2 and 9.3) and boosts the immune system to protect against infection and disease. The ensuing **resistance or adaptation stage** requires continued mobilization of the body's resources to cope and overcome a sustained challenge. The **exhaustion stage** (currently described as *allostatic overload*) occurs when the body's physiological and immune systems no longer effectively cope with the stressor and marks the onset of diseases such as cardiovascular and renal disease (**diseases of adaptation**).

In the mid-1950s, studies emerged to demonstrate that psychological stressors (e.g., repeated clicking noises and electric shock in monkeys,[11] the experience of unpleasant interviews in humans[12,13]) are also highly effective in activating adrenal hormone secretion. According to Mason, a number of psychological factors, such as degree of comfort, unpleasantness, or suddenness of an unanticipated stimulus, can modulate the magnitude of the stress response.[14]

The central nervous system (CNS) and endocrine system are remarkably sensitive to emotional, psychological, and social influences. Psychological stressors can elicit a reactive or anticipatory stress response. For example, an examination with no physical stressor may elicit a **reactive response** (or **white coat syndrome**) involving physiological changes, such as increased heart rate and dry mouth. **Anticipatory responses** occur when physiological responses develop in anticipation of psychological stress or threat. The fear of a potential encounter with a dangerous, unknown stimulus (such as a predator) or more conditioned situations that bring up unpleasant emotions can generate anticipatory responses.[15] Anticipation of re-exposure to these unwanted events produces a physiological stress response. For example, a child with a history of parental abuse may experience a physiological stress response in anticipation of further abuse when that parent enters the room. Another well-known example of a conditioned emotional response is the development of post-traumatic stress disorder (PTSD) in some military veterans and survivors of natural disasters.

Psychoneuroimmunology (PNI) is the study of how consciousness (*psycho*), mediated by the CNS (*neuro*), interacts with the immune system (*immunology*) to defend the body against infection. Psychoneuroimmunology assumes that immune-mediated diseases result from complex interrelationships among psychosocial, emotional, genetic, neurological, endocrine, immunological, and behavioural factors.[16–18] The immune system is integrated with other physiological

CHAPTER 9 Stress and Disease

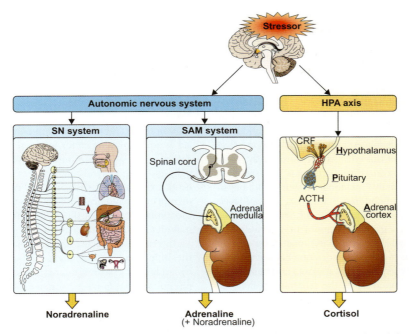

FIGURE 9.2 Effector Systems of the Stress Response. A stressor elicits rapid activation of the autonomic nervous system with its sympathoneuronal *(SN)* and sympatho-adrenomedullary *(SAM)* limbs releasing their main effectors, noradrenaline and adrenaline, respectively. Activation of the hypothalamic–pituitary–adrenocortical *(HPA)* axis results in synthesis and release of its main effector, cortisol or corticosterone, in rodents. *ACTH,* Adrenocorticotropic hormone; *CRF,* corticotropin-releasing factor. (From Deussing, J. M., & Chen. A. [2018]. The corticotropin-releasing factor family: physiology of the stress response. *Physiological Reviews, 98,* 2225–2286 [Figure 1]. https://journals.physiology.org/doi/full/10.1152/physrev.00042.2017.)

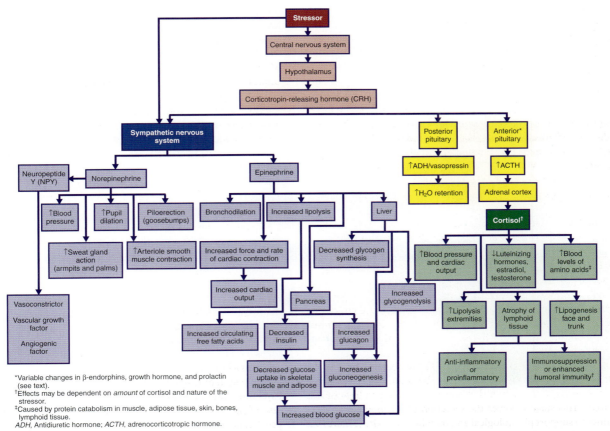

*Variable changes in β-endorphins, growth hormone, and prolactin (see text).
†Effects may be dependent on *amount* of cortisol and nature of the stressor.
‡Caused by protein catabolism in muscle, adipose tissue, skin, bones, lymphoid tissue.
ADH, Antidiuretic hormone; *ACTH,* adrenocorticotropic hormone.

FIGURE 9.3 The Stress Response.

processes and sensitive to changes in CNS and endocrine functioning linked to psychological states. Stressors include a broad range of physical and emotional sources—for example, infection, noise, decreased oxygen supply, pain, malnutrition, heat, cold, trauma, prolonged exertion, radiation, responses to life events (including anxiety, depression, anger, fear, loss, and excitement), obesity, advanced age, medications, disease, surgery, and medical treatment.

The study of PNI is ongoing, especially with respect to the causal role of personality and emotional factors in cancer mortality and morbidity. For example, mouse models suggest a strong link between stress and breast cancer progression, but this effect is not consistently found in humans.[19,20] What is becoming increasingly clear is that secretion of stress hormones influences many metabolic systems and physiological events in both adults and children.[21] Maternal cortisol levels greatly impact the intrauterine development of the fetus. Increased maternal cortisol levels during sensitive developmental periods may produce alterations in physiological systems that impact obesity risk.[22] Furthermore, studies now point to a strong association between modulation of the immune system by psychosocial stressors and health outcomes.[23] With increased understanding of the relationship between stress and human diseases, new strategies are emerging to treat stress-related disorders.

Stress Overview: Allostasis, Multiple Mediators, and Systems

Allostasis refers to "stability through change" and describes the link between stress and disease.[24] Instead of the "fixed homeostasis model" in which physiological regulation revolves around an unchanging set point (e.g., return of cortisol to basal levels after a stress response), allostasis involves a dynamic strategy with the brain continuously monitoring many parameters to anticipate what is required from the neuroendocrine and autonomic systems to meet the challenges of future events.[3,25,26] A return to initial basal hormone levels may not be the most adaptive strategy to cope with anticipated stress encounters. When chronic activation of regulatory systems taxes the body and brain, however, diseases and disorders may emerge. Allostatic overload is the term used to describe overactivation of these adaptive regulatory physiological systems that may lead to clinical pathophysiology and increase of the chance of disease.

Moreover, allostasis and allostatic overload are highly individualized; that is, an event or situation that is normal for one person may be stressful for another.[27,28] The experience of allostatic overload exacts a "wear and tear" toll on the body. The brain is also a key player in determining the extent of allostatic overload. Psychological stress can both act as a precipitating factor for some diseases, as well as a contributor that worsens symptoms and negative outcomes in anxiety, persistent pain and fatigue syndromes, ulcers, asthma, obesity, metabolic syndrome, essential hypertension, and type 2 diabetes. In addition, stress disrupts the biological process of sleep and growth and reproductive functions.[29-33] Some of these disorders are the leading causes of death in both Canada and the United States (Table 9.1).

In response to acute and chronic stress, brain regions, including the hippocampus, amygdala, and prefrontal cortex, may respond by undergoing structural remodelling that alters behavioural and physiological responses to increase the risk of developing cognitive impairments and depression.[1,26] Key physiological systems involved in allostatic overload include exaggerated secretion of cortisol, catecholamines of the sympathetic nervous system, and proinflammatory cytokines, as well as a decline in parasympathetic activity. A prevalent example is sleep deprivation from being "stressed out." Sleep deprivation and disturbances, such as sleep apnea, short sleep duration, and insomnia, have significant associations with allostatic load, leading to damaging effects including elevated evening cortisol concentration; elevated insulin and blood glucose levels; increased blood pressure; reduced parasympathetic activity; increased levels of proinflammatory cytokines; and increased secretion of the hormone ghrelin (primarily by cells of the stomach and pancreas), which increases appetite.[34,35] Overall, the dynamic and damaging effects of allostatic overload can induce sleep deprivation, which then facilitates increased caloric intake, depressed mood, cognitive deficits, and a host of other unhealthy responses.

TABLE 9.1 Examples of Stress-Related Diseases and Conditions

Target Organ or System	Disease or Condition	Target Organ or System	Disease or Condition
Cardiovascular system	Coronary artery disease Hypertension Stroke Disturbances of heart rhythm	Gastro-intestinal system	Ulcer Irritable bowel syndrome Diarrhea Nausea and vomiting Ulcerative colitis
Muscle	Tension headaches Muscle contraction backache	Genitourinary system	Diuresis Impotence Frigidity
Connective tissues	Rheumatoid arthritis (autoimmune disease) Related inflammatory diseases of connective tissue	Skin	Eczema Neurodermatitis Acne
Pulmonary system	Asthma (hypersensitivity reaction) Hay fever (hypersensitivity reactions)	Endocrine system	Type 2 diabetes mellitus Amenorrhea
Immune system	Immunosuppression or deficiency Autoimmune diseases	Central nervous system	Fatigue and lethargy Type A behaviour Overeating Depression Insomnia

THE STRESS RESPONSE

> ✓ **QUICK CHECK 9.2**
> 1. Define the *hypothalamic–pituitary–adrenal* axis.
> 2. Define *psychoneuroimmunology*.
> 3. How does the immune system participate in stress-related diseases?
> 4. Why do stress-related diseases occur?
> 5. What intervention or prevention activities reduce stress-related diseases?

Because of the important role that stress plays in many disease processes, research has begun to focus on physiological mechanisms underlying mind–body interactions to understand and prevent stress-related diseases (see also the *Geriatric Considerations: Aging and the Stress–Age Syndrome* box at the end of the chapter). Using a multidisciplinary approach involving molecular biology, immunology, neurology, endocrinology, and behavioural science, researchers are investigating how stressful life events occurring over a prolonged period of time impair immune functions. Knowledge emerging from the various disciplines offers a holistic and complex model of the biochemical relationships among the CNS, autonomic nervous system (ANS), endocrine system, and immune system.

Regulation of the Hypothalamic–Pituitary–Adrenal System

A key stress hormone relationship is the regulation of the **hypothalamic–pituitary–adrenal (HPA) system** (Figure 9.2). In sequence, the perception of stress activates the hypothalamus to secrete **corticotropin-releasing hormone (CRH)**, which binds to specific receptors on anterior pituitary cells that, in turn, produce **adrenocorticotropic hormone (ACTH)**. ACTH circulates through the blood to the adrenal glands located on the top of the kidneys. Binding to specific receptors on the cortex of the adrenal glands results in the release of glucocorticoid hormones (primarily **cortisol**).

Physiological Effects of Cortisol

During stress, the secretion of glucocorticoid hormones, primarily **cortisol** (cortisol is known outside the body as *hydrocortisone*), reaches all tissues, including the brain, easily penetrates cell membranes, and reacts with numerous intracellular glucocorticoid receptors (see Figure 9.3). Glucocorticoids exert an effect on almost all tissues and organs. Similarly, their influence on a large proportion of the human genome also results in significant diverse biological actions.[29] They regulate many functions of the CNS, including arousal, cognition, mood, sleep, as well as metabolism, maintenance of cardiovascular tone, the immune and inflammatory reaction, and growth and reproduction.

Cortisol mobilizes substances needed for cellular metabolism and stimulates gluconeogenesis or the formation of glucose from noncarbohydrate sources, such as amino acids or free fatty acids in the liver. In addition, cortisol enhances the elevation of blood glucose levels along with other counter-regulatory hormones, such as epinephrine, glucagon, and growth hormone. Cortisol also inhibits the uptake and oxidation of glucose by many body cells. Overall, cortisol's actions on carbohydrate metabolism result in increased blood glucose levels, thereby energizing the body to combat the stressor. Table 9.2 summarizes the effects of cortisol.

Cortisol also affects protein metabolism. It has an *anabolic* effect by increasing the rate of protein synthesis and RNA in the liver. This effect is countered by its *catabolic* effect on protein stores in other tissues. Protein catabolism acts to increase levels of circulating amino acids; therefore, chronic exposure to excess cortisol can severely deplete protein stores in muscle, bone, connective tissue, and skin.

Another important adaptive function of cortisol is to enhance immunity during acute stress.[36] Cortisol exerts beneficial effects by inhibiting initial inflammatory effects, for example, vasodilation and increased capillary permeability. Cortisol also promotes resolution and repair. These actions are mainly accomplished by facilitating the effects of glucocorticoid receptor, namely, the transcription of genetic material (through DNA binding) within leukocytes.[37]

Pathophysiological Effects of Cortisol

Chronic dysregulation of the HPA axis, especially abnormal elevated levels of cortisol, contributes to a wide variety of disorders, including obesity, sleep deprivation, lipid abnormalities, hypertension, diabetes, atherosclerosis, and loss of bone density.[3,28,29,38] In the brain, chronic glucocorticoid secretion may (1) reduce hippocampal volume, (2) enlarge the ventricles, and (3) modulate reversible cortical atrophy.[1,29] Furthermore, these CNS changes may contribute to cognitive impairments and emotional disorders.

In the periphery, heightened stress-induced cortisol levels promote gastric secretion by the parietal cells of the stomach. This increased acid secretion along with *Helicobacter pylori* infection, which effectively erodes the protective mucosal layer of the stomach, may account for the gastro-intestinal ulceration observed by Selye in his experiments with stress. Furthermore, glucocorticoids contribute to the development of metabolic syndrome and the pathogenesis of obesity (see *Health Promotion: Glucocorticoids, Insulin, Inflammation, and Obesity*) by directly causing insulin resistance and influencing genetic variations that predispose to obesity.[39–41]

Cortisol also has effects on fetal development. High maternal cortisol levels during pregnancy often result in low birth weight.[42,43] The consequences of cortisol-induced low birth weight now extend to disease risk in later life. Such diseases include obesity, cardiovascular conditions (e.g., hypertension), and behavioural disorders (because of altered brain structure).[42,44,45] Thus, glucocorticoids can have a dramatic effect on both human pathophysiology and consequential lifespan.[3,29,38]

The feedback mechanisms of the HPA axis actually sense and determine the circulating glucocorticoid levels by stimulating or inhibiting their release from the adrenal cortex, in contrast to other tissues, which only passively respond to the circulating glucocorticoids.[29] Changes in the sensitivity of the HPA axis and peripheral tissues could possibly produce peripheral effects in tissue cortisol (hyper- or hypocortisolism). For example, both high HPA axis reactivity to stress and increased peripheral tissue sensitivity to glucocorticoids are associated with the severity of coronary artery disease (see *Health Promotion: Psychosocial Stress and Progression to Coronary Heart Disease*).[46,47]

Cortisol secretion during stress exerts beneficial effects by inhibiting initial inflammatory effects, for example, vasodilation and increased capillary permeability.[37] Cortisol also promotes resolution and repair. These actions are mainly accomplished by facilitating the effects of glucocorticoid receptor, namely, the transcription of genetic material (through DNA binding) within leukocytes.[37] Because glucocorticoids are so widely expressed, they influence virtually all immune cells. The adaptiveness or destructiveness of cortisol-induced effects may depend on the intensity, type, and duration of the stressor; the tissue involved; and the subsequent concentration and length of cortisol exposure. Finally, glucocorticoids can induce T lymphocyte (T-cell) apoptosis.[37,48]

TABLE 9.2 Physiological Effects of Cortisol

Functions Affected	Physiological Effects
Carbohydrate and lipid metabolism	It diminishes peripheral uptake and utilization of glucose; promotes gluconeogenesis in liver metabolism cells; and enhances gluconeogenic response to other hormones. It promotes lipolysis in adipose tissue.
Protein metabolism	It increases protein synthesis in liver and decreases protein synthesis (including immunoglobulin synthesis) in muscle, lymphoid tissue, adipose tissue, skin, and bone. It increases plasma level of amino acids; stimulates deamination in liver.
Anti-inflammatory effects (systemic effects)	High levels of cortisol used in medication therapy suppress inflammatory response and inhibit proinflammatory activity of many growth factors and cytokines; however, over time, some individuals may develop tolerance to glucocorticoids, causing an increased susceptibility to both inflammatory and autoimmune diseases.
Proinflammatory effects (possible local effects)	Cortisol levels released during stress response may increase proinflammatory effects.
Lipid metabolism	Lipolysis takes place in extremities, and lipogenesis takes place in the face and trunk.
Immune effects	*Treatment* levels of glucocorticoids are immunosuppressive; thus they are valuable agents used in numerous diseases/conditions. T-cell or innate immune system is particularly affected by these larger doses of glucocorticoids, with suppression of Th1 function or innate immunity. *Stress* can cause a different pattern of immune response. These nontherapeutic levels can suppress innate (Th1) and increase adaptive (Th2) immunity—the so-called Th2 shift. Several factors influence this complex physiology and include long-term adaptations, reproductive hormones (i.e., overall, androgens suppress and estrogens stimulate immune responses), defects of the hypothalamic–pituitary–adrenal axis, histamine-generated responses, and acute versus chronic stress. Thus, stress seems to cause a Th2 shift *systemically*, whereas *locally*, under certain conditions, it can induce proinflammatory activities and by these mechanisms may influence onset or course of infections, autoimmune/inflammatory, allergic, and neoplastic diseases.
Digestive function	It promotes gastric secretion.
Urinary function	It enhances excretion of calcium.
Connective tissue function	It decreases proliferation of fibroblasts in connective tissue (thus delaying healing).
Muscle function	It maintains normal contractility and maximal work output for skeletal and cardiac muscle.
Bone function	It decreases bone formation.
Vascular system/myocardial function	It maintains normal blood pressure; permits increased responsiveness of arterioles to constrictive action of adrenergic stimulation; and optimizes myocardial performance.
Central nervous system function	It somehow modulates perceptual and emotional functioning. It is essential for normal arousal and initiation of daytime activity.
Possible synergism with estrogen in pregnancy?	It may suppress the maternal immune system to prevent rejection of the fetus.

Effects of Exogenous Glucocorticoids

Stress hormones, especially glucocorticoids (cortisol), are powerful anti-inflammatory/immunosuppressive agents. The synthetic forms of glucocorticoid hormones (exogenous types of anti-inflammatory glucocorticoids administered for a pharmaceutical reaction) are poorly metabolized when compared with endogenous glucocorticoids. As such, synthetic glucocorticoids have a longer half-life and exert no circadian rhythm. Moreover, these synthetic compounds bind with different targets, resulting in a unique effect for each agent.[49]

Elevated levels of glucocorticoids and catecholamines (epinephrine and norepinephrine), both endogenous and exogenously administered, may decrease innate immunity (e.g., inflammatory response) and increase autoimmune responses (e.g., hypersensitivity reactions). Cortisol *modulates* the immune system by inducing T-cell apoptosis,[37,48] rather than suppressing it completely. The prolonged effects of cortisol contribute further to the dysregulation of the immune response and might even accentuate the inflammatory response (e.g., stroke).[49]

Initially, immune responses are regulated by cells of innate immunity called antigen-presenting cells (APCs), such as monocytes/macrophages (see Chapter 7), dendritic cells, and other phagocytic cells, as well as Th1 and Th2 lymphocytes (T-helper cells involved in adaptive immunity; see Chapter 7). Th1 and Th2 each have slightly different functions: the Th1 branch fights viruses, cancer and intracellular bacteria and initiates more of a cellular response, whereas the Th2 branch fights extracellular bacteria and parasites and initiates more of a humoral response. The Th2 branch is also responsible for allergic reactions.

The overall effect of cortisol secretion and the stress response is a shift from Th1 (cell-based immunity) towards the Th2 humoral response (antibodies), also known as **a Th1 to Th2 shift**. Cytokines secreted by Th2 cells also act to inhibit Th1 cells and can promote adaptive immunity by stimulating growth and activating mast cells and eosinophils, as well as the differentiation of B lymphocyte (B-cell) immunoglobulins (see Figure 9.4). This shift serves a protective function during acute short-term stress by preventing an overactivation of the inflammatory response. During prolonged or chronic stress, however, this shift to the Th2 response results in a decreased ability of the organism to fight viral infections, as well as an increased susceptibility to allergies. A short-term suppression of the Th1 branch of the immune system during a stressful situation actually promotes survival and benefits the organism because the immune system uses a large amount of energy which is better channelled to the fight-or-flight response during acute stress.

Neuroendocrine Regulation: Autonomic Nervous System
Sympathetic Nervous System

Arousal of the sympathetic nervous system occurs simultaneously with the HPA system during stress, resulting in a release of norepinephrine (adrenergic stimulation) and a stimulation of the adrenal medulla to release catecholamines (80% epinephrine and 20% norepinephrine) into the bloodstream. Stress also plays a role in the gut–brain axis (See *Health Promotion: Stress and the Gut–Brain Axis*).

HEALTH PROMOTION

Glucocorticoids, Insulin, Inflammation, and Obesity

The signs and symptoms of Cushing's syndrome (e.g., excess glucocorticoids) include truncal obesity, relatively thin extremities, a "moon face," and a "buffalo [neck] hump." In such individuals, the possibility of associated hypertension is high, and the risk of infection and metabolic syndrome or type 2 diabetes is increased. The likelihood of an elevated ratio of intra-abdominal subcutaneous fat mass to nonabdominal fat mass is high because the glucocorticoids mediate the redistribution of stored calories (in the form of fat) into the abdominal region. The specific increase in abdominal fat stores is a consequence of elevated levels of glucocorticoids combined with increased insulin action. However, the increased levels of glucocorticoids need not be present in the circulation; instead, they can be generated locally in fat by conversion of inactive cortisone to active cortisol through the action of the isoenzyme 11β-hydroxysteroid dehydrogenase (11β-HSD) type 1. This conversion is referred to as "pre-receptor" metabolism of cortisol. The active steroid is secreted directly to the liver through the portal vein. Glucocorticoids inhibit *in vitro* insulin synthesis as well as secretion of insulin by the pancreas. However, increasing levels of glucocorticoids in vivo contribute to insulin resistance in the tissues and increased insulin secretion (as a result of suppression of insulin action on the liver). Hepatic insulin resistance is strongly associated with abdominal obesity.

The plasma concentration of inflammatory mediators, such as tumour necrosis factor-alpha (TNF-α) and interleukin-6 (IL-6), is actually increased in the insulin-resistant states of obesity and type 2 diabetes. Two mechanisms might be involved in the pathogenesis of inflammation: (1) glucose and macronutrient intake (i.e., which can increase as a result of chronic stress and corticosteroid secretion) cause oxidative stress (via the processes of metabolism); and (2) the increased concentrations of TNF-α and IL-6 associated with obesity and type 2 diabetes might interfere with insulin signal transduction. This interference might promote inflammation. Chronic overnutrition (obesity) might thus be a proinflammatory state with oxidative stress.

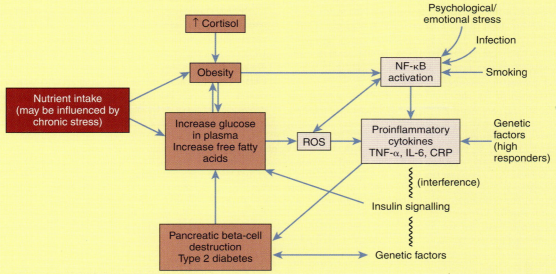

Stress, Inflammation, Obesity, and Type 2 Diabetes. The induction of reactive oxygen species *(ROS)* generation and inflammation through the proinflammatory transcription factor NF-κB activates most proinflammatory genes. Macronutrient intake, obesity, free fatty acids, infection, smoking, psychological stress, and genetic factors increase the production of ROS. Interference with insulin signalling (insulin resistance) leads to hyperglycemia and proinflammatory changes. Proinflammatory changes increase levels of TNF-α and IL-6, and also lead to the inhibition of insulin signalling and insulin resistance. Inflammation in pancreatic beta cells leads to beta-cell dysfunction, which in combination with insulin resistance leads to type 2 diabetes. *CRP*, C-reactive protein; *IL-6*, interleukin-6; *TNF-α*, tumour necrosis factor-alpha.

Data from Dallman, M. F., la Fleur, S. E., Pecoraro, N. C., et al. (2004). *Endocrinology, 145*(6), 2633–2638; Dandona, P., Aljada, A., & Bandyopadhyay, A. (2004). *Trends in Immunology, 25*(1), 4–7; Khadir, A., Tiss, A., Kavalakatt, S., et al. (2015). *Mediators of Inflammation, 2015*, 512603; Kim, S. P., Ellmerer, M., Van Citters, G. W., et al. (2003). *Diabetes, 52*, 2453–2460; Masuzaki, H., Paterson, J., Sinyama, H., et al. (2001). *Science, 294*, 2166–2170; Padgett, D. A., & Glaser, R. (2003). *Trends in Immunology, 24*(8), 444–448; Shimanoe, C., Hara, M., Nishida, Y., et al. (2015). *PLoS One, 10*(2), e0118105; Spencer, S. J., & Tilbrook, A. (2011). *Stress, 14*(3), 233–246; Strack, A. M., Sebastian, R. J., Schwartz, M. W., et al. (1995). *American Journal of Physiology, 268*, R142–R149; Wagen Knecht, L. E., Langefeld, C. D., Scherzinger, A. L., et al. (2003). *Diabetes, 52*(10), 2490–2496.

Circulating catecholamines essentially mimic direct sympathetic stimulation and cannot cross the blood–brain barrier. The brain synthesizes them locally via the sympathetic nervous system. Table 9.3 summarizes the effects of catecholamines on organs and tissues. Norepinephrine's actions include the regulation of blood pressure, promotion of arousal, and increased vigilance, anxiety, and other protective emotional responses.

The catecholamines stimulate two major classes of receptors: α-adrenergic receptors ($α_1$ and $α_2$) and β-adrenergic receptors ($β_1$ and $β_2$). Table 13.7 summarizes the actions of the two subclasses of adrenergic receptors. (Chapters 1, 18, and 23 discuss the receptors of the sympathetic nervous system further.) Epinephrine binds with and activates both α and β receptors, whereas norepinephrine binds primarily with α receptors.

HEALTH PROMOTION

Psychosocial Stress and Progression to Coronary Heart Disease

There is a physiological link between stress and coronary heart disease. One of the primary risk factors for coronary heart disease is hypertension. In fact, the condition of prehypertension is a good predictor for future cardiovascular events.[a] Prehypertension is defined as a systolic blood pressure of 120 to 139 mm Hg or a diastolic blood pressure of 80 to 90 mm Hg. Individuals with prehypertension are much more likely to develop actual hypertension and, eventually, coronary heart disease.

People with a highly reactive personality type who experience high levels of anxiety with stress are much more likely to progress from prehypertension to hypertension and then to develop cardiac disease, specifically coronary heart disease, than those who have better coping abilities. Further long-term psychological stress, such as that experienced in a strained marriage or an unhappy work environment, not only can accelerate the progression of hypertension and coronary heart disease but it contributes to higher mortality rates from coronary heart disease.

Trait anger, defined as a stable personality trait characterized by frequency, intensity, and duration of anger, is also a factor in the development of coronary heart disease at higher rates than in the general population. Individuals with trait anger also have more strokes. Furthermore, hostile individuals with advanced cardiovascular disease may be particularly susceptible to stress-induced increases in sympathetic activity and inflammation.

One popular mechanism for the interaction between psychosocial stress and cardiovascular disease suggests that stress triggers an inflammatory response that, over time, increases the chances of developing coronary heart disease. The primary mechanisms proposed are chronically elevated cortisol levels and dysregulation of the circadian rhythm for cortisol release. Chronic stress also alters HPA function, resulting in an abnormal stress response pattern. Persons with coronary heart disease along with increased inflammatory markers exhibited this alteration in HPA activity. The involvement of T-regulatory cells (Treg cells) is now an emerging mechanism of this response. Treg cells play an important role in maintaining peripheral tolerance of tissue antigens, preventing autoimmune diseases, and decreasing chronic inflammatory diseases. Naturally occurring CD4+CD25+ Treg cells are actually downregulated in individuals with acute coronary syndrome (ACS). Additionally, the sympathetic nervous system plays an important role in immune homeostasis by maintaining the number of Treg cells in the periphery, and this may be affected by psychological stress. The Treg-cell lineage, however, is quite diverse.

Because coronary heart disease is one of the major causes of death in industrialized countries, development of successful interventional programs is of high priority. Programs in which dietary changes, exercise, stress management, and positive support systems are implemented continue to show positive results for slowing the progression of heart disease and decreasing the risk factors for disease development. Mindfulness intervention training as part of cardiac rehabilitation programs has potential for reducing the progression of coronary heart disease. Furthermore, individuals in these programs report decreased levels of depression and stress, as well as overall improvement in mental health.

[a]Hypertension Canada. (2020). *Hypertension & you: associated health risks.* https://hypertension.ca/hypertension-and-you/about-hypertension/associated-health-risks/.
Data from Albuquerque, N. L. S., de Araujo, T. L., de Oliveira Lopes, M. V., et al. (2020). Hierarchical analysis of factors associated with hospital readmissions for coronary heart disease: a case–control study. *Journal of Clinical Nursing, 29*(13–14), 2329–2337, https://doi.org/10.1111/jocn.15244; Almuwaqqat, Z., O'Neal, W. T., Hammadah, M., et al. (2020). Abnormal P-wave axis and myocardial ischemia development during mental stress. *Journal of Electrocardiology, 60,* 3–7, https://doi.org/10.1016/j.jelectrocard.2020.02.019; Bremner, J. D., Fani, N., Cheema, F. A., et al. (2019). Effects of a mental stress challenge on brain function in coronary artery disease patients with and without depression. *Health Psychology, 38*(10), 910–924, https://doi.org/10.1037/hea0000742; Zuraida, E., & Syahrul, S. (2019). The effectiveness of mindfulness-based intervention on reducing clinical outcomes among heart disease outpatients: a systematic review. *International Journal of Caring Sciences, 12*(3), 1506–1519. http://www.internationaljournalofcaringsciences.org/docs/21_eli_original_12_3.pdf

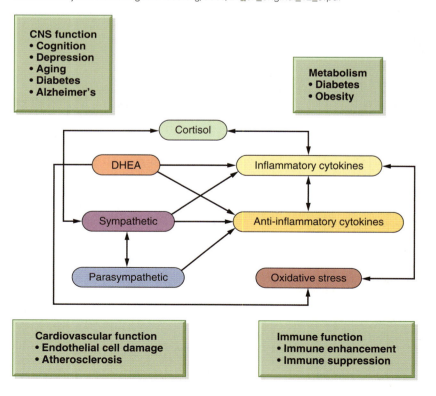

FIGURE 9.4 Stress Interactions Are Nonlinear and Complex. Nonlinearity means that when one mediator is increased or decreased, the subsequent compensatory changes in other mediators depend on time and level of change, causing multiple interacting variables. The inevitable consequences from adapting to daily life over time include changes in behavioural responses. For example, these changes include sleeping patterns, smoking, alcohol consumption, physical activity, and social interactions. These behavioural patterns are a part of the allostatic overload with chronic elevations in cortisol level, sympathetic activity, and levels of proinflammatory cytokines, and a decrease in parasympathetic activity. *CNS,* Central nervous system; *DHEA,* dehydroepiandrosterone. (Reprinted with permission from McEwen, B. S. [2008]. Central effects of stress hormones in health and disease: understanding the protective and damaging effects of stress and stress mediators. *European Journal of Pharmacology, 583*[2–3], 174–185.)

TABLE 9.3 Physiological Effects of Catecholamines[a]

Organ/Tissue	Process or Result
Brain	Increased blood flow; increased glucose metabolism
Cardiovascular system	Increased rate and force of contraction
	Peripheral vasoconstriction
Pulmonary system	Bronchodilation
Skeletal muscle	Increased glycogenolysis
	Increased contraction
	Increased dilation of muscle vasculature
	Decreased glucose uptake and utilization (decreases insulin release)
Liver	Increased glucose production
	Increased glycogenolysis
Adipose tissue	Increased lipolysis
	Decreased glucose uptake
Skin	Decreased blood flow
Gastro-intestinal and genitourinary tracts	Decreased protein synthesis
	Decreased smooth muscle contraction
	Increased renin release
	Increased gastro-intestinal sphincter tone
Lymphoid tissue	Acute and chronic stress inhibits several components of innate immunity, particularly decreasing natural killer cells
Macrophages	Inhibited and stimulated macrophage activity
	Depends on availability of type 1/proinflammatory cytokines, presence or absence of antigenic stressors, and peripheral corticotropin-releasing hormone (CRH)

[a]Some of these responses require glucocorticoids (e.g., cortisol) for maximal activity (see text for explanation).
Data from Elenkov, I. J., & Chrousos, G. P. (2002). *Annals of the New York Academy of Sciences*, 966, 290–303; Granner, D. K. (2018). Rodwell, V. W., Bender, D. A., et al. (Eds.). *Harper's illustrated biochemistry* (31st ed.). McGraw-Hill; Kvetnansky, R., Lu, X., & Ziegler, M. G. (2013). Stress-triggered changes in peripheral catecholaminergic systems. In L.E. Eiden (Ed.), *Advances in pharmacology: a new era of catecholamines in the laboratory and clinic*, volume 68 (pp. 359–397). Elsevier Inc.

The liver and skeletal muscles rapidly metabolize epinephrine, and epinephrine has numerous effects on a variety of body organs. Epinephrine influences cardiac action by enhancing myocardial contractility (causing an inotropic effect), increasing heart rate (causing a chronotropic effect), and increasing venous return to the heart, ultimately increasing both cardiac output and blood pressure. Epinephrine also dilates blood vessels supplying skeletal muscles, allowing for greater blood flow and subsequent oxygenation of the tissue. Metabolically, epinephrine causes transient hyperglycemia (high blood sugar), reduces glucose uptake in the muscles and other organs, and decreases insulin release from the pancreas, thus preventing glucose uptake by peripheral tissue and preserving it for the CNS. Epinephrine also mobilizes free fatty acids and cholesterol.

Catecholamine secretion additionally increases proinflammatory cytokine production, which elevates heart rate and blood pressure and impairs wound healing.[50] Chronic stress-induced increases in norepinephrine levels can ultimately result in increased production of inflammatory leukocytes that adhere to vessel walls and promote the development of plaque.[47,51] Proteases released from these inflammatory leukocytes further promote risk of myocardial infarction and stroke by weakening the fibrous cap of the plaque, which can advance plaque rupture.[47] In addition to a stress-induced increased risk of cardiovascular disease, the effects of stress on inflammatory cytokine secretion also influence depression, autoimmune disorders, and virally mediated cancers,[52,53] and may be important in functional decline that leads to frailty, disability, and untimely death.[31,54] Finally, stress-induced excessive levels of inflammatory cytokines during infection or inflammatory illness can stimulate the formation of prostaglandins that bind to various areas in the brain and activate a collection of nonspecific symptoms (i.e., fever, achiness, sleepiness, and anorexia) called the "sickness syndrome."[55]

Parasympathetic Nervous System

The parasympathetic system balances the sympathetic nervous system and influences adaptation or maladaptation to stressful events. The parasympathetic system generally opposes the sympathetic system; for example, the parasympathetic nervous system slows the heart rate via the vagus nerve. The parasympathetic system also has anti-inflammatory effects.[49] Under conditions of allostatic overload, the parasympathetic system may decrease its response relative to the sympathetic system, resulting in increased or prolonged inflammatory responses.[3] Researchers are able

HEALTH PROMOTION

Stress and the Gut–Brain Axis

The gut–brain axis (GBA) combines the sympathetic and parasympathetic components of the autonomic nervous system in both the afferent and efferent nerve pathways of the gut. The microbiome of the gut is a key player in this gut–brain axis, and diet is one of the main ways of influencing this gut–brain axis to reduce the effects of stress on the body. The neuro-immuno-endocrine mediators of the GBA allow the brain to influence intestinal function, but the microbiome of the gut plays a key role in the GBA structure as well. There are many ways in which the brain communicates with the gut, including the vagus nerve, gut hormones (often related to glucose metabolism), the immune system, tryptophan signalling, and metabolites such as free-fatty acids. The genetic material in the microbiome is approximately 150 times greater than the actual human genome, leading some scientists to label the gut microbiome as a "superorganism". The gut microbiome has been implicated in a variety of stress-related conditions including anxiety, depression, and irritable bowel syndrome. Disruptions in the microbiome are also associated with numerous allergies, autoimmune disorders, metabolic disorders, and neuropsychiatric disorders. Stress can perturb this microbiome. Moreover, the changes in the flora of the gut can actually change behaviour, and the microbiome can influence the brain during critical phases of development.

It is possible to manipulate the gut flora to maintain health and help prevent and treat disease. Administration of probiotics such as lactobacillus to mice reduced their anxiety and depression-like behaviour. Antibiotics can also reduce the number of commensal bacteria that allow for invasion of parasites and other pathogens in the gut. Though probiotics and antibiotics both aid in promoting the health of the GBA, diet (i.e., reduction in gluten) and lifestyle (i.e., reduced stress) are among the most critical factors that can influence this microbiome.

Data from Rege, S., & Graham, J., (2017). *The simplified guide to the gut-brain axis—how the gut and the brain talk to each other*. PsychSceneHub, https://psychscenehub.com/psychinsights/the-simplified-guide-to-the-gut-brain-axis/; Foster, J. A., Rinaman, L., & Cryan, J. F. (2017). Stress & the gut-brain axis: regulation by the microbiome. *Neurobiology of Stress*, 7, 124–136. https://doi.org/10.1016/j.ynstr.2017.03.001.

to evaluate the relative balance of the parasympathetic and sympathetic nervous systems using a technique known as heart rate variability (the measurement of R wave variability from heartbeat to heartbeat).

Histamine and Other Hormones

The immune system is integrated with other physiological processes and is sensitive to changes in CNS and endocrine functioning, such as those that accompany psychological states.[55] Stressors can elicit the stress response through the action of the nervous and endocrine systems, specifically CRH from the hypothalamus and from peripheral inflammatory sites (called *peripheral [immune] CRH*).[56,57] **Peripheral (immune) CRH** is proinflammatory, causing an increase in vasodilation and vascular permeability. Mast cells are the target of peripheral CRH, and they release histamine, which is a well-known mediator of acute inflammation and allergic reactions (Figure 9.5). Histamine induces acute inflammation and allergic reactions while suppressing Th1 activity (decreasing innate immunity) and promoting Th2 activity (increasing adaptive immunity).[58–61]

Stress also suppresses thyroid hormone synthesis. Thyroid hormone is involved in growth and reproduction, and decreased synthesis of this hormone conserves energy. **Neuropeptide Y (NPY)**, a sympathetic neurotransmitter, is another stress mediator. Because NPY is a growth factor for many cells, increased levels of NPY have a significant impact on atherosclerosis and tissue remodelling. Table 9.4 lists other hormones involved with the stress response.

Locally, stress can exert both proinflammatory or anti-inflammatory effects. Moreover, some evidence indicates that stress is not a uniform, nonspecific reaction.[62] Different types of stressors might have variable effects on the immune response. Thus, stress may systemically cause a decrease in innate immunity and enhance adaptive immunity, whereas locally, under certain conditions, it can induce proinflammatory activities that may influence the onset and cause of infection, autoimmune/inflammatory, and allergic responses. In summary, stress can activate an excessive immune response and, through cortisol and the catecholamines, suppress Th1 responses while enhancing Th2 responses.

Role of the Immune System

The immune, nervous, and endocrine systems communicate through similar (and highly complex) pathways using hormones, neurotransmitters, neuropeptides, and immune cell products.[37] Neuroendocrine-produced factors affect various components of immune system responses involved in the stress reaction. Similarly, immune cell–derived cytokines

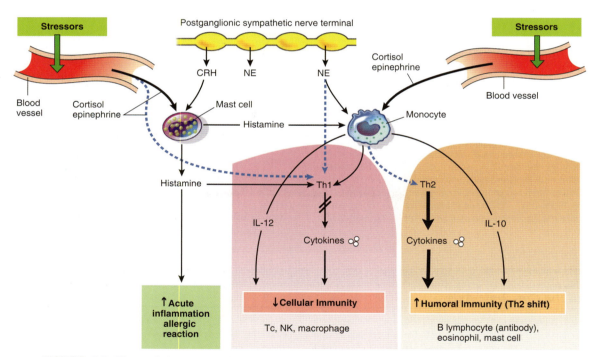

FIGURE 9.5 Effect of Corticotropin-Releasing Hormone–Mast Cell–Histamine Axis, Cortisol, and Catecholamines on the Th1/Th2 Balance—Innate and Adaptive Immunity. Adaptive immunity provides protection against multicellular parasites, extracellular bacteria, some viruses, soluble toxins, and allergens. Innate immunity provides protection against intracellular bacteria, fungi, protozoa, and several viruses. Type 1 cytokines or proinflammatory cytokines include IL-12, IFN-γ, and TNF-α. Type 2 cytokines or anti-inflammatory cytokines include IL-10 and IL-4. Solid lines (*black*) represent stimulation, whereas dashed lines (*blue*) represent inhibition (i.e., Th1 and Th2 are mutually inhibitory, IL-12 and IFN-γ inhibit Th2, and vice versa; IL-4 and IL-10 inhibit Th1 responses). Stress and CRH modulate inflammatory/immune and allergic responses by stimulating cortisol (glucocorticoid), catecholamines, and peripheral (immune) CRH secretion and by changing the production of regulatory cytokines and histamines. CRH (peripheral, immune), Corticotropin-releasing hormone; *IFN-γ*, interferon-gamma; *IL*, interleukin; *NE*, norepinephrine; *NK*, natural killer cell; *Tc*, T-cytotoxic cell; *Th*, T-helper cell; *TNF-α*, tumour necrosis factor-alpha; *dashed lines,* decreased (inhibited); *solid lines,* increased (stimulation). (Reprinted with permission from Elenkov, I. J., & Chrousos, G. P. [1999]. Stress hormones, Th1/Th2 patterns, pro/anti-inflammatory cytokines and susceptibility to disease. *Trends in Endocrinology & Metabolism, 10*[9], 359–368.)

TABLE 9.4 Other Hormones That Influence the Stress Response

Hormone	Source	Action
β-Endorphins (endogenous opiates)	Pituitary and hypothalamus	They activate endorphin (opiate) receptors on peripheral sensory nerves, leading to pain relief or analgesia. Hemorrhage increases levels to inhibit blood pressure or delay compensatory changes that would increase blood pressure.[a]
Growth hormone (somatotropin)	Anterior pituitary gland	It affects protein, lipid, and carbohydrate metabolism. It counters the effects of insulin. It is involved in tissue repair. It may participate in growth and function of immune system, and its effects are mediated through insulin-like growth factor.[b] Levels increase after a variety of stressful stimuli (cardiac catheterization, electroshock therapy, gastroscopy, surgery, fever, physical exercise). Increased levels are associated with psychological stimuli (taking examinations, viewing violent or sexually arousing films, participating in certain psychological performance tests). Prolonged stress (chronic stress) suppresses growth hormone.
Prolactin	Anterior pituitary gland; numerous extrapituitary tissue sites[c]	It increases in response to many stressful stimuli (including procedures such as gastroscopy, proctoscopy, pelvic examination, and surgery).[d] It is increased for in situ breast cancer.[e] It requires more intense stimuli than those leading to increases in catecholamine or cortisol levels. Levels show little change after exercise.
Oxytocin	Hypothalamus	It promotes bonding and social attachment.[f] In animals, it is associated with reduced hypothalamic–pituitary–adrenal activation levels and reduced anxiety.[f]
Testosterone	Leydig cells in testes	It regulates male secondary sex characteristics and libido. Levels decrease after stressful stimuli (anaesthesia, surgery, marathon running, mountain climbing).[g] It is decreased by psychological stimuli; however, some data indicate that psychological stress associated with competition (e.g., pistol shooting) increases both testosterone and cortisol levels, especially in athletes older than 45 years.[h] It is markedly reduced in individuals with respiratory failure, burns, and heart failure.[i] Decreased levels occur during aging and are associated with lowered cortisol responsiveness to stress-induced inflammation.[j]
Estrogen	Ovaries	It works in concert with oxytocin, exerting calming effect during stressful situations.[k]
Melatonin	Produced by pineal gland	It increases during stress response. Release is suppressed by light and increased in dark. Receptors have been identified on lymphoid cells, possibly higher density of receptors on T cells than on B cells. Suppression of lymphocyte function by trauma was reversed by melatonin.[l]
Somatostatin (SOM)	Produced by sensory nerve terminals found in and released from lymphoid cells and hypothalamus	Natural killer function and immunoglobulin synthesis are decreased by SOM. Growth hormone secretion is decreased by SOM.
Vasoactive intestinal peptide (VIP)	Found in neurons of CNS and in peripheral nerves	VIP increases during stress. VIP-containing nerves are located in both primary and secondary lymphoid tissues, around blood vessels, and in gastro-intestinal tract. VIP receptors are on both T and B cells; VIP may influence lymphocyte maturation. Cytokine production by T cells is modified by VIP; and B-cell and antibody production is influenced by VIP.
Calcitonin gene–related peptide (CGRP)	Found in spinal cord motor neurons and in sensory neurons near dendritic cells of skin and in primary and secondary lymphoid tissues	CGRP receptors are present on T and B lymphocytes (T cells and B cells); thus it is likely that CGRP can modulate immune function. CGRP may enhance acute inflammatory response because it is a vasodilator. Maturation of immune B cells is inhibited by CGRP; and IL-1 is inhibited by CGRP, which is important for activation of T cells. It has been shown to interfere with lymphocyte activation.

Continued

TABLE 9.4 Other Hormones That Influence the Stress Response—cont'd

Hormone	Source	Action
Neuropeptide Y (NPY)	Present in neurons of CNS and in neurons throughout body; colocalized in nerve terminals in lymphatic tissues with norepinephrine	Lymphocytes have receptors for NPY and thus may modulate their function.[m] Several lines of evidence suggest that NPY is a neurotransmitter and neurohormone involved in stress response. Increased levels of NPY occur in plasma in response to severe or prolonged stress; may be responsible for stress-induced regional vasoconstriction (splanchnic, coronary, and cerebral); and may also increase platelet aggregation.[b] It may be important in preventing depression.
Substance P (SP)	Produced by neuropeptide classified as tachykinin (increases heart rate subsequent to lowering blood pressure) found in brain, as well as nerves innervating secondary lymphoid tissues	SP increases in response to stress. Receptors for SP are found on membranes of both T and B cells, mononuclear phagocytic cells, and mast cells. Proinflammatory activity induces release of histamine from mast cells during stress response. It causes smooth muscle contraction, causes macrophages and T cells to release cytokines, and increases antibody production.
Ghrelin	Produced by enteroendocrine cells of the GI tract, particularly in the stomach, in response to stress	It is often called the "hunger hormone" because of its effects on food intake. It increases gastric motility and gastric acid secretion. Ghrelin also activates cells in the anterior pituitary gland and hypothalamus, as well as neuropeptide Y neurons, to increase appetite.[n]
Thyroid hormone (thyroxine and tri-iodothyronine)	Produced in the thyroid gland in response to thyroid stimulating hormone from the anterior pituitary gland	These hormones are decreased during the stress response because the impact of stress on the thyroid is to slow body metabolism.[o]
Adipokines and oxidative stress	Derived from adipose tissue	These hormones regulate appetite, metabolism, fat distribution, insulin activity, and inflammation. *Adiponectin* increases insulin sensitivity, reduces inflammation, and oxidative stress. *Leptin* stimulates the inflammatory response and oxidative stress. *Resistin* is a pro-inflammatory cytokine that increases oxidative stress. Increased oxidative stress occurs with increased blood glucose levels.[p]

[a]Amico, J. A., Mantella, R. C., Vollmer, R. R., et al. (2004). Anxiety and stress responses in female oxytocin deficient mice. *Journal of Neuroendocrinology, 16*(4), 319–324. https://doi.org/10.1111/j.0953-8194.2004.01161.x. [Seminal Reference]

[b]Rabin, B. S. (1999). The nervous system—immune system connection. In B. S. Rabin (Ed.), *Stress, immune function, and health: the connection*. Wiley-Liss. [Seminal Reference]

[c]Cacioppo, J. T., Berntson, G. G., Malarkey, W. B., et al. (1998). Autonomic, neuroendocrine, and immune responses to psychological stress: the reactivity hypothesis. *Annals of the New York Academy of Science, 840*, 664–673. https://doi.org/10.1111/j.1749-6632.1998.tb09605.x. [Seminal Reference]

[d]Rohleder, N., Kudielka, B. M., Hellhammer, D. H., et al. (2002). Age and sex steroid-related changes in glucocorticoid sensitivity of pro-inflammatory cytokine production after psychosocial stress. *Journal of Neuroimmunology, 126*(1–2), 69–77. https://doi.org/10.1016/s0165-5728(02)00062-0. [Seminal Reference]

[e]Tikk, K., Sookthai, D., Fortner, R. T., et al. (2015). Circulating prolactin and in situ breast cancer risk in the European EPIC cohort: a case-control study. *Breast Cancer Research, 17*(1), 49. https://doi.org/10.1186/s13058-015-0563-6.

[f]Lieberwirth, C., & Wang, Z. (2014). Social bonding: regulation by neuropeptides. *Frontiers in Neuroscience, 8*, 171. https://doi.org/10.3389/fnins.2014.00171.

[g]Chesnokova, V., & Melmed, S. (2002). Minireview: Neuro-immuno-endocrine modulation of the hypothalamic-pituitary-adrenal (HPA) axis by gp130 signaling molecules. *Endocrinology, 143*(5), 1571–1574. https://doi.org/10.1210/endo.143.5.8861. [Seminal Reference]

[h]Guezennec, C. Y., Lafarge, J. P., Bricout, V. A., et al. (1995). Effect of competition stress on tests used to assess testosterone administration in athletes. *International Journal of Sports Medicine, 16*(6), 368–372. https://doi.org/10.1055/s-2007-973022. [Seminal Reference]

[i]Volterrani, M., Rosano, G., & Iellamo, F. (2012). Testosterone and heart failure. *Endocrine, 42*(2), 272–277. https://doi.org/10.1007/s12020-012-9725-9.

[j]Bauer-Wu, S. M. (2002). Psychoneuroimmunology. Part II: Mind-body interventions. *Clinical Journal of Oncology Nursing, 6*(4), 243–246. https://doi.org/10.1055/s-2007-973022. [Seminal Reference]

[k]Kudwa, A. E., McGivern, R. F., & Handa, R. J. (2014). Estrogen receptor β and oxytocin interact to modulate anxiety-like behavior and neuroendocrine stress reactivity in adult male and female rats. *Physiology & Behavior, 129*, 287–296. https://doi.org/10.1016/j.physbeh.2014.03.004.

[l]Maestroni, G. J. (1999). MLT and the immune-hematopoietic system. *Advances in Experimental Medicine and Biology, 460*, 395-405. https://doi.org/10.1007/0-306-46814-x_47.

[m]Petitto, J. M., Huang, Z., & McCarthy, D. B. (1994). Molecular cloning of NPY-Y1 receptor cDNA from rat splenic lymphocytes: Evidence of low levels of mRNA expression and NPY binding sites. *Journal of Neuroimmunology, 54*, 81–86. https://doi.org/10.1016/0165-5728(94)90234-8. [Seminal Reference]

[n]Müller, T. D., Nogueiras, R., Andermann, M. L., et al. (2015). Ghrelin. *Molecular Metabolism, 4*(6), 437–60. https://doi.org/10.1016/j.molmet.2015.03.005.

[o]Chatzitomaris, A., Hoermann, R., Midgley, J. E., et al. (2017). Thyroid allostasis–adaptive responses of thyrotropic feedback control to conditions of strain, stress, and developmental programming. *Frontiers in Endocrinology, 8*. https://doi.org/10.3389/fendo.2017.00163.

[p]Li, J., & Shen, X. (2019). Oxidative stress and adipokine levels were significantly correlated in diabetic patients with hyperglycemic crises. *Diabetology & Metabolic Syndrome, 11*, 13. https://doi.org/10.1186/s13098-019-0410-5.

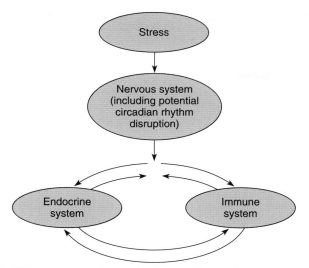

FIGURE 9.6 Nervous System/Endocrine System/Immune System Interactions. Interconnections or pathways of communication among the immune, nervous, and endocrine systems.

and other products affect neurocrine and endocrine cells.[55,63,64] Several pathways regulate communication among these systems, linking the signals together (Figure 9.6).

Stress-induced secretion of HPA hormones and catecholamines of the ANS sympathetic branch directly influence the immune system. Immune cells have receptors for ACTH, CRH, endorphins, norepinephrine, growth hormone, steroids, and other products of the stress response. Cholinergic, adrenergic, and peptidergic nerves also innervate lymphoid organs, such as the thymus, spleen, lymph nodes, and bone marrow.[63] Exposure to stress increases endogenous opiate secretion to enhance or suppress immune cell functions in a concentration-dependent manner (see Table 9.4).[63,65–68]

Lymphocytes also produce ACTH and endorphins in small amounts that influence the immune response in an autocrine (same cell stimulation) or paracrine (cell to cell) manner in ongoing immune and memory cytotoxic responses.[63,69,70] The T-cell growth factor, interleukin-2 (IL-2), for instance, can upregulate pituitary ACTH. Immune-derived cytokines have both direct and indirect effects on the HPA and adrenal cell functions. As such, the immune system has an adaptive role to signal and alert other systems of internally threatening stimuli (e.g., infection, tissue damage, tumour cells). Bacterial and viral infections, as well as cancer, tissue injury, and other stressors trigger the release of immune inflammatory mediators (IL-6, tumour necrosis factor-beta [TNF-β], interferon) that, in turn, initiate a stress response through the HPA pathway. Enhanced systemic production of these cytokines can also induce other CNS and behaviour changes during an acute infectious episode.[71–74]

Although acute stress activates HPA hormone secretion and immune system products, such as interleukin-1 (IL-1), continued stress-induced secretion of glucocorticoids inhibits production of IL-1 by activated macrophages and monocytes.[63,75] Prolonged severe stress may lead to enlargement of the adrenal gland with simultaneous involution or destruction of the thymus and lymph nodes. Increased secretion of glucocorticoids may be an important mechanism underlying stress-related immune structure alterations and suppression of the immune response.[55]

In addition to the HPA and sympathetic nervous system, the pineal gland regulates the immune response and mediates the effects of circadian rhythm on immunity. Blocked production of melatonin by the pineal gland (because of disrupted light-dark cycles and pharmacological means) suppresses the immune response, whereas administration of melatonin reverses these effects.[76] This immunomodulation pathway may effect immune changes found with sleep disturbance and dysregulated circadian rhythm,[77] which are common among acutely ill, stressed persons.

In summary, neuropeptides and hormones have significant effects on the immune system. Whether this impact on immune system functions is suppressive or potentiating depends on the type of factor secreted (some factors enhance, some suppress, and some both enhance and suppress), the concentration and length of exposure, and the target cell.[74] Neuropeptides and neuroendocrine hormones may directly control biochemical events affecting cell proliferation, differentiation, and function or may indirectly control immune cell behaviour by affecting the production or activity of cytokines.[63,64] Chronic stress affects many immune cell functions, and can lead to decreased natural killer (NK)-cell and T-cell cytotoxicity and impaired B-cell function.[32,70] Importantly, these impairments in the immune system may have negative health consequences for stressed individuals, such as increased risk of infection and some types of cancer.[78,79] Common pathophysiological origins related to chronic inflammatory processes include cardiovascular disease, osteoporosis, arthritis, type 2 diabetes mellitus, chronic obstructive pulmonary disease, other diseases associated with aging, and some cancers; all are characterized by the prolonged presence of proinflammatory cytokines.[15,80]

Although inflammation is a normal response and is most often beneficial, excessive inflammation can damage tissue. Stress and negative emotions are associated directly with the production of increased levels of proinflammatory cytokines, providing a link between stress, immune function, and disease.[81–83]

STRESS, PERSONALITY, COPING, AND ILLNESS

Extreme physiological stressors, such as severe burn injury, represent a predictable stimulus for stress responses. A less severe and defined event or situation, however, can be a stressor for one person and not for another. Stress itself is not an independent entity but a system of interdependent processes, moderated by the nature, intensity, and duration of the stressor and the perception, appraisal, and coping efficacy of the affected individual, all of which in turn, mediate the individual's psychological and physiological response to stress. A person's appraisal of a situation facilitates their own particular adjustment to repetitive stressors.[27] In fact, the influence of an individualized stress appraisal on physiological processes reduces Tc-cell cytotoxicity, but has a limited effect on the number of circulating Th cells or Tc cells.

Psychosocial distress may be predictive of psychological, social, and physical health outcomes (see *Health Promotion:* Acute Emotional Stress and Adverse Heart Effects). A psychologically distressed individual may experience a general stress-induced state of unpleasant arousal that manifests as physiological, emotional, cognitive, and behaviour changes.[84] Periods of depression and emotional upheaval associated with adverse life events may place the affected individual at increased risk for immunological deficits accompanied by ill health.[55] For example, there is a relationship between depression and reduction in lymphocyte proliferation and NK-cell activity.[85] Multiple moderating factors may be important in immune modulation in depressed individuals, including alcoholism and other lifestyle factors, such as social support. Examples of triggering circumstances include bereavement, academic pressures, and marital conflict. Aging also may increase psychosocial distress and is associated with immune changes (see *Health Promotion:* Partner's Survival and Spouse's Hospitalizations and/or Death).[80,81]

HEALTH PROMOTION
Acute Emotional Stress and Adverse Heart Effects

Myocardial Ischemia
- Individuals with coronary heart disease may develop myocardial ischemia during mental or acute emotional stress even though their exercise or chemical nuclear test results are negative.
- Systemic vascular resistance increases during periods of mental or acute emotional stress with concomitant increased myocardial oxygen demand.

Left Ventricular Dysfunction
- More evidence for left ventricular dysfunction exists in older women.
- After acute emotional stress or trauma, there is an increase in sudden chest pain and shortness of breath.
- Left ventricular dysfunction is more common in the cardiac apex.
- Alterations are possibly a result of increased levels of catecholamines.

Ventricular Dysrhythmias
- Intense or unusual acute stress precipitates about 20% of serious ventricular dysrhythmias or sudden cardiac death.
- Altered brain activity may lead to changes in ventricular repolarization and electrical instability of the cardiac muscle.

Data from Pimple, P., Shah, A., Rooks, C., et al. (2015). *American Heart Journal, 169*(1), 115–121; Ramadan, R., Sheps, D., Esteves, F., et al. (2013). *Journal of the American Heart Association, 2*(5), e000321; Wei, J., Rooks, C., Ramadan, R., et al. (2014). *American Journal of Cardiology, 114*(2), 187–192; Wittstein, I. S., Thiemann, D. R., Lima, J. A. C., et al. (2005). *New England Journal of Medicine, 352*(6), 539–548; Ziegelstein, R. C. (2007). *JAMA, 298*(3), 324–329.

HEALTH PROMOTION
Partner's Survival and Spouse's Hospitalizations and/or Death

A Harvard study shows that a spouse's chances of dying increase not only when the partner dies but also when that partner becomes seriously ill. The 9-year follow-up study consisted of 518 240 older couples. Mortality after the partner's hospitalization varied according to the spouse's diagnosis. For older persons whose spouse had been hospitalized, the short-term risk of dying approached that of an older person after his or her spouse's death. A wife's hospitalization increased her husband's chances of dying within 1 month by 35%; a husband's hospitalization increased his wife's chances of dying by 44%. Likewise, a wife's death increased her partner's 1-month mortality risk by 53%, and a husband's death raised his partner's risk by 61%. The researchers commented that a spouse's illness or death can increase a partner's mortality by causing severe stress and removing a primary source of emotional, psychological, practical, and financial support.

Data from Carey, F. M., Shah, S. M., DeWilde, S., et al. (2014). *JAMA Internal Medicine, 174*(4), 598–605; Christakis, N. A., & Allison, P. D. (2006). *New England Journal of Medicine, 354*(7), 719–730.

Personality characteristics are also associated with differences in appraisal and response to stressors. Specific personality characteristics, such as academic achievement, motivation, optimism, and aggression, are correlated with immunological alterations. For example, aggression is positively associated with changes in T- and B-cell numbers in male military personnel. In addition, optimism, perceived stress, and anxiety enhance responses to influenza vaccinations after age 50.[68,86]

Stressful life events and mood are important factors that exacerbate symptoms in acquired immunodeficiency syndrome (AIDS) infection, diabetes, and multiple sclerosis.[64,87,88] In addition, the interaction with health care providers in a clinical setting, the diagnosis of a major illness,

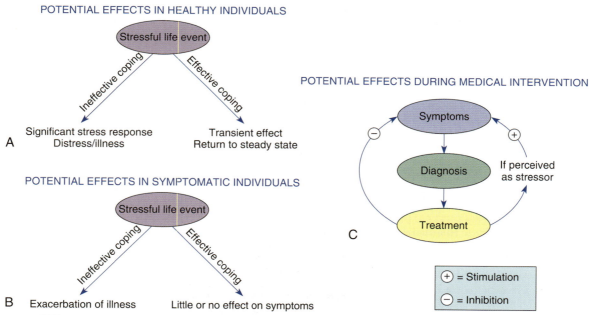

FIGURE 9.7 Numerous Factors Moderate Health Outcome Determination in Stressful Life Situations. Whether a life-challenged individual experiences distress or illness depends on the person's appraisal of the event and the coping strategies used during the stressful period. Models (**A**) and (**B**) reflect possible outcomes in stressed healthy and symptomatic individuals. Model (**C**) illustrates the dynamic clinical setting in which the diagnosis of a serious illness and subsequent medical interventions may be perceived as stressful challenges and have potentially detrimental influences on physical outcome.

and the process of undergoing various clinical procedures (e.g., blood sampling, injections, examinations, surgical procedures) may represent significant negative life events to many individuals (Figure 9.7). These additional stresses may interfere with the efficacy of the medical intervention. Identifying and reducing stress in the clinical setting have particular applicability for both preventing disease and managing illness.

Many studies have linked severe psychosocial stress resulting from negative life events to chronic disorders with mental and physical consequences. A life-threatening event may lead to the development of PTSD.[89–92] Early research with breast cancer survivors demonstrates a link between sympathetic activity and HPA-axis activation, noting that some women reported symptoms of PTSD (heart palpitations, panic, shakiness, nausea) when they thought about cancer recurrence or when they found themselves near the hospital where treatment began.[93] Furthermore, the threat of cancer recurrence (using a simulated mammography event as a stressor to elicit thoughts of cancer recurrence) elicited greater alterations in heart rate variability when compared with another simulated controlled stressor.[94] These studies show a connection between re-exposure to mammography, which occurred repeatedly throughout breast cancer survivorship, and activation of the ANS.

These uncontrolled stressful events may negatively affect the course of illness and interfere with the efficacy of the medical intervention. Identifying and reducing stress in the clinical setting have particular applicability in both disease prevention and illness management. In addition to medical procedures, patient–provider communication provides an important area for future research. Recent studies of cancer communication and patient–provider interaction indicate a link between communication events and emotional outcomes, such as uncertainty and mood state in breast cancer survivors.[95,96]

Coping

Coping is the process of managing stressful challenges that tax the individual's resources.[67] Coping responses may be adaptive or maladaptive, and the extent to which an individual responds to distress, using effective

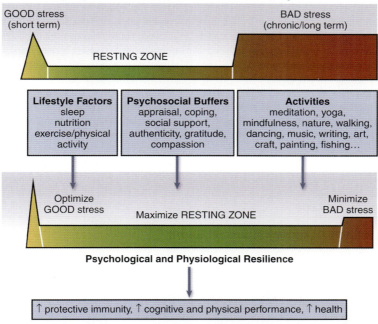

FIGURE 9.8 Staying on the Good Side of the Stress Spectrum. GOOD stress is on the left of the spectrum and involves a rapid biological response to the stressor, followed by a rapid shutdown of the response upon cessation of the stressor. These responses support physiological conditions that are likely to enhance protective immunity, cognitive and physical performance, and overall health. BAD stress, represented on the right of the spectrum, involves exposure to chronic or long-term biological changes that are likely to result in dysregulation or suppression of immune function, a decrease in cognitive and physical performance, and an increased likelihood of disease. Short-term stress or long-term stress (or both) is generally superimposed on a psychophysiological RESTING ZONE of low/no stress that also represents a state of health maintenance/restoration. To maintain health, one needs to optimize GOOD stress, maximize the RESTING ZONE, and minimize BAD stress. Achieving psychological and physiological resilience involves a multipronged approach. Sleep of a quality and duration that helps one feel rested in the morning, a moderate and healthy diet, and consistent and moderate exercise or physical activity are three LIFESTYLE FACTORS that are likely to enable one to stay on the "good" side of the stress spectrum. Effective appraisal and coping mechanisms, genuine gratitude, social support, and compassion toward others and oneself are likely to provide PSYCHOSOCIAL BUFFERS against bad stress and enable one to stay on the GOOD side of the stress spectrum. Additionally, depending on individual preferences, ACTIVITIES, such as meditation, yoga, being in nature, exercise/physical activity, music, art, craft, dance, fishing, painting, also may reduce BAD stress, extend the RESTING ZONE, and optimize GOOD stress. Such personal activities are likely to involve different strokes for different folks and need not always be meditative or reflective in nature. (Adapted from Dhabhar, F. S., & McEwen, B. S. [2007]. Bidirectional effects of stress on immune function: possible explanations for salubrious as well as harmful effects. In R. Ader [Ed.], *Psychoneuroimmunology IV.* Elsevier.)

positive coping strategies, determines the degree of successful moderation of the stress challenge. For example, studies are beginning to support a role for stress reduction in slowing human immunodeficiency virus (HIV) progression.[42,46,52,97] Similarly, the COVID-19 pandemic indicates a need for programs to facilitate coping and positive mental health due to increased stress.[98] Other investigations are under way to determine the benefits offered by exercise and mindfulness, as well as others, such as inclusion of green space in urban environments.[31] Studies are also focusing on mediating factors that influence stress susceptibility or resilience, such as age, socioeconomic status, gender, social support, religious or spiritual factors, personality, self-esteem, genetics, past experiences, and current health status (Figure 9.8).[99]

Coping strategies are especially beneficial when they are problem-focused and individuals seek social support.[67,76] Evidence suggests that effective interventions may result in greater stress resilience and improved psychological and physiological outcomes.[100] For example, women with recurrent metastatic breast cancer and weekly group counselling in conjunction with routine medical treatment lived an average of 19 months longer than control subjects, suggesting a positive influence of group support for these women.[74,76]

Maladaptive coping can result in a change in behaviour contributing to potentially adverse health effects (e.g., increased smoking, change in eating habits). Serious disturbances of the sleep–wake cycle (observed in many stressed people and in experimental and many clinical settings)[34,101] may exacerbate the pathophysiological status of some individuals.[102-104] Sleep deprivation and circadian disruption, even in young, otherwise healthy individuals, have detrimental influences on respiratory and immune system function. Even partial sleep deprivation can be associated with reduced NK-cell activity in healthy subjects, and only recently have seriously ill individuals been assessed for adequacy and structure of sleep during recovery.[102]

Behavioural styles, such as overcommitment to employment-related tasks, repression, denial, escape–avoidance, and concealment, are associated with altered immune functions.[105] Repression is associated with lower monocyte counts, higher eosinophil counts, higher serum glucose levels, and more self-reported medication reactions in medical outpatients,[77] and with higher Epstein-Barr virus antibody titres in students.[75] A prospective long-term study also found increased markers of accelerated HIV infection in gay men who concealed their homosexual identity.[64] Schoolteachers who devoted long hours without reward and who were unable to disengage from work-related tasks also had lowered innate immune responses.[106]

The importance of social support for seriously ill individuals also needs to be considered in the health of caregivers. Significant stress manifested as depression, anxiety, and fatigue is present in family caregivers of those with cancer, Alzheimer's disease, and burn trauma.[107] Enhanced social support of caregivers improves measures of immune function.[65,66,76,108,109]

Interventions to potentially prevent or manage stress-related psychological or physical problems include both short- and long-term education on evaluating and adopting effective coping strategies. Approaches may be used or investigated on an individual or group basis. Incorporation of effective stress management approaches into clinical education facilitates their use in the clinical arena. Future research could focus on the efficacy of such approaches with different populations because it is clear one size does not fit all (coping of cancer survivors may be vastly different from coping of combat veterans).

In summary, the mind and body are connected through a multitude of complex physical and emotional interactions.[110] Understanding the complexity of these interactions is a challenge for researchers. Areas of promise include investigating relationships between the effects of stress on illness, as well as developing effective stress management techniques and approaches that improve health outcomes.

GERIATRIC CONSIDERATIONS
Aging and the Stress–Age Syndrome

With aging, sometimes a set of neurohormonal and immune alterations, as well as tissue and cellular changes, develop. These changes have been defined as stress–age syndrome and include:
- Alterations in the excitability of structures of the limbic system and hypothalamus
- Increase of the blood concentrations of catecholamines, ADH, ACTH, and cortisol
- Decrease of the concentrations of testosterone, thyroxine, and others
- Alterations of opioid peptides
- Immunodepression and pattern of chronic inflammation
- Alterations in lipoproteins
- Hypercoagulation of the blood
- Free radical damage of cells

Some of the alterations are adaptational, whereas others are potentially damaging. These stress-related alterations of aging can influence the course of developing stress reactions and lower adaptive reserve and coping capacity.

ACTH, Adrenocorticotropic hormone; *ADH*, antidiuretic hormone.
Data from Frolkis, V. V. (1998). Stress-age syndrome. *Mechanisms of Ageing and Development, 69*(1–2), 93–107.

CASE STUDY

Stella is a 39-year-old woman who has just been admitted to the nurse's unit for elective hip surgery, for which she has waited 9 months. She has lived a very active outdoor lifestyle up until this point. She is a healthy person with no other comorbidities and has three school-aged children at home. When the nurse's shift occurs, Stella is 14 hours postoperative. Her pain is 4/10.

Consider what the nurse needs to know in order to care for her properly and anticipate her response postsurgery. How does the nurse understand her context?

Critical Thinking and Clinical Judgement Questions

1. a) What is stress? b) Given Stella's age, identify some stressors that could be impacting Stella.

2. a) How does stress impact the body? b) Is it possible to control stress? If so, how? c) What clinical manifestations would the nurse monitor for in this patient?
   - Stella develops pneumonia on her second postoperative day. Her initial vital signs are:
   - Temperature 39.3° C
   - Heart rate 123
   - Respiratory rate 34
   - BP 90/40
   - O_2 saturation 90% on room air

   What would be the nurse's best course of action considering these values?

DID YOU UNDERSTAND?

Overview
1. Stress is broadly defined as a threat that is perceived or anticipated, resulting in interactions between the body and the brain (the stress response).

Historical Background and General Concepts
1. Cannon used the term *stress* in both a physiological and a psychological sense in 1914. The idea that stressful events could cause physiological responses was further developed by Selye in 1946. Selye's work demonstrated that internal or external stressors could result in adrenal gland enlargement, immune alterations (increased leukocytes), and gastro-intestinal manifestations (ulcers). These global physiological responses were labelled the general adaptation syndrome (GAS).
2. GAS occurs in three stages: the alarm stage, the resistance or adaptation stage, and the exhaustion stage (now referred to as *allostatic overload*). Diseases of adaptation develop if the resistance or adaptation stage does not restore homeostasis. Although important, the concept that stress is entirely the result of a physical disturbance is greatly oversimplified.
3. Continuing the evolution of this research, adrenal gland hormone responses to stressors were suggested in the 1950s and central nervous system (CNS) and endocrine responses were proposed in the 1970s.
4. Psychological stressors can be anticipatory and triggered by expectations of an upcoming stressor or can be reactive to a stressor. Both of these psychological stressors are capable of eliciting a physiological stress response.
5. The study of the body's response to stressors continues to evolve and has become known by the term *psychoneuroimmunology* (PNI).
6. The concepts of allostasis (stability through change; monitoring the environment for adaptive response) and homeostasis (return to base levels reflecting an unchanging set point) both indicate physiological responses. Allostatic overload can occur when there is overactivation of adaptive responses that may in turn increase susceptibility to disease.
7. The stress response is initiated when a stressor is present in the body or perceived by the mind. Psychological stress may cause or worsen several diseases or disorders, including anxiety, depression, insomnia, persistent pain and fatigue syndromes, obesity, metabolic syndrome, essential hypertension, type 2 diabetes, atherosclerosis and its cardiovascular consequences, osteoporosis, and autoimmune inflammatory and allergic disorders. A classic example of stress and allostatic overload is sleep alteration and the associated damaging effects of elevated evening cortisol, insulin, and glucose.

The Stress Response
1. The stress response involves the nervous system (sympathetic branch of the autonomic nervous system), the endocrine system (pituitary and adrenal glands), and the immune system. More simply, these relationships are often cited together as the hypothalamic–pituitary–adrenal (HPA) axis.
2. The physiology of managing stressful events is complex, involving mechanisms of both protection and injury. The two major stress regulation systems are the autonomic nervous system (ANS) and the HPA system.
3. Activation of the ANS consists of sympathetic stimulation of the adrenal medulla and nerve endings to rapidly secrete catecholamines (norepinephrine, epinephrine, neuropeptide Y).
4. Activation of the HPA system involves sequential secretion of corticotropin-releasing hormone from the hypothalamus, which stimulates receptors in the anterior pituitary to secrete adrenocorticotropic hormone (ACTH) that, in turn, stimulates the adrenal cortex to secrete glucocorticoids, particularly cortisol.
5. Glucocorticoids reach all tissues, including the brain, easily penetrate cell membranes, and react with numerous intracellular glucocorticoid receptors. Because they spare almost no tissue or organ and influence a large proportion of the human genome, they broadly exert diverse biological actions. For example, glucocorticoids have an important modulatory role in the CNS. These hormones regulate memory, cognition, mood, and sleep and influence many other body systems.
6. In general, catecholamines of the sympathetic system prepare the body to act; for example, cortisol mobilizes glucose (for energy) and other substances.
7. Cortisol is the primary glucocorticoid produced during stress.
8. Cortisol's chief effects involve metabolic processes. By inhibiting the use of metabolic substances while promoting their formation, cortisol mobilizes glucose, amino acids, lipids, and fatty acids and delivers them to the bloodstream. As an example, anabolic effects of cortisol increase the rate of protein synthesis in the liver, whereas the catabolic effects of cortisol increase levels of amino acids, ultimately depleting protein stores in muscle, bone, skin, and connective tissue.
9. Cortisol contributes to elevated blood glucose and inhibits glucose uptake by body cells providing energy to combat perceived or anticipated stressors.
10. Chronic dysregulation of the HPA axis, especially abnormal elevated levels of cortisol, has been linked to a wide variety of disorders, including obesity, sleep deprivation, lipid abnormalities, hypertension, diabetes, atherosclerosis, and loss of bone density.
11. Glucocorticoids contribute to the development of metabolic syndrome and the pathogenesis of obesity. They can directly cause insulin resistance and influence genetic variations that predispose to obesity.
12. Elevated levels of glucocorticoids and catecholamines (epinephrine and norepinephrine), both endogenous and exogenous (synthetic pharmaceuticals), may decrease innate immunity and increase autoimmune responses. However, prolonged effects of cortisol may accentuate inflammation. Overall, stress activates an excessive immune response and, through cortisol and the catecholamines, suppresses Th1 responses while enhancing Th2 responses.
13. Glucocorticoids from the adrenal cortex, in response to ACTH from the pituitary gland, comprise the major stress hormones along with the catecholamines epinephrine and norepinephrine.
14. Norepinephrine's chief effects complement those of epinephrine. Norepinephrine constricts blood vessels of the viscera and skin; this has the effect of shifting blood flow to the vessels dilated by epinephrine. Norepinephrine also increases mental alertness.
15. Epinephrine exerts its chief effects on the cardiovascular system. Epinephrine increases cardiac output and increases blood flow to the heart, brain, and skeletal muscles by dilating vessels that supply these organs. It also dilates the airways, thereby increasing delivery of oxygen to the bloodstream.
16. The parasympathetic system balances or restrains the sympathetic system, resulting in slowed heart rates, and anti-inflammatory effects. During prolonged stress (allostatic overload) the parasympathetic system is less effective in opposing the sympathetic system.

17. Other hormones, including β-endorphins, growth hormone, prolactin, oxytocin, the steroid sex hormones, and antidiuretic hormone, influence the stress response by their diverse actions.

Stress, Personality, Coping, and Illness

1. Stress is a system of interdependent processes that are moderated by the nature, intensity, and duration of the stressor and the coping efficacy of the affected individual, all of which in turn mediate the psychological and physiological response to stress.
2. Personality characteristics are associated with individual differences in appraisal and response to stressors. Further, the appraisal of events as distressful may be predictive of psychological, social, and physical health outcomes (maladaptive coping, depression, post-traumatic stress disorder, heart disease, altered immunity).
3. Coping styles associated with altered immunity include repression, denial, escape–avoidance, and concealment. Coping strategies are more beneficial when they are problem-focused and may result in improved resilience and better psychological and physiological outcomes.

Geriatric Considerations: Aging and the Stress–Age Syndrome

1. With aging, often a set of neurohormonal and immune alterations, including tissue and cellular changes, occur. These changes are collectively called *stress–age syndrome*.
2. The changes are numerous, with some being adaptive whereas others are potentially damaging.
3. Coping techniques for managing stress may mitigate the effects of stress on maladaptive behaviours such as excessive alcohol ingestion and smoking, and, by extension, impact the effects of existing chronic illness.

10

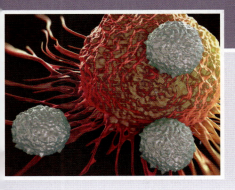

Biology of Cancer

Stephanie Zettel, with originating chapter contributions by Kathryn L. McCance and Neal S. Rote

Additional resources are available online at http://evolve.elsevier.com/Canada/Huether/pathophysiology

CHAPTER OUTLINE

- Cancer Terminology and Characteristics, 234
  - Tumour Classification and Nomenclature, 234
- The Biology of Cancer Cells, 235
  - Sustained Proliferative Signalling, 239
  - Evading Growth Suppressors, 242
  - Genomic Instability, 244
  - Enabling Replicative Immortality, 246
  - Inducing Angiogenesis, 246
  - Reprogramming Energy Metabolism, 247
  - Resisting Apoptotic Cell Death, 248
  - Tumour-Promoting Inflammation, 249
  - Evading Immune Destruction, 251
  - Activating Invasion and Metastasis, 252
- Clinical Manifestations of Cancer, 255
  - Paraneoplastic Syndromes, 255
- Pain, 255
- Fatigue, 255
- Cachexia, 255
- Anemia, 258
- Leukopenia and Thrombocytopenia, 258
- Infection, 258
- Gastrointestinal Tract, 258
- Hair and Skin, 258
- Diagnosis, Characterization, and Treatment of Cancer, 259
  - Diagnosis and Staging, 259
  - Classification of Tumours: Classic Histology and Modern Genetics, 261
  - Treatment, 261
- CASE STUDY, 263

LEARNING OBJECTIVES

1. Differentiate benign from malignant tumours.
2. Identify and differentiate among types of cancers based on cell type, such as adenocarcinoma, lymphoma, or sarcoma.
3. Identify the importance of tumour markers.
4. Identify the two mutational routes resulting in uncontrolled cellular proliferation.
5. Describe the properties of autonomy and anaplasia.
6. Discuss in general cell surface changes and their functional importance in cancer.
7. Define proto-oncogene, cellular oncogene, viral oncogene, and tumour suppressor gene.
8. Discuss the idea of cancer-prone families.
9. Describe the function of stem cells in cancer.
10. Discuss the role of chronic inflammation and the development of cancer cells.
11. Describe bacterial and viral causes of cancer.
12. Discuss the factors implicated in metastasis of tumours: rate of growth, angiogenesis, lack of cellular adhesion, and absence of cellular barriers.
13. Discuss mechanisms that favour or inhibit the metastasis of cancer cells.
14. Describe the manifestations of cancer that lead to diagnosis.
15. Describe the treatment strategies for cancer.
16. Describe the side effects associated with cancer treatment.

KEY TERMS

Adenocarcinoma, 234
Adjuvant chemotherapy, 262
Aerobic glycolysis, 248
Anaplasia, 234
Angiogenesis, 246
Angiogenic factor, 246
Apoptosis, 248
Autocrine stimulation, 239
Benign tumour, 234
Brachytherapy, 261
Cachexia, 255
Cancer, 234
Cancer-associated fibroblasts (CAFs), 251
Carcinoma, 234
Carcinoma in situ (CIS), 235
Caretaker gene, 244
Chromosome instability, 246
Chromosome translocation, 237
Clonal expansion, 238
Clonal proliferation, 238
DNA methylation, 237
Dormancy, 253
Epigenetic silencing, 245
Epithelial-mesenchymal transition (EMT), 252
Fas/CD95, 248
Gene amplification, 237
Germ cell mutation, 242
Human T-cell lymphotropic virus type 1 (HTLV-1), 251
Hypoxia-inducible factor-1 alpha (HIF-1α), 246
Induction chemotherapy, 262
Leukemia, 235
Lymphoma, 235
Malignant tumour, 234
Matrix metalloproteinase (MMP), 247
Metastasis 252
MicroRNA (miRNA), 245
Neoadjuvant chemotherapy, 262
Neoplasm, 234
Neovascularization, 246

CHAPTER 10 Biology of Cancer

Noncoding RNA (ncRNA), 237
Oncogene, 239
Oncomir, 245
Paraneoplastic syndrome, 255
Personalized medicine, 261
Pleomorphic, 234
Point mutation, 237
Proto-oncogene, 239
RAS, 239
Receptor tyrosine kinase, 241
Retinoblastoma *(RB)* gene, 244
Reverse Warburg effect, 248
Sarcoma, 235
Silencing, 245
Somatic cell mutation, 244
Staging of cancer, 260
Stroma, 234
Telomerase, 246
Telomere, 246
Thrombospondin-1 (TSP-1), 247
Transformation, 238
Tumour, 234
Tumour-associated macrophage (TAM), 250
Tumour-initiating cells (TIC), 253
Tumour initiation, 235
Tumour marker, 260
Tumour progression, 236
Tumour promotion, 236
Tumour protein p53 *(TP53)*, 244
Tumour-suppressor gene, 242
Warburg effect, 248

Cancer is a leading cause of suffering and death in the developed world. Over the past 35 years, intensive research has led to a significantly enhanced understanding of this complex and frightening disease. Cancer is now a collection of more than 100 different diseases, each caused by a specific and often unique age-related accumulation of genetic and epigenetic alterations. Environment, heredity, and behaviour interact to modify the risk of developing cancer and the response to treatment. Improvements in treatment strategies and supportive care, coupled with new, often individualized therapies based on advances in our fundamental understanding of the basic pathophysiology of malignancy, have contributed to an increasing number of effective options for these diverse, often lethal, disorders collectively called cancer.

CANCER TERMINOLOGY AND CHARACTERISTICS

> **QUICK CHECK 10.1**
> 1. What is cancer?
> 2. Identify the major differences between benign and malignant tumours.
> 3. What is carcinoma in situ?

The term **cancer** comes from the Latin translation of the Greek word for crab, *karkinoma*, which the physician Hippocrates used to describe the appendagelike projections extending from tumours into adjacent tissue. The word **tumour** originally referred to any swelling caused by inflammation but is now generally reserved for describing a new growth, or **neoplasm**.

Tumour Classification and Nomenclature

The careful evaluation of each cancer is important for many reasons. Different cancers will have different causes, different rates and patterns of progression, and different responses to treatment. The classification starts with knowing the tissue and organ of origin, the extent of distribution to other sites, and the microscopic appearance of the lesion. Increasingly, classification of cancer also includes a detailed description of its critical genetic changes. (See Figure 10.1 for a flow chart showing how cancer begins and spreads.)

Benign and Malignant

Not all tumours or neoplasms, however, are cancer; tumours and neoplasms can be benign or malignant (cancerous). **Benign tumours** are usually encapsulated with connective tissue and contain fairly well-differentiated cells and well-organized **stroma** (i.e., connective tissue) (Figure 10.2). They retain recognizable normal tissue structure and do not invade beyond their capsule, nor do they spread to regional lymph nodes or distant locations. Mitotic cells are very rarely present during microscopic analysis. Benign tumours are generally named according to the tissues from which they arise with the suffix "-oma," which indicates a tumour or mass. For example, a benign tumour of the smooth muscle of the uterus is a *leiomyoma*, and a benign tumour of fat cells is a *lipoma*. Benign tumours can become extremely large and, depending on their location in the body, can cause morbidity or be life-threatening. For example, a benign meningioma at the base of the skull may cause symptoms by compressing adjacent normal brain tissue.

Some benign tumours can progress to cancer and then are referred to as **malignant tumours**, which are distinguished from benign tumours by more rapid growth rates and specific microscopic alterations, including loss of differentiation and absence of normal tissue organization (Figure 10.3). One of the microscopic hallmarks of cancer cells is **anaplasia**, the loss of cellular differentiation. Malignant cells are also **pleomorphic**, with marked variability of size and shape. They often have large darkly stained nuclei, and mitotic cells are common. Malignant tumours may have a substantial amount of stroma, but it is disorganized, with loss of normal tissue structure. Malignant tumours also lack a capsule and grow to invade nearby blood vessels, lymphatics, and surrounding structures. Moreover, the most important and most deadly characteristic of malignant tumours is their ability to spread far beyond the tissue of origin, a process known as *metastasis*.

Unlike benign tumours, which take their name relative to the tissue of origin, cancers take their name from their original cell type. In other words, cancers arising in epithelial tissue are **carcinomas**, and if they arise from or form ductal or glandular structures, they are **adenocarcinomas**. Hence, a malignant tumour arising from breast glandular

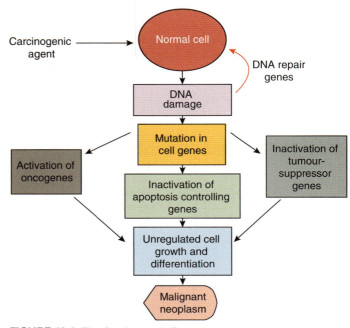

FIGURE 10.1 The Carcinogenic Process.

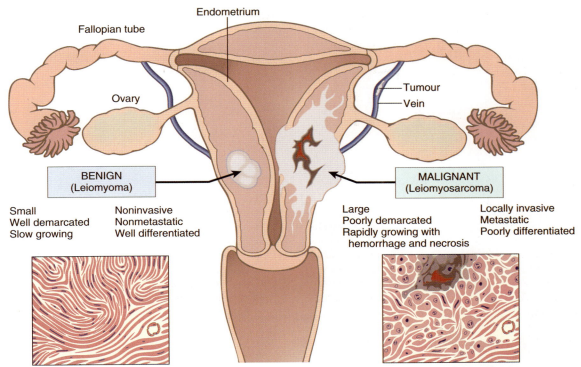

FIGURE 10.2 Comparison Between a Benign Tumour and a Malignant Tumour of the Same Origin. (From Kumar, V., Abbas, A. K., & Aster, J. C. [Eds.]. [2021]. *Robbins and Cotran pathologic basis of disease* [10th ed.]. Elsevier.)

tissue is a mammary adenocarcinoma, whereas an example of a benign breast tumour is a fibroadenoma. Cancers arising from mesenchymal tissue (including connective tissue, muscle, and bone) usually have the suffix **sarcoma**. For example, malignant cancers of skeletal muscle are rhabdomyosarcomas. Cancers of lymphatic tissue are **lymphomas**, whereas cancers of blood-forming cells are **leukemias**. However, many cancers, such as Hodgkin's disease and Ewing sarcoma, do not follow this nomenclature convention.

Carcinoma in Situ

Carcinoma in situ (often abbreviated **CIS**) refers to preinvasive epithelial tumours of glandular or squamous cell origin. Cancers develop incrementally as they accumulate specific genetic lesions. Careful surveillance for cancer often detects abnormal growths in epithelial tissues that have atypical cells and increased proliferation rate compared with normal surrounding tissues. These early-stage cancers are only in the epithelium and have not penetrated the local basement membrane or invaded the surrounding stroma. Based on these characteristics, they are not malignant. CIS occurs in a number of sites, including the cervix, skin, oral cavity, esophagus, and bronchus. In glandular epithelium, in situ lesions occur in the stomach, endometrium, breast, and large bowel. In the breast, ductal carcinoma in situ (DCIS) fills the mammary ducts but has not progressed to local tissue invasion.[1] DCIS lesions are readily treatable, although the optimal therapeutic approach is controversial. CIS lesions can have one of the following three fates: (1) they can remain stable for a long time, (2) they can progress to invasive and metastatic cancers, or (3) they can regress and disappear. CIS can vary from low-grade to high-grade dysplasia, with the high-grade lesions having the highest likelihood of becoming invasive cancers. The time that such preinvasive lesions remain in situ before becoming invasive is unknown. Some carcinomas of the cervix appear as preinvasive lesions in situ for several years before they progress to invasive carcinoma and metastatic tumours (Figure 10.4). Knowing how to best treat low-grade CIS lesions is challenging (i.e., removal versus "watchful waiting"), because the proportion that progress to cancer versus the proportion that will never cause clinical problems is usually not known.

THE BIOLOGY OF CANCER CELLS

> ✓ **QUICK CHECK 10.2**
> 1. Describe the differences between point mutations, chromosomal translocations, and gene amplification in the process of cancer.
> 2. Why is the tumour microenvironment important to cancer progression?

Although many types of cancer exist, and the course of the disease is complex because it affects different tissues, there are several traditional hallmarks of cancer.[2,3] Initially, there were six hallmarks, but with time and new research findings, there are now eight hallmarks and two traits that enable cancer progression. Furthermore, analysis of these hallmarks provides an accurate framework of why and how a cell becomes malignant. The following discussion is organized in the context of those 10 hallmarks/enablers (Figure 10.5).

Two fundamental concepts are the foundation for understanding the biology of cancer. (1) Cancer is a complex *genetic* disease arising from multiple mutations in genetic material; and (2) the *microenvironment* of a tumour is a heterogeneous mixture of cells, both cancerous and benign (often structural and related to connective tissue), as well as their secretions. These concepts affect every stage of cancer development and evolve during that development. **Tumour initiation**, the process that produces the initial cancer cells, is the first stage of cancer

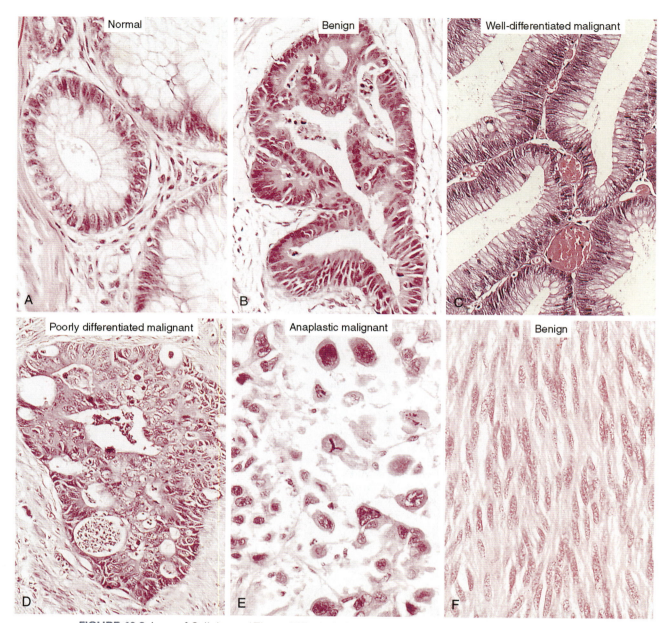

FIGURE 10.3 **Loss of Cellular and Tissue Differentiation During the Development of Cancer.** The cells of a benign neoplasm (B) resemble those of the normal colonic epithelium (A) in that they are columnar and have an orderly arrangement. Loss of some degree of differentiation is evident in that the neoplastic cells do not show much mucin vacuolization (large, clear cytoplasmic vacuoles in [A]). Cells of the well-differentiated malignant neoplasm (C) of the colon have a haphazard arrangement, and although gland lumina are formed they are architecturally abnormal and irregular. Nuclei vary in shape and size, especially when compared with those illustrated in (A). Cells in the poorly differentiated malignant neoplasm (D) have an even more haphazard arrangement, with very poor formation of gland lumina. Nuclei show greater variation in shape and size compared with the well-differentiated malignant neoplasm (C). Cells in anaplastic malignant neoplasms (E) bear no relation to the normal epithelium, with no recognizable gland formation. Tremendous variation is found in the size of cells and their nuclei, with very intense staining (hyperchromatic nuclei). Not knowing the site of origin makes it impossible to classify this tumour by microscopic appearance alone. Well-differentiated tumours often resemble their cell of origin, as shown in the example of a benign tumour of smooth muscles (F). (From Stevens, A., & Lowe, J. [2000]. *Pathology* [2nd ed.]. Mosby.)

development and depends on specific mutations and characteristics of the microenvironment to influence transformation of these cells. **Tumour promotion** is the next stage and is the process during which the population of cancer cells expands with diversity of cancer cell phenotypes and a gain in function. Additional mutations and a changing tumour microenvironment further enable this process. Finally, **tumour progression**, the process leading to spread of the tumour to adjacent and distal sites (metastasis), is governed by even more

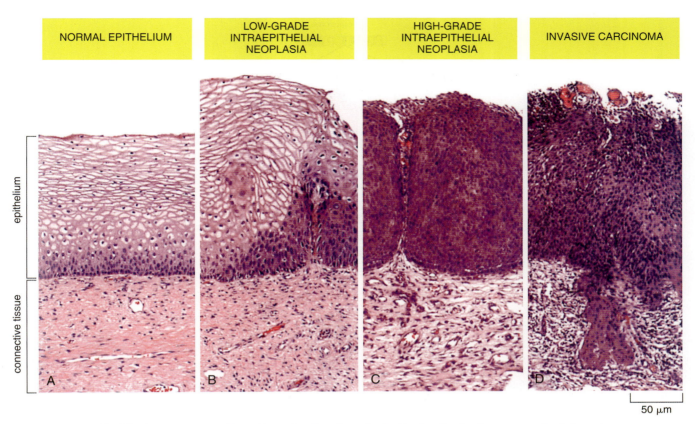

FIGURE 10.4 Progression From Normal to Neoplasm in the Uterine Cervix. A sequence of cellular and tissue changes progressing from low-grade to high-grade intraepithelial neoplasms (also called *carcinoma in situ*) and then to invasive cancer is seen often in the development of cancer. In this example of the early stages of cervical neoplastic changes, the presence of anaplastic cells and loss of normal tissue architecture signify the development of cancer. The high rate of cell division and the presence of local mutagens and inflammatory mediators all contribute to the accumulation of genetic abnormalities that lead to cancer. (Courtesy Andrew J. Connolly. From Alberts, B., Johnson, A., Lewis, J., et al. [2008]. *Molecular biology of the cell* [5th ed.]. Garland Publishing.)

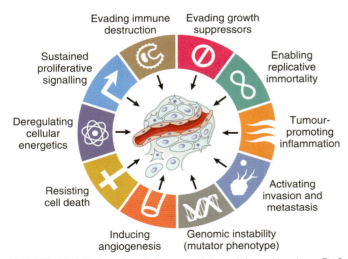

FIGURE 10.5 Hallmarks of Cancer. (Adapted from Hanahan, D. & Weinberg, R.A. (2011). Hallmarks of cancer: the next generation. *Cell, 144*[5], 646–674, with permission from Elsevier. Found in Kumar, V., Abbas, A. K., & Aster, J. C. [Eds.]. [2021]. *Robbins and Cotran pathologic basis of disease* [10th ed.]. Elsevier.)

mutations and changing microenvironments at the primary tumour and at sites of metastasis as disruption of blood and lymphatic circulation allow for invasion of the tumour at more distant sites.

Cancer is a disease of cumulative genetic changes during aging. The fraction of individuals who develop cancer increases dramatically with age. Genetic changes may occur by both mutational and epigenetic mechanisms. Mutation generally means an alteration in the DNA sequence affecting expression or function of a gene (Figure 10.6). Mutations include small-scale changes in DNA, such as **point mutations**: the alteration of one or a few nucleotide base pairs (see Chapter 2). This type of mutation can have profound effects on the activity of resultant proteins. **Chromosome translocations** are large changes in chromosome structure in which a piece of one chromosome translocates to another chromosome. **Gene amplification** is the result of repeated duplication of a region of a chromosome often known as a promoter sequence where instead of normal two copies of a gene, tens or even hundreds of copies are present. Epigenetic effects including **DNA methylation**, histone acetylation, or altered expression of **noncoding RNA (ncRNA)** also affect gene expression (see Chapter 3). Some mutations, referred to as *driver mutations*, "drive" the progression of cancer. There may be as many as 140 different driver mutations, although some are more critical than others, and each cancer only has a relatively small number of these.[4] Not all mutations in cancer

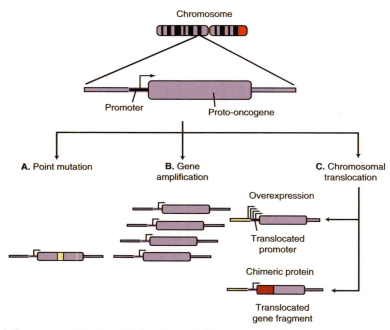

FIGURE 10.6 Oncogene Activation Mechanisms. Cellular genes may become cancerous oncogenes as a result of (**A**) point mutations that alter one or a few nucleotide base pairs, causing the production of a protein that is activated as a result of the altered sequence (e.g., RAS); (**B**) amplification of the cellular gene, resulting in higher levels of protein expression (e.g., MYCN [v-myc avian myelocytomatosis viral oncogene neuroblastoma derived homologue] in neuroblastoma); or (**C**) chromosomal translocations that either (1) lead to the juxtaposition of a strong promoter, causing increased protein expression (myelocytomatosis viral oncogene homologue in Burkitt lymphoma), or (2) produce a novel fusion protein that is derived from gene fragments normally present on different chromosomes (BCR-ABL in chronic myeloid leukemia). (From Haber, D. A. [2004]. Molecular genetics of cancer. In D. C. Dale, & D. D. Federman, [Eds.]. *ACP medicine*. New York: WebMD.)

contribute to the malignant phenotype. Some are just random events and are referred to as *passenger mutations*; they are just along for the ride. After a critical number of driver mutations have occurred, the cell becomes cancerous. The cancer cell has a selective advantage over its neighbours in that its progeny can accumulate faster than its nonmutant neighbours. This selective advantage is referred to as **clonal proliferation** or **clonal expansion** (Figure 10.7). As a clone with mutations proliferates, it may become an early-stage tumour, for example, a carcinoma in situ or a benign colonic polyp. The increasingly rapid cell division and impaired DNA repair mechanisms of cancer cells result in a continuing accumulation of mutations throughout the progression to the most aggressive metastatic lesion. Thus, **transformation**, the process by which a normal cell becomes a cancer cell, is directed by progressive accumulation of genetic changes that alter the basic nature of the cell and drive it to malignancy. The process of tumour development is a form of Darwinian evolution because cells with a heritable change that confers a survival advantage out-compete their neighbours. Each cancer cell may develop its own set of mutations, resulting in a genomically heterogeneous mixture of cells with subsets that have accumulated more and more mutations that then increase the cell's malignant potential.[5] Many cancer cells that do not accumulate a critical set of mutations lose the competition and die during this process.

The processes occurring during the development of cancer are, in many ways, analogous to wound healing. The initial proliferation of cancer cells and enlargement of the tumour elicit the synthesis of proinflammatory mediators by the cancer cells and adjacent nonmalignant cells. As with wound healing, mediators recruit inflammatory or immune cells (primarily T lymphocytes [T cells] and macrophages, but also B lymphocytes [B cells] and neutrophils) and cells normally associated with tissue repair (fibroblasts, adipocytes, mesenchymal stem cells, endothelial cells, and pericytes). These cells form the stroma (tumour microenvironment) that surrounds and infiltrates the tumour (Figure 10.8).[6] In some conditions, stromal cells may make up 90% of the tumour mass.[7] Extensive paracrine signalling among the stromal and cancer cells affects both populations; cancer cells increase proliferation and become more heterogeneous during tumour growth, and several populations of stromal cells undergo evolution to phenotypes that promote cancer progression and metastatic potential.[8] Cancer heterogeneity arises from ongoing proliferation and mutation. Tumour-associated endothelial cells, fibroblasts, and inflammatory cells develop different and distinct gene expression profiles with unique cell surface molecules and patterns of secreted molecules. During this process there is generally a great deal of cancer cell death, but the surviving cells are more aggressive, and many take on a metastatic phenotype. Because continuing somatic mutations may be random, cancer cells in different regions of the tumour may be genetically diverse. Additionally, a population of cancer stem cells may arise as cells become more and more undifferentiated from their original tissue. Although how cancer cells become undifferentiated remains unclear, many of the hallmarks of cancer are consequences of cancer–stromal interactions (discussed later in this chapter).

Several of the hallmarks or enablers are (1) *primarily genomic alterations that initiate and maintain development of cancer*. These genomic alterations are discussed first and include sustained proliferative signalling, evading growth suppressors, genomic instability, and enabling replicative immortality (see Figure 10.5). Other hallmarks or enablers are (2) *secondary to genomic change* and include inducing angiogenesis and reprogramming energy metabolism. A third group, (3) *tumour resistance to destruction* by the host's protective mechanisms, includes resistance to apoptotic cell death, tumour-promoting inflammation,

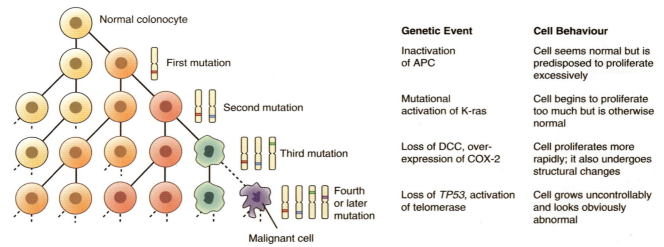

FIGURE 10.7 Clonal Proliferation Model of Neoplastic Progression in the Colon. During clonal proliferation, progressively altered populations of colon cells (colonocytes) arise over time. As genetic and epigenetic changes occur, different subclones (indicated by different colour cells) coexist for a time. Clones that grow the fastest out-compete other clones, producing even more malignant, and abnormal-appearing, growths. The sequential accumulation of mutations has been well studied in the progression from a normal colon cell to a benign intestinal polyp to a malignant colon cancer. One of the earliest mutations in colon cancer is loss of the tumour-suppressor gene *APC*. Additional mutations (often in the oncogene *RAS*), activation of COX-2, and loss of the tumour suppressors *DCC* and *TP53* occur as the lesion progresses from a benign polyp to an invasive carcinoma. *APC*, Adenomatous polyposis coli; *COX-2*, cyclo-oxygenase-2; *DCC*, deleted in colon cancer; *TP53*, tumour protein p53 gene. (Modified from Kumar, V., Cotran, R. S., & Robbins, S. L. [1997]. *Basic pathology* [6th ed.]. Saunders; and Mendelsohn, I., Howley, P., Israel, M. A., et al. [2001]. *The molecular basis of cancer* [2nd ed.]. Saunders.)

and evading immune destruction. The last hallmark is the culmination of the previous nine: activating invasion and metastasis.

Sustained Proliferative Signalling

The first and foremost hallmark of cancer is uncontrolled cellular proliferation. Normal cells generally only enter proliferative phases in response to growth factors that bind to specific receptors on the cell surface. The cytoplasmic components of the receptors are associated with signalling molecules that undergo activation and in turn, activate intracellular signalling pathways leading to induction or activation of regulatory factors affecting DNA synthesis, entrance into the cell cycle, and changes in expression of other genes related to cell metabolism for optimal growth (Figure 10.9). One example is initiation of proliferation by epidermal growth factor (EGF). EGF binds and cross-links two EGF receptors on the cell surface. The cytoplasmic portions of the receptors are tyrosine kinases that attach phosphorus to tyrosine in neighbouring proteins, including each other (autophosphorylation). Phosphorylation allows the receptor to attach to bridging protein, which links the EGF receptors to plasma membrane–associated inactive RAS. *RAS* is an acronym for "rat sarcoma," where it was found originally. Inactive RAS is associated with guanine diphosphate (GDP). Association between the EGF receptor and inactive RAS modifies the binding of GDP, which is replaced with guanosine triphosphate (GTP). GTP activates RAS, which is a GTPase that converts GTP to GDP, during which it can activate signalling pathways such as the mitogen-activated protein kinase (MAPK) pathway and the phosphatidylinositol-3-kinase (PI3K) pathway. These signalling pathways phosphorylate other cytoplasmic proteins and affect activity and nuclear localization of transcription factors, such as myelocytomatosis viral oncogene homologue (MYC), that govern the transcription of cell cycle regulators (i.e., G_1 phase of the cell cycle), such as cyclins, and entrance into cellular proliferation. Proliferation can be discontinued through this pathway by decreased levels of growth factors in the environment or inactivation of signalling pathway components. Targeting these cyclins that effectively "turn on" cell division has been a promising area for the development of monoclonal antibodies in novel research of the treatment of cancer.

The genes that encode components of receptor-mediated pathways designed to regulate normal cellular proliferation are collectively called **proto-oncogenes**. Cancerous cells characteristically express mutated or overexpressed proto-oncogenes, which are referred to as **oncogenes**. Oncogenes are also independent of normal regulatory mechanisms and undergo uncontrolled cell growth. Additionally, oncogenes can affect any portion of the growth factor pathways, such as described for EGF. For example, most growth factors originate from neighbouring cells, but some cancers acquire the ability to secrete growth factors that stimulate their own growth, a process known as **autocrine stimulation**. As described later in this chapter, noncancerous stromal cells within a tumour can also undergo slight modification in order to benefit the cancer. In some instances, stromal cells produce excessive growth factors that drive the proliferation of cancer cells. Other cancers increase the expression of growth factor receptors; for example, in breast cancer, production of the human epidermal growth factor receptor 2 (HER2, also known as the EGF receptor gene *[ERBB-2]*) is upregulated and is hyper responsive to low levels of EGF. Some breast and lung cancers are effectively treated by inhibitors of HER2 and other EGF receptors that block this pathway.[9]

Oncogenes may also lead to constant activation of the signal cascade from the cell surface receptor to the nucleus. Up to a third of all cancers have an activating mutation in the *RAS* gene resulting in a continuous cell growth signal, even when growth factors are missing (see Figure 10.9). Other mutations in the EGF receptor pathway include excessive proliferation signalling by hyperactivation of PI3K (and the increased production of transcription factors in the nucleus).

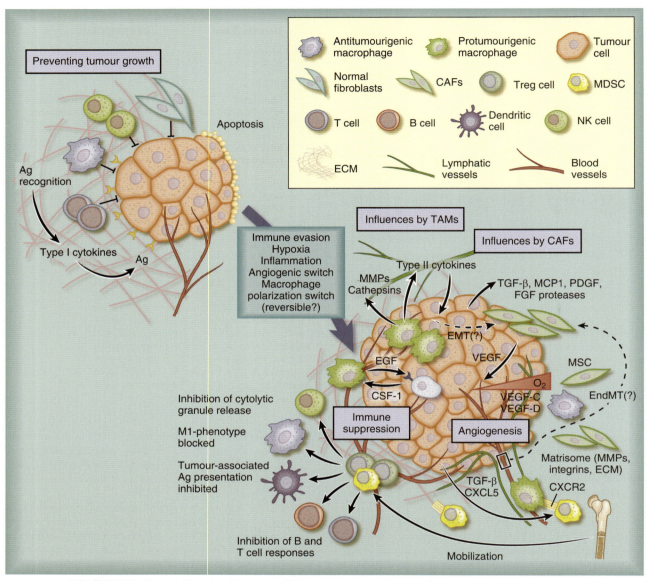

FIGURE 10.8 Cancers Live in a Complex Microenvironment. Cancer cells express tumour-specific antigens that ideally can be recognized by cells of the immune system and inflammatory systems (natural killer cells [*NK cells*], antitumourigenic M1 macrophages, T-cytotoxic cells) and destroyed by apoptosis or undergo growth suppression by type I cytokines. However, successful cancers produce a variety of cytokines and chemokines that are chemoattractants for stromal cells that infiltrate the tumour and undergo change to protumourigenic phenotypes. The affected cells include tumour-associated M2 macrophages, cancer-associated fibroblasts *(CAFs)*, mesenchymal stem cells *(MSCs)*, and immune suppressor cells of T-cell origin (T-regulatory cells *[Treg cells]*) and myeloid origin (myeloid-derived suppressor cells *[MDSC]*). Through multiple receptor-mediated interactions between other stromal cells and the cancer cells, the stromal cells, as well as the cancer cells, collectively produce a battery of additional cytokines (e.g., TGF-β, type II cytokines), chemokines (e.g., CXCL5), growth factors (e.g., VEGF, EGF, CSF-1, FGF, PDGF), and proteases (e.g., MMPs) and secrete components of the extracellular matrix *[ECM]*. The stromal reaction promotes tumour progression, including new blood vessel growth (angiogenesis), tumour cell proliferation and differentiation, suppression of immune rejection and tumour cell apoptosis, invasion, and commitment to metastasis. *Ag*, Antigen; *CSF-1*, colony-stimulating factor-1; *CXCL5*, C-X-C motif chemokine 5; *CXCR2*, C-X-C chemokine receptor type 2; *EGF*, epidermal growth factor; *EMT*, epithelial-mesenchymal transition; *FGF*, fibroblast growth factor; *MCP-1*, macrophage chemotactic protein-1; *MMPs*, matrix metalloproteinases; O_2, oxygen; *PDGF*, platelet-derived growth factor; *TAM*, tumour-associated macrophage; *TGFβ*, transforming growth factor-beta; *VEGF*, vascular endothelial growth factor. (Modified from Quail, D. F., & Joyce, J. A. [2013]. Microenvironmental regulation of tumor progression and metastasis. *Nature Medicine 19*[11], 1423–1437. https://doi.org/10.1038/nm.3394.)

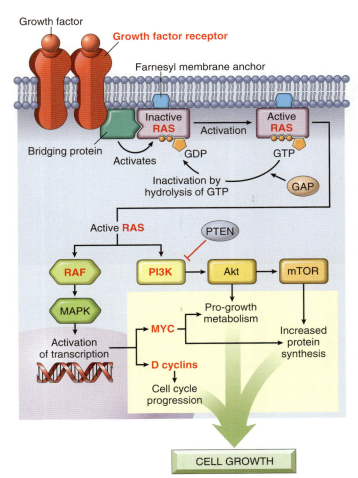

FIGURE 10.9 **Growth Factor Signalling Pathways in Cancer.** Growth factor receptors, RAS, PI3K, MYC, and D cyclins are oncoproteins that are activated by mutations in various cancers. GAPs apply brakes to *RAS* activation, and PTEN serves the same function for *PI3K*. *Akt,* Protein kinase B; *GAP,* GTPase-activating protein; *GDP,* guanosine diphosphate; *GTP,* guanosine triphosphate; *MAPK,* mitogen-activated protein kinase; *mTOR,* mammalian target of rapamycin; *MYC,* myelocytomatosis viral oncogene homologue; *PI3K,* phosphoinositidyl-3-kinase; *PTEN,* phosphatase and tensin homologue; *RAF,* rapidly accelerated fibrosarcoma. (From Kumar, V., Abbas, A. K., & Aster, J. C. [Eds.]. [2021]. *Robbins and Cotran pathologic basis of disease* [10th ed.]. Elsevier.)

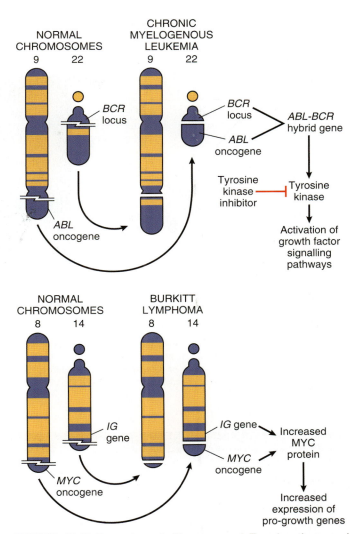

FIGURE 10.10 Examples of Chromosomal Translocations and Associated Oncogenes. See text for further explanation. *ABL,* Abelson gene; *BCR,* breakpoint cluster region gene; *IG,* immunoglobulin gene; *MYC,* myelocytomatosis viral oncogene homologue. (From Kumar, V., Abbas, A. K., & Aster, J. C. [Eds.]. [2021]. *Robbins and Cotran pathologic basis of disease* [10th ed.]. Elsevier.)

In turn, several types of genetic events can activate oncogenes. A point mutation that is frequently observed in lung cancer results in continuous activation of the EGF receptor tyrosine kinase. A point mutation in the *RAS* gene converts it from a regulated proto-oncogene to an unregulated oncogene. Activating point mutations in *RAS* are present in many cancers, especially pancreatic and colorectal cancer. Specialized tests, such as direct DNA sequencing, can detect such point mutations in clinical samples.

Similarly, translocations can activate oncogenes in one of two distinct mechanisms (Figure 10.10). First, a translocation can cause excess and inappropriate production of a proliferation factor. One of the best examples is the t(8;14) translocation found in many Burkitt lymphomas; t(8;14) designates a chromosome that has a piece of chromosome 8 fused to a piece of chromosome 14 (see Chapter 21).[10] Burkitt lymphoma is an aggressive cancer of B lymphocytes. The *MYC* proto-oncogene found on chromosome 8 is normally activated at low levels in proliferating lymphocytes and is inactivated in mature lymphocytes.

If the t(8;14) translocation occurs, the *MYC* gene is aberrantly placed under the control of a B-cell immunoglobulin gene *(IG)* present on chromosome 14. The *IG* gene is very active in maturing B cells. The t(8;14) translocation alters the control of *MYC*; its normal low-level expression is switched to high levels, as directed by an *IG* gene promoter. Hyperproduction of MYC protein drives proliferation and blocks differentiation.

Second, chromosome translocations can lead to the production of novel proteins with growth-promoting properties. In chronic myeloid (or *myelogenous*) leukemia (CML) a specific chromosome translocation is almost always present (see Figure 10.10). This translocation, t(9;22), was first identified in association with CML in Philadelphia in 1960 and is often referred to as the *Philadelphia chromosome*.[11] Translocation fuses two chromosomes in the middle of two different genes: *BCR* (breakpoint cluster region gene) on chromosome 9 and *ABL* (Abelson gene) on chromosome 22. The result is production of a *BCR-ABL* fusion protein containing the first half of BCR and the second

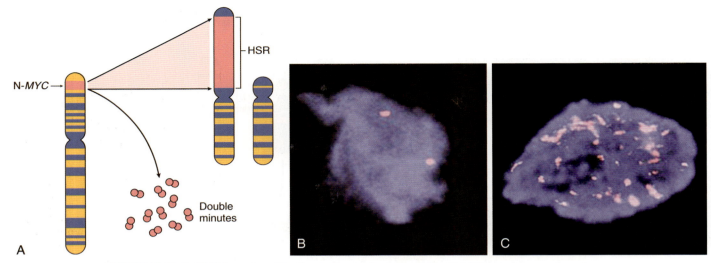

FIGURE 10.11 N-*MYC* Gene Amplification in Neuroblastoma. **A,** The N-*MYC* gene is present on chromosome 2, becomes amplified, and is seen either as extra chromosomal double minutes or as a chromosomal homologous staining region *(HSR)*. The N-*MYC* gene is detected in human neuroblastoma cells using a technique called FISH (fluorescent in situ hybridization). **B,** A single pair of N-*MYC* genes is detected in normal cells and in low-grade neuroblastoma. **C,** Multiple, amplified copies of the N-*MYC* gene are detected in some cases of neuroblastoma. Amplification of the N-*MYC* gene is strongly associated with a poor prognosis in childhood neuroblastoma. (**A,** from Kumar, V., Abbas, A. K., & Aster, J. C. [Eds.]. [2015]. *Robbins and Cotran pathologic basis of disease* [9th ed.]. Saunders. **B, C,** Courtesy Arthur R. Brothman, PhD, FACMG, University of Utah School of Medicine, Salt Lake City, Utah.)

TABLE 10.1 Comparison of Cancer Gene Types

Gene Type	Normal Function	Mutation Effect
Caretaker genes	Maintain DNA and chromosome stability	Chromosome instability leads to increased rates of mutation
Dominant oncogenes[a]	Encode proteins that promote growth (e.g., growth factors)	Overexpression or amplification causes gain of function
Tumour suppressors (recessive oncogenes)	Encode proteins that inhibit proliferation and prevent or repair mutations	Loss of function of both alleles increases cancer risk

[a]Nonmutant state referred to as proto-oncogene.

half of ABL (a nonreceptor tyrosine kinase). BCR-ABL is an unregulated protein tyrosine kinase that promotes growth of myeloid cells. *Imatinib* (Gleevec), a medication that specifically targets this tyrosine kinase, represents the first successful chemotherapy targeted against the product of a specific oncogenic mutation. Imatinib and related tyrosine kinase inhibitors (TKIs) are highly effective in the treatment of CML and, because of their specificity, lack the toxic adverse effects noted with nonspecific anticancer medications. However, imatinib is not effective in cancers that do not have the t(9;22) translocation or related mutations. In modern personalized cancer therapy, knowledge of the specific genetic alteration can dictate the optimal medications for the individual.

Oncogenes may also be activated by gene amplification (Figure 10.11). Gene amplification results in increased expression of an oncogene, or in some cases medication-resistance genes. The N-*MYC* oncogene, a member of the *MYC* family, is amplified in 25% of childhood neuroblastoma and confers a poor prognosis. The HER2 gene *(ERBB2)* is amplified in 20% of breast cancers.

Evading Growth Suppressors

Uncontrolled cancer cell proliferation is also related to inactivation of tumour-suppressor genes. **Tumour-suppressor genes** normally regulate the cell cycle, inhibit proliferation resulting from growth signals, stop cell division when cells are damaged, and prevent mutations. Hence, they also have been referred to as *antioncogenes*. Whereas oncogenes are *activated* in cancers, tumour suppressors must be *inactivated* to allow cancer to occur (Table 10.1 and Figure 10.12). Furthermore, a single genetic event can activate an oncogene because it can act in a dominant manner in the cell, but both copies of a tumour suppressor gene (i.e., one from each parent) must undergo mutations (i.e., become inactivated) in order for cancer to occur.

Because inactivation of tumour-suppressor genes requires at least two mutations (one in each allele), a single **germ cell mutation** (sperm or egg) results in the transmission of cancer-causing genes from one generation to the next, producing families with a high risk for specific cancers. These inherited mutations that predispose to cancer are almost invariably in tumour-suppressor genes because it only takes a

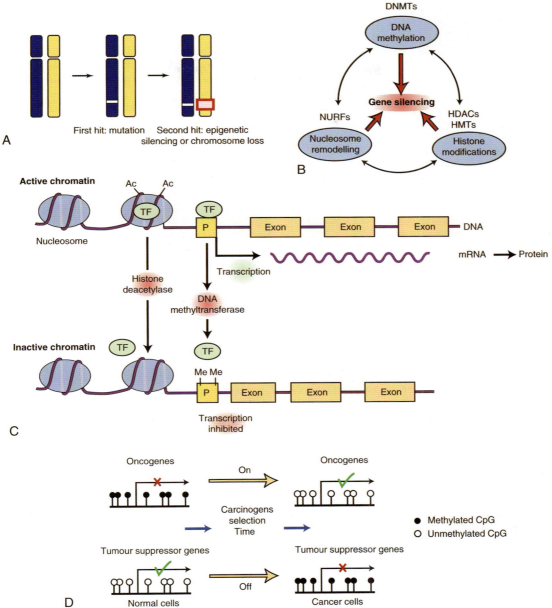

FIGURE 10.12 Silencing Tumour-Suppressor Genes. A variety of mechanisms can deactivate tumour-suppressor genes. **A,** In this example, the first instance is a point mutation in a tumour-suppressor gene *(white box)*, followed by either epigenetic silencing or chromosome loss of the second allele *(red box)*. **B,** Genes can normally be silenced by a variety of interacting processes, including DNA methylation, histone modification, nucleosomal remodelling, and microRNA changes (not shown). A number of cellular enzymes contribute to these modifications, including DNA methyltransferases *(DNMTs)*, histone deacetylases *(HDACs)*, histone methyltransferases *(HMTs)*, and complex nucleosomal remodelling factors *(NURFs)*. Gene silencing is essential for normal development and differentiation. **C,** Histone modification and promoter methylation *(Me)* regulate gene expression (exons code for resultant messenger *[mRNA]* after the introns are spliced out). Genes are transcribed when chromatin is modified by addition of acetyl *(Ac)* groups to specific lysine groups in histones. Gene expression can be turned off when specific acetyl groups are removed (by HDACs) or when the CpG-rich promoter regions of genes are modified by direct DNA methylation (by DNA methyltransferase). In addition, small endogenous RNA molecules (microRNAs) can bind to mRNA and reduce gene expression. **D,** Changes in promoter methylation turn cancer genes off and on. Oncogenes can be turned on by promoter hypomethylation, and tumour-suppressor genes can be turned off by promoter hypermethylation. Each of these changes can produce selective growth and survival advantages for the cancer cell. *P,* Promoter region; *TF,* transcription factor. (**B,** Reprinted from Jones, P. A., & Baylin, S. B. [2007]. The epigenomics of cancer. *Cell, 128*[4], 683–692, with permission from Elsevier. **C,** From Gluckman, P. D., Hanson, M. A., Cooper, C., et al. [2008]. Effect of in utero and early-life conditions on adult health and disease. *The New England Journal of Medicine, 359*[1], 61–73, reprinted with permission from Massachusetts Medical Society. **D,** from Shames, D. S., Minna, J. D., & Gazdar, A. F. [2007]. DNA methylation in health, disease, and cancer. *Current Molecular Medicine, 7*[1], 85–102.)

TABLE 10.2 Some Familial Cancer Syndromes Caused by Tumour-Suppressor Gene Function Loss

Syndrome	Gene
Retinoblastoma	RB1
Li-Fraumeni syndrome	p53 (TP53)
Familial melanoma	p16$^{INK\alpha}$ (CDKN2A)
Neurofibromatosis	Neurofibromin (NF1)
Familial adenomatous polyps	APC
Breast cancer	BRCA1

single additional mutation in any other cell (somatic cell mutation) to completely inactivate the tumour-suppressor gene (Table 10.2).[12]

The retinoblastoma (RB) gene is a prototypical tumour-suppressor gene. Normal cells receive diverse "antigrowth" signals from their normal environment. Similarly, contact with other cells, with basement membranes, and with some soluble factors normally signal cells to stop proliferating. Tumour-suppressor genes, such as RB, monitor antigrowth cellular signals and block activation of the growth and division phase in the cell cycle. RB essentially puts the brakes on cell division and is a key regulator of cellular metabolism. Mutations in RB lead to persistent cell growth.

The antiproliferative activity of RB depends on the degree of protein phosphorylation.[13] Phosphorylation of the RB protein inactivates the RB gene and allows cells to enter the cell cycle with increased production of transcription factors and corresponding production of DNA. Likewise, low levels of phosphorylation (or hypophosphorylation) have the opposite effect and inhibit cell growth because of the increased binding of RB to transcription factors and resultant inhibition of the cell cycle. Fewer cells pass through the cell cycle as a result. Growth factor–regulated kinases increase phosphorylation (hyperphosphorylation) and consequent inactivation of RB. A variety of genetic mutations in cancers also inactivate RB, resulting in unregulated and continuous cellular proliferation. For example, RB mutations exist in childhood retinoblastoma, and in many lung, breast, and bone cancers. The RB gene resides on chromosome 13, in a particular region referred to as q14 (13q14). Most individuals with RB mutations have a subtle mutation, such as a point mutation, in one allele (i.e., from one parent). The RB gene in the other chromosome may be inactivated through loss of the 13q14 region or epigenetic mechanisms (DNA methylation, histone modification, or microRNA, which modulates the efficiency of mRNA translation). The familial form of retinoblastoma is an example of how an increased risk for cancer can be inherited. A mutation in one RB allele is inherited, and only one additional mutation in the normal allele will lead to cancer (see Table 10.2). Approximately half of children with retinoblastoma have the inheritable form, and most will develop tumours in both eyes (bilateral retinoblastoma).

Another classic tumour-suppressor gene is tumour protein p53 (TP53). The protein, p53, has been called the *guardian of the genome*. TP53 monitors intracellular signals related to stress and activates caretaker genes—genes that are responsible for the maintenance of genomic integrity (Figure 10.13). Many types of cellular stress (e.g., anoxia, oncogene expression, nuclear damage) produce intracellular signals (e.g., levels of nucleotides and glucose, degree of oxygenation, DNA damage, and other indicators of cellular abnormalities) detectable by p53. Normally p53 is in an inactive complex with inhibitor molecules. Stress activates kinases that phosphorylate p53 into an active suppressor of cell division and activator of caretaker genes. Caretaker genes encode proteins that repair damaged DNA, such as occurs with errors in DNA replication, mutations caused by ultraviolet or ionizing radiation, and mutations caused by chemicals and medications. The p53 protein also controls initiation of cellular senescence or apoptosis and suppresses cell division until DNA repair or the correction of other effects of stress is complete. If the DNA damage is too great for sufficient repair and the effects of stress have taken their toll on the cell, the cell enters senescence or apoptosis, thus preventing further DNA damage and mutations. Loss of function of TP53 or caretaker genes leads to increased mutation rates and cancer.[14] Li-Fraumeni syndrome is a very rare inheritable loss-of-function mutation in TP53 in one allele resulting in a 25-fold increase of developing malignancy at early age (less than 50 years of age). These malignancies may include breast cancer, brain tumours, acute leukemia, soft tissue sarcomas, bone sarcoma, and adrenal cortical carcinoma.

Other familial cancers with inheritable mutations in tumour-suppressor genes include Wilms tumour, a childhood cancer of the kidney (WT1 gene); neurofibromatosis (NF1 gene); and familial polyposis coli or adenomas of the colon (APC gene). Characterization of cancer-causing genes and other genetic factors helps identify individuals prone to developing cancer and contributes to further understanding of sporadic cancers. Individuals known to carry mutations in tumour-suppressor genes are candidates for targeted cancer screening to facilitate early cancer detection and therapy.

Genomic Instability

> ✓ **QUICK CHECK 10.3**
> 1. What are the heritable changes in cells that contribute to cancer development?
> 2. Define *oncogene*, *proto-oncogene*, and *tumour-suppressor gene*.
> 3. Biologically, why do tumour-suppressor genes have to be inactivated to cause cancer?
> 4. Define *epigenetics* and *epigenetic silencing*.
> 5. Distinguish between mutations in somatic cells versus in germ cells.
> 6. Define *telomeres*, *telomerase*, and *senescence*, and describe their effects on cancer.

Genomic instability refers to an increased tendency of alterations—mutability—in the genome during the life cycle of cells. Inherited and acquired mutations in caretaker genes that protect the integrity of the genome and DNA repair increase the level of genomic instability and risk for developing cancer. In other words, these mutations cause stable cells to become more labile. Acquired mutations in "guardians of the genome," such as TP53, that detect DNA damage and activate repair mechanisms result in an increasing accumulation of mutations in the overall DNA as a whole. For example, xeroderma pigmentosum is a defect in the repair of DNA pyrimidine dimers created by ultraviolet (UV) light that increases the risk for skin cancers. Hereditary nonpolyposis colorectal cancer results from an inherited defect in repairing DNA base pair mismatches that occur occasionally during DNA replication. Affected individuals have an increased rate of small insertions and deletions in DNA (and more labile cells), leading to a high rate of colon and other cancers. Some inherited mutations threaten the integrity of entire chromosomes. Bloom's syndrome, caused by mutations in a DNA helicase, presents with an increased risk of several forms of cancer, and those with Fanconi aplastic anemia, caused by loss of function for repairing DNA double-strand breaks, have a particularly increased risk of acute myelogenous leukemia. These examples are autosomal recessive

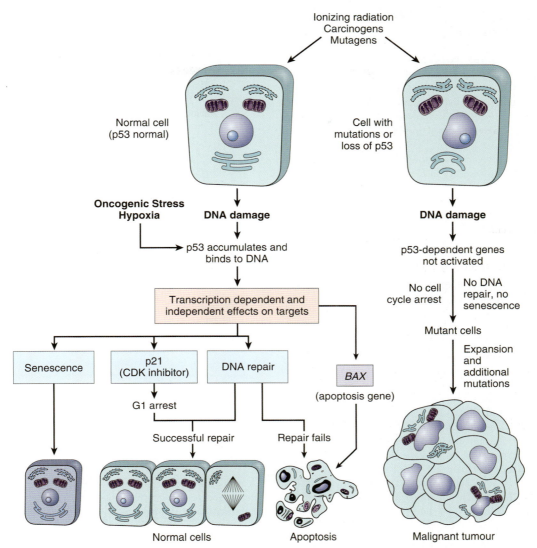

FIGURE 10.13 The Role of p53 in Maintaining the Integrity of the Genome. Activation of normal p53 by DNA-damaging agents or by hypoxia leads to cell cycle arrest in G_1 by upregulation of the cell cycle inhibitor p21 and induction of DNA repair transcriptional upregulation of the cyclin-dependent kinase inhibitor *CDKN1A* (encoding the cyclin-dependent kinase inhibitor p21) and the *GADD45* genes. Successful repair of DNA allows cells to proceed with the cell cycle. If DNA repair fails, p53 triggers either apoptosis or senescence. In cells with loss or mutation of the *p53* gene, DNA damage does not induce cell cycle arrest or DNA repair, and genetically damaged cells proliferate, giving rise eventually to malignant neoplasms. *BAX*, Bcl-2–associated X protein gene; *CDK*, cyclin-dependent kinase. (From Kumar, V., Abbas, A. K., & Aster, J. C. [Eds.]. [2021]. *Robbins and Cotran pathologic basis of disease* [10th ed.]. Elsevier.)

disorders in which affected individuals demonstrate marked chromosomal instability.

Genomic instability may also result from increased **epigenetic silencing** or modulation of gene function (Chapter 3). Many cancers have increased methylation of DNA in the promoter region of tumour-suppressor genes. They also have associated changes in the modification of histones in the chromatin, often correlated with methylation of DNA. These changes alter the promoter regions of genes, leading to their **silencing** or altered gene expression.

Changes in gene regulation can affect not just single genes but also entire intracellular signalling networks. Changes in **microRNAs** (**miRNAs**, or *miRs*) and other ncRNAs can regulate gene expression networks.[15] miRNAs regulate diverse signalling pathways, and the miRNAs that stimulate cancer development and progression are termed **oncomirs**.[16] miRNAs decrease the stability and expression of other genes by pairing with mRNA and decreasing the efficiency of translation.

Mutations in *BRCA1* and *BRCA2* (breast cancer 1 and 2, early-onset genes) are currently of clinical importance because of how common they are in the general population. Both are tumour suppressor genes and caretaker genes that repair double-stranded DNA breaks. Inherited mutations in either gene greatly increase the risk for a variety of tumours, especially breast cancer in both women and men, and ovarian or prostate cancers. Approximately 11% of women generally will develop breast cancer within their lifetime, whereas about 47 to 66% of women with a high-risk *BRCA1* mutation and 40 to 57% with a *BRCA2* mutation will develop breast cancer by age 70.[17] Ovarian cancer occurs in approximately 1.2% of the general population, but about 35 to 46% of women with an inherited mutation in *BRCA1* and about 13 to 23% with a mutation in *BRCA2* will develop ovarian cancer by age 70. At-risk women are currently offered prophylactic surgery to reduce the risk of cancer.

In addition to specific gene mutations and abnormal epigenetic silencing, chromosome instability also appears to be increased in malignant cells, resulting in a high rate of chromosome loss, as well as loss of heterozygosity and chromosome amplification. The underlying mechanism of this instability is not clear but there may be malfunctions in the cellular machinery that regulates chromosome segregation at mitosis.

Enabling Replicative Immortality

A hallmark of cancer cells is their immortality, in that they seem to have an unlimited lifespan and will continue to divide for years under appropriate laboratory conditions. One such example is HeLa cells, which came from a cervical cancer specimen obtained in 1951 that continues to grow and divide in laboratories around the world today.[18] Most normal cells are not immortal and can divide only a limited number of times (known as the *Hayflick limit*) before they either enter senescence (cease dividing) or enter crisis (apoptosis) and die. One major block to unlimited cell division (i.e., immortality) is the size of a specialized structure called the *telomere*. Telomeres are protective ends, or caps, of repeating hexanucleotides (six nucleotide units) on each chromosome and are placed and maintained by a specialized enzyme called telomerase (Figure 10.14).[19] As one might expect, telomerase is usually active only in germ cells (in ovaries and testes) and in stem cells. All other cells of the body lack telomerase activity. Therefore, when nongerm cells begin to proliferate abnormally, their telomere caps shorten with each cell division. Short telomeres normally signal the cell to cease cell division. If the telomeres become critically small, the chromosomes become unstable and fragment, and the cells die.

Cancer cells are very heterogeneous, and many cells die as the cancer develops. When they reach a critical age, most cancer cells activate telomerase to restore and maintain their telomeres, thereby allowing continuous division.[20] The trigger for re-expression of telomerase activity seems to require expression of specific oncogenes, such as *RAS* or *MYC*, and loss of function of certain tumour-suppressor genes, such as *p53* and *RB*. Restoration of telomerase activity occurs in about 90% of cancers. The remaining cancers appear to recruit or originate from stem cells, becoming cancer stem cells that maintain levels of telomerase activity characteristically found in somatic stem cells.[21] Because telomerase is specifically activated in cancer cells, and potentially in cancer stem cells, it is an attractive therapeutic target.

Inducing Angiogenesis

> ✓ **QUICK CHECK 10.4**
> 1. Why is the stroma important for cancer growth and invasion?
> 2. Identify cancers that are the result of chronic inflammation.
> 3. Why does inflammation fuel cancer development or invasion?
> 4. Identify common viruses that can cause cancer.
> 5. How do cancers protect themselves from cell death?
> 6. Why is angiogenesis important to cancer development?

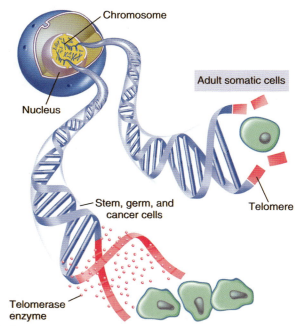

FIGURE 10.14 Control of Immortality: Telomeres and Telomerase. Normal adult somatic cells cannot divide indefinitely because telomeres cap the ends of their chromosomes. In the absence of the telomerase enzyme, telomeres become progressively shorter with each division until, when they are critically short, they signal to the cell to stop dividing. In germ cells, adult stem cells, and cancer cells, the telomerase gene is "switched on," producing an enzyme that rebuilds the telomeres. Thus, like germ cells, the cancer cell becomes immortal and able to divide indefinitely without losing its telomeres.

A major component of wound healing is the process of establishing new blood vessels within the tissue undergoing repair (called neovascularization or angiogenesis). Access to a blood supply is also obligatory to the growth and spread of cancer. Without a blood supply to deliver oxygen and nutrients, growth of a tumour is limited to about a millimetre in diameter.

Angiogenic factors and angiogenic inhibitors normally control development of new vessels. In cancerous tumours, several mechanisms increase and maintain secretion of angiogenic factors by the cancer cells, as well as prevent release of angiogenic inhibitors. Hypoxia-inducible factor-1 alpha (HIF-1α), an oxygen-sensitive transcription factor, is a major regulator of angiogenesis in normal tissue. HIF-1α is stabilized under hypoxic conditions and induces expression of proangiogenic factors, such as vascular endothelial growth factor (VEGF) and basic fibroblast growth factor (bFGF). Inactivation of tumour-suppressor genes (e.g., *p53*) or increased expression of oncogenes (e.g., *HER2*) leads to increased expression of HIF-1α–regulated angiogenic factors and increased vascularization. Increased expression of HIF-1α also is related to increased resistance to chemotherapy, increased tumour cell glycolysis, increased metastasis, and a poor prognosis. These effects may likely occur through an autocrine mechanism by which VEGF activates tumour-associated VEGF receptors. For example, in soft tissue sarcomas, VEGF induces increased expression of anti-apoptotic proteins (e.g., B-cell lymphoma 2 [Bcl-2]) and activation of intracellular survival signal pathways. Therefore, the use of angiogenic inhibitors targeting VEGF signalling can actually inhibit angiogenesis and diminish tumour growth.

Other routes of angiogenic factor *induction* include mutations in cancer oncogenes (e.g., *RAS*, *MYC*) that increase transcription of

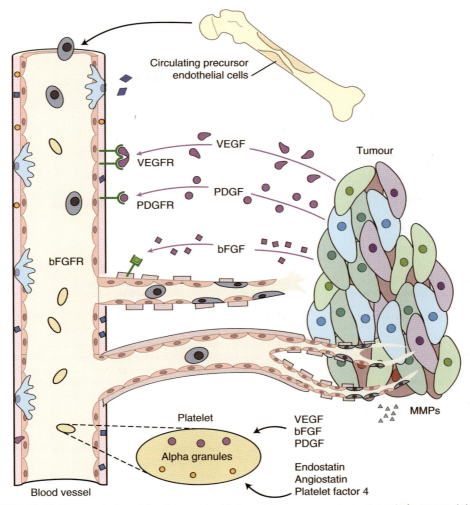

FIGURE 10.15 Tumour-Induced Angiogenesis. Malignant tumours secrete angiogenic factors and tissue-remodelling matrix metalloproteinases *(MMPs)* that actively induce formation of new blood vessels. New blood vessels are formed from both local endothelial cells and circulating precursor cells recruited from the bone marrow. Circulating platelets can also release regulatory proteins into the tumour. *bFGF* and *bFGFR*, Basic fibroblast growth factor and its receptor, respectively; *PDGF* and *PDGFR*, platelet-derived growth factor and its receptor, respectively; *VEGF* and *VEGFR*, vascular endothelial growth factor and its receptor, respectively. (Reprinted with permission from Macmillan Publishers Ltd: Folkman, J. [2007]. Angiogenesis: an organizing principle for drug discovery? *Nature Reviews Drug Discovery* 6[4], 273–286.)

VEGF by cancer cells. Moreover, most cells in the tumour microenvironment also secrete VEGF, including tumour-infiltrating monocytes, endothelial cells, adipocytes, and cancer-associated fibroblasts.

Angiogenesis inhibitors, such as thrombospondin-1 (TSP-1), normally bind to cellular surface receptors on inflammatory cells and negatively regulate angiogenesis in wound healing and tissue remodelling. The expression of angiogenesis inhibitors is under the control of *p53*, which is suppressed in cancer cells, thus diminishing the controls by stromal cells on inflammatory cell secretion of angiogenic factors.

Cancer cells and stromal cells may also increase production of matrix metalloproteinases (MMPs; e.g., MMP-9) (Figure 10.15). MMPs are zinc-dependent proteases that digest the surrounding extracellular matrix (ECM). The ECM contains stored latent (inactive) forms of some angiogenic factors (e.g., bFGF, transforming growth factor-beta [TGF-β]), and MMPs activate the stored forms into functional angiogenic factors.

The vessels formed within tumours differ from those in healthy tissue. They originate from endothelial tissue sprouting and irregular branching from existing capillaries, rather than regular branching seen in healthy tissue. The cell contact between each endothelial cell is less tight resulting in vessels that are more porous and prone to hemorrhage, and allow passage of tumour cells into the vascular system.

Reprogramming Energy Metabolism

Cancer cells live in a distinct environment from normal cells and have different nutritional requirements from nonproliferating cells. The successful cancer cell divides rapidly, with the consequent requirement for the building blocks to construct new cells. Nonmalignant cells in the presence of adequate oxygen normally generate adenosine triphosphate (ATP) by mitochondrial oxidative phosphorylation (OXPHOS), generating 36 ATP molecules from each glucose molecule that is broken down to water and carbon dioxide. In the absence of sufficient oxygen (hypoxia), normal cells perform glycolysis (anaerobic glycolysis),

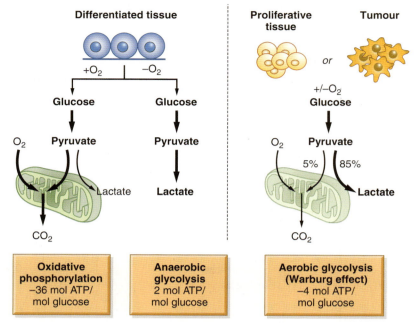

FIGURE 10.16 Cancers Have Altered Metabolism. Normal tissues use oxidative phosphorylation (OXPHOS) to turn glucose into carbon dioxide (CO_2) and energy (in the form of adenosine triphosphate [ATP]). Cancers take a different approach; even in the presence of oxygen (O_2), they do not use OXPHOS. Instead, they consume large quantities of glucose to make cellular building blocks, supporting rapid proliferation. (From Vander Heiden, M. G., Cantley, L. C., & Thompson, C. B. [2009]. Understanding the Warburg effect: the metabolic requirements of cell proliferation. *Science, 324*, 1029–1033.)

generating only two ATP molecules per molecule of glucose, with lactic acid and pyruvate as by products.

Interestingly, even in the presence of adequate oxygen, cancer cells may not use OXPHOS, but are reprogrammed to glycolysis (**Warburg effect**) (Figure 10.16). Thus, the Warburg effect is the use of glycolysis under normal oxygen conditions, hence the name **aerobic glycolysis**. Aerobic glycolysis is a highly regulated and beneficial adaptation for cancer cells rather than a result of cancer-specific mitochondrial dysfunction (as originally thought).[22] This is because the shift from OXPHOS to glycolysis allows lactate and other products of glycolysis to be used for more efficient production of lipids, nucleosides, amino acids, and other molecular building blocks needed for rapid cell growth.

A new model, the **reverse Warburg effect**, may play a role in certain cancers. Cancer cells may continue using the OXPHOS to generate large amounts of ATP. However, they also may manipulate the cancer-associated fibroblasts (CAFs), perhaps by inducing oxidative stress, to undergo aerobic glycolysis and secrete metabolites (e.g., lactate, pyruvate) that the cancer cells can use in the citric acid cycle (Krebs cycle) to feed OXPHOS and produce ATP.[23] Induction of autophagy in the CAFs is a secondary consequence and results both in consumption of the CAFs and the release of materials needed by the cancer cell in the synthesis of new organelles.

Promoters of aerobic glycolysis are activated by oncogenes and mutated tumour-suppressor molecules. Upregulation of glucose transporter 1 (GLUT1) under the control of oncogenes (e.g., *RAS*, *MYC*) and mutant tumour suppressors (e.g., *TP53*) increases transport of glucose into the cytoplasm. These and other oncogenes or mutant tumour-suppressor genes inhibit OXPHOS and promote the aerobic glycolytic pathway and related metabolic pathways that support the rapid growth of cancers.[24]

Clinically, the high glucose utilization of a cancer can be exploited for its detection.[25] For instance, ^{18}F-fluorodeoxyglucose (FDG) is incorporated into cells in the same way as glucose, with two key differences: (1) it cannot be broken down by glycolysis because it is missing a key hydroxyl group. FDG accumulates in cells as a result; (2) ^{18}F-FDG can be imaged by a positron emission tomography (PET) scan because it is tagged with [18]F. This means small metastatic tumour masses that are consuming huge amounts of glucose can readily be detected using this imaging method (Figure 10.17).

Resisting Apoptotic Cell Death

Programmed cell death (**apoptosis**) is a mechanism by which individual cells can self-destruct under conditions of tissue remodelling or as a protection against aberrant cell growth that may lead to malignancy. Two pathways may trigger apoptosis (Figure 10.18): (1) the intrinsic pathway (mitochondrial pathway) monitors cellular stress. Cellular stress may include DNA damage, genomic instability, aberrant proliferation, loss of adhesion to ECM or to adjacent cells, and other causes and characteristics of abnormal cellular physiology; (2) the extrinsic pathway is activated through a plasma membrane receptor complex linked to intracellular activators of apoptosis (known as the *death receptor*) (see Chapter 4).

The Bcl-2 family of genes regulates apoptosis and encodes for proteins that function in the mitochondrial membrane to either stimulate (e.g., Bcl-2–associated X protein [BAX] and Bcl-2–homologous antagonist/killer [BAK]) or inhibit (Bcl-2 protein) apoptosis. Both groups regulate mitochondrial release of proapoptotic molecules (e.g., cytochrome c). The expression of the BAX gene is also regulated by the *TP53* gene and is involved in P53-mediated apoptosis. Intracellular stress (i.e., DNA damage) affects the expression of the *TP53* gene, and if DNA damage is irreparable, phosphorylation of TP53 induces transcription of proapoptotic factors and BAX/BAK proteins.

The extrinsic pathway is relatively dormant until the death receptor is activated. The principal apoptotic receptor is **Fas/CD95** (the

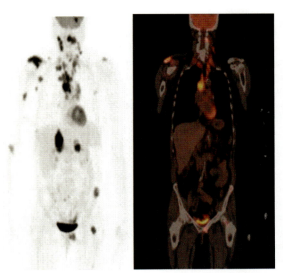

FIGURE 10.17 The Intense Glucose Requirement of Cancer Aids in Diagnosis. This 54-year-old woman had a non–small cell lung carcinoma (NSCLC) surgically removed. Five years later, these images were obtained. The positron emission tomography (PET) scan using ^{18}F-deoxyglucose shows metastatic lesions in the brain, right shoulder, and mediastinal and cervical lymph nodes as well as the liver, left pelvis, and proximal femur. *Left,* PET whole-body image; *right,* representative coronal image from the whole-body FDG-PET/CT–fused image of the same patient. The fused image consists of the computed tomography [CT] image with the metabolic information superimposed in colour. The pattern of distribution is most likely from the primary tumour to the large mediastinal lymph nodes, followed by lymphatic spread to cervical lymph nodes. Bloodborne dissemination produced the bone, brain, and liver metastases. Normally, only the heart, brain, and bladder show a strong signal on PET scan. *FDG,* Fluorodeoxyglucose. (Images courtesy John Hoffman, MD, Huntsman Cancer Institute, Salt Lake City, Utah.)

CD95 nomenclature is an alternative for Fas) (see Figure 10.18). Fas is a receptor for Fas ligand (FasL) and similar molecules, such as tumour necrosis factor (TNF). T-cytotoxic lymphocytes (Tc cells) and natural killer (NK) cells express surface and soluble FasL and can produce TNF, thus inducing apoptosis in target cells. The Fas receptor is linked to a complex of intracellular proteins (the Fas-associated death domain [FADD] signalling complex) that triggers apoptosis.

Both pathways activate a series of intracellular effector enzymatic molecules (caspases) that either directly cut DNA and other substrates or activate other enzymes that do. Regardless, cell death is the outcome.

Apoptotic pathways are dysregulated in most cancers. Most commonly, loss-of-function mutations to the *TP53* gene suppress activation of apoptosis during DNA damage. The balance between pro- and antiapoptotic molecules can also be affected by overexpression of antiapoptotic molecules or diminished expression of antiapoptotic molecules resulting from mutations. For example, overexpression of Bcl-2 occurs in the vast majority of follicular B-cell lymphomas. Excess expression of other antiapoptotic members of the Bcl-2 family also may provide increased resistance to chemotherapeutic medications, many of which act through induction of apoptosis. Other mechanisms of providing resistance to apoptosis include downregulation of caspases or production of caspase inhibitors. By whatever mechanism, or combination of mechanisms, successful cancers suppress apoptotic pathways and increase resistance to cell death.

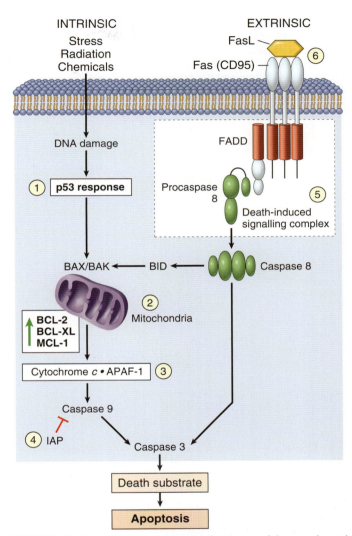

FIGURE 10.18 Extrinsic and Intrinsic Pathways of Apoptosis and Mechanisms Used by Tumour Cells to Evade Cell Death. (1) Loss of p53 leading to reduced function of proapoptotic factors, such as BAX. (2) Reduced egress of cytochrome *c* from mitochondria as a result of upregulation of antiapoptotic factors, such as Bcl-2. (3) Loss of apoptotic peptidase-activating factor 1 *(APAF1).* (4) Upregulation of inhibitors of apoptosis *(IAP).* (5) Reduced CD95 levels. (6) Inactivation of death domain signalling complex (Fas-associated death domain *[FADD]*). *BAK,* Bcl-2–homologous antagonist or killer; *Bcl-2,* B-cell lymphoma 2; *Bcl-XL,* B-cell lymphoma-extra-large; *BID,* BH3 interacting-domain death agonist (related to Bcl-2); *Fas,* apoptosis antigen 1 receptor; *FasL,* Fas ligand; *MCL-1,* myeloid leukemia cell differentiation protein. (From Kumar, V., Abbas, A. K., & Aster, J. C. [Eds.]. [2015]. *Robbins and Cotran pathologic basis of disease* [9th ed.]. Saunders.)

Tumour-Promoting Inflammation

Successful tumours generally evade the natural immune/inflammatory responses of the body to cancer, but the relationship between a cancer and the immune system is actually much more complex.[26] The inflammatory response may even contribute to the onset of cancer and be manipulated throughout the process to benefit tumour progression and spread.[27]

Chronic inflammation is an important factor in the development of cancer[28] and may result from many causes: for example, solar irradiation, asbestos exposure (mesothelioma), pancreatitis, and infection (Table 10.3). Additionally, some organs appear to be more susceptible

TABLE 10.3 Chronic Inflammatory Conditions Associated with Neoplasms

Pathological Condition	Associated Neoplasm(s)	Etiological Agent
Asbestosis, silicosis	Mesothelioma, lung carcinoma	Asbestos fibres, silica particles
Bronchitis	Lung carcinoma	Silica, asbestos, smoking (nitrosamines, peroxides)
Cystitis, bladder inflammation	Bladder carcinoma	Chronic indwelling, urinary catheters
Gingivitis, lichen planus	Oral squamous cell carcinoma	
Inflammatory bowel disease, Crohn's disease, chronic ulcerative colitis	Colorectal carcinoma	
Lichen sclerosus	Vulvar squamous cell carcinoma	
Chronic pancreatitis, hereditary pancreatitis	Pancreatic carcinoma	Alcoholism, mutation in trypsinogen gene
Reflux oesophagitis, Barrett's esophagus	Esophageal carcinoma	Gastric acids
Sialadenitis	Salivary gland carcinoma	
Sjögren's syndrome, Hashimoto's thyroiditis	MALT lymphoma	
Skin inflammation	Melanoma	Ultraviolet light
Cancers Associated with Infectious Agents		
Opisthorchiasis, cholangitis	Cholangiosarcoma, colon carcinoma	Liver flukes (*Opisthorchis viverrini*), bile acids, bacterial infection
Chronic cholecystitis	Gall bladder cancer	Bacteria, gall bladder stones
Gastritis/ulcers	Gastric adenocarcinoma, MALT	*Helicobacter pylori*
Hepatitis	Hepatocellular carcinoma	Hepatitis B and/or C virus
Mononucleosis	B-cell non-Hodgkin's lymphoma, Burkitt lymphoma	Epstein-Barr Virus
Acquired immunodeficiency syndrome (AIDS)	Non-Hodgkin's lymphoma, squamous cell carcinomas, Kaposi's sarcoma	Human immunodeficiency virus (HIV), human herpesvirus type 8
Osteomyelitis	Skin carcinoma in draining sinuses	Bacterial infection
Pelvic inflammatory disease, chronic cervicitis	Ovarian carcinoma, cervical/anal carcinoma	Gonorrhea, chlamydia, human papillomavirus
Chronic cystitis	Bladder, liver, rectal carcinoma, follicular lymphoma of the spleen	

Data from Coussens, L. M., & Werb, Z. (2002). Inflammation and cancer. *Nature, 420*(6917), 860–867.

to the oncogenic effects of chronic inflammation (e.g., the gastro-intestinal [GI] tract, prostate, thyroid gland). Individuals who have suffered with ulcerative colitis for 10 years or more have up to a 30-fold increase in the risk of developing colon cancer.[29] Chronic viral hepatitis caused by hepatitis B virus (HBV) or hepatitis C virus (HCV) infection markedly increases the risk of liver cancer.

A specific example is the association between gastric inflammation induced by infection with the bacterium *Helicobacter pylori* and the risk for gastric cancer. *H. pylori* is a bacterium that infects more than half of the world's population. Chronic infection with *H. pylori* is an important cause of peptic ulcer disease and is strongly associated with gastric carcinoma, a leading cause of cancer deaths worldwide. It is also associated with a less common cancer, gastric mucosa-associated lymphoid tissue (MALT) lymphomas.[30] *H. pylori* infection often occurs in childhood and disproportionately affects lower socioeconomic classes. Although most infections are asymptomatic, prolonged chronic inflammation can lead to increased gastric acid secretion, atrophic gastritis, and duodenal ulcers, or benign cellular proliferation that can, in a small fraction of individuals, progress to dysplastic changes and, finally, gastric adenocarcinoma. *H. pylori* infection can both directly and indirectly produce genetic and epigenetic changes in cells of infected stomachs, including mutations in *TP53* and alterations in the methylation of specific genes. Eradication of *H. pylori* from infected individuals before the development of dysplasia may prevent the development of cancer. However, there is no expert consensus on the value of population screening and treatment strategies. The MALT lymphomas associated with chronic *H. pylori* infections may depend on chronic inflammation and antigenic stimulation associated with infections, and therefore, treatment with antibiotics may be useful, even in cases of early lymphoma.

Once cells with malignant phenotypes have developed, additional complex interactions occur between the tumour and the surrounding stroma and cells of the immune and inflammatory systems. Cancers disrupt the environment, initiate or enhance inflammation, and, in turn, recruit local and distant cells (macrophages, lymphocytes, and other cellular components of inflammation). The acute inflammatory response is initially designed to eliminate infection but evolves to initiate and direct the healing process (see Chapter 6). Successful tumours appear capable of manipulating cells of the inflammatory response from a rejection response toward the phenotypes associated with wound healing and tissue regeneration; this process includes induction of cellular proliferation, neovascularization, and local immune suppression in the damaged tissue.[31] These activities benefit cancer progression, as well as increase resistance to chemotherapeutic agents.

One of the key cells that promote tumour survival is the **tumour-associated macrophage (TAM)**. Tumours commonly produce cytokines and chemokines that are chemotactic factors for monocytes/macrophages (e.g., colony-stimulating factor-1 [CSF-1; also known as *macrophage colony-stimulating factor*, or M-CSF], the chemokine ligand 2 [CCL2; also known as *macrophage chemotactic protein-1*, or MCP-1]). Levels of CCL2 in human breast cancer and cancers of the esophagus are related to the degree of macrophage infiltration and progression of the tumour. Most tumours have large numbers of TAMs, whose presence frequently correlates with a worse prognosis. Monocytes move from the blood and into the tumour, where they mature into macrophages. Monocytes also have the capacity to differentiate into several macrophage phenotypes, depending upon the conditions in the microenvironment. The classic proinflammatory macrophage (M1) is the primary macrophage in the acute inflammatory response and is responsible for removal and destruction of infectious agents. During healing, however, a different phenotype (M2) produces anti-inflammatory mediators to suppress ongoing inflammation and induce cellular proliferation, angiogenesis, and wound healing.[32] TAMs appear to phenotypically mimic the M2 phenotype.

TAMs have diminished cytotoxic response and develop the capacity to block Tc-cell and NK-cell functions, as well as produce cytokines that are advantageous for tumour growth and spread. TAMs secrete cellular growth factors (e.g., TGF-β and fibroblast growth factor-2 [FGF-2]) that favour tumour cell proliferation, angiogenesis, and tissue remodelling, similar to their activities in wound healing. They also secrete angiogenesis factors (e.g., VEGF) that induce neovascularization and MMPs that degrade intercellular matrix. The overall effect is increased tumour growth, invasion of the blood vessels, increased oxygen to the tumour, and invasion through the degraded matrix into the local tissue.

Cancer-associated fibroblasts (CAFs) synthesize the ECM that surrounds and permeates the tumour.[33] Cytokines and growth factors stored in the matrix, as well as growth factors, metalloproteases, proteoglycans, and other molecules secreted by CAFs contribute greatly to cancer progression, local spread, and metastasis.

Evading Immune Destruction

Many cancers express cell surface antigens that are not generally found on normal cells from the same tissue. Tumour-associated antigens include products of oncogenes, antigens from oncogenic viruses, oncofetal antigens (expressed in embryonic tissues and tumours) and altered glycoproteins and glycolipids.[34] The tumour cell processes viral and tumour antigens and presents them on the cell surface along with major histocompatibility complex (MHC) class I molecules that target CD8+ Tc cells (see Chapter 7).

NK cells recognize altered cell surface glycoproteins and glycolipids. As such, cancer cells should be recognized as foreign and destroyed by the immune system. Similarly, in the laboratory, T cells and NK cells recognize and kill cancer cells. This observation gave rise to two hypotheses: (1) immune surveillance and (2) immunotherapy. The immune surveillance hypothesis predicts that most developing malignancies are suppressed by an efficient immune response against tumour-associated antigens. The immunotherapy hypothesis predicts that the immune system could be used to target tumour-associated antigens and destroy tumours clinically. Immunotherapy could be either active, by immunization with tumour antigens to elicit or enhance the immune response against a particular cancer, or passive, by injecting the cancer patient with antibodies or lymphocytes directed against the tumour antigens. However, the interactions between cancer and the immune system are more complex than originally envisioned, and both hypotheses remain controversial.

What is the role of the immune system in protecting against cancer? The most clearly documented effective response of the immune system to cancer is in relation to identifying and destroying oncogenic viruses before they give rise to cancer. Several viruses have been associated with human cancer: human papillomavirus (HPV), Epstein-Barr virus (EBV; also known as *HHV4*), Kaposi sarcoma herpesvirus (KSHV; also known as HHV8), and hepatitis B and C viruses (HBV, HCV) are associated with about 15% of all human cancers worldwide (see Table 10.3).[35] Cancer of the cervix and hepatocellular carcinoma account for approximately 80% of virus-linked cancer cases.

A great example of this relationship is with HPV and cervical cancer. Virtually all cervical cancer is caused by infection with specific types of HPV, which infects basal skin cells and commonly causes warts. There are more than 120 HPV types, but only about 40 can infect human mucosal tissue, and only a few (HPV-16, -18, -31, and -45) are associated with the highest risk of developing cervical, anogenital, and penile cancer. Most HPV infection is handled effectively and rapidly by the immune system and does not cause cancer. Cancer is more common in people with prolonged infection with HPV (a decade or more), during which the viral DNA becomes integrated into the genomic DNA of the infected basal cell of the cervix and directs the persistent production of viral oncogenes. Early oncogenic HPV infection is readily detected by the Papanicolaou (Pap) test, an examination of cervical epithelial scrapings. Early detection of atypical cells in a Pap test alerts health care providers to the possibility of cervical carcinoma in situ, which can be effectively treated. The Pap test is probably the most effective cancer-screening test developed to date. For women age 30 to 65 years old, additional testing for HPV infection of cervical cells (HPV test) should be added.[36] Vaccines protecting against the common oncogenic HPV types (HPV-16 and HPV-18 [types that cause 70% of cervical cancers] and HPV-6 and HPV-11 [types that cause 90% of genital warts]) were approved for clinical use beginning in 2006; administration of these vaccines to young men and women before an initial HPV infection is likely to prevent many cases of cervical cancer.

Similarly, chronic hepatitis B infections are common in parts of Asia and Sub-Saharan Africa and confer up to a 200-fold increased risk of developing liver cancer. Chronic hepatitis C infections have become increasingly recognized in Western countries. Up to 80% of liver cancer cases worldwide are associated with chronic hepatitis caused either by HBV or by HCV. The initial infection with HBV or HCV is not associated with cancer; rather, it is the chronic nature of the infection in chronic viral hepatitis that markedly increases cancer risk. In both cases, it appears that a lifetime of chronic liver inflammation predisposes to the development of hepatocellular carcinoma. Widespread use of the HBV vaccine significantly decreases the incidence of chronic hepatitis B and hence hepatocellular carcinoma. A vaccine for HCV is not yet available because HCV is highly variable between strains and rapidly mutates. Although investigation into developing an HCV vaccine is underway and involves the induction of a T-cell response, there are still many questions about its overall effectiveness at eliminating HCV infection.[37]

For most other human tumour viruses, immunoprophylaxis is not yet available. EBV and HHV8 are members of the Herpesviridae family. EBV infects more than 90% of adults, usually as children and without symptoms. EBV infection during adolescence may cause infectious mononucleosis. The virus infects B cells and stimulates their limited proliferation and usually becomes latent throughout the individual's life. If the individual is immunosuppressed because of HIV infection or because of medications given for an organ transplant, persistent EBV infection can lead to the development of B-cell lymphomas. EBV infection also is associated with Burkitt lymphoma in areas of endemic malaria and with nasopharyngeal carcinoma, a cancer endemic in Chinese populations in Southeast Asia. HHV8 is linked to the development of Kaposi sarcoma, a cancer that was once seen primarily in older men but now occurs in a markedly more virulent form in immunosuppressed individuals, especially those with acquired immunodeficiency syndrome (AIDS). HHV8 also has been linked to several rare lymphomas. **Human T-cell lymphotropic virus type 1 (HTLV-1)** is an oncogenic retrovirus linked to the development of adult T-cell leukemia and lymphoma (ATLL). HTLV-1 is transmitted vertically (i.e., inherited by children from infected parents) and horizontally (e.g., by breastfeeding, sexual intercourse, blood transfusions, and exposure to infected needles). Infection with HTLV-1 may be asymptomatic, and only a small fraction of infected individuals develop ATLL, often many years after acquiring the virus.

Immunization does work to prevent viral-induced cancers. The immune surveillance hypothesis predicts that components of the immune system, especially T cells, monitor the body and destroy most nascent tumours, even those not caused by viruses. If the immune surveillance hypothesis is correct, compromise of the immune system by immunosuppressive medications or development of genetic or acquired immune deficiencies would result in increased incidences of all types of cancer.[38] Interestingly, defective immune responses generally only increase the risk for lymphoid cancers, many of which are associated with viral infections. For example, individuals taking chronic powerful immunosuppressive medications, such as those given for kidney, heart, or liver transplant, have a much higher risk of developing viral-associated cancers, with a 10-fold increased risk of non-Hodgkin's lymphoma (caused by EBV) and up to a 1 000-fold increased risk of Kaposi sarcoma (caused by HHV8). The same immunosuppressed individuals, however, have only a slight increase in the risk of common cancers such as lung and colon cancer (and this could well be because of increased inflammation at those sites), and no increase in the risk of breast or prostate cancer.

Many tumours also have an abundance of tumour-infiltrating lymphocytes (TILs). Cancers actively recruit an immune and stromal response to assist in the remodelling of tissues, formation of new blood vessels, and promotion of metastasis.[39] NK cells are generally in low amounts in tumours. The predominant TILs are T-regulatory (Treg) cells. Treg cells are CD4+ cells that differentiate under the control of specific cytokines, primarily TGF-β. The role of Treg cells during wound healing is to control or limit the immune response to protect the host's own tissues against autoimmune reactions, whereas tumours manipulate their function to prevent a destructive antitumour immune response and provide cytokines that facilitate tumour cell proliferation and spread. Treg cells and TAMs, as well as other stromal cells, produce very high levels of TGF-β and interleukin-10 (IL-10). IL-10 is an immunosuppressive cytokine, which generally decreases T-helper cell 1 (Th1) and Th2 activity, suppresses antigen recognition and cell proliferation by Th cells, and suppresses the capacity of CD8+ Tc cells to recognize, proliferate, and kill tumour cells.[40] The goal of current immunotherapy regimens is to reverse this relationship and facilitate T-cell–mediated cancer cell death (discussed later in this chapter).

The release of immunosuppressive factors into the tumour microenvironment also increases resistance of the tumour to chemotherapy and radiotherapy. Increased levels of Treg cells in blood and lymph nodes, as well as infiltrating the tumour, correlate with poor outcomes in breast and GI tumours. In advanced non–small cell lung cancer, an elevated ratio of Treg to Tc cells is related to a poor response to platinum-based chemotherapy. Immunosuppressive cytokines additionally lower the cancer cell's sensitivity to immune-mediated death (Figure 10.19). With increasing heterogeneity of cells within the tumour, subpopulations of antigen-negative cancer cell variants may selectively outgrow more immune-sensitive cells.[41] Variants may suppress the production of particular antigens or suppress levels of antigen-presenting MHC class I molecules. Other cytokines appear to increase the cancer cell's resistance to apoptosis. For example, the Th2 cytokine IL-4 increases the resistance of thyroid cancer to chemotherapy; IL-6 produced by Th cells, adipocytes, and fibroblasts activates survival pathways in breast cancer, leading to resistance to radiotherapy; and adipocytes enhance the transcription of the anti-apoptotic factor Bcl-2 in leukemia cells.

Activating Invasion and Metastasis

Metastasis is the spread of cancer cells from the site of the original tumour to distant tissues and organs through the body. Metastasis is a defining characteristic of cancer and is the major cause of death from cancer. Cancer that has not metastasized can often be cured by a combination of surgery, chemotherapy, and radiation. These same therapies are frequently ineffective against cancer that has metastasized.

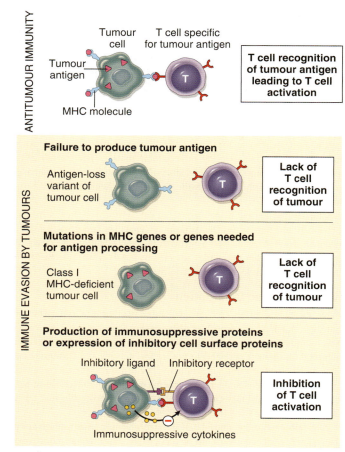

FIGURE 10.19 Mechanisms by Which Tumour Cells Evade the Immune System. Tumours may evade the immune response by losing expression of antigens or major histocompatibility complex (MHC) molecules or by producing immunosuppressive cytokines or ligands for inhibitory receptors on T cells. (From Kumar, V., Abbas, A. K., & Aster, J. C. [Eds.]. [2015]. *Robbins and Cotran pathologic basis of disease* [9th ed.]. Saunders.)

For example, in appropriately treated women with localized low-stage breast cancer, the 5-year survival rate is often greater than 90%. Tragically, less than 30% of women with metastatic breast cancer are still alive 5 years after diagnosis. A growing body of basic and clinical research is defining the biological principles of metastasis, with the hope that this improved understanding will lead to novel diagnostic approaches and better therapies to prevent and treat metastatic cancers.

How do cancer cells develop the ability to metastasize? Metastasis is a highly inefficient process. Cancer cells must surmount multiple physical and physiological barriers to spread, survive, and proliferate in distant locations, and the destination must be receptive to the growth of the cancer. Changes in the tumour microenvironment initiate the metastatic process and may include stromal cell adaptation to increase tumour mass and intratumour hypoxia.[42] As this diversity increases within the changing tumour microenvironment, some cancer cells evolve with multiple new abilities that can facilitate metastasis. The model for transition to metastatic cancer cells is called **epithelial-mesenchymal transition (EMT)**.[43]

Research with carcinomas provide much of what is known about epithelial-mesenchymal transition (EMT). Carcinomas originate from highly differentiated and polarized epithelial cells that form structured sheets stabilized by multiple adherences to neighbouring cells and to a basement membrane (an extracellular meshwork of collagens and other connective tissue proteins) along the cell's basal surface. Although the degree of malignant transformation resulting in a primary carcinoma may be adequate for local expansion of the tumour, neoplastic cells usually retain some epithelial-like characteristics that prevent dissociation from the ECM and preclude successful metastasis to distal sites. A greater degree of cellular "de-differentiation" is necessary to produce the phenotype that can separate from the primary tumour and flourish in a potentially hostile secondary site. This results from a programmed transition of the still partially epithelial-like carcinoma to a more undifferentiated mesenchymal-like phenotype (Figure 10.20). A similar process occurs with tumours of endothelial origin (endothelial-mesenchymal transition).

EMT is a process that occurs normally in embryonic development, as well as wound healing and tissue repair. Generally, cells that have transitioned into a mesenchymal-like phenotype have suppressed expression of adhesion molecules with a loss of polarity, increased migratory capacity, elevated resistance to apoptosis, and demonstrated the potential to redifferentiate into other cell types.[44] More importantly, the transition to a mesenchymal-like phenotype is, in most cases, driven by cytokines and chemokines produced within the tumour microenvironment.[45] IL-8 is an effective driver of carcinoma cells into EMT.

Invasion, or local spread, is a prerequisite for metastasis. In its earliest stages local invasion may occur by direct tumour extension. Eventually, however, cells migrate away from the primary tumour and invade the surrounding tissues (see Figure 10.20). Invasion is a multistep process within EMT that includes (1) diminished cell-to-cell adhesion, (2) digestion of the surrounding ECM, and (3) increased motility of individual cancer cells.

Recruitment of TAMs and other cells of inflammation is critical for invasion. Cells are normally attached to the ECM. TAMs and other stromal (or supporting) cells secrete proteases and protease activators that promote digestion of connective tissue capsules and other structural barriers. Degradation of the surrounding ECM creates pathways through which cells can move, while releasing bioactive peptides as digestion products that further stimulate tumour growth and mobility.

Normal cells, when separated from their ECM, undergo *anoikis*, a form of apoptosis. Tumour cells that have adapted to a hypoxic environment are already resistant to apoptosis, often by loss of normal cell death pathways. The process of EMT frequently increases resistance to apoptosis. For example, neuroblastomas with loss of the proapoptotic genes are able to avoid apoptosis after degradation of a normal ECM because they lack the enzymes (i.e., caspase 8) with which to initiate the apoptotic process and destroy DNA (and other substrates). These cells are more able to metastasize than the same cells with normal levels of these enzymes. Individuals with low levels of pro-apoptotic enzymes such as caspase 8 in neuroblastomas have a poor prognosis.

To transition from local to distant metastasis, the cancer cells must also be able to invade local blood and lymphatic vessels, a task facilitated by stimulation of neoangiogenesis and lymphangiogenesis by factors such as VEGF. After release from the ECM and digestion of basement membranes, mobile cancer cells gain access to the circulation, perhaps facilitated by the leaky newly made vessels and attraction of the cells because of chemoattractants coming from these new vessels. Once in the circulation, metastatic cells must be able to withstand the physiological stresses of travel in the blood and lymphatic circulation, including high shear rates and exposure to immune cells. One interesting mechanism is for tumour cells to bind to blood platelets, giving them a protective coat of nonmalignant blood cells that both shields the tumour cells and creates a small tumour embolus, or cancer clot, that can promote cancer cell survival in distant locations (see Figure 10.20).

Cancer cells spread through both vascular and lymphatic pathways. The neovascularization of a cancer offers malignant cells direct access into the venous blood and draining lymphatic vessels. The venous and lymphatic drainage networks associated with the primary tumour frequently determine the pattern of metastasis. Single cells, clumps, and even tumour fragments can disseminate by these routes. For instance, anatomical patterns of lymphatic and venous blood flow help determine how colon cancers spread to the liver, liver cancers spread through the portal vein to the lungs, lung cancers spread through the systemic circulation to the brain, and breast cancer spreads through the lymphatics to axillary lymph nodes. Cancers often spread first to regional lymph nodes through the lymphatics and then to distant organs through the bloodstream.

How different cancers select different sites for metastasis can be a mystery. Metastatic breast cancer often spreads through the bloodstream to bones but rarely to kidney or spleen, whereas lymphomas often spread to the spleen but uncommonly spread to bone. Different types of cancer cells injected into the carotid artery of mice,[46] in spite of identical blood flow–mediated distribution of the cancer cells, produced cancers of each cell type in very different parts of the brain. Specific interactions between the cancer cells and specific receptors on the small blood vessels in different organs likely causes this selectivity. Furthermore, experimental metastasis studies in mice are beginning to reveal additional molecular reasons for this tissue specificity. Examples include interaction between $\alpha 3\beta 1$ integrins binding to laminin-5 receptors in the lung, and the chemokine receptor CXCR4 on breast cancer cells promoting homing to lung tissues expressing the ligand CXCL12.[47]

A cancer's ability to establish a metastatic lesion in a new location requires that the cancer survive in the specific environment and be capable of forming complex and heterogeneous tumours. It only takes a few cancer cells to establish a tumour, and these cells are **tumour-initiating cells** (TICs) (or *cancer stem cells*).[47] The microenvironment is critical to the survival and propagation of these cells. The tumor-initiating and chemoresistant features of TICs highly encourage the development of specific TIC-targeting treatments. Interestingly, current research into the use of metformin to change the glycolytic phenotype of cancer cells (i.e., block the Warburg effect) shows some promise with tumours such as osteosarcoma, glioblastoma, and breast TICs.

The degree of de-differentiation may be variable, but most cells undergoing EMT acquire stem cell traits that facilitate initial growth in a new microenvironment.[48] The EMT is not a stable transition; after taking residence in the metastatic site, the tumour tends to regain some characteristics of the primary tumour, thus reverting somewhat to its epithelial origins. Because metastasis requires successful completion of each and every step, there may be many opportunities to interrupt this potentially lethal pathway when developing treatments for cancer.

However, metastasis does not universally result in proliferation at a new site. Some cancer cells survive at a new site but do not proliferate to form a clinically relevant metastatic site. These cancer cells appear to exist in a state of *dormancy*. **Dormancy** is cellular quiescence—a stable, nonproliferative state that is reversible. Cells may remain quiescent for years before initiating proliferation. About two thirds of breast cancer deaths occur after a 5-year disease-free interval. In other conditions, solitary tumour cells can be detected in the blood years after a complete clinical remission in individuals, and many people with detectable micrometastases will not develop clinically obvious metastases. Cancer cell dormancy may be extremely common, even without a history of

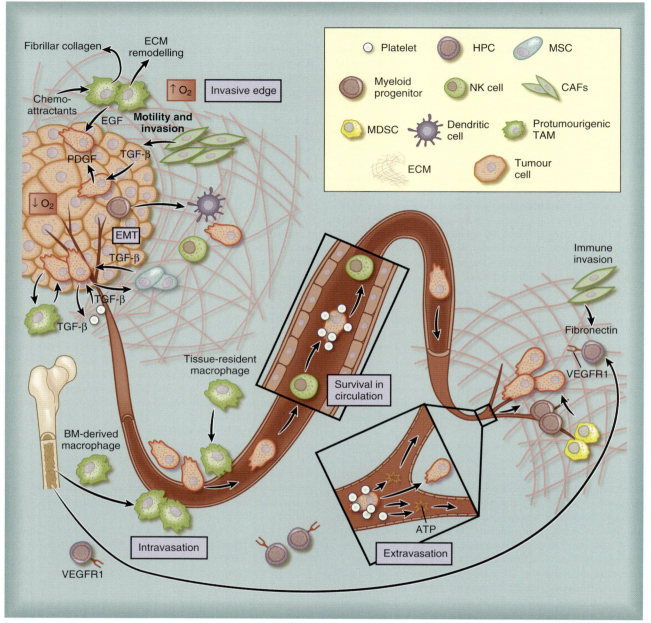

FIGURE 10.20 Epithelial-Mesenchymal Transition and Metastasis. The microenvironment supports metastatic dissemination and colonization at secondary sites. Stromal cells (e.g., mesenchymal stem cells *[MSC]*), possibly facilitated by a relative decrease in oxygen (O_2) levels in the tumour, contribute to the epithelial-mesenchymal transition *(EMT)* through which tumour cells develop a metastatic phenotype characterized by suppression of adhesion molecules and reduced adherence to adjacent cells and extracellular matrix *(ECM)*, increased local invasion, and access to the blood and lymphatic circulations. One major mediator of this process is transforming growth factor-beta *(TGF-β)*, which is secreted by the tumour stroma. Protumourigenic tumour-associated macrophage *(TAMs)*, and cancer-associated fibroblasts *(CAFs)* facilitate intravascularization of tumour cells into the circulation and tend to cluster at the leading edge of the invading cancer cells. They secrete matrix metalloproteinases that promote digestion and remodelling of the surrounding ECM. Their association with platelets promotes their survival in the circulation in addition to clotting factors that shield the cancer cells from cytotoxic immune cells (T-cytotoxic cells and natural killer cells *[NK cells]*) that are also suppressed by myeloid-derived suppressor cells *(MDSC)*. The induction of fibronectin provides a site for the influx of hematopoietic progenitor cells *(HPC)* that have receptors for vascular endothelial cell growth factor and sets the stage for the beginning of metastasis. HPC appear essential for establishment of a metastatic site. At a metastatic site, cancer cells will adhere to local vascular endothelium, undergo extravascularization facilitated by the effects of adenosine triphosphate *(ATP)* on the endothelium, and undergo mesenchymal-to-epithelial transition. Molecular signalling from the cancer and initiation of a favourable microenvironment help to prepare sites for metastasis. *BM*, Bone marrow; *EGF*, epidermal growth factor; *PDGF*, platelet-derived growth factor; *VEGFR1*, vascular endothelial cell growth factor receptor 1. (Reprinted with permission from Macmillan Publishers Ltd: Quail, D. F., & Joyce, J. A. [2013]. Microenvironmental regulation of tumor progression and metastasis. *Nature Medicine, 19*[11]: 1423–1437.)

clinical cancer. Studies of deceased individuals without any history of cancer suggest that most human beings have dormant cancer cells that never adjusted to form a malignant tumour.[49]

The causes of dormancy and, more importantly, escape from dormancy and development of a malignant cancer are largely unknown but have the potential to facilitate the development of cancer therapies. Dormancy may result from features of the cell or the environmental niche, or both. Individuals with clinical cancers may shed disseminated tumour cells very early from premetastatic lesions.[50] These early cells may have developed inadequately to a metastatic phenotype and thus, cannot recruit cells into a supportive stroma or initiated angiogenesis. Another consideration is the niche (or site) itself. It is not clear whether a developing cancer secretes factors that enter the bloodstream and prepare potential metastatic niches.[51] Early disseminated cancer cells may encounter nonsupportive niches that foster dormancy.

CLINICAL MANIFESTATIONS OF CANCER

QUICK CHECK 10.5
1. Describe the major clinical manifestations of cancer.
2. How is cancer diagnosed?
3. What are the most common treatments of cancer?

The clinical manifestations of cancer are numerous and depend on the localization and type of tumour; some are apparent before actual diagnosis of a malignancy. Generally, the variety and intensity of symptoms will increase as the malignancy progresses.

Paraneoplastic Syndromes

Paraneoplastic syndromes are symptom complexes that are triggered by a cancer but are not caused by direct local effects of the tumour mass. They are most commonly caused by biological substances released from the tumour (e.g., hormones, cytokines) or by an immune response triggered by the tumour. For example, a small fraction of carcinoid tumours release substances, including serotonin, into the bloodstream that cause flushing, diarrhea, wheezing, and rapid heartbeat. A number of cancers trigger an antibody response that attacks the nervous system, causing a variety of neurological disorders that can precede other symptoms of cancer by months.

Although infrequent, paraneoplastic syndromes are significant because they may be the earliest symptom of an unknown cancer and, in affected individuals, can be serious, often irreversible, and sometimes life-threatening. Table 10.4 presents the classifications of paraneoplastic syndromes.

Pain

Pain is one of the most feared complications of advanced cancer. Although pain can be one of the presenting symptoms of cancer, most commonly there is little or no pain during the early stages of malignant disease. Significant pain, however, occurs in a large fraction of those individuals who are terminally ill with cancer. Fear, anxiety, sleep loss, fatigue, and overall physical deterioration strongly influence the perception of pain. Pain is also the result of an interaction among physiological, cultural, and psychological aspects of being. (The neurophysiology of pain is discussed in Chapter 14.)

Cancer-associated pain can arise from a variety of direct and indirect mechanisms. Direct pressure, obstruction, invasion of a sensitive structure, stretching of visceral surfaces, tissue destruction, infection, and inflammation can all cause pain. Pain can occur at the site of the primary tumour or can result from a distant metastatic lesion. Furthermore, pain may be referred away from the involved site and manifest, for example, as back pain.

Specific sites are more prone to cancer-associated pain. Bone metastases, common in advanced breast and prostate cancer, can cause significant pain because of periosteal irritation, medullary pressure, vertebral collapse, and pathological fractures. Brain tumours (primary or metastatic) can, depending on the location, cause headache, seizures, or neurological deficits. Pain in the abdomen may be caused by bowel obstruction, or inflammation and infection. Hepatic malignancies can stretch the liver, resulting in a dull pain or a feeling of fullness over the right upper abdominal quadrant. Mucosal surfaces can develop painful ulcerative lesions from the cancer, chemotherapy, and radiation or leukopenia (or both).

The diagnosis and treatment of pain is one of the primary responsibilities of the medical team. The individual's perception and reporting of pain can vary widely and be affected by such factors as age and cultural background. The priority of treatment is to control pain rapidly and completely, as judged by the individual. The second goal is to prevent recurrence of pain. Objective measurements of pain are increasingly being included along with the reporting of more traditional vital signs. Many institutions are using specialized pain management teams that are trained to recognize different types of acute and persistent pain, as well as the individual's response to that pain. Many modalities are available to treat pain, ranging from combinations of nonsteroidal anti-inflammatory drugs (NSAIDs) and narcotics to palliative surgery and radiation therapy. Individual-controlled analgesia provides many benefits, not the least of which is regaining some control over one's own body. Although cancer pain is a complex problem arising from multiple sources, individuals should be assured that suffering is not inevitable, and that relief is attainable.

Fatigue

Fatigue, though a very general symptom and often present with a variety of pathophysiological conditions, is the most frequently reported symptom of cancer and cancer treatment. The exact mechanisms that produce fatigue, however, are poorly understood. Suggested causes include sleep disturbances, various biochemical changes secondary to disease and treatment, numerous psychosocial factors, and environmental and physical factors.

The *physiological* understanding of fatigue probably includes mechanisms for decreased muscle contractility. Overall, studies of muscle function suggest that some individuals with cancer may lose portions of muscle function needed to perform normal physical activities. Other areas of research include muscle function consequences from metabolic products of cancer treatment and associated muscle loss from circulating cytokines (e.g., TNF and IL-1). Similar to pain, fatigue is a subjective clinical manifestation. Individuals with cancer describe fatigue in many ways (e.g., weakness, lack of energy, depression). Some of these symptoms have been termed "chemo brain," or mild cognitive impairment. The changes in cognitive function can be caused by the cancer itself or by the stress associated with the diagnosis of cancer, because symptoms similar to "chemo brain" also occur in individuals who have not received chemotherapy.

Cachexia

The multiorgan syndrome of **cachexia** includes a constellation of clinical manifestations, including anorexia; wasting; thermogenesis; altered heart and liver function; gut malabsorption; early satiety (filling); taste alterations; and altered protein, lipid, and carbohydrate metabolism (Figure 10.21).

TABLE 10.4 Paraneoplastic Syndromes

Clinical Syndromes	Major Forms of Underlying Cancer	Causal Mechanism
Endocrinopathies		
Cushing's syndrome	Small cell lung carcinoma Pancreatic carcinoma Neural tumours	ACTH or ACTH-like substance
Syndrome of inappropriate antidiuretic hormone (SIADH) secretion	Small cell lung carcinoma; intracranial neoplasms	Antidiuretic hormone or atrial natriuretic hormones
Hypercalcemia	Squamous cell carcinoma of lung Breast carcinoma Renal carcinoma Adult T-cell leukemia or lymphoma Ovarian carcinoma	PTHRP, TGF-α, TNF, IL-1
Hypoglycemia	Fibrosarcoma Other mesenchymal sarcomas Hepatocellular carcinoma	Insulin or insulinlike substance
Carcinoid syndrome	Bronchial adenoma (carcinoid) Pancreatic carcinoma Gastric carcinoma	Serotonin, bradykinin
Polycythemia	Renal carcinoma Cerebellar hemangioma Hepatocellular carcinoma	Erythropoietin
Nerve and Muscle Syndromes		
Myasthenia	Bronchogenic carcinoma	Immunological
Disorders of central and peripheral nervous systems	Breast carcinoma	Unknown
Dermatological Disorders		
Acanthosis nigricans	Gastric carcinoma Lung carcinoma Uterine carcinoma	Immunological; secretion of epidermal growth factor
Dermatomyositis	Bronchogenic, breast carcinoma	Immunological
Osseous, Articular, and Soft Tissue Changes		
Hypertrophic osteoarthropathy and clubbing of fingers	Bronchogenic carcinoma	Unknown
Vascular and Hematological Changes		
Venous thrombosis (Trousseau phenomenon)	Pancreatic carcinoma Bronchogenic carcinoma Other cancers	Tumour products (mucins that activate clotting)
Nonbacterial thrombotic endocarditis	Advanced cancers	Hypercoagulability
Anemia	Thymic neoplasms	Unknown
Others		
Nephrotic syndrome	Various cancers	Tumour antigens; immune complexes

Adapted from Kumar, V., Abbas, A. K., & Aster, J. (Eds.). (2021). *Robbins and Cotran pathologic basis of disease* (10th ed.). Elsevier.
ACTH, Adrenocorticotropic hormone; *IL*, interleukin; *PTHRP*, parathyroid hormone–related protein; *TGF-α*, transforming growth factor-alpha; *TNF*, tumour necrosis factor.

Although several definitions of cachexia exist, two factors are significant: (1) weight loss and (2) inflammation. Severe weight loss is primarily from *loss of skeletal muscle and body fat*.[52] The wasting that occurs in muscle may be dependent on alterations in other organs or tissues, including white adipose tissue.[52] Cachexia as a syndrome is multifactorial, involving changes in many metabolic pathways. The cachectic syndrome involves (i) abnormalities in heart function, (ii) alterations in liver protein synthesis, (iii) changes in hypothalamic mediators, and (iv) activation of brown adipose tissue and GI function.[52] All of these changes result in a major decrease in quality of life and indirectly result in death in some individuals. The incidence of the syndrome among individuals with cancer is very high and varies by tumour type.[52]

Molecular Basis of Cachexia

Cachexia has been discussed as a type of *energy balance disorder* where energy intake is decreased, and energy expenditure is increased.[52] Energy intake and expenditure depends on the tumour type and its growth phase. Because individuals receiving total parenteral nutrition still lose weight, increased energy expenditure at rest may be the cause of the wasting syndrome.[52] Both the mitochondria and sarcoplasmic

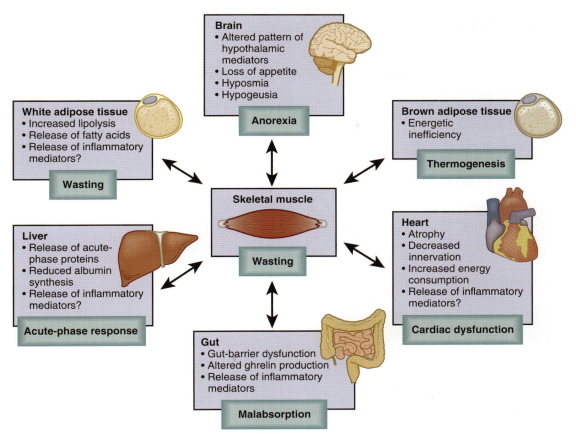

FIGURE 10.21 Cachexia: A Multiorgan Syndrome. Loss of skeletal muscle and of adipose tissue are major contributors to cachexia. But many other organs have a role in the cachexia syndrome, and the wasting that takes place in muscle may be dependent on alterations in these other organs or tissues. Changes in hypothalamic function and activation of brown adipose tissue, as well as alterations in liver and heart function, also are involved in the syndrome. Recent studies support a role for gut microbiota in cancer cachexia and the possibility of a gut-microbiota–skeletal muscle relationship. Recent data suggest that the conversion of white adipose tissue to brown adipose tissue is triggered by both humoral inflammatory mediators (such as interleukin-6) and tumour-derived compounds (such as parathyroid-hormone–related protein). (From Bindels, L. B., Beck, R., Schakman, O., et al. [2012]. Restoring specific lactobacilli levels decreases inflammation and muscle atrophy markers in an acute leukemia mouse model. *PLoS One, 7*[6], e37971; Bindels, L. B., & Delzenne, N. M. [2013]. Muscle wasting: the gut microbiota as a new therapeutic target? *International Journal of Biochemistry & Cell Biology, 45*[10], 2186–2190.)

reticulum (SR) as they work together in muscle function have a role in the development of cachexia. Some hypotheses related to these functions include increased production of peroxisome-proliferator–activated receptor-γ coactivator-1 alpha (PGC1α), a nuclear receptor that functions as a transcription factor in the regulation of genes. This transcription factor then activates a mitochondrial protein (mitofusin-2 [MFN2]) that interacts with muscle SR and controls calcium (Ca^{2+}) signalling between cellular organelles. The overexpression of PGC1α can activate MFN2 expression, leading to Ca^{2+} deregulation, which is closely associated with *muscle wasting*.[52] Muscle weakness and fatigue is related to loss of myofibrillar proteins in muscle cells. Abnormalities in protein and amino acid metabolism are noted in cachectic muscle (Figure 10.22).

Contributing further to muscle wasting is an increase in apoptosis and an impaired capacity for regeneration.[52] Increased protein turnover and the wasting process involves many signalling pathways. Similarly, increased inflammatory mediators including cytokines, myostatin, and tumour-derived factors activate these pathways. In addition to muscle wasting, miRNAs may be involved in stimulating the breakdown of adipose tissue.[53,54] In cancer cachexia, skeletal muscle loss includes major loss of white adipose tissue (WAT). The WAT loss is thought to be caused by (1) increased lipolysis, (2) decreased activity of lipoprotein lipase (LPL), and (3) decreased new or de novo lipogenesis in adipose tissue.[52] New data show that WAT cells undergo a "browning" process during cancer cachexia where they change to beige cells called brown adipose tissue-*(BAT-)like cells*.[55,56] Browning is associated with increased thermogenesis. Tumour-derived compounds, such as IL-6 (which also may be released by immune cells) and parathyroid-hormone–related protein (PTHRP), may be the drivers of thermogenesis.[55]

An unusual and frustrating component of cancer care is the person's early satiety, or a sense of being full after only a few mouthfuls of food. Brain mediators are involved in the regulation of food intake and include appetite, satiation, taste, and smell of food. Therefore, the brain is an important organ in anorexia and consequently altered energy balance. Profoundly altered are both *orexigenic* (appetite-stimulating) and *anorexigenic* (appetite-suppressing) brain pathways.[57] (Chapters 6 and 7 discuss cytokines in detail.)

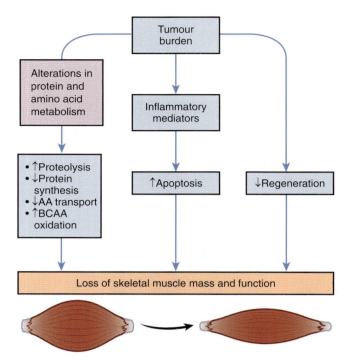

FIGURE 10.22 **Wasting of Skeletal Muscle.** Inflammation plays a major role in muscle wasting and is linked to alterations in protein and amino acid metabolism, activation of muscle cell apoptosis, and decreased regeneration. *AA*, Amino acid; *BCAA*, branched-chain amino acid. (Reprinted with permission from Macmillan Publishers Ltd: Argilés, J. M., Busquets, S., Stemmler, B., & López-Soriano, F. J. [2014]. Cancer cachexia: understanding the molecular basis. *Nature Reviews: Cancer, 14*[11], 754–762. https://doi.org/10.1038/nrc3829.)

Anemia

Anemia is commonly associated with malignancy; 20% of persons diagnosed with cancer have low hemoglobin levels. Mechanisms that cause anemia include (1) chronic bleeding (resulting in iron deficiency), (2) severe malnutrition, (3) cytotoxic chemotherapy, and (4) malignancy in blood-forming organs. Chronic bleeding and iron deficiency can accompany colorectal or genitourinary malignancy. People with gastric, pancreatic, or upper-intestinal cancer also have problems with the absorption of iron. There may also be a defect in the reutilization of iron because of lack of transfer of iron from the storage pool to blood cell precursors. Increased secretion of IL-6 and hepcidin (a hormone secreted by the liver that regulates the body's iron distribution) can cause this defect (see Chapter 20). Cancer also results in defects in erythropoietin production and shortened duration of red cell survival. In addition, anorexia can cause both iron and folate deficiency. Megaloblastic (large red cell) anemias may also develop after methotrexate treatment.

Administration of erythropoietin, which stimulates production of erythrocytes, can be effective in correcting anemia in people with cancer, as many subjects required fewer red blood cell transfusions in clinical trials. In addition, erythropoietin can successfully treat anemias occurring after chemotherapy or radiotherapy. However, recent studies indicate that aggressive use of erythropoietin increases the risk of blood clots and can decrease cancer survival.

Leukopenia and Thrombocytopenia

Direct tumour invasion of the bone marrow causes both leukopenia (a decreased total white blood cell count) and thrombocytopenia (a decreased number of platelets). More commonly, many chemotherapeutic medications, which primarily affect rapidly dividing cells, are toxic to the bone marrow, often causing granulocytopenia and thrombocytopenia. Granulocytopenia also can result from radiation therapy if it encompasses significant areas of the bone marrow. The duration of granulocytopenia, and the corresponding risk of serious infection, can be lessened by treatment with recombinant human granulocyte colony-stimulating factor (rhG-CSF, filgrastim). rhG-CSF stimulates white blood cell precursors in the marrow to proliferate and differentiate rapidly. Thrombocytopenia is a major cause of hemorrhage in people with cancer and platelet transfusions are effective treatment. Thrombocytopenia also is an accompanying disorder of disseminated intravascular coagulation that occurs in people with acute promyelocytic leukemia (see Chapter 21) and severe infections.

Infection

Infection is the most significant cause of complications and death in people with malignant disease. Advanced malignancies are highly immunosuppressive, as are the radiotherapy and chemotherapy used to treat it. (Table 10.5 summarizes the factors that predispose people with cancer to infection.) When the absolute granulocyte count falls below 500 cells per microlitre, the risk of serious microbial (bacterial and fungal) infection increases. Surgery also can lower resistance to infection because removal of large quantities of tissue, together with hemorrhage, dead spaces, and poor tissue perfusion, can create favourable sites for infection. Hospital-related (health care–associated) infections increase because of indwelling medical devices, inadequate wound care, and the introduction of microorganisms from visitors and other individuals.

Gastrointestinal Tract

The entire GI tract relies on rapidly growing cells to produce an effective barrier to trauma and infection and to provide an absorptive surface for nutrients. Both chemotherapy and radiation therapy may cause a decreased cell turnover, thereby leading to oral ulcers (stomatitis), malabsorption, and diarrhea. The disruption of barrier defences also increases the risk for infection, especially invasion by a person's own GI microbiome.

Therapy-induced nausea, thought to be caused by an agent's direct action upon the central nervous system's vomiting centres, historically has been a major obstacle for continuing therapy. Aggressive antinausea (antiemetic) therapy, including the centrally acting serotonin 5-hydroxytryptamine (5-HT3) antagonists (such as ondansetron [Zofran] or dolasetron [Anzemet]), enables better tolerance of chemotherapy-induced nausea. Other popular antiemetics include steroids and phenothiazines. Naturally occurring and synthetic cannabinoids, the active ingredients in marijuana, increase appetite in addition to having antinausea properties.

Increasing nutritional intake is important with cancer. Analgesia often includes opiate agents, vital in treating severe cases of mucosal lesions. Supplemental nutrition through enteral or parenteral routes may be needed to combat malnutrition. Good oral hygiene may help prevent complications arising from mucosal membrane breakdown.

Hair and Skin

Alopecia (hair loss) results from chemotherapy effects on hair follicles. Alopecia is usually temporary, although hair may regrow with a different texture initially. Not all chemotherapeutic agents cause alopecia. Decreased renewal rates of the epidermal layers in the skin may lead to skin breakdown and dryness, altering the normal barrier protection against infection. Radiation therapy may cause skin erythema (redness) and contribute to breakdown.

TABLE 10.5 Factors Predisposing Individuals With Cancer to Infection

Factor	Basis
Age	Many common malignancies occur mostly in older age. Immunological functions decline with age. General debility reduces immunocompetence. Immobility predisposes to infection. Far-advanced cancer often results in immobility and general debility that worsen with age. Older adults are predisposed to nutritional inadequacies. Malnutrition impairs immunocompetence.
Tumour	Nutritional derangements can result. Sites and circumstances favourable to growth of microorganisms (obstruction, serous or blood effusion, ulceration) can be created. Far-advanced disease predisposes individuals to debility and immobility. Humoral or cellular immune defects may result. Metastasis to bone marrow may cause leukopenia or other defects in immunity.
Leukemias	Inadequate granulocyte production (impaired phagocytosis) results. Thrombocytopenia (bleeding) can occur. Late effect: chronic lung disease from *Pneumocystis carinii* pneumonia can develop during therapy.
Lymphomas and other mononuclear phagocyte malignancies	Humoral and cellular immune defects (anergy, altered immunoglobulin production) result. Late effect: splenectomy in children can cause increased susceptibility to infection.
Surgical treatment	Invasive procedure interrupts first lines of defence. Radical nature of surgery (removal of large blocks of tissue in lengthy procedures) causes hemorrhage, decreased tissue perfusion, creation of dead spaces, devitalization of tissues. Procedure may be "dirty" surgery (bowel, infected or contaminated areas). Surgery patients are often older and at poor risk. Long preoperative hospitalization often precedes surgery. Patients may have received previous adrenocorticosteroid therapy. Patients may have infections at sites remote from operative area. Nutritional derangements (especially important in head and neck surgery) may result. Lymph node dissection may predispose patient to local infection and impair containment to area. Gynecological surgery may result in fistulae. Lung surgery may cause bronchopleural fistulae. Debility and immobility may result.

Data from Donovan, M. I., & Girton, S. F. (1984). *Cancer care nursing* (2nd ed.). Appleton-Century-Crofts; Murphy, G. P., Lawrence, W., & Lenhard, R. E. (Eds.). (1995). *Clinical oncology* (2nd ed.). American Cancer Society. [Seminal Reference]

DIAGNOSIS, CHARACTERIZATION, AND TREATMENT OF CANCER

The diagnosis of cancer has a profound effect on individuals and their families. Responses range from depression to resigned fatalism to an aggressive no-holds-barred pursuit of therapy. The choice of therapy should be based on full consideration by the individual, the family, and the medical team of the individual's diagnosis, prognosis, and therapeutic options. Chemotherapy, radiotherapy, surgery, and combinations of these modalities can be effective at treating cancer. Caregivers must recognize that many individuals seek additional non–science-based explanations and therapies and often use these therapies, either concurrently or sequentially.

Diagnosis and Staging
Histological Staging

Screening tests, routine examinations, and investigation of symptoms are all ways to discover the presence of cancer in the body. The symptoms of a cancer are as diverse as the types of cancer themselves. The location of the cancer can determine symptoms by physical pressure, obstruction, and loss of normal function, or a cancer can cause problems far away from its source by pressing on nerves or secreting bioactive compounds. Upon diagnosis, it is important to obtain a tissue sample from the tumour in order to correctly classify the condition and reach a definitive diagnosis for maximal therapy and treatment. Table 10.6 describes various methods of obtaining tissue.

The pathologist then examines the tissue microscopically for the histological hallmarks of cancer detailed in the beginning of this chapter. A variety of clinically available tests further facilitate the classification of cancer, including immunohistochemical stains, flow cytometry, electron microscopy, chromosome analysis, and genetic studies.

Staging a cancer initially involves determining the size of the tumour, the degree to which it has locally invaded, and the extent to which it has spread (metastasized) (Figure 10.23). Staging uses many specific molecular tests and can be diverse, depending on the tumour. Staging generally consists of 4 stages with carcinoma in situ regarded as a special case: cancer confined to the organ of origin is stage 1; cancer that is locally invasive is stage 2; cancer that has spread to regional structures, such as lymph nodes, is stage 3; and cancer that has spread to distant sites, such as a liver cancer spreading to lung or a prostate cancer spreading to bone, is stage 4. The World Health Organization's TNM system: *T* indicates tumour spread, *N* indicates node involvement, and *M* indicates the presence of distant metastasis (see Figure 10.23) is a

TABLE 10.6 Obtaining Tissue: The Biopsy

Procedure	Purpose	Example
Excisional biopsy	The complete removal of area of interest, usually with a margin of normal tissue	Full resection (e.g., mastectomy, partial colectomy)
Incisional biopsy	The removal of a portion of a lesion	Lymph node biopsy, muscle mass biopsy
Core needle biopsy	The removal of tissue with a needle; often performed with direct vision, or guided with ultrasound or CT; provides an intact core tissue sample	Needle biopsy of prostate or liver mass
Fine needle aspirate	The removal of dissociated cells with a small-gauge needle for cytological study; does not preserve tissue structure	Thyroid, breast mass
Exfoliative cytology	The removal of cells shed from surface (e.g., from cervix, sputum [lung], or urine)	Brushings from lung or colon endoscopy

CT, Computed tomography.

TNM system for Staging Breast Cancer

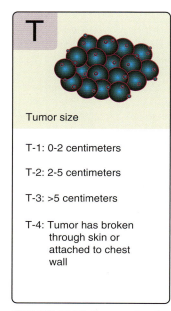
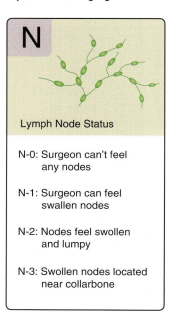
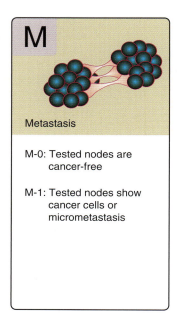

Tumor size
- T-1: 0-2 centimeters
- T-2: 2-5 centimeters
- T-3: >5 centimeters
- T-4: Tumor has broken through skin or attached to chest wall

Lymph Node Status
- N-0: Surgeon can't feel any nodes
- N-1: Surgeon can feel swollen nodes
- N-2: Nodes feel swollen and lumpy
- N-3: Swollen nodes located near collarbone

Metastasis
- M-0: Tested nodes are cancer-free
- M-1: Tested nodes show cancer cells or micrometastasis

FIGURE 10.23 Tumour Staging Using the TNM System. Example of staging for breast cancer. See figure for explanation of the abbreviations.

common scheme for standardizing the staging of cancer. The prognosis generally worsens with increasing tumour size, lymph node involvement, and metastasis. Staging may also alter the choice of therapy, with more aggressive therapy to treat and manage a more invasive disease.

Tumour Markers

Specific biochemical markers of tumours help with both cancer surveillance and its diagnosis. **Tumour markers** are substances produced by both benign and malignant cells that are either present in or on tumour cells or found in blood, spinal fluid, or urine. Tumour markers include hormones, enzymes, genes, antigens, and antibodies (Table 10.7). If the tumour marker itself has biological activity, then it can cause symptoms, such as those described in Table 10.7. For example, the adrenal medulla normally secretes the catecholamine epinephrine (adrenaline). Benign tumours of the adrenal medulla (pheochromocytoma) can produce catecholamines (e.g., adrenaline) in vast excess, leading to rapid pulse rate, high blood pressure, diaphoresis (i.e., sweating), and tremors. Detection of elevated blood or urine levels of catecholamines helps to confirm the diagnosis, and treatment of the disease relieves the symptoms. Tumour markers have three functions: (1) to screen and identify individuals at high risk for cancer; (2) to help diagnose the specific type of tumour in individuals with clinical manifestations relating to their tumour, as in adrenal tumours or enlarged liver or prostate; and (3) to follow the clinical course of a tumour.

There is still no tumour marker that can screen populations of healthy individuals for cancer.[58] A few normal individuals with test results at the high end of the normal distribution ("false positives") can lead to expensive and invasive additional tests (and unnecessary concern). Similarly, some individuals with the disease will have test results in the normal range (or "false negatives") and not receive the required therapy. More importantly, some nonmalignant conditions can also produce tumour markers. As such, the presence of an elevated tumour marker may suggest a specific diagnosis, but it is not a definitive diagnostic test. For example, prostate tumours secrete prostate-specific antigen (PSA) into the blood, but most men (approximately 75%) with elevated levels of PSA do not have cancer upon biopsy.[59] For every 1 000 men (ages 55 to 69) screened repeatedly, only zero to one prostate cancer–related death would be avoided, 100 to 120 men would undergo

TABLE 10.7 Examples of Tumour Markers

Marker Name	Nature	Type of Tumour
Adrenocorticotropic hormone (ACTH)	Peptide hormone	Pituitary adenomas
Alpha fetoprotein (AFP)	70-kDa protein	Hepatic, germ cell
Beta-human chorionic gonadotropin (β-HCG)	Glycopeptide hormone	Germ cell
Cancer agent (CA)15-3/CA27.29	Protein antigen	Breast
CA-125	Glycoprotein antigen	Ovary
Carcinoembryonic antigen (CEA)	200-kDa glycoprotein	Gastro-intestinal, pancreas, lung, breast, etc.
Catecholamines	Epinephrine and precursors	Pheochromocytoma (adrenal medulla)
Estrogen receptor (ER)/progesterone receptor (PR)	Extracted receptor	Breast
Homovanillic acid/vanillylmandelic acid (HVA/VMA)	Catecholamine metabolites	Neuroblastoma
Prostate-specific antigen (PSA)	33-kDa glycoprotein	Prostate
Urinary Bence Jones protein	Immunoglobulin light chain	Multiple myeloma

> **BOX 10.1 Types of Genetic Lesions in Cancer**
>
> 1. Point mutations
> 2. Subtle alterations (insertions, deletions)
> 3. Chromosome changes (aneuploidy and loss of heterozygosity)
> 4. Amplifications
> 5. Gene silencing (DNA methylation, histone modification, microRNAs)
> 6. Exogenous sequences (tumour viruses)

unnecessary biopsies with some complications, and 110 men would be diagnosed with prostate cancer (frequently slow growing and not life-threatening), and 50 of these would have major complications related to treatment.[60] However, falling levels of PSA after radiation or surgical therapy may actually indicate successful treatment for prostate cancer, and a later rise may indicate a recurrence. Identification of ideal sensitive and specific tumour markers of common cancers remains a high priority because the early detection of cancer often improves the treatment outcome.

Classification of Tumours: Classic Histology and Modern Genetics

Classification of cancer helps to identify the types of genetic lesions in cancer and influences the choice of therapy (Box 10.1). Gross and light microscopic appearance initially dictated treatment decisions, and now incorporates immunohistochemical analysis of protein expression as well. Increasingly, this immunohistochemical analysis involves more extensive genetic analysis of the tumours. The range of genetic analysis is expanding rapidly. A single gene may be examined (e.g., to determine whether there is a characteristic chromosomal translocation diagnostic of CML), or a panel of genes and proteins may be examined (e.g., in breast cancer) to determine if the tumour expresses estrogen receptor, progesterone receptor, and the EGF receptor HER2, or if there are mutations in specific genes that modify response to therapy. In a research setting and increasingly in clinical settings, the polymerase chain reaction (PCR) (amplifying small amounts of DNA for further study), microarray (which can detect thousands of genes at the same time), or advanced DNA sequencing technology can measure global gene expression and mutation analysis. These analyses classify tumours more precisely and may predict the most effective therapy. This detailed analysis of each tumour is a form of personalized medicine that offers therapy based on a very detailed knowledge of the characteristics of each individual's specific cancer.[61] This enhanced molecular characterization subdivides cancers into therapeutically and prognostically relevant smaller groups. As an example, there are now four types of breast cancers (luminal A, luminal B, basal-like, and others) based on their expression of specific markers, such as estrogen receptor, HER2/neu (a type of receptor tyrosine kinase), and other specific genes and proteins. Each subtype has a different response to therapy and a different prognosis.

Treatment

Until late in the last century, the mainstays of cancer therapy have been surgery, chemotherapy, and radiation therapy. These approaches have been highly successful for certain types of cancer but have many limitations. Cancer therapy is now in a process of rapid evolution. Armed with a clearer understanding that cancer is, in fact, multiple diseases that share general hallmarks and enablers, and that the specific mechanisms underlying each hallmark may vary considerably among cancers (e.g., the large variety of oncogenes that may be used to differentiate cancers), modern cancer therapy is reaching a stage where complete genetic analysis of an individual cancer may determine the appropriate combination of therapies (e.g., immunotherapy and targeted monoclonal antibodies for tumour markers). Thus, effective therapy may include a combination of reagents targeting several hallmarks and under constant modification to target the evolving cancer cells.

Surgery

Surgery plays many roles in the care of individuals with cancer. Surgery is often the definitive treatment of cancers that do not spread beyond the limits of surgical excision. It also is indicated for the relief of symptoms, for example, those caused by tumour mass obstruction. In selected high-risk diseases, surgery also plays a role in the prevention of cancer. For example, individuals with familial adenomatous polyposis because of germline mutations of the *APC* gene have close to a 100% lifetime risk of colon cancer, so a prophylactic colectomy is indicated. Similarly, women with *BRCA1/2* mutations have a markedly increased risk of breast and ovarian cancer and often choose prophylactic mastectomy or bilateral salpingo-oophorectomy (removal of ovaries and fallopian tubes), or both.

Key principles apply specifically to cancer surgery, including obtaining adequate surgical margins during a resection to prevent local recurrences, placing needle tracks and biopsy incision scars (that may be contaminated with cancer cells) carefully so they can be removed in subsequent incisions, avoiding the spread of cancer cells during surgical procedures through careful technique, and paying attention to obtaining adequate tissue specimens during biopsies so that the pathologist can be confident of the diagnosis. Additionally, the surgeon provides critical staging information by inspection, sampling, and removal of local and regional lymph nodes during procedures.

Radiation Therapy

Radiation therapy is used to kill cancer cells while minimizing damage to normal structures. Ionizing radiation damages cells by imparting enough energy to cause molecular damage, especially to DNA. The damage may be (1) lethal, in which the cell is killed by radiation; (2) potentially lethal, in which the cell is so severely affected by radiation that modifications in its environment will cause it to die; or (3) sublethal, in which the cell can subsequently repair itself. Cellular compartments with rapidly renewing cells are, in general, more radiosensitive. Effective cell killing by radiation also requires good local delivery of oxygen, something not always present in large cancers. Radiation produces slow changes in most cancers and irreversible changes in normal tissues as well. Because of these irreversible changes, each tissue has a maximum lifetime dose of radiation it can tolerate. Radiation is well suited to treat localized disease in areas that are hard to reach surgically: for example, in the brain and pelvis. A number of radiation delivery methods are available, with external beam being the most common. Radiation sources, such as small ^{125}I-labelled capsules (also called *seeds*), can also be temporarily placed into body cavities, a delivery method termed brachytherapy. Brachytherapy is useful in the treatment of cervical, prostate, and head and neck cancers.

Chemotherapy

The era of modern chemotherapy began with the observation in World War II that mustard gas exposure caused suppression of the bone marrow. Furthermore, related compounds, such as nitrogen mustard and cyclophosphamide (Procytox), produced clinical responses in hematological malignancies, including lymphomas. Also, in the late 1940s, the remarkable clinical observation that the vitamin folic acid could *increase* leukemia growth led to the development of antifolate medications (leading ultimately to methotrexate [Apo-Methotrexate]) that produced remissions in previously untreatable leukemia.

All chemotherapeutic agents take advantage of specific vulnerabilities in target cancer cells. *Antimetabolites*, such as methotrexate and L-asparaginase (Elspar), block normal growth pathways in all cells, but leukemia and other cancer cells are exquisitely sensitive to folic acid and asparagine deprivation, whereas nonmalignant cells are far less sensitive. Similarly, some cancer cells are highly sensitive to *DNA-damaging agents*, such as cyclophosphamide and anthracyclines, because of the oncogenic mutations that accelerate the cell cycle and DNA synthesis. Vincristine (Oncovin) and the taxanes block the formation of the microtubule that is required for mitosis, thus preventing the cancer cell from undergoing further replication (see Chapter 1).

Single chemotherapeutic agents often shrink cancers, but these medications given alone rarely, if ever, provide a cure. Hence, chemotherapy medications are usually given in combinations designed to attack a cancer from many different weaknesses at the same time and to limit the dose and the toxicity of any single agent. Cancers contain a very large number of cells, and commonly a small fraction of those cells may be resistant to a particular medication. However, those cells are likely to be sensitive to the second or third medication in a chemotherapy cocktail. Scheduling of medication administration is also very important, with many studies showing cancers are more likely to develop medication resistance if there are significant delays between planned courses of chemotherapy.

There are many distinct purposes of chemotherapy. **Induction chemotherapy** seeks to cause shrinkage or disappearance of tumours. In Hodgkin's disease, for example, chemotherapy alone can be used in some cases to cure the disease. In other settings, chemotherapy may shrink the tumour and improve symptoms without ultimately providing a cure. **Adjuvant chemotherapy** is given after surgical excision of a cancer with the goal of eliminating micrometastases. **Neoadjuvant chemotherapy** is given before localized (surgical or radiation) treatment of a cancer. As with induction chemotherapy, the effectiveness, or lack thereof, of neoadjuvant therapy can be measured (e.g., with follow-up scans). Neoadjuvant therapy can shrink a cancer so that surgery may spare more normal tissue. For example, in the bone cancer osteogenic sarcoma, neoadjuvant therapy often converts a large tumour mass into a much smaller mass, allowing the surgeon to perform a limb-sparing excision rather than an amputation.

Immunotherapy

The expression of unique antigens on cancer cells that can be targeted by T cells has driven the quest for effective therapies to initiate an immune response, boost a currently inadequate immune response, or convert a tumour-protective immune response to a destructive one. Since the 1950s this quest has been characterized by promises and frustrations. The Nobel Prize in Physiology or Medicine 2018 was awarded jointly to James P. Allison and Tasuku Honjo for their discovery of cancer therapy by inhibition of negative immune regulation.[62]

Vaccines have also been extremely effective in protecting us against infective agents. Although they generally induce a prophylactic immune response, at least one vaccine (against rabies) is administered after the infection. Vaccines against oncogenic viruses provide protection and prevent the onset of viral-induced tumours. For approximately 50 years, numerous potential therapeutic vaccines have been tested with little success. Initially, whole tumour cell vaccines prepared from an individual's own cancer (autologous) or from cancers from other individuals (allogeneic) were used, with or without adjuvants that induced inflammatory responses (e.g., bacille Calmette-Guérin [BCG]) or augmented the vaccine's immunogenicity. Several allogeneic cancer cell vaccines continue to be tested. So far, none has been shown to be effective enough to be licensed. Other approaches have included immunization with:

- Protein extracts from cancers
- Peptides that represented the epitope from these proteins
- Dendritic cells that have processed and present cancer antigens
- DNA containing the genetic sequence for cancer antigens that transfects the recipient's cells and expresses that antigen
- Viral vectors that contain the genetic information for cancer antigens[63]

Sipuleucel-T (Provenge) is one such drug that has been approved for the treatment of metastatic prostate cancer that is resistant to conventional therapy and has been available in Canada since February 2015. Dendritic cells are obtained from an individual with prostate cancer and incubated with a protein resulting from the fusion of prostatic acid phosphatase, a cancer antigen found in 95% of prostate cancers, and granulocyte-macrophage colony-stimulating factor, an immune cell stimulating cytokine. The dendritic cells process and present the antigen and are infused back into the patient. In clinical trials, treatment with sipuleucel-T extended the lives of patients by 4.1 months. These results may not seem spectacular, but they were meaningful in this group of patients with very advanced and terminal disease. The medication is extremely costly, at over $100 000 per treatment. Other vaccine approaches against B-cell lymphoma and melanoma have shown promising results.[64]

Passive immunotherapy using lymphocytes against cancer cell antigens is also available but with limited success. In recent years, passive administration of tumour-targeting lymphocytes (adoptive cell therapy [ACT]) has improved the effectiveness of cancer treatment as well. A major source of patient's lymphocytes is those that have infiltrated the tumour.[65] The efficacy of these cells is increased by depleting the Treg cells within the population or by engineering the T-cell receptor for greater specificity against the tumour.[66]

A family of monoclonal antibodies, called *checkpoint inhibitors*, is under investigation. These antibodies are directed against costimulatory molecules involved in repressing T-cell immune responses (see Chapter 7). By blocking inhibitory signals, Tc cells may retain tumour-killing capacity.

Targeted Disruption of Cancer

As discussed previously, cancers appear to share a variety of hallmarks that contribute to the malignant phenotype. Recent molecular and genetic analyses of groups of cancer can classify an individual's cancer by the spectrum of mutations underlying the cancer phenotype.[67] However, each of the therapeutic approaches described previously generally treats specific vulnerabilities of the cancer rather than a variety of contributing factors. That approach is not successful in most invasive cancers because some cancer cells may undergo further mutation, leading to therapeutic resistance.

Exceptions include targeted medications, used in combination with conventional chemotherapy, against very specific characteristics of selected cancers. For example, imatinib is a competitive inhibitor of tyrosine kinases, primarily the BCR-ABL tyrosine kinase (Table 10.8). It is highly effective in treating CML but ineffective in virtually all other cancers. Monoclonal antibodies against the CD20 antigen expressed on some B-cell lymphomas, the EGF receptor on colon cancers and head and neck cancers, and the EGF receptor HER2 on breast cancer are relatively successful.[68] These medications are so tightly targeted they have much less toxicity than conventional chemotherapies that have targets in virtually all cells.

Tumour growth and progression is dependent on a variety of mutations leading to expression of oncogenes, inactivation of tumour-suppressor molecules, and interactions with inflammatory cells in the tumour microenvironment that foster angiogenesis, resistance to apoptosis and immune-mediated cancer cell death, altered tumour cell

TABLE 10.8 Examples of Molecular-Era Anticancer Medications

Medication (Trade Name)	Type of Medication	Molecular Target	Disease
Imatinib (Gleevec)	Small molecule TKI	BCR-ABL tyrosine kinase, FGF receptor tyrosine kinase	Chronic myeloid leukemia, gastro-intestinal stromal tumour
Erlotinib (Tarceva)	Small molecule TKI	EGF receptor tyrosine kinase	Subset of lung cancer
Trastuzumab (Herceptin)	Monoclonal antibody	HER2 receptor tyrosine kinase	HER2-positive breast cancer
Bevacizumab (Avastin)	Monoclonal antibody	VEGFR	Advanced colorectal cancer
Rituximab (Rituxan)	Monoclonal antibody	CD20 antigen on B lymphocytes	B-cell malignancies

EGF, Epidermal growth factor; *FGF*, fibroblast growth factor; *HER2*, human epidermal growth factor receptor 2; *TKI*, tyrosine kinase inhibitor; *VEGFR*, vascular endothelial growth factor receptor.

metabolism, and metastasis. A more efficacious therapeutic approach, therefore, may be a combination of medications highly targeted to cancer hallmarks.[69]

The National Cancer Institute lists more than 25 medications as cancer-targeting agents that inactivate oncogenes, block angiogenesis, and affect cancer cell metabolism.[70] Monoclonal antibodies are available that induce apoptosis in tumour-infiltrating cells such as TAM, Treg cells, and tumour endothelium.[71] Additionally, specific antagonists may neutralize the effects of cytokines, chemokines, and other tumour-enhancing mediators produced in the tumour microenvironment.[72] These antagonists are usually in the form of monoclonal antibodies, which are available against TNF-α, VEGF, HER2, and other ligands and their receptors. Such highly specific targeting would minimize secondary toxic effects.

CASE STUDY

Mrs. Haines, age 35, has been coughing up blood for a month. A biopsy confirms small cell lung cancer (SCLC) Stage III as a diagnosis. Treatment will consist of chemotherapy for three cycles, starting next week. In addition, she will start radiation therapy after one cycle of chemotherapy.

Critical Thinking and Clinical Judgement Questions
1. What information do you think the patient needs to know?
2. What are some clinical manifestations of cancer the nurse would expect to see with their assessment?
3. a) What does Stage III mean? b) What is the purpose of staging a cancer?

DID YOU UNDERSTAND?

Cancer Terminology and Characteristics
1. Benign tumours are usually encapsulated and well differentiated and do not spread to distant locations.
2. Malignant tumours, compared with benign tumours, have more rapid growth rates, specific microscopic alterations (anaplasia, loss of differentiation), absence of normal tissue organization, and no capsule. They invade blood vessels and lymphatics and have distant metastases.
3. Carcinomas arise from epithelial tissue, and leukemias are cancers of blood-forming cells. Carcinoma in situ (CIS) refers to noninvasive epithelial tumours of glandular or squamous cell origin.

The Biology of Cancer Cells
1. Genetic changes are the basis of cancer. These changes include small and large DNA mutations that alter genes, chromosomes, and noncoding RNAs, as well as epigenetic changes because of altered chemical modifications of DNA and histones.
2. The incidence of cancer increases with age as the individual acquires genetic hits or mutations with time. Mutations activate growth-promotion pathways, block antigrowth signals, prevent apoptosis, stimulate telomerase and new blood vessel growth, and allow tissue invasion and distant metastasis.
3. Some mutations are more important for cancer progression. These mutations can be called *driver mutations*. *Passenger mutations* are random mutations that presumably do not contribute to cancer progression.
4. Key genetic mechanisms have a role in human carcinogenesis: (a) mutations of proto-oncogenes, resulting in hyperactivity of growth-related gene products (such genes are called *oncogenes*); (b) mutation of genes, resulting in loss or inactivity of gene products that normally would inhibit growth (such genes are called *tumour-suppressor genes*); and (c) mutation of caretaker genes that normally prevent mutations.
5. Oncogenes are independent of normal regulatory mechanisms and signal uncontrolled proliferation.
6. Some oncogenes, such as *RAS*, result from point mutations.
7. Oncogenes can result from genetic translocations. The Philadelphia chromosome in chronic myeloid leukemia (CML) results from a translocation that creates a novel protein fusion of the *BCR* and *ABL* genes and expression of an unregulated promoter of cell growth.
8. Tumour-suppressor genes must be inactivated in cancer cells by mutations to each allele, one from each parent.
9. A common mutation in cancer cells is inactivation of the tumour-suppressor gene tumour protein p53 *(TP53)*, which controls expression of many genes that repair DNA damage, suppression of cellular proliferation during genomic repair, and initiation of apoptosis. Inactivation of p53 results in increased mutation rates and cancer.
10. Caretaker genes are responsible for maintaining genomic integrity. Inherited mutations can disrupt caretaker genes and cause chromosome instability.

11. Abnormal gene silencing is emerging as a major factor in cancer progression. Gene expression can be regulated in a heritable manner (i.e., passed from a parent to a child or from a single cell to its progeny) by an "epigenetic" mechanism called *silencing*.
12. In rare families, an initial inheritable mutation in a tumour-suppressor gene, such as *TP53*, the retinoblastoma gene *(RB)*, or the breast cancer genes *(BRCA1* and *BRCA2)*, may lead to a greatly increased risk of developing particular cancers.
13. Changes in gene regulation can affect not just single genes but entire networks of signalling. Gene expression networks can be regulated by changes in microRNAs (miRNAs or miRs) and other ncRNAs.
14. Cancer cells are immortal.
15. When they reach a critical age, cancer cells activate telomerase to restore and maintain their telomeres, thereby allowing cancer cells to divide repeatedly or become immortal.
16. Like many normal adult tissues, cancers can contain rare stem cells that provide a source of immortal cells. To fully eradicate a cancer, it may be necessary to target the cancer stem cell.
17. Access to the vascular system is essential for tumour growth.
18. Stromal cells and cancer cells can secrete multiple factors, such as vascular endothelial growth factor (VEGF), that stimulate new blood vessel growth (called *neovascularization* or *angiogenesis*).
19. The successful cancer cell divides rapidly, with the consequent requirement for the building blocks of new cells; cancer cell division often occurs in a hypoxic and acidic environment. Many cancer genes also encourage aerobic glycolysis and promote high glucose utilization of a cancer.
20. In cancer, defects in the intrinsic or extrinsic pathways, or both, provide resistance to apoptotic cell death.
21. Overexpression of B-cell lymphoma 2 (Bcl-2) blocks apoptosis in most follicular B-cell lymphomas.
22. Some conditions of chronic inflammation increase the risk of developing cancer. A prime example is the association between gastric cancer and infection with *Helicobacter pylori*.
23. Cells recruited to the tumour microenvironment are essential to the growth and spread of cancer and are active participants in induction of cellular proliferation, angiogenesis, degradation of extracellular matrix (ECM), suppression of infiltrating immune cells, and the development and spread of metastatic cells.
24. Unique antigens and other markers on tumour cells can be recognized by T lymphocytes and natural killer cells of the immune system, leading to destruction of the tumour cell.
25. Cancer cells can evade rejection by the immune system by production of immunosuppressive factors, induction of immunosuppressive T-regulatory cells, evolution of tumour–antigen-negative variants, or suppressed expression of antigen-presenting MHC class I molecules.
26. Antibodies induced by vaccines against oncogenic viruses, such as human papillomavirus (HPV) and hepatitis B virus (HBV), protect against initial infection and development of cervical and liver tumours, respectively.
27. Defects in the immune system increase the risk of viral-associated cancers but have a minimal effect on the risk of other cancers.
28. Metastasis is the major cause of death from cancer.
29. Metastasis is a complex process that requires cells to have many new abilities, including the ability to invade, survive, and proliferate in a new environment.
30. Carcinomas undergo a process of epithelial-mesenchymal transition (EMT) during which many epithelial-like characteristics are lost (e.g., polarity, adhesion to basement membrane), resulting in increased migratory capacity, increased resistance to apoptosis, and a dedifferentiated stem cell–like state that favours growth in foreign microenvironments and establishment of metastatic disease.
31. Invasion consists of loss of cell-to-cell contact, degradation of the ECM, and migration of tumour cells to the vascular or lymphatic systems. Stromal cells, particularly tumour-associated macrophages (TAMs), are essential to this process.
32. Some cancers appear to selectively home to particular metastatic sites, which may be a result of expression of particular receptors for ligands expressed by cells at the site.

Clinical Manifestations of Cancer

1. Paraneoplastic syndromes are rare symptom complexes, often caused by biologically active substances released from a tumour or by an immune response triggered by a tumour, that manifest as symptoms not directly caused by the local effects of the cancer.
2. Clinical manifestations of cancer include pain, fatigue, cachexia, anemia, leukopenia, thrombocytopenia, and infection.
3. Pain is generally associated with the late stages of cancer. It can be caused by pressure, obstruction, invasion of a structure sensitive to pain, stretching, tissue destruction, and inflammation.
4. Fatigue is the most frequently reported symptom of cancer and cancer treatment.
5. Cachexia is a multiorgan syndrome with many clinical manifestations including anorexia; muscle wasting; thermogenesis; altered heart and liver function; gut malabsorption; early satiety; taste alterations; and altered protein, lipid, and carbohydrate metabolism. Two factors are most significant: muscle loss and inflammation. Muscle wasting involves many protein signalling pathways and inflammatory mediators. Profoundly altered are both appetite-stimulating and appetite-suppressing brain pathways.
6. Anemia associated with cancer usually occurs because of malnutrition, chronic bleeding and resultant iron deficiency, chemotherapy, radiation, and malignancies in the blood-forming organs.
7. Leukopenia is usually a result of chemotherapy (which is toxic to bone marrow) or radiation (which kills circulating leukocytes).
8. Thrombocytopenia is usually the result of chemotherapy or malignancy in the bone marrow.
9. Infection may be caused by leukopenia, immunosuppression, or debility associated with advanced disease. It is the most significant cause of complications and death.
10. The gastro-intestinal tract relies on rapidly growing cells to provide an absorptive surface for nutrients. Both chemotherapy and radiation therapy may cause decreased cell turnover, thereby leading to oral ulcers (stomatitis), malabsorption, and diarrhea.
11. Alopecia (hair loss) results from chemotherapy effects on hair follicles. Alopecia is usually temporary, although hair may initially regrow with a different texture. Not all chemotherapeutic agents cause alopecia. Decreased renewal rates of the epidermal layers in the skin may lead to skin breakdown and dryness, altering the normal barrier protection against infection.

Diagnosis, Characterization, and Treatment of Cancer

1. The diagnosis of cancer requires a biopsy and examination of tumour tissue by a pathologist. Cancer classification is established by a variety of tests.
2. Tumour staging involves the size of the tumour, the degree to which it has locally invaded, and the extent to which it has spread. A standard scheme for staging is the T (tumour spread), N (node involvement), and M (metastasis) system.

3. The classification, and hence the treatment decisions, of cancers was originally based on gross and light microscopic appearance and is now commonly accompanied by immunohistochemical analysis of protein expression. Increasingly, staging is supplemented by a more extensive molecular analysis of the tumours.
4. Tumour markers are substances (i.e., hormones, enzymes, genes, antigens, antibodies) found in cancer cells and in blood, spinal fluid, or urine. They are used to screen and identify individuals at high risk for cancer, to help diagnose specific types of tumours, and to follow the clinical course of cancer.
5. Cancer is treated routinely with surgery, radiation therapy, chemotherapy, and combinations of these modalities.
6. Surgical therapy is used for nonmetastatic disease (in which cure is possible by removing the tumour) and as a palliative measure to alleviate symptoms.
7. Ionizing radiation causes cell damage; therefore, the goal of radiation therapy is to damage the tumour without causing excessive toxicity or damage to nondiseased structures.
8. The theoretical basis of chemotherapy is the vulnerability of tumour cells in various stages of the cell cycle.
9. Modern chemotherapy uses combinations of medications with different targets and different toxicities.
10. Immunotherapy attempts to modify the immune system from a cancer-protective state to a destructive condition.
11. Future treatment of tumours will, most likely, use a careful histological and genetic analysis of individual cancers that prescribes a combination of tumour-targeting medications to simultaneously disrupt multiple hallmarks of that particular cancer.

11

Cancer Epidemiology

Stephanie Zettel, with originating chapter contributions by Kathryn L. McCance and Lois E. Brenneman

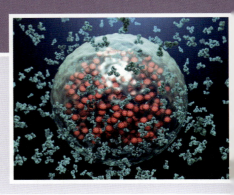

Additional resources are available online at https://evolve.elsevier.com/Canada/Huether/pathophysiology.

CHAPTER OUTLINE

Genetics, Epigenetics, and Tissue, 266
Incidence and Mortality Trends, 272
In Utero and Early Life Conditions, 272
Environmental and Lifestyle Factors, 274
  Tobacco Use, 274
  Diet, 276
  Nutrition, Obesity, Alcohol Consumption, and Physical Activity: Impacts on Cancer, 276

Ionizing Radiation, 282
Ultraviolet Radiation, 285
Electromagnetic Radiation, 287
Infection, and Sexual and Reproductive Behaviour, 288
Other Viruses and Microorganisms, 288
Air Pollution, 289
Chemical and Occupational Hazards as Carcinogens, 289

LEARNING OBJECTIVES

1. Describe why smoking and exposure to radiation are major risk factors for cancer and how they alter cellular structure and function.
2. Identify why lifestyle factors and environment are thought to be more important than genetics for the development of cancer.
3. Describe how effects in utero and early in life can lead to future cancer diagnoses.
4. Discuss the importance of diet in relation to cancer.
5. Identify why obesity increases mortality rates in some cancer types.
6. Discuss the effects of alcohol consumption on cancer risk.
7. Describe the bystander effect.
8. Describe the effects of ultraviolet radiation on the skin.
9. Identify potential sources of electromagnetic radiation and why they might be controversial.
10. Identify risk factors for HPV and cervical cancer.

KEY TERMS

Abscopal, 284
Asbestos-silicate mineral, 290
Basal cell carcinoma (BCC), 285
Bystander effect, 284
Developmental plasticity, 272
Environmental tobacco smoke (ETS), 274
Genomic instability, 284
Individual carcinogen, 266
Melanoma, 285
Methylome, 273
Nontargeted effect, 284
Nutrigenomics, 276
Particulate matter (PM), 289
Phase I activation enzymes, 278
Phase II detoxification enzymes, 278
Radiofrequency electromagnetic radiation (RF-EMR), 287
Radon, 289
Squamous cell carcinoma (SCC), 285
UV radiation, 285
Xenobiotic, 278

Although cancer has multiple etiologies, avoiding high-risk behaviours and exposure to **individual carcinogens** (cancer-causing substances) can prevent many types of cancer (Figure 11.1). Lifestyle behaviours, dietary and environmental factors, and occupational exposure contribute to the number of cancer cases and death[1–3] and any of the following factors can contribute to the development of cancer:[4–6]
- Lifestyle choices, such as smoking, alcohol use, and nutritional intake
- Lack of physical exercise; overweight, obesity
- Infections, sexual practices
- Environmental conditions, including exposure to sunlight, natural and medical radiation, workplace exposures, and involuntary or unknown exposures
- Prescribed and illicit medications
- Socioeconomic factors that affect exposures and susceptibility
- Carcinogenic substances present in air, water, and soil

There is much variation in environmental factors and their attributable risk for cancer. The International Agency for Research on Cancer (IARC) completed a review of the more than 100 chemicals, occupations, physical agents, biological agents, and other agents classified as carcinogenic to humans.[4] Table 11.1 contains a simplified table with a list of classifications by cancer sites.

GENETICS, EPIGENETICS, AND TISSUE

> ✓ **QUICK CHECK 11.1**
> 1. Describe what is meant by the statement "environment is the main cause of cancer."
> 2. What is the role of the microenvironment in cancer development and progression?

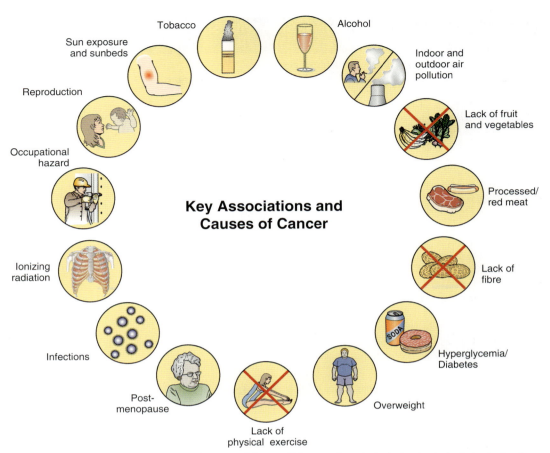

FIGURE 11.1 Key Associations and Causes of Cancer. Tobacco, diet, alcohol, obesity, lack of physical activity, hormones, infections, ionizing radiation, occupational hazards, reproductive factors, and ultraviolet light are key factors for cancer. Although diet is key and known to affect cancer risk, identifying specific dietary factors that elevate risk has been very difficult.

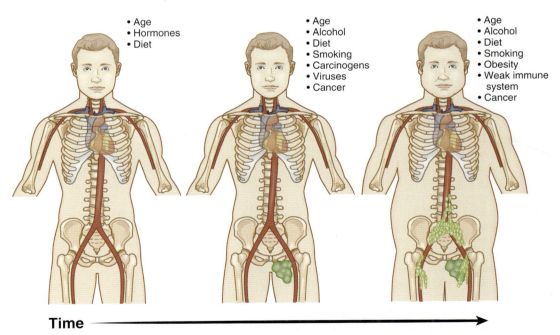

FIGURE 11.2 Environmental Factors and Genetic, Epigenetic, and Other Host Factors. Over time a person's internal genetic makeup persistently interacts with external or environmental factors. Environmental factors (e.g., diet, smoking, alcohol use, hormones, certain viruses, chemical carcinogens) collectively interact with internal epigenetic factors and genetic mutations to destabilize normal biological factors including immune factors for balancing growth and maturation. (Adapted from National Cancer Institute. [2007]. *Understanding cancer series: cancer: inside and outside factors*. National Cancer Institute, National Institutes of Health.)

TABLE 11.1 List of Classifications by Cancer Sites With Sufficient or Limited Evidence in Humans

Cancer Site	Carcinogenic Agents With Sufficient Evidence in Humans	Agents With Limited Evidence in Humans
Lip, Oral Cavity, and Pharynx		
Lip		Solar radiation
Oral cavity	Alcoholic beverages Betel quid with tobacco Betel quid without tobacco Human papillomavirus (HPV) type 16 Tobacco, smokeless Tobacco smoking	
Salivary gland	X-radiation, γ-radiation	Radioiodines, including iodine-131
Tonsil	HPV-16	
Pharynx	Alcoholic beverages Betel quid with tobacco HPV-16 Tobacco smoking	Asbestos (all forms) Mate drinking, hot Printing presses Tobacco smoke, secondhand
Nasopharynx	Epstein-Barr virus (EBV) Formaldehyde Salted fish, Chinese style Wood dust	
Digestive tract, upper	Acetaldehyde associated with consumption of alcoholic beverages	
Digestive Organs		
Esophagus	Acetaldehyde associated with consumption of alcoholic beverages Alcoholic beverages Betel quid with tobacco Betel quid without tobacco Tobacco, smokeless Tobacco smoking X-radiation, γ-radiation	Dry cleaning Mate drinking, hot Pickled vegetables (traditional Asian) Rubber production industry Tetrachloroethylene
Stomach	*Helicobacter pylori* Rubber production industry Tobacco smoking X-radiation, γ-radiation	Asbestos (all forms) EBV Lead compounds, inorganic Nitrate or nitrite (ingested) under conditions that result in endogenous nitrosation Pickled vegetables (traditional Asian) Salted fish (Chinese style)
Colon and rectum	Alcoholic beverages Tobacco smoking X-radiation, γ-radiation	Asbestos (all forms) *Schistosoma japonicum*
Anus	Human immunodeficiency virus type 1 (HIV-1) HPV-16	HPV-18, HPV-33
Liver and bile duct	Aflatoxins Alcoholic beverages *Clonorchis sinensis* Estrogen-progestogen contraceptives Hepatitis B virus (HBV) Hepatitis C virus (HCV) *Opisthorchis viverrini* Plutonium Thorium-232 and its decay products Tobacco smoking (in smokers and in smokers' children) Vinyl chloride	Androgenic (anabolic) steroids Arsenic and inorganic arsenic compounds Betel quid without tobacco HIV-1 Polychlorinated biphenyls *S. japonicum* Trichloroethylene X-radiation, γ-radiation
Gallbladder	Thorium-232 and its decay products	
Pancreas	Tobacco, smokeless Tobacco smoking	Alcoholic beverages Thorium-232 and its decay products X-radiation, γ-radiation
Digestive tract, unspecified		Radioiodines, including iodine-131

TABLE 11.1 **List of Classifications by Cancer Sites With Sufficient or Limited Evidence in Humans—cont'd**

Cancer Site	Carcinogenic Agents With Sufficient Evidence in Humans	Agents With Limited Evidence in Humans
Respiratory Organs		
Nasal cavity and paranasal sinus	Isopropyl alcohol production Leather dust Nickel compounds Radium-226 and its decay products Radium-228 and its decay products Tobacco smoking Wood dust	Carpentry and joinery Chromium (VI) compounds Formaldehyde Textile manufacturing
Larynx	Acid mists, strong inorganic Alcoholic beverages Asbestos (all forms) Tobacco smoking	HPV-16 Mate drinking, hot Rubber production industry Sulphur mustard Tobacco smoke, secondhand
Lung	Aluminum production Arsenic and inorganic arsenic compounds Beryllium and beryllium products Bis(chloromethyl) ether; chloromethyl methyl ether (technical grade) Cadmium and cadmium compounds Chromium (VI) compounds Coal, indoor emissions from household combustion Coal gasification Coal-tar pitch Coke production Hematite mining (underground) Iron and steel founding MOPP (vincristine-prednisone-nitrogen mustard-procarbazine mixture) Nickel compounds Painting Plutonium Radon-222 and its decay products Rubber production industry Silica dust, crystalline Soot Sulphur mustard Tobacco smoke, secondhand Tobacco smoking X-radiation, γ-radiation	Acid mists, strong inorganic Art glass, glass containers, and pressed ware (manufacture of) Biomass fuel (primarily wood), indoor emissions from household combustion of Bitumens, oxidized, and their emissions during roofing Bitumens, hard, and their emissions during mastic asphalt work Carbon electrode manufacture α-Chlorinated toluenes and benzyl chloride (combined exposure) Cobalt metal with tungsten carbide Creosotes Engine exhaust, diesel Frying, emissions from high-temperature Insecticides, nonarsenical (occupational exposures in spraying and application) Printing processes 2,3,7,8-Tetrachlorodibenzo-*para*-dioxin Welding fumes
Bone, Skin, Mesothelium, Endothelium, and Soft Tissue		
Bone	Plutonium Radium-224 and its decay products Radium-226 and its decay products Radium-228 and its decay products X-radiation, γ-radiation	Radioiodines, including iodine-131
Skin (melanoma)	Solar radiation Ultraviolet-emitting tanning devices	
Skin (other malignant neoplasms)	Arsenic and inorganic arsenic compounds Azathioprine Coal-tar distillation Coal-tar pitch Cyclosporine Methoxypsoralen plus ultraviolet A Mineral oils, untreated or mildly treated Shale oils Solar radiation Soot X-radiation, γ-radiation	Creosotes HIV-1 HPV-5 and HPV-8 (in individuals with epidermodysplasia verruciformis) Nitrogen mustard Petroleum refining (occupational exposures) Ultraviolet-emitting tanning devices Merkel cell polyomavirus (MCPyV)

Continued

TABLE 11.1 **List of Classifications by Cancer Sites With Sufficient or Limited Evidence in Humans—cont'd**

Cancer Site	Carcinogenic Agents With Sufficient Evidence in Humans	Agents With Limited Evidence in Humans
Mesothelium (pleura and peritoneum)	Asbestos (all forms) Erionite Painting	
Endothelium (Kaposi sarcoma)	HIV-1 Kaposi sarcoma herpesvirus	
Soft tissue		Polychlorophenols or their sodium salts (combined exposures) Radioiodines, including iodine-131 2,3,7,8-Tetrachlorodibenzo-*p*-dioxin
Breast and Female Genital Organs		
Breast	Alcoholic beverages Diethylstilbestrol Estrogen–progestogen contraceptives Estrogen–progestogen menopausal therapy X-radiation, γ-radiation	Estrogen menopausal therapy Ethylene oxide Shiftwork that involves circadian disruption Tobacco smoking
Vulva	HPV-16	HIV-1
Vagina	Diethylstilbestrol (exposure in utero) HPV-16	HIV-1
Uterine cervix	Diethylstilbestrol (exposure in utero) Estrogen–progestogen contraceptives HIV-1 HPV-16, 18, 31, 33, 35, 39, 45, 51, 52, 56, 58, 59 Tobacco smoking	HPV-26, 53, 66, 67, 68, 70, 73, 82 Tetrachloroethylene
Endometrium	Estrogen menopausal therapy Estrogen–progestogen menopausal therapy Tamoxifen	Diethylstilbestrol
Ovary	Asbestos (all forms) Estrogen menopausal therapy Tobacco smoking	Talc-based body powder (perineal use) X-radiation, γ-radiation
Male Genital Organs		
Penis	HPV-16	HIV-1 HPV-18
Prostate		Androgenic (anabolic) steroids Arsenic and inorganic arsenic compounds Cadmium and cadmium compounds Rubber production industry Thorium-232 and its decay products X-radiation, γ-radiation
Testis		Diethylstilbestrol exposure in utero
Urinary Tract		
Kidney	Tobacco smoking X-radiation, γ-radiation	Arsenic and inorganic arsenic compounds Cadmium and cadmium compounds Printing processes
Renal pelvis and ureter	Aristolochic acids, plants containing phenacetin Phenacetin, analgesic mixtures containing Tobacco smoking	Aristolochic acids
Urinary bladder	Aluminum production 4-Aminobiphenyl Arsenic and inorganic arsenic compounds Auramine production Benzidine Chlornaphazine Cyclophosphamide Magenta production 2-Naphthylamine	4-Chloro-*ortho*-toluidine Coal-tar pitch Coffee Dry cleaning Engine exhaust, diesel Hairdressers and barbers (occupational exposure) Printing processes Soot Textile manufacturing

TABLE 11.1 List of Classifications by Cancer Sites With Sufficient or Limited Evidence in Humans—cont'd

Cancer Site	Carcinogenic Agents With Sufficient Evidence in Humans	Agents With Limited Evidence in Humans
	Painting	
	Rubber production industry	
	Schistosoma haematobium	
	Tobacco smoking	
	ortho-Toluidine	
	X-radiation, γ-radiation	
Eye, Brain, and Central Nervous System		
Eye	HIV-1	Solar radiation
	Ultraviolet-emitting tanning devices	
	Welding	
Brain and central nervous system	X-radiation, γ-radiation	Radiofrequency electromagnetic fields (including from wireless phones)
Endocrine Glands		
Thyroid	Radioiodines, including iodine-131	
	X-radiation, γ-radiation	
Lymphoid, Hematopoietic, and Related Tissue		
Leukemia and lymphoma, or both	Azathioprine	Bis(chloroethyl)nitrosourea
	Benzene	Chloramphenicol
	Busulfan	Ethylene oxide
	1,3-Butadiene	Etoposide
	Chlorambucil	HBV
	Cyclophosphamide	Magnetic fields, extremely low frequency (childhood leukemia)
	Cyclosporine	Mitoxantrone
	EBV	Nitrogen mustard
	Etoposide with cisplatin and bleomycin	Painting (childhood leukemia from maternal exposure)
	Fission products, including strontium-90	Petroleum refining (occupational exposures)
	Formaldehyde	Polychlorophenols or their sodium salts (combined exposures)
	H. pylori	Radioiodines, including iodine-131
	HCV	Radon-222 and its decay products
	HIV-1	Styrene
	Human T-cell lymphotropic virus type 1	Teniposide
	Kaposi sarcoma herpesvirus	Tetrachloroethylene
	Melphalan	Trichloroethylene
	MOPP (vincristine-prednisone-nitrogen mustard-procarbazine mixture)	2,3,7,8-Tetrachlorodibenzo-*para*-dioxin
	Phosphorus-32	Tobacco smoking (childhood leukemia in smokers' children)
	Rubber production industry	Malaria (caused by infection with *Plasmodium falciparum* in holoendemic areas)
	Semustine (methyl-CCNU)	
	Thiotepa	
	Thorium-23 and its decay products	
	Tobacco smoking	
	Treosulfan	
	X-radiation, γ-radiation	
Multiple or Unspecific Sites		
Multiple sites (unspecified)	Cyclosporine	Chlorophenoxy herbicides
	Fission products, including strontium-90	Plutonium
	X-radiation, γ-radiation (exposure in utero)	
All cancer sites (combined)	2,3,7,8-Tetrachlorodibenzo-*para*-dioxin	

NOTE: This table does not include factors not covered in the IARC monographs, notably genetic traits, reproductive status, and some nutritional factors. Adapted from Cogliano, V. J., Baan, R., Straif, K., et al. (2011). Preventable exposures associated with human cancers. *Journal of the National Cancer Institute, 103*, 1–13. https://jnci.oxfordjournals.org/content/early/2011/12/11/jnci.djr483.short?rss=1.

Both environmental and lifestyle factors, as well as genetic and epigenetic factors, cause cancer (Figure 11.2). Moreover, *patterns* of cancer incidence around the world are environmental in origin—and *not* primarily genetic. At the level of the cell, cancer is *driven* by genetic alterations and epigenetic abnormalities, and a weaker immune system and differences in hormone levels and metabolic factors tend to add to this risk (see Chapter 10). The greater external environment and the cell's immediate environment can influence the immune system, hormones, and metabolic factors even further because the biological environment that surrounds cells includes metabolic and hormonal factors (e.g., excess estrogen production from paraneoplastic sources, inflammatory mediators from tumour-mediated inflammation, and products from disordered glucose and lipid metabolism). Metabolic requirements, physical activity, infections, nutrition, occupational carcinogens, air pollution, and many other environmental factors all play a role in modifying the biological environment. The challenge is to connect the complex web between genotype, phenotype, and the environment to understand a person's relative risk of developing cancer.

Cancer development and progression involve the tissue microenvironment, or stroma. The microenvironment's interaction with environmental factors is becoming more important because stromal tissue has various immune cells that can promote inflammation. Chronic inflammation, such as that caused by environmental factors, includes inhaled tobacco smoke, asbestos fibres, or fine particles in the air from diesel engine exhaust and other industrial sources, and is also at the interface of environmental factors and genetics. These sources are major factors in lung and other respiratory tract cancers.[7,8] Complex interactions occur between the tumour, the surrounding stroma, and the cells of the immune and inflammatory systems after the development of malignant phenotypes (see Chapter 10).

INCIDENCE AND MORTALITY TRENDS

> **QUICK CHECK 11.2**
> 1. Briefly describe the incidence rates and death rates of common cancers in developing and developed countries.
> 2. Define *developmental plasticity*.
> 3. Describe how epigenetic processes can be modified by environmental factors.
> 4. Define the *developmental basis of health and disease*.

Cancer is a major cause of morbidity and mortality in all regions of the world.[9] According to GLOBOCAN, in 2018 worldwide, there were 18 078 957 million new cancer cases (2.4 cases per 1 000 people) and 9 555 027 million cancer deaths, and 43 841 302 million people were living with cancer (diagnosed in the past 5 years).[10] The global cancer burden is shifting from the more developed countries to economically disadvantaged countries.[11]

The Government of Canada compiles Canadian cancer statistics annually (see https://www.cancer.ca).[12] Approximately 2 in 5 Canadians will develop cancer within their lifetime, and about 1 in 4 Canadians will die of cancer. In 2020, estimates for new cancer diagnoses in Canada ranged about 225 800, with about 83 300 dying from it.[13] Most of the new cancer cases (48%) were predicted to be lung, breast, colorectal, and prostate cancer. Lung cancer is the leading cause of cancer death in Canada. The lung cancer death rate has actually dropped (especially for men) over the past 25 years. This drop is possibly related to changes in lifestyle habits (i.e., smoking cessation), which have resulted in a decline in the cancer death rate since the early 1990s overall.

HEALTH PROMOTION

World Health Organization Cancer Prevention Strategies

The World Health Organization suggests that prevention offers the most cost-effective, long-term strategy for controlling cancer and other noncommunicable diseases. Reducing the risk of developing cancer can be achieved through the following approaches, among other measures:

- *Avoid smoking*—Tobacco is responsible for nearly one-quarter of cancer deaths worldwide, making it the single greatest avoidable risk factor for cancer.
- *Follow a healthy lifestyle*—Eating a diet high in vegetables, fruit, and fibre, and low in red and processed meat, maintaining a healthy body weight, and being physically active can prevent about one-third of the 12 major cancers worldwide, according to the American Institute for Cancer Research and the World Cancer Research Fund.
- *Reduce alcohol consumption*—Reducing alcohol can be a factor for many different types of cancer, and the risk for cancer increases with the amount of alcohol consumed.
- *Avoid overexposure to sunlight and do not use tanning beds or sun lamps*—Limiting time in mid-day sun, wearing protective clothing, seeking shade, and using sunscreen can help reduce the risk for skin cancer, while still allowing people to receive the health benefits of sun exposure. Indoor tanning does not provide a safe alternative to the sun and should be avoided.
- *Avoid infections*—Certain vaccines can help reduce the risk for some infections associated with cancer (e.g., human papillomavirus, and hepatitis B and C).
- *Avoid environmental and occupational carcinogens*—Testing and awareness can help reduce the risk for some environmental causes of cancer (e.g., radon), and occupational carcinogens (e.g., industrial chemicals).

Data from World Health Organization. (2017). *Cancer prevention*. http://www.who.int/cancer/prevention/en/.

An estimated 86% of lung cancers are preventable and 72% are attributable to tobacco smoke, providing evidence that there is a lot of room for improvement in prevention. Moreover, with a 5-year net survival of only 19%, further improvements in treatment are paramount for reducing mortality for this disease. Lung cancer screening programs for high-risk populations are also on the horizon in Canada.[13]

Measuring the cancer burden in Canada is very important because it informs both research priorities and the allocation of appropriate resources for the effective treatment and management of its various forms. The World Health Organization (WHO) has suggested that prevention is the most effective long-term strategy for preventing cancer (see *Health Promotion:* World Health Organization Cancer Prevention Strategies).

IN UTERO AND EARLY LIFE CONDITIONS

A long latency period generally precedes the onset of adult cancers. Similarly, early life events can influence later susceptibility to certain chronic diseases (Figure 11.3).[14] **Developmental plasticity** is the degree to which an organism's development is contingent (external cues) on its environment. Specifically, the developmental origins hypothesis postulates that nutrition and other environmental factors affect cellular pathways during gestation, enabling a single genotype to produce a broad range of adult phenotypes.[15] Plasticity refers to the ability of genes to organize physiologically or structurally in response to environmental conditions during fetal development. The hypothesis also suggests that persistent epigenetic adaptations that occur early in development in response to maternal nutrition and the environment are associated with increased susceptibility to cancer and other adult-onset chronic diseases.[16] Throughout in utero development, the placenta plays a major role in controlling growth and development.[17] Because the placenta is a regulator of the intrauterine environment and can be influenced by exposures throughout pregnancy,[17] much research is being done with DNA methylation linking environmental cues to placental pathologies and adult life. The Dutch Famine Birth Cohort is a well-known study of the effects of prenatal undernutrition in humans. Undernutrition was linked to increased heart disease, metabolic disorders, and a possible link with breast cancer decades later.[18] Early versus late undernutrition in pregnancy indicated that the first trimester of pregnancy is particularly vulnerable to disease outcome in adulthood.[19] Much research is needed to understand nutrition in pregnancy and child vulnerabilities later in life. More recently, extra vitamin doses in the diet of pregnant mice changed the fur colour of pups.[20] This was the first study to show how maternal nutrition results in subsequent phenotype changes. The nutrients (B_{12}, folic acid, choline, and betaine) silenced the gene that rendered mice fat and yellow but did not alter its DNA sequence. As such, silencing, or switching the gene off, linked prenatal diet to diseases like diabetes, obesity, and cancer. These concepts, called the *developmental basis of health and disease*, are defining the hypothesis of disease onset. The focus of disease prevention and intervention needs to include the decades before onset—that is, in utero and neonatal periods. Emerging studies on epigenetic mechanisms in dietary-associated transgenerational human disease have the potential to benefit health outcomes in the next generation.[19]

Perhaps one of the best examples of early life events and future cancer is the chemical exposure to diethylstilbestrol (DES), a synthetic nonsteroidal estrogen. This medication was prescribed between 1938 and 1971 in an attempt to prevent multiple pregnancy-related problems, such as miscarriage, premature birth, and abnormal bleeding.[21] By the 1950s, it became clear that DES interfered with the *development* of the reproductive system in the fetus and did not prevent miscarriage. Data also suggest a DES-associated increase in cancer of the female genital tract throughout a woman's reproductive years.[22,23] More recent studies suggest that daughters of women who took DES during pregnancy may have a slightly increased risk for breast cancer before age 40 (i.e., 1.9 times the risk compared with unexposed women at age 40).[24] For every 1 000 DES-exposed women ages 45 to 49, 4 will most likely be diagnosed with breast cancer.

Animal studies have also linked DES exposure with an increased rate of a rare type of testicular cancer (rete testis) and prostate cancer.[25] Meta-analysis provides evidence that testicular cancer, hypospadias (urethral opening is on the underside of the penis and not the tip), and cryptorchidism (absence of one of both of the testes from the scrotum) are all positively associated with prenatal exposure to DES.[26] DES inhibits the hypothalamic–pituitary–gonadal axis, thereby blocking testicular synthesis of testosterone, lowering plasma testosterone levels, and inducing a chemical castration.[23] Testicular cancer is becoming more common in low- and middle-income countries where optimal treatment may not exist.[27]

In summary, fetal programming defines, in part, the developmental origins of health and disease.[28,29] The evidence for specific DNA methylation marks in utero environments and future phenotypes is growing. Genotype and gene–environmental interactions explain substantial proportions of interindividual variation in the **methylome** (set of nucleic acid methylation modifications in the genome or cell) at birth.[30] Modifications in volume, microstructure, and connectivity in specific brain regions, including the amygdala and the hippocampus, can result from exposure to early life adversity. These differences affect socioemotional outcomes in childhood and the risk for developing psychopathology later in life. Different phenotypes can also be passed on from one generation to the next, depending on which gene is modified (i.e., methylated).[31] (Tables 11.2 and 11.3).

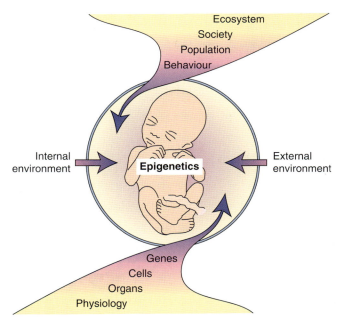

FIGURE 11.3 Fetal Vulnerability to External and Internal Environments. The fetus is particularly vulnerable to changes in the external and internal environments, which can have immediate and lifelong consequences. Such environmentally induced changes can occur at multiple levels, including molecular and behavioural. Ultimately these alterations may be epigenetic, inducing mitotically heritable alterations in gene expression without changing the DNA. (Adapted from Crews, E., & McLachlan, J. A. [2006]. Epigenetics, evolution, endocrine disruption, health, and disease. *Endocrinology, 147*[6 Suppl.], S4–S10.)

TABLE 11.2 Differences Between Multigenerational and Transgenerational Phenotypes

Phenotype	Exposure	Definition
Multigenerational	Direct	Simultaneous exposure of multiple generations to an environmental factor
Transgenerational	Initial germline exposure (ancestral)	Transgenerational phenotype that is transmitted to future generations via germline inheritance

TABLE 11.3 Somatic Versus Germ Cell Inheritance

Cell Type	Biological Response
Somatic cells	It is critical for adult-onset disease in an exposed individual; it is not transmitted to future generations as transgenerational effect.
Germ cells	It allows transmission between generations; it promotes transgenerational phenotype.

ENVIRONMENTAL AND LIFESTYLE FACTORS

> **QUICK CHECK 11.3**
> 1. What are the cancers associated with cigarette smoking?
> 2. How are dietary components related to cancer?
> 3. What are the possible pathophysiological mechanisms of obesity-associated cancer risk?
> 4. How does ionizing radiation contribute to carcinogenesis? Ultraviolet radiation?
> 5. Discuss the difficulty in determining cancer risks with electromagnetic radiation (EMR).

Tobacco Use

Cigarette smoking is carcinogenic and remains the most important cause of cancer. Tobacco smoking causes cancer in more than 15 organ sites, and exposure to secondhand smoke and parental smoking causes cancer in daughters and sons and in other nonsmokers.[32,33] Tobacco use is the largest preventable cause for cancer, and the risk is greatest for those who begin to smoke at a young age and continue to smoke throughout their lifetimes. More importantly, vaping (the act of inhaling and exhaling vapour produced by an e-cigarette), which was originally marketed to smokers as a way to help quit smoking, has become a worrisome trend in Canadian youth because it can also lead to nicotine addiction and expose the user to other harmful chemicals. According to the 2019 Canadian Tobacco and Nicotine Survey, among users aged 15 to 19, 31% vaped on a daily basis, compared with 38% of those aged 20 to 24, and over 50% of those aged 25 years and older.[35] In Canada in 2019, 4 684 400 people over the age of 12 smoked (daily or occasional smoking). This was 14.8% of the population but also represents a decline from 2018, where 4 926 800 (15.8% of the population) admitted to smoking on the same survey.[36] Asia is now considered to be the largest tobacco producer and consumer in the world.[34] The WHO reports that tobacco use caused an estimated 9.6 million deaths from cancer globally in 2018.[37] On average, smokers die 13 to 14 years earlier than nonsmokers;[38] about 25% will die prematurely during middle age (35 to 69 years).[39]

Cigarette smoking is a leading cause of death in Canada.[40] The incidence of smoking is highest within the group 20 to 34 years of age. Figure 11.4 shows a downward trend in smoking rates in Canada between 1965 and 2017.[40] In 2017, cigarette smoking was more common among men (16.7%) than women (13.5%), and there is a negative correlation between mental health and smoking rates, especially among youth.[41] Smoking rates tend to also be higher with lower socioeconomic conditions. The average consumption of cigarettes has decreased by more than three cigarettes per day since 1999. The quit ratio for smoking in 2019 was 63.1%, with 57.9% of current smokers planning to quit within the next 6 months and 26.9% considering quitting within the next month.[40]

Smoking affects nearly every organ of the body[42] (Figure 11.5). Nonsmokers are also affected by secondhand smoke. Every year in Canada, secondhand smoke causes 800 deaths from lung cancer and heart disease in nonsmokers.[43] In Canada in 2017, 63.6% of respondents to a survey on tobacco use had been exposed within the last month, and 13.3% were exposed to secondhand smoke on a daily basis.[40] Secondhand smoke, also called **environmental tobacco smoke (ETS)**, is the combination of sidestream smoke (burning end of a cigarette, cigar, or pipe) and mainstream smoke (exhaled by the smoker). More than 7 000 chemicals have been identified in mainstream tobacco smoke. Nonsmokers who live with smokers are at greatest risk for lung cancer, as well as numerous other noncancerous conditions.[44] Additionally, secondhand smoke results in infant deaths due to sudden unexpected infant death (SUID) or complications from low birth

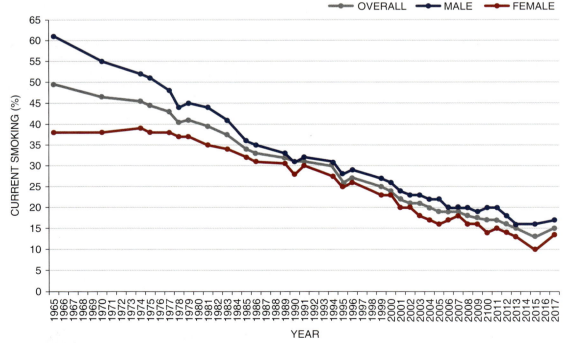

FIGURE 11.4 Smoking Prevalence in Canada, Adults Aged 15+, 1965–2017. NOTE: Includes daily and non-daily smokers. (From Reid, J. L., Hammond, D., Tariq, U., et al. [2019]. *Tobacco use in Canada: patterns and trends, 2019 edition*. Propel Centre for Population Health Impact, University of Waterloo. https://uwaterloo.ca/tobacco-use-canada/adult-tobacco-use/smoking-canada/historical-trends-smoking-prevalence.)

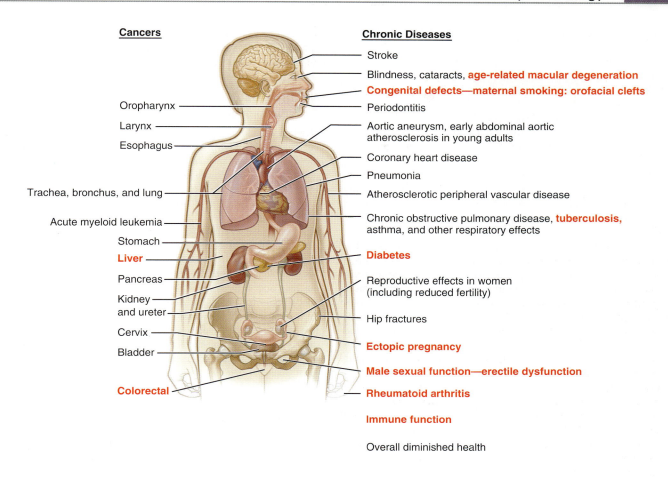
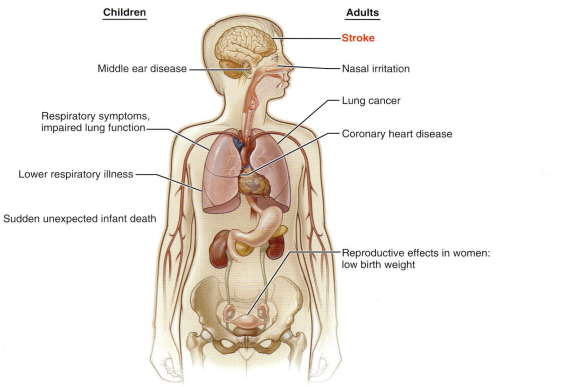

FIGURE 11.5 The Health Consequences Linked to Smoking. **NOTE:** The conditions in *red* are new diseases that have causally been linked to smoking. See text for discussion.

weight or other conditions as a result of parental smoking, particularly by the mother.

Smoking tobacco is linked to cancers of the lung, upper aerodigestive tract (oral cavity, pharynx, larynx, nasal cavity, paranasal sinuses, esophagus, and stomach), lower urinary tract (renal pelvis, penis, and bladder), kidney, pancreas, cervix, and uterus, as well as acute myeloid leukemia (see Figure 11.5). The new list of disease risks includes liver cancer and colorectal cancer. Secondhand smoke is a cause of stroke; increases the risk of death in people with cancer and cancer survivors, as well as those with age-related macular degeneration, tuberculosis, ectopic pregnancy, and diabetes mellitus; increases inflammation; impairs immunity; and is a cause of rheumatoid arthritis. Smoking causes even more deaths from vascular, respiratory, and other diseases than from cancer. The epidemic of smoking ranks among the greatest health catastrophes of the century and has caused an enormous avoidable public health tragedy.

Cigar or pipe smoking, or both, is strongly and causally related to cancers of the oral cavity, oropharynx, hypopharynx, larynx, esophagus, and lung. Cigar smokers who inhale deeply may be at increased risk of developing coronary heart disease and chronic obstructive pulmonary disease.[45] Pipe smokers have an increased risk of dying from cancers of the lung, lip, throat, esophagus, larynx, pancreas, colon, and rectum. Consumption of e-cigarettes and vaping has increased substantially since 2018, with the highest occurrence being among young people aged 15 to 24.[35]

The Tobacco Control Liaison Committee (created in 2000 by the federal, provincial, and territorial Advisory Committee on Population Health and Health Security [ACPHHS] to enable collaboration around implementation of the New Directions for Tobacco Control in Canada—A National Strategy) and the WHO Framework Convention on Tobacco Control (WHO FCTC) are national and global tobacco control initiatives for reducing both the demand for and supply of tobacco products. Control policies enforce bans on tobacco advertising, promotion, and sponsorship and provide evidence that calls for dramatic action.

Diet

Understanding dietary factors that increase the risk for cancer is most important but can be difficult. The ways in which diet affects one's likelihood of developing cancer are complicated by the variety of foods consumed, the many constituents of foods, the metabolic consequences of eating, and the temporal changes in the patterns of food use. Cancer risks in older adults may depend as much on diet in early life as on current eating practices.[46] In addition, studies in humans targeting diet and disease associations face a variety of challenges, including measurements of specific nutrients, food types, and dietary patterns.

Dietary sources of carcinogenic substances include compounds produced in the cooking of fat, meat, or protein and naturally occurring carcinogens associated with plant food substances, such as alkaloids or mould byproducts.[47] Figure 11.6 is a summary of convincing and probable judgements related to food and physical activity risk factors and the prevention of cancer.[47] Dietary components can act directly as mutagens or interfere with mutagen elimination. Abundant evidence exists that nutritional factors in many metabolic processes are related to cancer development.

Research is ongoing to understand the complexity of genomics, epigenomics, transcription factors (transcriptomics), proteomics, and metabolic factors (metabolomics) and the way that modifying any one or more of these factors influences cancer risk. **Nutrigenomics** is the study of the effects of nutrition on the phenotypic variability of individuals based on genomic differences. Investigators are focusing on the sequence and functions of genes, single nucleotide polymorphisms (SNPs), and amplifications and deletions within the DNA sequences as modifiers of the response to foods and drinks and their components.[47]

Nutrition, Obesity, Alcohol Consumption, and Physical Activity: Impacts on Cancer

What we eat, how much we weigh, and how much we move influence our risks of developing cancer. Mounting evidence is clear—everyday *choices* impact our chances of getting or preventing cancer. Ongoing tedious and comprehensive investigative work is linking diet, body weight, and exercise to risk for specific cancers.

Nutrition

The implementation of dietary patterns (e.g., Mediterranean dietary pattern) and the promotion of specific dietary recommendations (e.g., dietary approaches to lower blood pressure) are more widespread for fostering lifelong health.[48] The results of decades of research activity on the association of *specific* nutrients and foods and many forms of cancer is controversial. For example, much of the geological variation in incidence across the world for colorectal cancer has been attributed to differences in diet, particularly the consumption of red and processed meat, fibre, and alcohol, as well as body weight and physical activity.[49,50] With migration, these changes in risk are rapid, and the most plausible determinants of such changes are the adoption of the so-called "Western" diet. Japan has seen a rapid increase in the incidence of colorectal cancer with westernization of their diet.[51] Focusing on dietary patterns and meaningful biomarkers reflecting specific nutritional factors relevant to carcinogenesis may be a more successful approach to treating cancer. For instance, the following important cellular processes are affected by nutrition:

- The cell cycle
- The balance between cell proliferation and cell death (e.g., apoptosis)
- Cell differentiation
- Genes, including oncogenes and tumour-suppressor genes
- Cell signalling
- Gene expression
- Cellular microenvironment that influences gene expression
- Epigenetic regulation
- Hormonal regulation
- DNA damage and repair
- Carcinogen metabolism
- Inflammation and immunity

Epigenetic processes such as DNA methylation or acetylation (addition of an acetyl group) influence gene expression (see Chapters 3 and 10). Dietary sources of methyl groups, including folate, methionine, betaine, serine, and choline, are primary potential donors as modulators of DNA methylation[52] (Figure 11.7). Interestingly, individuals with high plasma concentrations of methionine, choline, and betaine may be at reduced risk for colorectal cancer.[53]

B vitamins, coenzymes in one-carbon metabolism (vitamins B_2, B_6, B_{12}), also are modulators of DNA methylation.[54] To date, there are limited human studies of the effects of methyl donor supply on methylation of specific genomic sequences.[55] Periconceptional maternal supplementation with 400 μg of folic acid per day, however, was associated with increased methylation in offspring aged 17 months.[55] Maternal diet during the periconceptional period established DNA methylation in the offspring with permanent phenotypic changes in experimental animals.[56] Methylation effects are similar in all tissues, suggesting that the methylating mechanism may alter markings in stem cells early in embryogenesis before tissue differentiation and persist into adult life.[57] Choline deficiency in pregnancy also results in hypermethylation of

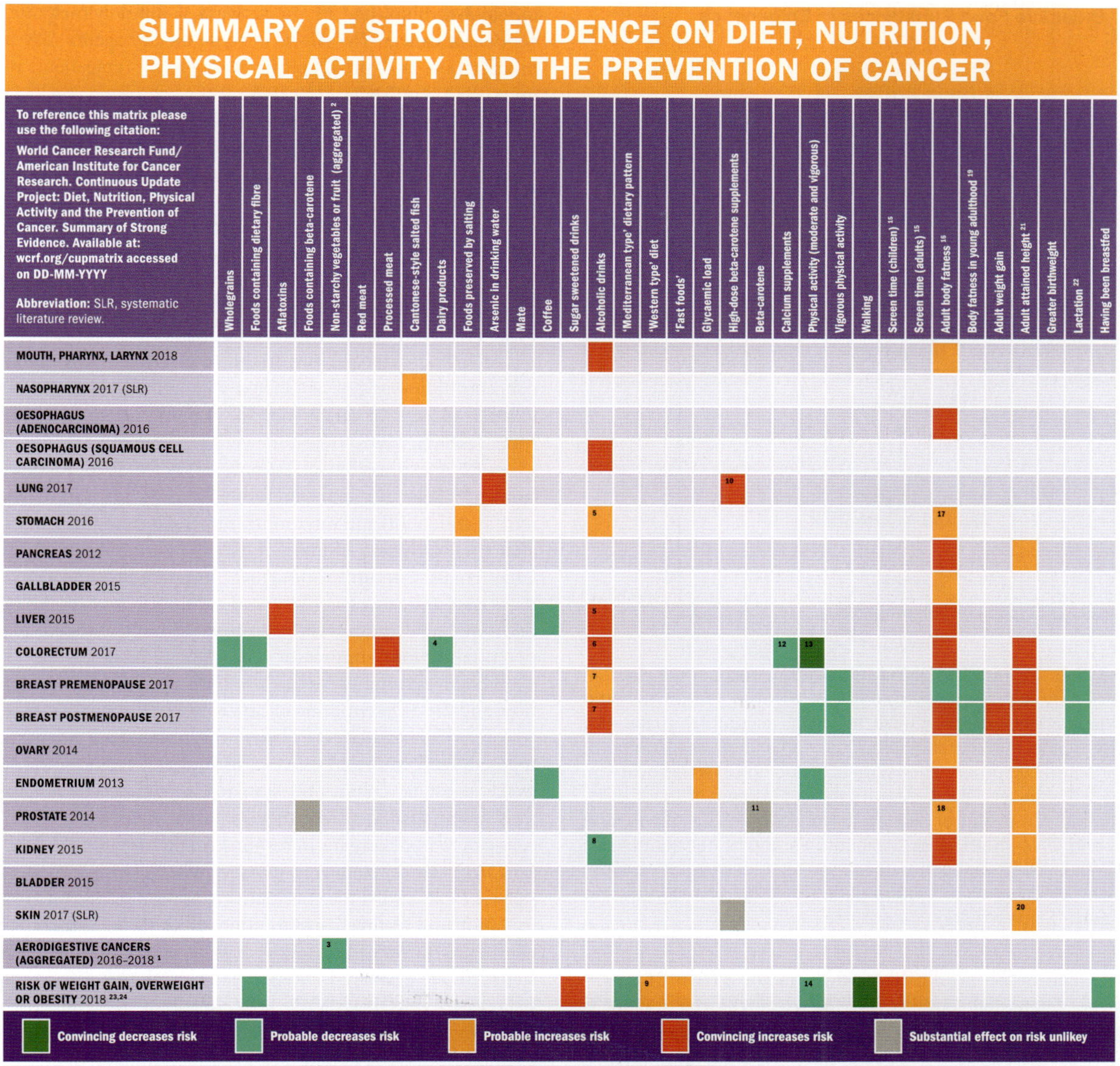

1 Includes mouth, pharynx and larynx, nasopharynx, oesophagus (squamous cell carcinoma and adenocarcinoma), lung, stomach and colorectal cancers.
2 Aggregated exposure which contains evidence for non-starchy vegetables, fruit and citrus fruit.
3 The Panel notes that while the evidence for links between individual cancers and non-starchy vegetables or fruits is limited, the pattern of association is consistent and in the same direction, and overall the evidence is more persuasive of a protective effect.
4 Includes evidence on total dairy, milk, cheese and dietary calcium intakes.
5 Stomach and liver: Based on intakes above approximately 45 grams of ethanol per day (about 3 drinks).
6 Based on intakes above approximately 30 grams of ethanol per day (about 2 drinks per day).
7 No threshold level of intake was identified.
8 Based on intakes up to 30 grams of ethanol per day (about 2 drinks per day). There is insufficient evidence for intake greater than 30 grams per day.
9 Such diets are characterised by high intakes of free sugars, meat and dietary fat; the overall conclusion includes all these factors.
10 Evidence is from studies of high-dose supplements in smokers.
11 Includes both foods naturally containing the constituent and foods which have the constituent added and includes studies using supplements.
12 Evidence derived from studies of supplements at dose >200 milligrams per day.
13 Colon cancer only.
14 Aerobic physical activity only.
15 Screen time is a marker of sedentary behaviour.
16 Body fatness is marked by body mass index (BMI) and where possible waist circumference and waist-hip ratio.
17 Stomach cardia cancer only.
18 Advanced prostate cancer only.
19 Young women aged about 18 to 30 years; body fatness is marked by BMI.
20 Malignant melanoma only.
21 Adult attained height is unlikely to directly influence the risk of cancer. It is a marker for genetic, environmental, hormonal and nutritional factors affecting growth during the period from preconception to completion of growth in length.
22 Evidence relates to effects on the mother who is breastfeeding and not to effects on the child who is being breastfed. Relates to overall breast cancer (unspecified).
23 The factors identified as increasing or decreasing risk of weight gain, overweight or obesity do so by promoting positive energy balance (increased risk) or appropriate energy balance (decreased risk), through a complex interplay of physiological, psychological and social influences.
24 Evidence comes mostly from studies of adults but, unless there is evidence to the contrary, also apply to children (aged 5 years and over).

FIGURE 11.6 Summary of Convincing and Probable Judgements. (This material has been reproduced from the World Cancer Research Fund/American Institute for Cancer Research: Diet, Nutrition, Physical Activity and Cancer: A Global Perspective. Continuous Update Project Expert Report 2018. *Recommendations and public health and policy implications*. Available at https://www.wcrf.org/sites/default/files/Recommendations.pdf.)

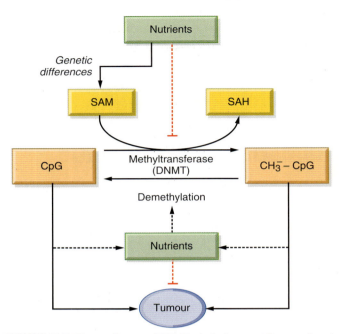

FIGURE 11.7 **Dietary Factors, DNA Methylation, and Cancer.** Certain dietary factors may supply methyl groups ($^+CH_3$) that can be donated through *S*-adenosylmethionine *(SAM)* to many acceptors in the cell (DNA, proteins, lipids, and metabolites). Donation and removal (demethylation) are affected by numerous enzymes, including DNA methyltransferase *(DNMT)*. Increased DNMT activity occurs in many tumour cells. Hypermethylation can inhibit or silence tumour-suppressor genes (see Chapter 10), and DNA methylation inhibitors as anticancer agents can block DNMT, thus reactivating tumour-suppressor genes. DNA hypomethylation can reactivate and mutate genes, including cancer-causing oncogenes. *SAH, S*-adenosylhomocysteine.

genomic DNA and of the insulin-like growth factor 2 (*IGF-2*) gene.[58] Similarly, severe folate deficiency (which increases the risk for hepatocellular cancer) induces hypomethylation of the *p53* tumour-suppressor gene (e.g. turns it off).[59–61] Several bioactive food components, including tea polyphenols and bioflavonoids, inhibit DNA methyltransferase (DNMT)-mediated DNA methylation (in vitro) in a dose-dependent manner[62] (see Figure 11.7). Enzyme histones, such as histone acetyl transferase (HAT) and histone deacetylase (HDAC), mediate acetylation and deacetylation and the resulting modification of genetic expression. Dietary components can act as regulators of gene expression by epigenetic mechanisms.[63,64] For example, there is strong evidence for the epigenetic effects of organosulphur (OSC) compounds from garlic and of isothiocyanates from cruciferous vegetables.[63] OSC agents are direct antioxidants, trapping electrons. But they can also have nonantioxidant effects (e.g., antiplatelet, fibrinolytic, anti-inflammatory, immunomodulatory, and antiaging actions) which are useful in the prophylaxis and treatment of various pathological states, such as cardiovascular diseases, cancer, neurodegenerative disorders, and diabetes. They also have antibacterial, antiviral, and some other activities. Similarly, butyrate produced in the colon by bacterial fermentation of nonstarch polysaccharide (fibre), diallyl disulphide from garlic and other allium vegetables, and sulforaphane from cruciferous vegetables can act as HDAC inhibitors to maintain DNA stability or modify transcription.[47]

There is a potential protective role of dietary polyphenols, such as curcumin, resveratrol, genistein, epigallocatechin-3-gallate, and indole-3-carbinol and its derivative 3,3′-diindolylmethane in the prevention of cancer. The effects of these dietary agents may include antiproliferation and proapoptosis through the epigenetic regulation of microRNAs (miRNAs).[65] Because of the promising results from these in vitro and in vivo studies, clinical trials are currently investigating the efficacies of these natural agents in cancer therapies (see http://www.canadiancancertrials.ca). Interest in resveratrol, a polyphenolic compound with anti-inflammatory, antioxidant, and anticancer activities, is growing because of its demonstrable role in possibly delaying age-related diseases, including cancers.[66] For example, feeding mice a diet supplemented with human equivalent doses of 105 and 210 mg of resveratrol daily resulted in inhibition of colorectal tumours through an epigenetic mechanism (miR-96, an miRNA).[66] Yet, a recent prospective cohort study in community-dwelling older persons found total urinary resveratrol metabolite concentration was not associated with inflammatory markers, cardiovascular disease, or cancer, nor was it predictive of all-cause mortality.[67] More research needs to be done with resveratrol, specifically.

miRNA expression in response to diet may be involved in several cancers.[47] Several dietary factors, including macronutrients (fat, protein, and alcohol) and micronutrients (folate and vitamin E, curcumin), alter the expression of many miRNAs in animals and humans[52,68] (see Chapter 10). Curcumin analogues (compared with just curcumin) with increased anticancer activity and solubility, such as EF24 (3,5-bis[2-fluorobenzylidene]piperidin-4-one), show enhanced expression of potential tumour-suppressor miRNAs.[69]

Bioactive components can also have a profound effect on differentiation, and the differentiation of cancer stem cells is a major area of current research. Cancer stem cells have been isolated and identified in hematopoietic and epithelial cancers, including cancers of the brain, breast, ovary, prostate, colon, and stomach.[47,70] Stem cells are found among most adult tissues, where they maintain and regenerate tissues. Stem cells can remodel organs in response to physiological triggers—*adaptive resizing*.[71] Cancer stem cells use several developmental mechanisms for self-renewal, and these mechanisms appear to be fundamental to the initiation and recurrence of tumours. Even if chemotherapy or radiation eliminates cancer cells, a full recovery is only achievable once the cancer stem cells are destroyed.[70] Repopulation with radioresistant or chemoresistant stem cells may significantly contribute to therapy resistance. Both medicine and food can modify the ability of a cancer cell to divide; for example, retinoic acid may promote differentiation of breast cancer stem cells.[72] Similarly, adequate consumption of specific food compounds, including vitamins A and D, genistein, green tea, epigallocatechin gallate (EGCG), sulforaphane, theanine, curcumin, choline, and possibly many others, may suppress cancer stem cell renewal.[72] Abnormal developmental signals that come from the extracellular microenvironment known as "niches" can initiate an uncontrolled self-renewal process. The loss of regulation in self-renewal signals, including Wnt, Notch, and hedgehog pathways, is a characteristic of cancer stem cells,[70] and various food bioactive components can modulate the signalling pathway.

A variety of food constituents may influence DNA repair.[47,73] Malnutrition can actually reduce DNA repair from damage,[74] whereas consumption of kiwi fruits, cooked carrots, or supplemental coenzyme Q_{10} in healthy adults can improve DNA repair.[47] Similarly, consumption of lycopene-rich vegetable juice can result in significantly decreased damage to the DNA of lung epithelial cells in healthy adults.[75]

Humans are constantly exposed to a variety of compounds termed **xenobiotics** (the Greek word *xenos* means "foreign"; *bios* means "life") that include toxic, mutagenic, and carcinogenic chemicals. Many of these chemicals are found in the human diet. Most xenobiotics are transported in the blood by lipoproteins and penetrate lipid membranes (see Chapter 4). The body has two main defence systems for counteracting these effects: (1) detoxification enzymes and (2) antioxidant systems (see Chapter 4). Enzymes that activate xenobiotics are called **phase I activation enzymes**. **Phase II detoxification enzymes** then protect further against a large array of reactive intermediates and nonactivated xenobiotics.[47] These enzymes are located predominantly in the liver and provide clearance of compounds through the portal circulation, thereby preventing the potentially carcinogenic agent(s) from entering the body through the gastro-intestinal tract and portal circulation. They also occur in the skin epithelia and can be induced in other extrahepatic tissue, such as the lung. They represent a potential target to influence carcinogen metabolism. Isothiocyanates from cruciferous vegetables induce the expression of phase II detoxification enzymes. Food and nutrition modify carcinogen metabolism and may modify carcinogenesis.

Glutathione-S-transferases (GSTs) are enzyme housekeepers involved in the metabolism of environmental carcinogens and reactive oxygen species (ROS). Individuals who lack these enzymes may be at higher risk for cancers because of decreased capacity to dispose of activated carcinogens. For example, the fungi that produce aflatoxins can grow on certain crops such as peanuts and some cereals (e.g., grains). Aflatoxins are carcinogens triggered by phase I activation enzymes in the liver that can produce DNA adducts. Individuals lacking these enzymes are at a higher risk for colon cancer. Diets high in isothiocyanates (from cruciferous vegetables) may decrease this risk.[76] Individuals who consume diets high in red meat and processed meat and who carry certain genetic polymorphisms have an increased risk of developing colorectal cancer.[47,77–79] Processed meats include those treated by preservatives or by smoking, curing, or salting. The EPIC study, which included 478 040 people from 10 countries, reported that the most convincing data are from meats, including sausages, bratwursts, frankfurters, and hot dogs, all of which have nitrites, nitrates, or other preservatives. These N-nitroso compounds can increase nitrogenous residues in the colon and cause DNA damage.[47] Dietary components either can be activated into potential carcinogens through metabolic processes or can be inactivated and prevent DNA damage.[47] High intake of red meat may result in the synthesis of higher levels of heme iron; iron can activate oxidative stress and inflammation in the colon. Meat may also have certain thermoresistant oncogenic bovine viruses (e.g., polyoma or papilloma virus) or possible single-stranded DNA viruses.[80] Cooking meat at high temperatures can result in the activation of heterocyclic amines that can increase the risk for colon cancer.[47]

Red cabbage contains the powerful antioxidant anthocyanin, which gives it its brilliant red colour. In the laboratory setting, anthocyanins can slow cancer cell proliferation, destroy already formed cancer cells, and stop the formation of new tumor growths.[47] Flavonoids found in plants may alter carcinogen metabolism, and dietary indole-3-carbinol can inhibit spontaneous occurrence of endometrial adenocarcinomas in rats.[47]

Chronic inflammation and immune function may help explain patterns of cancer around the world. People who are undernourished or live in poverty may have impaired immune status, which can be a factor in cancers caused by infectious agents, for example, cancers of the liver and cervix.[47]

Diet affects many pathways to cancer, and many of these processes are likely influenced, if not regulated, by DNA methylation, an epigenetic mechanism that affects gene function (see also Chapter 3). Figure 11.8 illustrates that many environmental factors may interact with the genome to produce altered epigenetic markers that change the expression of cancer-causing genes, tumour-suppressor genes, and oncogenes. Future research is needed to define robust biomarkers of cancer risk.

Obesity

Obesity in most developed countries (and in urban areas of many developing countries) has been increasing rapidly over the past 20 years. Obesity in Canada is an epidemic and constitutes a startling setback to major improvements in other areas of health.[81] In 2018, 26.8% of Canadians 18 and older (roughly 7.3 million adults) were clinically obese (based on current guidelines) whereas another 9.9 million adults (36.3%) were classified as overweight.[82] This means an alarming 63.1% of the Canadian population had health risks related to excess weight in 2018 compared with 61.9% of Canadians aged 18 and older in 2015. One in four adult Canadians and 1 in 10 children suffer from clinical obesity, which means that there are millions of Canadians living with obesity who may require immediate support in managing and controlling their weight. As a leading cause of type 2 diabetes, high blood pressure, heart disease, stroke, arthritis, and cancer, the condition impacts the entire community.

Numerous health conditions are linked to obesity and physical inactivity. The substantial suffering and long-term human and societal costs of obesity underlie the urgency to accelerate progress in obesity prevention.[83] Studies have significantly improved the understanding of the relationship between overweight or obesity, energy balance and cancer risk, cancer recurrence, and survival.[47,84,85] Consensus now exists that obesity is a risk factor for cancers of the endometrium, colorectum, kidney, esophagus, breast (postmenopausal), and pancreas. The association between obesity and cancers of the thyroid, gallbladder, liver, and ovary, as well as aggressive types of prostate cancer and non-Hodgkin's lymphoma, is now well-established.[47,84] Obesity is also recognized as a poor prognostic factor for several cancers.[86–88]

The 2020 Canadian Obesity Guidelines now define obesity as a chronic disease characterized by abnormal and/or excessive body fat (adiposity) that impairs health.[89] Assessment of obesity is not based on BMI alone. According to the WHO, worldwide obesity has nearly tripled since 1975, and more than 1.9 billion adults, 18 years of age and older, were overweight in 2016. Of these, more than 650 million were obese. Worldwide, 38 million children younger than age 5 were overweight or obese in 2019.[90]

The mechanisms of obesity-associated cancer risks are unclear and may vary by type of tumour and distribution of body fat. Emerging, however, are three main factors related to obesity and cancer: (1) the insulin–insulin-like growth factor 1 (IGF-1) axis, (2) sex hormones, and (3) adipokines or adipocyte-derived cytokines.[91] These three factors are linked to metabolic dysregulation of adipose tissue and endocrine and paracrine altered signalling of adipose tissue in obesity.[91,92] Metabolic changes in adipose tissue from obesity result in several alterations and include insulin resistance, hyperglycemia, dyslipidemia, hypoxia, and chronic inflammation.[91,93] Because tumour growth is regulated by interactions between tumour cells and their tissue microenvironment or stromal compartments that are rich in adipose tissue, adipocytes function as endocrine cells and critically shape the tumour microenvironment. Dysfunctional adipose tissue can create altered signalling pathways that involve proinflammatory mediators, macrophages, and cancer-associated fibroblasts. All of these cells are tumour-promoting cell types and, with insulin resistance and hypoxia, they can trigger compensatory angiogenesis and an energy reservoir for the embedded cancer cells.[91] The cancer-associated adipocytes (CAAs) undergo both structural and functional alterations during cancer progression that altogether create an environment toward increased cancer invasiveness and aggression[91] (Figure 11.9).

Alcohol Consumption

Alcohol is classified by the IARC as a human carcinogen. Excessive alcohol plays a contributory role in several common cancers.[47] Overall, there are strong data linking alcohol with cancers of the mouth, pharynx, larynx, esophagus, liver, colorectum, and breast.[94] The evidence does not show any "safe limit" of alcohol intake, and the health effect is from ethanol, regardless of the type of drink.

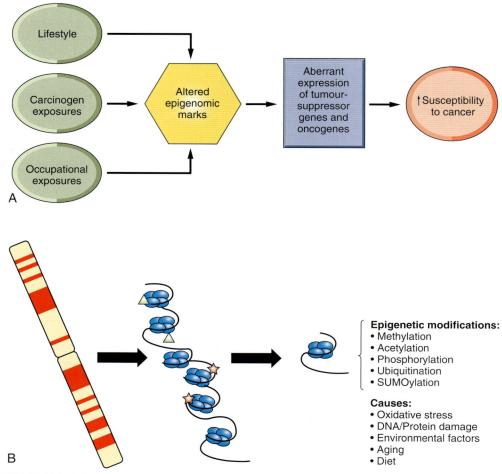

FIGURE 11.8 Epigenetic Modulation and Modifications. A, Overview of the potential role of epigenetic modulation by dietary and other environmental factors in cancer development. B, Epigenetic modulation model according to current knowledge. The different types of chemical modifications, such as methylation or acetylation, of promoter regions and/or other regulatory DNA sequences outside the gene can have a severe impact on gene transcription and translation and a resultant high modulation of gene expression and product (protein) functionality. (B, Reprinted with permission from Nowsheen, S., Aziz, K., Tran, P. T., et al. [2014]. Epigenetic inactivation of DNA repair in breast cancer. *Cancer Letters*, 342(2), 213–222.)

Mechanisms involved in alcohol-related carcinogenesis include (1) the effect of acetaldehyde, the first metabolite of ethanol oxidation; (2) the induction of cytochrome P-450 2E1 (genetic variant CYP2E1), leading to the generation of ROS; (3) increased procarcinogen activation (e.g., nitrosamines); (4) modulation of cellular regeneration (cell cycle); (5) nutritional deficiencies (retinol, retinyl esters, folic acid, other vitamins) that may predispose to altered mucosal integrity and enzyme and metabolic dysfunction; and (6) other structural abnormalities. Inherited factors also put some individuals at increased risk in DNA repair ability, carcinogen metabolism, and cell cycle control.[80] Recent investigation is concerned with epigenetic mechanisms and alcohol metabolism.[95,96] Figure 11.10 summarizes some of these epigenetic mechanisms and the effects of alcohol metabolism that may be important for cancer pathogenesis.

Physical Activity

Physical activity reduces the risk for breast and colon cancers and may reduce the risk for other cancers, including endometrial, lung, and prostate cancers.[97] Several biological mechanisms causing this effect include (1) decreasing insulin and IGF levels; (2) decreasing obesity; (3) increasing free radical scavenger systems; (4) altering inflammatory mediators; (5) decreasing levels of circulating sex hormones and metabolic hormones; (6) improving immune function; (7) enhancing cytochrome P-450, thus modifying carcinogen activation; and (8) increasing gut motility.[98-100] For colon cancer, physical activity increases gut motility, which reduces the length of time (transit time) that the bowel lining is exposed to potential mutagens.[101] For breast cancer, vigorous physical activity may decrease exposure of breast tissue to ovarian hormones, insulin, and IGF. A randomized trial found that after 12 months of moderate-intensity exercise, postmenopausal women had significantly decreased levels of serum estrogens.[102] Physical activity also helps prevent type 2 diabetes, which has been associated with risk for cancer of the colon and pancreas.[101,103]

Many questions are unanswered regarding the effect of frequency, intensity, and duration of exercise on decreasing the risk of cancer. Much of the literature suggests that between 3.5 and 4 hours of vigorous activity per week are necessary to optimize protection for colon cancer.[100] There is likely a dose–response relationship for colon cancer

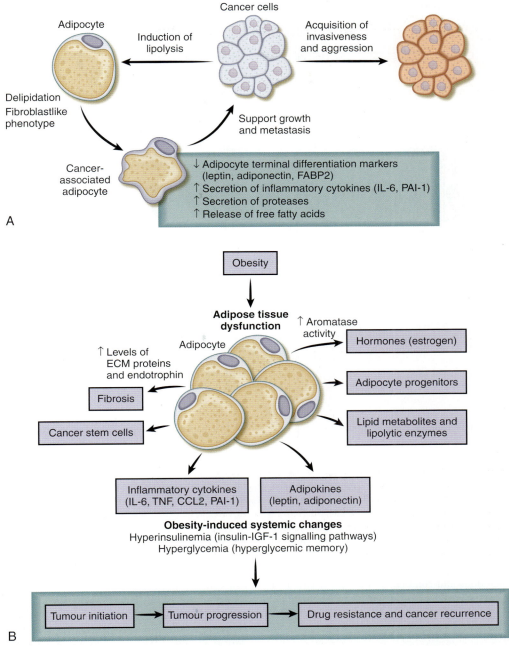

FIGURE 11.9 Structural and Functional Changes in Adipocytes and Interaction With the Microenvironment Contribute to Cancer Progression and Metastases: A Working Model. **A**, Signalling interactions occur between cancer cells and cancer-associated adipocytes. This interaction within the tumour microenvironment creates a place, or *niche*, permissive for cancer growth. Cancer cells stimulate the breakdown of lipids in adipocytes, leading to *delipidation* and the emergence of a fibroblastlike phenotype in adipocytes. The continuing alterations are associated with functional changes in the cells and include increased secretion of inflammatory mediators (cytokines) and proteases, and increased release of free fatty acids. All of these changes can support tumour growth and invasiveness. **B**, Obesity leads to excessive levels of proinflammatory cytokines, sex hormones, lipid metabolites, and altered adipokines. The altered adipose tissue becomes a source of various extracellular matrix proteins, cancer stem cells, and cancer-associated adipokines. Collectively these alterations contribute to tumour initiation, growth, and recurrence. The systemic metabolic changes of obesity—hyperinsulinemia and hyperglycemia—can further contribute to a tumour-permissive environment. *CCL2*, Chemokine ligand 2; *ECM*, extracellular matrix; *FABP2*, fatty acid binding protein 2; *IGF-1*, insulinlike growth factor 1; *IL-6*, interleukin-6; *PAI-1*, plasminogen activator inhibitor-1; *TNF*, tumour necrosis factor. (Reprinted with permission from Park, J., Morley, T. S., Kim, M., et al. [2014]. Obesity and cancer—mechanisms underlying tumour progression and recurrence. *Nature Reviews. Endocrinology, 10*[8], 455–465.)

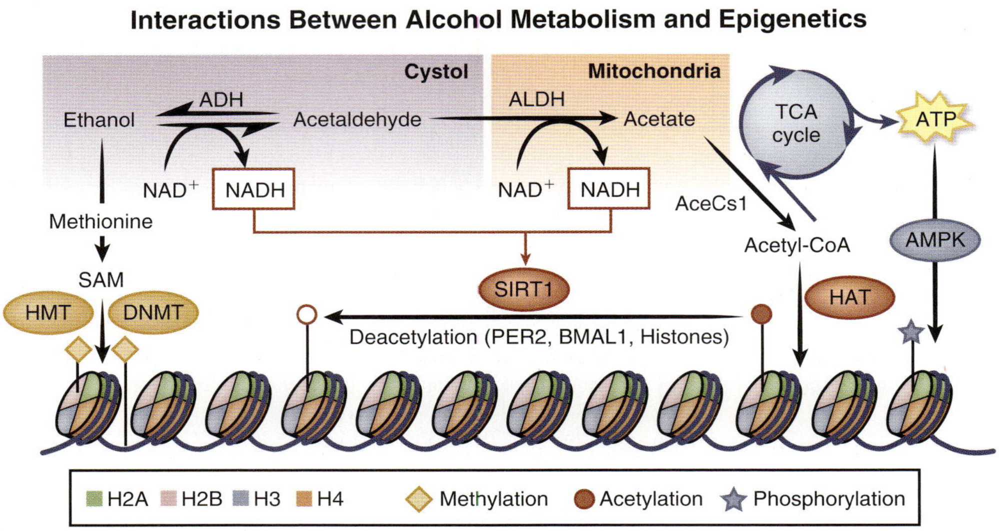

Interactions Between Alcohol Metabolism and Epigenetics

FIGURE 11.10 Alcohol Metabolism and Epigenetics. Chronic alcohol intake leads to decreased methylation called *hypomethylation* by decreasing *S*-adenosylmethionine *(SAM)* that is used by DNA enzymes called methyltransferases *(DNMTs)* and histone enzymes called methyltransferases *(HMTs)* to methylate DNA and histones. Additionally, alcohol metabolism increases the ratio of the coenzyme reduced nicotinamide adenine dinucleotide *(NADH)* to the oxidized nicotinamide adenine dinucleotide *(NAD+)*; this step inhibits the sirtuin enzyme *SIRT1*, which interferes with normal histone acetylation patterns. *AceCs1*, Acetyl-coenzyme A synthetase 1; *Acetyl-CoA*, acetyl-coenzyme A; *ADH*, alcohol dehydrogenase; *ALDH*, aldehyde dehydrogenase; *AMPK*, adenosine monophosphate–activated protein kinase; *ATP*, adenosine triphosphate; *BMAL1*, brain and muscle-like aryl hydrocarbon receptor nuclear translocator-like protein 1; *HAT*, histone acetyltransferase; *PER2*, period 2; *TCA*, tricarboxylic acid. (Adapted from Zakhari, S. [2013]. Alcohol metabolism and epigenetics changes. *Alcohol Research, 35*[1], 6–16.)

and breast cancer, and 30 to 60 minutes per day of moderate to vigorous intensity activity decreases breast cancer risk.[104] The *Canadian 24-Hour Movement Guidelines* (https://www.csep.ca/home) suggest that limiting sedentary behaviour and being physically active each day and for an accumulation of at least 150 minutes per week can help reduce the risk for many conditions, including certain types of cancer. Physical activity can also result in improved fitness, strength, and mental health.[105]

Aerobic exercise can also be beneficial for adults with cancer-related fatigue during and after cancer treatment.[106] Furthermore, exercise in children with cancer results in improved body composition, flexibility, and cardiorespiratory fitness.[107] The effects of exercise in the prevention of cancer for both adults and children, as well as the effects of postcancer treatment and the experience of survivors, are key areas for further research.

Ionizing Radiation

Much of the knowledge of the effects of ionizing radiation (IR) on human cancer comes from observations of the Hiroshima and Nagasaki atomic bomb exposures. These data provide the best estimate of human cancer risk over the dose range from 20 to 250 cGy for low linear energy transfer (LET) radiation, such as X-rays or γ-rays. Other evidence comes from groups exposed for medical reasons, underground miners exposed to radon gas, and other occupational exposures (Table 11.4). The atomic bomb exposures in Japan caused acute leukemias in adults and children and increased frequencies of thyroid and breast carcinomas. Lung, stomach, colon, esophageal, and urinary tract cancers, and multiple myeloma are all on the list. At Nagasaki and Hiroshima, leukemia incidence in individuals 15 years or younger reached its peak 6 to 7 years after the explosions and has steadily declined since 1952. People 45 years and older at the time of exposure had a latent period of 20 years before developing acute leukemia.

Interestingly, epidemiological data from Japanese atomic bomb survivors and from children exposed to radiation for medical intervention suggest that excess relative risks (ERRs) for radiation-induced cancers at a given age are exceptionally higher for individuals exposed during childhood than for those exposed at older ages.[108] Recent analyses of Japanese bomb survivors suggest that the ERR for cancer induction decreases with increasing age at exposure only until exposure ages of 30 to 40 years; with radiation exposure at older ages, the ERR does not decrease further, and for many individual cancer sites (liver, colon, lung, stomach, and bladder) the ERR may actually increase in all solid cancers combined.[110,111,118] These new data present a challenge to the conceptual understanding of the mechanisms of cancer induction.[111] Biological models of cancer development all predict that ERRs should decrease continuously with increasing age of radiation exposure. However, recent models of radiation carcinogenesis show IR acts not only as an *initiator* of premalignant cell clones but also as a *promoter* of pre-existing premalignant cell alterations.[109–111] Promotion is used here to mean the process by which an initiated cell clonally expands. Therefore, promotional processes from radiation can result in increasing excess lifetime cancer risks with increasing age at exposure. From these new data, investigators propose that radiation-induced cancer risks after exposure in middle age may be almost twice as high as previously estimated.[110]

Human exposure to IR includes emissions from the environment (e.g., radon), X-rays, computed tomography (CT) scans, radioisotopes, and other radioactive sources. Health risks involve not only neoplastic diseases but also cardiovascular disease and stroke following high doses in therapeutic medicine and lower doses in A-bomb survivors.[112,113] Late effects of radiation in A-bomb survivors show persistent elevations of inflammatory markers, implying immunological damage may be the cause of later cardiovascular effects.[114] For the first time, investigators using a model of umbilical vein endothelial cells have shown that low doses (0.05 Gy) of X-rays induce DNA damage and apoptosis in endothelial cells. These findings will need continued research.[115] Cardiac and blood vessel damage may manifest years after completion of radiation therapy.[116] Other risks include somatic mutations that may contribute to other diseases (e.g., birth defects and eye maladies) and, from animal studies, inherited mutations that may affect the incidence of diseases in future generations. Exposure to diagnostic radiography in utero has been associated with childhood cancer, particularly leukemia.[117–119] The link or association between in utero irradiation and childhood cancer is, however, controversial and varies with study methodology.[120] Heritable mutations are of particular concern for women because the number of oocytes is presumably fixed at birth and mutations, if not repaired, are cumulative.[121] The concern from high-dose medical exposure, for example, CT scans is very real.[112] In 2009 the US National Council on Radiation Protection and Measurements (NCRP)[122] reported that Americans were exposed to more than seven times as much IR from medical procedures as compared with that in the 1980s. The increased exposure is mostly because of the rapid increase in the use of CT imaging.[123] Several factors likely drive this increase in imaging, including improvements in the technology, that have led to increased clinical applications, patient demand, physician demand, defensive medical practices, and medical uncertainty.[124] Similarly, in Canada, the Canadian Nuclear Safety Commission has reported that medical procedures account for roughly 40% of the total annual radiation dose received by Canadians.[125]

Radiobiologists, geneticists, physicists, and others are debating the risks associated with low-dose radiation because of the potential effect on the health of current and future generations.[126] The expression of radiation-induced damage depends not only on dose, fractionation, and protraction but also on repair mechanisms, bystander effects, radioprotective substances (i.e., antioxidants), and the mechanism of radiation delivery.[121]

Radiation-Induced Cancer

IR is a mutagen and carcinogen and can penetrate cells and tissues and deposit energy in tissues at random in the form of ionizations (e.g., excitation or removal of an electron from the target atom). These ionizations can lead to irreversible or indirect damage from formation and attack by water-based free radicals (radiolysis).[126] The *general* characteristics of IR-induced carcinogenesis are well established.[127] The past two decades have focused on *specific* cellular and molecular mechanisms that relate to the induction of cancer, including dose–response relationships for chromosome aberrations, cell transformation, gene expression (genetic and epigenetic), alternative targets, mutagenesis in somatic cells, the biological effects that occur in nonirradiated cells (i.e., nontargeted effects), and effects on the microenvironment.[128] IR is a potent DNA-damaging agent causing cross-linking, nucleotide base damage, and single-strand breaks (SSBs) and double-strand breaks (DSBs)[129] to DNA, and disrupted cellular regulation processes can lead to carcinogenesis.[129] The DSB (Figure 11.11) is considered the characteristic lesion observed for the effects of IR. In certain experimental systems, one DSB may lead to cell cycle arrest and possible arrest of further repair. Yet many DSBs appear to result from clustered damage, a consequence of the pattern of distribution of ionizations with DNA. These patterns of clustered damage may be more difficult to accurately repair.[130] Furthermore, the nonhomologous end joining (NHEJ) pathway repairs most DSBs, and although this pathway is efficient for

TABLE 11.4 Cancer Associated With Exposure to Ionizing Radiation

Cancer Type	AB	AS	PM	TC	TH	RP	UM	RD
Leukemia	x	x			x			x
Thyroid	x			x				
Breast	x		x					
Lung	x	x			x		x	
Bone						x		
Stomach	x	x						
Esophagus	x	x						
Lymphoma	x	x						x
Brain			x				x	
Liver					x			
Skin				x			x	x

AB, Atomic bomb survivors; *AS*, ankylosing spondylitis patients; *PM*, postpartum mastitis patients; *RD*, radiologists; *RP*, radium dial painters; *TC*, tinea capitis patients; *TH*, individuals receiving Thorotrast; *UM*, underground miners.
Data from Jones, J. A., Casey, R. C., & Karouia, F. (2010). Ionizing radiation as a carcinogen. In C. A. McQueen (Ed.), *Comprehensive toxicology* (2nd ed.). Elsevier.

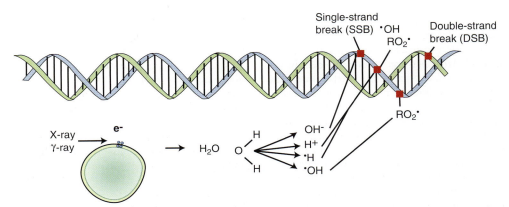

FIGURE 11.11 Free Radicals. Free radicals formed by water nearby and around DNA cause indirect effects. These effects have a short life of single free radicals. Oxygen can modify the reaction, enabling longer lifetimes of oxidative free radicals. *H*, Hydrogen; *H⁺*, hydrogen ion; •*H*, hydrogen free radical; *H₂O*, water; *O*, oxygen; *OH⁻*, hydroxyl ion; •*OH*, hydroxyl free radical; *RO₂•*, reactive oxygen species.

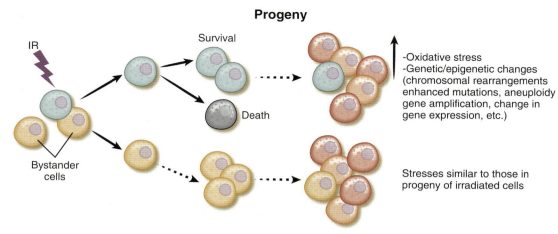

FIGURE 11.12 Radiation: Targeted and Nontargeted or Bystander Effects. Signalling from cells exposed to irradiation causes stressful effects, including oxidative stress, to those cells not directly radiated (called bystander cells) and their progeny. These induced effects may be similar to those reported in the progeny of irradiated cells. *IR*, Ionizing radiation. (Reprinted with permission from Azzam, E. I., Jay-Gerin, J. P., & Pain, D. [2012]. Ionizing radiation-induced metabolic oxidative stress and prolonged cell injury. *Cancer Letters, 327*[1–2], 48–60.)

joining the DNA broken ends, errors can occur, and repair may decline with age.[131] Irradiated human cells unable to execute the NHEJ pathway are supersensitive to the introduction of large-scale mutations and chromosomal aberrations.[126]

Although evidence suggests that interindividual differences in radiation responses may be attributed to certain genes, IR can activate oncogenes, resulting in uncontrolled cell growth[128,132] (see Chapter 10). Tumour-suppressor genes are also sensitive to IR. Several tumour-suppressor genes are deactivated by IR that promotes carcinogenesis.[128,132] Cells can detect and respond epigenetically, altering gene expression after low doses of radiation.[128] Gene expression can change as a function of radiation dose and radiation type.[128]

Nontargeted Effects

The progeny of irradiated cells from previous cell divisions (even though they did not receive the radiation directly) may also express a high level of gene mutations, cell lethality, and chromosomal aberration. Altogether these effects are called **genomic instability**. Genomic instability may contribute to secondary cancers. Similarly, the directly irradiated cells can also lead to genetic effects in so-called bystander cells or innocent cells (called **bystander effects**), even though they themselves received no direct radiation exposure.[126] For example, localized radiation to the head in an in vivo mouse model led to induced bystander effects in the lead-shielded distant spleen tissue, as well as medulloblastomas in the cerebellum.[133] The bystander effect is also evident in three-dimensional human tissues and in other whole animal organisms.[99] Bystander effects induced both DSBs and apoptotic cell death, supporting the role of signalling between the irradiated cells (the targeted cells) and unirradiated cells (the nontargeted, or bystander, cells) (Figure 11.12). The direct physical connection between cells or gap junctions, called gap junctional intercellular communication, and signalling pathways enable such communication to occur. Numerous intercellular and intracellular signalling pathways are implicated in the bystander response, and these effects are transmitted to the bystander cell descendants. These various effects demonstrated in vivo may reflect an ongoing inflammatory response (oxidative stress response) to the initial radiation-induced injury[134] (Box 11.1). One hypothesis is the stress response is due to elevated ROS affecting genomic instability. Importantly, therapeutic interference with specific signalling pathways (e.g., p38MAPK) may result in genome stabilization.[135] Both the *bystander* and the *genomic instability* effects are **nontargeted effects**.

Acute, Latent, and Microenvironmental Effects

IR causes acute and persistent short- and long-term effects.[100-102] Acute exposure to IR can cause damage to several organ systems, especially those with highly proliferative cells such as the hematopoietic system,

---

> **BOX 11.1** **A Paradigm Shift? Responses to Ionizing Radiation Mediated by Inflammatory Mechanisms**
>
> The conventional paradigm suggests that the consequences of exposure to IR are solely due to mutational DNA damage or cell death induced in irradiated cells at the time of exposure. There are, however, recent challenges to this paradigm: (1) **abscopal**, or "out-of-field," effects, where radiation treatment to one local area of the body results in an antitumour effect distant to the radiation site; (2) detection of plasma factors in vivo (clastogenic [or capable of chromosome damage] factors) that can affect the survival and function of irradiated cells; and (3) effects in nonirradiated cells that are in the vicinity of irradiated cells (bystander effects) or in the descendants of irradiated cells several generations after the initial radiation exposure (genomic instability). These nontargeted effects are different than the targeted effects that arise in cells upon immediate deposition of energy at the time of radiation exposure. The nontargeted effects arise as a result of intracellular signalling and appear to represent a genotype-dependent balance (and various epigenetic influences) of toxic factors and cellular responses that may involve both oxidative stress and inflammatory type processes (see Figure 11.12).
>
> Data from Azzam, E. I., Jay-Gerin, J. P., & Pain, D. (2012). Ionizing radiation-induced metabolic oxidative stress and prolonger cell injury. *Cancer Letters, 327*(1–2), 48–60; Mukherjee, D., Coates, P. J., Lorimore, S. A., et al. (2014). Responses to ionizing radiation mediated by inflammatory mechanisms. *Journal of Pathology, 232*(3), 289–299.

> **BOX 11.2** **Theoretical Models to Understand Low-Dose Ionizing Radiation**
>
> Several models estimate the risk of low-dose ionizing radiation. They include the **linear no-threshold (LNT) model**, which assumes that any dose, including very low doses, has the potential to cause mutations (see [A] in figure). Another model, the **linear-quadratic dose–response model**, illustrates a relationship between dose and biological response that is curved (i.e., response=dose^2) and implies that the rate of change in response is different at different doses; the response may change slowly at low doses, for example, but rapidly at high doses, (see [B]). The threshold model proposes a threshold dose below which radiation may not cause cancer in humans (see [C]). Proponents of this model argue that such thresholds are derived, for example, from the ability to repair damage caused by lower doses of radiation. There is some evidence that low doses may actually produce a higher level of risk per unit of dose, which is called the supralinear hypothesis (see [D]). The stochastic (or random probability) model (see [E]) is a major model for understanding low-dose radiation. Currently, the shape of the response curve for the low-dose region is really unknown.
>
>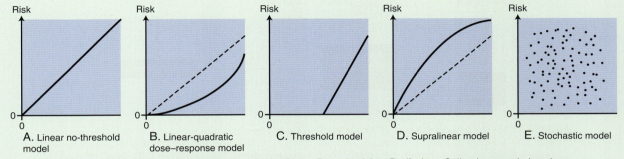
>
> A. Linear no-threshold model B. Linear-quadratic dose–response model C. Threshold model D. Supralinear model E. Stochastic model
>
> **Theoretical Models for Estimating the Risk of Low-Dose Ionizing Radiation.** Collective population dose is expressed as a person-rem (roentgen equivalent, man). Estimating a collective dose then enables an application of a "constant risk factor" to obtain a statistical estimate of the number of additional cancers (above background radiation) from that exposure. These computations apply to low doses–low-dose rates only. Many propose the best fit is the linear no-threshold (LNT) model (A). The most common alternative to the LNT model is the linear-quadratic model (B). The quadratic term is the square of the dose. The linear term is equal to zero. The threshold model (C) is a threshold below which there is *no* increase in cancer risk. Proponents of this model argue that because some toxic chemicals and materials exhibit such thresholds, radiation must also have a threshold. Their arguments are related to repair of the radiation damage caused by lower doses of radiation. Some evidence exists that low levels of radiation produce a higher level of risk per unit dose, which is called the *supralinear model* (D). The stochastic model (E) describes effects that are random and proposes that events cannot be predicted. (Adapted from Makhijani, A., Smith, B., & Thorne, M. C. [2006]. *Science for the vulnerable: setting radiation and multiple exposure environmental health standards to protect those at most risk*. Institute for Energy and Environmental Research.)

the skin, and the gastro-intestinal system[103] (see Chapter 4). Radiation's carcinogenic potential persists because of nontargeted radiation effects that alter cell and tissue signalling and change the microenvironment.[104,136] The brain's innate immune system is very vulnerable to cranial irradiation, altering the microenvironment and causing the recruitment and infiltration of macrophages.[137] With improvement in cancer survival, the long-term risks for a second cancer developing from treatment become more important.[138]

Low Dose and Dose Rate

The 2011 Fukushima nuclear accident in Japan, terrorist attacks, and exposure to radiation from medical procedures have increased the need to understand the human health effects of exposure to low-level IR.[139] Accurate measurements of risks from low doses of radiation are statistically difficult because they require such large populations. Interestingly, researchers have developed an in silico simulation model of a population-based cohort study for conducting future epidemiological studies of excess cancer risks in CT-exposed individuals.[140] Simulation models like these may provide reasonable approximations, and theoretical models are still used to estimate response curves (Box 11.2).

Ultraviolet Radiation

Ultraviolet radiation (**UV radiation**) comes from sunlight. Other sources of UV radiation include electric lights, black lights, and tanning lamps.[141] UV radiation is divided into three major wavelengths: UVA, UVB, and UVC radiation. UVA is the most abundant source of UV radiation received on earth, whereas most UVB and all UVC rays are absorbed by the earth's ozone layer.[141] UVA radiation is weaker than UVB, but UVA penetrates deeper into the skin and is more constant throughout the year, despite the weather.[141] UVB affects the outer layer of the skin, and UVC radiation does not increase health risks as much as UVB.[141] UV radiation can also be important to health because it produces vitamin D that helps in the absorption of calcium and phosphorus from food, and these compounds are all important for bone development. The WHO recommends 5 to 15 minutes of sun exposure two to three times a week; however, overexposure can result in acute and chronic health effects on the skin, eyes, and immune system.[142]

There are three main types of skin cancer: cancer that forms in melanocytes (pigment cells) called **melanoma**, cancer in the lower part of the epidermis or outer layer of the skin called **basal cell carcinoma (BCC)**, and cancer in the flat cells that form the surface of the skin called **squamous cell carcinoma (SCC)** (see Chapter 41). Melanoma, the most lethal form of skin cancer, can occur on any skin surface; however, in men, it is often found on the skin on the head, the neck, between the shoulders, and the hips. In women, it is more commonly found on the skin on the lower legs, between the shoulders, and the hips. Although rare in people with dark skin, melanoma is usually found under the fingernails, under the toenails, on the palms of the hands, or on the soles of the feet.[143] BCC commonly occurs on the head

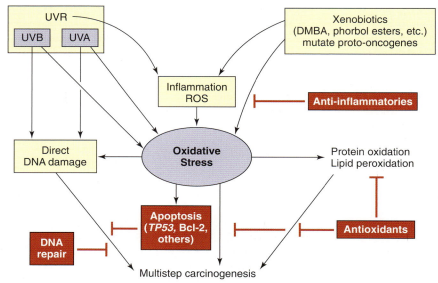

FIGURE 11.13 Theoretical Scheme of Multistep Skin Carcinogenesis. Ultraviolet radiation (UVR), inflammation, and xenobiotics lead to oxidative stress, resulting in direct DNA damage, protein oxidation, lipid peroxidation, and apoptosis. The protective mechanisms shown in red include apoptosis, DNA repair, and antioxidants. Bcl-2, B-cell lymphoma 2; DMBA, 7,12-dimethylbenz[a]anthracene; ROS, reactive oxygen species; TP53, tumour protein p53 gene; UVA, ultraviolet A; UVB, ultraviolet B. (Adapted from Sander, C. S., Chang, H., Hamm, F., et al. [2004]. Role of oxidative stress and the antioxidant network in cutaneous carcinogenesis. International Journal of Dermatology, 43[5], 326–335.)

and neck. SCC is found more commonly in men who work outdoors but can occur in anyone. SCC occurs on sun-exposed areas of the skin, including the nose, ears, lower lip, and dorsa of the hand. SCCs are composed of keratinizing cells and are more aggressive than BCC, but the development into invasive SCC is low.[144] For a more complete discussion about these skin cancers, see Chapter 41.

The incidence of BCC and SCC is strongly correlated with lifetime sunlight exposure (i.e., photocarcinogenesis). Specific patterns of sunlight exposure, intermittent or chronic, confer different host effects, acute or cumulative. Intense intermittent recreational sun exposure correlates with increased incidence of melanoma and BCC. Similarly, chronic occupational sun exposure correlates with increased SCC. Tanning bed use is yet another increased risk for BCC.[145] For other occupational factors linked to skin cancers, see Chapter 41. Depending on the time of day and a person's skin type, acute sun exposure may result in sunburn.[143] A sunburn is defined as a burn or pain and possible blistering that lasts for 2 or more days.[143] Cumulative sun exposure is the additive effects of intermittent sun exposure, chronic sun exposure, or both. Other skin cancer risk factors include IR, chronic arsenic ingestion, immunosuppression, and genetic factors. These skin cancers have a higher incidence among people with a light or fair skin tone, but they can occur in anyone and in those who do not burn from sunlight.[145]

UV radiation is known to cause specific gene mutations; for example, SCC involves mutation in the tumour protein p53 (TP53) gene, BCC in the patched 1 tumour-suppressor gene (PTCH1), and melanoma in the p16 gene.[146] The patched or hedgehog intracellular signalling pathway plays a central role in both sporadic BCCs and nevoid basal cell carcinoma syndrome (Gorlin syndrome) tumour growth.[147] Aberrant DNA methylation and histone modifications are present in tumour tissues and cell lines for skin cancers.[148–150] In addition, UV light induces the release of tumour necrosis factor-alpha (TNF-α) in the epidermis, which may reduce immune surveillance against skin cancer.[151] The identification of transcription factors and chemokine receptors suggests a critical role of inflammation in skin carcinogenesis.[152]

Skin exposure to UV radiation and IR, as well as chemical (xenobiotic) agents or medications, produces large quantities of ROS.[153] Uncontrolled release of ROS is an important contributor to skin carcinogenesis.[153] Imbalances in ROS and antioxidants can lead to oxidative stress, tissue injury, and direct DNA damage (Figure 11.13). ROS can induce a number of transcription factors (e.g., activator protein-1 [AP-1] and NF-κB)[154] and increase regulating genes that induce inflammation.[153,155] *Inflammation is a critical component of tumour progression.*

The incidence of melanoma has been increasing annually at rates of 2 to 7% in White populations since the 1980s.[156] Incidence is increasing worldwide, and in Canada incidence increased by 3.8% for men and 3.3% for women in 2019.[157] Pediatric melanoma is rare, but its incidence has been rising.[158] Therefore, health programs need to continue to encourage sun protective behaviour (protective clothing, sunscreen use, decreased time spent outside, decreased indoor tanning) to reduce melanoma incidence. Because death rates from melanoma have not risen as rapidly as incidence rates, controversy still exists about whether some of the incidence is a result of overdiagnosis.[159,160] Melanomas can appear suddenly and without warning, and can arise from or near a mole (melanocytic nevus) and freckles.[161] Complex interactions between UV exposure profiles and genotype combinations determine nevus numbers and size, as well as facial freckling.[161] When detected in the early stages, melanoma is highly curable.[162] Early-stage melanoma is classified as radial growth phase (RGP). Later-stage melanoma, called vertical growth phase (VGP), is characterized by invasion into the dermal layer and is frequently metastatic.[163] Much research is ongoing to understand the mechanisms that promote progression from less invasive RGP melanoma to aggressive VGP melanoma. Recent progress in understanding the molecular alterations in melanoma will likely advance its diagnosis, prognosis, and treatment.

The pathogenesis of melanoma is very complex, involving genetic and environmental factors. The genetic factors can be inherited: for example, in high-susceptibility genes (i.e., *cyclin-dependent kinase inhibitor 2A [CDKN2A]*) or in low-susceptibility genes (i.e., *melanocortin-1*). About 10 to 15% of melanomas are inherited as an autosomal dominant trait with variable penetrance.[164] The majority of melanomas are sporadic and seem to involve UV radiation damage.[165] UV radiation is correlated with DNA damage. Epidemiological and case-control studies suggest that UV radiation exposure is the most significant factor for the development of melanoma (episodes of intense, intermittent exposure [measured as history of sunburn]). Other evidence, however, reports that rates of melanoma are uncommon in persons with outdoor occupations. Furthermore, because melanomas sometimes occur in dark-skinned individuals, other environmental factors may be important. Recent analyses in Iceland and Italy and a previous large prospective study in Norway and Sweden suggest sunbed use as a reason for increased melanoma, especially in women.[165-167] Indoor tanning (sunbed use) is a risk factor for melanoma[168] (i.e., frequent indoor tanning increases melanoma risk). Certain skin conditions also are treated with UVA and UVB light therapy. Family history (i.e., genetic factors), skin type, and the density of moles are important in determining the risk of developing melanoma. Traits associated with a high risk for melanoma are light-coloured hair, eyes, and skin; an inability to tan; and a tendency to freckle, sunburn, and develop nevi.

The emerging molecular changes associated with melanoma emphasize that melanoma, like many other cancers, is not a single disease but a diverse group of disorders. The most frequent driver mutations in melanoma involve cell cycle control, progrowth pathways, and telomerase.[164] Although other genes may be involved, melanoma progression is often associated with a mutation in the *BRAF* oncogene.[163] The most common mutation in *BRAF*[V600E] promotes the progression of melanoma through activation of the mitogen-activated protein kinase (MAPK) signalling cascade.[163] Disease progression may involve factors secreted by the melanoma cells that activate extracellular matrix enzymes (matrix metalloproteinase-1 [MMP-1]) and adjacent stromal fibroblasts in the tumour microenvironment.[163]

Although avoiding sunlight by keeping in the shade and covering up is very important for protection, more data are needed to understand whether sunscreen prevents melanoma. A significant benefit from regular sunscreen use has not yet demonstrated primary prevention for BCC and melanoma.[169] Increased knowledge of the intricate cellular interactions in melanoma will increase understanding of melanoma etiology and pathogenesis. This knowledge is essential for early detection and treatment.

Electromagnetic Radiation

Health risks associated with **radiofrequency electromagnetic radiation (RF-EMR)** are very controversial. RF-EMR is in the frequency range of 30 kHz to 300 GHz. Electromagnetic fields (EMFs) generated by RF sources couple with the body and result in induced electric and magnetic fields with associated currents inside tissue.[170] Exposure to electric and magnetic fields is widespread. Microwaves, radar, mobile phones (e.g., cellphones and smartphones), cordless phones, cellphone towers (base stations), power frequency radiation associated with electricity and radio waves, fluorescent lights, computers, and other electric equipment create EMRs of varying strength. Despite the breadth of literature on microwaves (MW), the impact of EMR on human health is largely unknown. Scientific evidence is accumulating, although it has been hampered by the scarcity of methods to accurately measure exposure, the lack of a clear dose–response relationship, and the difficulty in reproducing effects. In addition, with competing priorities such as convenience, financial interest, and health necessity, a consensus on the risk–benefit ratio of EMR exposure may be difficult to achieve, and safety standards vary significantly, up to 1 000 times among countries.[171,172] Overall, there is limited evidence that magnetic fields cause childhood leukemia and insufficient evidence for other cancers in children.[173-176] A recent large census-cohort study from Switzerland did not suggest an association between predicted RF-EMF exposure from broadcast transmitters and childhood leukemia.[177] Studies of magnetic field exposure from power lines and electric blankets in adults reveal little evidence of an association with leukemia, brain tumours, or breast cancer.[173]

The most extensively studied exposure is from the use of wireless telephones (mobile and cordless phones); other exposures include occupational settings and sources from the general environment.[170] The INTERPHONE study,[178] a multicentre case-control study, is the largest study so far that studies the relationship between mobile phone use and brain tumours (i.e., glioma, acoustic neuroma, and meningioma). The pooled analyses included 2 708 glioma cases and 2 972 controls. The odds ratios (ORs) in terms of time spent on the phone showed that the highest time spent on the phone (greater than 1 640 hours of use) was related to glioma risk (OR 1.40; 95% confidence interval [CI] 1.03 to 1.89). There was a suggestion of increased risk for tumours on the same side of the head as the phone use (ipsilateral exposure) in the temporal lobe, where RF-EMF exposure is highest.[170] The OR for glioma increased with an increasing RF dose for exposures 7 years or more before diagnosis, but there was no association with estimated dose for exposures less than 7 years before diagnosis.[170] A Swedish investigative group performed a pooled analysis of two similar studies between the relationship of glioma, acoustic neuroma, and meningioma manifestation and mobile and cordless phone use.[179] Study participants who used a mobile phone for more than 1 year had an OR for glioma of 1.3 (95% CI 1.1 to 1.6). The OR increased with increasing time since first use and with total call time, attaining 3.2 (2.0 to 5.1) for more than 2 000 hours of use.[170] Ipsilateral use of the phone was associated with higher risk.[170] Similar findings were reported for cordless phones.[170] Although the INTERPHONE and Swedish studies were judged susceptible to bias, the WHO IARC Monograph Working Group concluded that the findings could not be dismissed because of bias alone and a causal relationship between mobile phones and glioma is possible.[170] The WHO Working Group concluded that there is "limited evidence in humans" for the carcinogenicity of RF-EMF based on associations between glioma and acoustic neuroma and exposure to RF-EMF from wireless phones.[170]

The WHO Working Group reviewed numerous mechanisms of carcinogenicity from RF-EMF.[170] The mechanisms included genotoxicity, effects on immune function, gene and protein expression, cell signalling, oxidative stress, apoptosis, and the blood–brain barrier. Other suggested mechanisms may include altered DNA repair mechanisms and epigenetic changes to DNA.[180] The WHO Working Group classified RF-EMF as "possibly carcinogenic to humans" (a Group 2B carcinogen, per IARC classification).

EMR from a cellphone can penetrate the skull and deposit energy 4 to 6 cm into the brain (Figure 11.14).[181] For example, a 50-minute cellphone exposure is associated with increased brain glucose metabolism in the region closest to the antenna.[182] Children have a smaller head and thinner skull bone than adults and a higher conductivity and higher absorption from RF-EMF than adults.[183-185] Concern is for children in whom the effects may be compounded because of increased vulnerability to radiation and their longer use of cellphones into adulthood. Advice about reducing exposures through simple precautions is increasing; for example, individuals should not hold a cellphone directly to their head, pregnant women should keep cellphones away from their abdomen, and children should not be allowed to play with or use a cellphone. Mobile phone manufacturers themselves are issuing advice on reducing exposure.[186] Ongoing unbiased research is desperately needed. Absolute proof of causation may be hindered because of

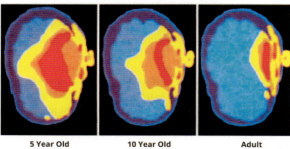

FIGURE 11.14 Electromagnetic Radiation From a Cellphone Can Penetrate the Skull. Electromagnetic radiation from a cellphone can penetrate the skull and deposit energy 4 to 6 cm into the brain. A 50-minute cellphone exposure was associated with increased brain glucose metabolism in the region closest to the antenna. This finding is of unknown clinical significance. (From Volkow, N. D., Tomasi, D., Wang, G.-J., et al. [2011]. *Journal of the American Medical Association, 305*[8], 808–813.)

TABLE 11.5 Number of New Cancer Cases[a] in 2018 Attributable to Infection, by Infectious Agent, and Development Status[b]

	Eastern Asia	Sub-Saharan Africa	Northern Europe
Hepatitis B virus	270 000 (10.5%)	15 000 (2.6%)	<1 000 (0.2%)
Hepatitis C virus	41 000 (1.5%)	8 500 (1.4%)	2 000 (0.9%)
Helicobacter pylori	480 000 (17.6%)	120 000 (19.3%)	12 000 (8%)
Human papillomavirus	140 000 (5.8%)	120 000 (19.3%)	12 000 (8%)
All infectious pathogens	**990 000 (37.9%)**	**210 000 (33.1%)**	**24 000 (13.6%)**

[a]Numbers are rounded to two significant digits.
[b]Data are the number of new cancer cases attributed to a particular infectious agent (proportion of the total number of new cases attributed to infection that is due to a specific agent).
Data from de Martel, C., Ferlay, J., Franceschi, S., et al. (2020). *Lancet Global Health, 8*(2), E180–E190.

the ethical questions associated with exposing individuals to potentially harmful interventions.

Infection, and Sexual and Reproductive Behaviour

Infection is an important contributor to cancer worldwide. The prevalence of cancer cases attributable to infections varies widely by region. In 2018, there were approximately 2.2 million cases of cancer from infection worldwide.[187] The highest prevalence occurred in Eastern Asia, at 37.9%, followed by sub-Saharan Africa at 33.1%, whereas the lowest incidence was in Northern Europe (13.6%) and Western Asia (13.8%).[188] The top four notable infections associated with new cancer cases are *Helicobacter pylori* (*H. pylori*), human papillomavirus (HPV), hepatitis B virus (HBV), and hepatitis C virus (HCV) (Table 11.5). Hepatitis B and hepatitis C can infect the liver and together, they account for a large majority of liver cancer cases (see Chapter 36); *H. pylori* accounts for the majority of all stomach cancers. Additional sources of cancer include the Epstein-Barr virus (EBV), which is linked to cancers of the nasopharynx, Hodgkin's disease, and non-Hodgkin's lymphoma; the human herpes virus type 8, which is linked to Kaposi sarcoma; and human T-cell lymphotropic virus type 1, which is linked to leukemia and lymphoma.

Large-scale prevention efforts to curb the incidence of HPV have increased over the years. At least 50% of sexually active people will have genital HPV at some time in their lives.[188] HPVs are a group of more than 150 related viruses. More than 40 of these viruses can easily spread from direct skin contact or through vaginal, rectal, or oral sex.[189] Low-risk HPVs do not cause cancer but can cause skin warts, called *condylomata acuminata*. High-risk HPVs, or oncogenic HPVs, can cause cancer. Even though about a dozen HPVs have been identified, HPV types 16 and 18 are responsible for the majority of cancers.[189] However, most high-risk HPV infections may cause cytological abnormalities or abnormal cell changes that disappear unexpectedly. Persistence of infection with high-risk HPV is a prerequisite for the development of cervical intraepithelial neoplasia (CIN) lesions (see Figure 33.16) and invasive cervical cancers.[12] HPV infection is a definite carcinogen for six types of cancer: cervix, penis, vulva, anus, and some oropharynx (including the base of the tongue and tonsils).[190] The incidence of HPV-associated oropharyngeal cancer has increased during the past 20 years, especially among men. Factors that may increase the risk of developing cancer following a high-risk HPV infection include smoking, decreased immunity, having many children (increased risk for cervical cancer), long-term oral contraceptive use (increased risk for cervical cancer), poor oral hygiene (increased risk for oropharyngeal cancer), and chronic inflammation.[191] Although the main mode of HPV transmission occurs through genital contact (oral, touching, or sexual intercourse), HPV can exist in virginal women before first intercourse.[192] Consensus is that newborn babies can be exposed to cervical HPV infection from the mother.[192] The possible modes of transmission in children, however, are controversial.[193]

Current guidelines (2013) from the Canadian Task Force on Preventive Health Care recommend that women should have a Papanicolaou smear (Pap test) every 3 years from age 25 up to the age of 70. There is little evidence to suggest when women should stop screening. Women who have received the HPV vaccine still need regular cervical screening[189,194] (see Chapter 33 for a discussion on the HPV vaccine). HPV vaccines protect males and females against diseases, including cancers, when given to the recommended age groups. HPV vaccines are given in three shots over 6 months.[195]

Other Viruses and Microorganisms

> **✓ QUICK CHECK 11.4**
> 1. Identify the high-risk types of HPV that are carcinogenic.
> 2. What components of air pollution are considered most important for carcinogenesis?
> 3. Why do certain chemicals present a notable challenge to the environment and cancer?

A discussion of the relationship between viruses, bacteria, and cancer appears in Chapter 10 and appropriate chapters in Unit 2. Other microorganisms involved in carcinogenesis include parasites such as

Opisthorchis viverrini (bile duct cancer) and *Schistosoma haematobium* (bladder cancer). Their specific roles in carcinogenesis are reported to be related to cofactors or carcinogens, or both.

Air Pollution

Outdoor air pollution is a complex mixture of many known carcinogens, and it is closely related to the incidence of lung cancer.[196] Past reviews of outdoor and household air pollution indicated that both were associated with increased rates of lung cancer, most particularly with exposures to increased levels of particles called **particulate matter (PM)**. Particulate matter, also known as *particle pollution*, is a mixture of extremely small particles and liquid droplets. PM consists of a complex mix of acids (such as nitrates and sulphates), organic chemicals, metals, and soil or dust particles. The IARC recently concluded that exposure to outdoor air pollution and to PM in outdoor air is "carcinogenic to humans" (IARC Group 1 carcinogen) and causes lung cancer.[197,198] The IARC's evaluation came from long-term epidemiological studies of residential exposure to air pollution. Specifically, focused reviews of lung cancer risk are with prominent components of PM in outdoor air ($PM_{2.5}$ particles with aerodynamic diameter equal to or less than 2.5 μm, or fine particles and PM_{10} [equal to or less than 10 μm, or inhalable particles]) (Figure 11.15).

$PM_{2.5}$ includes a higher proportion of mutagenic agents.[199] Importantly, analyses by continent of study (including North America, Europe, and others) yielded consistent, positive associations between $PM_{2.5}$ and lung cancer.[196] *Primary particles* are emitted directly from a source, for example, construction sites, unpaved roads, fields, smokestacks, or fires. *Secondary particles* are emitted from power plants, industries, and automobiles. These particles are a complex of chemicals including sulphur dioxide and nitrogen oxides and make up most of the fine particle pollution in Canada.[200] The lung easily absorbs fine or ultrafine particles, and macrophages and neutrophils that release tissue-damaging inflammatory mediators engulf these particles. Acute exposure to diesel exhaust that contains fine particles is linked to lung, throat, and eye irritations; asthma attacks; and myocardial ischemia (Figure 11.16).[201] Importantly, according to the WHO, diesel exhaust is carcinogenic and causes lung cancer.[202] The central hypothesis, based on rat studies, for the mechanisms related to particle-induced lung carcinogenesis is that insoluble particles cause pulmonary inflammation (e.g., cytokine release, ROS), which leads to oxidative stress and oxidation of DNA, proliferative response, and tissue remodelling that progresses toward fibrosis and tumour development.

Living close to certain industries is a recognized cancer risk factor.[203] Overall, fine particle pollution is also linked to other health problems and includes (1) premature death in people with heart or lung disease; (2) nonfatal heart attacks; (3) irregular heartbeat; (4) aggravated asthma; (5) decreased lung function; and (6) respiratory symptoms, including irritation of the airways, coughing, and shortness of breath.[200] In addition, other effects of particle pollution include reduced visibility (haze); environmental damage in lakes and streams, coastal waters, and river basins; depletion of nutrients in soil; and damage to forests and food crops.[200]

Indoor air pollution is generally considered worse than outdoor air pollution, partly because of cigarette smoke. ETS (secondhand smoke) can cause the formation of reactive oxygen free radicals and consequent DNA damage. The IARC has classified ETS as a human carcinogen. Another significant indoor air pollutant is radon gas. **Radon** is a natural radioactive gas derived from the radioactive decay of uranium that is ubiquitous in rock and soil; it can become trapped in houses and form radioactive decay products known to be carcinogenic to humans. The most hazardous houses can be identified by testing and then be modified to prevent further radon contamination. Exposure levels are

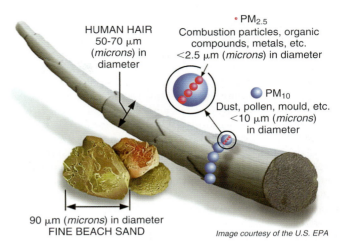

FIGURE 11.15 Particle Sizes and Pollution. *PM*, Particulate matter. (From Environmental Protection Agency. [2013]. *Particulate matter.* Updated March 18, 2013. Author.)

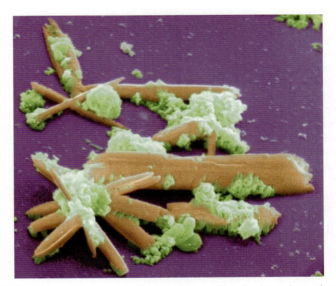

FIGURE 11.16 Exhaust Particulate Matter. Diesel exhaust is carcinogenic and causes lung cancer. *Green*, cancer cells; *brown rods*, exhaust particulate matter. (Thomas Deerinck, NCMIR/Science Source.)

greater from underground mines than from houses. Most of the lung cancers associated with radon are bronchogenic; however, small cell carcinoma does occur with greater frequency in underground miners. Radon increases the risk for lung cancer in underground miners in spite of their smoking status.

In China, some regions report very high levels of lung cancer in women who spend much of their time indoors. Exposures from heating and cooking combustion sources (e.g., oil vapours) and asbestos are identified as risk factors for lung cancer.[204] In addition, domestic coal use and ETS increase the risk for lung cancer in women and men.[205,206]

Chemical and Occupational Hazards as Carcinogens

Exposure to chemicals occurs every day—chemicals are present in air, soil, food, water, household products, toys, personal care products, workplaces, and homes. The number of known carcinogens in experimental animals is large. Most of these chemical carcinogens are potentially carcinogenic in humans, but there is a need for further research. Table 11.1 provides a summary of the chemicals according to sufficient or limited evidence in humans by cancer site. The IARC routinely updates known and probable carcinogenic agents.

Chemical carcinogenesis involves the classic genotoxic mechanisms, and exposure to genotoxic carcinogens might also involve a variety of nongenotoxic effects in cells.[207] The carcinogenic effects induced by several chemicals, including 2-acetylaminofluorene, tamoxifen, trichloroethylene, aflatoxin B_1, ochratoxin, nickel, and chromium, do not follow a classic genotoxic carcinogenesis model, but rather involve a spectrum of cellular alterations encompassing epigenetic alterations.[208] These epigenetically reprogrammed cells show an epigenetic profile similar to that frequently observed in cancer cells, including altered histone patterns, hypomethylation of DNA repetitive elements, alterations in proto-oncogenes, and hypermethylation of tumour-suppressor genes. Altered epigenetic status confers genome instability and loss of controlled growth signals, typically observed in cancer cells.[209] According to the director of the US National Institute of Environmental Health Sciences, "exposure to gene-altering substances, particularly in the womb and shortly after birth can lead to increased susceptibility to disease. There is a huge potential impact from these exposures, partly because the changes may be inherited across generations."[210]

Occupation factors account for a substantial percentage of cancers of the upper respiratory passages, lung, bladder, and peritoneum; however, fewer studies of nonsmokers exist.[211] One notable occupational factor is **asbestos-silicate mineral** woven into fabrics, used in fire-resistant, insulating materials, and many other industrial sources. Chrysotile asbestos, more than any other type, accounts for a majority of asbestos in buildings in North America. Asbestos increases the risk for mesothelioma and lung cancer and possibly other cancers. Benign conditions of asbestos exposures include pleural plaques, diffuse pleural thickening, and pulmonary fibrosis. The asbestos-related disorders (ARDs) are currently of significant occupational and public health concern.[212] Asbestos was used in homes and buildings built before the 1970s to insulate ceiling tiles, flooring, and pipe covers. In Western Europe, the epidemic of mesothelioma in building workers and other workers born after 1940 did not become apparent until the 1990s because of long latency. Asbestos usage has been banned in most developed countries, but it is still used in many developing countries and the incidence of cases of ARDs is rising.[212] No exposure to asbestos is without risk.

Inorganic arsenic, found principally in underground water (at levels ranging from 1 000 to 4 000 µg/L), is found in many regions of the world. According to the IARC, strong evidence indicates an increased risk for bladder, skin, and lung cancers following consumption of water with high levels of arsenic (generally greater than 200 µg/L).[213] Evidence for cancers of the liver, colon, and kidney is weaker. Other sources of inorganic arsenic are related to occupational exposures (see Table 11.1).

Carcinoma of the bladder has been linked with the manufacture of dyes, rubber, paint, and aromatic amines, especially β-naphthylamine and benzidine. Benzol inhalation is linked to leukemia in shoemakers and in workers in the rubber cement, explosives, and dyeing industries. Other notable occupational hazards include heavy metals (e.g., high-nickel alloy, chromium VI compounds, inorganic arsenic), silica, polycyclic aromatic hydrocarbons, sulphuric acid, and chloromethyl ether. Data from the Nurses' Health Study in the United States showed an increased risk of lung cancer associated with PM air pollution exposure.[214] Data from the European Study of Cohorts for Air Pollution Effects indicated that PM contributes to lung cancer incidence in Europe.[215] Studies of occupational exposure to diesel exhaust found an increased risk for lung cancer.[216] Other important exposures are included in Table 11.1. Disentangling data related to lung cancer, air pollution, and occupational risks is complex, especially in combination with active and passive smoking and the interplay of environmental factors and genetic polymorphisms at multiple loci.

DID YOU UNDERSTAND?

Overview
1. Cancer arises from a complicated and interacting web of multiple etiologies. Avoiding high-risk behaviours and exposure to individual carcinogens will prevent development of many types of cancers.
2. Lifestyle behaviours, dietary and environmental factors, and occupational exposure contribute to the number of cancer cases and deaths.

Genetics, Epigenetics, and Tissue
1. Cancers are caused by environmental and lifestyle factors, and genetic and epigenetic factors. Driven by genetic alterations and epigenetic abnormalities, biological processes also include variations in detoxifying enzymes or DNA repair genes. Interacting factors are weaker immune systems, differences in hormone levels, and metabolic factors. These factors are influenced by the surrounding microenvironment, or stroma.
2. Altogether, the biological environment is modified by metabolic and hormonal factors, inflammation, and disordered glucose and lipid metabolism. Once malignant phenotypes have developed, complex interactions occur between the tumour, the surrounding stroma, and the cells of the immune and inflammatory systems.

Incidence and Mortality Trends
1. Cancer is predicted to become a major cause of morbidity and mortality in the coming decades in all regions of the world.
2. The global cancer burden is shifting from the more developed countries to economically disadvantaged countries.
3. Overall, cancer death rates have been declining since the early 1990s for both men and women.

In Utero and Early Life Conditions
1. Emerging data suggest that early life events influence later susceptibility to chronic diseases.
2. Developmental plasticity is the degree to which an organism's development is contingent on its environment. Plasticity refers to the ability of genes to organize physiologically or structurally in response to environmental conditions during fetal development.
3. Studies of early versus late undernutrition in pregnancy indicate that the first trimester of pregnancy is particularly vulnerable to disease outcome in adulthood.
4. Research on DNA methylation marks, in utero environments, and future phenotypes is growing.

Environmental and Lifestyle Factors
Tobacco Use
1. Cigarette smoking is carcinogenic and the most important cause of cancer. Tobacco smoking causes cancer in more than 15 organ sites, and exposure to secondhand smoke and parental smoking causes cancer in daughters and sons and in other nonsmokers. The risk is greatest in those who begin to smoke when young and continue

smoking throughout life. However, smoking is pandemic, affecting all ages.
2. Smoking tobacco is linked to cancers of the lung, upper aerodigestive tract, lower urinary tract, kidney, pancreas, cervix, uterus, and myeloid leukemia. Recently added to the list are liver cancer and colorectal cancer.
3. Secondhand smoke is a cause of stroke, and 800 people in Canada die of lung cancer and heart disease related to secondhand smoke every year. Secondhand smoke increases the risk of death in people with cancer and cancer survivors as well as those with age-related macular degeneration, tuberculosis, ectopic pregnancy, and diabetes mellitus. Smoking increases inflammation, impairs immunity, and is a cause of rheumatoid arthritis. Smoking causes even more deaths from vascular and respiratory diseases.
4. Cigar or pipe smoking is causally related to cancers of the oral cavity, oropharynx, hypopharynx, larynx, esophagus, and lung. Pipe smokers have an increased risk of dying from cancers of lung, lip, throat, esophagus, larynx, pancreas, colon, and rectum.
5. Bidi smoking can cause cancers of the respiratory and digestive sites.

Diet
1. Understanding diet as a factor for increasing the risk for cancer is difficult yet essential. The complexity is due to the variety of foods consumed, the many constituents of foods, the metabolic consequences of eating, and the temporal changes in the patterns of food use.
2. Carcinogenic substances from diet can develop from the cooking of fat, meat, or protein (e.g., heterocyclic aromatic amines), and from naturally occurring compounds associated with plant foods.
3. Nutrigenomics is the study of the effects of nutrition on the phenotypic variability of individuals based on genomic differences. Investigators are focused on genes, single nucleotide polymorphisms, amplifications, and deletions within the DNA sequences as modifiers of the response to foods and drinks.

Nutrition, Obesity, Alcohol Consumption, and Physical Activity: Impacts on Cancer
1. Results from decades of research on specific nutrients and foods and cancers have been controversial. Less controversial are the implementation of dietary patterns, for example, the Mediterranean dietary pattern, and the promoting of specific dietary recommendations, for example, approaches to lower blood pressure.
2. The importance of diet has been illustrated by data showing changes in cancer risk among individuals in low-risk countries compared with those in high-risk countries. With migration, these changes (low risk becomes high risk) are rapid, and a plausible determinant of such changes is the adoption of the "Western" diet.
3. Most relevant to carcinogenesis, because many cellular functions are affected by nutrition (i.e., cell cycle, cell differentiation, proliferation, microRNA expression, self-renewal, DNA repair, hormonal axes), is focusing on dietary patterns and meaningful biomarkers specific to nutritional factors.
4. Nutrition may directly influence epigenetic factors that silence genes that should be active or activate genes that should be silent.
5. Dietary components can act directly as mutagens or interfere with their elimination.
6. Obesity has been increasing in developed countries and in urban areas of developing countries. Obesity in Canada is an epidemic. Studies have significantly improved the understanding of the relationship between overweight or obesity, energy balance and cancer risk, cancer recurrence, and survival.
7. Obesity is a risk factor for cancers of the endometrium, colorectum, kidney, esophagus, breast (postmenopausal), and pancreas. Evidence is growing for other cancers.
8. The mechanisms of obesity-associated cancer risks are unclear and vary by type of tumour and distribution of body fat. Emerging are three main factors related to obesity and cancer: (a) insulin–insulinlike growth factor (IGF) 1 axis, (b) sex hormones, and (c) adipokines or adipocyte-derived cytokines.
9. Metabolic changes in adipose tissue from obesity result in several alterations and include insulin resistance, hyperglycemia, dyslipidemia, hypoxia, and chronic inflammation. Tumour growth is regulated by interactions between tumour cells and stromal compartments that are rich in adipose tissue; adipocytes function as endocrine cells and shape the tumour microenvironment.
10. Alcohol plays a contributory role in several common cancers. Strong data link alcohol with cancers of the mouth, pharynx, larynx, esophagus, liver, colorectum, and breast. The evidence does not show any "safe limit" of alcohol intake, and the health effect is from ethanol, regardless of the type of drink.
11. Alcohol-related carcinogenesis involves acetaldehyde; reactive oxygen species; increased procarcinogen activation; modulation of cellular regeneration; nutritional deficiencies that may predispose to altered mucosal integrity, and enzyme and metabolic dysfunction; and other structural abnormalities. Under investigation are epigenetic alterations and the effects of alcohol metabolism.
12. Physical activity reduces the risk for breast and colon cancers and may reduce the risk for other cancers.
13. Biological mechanisms for the protective effects of physical activity include decreasing insulin and IGF levels, decreasing obesity, increasing free radical scavenger systems, altering inflammatory mediators, decreasing levels of circulating sex hormones and metabolic hormones, improving immune function, enhancing cytochrome P-450 activity (thus modifying carcinogen activation), and increasing gut motility.
14. Physical activity helps prevent type 2 diabetes, which has been associated with risk for cancer of the colon and pancreas.
15. Many unanswered questions remain regarding frequency, intensity, and duration of exercise and its protective effects.
16. The *Canadian 24-Hour Movement Guidelines* suggest that being active every day, and for at least 150 minutes per week, can help reduce the risk for many conditions, including certain types of cancer.
17. Exercise in children with cancer was associated with improved body composition, flexibility, and cardiorespiratory fitness.

Ionizing Radiation
1. Much of the knowledge of the effects of ionizing radiation (IR) on human cancer has come from Hiroshima and Nagasaki atomic bomb exposures, particularly data from the Life Span Study. Other evidence is from exposure to radiation for medical reasons, underground miners, and other occupational exposures. Human exposure includes emissions from the environment, X-rays, computed tomography (CT) scans, radioisotopes, and other radioactive sources.
2. From the atomic bomb exposures in Japan, increased frequencies of cancers occurred in thyroid and breast tissue, and lung, stomach, colon, esophageal, and urinary tract cancers increased, as did multiple myeloma.
3. Excess relative risks (ERRs) for radiation-induced cancers at a given age are much higher for individuals exposed during childhood. What is in question now is the ERRs of radiation exposure in adulthood.

4. New models of carcinogenesis identify IR not only as an initiator of premalignant cell clones but also as a promoter of pre-existing premalignant damage.
5. Other health risks from radiation include cardiovascular effects and somatic mutations that may contribute to other diseases. These effects may manifest years after completion of radiation therapy.
6. The risks from low-dose radiation are being debated among radiobiologists, geneticists, physicists, and others because of the potential effect on the health of current and future generations.
7. IR is a mutagen and carcinogen; it can penetrate cells and tissues and deposit energy in tissues at random in the form of ionizations.
8. IR affects many cellular processes, including gene expression, mitochondrial function, nucleotide base damage, and single-strand breaks and double-strand breaks to DNA. These changes can lead to carcinogenesis.
9. It is now known that radiation may induce a type of genomic instability to the progeny of the directly irradiated cells over many generations of cell divisions and can affect so-called bystander cells. Investigators are studying genomic instability as it may contribute to secondary cancers.
10. Epigenetic events after radiation include alterations in pathways affecting cell adhesion, extracellular matrix interactions, and cell-to-cell communication.

Ultraviolet Radiation

1. Ultraviolet (UV) radiation comes from sunlight. Other sources of UV radiation include electric lights, black lights, and tanning lamps. Most of the UV radiation received on earth is UVA and some UVB. UVA radiation is weaker than UVB, but UVA penetrates deeper into the skin and is more constant throughout the year despite the weather.
2. The incidence of basal cell carcinoma (BCC) and squamous cell carcinoma (SCC) is strongly correlated with lifetime sunlight exposure. Intense intermittent recreational sun exposure has been associated with melanoma and BCC. Tanning bed use has been associated with an increased risk for BCC and data suggest sun-bed use as a reason for increased melanoma, especially in women. Chronic occupational sun exposure has been associated with SCC.
3. Cumulative sun exposure is the additive effects of intermittent sun exposure, chronic sun exposure, or both.
4. UV radiation is known to cause specific gene mutations: for example, SCC involves mutation in the *TP53* gene, BCC in the patched 1 tumour-suppressor gene (*PTCH1*), and melanoma in the *p16* gene. Investigators are identifying epigenetic alterations in tumour tissues and cell lines for skin cancers.
5. Skin exposure to UV radiation produces ROS in large quantities that can overwhelm tissue antioxidants and other oxygen-degrading pathways. Imbalances in ROS can lead to oxidative stress, tissue injury, and direct DNA damage.
6. UV radiation can activate the transcription factor NF-κB and other free radicals important in regulating genes that induce inflammation. Inflammation is a critical component of tumour progression.
7. Melanoma is the most lethal skin cancer and the incidence of melanoma has been increasing worldwide. The pathogenesis of melanoma is complex, including genetic and environmental factors.

Electromagnetic Radiation

1. Radiofrequency electromagnetic radiation (RF-EMR) is a type of nonionizing and low-frequency radiation. Health risks associated with RF-EMR are controversial. Exposure to electric and magnetic fields is widespread.
2. RF-EMR sources include microwaves, radar, mobile phones, cordless phones, cellphone towers (base stations), power frequency radiation associated with electricity and radio waves, fluorescent lights, computers, and other electric equipment.
3. Data regarding the effects of RF-EMR have been slow to emerge because of lack of methods to accurately measure exposure, lack of clear dose–response relationships, reproducing effects, financial interests, and other priorities, such as convenience.
4. Overall, there is limited evidence that magnetic fields cause childhood leukemia and insufficient evidence for other cancers in children.
5. The WHO International Agency for Research on Cancer (IARC) Monograph Working Group classified RF-EMF as "possibly carcinogenic to humans" (a Group 2B carcinogen, per IARC classification).

Infection, and Sexual and Reproductive Behaviour

1. Infection is an important contributor to cancer worldwide. The top four notable infections associated with new cancer cases are human papillomavirus (HPV), *Helicobacter pylori*, hepatitis B virus (HBV), and hepatitis C virus (HCV).
2. Although about a dozen HPVs have been identified, HPV types 16 and 18 are responsible for the majority of cancers. Persistence of infection with high-risk HPV is a prerequisite for the development of cervical intraepithelial neoplasia (CIN) lesions and invasive cancer.
3. HPV infection has been identified as a definite carcinogen for six types of cancer: cervix, penis, vulva, anus, and some oropharynx (including the base of the tongue and tonsils).
4. The incidence of HPV-associated oropharyngeal cancer has increased during the past 20 years, especially among men.
5. Biological factors that may interact with HPV infection to increase cancer risk include long-term oral contraceptive use, smoking, decreased immunity, having many children, poor oral hygiene (increased risk for oropharyngeal cancer), and chronic inflammation.
6. HPV may be transmitted by genital contact (oral, touching, or sexual intercourse). The possible modes of transmission in children are controversial; newborn babies can be exposed to cervical HPV infection from the mother.

Air Pollution

1. Indoor and outdoor air pollution are both associated with increased rates of lung cancer. The IARC concluded that exposure to outdoor air pollution and to particulate matter (PM) in outdoor air is carcinogenic to humans.
2. $PM_{2.5}$ includes a higher proportion of mutagenic agents. Primary particles are emitted directly from a source, for example, construction sites, unpaved roads, or smokestacks. Secondary particles are emitted from power plants, industries, and automobiles. Diesel exhaust is carcinogenic and causes lung cancer.
3. Acute exposure to diesel exhaust that contains fine particles is linked to lung, throat, and eye irritations; asthma attacks; and myocardial ischemia.
4. The hypothesis for the mechanisms related to particle-induced lung carcinogenesis is that insoluble particles cause pulmonary inflammation, which leads to oxidative stress and oxidation of DNA, proliferative response, tissue remodelling that progresses toward fibrosis, and tumour development.
5. Fine particle pollution also is linked to premature death in people with heart or lung disease, nonfatal heart attacks, irregular heartbeat, and decreased lung function.

6. Indoor air pollution is generally considered worse than outdoor air pollution. Sources of indoor air pollution include secondhand smoke, heating and cooking combustion sources, radon, and coal use.

Chemicals and Occupational Hazards as Carcinogens

1. An estimated 100 000 synthetic chemicals are used in North America; only about 7% have been tested for their health effects.
2. Exposure to chemicals occurs from air, soil, food, water, household products, toys, personal care products, medications, workplaces, and homes.
3. The IARC has classified carcinogenic agents as known and probable.
4. Chemical carcinogenesis involves genotoxic and epigenetic alterations. Other mechanisms include hormonal disruption, interference with cell signalling mechanisms, and other unknown effects.
5. Exposure to gene-altering substances, particularly in the womb and shortly after birth, can lead to increased susceptibility to disease.
6. A substantial percentage of cancers of the upper respiratory passages, lung, bladder, and peritoneum are attributed to occupational factors.
7. Asbestos is linked to an epidemic of mesothelioma in Western Europe. Asbestos usage has been banned in most developed countries, but it is still used in many developing countries.

12

Cancer in Children and Adolescents

Stephanie Zettel, with originating chapter contributions by Lauri A. Linder

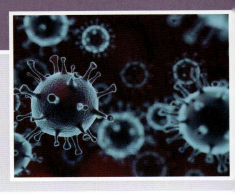

Additional resources are available online at https://evolve.elsevier.com/Canada/Huether/pathophysiology

CHAPTER OUTLINE

Incidence, Etiology, and Types of Childhood Cancer, 294
 Etiology, 295
 Genetic and Genomic Factors, 295

 Environmental Factors, 296
Prognosis, 297

LEARNING OBJECTIVES

1. Describe the incidence and types of childhood cancer.
2. Discuss some of the characteristic differences between cancer in children and cancer in adults.
3. Discuss the relative importance of host, genetic, and environmental factors in the occurrence, identification, and treatment of childhood cancer.
4. Discuss the prognosis factors in childhood cancer.

KEY TERMS

Embryonic tumour, 295
Li-Fraumeni syndrome (LFS), 295
Mesodermal germ layer, 294

Multiple causation, 295
Wilms tumour, 296

Cancer can occur at any age, but its impact at a younger age can be particularly devastating. While cancer in children and adolescents is rare, according to Statistics Canada, in 2019, cancer was the second leading cause of disease-related death in children under the age of 15 years.[1] Survival rates among children and adolescents with cancer have dramatically improved since the 1960s. Combination chemotherapy, the incorporation of research data obtained from clinical trials, and the use of multimodal treatment for solid tumours are among the factors contributing to improved cure rates.

INCIDENCE, ETIOLOGY, AND TYPES OF CHILDHOOD CANCER

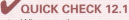 **QUICK CHECK 12.1**
1. What are the most common childhood cancers, and how do they differ from adult cancers?
2. Why are children less likely to develop carcinomas?
3. Compare and contrast different etiological factors associated with the development of childhood cancer.

In 2019, an estimated 1 000 children under the age of 14 years were diagnosed with cancer.[2] Childhood cancer accounts for less than 1% of all new cancer cases in Canada. The three types of cancer that account for most of the cases between birth and 14 years of age are leukemia, brain and central nervous system cancers, and lymphoma. Similarly, most cancer deaths in children from birth to 14 years of age are related to brain and central nervous system cancers, leukemia, and neuroblastoma and other peripheral nervous cell tumours. Young men are more likely to die from cancer than young women.

The types of malignancies that occur in children are vastly different from those that affect adults. The most common types of cancer among adults include prostate, breast, lung, and colon cancer. In contrast, children tend to develop leukemias, brain tumours, and sarcomas. Although many adult cancers have associated environmental and lifestyle factors that could theoretically be avoided, such as sun exposure and smoking, very few such factors have been linked to pediatric malignancies. More data are emerging that the developing child may be affected by epigenetic modifications resulting from parental exposures before conception, exposures in utero, and nutrition during early life.[3,4]

Most childhood cancers originate from the **mesodermal germ layer**, which develops into connective tissue, bone, cartilage, muscle, blood, blood vessels, gonads, kidney, and the lymphatic system (Figure 12.1). Thus, the more common childhood cancers are leukemias, sarcomas, and embryonic tumours.

Leukemias are circulating tumours that primarily involve the blood and bone marrow, whereas lymphoma tends to localize to lymph tissue. Common manifestations of these disorders are related to myelosuppression or organ dysfunction secondary to the infiltration of white blood cells. These malignancies also tend to present with nonspecific symptoms (i.e., "B symptoms" as opposed to absence of symptoms, or "A symptoms") such as malaise, weakness, unexplained fever, night sweats, and recurrent infections (those affected will often have large, nontender lymph nodes). Classification of hematological neoplasms is based on the cell type of the neoplasm, rather than its location in the body. Myeloid

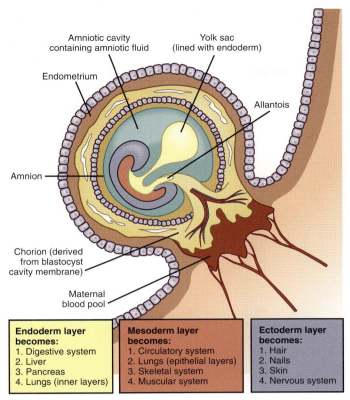

FIGURE 12.1 Mesodermal Germ Layer.

cancers involve cells from the myeloid lineage (e.g., erythrocytes, granulocytes, platelets, and monocytes), and lymphoid cancers are derived from B lymphocytes, T lymphocytes, and natural killer cells. Hodgkin's lymphoma is another example of a lymphoid cancer.[5]

Embryonic tumours originate during intrauterine life and contain abnormal cells that appear to be immature embryonic tissue unable to mature or differentiate into fully developed functional cells. Embryonic tumours are most often diagnosed early in life (usually by 5 years of age) and are rare in older children, adolescents, and adults. The names of these tumours often include the root term *blast* (e.g., neuroblastoma, retinoblastoma), which indicates the embryonic stage of development.

Sarcomas, leukemias, and lymphomas are cancers observed in childhood and also may occur in adults. Most adult cancers, however, involve epithelial tissue and are, therefore, *carcinomas*. Carcinomas rarely occur in children because these cancers most commonly result from environmental carcinogens and require a long period from exposure to the appearance of the carcinoma. Carcinomas begin to increase in incidence between the ages of 15 and 19 years, becoming the most common cancer tissue type observed after adolescence.[6]

Childhood cancers are often diagnosed during peak times of physical growth and maturation, accounting for the bimodal distribution in their incidence. In general, they are extremely fast-growing cancers, resulting in a relatively short *latency period* (the time from the initial exposure to the onset of symptoms). The distribution of cancer types also changes during childhood and adolescence. Leukemias and embryonal tumours have a peak incidence before the child is 5 years of age. Brain tumours, the second leading type of childhood cancer overall, have a peak incidence among children less than 15 years of age. The incidence of specific subtypes of brain tumours does, however, vary across childhood and adolescence. Lymphomas, both Hodgkin's and non-Hodgkin's, represent the third most common type of childhood cancer. Lymphoma is rare in children under 5 years of age and occurs with increasing frequency in children and adolescents 10 years of age and older. Rhabdomyosarcoma is the most common soft tissue sarcoma of childhood. Rhabdomyosarcoma has a bimodal age distribution with two thirds of cases occurring in children less than 6 years of age and one third occurring in children and adolescents 10 years of age and older. The two most common types of bone tumours are osteosarcoma and Ewing sarcoma. These cancers are more likely to occur in adolescents ages 15 and older.

Etiology

The causes of cancer in children are largely unknown. A few environmental factors are known to predispose a child to cancer, but there are relatively few causal factors for most childhood cancers. A number of host factors, many of which are genetic risk factors or congenital conditions, influence the development of childhood cancer (Table 12.1).

Because of their relatively short latency period, most childhood cancers do not lend themselves to early cancer warning signs. The CAUTION acronym from the American Cancer Society (and adopted by Canada), which outlines the seven warning signs of cancer, does not apply because it describes adult, environmentally caused carcinomas. Likewise, early screening strategies for childhood cancers are not available. Although host factors are important in identifying populations of children at risk for cancer, most children who are diagnosed with cancer do not have known predisposing environmental or host factors.

Multiple causation theory provides a useful framework for interpreting the results of epidemiological studies. For example, laboratory and epidemiological studies may indicate that exposure to a certain chemical can cause leukemia, but not all children exposed to that chemical will develop leukemia. Determining what other host and environmental factors must interact with chemical exposure to cause the disease requires further research.

Genetic and Genomic Factors

Acquired or inherited mutations in individual genes may contribute to the development of cancer in children and adolescents. Mutations in more than 150 oncogenes and tumour-suppressor genes have been associated with the subsequent development of both childhood and adult cancers (Table 12.2). Fanconi anemia and Bloom's syndrome are two autosomal recessive conditions that result in impaired DNA repair and are risk factors for the development of acute leukemia.[7] Retinoblastoma, a malignant embryonic tumour of the eye, occurs either as an inherited defect in the *RB1* gene or as an acquired mutation (see Chapter 17).

Although leukemia is not inherited as a genetic condition, siblings of children with leukemia have a two to four times increased risk for the development of leukemia relative to that of siblings of healthy children. The occurrence of leukemia in monozygous twins is estimated to be as high as 25%.

Li-Fraumeni syndrome (LFS) is an autosomal dominant disorder involving the *TP53* tumour-suppressor gene. For individuals with a mutation in the *TP53* gene, the risk of developing cancer as a child or adult is significantly higher than the risk in the unaffected population. Children and adults in families affected by LFS are at risk for soft tissue sarcoma, breast cancer, leukemia, osteosarcoma, melanoma, and cancer of the colon, pancreas, adrenal cortex, and brain. Individuals with LFS also are at increased risk of developing multiple primary cancers.[8]

Chromosomal abnormalities also may contribute to the development of childhood cancer. Chromosomal abnormalities include aneuploidy, deletions, amplifications, translocations, and fragility (see Chapter 2). These abnormalities may occur within the affected cancer cells as a consequence of malignant transformation or may be present as the consequence of a congenital syndrome.

TABLE 12.1 Congenital Factors Associated With Childhood Cancer

Syndrome	Associated Childhood Cancer
Chromosome Alterations	
Down syndrome	Acute leukemia
13q syndrome	Retinoblastoma
Chromosome Instability	
Ataxia-telangiectasia	Lymphoma
Bloom's syndrome	Acute leukemia, lymphoma, Wilms tumour
Fanconi anemia	Acute myelogenous leukemia, myelodysplastic syndrome, hepatic tumours
Hereditary Syndromes	
Beckwith-Wiedemann syndrome	Wilms tumour, sarcoma, brain tumours, neuroblastoma, hepatoblastoma
Neurofibromatosis type I	Brain tumour, sarcomas, neuroblastomas, Wilms tumour, nonlymphocytic leukemia
Neurofibromatosis type II	Meningioma (malignant or benign), acoustic neuroma or schwannoma, gliomas, ependymomas
Tuberous sclerosis	Glial tumours
Li-Fraumeni syndrome	Sarcoma, adrenocortical carcinoma
Von Hippel-Lindau disease	Cerebellar hemangioblastoma, retinal angioma, renal cell carcinoma, pheochromocytomas
Ataxia-telangiectasia	Leukemia, lymphoma, brain tumours
Gorlin syndrome	Medulloblastoma, skin tumours
Immunodeficiency Disorders	
Congenital	
Agammaglobulinemia	Lymphoma, leukemia, brain tumours
Immunoglobulin A (IgA) deficiency	Lymphoma, leukemia, brain tumours
Wiskott-Aldrich syndrome	Leukemia, lymphoma
Acquired	
Aplastic anemia	Leukemia
HIV/AIDS	
Organ transplantation	Leukemia, lymphoma
Congenital Malformation Syndromes	
Aniridia, hemihypertrophy, hamartoma, genitourinary anomalies	Wilms tumour
Cryptorchidism	Testicular tumour
Gonadal dysgenesis	Gonadoblastoma
Family Susceptibility	
Twin or sibling with leukemia	Leukemia

HIV/AIDS, Human immunodeficiency virus/acquired immunodeficiency syndrome.

TABLE 12.2 Selected Oncogenes and Tumour-Suppressor Genes Associated With Childhood Cancer

Gene	Associated Pediatric Tumour
Oncogenes	
ABL	Acute lymphoblastic leukemia
MYCN	Neuroblastoma
MYB	Neural tumours, leukemia, lymphoma, rhabdomyosarcoma, Wilms tumour, neuroblastoma
erbB	Glioblastomas
NRAS	Neuroblastoma, leukemia
HRAS/KRAS	Neuroblastoma, rhabdomyosarcoma, leukemia
ATM	Lymphoma, leukemia
Tumour-Suppressor Genes	
RB1	Retinoblastoma, sarcoma
WT1, WT2	Wilms tumour, leukemia
NF-1	Sarcoma, primitive neuroectodermal tumour, juvenile chronic myelocytic leukemia
NF-2	Brain tumours, melanoma, meningiomas
p16	Brain tumours, leukemia
TP53	Sarcoma, leukemia, brain tumours, lymphoma
DCC	Ewing sarcoma, rhabdomyosarcoma
CDKN2A	Glioblastoma, acute lymphoblastic leukemia
CDC2L1	Non-Hodgkin's lymphoma, neuroblastoma

Data from Beamer, L. C., Linder, L., Wu, B., et al. (2013). The impact of genomics on oncology nursing. *Nursing Clinics of North America, 48*(4), 585–626; Esparza, S. D., Sakamoto, K. M., Milton, B. A., et al. (2016). *Childhood cancer genetics.* http://emedicine.medscape.com/article/989983-overview#a1.

A chromosomal translocation results from the rearrangement of two nonhomologous chromosomes. Translocations may result in the creation of a fusion gene in which the two previously separate gene regions unite. Two fusion genes associated with acute lymphocytic leukemia (ALL) in children are the *BCR-ABL* gene, resulting from a translocation between chromosomes 9 and 22, and the *TEL-AML1* gene, resulting from a translocation between chromosomes 12 and 21.[9,10]

Several syndromes associated with specific congenital malformations are linked to a higher incidence of cancer development. In some cases, these children may be carefully followed and screened for tumour development. One of the more recognized syndromes is trisomy 21 (Down syndrome), which has an increased susceptibility to acute leukemia. The risk of developing leukemia is 10 to 20 times greater among children with Down syndrome than in children without Down syndrome. The age distribution for developing ALL among children with Down syndrome is similar to that of children without Down syndrome.[11]

Wilms tumour, a malignant tumour of the kidney, is particularly recognized for its association with a number of congenital anomalies, including genitourinary anomalies, aniridia (congenital absence of the iris), hemihypertrophy (muscular overgrowth of half of the body or face), and intellectual disabilities. Identifiable malformations and congenital predisposition syndromes are present in approximately 17% of children diagnosed with Wilms tumour.[12]

Environmental Factors

Finding the cause of any disease is typically a long, slow process. Epidemiological studies require many years to determine whether a risk factor is possibly related to the development of childhood cancer. No single factor determines whether an individual will develop cancer, even if a specific environmental exposure explains a high proportion of the occurrence of a specific cancer (Box 12.1).

Prenatal Exposure

Prenatal exposure to some medications and to ionizing radiation has been linked to childhood cancers. The most well-described medication is diethylstilbestrol (DES), which was prescribed by physicians to prevent spontaneous miscarriage (in women with previous miscarriage). In 1971, DES was identified as a transplacental chemical

BOX 12.1 Factors That May Contribute to the Development of Childhood and Adolescent Cancer

- Genetic and epigenetic factors
- Diet
- Immune function
- Occupational exposure
- Ionizing radiation
- Hormonal variations
- Viral illnesses
- Individual characteristics, such as the biological, social, and physical environment

TABLE 12.3 Medications That May Increase Risk for Childhood Cancer

Medication Class	Uses	Cancer Risk
Anabolic androgenic steroids	To stimulate bone growth and appetite; induce puberty; increase muscle mass and physical strength	Hepatocellular carcinoma
Epipodophyllotoxin and anthracycline chemotherapy agents	To treat cancer	Leukemia
Immunosuppressive agents	To prevent organ rejection following transplantation surgery	Lymphoma

HEALTH PROMOTION

Magnetic Fields and Development of Pediatric Cancer

Several recent reports have suggested an association between environmental sources and the development of cancer in children. The presence of low-frequency magnetic fields has been a concern for many years as causing leukemia in children. Several meta-analyses dating from 2000 all report significant associations between exposure and risk of leukemia. Based on pooled or meta-analyses, as well as subsequent peer-reviewed studies, there is strong evidence that excessive exposure to magnetic fields increases risk of adult leukemia, male and female breast cancer, and brain cancer. There is also some evidence that both paternal and maternal prenatal exposure to magnetic fields results in an increased risk of leukemia and brain cancer in offspring.

Ongoing research needs to be done in this area because environmental factors may require many years of exposure to cause disease. Additionally, an association between an environmental factor and childhood cancer does not establish causality. Ongoing research is needed to better understand the relationships between environmental factors and other factors associated with childhood cancer, as well as potential underlying mechanisms by which environmental factors may contribute to the development of childhood cancer.

Data from Carpenter, D. O. (2019). Extremely low frequency electromagnetic fields and cancer: how source of funding affects results. *Environmental Research, 178*, 108688. https://doi.org/10.1016/j.envres.2019.108688.

---

carcinogen because a small percentage of the daughters of women who took DES developed adenocarcinomas of the vagina. Since then, other studies have attempted to identify other medications taken by pregnant women that may cause cancer in their offspring, but no other medications have been found to have this effect. Current evidence suggests that an increased risk for childhood leukemia is associated with low levels of exposure to antenatal X-rays.[13] An association between antenatal X-ray exposure and childhood brain tumours has not been identified.[14] Other current areas of research include exploring epigenetic modifications resulting from prenatal exposures and their role in future cancer development.[7]

Childhood Exposure

Childhood exposure to ionizing radiation, medications, electromagnetic fields, or viruses has been associated with the risk of developing cancer. Retrospective research has shown a significant correlation between radiation-induced malignancies and either radiotherapy (cancer treatment) or radiation exposure from diagnostic imaging.[15] A few medications, in particular, may increase cancer risk during childhood (in addition to the medications and environmental agents that cause cancer in adults and increase risk for exposure during childhood). Table 12.3 highlights many of these medications.

The relationship between childhood cancer and other environmental factors (e.g., electromagnetic fields, small appliances, radon) has been the focus of many epidemiological studies. Although there are some associations between environmental exposures and acute leukemia, no conclusive causal evidence exists[16–18] (see *Health Promotion: Magnetic Fields and Development of Pediatric Cancer*).

The strongest association between viruses and the development of cancer in children has been the Epstein-Barr virus (EBV), which is linked to Burkitt lymphoma, nasopharyngeal carcinoma, and Hodgkin's disease.[19] Children with acquired immunodeficiency syndrome (AIDS), caused by human immunodeficiency virus (HIV), have an increased risk of developing non-Hodgkin's lymphoma and Kaposi sarcoma. However, with the use of highly active antiretroviral therapy in the developed world, the incidence of AIDS-related malignancies has declined dramatically.[20]

PROGNOSIS

More than 70% of children diagnosed with cancer are cured. Some of the factors leading to improved cure rates in pediatric oncology include the use of combination chemotherapy or multimodal treatment for solid childhood tumours and improvements in nursing and supportive care. The development of research centres for comprehensive childhood cancer treatment and cooperative study groups also have facilitated refinements in treatment protocols and data sharing, leading to improved survival rates.

The management of hematological malignancies in children and adolescents focuses on the use of combination chemotherapy to kill the malignant cells, followed by a stem cell transplant to rescue and restore bone marrow function[5] (see *Health Promotion*: Bone Marrow Transplantation: Improving Outcomes for Canadian Children and Adolescent Cancer Patients). *Induction* chemotherapy removes as many of the neoplastic cells as possible and is followed by the *consolidation* phase, aimed at eliminating nondetectable cells. *Maintenance* chemotherapy prolongs remission of the cancer. Administration of chemotherapy is often into the cerebrospinal fluid intrathecally because malignant blood and lymph cells can migrate across the blood–brain barrier to the central nervous system. The donor and host cells must be extensively cross-matched to ensure the transplantation is successful. There is a possibility of the transplanted donor cells mounting an

HEALTH PROMOTION

Bone Marrow Transplantation: Improving Outcomes for Canadian Children and Adolescent Cancer Patients

Allogeneic bone marrow transplantation (BMT) provides the chance of a cure to patients with potentially fatal leukemias and lymphomas. *Allogeneic* transplants involve the donation of bone marrow from an otherwise healthy donor and have dramatically improved patient outcomes in a number of ways. However, there are risks and side effects associated with BMT. Treatments include antimicrobials with greater specificity for bacterial and fungal infections that result from prolonged neutropenia, as well as the use of growth factors such as granulocyte colony-stimulating factors in the supportive care of patients with infections associated with transplantation.

While research continues into mechanisms that explain why some BMTs fail (i.e., due to graft-versus-host disease), efforts to identify the best possible marrow donors in Canada also have the potential to dramatically improve transplant outcomes. Extensive human leukocyte antigen (HLA) typing is essential for the "best" match and the "best" outcomes. Signing up to be a marrow donor is easy, and it is voluntary. Increasing the number of donors in the registry and the specificity of HLA typing ensures the usefulness of this registry (https://www.cttcanada.org/donations/fund.asp?id=5198) for both recipients and donors in years to come.

Data from Cell Therapy Transplant Canada. (2020). *About CTTC.* https://www.cttcanada.org/page/AboutCTTC.

immune attack on the host's tissues, resulting in *graft-versus-host disease*, which can be life-threatening.

Today, 83% of children diagnosed with cancer in Canada will survive, and this is partly due to increased efforts in research.[21] Childhood cancer is consistently underfunded, accounting for only 5% of all cancer research funding in Canada today. Survivors of childhood cancer are at increased risk of developing a second malignancy during their lifetime. This risk may be associated with a variety of factors, including previous chemotherapy or radiotherapy, genetic factors, and type of primary cancer (e.g., soft tissue sarcoma, neuroblastoma). Because childhood cancer should be viewed as a chronic disease instead of a fatal illness, treatment includes attention to quality of life and symptom management. Even those cancers that cannot be cured generally can be treated, resulting in significantly improved quality of life. Children and adolescents whose cancers are regarded as cured still face residual and late effects of their treatment. These late effects are more significant in children than in adults because treatment given during childhood occurs in a physically immature, growing individual. Late effects that need further study include physical impairments, reproductive dysfunction, soft tissue and bone atrophy, learning disabilities, secondary cancers, and psychological sequelae. More must be learned about the genetic factors associated with childhood malignancies and about the genetic consequences of treatment. A referral to genetic services is appropriate for families of children whose cancer is known to be transmitted genetically (e.g., retinoblastoma, LFS).

DID YOU UNDERSTAND?

Overview
1. Childhood cancer is a rare disease, but it remains the leading cause of death that is attributable to disease in children.

Incidence, Etiology, and Types of Childhood Cancer
1. The most common type of childhood cancer is leukemia, and the second most common type is cancer involving the brain or central nervous system.
2. Although many adult cancers are associated with environmental and lifestyle factors, very few such factors have been linked to pediatric malignancies because children have not lived long enough to be affected by them.
3. Children with immunodeficiencies are at increased risk of developing cancer because of an ineffective immune system.
4. Children with Down syndrome are at increased risk of developing leukemia.
5. Risk factors that may be associated with the development of childhood cancer include inherited and acquired genetic and epigenetic factors, diet, immune function, occupational exposure, ionizing radiation, hormonal variations, viral illnesses, and other individual characteristics (e.g., the biological, social, or physical environment).

Prognosis
1. Survivors of childhood cancer are at increased risk of developing a second malignancy during their lifetime, compared with the general population.

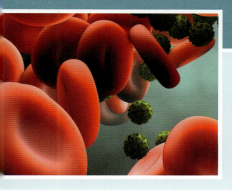

13

Structure and Function of the Neurological System

Kelly Power-Kean, with originating chapter contributions by Sue E. Huether

Additional resources are available online at https://evolve.elsevier.com/Canada/Huether/pathophysiology

CHAPTER OUTLINE

Overview and Organization of the Nervous System, 300
Cells of the Nervous System, 301
    The Neuron, 301
    Neuroglia and Schwann Cells, 302
    Nerve Injury and Regeneration, 302
The Nerve Impulse, 304
    Synapses, 304
    Neurotransmitters, 304
The Central Nervous System, 305
    The Brain, 305
    The Spinal Cord, 311
    Motor Pathways, 311

Sensory Pathways, 312
Protective Structures of the Central Nervous System, 313
Blood Supply of the Central Nervous System, 316
The Peripheral Nervous System, 318
The Autonomic Nervous System, 319
    Anatomy of the Sympathetic Nervous System, 319
    Anatomy of the Parasympathetic Nervous System, 322
    Neurotransmitters and Neuroreceptors, 322
    Functions of the Autonomic Nervous System, 322
GERIATRIC CONSIDERATIONS: **Aging and the Nervous System, 326**

LEARNING OBJECTIVES

1. Name the functional divisions of the nervous system.
2. List the parts of the central and peripheral nervous systems.
3. Explain the difference between a dendrite and an axon.
4. Discuss the importance of myelin and the nodes of Ranvier.
5. Describe the factors affecting nerve repair and regeneration after injury.
6. Discuss synaptic transmission of signals by neurotransmitters. Include an explanation of the regulation mechanisms of the process.
7. Develop a chart describing the three regions of the brain. Focus on the location, structures, function, and outputs of each region.
8. Discuss the function of the upper and lower motor neurons.
9. Name the different levels of the vertebral column.
10. Discuss the differences between the motor and sensory pathways of the spinal cord.
11. Discuss the purpose of the blood–brain barrier.
12. Draw the circulation path of blood and cerebrospinal fluid through the brain and spinal cord.
13. Describe the sensory and motor functions of the peripheral nervous system.
14. Discuss the effects of sympathetic and parasympathetic stimulation on the body systems.
15. Describe tests performed to assess the function of the nervous system.

KEY TERMS

Acetylcholine, 322
Adrenergic transmission, 322
Afferent pathway (ascending pathway), 301
Afferent (sensory) neuron, 311
α-Adrenergic receptor, 322
Anterior column, 311
Anterior fossa, 313
Anterior horn (ventral horn), 311
Anterior spinal artery, 318
Anterior spinothalamic tract, 312
Arachnoid, 314
Arachnoid villi, 315
Association fibre, 308

Associational neuron (interneuron), 302
Astrocyte, 302
Autonomic nervous system (ANS), 301
Axon, 301
Axon hillock, 301
Basal ganglia (basal nuclei), 308
Basal ganglia system (extrapyramidal system), 306
Basilar artery, 316
Basis pedunculi, 310
β-Adrenergic receptor, 322
Bipolar neuron, 301

Blood–brain barrier (BBB), 318
Brachial plexus, 319
Brain network, 305
Brainstem, 305
Broca area (Brodmann areas 44, 45), 307
Cauda equina, 311
Caudate nucleus, 308
Cavernous sinus, 316
Celiac, 319
Central canal, 311
Central nervous system (CNS), 301
Central sulcus (fissure of Rolando), 306
Cerebellum, 305

Cerebral aqueduct (aqueduct of Sylvius), 310
Cerebral cortex, 306
Cerebral nuclei, 308
Cerebral peduncle, 310
Cerebrospinal fluid (CSF), 314
Cholinergic transmission, 322
Choroid plexus, 314
Circle of Willis, 317
Collateral ganglia, 319
Contralateral control, 307
Conus medullaris, 311
Convergence, 304
Corpora quadrigemina, 310
Corpus callosum (transverse or commissural fibres), 308

Corticobulbar tract, 307
Corticobulbar tract axon, 311
Corticospinal tract (pyramidal system), 307
Cranial nerve, 301
Craniosacral division, 322
Dendrite, 301
Dermatome, 319
Diencephalon (interbrain), 309
Divergence, 304
Dopamine, 310
Dura mater, 313
Effector organ, 301
Efferent (motor) neuron, 311
Efferent pathway (descending pathway), 301
Ependymal cell, 302
Epicritic information, 312
Epithalamus, 309
Excitatory postsynaptic potential (EPSP), 304
Extradural space, 314
Extrapyramidal system, 308
Facilitation, 304
Falx cerebri, 314
Fascicle, 318
Filum terminale, 311
Frontal lobe, 306
Galea aponeurotica, 313
Ganglia (plexus), 301
Globus pallidus, 308
Grey matter, 306
Hypothalamus, 309
Inferior colliculi, 310
Inferior mesenteric, 319
Inhibitory postsynaptic potential (IPSP), 304
Inner dura (meningeal layer), 313
Insula (insular lobe), 308
Internal capsule, 308
Internal carotid artery, 316
Interventricular foramen (foramen of Monro), 315
Intervertebral disc, 316
Lateral aperture (foramen of Luschka), 315

Lateral column, 311
Lateral corticospinal tract, 311
Lateral horn, 311
Lateral spinothalamic tract, 312
Lateral sulcus (Sylvian fissure, lateral fissure), 306
Lentiform nucleus, 308
Limbic system, 308
Longitudinal fissure, 306
Lower motor neuron, 311
Lumbar plexus, 319
Median aperture (foramen of Magendie), 315
Meninges, 313
Metencephalon, 310
Microfilament, 301
Microglia, 302
Microtubule, 301
Midbrain (mesencephalon), 310
Middle fossa (temporal fossa), 313
Mixed nerves, 319
Motor unit, 311
Multipolar neuron, 301
Myelencephalon (medulla oblongata), 311
Myelin, 301
Myelin sheath, 301
Neurofibril, 301
Neurogenesis, 304
Neuroglia, 302
Neuroglial cell, 301
Neuromuscular (myoneural) junction, 302
Neuron, 301
Neuroplasticity, 304
Neurotransmitter, 304
Neurotrophic factors, 304
Nissl substance, 301
Nodes of Ranvier, 301
Nonmyelinating Schwann cell, 302
Norepinephrine, 322
Nucleus pulposus, 316
Occipital lobe, 308

Oligodendroglia (oligodendrocyte), 302
Parasympathetic nervous system, 319
Parietal lobe, 308
Pelvic nerve, 322
Periosteum (endosteal layer), 313
Peripheral nervous system (PNS), 301
Pia mater, 314
Plexus, 319
Pons, 311
Postcentral gyrus, 308
Posterior column (fasciculus gracilis, fasciculus cuneatus), 312
Posterior fossa, 313
Posterior horn, 311
Posterior root ganglion, 311
Posterior spinal artery, 318
Postganglionic neuron, 319
Postsynaptic neuron, 304
Precentral gyrus, 307
Prefrontal area, 306
Preganglionic neuron, 319
Premotor area (Brodmann area 6), 306
Presynaptic neuron, 304
Primary motor area (Brodmann area 4), 307
Primary voluntary motor area, 307
Protopathic, 312
Pseudounipolar neuron, 301
Putamen, 308
Pyramidal system, 307
Red nucleus, 310
Reflex arc, 311
Reticular activating system (RAS), 305
Reticular formation, 305
Reticulospinal tract, 311
Rubrospinal tract, 311
Sacral plexus, 319
Saltatory conduction, 301
Satellite cell, 301

Schwann (neurilemma) cell, 301
Sensory neuron, 302
Somatic nervous system, 301
Spatial summation, 304
Spinal cord, 311
Spinal tract, 311
Splanchnic nerve, 319
Striatum, 308
Subarachnoid space, 314
Subdural space, 314
Substantia gelatinosa, 311
Substantia nigra, 310
Subthalamus, 309
Sulci, 306
Summation, 304
Superior colliculi, 310
Superior mesenteric, 319
Sympathetic nervous system, 319
Sympathetic (paravertebral) ganglia, 319
Synapse, 304
Synaptic bouton, 304
Synaptic cleft, 304
Tegmentum, 310
Telencephalon (cerebral hemisphere), 306
Temporal lobe, 308
Temporal summation, 304
Tentorium cerebelli, 314
Thalamus, 309
Thoracolumbar division, 319
Unipolar neuron, 301
Upper motor neuron, 311
Ventricle, 314
Vermis, 310
Vertebral artery, 316
Vertebral column, 311
Vestibulospinal tract, 311
Wallerian degeneration, 302
Wernicke area, 308
White matter, 306

The human nervous system is an amazing structure responsible for decision making and for the body's ability to interact with the environment. This structure is also involved in the regulation and control of activities affecting our internal organs. It is a network composed of complex structures that send electrical and chemical signals between the brain and the body's many organs and tissues. Aging changes occur throughout life and vary among persons (see the Geriatric Considerations: Aging and the Nervous System box). This chapter provides a basic overview of the structure and function of the nervous system and supports the understanding of nervous system pathophysiology in the following chapters.

OVERVIEW AND ORGANIZATION OF THE NERVOUS SYSTEM

 QUICK CHECK 13.1
1. How do the functions of the somatic and autonomic nervous systems differ?
2. What are the three parts of a neuron?
3. How does myelin affect nerve signals?
4. Name and describe the process through which injured axons undergo repair.

Although the nervous system functions as a unified whole, structures and functions have been divided here to help understanding. The nervous system is divided into the central nervous system and the peripheral nervous system. The **central nervous system (CNS)** consists of the brain and spinal cord, enclosed within the protective cranial vault and vertebrae, respectively. The **peripheral nervous system (PNS)** includes the **cranial nerves**, the spinal nerves, and their ganglia. There are two peripheral nerve pathways. **Afferent pathways (ascending pathways)** carry sensory signals toward the CNS. **Efferent pathways (descending pathways)** innervate skeletal muscle and effector organs by sending motor signals away from the CNS.

Functionally, the PNS is divided into the somatic nervous system and the autonomic nervous system. The **somatic nervous system** consists of pathways that control voluntary motor movement (e.g., skeletal muscle). The **autonomic nervous system (ANS)** is involved with regulation of the body's internal environment (viscera) through involuntary control of organ systems. The ANS is further divided into sympathetic and parasympathetic divisions. **Effector organs** have a nervous supply provided by the nervous system.

CELLS OF THE NERVOUS SYSTEM

Two types of cells form the nervous tissue: neurons and supporting cells. The **neuron** is the primary cell of the nervous system. It is an electrically excitable cell and transmits information. **Neuroglial cells** (astrocytes, microglia, and oligodendrocytes in the CNS) and **Schwann (neurilemma) cells** and **satellite cells** (in the PNS) supply neurons with structural support, protection, and nutrition.

The Neuron

Working alone or in units, neurons detect environmental changes and start body responses to support a steady state. The size and structure of neurons vary greatly so that each neuron is adapted to perform specific functions. The fuel source for the neuron is mainly glucose. Cells in the CNS do not require insulin for glucose uptake. The cellular parts of neurons include four main components. **Microtubules** transport substances within the cell. **Neurofibrils** are very thin supportive fibres that extend throughout the neuron. It is thought that **microfilaments** help transport cellular products. **Nissl substances** consist of endoplasmic reticulum and ribosomes that are involved in protein synthesis.

A neuron (Figure 13.1) has three parts: a cell body (soma), the dendrites (thin branching fibres of the cell), and the axons. Most cell bodies are found within the CNS. Cell bodies found in the PNS usually are found in groups called **ganglia** (or **plexuses**—a group of relay nerves). The **dendrites** are extensions that carry nerve signals toward the cell body. **Axons** are long projections that carry nerve signals away from the cell body. The **axon hillock** is the cone-shaped process where the axon leaves the cell body. The first part of the axon hillock has the lowest threshold for stimulation, so action potentials begin there. A typical neuron has one axon, which may be wrapped with a layer of lipid material called **myelin**. Myelin is an insulating substance that speeds impulse spread. The entire membrane is the **myelin sheath** (Figures 13.2 and 13.25B). The **nodes of Ranvier** are regular gaps or interruptions in the myelin sheath. Axons can branch at the nodes of Ranvier. In the CNS, oligodendrocytes make myelin. In the PNS, Schwann cells make myelin. Telodendria form presynaptic vesicles for neurotransmission.

The principle of *divergence* refers to the ability of axonal branches to affect many different neurons. *Convergence* occurs when branches of various numbers of neurons "converge" on and affect a single neuron. Nutrient exchange is not possible through the myelin sheath. It can occur at the nodes of Ranvier where the axon is not insulated. Where there is

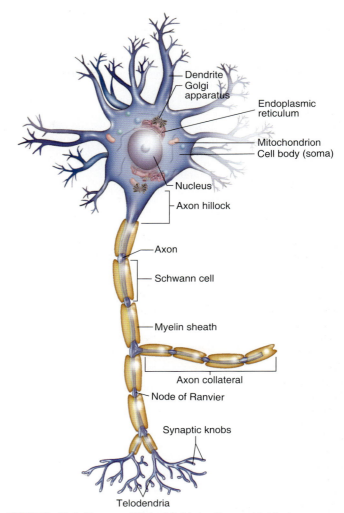

FIGURE 13.1 Neuron With Multiple Parts. Multipolar neuron: Peripheral nervous system neuron with multiple extensions from the cell body. (Modified from Patton, K. T., & Thibodeau, G. A. [2018]. *The human body in health & disease* [7th ed.]. Elsevier.)

myelin, the speed of nerve signals increase. Myelin acts as an insulator that allows an action potential to jump between segments rather than flow along the entire length of the membrane. This process creates an increase in speed and is called **saltatory conduction**. Disorders of the myelin sheath (demyelinating diseases), such as multiple sclerosis and Guillain-Barré syndrome, show the important role myelin plays in nerve conduction (see Chapter 16). Conduction speeds depend on the myelin coating and on the diameter of the axon. Larger axons send signals at a faster rate.

Structurally, neurons are classified based on the number of processes (projections) extending from the cell body. There are four types of cell structures: (1) unipolar, (2) pseudounipolar, (3) bipolar, and (4) multipolar. **Unipolar neurons** have one process that branches shortly after leaving the cell body. The retina is an example of this type. **Pseudounipolar neurons** (also called *unipolar*) also have one process. The dendritic part of each of these neurons extends away from the CNS, and the axon part projects into the CNS (see Figure 13.2). This makeup is typical of sensory neurons in cranial and spinal nerves. **Bipolar neurons** have two processes arising from the cell body. This type of neuron connects the rod and cone cells of the retina. **Multipolar neurons** are the most common and have many processes capable of wide branching. A motor neuron is typically multipolar (see Figure 13.2).

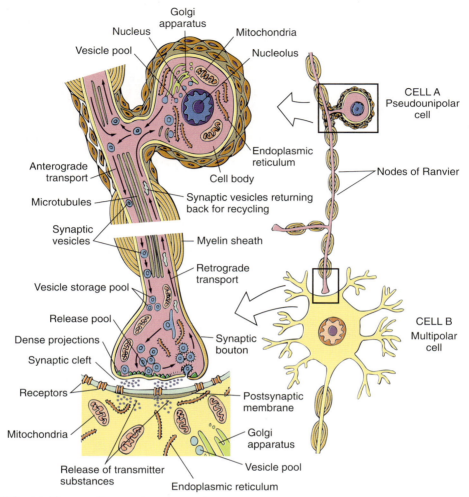

FIGURE 13.2 Neuronal Transmission and Synaptic Cleft. Electrical impulse travels along axon of first neuron (presynaptic cell) to synapse. Chemical transmitter is secreted into synaptic space to depolarize membrane (dendrite or cell body) of next neuron (postsynaptic cell) in the pathway. *Cell A* represents pseudounipolar cell; *cell B* represents multipolar cell.

Functionally, there are three types of neurons (their direction of transmission and typical makeup are noted in parentheses): (1) sensory (afferent, mostly pseudounipolar), (2) associational (interneurons, multipolar), and (3) motor (efferent, multipolar). **Sensory neurons** carry signals from peripheral sensory receptors to the CNS. **Associational neurons (interneurons)** send signals from neuron to neuron—that is, from sensory to motor neurons. They are found within the CNS. Motor neurons send signals away from the CNS to an effector (i.e., skeletal muscle or organs). In skeletal muscle, the end processes form a **neuromuscular (myoneural) junction** (see Figure 13.15).

Neuroglia and Schwann Cells

Neuroglia ("nerve glue") is the category of non-neuronal cells that support the neurons of the CNS. They include about half of the total brain and spinal cord volume and are 5 to 10 times more numerous than neurons. Different types of neuroglia serve different functions. **Astrocytes** surround blood vessels, fill the spaces between neurons, and add to synaptic function in the CNS.[1] **Oligodendroglia (oligodendrocytes)** form myelin sheaths within the CNS. **Ependymal cells** line the cerebrospinal fluid (CSF)–filled cavities of the CNS. **Microglia** remove debris (phagocytosis) in the CNS. Schwann cells form the myelin sheath around axons and direct axonal regrowth and functional recovery in the PNS.[2] **Nonmyelinating Schwann cells** supply metabolic support. (Figure 13.3 and Table 13.1 feature neuroglia and Schwann cells.)

Nerve Injury and Regeneration

Mature nerve cells do not divide. As such, injury can cause permanent loss of function. When an axon is severed or cut, **Wallerian degeneration** occurs in the distal axon: (1) typical swelling appears at the axon distal to the cut; (2) the neurofilaments hypertrophy; (3) the myelin sheath shrinks and breaks down; and (4) the axon collapses and disappears. The myelin sheaths re-form into Schwann cells that line up in a column between the severed part of the axon and the effector organ.

At the proximal end of the injured axon, similar changes occur but only back to the next node of Ranvier. In response to trauma, the cell body swells and dies by the process called chromatolysis (dispersing the Nissl substance) or apoptosis. During the repair process, the cell increases protein synthesis and mitochondrial activity. About 7 to 14 days after the injury, new terminal sprouts project from the proximal segment and may enter the remaining Schwann cell pathway. (Figure 13.4 shows a detailed

CHAPTER 13 Structure and Function of the Neurological System

CENTRAL NERVOUS SYSTEM NEUROGLIA

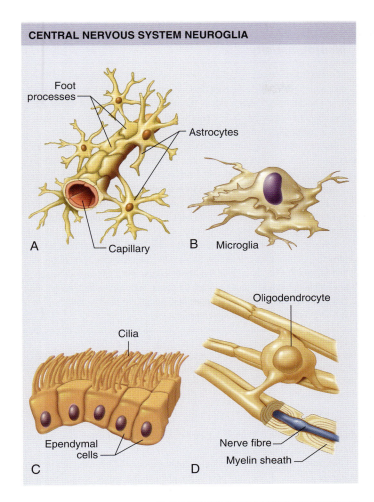

TABLE 13.1	Support Cells of the Nervous System
Cell Type	**Primary Functions**
Astrocytes	Form specialized contacts between neuronal surfaces and blood vessels
	Provide quick transport for nutrients and metabolites
	Form a key part of the blood–brain barrier
	Appear to be scar-forming cells of CNS, which may be a focus for seizures
	Appear to work with neurons in processing information and memory storage
Oligodendroglia (oligodendrocytes)	Form the myelin sheath in the CNS
Schwann cells	Form the myelin sheath in the PNS
Nonmyelinating Schwann cells	Provide metabolic support and regeneration of neurons in the PNS
Microglia	Clear cellular debris (phagocytic properties)
Ependymal cells	Line the ventricles and choroid plexuses involved in making cerebrospinal fluid

Data from Banaclocha, M. A. (2005). Neuromagnetic dialogue between neuronal minicolumns and astroglial network: a new approach for memory and cerebral computation. *International Journal of Neuroscience, 115*(3), 329–337; Sofroniew, M. V., & Vinters, H. V. (2010). Astrocytes: biology and pathology. *Acta Neuropathologica, 119*(1), 7–35; Vanderah, T., & Gould, D. (2015). *Nolte's the human brain: an introduction to its functional anatomy* (7th ed.). Mosby. *CNS,* Central nervous system; *PNS,* peripheral nervous system.

PERIPHERAL NERVOUS SYSTEM NEUROGLIA

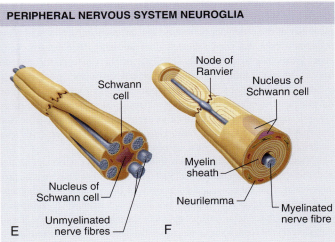

FIGURE 13.3 Types of Neuroglial Cells. Central nervous system (CNS) neuroglia: **A,** Astrocytes attached to the outside of a capillary blood vessel in the brain. **B,** A phagocytic microglial cell. **C,** Ciliated ependymal cells forming a sheet that usually lines fluid cavities in the brain. **D,** An oligodendrocyte with processes that wrap around nerve fibres in the CNS to form myelin sheaths. PNS neuroglia: **E,** A Schwann cell supporting a bundle of nerve fibres in the PNS. **F,** Another type of Schwann cell surrounding a peripheral nerve fibre to form a thick myelin sheath. (From Patton, K. T. [2019]. *Anatomy & physiology* [10th ed.]. Elsevier.)

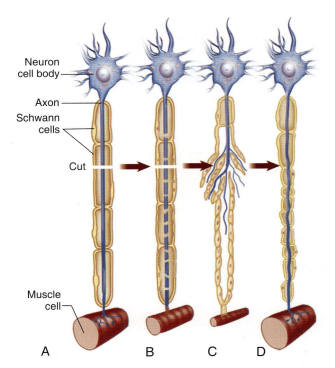

FIGURE 13.4 Repair of a Peripheral Nerve Fibre. When cut, a damaged motor axon can regrow to its distal end only if the Schwann cells still are intact (to form a guiding tunnel) and if scar tissue does not block its way. (From Patton, K. T., & Thibodeau, G. A. [2013]. *Anatomy & physiology* [8th ed.]. Mosby.)

version of these events.) This process occurs with myelinated fibres only, and normally occurs only in the PNS. An increased rate of scar formation and the different kind of myelin formed by the oligodendrocyte limits CNS axonal part renewal.

Nerve renewal depends on many factors. These factors include the site of the injury, the type of injury, the presence of inflammation, and the process of scarring. The closer the injury is to the nerve cell body, the greater the chance is that the nerve cell will die and not regenerate. A crushing injury allows better renewal than a cut injury. Crushed nerves can recover fully, but cut nerves form connective tissue scars that block or slow renewal of axonal branches. Recovery of peripheral nerves injured close to the spinal cord is poor and slow. This occurs because of the long distance between the cell body and the peripheral end of the axon.[3]

THE NERVE IMPULSE

QUICK CHECK 13.2
1. Explain the process of chemical impulse conduction.
2. What are neurotransmitters? Give two examples.
3. Compare summation and facilitation.

Neurons produce and conduct electrical and chemical impulses. The neurons selectively change the electrical potential of the plasma membrane and affect other nearby neurons by releasing chemicals (**neurotransmitters**). An unexcited neuron keeps a resting membrane potential. An action potential is created with an adequately raised membrane potential. The nerve impulse then flows to all parts of the neuron. The action potential response occurs only when the stimulus is strong enough. If the stimulus is too weak, the membrane stays unexcited. This property is termed the *all-or-none response* (see Chapter 1 for a review of electrical impulse conduction).

Synapses

Neurons are not physically continuous with one another. The space between adjacent neurons is a **synapse** (see Figure 13.2). Chemical and electrical conduction sends impulses across the synapse (see Figure 13.2). Here we will only discuss chemical conduction. Chapter 1 reviews information on electrical conduction (see Figure 1.28). The names of neurons that conduct a nerve impulse correspond to whether they relay signals toward the synapse (**presynaptic neurons**) or away from the synapse (**postsynaptic neurons**). When an impulse begins in a presynaptic neuron, the impulse reaches the vesicles, and the **synaptic bouton** stores the chemicals (neurotransmitters). Once released from the vesicles, the neurotransmitters diffuse across the **synaptic cleft** (the space between the neurons). They then bind to specific neurotransmitter (protein) receptor sites on the plasma membrane of the postsynaptic neuron, sending the impulse (see Figure 13.2). Brain synapses can change in strength and number throughout life. This ability is known as synaptic plasticity or **neuroplasticity** (see *Health Promotion:* Neuroplasticity).

Neurotransmitters

Neurotransmitters are chemicals made in the neuron and found in the presynaptic terminal (synaptic bouton). When released into the synaptic cleft, neurotransmitters bind to a receptor site (binding site) on the postsynaptic membrane of another neuron or effector. It is here that they affect ion channels (see Figure 13.2). Each neurotransmitter is removed by a specific process from its site of action. Many substances are neurotransmitters, including norepinephrine, acetylcholine, dopamine, histamine, and serotonin. Many of these transmitters have more than one function.[4] Table 13.2 reviews neurotransmitter and neuromodulator substances.

Because neurotransmitters are normally stored on one side of the synaptic cleft and the receptor sites are on the other side, chemical synapses work in one direction. Therefore, the transmission of action potentials occurs in one direction along a multineuronal pathway. The binding of the neurotransmitter at the receptor site changes the permeability of the postsynaptic neuron and its membrane potential. Two possible events can then follow: (1) excitement (depolarized; **excitatory postsynaptic potentials [EPSPs]**) of the postsynaptic neuron may occur, or (2) inhibition (hyperpolarized; **inhibitory postsynaptic potentials [IPSPs]**) of the postsynaptic neuron's plasma membrane may occur. The release of cannabinoid transmitters occurs from postsynaptic neurons. They modulate neurotransmitter release from the presynaptic neurons (retrograde transmission).[5] (Chapter 1 reviews electrical impulses and membrane potentials.)

Usually, a single EPSP cannot induce a neuron's action potential and the spread of the nerve impulse. Whether this response occurs depends on the number and frequency of potentials the postsynaptic neuron receives. This concept is known as **summation**. **Temporal summation** (time relationship) refers to the effects of successive, rapid signals received from a single neuron at the same synapse. **Spatial summation** (spacing effect) is the joint effect of signals from several neurons onto a single neuron at the same time. **Facilitation** refers to the effect of EPSP on the plasma membrane potential. The plasma membrane is helped when summation brings the membrane closer to the threshold potential and decreases the stimulus required to induce an action potential. The effect that a chemical neurotransmitter has on the plasma membrane potential depends on the balance of these effects. The mechanisms of **convergence** (many neurons firing and meeting on one neuron), **divergence** (one neuron firing and diverging on many neurons), summation, and facilitation allow for the joint processes of the nervous system.

HEALTH PROMOTION
Neuroplasticity

Scientists studying neuroplasticity explore ways to help the process of brain restructuring. Research supplies key information for the improvement of health related to diseases of aging. Researchers have found that as we age, the adult brain continues to form new neural connections and grow new neurons in response to learning or training.

Recent research suggests that physical activity can have a major impact on brain function. Research shows that sustained, regular, aerobic exercise produces major improvements in thinking processes and brain growth. It promotes **neurogenesis** by increasing the production of **neurotrophic factors**. It is also associated with improvements in spatial memory. New research aims to identify lifestyle behaviours that could improve normal brain growth and repair damaged brains.

Although the benefits of aerobic exercise have yet to be fully studied, many data support the value of exercise. Benefits include promoting brain plasticity and improving CNS function in the aging process and dementia. Behaviour, environmental issues, thought, and emotions may also affect neoplastic change. These factors have important implications for healthy development, learning, memory, and brain injury recovery.

Based on Cramer, S. A., Sur, M., Dobkin, B. H., et al. (2011). Harnessing neuroplasticity for clinical applications. *Brain, 134*(6), 1591–1609. doi:10.1093/brain/awr039; Liou, S. (2010, June 26). *Neurobiology* [Blog post]. http://web.stanford.edu/group/hopes/cgi-bin/hopes_test/neuroplasticity/.

TABLE 13.2 Substances That Are Neurotransmitters or Neuromodulators

Substance	Location	Effect	Clinical Example
Acetylcholine	Many parts of the brain, spinal cord, neuromuscular junction of skeletal muscle, and many ANS synapses	Excitatory or inhibitory	Alzheimer's disease (a type of dementia) is associated with a decrease in acetylcholine-secreting neurons. Myasthenia gravis (weakness of skeletal muscles) results from a decrease in acetylcholine receptors.
Monoamines			
Norepinephrine	Many areas of the brain and spinal cord; also, in some ANS synapses	Excitatory or inhibitory	Cocaine and amphetamines[a] result in overstimulation of postsynaptic neurons.
Serotonin	Many areas of the brain and spinal cord	Generally inhibitory	Involved with mood, anxiety, and sleep induction. Levels of serotonin are elevated in schizophrenia (delusions, hallucinations, withdrawal).
Dopamine	Some areas of brain and ANS synapses	Generally excitatory	Parkinson's disease (depression of voluntary motor control) results from the damage of dopamine-secreting neurons. Medications used to increase dopamine production cause vomiting and schizophrenia.
Histamine	Posterior hypothalamus	Excitatory (H1 and H2 receptors) and inhibitory (H3 receptors)	No clear cause exists for histamine-associated pathological conditions. Histamine is involved with arousal and attention, and links to other brain transmitter systems.
Amino Acids			
Gamma-aminobutyric acid (GABA)	Most neurons of CNS have GABA receptors	Most postsynaptic inhibition in the brain	Medications that increase GABA function have been used to treat epilepsy by reducing excessive discharge of neurons.
Glycine	Spinal cord	Most postsynaptic inhibition in the spinal cord	Glycine receptors are inhibited by strychnine.
Glutamate and aspartate	Widespread in the brain and spinal cord	Excitatory	Medications that block glutamate or aspartate, such as riluzole, are used to treat amyotrophic lateral sclerosis. These medications might prevent overexcitation from seizures and neural degeneration.
Neuropeptides			
Endorphins and enkephalins	Widely distributed in CNS and PNS	Generally inhibitory	Morphine and heroin bind to endorphin and enkephalin receptors on presynaptic neurons and reduce pain by blocking the release of neurotransmitters.
Substance P	The spinal cord, brain, and sensory neurons associated with pain, gastro-intestinal tract	Generally excitatory	Substance P is a neurotransmitter in pain transmission pathways. Blocking release of substance P by morphine reduces pain.

[a]They increase the release, and block the reuptake of, norepinephrine.
From Daroff, R. B., Fenichel, G. M., Jankovic, J., et al. (2012). *Bradley's neurology in clinical practice* (6th ed.). Saunders.
ANS, Autonomic nervous system; *CNS*, central nervous system; *PNS*, peripheral nervous system.

THE CENTRAL NERVOUS SYSTEM

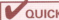

QUICK CHECK 13.3
1. Name the three major divisions of the brain and their parts.
2. Describe the limbic system's functions.
3. What are the two major functions of the hypothalamus?

The Brain

The brain is a functionally joined path of millions of neurons. These neurons have different genomes, structures, molecular structures, networks, and connections. The brain weighs about 1.4 kg (3 pounds) and receives 15 to 20% of the total cardiac output. The brain allows a person to reason, function intellectually, express personality and mood, and perceive and interact with the environment.

The brain is composed of three major structural divisions. These divisions are (1) the forebrain (prosencephalon), which includes the telencephalon and diencephalon; (2) the midbrain (mesencephalon), which connects the pons to the diencephalon; and (3) the hindbrain (rhombencephalon), which includes the cerebellum, pons, and medulla (Table 13.3 and Figure 13.5). The midbrain, medulla, and pons make up the brainstem. The brainstem connects the hemispheres of the brain, cerebellum, and spinal cord. A group of nerve cell bodies (nuclei) within the brainstem is called the reticular formation (Figure 13.6). The reticular formation is a large network of diffuse nuclei that connect the brainstem to the cortex. This formation controls vital reflexes, such as cardiovascular function and respiration. It also helps support wakefulness and attention and, therefore, is referred to as the reticular activating system (RAS) (see Figure 13.6). Some nuclei within the reticular formation control certain motor movements, such as balance and posture.[4]

Each part of the brain is associated with a different function. However, assigning specific functions to distinct regions of the brain is not exact. For clinical matters, functional specificity is very useful for pinpointing pathological conditions in various nervous system regions. Dr. Brodmann, a German neuropsychiatrist, first proposed that various actions are linked to many regions of the cerebral cortex.[6] (Figure 13.7C shows these regions and describes some of the areas.) The mapping of brain networks is also helpful in learning how varying parts of the brain interact when performing a given function[7,8] (Box 13.1).

TABLE 13.3 Divisions of the Central Nervous System

Primary Brain Vesicles	Secondary Vesicles	Structures in Secondary Vesicles
Forebrain (prosencephalon)	Telencephalon	Cerebral hemispheres Cerebral cortex Basal ganglia
	Diencephalon	Epithalamus Thalamus Hypothalamus Subthalamus
Midbrain (mesencephalon)	Mesencephalon	Corpora quadrigemina (tectum—superior and inferior colliculi) Cerebral peduncles
Hindbrain (rhombencephalon)	Metencephalon	Cerebellum Pons
	Myelencephalon	Medulla oblongata
Spinal cord	Spinal cord	Spinal cord

BOX 13.1 Brain Networks

The structure and joint function of neural nodes, networks, and interconnected pathways within the brain are being mapped in the advancing field of human connectomics. Several imaging techniques are available that use mathematical and computational models. Positron emission tomography (PET) measures pairs of gamma rays emitted by an introduced positron-emitting radionuclide. Tracer diffusion tensor magnetic resonance imaging (MRI) measures the diffusion of water in tissue and functional MRI measures changes in blood flow. Magnetoencephalography (MEG) measures magnetic fields produced by electric currents made by neurons. Finally, electroencephalography (EEG) measures voltage changes in brain neurons.

The figure that follows supplies an image of brain connectivity showing interconnecting cortical pathways using diffusion tensor imaging tracking technology. Such mapping of the brain adds to an understanding of the similarities and differences of the normally functioning brain. It can also be used to understand changes associated with aging and disease (i.e., degenerative brain disease, epilepsy, schizophrenia, and brain tumours).

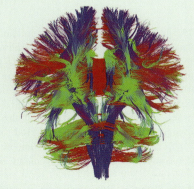

(Image reprinted with permission from Filippi, M. [2013]. Assessment of system dysfunction in the brain through MRI-based connectomics. *The Lancet Neurology, 12*[12], 1189–1199.)

From Park, H. J., & Friston, K. (2013). *Science, 342*(6158), 1238411; Pollock, J. D., Wu, D.-Y., & Satterlee, J. (2014). *Trends Neurosci, 37*(2), 106–123; Sporns, O. (2013). *Neuroimage, 80*, 53–61; see also the Human Connectome Project at https://www.humanconnectome.org/study/hcp-young-adult.

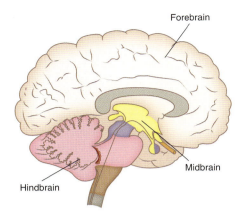

FIGURE 13.5 Structural Divisions of the Brain. (From Standring, S., [Ed.]. [2008]. *Gray's anatomy: the anatomical basis of clinical practice* [40th ed.]. Churchill Livingstone.)

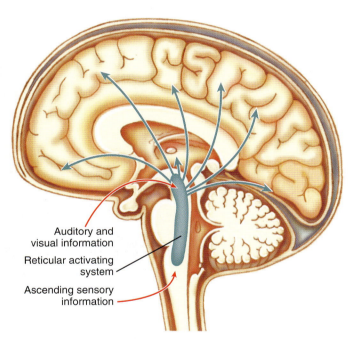

FIGURE 13.6 Reticular Activating System. Nuclei in the brainstem reticular formation make up the reticular activating system (RAS). It also includes fibres that conduct sensory information to the nuclei and fibres that conduct from the nuclei to widespread areas of the cerebral cortex. Functioning of the RAS is vital for consciousness.

Forebrain

Telencephalon. The cerebral cortex (the largest part of the brain) and the basal ganglia (made of several *nuclei*) make up the **telencephalon (cerebral hemispheres)**. Ridges called *gyri* cover the surface of the cerebral cortex (see Figure 13.7). These gyri increase the surface area of the cortex and the number of neurons. **Sulci** are the grooves on both sides of a gyrus and *fissures* are the deeper grooves. The **cerebral cortex** has an outer layer of cell bodies of neurons (**grey matter**). The **white matter** consists of myelinated nerve fibres that lie below the cerebral cortex.

A deep groove called the **longitudinal fissure** divides the two cerebral hemispheres. The surface of each hemisphere is divided into lobes named after the region of the skull under which each lobe lies. The

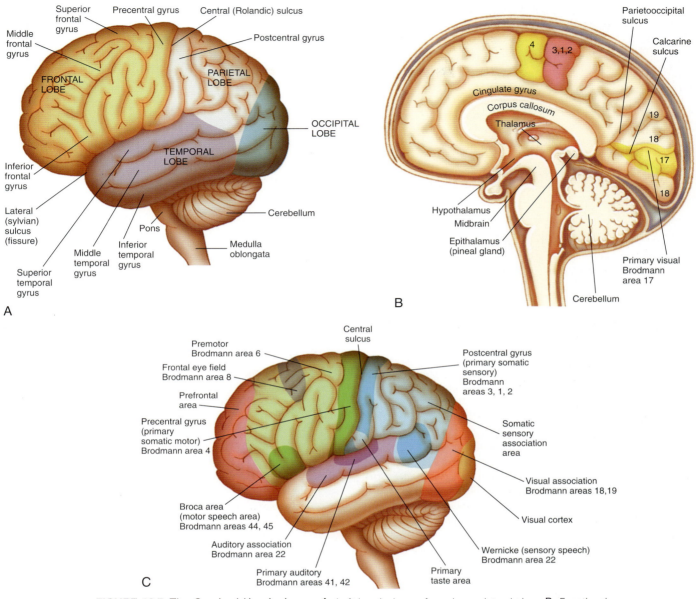

FIGURE 13.7 The Cerebral Hemispheres. **A**, Left hemisphere of cerebrum, lateral view. **B**, Functional areas of the cerebral cortex, midsagittal view. **C**, Functional areas of the cerebral cortex, lateral view.

posterior edge of the **frontal lobe** is on the **central sulcus (fissure of Rolando)**, and it borders inferiorly on the **lateral sulcus (Sylvian fissure, lateral fissure)** (see Figure 13.7). Dr. Brodmann created a map of about 50 different areas of the cerebral cortex. This map numbered the areas according to function and histology. Those who study the functions of the cortex use this map (e.g., Brodmann area 6 is involved in premotor movements). Goal-oriented behaviour (e.g., the ability to concentrate), short-term memory, the expansion of thought, and inhibition of the limbic areas of the CNS occur in the **prefrontal area**. Programming motor movements occurs in the **premotor area (area 6)** (see Figure 13.7C). This area holds the cell bodies that form part of the **basal ganglia system**, also called the **extrapyramidal system**. Efferent pathways outside the pyramids of the medulla oblongata make up this system. The middle frontal gyrus contains the frontal eye fields (part of area 8), which are involved in controlling eye movements.

The **primary motor area (area 4)**, found along the **precentral gyrus** forming the **primary voluntary motor area**, has a somatotopic structure that is often called a *homunculus* (little human) (Figure 13.8). Electrical stimulation of certain areas of this cortex causes specific muscles of the body to move. For example, stimulation of area 4 in the medial longitudinal fissure affects the lower limb and foot. Stimulation of the superior lateral surface of the precentral gyrus affects the trunk and arm, the middle third of the hand, and the lower third of the face and the mouth and throat. The axons travelling from the cell bodies in and on either side of this gyrus project fibres (axons) that form the **pyramidal system**. This system includes two tracts: (1) the **corticobulbar tract** synapses in the brainstem and supplies voluntary control of muscles in the head and neck; (2) the **corticospinal tracts (pyramidal system)** descend into the spinal cord and supply voluntary control of muscles throughout the body. Cerebral signals control function on the opposite

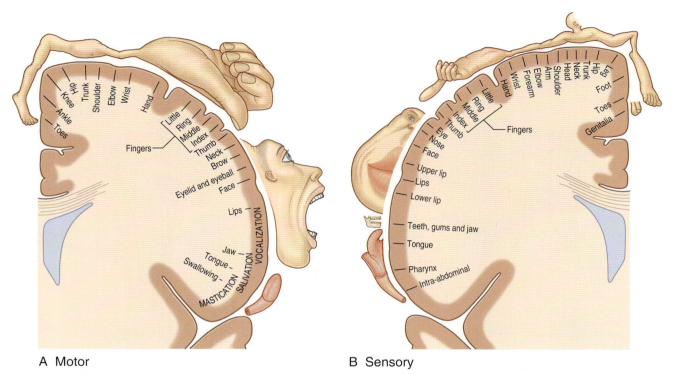

FIGURE 13.8 Primary Somatic Motor and Sensory Areas of the Cortex. A, The motor homunculus shows relative somatotopical representation in the main motor area. B, The sensory homunculus shows relative somatotopical representation in the somaesthetic cortex. (From Standring, S. [Ed.]. [2008]. *Gray's Anatomy: the anatomical basis of clinical practice* [40th ed.]. Churchill Livingstone.)

side of the body and is called contralateral control (Figure 13.9A). The Broca area (areas 44, 45) is anterior on the inferior frontal gyrus. It is usually on the left hemisphere and controls the motor aspects of speech. Damage to this area, commonly because of a cerebrovascular accident (stroke), results in being unable to, or having difficulty forming words (expressive aphasia or dysphasia) (see Chapter 15).

The parietal lobe lies within the borders of the central, parietooccipital, and lateral sulci. This lobe holds the major area for somatic sensory input. It is found mainly along the postcentral gyrus (areas 3, 1, 2) (see Figure 13.7), which is next to the primary motor area. Association fibres supply communication between the motor and sensory areas (and other regions in the cortex). Much of this region is involved in sensory association (storage, analysis, and interpretation of stimuli). (Figure 13.8 shows the distribution of functions linked with both the primary motor area and the primary sensory area of the cerebral cortex.)

The occipital lobe is below the parietooccipital sulcus and is superior to the cerebellum. The primary visual cortex (area 17) is in this region and receives input from the retinas. Much of this lobe is involved in visual association (areas 18, 19). The temporal lobe lies inferior to the lateral fissure and is composed of the superior, middle, and inferior temporal gyri. The primary auditory cortex (area 41) and its related association area (area 42) lie deep within the lateral sulcus on the superior temporal gyrus. The Wernicke area, along with adjacent portions of the parietal lobe, forms a *sensory speech area*. This area handles delivery and understanding of speech. Dysfunction in this area may result in receptive aphasia or dysphasia. The temporal lobe also is involved in memory recall and smell.

The insula (insular lobe) lies in the lateral sulci between the temporal and frontal lobes of each hemisphere. The insula processes sensory and emotional information and routes the information to other areas of the brain. Lying right below the longitudinal fissure is a mass of white matter pathways called the corpus callosum (transverse or commissural fibres). This structure connects and is essential in coordinating activities between the two cerebral hemispheres (see Figure 13.7).

Inside the cerebrum are many tracts (white matter) and nuclei (grey matter). The major cerebral nuclei are called the basal ganglia (basal nuclei) system. The basal ganglia system is a group of nuclei that includes the caudate nucleus, putamen, and globus pallidus. The putamen and globus pallidus together form the lentiform nucleus. The caudate nucleus and putamen together form the striatum[6] (Figure 13.10). Other structures in the basal ganglia include the *substantia nigra*, the *nucleus accumbens*, and the *subthalamic nucleus*. The nuclei of the basal ganglia are important for voluntary movement and cognitive and emotional functions.

The internal capsule is a thick layer of white matter in which axons of afferent (sensory) and efferent (motor) pathways pass to and from the cerebral cortex. This passage occurs through the centre of the cerebral hemispheres and between the caudate and lentiform nuclei (Figure 13.10B).

The basal ganglia and their interconnections with the thalamus, premotor cortex, red nucleus, reticular formation, and spinal cord are part of the extrapyramidal system. The extrapyramidal system is a part of the motor control system that causes involuntary reflexes and movement and has a steadying effect on motor control. Various involuntary or exaggerated motor movements occur in Parkinson's disease (substantia nigra) and Huntington's disease (striatum) (see Chapter 15).

The limbic system is a group of interconnected structures found between the telencephalon and diencephalon and surrounding the corpus callosum. It is composed of the amygdala, hippocampus, fornix, hypothalamus, and related autonomic nuclei (see Figure 13.10). It is an

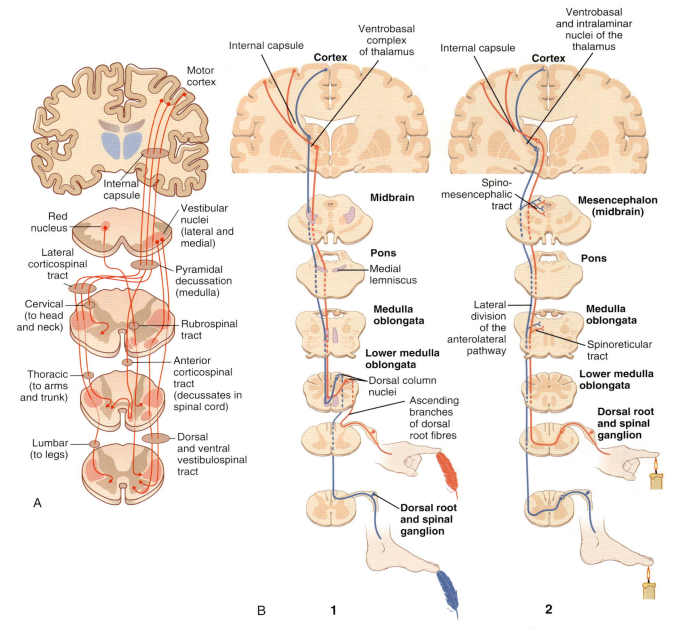

FIGURE 13.9 Examples of Somatic Motor and Sensory Pathways. A, Motor tracts. The pyramidal pathway through the lateral corticospinal tract and the extrapyramidal pathways through the rubrospinal, reticulospinal, and vestibulospinal tracts. **B,** Sensory tracts. (1) The posterior column-medial lemniscal pathway for sending key types of tactile signals: touch and proprioception. Note the lateral corticospinal tract decussation is in the lower medulla. (2) Anterior and lateral parts of the anterolateral sensory pathway: pain and temperature. Note the decussation is in the spinal cord. ([A], from Compston, A., McDonald, I., Noseworthy, J., et al. [2006]. *McAlpine's multiple sclerosis* [4th ed.]. Churchill Livingstone. [B], from Hall, J. E. [2016]. *Guyton and Hall textbook of medical physiology* [13th ed.]. Saunders.)

extension or modification of the olfactory system and affects the autonomic and endocrine systems. The limbic system mediates emotion and long-term memory through connections in the prefrontal cortex (limbic cortex). Its primary effects are involved in primitive behavioural responses, visceral reaction to emotion, motivation, mood, feeding behaviours, biological rhythms, and the sense of smell.

Diencephalon. The cerebrum surrounds the **diencephalon (interbrain)** and sits on top of the brainstem. It has four divisions: **epithalamus**, **thalamus**, **hypothalamus**, and **subthalamus** (see Table 13.3 and Figure 13.7). The epithalamus forms the roof of the third ventricle (a brain cavity) and makes up the most superior part of the diencephalon. The diencephalon controls vital functions and visceral activities and is closely related to those of the limbic system.

The thalamus borders and surrounds the third ventricle. It is a major integrating centre for afferent signals to the cerebral cortex. Many sensations are felt at this level, but cortical processing is needed

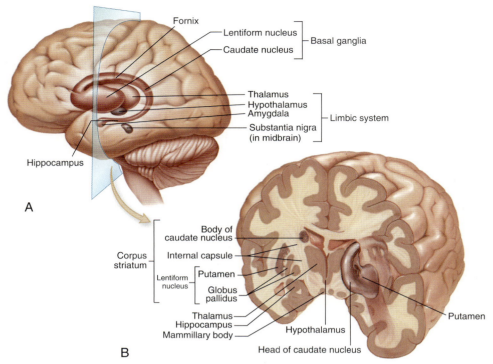

FIGURE 13.10 Basal Ganglia. **A**, The basal ganglia seen through the cortex of the left cerebral hemisphere. **B**, The basal ganglia seen in a frontal section of the brain. (From Patton, K. T., & Thibodeau, G. A. [2016]. *Anatomy & physiology* [9th ed.]. Mosby.)

BOX 13.2 Functions of the Hypothalamus

- Visceral and somatic responses
- Affectual responses
- Hormone synthesis
- Sympathetic and parasympathetic activity
- Temperature control
- Fluid balance
- Appetite and feeding responses
- Physical expression of emotions
- Sexual behaviour
- Pleasure–punishment centres
- Level of arousal or wakefulness

for interpretation. The thalamus serves also as a relay centre for information from the basal ganglia and cerebellum to the right motor area.

The hypothalamus forms the base of the diencephalon. The hypothalamus functions to (1) support a constant internal environment and (2) carry out behavioural patterns. Integrative centres control ANS function, regulate body temperature and endocrine function, and adjust emotional expression. The hypothalamus exerts its effect through the endocrine system, as well as through neural pathways (Box 13.2). The subthalamus lines the hypothalamus laterally. It serves as an important basal ganglia centre for motor functions.

Midbrain

Mesencephalon. Many structures make up the **midbrain (mesencephalon)**. The **corpora quadrigemina** is found on the ceiling of the midbrain. Two pairs of superior colliculi and two pairs of inferior colliculi make up this structure. The red nucleus, substantia nigra, and the basis pedunculi make up the **tegmentum** (the floor of the midbrain). Together the tegmentum and basis pedunculi make up the **cerebral peduncles**.

The **superior colliculi** are involved with voluntary and involuntary visual-motor movements (e.g., the ability of the eyes to track moving objects in the visual field). The **inferior colliculi** achieve similar motor activities but involve movements affecting the auditory system (e.g., positioning the head to improve hearing). The **red nucleus** receives ascending sensory information from the cerebellum and projects a minor motor pathway, the rubrospinal tract, to the cervical spinal cord. The last part of the basal ganglia is the **substantia nigra**, which makes the neurotransmitter **dopamine**. Its dysfunction is associated with Parkinson's disease and schizophrenia. Efferent fibres of the corticospinal, corticobulbar, and corticopontocerebellar tracts make up the **basis pedunculi**.

Other structures of this region are the nuclei of the cranial nerves III and IV. The **cerebral aqueduct (aqueduct of Sylvius)**, which carries CSF, also crosses this structure. Blockage of this aqueduct is often the cause of hydrocephalus.

Hindbrain

Metencephalon. The major structures of the **metencephalon** are the cerebellum and the pons. The cerebellum (see Figure 13.7) is made of grey and white matter. Its ridged cortical surface is like the surface of the cerebrum. A central fissure divides it into two lobes connected by the **vermis**.

The cerebellum handles two main functions. It controls reflexive, involuntary fine-tuning of motor control. It is also responsible for maintaining supporting balance and posture through widespread neural connections with the medulla and with the midbrain. The middle cerebellar peduncles connect the two hemispheres to the pons. These connections allow widespread sampling of visual, vestibular, and proprioceptive data from other regions of the CNS and periphery.

The **pons** (bridge) has a bulging appearance and is located below the midbrain and above the medulla. It transmits information from the cerebellum to the brainstem and between the two cerebellar hemispheres. This structure holds the nuclei of cranial nerves V through VIII.

Myelencephalon. The **myelencephalon** (usually called the **medulla oblongata**) forms the lowest part of the brainstem. This area controls reflex activities such as heart rate, breathing, blood pressure, coughing, sneezing, swallowing, and vomiting. The nuclei of cranial nerves IX through XII are in this region.

Major parts of the descending motor pathways (i.e., corticospinal tracts) cross to the other side at the medulla (see Figure 13.9). These pathways, together with other areas of crossing over in the CNS, are the basis for the phenomenon of *contralateral control*. The neural effects from lower brain centres process sleep–wake rhythms and link complex groups of diffuse structures and functions (see Chapter 14), including the RAS. Cells in the RAS receive same-sided signals from the afferent sensory pathways and send the signals to the higher brain centres, thus controlling CNS activity (see Figure 13.6).

The Spinal Cord

QUICK CHECK 13.4
1. What information do the ascending and descending spinal tracts send?
2. Contrast the functions of upper and lower motor neurons.
3. Name and describe the protective structures of the central nervous system.

The **spinal cord** is the part of the CNS that lies within the vertebral canal. The **vertebral column** surrounds and protects this structure. The spinal cord has many functions. This long nerve cable connects the brain and body, somatic and autonomic reflexes, motor pattern control centres, and sensory and motor modulation. It begins in the medulla oblongata and ends at the level of the first or second lumbar vertebra in adults (Figure 13.11). The end of the spinal cord, the **conus medullaris**, is cone shaped. Spinal nerves continue from the end of the spinal cord and form a nerve bundle called the **cauda equina**. The filament anchor from the conus medullaris to the coccyx is the **filum terminale** (see Figure 13.11). Figure 13.12 shows the coverings of the spinal cord.

The spinal cord is divided into vertebral sections (8 cervical, 12 thoracic, 5 lumbar, 5 sacral, and 1 coccygeal) that match paired nerves (see Figure 13.11). A cross-section of the spinal cord (Figure 13.13) is portrayed by a butterfly-shaped inner core of grey matter that holds nerve cell bodies. The **central canal** lies in the centre of this region and extends through the spinal cord from its origin in the fourth ventricle. The grey matter of the spinal cord divides into three regions. These regions include the **posterior horn**, or **dorsal horn** which is composed mainly of interneurons and axons from sensory neurons whose cell bodies lie in the **dorsal root ganglion**. At the tip of the posterior horn is the **substantia gelatinosa**, a structure involved in pain transmission (see Chapter 14). The **lateral horn** holds cell bodies involved with the ANS. The **anterior horn (ventral horn)** holds the nerve cell bodies for efferent pathways that leave the spinal cord by way of spinal nerves.

Surrounding the grey matter is white matter that forms ascending and descending pathways called **spinal tracts**. The names of the spinal tracts denote their beginning and ending points. For example, the spinothalamic tract (see Figure 13.13) carries nerve signals from the spinal cord to the thalamus. The names of grouped columns of spinal tracts denote their location within the white matter. These columns include the **anterior columns**, **lateral columns**, and posterior columns (see Figure 13.13).

Activated neural circuits in the spinal cord display specific motor responses. **Reflex arcs** form basic units that respond to stimuli and supply protective circuitry for motor output. Structures needed for a reflex arc are a receptor, an **afferent (sensory) neuron**, an **efferent (motor) neuron**, and an effector muscle or gland. A simple reflex arc may hold only two neurons (Figure 13.14). Interneurons are usually present and supply a link between sensory and motor neurons. The motor effects of reflex arcs mostly occur before the brain's higher centres sense the event. Reflex activity involving the ANS mediates much of the internal environmental control.

Afferent pathways send information from peripheral receptors and end in the cerebral or cerebellar cortex or both. Efferent pathways relay information from the cerebrum to the brainstem or spinal cord. The CNS fully contains the **upper motor neurons**. Their main roles are controlling fine motor movement and affecting or changing spinal reflex arcs and circuits. Generally, upper motor neurons form synapses with interneurons, which then form synapses with lower motor neurons that project into the periphery. **Lower motor neurons** directly influence muscles. Their cell bodies lie in the grey matter of the brainstem and spinal cord, but their processes extend out of the CNS and into the PNS. Damage to upper motor neurons usually results in initial paralysis followed within days or weeks by partial recovery. Damage to lower motor neurons leads to paralysis unless nerve renewal and recovery follows peripheral nerve damage (see Figure 13.4).

Nerve signals control muscle activity (i.e., stimulation and contraction). Motor neurons innervate one or more muscle cells, forming **motor units**. These units consist of a neuron and the skeletal muscles it stimulates. The *neuromuscular (myoneural) junction* is the space between the axon of the motor neuron and the plasma membrane of the muscle cell (Figure 13.15). (Chapter 16 discusses injury to motor neurons.)

Motor Pathways

Clinically relevant motor pathways are the lateral corticospinal and corticobulbar pyramidal tracts; and the extrapyramidal reticulospinal, vestibulospinal, and rubrospinal tracts. The corticospinal and corticobulbar pathways are basically the same tract and consist of a two-neuron chain. The cell bodies (upper motor neurons) begin in and around the precentral gyrus. They then pass through the corona radiata of the cerebrum, the internal capsule, middle three-fifths of the cerebral pedunculus, pons, and pyramid. They next cross contralaterally in the medulla oblongata and form the lateral corticospinal tract of the spinal cord (see Figures 13.9A and 13.13) and control the opposite side of the body. The **corticobulbar tract axons** synapse on motor cranial nuclei within the brainstem that control muscles of the face, head, and neck. The lateral corticospinal tract axons leave the tract to go to interneurons or motor neurons in the anterior horn. The **lateral corticospinal tract** has the same somatotopic organization as the body (see Figure 13.8). These lower motor neurons project through nerves to specific muscles. These tracts are involved in precise motor movements. The **reticulospinal tract** (see Figure 13.13) inhibits and excites spinal activity, thus controlling motor movement. The **vestibulospinal tract** arises from a vestibular nucleus in the pons and causes the extensor muscles of the body to rapidly contract. When a person starts to fall backward, this action occurs. The **rubrospinal tract** starts in the red nucleus, crosses over, and ends in the cervical spinal cord. It is important for muscle movement and fine muscle control in the upper limbs.

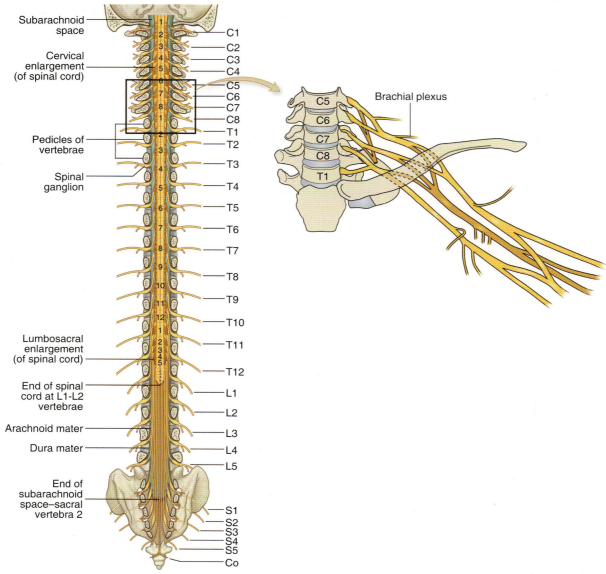

FIGURE 13.11 Vertebral Canal, Spinal Cord, and Spinal Nerves and an Enlarged Diagram of the Brachial Plexus Are Shown. (From Drake, R., Vogl, A. W., & Mitchell, A. W. M. [2015]. *Gray's anatomy for students* [3rd ed.]. Churchill Livingstone. **Inset,** from Chung, K. C., Yang, L. J.-S., & McGillicuddy, J. E. [Eds.]. [2012]. *Practical management of pediatric and adult brachial plexus palsies.* Saunders.)

Sensory Pathways

The three clinically important spinal afferent pathways are the posterior column, **anterior spinothalamic tract**, and lateral spinothalamic tract (see Figures 13.9B and 13.13). The **posterior (dorsal) column (fasciculus gracilis and fasciculus cuneatus)** carries fine-touch sensation, two-point discrimination, and proprioceptive information (i.e., **epicritic information**). A three-neuron chain forms the posterior column. The first neuron of the chain is the primary afferent neuron. It also is the sensory neuron of the reflex arc. After entering the spinal cord, it sends its axon on the same side up the spinal cord to a specific part of the posterior column. It then synapses in the three posterior column nuclei in the medulla oblongata. A basketball player has primary afferent neurons that could be more than 2 m long, running from the great toe up to the medulla oblongata. The axon of the second-order neuron crosses on the opposite side at the medial lemniscus, ascends and synapses with a specific nucleus of the thalamus. The third-order neuron, originating in the thalamus, continues the tract into the internal capsule, corona radiata, and postcentral gyrus (areas 3, 1, 2) (see Figures 13.7 and 13.9B).

The **anterior** and **lateral spinothalamic tracts** handle the sense of vague touch, and pain and temperature sense, respectively (see Figure 13.9B). The term **protopathic** describes these sensations. These tracts also form a three-neuron chain. Their primary afferent neurons synapse in the posterior horn of the spinal cord in several spinal segments above and below their point of entry, not just at the level they enter the intervertebral foramen. This action is an example of divergence. The axons of the second-order neurons in the posterior horn cross to the opposite side in the spinal cord in the lateral column and ascend to the same thalamic nucleus as the posterior column pathway. They then continue with the posterior column pathway to the postcentral gyrus.

CHAPTER 13 Structure and Function of the Neurological System

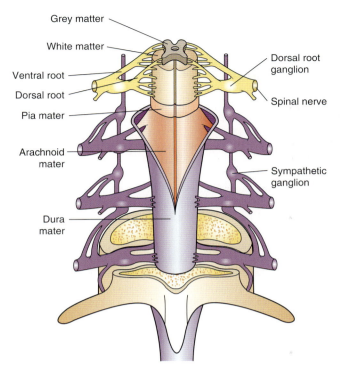

FIGURE 13.12 Coverings of the Spinal Cord. The dura mater is shown in purple. Note how it extends to cover the spinal nerve roots and nerves. The arachnoid is highlighted in red and the pia mater in pink. (From Patton, K.T., & Thibodeau, G.A. [2019]. *The human body in health & disease* [7th ed.]. Elsevier.)

Protective Structures of the Central Nervous System

Cranium

The cranium is composed of eight bones. The cranial vault covers and protects the brain and its structures. The *scalp* is the soft tissue that surrounds the cranium. The scalp consists of five layers: skin, connective tissue, epicranial aponeurosis, loose areolar tissue, and pericranium. The galea aponeurotica, which is a part of the epicranial aponeurosis, is a thick, fibrous band of tissue covering the cranium between the frontal and occipital muscles. This tissue supplies added protection to the skull. The subgaleal space has venous connections with the dural sinuses. If required, blood shunts to this space with increased intracranial pressure thus reducing pressure in the intracranial cavity. The subgaleal space is also a common site for wound drains after intracranial surgery.

The floor of the cranial vault is irregular and contains many foramina (openings) for cranial nerves, blood vessels, and the spinal cord to exit. Three fossae (depressions) comprise the cranial floor. The frontal lobes lie in the anterior fossa. The temporal lobes and base of the diencephalon lie in the middle fossa (temporal fossa). The cerebellum lies in the posterior fossa. These terms are commonly used as landmarks to describe the location of lesions within the cranium.

Meninges

Surrounding the brain and spinal cord are three protective membranes: the dura mater, the arachnoid, and the pia mater. Together they make up the meninges (Figure 13.16C). The dura mater (meaning literally "hard mother") is made of two layers, with the venous sinuses formed between them. The outermost layer forms the periosteum (endosteal layer) of the skull. The inner dura (meningeal

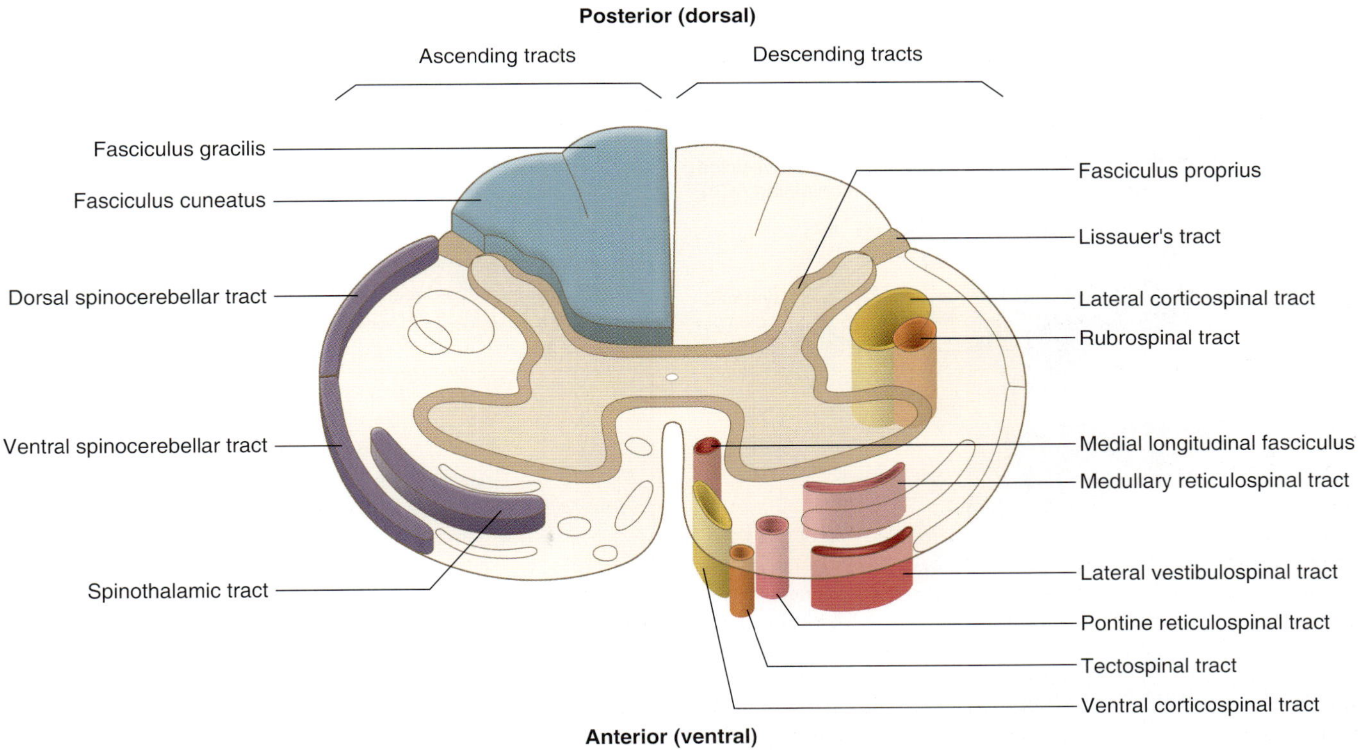

FIGURE 13.13 Ascending and Descending Tracts of the Spinal Cord. All ascending *(sensory)* and descending *(motor)* tracts are present on both the left and right side. In this figure, the left side shows the ascending tracts, and the right side shows the descending tracts. The location of Lissauer's tract and the fasciculus proprius (which hold both ascending and descending fibres) are also shown. (From Crossman, A. R., & Neary, D. [2015]. *Neuroanatomy: an illustrated colour text* [4th ed.]. Churchill Livingstone.)

layer) forms rigid membranes that support and separate the many brain structures.

One of these membranes, the falx cerebri, dips between the two cerebral hemispheres along the longitudinal fissure. The falx cerebri is attached anteriorly to the base of the brain at the crista galli of the ethmoid bone. The tentorium cerebelli is a membrane that separates the cerebellum below from the cerebral structures above. Internal to the dura mater is the location of the arachnoid, a spongy, weblike structure that loosely follows the contours of the cerebral structures.

The subdural space lies between the dura and arachnoid. Many small bridging veins that have little support cross the subdural space. Their disruption results in a subdural hematoma (see Chapter 16). The subarachnoid space lies between the arachnoid and the pia mater and holds CSF (Figure 13.16A,C). Unlike the dura mater and arachnoid, the fragile pia mater holds onto the contours of the brain and spinal cord. It supplies support for blood vessels serving brain tissue. The CSF producing choroid plexuses arise from the pial membrane (Figure 13.16B). The spinal cord attaches to the vertebrae by extension of the meninges. The meninges continue beyond the end of the spinal cord (at vertebrae levels L1 and L2) to the lower part of the sacrum. CSF found within the subarachnoid space also circulates inferiorly to about the second sacral vertebra.

The meninges form potential and real spaces important to understanding functional and pathological mechanisms. For example, between the dura mater and skull lies a potential space called the extradural space (see Figure 13.16C). The arterial supply to the meninges consists of blood vessels that lie within grooves in the skull. A skull fracture can sever one of these vessels and produce an epidural hematoma.

Cerebrospinal Fluid and the Ventricular System

Cerebrospinal fluid (CSF) is a clear, colourless fluid like blood plasma and interstitial fluid. The floating properties of CSF partially protect the intracranial and spinal cord structures from jolts and blows. The CSF also prevents the brain from tugging on meninges, nerve roots, and blood vessels. (Table 13.4 lists the elements of CSF.) Between 125 and 150 mL of CSF circulates within the ventricles (small cavities) and subarachnoid space at any given time. About 600 mL of CSF is made daily.

The choroid plexuses in the lateral, third, and fourth ventricles produce a major part of CSF. (Figure 13.16 shows the ventricles.) These plexuses have a rich network of blood vessels, supplied by the pia mater, which lie close to the ependymal cells of the ventricles. The tight

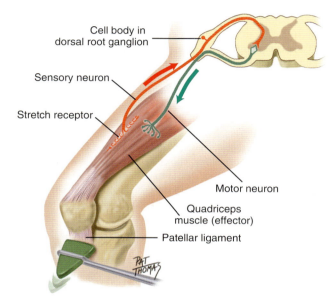

FIGURE 13.14 Cross-section of Spinal Cord Showing Simple Reflex Arc. (From Jarvis, C. [2016]. *Physical examination & health assessment* [7th ed.]. Saunders.)

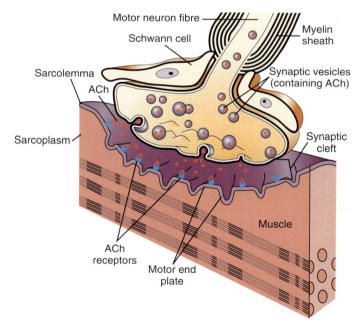

FIGURE 13.15 Normal Neuromuscular Junction. This figure shows how the distal end of a motor neuron fibre forms a synapse, or "chemical junction," with an adjacent muscle fibre. The neuron's synaptic vesicles release neurotransmitters (specifically, acetylcholine [ACh]) and they diffuse across the synaptic cleft. There, they stimulate receptors in the motor end-plate region of the sarcolemma. (From Damjanov, I. [2012]. *Pathology for the health professions* [4th ed.]. Saunders.)

TABLE 13.4 Composition of Cerebrospinal Fluid	
Constituent	**Normal Value**
Na^+	135–150 mmol/L of CSF
K^+	2.7–3.9 mmol/L of CSF
Cl^-	116–127 mmol/L of CSF
HCO_3^-	22.9 mmol/L of CSF
Glucose (fasting)	2.8–4.2 mmol/L of CSF (60–70% of blood glucose)
pH	7.28–7.32
Protein	0.15–0.45 g/L of CSF to 0.7 g/L
Albumin	56–76%
Globulin	6–19%
Cells	
White (lymphocyte)	$0–5 \times 10^6$ WBCs/L (0–10 cells/μL)
Red	0

From Sofronescu, A., & Wheeler, T. (2015). *Cerebrospinal fluid analysis*. https://emedicine.medscape.com/article/2093316-overview.
Cl^-, Chloride; *CSF*, cerebrospinal fluid; HCO_3^-, bicarbonate; K^+, potassium; Na^+, sodium; *WBC*, white blood cell.

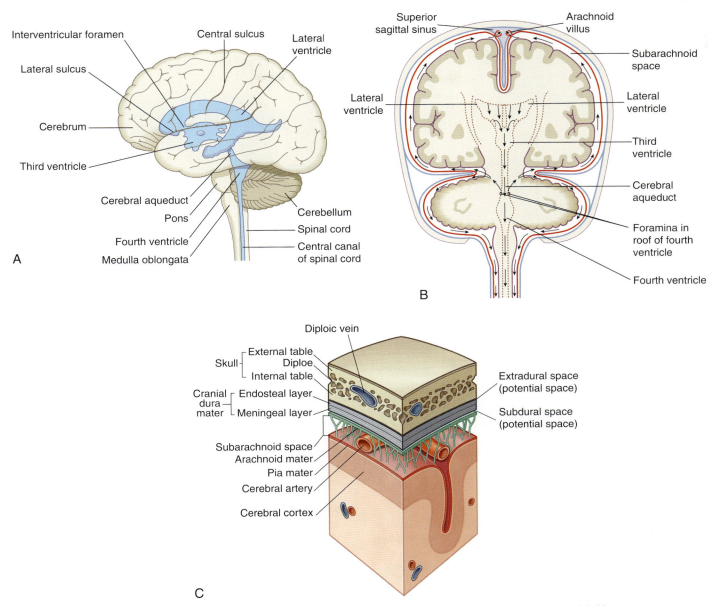

FIGURE 13.16 Flow of Cerebrospinal Fluid and Meninges of the Brain. A, Ventricles noted in blue within a translucent brain in a left lateral view. B, Flow of cerebrospinal fluid (CSF). The fluid produced by filtration of blood by the choroid plexus of each ventricle flows inferiorly through the lateral ventricles, interventricular foramen, third ventricle, cerebral aqueduct, fourth ventricle, and subarachnoid space to the blood. C, Meninges of the brain in relation to CSF and venous blood flow. ([A, B], from Waugh, A., & Grant, A. [2012]. *Ross and Wilson anatomy and physiology in health and illness* [12th ed.]. Churchill Livingstone. [C] from Drake, R., Vogl, A. W., & Mitchell, A. W. M. [2015]. *Gray's anatomy for students* [3rd ed.]. Churchill Livingstone.)

junctions of the choroid blood vessels provide a barrier between the CSF and blood that functions like the blood–brain barrier (see Figure 13.16B,C).

The CSF exerts pressure within the brain and spinal cord. When a person is supine, CSF pressure is about 80 to 180 mm of water pressure or about 5 to 14 mm of mercury pressure. This pressure doubles when the person moves to an upright position. CSF flow results from the pressure gradient between the arterial system and the CSF-filled cavities. Beginning in the lateral ventricles, the CSF flows through the interventricular foramen (foramen of Monro) into the third ventricle and then passes through the cerebral aqueduct (aqueduct of Sylvius) into the fourth ventricle. From the fourth ventricle, the CSF may pass through either the paired lateral apertures (foramen of Luschka) or the median aperture (foramen of Magendie) before linking with the subarachnoid spaces of the brain and spinal cord. The CSF does not, however, accumulate. It is reabsorbed into the venous circulation through the arachnoid villi. The arachnoid villi protrude from the arachnoid space, through the dura mater, and lie within the blood

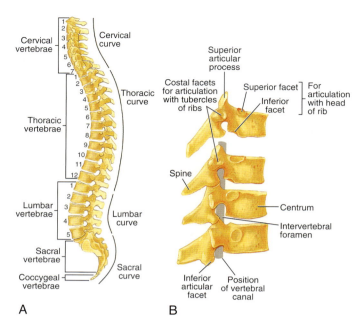

FIGURE 13.17 Vertebral Column. **A,** The normal curves and regions of the vertebral column. Numbers show the vertebrae in each region. **B,** Lateral view of several vertebrae showing how they articulate. (From Solomon, E. [2016]. *Introduction to human anatomy and physiology* [4th ed.]. Saunders.)

flow of the venous sinuses (see Figure 13.16B). The pressure gradient between the arachnoid villi and the cerebral venous sinuses allows the reabsorption of CSF. The villi act as one-way valves guiding CSF outflow into the blood but preventing blood flow into the subarachnoid space. The blood forms the CSF, and after circulating throughout the CNS, it returns to the blood.

Vertebral Column

The vertebral column (Figure 13.17) consists of 33 vertebrae: 7 cervical, 12 thoracic, 5 lumbar, 5 fused sacral, and 4 fused coccygeal. Between each interspace (except for the fused sacral and coccygeal vertebrae) is an **intervertebral disc** (Figure 13.18). At the centre of the intervertebral disc is the **nucleus pulposus**, a pulpy mass of elastic fibres. The intervertebral disc absorbs shocks, preventing damage to the vertebrae. The intervertebral disc is a common source of back problems. If the vertebral column receives too much stress, the disc may rupture and bulge into the spinal canal. The bulge may cause compression of the spinal cord or nerve roots.

Blood Supply of the Central Nervous System

> **QUICK CHECK 13.5**
> 1. Describe the circle of Willis and explain its role in supplying blood to the brain.
> 2. What is the source of the spinal cord's blood supply?
> 3. Describe the anatomy and function of the peripheral nervous system (PNS).
> 4. What are the plexuses? Give two examples in the PNS.
> 5. What are the cranial nerves? Give three examples.

Blood Supply to the Brain

The brain receives about 20% of the cardiac output or 800 to 1 000 mL of blood flow per minute. Carbon dioxide is a main regulator for blood

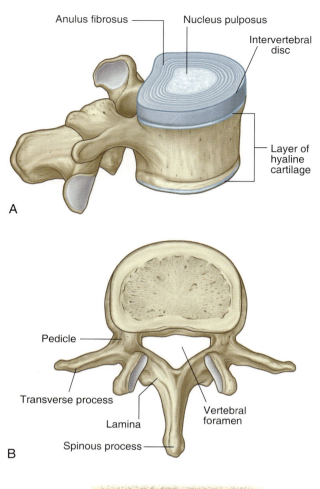

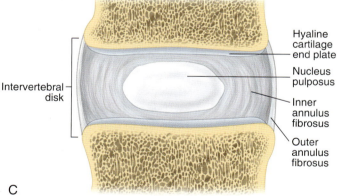

FIGURE 13.18 Intervertebral Disc. **A,** Sagittal image. **B,** Superior view of the structures of a typical vertebra. **C,** Magnified image. ([A,B], from Drake, R., Vogl, A. W., & Mitchell, A. W. M. [2015]. *Gray's anatomy for students* [3rd ed.]. Churchill Livingstone. [C] from Lawry, G. V., Kreder, H., Hawker, G., et al. [2010]. *Fam's musculoskeletal examination and joint injection techniques* [2nd ed.]. Mosby.)

flow within the CNS. It is a potent vasodilator, and its effects ensure adequate blood supply.

The brain gets its arterial supply from two systems: the **internal carotid arteries** and the **vertebral arteries** (Figure 13.19). The internal carotid arteries supply a greater amount of blood flow. They begin at the common carotid arteries, enter the cranium through the base of the

CHAPTER 13 Structure and Function of the Neurological System

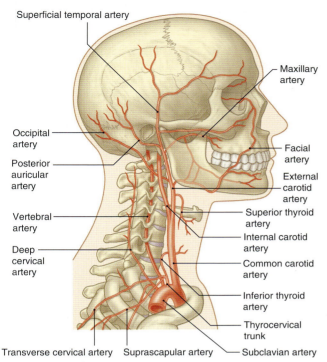

FIGURE 13.19 Major Arteries of the Head and Neck. (From Moses, K. P., Nava, P., Banks, J., et al. [2013]. *Atlas of clinical gross anatomy* [2nd ed.]. Saunders.)

skull, and pass through the cavernous sinus. After forming some small branches, these arteries divide into the anterior and middle cerebral arteries. The vertebral arteries begin at the subclavian arteries and pass through the transverse foramina of the cervical vertebrae, entering the cranium through the foramen magnum. They join at the junction of the pons and medulla to form the basilar artery (Figure 13.20). The basilar artery divides at the level of the midbrain to form two posterior cerebral arteries.

The circle of Willis (see Figure 13.20) supplies another route for blood flow when one of the contributing arteries is blocked (collateral blood flow). The posterior cerebral arteries, posterior communicating arteries, internal carotid arteries, anterior cerebral arteries, and anterior communicating artery form the circle of Willis. The anterior cerebral, middle cerebral, and posterior cerebral arteries leave the circle of Willis and spread to many brain structures. The border zone is the area between the major arterial regions. (Table 13.5 and Figure 13.21 show the structures served, functional relationships, and pathological factors related to blockage of cerebral arteries.)

Cerebral venous drainage does not match its arterial supply, while the venous drainage of the brainstem and cerebellum does match the arterial supply of these structures. The cerebral veins are classified as superficial veins and deep veins. The veins drain into venous plexuses and dural sinuses formed between the dural layers. They then empty into the internal jugular veins at the base of the skull (Figure 13.22). Adequacy of venous outflow can notably affect intracranial pressure. For example, head-injured persons who turn or let their heads fall to the side in part occlude venous return. As a result, the intracranial pressure can increase because of decreased flow through the jugular veins.

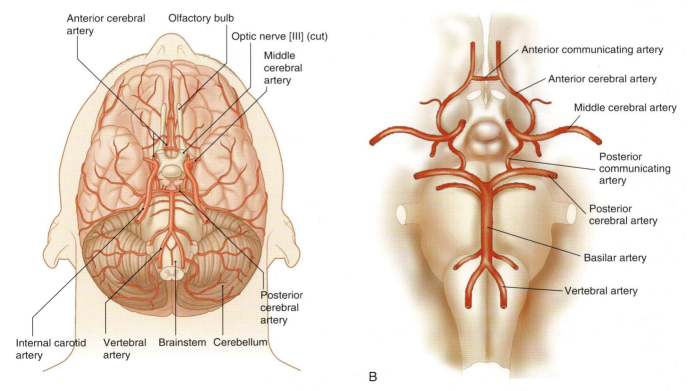

FIGURE 13.20 Arteries at the Base of the Brain. The arteries that make up the circle of Willis are the two anterior cerebral arteries, joined to each other by the anterior communicating artery and two short parts of the internal carotids. The posterior communicating arteries connect to the posterior cerebral arteries. ([A], from Moses, K. P., Nava, P., Banks, J., et al. [2013]. *Atlas of clinical gross anatomy* [2nd ed.]. Saunders. [B], from Hagen-Ansert, S. [2012]. *Textbook of diagnostic sonography* [7th ed.]. Mosby.)

CHAPTER 13 Structure and Function of the Neurological System

TABLE 13.5 Arterial Systems Supplying the Brain

Arterial Origin	Structures Served	Conditions Caused by Occlusion
Anterior cerebral artery	Basal ganglia; corpus callosum; medial surface of cerebral hemispheres; superior surface of frontal and parietal lobes	Hemiplegia on opposite side of the body, greater in lower than in upper limbs
Middle cerebral artery	Frontal lobe; parietal lobe; temporal lobe (mostly cortical surfaces)	Aphasia in dominant hemisphere and opposite side hemiplegia (see Chapter 15)
Posterior cerebral artery	Part of the diencephalon (thalamus, hypothalamus) and temporal lobe; occipital lobe	Visual loss; sensory loss; opposite side hemiplegia if cerebral peduncle affected

Data from Pagana, K. D., Pagana, T. J., & Pike-MacDonald, S. A. (2019). *Mosby's Canadian manual of diagnostic and laboratory tests* (2nd Cdn. ed.). Elsevier Inc.

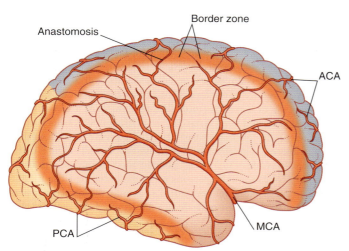

FIGURE 13.21 Areas of the Brain Affected by Blockage of the Anterior, Middle, and Posterior Cerebral Artery Branches. *ACA*, Grey area affected by blockage of branches of anterior cerebral artery; *MCA*, pink area affected by blockage of branches of middle cerebral artery; *PCA*, orange area affected by blockage of branches of posterior cerebral artery. Blockages can occur in the cortical or deep areas of the border zone. (From Fitzgerald, M. J. T., Gruener, G., & Mtui, E. [2012]. *Clinical neuroanatomy and neuroscience* [6th ed.]. Saunders.)

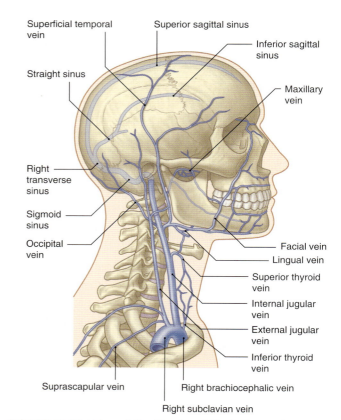

FIGURE 13.22 Veins of the Head and Neck. Deep veins and dural sinuses are projected on the skull. Note two superficial veins in the face are tributaries that send blood through emissary veins in the skull foramen into deep veins inside the skull ending in the internal jugular vein. (From Moses, K. P., Nava, P., Banks, J., et al. [2013]. *Atlas of clinical gross anatomy* [2nd ed.]. Saunders.)

Blood–Brain Barrier

The **blood–brain barrier (BBB)** describes cellular structures that selectively reduce certain potentially harmful substances in the blood from entering the interstitial spaces of the brain or CSF. This protective function allows neurons to work normally. Endothelial cells in brain capillaries with their intracellular tight junctions are the site of the BBB. Supporting cells include astrocytes, pericytes, and microglia[9] (Figure 13.23, and see Chapter 1). The exact nature of this process is debated, but it appears that some metabolites, electrolytes, and chemicals can cross into and out of the brain to varying degrees. This exchange has important implications for medication therapy because certain types of antibiotics and chemotherapeutic medications show a greater ability than others for crossing this barrier. Breakdown of the BBB can lead to inflammation and degeneration of neurons.

Blood Supply to the Spinal Cord

The spinal cord gets its blood supply from branches off the vertebral arteries and from branches from many regions of the aorta (Figure 13.24). The **anterior spinal artery** and the **posterior spinal arteries** branch from the vertebral artery at the base of the cranium and descend alongside the spinal cord. Arterial branches from vessels exterior to the spinal cord follow the spinal nerve through the intervertebral foramina, pass through the dura, and divide into the anterior and posterior radicular arteries.

The radicular arteries eventually connect to the spinal arteries. Branches from the radicular and spinal arteries form plexuses whose branches enter the spinal cord, supplying the deeper tissues. Venous drainage matches the arterial supply closely and drains into venous sinuses found between the dura and periosteum of the vertebrae.

THE PERIPHERAL NERVOUS SYSTEM

The cranial and spinal nerves, including their branches and ganglia, form the peripheral nervous system (PNS). Individual axons wrapped

CHAPTER 13 Structure and Function of the Neurological System

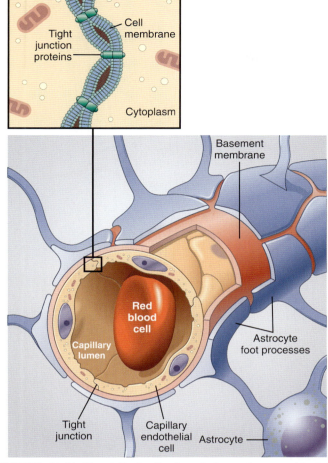

FIGURE 13.23 Blood–Brain Barrier. Cell membranes with tight junctions create a physical barrier between capillary blood and the cytoplasm of astrocytes. (From Bradley, W. G. [Ed.]. [2007]. *Neurology in clinical practice* [5th ed.]. Butterworth-Heinemann.)

(L5 to S5) hold nerves that innervate the anterior and posterior portions of the lower body, respectively.

The posterior rami of each spinal nerve, with their many processes, supply to a specific area in the body. Sensory signals thus arise from specific sites linked with a specific spinal cord segment. **Dermatomes** are specific areas of cutaneous innervation at these spinal cord segments (Figure 13.25C).

Like spinal nerves, cranial nerves are classified as peripheral nerves. Most cranial nerves are mixed nerves, although some are purely sensory or purely motor. Cranial nerves (Figure 13.25A) connect to nuclei in the brain and brainstem. Table 13.6 describes structural and functional features of the cranial nerves.

THE AUTONOMIC NERVOUS SYSTEM

> ✓ **QUICK CHECK 13.6**
> 1. What are the structural and functional divisions of the autonomic nervous system?
> 2. Compare cholinergic and adrenergic transmission.
> 3. What are the functions of the autonomic nervous system?

The structure and function of the autonomic nervous system (ANS) are complex and not well understood. Parts of the ANS are in both the CNS and the PNS; however, the ANS is part of the efferent division of the PNS, even though visceral afferent neurons are an important part of this system. Many neurons of the ANS travel in the spinal nerves and certain cranial nerves. The widespread activity of this system shows that its parts are found all over the body. The peripheral autonomic nerves carry mainly efferent fibres. The motor part of the ANS is a two-neuron system consisting of myelinated **preganglionic neurons** and unmyelinated **postganglionic neurons** (Figure 13.26). This layout differs from the somatic nervous system, where a single motor neuron travels from the CNS to the innervated structure. Visceral afferent neurons have their cell bodies in some sensory and cranial ganglia and their fibre processes travelling in peripheral nerves.

The CNS has autonomic areas in the: (1) intermediolateral horns of the spinal cord, (2) cardiovascular and respiratory centres in the reticular formation, and (3) both sympathetic and parasympathetic areas in the hypothalamus. CNS pathways connect all these areas.

The ANS directs and supports a steady state among internal organs. This includes control of cardiac muscle, smooth muscle, and the glands of the body. The ANS is considered an involuntary system because a person cannot *will* these functions to happen. The ANS divides structurally and functionally into two divisions: (1) the **sympathetic nervous system** and (2) the **parasympathetic nervous system** (Figure 13.27).

Anatomy of the Sympathetic Nervous System

The sympathetic nervous system mobilizes energy stores in times of need (e.g., in the "fight-or-flight response" or acute stress response) (see Figure 9.3; see also Chapter 9). Cell bodies found from the first thoracic (T1) through the second lumbar (L2) regions of the spinal cord innervate the sympathetic division. It is called the **thoracolumbar division**. The preganglionic axons of the sympathetic division form synapses shortly after leaving the spinal cord in the **sympathetic (paravertebral) ganglia**. These preganglionic axons travel several different ways: (1) directly synapsing with postganglionic neurons in the sympathetic chain ganglion at their level; (2) up or down the sympathetic chain ganglion before forming synapses with a higher or lower postganglionic neuron; or (3) through the sympathetic chain ganglion,

in a myelin sheath make up a peripheral nerve (cranial or spinal). **Fascicles** are axons that are arranged in bundles (Figure 13.25B).

The 31 pairs of spinal nerves get their names from the vertebral level from which they exit. There are 8 cervical, 12 thoracic, 5 lumbar, and 5 sacral pairs, and 1 coccygeal pair. The first cervical nerve exits above the first cervical vertebra, and the rest of the spinal nerves exit below their related vertebrae. From the thoracic region (and inferiorly), nerves relate to the vertebral level above their exit.

Mixed nerves are spinal nerves that have both sensory and motor neurons. They arise as rootlets lateral to anterior and posterior horns of the spinal cord. These two spinal nerve roots join in the region of the intervertebral foramen to form the spinal nerve trunk. Shortly after joining, the spinal nerve divides into anterior and posterior rami (branches). The anterior rami (except the thoracic) initially form **plexuses** (networks of nerve fibres), which then branch into the peripheral nerves. Instead of forming plexuses, the thoracic nerves pass through the intercostal spaces and innervate regions of the thorax.

The main spinal nerve plexuses innervate the skin and the underlying muscles of the limbs. For example, the last four cervical nerves (C5 to C8) and the first thoracic nerve (T1) form the **brachial plexus** (see Figure 13.11). The brachial plexus innervates the nerves of the arm, wrist, and hand. The **lumbar plexus** (L1 to L4) and **sacral plexus**

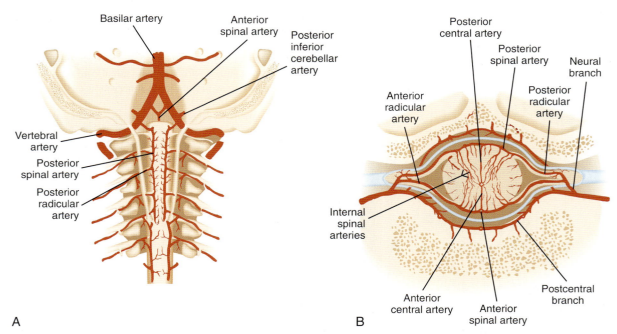

FIGURE 13.24 Arteries of the Spinal Cord. **A,** Arteries of cervical cord exposed from the rear. **B,** Arteries of spinal cord shown in horizontal section. (Redrawn from Rudy, E. B. [Ed.]. [1984]. *Advanced neurological and neurosurgical nursing.* Mosby.)

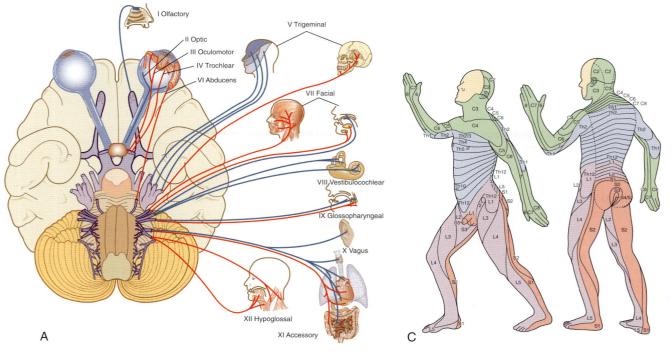

FIGURE 13.25 Cranial and Peripheral Nerves and Skin Dermatomes. **A,** Ventral surface of the brain showing attachment of the cranial nerves. The *red lines* indicate motor function, and the *blue lines* show sensory function. **B,** Peripheral nerve trunk and coverings. **C,** Dermatome map, anterolateral view *(left)* and posterolateral view *(right).* ([A], from Applegate, E. [2011]. *The anatomy and physiology learning system* [4th ed.]. Saunders. [C], from Salvo, S. G. [2014]. *Mosby's pathology for massage therapists* [3rd ed.]. Mosby.)

TABLE 13.6 The Cranial Nerves

Number and Name	Origin and Course	Function	How Tested
I. Olfactory	Fibres arise from nasal olfactory epithelium and form synapses with olfactory bulbs, which send signals to temporal lobe.	Purely sensory; carries signals for the sense of smell.	Person is asked to sniff and name scented substances, such as oil of cloves and vanilla.
II. Optic	Fibres arise from the retina of the eye to form the optic nerve, which passes through sphenoid bone; two optic nerves then form optic chiasma (with partial crossover of fibres) and eventually end in the occipital cortex.	Purely sensory; carries signals for vision.	Vision and visual fields are tested with an eye chart and by testing the point at which the person first sees an object (finger) moving into the visual field; inside of the eye is viewed with an ophthalmoscope to observe interior structures of the eye.
III. Oculomotor	Fibres emerge from the midbrain and exit from the skull to run to the eye.	Contains motor fibres to the inferior oblique and to superior, inferior, and medial rectus extraocular muscles that direct the eyeball; levator muscles of the eyelid; smooth muscles of iris and ciliary body; and proprioception (sensory) to the brain from extraocular muscles.	Pupils are examined for size, shape, and equality; pupillary reflex is tested with a penlight (pupils should constrict when illuminated), and the ability to follow moving objects is tested.
IV. Trochlear	Fibres arise from the posterior midbrain and exit from the skull to run to the eye.	Proprioceptor and motor fibres for superior oblique muscle of eye (extraocular muscle).	It is tested in common with cranial nerve III on the ability to follow moving objects.
V. Trigeminal	Fibres arise from the pons, form three divisions that exit from the skull and run to the face and cranial dura mater.	Supplies both motor and sensory signals for the face; conducts sensory signals from the mouth, nose, surface of the eye, and dura mater; also contains motor fibres that stimulate chewing muscles.	Sensations of pain, touch, and temperature are tested with a safety pin and hot and cold objects; corneal reflex is tested with a wisp of cotton; motor branch is tested by asking subject to clench teeth, open mouth against resistance, and move the jaw from side to side.
VI. Abducens	Fibres leave the inferior pons and exit from the skull to run to the eye.	Has motor fibres to lateral rectus muscle and proprioceptor fibres from the same muscle to the brain.	It is tested in common with cranial nerve III on the ability to move each eye laterally.
VII. Facial	Fibres leave the pons and travel through temporal bone to reach face.	Mixed: (1) supplies motor fibres to muscles of facial expression and to lacrimal and salivary glands, and (2) carries sensory fibres from taste buds of anterior part of the tongue.	Anterior two-thirds of the tongue is tested for the ability to taste sweet (sugar), salty, sour (vinegar), and bitter (quinine) substances; symmetry of face is checked; the subject is asked to close eyes, smile, whistle, and so on; tearing is tested with ammonia fumes.
VIII. Vestibulocochlear (acoustic)	Fibres run from the inner ear (hearing and equilibrium receptors in temporal bone) to enter the brainstem just below the pons.	Purely sensory; the vestibular branch transmits signals for the sense of equilibrium; cochlear branch transmits signals for the sense of hearing.	Hearing is checked by air and bone conduction by use of a tuning fork; vestibular tests: Bárány and caloric tests.
IX. Glossopharyngeal	Fibres arise from the medulla and leave the skull to run to the throat.	Mixed: (1) motor fibres serve pharynx (throat) and salivary glands, and (2) sensory fibres carry signals from the pharynx, posterior tongue (taste buds), and pressure receptors of the carotid artery.	Gag and swallow reflexes are checked; the subject is asked to speak and cough; the posterior one-third of the tongue may be tested for taste.
X. Vagus	Fibres arise from the medulla, pass through the skull, and descend through the neck region into the thorax and abdominal region.	Fibres carry sensory and motor signals for pharynx; a large part of this nerve is parasympathetic motor fibres, which supply smooth muscles of abdominal organs; receives sensory signals from viscera.	The test is the same as for cranial nerve IX (IX and X are tested in common) as they both serve muscles of the throat.
XI. Spinal accessory	Fibres arise from the medulla and superior spinal cord and travel to muscles of neck and back.	Supplies sensory and motor fibres for sternocleidomastoid and trapezius muscles, and muscles of soft palate, pharynx, and larynx.	Sternocleidomastoid and trapezius muscles are checked for strength by asking the subject to rotate head and shrug shoulders against resistance.
XII. Hypoglossal	Fibres arise from the medulla and exit from the skull to travel to the tongue.	Carries motor fibres to muscles of the tongue and sensory signals from the tongue to the brain.	The subject is asked to stick out tongue, and any position defects are noted.

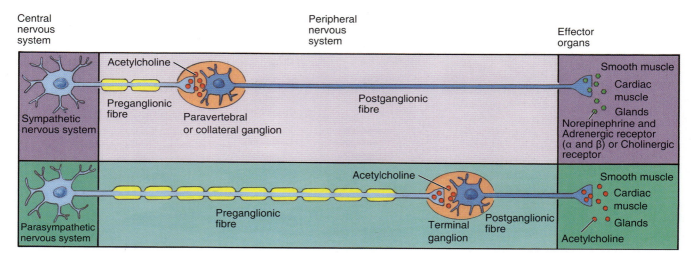

FIGURE 13.26 Preganglionic and Postganglionic Fibres of the Autonomic Nervous System. (From Applegate, E. [2011]. *The anatomy and physiology learning system* [4th ed.]. Saunders.)

postganglionic neurons within collateral ganglia (see Figure 13.27). Some preganglionic axons form pathways called **splanchnic nerves**, which lead to **collateral ganglia** on the front of the aorta. The closest branches of the aorta depict the collateral ganglia names. These include the **celiac**, **superior mesenteric**, and **inferior mesenteric**. The preganglionic neurons synapse with postganglionic neurons within the collateral ganglia. These postganglionic neurons leave the collateral ganglia and innervate the viscera below the diaphragm.

Preganglionic sympathetic neurons that innervate the adrenal medulla also travel in the splanchnic nerves and *do not* synapse before reaching the gland. The secretory cells in the adrenal medulla are considered modified postganglionic neurons. Because preganglionic sympathetic fibres are all myelinated, travel to the adrenal medulla is quick. This innervation causes the rapid release of epinephrine and norepinephrine. Epinephrine and norepinephrine are mediators of the fight-or-flight response (see Chapter 9).

Anatomy of the Parasympathetic Nervous System

The parasympathetic nervous system conserves and restores energy. The nerve cell bodies of this division are in the cranial nerve nuclei and in the sacral region of the spinal cord and therefore constitute the **craniosacral division**. Unlike the sympathetic branch, the preganglionic fibres in the parasympathetic division travel close to the organs they innervate before forming synapses with the relatively short postganglionic neurons (see Figure 13.27). Parasympathetic nerves arising from nuclei in the brainstem travel to the viscera of the head, thorax, and abdomen within cranial nerves. This includes the oculomotor (III), facial (VII), glossopharyngeal (IX), and vagus (X) nerves.

Preganglionic parasympathetic nerves that arise from the sacral region of the spinal cord run separately or together with some spinal nerves. The preganglionic axons unite to form the **pelvic nerve**, which innervates the viscera of the pelvic cavity. These preganglionic axons synapse with postganglionic neurons in terminal ganglia found close to the organs they innervate.

Neurotransmitters and Neuroreceptors

Sympathetic preganglionic fibres and parasympathetic preganglionic and postganglionic fibres release **acetylcholine**. Acetylcholine is the same neurotransmitter released by somatic efferent neurons (see Figure 13.26). These fibres are characterized by **cholinergic transmission**. Most postganglionic sympathetic fibres release **norepinephrine** (adrenaline) and function by **adrenergic transmission**. A few postganglionic sympathetic fibres, such as those that innervate the sweat glands, release acetylcholine.

The action of catecholamines varies with the type of neuroreceptor stimulated. It is important to remember that the adrenal medulla gland also releases catecholamines that physiologically and biochemically resemble the sympathetic nervous system. Two types of adrenergic receptors exist, α and β. Cells of the effector organs may have one or both types of adrenergic receptors. The **α-adrenergic receptors** are further subdivided according to the action produced. $α_1$-Adrenergic activity is related mostly to excitation or stimulation. $α_2$-Adrenergic activity is related to relaxation or inhibition. Most of the α-adrenergic receptors on effector organs belong to the $α_1$ class. There are two types of **β-adrenergic receptors**. $β_1$-Adrenergic receptors aid increased heart rate and contractility and cause the release of renin from the kidney. $β_2$-Adrenergic receptors aid all remaining effects attributed to β receptors).[10] Norepinephrine stimulates all $α_1$ and $β_1$ receptors and only certain $β_2$ receptors. The primary response from norepinephrine, however, is stimulation of the $α_1$-adrenergic receptors that cause vasoconstriction. Epinephrine strongly stimulates all four types of receptors and induces general vasodilation because of the large number of β receptors in muscle vasculatures. (Table 13.7 reviews the effects of neuroreceptors on their effector organs.)

Functions of the Autonomic Nervous System

The sympathetic and parasympathetic nervous systems together innervate many body organs. The two divisions often cause opposite responses. As an example, sympathetic stimulation of the stomach causes decreased peristalsis, whereas parasympathetic stimulation of the intestine increases peristalsis while sympathetic stimulation promotes responses for the protection of the person. For example, sympathetic activity increases blood glucose levels and temperature and raises blood pressure. In emergencies, a widespread discharge of the sympathetic system occurs, the fight-or-flight response, or acute stress response (see Chapter 9). An increased firing rate of sympathetic fibres

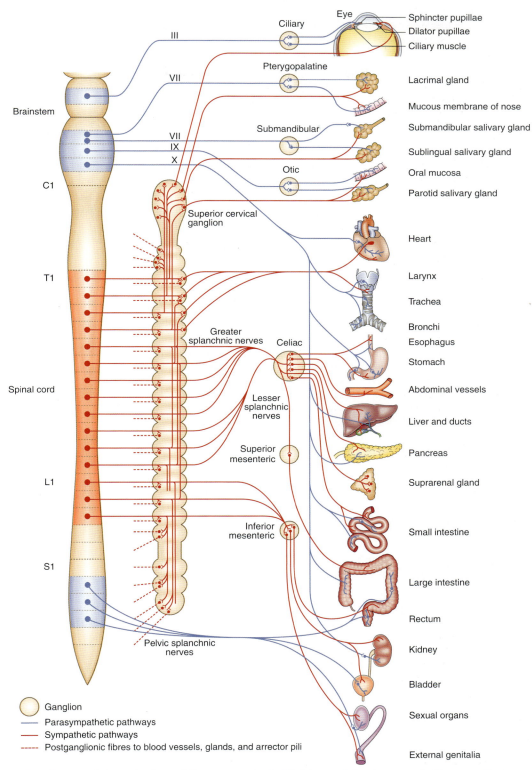

FIGURE 13.27 Sympathetic and Parasympathetic Divisions of the Autonomic Nervous System. Preganglionic neuron cell bodies are in the brainstem and sacral cord segments (parasympathetic or "craniosacral" division) and thoracic and upper lumbar cord segments (sympathetic or "thoraco-lumbar" division). The axons of these neurons synapse with postganglionic neurons, which innervate smooth muscle, cardiac muscle, and glands of the body. The postganglionic neuron cell bodies may be in distinct autonomic ganglia (represented with *circles*), or in or very near the wall of the innervated visceral organ. Note that sympathetic fibres supply the only innervation to peripheral effectors (sweat glands, arrector pili muscles, adipose tissue, and blood vessels). (From Cramer, D., & Darby, S. [2005]. *Basic and clinical anatomy of the spine, spinal cord, and ANS* [2nd ed.]. Elsevier/Mosby.)

TABLE 13.7 Actions of Autonomic Nervous System Neuroreceptors

Effector Organ or Tissue	Adrenergic Receptors	Adrenergic Effects	Cholinergic Effects (Nicotine and Muscarinic[a] Receptors)
Eye, iris			
Radial muscle	α_1	Dilation	—
Sphincter muscle	—	—	Constriction
Eye, ciliary muscle	β_2	Relaxation for far vision	Contraction for near vision
Lacrimal glands	α_1	Secretion	Secretion
Nasopharyngeal glands	—	—	Secretion
Salivary glands	α_1	Secretion of potassium and water	Secretion of potassium and water
	β	Secretion of amylase	—
Heart			
Sinoatrial (SA) node	β_1, β_2	Increase heart rate	Decrease heart rate; vagus arrest
Atrial	β_1, β_2	Increase contractility and conduction speed	Decrease contractility; shorten action potential duration
Atrioventricular (AV) junction	β_1, β_2	Increase automaticity and propagation speed	Decrease automaticity and propagation speed
Purkinje system	β_1, β_2	Increase automaticity and propagation speed	—
Ventricles	β_1, β_2	Increase contractility	Slight decrease in contraction
Arterioles			
Coronary	$\alpha_1, \alpha_2, \beta_2$	Constriction, dilation	Dilation
Skin and mucosa	α_1, α_2	Constriction	Dilation
Skeletal muscle	α, β_2	Dilation, constriction	Dilation
Cerebral	α_1	Constriction (slight)	Dilation
Pulmonary	α_1, β_2	Constriction, dilation	Dilation
Mesenteric	α_1	Constriction	Dilation
Renal	$\alpha_1, \beta_1, \beta_2$	Constriction, dilation	Dilation
Salivary glands	α_1, α_2	Constriction	Dilation
Veins, systemic	$\alpha_1, \alpha_2, \beta_2$	Constriction, dilation	—
Lung			
Bronchial muscle	α_2	Relaxation	Contraction
Bronchial glands	α_1, β_2	Decrease secretion; increase secretion	Stimulation
Stomach			
Motility	$\alpha_1, \alpha_2, \beta_1, \beta_2$	Decrease (usually)	Increase
Sphincters	α_1	Contraction (usually)	Relaxation (usually)
Secretion	α_2	Inhibition	Stimulation
Liver	α_1, β_2	Glycogenolysis and gluconeogenesis	—
Gallbladder and ducts	β_2	Relaxation	Contraction
Pancreas			
Acini	α	Decrease secretion	Secretion
Islet cells	α_2, β_2	Decrease secretion; increase secretion	—
Intestine			
Motility and tone	$\alpha_1, \alpha_2, \beta_1, \beta_2$	Decrease	Increase
Sphincters	α_1	Contraction	Relaxation (usually)
Secretion	α_2	Inhibition	Stimulation
Adrenal medulla	—	Secretion of epinephrine and norepinephrine (nicotinic effect)	
Kidney			
Renin secretion	α_1, β_1	Decrease; increase	—
Ureter			
Motility and tone	β_1	Increase	Increase (?)
Urinary bladder			
Detrusor	β_2	Relaxation	Contraction
Trigone and sphincter	α_1	Contraction	Relaxation
Sex organs, male	α_1	Ejaculation	Erection
Skin			
Pilomotor muscles	α_1	Contraction	—
Sweat glands	α_1	Localized secretion	—
Fat cells	$\alpha_2, \beta_1, \beta_2, \beta_3$	Inhibition of lipolysis; stimulation of lipolysis	—
Pineal gland	β	Melatonin synthesis	—

[a]Muscarinic receptors respond to circulating muscarinic antagonists.
Modified from Brunton, L. L., Chabner, B. A., & Knollmann, B. C. (Eds.). (2011). *Goodman & Gilman's the pharmacological basis of therapeutics* (12th ed.). McGraw-Hill; Yagiela, J. A., Dowd, F., Johnson, B., et al. (2011). *Pharmacology and therapeutics for dentistry* [6th ed.]. Mosby.

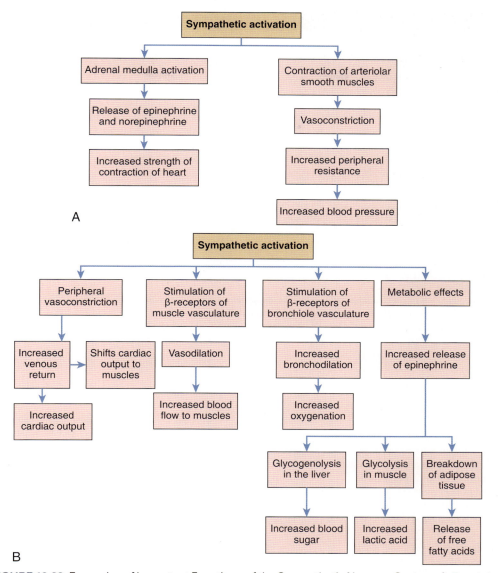

FIGURE 13.28 Examples of Important Functions of the Sympathetic Nervous System. A, Regulation of vasomotor tone. **B**, Regulation of strenuous muscular exercise ("fight-or-flight response," or acute stress response). (See also Chapter 9 and Figure 9.3 for more details on the stress response.)

and activation of sympathetic fibres normally silent and at rest (fibres to the sweat glands, pilomotor muscles, and the adrenal medulla, and vasodilator fibres to muscle) achieve this response. Control of vasomotor tone is thought to be the single most important function of the sympathetic nervous system. (Figure 13.28 shows some of the most important functions of the sympathetic nervous system.)

Increased parasympathetic activity promotes rest and calmness. A reduced heart rate and enhanced digestive visceral functions occur with parasympathetic activity. Stimulation of the vagus nerve (cranial nerve X) in the gastrointestinal tract increases peristalsis and secretion, as well as the relaxation of sphincters. Activation of parasympathetic fibres in the head, provided by cranial nerves III, VII, and IX, causes constriction of the pupil, tear secretion, and increased salivary secretion. Stimulation of the sacral division of the parasympathetic system contracts the urinary bladder and aids the process of genital erection.

The parasympathetic system lacks the widespread response of the sympathetic system. Activation of specific parasympathetic fibres regulates certain functions. Although the actions of the parasympathetic and sympathetic systems are usually opposite, there are exceptions. Peripheral vascular resistance, for example, increases markedly by sympathetic activation but is not altered noticeably by activity of the parasympathetic system. Sympathetic nerves innervate most blood vessels involved in the control of blood pressure. To decrease blood pressure, therefore, it is more important to block or halt the continuous discharge of the sympathetic system than to promote parasympathetic activity.

GERIATRIC CONSIDERATIONS
Aging and the Nervous System

Structural Changes with Aging
- Decrease in brain weight and size, markedly frontal regions
- Increase in ventricular volume
- Fibrosis and thickening of the meninges
- Narrowing of gyri and widening of sulci
- Increase in size of ventricles

Cellular Changes with Aging
- Decrease in the number of neurons not always related to changes in mental function
- Decrease in myelin
- Lipofuscin deposition (a pigment resulting from cellular autodigestion)
- Decrease in number of dendritic processes and synaptic connections
- Intracellular neurofibrillary tangles: a significant increase in cortex linked with Alzheimer's dementia
- Imbalance in amount and distribution of neurotransmitters
- Decrease in glucose metabolism

Cerebrovascular Changes with Aging
- Arterial atherosclerosis (may cause infarcts and scars)
- Increase in the permeability of the blood–brain barrier
- Decrease in vascular density

Functional Changes with Aging*
- Decrease in tendon reflexes
- Gradual deficit in taste and smell
- Decrease in vibratory sense
- Decrease in accommodation and colour vision
- Decrease in neuromuscular control with a change in gait and posture
- Sleep disturbances
- Memory impairments
- Cognitive changes linked with chronic disease

*Functional changes and nervous system aging have significant individual variation.
Data from Chételat, G., Landeau, B., Salmon, E., et al. (2013). *Neuroimage, 76*, 167–177; Fjell, A. M., McEvoy, L., Holland, D., et al. (2014). *Prog Neurobiol, 117*, 20–40; Fjell, A. M., & Walhovd, K. B. (2010). *Rev Neurosci, 21*(3), 187–221; Xekardaki, A., Kövari, E., Gold, G., et al. (2015). *Adv Exp Med Biol, 821*, 11–17.

DID YOU UNDERSTAND?

Overview and Organization of the Nervous System
1. The divisions of the nervous system are categorized as structural (CNS, PNS) or functional (somatic nervous system and ANS).
2. The CNS consists of the brain and spinal cord.
3. The PNS is composed of the cranial and spinal nerves. These nerves carry signals toward the CNS (afferent—sensory) and away from the CNS (efferent—motor) to and from target organs or skeletal muscle.

Cells of the Nervous System
1. The neuron and neuroglial cells form nervous tissue. The neuron is specialized in sending and receiving electrical and chemical signals. The neuroglial cell supplies support and maintenance functions.
2. The neuron is made of a cell body, dendrite(s), and an axon. A myelin sheath around some axons forms insulation that allows faster nerve impulse conduction.

The Nerve Impulse
1. The region between the neurons is the synapse. The region between the neuron and muscle is the myoneural junction.
2. Neurotransmitters are responsible for chemical conduction across the synapse.

The Central Nervous System
1. The cranial vault holds the brain and is divided into three distinct regions: (1) forebrain, (2) midbrain, and (3) hindbrain.
2. The forebrain includes the two cerebral hemispheres. It allows conscious awareness of internal and external stimuli, thought and memory processes, and voluntary control of skeletal muscles. The deep part of the forebrain is termed the *diencephalon* and processes incoming sensory data. The centre for control of skeletal muscle movements is in the frontal lobe. The centre for perception is in the parietal lobe. The Broca area and Wernicke area are major speech centres.
3. The midbrain is mainly a relay centre for motor and sensory tracts and a centre for auditory and visual reflexes.
4. The hindbrain allows sampling and comparison of sensory data, which are received from the periphery and motor signals of the cerebral hemispheres. It helps with coordination and skeletal muscle movement.
5. The spinal cord holds most of the nerve fibres that connect the brain with the periphery. The corticospinal tracts are descending pyramidal pathways from the motor cortex. The rubrospinal and reticulospinal tracts are descending extrapyramidal tracts that coordinate movement. The posterior column and anterior and lateral spinothalamic tracts carry sensory information to the brainstem, thalamus, and sensory cortex, respectively. Reflex arcs are sensory and motor circuits completed in the spinal cord and affected by the higher centres in the brain.
6. The scalp, cranium, meninges (dura mater, arachnoid, and pia mater), cerebrospinal fluid (CSF), and vertebral column protect the CNS. CSF is formed from blood components in the choroid plexuses of the ventricles and is reabsorbed in the arachnoid villi after circulating through the brain and subarachnoid space.
7. The carotid and vertebral arteries supply blood to the brain and connect to form the circle of Willis. The major branches projecting from the circle of Willis are the anterior, middle, and posterior cerebral arteries. Drainage of blood occurs through the venous sinuses and jugular veins.
8. Tight junctions between the cells of brain capillary endothelial cells and surrounding supporting cells form the blood–brain barrier.
9. Blood supply to the spinal cord comes from the vertebral arteries and branches arising from the aorta.

The Peripheral Nervous System

1. The cranial and spinal nerves make up the PNS. The PNS sends information from the CNS to muscle and effector organs through cranial and spinal nerve tracts arranged in fascicles. Multiple fascicles bound together form the peripheral nerve.

The Autonomic Nervous System

1. The ANS handles supporting a steady state in the internal environment. Two opposing systems make up the ANS: (a) the sympathetic nervous system responds to stress by mobilizing energy stores and prepares the body to defend itself, and (b) the parasympathetic nervous system conserves energy and the body's resources. Both systems function, more or less, at the same time.

14

Pain, Temperature, Sleep, and Sensory Function

Kelly Power-Kean, with originating chapter contributions by George W. Rodway and Sue E. Huether

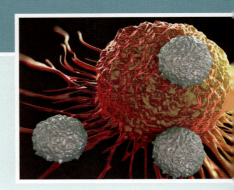

Additional resources are available online at https://evolve.elsevier.com/Canada/Huether/pathophysiology.

CHAPTER OUTLINE

Pain, 329
    Theories of Pain, 329
    Neuroanatomy of Pain, 330
    Pain Modulation, 331
    Clinical Descriptions of Pain, 333
Temperature Regulation, 334
    Control of Body Temperature, 335
    Temperature Regulation in Infants and Older Persons, 336
    Pathogenesis of Fever, 336
    Benefits of Fever, 337
    Disorders of Temperature Regulation, 337
Sleep, 338
    Sleep Disorders, 339

The Special Senses, 340
    Vision, 340
    Hearing, 344
    Olfaction and Taste, 347
Somatosensory Function, 347
    Touch, 347
    Proprioception, 347
GERIATRIC CONSIDERATIONS: Aging and Changes in Vision, 348
GERIATRIC CONSIDERATIONS: Aging and Changes in Hearing, 348
GERIATRIC CONSIDERATIONS: Aging and Changes in Olfaction and Taste, 348

LEARNING OBJECTIVES

1. Describe the difference between the two major types of nociceptors.
2. Describe the gate control theory of pain.
3. Name the three systems involved in pain perception.
4. Describe the effect that endorphins have on the transmission of pain signals.
5. Compare acute and persistent pain.
6. Compare somatic, visceral, and referred pain.
7. Compare neuropathic, peripheral, and central pain.
8. Describe the process of normal thermoregulation.
9. Describe the mechanisms of heat production, loss, and heat conservation.
10. Discuss the effects of fever, hyperthermia, and hypothermia.
11. Describe the normal sleep cycle.
12. Describe the types of sleep disorders. Give an example of each.
13. List the structures of the eye and explain their functions.
14. Describe the cause, manifestations, and complications of common ocular disorders.
15. Explain conductive and sensorineural hearing losses.
16. Differentiate acute otitis media from otitis media with effusion.
17. Describe the cause and effect of changes in smell and taste.
18. Define normal proprioception. Name the effects of altered proprioception.

KEY TERMS

A beta (Aβ) fibres, 330
A delta (Aδ) fibres, 330
Accidental hyperthermia, 337
Accommodation, 340
Acute bacterial conjunctivitis (pinkeye), 344
Acute otitis media (AOM), 346
Acute pain, 333
Affective-motivational system, 330
Age-related macular degeneration (AMD), 343
Ageusia, 347
Allergic conjunctivitis, 344
Allodynia, 334
Amblyopia, 341

Anosmia, 347
Aqueous humor, 340
Astigmatism, 343
Blepharitis, 344
C fibres, 330
Cannabinoid, 333
Cannabis, 333
Cataract, 341
Central fever, 338
Central neuropathic pain, 334
Central sensitization, 334
Chalazion, 344
Choroid, 340
Chronic conjunctivitis, 344
Circadian rhythm sleep disorder, 339

Cochlea, 345
Cognitive-evaluative system, 330
Colour blindness, 343
Conductive hearing loss, 345
Cone, 340
Conjunctivitis, 344
Cornea, 340
Crista ampullaris, 345
Descending facilitatory pathway, 333
Descending inhibitory pathway, 333
Diffuse noxious inhibitory control (DNIC), 333
Diplopia, 341
Dynorphin, 332

Dysgeusia, 347
Endocannabinoid, 333
Endogenous opioid, 331
Endogenous pyrogen, 336
Endomorphin, 332
Endorphin, 332
Enkephalin, 332
Entropion, 344
Equilibrium receptor, 345
Eustachian (pharyngotympanic) tube, 345
Excitatory neurotransmitter, 331
Exogenous pyrogen, 336
Expectancy-related cortical activation, 333
External auditory canal, 345

Fever, 336
Fever of unknown origin (FUO), 337
Fovea centralis, 340
Functional hearing loss, 346
Gate control theory, 330
Glaucoma, 341
Hair cell, 345
Heat cramp, 337
Heat exhaustion, 337
Heat stroke, 337
Heterosegmental pain inhibition, 333
Hordeolum (stye), 344
Hyperopia, 343
Hypersomnia, 339
Hyperthermia, 337
Hypogeusia, 347
Hyposmia, 347
Hypothermia, 338
Incus (anvil), 345
Inhibitory neurotransmitter, 331
Insomnia, 339
Intractable pain, 334
Iris, 340
Jerk nystagmus, 341
Keratitis, 344
Lens, 340
Macula lutea, 340
Maculae, 345
Malignant hyperthermia, 338
Malleus (hammer), 345
Mastoid air cell, 345
Mastoid process, 345
Meissner corpuscle, 347
Ménière's disease, 346
Merkel disc, 347
Mixed hearing loss, 346
Myopia, 343
Narcolepsy, 339
Neuromatrix theory, 330
Neuropathic pain, 334
Night terrors, 340
Nociceptin/orphanin FQ, 332
Nociception, 330
Nociceptive pain, 330
Nociceptive transmissions, 330
Nociceptor, 330
Non-nociceptive stimulation, 330
Non–rapid eye movement (NREM) sleep, 339
Nystagmus, 341
Obesity hypoventilation syndrome, 339
Obstructive sleep apnea syndrome (OSAS), 339
Olfaction, 347
Olfactory hallucination, 347
Optic chiasm, 340
Optic disc, 340
Optic nerve, 340
Organ of Corti, 345
Otitis externa, 346
Otitis media, 346
Otitis media with effusion (OME), 346
Otolith, 345
Oval window, 345
Pacinian corpuscle, 347
Pain modulation, 331
Pain perception, 330
Pain threshold, 331
Pain tolerance, 331
Pain transduction, 330
Pain transmission, 330
Parasomnia, 340
Parosmia, 347
Pattern theory, 329
Pendular nystagmus, 341
Perceptual dominance, 331
Perilymph, 345
Peripheral neuropathic pain, 334
Peripheral sensitization, 334
Persistent pain, 334
Pinna, 345
Presbycusis, 346
Presbyopia, 343
Proprioception, 347
Pupil, 340
Rapid eye movement (REM) sleep, 338
Referred pain, 333
Restless legs syndrome (RLS), 340
Retina, 340
Rod, 340
Ruffini ending, 347
Sclera, 340
Segmental pain inhibition, 333
Semicircular canal, 345
Sensorineural hearing loss, 346
Sensory-discriminative system, 330
Shift work sleep disorder, 339
Sleep, 338
Somatic pain, 333
Somnambulism (sleepwalking), 340
Specificity theory, 329
Stapes (stirrup), 345
Strabismus, 341
Suprachiasmatic nucleus (SCN), 340
Taste, 347
Therapeutic hyperthermia, 337
Thermoregulation, 334
Tinnitus, 346
Touch, 347
Trachoma, 344
Tympanic cavity, 345
Tympanic membrane, 345
Vertigo, 347
Vestibular nystagmus, 347
Vestibule, 345
Viral conjunctivitis, 344
Visceral pain, 333
Vitreous humor, 340
Willis-Ekbom disease, 340

Changes in sensory function may involve dysfunctions of the general or the special senses. Dysfunctions of the general senses include persistent pain (also referred to as *chronic pain*), abnormal temperature regulation, and tactile or proprioceptive dysfunction. Pain is an unpleasant but protective event that is uniquely experienced by everyone. It cannot be adequately defined, identified, or measured by an observer. Like pain, changes in temperature can signal disease. Fever is a common symptom of dysfunction. It is often the first sign in an infectious or inflammatory condition.

Sleep is a normal process that restores the body's energy and supports normal functioning. Sleep is so vital to both physiological and psychological functions that a lack of sleep causes a wide range of symptoms.

The special senses are vision, hearing, touch, smell, and taste. These senses are responsible for how persons perceive stimuli that are vital in interacting with the environment. Dysfunctions of the special senses include visual, auditory, vestibular (balance), olfactory (smell), and gustatory (taste) disorders.

PAIN

> ✓ **QUICK CHECK 14.1**
> 1. What is the difference between A delta (Aδ) and C fibres?
> 2. Give two examples of pain excitatory and inhibitory neurotransmitters.
> 3. How do A beta (Aβ) fibres prevent and cause pain?
> 4. What are two differences between nociceptive and neuropathic pain?

Pain is a complex experience. It involves complex interactions between physical, cognitive, spiritual, emotional, and environmental factors. Pain is more than a response to injury. McCaffery defined *pain* as "whatever the experiencing person says it is, existing whenever he says it does."[1] The Canadian Pain Coalition agrees with the International Association for the Study of Pain definition of *pain*, which is "an unpleasant sensory and emotional experience associated with actual or potential tissue damage or described in terms of such damage."[2] Acute pain is protective and promotes pulling away from painful stimuli. It allows the injured part to heal and teaches an individual to avoid painful stimuli.

Theories of Pain

The theories of pain include the specificity theory, pattern theory, gate control theory, and neuromatrix theory.

Specificity theory suggests that injury triggers specific pain receptors and fibres that project to the brain. *Intensity of pain* is directly related to the amount of associated tissue injury (i.e., pricking one's finger with a needle would cause slight pain, while cutting one's hand with a knife would produce more pain). The theory is useful when related to specific injuries and the acute pain associated with them. It does not account for persistent pain or cognitive and emotional causes that add to more complex types of pain.[3]

Pattern theory describes the role of impulse strength and the repatterning of the central nervous system (CNS) in starting the feeling of pain. The pattern theory does not account for all types of pain events.[3]

Gate control theory combines and builds upon parts of the other theories to explain the complex multidimensional aspects of pain perception and pain modulation.[3] Pain transmission is altered by a balance of signals sent to the spinal cord where cells in the substantia gelatinosa work as a "gate." The spinal gate controls pain transmission to higher centres in the CNS. Large myelinated A delta (Aδ) fibres and small unmyelinated C fibres respond to a wide range of painful stimuli (mechanical, thermal, and chemical). These fibres end on the interneurons in the substantia gelatinosa (laminae in the posterior horn of the spinal cord). Nociceptive transmissions on these fibres "open" the spinal gate and increase the feeling of pain. Closure or partial closure of the spinal gates can occur from non-nociceptive stimulation (i.e., from touch sensors in the skin). The non-nociceptive larger A beta (Aβ) fibres (large myelinated fibres that send touch and vibration sensations) carry these signals and decrease pain perception. The closure or partial closure of spinal gates through non-nociceptive stimulation (e.g., rubbing a painful area) explains the easing of some pain or discomfort. Other efferent CNS pathways descend to the spinal cord and may close, partially close, or open the gate modulation of the pain experience. The gate control theory, supported by progress in understanding neuronal pathways in the peripheral and central nervous systems, has improved our understanding of pain. As good as the gate control theory has been, there are factors about pain in paraplegics that "do not fit the theory."

Neuromatrix theory suggests that the brain makes patterns of nerve signals drawn from various inputs. These inputs include genetic, psychological, and cognitive experiences.[3] The sensations we normally feel from the body, including pain, also can be felt when inputs from the body are absent (as noted with phantom limb pain). Stimuli may trigger the patterns but do not produce them. Sensory inputs from the periphery normally start neuromatrix patterns, but these may also start freely in the brain with no outside input.[3] The neuromatrix theory shows the plasticity (adaptable change in structure and function) of the brain. It does not replace our understanding of gate control theory, and what we know about peripheral inflammation, spinal modulation, and midbrain descending control of pain. The neuromatrix theory builds upon gate control theory by explaining an integrated body-self. This provides a holistic and dynamic view of pain. However, there are many kinds of pain, and no single theory can explain the complex dynamics of the pain experience. Ongoing research is helping our understanding of the neural mechanisms of pain.[3]

Neuroanatomy of Pain

Three parts of the nervous system handle the sensation, perception, and response to pain:

1. *Afferent pathways* begin in the peripheral nervous system (PNS). These pathways travel to the spinal gate in the posterior horn and then ascend to higher centres in the CNS.
2. *Interpretive centres* found in the brainstem, midbrain, diencephalon, and cerebral cortex.
3. *Efferent pathways* descend from the CNS back to the posterior horn of the spinal cord.

Nociception is the processing of possibly harmful (noxious) stimuli through a normally working nervous system.[2] Nociceptors, or pain receptors, are free nerve endings in the afferent PNS. When they are simulated, nociceptive pain occurs. The cell bodies of nociceptors are in the posterior root ganglia for the body and in the trigeminal ganglion for the face. Nociceptors have a peripheral and central axonal branch that supply nerve stimulation to their target organ and the spinal cord, respectively. The sensitivity to pain differs according to nociceptor location. This is a result of uneven distribution of nociceptors throughout the body (Table 14.1).

TABLE 14.1 Stimuli That Activate Nociceptors (Pain Receptors)

Location of Receptor	Provoking Stimuli
Skin	Pricking, cutting, crushing, burning, freezing
Gastro-intestinal tract	Swollen or inflamed mucosa, enlargement or spasm of smooth muscle, traction on mesenteric attachment
Skeletal muscle	Ischemia, injuries of connective tissue sheaths, necrosis, bleeding, prolonged contraction, injection of irritating solutions
Joints	Synovial membrane inflammation
Arteries	Piercing, inflammation
Head	Traction, inflammation, or displacement of arteries, meningeal structures, and sinuses; prolonged muscle contraction
Heart	Ischemia and inflammation
Bone	Periosteal injury: fractures, tumour, inflammation

Nociceptors respond to different types of noxious (harmful) stimuli: mechanical (pressure or distortion), thermal (extreme temperatures), or chemical (acids or chemicals of inflammation such as bradykinin, histamine, leukotrienes, or prostaglandins). Nociception includes four phases: transduction, transmission, perception, and modulation.[3]

Pain transduction begins when nociceptors are triggered by a noxious stimulus. This process causes ion channels (sodium, potassium, calcium) on nociceptors to open, creating electrical signals. The impulses travel through axons of two main types of nociceptors that are sent to the spinal cord, brainstem, thalamus, and cortex (see Figure 13.9).[4] There are two main types of nociceptors: Aδ fibres and C fibres. Aδ fibres are larger myelinated fibres that quickly send sharp, well-localized "fast" sensations. Examples of this pain include a burn or pinprick to the skin. Activation of these fibres causes a spinal reflex withdrawal of the affected body part from the stimulus before a pain sensation is felt.[3] C fibres are the most numerous, are smaller and unmyelinated. They are found in muscle, tendons, body organs, and the skin. C fibres slowly send dull, aching, or burning sensations that are often constant and difficult to pinpoint.[3,5]

Pain transmission is the transfer of pain signals along the Aδ and C fibres (first-order neurons) into the posterior horn of the spinal cord (Figure 14.1). Here they form synapses with excitatory or inhibitory interneurons (second-order neurons) in the substantia gelatinosa of the posterior horn. The signals then synapse with projection neurons (third-order neurons) and cross the midline of the spinal cord. From there, the signals ascend to the brain through two lateral spinothalamic tracts. The neospinothalamic tract (anterior spinal thalamic tract) carries fast signals for acute sharp pain. The paleospinothalamic tract (lateral spinothalamic tract) carries slow signals for dull or persistent pain. The fast-sharp pain is felt first, followed by dull, throbbing pain. These tracts connect to the reticular formation, hypothalamus, thalamus (the major relay station of sensory information), and the limbic system. The signals are sent to the somatosensory cortex for interpretation of location and strength of pain (see Figure 14.1). They are also sent to other areas of the brain for an integrated response to pain.

Pain perception is the conscious awareness of pain. Perception occurs mainly in the reticular and limbic systems and the cerebral cortex. Many factors influence pain interpretation. These factors include genetics, cultural influences, gender roles, and life experience, including past pain events and level of health.[3] Three systems work together

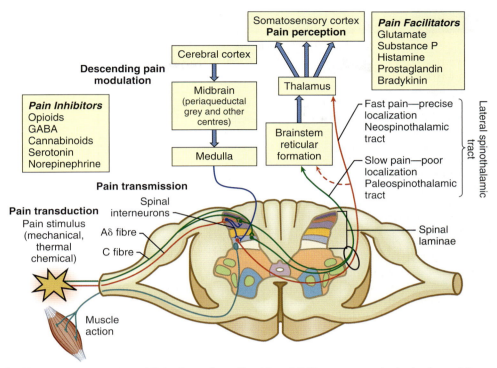

FIGURE 14.1 Transmission of Pain Sensations. The Aδ and C fibres synapse in the laminae of the posterior horn. They then cross over to the contralateral spinothalamic tract, and then ascend to synapse in the midbrain through the neospinothalamic and paleospinothalamic tracts. The sensory cortex then receives the signals. Descending pain inhibition is started in the cerebral cortex or from the midbrain and medulla. *GABA*, Gamma-aminobutyric acid.

to produce the perception of pain.[3] The **sensory-discriminative system** is mediated by the somatosensory cortex and is responsible for identifying the presence, character, location, and intensity of pain. The **affective-motivational system** determines a person's learned avoidance behaviours and emotional responses to pain. Mediation of these responses occurs through the reticular formation, limbic system, and brainstem. The **cognitive-evaluative system** guides the person's learned behaviour about the experience of pain. This system can modulate the feeling of pain. The cerebral cortex mediates this process. The "pain matrix" is a combination of these three systems.[6]

Pain threshold and tolerance are subjective events that affect a person's perception of pain. Genetics, gender, cultural beliefs, expectations, role socialization, physical and mental health, and age can impact pain perception[3] (Table 14.2). Health care providers often find it helpful to use pain scales to assess their patients' pain. Many pain scales are available for use with neonates, infants, children, adolescents, adults, older persons, and persons who have impaired communication skills.

The lowest amount of pain that a person can recognize is the **pain threshold**.[3] Strong pain at one location may increase the threshold in another location. For example, a person with severe pain in one knee is more likely to experience less intense persistent back pain (called **perceptual dominance**). Because of perceptual dominance, pain at one site may mask other painful areas. Stress, excessive physical exertion, acupuncture, sexual activity, and other factors can increase the levels of circulating neuromodulators. This increase raises the pain threshold.

The greatest amount of pain that a person can endure is called **pain tolerance**.[3] It differs greatly among people. It can also differ in the same person over time because of the body's ability to respond differently to noxious stimuli (see Table 14.2). Pain tolerance usually *decreases* with repeated exposure to pain, fatigue, anger, boredom, worry, and lack of sleep. Pain tolerance may *increase* with alcohol intake, persistent use of opioid medications, hypnosis, distracting activities, and strong beliefs or faith.

Pain Modulation

Pain modulation involves many different mechanisms that increase or decrease the transmission of pain signals throughout the nervous system. Depending on the mechanism, modulation can occur before, during, or after pain is felt.[7]

Neurotransmitters of Pain Modulation

A wide range of neurotransmitters act to modulate control over transmission of pain signals in the periphery, spinal cord, and brain.[3] The peripheral triggering mechanisms that start the release of **excitatory neurotransmitters** include tissue injury (prostaglandins, histamine, bradykinin) and chronic inflammatory injury (lymphokines). Glutamate, aspartate, substance P, and calcitonin are common excitatory neurotransmitters in the brain and spinal cord. These substances sensitize nociceptors by reducing the activation threshold, leading to increased responsiveness of nociceptors.[3]

Inhibitory neurotransmitters in the spinal cord include gamma aminobutyric acid (GABA) and glycine. Norepinephrine and 5-hydroxytryptamine (serotonin) play a role in pain inhibition in the medulla and pons but can excite peripheral nerves.[3]

Endogenous opioids are a family of morphine like neuropeptides that prevent transmission of pain signals in the periphery, spinal cord, and brain. This occurs when the endogenous opioids bind with certain opioid receptors (mu [μ], kappa [κ], and delta [δ]) on neurons. They hinder ion channels, preventing the release of excitatory neurotransmitters in the posterior horn. In the midbrain they affect descending inhibitory pathways[8] (Figure 14.2). In peripheral inflamed tissue,

TABLE 14.2 Pain Perception in Infants, Children, and Older Persons

	Infants	Children	Older Persons
Pain threshold	Painful neonatal experiences increase pain sensitivity (lower threshold); pain may increase with future procedures	Lower or same as adults	Individual responses, which vary, but pain threshold may be lower
Physiological symptoms	Increased heart rate, blood pressure, and respiratory rate; flushing or pallor, sweating, and decreased oxygen saturation	Same as infants; nausea and vomiting	Same as infants and children; nausea and vomiting; may decrease in persons with cognitive impairment
Behavioural responses	Changes in facial expression, crying, and body movements, with lowered brows drawn together; vertical bulge and furrows in forehead between brows; broadened nasal root; tightly closed eyes; angular, square-shaped mouth, chin quiver; withdrawal of affected limbs, rigidity, flailing	Individual responses, which vary	Individual responses, which vary, and may be influenced by presence of painful chronic diseases and decline in renal, intestinal, hepatic, cardiovascular, and neurological function; persons with cognitive impairment may demonstrate changes in behaviour (e.g., combative or withdrawn, increased confusion)

Data from Maxwell, L. G., Malavolta, C. P., & Fraga, M. V. (2013). *Clinics in Perinatology, 40*(3), 457–469; Molton, I. R., & Terrill, A. L. (2014). *American Psychologist, 69*(2), 197–207; Tracy, B., & Morrison, R. S. (2013). *Clinical Therapeutics, 35*(11), 1659–1668; Walker, S. M. (2014). *Paediatric Anaesthesia, 24*(1), 39–48.

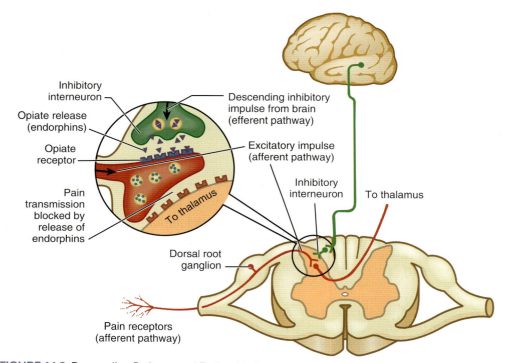

FIGURE 14.2 Descending Pathway and Endorphin Response. In this figure, a descending inhibitory signal is sent from the brain to an inhibitory interneuron in the posterior horn, causing the release of endorphin. The endorphin activates a μ opioid receptor and results in inhibition of pain transmission to ascending pathways.

opioids are made and released from immune cells and activate opioid receptors on sensory nerve terminals.[9] Opioid receptors are widely distributed throughout the body and are responsible for general sensations of well-being and modulation of many physiological processes. These processes include control of respiratory and cardiovascular functions, stress and immune responses, gastro-intestinal function, reproduction, and neuroendocrine control.[10]

Enkephalins are the most numerous of the natural opioids and bind to δ opioid receptors. The brain produces **endorphins** (endogenous morphine). The best-studied endorphin is β-endorphin, which binds to μ receptors and creates the greatest sense of excitement and substantial natural pain relief. **Dynorphins** are the strongest of the endogenous opioids. They bind firmly with κ receptors to decrease pain signals. Surprisingly, they play a role in neuropathic pain, in mood disorders and medication addiction.[11] **Endomorphins** bind with μ receptors and have strong pain relief effects.[3] **Nociceptin/orphanin FQ** is an opioid that *causes* pain or hyperalgesia but does not interact with opioid receptors. Nociceptin is also associated with inflammation, immune regulation, mood, and emotion. The nociceptin receptors are distributed widely throughout the PNS and CNS.[12]

Man-made and natural opiates have pharmacological actions like morphine. They bind as direct agonists to the opioid receptors. Morphine has 50 times higher attraction for μ receptors compared with other opioids. Naloxone (Narcan) is the only opioid receptor antagonist, with a higher attraction for the μ receptors than for the other receptors.[13] It is a life-saving drug that is used to counteract the effects of opioid overdose.

Endocannabinoids are made from phospholipids and are classified as eicosanoids. They activate cannabinoid CB_1 (mainly in the CNS) and CB_2 receptors (mainly in immune tissue [e.g., the spleen]) to modulate pain and other functions. These functions include memory, appetite, immune function, sleep, stress response, thermoregulation, and addiction. CB_1 receptors decrease pain transmission. This is done by inhibiting release of excitatory neurotransmitters in the spinal posterior horn, periaqueductal grey, thalamus, rostral ventromedial medulla (RVM), and amygdala. Cannabis (marijuana) makes a resin containing cannabinoid. Cannabinoids are pain relieving in humans, but their psychoactive and addictive properties limit their use. In 2020, the use of recreational cannabis was legalized in Canada. Research is in progress to develop cannabinoid receptor agonists that do not have addictive side effects.[14,15]

Pathways of Modulation

Descending inhibitory pathways, descending facilitatory pathways, and nuclei prevent or ease pain. Afferent stimulation of the ventromedial medulla and periaqueductal grey (PAG) (grey matter surrounding the cerebral aqueduct) in the midbrain stimulates efferent pathways. This stimulation inhibits afferent pain signals at the posterior horn.[8] The RVM stimulates efferent pathways that facilitate or inhibit pain in the posterior horn.[8] Inhibitory pathways can: (1) activate opioid receptors and inhibit release of excitatory neurotransmitters, (2) facilitate release of inhibitory neurotransmitters, or (3) stimulate inhibitory interneurons.

Aβ-fibre stimulation results in segmental pain inhibition. The signals arrive at the same spinal level as signals from Aδ or C fibres. They stimulate an inhibitory interneuron and decrease pain transmission. An example of this is rubbing an injured area to relieve pain.[8]

Diffuse noxious inhibitory control (DNIC) is an inhibitory pain system that involves a spinal-medullary-spinal pathway. Pain is relieved when two noxious stimuli occur at the same time from different sites (pain inhibiting pain). This system also is known as heterosegmental pain inhibition. Examples for this pain relief include acupuncture, deep massage, or intense cold or heat.[16]

Expectancy-related cortical activation (placebo effect [beneficial expectations] or nocebo effect [adverse expectations]) can exert control over pain-relieving systems to lessen or increase pain.[17] In other words, cognitive expectations can cause real, measurable physiological effects that share some of the same descending pain pathways as the pain modulatory systems.

Clinical Descriptions of Pain

Pain is described in a variety of ways. Because of the complex nature of pain, many terms overlap, and more than one description is often used. Box 14.1 reviews the broad categories of pain. A review of some of the most common clinical pain categories follows.

Acute pain (nociceptive pain) is a normal protective mechanism that alerts the person to a condition or experience that is instantly harmful to the body. Acute pain also causes the person to take quick action to relieve it. Acute pain is temporary, usually lasting minutes to several weeks.[18] It begins suddenly and is relieved after the chemical mediators that stimulate pain receptors are removed.[3] Stimulation of the sympathetic division of the autonomic nervous system results in physical symptoms including increased heart rate, hypertension, diaphoresis, and dilated pupils. It is common to experience anxiety related to the pain experience, its cause, treatment, and prognosis. Hope of recovery and expectation of limited duration is also common.[3]

BOX 14.1 Categories of Pain

I. Neurophysiological Pain
A. **Nociceptive pain**
  1. Somatic (e.g., skin, muscle, bone)
  2. Visceral (e.g., intestine, liver, stomach)
  3. Referred
B. **Neuropathic (non-nociceptive)**
  1. Central pain (injury in brain or spinal cord)
  2. Peripheral pain (injury in peripheral nervous system)

II. Neurogenic Pain
A. **Neuralgia (pain in the distribution of a nerve)**
B. **Constant**
  1. Sympathetically independent
  2. Sympathetically dependent

III. Temporal Pain (time related, duration)
A. **Acute pain**
  1. Somatic (e.g., pain resulting from skin laceration)
  2. Visceral (e.g., pain resulting from inflammation associated with appendicitis)
  3. Referred (e.g., shoulder pain referred from inflammation of the gallbladder)
B. **Persistent pain**

IV. Pain Location
A. **Abdominal pain**
B. **Chest pain**
C. **Headache**
D. **Low back pain**
E. **Orofacial pain**
F. **Pelvic pain**

V. Etiological Pain
A. **Cancer pain**
B. **Dental pain**
C. **Inflammatory pain**
D. **Ischemic pain**
E. **Vascular pain**

Adapted from Mersky, H. (2014). Taxonomy and classification of chronic pain syndromes. In H. T. Benzon, J. P. Rathmell, C. L. Wu, et al. (Eds.), *Practical management of pain* (5th ed., pp. 13–18). Mosby.

Acute pain results from cutaneous, deep somatic, or visceral structures and is classified as (1) somatic, (2) visceral, or (3) referred. Somatic pain starts with the skin, joints, and muscles. It is either sharp and easily located (especially fast pain carried by Aδ fibres) or dull, aching, throbbing, and poorly located as seen in polymodal C fibre transmissions. Visceral pain refers to pain in internal organs and the lining of body cavities. C fibres send this pain. Visceral pain tends to be poorly located and has an aching, gnawing, throbbing, or intermittent cramping quality. Nausea, vomiting, hypotension, and, in some cases, shock occur with visceral pain. Visceral pain often radiates (spreads away from the actual site of the pain) or is referred. Pain felt in an area removed or distant from its point of origin is referred pain. The same spinal segment as the actual site of pain supplies the area of referred pain. Signals from many skin and visceral neurons meet on the same ascending neuron, and the brain cannot identify between the different

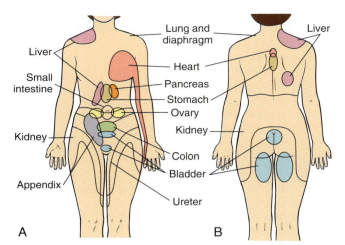

FIGURE 14.3 Sites of Referred Pain. **A**, Anterior view. **B**, Posterior view.

sources of pain. Because the skin has more receptors, the painful sensation is experienced at the referred site instead of at the site of origin.[19] Referred pain can be acute or persistent. Figure 14.3 shows common areas of referred pain and their related sites of origin. (Figure 13.25 shows cranial and peripheral nerves and skin dermatomes; see also Box 14.1.)

Pain lasting for more than 3 to 6 months is persistent pain (intractable pain). Persistent pain is also considered to be pain that lasts beyond the expected normal healing time. It varies with type of injury.[3] Persistent pain is poorly understood, serves no purpose, and causes suffering. It often appears to be out of proportion to any visible tissue injury. It may be ongoing (e.g., low back pain) or intermittent (e.g., migraine headaches). It is thought that changes in the PNS and CNS cause impairment in the regulation of nociception and pain modulation processes (peripheral and central sensitization) and lead to persistent pain[3] (see the discussion of neuropathic pain, described later in this section).

Neuroimaging studies have shown brain changes in persons with persistent pain. These brain changes may lead to cognitive deficits and decreased ability to cope with pain.[3] These negative symptoms of persistent pain are thought to be due, in part, to the stress of coping with continuous pain. The symptoms may be reversible when pain is controlled.[20] Because it is not possible to predict when acute pain will develop into persistent pain, early treatment of acute pain is encouraged.

Physiological responses to intermittent persistent pain are like those for acute pain. Persistent pain, however, allows for physiological adaptation, producing normal heart rate and blood pressure. This normalization may lead many to wrongly conclude that people with persistent pain are malingering because they do not appear to be in pain. As persistent pain progresses, certain behavioural and psychological changes often occur. These changes include depression, difficulty eating and sleeping, fixation with the pain, and avoiding pain-causing stimuli.[20] The desire to relieve pain and the need to hide it become conflicting drives for those with persistent pain. These persons fear being called complainers.[21] Persistent pain is considered meaningless. It is often associated with a sense of hopelessness as time passes and no cure seems possible. Table 14.3 lists some common chronic pain syndromes. Table 14.4 compares acute and persistent pain. Later chapters discuss persistent pain as it relates to specific organ systems.

Neuropathic pain is persistent pain started or caused by a primary injury or dysfunction in the nervous system. Neuropathic pain leads to long-term changes in pain pathway structures (neuroplasticity) and abnormal processing of sensory information.[22] There is an increase of pain without stimulation by injury or inflammation. Neuropathic pain is described as burning, shooting, shock like, or tingling. It is associated with increased sensitivity to painful or nonpainful stimuli with hyperalgesia, allodynia (the creation of pain by normally nonpainful stimuli), and the development of spontaneous pain.[23] Neuropathic pain is classified as either peripheral or central. It is associated with central and peripheral sensitization.[23] Peripheral neuropathic pain is caused by peripheral nerve injuries and an increase in the sensitivity and excitability of primary sensory neurons and cells in the posterior root ganglion (peripheral sensitization). Examples include nerve entrapment, diabetic neuropathy, or chronic pancreatitis.

An injury or dysfunction in the brain or spinal cord causes central neuropathic pain. A gradual repeated stimulation of group C neurons (wind-up) in the posterior horn leads to increased sensitivity of central pain signalling neurons (central sensitization). This central sensitization results in pathological changes in the CNS that cause persistent pain.[24] Examples include brain or spinal cord trauma, tumours, vascular injuries, multiple sclerosis, Parkinson's disease, postherpetic neuralgia, and phantom limb pain.[23,24]

The causative mechanisms of neuropathic pain include:[22]
- Changes in sensitivity of neurons—lower threshold with peripheral and central sensitization
- Spontaneous signals from regenerating peripheral nerves
- Changes in the posterior root ganglion and spinothalamic tract in response to peripheral nerve injury (i.e., deafferentation pain—loss of pain-related afferent information to the brain)
- Loss of pain inhibition and stimulation of pain easing by excitatory neurotransmitters in the posterior horn (e.g., release of glutamate by stimulation of N-methyl-D-aspartate [NMDA] receptors)
- Loss of descending inhibitory pain modulation
- Hyperexcitable spinal interneurons stimulated by Aβ fibres (nonpainful stimulation of pain)
- Release of nociceptive inflammatory cytokines, chemokines, and growth factors by activated glial cells
- Structural and functional changes in brain processing neural networks.

Because of the complexity of the causes of neuropathic pain syndromes, they are difficult to treat. Treatment often includes multiple therapies, including nonmedication options.[25]

TEMPERATURE REGULATION

> **QUICK CHECK 14.2**
> 1. Why is temperature regulation important?
> 2. What are the main heat-production methods? Heat-loss methods?
> 3. How does the hypothalamus alter its set point to change body temperature?
> 4. Compare and contrast hyperthermia and hypothermia and their effects on the body.

The balancing of heat production, heat conservation, and heat loss achieves human temperature regulation (thermoregulation). The normal range of body temperature is 36.2° to 37.7°C (96.2° to 99.4°F), but a person's individual body parts will vary in temperature. Body temperature rarely exceeds 41°C. The extremities are generally cooler than the trunk. The temperature at the core of the body (as measured by rectal temperature) is generally 0.5°C higher than the surface temperature (as measured by oral temperature). Internal temperature varies in response to activity, environmental temperature, and daily fluctuation (circadian rhythm). Oral temperatures vary within 0.2° to 0.5°C during

TABLE 14.3 Common Chronic Pain Syndromes

Condition	Description
Persistent low back pain	Most common chronic pain condition
	Results from poor muscle tone, inactivity, muscle strain, or sudden, vigorous exercise
Myofascial pain syndromes	Pain results from muscle spasm, tenderness, stiffness, or injury to muscle and fascia with peripheral and central sensitization
	Examples include myositis, fibrositis, myalgia, fibromyalgia, and muscle strain
	Trigger points—small hypersensitive regions in muscle or connective tissues that, when stimulated, produce pain in a specific area
	As disorder progresses, pain becomes increasingly generalized
Chronic postoperative pain	Persistent pain that can occur with disruption or cutting of sensory nerves; examples include post-thoracotomy, postmastectomy; risk factors may include pre-existing pain and genetic susceptibility
Cancer pain	Attributed to advance of disease, treatment, or coexisting disease entities
Deafferentation pain	Pain because of change of sensory input into central nervous system that is caused by damage to peripheral nerves
	Common types include severe burning pain caused by various stimuli, such as cold, light touch, or sound, and complex regional pain syndromes (occur after peripheral nerve injury and are characterized by continuous, severe, burning pain associated with vasomotor changes and muscle wasting)
Hyperalgesia	Increased sensitivity and decreased pain threshold to tactile and painful stimuli
	Pain is diffuse, modified by fatigue and emotion, and mixed with other sensations
	May result from chronic irritation of central nervous system areas
Hemiagnosia	Loss of ability to identify source of pain on one side of body
	Painful stimuli on that side produce discomfort, anxiety, moaning, agitation, and distress but no attempt to withdraw from stimulus
	Associated with stroke
Phantom limb pain	Pain experienced in amputated limb after stump has completely healed; may be immediate or occur months later; associated with preamputation pain, acute postoperative pain
	Exact cause is unknown, thought to originate in brain; can be influenced by emotions/sympathetic stimulation
Complex regional pain syndrome	Chronic pain is usually associated with limb injury, surgery, or fractures
	Characterized by autonomic and neuro-inflammatory features and pain out of proportion to expected pain

TABLE 14.4 Comparison of Acute and Persistent Pain

Characteristic	Acute Pain	Persistent Pain
Experience	An event	A situation; state of existence
Source	Outside agent or internal disease, injury, or inflammation	Unknown; if known, treatment is prolonged or ineffective
Onset	Usually sudden	May be sudden or develop gradually
Duration	Transient (up to 3 months); usually of short duration	Prolonged (months to years); lasts beyond expected normal healing time
	Resolves with treatment and healing	
Pain identification	Painful and nonpainful areas generally well identified	More difficult to tell painful and nonpainful areas apart, change in sensations becomes more difficult to assess
Clinical signs	Typical response pattern with more visible signs	Response patterns vary; fewer clear signs (adaptation)
	Anxiety and emotional distress common	Pain can interfere with sleep, productivity, and quality of life
Significance	Significant (informs person something is wrong); protective	Person looks for significance and meaning; serves no useful purpose
Pattern	Self-limiting or quickly corrected	Continuous or intermittent; strength may vary or remain constant
Course	Suffering usually decreases over time	Suffering usually increases over time
Actions	Leads to actions to relieve pain	Leads to actions to change pain experience
Prognosis	Eventual complete relief is likely	Complete relief is usually not possible

a 24-hour period. Women tend to have wider fluctuations that follow the menstrual cycle, with a quick rise in temperature just before ovulation. The daily fluctuating temperature in both genders peaks around 6 p.m. and is at its lowest during sleep. Maintenance of body temperature within the normal range is needed for life.

Control of Body Temperature

The hypothalamus and endocrine system are the primary mediators of thermoregulation. Peripheral thermoreceptors in the skin and abdominal organs (unmyelinated C fibres and thinly myelinated Aδ fibres) and central thermoreceptors in the hypothalamus, spinal cord, and other central locations provide the hypothalamus with information about skin and core temperatures. If these temperatures are low or high, the hypothalamus triggers heat production and heat conservation or heat loss mechanisms.

The chemical reactions of metabolism and skeletal muscle tone and contraction produce body heat. The heat-producing mechanism (chemical or nonshivering thermogenesis) begins with hypothalamic thyrotropin-stimulating hormone-releasing hormone (TSH-RH). It stimulates the anterior pituitary to release thyroid-stimulating hormone (TSH), which acts on the thyroid gland and stimulates the release of thyroxine. Thyroxine then acts on the adrenal medulla, causing the release of epinephrine into the bloodstream. Epinephrine causes vasoconstriction, stimulates glycolysis, and increases metabolic rate, thus

TABLE 14.5 Mechanisms of Heat Production and Heat Loss

Condition	Description
Heat Production	
Chemical reactions of metabolism	Reactions occur during intake and digestion of food and while supporting body at rest (basal metabolism); occur in body core (e.g., liver)
Skeletal muscle contraction	Gradual increase in muscle tone or rapid muscle oscillations (shivering)
Chemical thermogenesis	Release of epinephrine produces rapid, temporary increase in heat production by raising basal metabolic rate; quick, brief effect that offsets heat lost through conduction and convection; involves brown adipose tissue, which decreases significantly in older persons; thyroid hormone increases metabolism
Heat Loss	
Radiation	Heat loss through electromagnetic waves coming from surfaces with temperature higher than surrounding air
Conduction	Heat loss by direct molecule-to-molecule transfer from one surface to another, so that warmer surface loses heat to cooler surface
Convection	Transfer of heat through currents of gases or liquids; exchanges warmer air at body's surface with cooler air in surrounding space
Vasodilation	Diversion of core-warmed blood to surface of body, with heat transferred by conduction to skin surface and from there to surrounding environment; occurs in response to autonomic stimulation under control of hypothalamus
Evaporation	Body water evaporates from surface of skin and linings of mucous membranes; major source of heat reduction connected with increased sweating in warmer surroundings
Decreased muscle tone	Exhausted feeling caused by moderately reduced muscle tone and limited voluntary muscle activity
Increased respiration	Air is exchanged with environment through normal process; minimal effect
Voluntary mechanisms	"Stretching out" and "slowing down" in response to high body temperatures; increasing body surface area available for heat loss; dressing in light-coloured, loose-fitting garments
Adaptation to warmer climates	Gradual process beginning with lethargy, weakness, and faintness; proceeding through increased sweating, lowered sodium content, decreased heart rate, and increased stroke volume and extracellular fluid volume, ending with improved warm weather functioning and decreased symptoms of heat intolerance (work output, endurance, and coordination increase; subjective feelings of discomfort decrease)

increasing body heat. Norepinephrine and thyroxine activate brown fat thermogenesis. In this process, heat instead of adenosine triphosphate (ATP) is the source of energy. The circulatory system distributes the heat.[26]

The hypothalamus also triggers heat conservation by stimulating the sympathetic nervous system. This then stimulates the adrenal cortex and results in increased skeletal muscle tone, starting the shivering response and causing vasoconstriction. By constricting peripheral blood vessels, centrally warmed blood shunts away from the periphery to the core of the body where heat can be kept. This involuntary mechanism takes advantage of the insulating layers of the skin and subcutaneous fat to protect core temperature. The hypothalamus sends information to the cerebral cortex about cold, and voluntary responses result. Persons usually bundle up, keep moving, or curl up in a ball. These types of voluntary physical activities supply insulation, increase skeletal muscle activity, and decrease the amount of skin surface available for heat loss through radiation, convection, and conduction.[3]

The hypothalamus responds to warmer core and peripheral temperatures by reversing the same mechanisms, resulting in heat loss. Heat loss is achieved through (1) radiation, (2) conduction, (3) convection, (4) vasodilation, (5) evaporation of sweat, (6) decreased muscle tone, (7) increased respiration, (8) voluntary measures, and (9) adaptation to warmer climates (i.e., increasing or decreasing the volume of sweat). Table 14.5 reviews further information about mechanisms of heat production and heat loss.

Temperature Regulation in Infants and Older Persons

Infants (particularly low-birth-weight infants) and older persons require special attention to maintenance of body temperature. Term infants produce enough body heat, mainly through metabolism of brown fat. These infants cannot save heat produced because of their small body size, greater ratio of body surface to body weight, and inability to shiver. Infants also have little subcutaneous fat and are not as well insulated as adults.[27,28] Children also have a greater ratio of body surface to body weight. This factor lowers the sweating rate, creates a higher peripheral blood flow in the heat, and a greater extent of vasoconstriction in the cold than adults. They can adjust to changes in environmental temperatures but do so at a lower rate than adults.[27,28]

Older persons respond poorly to environmental temperature extremes. This response is attributed to their slowed blood circulation, structural and functional skin changes, overall decreased heat-producing activities, and the presence of disease (i.e., heart failure, chronic lung disease, diabetes mellitus, or peripheral vascular disease). Cold stress in older persons also decreases coronary perfusion.[27,28] Older persons also have a decreased shivering response (delayed onset and decreased effectiveness), slowed metabolic rate, decreased vasoconstrictor response, reduced or absent ability to sweat, decreased peripheral sensation, altered circadian rhythm, decreased perception of heat and cold, decreased thirst, decreased nutritional stores, and decreased brown adipose tissue.[27,28]

Pathogenesis of Fever

Fever (febrile response) is a temporary resetting of the hypothalamic thermostat to a higher level in response to exogenous or endogenous pyrogens. **Exogenous pyrogens** (endotoxins produced by pathogens; see Chapter 8) stimulate the release of **endogenous pyrogens** from phagocytic cells. Endogenous pyrogens include tumour necrosis factor-alpha (TNF-α), interleukin-1 (IL-1), interleukin-6 (IL-6), and interferon (IFN). These pyrogens raise the thermal set point by causing the hypothalamic creation of prostaglandin E_2 (PGE_2). The release of PGE_2 produces a combined response that raises body temperature through an increase in heat production and conservation (Figure 14.4). The person feels colder, dresses more warmly, decreases body surface area by curling up, and may go to bed to get warm. Body temperature is supported at the new level until the fever "breaks". It is then that the set point begins to return to normal with decreased heat production and increased heat reduction mechanisms. The person feels very warm, wears cooler clothes, throws off the covers, and stretches out. Once the body has returned to a normal temperature, the person feels more comfortable, and the hypothalamus adjusts thermoregulatory mechanisms to support the new temperature.

Fever of unknown origin (FUO) is a body temperature greater than 38.3°C [101°F]) for longer than 3 weeks' duration that is undiagnosed after 3 days of hospital investigation, 3 outpatient visits, or 1 week of ambulatory investigation. The categories of FUO include infectious, rheumatic or inflammatory, neoplastic, human immunodeficiency virus (HIV)-associated, and miscellaneous disorders.[29]

Benefits of Fever

Moderate fever helps the body respond to infectious processes in several ways:[30,31]

- Raising of the body temperature kills many microorganisms and adversely affects their growth and replication
- Higher body temperatures decrease serum levels of iron, zinc, and copper—minerals needed for bacterial replication
- Increased temperature causes lysosomal breakdown and autodestruction of cells, preventing viral replication in infected cells
- Heat increases lymphocytic change and motility of polymorphonuclear neutrophils, helping the immune response
- Enhanced phagocytosis and increased production of antiviral interferon

Effective suppression of fever can be achieved with the cautious use of antipyrogenic medications.[32] Infection and fever responses in older persons and children may vary. Box 14.2 lists the main features associated with fever at the extremes of age.[33]

Disorders of Temperature Regulation

Hyperthermia

Hyperthermia is elevation of the body temperature without an increase in the hypothalamic set point. Hyperthermia can produce nerve damage, coagulation of cell proteins, and death. At 41°C (105.8°F), nerve damage produces convulsions in the adult. Death results at 43°C (109.4°F). Hyperthermia may be therapeutic, accidental, or associated with stroke or head trauma. Prevention of hyperthermia in stroke and head trauma helps in limiting brain injury.[34]

Therapeutic hyperthermia is a form of local, regional, or whole-body hyperthermia used to destroy pathological microorganisms or tumour cells by helping the host's natural immune process or tumour blood flow.[34,35]

This is a summary of the forms of accidental hyperthermia:[3,36–38]

- Heat cramps are severe, spasmodic cramps in the abdomen and extremities that follow prolonged sweating and linked sodium loss. They usually occur in those not used to heat or those performing strenuous work in very warm climates. Fever, rapid pulse rate, and increased blood pressure occur with the cramps.
- Heat exhaustion results from prolonged high core or environmental temperatures. The high temperatures cause extreme vasodilation and profuse sweating. These factors lead to dehydration, decreased plasma volumes, hypotension, decreased cardiac output, and tachycardia. Symptoms include weakness, dizziness, confusion, nausea, and fainting.
- Heat stroke is a potentially fatal result of an overstressed thermoregulatory centre. Exertion, overexposure to environmental heat, or impaired physiological mechanisms for heat loss can cause heat stroke. With very high core temperatures (greater than 40°C [104°F]), the regulatory centre stops working, and the body's heat loss mechanisms fail. Symptoms include high core temperature, absence of sweating, rapid pulse rate, confusion, agitation, and coma. If not treated, complications such as cerebral edema, degeneration of the CNS, swollen dendrites, renal tubular necrosis, and liver failure with delirium, coma, and eventually death may occur.

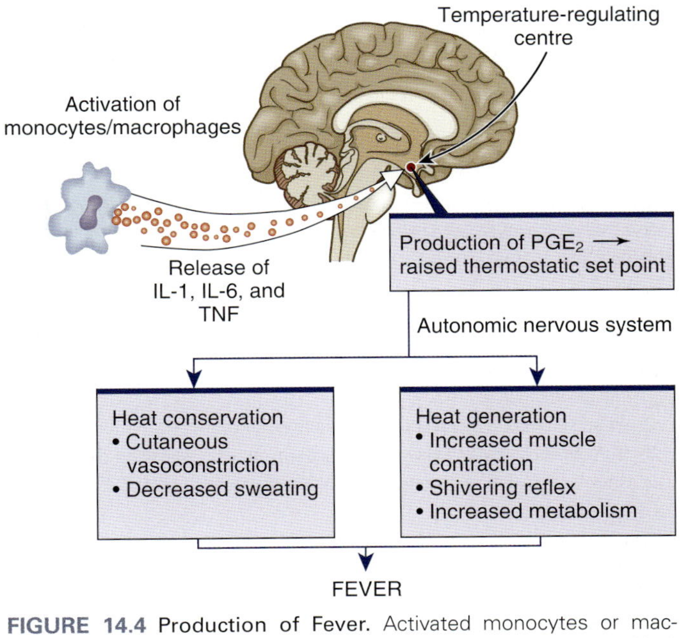

FIGURE 14.4 Production of Fever. Activated monocytes or macrophages secrete cytokines such as interleukin-1 (*IL-1*), interleukin-6 (*IL-6*), and tumour necrosis factor (*TNF*). These cytokines reach the hypothalamic temperature-regulating centre. They also promote the synthesis and secretion of prostaglandin E_2 (*PGE_2*) in the anterior hypothalamus. PGE_2 increases the thermostatic set point, which stimulates the autonomic nervous system. This stimulation results in shivering, muscle contraction, peripheral vasoconstriction, and increased metabolism mediated by thyroid hormone. (From Lewis, S. M., Bucher, L., Heitkemper, M. M., et al. [2014]. *Medical-surgical nursing: assessment and management of clinical problems* [9th ed.]. Mosby.)

BOX 14.2 Effects of Fever at the Extremes of Age

Older Persons
They show decreased or no fever response to infection; therefore, a decreased benefit of fever.
High morbidity and mortality result from lack of helpful aspects.

Children
They develop higher temperatures than adults do for relatively minor infections.
Febrile seizures before age 5 years are common.

- **Malignant hyperthermia** is a potentially fatal hypermetabolic complication of a rare inherited muscle disorder. The disorder may be triggered by inhaled anaesthetics and depolarizing muscle relaxants. The syndrome involves altered calcium function in muscle cells. This altered function causes hypermetabolism, uncoordinated muscle contractions, increased muscle work, increased oxygen consumption, and a raised level of lactic acid production. Acidosis develops, and body temperature rises. This results in tachycardia and cardiac dysrhythmias, hypotension, decreased cardiac output, and cardiac arrest. Signs look like those of coma—unconsciousness, absent reflexes, fixed pupils, apnea, and occasionally a flat electroencephalogram (EEG). Oliguria and anuria are common. It is most common in children and adolescents.

Hypothermia

Hypothermia (core body temperature less than 35°C [95°F]) produces depression of the CNS and the respiratory system, vasoconstriction, changes in microcirculation and coagulation, and ischemic tissue damage. Hypothermia may be accidental or therapeutic (Box 14.3). Most tissues can tolerate low temperatures in controlled situations, such as surgery. However, in severe hypothermia, ice crystals form on the inside of the cell, causing cells to rupture and die. Tissue hypothermia slows cell metabolism, increases the blood thickness, slows microcirculatory blood flow, helps blood coagulation, and stimulates extreme vasoconstriction (see the discussion of frostbite in Chapter 41).

Trauma and Temperature

Major body trauma can affect temperature regulation through various mechanisms. Damage to the CNS, inflammation, increased intracranial pressure, or intracranial bleeding typically produces a body temperature of greater than 39°C (102.2°F). This constant noninfectious fever, often called a "**central fever**," appears with or without bradycardia. A central fever does not cause sweating and is very resistant to antipyretic therapy.[39] Other traumatic mechanisms that produce temperature changes include accidental injuries, hemorrhagic shock, major surgery, and thermal burns. The severity and type of change (hyperthermia or hypothermia) vary with the severity of the cause and the body system affected.

SLEEP

> ✓ **QUICK CHECK 14.3**
> 1. Describe REM and non-REM sleep.
> 2. What is the major difference between the dyssomnias and parasomnias?

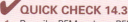 is an active multiphase process that provides restorative functions and promotes memory consolidation. Complex neural circuits, interacting hormones, and neurotransmitters involving the hypothalamus, thalamus, brainstem, and cortex control the timing of the sleep–wake cycle. They also coordinate this cycle with circadian rhythms (24-hour rhythm cycles).[40] Normal sleep has two phases that can be documented by EEG: **rapid eye movement (REM) sleep** (20 to 25% of sleep time) and slow-wave (non-REM) sleep. Non-REM sleep is divided into three stages (N1, N2, N3) from light to deep sleep followed by REM sleep. Four to six cycles of REM and non-REM sleep occur each night in an adult.[41]

The hypothalamus is a major sleep centre. The hypocretins (orexins), acetylcholine, and glutamate are neuropeptides secreted by the hypothalamus that promote wakefulness. Prostaglandin D_2, adenosine, melatonin, serotonin, l-tryptophan, GABA, and growth factors promote sleep. The pontine reticular formation is mainly responsible for creating REM sleep. The projections from the thalamocortical network produce non-REM sleep.[41]

REM sleep is started by *REM-on* and *REM-off* neurons in the pons and mesencephalon. REM sleep occurs about every 90 minutes starting 1 to 2 hours after non-REM sleep begins. This sleep is known as *paradoxical sleep* because the EEG pattern is like that of the normal awake

---

BOX 14.3 Defining Characteristics of Hypothermia

Accidental Hypothermia
The accidental decrease in core temperature to less than 35°C (95°F) results from sudden immersion in cold water, prolonged exposure to cold environments, diseases that reduce the ability to produce heat, or altered thermoregulatory mechanisms. It is most common among young people and older persons.

Factors That Increase Risk
1. Hypothyroidism
2. Hypopituitarism
3. Malnutrition
4. Parkinson's disease
5. Rheumatoid arthritis
6. Chronic increased vasodilation
7. Failure of thermoregulatory control resulting from cerebral injury, ketoacidosis, uremia, sepsis, and drug overdose

Response Mechanisms
1. Peripheral vasoconstriction—moves blood away from cooler skin to core to decrease heat loss and creates peripheral tissue ischemia
2. Intermittent reperfusion of extremities (Lewis phenomenon) helps preserve peripheral oxygenation until core temperature drops significantly
3. Hypothalamic centre causes shivering; thinking becomes sluggish, and coordination is reduced
4. Stupor; heart rate and respiratory rate decline; cardiac output decreases; metabolic rate falls; acidosis; eventual ventricular fibrillation and asystole occur at 30°C (86°F) and lower

Treatment
1. Most changes are reversible with rewarming
2. Core temperature greater than 30°C (86°F)—active rewarming (external)
3. Core temperature less than 30°C (86°F) or with severe cardiovascular problems—active core rewarming (internal)

Therapeutic Hypothermia
This process slows metabolism and preserves ischemic tissue during surgery (e.g., limb reimplantation), postcardiac arrest management of patients presenting with ventricular fibrillation or ventricular tachycardia or following neurological injury.

Effects and Cautions
1. Stresses the heart, leading to ventricular fibrillation and cardiac arrest (when the heart must be stopped during open heart surgery, this may be the desired outcome).
2. Exhausts liver glycogen stores by prolonged shivering.
3. Surface cooling may cause burns, frostbite, and fat necrosis.
4. May lead to immunosuppression with increased infection risk.
5. Slows drug metabolism.

From Corneli, H. M. (2012). *Pediatric Emergency Care, 28*(5), 475–480; Frink, M., Flohé, S., van Griensven, M., et al. (2012). *Mediators of Inflammation, 2012*, 762840; Lantry, J., Dezman, Z., & Hirshon, J. M. (2012). *British Journal of Hospital Medicine (London), 73*(1), 31–37.

pattern and the brain is very active with dreaming. REM and non-REM sleep alternate throughout the night, with lengthening periods of REM sleep and fewer periods of deeper stages of non-REM sleep toward morning. The changes associated with REM sleep include increased parasympathetic activity and variable sympathetic activity. Associated manifestations include rapid eye movement; muscle relaxation; loss of temperature regulation; altered heart rate, blood pressure, and respiration; penile erection in men and clitoral engorgement in women; release of steroids; and many memorable dreams. Respiratory control appears largely independent of metabolic requirements and oxygen variation. Loss of normal voluntary muscle control in the tongue and upper pharynx may produce some respiratory obstruction. Cerebral blood flow increases.

Non–rapid eye movement (NREM) sleep accounts for 75 to 80% of sleep time in adults. NREM sleep starts when inhibitory signals are released from the hypothalamus. During NREM sleep sympathetic tone decreases, and parasympathetic activity increases, creating a state of reduced activity. The basal metabolic rate falls by 10 to 15%; temperature decreases 0.5° to 1.0°C (0.9° to 1.8°F); heart rate, respiration, blood pressure, and muscle tone decrease; and knee jerk reflexes are absent. Pupil constriction occurs. During the various stages, cerebral blood flow to the brain decreases and growth hormone is released, with corticosteroid and catecholamine levels depressed. Box 14.4 reviews the sleep characteristics of infants and older persons.

Sleep Disorders

The International Classification of Sleep Disorders III (ISCD-3) includes six classifications of sleep disorders: (1) insomnia, (2) sleep-related breathing disorders, (3) central disorders of hypersomnolence, (4) circadian rhythm sleep–wake disorders, (5) parasomnias, and (6) sleep-related movement disorders.[42] The most common disorders are discussed here.

Common Dyssomnias

Insomnia is the inability to fall or stay asleep. Fatigue during wakefulness occurs and may be mild, moderate, or severe. It may be temporary, lasting a few days or months (primary insomnia), and related to travel across time zones or caused by acute stress.[43] Chronic insomnia can be idiopathic, start at an early age, and be associated with many factors. These factors include drug or alcohol abuse, persistent pain disorders, stress, chronic depression, the use of certain medications, obesity, aging, genetics, and environmental factors that result in hyperarousal.[44] (See Chapter 9 discussion of maladaptive coping related to sleep deprivation).

Obstructive sleep apnea syndrome (OSAS) is the most diagnosed sleep disorder. The Public Health Agency of Canada states that 6.4% of Canadians over the age of 18 years reported being diagnosed with sleep apnea. In addition, more than one in four Canadian adults (30%) were at high risk of developing OSAS, based on the presence of identified risk factors. Major risk factors include obesity, male gender, and older age.[44] A lack of daytime sleepiness often lessens awareness of a potential sleep disorder, and many persons are never properly diagnosed and treated.[45] OSAS results from partial or total upper airway collapse with obstruction to airflow recurring during sleep. Related symptoms include excessive loud snoring, gasping, and multiple apneic episodes (temporary pause of breathing) that last 10 seconds or longer. The periodic breathing eventually produces arousal, which disrupts the sleep cycle. This disruption reduces total sleep time and produces sleep and REM deprivation. Related conditions include decreased sensitivity to carbon dioxide and oxygen tensions, upper airway obstruction, a small airway, and decreased airway dilator muscle activation. Obesity hypoventilation syndrome may be related to leptin resistance because leptin also is a respiratory stimulant. Sleep apnea produces hypercapnia and low oxygen saturation. These factors eventually lead to polycythemia, pulmonary hypertension, systemic hypertension, stroke, right-sided heart failure, dysrhythmias, liver congestion, cyanosis, and peripheral edema.[3] Hypersomnia (excessive daytime sleepiness) is associated with OSAS. Persons may fall asleep while driving a car, working, or even while talking, with resulting safety concerns.[46] Sleep deprivation also can result in impaired mood and cognitive function. Symptoms include impairment of attention, episodic memory, working memory, and executive functions.[47]

To diagnose OSAS a polysomnography is needed, in addition to a history and physical examination. Treatments include use of nasal continuous positive airway pressure and dental devices, surgery of the upper airway and jaw in selected persons, and management of obesity.[48] Adenotonsillar hypertrophy is the major cause of OSAS in children, and obesity increases the risk. Adenotonsillectomy is the treatment of choice.[49]

Narcolepsy is a primary hypersomnia characterized by hallucinations, sleep paralysis, and, rarely, cataplexy (brief spells of muscle weakness). Narcolepsy is usually periodic or can occur in families. Narcolepsy without cataplexy is associated with immune-mediated damage of hypocretin (orexin)-secreting cells in the hypothalamus. Orexins stimulate wakefulness.[50]

Circadian rhythm sleep disorders are common disorders of the 24-hour sleep–wake schedule (circadian rhythm sleep disorders). They can result from having rapid time-zone changes (or jet-lag syndrome), changing the sleep schedule (rotating work shifts) involving 3 hours or more in sleep time, or changing the total sleep time from

---

BOX 14.4 Sleep Characteristics of Infants and Older Persons

Infants
- Infants sleep 10 to 16 hours per day: 50% REM (active) sleep, 25% non-REM (inactive) sleep.
- Infant sleep cycles are 50 to 60 minutes in length; 10 to 45 minutes of REM sleep accompanied by movement of the arms, legs, and facial muscles followed by about 20 minutes of non-REM sleep.
- At 1 year, REM and non-REM sleep cycles are about equal in length and infants sleep through the night with about two naps per day.

Older Persons
- Total sleep time lessens with a longer time to fall asleep and poorer quality sleep.
- Total time in slow-wave and final phase of non-REM sleep decreases by 15 to 30%.
- Increases occur in stage 1 and 2 non-REM sleep, related to an increased number of spontaneous arousals.
- Older persons tend to go to sleep earlier in the evening and wake earlier in the morning because of a phase advance in their normal circadian sleep cycle.
- Changes in sleep patterns occur about 10 years later in women than in men.
- Sleep disorders are more likely in older persons and increase the risk for morbidity and mortality.

REM, Rapid eye movement.
From Edwards, B. A., O'Driscoll, D. M., Asad, A., et al. (2010). *Seminars in Respiratory and Critical Care Medicine, 31*(5), 618–633; Galland, B. C., Taylor, B. J., Elder, D. E., et al. (2012). *Sleep Medicine Reviews, 16*(3), 213–222; Neikrug, A. B., & Ancoli-Israel, S. (2010). *Gerontology, 56*(2), 181–189; Ng, D. K., & Chan, C. H. (2013). *Pediatrics & Neonatology, 54*(2), 82–87.

day to day. They can also result from being diagnosed with one of two disorders. Advanced sleep phase disorder (early morning waking–early evening sleeping) results in sleep loss if social requirements lead to later bedtime. Delayed sleep phase disorder (late morning waking–late night to early morning sleeping) results in sleep loss because of required early morning rising (common in adolescents). These changes desynchronize the circadian rhythm. This alteration can depress the degree of vigilance, performance of psychomotor tasks, and arousal.[51,52] A circadian rhythm sleep disorder known as **shift work sleep disorder** affects many shift workers who rotate or work long shifts (such as nurses), particularly between the hours of 2200 (10:00 p.m.) and 0600 (6:00 a.m.).[51,52] Our sleep–wake cycle is driven by circadian rhythms. The disruption of this circadian influence may cause short-term problems such as cognitive deficits and difficulty concentrating. However, long-term health effects of shift work sleep disorder may be quite serious. These effects include depression, anxiety, increased risk for cardiovascular disease, and increased all-cause mortality.[51,52] Sleep cycle phenotype has a genetic basis and impacts the timing and cycles of sleep and can affect advances or delays in sleep–wake times.[51,52]

Common Parasomnias

Parasomnias are unusual behaviours occurring during NREM sleep.[3] These behaviours include sleepwalking, having night terrors, rearranging furniture, eating food, exhibiting sleep sex or violent behaviour, and having restless legs syndrome. The loss of REM paralysis, leading to possible harmful dream enactment, is a REM sleep behaviour disorder.[53]

Two dysfunctions of sleep (somnambulism and night terrors) are common in children and may be related to CNS immaturity. **Somnambulism (sleepwalking)** is a disorder primarily of childhood and appears to resolve within a few years. Sleepwalking is not associated with dreaming, and the child has no memory of the event when they wake up. Sleepwalking in adults is often associated with sleep-disordered breathing. Sudden episodes of apparent arousal, where the child expresses strong fear or emotion, are **night terrors**. However, the child is not awake and can be difficult to arouse. Once awake, the child has no memory of the night terror event. Night terrors are not associated with dreams. Although this problem occurs most often in children, adults also may experience it with related daytime anxiety.

Restless Legs Syndrome

Restless legs syndrome (RLS), or **Willis-Ekbom disease**, is a common sensorimotor disorder associated with unpleasant sensations (prickling, tingling, and crawling) and undesired periodic leg movements. These movements occur at rest and are worse in the evening or at night. There is a powerful urge to move the legs for relief with a significant effect on sleep and quality of life. The disorder is more common in women, during pregnancy, older persons, and persons with iron deficiency. RLS has a familial tendency and is associated with a circadian fluctuation of dopamine in the substantia nigra. Iron is a cofactor in dopamine production, and some persons respond to iron supplements as well as dopamine agonists.[54] Diagnostic and treatment guidelines have been created to aid with disease management.[54]

THE SPECIAL SENSES

> **QUICK CHECK 14.4**
> 1. Name the categories of visual disorders.
> 2. How does fluid accumulate in the middle ear during otitis media?
> 3. What factors are involved in the sensation of flavour?

Vision

The eyes are complex sense organs responsible for vision. Within a protective casing, each eye has receptors, a lens system for focusing light on the receptors, and a system of nerves for conducting signals from the receptors to the visual cortex of the occipital lobe of the brain. Abnormal ocular movements or changes in visual acuity, refraction, colour vision, or accommodation all may cause visual dysfunction. Visual dysfunction also may be the effect of another neurological disorder.

The Eye

The wall of the eye consists of three layers: (1) sclera, (2) choroid, and (3) retina (Figure 14.5). The **sclera** is the thick, white, outermost layer. It becomes transparent at the **cornea**—the part of the sclera in the central anterior region that allows light to enter the eye. The **choroid** is the deeply pigmented middle layer that prevents light from scattering inside the eye. The **iris**, part of the choroid, has a round opening, the **pupil**, through which light passes. Smooth muscle fibres control the size of the pupil so that it adjusts to bright light or dim light and to close or distant vision.

The **retina** is the innermost layer of the eye and has millions of rods and cones—special photoreceptors that change light energy into nerve signals. **Rods** mediate peripheral and dim light vision and are densest at the periphery of the retina. **Cones**, densest in the centre of the retina, are colour and detail receptors. There are no photoreceptors where the optic nerve leaves the eyeball. This point of exit creates the **optic disc**, or blind spot. Lateral to the optic disc is the **macula lutea**, the area of most distinct vision. In the centre is the **fovea centralis**, a tiny area that has only cones and provides the greatest visual acuity (see Figure 14.5).

As shown in Figure 14.11, nerve signals pass through the **optic nerves** (cranial nerve II) to the **optic chiasm**. The nerves from the inner (nasal) halves of the retinas cross to the opposite side and join fibres from the outer (temporal) halves of the retinas to form the optic tracts. The fibres of the optic tracts synapse in the posterior lateral geniculate nucleus and pass by way of the optic radiation (or geniculocalcarine tract) to the primary visual cortex in the occipital lobe of the brain. Some fibres terminate in the **suprachiasmatic nucleus (SCN)** (found above the optic chiasm) and are involved in regulating the sleep–wake cycle. The **lens**—a flexible, biconvex, crystal-like structure—focuses light entering the eye on the retina. The flexibility of the lens allows

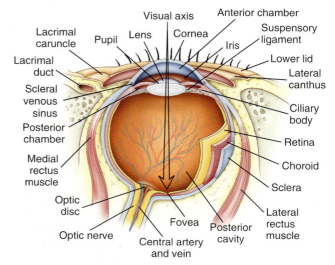

FIGURE 14.5 Internal Anatomy of the Eye. (Adapted from Patton, K. T. [2019]. *Anatomy and physiology* [10th ed.]. Elsevier.)

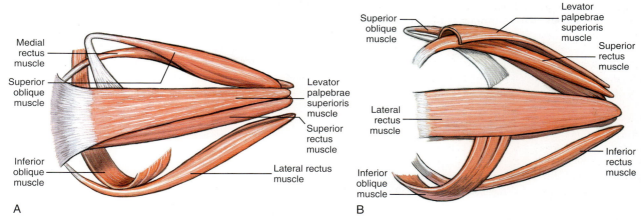

FIGURE 14.6 Extrinsic Muscles of the Right Eye. **A**, Superior view. **B**, Lateral view. (From Dutton, J. J. [2011]. *Atlas of clinical and surgical orbital anatomy* [2nd ed.]. Saunders.)

a change in curvature with contraction of the ciliary muscles, called **accommodation**. Accommodation allows the eye to focus on objects at different distances. The lens divides the anterior chamber into (1) the aqueous chamber and (2) the vitreous chamber. **Aqueous humor** fills the aqueous chamber and helps keep pressure inside the eye, as well as supply nutrients to the lens and cornea. The ciliary processes continuously secrete aqueous humor, and it is reabsorbed into the *scleral venous sinus*. Intraocular pressure (IOP) increases if a blockage occurs (causing glaucoma). **Vitreous humor** is a gel-like substance that fills the vitreous chamber. Vitreous humor is not replaced and helps to prevent the eyeball from collapsing inward.

The central retinal artery supplies blood to the inner retinal surface. The choroid supplies nutrients to the outer surface of the retina. Six extrinsic (extraocular) eye skeletal muscles allow gross eye movements and permit eyes to follow a moving object (Figure 14.6).

Visual Dysfunction

Alterations in ocular movements. Abnormal ocular movements result from oculomotor (III), trochlear (IV), or abducens (VI) cranial nerve dysfunction (see Table 13.6). The three types of eye movement disorders are (1) strabismus, (2) nystagmus, and (3) paralysis of individual extraocular (extrinsic) muscles.

In **strabismus**, one eye deviates from the other when the person is looking at an object. A weak or hypertonic muscle in one eye causes this disorder. The deviation may be upward, downward, inward (entropia), or outward (extropia). Strabismus in children requires early intervention to prevent **amblyopia** (reduced vision in the affected eye caused by cerebral blockage of the visual stimuli). The primary symptom of strabismus is **diplopia** (double vision). Causes include neuromuscular disorders of the eye muscle, diseases involving the cerebral hemispheres, or thyroid disease.

Nystagmus is an involuntary unilateral or bilateral rhythmic movement of the eyes. It may be present at rest or when the eye moves. A regular back-and-forth movement of the eyes is **pendular nystagmus**. In **jerk nystagmus**, one phase of the eye movement is faster than the other. Imbalanced reflex activity of the inner ear, vestibular nuclei, cerebellum, medial longitudinal fascicle, or nuclei of the oculomotor, trochlear, or abducens cranial nerves may cause nystagmus (see Table 13.6 and Figure 13.25). Drugs, retinal disease, and diseases involving the cervical spinal cord also may produce nystagmus.

Paralysis of specific extraocular muscles may cause limited abduction, abnormal closure of the eyelid, ptosis (drooping of the eyelid), or diplopia (double vision) because of unopposed muscle activity. Trauma or pressure around the cranial nerves or diseases such as diabetes mellitus and myasthenia gravis also paralyze specific extraocular muscles.

Alterations in visual acuity. Visual acuity is the ability to see objects in sharp detail. With advancing age, the lens of the eye becomes less flexible and adjusts slowly, causing a change of the refraction of light by the cornea and lens. Thus, visual acuity declines with age. Table 14.6 has a summary of changes in the eye caused by aging. Specific causes of visual acuity changes are (1) amblyopia, (2) presbyopia, (3) scotoma, (4) cataracts, (5) papilledema, (6) dark adaptation, (7) glaucoma, (8) retinal detachment (Figure 14.7), and (9) macular degeneration (Table 14.7).

A **cataract** is a cloudy or opaque area in the ocular lens and leads to visual loss when found on the visual axis. It is the leading cause of blindness in the world. The incidence of cataracts increases with age as the lens enlarges. Cataracts develop because of changes of metabolism and transport of nutrients within the lens. Although the most common form of cataract is degenerative, cataracts also may occur congenitally or because of infection, radiation, trauma, medications, or diabetes mellitus. Cataracts cause decreased visual acuity, blurred vision, glare, and decreased colour sense. The treatment for cataracts includes the removal of the entire lens and replacement with an intraocular artificial lens.[55]

Glaucomas are the second leading cause of blindness. Intraocular pressures greater than 12 to 20 mm Hg with death of retinal ganglion cells and their axons occur.[3]

There are three primary types of glaucoma (Figure 14.8).[56]
1. *Open angle.* Outflow obstruction of aqueous humor at the trabecular meshwork or scleral venous sinus, even though there is adequate space for drainage, is seen with this type of glaucoma. This is often an inherited disease and is a leading cause of blindness with few preliminary symptoms.
2. *Angle closure.* In this type of glaucoma there is displacement of the iris toward the cornea with obstruction of the trabecular meshwork and obstruction of outflow of aqueous humor from the anterior chamber; it may occur acutely with a sudden rise in intraocular pressure, causing pain and visual disturbances.
3. *Congenital closure.* This is a rare disease associated with congenital malformations and other genetic anomalies.

Glaucoma is often asymptomatic, and diagnosis may not occur until a late stage of disease. Both medical and surgical therapies are available.[56]

TABLE 14.6 Changes in the Eye Caused by Aging

Structure	Change	Consequence
Cornea	Thicker and less curved	Increase in astigmatism
Formation of grey ring at edge of cornea (arcus senilis)	Not harmful to vision	
Anterior chamber	Decrease in size and volume caused by thickening of lens	Occasionally puts pressure on *scleral venous sinuses* and may lead to increased intraocular pressure and glaucoma
Lens	Increase in opacity	Decrease in refraction with increased light scattering (blurring) and decreased colour vision (green and blue); can lead to cataracts
	Hardening	Lens becomes less flexible and can no longer change shape to focus on close-up images (presbyopia)
Ciliary muscles	Decease in pupil diameter, atrophy of radial dilation muscles	Constant constriction (senile miosis); decrease in critical flicker frequency[a]
Retina	Decrease in number of rods at periphery, loss of rods and associated nerve cells	Increase in least amount of light necessary to see an object

[a]The rate at which consecutive visual stimuli can be presented and still be perceived as separate.

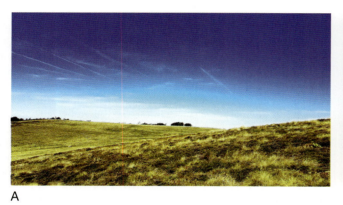
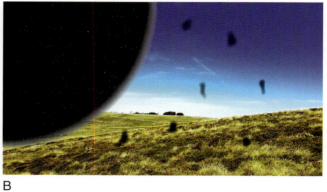

A   B

FIGURE 14.7 Perceived Visual Field of a Person With a Retinal Detachment. (iStockphoto/YuricBel.)

TABLE 14.7 Causes of Visual Acuity Changes

Disorder	Description
Amblyopia	Reduced or dimmed vision; cause unknown
	Associated with strabismus
	Accompanies such diseases as diabetes mellitus, renal failure, and malaria and use of drugs such as alcohol and tobacco
Presbyopia	Images appear to be out of focus; cause is related to the hardening of the lens
	Occurrence increases with age
	The less flexible lens cannot change shape to focus on close images
Scotoma	Circumscribed defect of central field of vision
	Often associated with retrobulbar neuritis and multiple sclerosis, pressure on optic nerve by tumour, inflammation of optic nerve, pernicious anemia, methyl alcohol poisoning, and use of tobacco
Cataracts	Cloudy or opaque area in ocular lens
	Incidence increases with age most commonly a result of degeneration; other causes are congenital
Papilledema	Edema and inflammation of optic nerve where it enters eyeball
	Caused by obstruction of venous return from retina by one of three main sources: increased intracranial pressure, retrobulbar neuritis, or changes in retinal blood vessels
Dark adaptation	With age, eye does not adapt as readily to dark
	Also, caused by changes in quantity and quality of rhodopsin; vitamin A deficiencies can produce this at any age
Glaucoma	Increased intraocular pressures (>12–20 mm Hg)
	Loss of acuity results from pressure on optic nerve, which blocks flow of nutrients to optic nerve fibres, leading to their death; sixth leading cause of blindness
Retinal detachment	Tear or break in retina with buildup of fluid and separation from underlying tissue; seen as floaters, flashes of light, or a curtain over visual field; risks include extreme myopia, diabetic retinopathy, sickle cell disease

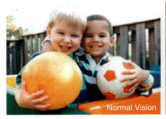
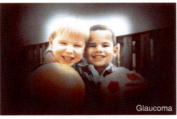

FIGURE 14.8 Glaucoma Vision. From National Eye Institute, retrieved from a webpage formerly available at https://www.flickr.com/photos/nationaleyeinstitute/7544734516/in/album-72157646474384400/.

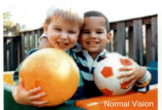
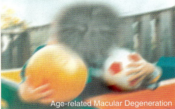

FIGURE 14.9 Age-related Macular Degeneration. From National Eye Institute, retrieved from a webpage formerly available at https://www.flickr.com/photos/nationaleyeinstitute/7544733860/sizes/l/.

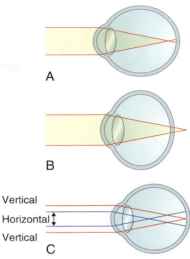

FIGURE 14.10 Changes in Refraction. **A,** Myopic eye. Parallel rays of light focus in front of the retina. **B,** Hyperopic eye. Parallel rays of light come to a focus behind the retina in the unaccommodated eye. **C,** Simple myopic astigmatism. The vertical bundle of rays focuses on the retina; the horizontal rays focus in front of the retina. (From Stein, H. A., Stein, R. M., & Freeman, M. I. [2013]. *The ophthalmic assistant: a text for allied and associated ophthalmic personnel* [9th ed.]. Saunders.)

Age-related macular degeneration (AMD) (Figure 14.9) is a severe and irreversible loss of vision and a major cause of blindness in older persons. Hypertension, cigarette smoking, diabetes mellitus, and family history of AMD are risk factors. The degeneration usually occurs after the age of 60 years. There are two forms: atrophic (dry, nonexudative) and neovascular (wet, exudative). The atrophic form is more common, is slowly progressive, with inflammation and accumulation of lipofuscin (a lysosomal pigmented residue) and drusen (waste products from photoreceptors) in the retina and may include limited night vision and difficulty reading. The neovascular form includes accumulation of drusen and lipofuscin, abnormal choroidal blood vessel growth, leakage of blood or serum, retinal detachment, fibrovascular scarring, loss of photoreceptors, and more severe and rapid loss of central vision. Treatment includes antivascular endothelial growth factor (anti-VEGF) injection for wet macular degeneration and antioxidant vitamins for dry macular degeneration.[58] Two carotenoids, lutein, and zeaxanthin, are antioxidants that selectively accumulate in the retina and may protect the eye from AMD.[57]

Alterations in accommodation. *Accommodation* refers to changes in the thickness of the lens. The oculomotor (III) cranial nerve mediates clear vision and controls accommodation. Pressure, inflammation, age, and disease of the oculomotor nerve may alter accommodation, causing diplopia, blurred vision, and headache.

Loss of accommodation with advancing age is termed **presbyopia**. With this condition the ocular lens becomes larger, firmer, and less elastic. A decrease in near vision is the major symptom, causing the person to hold reading material at arm's length. Treatment includes corrective forward, contact, and intraocular lenses or laser refractive surgery for monovision.[59]

Alterations in refraction. Changes in refraction are the most common visual problem. Causes include irregularities of the corneal curvature, the focusing power of the lens, and the length of the eye. The major symptoms of refraction changes are blurred vision and headache. The three most common types of refraction are (Figure 14.10):

1. **Myopia** (nearsightedness). When a person has an irregularly shaped cornea or eyeball; when they are looking at a distant object, the light rays focus in front of the retina.
2. **Hyperopia** (farsightedness). When a person has an irregularly shaped cornea or eyeball; when they are looking at a near object, the light rays focus behind the retina.
3. **Astigmatism** (unequal curvature of the cornea). Light rays bend unevenly and do not come to a single focus on the retina. Astigmatism may coexist with myopia, hyperopia, or presbyopia.

Alterations in colour vision. Normal sensitivity to colour diminishes with age because of the progressive yellowing of the lens that occurs with aging. All colours become less intense and a decrease in colour discrimination for blue and green occurs. (See the *Geriatric Considerations: Aging and Changes in Vision* box.) Colour vision deteriorates more rapidly for persons with diabetes mellitus than for the general population.

Colour blindness, an X-linked genetic trait, may also cause abnormal colour vision. Colour blindness affects about 8% of the male population and about 0.4% of the female population. Although many forms of colour blindness exist, most commonly the affected person cannot distinguish red from green.[69] In the most severe form persons see only shades of grey, black, and white.

Neurological disorders causing visual dysfunction. A disruption in vision may occur at many points along the visual pathway, causing various defects in the visual field. Visual changes may cause defects or blindness in the entire visual field or in half of a visual field (hemianopia). (Figure 14.11 shows the many areas along the visual pathway that may be damaged and the associated visual changes.) Injury to the optic nerve causes same-side blindness. Injury to the optic chiasm (the X-shaped crossing of the optic nerves) can cause various defects, depending on the location of the injury. Possible causes of optic tract damage include stroke, congenital defects, tumours, infection, and surgery.

External Eye Structure and Disorders

Protective external eye structures include the eyelids (palpebrae), conjunctivae, and lacrimal apparatus. The eyelids control the amount of light reaching the eyes, and the conjunctiva lines the eyelids. Tears released from the lacrimal apparatus bathe the surface of the eye and prevent friction, support hydration, and wash out foreign bodies and other irritants (Figure 14.12).

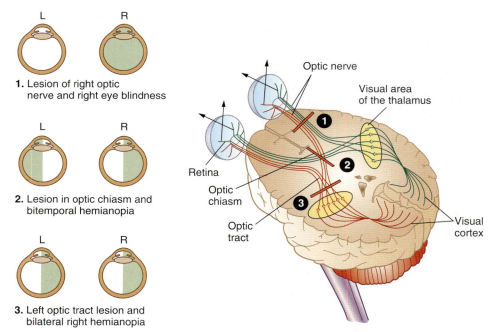

FIGURE 14.11 Visual Pathways and Defects. (Modified from Thompson, J. M., McFarland, G. K., Hirsch, J. E., et al. [2002]. *Mosby's clinical nursing* [5th ed.]. Mosby.)

Infection and inflammatory responses are the most common conditions affecting the supporting structures of the eyes. **Blepharitis** is an inflammation of the eyelids caused by *Staphylococcus* or seborrheic dermatitis. A **hordeolum (stye)** is an infection (usually staphylococcal) of the sebaceous glands of the eyelids usually centred near an eyelash. A **chalazion** is a noninfectious lipogranuloma of the meibomian (oil-secreting) gland that often occurs in association with a hordeolum and appears as a deep nodule within the eyelid. These conditions present with redness, swelling, and tenderness and are treated symptomatically. **Entropion** is a common eyelid malposition in which the lid margin turns inward against the eyeball. There are both surgical and nonsurgical treatments to reposition the lid margin.

Conjunctivitis is an inflammation of the conjunctiva (mucous membrane covering the front part of the eyeball) caused by viruses (most common), bacteria, allergies, or chemical irritants.[3] **Acute bacterial conjunctivitis (pinkeye)** is highly contagious and often caused by *Staphylococcus*, *Haemophilus*, *Streptococcus pneumoniae*, and *Moraxella catarrhalis*, although other bacteria may be involved. In children younger than 6 years, *Haemophilus* infection often leads to otitis media (conjunctivitis–otitis syndrome). Preventing the spread of the microorganism with meticulous handwashing and use of separate towels is important. Antibiotics are used to treat the disease.

An adenovirus causes **viral conjunctivitis**. It is contagious, with symptoms of watering, redness, and photophobia. **Allergic conjunctivitis** is associated with a variety of antigens, including pollens. **Chronic conjunctivitis** results from any persistent conjunctivitis. *Chlamydia trachomatis* causes **trachoma** (chlamydial conjunctivitis) and often is associated with poor sanitary conditions. It is the leading cause of preventable blindness in the world.

Keratitis is an infection of the cornea caused by bacteria or viruses. Bacterial infections can cause corneal ulceration, and type 1 herpes simplex virus can involve both the cornea and the conjunctiva. *Acanthamoeba* keratitis can occur from contact lens wear because of poor hygiene. Severe ulcerations with residual scarring require corneal transplantation.

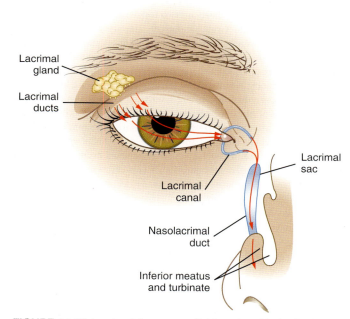

FIGURE 14.12 Lacrimal Apparatus. Fluid produced by lacrimal glands (tears) streams across the eye surface, enters the canals, and then passes through the nasolacrimal duct to enter the nose. (From Applegate, E. [2011]. *The anatomy and physiology learning system* [4th ed.]. Saunders.)

Hearing

Age-related hearing loss usually occurs gradually as we grow older. The loss of hearing usually arises from inner ear changes, but it may also involve the middle ear or changes in neural pathways between the ear and the brain.

The Normal Ear

The ear is divided into three areas: (1) the external ear, involved only with hearing; (2) the middle ear, involved only with hearing; and (3) the inner ear, involved with both hearing and equilibrium.

The external ear is composed of the **pinna** (auricle), which is the visible part of the ear, and the **external auditory canal**, a tube that leads to the middle ear (Figure 14.13). The temporal bones surround the external auditory canal. The opening (meatus) of the canal is just above the **mastoid process**. The air-filled sinuses, called **mastoid air cells**, of the mastoid process promote conductivity of sound between the external and the middle ear. The **tympanic membrane** separates the external ear from the middle ear. Sound waves entering the external auditory canal hit the tympanic membrane (eardrum) and cause it to vibrate.

The middle ear is composed of the **tympanic cavity**, a small chamber in the temporal bone. Three ossicles (small bones known as the **malleus [hammer]**, **incus [anvil]**, and **stapes [stirrup]**) send the vibration of the tympanic membrane to the inner ear. When the tympanic membrane moves, the malleus moves with it and transfers the vibration to the incus, which passes it on to the stapes. The stapes presses against the **oval window**, a small membrane at the entrance of the inner ear. The movement of the oval window sets the fluids of the inner ear in motion (Figure 14.14).

The **eustachian (pharyngotympanic) tube** connects the middle ear with the pharynx. Normally flat and closed, the eustachian tube opens briefly when a person swallows or yawns, and it equalizes the pressure in the middle ear with atmospheric pressure. Equalized pressure allows the tympanic membrane to vibrate freely. Through the eustachian tube, the mucosa of the middle ear is continuous with the mucosal lining of the throat.

The inner ear is a system of osseous labyrinths (bony, mazelike chambers) filled with **perilymph**. The **cochlea**, the **vestibule**, and the **semicircular canals** make up the bony labyrinth (see Figure 14.13). Suspended in the perilymph is the endolymph-filled membranous labyrinth that follows the shape of the bony labyrinth.

Within the cochlea is the **organ of Corti**, which has **hair cells** (hearing receptors). Sound waves that reach the cochlea through vibrations of the tympanic membrane, ossicles, and oval window set the cochlear fluids into motion. The hairs on the basilar membrane receptor cells are stimulated when bent or pulled by fluid movement. Once stimulated, hair cells transmit signals along the cochlear branch of the vestibulocochlear (VIII) cranial nerve to the auditory cortex of the temporal lobe in the brain (see Figure 14.14 and view an animation at https://www.youtube.com/watch?v=46aNGGNPm7s). The auditory cortex of the temporal lobe is where interpretation of the sound occurs.

The semicircular canals and vestibule of the inner ear have **equilibrium receptors**. In the semicircular canals, the dynamic equilibrium receptors respond to changes in direction of movement. Within each semicircular canal is the **crista ampullaris**, a receptor region composed of a tuft of hair cells covered by a gelatinous cupula. Rotation of the head causes the endolymph in the canals to lag and move in the direction opposite to the head's movement. Stimulation of the hair cells results in signals being transmitted through the vestibular branch of the vestibulocochlear (VIII) nerve to the cerebellum.

The vestibule in the inner ear has **maculae**—receptors essential to the body's sense of static equilibrium. As the head moves, **otoliths** (small pieces of calcium salts) move in a gel-like material in response to changes in the pull of gravity. The otoliths pull on the gel, which in turn pulls on the hair cells in the maculae. The triggering and transmissions of nerve signals in the hair cells travel to the brain (see Figure 14.14). Thus, the ear not only permits the hearing of a large range of sounds but also assists with maintaining balance through the sensitive equilibrium receptors (see an animation at https://www.youtube.com/watch?v=YMIMvBa8XGs).

Auditory Dysfunction

Between 5 and 10% of the general population have impaired hearing. It is the most common sensory defect. The major categories of auditory dysfunction are conductive hearing loss, sensorineural hearing loss, mixed hearing loss, and functional hearing loss. Hearing loss may range from mild to profound. Auditory changes caused by aging are common and incremental (see the *Geriatric Considerations:* Aging and Changes in Hearing box).

Conductive hearing loss. A **conductive hearing loss** occurs when a change in the outer or middle ear impairs conduction of sound from the outer to the inner ear. Many conditions commonly cause a conductive hearing loss. These conditions include impacted cerumen, foreign bodies lodged in the external auditory canal, benign tumours of the middle ear, carcinoma of the external auditory canal or middle ear, eustachian tube dysfunction, otitis media, acute viral otitis media,

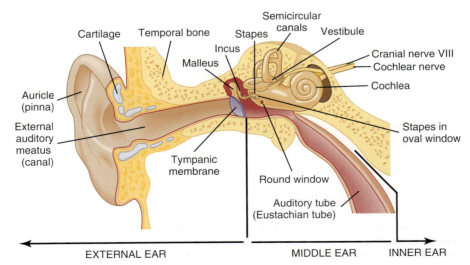

FIGURE 14.13 The Ear. External, middle, and inner ears. (Anatomical structures are not drawn to scale.) (From Applegate, E. [2011]. *The anatomy and physiology learning system* [4th ed.]. Saunders.)

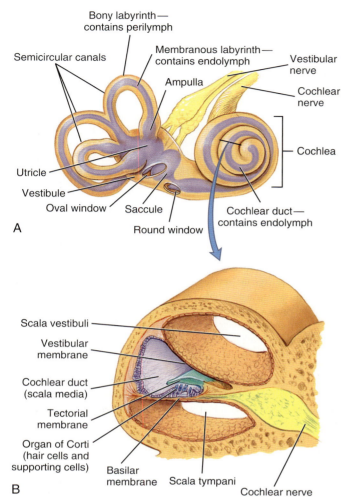

FIGURE 14.14 The Inner Ear. **A,** The bony labyrinth *(tan)* is the hard outer wall of the entire inner ear and includes the semicircular canals, vestibule, and cochlea. Within the bony labyrinth is the membranous labyrinth *(purple).* Perilymph surrounds and endolymph fills the labyrinth. Each ampulla in the vestibule has a crista ampullaris that detects changes in head position and sends sensory signals through the vestibular branch of the vestibulocochlear (VIII) cranial nerve to the brain. **B,** Section of the membranous cochlea. Hair cells in the organ of Corti detect sound and send the information through the cochlear nerve. The vestibular and cochlear branches join to form the vestibulocochlear cranial nerve (VIII). (From Applegate, E. [2011]. *The anatomy and physiology learning system* [4th ed.]. Saunders.)

chronic suppurative otitis media, cholesteatoma (accumulation of keratinized epithelium), and otosclerosis.

Symptoms of conductive hearing loss include diminished hearing and soft speaking voice. The voice is soft because often the person hears his or her voice, conducted by bone, as loud.

Sensorineural hearing loss. Impairment of the organ of Corti or its central connections causes a sensorineural hearing loss. The loss may occur gradually or suddenly. Conditions causing sensorineural loss include congenital and hereditary factors, noise exposure, aging, Ménière's disease, ototoxicity, systemic disease (syphilis, Paget's disease, collagen diseases, diabetes mellitus), neoplasms, and autoimmune processes.[60] Congenital and neonatal sensorineural hearing loss may be caused by maternal rubella, ototoxic medications, prematurity, traumatic delivery, erythroblastosis fetalis, bacterial meningitis, and congenital hereditary malfunction. A noted delay in speech development assists diagnosis. Sudden-onset bilateral sensorineural hearing loss is a medical emergency.

Presbycusis is the most common form of sensorineural hearing loss in older persons. Its cause may be atrophy of the basal end of the organ of Corti, loss of auditory receptors, changes in vascularity, or stiffening of the basilar membranes. Ototoxic components (substances that cause destruction of auditory function) have been observed after exposure to various medications and chemicals. Examples include antibiotics such as streptomycin, neomycin, gentamicin, and vancomycin; diuretics such as ethacrynic acid (Edecrin) and furosemide (Apo-Furosemide); and chemicals such as salicylate, quinine, carbon monoxide, nitrogen mustard, arsenic, mercury, gold, tobacco, and alcohol. In most instances, the medications and chemicals listed initially cause tinnitus (ringing in the ear), followed by an ongoing high-tone sensorineural hearing loss that is permanent.

Mixed and functional hearing loss. A combination of conductive and sensorineural losses is a mixed hearing loss. With functional hearing loss, which is rare, the person does not respond to voice and appears not to hear. Emotional or psychological factors are thought to be the cause.

Ménière's disease. Ménière's disease (endolymphatic hydrops) is an episodic disorder of the middle ear with an unknown etiology that can be unilateral or bilateral. There is excessive endolymph and pressure in the membranous labyrinth that disrupts both vestibular (equilibrium) and hearing functions. There are four symptoms: recurring episodes of vertigo (often accompanied by severe nausea and vomiting), hearing loss, ringing in the ears (tinnitus), and a feeling of fullness in the ear. Treatment is symptomatic with medical management or surgical management when medications fail.[61]

Ear Infections

Otitis externa. Otitis externa is the most common inflammation of the outer ear and may be acute or persistent, infectious or noninfectious. The most common origins of acute infections are bacterial microorganisms including *Pseudomonas*, *Staphylococcus aureus*, and, less commonly, *Escherichia coli*. Fungal infections are less common. Infection usually follows prolonged exposure to moisture (swimmer's ear). The earliest symptoms are inflammation with pruritus, swelling, and clear drainage progressing to purulent drainage with obstruction of the canal. Tenderness and pain with earlobe retraction accompany inflammation. Early treatment such as acidifying solutions and topical antimicrobials usually provide effective treatment for later stages of disease.[62] Chronic infections are more often related to allergy or skin disorders.

Otitis media. Otitis media is a common infection of infants and children. Most children have one episode by 3 years of age. The most common pathogens are *S. pneumoniae*, *Haemophilus influenzae*, and *M. catarrhalis*. Predisposing factors include allergy, sinusitis, submucosal cleft palate, adenoidal hypertrophy, eustachian tube dysfunction, and immune deficiency. Breastfeeding is a protective factor. Recurrent acute otitis media may be genetically determined.[63]

Acute otitis media (AOM) is associated with ear pain, fever, irritability, inflamed tympanic membrane, and fluid in the middle ear. The appearance of the tympanic membrane progresses from erythema to opaqueness with bulging as fluid accumulates. There is an increasing prevalence of AOM caused by penicillin-resistant microorganisms. Otitis media with effusion (OME) is the presence of fluid in the middle ear without symptoms of acute infection.

Treatment includes symptom management, particularly of pain, with watchful waiting, and antimicrobial therapy for severe illness. The placement of tympanostomy tubes may be required when there is persistent bilateral effusion and significant hearing loss. Complications include mastoiditis, brain abscess, meningitis, and chronic otitis media with hearing loss. Persistent middle ear effusions may affect speech, language, and cognitive abilities. Multivalent vaccines for prevention of otitis media are effective for reducing disease incidence.[64]

Olfaction and Taste

Olfaction (smell) is a function of the olfactory (I) cranial nerve and part of the trigeminal (V) cranial nerve. Taste (gustation) is a function of multiple nerves in the tongue, soft palate, uvula, pharynx, and upper esophagus which are innervated by the facial (VII) and glossopharyngeal (IX) cranial nerves. Hormones influence both cranial nerves within the sensory cells. Dysfunctions of smell and taste may occur separately or jointly. The strong relationship between smell and taste creates the sensation of flavour. If either sensation is impaired, the perception of flavour is altered. Figure 14.15 shows the olfactory structures.

Olfactory cells, found in the olfactory epithelium, are the receptor cells for smell. Seven different primary classes of olfactory stimulants have been found: (1) camphoraceous, (2) musky, (3) floral, (4) peppermint, (5) ethereal, (6) pungent, and (7) putrid. The primary sensations of taste are (1) sour, (2) salty, (3) sweet, (4) bitter, and (5) umami (savouriness). Taste buds (fungiform, foliate, and circumvallate) sensitive to each of the primary sensations are found in specific areas of the tongue.

Sensitivity to odours declines steadily with aging. See the *Geriatric Considerations: Aging and Changes in Olfaction and Taste* box for a summary of changes in olfaction and taste with aging.

Olfactory and Taste Dysfunctions

Olfactory dysfunctions include:
- Hyposmia—impaired sense of smell
- Anosmia—complete loss of sense of smell
- Olfactory hallucinations—smelling odours that are not present
- Parosmia—abnormal or perverted sense of smell

Cranial nerve injury can impair the sense of smell. Impaired smell associated with injury near the hippocampus may alter taste.

Hypogeusia is a decrease in taste sensation, while ageusia is an absence of the sense of taste. These disorders result from cranial nerve injuries and can be specific to the area of the tongue innervated. Dysgeusia is a perversion of taste in which substances have an unpleasant flavour (i.e., metallic). Changes in taste may compromise adequate nutrition or cause anorexia.[65]

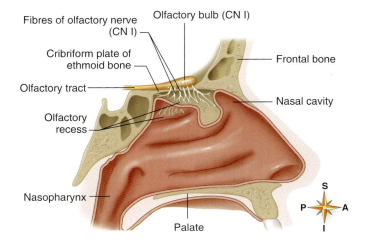

FIGURE 14.15 Olfaction. Midsagittal section of the nasal area shows the location of major olfactory sensory structures. (From Patton, K. T. [2019]. *Anatomy & physiology* [10th ed.]. Elsevier.)

SOMATOSENSORY FUNCTION

> **QUICK CHECK 14.5**
> 1. How are different touch receptors distributed over the body?
> 2. What are two common causes of changes in proprioception?

Touch

The sensation of touch involves four afferent fibre types that mediate tactile sensation, and there may be an added sensory nerve that transmits pleasurable touch.[66] Receptors sensitive to touch are present in the skin with high densities in the fingers and lips. Meissner corpuscles and Pacinian corpuscles are fast-adapting receptors and sense movement across the skin and vibration, respectively. The slowly adapting Merkel discs sense sustained light touch, and Ruffini endings respond to deep sustained pressure, stretch, and joint position. The posterior column of the spinal cord and the anterior spinothalamic tract carry specific sensory input to the higher levels of the CNS.

The cutaneous senses develop before birth, but structural growth continues into early adulthood. Then a gradual decline occurs, with loss in tactile discrimination with advancing age.[67] Alterations at any level of the nervous system, from the receptor to the cerebral cortex can cause an abnormal tactile sense. Factors that interrupt or impair reception, transmission, perception, or interpretation of touch may cause tactile dysfunction. These factors include trauma, tumour, infection, metabolic changes, vascular changes, and degenerative diseases. In addition, most tactile sensations evoke affective responses that determine whether the sensation is unpleasant, pleasant, or neutral.

Proprioception

Proprioception is the awareness of the position of the body and its parts. It depends on signals from the inner ear and from receptors in joints and ligaments. The posterior columns and the spinocerebellar tracts send sensory data to higher centres, with some data passing through the medial lemnisci and thalamic radiations to the cortex. These stimuli are necessary for the coordination of movements, the grading of muscular contraction, and the maintenance of equilibrium.

A progressive loss of proprioception has been reported in older persons and is associated with an increased risk for falls and injury.[68] As with tactile dysfunction, any factor that interrupts or impairs the reception, transmission, perception, or interpretation of proprioceptive stimuli also alters proprioception and increases risk for falls and injury. Two common causes of changes in proprioception are vestibular dysfunction and neuropathy.

Specific vestibular dysfunctions are vestibular nystagmus and vertigo. Vestibular nystagmus is the constant, involuntary movement of the eyeball and develops when the vestibular system within the semicircular canals is overstimulated. Vertigo is the sensation of spinning that occurs with inflammation of the semicircular canals in the inner ear. The person may feel either that he or she is moving in space or that the world is revolving. Vertigo often causes loss of balance, and nystagmus may occur. Ménière's disease can cause loss of proprioception during an acute attack, so that standing or walking is impossible.

Peripheral neuropathies also can cause proprioceptive dysfunction. Conditions commonly associated with renal disease and diabetes mellitus may cause neuropathies. Although the exact sequence of events is unknown, neuropathies cause a diminished or absent sense of body position or position of body parts. Gait changes often occur.

GERIATRIC CONSIDERATIONS
Aging and Changes in Vision

- The incidence of cataracts increases with age.
- Age-related macular degeneration (AMD) is a major cause of blindness in older persons. It is a severe and irreversible loss of vision.
- Presbyopia is the loss of visual accommodation associated with advancing age.
- Colour discrimination diminishes with age, with blue and green most commonly affected.
- See Tables 14.6 and 14.7 for more information.

GERIATRIC CONSIDERATIONS
Aging and Changes in Hearing[a]

Cochlear hair cell degeneration	Inability to hear high-frequency sounds (presbycusis, sensorineural loss); interferes with understanding speech; both ears may lose hearing at different times
Loss of auditory neurons in spiral ganglia of organ of Corti	Inability to hear high-frequency sounds (presbycusis, sensorineural loss); interferes with understanding speech; both ears may lose hearing at different times
Degeneration of basilar (cochlear) conductive membrane of cochlea	Inability to hear at all frequencies but worse at higher frequencies (cochlear conductive loss)
Decreased vascularity of cochlea	Equal loss of hearing at all frequencies (strial loss); inability to disseminate localization of sound
Loss of cortical auditory neurons	Equal loss of hearing at all frequencies (strial loss); inability to disseminate localization of sound

[a]Hearing loss affects about 33% of older persons.
Data from Frisina, R. D. (2009). *Annals of the New York Academy of Sciences, 1170*, 708–717; Roth, T. N. (2015). *Handbook of Clinical Neurology, 129*, 357–373.

GERIATRIC CONSIDERATIONS
Aging and Changes in Olfaction and Taste

- Decline in sensitivity to odours, usually after age 80, occurs.
- Loss of olfaction may diminish appetite, taste, and food choice and may affect nutrition.
- Inability to smell toxic fumes or gases can pose a safety hazard.
- Decrease in taste sensitivity is more gradual than decline in sense of smell.
- Higher concentrations of flavours are required to stimulate taste.
- Decreased salivary secretion may affect taste.

DID YOU UNDERSTAND?

Pain

1. Pain (nociception) is a complex, unpleasant sensory experience that involves dynamic interactions between physical, cognitive, spiritual, emotional, and environmental factors. Pain is protective.
2. Three portions of the nervous system are responsible for sensation, perception, and response to pain: (a) the afferent pathways, (b) the interpretive centres of the central nervous system, and (c) the efferent pathways.
3. Nociception involves four phases: transduction, transmission, perception, and modulation.
4. There are two primary types of nociceptors: Aδ fibres and C fibres. Myelinated Aδ fibres send sharp, well-localized "fast" pain. Smaller, unmyelinated C fibres more slowly send dull, aching, or burning sensations that are less localized.
5. The somatosensory cortex mediates localization and intensity of pain. The reticular formation, limbic system, and brainstem control emotional and affective responses to pain. The cortex coordinates the meaning an experience of pain.
6. Pain threshold is the lowest intensity of pain that a person can recognize. Pain tolerance is the greatest intensity of pain that a person can endure. Both are subjective and influenced by many factors.
7. Neuromodulators of pain include substances that (a) stimulate pain nociceptors (e.g., prostaglandins, bradykinins, lymphokines, substance P, and glutamate) and (b) suppress pain (e.g., GABA, endogenous opioids, endocannabinoids). Some substances excite peripheral nerves but inhibit central nerves (e.g., serotonin, norepinephrine).
8. The central nervous system produces endogenous opioids that inhibit pain transmission. They include enkephalins, endorphins, dynorphins, and endomorphins.
9. Descending inhibitory and facilitatory pathways and nuclei inhibit or ease pain. Efferent pathways from the ventromedial medulla and periaqueductal grey inhibit pain signals at the posterior horn. The rostroventromedial medulla stimulates efferent pathways that ease or inhibit pain in the posterior horn.
10. Segmental pain inhibition occurs when signals from Aβ fibres (touch and vibration sensations) arrive at the same spinal level as signals from Aδ or C fibres.
11. Diffuse noxious inhibitory control occurs when two different sites simultaneously transmit pain signals and inhibit pain through a spinal-medullary-spinal pathway.
12. Classifications of pain include nociceptive pain, non-nociceptive pain, acute pain, and persistent pain.

13. Acute pain may be (a) somatic (superficial), (b) visceral (internal), or (c) referred (present in an area distant from its origin). The same spinal segment as the actual site of pain supplies the area of referred pain.
14. Persistent pain is pain lasting beyond the expected normal healing time and may be intermittent or persistent.
15. Psychological, behavioural, and physiological responses to persistent pain include depression, sleep disorders, preoccupation with pain, lifestyle changes, and physiological adaptation.
16. Neuropathic pain is increased sensitivity to painful stimuli and results from abnormal processing of pain information in the peripheral or central nervous system.

Temperature Regulation

1. A precise balancing of heat production, heat conservation, and heat loss achieves temperature regulation. The normal range of body temperature is 36.2° to 37.7°C (96.2° to 99.4°F).
2. Temperature regulation is mediated by the hypothalamus through central thermoreceptors in the skin, hypothalamus, spinal cord, abdominal organs, and other central locations.
3. Chemical reactions of metabolism and skeletal muscle tone and contraction produce body heat.
4. Vasoconstriction and voluntary mechanisms conserve heat.
5. Radiation, conduction, convection, vasodilation, evaporation of sweat, decreased muscle tone, increased respiration, voluntary measures, and adaptation to warmer climates are causes of body heat loss.
6. Infants do not conserve heat well because of their greater body surface to body weight ratio and low amount of subcutaneous fat. Older persons have poor responses to environmental temperature extremes because of slowed blood circulation, structural and functional changes in the skin, and overall decreased heat-producing activities.
7. The release of exogenous pyrogens from bacteria or the release of endogenous pyrogens from phagocytic cells trigger fever. Fever is both a normal immunological mechanism and a symptom of disease.
8. Fever involves the "resetting of the hypothalamic thermostat" to a higher level. When the fever breaks, the set point returns to normal.
9. Fever of unknown origin is a body temperature greater than 38.3°C (101°F) for longer than 3 weeks' duration that is still undiagnosed after 3 days of hospital investigation, 3 outpatient visits, or 1 week of ambulatory investigation.
10. Fever production aids responses to infectious processes. Higher temperatures kill many microorganisms, promote immune responses, and decrease serum levels of iron, zinc, and copper. Bacteria require these substances for replication.
11. Hyperthermia can produce nerve damage, coagulation of cell proteins, and death. Forms of accidental hyperthermia include heat cramps, heat exhaustion, heat stroke, and malignant hyperthermia. Heat stroke and malignant hyperthermia may cause death.
12. Hypothermia slows the rate of chemical reaction (tissue metabolism), increases the viscosity of the blood, slows blood flow through the microcirculation, helps blood coagulation, and stimulates profound vasoconstriction. Hypothermia may be accidental or therapeutic.

Sleep

1. Sleep is an active multiphase process divided into rapid eye movement (REM) and non–rapid eye movement (non-REM) sleep, each of which has its own series of stages. While asleep, a person progresses through REM and non-REM sleep in a predictable cycle.
2. Mechanisms in the pons and mesencephalon control REM sleep. Release of inhibitory signals from the hypothalamus control non-REM sleep. Non-REM sleep accounts for 75 to 80% of sleep time.
3. The sleep patterns of infants, young children, and older persons vary in total sleep time, cycle length, and percentage of time spent in each sleep cycle. Older persons experience a decrease in total sleep time.
4. Sleep disorders include (a) dyssomnias (disorders of initiating sleep) and (b) parasomnias (sleepwalking or night terrors and restless legs syndrome).
5. The restorative, reparative, and growth processes occur during non-REM sleep. Sleep dyssomnias can cause significant changes in personality and functioning.

The Special Senses

1. The wall of the eye has three layers: sclera, choroid, and retina. The retina has millions of photoreceptors known as rods and cones that receive light through the lens and then convey signals to the optic nerve and then to the visual cortex of the brain.
2. Vitreous and aqueous humor fill the eye chambers and prevent the eye from collapsing.
3. The major changes in ocular movement include strabismus, nystagmus, and paralysis of specific extraocular muscles.
4. Structural eye changes caused by aging result in decreased visual acuity.
5. Amblyopia, scotoma, cataracts, papilledema, glaucoma, and macular degeneration are causes of visual acuity changes.
6. A cataract is a cloudy or opaque area in the ocular lens and leads to visual loss when found on the visual axis.
7. Intraocular pressures greater than 12 to 20 mm Hg with death of retinal ganglion cells and their axons are characteristics of glaucoma.
8. Age-related macular degeneration is irreversible loss of vision with dry or wet forms.
9. Changes in accommodation develop with increased intraocular pressure, inflammation, and disease of the oculomotor nerve. Presbyopia is loss of accommodation caused by loss of elasticity of the lens with aging.
10. Changes in refraction, including myopia, hyperopia, and astigmatism, are the most common visual disorders.
11. Changes in colour vision can be related to yellowing of the lens with aging and colour blindness, an inherited trait.
12. The eyelids, conjunctivae, and lacrimal apparatus protect the eye. Infections are the most common conditions affecting the supporting structures of the eyes; they include blepharitis, conjunctivitis, chalazion, and hordeolum.
13. Trauma or disease of the optic nerve pathways, or optic radiations, can cause blindness in the visual fields.
14. Blepharitis is an inflammation of the eyelid. A hordeolum (stye) is an infection of the eyelid's sebaceous gland. A chalazion is an infection of the eyelid's meibomian gland.
15. Conjunctivitis can be acute or chronic, bacterial, viral, or allergic. Redness, edema, pain, and lacrimation are common symptoms. Chlamydial conjunctivitis is the leading cause of blindness in the world and is associated with poor sanitary conditions.
16. Keratitis is a bacterial or viral infection of the cornea that can lead to corneal ulceration. Photophobia, pain, and tearing are common symptoms.
17. The ear is composed of the external ear, middle ear, and inner ear. The external structures are the pinna, auditory canal, and tympanic membrane. The tympanic cavity, oval window, eustachian tube, and fluid compose the middle ear and send sound vibrations to the inner ear.

18. The inner ear includes the bony and membranous labyrinths that send sound waves through the cochlea to the acoustic division of the cranial nerve VIII. The semicircular canals and vestibule help support balance through the equilibrium receptors.
19. Hearing loss is classified as conductive, sensorineural, mixed, or functional.
20. Conductive hearing loss occurs when sound waves cannot be conducted through the middle ear.
21. Sensorineural hearing loss develops with impairment of the organ of Corti or its central connections. Presbycusis is the most common form of sensorineural hearing loss in older persons.
22. A combination of conductive and sensorineural loss is a mixed hearing loss.
23. Loss of hearing with no known organic cause is a functional hearing loss.
24. Ménière's disease is a disorder of the middle ear that affects hearing and balance.
25. Otitis externa is an infection of the outer ear associated with prolonged exposure to moisture.
26. Otitis media is an infection of the middle ear that is common in children. Accumulation of fluid behind the tympanic membrane is a common finding.
27. Dysfunction of olfaction or taste alters the perception of flavour. Sensitivity to odour and taste decreases with aging.
28. Hyposmia is a decrease in the sense of smell, and anosmia is the complete loss of the sense of smell. Inflammation of the nasal mucosa and trauma or tumours of the olfactory nerve lead to a decreased sense of smell.
29. Hypogeusia is a decrease in taste sensation. Ageusia is the absence of the sense of taste. Loss of taste buds or trauma to the facial or glossopharyngeal nerves decreases taste sensation.

Somatosensory Function
1. Tactile sensation is a function of receptors present in the skin (Pacinian corpuscles). The posterior column and anterior spinothalamic tract conduct the sensory response to the brain.
2. Changes in touch can result from disruption of skin receptors, sensory transmission, or central nervous system perception.
3. Proprioception is the awareness of the position and location of the body and its parts. Proprioceptors are found in the inner ear, joints, and ligaments. Proprioceptive stimuli are necessary for balance, coordinated movement, and grading of muscular contraction.
4. Disorders of proprioception can occur at any level of the nervous system and result in impaired balance and lack of coordinated movement.

Geriatric Considerations: Aging and Changes in Vision
1. Factors affecting altered vision of older people include cataract formation, macular degeneration, presbyopia, and diminished colour discrimination.

Geriatric Considerations: Aging and Changes in Hearing
1. About one third of older persons have hearing loss.
2. Factors affecting altered hearing of older people include cochlear hair cell degeneration, loss of auditory neurons, degeneration of conductive membranes, and decreased vascularity.

Geriatric Considerations: Changes in Olfaction and Taste
1. Loss of olfaction usually occurs after the age of 80 years.
2. Decrease in taste is a gradual occurrence.
3. Changes in olfaction and taste may affect appetite, food choices and nutrition.

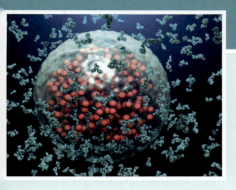

15

Alterations in Cognitive Systems, Cerebral Hemodynamics, and Motor Function

Kelly Power-Kean, with originating chapter contributions by Barbara J. Boss and Sue E. Huether

Additional resources are available online at https://evolve.elsevier.com/Canada/Huether/pathophysiology.

CHAPTER OUTLINE

Alterations in Cognitive Systems, 352
 Alterations in Arousal, 352
 Alterations in Awareness, 358
 Data-Processing Deficits, 360
 Seizure Disorders, 365
 Types of Seizure, 366
Alterations in Cerebral Hemodynamics, 367
 Increased Intracranial Pressure, 367
 Cerebral Edema, 368
 Hydrocephalus, 369
Alterations in Neuromotor Function, 369
 Alterations in Muscle Tone, 369
 Alterations in Muscle Movement, 371
 Upper and Lower Motor Neuron Syndromes, 374
 Motor Neuron Diseases, 376
 Amyotrophic Lateral Sclerosis, 377
Alterations in Complex Motor Performance, 378
 Disorders of Posture (Stance), 378
 Disorders of Gait, 378
 Disorders of Expression, 378
Extrapyramidal Motor Syndromes, 378
CASE STUDY: Seizure, 379

LEARNING OBJECTIVES

1. Describe how the brain affects the level of consciousness, pattern of breathing, vomiting, pupillary changes, oculomotor responses, and motor responses.
2. Describe the differences between brain death and cerebral death.
3. Describe the differences between persistent vegetative state, minimally conscious state, and locked-in syndrome.
4. Differentiate among the different types of seizures.
5. Define retrograde amnesia, anterograde amnesia, and executive attention deficits.
6. Compare and contrast the different data processing deficits.
7. Describe the pathophysiology of Alzheimer's disease.
8. Define cerebral perfusion pressure.
9. List the causes of increased intracranial pressure (ICP). Discuss the associated clinical manifestations.
10. Describe the normal process of autoregulation in the cerebral blood vessels. Explain how autoregulation fails when ICP rises dramatically.
11. Describe the mechanisms and manifestations of the herniation syndromes.
12. List the causes of cerebral edema. Give examples of the pathophysiology producing each cause.
13. Describe the causes and manifestations of hydrocephalus.
14. Compare and contrast the major motor syndromes including CNS motor, motor unit, pyramidal, extrapyramidal, cerebellar, and upper and lower motor neuron.
15. Explain the pathophysiology of amyotrophic lateral sclerosis (ALS).
16. Identify the areas of the brain in which alterations in emotions and behaviours occur when damaged.
17. Match the major cerebral function deficits to cognitive descriptions of behaviours.
18. Compare and contrast the various forms of dyspraxia.

KEY TERMS

Acute confusional state, 360
Acute hydrocephalus, 369
Agnosia, 360
Akinesia, 373
Alzheimer's disease (AD) (dementia of Alzheimer's type [DAT], senile disease complex), 363
Amnesia, 358
Amyotrophic lateral sclerosis, 377
Anterograde amnesia, 358
Aphasia, 360
Apraxia or dyspraxia, 378
Areflexia, 375
Arousal, 352
Autoregulation, 367
Awareness, 358
Basal ganglia motor syndrome, 379
Basal ganglion gait, 378
Basal ganglion posture, 378
Bradykinesia, 373
Brain death (total brain death), 357
Bulbar palsy, 377
Cerebellar (ataxic) gait, 378
Cerebellar motor syndrome, 379
Cerebral blood flow (CBF), 366
Cerebral blood oxygenation, 367
Cerebral blood volume (CBV), 367
Cerebral death (irreversible coma), 357

CHAPTER 15: Alterations in Cognitive Systems, Cerebral Hemodynamics, and Motor Function

Cerebral edema, 368
Cerebral perfusion pressure (CPP), 367
Clonic phase, 366
Communicating hydrocephalus, 369
Consciousness, 352
Convulsion, 365
Cytotoxic (metabolic) edema, 369
Decerebrate posture/response, 378
Decorticate posture/response (antigravity posture, hemiplegic posture), 378
Delirium (hyperactive confusional state), 362
Dementia, 362
Diplegia, 375
Dysphasia, 360
Dyspraxia, 364
Dystonia, 378
Dystonic movement, 378
Dystonic posture, 378
Epilepsy, 365
Epileptogenic focus, 366
Excited delirium syndrome (ExDS), 362
Executive attention deficit, 358
Extinction, 358
Extrapyramidal motor syndrome, 379
Fasciculation, 375
Fibrillation, 375
Flaccid paresis/paralysis, 375
Frontal lobe ataxic gait, 378
Frontotemporal dementia (FTD) (Pick disease), 365
Guillain-Barré syndrome, 377
Hemiparesis, 375
Hemiplegia, 375
Hiccup, 356
Huntington's disease (HD), 371
Hydrocephalus, 369
Hyperkinesia, 371
Hypermimesis, 378
Hypertonia, 370
Hypoactive delirium (hypoactive confusional state), 362
Hypokinesia, 373
Hypomimesis, 378
Hypotonia, 369
Ictus, 366
Image processing, 358
Increased intracranial pressure (increased ICP), 367
Interstitial edema, 369
Intracranial pressure (ICP), 367
Level of consciousness, 353
Locked-in syndrome, 358
Lower motor neuron syndromes, 375
Memory, 358
Memory disorder, 358
Minimally conscious state (MCS), 358
Mirror focus, 366
Motor response, 356
Neglect syndrome, 358
Neuritic plaques, 363
Neurofibrillary tangle, 363
Noncommunicating hydrocephalus (internal hydrocephalus, intraventricular hydrocephalus), 369
Normal-pressure hydrocephalus, 369
Oculomotor response, 356
Paralysis, 374
Paraparesis, 375
Paraplegia, 375
Paratonia (gegenhalten), 370
Paresis, 374
Parkinsonism (Parkinson's syndrome, parkinsonian syndrome, paralysis agitans), 373
Parkinson's disease (PD), 373
Paroxysmal dyskinesia, 371
Patterns of breathing, 353
Persistent vegetative state (VS), 358
Postictal phase, 366
Preictal phase, 366
Prodroma, 366
Progressive bulbar palsy, 377
Progressive spinal muscular atrophy, 377
Psychogenic alterations in arousal (unresponsiveness), 353
Pupillary change, 353
Pyramidal motor syndrome, 374
Quadriparesis, 375
Quadriplegia, 375
Retrograde amnesia, 358
Rigidity, 370
Secondary parkinsonism, 373
Seizure, 365
Selective attention, 358
Selective attention deficit, 358
Sensory inattentiveness, 358
Spasticity, 370
Spinal shock, 374
Status epilepticus, 366
Structural alterations in arousal, 352
Tardive dyskinesia, 371
Tentorium cerebelli, 352
Tonic phase, 366
Tourette syndrome, 371
Upper motor neuron gait, 378
Upper motor neuron paresis or paralysis, 374
Vasogenic edema, 368
Vomiting, 356
Yawning, 356

A person achieves cognitive and behavioural functional competence by integrated processes of cognitive systems, sensory systems, and motor systems. The purpose of this chapter is to present the concepts and processes of alterations in these systems to understand the manifestations of neurological dysfunction and disease.

The neural systems that are essential to cognitive function are (1) attentional systems that provide arousal and maintenance of attention over time; (2) memory and language systems by which information is communicated; and (3) affective or emotive systems that mediate mood, emotion, and intention. These core systems are fundamental to the processes of abstract thinking and reasoning. The organization and operationalization of products of abstraction and reasoning occurs through the executive attentional networks. The normal functioning of these networks manifests through the motor network in a behavioural array viewed by others as appropriate to human activity and successful living.

ALTERATIONS IN COGNITIVE SYSTEMS

QUICK CHECK 15.1
1. Why are structural and metabolic factors capable of producing coma?
2. Why is level of consciousness the most critical index of central nervous system function?
3. Why does Cheyne-Stokes respiration appear in a comatose individual?
4. Why are oculomotor changes associated with levels of brain injury?

Full **consciousness** is a state of awareness of oneself and the environment, and a set of responses to that environment. The fully conscious individual starts spontaneous, purposeful activity independently to a perceived stimulus. Any decrease in this state of awareness and varied responses is a decrease in consciousness.

Consciousness has two components: arousal (state of awakeness) and awareness (content of thought). Mediation of **arousal** occurs by the reticular activating system. This system regulates aspects of attention and information processing and maintains consciousness. Awareness encompasses all cognitive functions. Mediation of these functions is by attentional systems, memory systems, language systems, and executive systems.

Alterations in Arousal

The causes of alterations in level of arousal can be structural, metabolic, or psychogenic (functional) disorders.

PATHOPHYSIOLOGY **Structural alterations in arousal** are divided according to the original location of the pathological condition. Causes include infection, vascular alterations, neoplasms, traumatic injury, congenital alterations, degenerative changes, polygenic traits, and metabolic disorders.

Supratentorial disorders (above the tentorium cerebelli) produce changes in arousal by either diffuse or localized dysfunction. The **tentorium cerebelli** is an extension of the dura mater that separates the cerebellum from the inferior portion of the occipital lobes. The cause of diffuse dysfunction may be by disease processes affecting the cerebral cortex or the underlying subcortical white matter (e.g., encephalitis). Disorders outside the brain but within the cranial vault (extracerebral) can produce diffuse dysfunction. This dysfunction includes neoplasms, closed-head trauma with subsequent subdural bleeding, and accumulation of pus in the subdural space. Disorders within the brain substance (intracerebral)—such as bleeding, infarcts, emboli, and tumours—function mainly as masses. Such localized destructive processes directly impair function of the thalamic or hypothalamic activating systems. They may also secondarily compress these structures in a process of herniation.

Infratentorial disorders (below the tentorium cerebelli) produce a decline in arousal by (1) direct destruction or compression of the reticular activating system and its pathways (e.g., accumulations of blood or pus, neoplasms, and demyelinating disorders) or (2) destruction of the brainstem (midbrain, pons, medulla) either by direct invasion or by indirect impairment of its blood supply.

Metabolic disorders produce a decline in arousal by alterations in delivery of energy substrates. This decline occurs with hypoxia, electrolyte disturbances, or hypoglycemia. Metabolic disorders caused by liver or renal failure cause alterations in neuronal excitability. This occurs because of failure to metabolize or eliminate medications and toxins. All the systemic diseases that eventually produce nervous system dysfunction are part of this metabolic category.

Psychogenic alterations in arousal (unresponsiveness) may signal general psychiatric disorders. Despite apparent unconsciousness, the person is physiologically awake, and the neurological examination reflects normal responses.

CLINICAL MANIFESTATIONS AND EVALUATION Five patterns of neurological function are critical to the evaluation process. These patterns include (1) level of consciousness, (2) pattern of breathing, (3) pupillary reaction, (4) oculomotor responses, and (5) motor responses. Patterns of clinical manifestations help in determining the extent of brain dysfunction. They also serve as indexes for identifying increasing or decreasing central nervous system (CNS) function. (Table 15.1) presents the distinctions between metabolically induced and structurally induced manifestations. The types of manifestations suggest the cause of the altered arousal state (Table 15.2).

Level of consciousness is the most critical clinical index of nervous system function. Changes indicate either improvement or deterioration of the individual's condition. A person who is alert and oriented to self, others, place, and time is functioning at the highest level of consciousness. This functioning implies full use of all the person's cognitive capacities. From this normal alert state, levels of consciousness diminish in stages from confusion and disorientation (which can occur simultaneously) to coma. (Table 15.3) defines each of these states.

Patterns of breathing help evaluate the level of brain dysfunction and coma (Figure 15.1). Evaluation of rate, rhythm, and pattern should occur. Categorization of breathing patterns can be hemispheric or brainstem patterns (Table 15.4).

With normal breathing, a neural centre in the forebrain (cerebrum) produces a rhythmic pattern. When consciousness decreases, lower brainstem centres regulate the breathing pattern by responding only to changes in partial pressure of carbon dioxide in arterial blood ($PaCO_2$) levels. This breathing pattern is called *posthyperventilation apnea*. *Cheyne-Stokes respiration* is an abnormal rhythm of ventilation with alternating periods of tachypnea and apnea (crescendo–decrescendo pattern). Increases in $PaCO_2$ levels lead to tachypnea. The $PaCO_2$ level then decreases to below normal and breathing stops (apnea) until the carbon dioxide reaccumulates and again stimulates tachypnea (see Figure 15.1). In cases of opiate or sedative medication overdose, the respiratory centre is depressed so the rate of breathing gradually decreases until respiratory failure occurs.

Pupillary changes indicate the presence and level of brainstem dysfunction. This occurs because brainstem areas that control arousal are adjacent to areas that control the pupils (Figure 15.2). For example, severe ischemia and hypoxia usually produce dilated, fixed pupils. Hypothermia may cause fixed pupils.

Some drugs affect pupils and must be considered in evaluating individuals in comatose states. Large doses of atropine and scopolamine fully dilate and fix pupils. Doses of sedatives (e.g., benzodiazepines) in sufficient amounts to produce coma, and taken in combination with other CNS-depressant agents (e.g., alcohol or barbiturates), cause the pupils to become midposition or moderately dilated, unequal, and

TABLE 15.1 Clinical Manifestations of Metabolic and Structural Causes of Altered Arousal

MANIFESTATIONS	METABOLICALLY INDUCED	STRUCTURALLY INDUCED
Blink to threat (cranial nerves II, VII)	Equal	Asymmetrical
Optic discs (cranial nerve II)	Flat, good pulsation	Papilledema
Extraocular movement (cranial nerves III, IV, VI)	Roving eye movements; normal oculocephalic reflex (doll's eyes phenomenon) and oculovestibular reflex (caloric ice water test)	Gaze paresis, nerve palsy
Pupils (cranial nerves II, III)	Equal and reactive; may be dilated (e.g., atropine), pinpoint (e.g., opiates), or midposition and fixed (e.g., benzodiazepines combined with other central nervous system–depressant agents)	Asymmetrical or nonreactive; may be midposition (midbrain injury), pinpoint (pons injury), large (tectal injury)
Corneal reflex (cranial nerves V, VII)	Symmetrical response	Asymmetrical response
Grimace to pain (cranial nerve VII)	Symmetrical response	Asymmetrical response
Motor function movement	Symmetrical	Asymmetrical
Muscle tone	Symmetrical	Paratonic (rigid), spastic, flaccid, especially if asymmetrical
Posture	Symmetrical	Decorticate, especially if symmetrical; decerebrate, especially if asymmetrical (see Figure 15.6)
Deep tendon reflexes	Symmetrical	Asymmetrical
Babinski sign	Absent or symmetrical response	Present
Sensation	Symmetrical	Asymmetrical

TABLE 15.2 Differential Characteristics of States Causing Altered Arousal

MECHANISM	MANIFESTATIONS
Supratentorial mass lesions compressing or displacing diencephalon or brainstem	Initiating signs usually of focal cerebral dysfunction: vomiting, headache, hemiparesis, ocular signs, seizures, coma Signs of dysfunction progress rostral to caudal Neurological signs at any given time point to one anatomical area (e.g., diencephalon, mesencephalon, medulla) Motor signs often asymmetrical
Infratentorial mass of destruction causing coma	History of preceding brainstem dysfunction or sudden onset of coma Localizing brainstem signs precede or accompany onset of coma and always include oculovestibular abnormality Cranial nerve palsies usually manifest "bizarre" respiratory patterns that appear at onset
Metabolic coma Exogenous toxins (medications) Endogenous toxins (organ system failure)	Confusion and stupor commonly precede motor signs Motor signs usually are symmetrical Preservation of pupillary reactions usually occurs Asterixis, myoclonus, tremor, and seizures are common Acid–base imbalance with hyperventilation or hypoventilation is common
Psychiatric unresponsiveness	Lids close actively; pupils reactive or dilated (cycloplegics) Oculocephalic reflexes are unpredictable; oculovestibular reflexes are physiological (nystagmus is present) Motor tone is inconsistent or normal Eupnea or hyperventilation is usual No pathological reflexes are present Electroencephalogram (EEG) is normal

TABLE 15.3 Levels of Altered Consciousness

STATE	DEFINITION
Confusion	Loss of ability to think rapidly and clearly; impaired judgement and decision making
Disorientation	The person may exhibit restlessness, anxiety, and irritation; disorientation to time occurs first, followed by disorientation to place and familiar others (family members) and impaired memory; recognition of self is lost last
Lethargy	Limited spontaneous movement or speech; easy arousal with normal speech or touch; orientation to time, place, or person may or may not occur
Obtundation	Mild to moderate reduction in arousal (awakeness) with limited response to environment; falls asleep unless stimulated verbally or tactilely; answers questions with minimal response
Stupor	Condition of deep sleep or unresponsiveness from which person may be aroused or caused to open eyes only by vigorous and repeated stimulation; response is often withdrawal or grabbing at stimulus
Light coma	Associated with purposeful movement on stimulation
Coma	Associated with nonpurposeful movement only on stimulation
Deep coma	Associated with unresponsiveness or no response to any stimulus

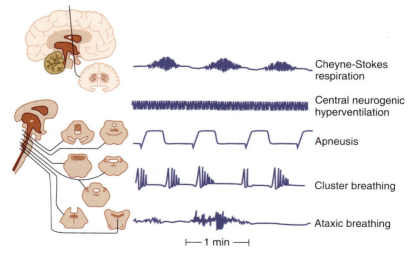

FIGURE 15.1 Abnormal Respiratory Patterns With Corresponding Level of Central Nervous System Activity. (From Urden, L. D., Stacy, K. M., & Lough, M. E. [2010]. *Critical care nursing: diagnosis and management* [6th ed.]. Mosby.)

TABLE 15.4 Patterns of Breathing

BREATHING PATTERN	DESCRIPTION	LOCATION OF INJURY
Hemispheric Breathing Patterns		
Normal	After a period of hyperventilation that lowers partial pressure of carbon dioxide in arterial blood ($PaCO_2$), the individual continues to breathe regularly but with reduced depth.	Response of nervous system to an external stressor—not associated with injury to central nervous system (CNS)
Posthyperventilation apnea	Respirations stop after hyperventilation has lowered partial pressure of carbon dioxide (PCO_2) level below normal. Rhythmic breathing returns when PCO_2 level returns to normal.	Associated with diffuse bilateral metabolic or structural disease of cerebrum
Cheyne-Stokes respirations	Breathing pattern has a smooth increase (crescendo) in rate and depth of breathing (hyperpnea), which peaks. A gradual smooth decrease (decrescendo) in rate and depth of breathing to the point of apnea follows when the cycle repeats itself. The hyperpneic phase lasts longer than the apneic phase.	Bilateral dysfunction of deep cerebral or diencephalic structures; seen with supratentorial injury and metabolically induced coma states
Brainstem Breathing Patterns		
Central neurogenic hyperventilation	A sustained, deep, rapid, but regular pattern (hyperpnea) occurs, with a decreased $PaCO_2$ and a corresponding increase in pH and PO_2.	May result from CNS damage or disease that involves midbrain and upper pons; seen after increased intracranial pressure and blunt head trauma
Apneusis	A prolonged inspiratory cramp (a pause at full inspiration) occurs; a common variant of this is a brief end-inspiratory pause of 2 or 3 seconds, often alternating with an end-expiratory pause.	Indicates damage to respiratory control mechanism located at pontine level; most associated with pontine infarction but documented with hypoglycemia, anoxia, and meningitis
Cluster breathing	A cluster of breaths has a disordered sequence with irregular pauses between breaths.	Dysfunction in lower pontine and high medullary areas
Ataxic breathing	Completely irregular breathing occurs, with random shallow and deep breaths and irregular pauses. The rate is often slow.	Originates from a primary dysfunction of medullary neurons controlling breathing
Gasping breathing pattern (agonal gasps)	A pattern of deep "all-or-none" breaths accompanied by a slow respiratory rate.	Indicative of a failing medullary respiratory centre

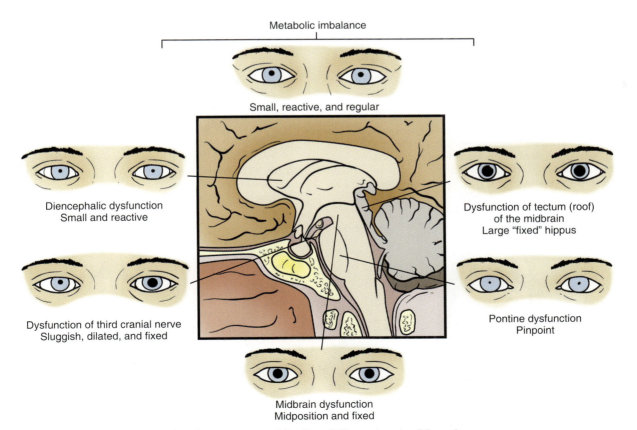

FIGURE 15.2 Appearance of Pupils at Different Levels of Consciousness.

commonly fixed to light. Opiates cause pinpoint pupils. Severe barbiturate intoxication may produce fixed pupils.

Oculomotor responses (resting, spontaneous, and reflexive eye movements) change at various levels of brain dysfunction in comatose individuals. Persons with metabolically induced coma, except with barbiturate-hypnotic and phenytoin poisoning, generally retain ocular reflexes even when other signs of brainstem damage are present. Destructive or compressive injury to the brainstem causes specific abnormalities of the oculocephalic and oculovestibular reflexes (Figures 15.3 and 15.4). Injuries that involve an oculomotor nucleus or nerve cause the involved eye to deviate outward. This deviation produces a resting dysconjugate lateral position of the eye.

Assessment of **motor responses** helps to evaluate the level of brain dysfunction. It also determines the most severely damaged side of the brain. The pattern of response noted may be (1) purposeful; (2) inappropriate, generalized motor movement; or (3) not present. Motor signs indicating loss of cortical inhibition that are commonly associated with decreased consciousness include primitive reflexes and rigidity (**paratonia**) (Figure 15.5). Primitive reflexes include grasping, reflex sucking, snout reflex, and palmomental reflex. All of these reflexes are normal in the newborn but disappear in infancy. Table 15.5 defines abnormal flexor and extensor responses in the upper and lower extremities and illustrated in Figure 15.6.

Vomiting, **yawning**, and **hiccups** are complex reflex-like motor responses that are integrated by neural mechanisms in the lower brainstem. Compression or diseases involving tissues of the medulla oblongata (e.g., infection, neoplasm, infarction) produce these responses but also occur relative to other more benign stimuli to the vagal nerve. Most CNS disorders produce nausea and vomiting. Vomiting without nausea indicates direct involvement of the central neural mechanism (or pyloric obstruction; see Chapters 36 and 37). Vomiting often accompanies CNS injuries that (1) involve the vestibular nuclei or its

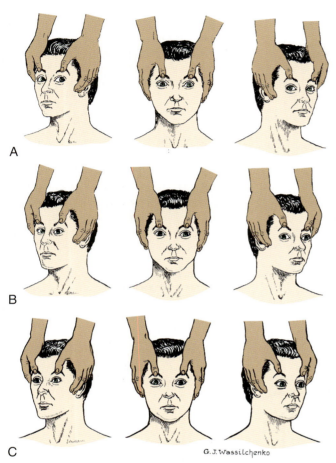

FIGURE 15.3 Test For Oculocephalic Reflex Response (Doll's Eyes Phenomenon). **A**, Normal response—eyes turn together to side opposite from turn of head. **B**, Abnormal response—eyes do not turn in conjugate manner. **C**, Absent response—eyes move in direction of head movement (brainstem injury). (From Rudy, E. B. [1984]. *Advanced neurological and neurosurgical nursing*. Mosby.)

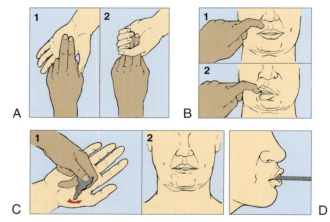

FIGURE 15.5 Pathological Reflexes. **A**, Grasp reflex. **B**, Snout reflex. **C**, Palmomental reflex (contraction of the mentalis muscle of the chin caused by stimulation of the thenar eminence at the base of the thumb). **D**, Suck reflex.

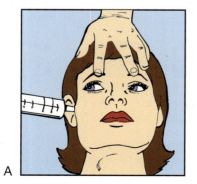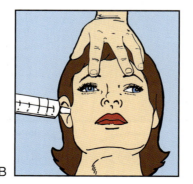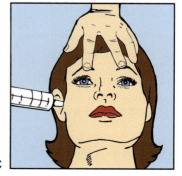

FIGURE 15.4 Test For Oculovestibular Reflex (Caloric Ice Water Test). **A**, Ice water is injected into the ear canal. Normal response—conjugate eye movements. **B**, Abnormal response—dysconjugate or asymmetrical eye movements. **C**, Absent response—no eye movements.

TABLE 15.5 Abnormal Motor Responses With Decreased Responsiveness

MOTOR RESPONSE	DESCRIPTION	LOCATION OF INJURY
Decorticate posturing/rigidity: upper extremity flexion, lower extremity extension	Slowly developing flexion of arm, wrist, and fingers with adduction in the upper extremity and extension, internal rotation, and plantar flexion of lower extremity	Hemispheric damage above midbrain releasing medullary and pontine reticulospinal systems
Decerebrate posturing/rigidity: upper and lower extremity extensor responses	Opisthotonos (hyperextension of vertebral column) with clenching of teeth; extension, abduction, and hyperpronation of arms; and extension of lower extremities	Associated with severe damage involving midbrain or upper pons
	In acute brain injury, shivering and hyperpnea may accompany unelicited recurrent decerebrate spasms	Acute brain injury often causes limb extension regardless of location
Extensor responses in upper extremities accompanied by flexion in lower extremities		Pons
Flaccid state with little or no motor response to stimuli		Lower pons and upper medulla

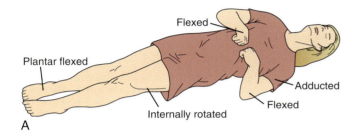

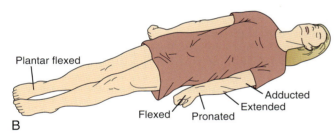

FIGURE 15.6 Decorticate and Decerebrate Posture/Responses. **A**, Decorticate posture/response. Flexion of arms, wrists, and fingers with adduction in upper extremities. Bilateral extension, internal rotation, and plantar flexion in lower extremities. **B**, Decerebrate posture/response. All four extremities in rigid extension with hyperpronation of forearms and plantar extension of feet. (From deWit, S. C., & Kumagai, C. K. [2013]. *Medical-surgical nursing* [2nd ed.]. Saunders.)

BOX 15.1 Canadian Minimal Criteria for Neurological Determination of Death

1. Established etiology capable of causing neurological death in the absence of reversible conditions capable of mimicking neurological death
2. Unresponsive coma with bilateral absence of motor responses, excluding spinal reflexes
3. No spontaneous respiration (apnea)
4. No brainstem functions, defined by absent gag and cough reflexes and the bilateral absence of corneal responses, pupillary responses to light, with pupils at mid-size or greater, and ocular responses to head turning or caloric stimulation (see Figures 15.3 and 15.4)
5. Absent confounding factors

From Shemie, S. D., Doig, C., Dickens, B., et al. (2006). Severe brain injury to neurological determination of death: Canadian forum recommendations. *Canadian Medical Association Journal, 174*(6), S1–S12. doi:10.1503/cmaj.045142. Copied under licence from Access Copyright. Further reproduction, distribution or transmission is prohibited except as otherwise permitted by law.

immediate projections, particularly when double vision (diplopia) also is present; (2) impinge directly on the floor of the fourth ventricle; or (3) produce brainstem compression secondary to an increase in intracranial pressure.

Outcomes of Alterations in Arousal

Outcomes of alterations in arousal fall into two categories: *extent of disability* (*morbidity*) and *mortality*. Outcomes depend on the cause and extent of brain damage and the duration of coma. Some individuals may recover consciousness and an original level of function. Some individuals may have permanent disability. Some individuals may never regain consciousness and experience neurological death. Two forms of neurological death—brain death and cerebral death—result from severe pathological conditions and are associated with irreversible coma. Other possible outcomes are a vegetative state, a minimally conscious state, or locked-in syndrome. The extent of disability has four subcategories: recovery of consciousness, residual cognitive function, psychological function, and vocational function.

Brain death (**total brain death**) occurs when the brain is damaged so completely that it can never recover (irreversible) and cannot maintain the body's internal homeostasis. Canadian guidelines define *brain death*, or *neurological determination of death* (NDD), as the irreversible cessation of all brainstem functions. Clear medical standards, including criteria and minimal testing for the determination of NDD, have been established. The abnormality of brain function must result from structural or known metabolic disease and must *not* be caused by a depressant medication, alcohol poisoning, or hypothermia.[1] Box 15.1 presents the clinical criteria used to determine brain death. When confirmation of any of the minimal clinical criteria does not occur, additional tests are required. Accepted additional tests include cerebral radiocontrast angiography and radionuclide angiography. The NDD in neonates, infants, and children includes the same criteria as for adults, with some additional recommendations.[2]

Cerebral death, or **irreversible coma**, is death of the cerebral hemispheres exclusive of the brainstem and cerebellum. Brain damage is permanent. The individual is forever unable to respond behaviourally in any significant way to the environment. The brainstem may continue to maintain internal homeostasis (i.e., body temperature, cardiovascular functions, respirations, and metabolic functions). The survivor of cerebral death may remain in a coma or emerge into a persistent vegetative state or a minimally conscious state. In coma, the eyes are usually closed with no eye opening. The person does not follow commands, speak, or have voluntary movement.[1]

A **persistent vegetative state (VS)** is complete unawareness of the self or surrounding environment and complete loss of cognitive function. The individual does not speak any comprehensible words or follow commands. Sleep–wake cycles are present, eyes open spontaneously, and blood pressure and breathing are maintained without support. Brainstem reflexes (pupillary, oculocephalic, chewing, swallowing) are intact but cerebral function is absent. There is bowel and bladder incontinence. Recovery is unlikely if the state persists for 12 months. In a **minimally conscious state (MCS)** individuals may follow simple commands, manipulate objects, gesture, or give yes/no responses, have intelligible speech, and have movements such as blinking or smiling.[1]

With **locked-in syndrome** there is complete paralysis of voluntary muscles except for eye movement. Content of thought and level of arousal are intact. A disruption of the efferent pathways occurs (injury at the base of the pons with the reticular formation intact, often caused by basilar artery occlusion).[3] Thus, the individual cannot communicate through speech or body movement but is fully conscious, with intact cognitive function. Vertical eye movement and blinking are a means of communication.

Alterations in Awareness

> **✓ QUICK CHECK 15.2**
> 1. Why is irreversible coma different from brain death?
> 2. What is the difference between anterograde and retrograde amnesia?
> 3. What is an example of neglect syndrome?

Awareness (content of thought) encompasses all cognitive functions. This includes awareness of self, environment, and affective states (i.e., moods). Awareness is mediated by all the core networks under the guidance of executive attention networks. These networks include selective attention and memory. Executive attention networks involve abstract reasoning, planning, decision making, judgement, error correction, and self-control. Each attentional function is a network of interconnected brain areas and not localized to a single brain area.

Selective attention (orienting) refers to the ability to select specific information to be processed from available, competing environmental and internal stimuli, and to focus on that stimulus (i.e., to concentrate on a specific task without being distracted).[4] *Selective visual attention* is the ability to select objects from multiple visual stimuli and process them to complete a task. *Selective auditory* or *hearing attention* is the ability to select or filter specific sounds and process them to complete a task. Multiple areas of the brain are involved in selective attention including cortical areas, thalamic nuclei, and the limbic system. **Selective attention deficits** can be temporary, permanent, or progressive. Disorders associated with selective attention deficits include seizure activity, parietal lobe contusions, subdural hematomas, stroke, gliomas or metastatic tumour, late Alzheimer's dementia, frontotemporal dementia, and psychotic disorders.

Memory is the recording, retention, and retrieval of information. **Amnesia** is the loss of memory and can be mild or severe. Two types of amnesia are retrograde amnesia and anterograde amnesia. The person experiencing **retrograde amnesia** has difficulty retrieving past personal history memories or past factual memories. **Anterograde amnesia** is the inability to form new personal or factual memories. The retention and retrieval of memories of the distant past can occur. **Image processing** is a higher level of memory function and includes the ability to use sensory data and language to form concepts, assign meaning, and make abstractions. Alterations in image processing include an inability to form concepts and generalizations or to reason. Thinking is very concrete. These **memory disorders** may be temporary (e.g., after a seizure) or permanent (e.g., after severe head injury or in Alzheimer's disease). There may be only the memory disorder, or the memory disorder may be associated with other cognitive disorders.

Executive attention deficits include the inability to maintain sustained attention and a working memory deficit. Sustained attention deficit is an inability to set goals and recognize when an object meets a goal. A working memory deficit is an inability to remember instructions and information needed to guide behaviour. Executive attention deficits may be temporary, progressive, or permanent. Attention-deficit/hyperactivity disorder (ADHD) is a common disorder of childhood that can continue through adulthood (Box 15.2). Table 15.6 summarizes alterations in attention and memory.

PATHOPHYSIOLOGY Generally, the primary pathophysiological mechanisms that operate in disorders of awareness are (1) direct destruction caused by ischemia and hypoxia or indirect destruction resulting from compression and (2) the effects of toxins and chemicals or metabolic disorders. Disorders of selective attention, at least as they relate to visual orienting behaviour, are produced by disease that involves portions of the midbrain. Disease affecting the superior colliculi manifests as a slowness in orienting attention. Parietal lobe disease may produce *unilateral neglect syndrome* or lack of awareness of one side of the body or lack of response to stimuli on one side of the body. This disease can occur after a stroke. An individual may groom or dress on only one side or eat food from only one side of the plate. **Sensory inattentiveness** is a form of neglect. The person can recognize individual sensory input from the dysfunctional side when asked but ignores the sensory input from the dysfunctional side when stimulated from both sides (**extinction**). The entire complex of denial of dysfunction, loss of recognition of one's own body parts, and extinction sometimes is referred to as hemineglect or **neglect syndrome**.

> **BOX 15.2   Attention-Deficit/Hyperactivity Disorder**
>
> Initially attention-deficit/hyperactivity disorder (ADHD) was considered a neurodevelopmental disorder of childhood. It is now known that 50 to 75% of persons diagnosed in childhood have continuing symptoms into adulthood. Often the diagnosis is made in adolescence or young adulthood at the time expected behavioural control and self-organization occurs. The ability to function at work, at home, and in social situations is often impaired. This impairment is related to inattentiveness, hyperactivity, impulsivity, and problems with executive function. Continued treatment including medications for symptomatic adults is supported. Substance abuse, which is more common in persons with ADHD, is reduced with continued treatment. The multifactorial patterns of inheritance and gene–environment interactions and the pathogenesis and pathophysiology of this complex disorder are under investigation. Findings from structural and functional neuroimaging suggest the involvement of developmentally abnormal brain networks related to cognition, attention, emotion, and sensorimotor functions. It is hoped that new findings will lead to improved prevention, diagnosis, treatment options, and functional outcomes.

Data from Baroni, A., & Castellanos, F. X. (2015). *Current Opinion in Neurobiology, 30*, 1–8; Harstad, E., & Levy, S. (2014). *Pediatrics, 134*(1), e293–e301; Matthews, M., Nigg, J. T., & Fair, D. A. (2014). *Current Topics in Behavioral Neurosciences, 16*, 235–266; Sharma, A., & Couture, J. (2014). *Annals of Pharmacotherapy, 48*(2), 209–225.

TABLE 15.6 Clinical Manifestations of Alterations in Attention and Memory

Deficit	Clinical Signs	Symptoms
Attention		
Selective attention (orienting)	Inability to focus attention; decreased eye, head, and body movements associated with focusing on stimuli; decreased search and scanning; faulty orientation to stimuli, causing safety problems	Person reports inability to focus attention, failure to perceive objects and other stimuli (history of injuries, falls, safety problems); can exhibit neglect syndrome (i.e., unilateral neglect with failure to groom or recognize one side of the body)
Memory		
Antegrade amnesia (inability to form new memories)	*Left hemisphere:* disorientation to time, situation, place, name, person (verbal identification); impaired language memory (e.g., names of objects); impaired semantic memory *Right hemisphere:* disorientation to self, person (visual), place (visual); impaired episodic memory (personal history); impaired emotional memory *Either or both hemispheres:* confusion; behavioural change	Person reports disorientation, confusion, "not listening," "not remembering"; reports by others of disorientation, not able to remember, not able to learn new information
Retrograde amnesia (loss of memories)	*Left hemisphere:* inability to retrieve personal history, past medical history; unaware of recent current events *Right hemisphere:* inability to recognize persons, places, objects, music, and so on from past	Person reports remote memory problems; others report that person cannot recall formerly known information
Image processing	Inability to categorize (identify similarities and differences) or sort; inability to form concepts; inability to analyze relationships; misinterpretations; inability to interpret proverbs	Reports by others of frequent misinterpretation of data, failure to conceptualize or generalize information
	Inability to perform deductive reasoning (convergent reasoning); inability to perform inductive reasoning (divergent reasoning); inability to abstract; concrete reasoning demonstrated; delusions	Reports by others of predominantly concrete thinking; lack of understanding of everyday situations, health care regimens, and such; delusional thinking
Executive Attention Deficits		
Vigilance	Failure to stay alert and orient to stimuli	Person reports decreased alertness or ability to orient
Detection	Lack of initiative (anergy); lack of ambition; lack of motivation; flat affect; no awareness of feelings; appears depressed, apathetic, and emotionless; fails to appreciate deficit; disinterested in appearance; lacks concern about childish or crude behaviour	Reports by others of laziness or apathy, flat affect, or lack of emotional expression; failure to exhibit or be aware of feelings
Mild	Responds to immediate environment but no new ideas; grooming and social graces are lacking	Reports by others of lack of ambition, motivation, or initiative; failure to carry out adult tasks; lack of social graces and new ideas
Severe	Motionless; lack of response to even internal cues; does not respond to physical needs; does not interact with surroundings	Reports by others of failure to groom or toilet self, unawareness of surroundings and own physical needs
	Inability to use feedback regarding behaviour; failure to recognize omissions and errors in self-care, speech, writing, and arithmetic; impaired cue utilization; overestimation of performance	Reports by others of not changing behaviour when requested; unawareness of limitations; does not recognize and correct errors in dressing, grooming, toileting, eating, and such; fails to recognize speech and arithmetic errors; careless speech
	Failure to shift response set; failure to change behaviour when conditions change; cue utilization may be impaired	Reports by others of failure to use feedback; inability to incorporate feedback (does not correct when feedback is given)
Working memory (recent or short-term memory)	Inability to set goals or form goals; indecisiveness	Reports by others of failure to set goals, indecisiveness
	Failure to make plans; inability to produce a complete line of reasoning; inability to make up a story; appears impulsive	Reports by others of failure to plan, impulsiveness, "does not think things through"
	Failure to initiate behaviour; failure to maintain behaviour; failure to discontinue behaviour; slowness to alternate response for the next step; motor perseveration	Reports by others of not knowing where to begin, inability to carry out sequential acts (maintain a behaviour), inability to cease a behaviour

A disorder in vigilance may be produced by disease in the prefrontal areas. Dysfunction in the right anterior cingulate gyrus and basal ganglia may cause detection problems. Problems with working memory may be produced with left lateral frontal injury. Anterograde amnesia originates from pathological conditions in the hippocampus and related temporal lobe structures; the diencephalic region including the thalamus; and the basal forebrain. Retrograde amnesia and higher-level memory deficits originate from pathological conditions in the widely distributed association areas of the cerebral cortex (Figure 13.7 C). Executive attention deficits are associated with alterations in the frontal and prefrontal cortex. This includes the anterior cingulate gyrus, supplementary motor area, and portions of the basal ganglia.

CLINICAL MANIFESTATIONS Table 15.6 presents the clinical manifestations of selective attention deficits, memory deficits, and executive attention function deficits.

EVALUATION AND TREATMENT Immediate medical management is directed at diagnosing the cause and treating reversible factors. Rehabilitative measures generally focus on compensatory or restorative activities. These measures have been assisted by computer technology and other electronic devices.

Data-Processing Deficits

> ✓ **QUICK CHECK 15.3**
> 1. What are two types of dysphasia?
> 2. How does dysphasia differ from dysarthria?
> 3. What are some causes of delirium?

Data-processing deficits are problems associated with recognizing and processing sensory information. This includes agnosia, dysphasia, and acute confusional states and delirium.

Agnosia

Agnosia is a defect of pattern recognition. It is a failure to recognize the form and nature of objects. Agnosia can be tactile, visual, or auditory, but generally only one sense is affected. For example, an individual may be unable to identify a safety pin by touching it with a hand but is able to name it when looking at it. Agnosia may be as minimal as a finger agnosia (failure to identify by name the fingers of one's hand) or more extensive, such as a colour agnosia. Although agnosia is associated most with cerebrovascular accidents, it may arise from any pathological process that injures specific areas of the brain.

Dysphasia

Dysphasia is impairment of comprehension or production of language with impaired communication. Comprehension or use of symbols, in either written or verbal language, is disturbed or lost. Aphasia is a more severe form of dysphasia and an inability to communicate using language. Often the terms *dysphasia* and *aphasia* are used interchangeably. Dysphasia results from dysfunction in the left cerebral hemisphere (i.e., Broca area [inferior frontal gyrus] and Wernicke area [superior temporal gyrus]) and the subcortical and cortical connecting networks (Figure 15.7 and see Figure 13.7). Dysphasias usually are associated with a cerebrovascular accident involving the middle cerebral artery or one of its many branches. Language disorders, however, may arise from a variety of injuries and diseases. This includes vascular, neoplastic, traumatic, degenerative, metabolic, or infectious causes. Most language disorders result from acute processes or a chronic residual deficit of the acute process.

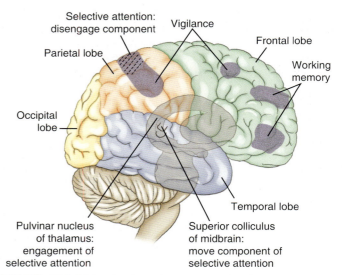

FIGURE 15.7 Right Cortical, Subcortical, and Brainstem Areas of the Brain Mediating Cognitive Function. (From Boss, G. J., & Wilkerson, R. [2008]. Communication: language and pragmatics. In S. P. Hoeman [Ed.], *Rehabilitation nursing: prevention, intervention & outcomes* [4th ed., p. 508]. Mosby.)

Classifications of dysphasias are anatomical (i.e., Wernicke or Broca area dysphasias) or functional as disorders of fluency (quality and content of speech). *Expressive dysphasia* (also known as Broca, motor, or nonfluent dysphasia) involves loss of ability to produce spoken or written language, with slow or difficult speech. Verbal comprehension is usually present. Expressive dysphasia is differentiated from *dysarthria*, in which words cannot be spoken clearly because of cranial nerve damage or muscle impairment. *Receptive dysphasia* (also known as Wernicke, sensory, or fluent dysphasia) involves an inability to understand written or spoken language. Speech is fluent, flowing at a normal rate, but words and phrases have no meaning. *Anomic aphasia* is a sensory aphasia distinguished by difficulty finding words and naming a person or object. Circumlocution, or describing an object as a way of trying to name something, is common in anomic aphasia. Auditory comprehension is present in *conductive dysphasia*, but there is impaired verbatim repetition. Naming also can be impaired. The person recognizes the errors and tries to correct them. Speech is fluent but words and sounds may be transposed. Damage is in the left hemisphere to networks that connect Broca and Wernicke areas. *Transcortical dysphasias* are rare and can be motor, sensory, or mixed. They involve areas of the brain that connect into the language centres. *Global dysphasia* is the most severe dysphasia and involves both expressive and receptive dysphasia. The individual is nonfluent or mute; cannot read or write; and has impaired comprehension, naming, reading, and writing. Global dysphasia is usually associated with a cerebrovascular accident involving the middle cerebral artery. Table 15.7 compares types of dysphasias, and Table 15.8 illustrates some of the language disturbances. Pure dysphasias are rare and are often mixed, making diagnosis difficult. All types of dysphasia usually improve with speech rehabilitation.

Acute Confusional States and Delirium

Acute confusional states (also may be known as *acute organic brain syndromes*) are transient disorders of awareness and may have either a sudden or a gradual onset. Delirium is a type of acute confusional state, but for this discussion acute confusional states and delirium are synonymous. Box 15.3 summarizes the many medical conditions associated with delirium.

TABLE 15.7 Major Types of Dysphasia

Type	Expression	Verbal Comprehension	Repetition	Reading Comprehension	Writing	Location of Lesion	Cause of Lesion
Expressive							
Broca, nonfluent or motor aphasia	Cannot find words, difficulty writing	Relatively intact	Impaired	Variable	Impaired	Left posteroinferior frontal lobe (Broca area)	Occlusion of one or several branches of left middle cerebral artery supplying inferior frontal gyrus
Transcortical motor, nonfluent dysphasia	Halting speech	Intact	Intact	Impaired	Impaired	Anterior superior frontal lobe	Occlusion at the border zone between two arterial territories
Receptive							
Wernicke, receptive fluent or sensory dysphasia	Meaningless verbal language, inappropriate words or unable to monitor language for correctness so errors are not recognized. Intonation, accent, cadence, rhythm, and articulation normal	Impaired; disturbance in understanding all language	Impaired	Impaired	Impaired	Left posterosuperior temporal lobe (Wernicke area)	Occlusion of inferior division of left middle cerebral artery
Conductive dysphasia	Difficulty repeating words, phrases spoken to them; naming is impaired	Intact	Severely impaired	Variable	Variable	Inferior and posterior temporal lobe; parietotemporal junction	Occlusion in distributions of left middle cerebral artery
Anomic dysphasia	Hesitancy, difficulty recalling names, objects, or numbers	Intact	Impaired	Variable	Intact except for anomia	Left temporoparietal zones; arcuate fasciculus	Diffuse left hemisphere brain disease
Transcortical sensory, fluent dysphasia	Repeats words and phrases spoken to them	Poor	Intact	Impaired	Impaired	Posterior temporal lobe	Occlusion at the border zone between two cerebral arterial territories
Other							
Transcortical mixed motor and sensory, nonfluent	Repeats words and phrases spoken to them	Impaired	Intact	Impaired	Impaired	Left cerebral hemisphere; spares the perisylvian cortex	Occlusion at the border zone between two cerebral arterial territories
Global or nonfluent; summation of motor and sensory aphasia	Mute	Impaired	Impaired	Impaired	Impaired	Large areas of the left cortex and subcortical regions	Occlusion of left middle cerebral artery of left internal carotid artery, tumours, other mass lesions, hemorrhage, embolic occlusion of ascending parietal or posterior temporal branch of middle cerebral artery

TABLE 15.8 Examples of Dysphasia

Disorder	Example
Receptive Dysphasia	
Wernicke/Fluent/Sensory Dysphasia	
Verbal paraphasia	*Question:* What did the car do?
	Patient: The car would spit sweetly down the road. (The car sped swiftly down the road.)
Conductive	*Request:* Say, "Persistence is essential to success."
	Patient: Mesastence is instans to success.
Neologism	*Question:* What do you call this? (Pointing to a plant.)
	Patient: It's a logper.
Anomic aphasia (circumlocution example)	*Question:* What do you call this? (Pointing to a plant.)
	Patient: Something that grows.
	Patient: It's …
	Or
	Question: What did you do this morning?
	Patient: Reading.
	Question: Were you reading a book or newspaper?
	Patient: One of those.
Expressive Dysphasia	
Nonfluent/Broca/Motor Dysphasia	
Telegraphic style	*Question:* Where is your daughter? *Patient:* Calgary … home … Monday.

From Boss, B. J. (1984). Dysphasia, dyspraxia, and dysarthria: distinguishing features, Part I. *Journal of Neurosurgical Nursing*, 16(3), 151–160.

BOX 15.3 Conditions Causing Acute Confusional States or Delirium

- Drug intoxication
- Alcohol or drug withdrawal
- Metabolic disorders (e.g., hypoglycemia, thyroid storm)
- Brain trauma or surgery
- Post anaesthesia
- Febrile illnesses or heat stroke
- Electrolyte imbalance, dehydration
- Heart, kidney, or liver failure

PATHOPHYSIOLOGY Acute confusional states arise from disruption of a widely distributed neural network. This network involves the reticular activating system of the upper brainstem and its projections into the thalamus, basal ganglion, and specific association areas of the cortex and limbic areas. Delirium (hyperactive confusional state) is associated with autonomic nervous system overactivity. This condition typically develops over 2 to 3 days. It most commonly occurs in Critical Care Units, following surgery, or during withdrawal from CNS depressants (i.e., alcohol or narcotic agents). Delirium is associated with right-upper middle-temporal gyrus or left temporal-occipital junction disruption, and several neurotransmitters (i.e., acetylcholine and dopamine) are involved.[5] Excited delirium syndrome (ExDS), is also known as *agitated delirium*. It is a type of hyperkinetic delirium that can lead to sudden death. Its symptoms include altered mental status, combativeness, aggressiveness, tolerance to significant pain, rapid breathing, sweating, severe agitation, elevated temperature, noncompliance, or poor awareness in following direction, inability to become fatigued, unusual or superhuman strength, and inappropriate clothing for the current environment. Hypoactive delirium (hypoactive confusional state) is more likely to be associated with right-sided frontal-basal ganglion disruption.

Most metabolic disturbances (i.e., hypoglycemia, thyroid disorders, liver, or kidney disease) that produce delirium interfere with neuronal metabolism or synaptic transmission. Many drugs and toxins also interfere with neurotransmission function at the synapse.

CLINICAL MANIFESTATIONS Delirium initially manifests as difficulty in concentrating, restlessness, irritability, insomnia, tremulousness, and poor appetite. Some persons experience seizures. Unpleasant, even terrifying, dreams or hallucinations may occur. In a fully developed delirium state, the individual is completely inattentive, and gross alteration of perceptions occurs with extensive misperception and misinterpretation. The person appears distressed and often perplexed. Conversation is incoherent. Frank tremor and high levels of restless movement are common. Violent behaviour may be present. The individual cannot sleep, experiences flushing, has dilated pupils, a rapid pulse rate (tachycardia), elevated temperature, and profuse sweating (diaphoresis). Delirium typically abates suddenly or gradually in 2 to 3 days. Occasionally delirium states persist for weeks.

Hypoactive delirium is associated with underactivity. This condition may occur in individuals who have fevers or metabolic disorders (i.e., chronic liver or kidney failure) or who are under the influence of CNS depressants. The individual exhibits decreases in mental function, specifically alertness, attention span, accurate perception, interpretation of the environment, and reaction to the environment. Forgetfulness and apathy are prominent, speech may be slow, and the individual dozes frequently.

EVALUATION AND TREATMENT The initial goals are to (1) establish that the individual is confused and (2) determine the cause of the confusion (organic or functional) (Table 15.9). The next step is to differentiate whether the confusion is delirium or an underlying dementia. Individuals with dementia are at increased risk of developing delirium. A complete history, physical examination, and laboratory tests (electrocardiogram and blood, urine, cerebrospinal fluid [CSF], and radiological studies) are needed. Several assessment scales are available to guide evaluation (such as Clinical Assessment of Confusion A and B, Confusion Assessment Method for the Intensive Care Unit [CAM-ICU], and Intensive Care Delirium Screening Checklist).[6–9] After the cause is identified, treatment is directed at controlling the primary disorder with supportive measures used as appropriate. Delirium is preventable in some individuals.[1] Table 15.10 contains a comparison of the features differentiating delirium and dementia.

Dementia

Dementia is an acquired deterioration and a progressive failure of many cerebral functions. Symptoms include impairment of intellectual processes with a decrease in orienting, memory, language, judgement, and decision making. Because of declining intellectual ability, the individual may exhibit alterations in behaviour. Examples of these alterations include agitation, wandering, and aggression.

PATHOPHYSIOLOGY Mechanisms leading to dementia include neuron degeneration, compression of brain tissue, atherosclerosis of cerebral vessels, and brain trauma. Genetic predisposition is associated with the neuro-degenerative diseases. These diseases include Alzheimer's, Huntington's, and Parkinson's diseases. CNS infections, including the human immunodeficiency virus (HIV) and slow-growing viruses

TABLE 15.9 Differences Between Organic and Functional Confusion

Factor	Organic Confusion	Functional Confusion
Memory impairment	Recent more impaired than remote	No consistent difference between recent and remote
Disorientation		
Time	Within own lifetime or reasonably near future	May not be related to person's lifetime
Place	Familiar place or one where person might easily be found	Bizarre or unfamiliar places
Person	Sense of identity usually preserved	Sense of identity diminished
	Misidentification of others as familiar	Misidentification of others based on delusion system
Hallucinations	Visual, vivid	Auditory more frequent
	Animals and insects common	Bizarre and symbolic
Illusions	Common	Not prominent
Delusions	Concern everyday occurrences and people	Bizarre and symbolic
Confused	Spotty confusion	More consistent
	Clear intervals mixed with confused episodes	No tendency to become worse at night
	Worse at night	

From Morris, M., & Rhodes, M. (1972). Guidelines for the care of confused patients. *American Journal of Nursing, 72*(9), 1632.

TABLE 15.10 Comparison of Delirium and Dementia

FEATURE	DELIRIUM	DEMENTIA
Age	Usually older	Usually older
Onset	Acute—common during hospitalization	Usually insidious; acute in some cases of strokes/trauma
Associated conditions	Urinary tract infection, thyroid disorders, hypoxia, hypoglycemia, toxicity, fluid–electrolyte imbalance, renal insufficiency, trauma, postsurgical anaesthesia	May have no other conditionsBrain trauma
Course	Fluctuating/reversible with treatment	Chronic slow decline
Duration	Hours to weeks	Months to years
Attention	Impaired	Intact early; often impaired late
Sleep–wake cycle	Disrupted	Usually normal
Alertness	Impaired	Normal
Orientation	Impaired	Intact early; impaired late
Behaviour	Agitated, withdrawn or depressed	Intact early
Speech	Incoherent, rapid, or slowed	Word-finding problems
Thoughts	Disorganized, delusions	Impoverished
Perceptions	Hallucinations/illusions	Usually intact early

Adapted from Caplan, J. P., & Rabinowitz, T. (2010). An approach to the patient with cognitive impairment: delirium and dementia. *Medical Clinics of North America, 94*(6), 1103–1116, ix.

associated with Creutzfeldt-Jakob disease, also lead to nerve cell degeneration and brain atrophy.

CLINICAL MANIFESTATIONS Table 15.11 presents clinical manifestations of the major dementias.

EVALUATION AND TREATMENT Establishing the cause for dementia may be complicated. Evaluation of individuals with clinical manifestations of dementia should include laboratory and neuropsychological testing to identify underlying conditions that may be treatable. Unfortunately, no specific cure exists for most progressive dementias. Therapy is directed at maintaining and maximizing use of the remaining capacities, restoring functions if possible, and accommodating to lost abilities. Helping the family to understand the process and to learn ways to assist the individual is essential.

Alzheimer's Disease

Alzheimer's disease (AD) (dementia of Alzheimer's type [DAT], senile disease complex) is the leading cause of severe cognitive dysfunction in older adults. The three forms of AD are nonhereditary sporadic or late-onset AD (70 to 90%), early-onset familial AD (FAD), and early-onset AD (very rare). More than 500 000 Canadians have AD or another form of dementia. Expectations are that the numbers will increase to 912 000 by 2030.[10]

PATHOPHYSIOLOGY The exact cause of AD is unknown. Early-onset FAD has been linked to three genes with mutations on chromosome 21 (abnormal amyloid precursor protein 14 *[APP14]*, abnormal presenilin 1 *[PSEN1]*, and abnormal presenilin 2 *[PSEN2]*). Late-onset AD may be related to the involvement of chromosome 19 with the apolipoprotein E gene-allele 4 *(APOE4)*. Studies are ongoing to classify the genetic variations of AD.[11] DNA methylation is an epigenetic marker for AD.[12] Sporadic late-onset AD is the most common form and does not have a specific genetic association. However, the cellular pathology of sporadic late-onset AD is the same as that for gene-associated early- and late-onset AD.[13] Pathological alterations in the brain include accumulation of extracellular neuritic plaques containing a core of amyloid beta protein, intraneuronal neurofibrillary tangles, and degeneration of basal forebrain cholinergic neurons with loss of acetylcholine. Failure to process and clear amyloid

TABLE 15.11 Clinical Manifestations of the Major Degenerative Dementias

Disease	First Symptom	Mental Status	Neurobehaviour	Neurological Examination
Alzheimer's disease	Memory loss; impaired learning	Episodic memory loss	Initially normal, progressive cognitive impairment	Initially normal
Creutzfeldt-Jakob disease	Dementia, mood, anxiety, movement disorders	Variable, frontal/executive, focal cortical, memory	Depression, anxiety	Myoclonus, rigidity, parkinsonism
Dementia with Lewy body	Visual hallucinations; delusions that family members/friends are someone else; REM sleep disorder; delirium; parkinsonism	Drawing and frontal/executive; spares memory; delirium prone	Visual hallucinations, depression, sleep disorder, delusions	Parkinsonism
Frontotemporal dementia	Apathy; poor judgement/reasoning, speech/language	Frontal/executive, language; spares drawing	Apathy, decline in person or social conduct, euphoria, depression	Due to PSP/CBD overlap; vertical gaze palsy, axial rigidity, dystonia, alien hand
Vascular dementia	Often but not always sudden, usually within 3 months of a stroke; variable: apathy, falls, focal weakness	Frontal/executive, cognitive slowing; memory can be intact	Apathy, delusions, anxiety	Usually motor slowing; can be normal

CBD, Cortical basal degeneration; *PSP*, progressive supranuclear palsy; *REM*, rapid eye movement.
Adapted from Bird, T. D., & Miller, B. L. (2008). Dementia. In A. S. Fauci, E. Braunwald, D. L. Kasper, et al. (Eds.), *Harrison's principles of internal medicine* (17th ed., p. 2538). McGraw-Hill.

precursor protein results in the accumulation of toxic fragments of amyloid beta protein. This accumulation leads to formation of diffuse neuritic plaques, disruption of nerve impulse transmission, and death of neurons. The tau protein, a microtubule-binding protein in neurons, detaches and forms an insoluble filament called a **neurofibrillary tangle**, contributing to neuronal death (Figure 15.8). Neuritic plaques and neurofibrillary tangles are more concentrated in the cerebral cortex and hippocampus. The loss of neurons results in brain atrophy with widening of sulci and shrinkage of gyri (see Figure 15.8). Loss of synapses, acetylcholine, and other neurotransmitters contributes to the decline of memory and attention, and to the loss of other cognitive functions associated with AD.[14]

CLINICAL MANIFESTATIONS AD has a long preclinical and prodromal course. Pathophysiological changes can occur decades before the appearance of the clinical dementia syndrome. The disease progresses from mild short-term memory deficits culminating in total loss of cognitive and executive functions. Initial clinical manifestations are insidious. These manifestations are often attributed to forgetfulness, emotional upset, or other illness. The individual becomes progressively more forgetful over time, particularly in relation to recent events. Memory loss increases as the disorder advances. The person becomes disoriented and confused and loses the ability to concentrate. Abstraction, problem solving, and judgement gradually deteriorate with failure in mathematical calculation ability, language, and visuospatial orientation. **Dyspraxia** may appear. The mental status changes induce behavioural changes, including irritability, agitation, and restlessness. Mood changes also result from the deterioration in cognition. The person may become anxious, depressed, hostile, emotionally labile, and prone to mood swings. Motor changes may occur if the posterior frontal lobes are involved. The motor changes cause rigidity and flexion posturing. Weight loss can be significant. Great variability in age of onset, intensity and sequence of symptoms, and location and extent of brain abnormalities is common. Table 15.12 summarizes the stages for the progression of AD.

EVALUATION AND TREATMENT The diagnosis of AD is made by ruling out other causes. Clinical criteria have been developed to assist diagnosis.[15] The clinical history, including mental status examinations

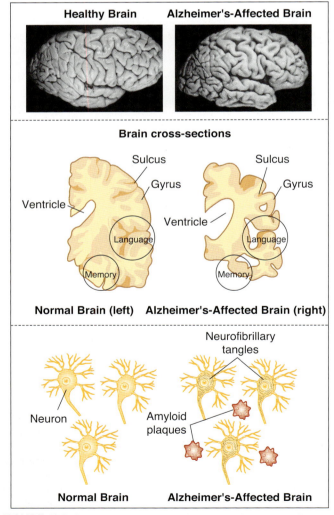

FIGURE 15.8 Common Pathological Findings in Alzheimer's Disease. The middle panel represents coronal slices through the left brain (facing anterior).

TABLE 15.12 Progression of Alzheimer's Disease

Stage	Mild Cognitive Impairment	Early Stage	Middle Stage	Late Stage	End Stage
Cognitive	Mild memory loss	Measurable short-term memory loss; difficulty with word finding; other cognition problems compared with previous behaviour	Moderate to severe cognitive problems: impaired reasoning, judgement, and problem solving; disorientation to time, place, and person; difficulty planning and organizing; progressive memory loss	Little cognitive ability; language not clear	No significant cognitive function; loss of orientation to self
Functional	Possibly depression (versus apathy); mild anxiety	Mild IADL problems	IADL-dependent; some ADL problems	ADL-dependent; incontinent	Nonambulatory/bedbound; unable to eat related to failure to sense hunger or thirst, difficulty swallowing

ADL, (Basic) activities of daily living; IADL, instrumental activities of daily living.
Adapted from National Conference of Gerontological Nurse Practitioners and the National Gerontological Nursing Association. (2008). Current treatment options and management strategies in Alzheimer's disease and related dementias. *Counseling Points, 1*(1), 4–13. https://www.gapna.org/sites/default/files/download/CounselingPoints/cp2008Vol1Num2.pdf; Peña-Casanova, J., Sánchez-Benavides, G., de Sola-Llopis, S., et al. (2012). Neuropsychology of Alzheimer's disease. *Archives of Medical Research, 43*(8), 686–693.

(Mini–Mental Status Examination, clock drawing, and Geriatric Depression Scale), laboratory tests, brain imaging of structure, blood flow and metabolism, and the course of the illness (which may span 5 years or more), is used to assess progression of the disease. Efforts are in progress to identify imaging and biochemical markers for risk assessment and early diagnosis and progression of Alzheimer's type and other neuro-degenerative causes of dementia.[16,17] See *Health Promotion: Reducing Risk Factors Associated With Alzheimer's Disease.*

HEALTH PROMOTION
Reducing Risk Factors Associated with Alzheimer's Disease

When considering risk factors and the likelihood of becoming affected by a certain disease, four main characteristics are identified: (1) the characteristics of the person, (2) lifestyle, (3) environment, and (4) genetic background. When considering Alzheimer's disease, risk factors do not cause the disease but rather increase the chance of being affected by the disease. Nonmodifiable risk factors include age and genetic makeup. However, some risk factors are modifiable. The Alzheimer Society of Canada states that maintaining a healthy lifestyle can help reduce the risk for Alzheimer's disease and other dementias. Several key modifiable risk factors include: (1) diabetes, (2) hypertension, (3) obesity, (4) smoking, (5) depression, (6) cognitive inactivity or low education, (7) physical inactivity, (8) poor diet, (9) high alcohol intake, (10) head injuries, (11) hearing loss, and (12) social isolation.

Data from Alzheimer Society Canada. (2021). *Risk factors.* https://alzheimer.ca/en/about-dementia/how-can-i-prevent-dementia/risk-factors-dementia.

Treatment is directed at using devices to compensate for the impaired cognitive function. These devices include memory aids; maintaining unimpaired cognitive functions; and maintaining or improving the general state of hygiene, nutrition, and health. Cholinesterase inhibitors have shown a modest effect on cognitive function in mild to moderate AD. An N-methyl-D-aspartate (NMDA) receptor antagonist blocks glutamate activity and may slow progression of disease in moderate to severe AD. The development of treatments, beginning in the preclinical stage to prevent, modify, or halt disease pathology are underway.[18,19]

Frontotemporal Dementia

Frontotemporal dementia (FTD), previously known as **Pick disease**, is the second most common form of dementia. FTD is a degenerative disease of the frontal and anterior frontal lobes. There is a familial association with an age of onset less than 60 years and an estimated incidence of 15 per 100 000. Most cases involve mutations of genes encoding tau protein. There are three distinct clinical syndromes identified in frontotemporal degeneration, depending on the site of atrophy: (1) behavioural variant of FTD, (2) progressive nonfluent aphasia, and (3) semantic dementia. Differentiating pathological and clinical diagnostic criteria are in development.[20,21] There is no specific treatment.

Seizure Disorders

Seizure disorders represent a manifestation of disease and not a specific disease entity. A **seizure** is a sudden, transient disruption in brain electrical function caused by abnormal excessive discharges of cortical neurons. **Epilepsy** is the recurrence of seizures and a type of seizure disorder for which no underlying, correctable cause for the seizure can be found. The use of the term **convulsion** sometimes is used to describe seizures and refers to the tonic-clonic (jerky, contract-relax) movement associated with some seizures. Chapter 17 presents seizures in children.

Conditions Associated With Seizure Disorders

Any disorder that alters the neuronal environment may cause seizure activity. There are many conditions that may produce a seizure. These conditions include metabolic disorders, congenital malformations, genetic predisposition, perinatal injury, postnatal trauma, myoclonic syndromes, infection, brain tumour, vascular disease, and medication or alcohol abuse. The onset of seizures also may indicate the presence of an ongoing primary neurological disease. Table 15.13 summarizes the structural and metabolic causes of recurrent seizures in adults. The cause of seizures is often unknown.

Several factors may lower the threshold for seizures. These factors include hypoglycemia, fatigue, or lack of sleep, emotional or physical stress, fever, large amounts of water ingestion, constipation, use of antipsychotic medications (i.e., chlorpromazine [Largactil] and clozapine [Clozaril]) especially when combined with alcohol, withdrawal from depressant medications (including alcohol), or hyperventilation (respiratory alkalosis). Some environmental stimuli, such as blinking lights, a poorly adjusted television screen, loud noises, certain music, certain odours, or being startled, have been known to initiate a seizure. Women may have increased seizure activity immediately before or during menses.

Types of Seizure

> ✓ **QUICK CHECK 15.4**
> 1. What is an epileptogenic focus?
> 2. Why can so many conditions trigger seizures?
> 3. Why is a continued seizure dangerous?

The classification of seizures occurs by clinical manifestations, site of origin, electroencephalogram (EEG) correlates, or response to therapy. Chapter 17 presents the types of seizures and clinical manifestations (see Table 17.6). Table 15.14 defines the terms used to describe seizure activity.

TABLE 15.13 Structural and Metabolic Causes of Recurrent Seizures in Adults

Age At Onset	Probable Cause
Young adults (18 to 35 years)	Alcohol or drug withdrawal (e.g., barbiturates, benzodiazepines)
	Brain tumour
	Idiopathic
	Illicit drug use (e.g., cocaine, amphetamine)
	Post-traumatic brain injury
	Perinatal insults
Older adults (>35 years)	Alcohol or drug withdrawal (e.g., barbiturates, benzodiazepines)
	Brain tumour
	Cerebrovascular disease (e.g., stroke, aneurysm, arteriovenous malformations, infection)
	Central nervous system degenerative diseases (e.g., Alzheimer's disease, multiple sclerosis)
	Idiopathic
	Metabolic disorders (e.g., uremia, hepatic failure, electrolyte abnormalities, hypoglycemia)
	Post-traumatic brain injury

Data from Daroff, R. B., Fenichel, G. M., Jankovic, J., et al. (2012). *Bradley's neurology in clinical practice* (6th ed.). Saunders.

TABLE 15.14 Terminology Applied to a Seizure Disorder

Term	Definition
Preictal Phase	
Prodroma	Early clinical manifestation (such as malaise, headache, or sense of depression) that may occur a few days to hours before onset of a seizure
Aura	A partial seizure experienced as a peculiar sensation preceding onset of generalized seizure that may take the form of gustatory, visual, or auditory experience or a feeling of dizziness, numbness, or just "a funny feeling"
Ictal Phase	The event of the seizure
Tonic phase	A state of muscle contraction in which there is excessive muscle tone
Clonic phase	A state of alternating contraction and relaxation of muscles
Postictal Phase	Time period immediately following cessation of seizure activity

Epilepsy is the result of the interaction of complex genetic mutations with environmental effects that cause abnormalities in synaptic transmission, an imbalance in the brain's neurotransmitters, or the development of abnormal nerve connections after injury.[22] A group of neurons may exhibit a paroxysmal depolarization shift and function as an **epileptogenic focus**. These neurons are hypersensitive and are more easily activated by hyperthermia, hypoxia, hypoglycemia, hyponatremia, repeated sensory stimulation, and certain sleep phases. Epileptogenic neurons fire more frequently and with greater amplitude. When the intensity reaches a threshold point, cortical excitation spreads. Excitation of the subcortical, thalamic, and brainstem areas corresponds to the **tonic phase** (muscle contraction with increased muscle tone) and is associated with loss of consciousness. The **clonic phase** (alternating contraction and relaxation of muscles) begins when inhibitory neurons in the cortex, anterior thalamus, and basal ganglia react to the cortical excitation. The seizure discharge is interrupted, producing intermittent muscle contractions that gradually decrease and finally cease. The epileptogenic neurons are exhausted.

During seizure activity, consumption of oxygen is high—about 60% greater than normal. Although **cerebral blood flow (CBF)** also increases, oxygen and glucose are rapidly depleted, and lactate accumulates in brain tissue. Continued severe seizure activity has the potential for progressive brain injury and irreversible damage. In addition, if a seizure focus in the brain is active for a prolonged period, a **mirror focus** may develop in contralateral normal tissue and cause seizure activity.

CLINICAL MANIFESTATIONS The clinical manifestations associated with seizure depend on its type (see Table 17.6). Two types of symptoms signal the **preictal phase** of a generalized tonic-clonic seizure. The **prodroma** is early manifestations occurring hours to days before a seizure and may include anxiety, depression, or inability to think clearly; and a partial seizure that immediately precedes the onset of a generalized tonic-clonic seizure. Both may become familiar to the person experiencing recurrent generalized seizures and may enable the person to prevent injuries during the seizure. The **ictus** is the episode of the epileptic seizure with tonic-clonic activity. Relaxation of urinary and bowel sphincters may occur, leading to bladder and bowel incontinence. The maintenance of an airway is essential. **Status epilepticus** in adults is (1) a state of continuous seizures lasting more than 5 minutes, or (2) rapidly recurring seizures before the person has fully regained consciousness from the preceding seizure, or (3) a single seizure lasting more than 30 minutes. The **postictal phase** follows an epileptic seizure. Symptoms include headache, confusion, dysphasia, memory loss, and paralysis that may last hours or a day or two. Deep sleep also is common.[1]

EVALUATION AND TREATMENT The health history, physical examination, and laboratory tests of blood and urine can identify systemic diseases known to promote seizures. These tests include concentrations of blood glucose, serum calcium, blood urea nitrogen, and urine sodium, and creatinine clearance. Brain imaging and CSF examination help identify neurological diseases associated with seizures. The type of seizure and location in the brain tissue is identified using an EEG.

Treatment for a seizure disorder is to first correct or control its cause. If this treatment is not possible, the major means of management is the judicious administration of antiseizure medications. Dietary treatments (e.g., ketogenic and Atkins diet) are effective for some individuals. Surgical interventions can improve seizure control and quality of life in people with medication-resistant epilepsy.[23] Vagus nerve stimulation can reduce seizure frequency in persons with drug resistant focal seizures.[23]

CHAPTER 15 Alterations in Cognitive Systems, Cerebral Hemodynamics, and Motor Function

ALTERATIONS IN CEREBRAL HEMODYNAMICS

> **QUICK CHECK 15.5**
> 1. What are the four stages of increased intracranial pressure?
> 2. How does supratentorial herniation differ from infratentorial herniation?
> 3. What are the different types of cerebral edema?
> 4. How is communicating hydrocephalus different from noncommunicating hydrocephalus?

An injured brain reacts with structural, chemical, and pathophysiological changes. Primary brain injury is the original trauma. Secondary brain injury is a consequence of alterations in CBF, **intracranial pressure (ICP)**, and oxygen delivery (Box 15.4 and see Chapter 16).

Alterations in CBF may be related to three injury states: (1) inadequate cerebral perfusion, (2) normal cerebral perfusion but with an elevated ICP, and (3) excessive **cerebral blood volume (CBV)**. Treatments for these injury states aim to improve or maintain **cerebral perfusion pressure (CPP)** and control ICP.

BOX 15.4 Cerebral Hemodynamics

Cerebral blood flow to the brain is normally maintained at a rate that matches local metabolic needs of the brain.
Cerebral perfusion pressure (70 to 90 mm Hg) is the pressure required to perfuse the cells of the brain.
Cerebral blood volume is the amount of blood in the intracranial vault at a given time.
Cerebral blood oxygenation is measured by oxygen saturation in the internal jugular vein.
Intracranial pressure normally is 1 to 15 mm Hg, or 60 to 180 cm H_2O.

Increased Intracranial Pressure

Increased intracranial pressure (increased ICP) may result from an increase in intracranial content (as occurs with tumour growth), edema, excess CSF, or hemorrhage. It requires an equal reduction in volume of the other cranial contents. The most readily displaced content is CSF. If ICP remains high after CSF displacement out of the cranial vault, the alteration of CBV and blood flow occurs.

In *stage 1 of intracranial hypertension*, vasoconstriction and external compression of the venous system occur to further decrease the ICP. During the first stage of intracranial hypertension, ICP may not change because of the effective compensatory mechanisms. As a result, there may no detectable symptoms (Figure 15.9). Small increases in volume, however, cause an increase in pressure, and the pressure may take longer to return to baseline. Detection of this pressure change occurs with ICP monitoring.

In *stage 2 of intracranial hypertension*, continued expansion of intracranial contents. The resulting increase in ICP may exceed the ability of the brain's compensatory mechanisms to adjust. The pressure begins to compromise neuronal oxygenation. As a result, systemic arterial vasoconstriction occurs to elevate the systemic blood pressure sufficiently to overcome the increased ICP. Clinical manifestations at this stage usually are subtle and transient. The manifestations include episodes of confusion, restlessness, drowsiness, and slight pupillary and breathing changes (see Figure 15.9). Interventions at this stage reduce ICP and promote better clinical outcomes.

In *stage 3 of intracranial hypertension*, ICP begins to approach arterial pressure. The brain tissues begin to experience hypoxia and hypercapnia, and the individual's condition rapidly deteriorates. Clinical manifestations include decreasing levels of arousal or central neurogenic hyperventilation, widened pulse pressure, bradycardia, and small, sluggish pupils (see Figure 15.9).

Dramatic sustained rises in ICP are not seen until all compensatory mechanisms have been exhausted. Then dramatic rises in ICP occur over a very short period. **Autoregulation**, the compensatory alteration in the

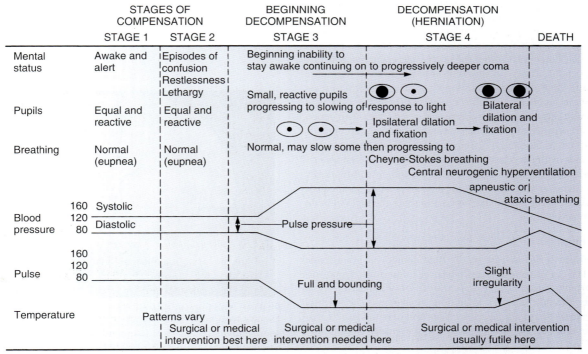

FIGURE 15.9 Clinical Correlates of Compensated and Uncompensated Stages of Intracranial Hypertension. (From Beare, P. G., & Myers, J. L. [1998]. *Principles and practice of adult health nursing* [3rd ed.]. Mosby.)

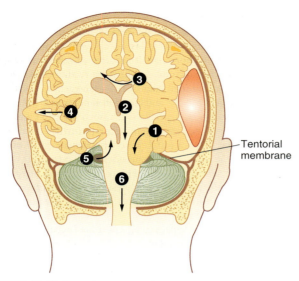

FIGURE 15.10 Brain Herniation Syndromes. Herniations can occur both above and below the tentoria membrane. Supratentorial: **1**, uncal (transtentorial); **2**, central; **3**, cingulate; **4**, transcalvarial (external herniation through an opening in the skull). Infratentorial: **5**, upward herniation of cerebellum; **6**, cerebellar tonsillar move down through foramen magnum.

diameter of the intracranial blood vessels designed to maintain a constant blood flow during changes in CPP, is lost with progressively increased ICP. Accumulating carbon dioxide may still cause vasodilation locally. Without autoregulation this vasodilation causes the blood pressure in the vessels to drop and the blood volume to increase. The brain volume is further increased and ICP continues to rise. Small increases in volume cause dramatic increases in ICP, and the pressure takes much longer to return to baseline. As the ICP begins to approach systemic blood pressure, CPP falls, and cerebral perfusion slows dramatically. The brain tissues experience severe hypoxia, hypercapnia, and acidosis.

In *stage 4 of intracranial hypertension*, brain tissue shifts (herniates) from the compartment of greater pressure to a compartment of lesser pressure. An increased ICP in one compartment of the cranial vault is not evenly distributed throughout the other vault compartments (see Figures 15.9 and 15.10). With this shift in brain tissue, compromise of the herniating brain tissue's blood supply occurs. This factor causes further ischemia and hypoxia in the herniating tissues. The volume of content within the lower pressure compartment increases. This action exerts pressure on the brain tissue that normally occupies that compartment. As a result, its blood supply is impaired. For example, herniation into the brainstem impairs the vital cardiovascular and respiratory regulatory centres and can cause death. The herniation process markedly and rapidly increases ICP. Mean systolic arterial pressure soon equals ICP, and CBF ceases at this point. Box 15.5 outlines the types of brain herniation syndromes.

Cerebral Edema

Cerebral edema is an increase in the fluid content of brain tissue (Figure 15.11). An increase in extracellular or intracellular tissue volume is the result. It occurs after brain insult from trauma, infection, hemorrhage, tumour, ischemia, infarction, or hypoxia. The harmful effects of cerebral edema are caused by distortion of blood vessels, displacement of brain tissues, increase in ICP, and eventual herniation of brain tissue to a different brain compartment.

Three types of cerebral edema are (1) vasogenic edema, (2) cytotoxic (metabolic) edema, and (3) interstitial edema. Vasogenic edema

BOX 15.5 Brain Herniation Syndromes

Supratentorial Herniation

1. *Uncal herniation.* It occurs when the uncus or hippocampal gyrus, or both, shifts from the middle fossa through the tentorial notch into the posterior fossa, compressing the ipsilateral third cranial nerve, the contralateral third cranial nerve, and the mesencephalon. Uncal herniation generally is caused by an expanding mass in the lateral region of the middle fossa. The classic manifestations of uncal herniation are a decreasing level of consciousness, pupils that become sluggish before fixing and dilating (first the ipsilateral, then the contralateral pupil), Cheyne-Stokes respirations (which later shift to central neurogenic hyperventilation), and the appearance of decorticate and then decerebrate posturing.
2. *Central herniation.* It occurs when there is a straight downward shift of the diencephalon through the tentorial notch. It may be caused by injuries or masses located around the outer perimeter of the frontal, parietal, or occipital lobes; extracerebral injuries around the central apex (top) of the cranium; bilaterally positioned injuries or masses; and unilateral cingulate gyrus herniation. The individual rapidly becomes unconscious; moves from Cheyne-Stokes respirations to apnea; develops small, reactive pupils and then dilated, fixed pupils; and passes from decortication to decerebration.
3. *Cingulate gyrus herniation.* It occurs when the cingulate gyrus shifts under the falx cerebri. Little is known about its clinical manifestations.
4. *Transcalvarial.* The brain shifts through a skull fracture or a surgical opening in the skull. This type of external herniation may occur during a craniectomy—surgery in which a removal of a flap of skull occurs. This type of herniation prevents replacement of the piece of skull.

Infratentorial Herniation

1. The most common syndrome is *cerebellar tonsillar*. The cerebellar tonsil shifts through the foramen magnum because of increased pressure within the posterior fossa. The clinical manifestations are an arched stiff neck, paresthesias in the shoulder area, decreased consciousness, respiratory abnormalities, and pulse rate variations. Occasionally the force produces an *upward transtentorial* herniation of a cerebellar tonsil or the lower brainstem. There is an increase in intracranial pressure, but no specific set of clinical manifestations associated with infratentorial herniation (see Figure 15.10).

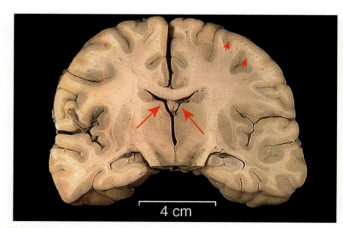

FIGURE 15.11 Brain Edema. This coronal section of the cerebrum demonstrates marked compression in the lateral ventricles *(long arrows)* and flattening of gyri *(short arrows)* from extensive bilateral cerebral edema. Edema increases intracranial pressure, leading to herniation. (From Klatt, E. C. [2010]. *Robbins and Cotran atlas of pathology* [2nd ed.]. Saunders.)

is clinically the most important type. It is caused by the increased permeability of the capillary endothelium of the brain after injury to the vascular structure. The selective permeability of capillaries that comprise the blood–brain barrier is disrupted. Plasma proteins leak into the extracellular spaces, drawing water to them and increasing the water content of the brain parenchyma. Vasogenic edema begins in the area of injury and spreads. Fluid accumulates in the white matter of the ipsilateral side because the parallel myelinated fibres separate more easily. Edema promotes more edema because of ischemia from the increasing ICP.

Clinical manifestations of vasogenic edema include focal neurological deficits, disturbances of consciousness, and a severe increase in ICP. Vasogenic edema resolves by slow diffusion.

In cytotoxic (metabolic) edema, toxic factors directly affect the cellular elements of the brain parenchyma (neuronal, glial, and endothelial cells). These factors cause failure of the active transport systems. The cells lose their potassium and gain larger amounts of sodium. Water follows by osmosis into the cells, so that the cells swell. Cytotoxic edema occurs principally in the grey matter and may increase vasogenic edema.

Interstitial edema is seen most often with noncommunicating hydrocephalus. Transependymal movement of CSF from the ventricles into the extracellular spaces of the brain tissues causes edema. The brain fluid volume increases mainly around the ventricles, with increased hydrostatic pressure within the white matter. Reduction in the size of the white matter occurs because of the rapid disappearance of myelin lipids.

Hydrocephalus

The term hydrocephalus refers to various conditions characterized by excess fluid in the cerebral ventricles, subarachnoid space, or both. Hydrocephalus occurs because of interference with CSF flow. Causes include increased fluid production, obstruction within the ventricular system, or defective reabsorption of the fluid. A tumour of the choroid plexus may, in rare instances, cause overproduction of CSF. Table 15.15 reviews the types of hydrocephalus.

Hydrocephalus may develop from infancy through adulthood. Communicating hydrocephalus is faulty resorption of CSF from the cerebral subarachnoid space. This defect occurs more often in adults. Noncommunicating hydrocephalus (internal hydrocephalus, intraventricular hydrocephalus) is obstruction within the ventricular system. This defect occurs more often in children (see Figure 17.6). Congenital hydrocephalus is ventricular enlargement before birth and is rare.

PATHOPHYSIOLOGY The obstruction of CSF flow associated with hydrocephalus produces increased pressure and dilation of the ventricles proximal to the obstruction. The increased pressure and dilation cause atrophy of the cerebral cortex and degeneration of the white matter tracts. Selective preservation of grey matter occurs. When excess CSF fills a defect caused by atrophy, a degenerative disorder, or a surgical excision, this fluid is not under pressure. As a result, atrophy and degenerative changes do not occur.

CLINICAL MANIFESTATIONS Most cases of hydrocephalus develop gradually and insidiously over time. Acute hydrocephalus presents with signs of rapidly developing increased ICP. The person quickly deteriorates into a deep coma if not promptly treated. Normal-pressure hydrocephalus (dilation of the ventricles without increased pressure) develops slowly, with the individual or family noting declining memory and cognitive function. The triad symptoms of an unsteady, broad-based gait with a history of falling; incontinence; and dementia are common.

EVALUATION AND TREATMENT The diagnosis is based on physical examination, computed tomography (CT) scan, and magnetic resonance imaging (MRI). The completion of a radio isotopic cisternogram may diagnose normal-pressure hydrocephalus. Treatment of hydrocephalus can include surgery to resect cysts, neoplasms, or hematomas or by ventricular bypass into the normal intracranial channel or into an extracranial compartment using a shunting procedure. Shunting is one of the three most common neurosurgical procedures. When a papilloma is present, excision or coagulation of the choroid plexus occasionally occurs. In normal-pressure hydrocephalus, reduction in CSF occurs through diuresis or placement of a ventriculoperitoneal shunt.[24]

ALTERATIONS IN NEUROMOTOR FUNCTION

TABLE 15.15 Types of Hydrocephalus

Type	Mechanism	Cause
Noncommunicating	Obstruction of CSF flow between ventricles	Congenital abnormality
	Aqueduct stenosis	
	Arnold-Chiari malformation (brain extension through foramen magnum)	
	Compression by tumour	
Communicating	Impaired absorption of CSF within subarachnoid space	Infection with inflammatory adhesions
	Compression of subarachnoid space by a tumour	
	High venous pressure in sagittal sinus	
	Head injury	
	Congenital malformation	
	Increased CSF secretion by choroid plexus	Secreting tumour

CSF, Cerebrospinal fluid.

> **QUICK CHECK 15.6**
> 1. Why are there so many causes of hypertonia?
> 2. How is chorea different from athetosis?
> 3. Why is paresis/paralysis a type of hypokinesia?
> 4. What structures are involved in alterations of complex motor performance?

Movements are complex patterns of activity controlled by the cerebral cortex, the pyramidal system, the extrapyramidal system, and the motor units. Dysfunction in any of these areas can cause motor dysfunction. General neuromotor dysfunctions are associated with changes in muscle tone, movement, and complex motor performance.

Alterations in Muscle Tone

Normal muscle tone involves a slight resistance to passive movement. Throughout the range of motion, the resistance is smooth, constant, and even. Table 15.16 presents the alterations of muscle tone and their characteristics and causes.

Hypotonia

In hypotonia (decreased muscle tone), passive movement of a muscle occurs with little or no resistance. Causes include cerebellar damage

TABLE 15.16 Alterations in Muscle Tone

Alterations	Characteristics	Cause
Hypotonia	Passive movement of a muscle mass with little or no resistance Muscles may be moved rapidly without resistance	Thought to be caused by decreased muscle spindle activity because of decreased excitability of neurons (e.g., muscular dystrophy, cerebral palsy)
Flaccidity	Associated with limp, atrophied muscles, and paralysis	Occurs typically when nerve impulses necessary for muscle tone are lost
Hypertonia	Increased muscle resistance to passive movement May be associated with paralysis May be accompanied by muscle hypertrophy	Results when lower motor unit reflex arc continues to function but is not mediated or regulated by higher centres (e.g., stroke, brain tumours, multiple sclerosis)
Spasticity	A gradual increase in tone causing increased resistance until tone suddenly diminishes, which results in clasp-knife phenomenon; increased deep tendon reflexes (hyperreflexia); clonus (spread of reflexes)	Exact mechanism unclear; appears to arise from an increased excitability of alpha motor neurons to any input because of absence of descending inhibition of pyramidal systems (e.g., multiple sclerosis, brain trauma, cerebral palsy)
Paratonia (gegenhalten)	Resistance to passive movement, which varies in direct proportion to force applied	Exact mechanism unclear; associated with frontal lobe injury (e.g., progressive Alzheimer's dementia)
Dystonia	Sustained involuntary muscle contraction with twisting movement	Produced by slow muscular contraction; lack of reciprocal inhibition of muscle (e.g., neuroleptic medication adverse effects, meningitis)
Rigidity	Muscle resistance to passive movement of a rigid limb that is uniform in both flexion and extension throughout the motion	Occurs because of constant, involuntary contraction of muscle—usually involves extrapyramidal tracts (e.g., Parkinson's disease)
Plastic or lead-pipe rigidity	Increased muscular tone relatively independent of degree of force used in passive movement; does not vary throughout the passive movement	Associated with basal ganglion damage (e.g., Parkinson's disease)
Cogwheel rigidity	Uniform resistance may be interrupted by a series of brief jerks, resulting in movements much like a ratchet, cogwheel phenomenon	Associated with basal ganglion damage
Gamma rigidity	Characterized by extensor posturing (decerebrate rigidity)	Loss of excitation of extensor inhibitory areas by cerebral cortex decreasing inhibition of alpha and gamma motor neurons
Alpha rigidity	Impaired relaxation characterized by extensor rigidity of skeletal muscle after contraction	Loss of cerebellum input to lateral vestibular nuclei

and pure pyramidal tract damage (a rare occurrence). The hypotonia contributes to the ataxia and intention tremor in cerebellar damage. Hypotonia manifests with minimal weakness and normal or slightly exaggerated reflexes. A pure pyramidal tract injury produces hypotonia and weakness. Hypotonia also occurs when the nerve impulses needed for muscle tone are lost. This can occur in spinal cord injury or cerebrovascular accident.

Individuals with hypotonia tire easily or are weak. They may have difficulty rising from a sitting position, sitting down without using arm support, walking up and down stairs, and an inability to stand on their toes. Because of their weakness, accidents during ambulatory and self-care activities are common. The joints become hyperflexible, so persons with hypotonia may be able to assume positions that require extreme joint mobility. The joints may appear loose. The muscle mass atrophies because of decreased input entering the motor unit. Muscles appear flabby and flat. Gradual replacement of muscle cells by connective tissue and fat occurs. Fasciculations may be present in some cases.

Hypertonia

In **hypertonia** (increased muscle tone), passive movement of a muscle occurs with resistance to stretch. It is caused by upper motor neuron damage (see Table 15.16). The four types of hypertonia are **spasticity** (usually corticospinal in origin) (Figures 15.12 and 15.13), **paratonia (gegenhalten)**, dystonia (Figure 15.14), and **rigidity** (usually extrapyramidal in origin). Four types of rigidity include: plastic or lead-pipe, cogwheel, gamma (independent of stretch reflex pathways), and alpha (dependent on stretch reflex pathways) (see Table 15.16).

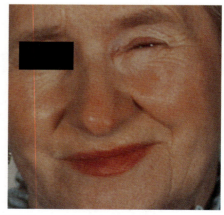

FIGURE 15.12 Paroxysm of Left-sided Hemifacial Spasm. (From Perkin, G. D. [2002]. *Mosby's color atlas and text of neurology* [2nd ed.]. Mosby.)

Individuals with hypertonia tire easily or are weak. Passive movement and active movement are affected equally, except in paratonia. In paratonia more active than passive movement is possible. As a result of hypertonia and weakness, accidents occur during ambulatory and self-care activities.

The muscles may atrophy because of decreased use. However, hypertrophy occasionally occurs because of the overstimulation of muscle fibres. Overstimulation occurs when the motor unit reflex arc remains intact and functioning. It is not inhibited by higher centres.

CHAPTER 15 Alterations in Cognitive Systems, Cerebral Hemodynamics, and Motor Function

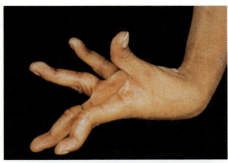
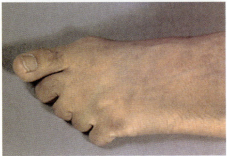

FIGURE 15.13 Dystonic Posturing of the Hand and Foot. (From Perkin, G. D. [2002]. *Mosby's color atlas and text of neurology* [2nd ed.]. Mosby.)

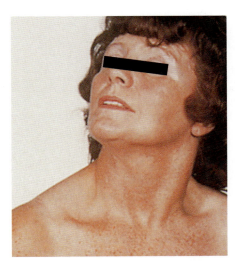

FIGURE 15.14 Spasmodic Torticollis. A characteristic head posture related to spasticity. (From Perkin, G. D. [2002]. *Mosby's color atlas and text of neurology* [2nd ed.]. Mosby.)

This lack of higher-centre inhibition causes continual muscle contraction, resulting in enlargement of the muscle mass and the development of firm muscles.

Alterations in Muscle Movement

Movement requires a change in the contractile state of muscles. Abnormal movements occur when CNS dysfunction alters muscle innervation. The neurotransmitter *dopamine* has a role in several movement disorders. Some movement disorders (e.g., the akinesias) result from too little dopaminergic activity. Other disorders (e.g., chorea, ballism, tardive dyskinesia) result from too much dopaminergic activity. Still others are not primarily related to dopamine function. Movement disorders are not necessarily associated with muscle mass, strength, or tone. Some disorders are neurological dysfunctions resulting in insufficient or excessive movement or involuntary movement.

Hyperkinesia is excessive, purposeless movement and represents the second broad category of abnormal movements. Within this category are several specific dysfunctions including tremors (Table 15.17). Also included under the general category of hyperkinesias are *dyskinesias* and abnormal involuntary movements. Huntington's disease symptoms are the hallmark of hyperkinesia.

Paroxysmal dyskinesias are abnormal, involuntary movements that occur as spasms. The type of dyskinesia varies depending on the specific disorder.

Tardive dyskinesia is the involuntary movement of the face, lip, tongue, trunk, and extremities. Although the condition occurs occasionally in individuals with Parkinson's disease, it usually occurs as an adverse effect of prolonged antipsychotic medication therapy. The most common symptom of tardive dyskinesia is rapid, repetitive, stereotypical movements. These movements include continual chewing with intermittent protrusions of the tongue, lip smacking, and facial grimacing. The symptoms are called *extrapyramidal symptoms* because the extrapyramidal system controls involuntary reflexes and coordination of movement and posture (see Table 15.19).

Other movement disorders in this category are (1) complex repetitive movements, including automatism (unconscious behaviour), stereotypy (ritualistic behaviour such as rocking), complex tics such as Tourette syndrome (see *Health Promotion*: Tourette Syndrome), compulsions, perseverations, and mannerisms; (2) excessive reactions to certain stimuli; and (3) paroxysmal excessive activity, including cataplexy and excessive startle reaction.

HEALTH PROMOTION
Tourette Syndrome

There is growing evidence that Tourette syndrome (TS) occurs worldwide and has common features across all races and cultures. The hallmark of TS is the presence of motor tics (sudden, rapid, repetitive nonrhythmic movements) and vocal tics. The tics may be either simple, involving only an individual muscle group (e.g., eye blinking or grunting), or complex, requiring coordinated movement of muscle groups (e.g., head banging or repeating of another person's words). The syndrome has a complex multifactorial etiology with undetermined genetic, environmental, immune, and hormonal factors. Recent research has indicated that exposure to certain environmental factors during the prenatal, perinatal, and postnatal periods may impact the onset and progression of TS. The pregnancy-related exposures include maternal smoking and prenatal life stressors. Other factors that may cause a worsening of TS-related tics include low birth weight and forceps use during delivery. Further studies have also indicated that exposure to certain pathogens may be linked to the disease. Additional studies exploring these relationships may hold promise for the improvement of the course of TS related to these modifiable risk factors.

Data from Hoekstra, P. J., Dietrich, A., Edwards, M. J., et al. (2013). *Neuroscience & Biobehavioral Reviews, 37*(6), 1040–1049.

Hypokinesia is decreased amplitude of movement. Bradykinesia is decreased speed of movement. Akinesia is absence of voluntary movement. All these terms represent a deficit of voluntary movement. Parkinson's disease symptoms are the hallmark of a lack of voluntary movement.

Huntington's Disease

Huntington's disease (HD), also known as *chorea*, is a relatively rare, hereditary, degenerative hyperkinetic movement disorder diffusely involving the basal ganglia and cerebral cortex. The onset of HD is usually between 25 and 45 years of age, when the trait may already have

TABLE 15.17	Types of Hyperkinesia and Tremor	
Type	Characteristics	Causes
Hyperkinesia		
Chorea[a]	Nonrepetitive muscular contractions, usually of extremities of face; random pattern of irregular, involuntary rapid contractions of groups of muscles; disappears with sleep, decreases with resting; increases with emotional stress and attempted voluntary movement	Associated with excess concentration of or super sensitivity to dopamine within basal ganglia
Athetosis[a]	Disorder of distal muscle postural fixation; slow, sinuous, irregular movements most obvious in distal extremities, more rhythmic than choreiform movements and always much slower; movements accompany characteristic hand posture; slowly fluctuating grimaces	Occurs most commonly as result of injury to putamen of basal ganglion; exact pathophysiological mechanism is not known
Ballism	Disorder of proximal muscle postural fixation with wild flinging movement of limbs; movement is severe and stereotyped, usually lateral; does not lessen with sleep; ballism is most common on one side of body, a condition termed *hemiballism*	Results from injury to subthalamic nucleus (one of nuclei that comprise basal ganglia); thought to be caused by reduced inhibitory influence in nucleus, a release phenomenon; hemiballism results from injury to contralateral subthalamic nucleus
Hyperactivity	State of prolonged, generalized, increased activity that is largely involuntary but may be subject to some voluntary control; not highly stereotyped but rather manifests as continuous changes in total body posture or in excessive performance of some simple activity, such as pacing under inappropriate circumstances	Frontal and reticular activating system injury may be the cause
Wandering	Tendency to wander without regard for environment	"Release phenomenon" associated with bilateral injury to globus pallidus or putamen
Akathisia	Special type of hyperactivity; mild compulsion to move (usually more localized to legs); severe, frenzied motion possible; movements are partly voluntary and may be transiently suppressed; carrying out movement brings sense of relief; frequent complication of antipsychotic medications	Dopaminergic transmission may be involved
Tremor at Rest		
Parkinsonian tremor	Rhythmic, oscillating movement affecting one or more body parts Regular, rhythmic, slower flexion–extension contraction; involves principally metacarpophalangeal and wrist joints; alternating movements between thumb and index finger described as "pill rolling"; disappears during voluntary movement	Caused by regular contraction of opposing groups of muscles Loss of inhibitory influence of dopamine in the basal ganglia, causing instability of basal ganglial feedback circuit within cerebral cortex
Postural Tremor		
Asterixis (tremor of hepatic encephalopathy)	Irregular flapping movement of hands accentuated by outstretching arms	Exact mechanisms responsible unknown; thought to be related to accumulation of products normally detoxified by liver (e.g., ammonia)
Metabolic	Rapid, rhythmic tremor affecting fingers, lips, and tongue; accentuated by extending body part; enhanced physiological tremor	Occurs in conditions associated with disturbed metabolism or toxicity, as in thyrotoxicosis (hyperthyroidism), alcoholism, and chronic use of barbiturates, amphetamines, lithium, or amitriptyline (Elavil); exact mechanism responsible unknown
Essential (familial)	Tremor of fingers, hands, and feet; absent at rest but accentuated by extension of body part, prolonged muscular activity, and stress	Not associated with any other neurological abnormalities; cause unknown
Intention Tremor		
Cerebellar	Tremor initiated by movement, maximal toward end of movement	Occurs in disease of dentate nucleus (one of deep cerebellar nuclei responsible for efferent output) and superior cerebellar peduncle (stalk-like structure connected to pons); caused by errors in feedback from periphery and errors in preprogramming goal-directed movement
Rubral	Rhythmic tremor of limbs that originates proximally by movement	Results from lesions involving dentatorubrothalamic tract (a spinothalamic tract connecting red nucleus in reticular formation and dentate nucleus in cerebellum)
Myoclonus	Series of shock-like, nonpatterned contractions of portion of a muscle, entire muscle, or group of muscles that cause throwing movements of a limb; usually appear at random but frequently triggered by sudden startle; do not disappear during sleep	Associated with an irritable nervous system and spontaneous discharge of neurons; structures associated with myoclonus include cerebral cortex, cerebellum, reticular formation, and spinal cord

[a]Choreoathetosis involves both chorea and athetosis; precise pathophysiology is unknown.

been passed to the person's children. Approximately 1 in 7 000 people in Canada has HD.[25]

PATHOPHYSIOLOGY HD is inherited from one or both parents who have the autosomal dominant trait with high penetrance. The genetic defect of HD is on the short arm of chromosome 4. There is an abnormally long polyglutamine tract in the huntingtin (htt) protein that is toxic to neurons caused by a cytosine-adenine-guanine (CAG) trinucleotide repeat expansion (40 to 70 repeats instead of 9 to 34) with abnormal protein folding. Age of symptom onset is related to the length of the repeat sequences and mechanisms of toxicity. Repeat lengths greater than 60 cause the juvenile form of the disease.[26] Fathers, but not mothers, with high normal alleles do not develop HD but are at risk of transmitting potentially penetrant HD alleles (greater than or equal to 36) to their offspring, who can develop HD.[27]

The principal pathological feature of HD is severe degeneration of the basal ganglia, particularly the caudate nucleus. Tangles of protein (htt protein) collect in the brain cells and chains of glutamine on the abnormal molecules stick to each other and contribute to neuronal loss. Basal ganglia and nigral depletion of gamma-aminobutyric acid (GABA), an inhibitory neurotransmitter, is the principal biochemical alteration in HD. It alters the integration of motor and mental function.[28]

CLINICAL MANIFESTATIONS Symptoms of HD progress slowly. Symptoms include involuntary fragmentary movements, such as chorea, athetosis, and ballism (see Table 15.17). Chorea, the most common type of abnormal movement, begins in the face and arms, eventually affecting the entire body. There is emotional lability and progressive dysfunction of intellectual and thought processes (dementia). Any one of these features may mark the onset of the disease. Cognitive deficits include loss of working memory and reduced capacity to plan, organize, and sequence. Thinking is slow, and apathy is present. Restlessness, disinhibition, and irritability are common. Euphoria or depression may be present.

EVALUATION AND TREATMENT The diagnosis of HD is based on family history and clinical presentation of the disorder. Demonstration of neuroradiological abnormalities can occur up to 15 years before clinical symptoms. No known treatment is effective in halting the degeneration or progression of symptoms, and the disease is fatal. Symptomatic medication therapies are available.[29]

Hypokinesia

Hypokinesia (decreased movement) is loss of voluntary movement despite preserved consciousness and normal peripheral nerve and muscle function. Types of hypokinesia include akinesia, bradykinesia, and loss of associated movement.

Akinesia and bradykinesia. *Akinesia* is a decrease in voluntary and associated movements. It is related to dysfunction of the extrapyramidal system. It is caused by either a deficiency of dopamine or a defect of the postsynaptic dopamine receptors, which occurs in parkinsonism. *Bradykinesia* is slowness of voluntary movements. All voluntary movements become slow, laboured, and deliberate, with difficulty in (1) initiating movements, (2) continuing movements smoothly, and (3) performing synchronous (at the same time) and consecutive tasks. Both akinesia and bradykinesia involve a delay in the time it takes to start to perform a movement.

Loss of associated movement. In hypokinesia, the normal, habitually associated movements that provide skill, grace, and balance to voluntary movements are lost. Decreased associated movements accompanying emotional expression cause an expressionless face, a statue-like posture, absence of speech inflection, and absence of spontaneous gestures. Decreased associated movements accompanying locomotion cause reduction in arm and shoulder movements, hip swinging, and rotary motion of the cervical spine.

Parkinson's Disease

Parkinson's disease (PD) is a complex motor disorder accompanied by systemic nonmotor and neurological symptoms. Etiological classification of parkinsonism includes primary parkinsonism and secondary parkinsonism. Primary PD begins after the age of 40 years, with the incidence increasing after age 60 years. It is more prevalent in males and a leading cause of neurological disability in individuals older than 60 years. From 2013 to 2014, approximately 84 000 Canadians aged 40 years and older were living with parkinsonism.[30] With an aging population, estimates state that the number of Canadians with parkinsonism will double between 2011 and 2031. The familial form represents about 10% of PD. Most cases are sporadic or idiopathic. *Secondary parkinsonism* is parkinsonism caused by disorders other than PD (i.e., head trauma, infection, neoplasm, atherosclerosis, toxins, medication intoxication). Medication-induced parkinsonism, caused by neuroleptics, antiemetics, and antihypertensives, is the most common secondary form and usually is reversible.

PATHOPHYSIOLOGY The pathogenesis of primary PD is unknown. Several gene mutations have been identified that influence nerve function in PD. Gene–environment interactions are probable causes of neurodegeneration in PD. The primary pathology is degeneration of the basal ganglia (see Figure 13.10) with dysfunctional or misfolded α-synuclein protein and loss of dopamine-producing neurons in the substantia nigra and posterior striatum. The resulting depletion of dopamine, an inhibitory neurotransmitter, and relative excess of cholinergic (excitatory) activity in the feedback circuit are manifested by hypertonia (tremor and rigidity) and akinesia. These symptoms produce a syndrome of abnormal movement called *parkinsonism* (**Parkinson's syndrome, parkinsonian syndrome, paralysis agitans**) (Figure 15.15). Neuroimaging shows degeneration of dopaminergic neurons preceding the onset of motor symptoms by as long as 3 to 6 years.[31] Dementia may develop over decades with infiltration of Lewy bodies (accumulation of abnormal protein in nerve cells) and plaque formation like AD.[32] Loss of cholinergic subcortical input into the cortex is associated with nonmotor symptoms of PD.[33]

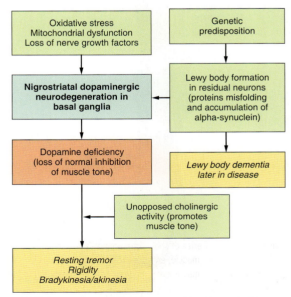

FIGURE 15.15 Pathophysiology of Parkinson's Disease.

CLINICAL MANIFESTATIONS The classic manifestations of PD are resting tremor, rigidity, bradykinesia or akinesia, postural disturbance, dysarthria, and dysphagia. They may develop alone or in combination. As the disease progresses, all symptoms are usually present. There is no true paralysis. The symptoms are always bilateral but usually involve one side early in the illness. Because the onset is insidious, the beginning of symptoms is difficult to document. Early in the disease, reflex status, sensory status, and mental status usually are normal. Loss of smell can be an early nonmotor symptom. Postural abnormalities (flexed, forward leaning), difficulty walking, and weakness develop as neurodegeneration progresses (Figure 15.16). Slurring of speech may occur.

Disorders of equilibrium result from postural abnormalities. The person with PD cannot make the appropriate postural adjustment to tilting or falling and falls like a post when starting to tilt. The festinating gait (short, accelerating steps) of the individual with PD is an attempt to maintain an upright position while walking. Individuals are also unable to right themselves when changing from a reclining or crouching position to a standing position, and when rolling over from a supine to a lateral or prone position. Sleep disorders and excessive daytime sleepiness are commonly experienced. Sensory disturbances (pain and impaired smell and vision), urinary urgency, difficulty concentrating, depression, and hallucinations are some of the nonmotor symptoms of PD.[37,38] Autonomic–neuroendocrine changes also contribute to nonmotor symptoms. These symptoms include inappropriate diaphoresis, orthostatic hypotension, drooling, gastric retention, constipation, and urinary retention.

Progressive dementia is more common in persons older than 70 years. Further compromise of mental status may occur by the adverse effects of the medication taken to control symptoms.

EVALUATION AND TREATMENT The diagnosis of PD is based on the history and the clinical features of the disease. Causes of secondary parkinsonism are first excluded. Specific gene panels and imaging studies are evolving for early diagnosis.[34] Treatment of PD is symptomatic with medication therapy to decrease akinesia. Because of troublesome adverse effects and loss of effectiveness, initiation of medication therapy may occur until the symptoms become incapacitating. Deep brain stimulation (i.e., subthalamic neurostimulation) is replacing surgery to treat persons unresponsive to medication therapy. Implants of stem cells and fetal cells, as well as gene therapy, are strategies for future treatments.[35] Dysphagia and general immobility are special problems of the individual with PD requiring interdisciplinary efforts to improve functional status.[36]

Upper and Lower Motor Neuron Syndromes

Paresis and paralysis are symptoms of upper and lower motor neuron syndromes (Table 15.18). **Paresis** (weakness) is partial paralysis with incomplete loss of muscle power. **Paralysis** is loss of motor function so that a muscle group is unable to overcome gravity.

Upper Motor Neuron Syndromes

Upper motor neuron syndromes are the result of damage to descending motor pathways at cortical, brainstem, or spinal cord levels. **Upper motor neuron paresis or paralysis** is known also as *spastic paresis/paralysis*. Different terms are used to describe the specific disorders (Box 15.6).

Upper motor neuron paresis or paralysis is associated with a **pyramidal motor syndrome**. This syndrome involves a series of motor dysfunctions resulting from interruption of the pyramidal system (Figures 15.17 and 15.18). The injury may be in the cerebral cortex, the subcortical white matter, the internal capsule, the brainstem, or the spinal cord. The clinical manifestations reflect muscle overactivity. This includes excessive movements, such as clonus and spasms, occurring regularly because of loss of higher motor centre control. There is great variation, depending on the suddenness of onset and the age of the individual.

Spinal shock is the temporary loss of all spinal cord functions below the lesion (below the level of the pons). Complete flaccid paralysis,

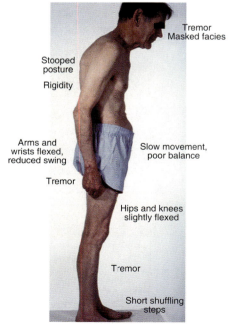

FIGURE 15.16 Stooped Posture of Parkinson's Disease. (From Perkin, D. G. [2002]. *Mosby's color atlas and text of neurology* [2nd ed.]. Mosby.)

TABLE 15.18 Upper and Lower Motor Neuron Syndromes Signs and Symptoms	
Upper Motor Neuron (Pyramidal Cells—Motor Cortex)	**Lower Motor Neuron (Cranial Nerve Nuclei—Brainstem; Ventral Horn—Spinal Cord)**
Muscle groups are affected	Individual muscles may be affected
Mild weakness	Mild weakness
Minimal disuse muscle atrophy	Marked muscle atrophy
No fasciculations	Fasciculations
Increased muscle stretch reflexes (clasp-knife spasticity; resistance to passive flexion that releases abruptly to allow easy flexion)	Decreased muscle stretch reflexes
Clonus may be present	Clonus not present
Hypertonia, spasticity	Hypotonia, flaccidity
	Hyporeflexia
Pathological reflexes (Babinski and Hoffmann signs, loss of abdominal reflexes)	No Babinski sign
Often initial impairment of only skilled movements	Asymmetrical and may involve one limb only in beginning to become generalized as disease progresses

absence of reflexes, and marked disturbances of bowel and bladder function are characteristics of this condition. Hypotension can occur from loss of sympathetic tone at higher levels of spinal cord injury. A major factor in spinal shock is the sudden destruction of the efferent pathways. If destruction occurs more slowly, spinal shock may not develop (see Chapter 16).

If an interruption of the pyramidal system occurs above the level of the pons, the hand and arm muscles are greatly affected. Paralysis rarely involves all the muscles on one side of the body, even when the hemiplegia results from complete damage to the internal capsule. Bilateral movements, such as those of the eye, jaw, and larynx, as well as those of the trunk, are affected only slightly, if at all. Influence of the limbs is predominant.

Paralysis associated with a pyramidal motor syndrome rarely remains flaccid for a prolonged time. After a few days or weeks, a gradual return of spinal reflexes marks the end of spinal shock. Reflexes then become hyperactive, and muscle tone increases significantly, particularly in antigravity muscles. *Spasticity* is common, although rigidity occasionally occurs (see Table 15.16). Most often, passive range-of-motion movements cause "clasp-knife" rigidity. This occurs probably by activating the stretch receptors in the muscle spindles and the Golgi tendon organ. (Chapter 38 discusses muscle function.) With pyramidal motor syndrome, predominantly the flexors of the arms and the extensors of the legs are affected.

Lower Motor Neuron Syndromes

Lower (primary, alpha) motor neurons are the large motor neurons in the anterior (or ventral) horn of the spinal cord and the motor nuclei of the brainstem. The axons from these nerve cell bodies bring nerve impulses from upper motor neurons to the skeletal muscles through the anterior spinal roots or cranial nerves (Figure 15.19). **Lower motor neuron syndromes** impair both voluntary and involuntary movement. The degree of paralysis or paresis is proportional to the number of lower motor neurons affected. If only some of the motor units that supply a muscle are affected, only partial paralysis (or paresis) results. If all motor units are affected, complete paralysis results. Other clinical manifestations also are proportional to the degree of dysfunction. The precise manifestations depend on the location of the dysfunction in the motor unit and in the CNS.

Normal motor movement requires small motor (gamma) neurons, which maintain muscle tone and protect the muscle from injury. They depend on input from the muscle spindle (arriving through an afferent limb rising to the cord). Dysfunction in this motor system (the gamma loop) impairs tone and reduces tendon reflexes, causing hyporeflexia. The muscles become susceptible to damage from hyperextensibility.

Generally, the large and small motor neuron systems are equally affected. Therefore, the muscle has reduced or absent tone. It is accompanied by hyporeflexia or **areflexia** (loss of tendon reflexes) and **flaccid paresis/paralysis**.

Denervated muscles (i.e., muscles that have lost their nervous system input) atrophy over weeks to months, mostly from disuse, and

> ### BOX 15.6 Upper Motor Neuron Paresis or Paralysis
>
> **Hemiparesis/hemiplegia** is paresis/paralysis of the upper and lower extremities on one side.
> Diplegia is paralysis of corresponding parts of both sides of the body because of cerebral hemisphere injuries.
> Paraparesis/paraplegia is weakness/paralysis of the lower extremities because of lower spinal cord injury.
> Quadriparesis/quadriplegia is paresis/paralysis of all four extremities because of upper spinal cord injury (Chapter 16 addresses spinal cord injury).

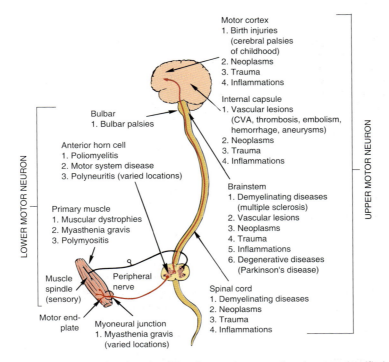

FIGURE 15.17 Motor Function Syndromes. Disturbances in motor function are classified pathologically along upper and lower motor neuron structures. It should be noted that the same pathological condition occurs at more than one site in an upper motor neuron *(top right)*. A few pathological conditions involve both upper and lower motor neuron structures, as in amyotrophic lateral sclerosis, for example. Other lesion sites include myoneural junction and primary muscle, making it possible to classify conditions as neuromuscular and muscular, respectively.

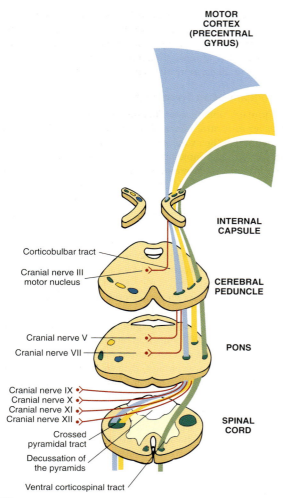

FIGURE 15.18 Structures of the Upper Motor Neuron, or Pyramidal, System. Pyramidal system fibres are shown to originate primarily in cells in the precentral gyrus of the motor cortex; to converge at the internal capsule; to descend to form the central third of the cerebral peduncle; to descend further through the pons, where small fibres supply cranial nerve motor nuclei along the way; to form pyramids at the medulla, where most of the fibres decussate; and then to continue to descend in the lateral column of white matter of the spinal cord. A few fibres descend without crossing at the level of the medulla (i.e., the ventral [anterior] corticospinal tract).

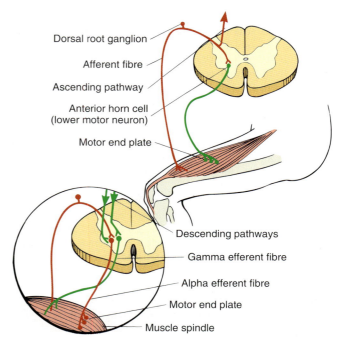

FIGURE 15.19 Structures Composing Lower Motor Neuron, Including Motor (Efferent) and Sensory (Afferent) Elements. *(Top)* Anterior horn cell (in anterior grey column of spinal cord and its axon), terminating in motor end plate as it innervates extrafusal muscle fibres in quadriceps muscle. *(Detailed enlargement)* Sensory and motor elements of gamma loop system. Gamma efferent fibres shown innervating the muscle spindle (sensory receptor of skeletal muscle). Contraction of muscle spindle fibres stretches the central portion of the spindle and causes the gamma afferent spindle fibre to transmit impulse centrally to the cord. Muscle spindle gamma afferent fibres in turn synapse on the anterior horn cell, and impulses are transmitted by way of alpha efferent fibres to skeletal (extrafusal) muscle, causing it to contract. Interruption of muscle spindle discharge occurs by active contraction of skeletal muscle fibres.

demonstrate **fasciculations** (muscle rippling or quivering under the skin). Occasionally, denervated muscles cramp. **Fibrillation** is isolated contraction of a single muscle fibre because of metabolic changes in denervated muscle and is not clinically visible.

Motor Neuron Diseases

Motor neuron diseases result from progressive degeneration of upper or lower motor neurons in the spinal cord, brainstem, or cortex. Amyotrophic lateral sclerosis and paralytic poliomyelitis (see Chapter 8) are examples of these diseases.

Several pathological processes may give rise to motor neuron diseases that can be sporadic or inherited. A virally induced or postinfectious or postvaccination inflammatory process may injure or destroy anterior horn cells or cranial nerve cell bodies. Most of these inflammatory processes are mild and experience rapid cellular recovery (Box 15.7).

In motor neuron disease, muscle strength, muscle tone, and muscle bulk are affected in the muscles innervated by the involved motor neurons. The paresis and paralysis associated with anterior horn cell injury are segmental. Because each muscle is supplied by two or more roots, the segmental character of the weakness may be difficult to recognize. When cranial nerve motor nuclei are affected (they lack nerve roots and have only small rootlets near the point of exit from the brainstem), the distribution of the motor weakness follows that of the peripheral nerve. The weakness may involve distal muscles, proximal muscles, and the muscles of midline structures. Hypotonia and hyporeflexia or areflexia are present.

The atrophy associated with motor neuron disease is segmental when the anterior horn cells of the spinal cord are involved. The atrophy follows the distribution of the peripheral nerve when the motor nuclei of the cranial nerves are affected. The atrophy may be in distal, proximal, or midline muscles. Fasciculations are particularly associated with primary motor neuron injury, and muscle cramps are common. Mild fatigue is a common complaint. If there is a limitation of the pathological process to the primary motor neuron, no sensory changes are evident.

Because degenerative disorders can cause loss of nerve cells in the anterior horn or motor nuclei, the surviving cells are small, shrunken, and filled with lipofuscin. Astrocytes replace lost neurons. The roots or rootlets are thin, and the muscles show denervation and atrophy.

Several brainstem syndromes involve damage to one or more of the cranial nerve nuclei. These syndromes are called *cranial nerve palsy*. The cause of these syndromes may be vascular occlusion, tumour, aneurysm, tuberculosis, or hemorrhage.

> **BOX 15.7 Bell's Palsy**
>
> The etiology of Bell's palsy (unilateral facial nerve palsy) remains unknown. There is usually an inflammatory reaction compressing the facial nerve, particularly in the narrowest segment, followed by demyelinating neural change. The most distressing signs are unilateral facial weakness and the inability to smile or whistle. Bell's palsy may be caused by reactivation of herpes viruses in cranial nerve VII (facial), geniculate ganglia, or an autoimmune response. The signs usually have an acute onset (within 72 hours). Herpes simplex type 1 has been detected in up to 78% of cases, and herpes zoster has been detected in 30% of cases. Severe pain with facial palsy and a vesicular rash in the ear or mouth suggest herpes zoster infection. Ramsay Hunt syndrome (herpes zoster oticus) is rare, but complete recovery is less than 50%. Recovery from Bell's palsy is usually complete. Treatment of both disorders may include combination antivirals and oral steroids. Individualization of treatment should occur according to severity of symptoms.

Data from Baugh, R. F., Basura, G. J., Ishii, L. E., et al. (2013). *Otolaryngology—Head and Neck Surgery, 149*(3 Suppl.), S1–S27. https://oto.sagepub.com/content/149/3_suppl/S1.full); De Ru, J. A., & Van Benthem, P. P. G. (2014). *Evidence-Based Medicine, 19*(1), 15; Glass, G. E., &Tzafetta, K. (2014). *Family Practice, 31*(6), 631–642; Greco, A., Gallo, A., Fusconi, M., et al. (2012). *Autoimmunity Reviews, 12*(2), 323–328.

The anterior horn cells and the motor nuclei of the cranial nerves may be affected secondarily in many severe pathological processes that primarily involve the peripheral nerves. The condition may extend proximally to affect the nerve roots or rootlets and the motor neurons themselves, a process commonly seen in **Guillain-Barré syndrome** (see Chapter 16). If the destruction of enough motor neurons occurs, permanent loss of motor function results because regeneration of the damaged axons requires a living neuronal cell body.

A group of degenerative disorders principally cause progressive motor cell atrophy. One of these disorders is **progressive spinal muscular atrophy**. In this condition the anterior horn cells of the spinal cord are the affected motor neurons that degenerate. This disorder occurs in adults and closely resembles the familial progressive muscular atrophies that occur in infants and children. These are inherited metabolic disorders (see Chapter 40). The disorder is a **progressive bulbar palsy** if the motor nuclei of the cranial nerves are affected instead of the anterior horn cells. It is given this name because the myelencephalon originally was called the *bulb* and a degenerative process causes a progressively more serious condition. The disorder is a **bulbar palsy** when any lower motor neuron syndrome involves the cranial nerves that arise from the bulb (i.e., cranial nerves IX, X, and XII).

The clinical manifestations of bulbar palsy include paresis or paralysis of the jaw, face, pharynx, and tongue musculature. Articulation is affected, especially articulation of the lingual *(r, n, l)*, labial *(b, m, p, f)*, dental *(d, t)*, and palatal *(k, g)* consonants. Modulation is impaired, making the voice rasping or nasal. A decrease or loss of pharyngeal reflexes occurs. Palate and vocal cord movement during phonation is impaired and chewing and swallowing are affected. The facial muscles are weak, and the face appears to droop. There is a decrease in the jaw jerk. Atrophy eventually becomes apparent, as do fasciculations. All these manifestations become progressively worse, leading to aspiration, malnutrition, possible dehydration, and an inability to communicate verbally.

Amyotrophic Lateral Sclerosis

Amyotrophic lateral sclerosis (ALS; sporadic motor neuron disease, sporadic motor system disease, motor neuron disease [MND], Lou Gehrig's disease) is a worldwide neuro-degenerative disorder. This disorder diffusely involves lower and upper motor neurons, resulting in progressive muscle weakness. *Amyotrophic* (without muscle nutrition or progressive muscle wasting) refers to the predominant lower motor neuron component of the syndrome. *Lateral sclerosis*, scarring of the corticospinal tract in the lateral column of the spinal cord, refers to the upper motor neuron component of the syndrome. ALS occurs in young adults or older adults, but it is most diagnosed in middle to late adulthood. It is estimated that 3 000 Canadians are currently living with ALS. It is estimated that 1 000 Canadians die each year from ALS and 1 000 persons are diagnosed annually with the disease.[37]

Most cases of ALS are sporadic. A subset (about 10%) of persons has a familial form with genetic mutations in superoxide dismutase (SOD) that contribute to the neurotoxicity affecting motor neurons. Mutated TAR RNA-binding protein 43 (TDP-43) is a major constituent of the neuronal protein inclusions in ALS. Evaluation of gene and environmental interactions as a cause of ALS is ongoing.[38]

PATHOPHYSIOLOGY The cause of ALS is unknown. Oxidative stress, mitochondrial dysfunction, defects in axonal transport, excitotoxicity and glutamate transport, neuronal cytoplasmic inclusions (i.e., TDP-43 protein), and neuro-inflammation as causes of neuron degeneration are under investigation.[39]

The principal pathological feature of ALS is degeneration of lower and upper motor neurons. There is a decrease in large motor neurons in the spinal cord, brainstem, and cerebral cortex (premotor and motor areas), with ongoing degeneration in the remaining motor neurons. Death of the motor neuron results in axonal degeneration and secondary demyelination with glial proliferation and sclerosis (scarring). Evidence shows widespread neural degeneration of nonmotor neurons in the spinal cord and motor cortices, as well as in the premotor, sensory, and temporal cortices.

Lower motor neuron degeneration denervates motor units. Adjacent, still viable lower motor neurons attempt to compensate by distal intramuscular sprouting, reinnervation, and enlargement of motor units.

CLINICAL MANIFESTATIONS The initial symptoms of the disease are heterogeneous and may be related to lower or upper motor neuron dysfunction or both. About 60% of individuals have a spinal form of the disease. Symptoms include focal muscle weakness beginning in the arms and legs and progressing to muscle atrophy, spasticity, and loss of manual dexterity and gait. No associated mental, sensory, or autonomic symptoms are present. ALS with progressive bulbar palsy presents with difficulty speaking and swallowing. Peripheral muscle weakness and atrophy usually occur within 1 to 2 years. These individuals have a poorer response to treatment with mechanical ventilation.[40] FTD may occur concurrently.[41]

EVALUATION AND TREATMENT Diagnosis of ALS is based predominantly on the history and physical examination with no evidence of other neuromuscular disorders. Electromyography and muscle biopsy results verify lower motor neuron degeneration and denervation. Imaging studies and CSF biomarkers can assist in making the diagnosis. Little treatment is available to alter the overall course of the ALS syndrome. The medication riluzole (Rilutek), an antiglutamate, has extended the length of time patients have before they require ventilatory assistance. Supportive and rehabilitative management are directed toward preventing complications of immobility. Psychological support of the affected individual and the family is extremely important.[1] ALS is fatal from respiratory failure, usually within 3 years of diagnosis. Approximately 80% of people with ALS die within 2 to 5 years of diagnosis.[37]

ALTERATIONS IN COMPLEX MOTOR PERFORMANCE

Alterations in complex motor performance include disorders of posture (stance), disorders of gait, and disorders of expression.

Disorders of Posture (Stance)

An inequality of tone in muscle groups, because of a loss of normal postural reflexes, results in a posturing of limbs. Disruption of equilibrium and balance occurs. Many reflex systems govern tone and posture, but the most important factor in posture control is the stretch reflex. During this reflex extensor (antigravity) muscle stretching causes increased extensor tone and inhibited flexor tone. Four types of disorders of posture are (1) dystonic posture, (2) decorticate posture/response, (3) decerebrate posture/response, and (4) basal ganglion posture.

Dystonia is the maintenance of an abnormal posture through muscular contractions. When muscular contractions are sustained for several seconds, they are called dystonic movements. When contractions last for longer periods, they are called dystonic postures. Dystonic postures may last for weeks, causing permanent, fixed contractures. Dystonia has been associated with basal ganglia abnormality, but the exact pathophysiological mechanisms are unknown. One dystonic posture is decorticate posture/response (striatal posture or upper motor neuron dysfunction posture), which may be unilateral or bilateral.

Decorticate posture/response (also referred to as antigravity posture or hemiplegic posture) presents as upper extremities flexed at the elbows and held close to the body and by lower extremities that are externally rotated and extended (see Figure 15.6). Decorticate posture/response is thought to occur when the brainstem is not inhibited by the cerebral cortex motor area. Upper motor neuron posture is commonly described as the arm flexed at the elbow with a wrist drop, the leg inadequately bent at the knee, the hip excessively circumabducted, and the presence of footdrop.

Decerebrate posture/response refers to increased tone in extensor muscles and trunk muscles, with active tonic neck reflexes. When the head is in a neutral position, all four limbs are rigidly extended (see Figure 15.6). Severe injury to the brain and brainstem causes the decerebrate posture. This results in overstimulation of the postural righting and vestibular reflexes.

Basal ganglion posture refers to a stooped, hyperflexed posture with a narrow-based, short-stepped gait. This posture abnormality results from the loss of normal postural reflexes and not from defects in proprioceptive, labyrinthine, or visual function. Dysfunctional equilibrium results when the individual loses stability and cannot make the appropriate postural adjustment to tilting or loss of balance, falling instead. Dysfunctional righting is the inability to right oneself when changing from a lying or crouching to a standing position or when rolling from the supine to the lateral or prone position. Dysfunctional postural fixation is the involuntary flexion of the head and neck. This flexion causes the person difficulty in maintaining an upright trunk position while standing or walking. Basal ganglion dysfunction accounts for this posture.

Disorders of Gait

Four predominant types of gait associated with neurological disorders are (1) upper motor neuron dysfunction gait, (2) cerebellar (ataxic) gait, (3) basal ganglion gait, and (4) frontal lobe ataxic gait. Equilibrium and balance affect posture and gait disturbances.[42]

Several types of upper motor neuron gait exist. With mild forms, the individual may have footdrop with fatigue and hip and leg pain. A spastic gait, which is associated with unilateral injury, manifests by a shuffling gait with the leg extended and held stiff. This gait causes a scraping over the floor surface. The leg swings improperly around the body rather than being lifted and placed. The foot may drag on the ground, and the person tends to fall to the affected side. A scissors gait is associated with bilateral injury and spasticity. Adduction of the legs occurs so they touch each other. As the person walks, the legs swing around the body but then cross in front of each other because of adduction. Injury to the pyramidal system accounts for these gaits (e.g., stroke, cerebral palsy, multiple sclerosis, spinal cord tumour).

A cerebellar (ataxic) gait is wide based, with the feet apart and often turned outward or inward for greater stability. The pelvis is stiff, and the individual staggers when walking. Cerebellar dysfunction with loss of coordination accounts for this gait.

A basal ganglion gait is a broad-based gait in which the person walks with small steps and a decreased arm swing. Flexion of the head and body occurs and the arms are semiflexed and abducted. The legs are flexed and rigid in more advanced states. Basal ganglion dysfunction accounts for this gait and is associated with PD.

A frontal lobe ataxic gait is wide based with increased body sway and falls, loss of control of truncal motion, gait ignition failure, start hesitation, shuffling, and freezing. The gait is associated with frontal lobe damage or degeneration. The pattern may change as the frontal disease progresses. The slowness of walking, lack of heel–shin or upper limb ataxia, dysarthria, or nystagmus distinguishes the wide stance from cerebellar ataxic gait.[42]

Balance, coordination, and sensory dysfunction that further alter mobility and increase risk for falls often accompany gait disorders. Assessment and intervention strategies are important for prevention of injury.

Disorders of Expression

Disorders of expression involve the motor aspects of communication and include (1) hypermimesis, (2) hypomimesis, and (3) apraxia or dyspraxia. Hypermimesis commonly manifests as pathological laughter or crying. Pathological laughter is associated with right hemisphere injury. Pathological crying is associated with left hemisphere injury. The exact pathophysiology is not known. Hypomimesis manifests as *aprosody*—the loss of emotional language. *Receptive aprosody* involves an inability to understand emotion in speech and facial expression. *Expressive aprosody* involves the inability to express emotion in speech and facial expression. Aprosody is associated with right hemisphere damage.

Apraxia or dyspraxia (the terms are often used interchangeably) is a disorder of learned skilled movements with difficulty planning and executing coordinated motor movements. It can be developmental, beginning at birth (developmental apraxia), or associated with vascular disorders (common in stroke), trauma, tumours, degenerative disorders, infections, or metabolic disorders. People with apraxia have difficulty performing tasks requiring motor skills. These skills include speaking, writing, using tools or utensils, playing sports, following instructions, and focusing.[43]

True apraxias occur when the connecting pathways between the left and right cortical areas are interrupted. Apraxias may result from any pathological process that disrupts the cortical areas necessary for the conceptualization and execution of a complex motor act or the communication pathways within the left hemisphere or between the hemispheres.[1]

EXTRAPYRAMIDAL MOTOR SYNDROMES

Because the extrapyramidal system encompasses all the motor pathways except the pyramidal system, two types of motor dysfunction

TABLE 15.19 Pyramidal Versus Extrapyramidal Motor Syndrome

Manifestions	Pyramidal Motor Syndrome	Extrapyramidal Motor Syndrome
Unilateral movement	Paralysis of voluntary movement	Little or no paralysis of voluntary movement
Tendon reflexes	Increased tendon reflexes	Normal or slightly increased tendon reflexes
Babinski sign	Present	Absent
Involuntary movements	Absence of involuntary movements	Presence of tremor, chorea, athetosis, or dystonia
Muscle tone	Spasticity in muscles (e.g., clasp-knife phenomenon)	Plastic rigidity (equal throughout movement) or intermittent—cogwheel rigidity (generalized but predominantly in flexors of limbs and trunk)
	Hypertonia present in flexors of arms and extensors of legs	Hypotonia, weakness and gait disturbances in cerebellar disease

make up the extrapyramidal motor syndromes: (1) basal ganglia motor syndromes and (2) cerebellar motor syndromes. Unlike pyramidal motor syndromes, both extrapyramidal motor syndromes result in movement or posture disturbance without significant paralysis, along with other distinctive symptoms (Table 15.19).

An imbalance of dopaminergic and cholinergic activity in the corpus striatum causes basal ganglia motor syndromes. A relative excess of cholinergic activity produces akinesia and hypertonia. A relative excess of dopaminergic activity produces hyperkinesia and hypotonia. Symptoms associated with Parkinson's and Huntington's diseases are exemplary of disorders of the basal ganglia. Cerebellar motor syndromes are associated with ataxia and other symptoms affecting coordinated movement. Cerebellar motor syndromes primarily influence the same side of the body. For example, damage to the right cerebellum generally causes symptoms on the right side of the body.

Short- or long-term use of certain medications may cause medication-induced extrapyramidal effects. The medications involved, including the antipsychotic haloperidol (Haldol) and the antiemetic metoclopramide (Metoclopramide), antagonize the dopamine D2 receptors, resulting in extrapyramidal adverse effects.

CASE STUDY

Jane Damiani is a 16-year-old girl who presented to the emergency department accompanied by her mother, cheerleading coach, and teammate. The patient was competing in a cheerleading event. Just after her team competed their routine, her teammate saw that Jane suddenly appeared to lose consciousness and fell to the ground. Her teammate described the event like her arms and legs were stiff in appearance, "like a board". She was observed moving on the ground with a series of violent, rhythmic, muscle contractions that gradually decreased until they stopped. Just before Jane fell to the ground, she let out a shrill cry and appeared to stop breathing. The coach stated that the whole experience took about 4 minutes from the time Jane fell to the ground to when she was lying motionless.

History of Present Illness: Jane's mother stated that in the morning Jane was feeling a bit lightheaded and shaky but attributed this to being nervous about the day's cheerleading competition and not having a good night's sleep. Just before the competition, Jane stated she felt "fine" and was ready to compete with her team. The gymnasium was extremely hot that day and all competitors were sweating profusely. When the nurse in the emergency department asked Jane if she could remember what had happened, she said that she could not. The last memory she had was lying on the ground with her coach and teammate standing over her and calling her name. She states that she feels very tired, has a headache, and just wants to go to sleep. Her next menses is due to start in 2 days.

Past Medical Hx: A healthy teenager with no previous seizure activity. She was a full-term baby with no adverse childhood events. She has been well for the last year and has not had any recent colds or flus.

Family Hx: Her older sister, age 17, was diagnosed with epilepsy at age 5. Her mother and father are in good health, with no diagnosed health problems.

Medications: Tri-Cyclen 28 (oral contraceptive) for treating dysmenorrhea, occasional OTC ibuprofen, no vitamin, or herbal supplements

Social history: A high-school student, nonsmoker, nondrinker, no recreational drugs; exercises for 45 minutes per day 4 times per week at the gym, has regularly participated in cheerleader practice and competitions, not sexually active, eats a well-balanced diet.

Review of Systems: Unremarkable with the exception of feeling tired and weak and having a mild frontal headache. No nausea, no vomiting, no bowel incontinence during episode, incontinence of urine experienced.

Physical Exam: Appears stated age, well-groomed, and sleepy when asked questions. Her cheerleading top is damp from perspiration and her skirt is wet from her incontinence episode. Her skin is moist, pale, and warm. There are no abrasions noted from her fall to the ground. HEENT unremarkable; ROM neck full, no lymphadenopathy or thyroidomegaly, JVP normal, no carotid bruits. Respiratory, cardiovascular, gastrointestinal, and musculoskeletal exams unremarkable. Neuro exam includes orientation to time, person, and place, sleepy, CN I-12 intact, 5/5 muscle strength, deep tendon reflexes 2+ bilaterally, sensation to touch intact, rapid alternating movements normal, negative Babinski, Romberg normal, gait and balance normal.

Vital signs: BP 128/74 LA sitting; pulse 78 regular; RR 14 unlaboured; temperature 36.8°C oral; BMI 26

Critical Thinking and Clinical Judgement Questions

1. The primary care provider suspects a diagnosis of generalized tonic-clonic seizure. Identify five possible contributing factors to this patient's seizure.
2. Based on the information provided, identify eight clinical signs and symptoms in this patient that are consistent with a diagnosis of a generalized clonic-tonic seizure.
3. Name the diagnostic tests the primary care provider could order to confirm the diagnosis of generalized clonic-tonic seizure. Indicate what each test is assessing.
4. Define and describe the terms *preictal phase*, *ictal phase*, and *postictal stage*. Identify what Jane experienced during each of these phases.

DID YOU UNDERSTAND?

Alterations in Cognitive Systems

1. Full consciousness is an awareness of oneself and the environment with an ability to respond to external stimuli with a wide variety of responses.
2. Consciousness has two components: arousal (level of awakeness) and awareness (content of thought).
3. An altered level of arousal occurs by diffuse bilateral cortical dysfunction, bilateral subcortical (reticular formation, brainstem) dysfunction, localized hemispheric dysfunction, and metabolic disorders.
4. An alteration in breathing pattern and the level of consciousness reflects the level of brain dysfunction.
5. Pupillary changes reflect changes in level of brainstem function, medication action, and response to hypoxia and ischemia.
6. Abnormal eye movements reflect alterations in brainstem function.
7. Level of brain function manifests by changes in generalized motor responses or no responses.
8. Loss of cortical inhibition associated with decreased consciousness produces abnormal flexor and extensor movements.
9. Brain death results from irreversible brain damage, with an inability to maintain internal homeostasis.
10. Cerebral death, or irreversible coma, represents permanent brain damage. The ability to maintain cardiac, respiratory, and other vital functions is maintained.
11. Arousal returns in vegetative states, but awareness is absent.
12. Alterations in awareness include alterations in executive attention (abstract reasoning, planning, decision making, judgement, error correction, and self-control) and memory.
13. With a deficit in selective attention, mediated by midbrain, thalamus, and parietal lobe structures, the individual cannot focus on selective stimuli and thus neglects those stimuli.
14. The loss of some memories occurs in retrograde amnesia. In anterograde amnesia, formation of new memories cannot occur.
15. Frontal areas mediate vigilance, detection, and working (short-term) memory.
16. With vigilance deficits, the person cannot maintain sustained concentration.
17. With detection deficits, the person is unmotivated and may be perceived by others as lazy or apathetic.
18. Data-processing deficits include agnosias, dysphasias, acute confusional states, and dementias.
19. Agnosias are defects of recognition and may be tactile, visual, or auditory. Dysfunction in the primary sensory area or the interpretive areas of the cerebral cortex cause agnosias.
20. Dysphasia (aphasia) is an impairment of comprehension or production of language. Most dysphasias are expressive or receptive.
21. Characteristics of acute confusional states include a loss of detection and, in the case of delirium, intense autonomic nervous system hyperactivity.
22. Alzheimer's disease is a chronic irreversible dementia that is related to altered production or failure to clear amyloid from the brain with plaque formation, formation of neurofibrillary tangles, and loss of basal forebrain cholinergic neurons.
23. Frontotemporal dementias are rare early-onset degenerative diseases like Alzheimer's disease.
24. Seizures represent a sudden, chaotic discharge of cerebral neurons with transient alterations in brain function. Seizures may be generalized or focal and can result from cerebral lesions, biochemical disorders, trauma, or epilepsy.

Alterations in Cerebral Hemodynamics

1. Alterations in cerebral blood flow are related to changes in cerebral perfusion pressure, changes in cerebral blood volume, and cerebral blood oxygenation.
2. ICP may result from edema, excess cerebrospinal fluid, hemorrhage, or tumour growth. When ICP approaches arterial pressure, hypoxia and hypercapnia produce brain damage.
3. Cerebral edema is an increase in the fluid content of the brain resulting from infection, hemorrhage, tumour, ischemia, infarction, or hypoxia. Cerebral edema can cause increased ICP.
4. The shifting or herniation of brain tissue from one compartment to another disrupts the blood flow of both compartments and damages brain tissue.
5. Supratentorial herniation involves the temporal lobe and hippocampal gyrus shifting from the middle fossa to posterior fossa. Transtentorial herniation involves a downward shift of the diencephalon through the tentorial notch; and shifting of the cingulate gyrus can occur under the falx cerebri.
6. The most common infratentorial herniation is a shift of the cerebellar tonsils through the foramen magnum.
7. Hydrocephalus comprises a variety of disorders characterized by an excess of fluid within the ventricles, subarachnoid space, or both. Hydrocephalus occurs because of interference with CSF flow caused by increased fluid production or obstruction within the ventricular system or by defective reabsorption of the fluid.

Alterations in Neuromotor Function

1. General neuromotor dysfunctions are associated with changes in muscle tone, movement, and complex motor performance.
2. Hypotonia and hypertonia are the main categories of altered tone.
3. Hypotonia is associated with pyramidal tract or cerebellar injury. Muscles are flaccid and weak with atrophy.
4. The four types of hypertonia are spasticity, paratonia (gegenhalten), dystonia, and rigidity.
5. Hyperkinesia, hypokinesia, paresis, and paralysis are the main categories of alterations in muscle movement.
6. Included in the category of hyperkinesia are chorea, athetosis, ballism, akathisia, tremor, and myoclonus.
7. Huntington's disease (chorea) is a rare hereditary disease involving the basal ganglia and cerebral cortex that commonly manifests between 25 and 45 years of age.
8. The major pathological feature of Huntington's disease is severe degeneration of the basal ganglia and the cerebral cortex with an excess of dopaminergic activity that causes involuntary, fragmentary hyperkinetic movements.
9. Types of hypokinesia include akinesia, bradykinesia, and loss of associated movement.
10. Parkinson's disease is a commonly occurring degenerative disorder of the basal ganglia (corpus striatum) involving degeneration of the dopamine-secreting nigrostriatal pathway.
11. Dopamine depletion in the basal ganglia and excess cholinergic activity in the cortex, basal ganglia, and thalamus cause tremor and rigidity in Parkinson's disease. Progressive dementia may be associated with an advanced stage of the disease.
12. Characteristics of an upper motor neuron syndrome include paresis or paralysis, hypertonia, and hyperreflexia.
13. Two subtypes of paresis or paralysis are upper motor neuron spastic paresis/paralysis and lower motor neuron flaccid paresis/paralysis.

14. Upper motor neuron syndromes are the result of damage to descending motor pathways at cortical, brainstem, or spinal cord levels and result in spastic paralysis.
15. Spinal shock is temporary loss of all spinal cord function below the lesion (below the level of the pons). Complete flaccid paralysis, absence of reflexes, and marked disturbances of bowel and bladder function are characteristics of this dysfunction.
16. Lower motor neuron syndromes manifest by impaired voluntary and involuntary movements and flaccid paralysis.
17. Partial paralysis occurs with only partial loss of alpha motor neurons. Total paralysis is complete loss of alpha motor neurons. Loss of gamma motor neurons impairs muscle tone and decreases tendon reflexes.
18. Lower (primary, alpha) motor neuron syndromes involve the large motor neurons in the anterior (or ventral) horn of the spinal cord and the motor nuclei of the brainstem and cause flaccid paralysis.
19. Amyotrophic lateral sclerosis involves degeneration of both upper and lower motor neurons with progressive muscle weakness and atrophy.

Alterations in Complex Motor Performance

1. Alterations in complex motor performance include disorders of posture (stance), disorders of gait, and disorders of expression.
2. Disorders of posture include dystonic posture, decerebrate posture/response, basal ganglion posture, and senile posture.
3. Disorders of gait include upper motor neuron gait, cerebellar (ataxic) gait, basal ganglion gait, and frontal lobe ataxic gait.
4. Disorders of expression include hypermimesis, hypomimesis, and apraxia (dyspraxia).
5. Apraxia is an impairment of the conceptualization or execution of a complex motor act.

Extrapyramidal Motor Syndromes

1. Extrapyramidal motor syndromes include basal ganglia and cerebellar motor syndromes.
2. Basal ganglia motor syndromes manifest by alterations in muscle tone and posture, including rigidity, involuntary movements, and loss of postural reflexes.
3. Cerebellar motor syndromes result in loss of muscle tone, difficulty with coordination, and disorders of equilibrium and gait.

16

Disorders of the Central and Peripheral Nervous Systems and Neuromuscular Junction

Kelly Power-Kean, with originating chapter contributions by Barbara J. Boss and Sue E. Huether

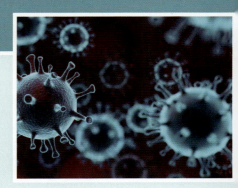

Additional resources are available online at https://evolve.elsevier.com/Canada/Huether/pathophysiology.

CHAPTER OUTLINE

Central Nervous System Disorders, 383
  Traumatic Brain and Spinal Cord Injury, 383
  Degenerative Disorders of the Spine, 391
  Cerebrovascular Disorders, 394
  Primary Headache Syndrome, 398
  Infection and Inflammation of the Central Nervous System, 400
  Demyelinating Disorders, 402

Peripheral Nervous System and Neuromuscular Junction Disorders, 403
  Peripheral Nervous System Disorders, 404
  Neuromuscular Junction Disorders, 404
Tumours of the Central Nervous System, 405
  Brain Tumours, 405
  Spinal Cord Tumours, 408

LEARNING OBJECTIVES

1. Define the different types of head injury. Give examples of the type of force needed to produce each.
2. Describe the four classifications of vertebral column injury.
3. Explain spinal shock and autonomic hyperreflexia.
4. Identify the causes of low back pain.
5. Describe the disorders produced by interruption to cerebral vascular flow. Include the location, manifestations, and rehabilitation potential of each.
6. Describe the differences between types of headaches.
7. Describe infectious processes that occur in the central nervous system.
8. Explain the pathophysiology of a brain abscess.
9. Explain how an HIV infection can affect the nervous system.
10. Explain the pathophysiology of the degenerative disorders of the spine.
11. Explain the pathophysiology and clinical manifestations of multiple sclerosis.
12. Describe the pathophysiology and clinical manifestations of myasthenia gravis.
13. Discuss the cellular pathophysiology, manifestations, and treatment of central nervous system tumours.

KEY TERMS

Arteriovenous malformation (AVM), 397
Astrocytomas, 406
Autonomic hyperreflexia (dysreflexia), 389
Bacterial meningitis, 400
Brain abscess, 401
Brudzinski sign, 398
Cauda equina syndrome, 393
Cerebral infarction, 395
Cerebrovascular accident (CVA), 394
Cholinergic crisis, 405
Chronic traumatic encephalopathy (CTE), 387
Closed brain injuries, 383
Cluster headache, 399
Compound skull fracture, 386
Compressive syndrome (sensorimotor syndrome), 408
Contrecoup injury, 383
Contusion, 383
Coup injury, 383
Degenerative disc disease (DDD), 393
Diffuse brain injury (diffuse axonal injury [DAI]), 386
Embolic stroke, 395
Encephalitis, 401
Ependymoma, 407
Epidural (extradural) hematoma, 384
Focal brain injury, 383
Fungal meningitis, 400
Fusiform aneurysm (giant aneurysm), 397
Glioblastoma multiforme, 406
Glioma, 406
Guillain-Barré syndrome, 404
Headache, 398
Hemorrhagic stroke (intracranial hemorrhage), 396
HIV-associated neurocognitive disorder (HAND), 402
Hypoperfusion, or hemodynamic stroke, 395
Intracerebral hematoma, 386
Intracranial aneurysm, 397
Irritative syndrome (radicular syndrome), 409
Ischemic penumbra, 396
Ischemic stroke, 395
Kernig sign, 398
Lacunar stroke (lacunar infarct or small vessel disease), 395
Low back pain (LBP), 391
Meningioma, 408
Meningitis, 400
Metastatic brain tumours, 408
Migraine, 398
Mild traumatic brain injury (mild concussion), 387
Moderate traumatic brain injury (moderate concussion), 387
Multiple sclerosis (MS), 402
Myasthenia gravis, 404
Myasthenic crisis, 405

Neurofibroma (benign nerve sheath tumour), 408
Neurofibromatosis type 1 (NF1), 408
Neurofibromatosis type 2 (NF2), 408
Neurogenic shock, 389
Ocular myasthenia, 404
Oligodendroglioma, 406
Open brain injury, 386
Open (penetrating) trauma, 383
Plexus injury, 404
Postconcussion syndrome, 387
Post-traumatic seizure, 387
Primary brain (intracerebral) tumour, 406
Primary spinal cord injury, 388
Purpura fulminans, 400
Radiculopathy, 394
Saccular aneurysm (berry aneurysm), 397
Secondary brain injury, 387
Secondary spinal cord injury, 388
Severe traumatic brain injury (severe concussion), 387
Spinal cord abscess, 401
Spinal cord tumours, 408
Spinal shock, 389
Spinal stenosis, 393
Spondylolisthesis, 393
Spondylolysis, 393
Subarachnoid hemorrhage (SAH), 397
Subdural hematoma, 385
Tension-type headache (TTH), 399
Thrombotic stroke (cerebral thrombosis), 395
Transient ischemic attack (TIA), 395
Traumatic brain injury (TBI), 383
Vertebral injury, 388
Viral meningitis (aseptic or nonpurulent meningitis), 400
West Nile virus (WNV), 402

There are many causes for alterations in the function of the central nervous system (CNS). These causes include traumatic injury, vascular disorders, tumour growth, infectious and inflammatory processes, and metabolic derangements (including those arising from nutritional deficiencies and medications or chemicals). Alterations in peripheral nervous system function involve the nerve roots, a nerve plexus or the nerves themselves, or the neuromuscular junction.

CENTRAL NERVOUS SYSTEM DISORDERS

> ✓ **QUICK CHECK 16.1**
> 1. How is a concussion different from a contusion?
> 2. Why do epidural, subdural, and intracerebral hematomas act like expanding masses?
> 3. Why is head motion the main cause of diffuse brain injury?

Traumatic Brain and Spinal Cord Injury
Traumatic Brain Injury

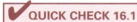Traumatic brain injury (TBI) is an alteration in brain function or other evidence of brain disease caused by an external force. In Canada, TBI is the primary cause of death and disability in persons under the age of 40. TBI occurs at a rate of 500 out of 100 000 persons annually. TBI has an annual incidence rate greater than all combined cases of multiple sclerosis (MS), spinal cord injury, human immunodeficiency virus (HIV)/acquired immune deficiency syndrome (AIDS), and breast cancer. Children and youth, many of them while participating in sports and recreational-related activities, sustain 30% of all TBIs. An estimate of the incidence of TBI among Indigenous people is four to five times the rate of the general population.[1]

In recent years, there have been improved survival outcomes of persons with TBI. The University of Calgary is involved in multiple research projects including the areas of concussion, and the assessment and management of mild TBI among children and adolescents (see https://ucalgary.ca/labs/brain-injury-research-children). Advancements have been made in improved safety measures (e.g., seatbelts, air bags, helmets), decreased transport time to hospitals or trauma centres, improved on-scene medical management, and prevention and management of secondary brain injury.

TBI is classified as either primary or secondary. A direct impact causes a primary brain injury. Injury can be focal, affecting one area of the brain, or diffuse (diffuse axonal injury [DAI]), involving more than one area of the brain.[2] Focal brain injury and DAI each account for half of all injuries. Focal brain injury is responsible for more than two thirds of head injury deaths. DAI is responsible for less than one third of deaths. More severely disabled survivors, including those surviving in an unresponsive state or decreased level of consciousness, have DAI. Secondary injury is an indirect result of the primary injury. Secondary injury includes systemic responses and a cascade of cellular and molecular cerebral events. TBI can be mild, moderate, or severe. Assessment using the Glasgow Coma Scale (GCS) determines the severity of the injury (Table 16.1). Most TBIs are mild. The key feature of a severe TBI is loss of consciousness for 6 hours or more.[3] Chapter 15 reviews information about increased intracranial pressure (ICP).

Primary brain injury.
Focal brain injury. Closed (blunt) trauma or open (penetrating) trauma causes a focal brain injury. Closed injury is more common. This injury involves either the head striking a hard surface, a rapidly moving object striking the head, or by blast waves. The dura remains intact, and no exposure of brain tissues to the environment occurs. Blunt trauma may result in focal brain injuries and diffuse axonal injuries. Both injuries can occur at the same time (Table 16.2). Open injury occurs with penetrating trauma or skull fracture. A break in the dura results in exposure of the cranial contents to the environment.[3]

Closed brain injuries are specific, clearly observable brain injuries that occur in a precise location. Seventy-five to ninety percent of blunt trauma injuries are mild. Injury to the vault, vessels, and supporting structures can produce more severe damage. These injuries include contusions and epidural, subdural, and intracerebral hematomas. The injury may be a coup injury (at the site of impact) or contrecoup injury (from the brain bouncing back and hitting the opposite side of the skull) (Figure 16.1). Compression of the skull at the point of impact produces contusions or brain bruising. This occurs from blood leaking from an injured vessel. The severity of contusion varies with the amount of force the skull has on the underlying brain tissue. The smaller the area of impact, the more severe the injury. This result occurs because of the intensity of force. Brain edema forms around and in damaged neural tissues. This edema contributes to increasing ICP (see Chapter 15). Hemorrhages, edema, infarction, and necrosis can occur within the contused areas. The tissue has a pulpy quality. The greatest effects of these injuries peak 18 to 36 hours after a severe head injury.

The frontal lobes are the most common location of contusions. Areas most affected include the poles and along the inferior orbital surfaces; in the temporal lobes, especially at the anterior poles and along the inferior surface; and at the frontotemporal junction. Contusions cause changes in attention, memory, affect, emotion, behaviour, and executive attention functions (see Chapter 15). Contusions occur in the parietal and occipital lobes less frequently. Focal cerebral contusions are usually superficial, involving just the gyri. Hemorrhagic contusions may join into one large intracranial hematoma.

A contusion may present with immediate loss of consciousness (lasting no longer than 5 minutes), loss of reflexes (person falls to the ground), a brief pause of breathing, a brief period of bradycardia, and a decrease in blood pressure (lasting 30 seconds to a few minutes). Increased cerebrospinal fluid (CSF) pressure and electrocardiogram (ECG) and electroencephalogram (EEG) changes occur on impact. Vital signs may stabilize to normal in a few seconds. Reflexes then return, and the person regains consciousness over minutes to days. Remaining deficits may continue, and some persons never regain a full level of consciousness.

Evaluation is based on results of the health history, level of consciousness according to the Glasgow Coma Scale (see Table 16.1), results of imaging studies (e.g., computed tomography [CT], magnetic resonance imaging [MRI], and positron emission tomography [PET] scans), and assessment of vital factors (e.g., ICP and EEG). Surgical removal of large contusions and areas of hemorrhage may be required. Controlling ICP and managing symptoms are goals of treatment.

Epidural (extradural) hematomas (bleeding between the dura mater and the skull) represent 1 to 2% of major head injuries. This type of injury occurs in all age groups, but most commonly in those 20 to 40 years old. An artery is the source of bleeding in 85% of epidural hematomas, usually occurring with a skull fracture. About 15% of these injuries result from injury to the meningeal vein or dural sinus (Figure 16.2). The temporal fossa is the most common site of epidural hematoma caused by injury to the middle meningeal artery or vein. The temporal lobe shifts towards the middle, causing uncal and hippocampal gyrus herniation (bulging) through the tentorial notch. At times, the subfrontal area experiences epidural hemorrhages. This occurs most often in young and older persons. This injury is the result of damage to the anterior meningeal artery or a venous sinus. In the occipital-suboccipital area, damage results in herniation of the posterior fossa contents through the foramen magnum (see Figure 15.10).

Persons with temporal epidural hematomas lose consciousness at injury. About one third of those affected then become aware for a few minutes to a few days (if a vein is bleeding). As the hematoma grows, a worsening headache, vomiting, drowsiness, confusion, seizure, and hemiparesis may develop. Because temporal lobe herniation occurs, the level of consciousness is rapidly lost. Ipsilateral (same side of the body) pupil dilation and contralateral (opposite side of the body) hemiparesis occurs. The diagnosis of epidural hematoma usually requires a CT scan or an MRI. The prognosis is good if treatment begins before dilation of both pupils occurs. Epidural hematomas are usually medical emergencies. Treatment includes monitoring and evaluation or surgical removal of the hematoma.[4]

TABLE 16.1 Glasgow Coma Scale[a]

Score[b]	Best Eye Response Score (4)	Best Verbal Response Score (5)	Best Motor Response Score (6)
1	No eye opening	No verbal response	No motor response
2	Eye opening to pain	Incomprehensible sounds	Extension to pain
3	Eye opening to verbal command	Inappropriate words	Flexion to pain
4	Eyes open spontaneously	Confused	Withdrawal from pain
5	NA	Oriented	Localizing pain
6	NA	NA	Obeys commands

[a]The Glasgow Coma Scale (GCS) is scored between 3 and 15, with 3 being the worst and 15 the best. It is composed of the sum of three parameters: Best Eye Response, Best Verbal Response, and Best Motor Response. Mild Brain Injury=13 or higher; Moderate Brain Injury = 9 to 12; Severe Brain Injury=8 or less.

[b]It is important to break the scoring report into its components, for example, E3V3M5=GCS 11. A total score is meaningless without this information. Age affects the GCS. Older persons with traumatic brain injury (TBI) have better GCS scores than younger persons with similar TBI severity (i.e., older persons have higher GCS scores than those of younger persons with TBI with similar anatomical TBI severity).
Data from Salottolo, K., Levy, A. S., Slone, D. S., et al. (2014). The effect of age on Glasgow Coma Scale score in patients with traumatic brain injury. *JAMA Surgery, 149*(7), 727–734; Teasdale, G., & Jennett, B. (1974). Assessment of coma and impaired consciousness. A practical scale. *Lancet, 2*, 81–84.

TABLE 16.2 Classification of Brain Injuries

Type of Injury	Mechanism
Primary Brain Injury	
Focal Brain Injury	Localized injury from impact
Closed injury	Blunt trauma
Coup	Injury is directly below the site of forceful impact
Contrecoup	Injury is on opposite side of the brain from the site of forceful impact
Epidural (extradural) hematoma	Motor vehicle accidents, minor falls, sporting accidents
Subdural hematoma	Forceful impact: motor vehicle accidents or falls, especially in older persons or persons with chronic alcohol misuse
Subarachnoid hemorrhage	Bleeding caused by forceful impact, usually motor vehicle accidents or long-distance falls
Open injury	Penetrating trauma: missiles (bullets) or sharp projectiles (knives, ice picks, axes, screwdrivers)
Compound fracture	Objects strike the head with great force, or the head strikes an object forcefully; temporal blows, occipital blows, upward impact of cervical vertebrae (basilar skull fracture)
Diffuse Axonal Injury (can occur with focal injury)	Traumatic shearing forces; tearing of axons from twisting and rotational forces with injury over widespread brain areas; the moving head strikes a hard, solid surface or a moving object strikes an unmoving head; twisting head motion without impact
Secondary Brain Injury	
Secondary brain injury	Decrease in CBF caused by edema, hemorrhage, increased ICP; neuro-inflammation
Cell death	Release of excitatory neurotransmitters (glutamate); failure of cell ion pumps, mitochondrial failure

CBF, Cerebral blood flow; *ICP*, intracranial pressure.

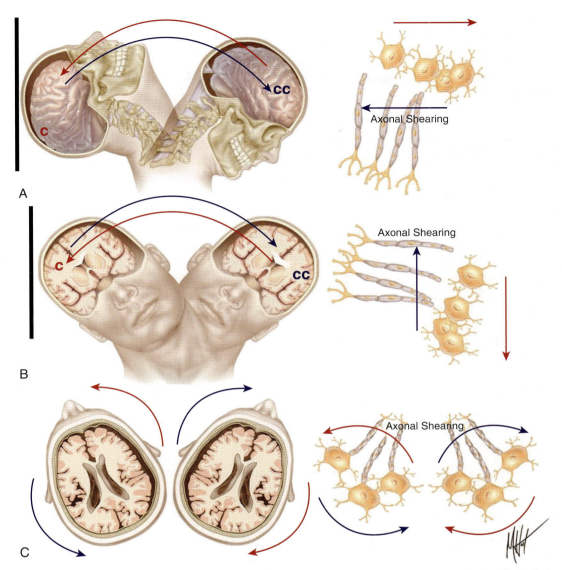

FIGURE 16.1 Coup and Contrecoup Focal Injury With Acceleration/Deceleration Axonal Shearing. **A,** Sagittal force causing coup *(c)* and contrecoup injury *(cc)*. **B,** Lateral force causing coup *(c)* and contrecoup *(cc)* injury. **C,** Axial or rotational injury with shearing of axons, mainly at the base of the brain. Acceleration/deceleration axonal shearing injury occurs throughout the brain (*red* and *blue directional arrows* in all three images). (Borrowed from Pascual, J. M., & Preito, R. [2012]. Surgical management of severe closed head injury in adults. In A. Quinones-Hinojosa [Ed.], *Schmidek and Sweet operative neurosurgical techniques* [6th ed., Vol. 2, pp. 1513–1538]. Saunders. Originally redrawn from Adams, J. H. [1990]. Brain damage in fatal nonmissile head injury in man. In R. Braakman [Ed.], *Handbook of clinical neurology, head injury* [Vol. 13, pp. 43–63]. Elsevier Science Publishers BV; Gennarelli, T. A., Thibault, L. E., Adams, J. H., et al. [1982]. Diffuse axonal injury and traumatic coma in the primate. *Annals of Neurology, 12,* 564–574.)

Subdural hematomas (bleeding between the dura mater and the brain) occur in 10 to 20% of persons with TBI. *Acute subdural hematomas* develop quickly, commonly within hours. They usually are found at the top of the skull (the cerebral convexities). Bilateral hematomas occur in 15 to 20% of persons. Subacute subdural hematomas develop more slowly, often over 48 hours to 2 weeks. *Chronic subdural hematomas* develop over weeks to months. They are usually found in older persons and persons who abuse alcohol. These persons usually have some degree of brain atrophy with a resulting increase in extradural space. As a result, bridging veins tear and this causes rapid and subacute development of subdural hematomas. Torn cortical veins or venous sinuses and bruised tissue also may be the source. These subdural hematomas act like growing masses, increasing ICP that eventually applies pressure to the bleeding vessels (see Figure 16.2). Brain herniation can result. With a chronic subdural hematoma, the existing subdural space slowly fills with blood. A vascular membrane forms around the hematoma in about 2 weeks. Further growth may take place.

In acute, rapidly developing subdural hematomas, the growing clots apply pressure to the brain. As ICP rises, pressure is applied to the bleeding veins. Bleeding is self-limiting, although pressure to the cerebrum and movement of brain tissue can cause temporal lobe herniation.

An acute subdural hematoma usually begins with a headache, drowsiness, restlessness or agitation, slowed thought, and confusion.

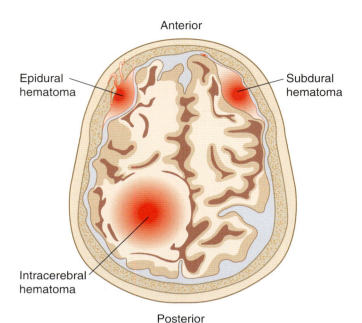

FIGURE 16.2 Brain Hematomas.

These symptoms worsen over time and progress to loss of consciousness, breathing pattern changes, and pupil dilation (i.e., the symptoms of temporal lobe herniation). Homonymous hemianopia (impaired vision in either the right or the left field [see Figure 14.11]), dysconjugate gaze (failure of the eyes to turn together in the same direction), and gaze palsies may occur.

Of persons affected by chronic subdural hematomas, 80% have chronic headaches and tenderness over the hematoma. Most persons appear to have a worsening dementia with generalized rigidity (paratonia). Chronic subdural hematomas require a craniotomy to remove the jelly-like blood. Percutaneous (through the skin) drainage for chronic subdural hematomas has been successful. However, reaccumulation often occurs unless the surrounding membrane is removed.

Intracerebral hematomas (bleeding within the brain) occur in 2 to 3% of persons with head injuries. These injuries may be single or multiple and are associated with contusions. They are found mainly in the frontal and temporal lobes but may also occur in the hemispheric deep white matter. Penetrating (going through the skull) injury or shearing forces injure small blood vessels. The intracerebral hematoma then acts as a growing mass. The growing mass increases ICP, applies pressure to brain tissues, and causes edema (see Figure 16.2). Delayed intracerebral hematomas may appear 3 to 10 days after the head injury. Intracerebral hematomas also can occur with nontraumatic brain injury, as seen in hemorrhagic stroke.

Intracerebral hematomas cause a decreasing level of consciousness. Coma or a confusional state from other injuries can make the cause of this increasing unresponsiveness difficult to notice. Contralateral (opposite side) hemiplegia also may occur. As ICP rises, temporal lobe herniation may appear. In delayed intracerebral hematoma, the presentation is like that of a hypertensive brain hemorrhage. Symptoms include sudden, rapidly decreased level of consciousness with pupil dilation, breathing pattern changes, hemiplegia, and bilateral positive Babinski reflexes.

History and physical examination help to form the diagnosis. CT scan, MRI, and cerebral angiography confirm the diagnosis. Removal of a single intracerebral hematoma has only occasionally been helpful and is usually used for subcortical white matter hematomas. Otherwise, treatment focuses on decreasing the ICP and letting the hematoma reabsorb slowly.

Open brain injury (trauma that penetrates the dura mater) creates both focal and diffuse injuries. This includes compound skull fractures and missile injuries (e.g., bullets, rocks, knives, and blunt instruments). A compound skull fracture opens a path between the cranial contents and the environment. Whenever cuts of the scalp, tympanic membrane, sinuses, eye, or mucous membranes are present, a compound skull fracture should be considered. Such fractures may involve the cranial vault or the base of the skull (basilar skull fracture). Cranial nerve damage and spinal fluid leak may occur with a basilar skull fracture.

The causes of open brain trauma are crush injury or stretch injury. A crush injury includes cutting and crushing of whatever the missile touches. A stretch injury includes blood vessels and nerves damaged without direct contact and is caused by stretching. Injury also occurs to the coverings and the brain (scalp and brain lacerations). This may include skull fractures and meningeal or cerebral lacerations from projectiles and debris driven into the brain matter.

Most persons become unconscious with an open brain injury. The location of injury, amount of damage and bleeding determine the depth and length of the coma. Open brain injury often requires the removal of injured tissues to prevent infection and removal of blood clots. These actions reduce ICP. Steroids, dehydrating agents, osmotic diuretics, or combinations of these medications are the usual treatment of ICP. The use of antibiotics aims to prevent infection.

A compound fracture is diagnosed using physical examination and skull X-rays. Basilar skull fracture is determined based on clinical findings, such as spinal fluid leaking from the ear or nose. Skull X-rays often do not show the fracture. Intracranial air or air in the sinuses on X-ray, CT scan, or MRI is indirect evidence of a basilar skull fracture. Treatment of a basilar skull fracture includes bed rest and close observation for meningitis and other complications.

Diffuse brain injury. Diffuse brain injury (diffuse axonal injury [DAI]) involves widespread areas of the brain. The physical effects from high levels of acceleration and deceleration, such as whiplash, or rotational forces, cause shearing of delicate axonal fibres and white matter tracts that project to the cerebral cortex (see Figure 16.1). The most severe axonal injuries are located more peripheral to the brainstem. These injuries cause extensive cognitive and affective impairments, as seen in survivors of TBI from motor vehicle accidents. Axonal damage reduces the speed of information processing and responding and disrupts the person's attention span.[5]

The use of an electron microscope is the only way to detect axonal damage. Detection of damage involves numerous axons, either alone or with actual tissue tears. Advanced imaging techniques help detect areas of injury. Areas where axons and small blood vessels are torn appear as small hemorrhages. These tears commonly occur in the corpus callosum and dorsolateral quadrant of the rostral brainstem at the superior cerebellar peduncle. More damaged axons are visible 12 hours to several days after the initial injury. The severity of diffuse injury relates to how much shearing force the brainstem experienced. DAI is not associated with intracranial hypertension immediately after injury. However, acute brain swelling caused by increased intravascular blood flow within the brain, vasodilation, and increased cerebral blood volume is seen often and can result in death. DAI may induce long-term neurodegenerative processes. These changes may continue for years after injury, with the development of chronic traumatic encephalopathy and Alzheimer disease–like pathological changes.[6]

Secondary Brain Injury. **Secondary brain injury** is an indirect result of primary brain injury, including trauma and stroke syndromes. Both systemic and cerebral processes are contributing factors. Systemic processes include hypotension, hypoxia, anemia, hypercapnia, and hypocapnia. Cerebral findings include inflammation, cerebral edema, increased intracranial pressure (IICP), decreased cerebral perfusion pressure, cerebral ischemia, and brain herniation. Cellular and molecular brain damage from the effects of primary injury develops hours to days later and causes disruption of the blood–brain barrier and neuronal death. Mechanisms include oxidative stress, excitotoxicity (excessive stimulation by excitatory neurotransmitters, such as glutamate), and mitochondrial failure.

The management of secondary brain injury is related to prevention of hypoxia and maintenance of cerebral perfusion pressure. Management includes removal of hematomas and treatment of hypotension, hypoxemia, anemia, intracranial pressure, fluid and electrolyte balance, body temperature, and ventilation. The development of neuroprotective agents is in progress but is difficult because of the complexity of multiple interacting secondary injury cascades.[7] Nutrition management has emerged as critically important in the care of individuals with severe brain injury.[8] Long-term recovery and mortality can be influenced by systemic complications, such as pneumonia, fever, infections, and immobility, that contribute to further brain injury and delays in repair and recovery.

Categories of Traumatic Brain Injury. Several categories of TBI exist and are presented here as mild, moderate, and severe. The terms *concussion* and *traumatic brain injury* are often used interchangeably. The severity of TBI commonly considers the duration of loss of consciousness, the GCS score, posttraumatic amnesia, and brain imaging results.[9]

Mild traumatic brain injury (mild concussion) is characterized by immediate but transitory clinical manifestations. There may be no loss of consciousness, or loss of consciousness may last less than 30 minutes. Most blunt trauma injuries cause mild concussion. The GCS score is 13 to 15. The initial confusional state lasts for 1 to several minutes, possibly with amnesia for events preceding the trauma (retrograde amnesia). Persons may experience headache, nausea, vomiting, impaired ability to concentrate, and difficulty sleeping for up to a few days. A blood test to evaluate for the presence of mild TBI in adults is available to determine if there is a need for a computed tomography (CT) scan.[10]

Moderate traumatic brain injury (moderate concussion) is any loss of consciousness lasting more than 30 minutes and up to 6 hours. The GCS score is 9 to 12. A basal skull fracture may be present, but there is no brainstem injury. There is transitory decerebration or decortication (see Figure 15.6). The person is confused and experiences post-traumatic amnesia that lasts for more than 24 hours. There often are permanent deficits in selective attention, vigilance, detection, working memory, data processing, vision or perception, and language. There may also be mood and affect changes ranging from mild to severe. Brain imaging is abnormal.

Severe traumatic brain injury (severe concussion) is loss of consciousness lasting more than 6 hours. The GCS is 3 to 8. Often there are associated signs of brainstem damage. These signs include changes in pupillary reaction, cardiac and respiratory symptoms, decorticate or decerebrate posturing (see Figure 15.6), and abnormal reflexes. Brain imaging is abnormal. IICP appears 4 to 6 days after injury. Pulmonary complications occur often, with severe sensorimotor and cognitive system deficits. Other signs include severely compromised coordinated movements and verbal and written communication, inability to learn and reason, and inability to modulate behaviour. Severe injury causes permanent neurological deficits, and some individuals remain in a vegetative state or die because of brain injury or secondary complications.

The goal of treating TBI is to maintain cerebral perfusion and oxygenation and promote neuroprotection. Implementation of management guidelines for TBI decreases death and improves neurological outcome. The Corticosteroid Randomization After Significant Head Injury (CRASH) trial showed corticosteroids increase mortality with acute TBI. As a result, these drugs are no longer used.[11]

Complications of Traumatic Brain Injury. Many complications are associated with TBI. The severity of injury and the parts of the brain that are affected determine the complications that occur. Altered states of consciousness can range from confusion to deep coma (see Table 15.3). Cognitive deficits; hydrocephalus; sensory-motor disorders, including pain, paresis, and paralysis; and loss of coordination may be present. A summary of the three most common post-traumatic brain syndromes follows.

Postconcussion syndrome may last for weeks to months after a concussion. Symptoms of this syndrome include headache, dizziness, fatigue, nervousness or anxiety, irritability, insomnia, depression, inability to concentrate, and forgetfulness. Treatment includes reassurance and symptomatic relief. It is also important to include 24 hours of close observation after the concussion in the event that bleeding or swelling in the brain occurs. Symptoms requiring further evaluation and treatment include drowsiness or confusion, nausea or vomiting, severe headache, memory deficit, seizures, drainage of CSF from the ear or nose, weakness or loss of feeling in the extremities, unequal pupil size, and double vision. Guidelines for the management of pediatric and adult concussion exist.[12-14] Guidelines also exist for the management of sports-related concussion.[15]

Post-traumatic seizures (epilepsy) occur in about 10 to 20% of TBIs.[16] The highest risk is among open brain injuries. Seizures can occur within days, and up to 2 to 5 years or longer after the trauma. The cause is poorly understood. Cellular and molecular changes in the brain associated with injury and repair may cause the hyperexcitable state that leads to seizure initiation. These changes include sprouting of new neurons with hyperexcitability and decreases in GABAergic inhibition. Seizure prevention medications should be started for moderate to severe TBI at the time of injury. Clinical trials are ongoing to test medications that prevent the development of post-traumatic seizures.[16]

Chronic traumatic encephalopathy (CTE) (previously called *dementia pugilistica*) is a progressive dementing disease that develops with repeated brain injury. CTE is associated with injury from contact sports such as hockey and football, blast injuries in soldiers, or work-related head trauma. Hyperphosphorylated tau neurofibrillary tangles are present in the brain, and research continues to discover the link between neurotrauma and CTE. CTE is associated with violent behaviours, loss of control, depression, suicide, memory loss, cognitive change, and change in motor function. It is diagnosed from history and clinical evaluation and at autopsy.[17]

Spinal Cord and Vertebral Injury

Each year, approximately 4 259 persons in Canada experience serious spinal cord injury. Male gender and ages 20 to 39 years are strong risk factors for experiencing a traumatic spinal cord injury. Motor vehicle accidents, sports activities, and violence are the leading cause of injury in this age group. A significant number of injuries also occur in persons aged 70 years and older. This is mainly because of falls.[18] Older persons are particularly at risk for trauma that results in serious spinal cord injury because of pre-existing degenerative vertebral disorders.

PATHOPHYSIOLOGY **Primary spinal cord injury** occurs with the initial mechanical trauma and immediate tissue damage. Table 16.3

TABLE 16.3 Spinal Cord Injuries

Injury	Description
Cord concussion	Results in temporary disruption of cord-mediated functions
Cord contusion	Bruising of neural tissue causes swelling and temporary loss of cord-mediated functions
Cord compression	Pressure on the spinal cord causes ischemia to tissues; must be relieved (decompressed) to prevent permanent damage to the spinal cord
Laceration	Tearing of neural tissues of the spinal cord; may be reversible if only slight damage sustained by neural tissues; may result in permanent loss of cord-mediated functions if the spinal tracts are disrupted
Transection	Severing of the spinal cord causes permanent loss of function
Complete	All tracts in the spinal cord are completely disrupted; all cord-mediated functions below injury are completely and permanently lost
Incomplete	Some tracts in the spinal cord remain intact, together with functions mediated by these tracts; has potential for recovery although function is temporarily lost
Preserved sensation only	Some sensation below level of injury
Preserved motor nonfunctional	Preserved motor function without useful purpose; sensory function may or may not be preserved
Preserved motor functional	Preserved voluntary motor function that is functionally useful
Hemorrhage	Bleeding into neural tissue because of blood vessel damage; usually no major loss of function
Damage or obstruction of spinal blood supply	Causes local ischemia

reviews injuries to the cord. Primary spinal cord injury occurs if an injured spine does not receive adequate immobilization immediately following injury. This injury also may occur with dislocation from longitudinal stretching of the cord with or without flexion or extension of the vertebral column. The stretching causes altered axon transport, edema, myelin degeneration, and retrograde or Wallerian degeneration (see Chapter 13).

Secondary spinal cord injury is a disease-causing process involving vascular, cellular, and biochemical events. These events begin within a few minutes after injury and continue for weeks. This injury includes edema, ischemia, excitotoxicity, inflammation, oxidative damage, and activation of necrotic and apoptotic cell death.

With secondary spinal cord injury, microscopic hemorrhages appear in the central grey matter. These hemorrhages increase in size until the entire grey matter is hemorrhagic and necrotic. Edema in the white matter occurs, impairing the microcirculation of the cord. Hemorrhages and edema are followed by decreased vascular perfusion and development of ischemic areas. These symptoms are greatest at the level of injury and two cord segments above and below it. Cellular and subcellular alterations and tissue necrosis occur. Cord swelling increases the person's degree of dysfunction. This dysfunction makes it difficult to distinguish functions permanently lost from those temporarily impaired. In the cervical region at C1 to C4, cord swelling may be life-threatening because cardiovascular and respiratory control functions can be lost. Circulation in the white matter tracts of the spinal cord returns to normal in about 24 hours.

Excitotoxicity (excessive stimulation by excitatory neurotransmitters, such as glutamate), excess intracellular calcium, oxidative damage, and cell death occur similarly to those described for TBI. Spared neurons continue to be chronically injured. Death of oligodendrocytes and myelin degeneration, axonal disruption, glial scarring, cystic cavitation, and release of inhibitory mediators results. The process results in a physical and chemical barrier to regeneration.[19]

Vertebral injuries result from acceleration, deceleration, or deformation forces occurring at impact. These forces cause vertebral fractures, dislocations, and bone fragments that can cause compression to the tissues. They may also pull or exert traction (tension) on the tissues, or cause shearing of tissues so they slide into one another (Figures 16.3 to 16.6). Vertebral injuries can be classified as (1) simple fracture—a single break usually affecting transverse or spinous processes; (2)

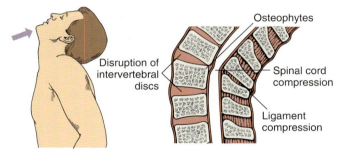

FIGURE 16.3 Hyperextension Injuries of the Spine. Hyperextension injuries of the spine can result in fracture or nonfracture injuries with spinal cord damage.

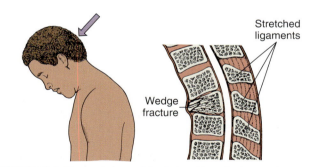

FIGURE 16.4 Flexion Injury of the Spine. Hyperflexion produces translation (subluxation) of vertebrae that compromises the central canal and compresses spinal cord parenchyma or vascular structures.

compressed (wedged) vertebral fracture—vertebral body compressed anteriorly; (3) comminuted (burst) fracture—vertebral body shattered into several pieces; and (4) dislocation.

The vertebrae fracture easily with direct and indirect trauma. When the supporting ligaments are torn, the vertebrae move out of alignment and dislocations occur. A horizontal force moves the vertebrae straight forward. If the person is in a flexed position at the time of injury, the vertebrae are then angulated. Flexion and extension injuries may result in dislocations. (Table 16.4 reviews bone, ligament, and joint injuries.)

Vertebral injuries in adults occur most often at vertebrae C1 to C2 (cervical), C4 to C7, and T10 (thoracic) to L2 (lumbar) (see Figure 13.11). These are the most moveable portions of the vertebral column. The spinal cord fills most of the vertebral canal in the cervical and lumbar regions. As a result, spinal cord injury can easily occur in these locations.

CLINICAL MANIFESTATIONS Spinal shock develops immediately after injury. This occurs because of loss of continuous tonic discharge from the brain or brainstem and decrease of suprasegmental signals. The decrease in signals is caused by cord hemorrhage, edema, or anatomical transection. Normal activity of spinal cord cells at and below the level of injury stops. This results in complete loss of reflex function, flaccid paralysis, absence of sensation, loss of bladder and rectal control,

temporary drop in blood pressure, and poor venous circulation. The condition also results in altered temperature control because of damage to the sympathetic nervous system. The hypothalamus cannot regulate body heat through vasoconstriction and increased metabolism. The person, therefore, assumes the temperature of the air (poikilothermia). Spinal shock generally lasts 7 to 20 days, with a range of a few days to 3 months. It ends with the reappearance of reflex activity, hyperreflexia, spasticity, and reflex emptying of the bladder. Table 16.5 reviews the signs of spinal cord injury.

Neurogenic shock, also called *vasogenic shock*, occurs with cervical or upper thoracic cord injury above T6. Neurogenic shock may occur in addition to spinal shock. The absence of sympathetic activity, through loss of supraspinal control and unopposed parasympathetic tone, caused by the intact vagus nerve, results in neurogenic shock. Symptoms include vasodilation, hypotension, bradycardia, and failure of body temperature regulation. Hypovolemic or cardiogenic shock may complicate neurogenic shock if there is coexisting heart failure or blood loss (see Chapter 24).

Loss of motor and sensory function depends on the extent and level of injury. Paralysis of the lower half of the body with both legs involved is termed *paraplegia*. Paralysis involving all four extremities is termed *quadriplegia* (tetraplegia). In complete quadriplegia, the level of injury is above C6 and all upper extremity function is lost. In incomplete quadriplegia, function at or above C6 is preserved, leaving the shoulder, upper arm, and some forearm muscle control intact. The initial clinical manifestations associated with acute spinal cord injury are related to spinal shock described above. The duration of this state is highly variable. In most persons, reflex activity returns in about a week. Return of spinal neuron excitability occurs slowly. Depending on the degree of damage, either of the following can occur: (1) motor, sensory, reflex, and autonomic functions return to normal; or (2) autonomic neural activity in the isolated segment develops. Spasticity is common, with hyperreflexia, clonus, and painful muscle spasms. Sometimes after several months, episodes of autonomic hyperreflexia occur.

Autonomic hyperreflexia (dysreflexia) is a syndrome of sudden, massive reflex sympathetic discharge associated with spinal cord injury at level T6 or above. Descending inhibition is blocked in this syndrome (Figure 16.7). It may occur after spinal shock resolves and be a recurrent complication. Characteristics involve many changes in the body's autonomic functions. These changes include sudden hypertension (up to 300 mm Hg, systolic), a pounding headache, blurred vision, sweating above the level of the lesion with flushing of the skin, nasal congestion, nausea, piloerection caused by pilomotor spasm, bradycardia (30 to 40 beats/min). The symptoms may develop singly or in combination. The condition can cause serious complications (stroke, seizures, myocardial ischemia, and death) and requires immediate treatment.

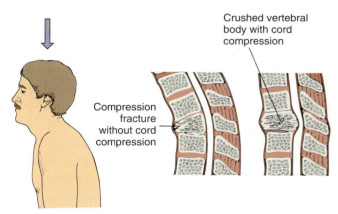

FIGURE 16.5 Axial Compression Injuries of the Spine. In axial compression injuries of the spine, contusion of the spinal cord occurs directly by pushing the bone or disc material into the spinal canal.

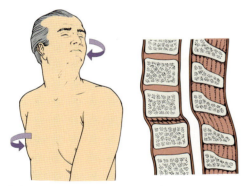

FIGURE 16.6 Flexion-rotation Injuries of the Spine.

TABLE 16.4	Mechanisms of Vertebral Injury Involving Bone, Ligaments, and Joints		
Mechanism of Injury	**Location of Vertebral Injury**	**Forces of Injury**	**Location of Injury**
Hyperextension	Fracture and dislocation of posterior elements, such as spinous processes, transverse processes, laminae, pedicles, or posterior ligaments	Results from forces of acceleration–deceleration and sudden decrease in anteroposterior diameter of the spinal cord	Cervical area
Hyperflexion	Fracture or dislocation of vertebral bodies, discs, or ligaments	Results from sudden and excessive force that pushes the neck forward or causes an exaggerated lateral movement of the neck to one side	Cervical area
Vertical compression (axial loading)	Shattering fractures	Results from a force applied along an axis from top of the cranium through vertebral bodies	T12 to L2
Rotational forces (flexion-rotation)	Rupture support ligaments in addition to producing fractures	Add shearing force to acceleration forces	Cervical area

TABLE 16.5 Clinical Manifestations of Spinal Cord Injury

Stage	Clinical Manifestations

Spinal Shock Stage Complete spinal cord transection	Loss of motor function
	  1. Quadriplegia with injuries of the cervical spinal cord
	  2. Paraplegia with injuries of the thoracic spinal cord
	Muscle flaccidity
	Loss of all reflexes below level of injury
	Loss of pain, temperature, touch, pressure, and proprioception below the level of injury
	Pain at the site of injury caused by zone of hyperesthesia above the injury
	Atonic bladder and bowel
	Paralytic ileus with distension
	Loss of vasomotor tone in lower body parts; low and unstable blood pressure
	Loss of perspiration below the level of injury
	Loss or extreme decrease of genital reflexes such as penile erection and bulbocavernous reflex
	Dry and pale skin; possible ulceration over bony prominences
	Breathing impairment

Partial spinal cord transection	Asymmetrical flaccid motor paralysis below level of injury
	Asymmetrical reflex loss
	Preservation of some sensation below the level of injury
	Vasomotor instability less severe than that seen with complete cord transection
	Bowel and bladder function damage less severe than that seen with complete cord transection
	Preservation of ability to perspire in some parts of the body below the level of injury
	Brown-Séquard's syndrome (associated with penetrating injuries, hyperextension and flexion, locked facets, and compression fractures)
	  1. Ipsilateral paralysis or paresis below the level of injury
	  2. Ipsilateral loss of touch, pressure, vibration, and position sense below the level of injury
	  3. Contralateral loss of pain and temperature sensations below the level of injury
	Central cervical cord syndrome (acute cord compression between bony bars or spurs anteriorly and thickened ligamentum flavum posteriorly associated with hyperextension)
	  1. Motor deficits in upper extremities, especially hands, denser than in lower extremities
	  2. Varying degrees of bladder dysfunction
	Burning hand syndrome (variant of central cord syndrome; in 50% of cases an underlying spine fracture/dislocation is present)
	  1. Severe burning paresthesias and dysesthesias in the hands or feet
	Anterior cord syndrome (compromise of the anterior spinal artery by occlusion or pressure effect of disc)
	  1. Loss of motor function below the level of injury
	  2. Loss of pain and temperature sensations below the level of injury
	  3. Touch, pressure, position, and vibration senses intact
	Posterior cord syndrome (associated with hyperextension injuries with fractures of the vertebral arch)
	  1. Impaired light touch and proprioception
	Conus medullaris syndrome (compression injury at T12 from disc herniation or burst fracture of body of T12)
	  1. Flaccid paralysis of the legs
	  2. Flaccid paralysis of the anal sphincter
	  3. Variable sensory deficits
	Cauda equina syndrome (compression of nerve roots below L1 caused by fracture and dislocation of spine or large posterocentral intervertebral disc herniation)
	  1. Lower extremity motor deficits
	  2. Variable sensorimotor dysfunction
	  3. Variable reflex dysfunction
	  4. Variable bladder, bowel, and sexual dysfunction
	Syndrome of neuropraxia (postathletic injury, associated with congenital spinal stenosis)
	  1. Dramatic but temporary neurological deficits, including quadriplegia
	Horner's syndrome (injury to preganglionic sympathetic trunk or postganglionic sympathetic neurons of superior cervical ganglion)
	  1. Ipsilateral pupil smaller than the contralateral pupil
	  2. Sunken ipsilateral eyeball
	  3. Ptosis of the affected eyeball
	  4. Lack of perspiration on the ipsilateral side of the face

Heightened Reflex Activity Stage	Emergence of Babinski reflexes, possibly progressing to a triple reflex; possible development of still later flexor spasms Reappearance of ankle and knee reflexes, which become hyperactive Contraction of the reflex detrusor muscle leading to urinary incontinence Appearance of reflex defecation Mass reflex with flexion spasms, profuse sweating, piloerection, and bladder emptying Occasional bowel emptying may be caused by autonomic stimulation of skin or from full bladder Episodes of hypertension Defective heat-induced sweating Eventual development of extensor reflexes, first in muscles of hip and thigh, later in the leg Possible paresthesias below the level of transection: dull, burning pain in the lower back, abdomen, buttocks, and perineum

In autonomic hyperreflexia, sensory receptors below the level of the cord injury are stimulated. The intact autonomic nervous system reflexively responds with an arteriolar spasm that increases blood pressure. Baroreceptors in the cerebral vessels, the carotid sinus, and the aorta sense the hypertension and stimulate the parasympathetic system. The heart rate decreases, but the visceral and peripheral vessels do not dilate. This occurs because efferent impulses cannot pass through the cord.

The most common cause of autonomic hyperreflexia is a distended bladder or rectum. Any sensory stimulation (i.e., skin or pain receptors), however, can cause autonomic hyperreflexia. Intravenous fluids may be needed to maintain blood pressure. Medication therapy may be needed to lower blood pressure and reduce complications. Bladder, bowel, and skin care management are important preventive strategies. Education of the person and family regarding triggers, acute management, and wearing a medic alert tag are important.[20]

EVALUATION AND TREATMENT Physical examination and imaging studies determine the diagnosis of spinal cord injury. Neurogenic shock must be differentiated from other kinds of shock (i.e., hypovolemic shock). For all suspected or confirmed vertebral fractures or dislocations, the immediate intervention is immobilization of the spine to prevent further injury. Decompression and surgical fixation may be necessary.

Therapeutic hypothermia has shown some encouraging evidence for improved outcomes, particularly for cervical cord injuries, but more research is needed. Clinical trials are in progress to treat acute spinal cord injury. These include cell-based therapies, immune modulators, vasculature selective treatments, and functional electrical stimulation. Nutrition, lung function, skin integrity, prevention of pressure ulcers, and bladder and bowel management must be addressed. Plans for rehabilitation need early attention.[21-23]

Degenerative Disorders of the Spine

Low Back Pain

Low back pain (LBP) affects the area between the lower rib cage and gluteal muscles and often radiates into the thighs. In Canada, back and neck pain is the leading cause of disability-adjusted life years, and it is the second leading cause overall in high-income countries.[24] LBP is the primary cause of disability worldwide.[25] The related problems of disability include psychological, financial, occupational, and social effects on the person and family members.

Risk factors include occupations that require repeated lifting in the forward bent-and-twisted position; exposure to vibrations caused by vehicles or industrial machinery; obesity; and cigarette smoking. Some people have a genetic predisposition for LBP.

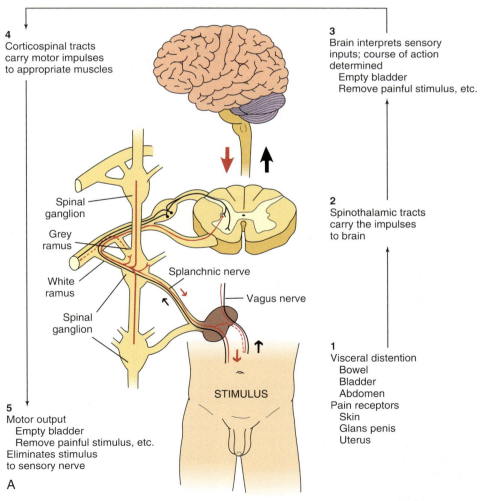

FIGURE 16.7 Autonomic Hyperreflexia. **A,** Normal response pathway. *(Continued)*

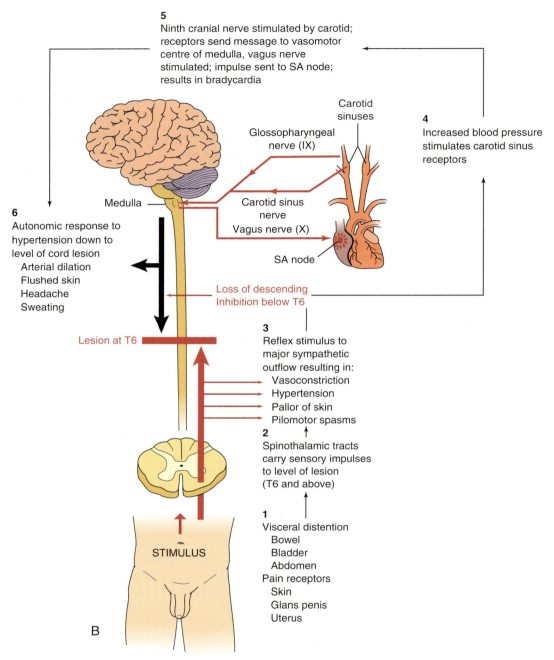

FIGURE 16-7, cont'd B, Autonomic dysreflexia pathway. *SA,* Sinoatrial. (Modified from Rudy, E. B. [1984]. *Advanced neurological and neurosurgical nursing.* Mosby.)

PATHOGENESIS Most cases of LBP are idiopathic or nonspecific, and no precise diagnosis is possible. *Acute* LBP is often associated with muscle or ligament strain. Acute LBP is more common in persons younger than 50 years of age without a history of cancer. Common causes of *chronic* LBP include degenerative disc disease (DDD), spondylolysis, spondylolisthesis (vertebra slides forward or slips in relation to a vertebra below), spinal osteochondrosis, spinal stenosis, and lumbar disc herniation. There are many other causes of chronic LBP. These include tension caused by tumours or disc prolapse, bursitis, synovitis, rising venous and tissue pressures (found in degenerative joint disease), abnormal bone pressures, spinal immobility, inflammation caused by infection (as in osteomyelitis), and pain referred from viscera or the posterior peritoneum. Systemic causes of LBP include bone diseases, such as osteoporosis or osteomalacia, and hyperparathyroidism. Anatomically, LBP must originate from innervated structures. Deep pain is widely referred and varies. The nucleus pulposus has no intrinsic innervation, but when herniated through a prolapsed disc, it irritates the spinal nerve dural membranes and causes pain referred to the segmental area (Figure 16.8).

The interspinous bursae can be a source of pain between L3, L4, L5, and S1 (sacral) but also may affect L1, L2, and L3 spinous processes. Many pain receptors supply the anterior and posterior longitudinal ligaments of the spine, the interspinous and supraspinous ligaments, and the ligamentum flavum. All these ligaments are at risk for traumatic tears (sprains) and fracture. Inflammation and nerve sprouting within the disc may cause pain.[26]

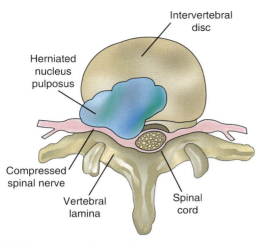

FIGURE 16.8 Herniated Nucleus Pulposus.

CLINICAL MANIFESTATIONS About 1% of persons with acute LBP have pain along the distribution of a lumbar nerve root (radicular pain). The most common involves the sciatic nerve (sciatica). Sensorineural and motor deficits, such as tingling, numbness, and weakness in various parts of the leg and foot often are experienced with sciatica. Major or gradual motor or sensory deficit may cause cauda equina syndrome. This syndrome includes new-onset bowel or bladder incontinence or urinary retention, loss of anal sphincter tone, and saddle anaesthesia. History of cancer metastasis to bone and suspected spinal infection can be associated with chronic LBP.

EVALUATION AND TREATMENT History and physical examination determine the diagnosis of LBP. Imaging and nerve conduction studies are obtained with severe neurological deficit or serious underlying disease. Diagnosis and treatment guidelines are available to plan therapy.[25,27] Most persons with acute LBP benefit from a nonspecific short-term treatment including pain relief medications, exercises, physiotherapy, and education. Treatment also includes advising individuals to stay active and continue their usual activity, including work, within the limits permitted by pain. Persons not responding to medical management or for emergency management of cauda equina syndrome may require surgical treatments. This may include discectomy and spinal fusions. Persons with chronic LBP may benefit from many therapies. This includes anti-inflammatory and muscle relaxant medications, exercise programs, massage, topical heat, spinal manipulation, acupuncture, cognitive-behavioural therapies, and interdisciplinary care.[27] There is little evidence for efficacy of opioids for chronic LBP, and a high risk for addiction.[27] The complexity of causes adds to the difficulty in defining the origins of the condition and clearly defining the most effective therapies.

Degenerative Joint Disease

Degenerative disc disease. Degenerative disc disease (DDD) is common in persons 30 years of age and older. It is a process of normal aging as a response to continuous vertical compression of the spine (axial loading). DDD includes a genetic component, involving genes that code the cartilage protein. The combination of environmental interactions and genetic predisposition increases susceptibility to lumbar disc disease. These factors disrupt the normal building and maintenance of cartilage.[28] Causes include biochemical (e.g., inflammatory mediators) and biomechanical alterations (e.g., mechanical loading and compression) of the intervertebral disc tissue. For example, loss of disc proteoglycans and collagen with disc dehydration and loss of hydrostatic pressure alters disc structure and function. The annulus (outer fibrous ring) can tear, and the disc can herniate, pinching nerves or placing strain on the spine. The findings in DDD include disc protrusion; spondylolysis and/or subluxation (spondylolisthesis); degeneration of vertebrae; and spinal stenosis. Lumbar disk disease commonly affects adults at some point in their lives. However, only a small percentage of people with DDD have any functional deficits because of pain.

Spondylolysis. Spondylolysis is a structural defect including degeneration, fracture, or developmental defect. It occurs in the pars interarticularis of the vertebral arch (the joining of the vertebral body to the posterior structures). This affects the lumbar spine at L5 most often. Mechanical pressure may cause an anterior or posterior displacement of the deficient vertebra (spondylolisthesis). Heredity plays a significant role. Spondylolysis is associated with an increased incidence of other congenital spinal defects. Symptoms include lower back and lower limb pain.

Spondylolisthesis. Spondylolisthesis is an osseous defect of the pars interarticularis. It allows a vertebra to slide anteriorly in relation to the vertebra below, commonly occurring at L5 to S1. Spondylolisthesis is graded from 1 to 4 based on the percentage of slip that occurs. Grades 1 and 2 have symptoms of pain in the lower back and buttocks, muscle spasms in the lower back and legs, and tightened hamstrings. Management includes exercise, rest, and back bracing. Vertebral slippage in grades 3 and 4 usually requires surgical treatment.

Spinal stenosis. Spinal stenosis is a narrowing of the spinal canal that causes pressure on the spinal nerves or cord. It can be congenital or acquired (more common) and associated with trauma or arthritis. The area of the spine affected determines its classification: cervical, thoracic, or lumbar. Acquired conditions include a bulging disc, facet hypertrophy, or a thick ossified posterior longitudinal ligament. Symptoms are related to the area of the spine affected. Symptoms may include pain; numbness; and tingling in the neck, hands, arms, or legs with weakness and difficulty walking. For those with chronic symptoms and those who do not respond to medical management, surgical decompression is recommended.

Herniated Intervertebral Disc

Herniation of an intervertebral disc is a displacement of the nucleus pulposus or annulus fibrosus beyond the intervertebral disc space (see Figure 16.8). Trauma and/or DDD usually cause rupture of an intervertebral disc. Risk factors are weight-bearing sports, light weightlifting, and certain work activities, such as repeated lifting. Men experience herniation more often than women, with the highest incidence in the 30- to 50-year age group. The discs most affected are the lumbosacral discs L4–L5 and L5–S1. Disc herniation occasionally occurs in the cervical area, usually at C5–C6 and C6–C7. Herniation at the thoracic level is rare. The herniation may occur instantly, within a few hours, or months to years after injury.

PATHOPHYSIOLOGY A tear in the ligament and posterior capsule of the disc are usually present in a herniated disc. The tear allows the nucleus pulposus to bulge and compress the nerve root. The vascular supply may be decreased and cause inflammatory changes in the nerve root (radiculitis). At times, the injury tears the entire disc loose. This causes the disc capsule and nucleus pulposus to bulge onto the nerve root or press on the spinal cord. Multiple nerve root compressions may be found at the L5–S1 level, where the cauda equina may be affected. This compression may cause cauda equina syndrome (see Table 16.5).

CLINICAL MANIFESTATIONS The location and size of the herniation into the spinal canal and the amount of space in the canal, determine

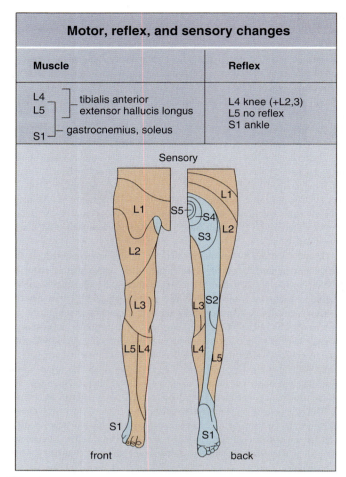

FIGURE 16.9 Clinical Features of a Herniated Nucleus Pulposus.

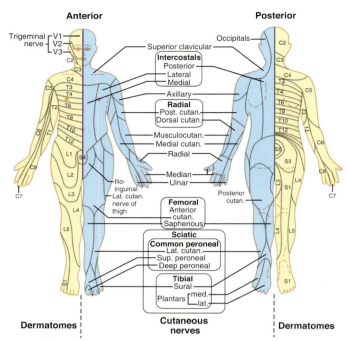

FIGURE 16.10 Sensory Nerve Distribution of Skin Dermatomes. *cutan.*, Cutaneous; *lat.*, lateral; *med.*, medial; *musculocutan.*, musculocutaneous; *post.*, posterior; *sup.*, superior. (Redrawn from Patton, H. D., Sundsten, J. W., Crill, W. E., et al. [Eds.]. [1976]. *Introduction to basic neurology*. Saunders. Borrowed from Canale, S. T., & Beaty, J. H. [2013]. *Campbell's operative orthopaedics* [12th ed.]. Mosby.)

the clinical signs associated with the injury (Figure 16.9). Compression and/or inflammation of a spinal nerve caused by disc herniation follows along the path of a dermatome. This process is called **radiculopathy** (Figure 16.10). A herniated disc in the lumbosacral area is associated with pain that radiates along the sciatic nerve path over the buttock and into the calf or ankle. The pain occurs with straining, coughing, and sneezing, and usually on straight leg raising. Other signs include limited range of motion of the lumbar spine; tenderness in the sciatic notch and along the sciatic nerve; impaired pain, temperature, and touch sensations in the L4–L5 or L5–S1 dermatomes of the leg and foot; decreased or absent ankle jerk reflex; and mild foot weakness. Rarely, there is development of cauda equina syndrome.

With the herniation of a lower cervical disc, paresthesias and pain are present in the upper arm, forearm, and hand along the affected nerve root path. Neck movement and straining, coughing, and sneezing, may increase neck and nerve root pain. Neck range of motion is decreased. Slight weakness and atrophy of biceps or triceps muscles may occur. The biceps or triceps reflex also may decrease. At times signs of corticospinal and sensory tract impairments appear. This includes motor weakness of the lower extremities, sensory disturbances in the lower extremities, and presence of a Babinski reflex.

EVALUATION AND TREATMENT History and physical examination, imaging, electromyelography, and nerve conduction studies all assist in the diagnosis of a herniated intervertebral disc. Evidence-based practice guidelines exist to guide treatment.[28] Most herniated discs heal on their own over time and do not require surgery. If there is evidence of severe compression (weakness or decreased deep tendon, bladder, or bowel reflexes) or if a conservative approach is unsuccessful, surgical treatment is indicated. Cauda equina syndrome rarely develops and requires emergency surgical evaluation and long-term follow-up.[29]

Cerebrovascular Disorders

> ✓ **QUICK CHECK 16.2**
> 1. Why is atherosclerosis a risk factor for thrombotic stroke?
> 2. Why do the signs and symptoms of a TIA resolve completely?
> 3. Why do lacunar strokes involve small infarcts?
> 4. How is an arteriovenous malformation (AVM) different from an aneurysm?

Cerebrovascular disease is any abnormality of the brain caused by a pathological process in the blood vessels. It is the most frequently occurring neurological disorder and often requires hospitalization. Included in this category are injuries of the vessel wall, blockage of the vessel lumen by thrombus or embolus, rupture of the vessel, and alteration in blood quality such as increased blood thickness.

The brain abnormalities caused by cerebrovascular disease are either (1) ischemia with or without infarction (death of brain tissues) or (2) hemorrhage. The common clinical sign of cerebrovascular disease is a **cerebrovascular accident (CVA)** or stroke. The symptoms occur suddenly and are focal (i.e., slurred speech, difficulty swallowing, limb weakness, or paralysis). In its mildest form, a CVA is so minimal that it is almost unnoticed. In its most severe form, hemiplegia, coma, and death result.

Cerebrovascular Accidents (Stroke Syndromes)

In Canada, cerebrovascular disease is the third highest cause of death. It is estimated that 13 480 Canadians died in 2018 related to cerebrovascular disease.[30] Approximately 80% of all CVAs can be prevented[31] (see *Health Promotion:* Prevention of Stroke in Women). Persons with hypertension and type 2 diabetes mellitus have a fourfold increase of CVA incidence and an eightfold increase in death from stroke.[32] Research has shown that Indigenous peoples are more likely to be diagnosed with hypertension and type 2 diabetes.[33] These factors put them at a higher risk for CVAs than the general population. The first stroke and all-cause mortality rates have shown a steady decline in recent years. This decrease is associated with improved control of hypertension, diabetes, and dyslipidemia, as well as smoking cessation.[34]

HEALTH PROMOTION

Prevention of Stroke in Women

Stroke is a leading cause of death in Canadian women. The number of women with stroke will outnumber men in the future. The Heart and Stroke Foundation of Canada recommends several ways women can decrease the risk for stroke. A summary of these recommendations is:
- Become and remain smoke-free
- Achieve and maintain a healthy body weight
- Be physically active with at least 150 minutes of moderate to vigorous-intensity aerobic physical activity per week
- Maintain a healthy blood pressure through lifestyle changes (such as increased physical activity) and, when needed, through medication
- Eat a healthy diet that is lower in fat and higher in fibre, and includes foods recommended in Canada's Dietary Guidelines
- Use medications to reduce the risk for stroke as prescribed by your health care provider; for example, medications for hypertension, dyslipidemia, and diabetes, or other medications such as acetylsalicylic acid (Aspirin)
- Identify causes of excess stress and use strategies to reduce them
- Be aware of a possible increased risk for stroke related to your family background
- Be aware of stroke risk factors (e.g., obesity, hypertension, and diabetes)
- Be aware that postmenopausal hormone therapy (conjugated equine estrogen) with or without medroxyprogesterone (Provera) should not be used for primary or secondary prevention of stroke

From Heart and Stroke Foundation of Canada. (2018). *Women's unique risk factors*. https://www.heartandstroke.ca/heart/risk-and-prevention/womens-unique-risk-factors.

CVAs (stroke syndromes) are classified as ischemic, hemorrhagic, or associated with hypoperfusion. Risk factors for stroke include:
- Poorly or uncontrolled arterial hypertension
- Smoking, which increases the risk for stroke by 50%
- Insulin resistance and diabetes mellitus
- Polycythemia and thrombocythemia
- High total cholesterol or low high-density lipoprotein (HDL) cholesterol, elevated lipoprotein-a
- Congestive heart disease and peripheral vascular disease
- Hyperhomocysteinemia
- Atrial fibrillation
- *Chlamydia pneumoniae* infection

Ischemic stroke. **Ischemic stroke** occurs when there is blockage to arterial blood flow to the brain. This occurs with thrombus formation, an embolus, or hypoperfusion related to decreased blood volume or heart failure. The inadequate blood supply results in ischemia (inadequate cellular oxygen) and can progress to infarction (death of tissue).

Transient ischemic attacks (TIAs) are episodes of neurological dysfunction lasting no more than 1 hour and resulting from focal cerebral ischemia. The signs of a TIA may include weakness, numbness, sudden confusion, loss of balance, or a sudden severe headache. The use of brain imaging tests often reveals a brain infarction. About 12% of persons who experience a TIA will have a stroke.[34]

Thrombotic strokes (cerebral thromboses) originate from arterial blockages caused by thrombi formation in arteries supplying the brain or intracranial vessels. Conditions causing increased coagulation or inadequate cerebral perfusion increase the risk for thrombosis. Dehydration, hypotension, and prolonged vasoconstriction from malignant hypertension can cause inadequate perfusion. Cerebral thrombosis develops most often from atherosclerosis and inflammatory disease processes that damage arterial walls. It may take as long as 20 to 30 years for blockage to develop at the branches and curvature found in the cerebral circulation (see Chapter 24 for a discussion of atherogenesis). The smooth stenotic area can degenerate, forming an ulcerated area of the vessel wall. Platelets and fibrin stick to the damaged wall, and a clot forms, gradually blocking the artery. The clot may grow both distally and proximally. Thrombotic strokes also occur when parts of a clot break away, travel upstream, and block blood flow, causing acute ischemia.

Embolic stroke involves pieces that break from a thrombus formed outside the brain. These thrombi usually develop in the heart, aorta, or common carotid artery. Other causes of embolism include fat, air, tumour, bacterial clumps, and foreign bodies. The embolus usually involves small brain vessels and blocks at a bifurcation or other point of narrowing, causing ischemia. An embolus may plug the lumen entirely and remain in place or break into fragments and become part of the vessel's blood flow. Risk factors for an embolic stroke include atrial fibrillation, left ventricular aneurysm or thrombus, left atrial thrombus, recent myocardial infarction, endocarditis, rheumatic valve disease, mechanical valvular prostheses, atrioseptal defects, patent foramen ovale, and primary cardiac tumours. In persons who experience an embolic stroke, a second stroke usually follows because the source of emboli continues to exist. The movement of the emboli is usually in the distribution of the middle cerebral artery (the largest cerebral artery). Ischemic strokes in children are associated with congenital heart disease, cerebral arteriovenous malformations, and sickle cell disease (see Chapter 17).

Lacunar strokes (lacunar infarcts or small vessel disease) are usually caused by blockage and breakage of a single, deep artery that supplies small subcortical vessels. This injury causes ischemic lesions (0.5 to 15 mm, or lacunes) usually in the basal ganglia, internal capsules, and pons. These strokes are rare, and, because of the location and small area of injury, they may have only motor or sensory deficits.[35] Lacunar strokes are associated with untreated high blood pressure.

Hypoperfusion, or hemodynamic stroke, is associated with *systemic* hypoperfusion caused by cardiac failure, pulmonary embolism, or bleeding that results in inadequate blood supply to the brain. Stroke may occur more readily if there is carotid artery blockage. Symptoms are usually bilateral and widespread.[36]

PATHOPHYSIOLOGY **Cerebral infarction** results when an area of the brain loses its blood supply because of vascular blockage. Causes include (1) abrupt vascular blockage (e.g., embolus or thrombi), (2) gradual vessel blockage (e.g., atheroma), and (3) partial blockage of stenotic vessels. Cerebral thrombi and cerebral emboli most commonly produce blockage, but atherosclerosis and hypertension are the most common causes.

There is a central core of irreversible ischemia and necrosis with cerebral infarction. The central core is surrounded by a zone of borderline ischemic tissue, the **ischemic penumbra**. Ischemia in the penumbra is not severe enough to result in structural damage. Quick restoration of blood flow in the penumbra by injection of thrombolytic agents assists perfusion and may prevent necrosis and loss of neurological function. The period for protecting the penumbra is about 3 hours.

Cerebral infarctions are ischemic or hemorrhagic. In *ischemic infarcts*, the affected area becomes pale and softens 6 to 12 hours after the blockage. Necrosis, swelling around the injury, and mushy breakdown appear by 48 to 72 hours after infarction. There is an influx of macrophages and phagocytosis of necrotic tissue. The necrosis resolves by about the second week, leaving a cavity surrounded by glial scarring.

Hemorrhagic transformation of an ischemic stroke is bleeding that occurs into the infarcted area through leaking vessels. Thrombolytic therapy may worsen the hemorrhagic transformation of ischemic stroke.[37] Guidelines are available for treatment.

CLINICAL MANIFESTATIONS Clinical signs of thrombotic and embolic stroke vary, depending on the artery blocked. Different sites of blockage create different syndromes. These syndromes include carotid artery syndromes (dysphasia and contralateral motor [i.e., paresis] sensory [i.e., numbness] deficits, conjugate ipsilateral eye deviation), middle cerebral artery syndromes (dysphasia and contralateral motor and sensory deficits), or vertebrobasilar system syndromes (dizziness and ataxia, can progress to quadriplegia and coma).[38] Contralateral motor and sensory signs occur on the opposite side of the body from the location of the brain lesion because motor tracts originate in the cortex and most cross over in the medulla. Sensory tracts originate in the periphery and cross over in the spinal cord. Ipsilateral signs occur on the same side as the brain lesion but are rare in stroke syndromes. See Figure 16.11 for the Heart and Stroke Foundation of Canada's assessment tool for persons presenting with signs and symptoms of stroke.

EVALUATION AND TREATMENT The diagnosis of stroke occurs with imaging. The focus of ischemic stroke treatment includes (1) restoring brain perfusion in a time frame that does not contribute to reperfusion injury, (2) reducing the ischemic cascade pathways, (3) lowering cerebral metabolic demand so that the susceptible brain tissue is protected against impaired perfusion, (4) preventing recurrent ischemic events, and (5) promoting tissue restoration. Intravenous thrombolysis, using tissue plasminogen activator (tPA), is given within 3 and up to 4.5 hours of start of symptoms. Other strategies include endovascular intra-arterial thrombolysis, thrombectomy, and placement of removable stents.[39] Supportive management is given to control cerebral edema and increased ICP, and to provide neuroprotection. Stopping the disease process by control of risk factors is critical. The use of antiplatelet therapy may be used. Guidelines are available for the assessment and management of acute ischemic stroke.[40]

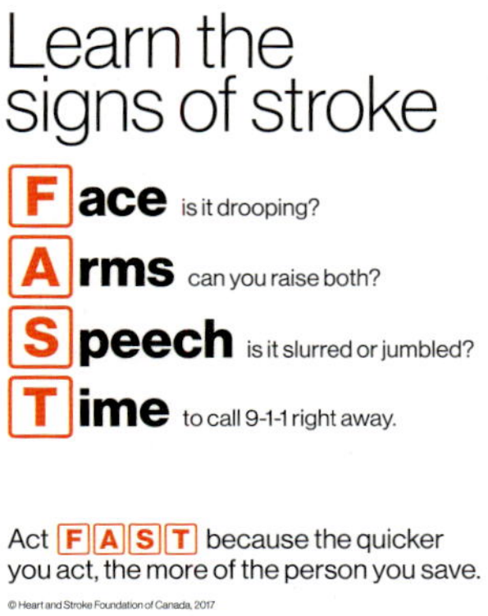

In embolic strokes, preventing further embolization by beginning anticoagulation therapy and correcting the primary problem is the goal of treatment. Persons experiencing ischemic strokes may undergo rehabilitation, and recovery of function is often possible.

Hemorrhagic stroke. Hemorrhagic stroke (intracranial hemorrhage) can occur within the brain tissue (intraparenchymal) or in the subarachnoid or subdural spaces. Hemorrhagic stroke is the third most common cause of CVA. The primary cause of intraparenchymal hemorrhagic stroke is chronic hypertension. Hypertensive causes of hemorrhagic stroke involve primarily smaller arteries and arterioles. This results in thickening of the vessel walls and increased cellularity of the vessels. Necrosis may be present. Microaneurysms in these smaller vessels or arteriolar necrosis may occur before the bleeding. Other causes include tumours, coagulation disorders, trauma, or illicit drug use, particularly cocaine. Prevention or control of hypertension decreases the incidence of hemorrhagic stroke.

Subarachnoid hemorrhage is associated with ruptured aneurysms or arteriovenous malformations or brain injury. Subdural hemorrhage (hematoma) is usually associated with brain trauma.

PATHOPHYSIOLOGY A mass of blood is formed as bleeding continues into the brain tissue. Adjacent brain tissue is deformed, compressed, and displaced. These factors produce ischemia, edema, increased ICP, and necrosis. Rupture or seepage of blood into the ventricular system often occurs and is associated with higher risk of death. Hemorrhages are large, small, slit, or petechial. The most common sites for hypertensive hemorrhages are in the putamen of the basal ganglia, the thalamus, the cortex and subcortex, the pons, the caudate nucleus, and the cerebellar hemispheres. Because neurons surrounding the ischemic or infarcted areas undergo changes that disrupt plasma membranes, cellular edema results. This causes further compression of capillaries. Maximal cerebral edema develops in about 72 hours and takes about 2 weeks to settle down. Most persons survive an initial hemispheric ischemic stroke unless there is massive cerebral edema, which is nearly always fatal. The cerebral hemorrhage resolves through reabsorption. A cavity surrounded by a dense gliosis (glial scar) forms after removal of the blood.

CLINICAL MANIFESTATIONS The symptoms of hemorrhagic stroke are like those for embolic and thrombotic stroke. The symptoms depend on the location and size of the bleed. They can occur suddenly and with activity. Once an unresponsive state occurs, the person rarely survives. The immediate prognosis is poor; however, if the person survives, recovery of function is possible.

It is difficult to differentiate ischemic from hemorrhagic stroke based on symptoms. Persons having intracranial hemorrhage from a ruptured or leaking aneurysm have one of three sets of symptoms: (1) onset of a severe generalized headache with an almost immediate progression into an unresponsive state, (2) headache but with consciousness maintained and seizures, nausea, and vomiting may occur, and (3) sudden progression into unconsciousness. If the hemorrhage occurs in the subarachnoid space, there may be no local signs. If bleeding spreads into the brain tissue, hemiparesis/paralysis, dysphasia, or homonymous hemianopia (visual field loss on the same side of both eyes) may be present. Warning signs of a future aneurysm rupture include headache, transient unilateral weakness, transient numbness and tingling, and transient speech disturbance. However, such warning signs are often absent.

EVALUATION AND TREATMENT The neurological exam and brain imaging are important to stroke diagnosis. Treatment of intracranial

FIGURE 16.11 Signs of Stroke. (From Heart and Stroke Foundation of Canada. [2018]. *Signs of stroke.* https://www.heartandstroke.ca/stroke/signs-of-stroke. © 2018, Heart and Stroke Foundation of Canada. Reproduced with the permission of the Heart and Stroke Foundation of Canada. www.heartandstroke.ca.)

bleeding, regardless of cause, focuses on stopping or reducing the bleeding, controlling blood pressure, edema, and increased ICP, preventing rebleeding, and preventing vasospasm. Surgical treatments, including endovascular approaches, are options for ruptured aneurysms, vascular malformations, and subarachnoid hemorrhage.[41]

Intracranial aneurysm. **Intracranial aneurysms** are a dilation or ballooning of a cerebral vessel from a weakness in the vessel wall. Risk factors include arteriosclerosis, congenital abnormality, cocaine use, trauma, inflammation, and smoking for family history. The size may vary from 2 mm to 2 or 3 cm. Most aneurysms are found at bifurcations in or near the circle of Willis, in the vertebrobasilar arteries, or within the carotid system. These locations have higher wall sheer stress (frictional force of blood against the endothelium of a blood vessel) and flow turbulence (see Figures 13.19 and 13.20). Aneurysms may be single, but at times more than one is present. In these instances, the aneurysms may be unilateral or bilateral. Peak incidence of rupture occurs in persons 50 to 59 years of age. The incidence in postmenopausal women is slightly higher than that in men.

PATHOPHYSIOLOGY No single pathological mechanism exists. Aneurysms rupture through thin areas of blood vessels, often at bifurcation sites. There is hemorrhage into the subarachnoid space that spreads rapidly, producing localized changes in the cerebral cortex and focal irritation of nerves and arteries (see the discussion of Laplace's law in Chapter 23). Bleeding ceases when a fibrin-platelet plug forms at the point of rupture and as a result of compression. Blood undergoes reabsorption through arachnoid villi, usually within 3 weeks.

Aneurysms are named based on their shape and form. **Saccular aneurysms (berry aneurysms)** occur frequently (in approximately 2% of the population). They result from congenital abnormalities in the tunica media of the arterial wall and wall weakening related to atherosclerosis and hypertension.[42] The sac gradually grows over time. A saccular aneurysm may be (1) round with a narrow stalk connecting it to the parent artery, (2) broad-based without a stalk, or (3) cylindrical (Figure 16.12). Their highest incidence of rupturing or bleeding (subarachnoid hemorrhage) is among persons 20 to 50 years of age.

Fusiform aneurysms (giant aneurysms) are less common. They occur because of diffuse arteriosclerotic changes. They most commonly occur in the basilar arteries or terminal portions of the internal carotid arteries. They act as space-occupying lesions.

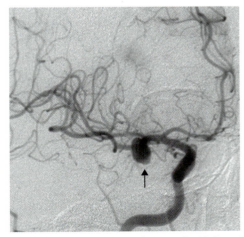

FIGURE 16.12 Berry Aneurysm, Angiogram. In this lateral view, with contrast filling a portion of the cerebral arterial circulation, a berry aneurysm *(arrow)* involving the middle cerebral artery of the circle of Willis at the base of the brain is shown. (From Klatt, E. C. [2015]. *Robbins and Cotran atlas of pathology* [3rd ed.]. Saunders.)

CLINICAL MANIFESTATIONS Aneurysms often are asymptomatic. Their presence is unknown until discovered incidentally or at autopsy. Symptoms include sudden severe headache, dizziness, and cranial nerve compression. The signs, however, vary depending on the location and size of the aneurysm. Most affected are cranial nerves III, IV, V, and VI (see Table 13.6) Unfortunately, the most common first sign of the presence of an aneurysm is an acute subarachnoid hemorrhage, intracerebral hemorrhage, or combined subarachnoid-intracerebral hemorrhage (see "Hemorrhagic Stroke").

EVALUATION AND TREATMENT Arteriography confirms diagnosis before a bleeding episode. After a subarachnoid or intracerebral hemorrhage, a diagnosis of an aneurysm is based on symptoms, history, and imaging. Treatments for intracranial aneurysm are both medical (i.e., control of hypertension) and surgical (i.e., external ventricular drain placement, microvascular clipping or placement of endovascular coils).[43]

Vascular malformation. Vascular malformations are rare congenital vascular lesions. An **arteriovenous malformation (AVM)** is a mass of dilated vessels between the arterial and venous systems (arteriovenous fistula) without an intervening capillary bed. AVMs may occur in any part of the brain and vary in size from a few millimetres to large malformations. They occur equally in males and females and occasionally occur in families. Although AVMs are usually present at birth, symptoms exhibit later in life and commonly occur before 30 years of age.

PATHOPHYSIOLOGY AVMs have abnormal blood vessel structure with abnormally thin walls.[44] There is direct shunting of arterial blood into the venous vasculature without disruption of the arterial blood pressure with an increased risk for rupture. One or several arteries may feed the AVM. Over time, they become twisted and dilated. With moderate to large AVMs, enough blood shunts into the malformation to rob surrounding tissue of adequate blood flow.

CLINICAL MANIFESTATIONS Twenty percent of persons with an AVM have a characteristic chronic, ordinary headache, although some experience migraine. Fifty percent of persons experience seizures. The other 50% experience an intracerebral, subarachnoid, or subdural hemorrhage with progressive neurological effects. Bleeding from an AVM into the subarachnoid space causes symptoms identical to those associated with a ruptured aneurysm. If bleeding is into the brain tissue, focal signs that develop resemble a stroke that is progressing in severity. Ten percent of persons experience hemiparesis or other focal signs. At times, noncommunicating hydrocephalus (see Chapter 15) develops with a large AVM that extends into the ventricular lining. Some AVMs never cause symptoms.

EVALUATION AND TREATMENT A systolic bruit over the carotid artery in the neck or the mastoid process, or the eyeball in a young person, representing audible turbulent blood flow, is usually diagnostic of an AVM. Imaging confirms diagnosis. Treatment options include direct surgical removal, endovascular embolization, or radiotherapy.[45]

Subarachnoid hemorrhage. **Subarachnoid hemorrhage (SAH)** is the escape of blood from a defective or injured vessel into the subarachnoid space. Persons at risk for a subarachnoid hemorrhage are those with intracranial aneurysm, intracranial AVM, hypertension, or a family history of SAH, and those who have experienced head injuries. Subarachnoid hemorrhages often recur, especially from a ruptured intracranial aneurysm.

PATHOPHYSIOLOGY When a vessel is leaking, blood oozes into the subarachnoid space. When a vessel tears, blood under pressure moves into the subarachnoid space. Autoregulation of blood flow is impaired, and there is a compensatory increase in systolic blood pressure.[46] The expanding hematoma acts like a space-occupying lesion. This causes compression and displacement of brain tissue with increased ICP, decreased cerebral blood flow, blood–brain barrier breakdown, brain edema, inflammation, and cell death. Secondary brain injury can occur as described for TBI. In addition, the escaped blood coats nerve roots; clogs arachnoid granulations, impairing CSF reabsorption; and obstructs foramina (passages) within the ventricular system, impairing CSF circulation. Granulation tissue is formed, and meningeal scarring with impairment of CSF reabsorption and secondary hydrocephalus often results. Death caused by subarachnoid hemorrhage is 50% at 1 month.

Delayed cerebral ischemia is a syndrome of progressive neurological deterioration. It is associated with *cerebral artery vasospasm*. It occurs in 3 to 14 days after a subarachnoid hemorrhage in about 50% of cases. Vasospasm may be related to the release of vasoactive substances during the hemorrhage, loss of autoregulation of blood flow, and neuron electrical activity that affects adjacent areas of the brain. Vasospasm with micro thrombosis causes decreased cerebral perfusion with extension of ischemic injury and increased risk of death.[47]

CLINICAL MANIFESTATIONS Early symptoms associated with leaking vessels are episodic. They include headache, changes in mental status or level of consciousness, nausea or vomiting, and focal neurological defects. A ruptured vessel causes a sudden, throbbing, "explosive" headache, nausea and vomiting, visual disturbances, motor deficits, and loss of consciousness related to a dramatic rise in ICP. Meningeal irritation and inflammation often occur, causing neck stiffness (nuchal rigidity), photophobia, blurred vision, irritability, restlessness, and low-grade fever. A positive **Kernig sign** (straightening the knee with the hip and knee in a flexed position produces pain in the back and neck regions) and a positive **Brudzinski sign** (passive flexion of the neck produces neck pain and increased rigidity) may appear. No localizing signs are present if the bleed occurs only in the subarachnoid space.

The Hunt and Hess SAH grading system is based on description of the clinical symptoms (Table 16.6).[48] Rebleeding is a significant risk with a high incidence of death (up to 70%). The period of greatest risk is during the first 72 hours and up to 2 weeks after the first bleed. Rebleeding causes a sudden increase in blood pressure and ICP, along with a deteriorating neurological status.

TABLE 16.6 Subarachnoid Hemorrhage Classification Scale

Category	Description
Grade I	Neurological status intact; mild headache, slight nuchal rigidity
Grade II	Neurological deficit shown by cranial nerve involvement; moderate to severe headache with more pronounced meningeal signs (e.g., photophobia, nuchal rigidity)
Grade III	Drowsiness and confusion with or without focal neurological deficits; pronounced meningeal signs
Grade IV	Stuporous with pronounced neurological deficits (e.g., hemiparesis, dysphasia); nuchal rigidity
Grade V	Deep coma state with decerebrate posturing and other brainstem functioning

From Tateshima, S., & Duckwiler, G. (2012). Vascular diseases of the nervous system. In R. B. Daroff, G. M. Fenichel, J. Jankovic, et al. (Eds.), *Bradley's neurology in clinical practice.* Saunders.

Seizures occur in 25% of persons with an SAH, and hydrocephalus after a bleed occurs in 20% of cases. Hypothalamic dysfunction, revealed by salt wasting, hyponatremia, and ECG changes, is common.

EVALUATION AND TREATMENT The diagnosis of an SAH is based on the clinical presentation, imaging, and CSF evaluation. Treatment is directed at controlling ICP, improving cerebral perfusion pressure, preventing ischemia and hypoxia of neural tissues, and avoiding rebleeding episodes. Surgical intervention is common. Treatment guidelines are available to guide therapy.[49]

Primary Headache Syndrome

> ✓ **QUICK CHECK 16.3**
> 1. What are two differences between the symptoms of migraine and cluster headaches?
> 2. How can bacterial meningitis lead to an amputation?
> 3. What are the autoimmune mechanisms that cause multiple sclerosis lesions?

Headache is a common neurological disorder and is usually a harmless symptom. However, it can be associated with serious disease such as brain tumour, meningitis, or cerebrovascular disease. The headache syndromes discussed here are the chronic, recurring type not associated with structural abnormalities or systemic disease. This includes migraine, cluster, and tension-type headaches. Characteristics of the major types of headache syndromes are reviewed in Table 16.7.

Migraine

Migraine is an episodic neurological disorder. It is characterized by a headache lasting 4 to 72 hours. It is diagnosed when any two of the following features occur: unilateral head pain, throbbing pain, pain worsens with activity, moderate or severe pain intensity; *and* at least one of the following: nausea and/or vomiting, or photophobia and phonophobia.[50] Migraine is classified as (1) *migraine with aura* with visual, sensory, or motor symptoms; (2) *migraine without aura* (most common), and (3) *chronic migraine*.

In Canada, it is estimated that migraine occurs in 25% of women, 8% of men, and 10% of children.[51] It is more common in those who are 25 to 55 years of age.[52] There often is a family history of migraine. In susceptible women, migraine occurs most frequently before and during menstruation. It is decreased during pregnancy and menopause. The cyclic withdrawal of estrogen and progesterone may trigger attacks of migraine.[53]

Migraine is caused by a combination of multiple genetic and environmental factors. Triggers may cause migraine. Triggers can be genetic or associated with many factors. These factors include fatigue, oversleeping, missed meals, overexertion, weather change, stress or relaxation from stress, hormonal changes (menstrual periods), excess afferent stimulation (bright lights, strong smells), and chemicals (alcohol or nitrates).

The pathophysiological basis for migraine is complex and not clearly understood. There is no identifiable pathology, but there are associated changes in brain metabolism and blood flow. Current theories include neurological, vascular, hormonal, and neurotransmitter components. Migraine aura is associated with cortical spreading depression (CSD). CSD is a spontaneous spreading wave of glial and neuronal depolarization resulting in hyperactivity that starts in the occipital region and spreads across the cortex. CSD starts the release of neurotransmitters that activate the trigeminal vascular system (afferent projections from cranial nerve V). This then stimulates vasodilation of dural blood

TABLE 16.7 Characteristics of Common Headaches

	Migraine		Cluster Headache/	Tension-Type
	Without Aura	**With Aura (25–30%)**	**Proximal Hemicrania**	**Headache**
Age of onset	Childhood, adolescence, or young adulthood	Childhood, adolescence, or young adulthood	Young adulthood, middle age	Young adulthood, middle age
Gender	Higher in females	Higher in females	Male	Not gender specific
Family history of headaches	Yes	Yes	No	Yes
Onset and evolution	Slow to rapid	Slow to rapid	Rapid	Slow to rapid
Time course	Episodic	Episodic	Clusters in time	Episodic, may become constant
Quality	Usually throbbing	Usually throbbing	Steady	Steady
Location	Variable, unilateral to bilateral	Variable, unilateral to bilateral	Orbit, temple, cheek	Variable
Associated features	Prodrome, vomiting	Aura: visual, sensory, language, and motor disturbance Prodrome, vomiting	Lacrimation, rhinorrhea, Horner's syndrome	None

vessels, activation of inflammation, peripheral and central sensitization of pain receptors (hypersensitivity to pain), and activation of areas of the brainstem and forebrain that modulate pain. Release of inflammatory mediators with sterile meningeal inflammation and edema of blood vessels may be an important part of migraine pain.[54] The clinical phases of a migraine attack are:

1. *Premonitory phase:* Up to one third of persons have premonitory symptoms hours to days before onset of aura or headache. These symptoms may include tiredness, irritability, loss of concentration, stiff neck, and food cravings.
2. *Migraine aura:* Up to one third of persons have aura symptoms at least some of the time that may last up to 1 hour. Symptoms can be visual, sensory, or motor.
3. *Headache phase:* Throbbing pain usually begins on one side and spreads to the entire head. Headache may be accompanied by fatigue, nausea and vomiting, or dizziness. There may be hypersensitivity to anything touching the head. Symptoms may last from 4 to 72 hours (usually about a day).
4. *Recovery phase:* Irritability, fatigue, or depression may take hours or days to resolve.

The features of the types of migraine headache are reviewed in Table 16.7. The diagnosis of migraine is made from medical history and physical examination. Imaging and EEG confirm diagnosis. The management of migraine includes avoidance of triggers (e.g., darkening the room, applying ice). Sleeping can provide some relief with the onset of acute migraine. Medication management for the treatment and prevention of migraine is available.[55] A transcutaneous electrical stimulation device providing trigeminal neurostimulation has been approved by Health Canada for the prevention of migraine.[56]

Chronic migraines usually begin as episodic migraines that increase in frequency over time. Chronic migraine occurs at least 15 days in a month (can occur daily or on a near-daily basis) for more than 3 months. Chronic migraines are associated with overuse of pain-relieving migraine medications (sometimes called *rebound headaches*), obesity, and caffeine overuse. Treatment is like that for episodic migraine.

Cluster Headache

Cluster headaches are one of a group of disorders referred to as *trigeminal autonomic cephalalgias* (headaches involving the autonomic division of the trigeminal nerve).[57] They occur in one side of the head, primarily in men between 20 and 50 years of age. The pain may alternate sides with each headache episode and is severe, stabbing, and throbbing. These uncommon headaches occur in clusters (up to 8 attacks per day) and last for minutes to hours for a period of days, followed by a long period of spontaneous remission. Cluster headache has an episodic and a chronic form with extreme pain intensity and short duration. If the cluster of attacks occurs more frequently without sustained spontaneous remission, they are classified as *chronic cluster headaches* (10 to 20% of cases) (see Table 16.7). Triggers are like those that cause migraine headache.

Trigeminal activation occurs but the mechanism is unclear. The pathogenic mechanism for pain is related to the release of vasoactive substances and the formation of neurogenic inflammation. Autonomic dysfunction is characterized by sympathetic underactivity and parasympathetic activation. There is unilateral trigeminal distribution of severe pain with ipsilateral autonomic manifestations. This includes tearing on affected side, ptosis of the ipsilateral eye, and congestion of the nasal mucosa. Preventative medications are used to treat cluster headache, as well as avoidance of triggers. Acute attacks are managed with oxygen inhalation, sumatriptan (Imitrex) or inhaled ergotamine tartrate (Medihaler Ergotamine), and nerve stimulation. New medications are under investigation.[58]

Tension-Type Headache

Tension-type headache (TTH) is the most common type of recurrent headache. The average age of onset is during the second decade of life. It is a gradual onset, mild to moderate bilateral headache with a sensation of a tight band or pressure around the head. The headache occurs in episodes and may last for several hours or several days. It is not aggravated by physical activity. Chronic tension-type headache (CTTH) develops from episodic TTH and represents headache that occurs at least 15 days per month for at least 3 months.

Both central and peripheral mechanisms operate in causing tension headaches. The central pain mechanism is associated with CTTH. The peripheral mechanism is associated with episodic TTH. The central pain mechanism probably involves hypersensitivity of pain fibres from the trigeminal nerve that leads to central sensitization. The peripheral sensitization of myofascial sensory nerves may contribute to muscular hypersensitivity and the development of CTTH. Headache sufferers have more localized pain and tenderness of pericranial muscles. Many persons have both TTHs and migraines.

Mild TTHs are treated with ice, and more severe forms are treated with Aspirin or nonsteroidal anti-inflammatory medications. CTTHs are best managed with a tricyclic antidepressant and behavioural and relaxation therapy. Some persons benefit from injection of botulinum toxin A. Long-term use of analgesics or other medications, such as muscle relaxants, antihistamines, tranquilizers, caffeine, and ergot alkaloids, should be avoided.[59]

Infection and Inflammation of the Central Nervous System

Bacteria, viruses, fungi, parasites, and mycobacteria may infect the CNS. The invading organisms enter the nervous system either by spreading through arterial blood vessels (Figure 16.13) or by invading the nervous tissue from another site of infection. Neurological infections produce disease in several ways: direct neuronal or glial infection, mass lesion formation, inflammation with resulting edema, interruption of CSF pathways, neuronal or vascular damage, and secretion of neurotoxins. An immune process may start an inflammatory reaction.

Meningitis

Meningitis is inflammation of the brain or spinal cord. Bacteria, viruses, fungi, parasites, or toxins may cause infectious meningitis. The infection may be acute, subacute, or chronic with the pathophysiology, symptoms, and treatment differing for each type of microorganism.

Fungal meningitis is a chronic, much less common condition than bacterial or viral meningitis. The infection most often occurs in persons with impaired immune responses or alterations in normal body flora. It develops slowly, usually over days or weeks. Fungi in the nervous system usually produce a granulomatous reaction, forming granulomata or gelatinous masses in the meninges at the base of the brain. Fungi also may extend along the perivascular sites in the subarachnoid space and into the brain tissue. Here, they produce arteritis with thrombosis, infarction, and communicating hydrocephalus. Meningeal fibrosis develops later in the inflammatory process. Cranial nerve dysfunction, caused by compression, often results from the granulomata and fibrosis. The first manifestations are often those of dementia (see Chapter 15) or communicating hydrocephalus (see Chapter 15). The person is usually afebrile.

Viral meningitis (aseptic or nonpurulent meningitis) is thought to be limited to the meninges. An identifiable bacterium cannot be found in the CSF. The most common viruses are enteroviral viruses (echovirus, coxsackievirus, and nonparalytic poliomyelitis), arboviruses, and herpes simplex type 2. Viruses enter the nervous system by crossing the blood–brain barrier, by direct spread along peripheral nerves, or through the choroid plexus epithelium. Recognition of viral antigens by immune cells activates the inflammatory response. The clinical symptoms of viral meningitis are like those of bacterial meningitis, but milder. Viral meningitis is managed with antiviral medications and steroids.

Bacterial meningitis is primarily an infection of the pia mater and arachnoid, the subarachnoid space, the ventricular system, and the CSF. Meningococci (*Neisseria meningitidis*) and pneumococci (*Streptococcus pneumoniae*) are the most common pathogens in adults. An increase of medication-resistant strains of *S. pneumoniae* is a developing problem worldwide. With pneumococcal meningitis, young persons and those more than 40 years of age are mostly affected. Outbreaks may occur in student residences and military bases. Predisposing conditions are otitis or sinusitis (25%), immunocompromised status (16%), and pneumonia (12%). The disease is spread by respiratory droplets and contact with contaminated saliva or respiratory tract secretions (kissing, coughing, sneezing, or sharing utensils, food, and drink).[60] Carriers of the meningococcal bacteria do not develop meningitis but may pass it on to others.

PATHOPHYSIOLOGY Meningococci and pneumococci are inhaled and attach to epithelial cells in the nasopharynx. Here the bacteria cross the mucosal barrier, enter the bloodstream, travel to cerebral blood vessels, cross the blood–brain barrier, and infect the meninges. With bacterial infection, large numbers of neutrophils are recruited to the subarachnoid space. Release of cytotoxic inflammatory agents and bacterial toxins change the blood–brain barrier, causing cerebral edema, and damage brain tissue. The inflammatory discharge thickens the CSF and interferes with normal CSF flow around the brain and spinal cord. It may obstruct arachnoid villi and produce hydrocephalus. Meningeal cells become edematous, and the combined discharge and edematous cells increase ICP. Engorged blood vessels and thrombi can alter blood flow, causing further injury.[61]

CLINICAL MANIFESTATIONS The clinical symptoms of bacterial meningitis can be grouped into infectious signs, meningeal signs, and neurological signs. The clinical symptoms of systemic infection include fever, tachycardia, and chills. The clinical symptoms of meningeal irritation are a severe throbbing headache, severe photophobia, nuchal rigidity, and positive Kernig and Brudzinski signs. The neurological signs include a decrease in consciousness, cranial nerve palsies, focal neurological deficits (such as hemiparesis/hemiplegia and ataxia), and seizures. Often there is projectile vomiting. As ICP increases, papilledema develops, and delirium may progress to unconsciousness and death. With meningococcal meningitis, a petechial or purpuric rash covers the skin and mucous membranes. A rare complication is acute infectious purpura fulminans. This is a rapidly progressive syndrome of hemorrhagic infarction of the skin and disseminated intravascular coagulation. This infection can lead to multiple organ failure, ischemic

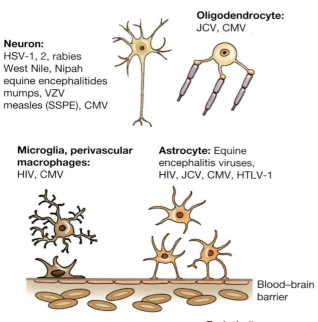

FIGURE 16.13 Viral Infection in the Central Nervous System. Viruses infect specific cell types within the central nervous system, depending on the properties of the virus together with individual cell membrane proteins expressed on permissive cell types. Normally the brain is protected from circulating pathogens and toxins by the blood–brain barrier. *CMV*, Cytomegalovirus; *HIV*, human immunodeficiency virus; *HSV*, herpes simplex virus; *HTLV-1*, human T-cell lymphotropic virus type 1 (causes T-cell leukemia); *JCV*, John Cunningham virus (a polyomavirus causing progressive multifocal leukoencephalopathy); *SSPE*, subacute sclerosing panencephalitis; *VZV*, varicella-zoster virus. (Adapted from Power, C., & Noorbakhsh, G. [2007]. Central nervous system viral infections: clinical aspects and pathogenic mechanisms. In S. Gilman [Ed.], *Neurobiology of disease* [p. 488]. Elsevier.)

necrosis of digits and limbs with amputation required, and death. It is caused by bacterial endotoxin and inflammatory cytokines.

EVALUATION AND TREATMENT Rapid diagnosis, antibiotic administration, and supportive treatment are important to prevent morbidity and mortality from bacterial meningitis. Diagnosis is based on physical examination, blood cultures, and the results of nasopharyngeal smear and antigen tests. CSF analysis and cultures are required for diagnosis. Serious complications, including septic shock, disseminated intravascular coagulation, purpura fulminans, limb damage, and multiple organ failure, require intensive multidisciplinary care. Vaccinations are available to prevent meningococcal, pneumococcal, and *Haemophilus influenzae* meningitis.[62]

Brain or Spinal Cord Abscess

Abscesses, localized collections of pus, may form within the parenchyma of the brain or spinal cord but are rare. Immunosuppressed persons are particularly at risk.

Brain abscesses are classified as epidural, subdural, or intracerebral. *Epidural brain abscesses (empyemas)* are associated with osteomyelitis in a cranial bone. *Subdural brain abscesses (empyemas)* arise from a sinus infection or a vascular source. *Intracerebral brain abscesses* arise from a vascular source. Spinal cord abscesses are rare and are classified as epidural or intramedullary (within the spinal cord). Epidural spinal abscesses usually begin as osteomyelitis in a vertebra. The infection then spreads into the epidural space. (Osteomyelitis is discussed in Chapter 39.)

PATHOPHYSIOLOGY Microorganisms enter the CNS by direct extension or distribution along the wall of a vein. Infective emboli carry organisms from distant sites. Illegal drug users who share needles are at risk, as are immunosuppressed persons. For example: *Toxoplasma gondii* is producing an ever-increasing number of CNS abscesses in persons with AIDS.[63] Streptococci, staphylococci, and *Bacteroides*, often combined with anaerobes, are the most common bacteria that cause abscesses. Yeast and fungi also may be involved.

Brain abscesses progress from localized inflammation to a necrotic core. The formation of a connective tissue capsule occurs, usually within 14 days or longer.[64] Existing abscesses also tend to spread and form daughter abscesses.

CLINICAL MANIFESTATIONS Early symptoms include low-grade fever, headache (most common symptom), nausea and vomiting, neck pain and stiffness, confusion, drowsiness, sensory deficits, and communication deficits. Later symptoms are associated with a growing mass and include decreased attention span, memory deficits, decreased visual acuity and narrowed visual fields, papilledema, ocular palsy, ataxia, dementia, and seizures. The development of symptoms may be very gradual, often making an abscess difficult to diagnose.[64]

Extradural brain abscesses are associated with localized pain, purulent drainage from the nasal passages or auditory canal, fever, localized tenderness, and neck stiffness. Clinical symptoms of spinal cord abscesses have four stages: (1) spinal aching; (2) severe root pain, accompanied by spasms of the back muscles and limited vertebral movement; (3) weakness caused by progressive cord compression; and (4) paralysis.

EVALUATION AND TREATMENT The diagnosis is suggested by clinical features and confirmed by imaging studies. Antibiotics and surgical aspiration or excision is usually indicated. Intracranial pressure may have to be managed. Spinal cord abscesses are treated with surgical decompression or aspiration, antibiotic therapy, and supportive therapy.

Encephalitis

Encephalitis is an acute febrile illness, usually of viral origin, with nervous system involvement. Bites of mosquitos, ticks, or flies cause the most common forms. Herpes simplex type 1 is the most common sporadic cause of encephalitis. Viruses infect specific cell types in the CNS, as shown in Figure 16.13. Referred to as *infectious viral encephalitides*, encephalitis may occur as a complication of systemic viral diseases. These diseases include poliomyelitis, rabies, or mononucleosis. It may also arise after recovery from viral infections such as rubella, varicella, rubeola, or yellow fever. Encephalitis also may follow vaccination with a live attenuated virus vaccine if the vaccine has an encephalitis component. Typhus, trichinosis, malaria, and schistosomiasis also are associated with encephalitis.

Except for the California viral encephalitis, which is common, the arthropod-borne encephalitides occur in epidemics, varying in geographic and seasonal incidence (Table 16.8 and *Health Promotion*: West Nile Virus). Eastern equine encephalitis is the most serious but least common of the encephalitides. The Powassan virus, Chikungunya

TABLE 16.8 Common Arboviruses of North America

Virus	Distribution	Insect Vector	Immediate Vertebrate Host
West Nile	United States, Canada, Mexico	Mosquito (*Culex* spp.)	Passerine birds (jays, blackbirds, crows, finches, sparrows)
St. Louis encephalitis	United States, Canada, Mexico	Mosquito (*Culex* spp.)	Passerine birds (sparrows, house finches)
Eastern equine encephalitis	Atlantic and Gulf Coast states, upper New York, Michigan, Eastern Canada	Mosquito (*Culex* spp.)	Fresh water swamp birds
Western equine encephalitis	Western United States, Canada	Mosquito (*Culex* spp.)	Passerine birds, jackrabbit
Venezuelan encephalitis	Mexico, Florida, Texas	Mosquito (*Culex* and *Aedes* spp.)	Rodents, aquatic birds
Powassan encephalitis	Northern United States, Canada	Ixodes ticks	Squirrels, mice, ground hogs, voles
La Crosse or Jamestown encephalitis	North central and northeast United States	Mosquito (*Aedes triseriatus*)	Chipmunks, squirrels
Colorado tick fever	Rocky Mountain states, Canada	Tick (*Dermacentor andersoni*)	Chipmunks, squirrels, small mammals
Dengue	Mexico and Florida	Mosquito (*Aedes* spp.)	Humans and nonhuman primates

From Davis, L. E., Beckham, J. D., & Tyler, K. L. (2008). North American encephalitic arboviruses. *Neurology Clinics, 26*(3), 727–757 (Table 2). doi:10.1016/j.ncl.2008.03.012.

HEALTH PROMOTION
West Nile Virus

West Nile virus (WNV), a *Flavivirus* transmitted predominantly by the *Culex* mosquito, appeared in New York State in 1999. It is the most common cause of epidemic meningoencephalitis and the leading cause of arboviral encephalitis in North America. The first human case of WNV infection in Canada was reported in 2002. Humans and horses, as well as other mammals, are secondary hosts. Birds and mosquitoes are life cycle hosts. In most parts of Canada, the risk of becoming infected with WNV starts mid-April and ends after the first hard frost. Besides mosquito transmission, WNV can be transmitted through blood transfusions and organ transplants. Health experts think that transmission from mother to unborn child and through breast milk is possible.

The most effective way to avoid infection with WNV is to prevent mosquito bites. Since mosquitoes are most active at dawn and dusk, avoiding outdoor activities during those times reduces the risk of bites. It is recommended during outdoor activities to wear long pants and long-sleeved loose shirts, socks, and a hat, and light-coloured clothing. In addition, the use of an insect repellant that contains DEET or icaridin is recommended. Since mosquitoes lay their eggs in standing water, removing any areas of standing water around the home is suggested. The use of window and door screens also helps in preventing mosquitoes from entering the home.

Data from Government of Canada. (2021). *Surveillance of West Nile virus*. https://www.canada.ca/en/public-health/services/diseases/west-nile-virus/surveillance-west-nile-virus.html; Government of Canada. (2016). *Prevention of West Nile virus*. https://healthycanadians.gc.ca/diseases-conditions-maladies-affections/disease-maladie/west-nile-nil-occidental/prevention-eng.php; Petersen, L. R., Brault, A. C., & Nasci, R. S. (2013). West Nile virus: review of the literature. *Journal of the American Medical Association, 310*(3), 308–315; Reisen, W. K. (2013). Ecology of West Nile virus in North America. *Viruses, 5*(9), 2079–2105.

virus, West Nile virus (WNV) and Zika virus have recently emerged in North America as increasing causes of neurological illness.[65] If Lyme disease—caused by the transmission of the spirochete *Borrelia burgdorferi* through tick bites—progresses to post-Lyme disease syndrome, encephalopathy and polyneuropathy may occur. As these viruses have become more prevalent in Canada, it is essential that health care professionals monitor for these illnesses to ensure swift diagnosis and treatment.

PATHOPHYSIOLOGY Viruses gain access to the CNS through the bloodstream, olfactory bulb, or choroid plexus, or from peripheral nerves. Meningeal involvement is present in all encephalitides. The various encephalitides may cause widespread nerve cell degeneration. Edema, necrosis with or without hemorrhage, and increased ICP develop.

CLINICAL MANIFESTATIONS Encephalitis ranges from a mild infectious disease to a life-threatening disorder. Mild symptoms include malaise, headache, body aches, nausea, and vomiting. Dramatic clinical symptoms include fever, delirium, or confusion progressing to unconsciousness, difficulty with word finding, seizure activity, cranial nerve palsies, paresis and paralysis, involuntary movement, and abnormal reflexes. Signs of marked ICP may be present.

EVALUATION AND TREATMENT Diagnosis is made by history and clinical presentation aided by CSF examination and culture, serological studies, white blood cell count, CT scan, or MRI. Treatment is specific to the type of virus and may include antiviral agents, antibiotics, and steroids. Herpes encephalitis is treated with antiviral agents, such as acyclovir (Zovirax). Measures to control ICP are essential.

Neurological Complications of Acquired Immunodeficiency Syndrome (AIDS)

The most common neurological disorder associated with AIDS is **human immunodeficiency virus (HIV)-associated neurocognitive disorder (HAND)**. HAND is a range of disorders that includes mild neurocognitive disorder and HIV-associated dementia, which is rare. Combined antiretroviral therapy (cART) with more efficient CNS drug penetration has reduced the prevalence and improved survival for individuals with HAND. Milder forms of the disease may persist because of longer life and the ability of the virus to survive within brain tissue in some individuals.

The onset of clinical manifestations includes neurocognitive impairment, behavioral disturbance, and motor abnormalities. Specific symptoms can include an organic psychosis with agitation, inappropriate behavior, and hallucinosis. Motor signs can include difficulty speaking, progressive loss of balance, gait disturbances, or paralysis. Diagnosis is difficult during early stages of manifestations. CSF analysis and imaging help establish the diagnosis. HIV antiretroviral treatment improves survival for individuals with severe HAND but does not reverse the impairment.[66]

Demyelinating Disorders

Demyelinating disorders result from damage to the myelin nerve sheath and affect neural transmission. They can occur in either the central (i.e., multiple sclerosis) or the peripheral (i.e., Guillain-Barré syndrome) nervous system. Contributing factors include genetics, infections, autoimmune reactions, environmental toxins, and unknown factors.

Multiple Sclerosis

Multiple sclerosis (MS) is a chronic immune-mediated inflammatory disease involving degeneration of CNS myelin, scarring (sclerosis or plaque formation), and loss of axons. Canada has one of the highest rates of MS in the world, with an estimated 77 000 Canadians living with the disease.[67] The cause of MS is unknown. MS is an autoimmune response to self or microbial antigens in genetically susceptible persons. The onset of MS is usually between 20 and 40 years of age and is more common in women. Men may have a more severe progressive course. The prevalence rate is higher in northern latitudes. Risk factors that may be involved include smoking, vitamin D deficiency, obesity, infection including Epstein-Barr virus infection, and genetic factors.[68]

PATHOPHYSIOLOGY MS is a diffuse and progressive disease with patches of damage that can occur throughout the brain and spinal cord. There are multiple focal areas of myelin loss within the CNS called *plaques*. The plaques form when autoreactive T lymphocytes (T cells) and B lymphocytes (B cells) cross the blood–brain barrier and attack myelin. This attack triggers a release of inflammatory mediators and loss of oligodendrocytes (myelin-producing cells). Activation of glia cells (brain macrophages) contributes to inflammation and injury. Loss of myelin disrupts nerve signals with resulting death of neurons and brain atrophy. Normal-appearing white matter can be microscopically very abnormal. Grey matter lesions and atrophy have been documented during later stages of the disease process.[69] These degenerative processes begin before symptom onset and progress throughout a person's life (Figure 16.14). Myelin degeneration also can present as *optic neuritis* or involve the spinal cord. *Spinal MS* can occur with or without the presence of brain lesions. The multifocal, multistage features of MS lesions in established disease produce symptoms that are multiple and variable.

CLINICAL MANIFESTATIONS The most common initial symptoms of MS are paresthesias of the face, trunk, or limbs; weakness; impaired gait;

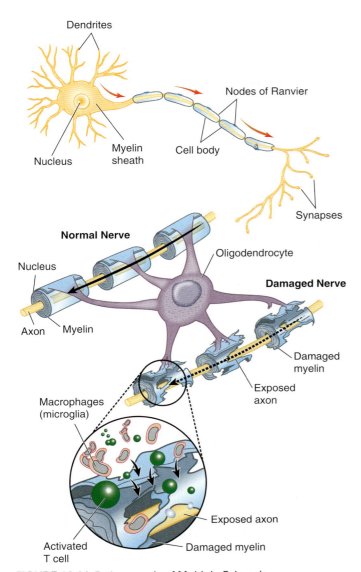

FIGURE 16.14 Pathogenesis of Multiple Sclerosis.

The MS Society of Canada identifies 4 types of MS: (1) *clinically isolated syndrome*, which is the earliest form of MS and refers to a single episode of neurological symptoms that are suggestive of MS; (2) *relapsing-remitting*, unpredictable but defined relapses where new symptoms appear or existing symptoms worsen; (3) *secondary-progressive*, initial remitting and relapsing symptoms with a steady decline in function; (4) *primary-progressive*, progressive course from onset without defined relapses. Without treatment, transition to the progressive types with insidious neurological decline occurs. Early cognitive changes are common and may include poor judgement, apathy, emotional changes, and depression.

EVALUATION AND TREATMENT There is no single test available to diagnose or rule out MS. Diagnosis includes the history and clinical examination in combination with MRI (most sensitive test), CSF findings, and evoked potentials.[71] Constantly elevated levels of CSF immunoglobulin G (IgG) are found in about two thirds of persons with MS. Oligoclonal IgG bands on electrophoresis are found in more than 90% of persons with MS. Evoked potential studies aid diagnosis by detecting decreased conduction velocity in visual, auditory, and somatosensory pathways. MRI is the most sensitive available method of detecting demyelinated plaques and monitoring disease.

The treatment goal in MS is prevention of exacerbations, prevention of permanent neurological damage, and control of symptoms. Disease-modifying medications are started with diagnosis and include corticosteroids, immunosuppressants, and immune system modulators.[72] Continuous monitoring is important because of the increased risk for infection when taking these medications. Plasma exchange may be used in persons who do not respond to steroids. Medications are also available for symptom control. The long-term benefit of these medications is under investigation.[73] Supportive care includes participation in a regular exercise program; cessation of smoking; and avoidance of overwork, extreme fatigue, and heat exposure. The administration of vitamin D to prevent disease progression is being evaluated.[74] Stem cell therapy is under investigation.[75]

A recent theory has emerged associating chronic cerebrospinal venous insufficiency (CCSVI) with the symptoms of MS. It has been suggested that the presence of a blockage or narrowing of the veins in the head and neck does not allow for efficient removal of blood from the CNS, causing these symptoms. Global clinical studies have been conducted on this treatment with conflicting results. The procedure is not approved for treatment of MS in Canada.[76]

Guillain-Barré Syndrome

Guillain-Barré syndrome is a rare demyelinating disorder caused by a humoral and cell-mediated immunological reaction directed at the peripheral nerves. It usually occurs after a respiratory tract or gastrointestinal infection. The clinical symptoms can vary from tingling and weakness to paralysis of the legs to complete quadriplegia, respiratory insufficiency, and autonomic nervous system instability. Intravenous immunoglobulin or plasmapheresis is used during the acute phase and followed by aggressive rehabilitation.[77] Recovery occurs within weeks to months or up to 2 years. About 30% of persons have residual weakness.

PERIPHERAL NERVOUS SYSTEM AND NEUROMUSCULAR JUNCTION DISORDERS

 QUICK CHECK 16.4
1. Where in the peripheral nervous system can disease occur?
2. Why do antibodies contribute to the symptoms of myasthenia gravis?
3. How do myasthenic crisis and cholinergic crisis differ?

or urinary incontinence indicating widespread CNS involvement. Visual impairment is associated with optic neuritis. Cerebellar and corticospinal involvement presents as nystagmus, ataxia, and weakness with all four limbs involved. Intention tremor and slurred speech may also occur.

The onset, duration, and severity of symptoms are different for each person. Disease exacerbations (also known as relapses or flares) are the temporary occurrence or worsening of symptoms. The symptoms may be mild or serious and may last for several days or weeks. They may also be followed by progressive symptoms, including paresthesias, difficulty speaking, ataxia, or visual changes. The mechanism of these exacerbations is related to delayed or blocked conduction caused by inflammation and demyelination. Various events can occur immediately before the exacerbation of symptoms. These events are regarded as precipitating factors or triggers, including trauma, emotional stress, and pregnancy. Painful sensory events, spastic paralysis, and bowel and bladder incontinence are common with spinal involvement.[70] Recovery from symptoms during remissions is caused by downregulation of inflammation and the restoration of axonal function. Restoration occurs either by remyelination, the resolution of inflammation, or the restoration of conduction to demyelinated axons.

Peripheral Nervous System Disorders

The peripheral nervous system is made up of motor anterior horn cells, nerve fibres, sensory axons of the posterior root ganglia, and peripheral autonomic ganglia and their axons. Acute or chronic disease processes, inflammation, or trauma may injure these peripheral nerves and cause a neuropathy. Disease processes may injure the axons travelling to and from the brainstem and spinal cord neuronal cell bodies. The injury may affect a distinct anatomical area on the axon. Spinal nerves may also be injured at the roots, at the plexus (plexus injuries) before peripheral nerve formation, or at the nerves themselves. The cranial nerves do not have roots or plexuses and are affected only within themselves. Autonomic nerve fibres may be injured. This injury occurs as they travel in certain cranial nerves and emerge through the ventral root and plexuses to pass through the peripheral nerves of the body. Peripheral nervous system disorders are reviewed in Table 16.9.

Neuromuscular Junction Disorders

Transmission of the nerve impulse at the neuromuscular junction requires the release of adequate amounts of neurotransmitter from the presynaptic terminals of the axon and effective binding of the released transmitter to the receptors on the membranes of muscle cells (see Figure 13.15). **Botulism** food poisoning results from the botulinum neurotoxin released from *Clostridium botulinum*. The toxin inhibits the release of acetylcholine at the myoneural junction and causes flaccid paralysis.

Myasthenia Gravis

Myasthenia gravis is the most common neuromuscular disorder. It is an acquired chronic autoimmune disease that is mediated by antibodies against the acetylcholine receptor (AChR) at the postsynaptic membrane of the neuromuscular junction. The Canadian prevalence is about 30 cases per 100 000 population,[78] and it is more common in women. Thymic tumours, pathological changes in the thymus, and other autoimmune diseases are associated with the disorder. (Autoimmune mechanisms are discussed in Chapter 8). Ocular myasthenia is more common in males. It involves weakness of the eye muscles and eyelids and may include swallowing difficulties and slurred speech.

PATHOPHYSIOLOGY Myasthenia gravis results from a defect in nerve impulse transmission at the neuromuscular junction. The postsynaptic AChRs on the muscle cell's plasma membrane are no longer recognized as "self" and elicit T-cell–dependent formation of IgG autoantibodies. The autoantibodies fix onto AChR sites, blocking the binding of acetylcholine. Eventually the antibody action destroys receptor sites. This loss of AChR sites causes decreased transmission of the nerve impulse across the neuromuscular junction and decreased muscle depolarization. Symptomatic persons without anti-AChR antibodies may have antibodies against muscle-specific kinase (MuSK), an enzyme required for maintenance of the neuromuscular junction, with similar symptoms. Why this autosensitization occurs is unknown. Thymomas occur in about half of myasthenia gravis cases. It is thought that they are associated with loss of self-tolerance, but the actual mechanism is unknown.[79]

CLINICAL MANIFESTATIONS Myasthenia gravis has a gradual onset. The variable distribution of AChR sites or the number of and different isoforms of antibodies may determine when and which muscle groups are affected first; generally, the muscles of the eyes, face, mouth, throat, and neck are the earliest to show signs. There can be drooling and difficulty chewing and swallowing food. These problems can affect nutrition and put the person at risk for respiratory aspiration. The muscles of the neck, shoulder girdle, and hip flexors are less frequently affected. Muscle fatigue is common after exercise and there can be progressive weakness. The respiratory muscles of the diaphragm and chest wall can become weak, causing impaired ventilation. Clinical symptoms may first appear during pregnancy, during the postpartum period, or with the administration of certain anaesthetic agents. The progression of myasthenia gravis varies. It may first appear as a mild case that spontaneously lessens, with a series of relapses and symptom-free intervals ranging from weeks to months. Over time, the disease can progress.

TABLE 16.9 Peripheral Nervous System Disorders

Disorder	Pathology	Clinical Manifestations
Radiculopathies	Involves injury to spinal roots as they exit or enter vertebral canal; caused by compression, inflammation, direct trauma	Strength, tone, and bulk of muscles innervated by involved roots affected; pattern is like that seen in amyotrophies, with tone and deep tendon reflexes decreased, rarely absent; fasciculations; mild fatigue; sensory alterations, pain
Plexus injuries	Involve nerve plexus distal to spinal roots but proximal to formation of peripheral nerves; caused by trauma, compression, infiltration, or iatrogenic (positioning or intramuscular injection)	Motor weakness, muscle atrophy, sensory loss in affected areas; paralysis common
Neuropathies	Called *sensorimotor* if sensory, motor, and reflex effects; pure sensory caused by leprosy, industrial solvents, chloramphenicol, and hereditary mechanisms; motor caused by Guillain-Barré syndrome, infectious mononucleosis, viral hepatitis, acute porphyria, or lead, mercury, and triorthocresyl phosphate (TCP) poisoning	Muscle strength, tone, and bulk affected; whole muscles or groups may be paretic or paralyzed; muscles of feet and legs first, then hands and arms; tone and deep tendon reflexes generally decreased with atrophy and fasciculation; mild fatigue; some specific symptoms of paresthesia and dysesthesia; altered reflexes; autonomic disturbances; deformities; metabolic changes
Guillain-Barré syndrome (several antibody subtypes have been identified)	Involves acute onset of motor, sensory, or autonomic symptoms caused by autoimmune inflammatory response, resulting in axonal demyelination; most commonly presents as ascending motor paralysis; often preceded by respiratory tract or gastro-intestinal viral infection	Clinical manifestations are related to antibody subtypes; manifestations can include paresis of legs to complete quadriplegia, paralysis of eye muscles, respiratory insufficiency, autonomic nervous system instability; sensory symptoms (pain, numbness, paresthesias); may progress to respiratory arrest or cardiovascular collapse

From Vucic, S., Kiernan, M. C., & Cornblath, D. R. (2009). Guillain-Barré syndrome: an update. *Journal of Clinical Neuroscience, 16*(6), 733–741.

Myasthenic crisis can develop as the disease progresses. This occurs when severe muscle weakness causes extreme quadriparesis or quadriplegia, respiratory insufficiency with shortness of breath, and extreme difficulty in swallowing. The person in myasthenic crisis is in danger of respiratory arrest.

Cholinergic crisis may arise from anticholinesterase medication toxicity. Symptoms include increased intestinal motility, episodes of diarrhea and complaints of intestinal cramping, bradycardia, pupillary constriction, increased salivation, and diaphoresis. These symptoms are caused by the smooth muscle hyperactivity secondary to excessive accumulation of acetylcholine at the neuromuscular junctions and excessive parasympathetic like activity. As in myasthenic crisis, the person is in danger of respiratory arrest.

EVALUATION AND TREATMENT The diagnosis of myasthenia gravis is made based on a response to edrophonium chloride (Tensilon), results of electromyogram studies, and detection of anti-AChR or MuSK antibodies. With the intravenous administration of medication, immediate improvement in muscle strength occurs and usually persists for several minutes. Imaging helps determine whether a thymoma is present. Current treatments for myasthenia gravis have improved prognosis, including in those who have ocular myasthenia.

Anticholinesterase medications, steroids, and immunosuppressant medications (e.g., azathioprine [Imuran] and cyclosporine [Sandimmune]) are used to treat myasthenia gravis and prevent myasthenic crisis. For persons with cholinergic crisis, anticholinergic medications are stopped until blood levels are nontoxic. In addition, ventilatory support is provided and breathing complications are prevented. Plasmapheresis may be lifesaving. Thymectomy is the treatment of choice in persons with a thymoma and those with anti-AChR antibodies. The removal of the thymus stops the production of self-reactive T cells and B cells that produce the antibodies.[80]

TUMOURS OF THE CENTRAL NERVOUS SYSTEM

> ✓ **QUICK CHECK 16.5**
> 1. How is an encapsulated central nervous system (CNS) tumour different from a nonencapsulated CNS tumour?
> 2. What are three types of spinal cord tumours?
> 3. What are some common signs and symptoms of compressive and irritative spinal cord tumour syndromes?

CNS tumours include both brain and spinal cord tumours. In 2019, the estimated number of new cases of brain and spinal cord tumours in Canada was 3 000. The estimated number of deaths was 2 400.[81] CNS tumours are the second most common type of cancer occurring in children.[82] About 70 to 75% of all intracranial tumours in children are located infratentorially (see Chapter 17). In adults 70% are located supratentorially. Peripheral nerve tumours are rare in children and common in adults. Carcinogenesis is discussed in Chapter 10, pituitary tumours are discussed in Chapter 19, and cerebral tumours in children are discussed in Chapter 17.

Brain Tumours

Tumours within the cranium can be either primary or metastatic. *Primary brain tumours* originate from brain substance, including neuroglia, neurons, cells of blood vessels, and connective tissue. *Extracerebral tumours* originate outside substances of the brain and include meningiomas, acoustic nerve tumours, and tumours of pituitary and pineal glands. *Metastatic (secondary) brain tumours* are the most common, arise in organ systems outside the brain, and spread to the brain. Common sites of intracranial tumours are illustrated in Figure 16.15.

Local effects of cranial tumours are caused by the destructive action of the tumour itself on a site in the brain and by compression causing decreased cerebral blood flow. Generalized effects result from increased ICP. Increased ICP is caused by growth of the tumour, blockage of the ventricular system, hemorrhages in and around the tumour, or cerebral edema (Figure 16.16). Symptoms include seizures, visual disturbances, unstable gait, and cranial nerve dysfunction.

Intracranial brain tumours do not metastasize as readily as tumours in other organs because there are no lymphatic channels within the brain substance. If metastasis does occur, it is usually through seeding of cerebral blood or CSF during cranial surgery or through artificial shunts.

Primary Brain (Intracerebral) Tumours

Primary brain (intracerebral) tumours, also called **gliomas** (cells that support brain neurons), include astrocytomas, oligodendrogliomas, and ependymomas. They make up 50 to 60% of all adult brain tumours and about 2% of all cancers in Canada (Table 16.10). The cause for primary brain tumours is not clear. Ionizing radiation is the only known environmental risk factor. The World Health Organization (WHO) divides gliomas into four grades based on histopathological features,

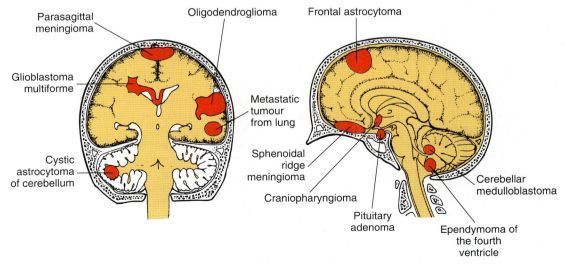

FIGURE 16.15 Common Sites of Intracranial Tumours.

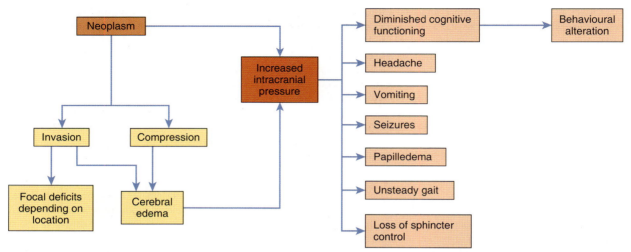

FIGURE 16.16 Origin of Clinical Manifestations Associated With an Intracranial Neoplasm.

cellular density, atypia, mitotic activity, microvascular proliferation, and necrosis (Table 16.11). Grades I and II are generally benign or slow growing. Grades III and IV are malignant tumours.

Surgical or radiosurgical excision, surgical decompression, chemotherapy, radiotherapy, and hyperthermia are treatment options for these tumours. Supportive treatment is directed at reducing edema. New treatment options are emerging. (Cancer treatment is discussed in Chapter 10.)

Astrocytoma. Astrocytomas are the most common glioma (75% of all tumours of the brain and spinal cord).[83] They are classified by grade and type (see Table 16.11). These tumour cells are thought to have lost normal growth restraint and thus multiply uncontrollably. Astrocytomas are graded I through IV, with grades I and II being slow-growing tumours that are most common in children. Grade I and II astrocytomas commonly progress to a higher grade, faster growing tumour. They may occur anywhere in the brain or spinal cord, and are generally located in the cerebrum, hypothalamus, or pons. Low-grade astrocytomas tend to be located laterally or supratentorially in adults and in a midline or near-midline position in children.

Headache and subtle neurobehavioural changes may be early signs, with other neurological symptoms evolving slowly. Increased ICP occurs late in the tumour's course. Onset of a focal seizure disorder between the second and sixth decade of life suggests an astrocytoma. Low-grade astrocytomas are treated with surgery or by external radiation. About 50% of persons survive 5 years when surgery is followed by radiation therapy.[83,84]

Grades III and IV astrocytomas are found mainly in the frontal lobes and cerebral hemispheres. They may also occur in the brainstem, cerebellum, and spinal cord. Men are twice as likely to have astrocytomas as women. In the 15- to 34-year-old age group they are the third most common brain cancer, whereas in the 35- to 54-year-old age group they are the fourth most common.

Grade IV astrocytoma, **glioblastoma multiforme**, is the most lethal and common type of primary brain tumour. This type is highly vascular and extensively irregular and infiltrative, making it difficult to remove surgically. Fifty percent of glioblastomas are bilateral or at least occupy more than one lobe at the time of death. The typical clinical presentation for a glioblastoma multiforme is that of diffuse, nonspecific clinical signs, such as headache, irritability, and "personality changes" that progress to more clear-cut symptoms. These symptoms include increased ICP, including headache on position change, papilledema, vomiting, or seizure activity. Symptoms may progress to include definite focal signs, such as hemiparesis, dysphasia, dyspraxia, cranial nerve palsies, and visual field deficits.

Higher grade astrocytomas are treated surgically and with radiotherapy and chemotherapy. Recurrence is common, and survival time is less than 5 years for grade III and IV tumours. Bevacizumab is an antiangiogenic monoclonal antibody that has been approved for the treatment of recurrent glioblastoma multiforme in Canada and the U.S.[85]

Oligodendroglioma. Oligodendrogliomas constitute about 2% of all brain tumours and 10 to 15% of all gliomas. They are usually slow-growing tumours (grade II). Most oligodendrogliomas are macroscopically indistinguishable from other gliomas and may be a mixed type of oligodendroglioma and astrocytoma. Most are found in the frontal and temporal lobes, often in the deep white matter. They may also be found in other parts of the brain and spinal cord. Malignant degeneration occurs in about one third of persons with oligodendrogliomas. These tumours are referred to as oligodendroblastomas (grade III). More than 50% of persons experience a focal or generalized seizure as the first symptom. Only half of those with an oligodendroglioma have increased ICP at the time of diagnosis and surgery. Only one third develop focal symptoms. Treatment includes surgery, radiotherapy, and chemotherapy.

Ependymoma. Ependymomas are nonencapsulated gliomas that arise from ependymal cells. They are rare in adults, usually occurring in the spinal cord.[86] However, in children ependymomas are typically located in the brain. They make up about 1.9% of all primary brain tumours in adults, 4% in children, and 5.7% in adolescents. Approximately 70% of these tumours occur in the fourth ventricle, with others found in the third and lateral ventricles and caudal portion of the spinal cord. Approximately 40% of infratentorial ependymomas occur in children younger than 10 years. Cerebral (supratentorial) ependymomas occur at all ages.

Fourth ventricle ependymomas present with difficulty in balance, unsteady gait, uncoordinated muscle movement, and difficulty with fine motor movement. The symptoms of a lateral and third ventricle ependymoma that involves the cerebral hemispheres are seizures, visual changes, and hemiparesis. Blockage of the CSF circulation produces hydrocephalus and presents with headache, nausea, and vomiting.

The time between first symptoms and surgery may be as short as 4 weeks or as long as 8 years. Ependymomas are treated with radiotherapy, radiosurgery, and chemotherapy. About 84% of persons aged 20 to 44 years survive 5 years.[87]

TABLE 16.10 Brain and Spinal Cord Tumours

Neoplasm	Location	Characteristics	Cell of Origin
Gliomas			
Astrocytoma	Anywhere in brain or spinal cord	Slow growing, invasive	Astrocytes
Glioblastoma multiforme	Predominantly in cerebral hemispheres	Highly invasive and malignant	Thought to arise from mature astrocytes
Oligodendrocytoma	Most commonly in frontal lobes deep in white matter; may arise in brainstem, cerebellum, and spinal cord	Relatively avascular; tends to be encapsulated; more malignant form called *oligodendroblastoma*	Oligodendrites
Ependymoma	Intramedullary: wall of ventricles; may arise in caudal tail of spinal cord	More common in children, variable growth rates; more malignant, invasive form is called *ependymoblastoma*; may extend into ventricle or invade brain tissue	Ependymal cells
Neuronal Cell			
Medulloblastoma	Posterior cerebellar vermis, roof of fourth ventricle	Well demarcated but infiltrating, rapid growing; fills fourth ventricle	Embryonic cells
Mesodermal Tissue			
Meningioma	Intradural, extramedullary: sylvian fissure region, superior parasagittal surface of frontal and parietal lobes, olfactory groove, wing of sphenoid bone, superior surface of cerebellum, cerebellopontine angle, spinal cord	Slow growing, circumscribed, encapsulated, sharply demarcated from normal tissues, compressive in nature	Arachnoid cells; may be from fibroblasts
Choroid Plexus			
Papillomas	Choroid plexus of ventricular system, lateral ventricle in children, fourth ventricle in adults	Usually benign; slow expansion inducing hemorrhage and hydrocephalus; malignant tumour is rare	Epithelial cells
Cranial Nerves and Spinal Nerve Roots			
Neurilemmoma	Cranial nerves (most commonly vestibular division of cranial nerve VIII)	Slow growing	Schwann cells
Neurofibroma	Extramedullary—spinal cord	Slow growing	Neurilemma, Schwann cells
Pituitary Tumours			
	Pituitary gland; may extend to or invade floor of third ventricle	Age linked, several types, slow growing, macroadenomas and microadenomas	Pituitary cells, pituitary chromophobes, basophils, eosinophils
Germ Cell Tumours			
	Neurohypophysis, hypothalamus, pineal region Primarily in adolescents More common in males than females Variable prognosis	Rare, 0.5% of all primary brain tumours	Several types—germinoma, embryonal carcinoma, yolk sac tumour, choriocarcinoma, teratoma, mixed germ cell tumour—with different cell origins
Pineal region	Pineal region; pineal parenchyma	Several types (germinoma, pineocytoma, teratoma)	Several types with different cell origins
Blood Vessel Tumours			
Angioma	Predominantly in posterior cerebral hemispheres	Slow growing	Arising from congenitally malformed arteriovenous connections
Hemangioblastomas	Predominantly in cerebellum	Slow growing	Embryonic vascular tissue

Primary Extracerebral Tumours

Meningioma. Meningiomas constitute about one third of all intracranial tumours. These tumours usually start from the arachnoidal (meningeal) cap cells in the dura mater. They rarely start from arachnoid cells of the choroid plexus of the ventricles. Meningiomas are located most commonly in the olfactory grooves, on the wings of the sphenoid bone (at the base of the skull), in the tuberculum sellae (next to the sella turcica), on the superior surface of the cerebellum, and in the cerebellopontine angle and spinal cord.[88] The cause of meningiomas is unknown.

A meningioma is sharply defined and adapts to the shape it occupies. It may extend to the dural surface and wear away the cranial bones or produce an osteoblastic reaction.

Meningiomas are slow growing, and symptoms occur when they reach a certain size and begin to indent the brain tissue. Focal seizures are often the first symptoms, and increased ICP is less common than with gliomas.

There is a 20% recurrence rate even with complete surgical removal. If only partial resection is possible, the tumour recurs. Radiation therapies also are used to slow growth.

Nerve sheath tumours. Neurofibromas (benign nerve sheath tumours) are a group of autosomal dominant disorders of the nervous system. They include **neurofibromatosis type 1 (NF1)** (previously known as von Recklinghausen's disease) and **neurofibromatosis type 2 (NF2)**. The two types are also known as *peripheral neurofibromatosis* and *central neurofibromatosis*, respectively.

TABLE 16.11 Grades of Astrocytomas

Grade[a]	Type	Description	Characteristics
I	Pilocytic astrocytoma	Common in children and young adults and people with neurofibromatosis type 1; common in cerebellum	Least malignant, well differentiated; grows slowly; near-normal microscopic appearance, noninfiltrating
II	Diffuse, low-grade astrocytoma (fibrillary, gemistocytic, protoplasmic) Oligodendroglioma	Common in young adults; more common in cerebrum but can occur in any part of brain	Abnormal microscopic appearance; grows slowly; infiltrates to adjacent tissue; may recur at higher grade
III	Anaplastic (malignant) astrocytoma Anaplastic oligodendroglioma	Common in young adults	Malignant; many cells undergoing mitosis; infiltrates adjacent tissue; frequently recurs at higher grade
IV	Glioblastoma (glioblastoma multiforme)	Common in older persons, particularly men Predominant in cerebral hemispheres	Poorly differentiated; increased number of cells undergoing mitosis; bizarre microscopic appearance; widely infiltrates; neovascularization; central necrosis

[a]World Health Organization Grading of Central Nervous System Tumours.
Data from American Brain Tumor Association. (2010). *Brain tumor primer* (9th ed.); Louis, D. N., Ohgaki, H., Wiestler, O. D., et al. (2007). The 2007 WHO classification of tumours of the central nervous system. *Acta Neuropathologica, 114*(2), 97–109.

NF1 is the most common type of nerve sheath tumour, with an incidence of about 1 in 3 500 people. It causes multiple cutaneous neurofibromas, cutaneous macular lesions (café-au-lait spots and freckles), and less commonly, bone and soft tissue tumours. Inactivation of the *NF1* gene results in loss of function of neurofibromin in Schwann cells and promotes tumourigenesis (neurofibromas). Learning disabilities are present in about 50% of affected persons.[89]

NF2 is rare and occurs in about 1 in 60 000 people. The *NF2* gene product is neurofibromin 2 (merlin), a tumour-suppressor protein. Mutations promote development of CNS tumours, particularly schwannomas, although other tumour types can occur (meningiomas, ependymomas, astrocytomas, and neurofibromas). Schwannomas of the vestibular nerves present with hearing loss and deafness. Other symptoms may include loss of balance and dizziness. Schwannomas also may develop in other cranial, spinal, and peripheral nerves, and cutaneous signs are less prominent.

Genetic testing is available for the management of families susceptible to NF, and prenatal diagnosis is possible. Diagnostic criteria based on symptoms and neuroimaging studies have been established for NF1.[90] Surgery is the major treatment. Persons with NF2 have high morbidity and reduced life expectancy, particularly with early age of onset. In the future genetically tailored medications are likely to provide personalized therapy for both devastating conditions.

Metastatic brain tumours. Metastatic brain tumours from systemic cancers are 10 times more common than primary brain tumours; 20 to 40% of persons with cancer have metastasis to the brain.[91] Common primary sites include lung, breast, skin (e.g., melanomas), kidney, colorectal, and other types of cancer. Metastasis to the brain is thought to be through vascular channels (see Chapter 10).

Metastatic brain tumours produce signs like those of glioblastomas, although several unusual syndromes do exist. Carcinomatous (metastatic cancer) encephalopathy causes headache, nervousness, depression, trembling, confusion, forgetfulness, and gait disorder. In carcinomatosis of the cerebellum, headache, dizziness, and ataxia are found. Carcinomatosis of the craniospinal meninges (also called *carcinomatous meningitis*) manifests with headache, confusion, and symptoms of cranial or spinal nerve root dysfunction. Metastatic brain tumours carry a poor prognosis. Treatment is guided by the pathology of the original tumour; number, size, and location of the brain metastasis; and prior cancer treatments. With the development of new medications that cross the blood–brain barrier, chemotherapy is increasingly recommended.[92] Survival is about 1 year.

Spinal Cord Tumours

Primary spinal cord tumours are rare and represent about 2% of CNS tumours. They may be extramedullary extradural, intradural extramedullary, or intradural intramedullary. Intramedullary tumours originate within the neural tissues of the spinal cord. Extramedullary tumours originate from tissues outside the spinal cord. Intramedullary tumours are primarily gliomas (astrocytomas and ependymomas). Gliomas are difficult to remove completely, and radiotherapy is required. Spinal ependymomas may be completely removed and are more common in adults. Extramedullary tumours are either peripheral nerve sheath tumours (neurofibromas or schwannomas) or meningiomas. Neurofibromas are generally found in the thoracic and lumbar region. Meningiomas are more evenly distributed through the spine. Complete removal of these tumours can be curative. Other extramedullary tumours are sarcomas, vascular tumours, chordomas, and epidermoid tumours. Intramedullary tumours include ependymoma, astrocytoma, and hemangioblastoma.

Metastatic spinal cord tumours are usually carcinomas (i.e., from breast, lung, or prostate cancer), lymphomas, or myelomas. Their location is often extradural, having spread to the spine through direct extension from tumours of the vertebral structures or from extraspinal sources extending through the interventricular foramen or bloodstream.

PATHOPHYSIOLOGY Intramedullary spinal cord tumours produce dysfunction by both invasion and compression. Extramedullary spinal cord tumours produce dysfunction by compressing adjacent tissue, not by direct invasion. Metastases from spinal cord tumours occur from direct extension or seeding through the CSF or bloodstream.

CLINICAL MANIFESTATIONS An acute onset of symptoms suggests a vascular blockage of vessels supplying the spinal cord. Gradual and progressive symptoms suggest compression. The compressive syndrome (sensorimotor syndrome) involves both the anterior and the posterior spinal tracts. Motor function and sensory function are affected as the tumour grows. Pain is usually an initial symptom.

The irritative syndrome (radicular syndrome) combines the symptoms of a cord compression with radicular pain that occurs in the sensory root distribution and indicates root irritation. The segmental symptoms include segmental sensory changes. These changes include paresthesias and impaired pain and touch perception; motor disturbances, including cramps, atrophy, fasciculations, and decreased or absent deep tendon reflexes, and continuous spinal pain.

CHAPTER 16 Disorders of the Central and Peripheral Nervous Systems

EVALUATION AND TREATMENT The diagnosis of a spinal cord tumour is made through imaging, CT-guided needle biopsy, or open biopsy. Involvement of specific cord segments is established. Any metastases also are identified. Treatment varies depending on the nature of the tumour and the person's clinical status. Surgery is essential for most spinal cord tumours.[93]

DID YOU UNDERSTAND?

Central Nervous System Disorders

1. Thirty percent of all traumatic brain injuries are experienced by children and youth.
2. Primary brain injury is caused by direct impact and involves neural injury, primary glial injury, and vascular responses.
3. Primary brain injuries can be focal or diffuse.
4. Focal brain injury can be caused by closed (blunt) trauma or open (penetrating) trauma. Open injury involves a skull fracture with exposure of the cranial vault to the environment.
5. Focal brain injury includes contusion, laceration, epidural (extradural) hematoma, subdural hematoma, intracerebral hematoma, and open brain injury.
6. Diffuse brain injury (diffuse axonal injury [DAI]) results from shearing forces that result in axonal damage ranging from mild concussion to severe DAI.
7. Secondary brain injury develops from systemic and intracranial responses to primary brain trauma that result in further brain injury and neuronal death.
8. Spinal cord injury involves damage to neural tissues by compressing tissue, pulling, or exerting tension on tissue, or shearing tissues so that they slide into one another.
9. Spinal cord injury may cause spinal shock with cessation of all motor, sensory, reflex, and autonomic functions below the transected area. Loss of motor and sensory function depends on the level of injury.
10. Neurogenic shock occurs with cervical or upper thoracic cord injury (above T5) and can occur concurrently with spinal shock.
11. Autonomic hyperreflexia (dysreflexia) is a syndrome of sudden, massive reflex sympathetic discharge associated with spinal cord injury at level T6 or above. Flexor spasms occur with profuse sweating, piloerection, and automatic bladder emptying.
12. Complete spinal cord transection results in paralysis. Paralysis of the lower half of the body with both legs involved is called *paraplegia*. Paralysis involving all four extremities is called *quadriplegia* or *tetraplegia*.
13. Return of spinal neuron excitability occurs slowly. Reflex activity can return in 1 to 2 weeks in most persons with acute spinal cord injury.
14. Low back pain is pain between the lower rib cage and gluteal muscles and often radiates into the thighs.
15. Most causes of low back pain are unknown. Some secondary causes are disc prolapse, tumours, bursitis, synovitis, degenerative joint disease, osteoporosis, fracture, inflammation, and sprain.
16. Degenerative disc disease is an alteration in intervertebral disc tissue and can be related to normal aging.
17. Spondylolysis is a structural defect of the spine with displacement of the deficient vertebra.
18. Spondylolisthesis involves forward slippage of a vertebra and can include a crack or fracture of the pars interarticularis, usually at the L5–S1 vertebrae.
19. Herniation of an intervertebral disc is a displacement of the nucleus pulposus or annulus fibrosus beyond the intervertebral disc space. Herniation most commonly affects the lumbosacral discs L5–S1 and L4–L5. The extruded pulposus compresses the nerve root, causing pain that radiates along the sciatic nerve.
20. Cerebrovascular disease is the most frequently occurring neurological disorder. Any abnormality of the blood vessels of the brain is referred to as a *cerebrovascular disease*.
21. Cerebrovascular disease is associated with two types of brain abnormalities: (a) ischemia with or without infarction and (b) hemorrhage.
22. Transient ischemic attacks are episodes of neurological dysfunction lasting no more than 1 hour and resulting from focal cerebral ischemia.
23. Cerebrovascular accidents (stroke syndromes) are classified as ischemic (thrombotic or embolic), hemorrhagic (intracranial hemorrhage), or associated with hypoperfusion.
24. Intracranial aneurysms result from defects in the vascular wall and are classified based on form and shape. They are often asymptomatic, but the signs vary depending on the location and size of the aneurysm.
25. An arteriovenous malformation is a mass of dilated blood vessels. Although usually present at birth, symptoms are delayed and usually occur before age 30.
26. A subarachnoid hemorrhage occurs when blood escapes from defective or injured vasculature into the subarachnoid space. When a vessel tears, blood under pressure is pumped into the subarachnoid space. The blood produces an inflammatory reaction in these tissues and increased intracranial pressure results.
27. Migraine is an episodic headache that can be associated with triggers. It may have an aura associated with a cortical spreading depression that alters cortical blood flow. Pain is related to over activity in the trigeminal vascular system.
28. Cluster headaches are a group of disorders that occur primarily in men. They occur in clusters over a period of days with extreme pain intensity, short duration and are associated with trigeminal activation.
29. Tension-type headache is the most common headache. Episodic-type headaches involve a peripheral pain mechanism. The chronic type involves a central pain mechanism and may be related to hypersensitivity to pain in craniocervical muscles.
30. Bacteria, viruses, fungi, protozoa, and rickettsiae can cause infection and inflammation of the central nervous system (CNS). Bacterial infections are fever or pus producing.
31. Meningitis (infection of the meninges) is classified as bacterial (i.e., meningococci), aseptic (viral or nonpurulent), or fungal. Bacterial meningitis mainly is an infection of the pia mater, the arachnoid, and the fluid of the subarachnoid space. Aseptic meningitis is thought to be limited to the meninges.
32. Brain abscesses often are caused by infections outside the CNS. Organisms gain access to the CNS from adjacent sites or spread along the wall of a vein. A localized inflammatory process develops with formation of exudate. After a few days, the infection becomes delimited with a centre of pus and a wall of granular tissue.
33. Encephalitis is an acute febrile illness of viral origin with nervous system involvement. Bites of mosquitos, ticks, or flies; viruses; and herpes simplex type 1 cause the most common encephalitis. Meningeal involvement appears in all encephalitides.
34. A common neurological complication of AIDS is HIV-associated neurocognitive disorder (HAND).

35. Multiple sclerosis is a chronic inflammatory demyelinating disorder with scarring (sclerosis) and loss of axons. Pathogenesis is unknown. The demyelination is thought to result from an immunogenetic-viral cause in genetically susceptible persons.
36. Guillain-Barré syndrome is a demyelinating disorder caused by a humoral and cell-mediated immunological reaction directed at the peripheral nerves.

Peripheral Nervous System and Neuromuscular Junction Disorders

1. With disorders of the roots of spinal cord nerves, the roots may be compressed, inflamed, or torn. Symptoms include local pain or paresthesias in the sensory root distribution. Treatment may involve surgery, antibiotics, steroids, radiation therapy, and chemotherapy.
2. Plexus injuries involve the plexus distal to the spinal roots. Paralysis can occur with complete plexus involvement.
3. When peripheral nerves are affected, axon and myelin degeneration may be present. These syndromes are classified as sensorimotor, sensory, or motor.
4. Myasthenia gravis is a disorder of voluntary muscles characterized by muscle weakness and fatigability. It is considered an autoimmune disease and is associated with an increased incidence of other autoimmune diseases.
5. Myasthenia gravis results from a defect in nerve impulse transmission at the postsynaptic membrane of the neuromuscular junction. Immunoglobulin G antibody is secreted against the "self" acetylcholine receptors and blocks the binding of acetylcholine. The antibody action destroys the receptor sites, causing decreased transmission of the nerve impulse across the neuromuscular junction.

Tumours of the Central Nervous System

1. Two main types of tumours occur within the cranium: primary and metastatic. Primary tumours are classified as intracerebral tumours (astrocytomas, oligodendrogliomas, and ependymomas) or extracerebral tumours (meningioma or nerve sheath tumours). Metastatic tumours can be found inside or outside the brain substance.
2. CNS tumours cause local and generalized manifestations. Local manifestations include seizures, visual disturbances, unstable gait, and cranial nerve dysfunction.
3. Spinal cord tumours are classified as intramedullary tumours (within the neural tissues) or extramedullary tumours (outside the spinal cord). Metastatic spinal cord tumours are usually carcinomas, lymphomas, or myelomas.
4. Extramedullary spinal cord tumours produce dysfunction by compression of adjacent tissue. Intramedullary spinal cord tumours produce dysfunction by both invasion and compression.

17

Developmental Alterations of Neurological Function

Kelly Power-Kean, with originating chapter contributions by Russell J. Butterfield and Sue E. Huether

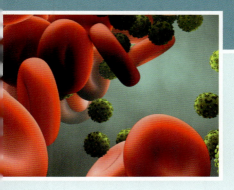

Additional resources are available online at https://evolve.elsevier.com/Canada/Huether/pathophysiology

CHAPTER OUTLINE

Development of the Nervous System in Children, 412
Structural Malformations, 413
    Defects of Neural Tube Closure, 413
    Craniostenosis, 414
    Malformations of Brain Development, 415
Alterations in Function: Encephalopathies, 416
    Static Encephalopathies, 416
    Inherited Metabolic Disorders of the Central Nervous System, 417
    Acute Encephalopathies, 419
    Infections of the Central Nervous System, 420
Cerebrovascular Disease in Children, 420
    Perinatal Stroke, 420
    Childhood Stroke, 420
    Epilepsy and Seizure Disorders in Children, 420
Childhood Tumours, 421
    Brain Tumours, 421
    Embryonal Tumours, 422

LEARNING OBJECTIVES

1. Explain the purpose of the two fontanelles that are present until the age of 18 months.
2. List the risk factors associated with neural tube defects.
3. Identify the structural malformations that occur because of defects of neural tube closure.
4. Identify the structural malformations that occur because of malformations in the axial skeleton.
5. List the most common factors that cause injury to the nervous system during the perinatal and postnatal periods.
6. Describe the forms of encephalopathy and discuss the causes, manifestations, treatment, and prognosis of each.
7. Identify metabolic disorders that result in neurological alterations in children.
8. Discuss the major types of seizures seen in children and describe their clinical manifestations.
9. List the common causes of bacterial and viral meningitis.
10. Discuss the significance of cerebrovascular disease in children.
11. Identify the common types of central nervous system tumours found in children.
12. List the common signs and symptoms of increased intracranial pressure in children.

KEY TERMS

Acute bacterial meningitis, 420
Anencephaly, 413
Aseptic meningitis, 420
Ataxic cerebral palsy, 416
Brainstem glioma, 422
Cerebellar astrocytoma, 421
Cerebral palsy, 416
Chiari II malformation (Arnold-Chiari malformation), 413
Congenital hydrocephalus, 415
Cortical dysplasia, 415
Craniopharyngioma, 422
Craniostenosis, 414
Cyclopia, 413
Dandy-Walker malformation (DWM), 416
Dystonic cerebral palsy, 416
Encephalitis, 420
Encephalocele, 413
Encephalopathy, 416
Ependymoma, 421
Epilepsy, 420
Extrapyramidal/nonspastic cerebral palsy, 416
Fontanelle, 412
Hemorrhagic stroke (intracranial hemorrhage), 420
Ischemic (occlusive) stroke, 420
Lead poisoning, 419
Lysosomal storage disease, 419
Macewen sign ("cracked pot" sign), 416
Medulloblastoma, 421
Meningitis, 420
Meningocele, 413
Microcephaly, 415
Myelomeningocele, 413
Neural tube defect (NTD), 413
Neuroblastoma, 422
Optic glioma, 422
Phenylketonuria (PKU), 419
Pica, 419
Pyramidal/spastic cerebral palsy, 416
Retinoblastoma, 423
Spina bifida (split spine), 413
Spina bifida occulta, 414
Tay-Sachs disease (GM_2 gangliosidosis), 419
Viral encephalitis, 420
Viral meningitis (aseptic or nonpurulent meningitis), 420

CHAPTER 17 Developmental Alterations of Neurological Function

Neurological disorders in children can occur from infancy through adolescence and include congenital malformations, genetic defects in metabolism, brain injuries, infection, tumours, and other disorders that affect neurological function.

DEVELOPMENT OF THE NERVOUS SYSTEM IN CHILDREN

> **QUICK CHECK 17.1**
> 1. When does development of neuronal myelination occur?
> 2. What is a major function of the fontanelles?
> 3. Why do many of the reflexes of infancy disappear by 1 year of age?

The nervous system develops from the embryonic ectoderm. This development involves a complex, sequential process that occurs in stages, which include (1) formation of the neural tube (3 to 4 weeks' gestation), (2) development of the forebrain from the neural tube (2 to 3 months' gestation), (3) neuronal proliferation and migration (3 to 5 months' gestation), (4) formation of network connections and synapses (5 months' gestation to many years postnatally), and (5) myelination (birth to many years postnatally). Critical periods must pass uninterrupted if the fetus is to develop normally. Genetic and environmental factors (e.g., nutrition, hormones, oxygen levels, toxins, alcohol, medications, drugs, maternal infections, and maternal disease) can have a significant effect on neural development[1] (see *Health Promotion: Prevention of Fetal Alcohol Spectrum Disorders*).

HEALTH PROMOTION
Prevention of Fetal Alcohol Spectrum Disorders

The term *fetal alcohol spectrum disorder* (FASD) describes the damage that prenatal alcohol exposure can cause in the unborn child. Alcohol crosses the placenta and the blood–brain barrier and exerts teratogenic effects on the developing brain. Damage includes physical defects and cognitive, behavioural, emotional, and adaptive functioning deficits. FASD includes diagnoses of fetal alcohol syndrome (FAS), partial FAS, alcohol-related neurodevelopmental disorder (ARND), and alcohol-related birth defects (ARBD).[a] ARND has neurobehavioural and cognitive deficiencies. It is among the most common causes of mental deficits that persist throughout adulthood. ARND is 100% preventable. It is estimated that in Canada nine in every 1,000 babies are born with FASD.[b] Studies indicate that the incidence of FAS in Canada is higher among Indigenous populations and in rural and remote communities.[b] As there is no known amount of alcohol that is safe to consume while pregnant; all medical guidelines on alcohol use in Canada advise that women not drink alcohol during pregnancy.[a]

References
1. Glauser, W., Tepper, J., & Petch, J. (2016). Alcohol and pregnancy: is it safe to have a little? *Healthy Debate*. https://healthydebate.ca/2016/05/topic/alcohol-pregnancy-guidelines.
2. Government of Canada. (2017). *Fetal alcohol spectrum disorder.* https://www.canada.ca/en/health-canada/services/healthy-living/your-health/diseases/fetal-alcohol-spectrum-disorder.html.

The growth and development of the brain occurs most rapidly from the third month of gestation through the first year of life, reflecting the proliferation of neurons and glial cells. Although all of the neurons that an individual will ever have are present at birth, development of skills, such as walking, talking, and thinking, depends on these cells making

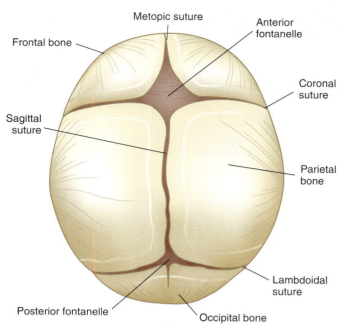

FIGURE 17.1 Cranial Sutures and Fontanelles in Infancy. Fibrous union of suture lines and interlocking of serrated edges (occurs by 6 months; solid union requires approximately 12 years).

correct connections with other cells. By the first year one half of postnatal brain growth occurs and is 90% complete by age 6 years. Cerebral blood flow and oxygen consumption during these years are about twice those of the adult brain.

A separation of the bones of the infant's skull occurs at the suture lines, forming two **fontanelles**, or "soft spots". One is the diamond-shaped anterior fontanelle and one triangular-shaped posterior fontanelle. The sutures allow for expansion of the growing brain. The posterior fontanelle may be open until 2 to 3 months of age; the anterior fontanelle normally does not fully close until 18 months of age (Figure 17.1). Head growth usually reflects brain growth. Monitoring the fontanelles and careful measurement and recording of the head circumference on standardized growth charts are important aspects of the pediatric examination. A common cause of accelerating head growth and macrocephaly is hydrocephalus. This condition presents with an enlargement of the cerebrospinal fluid (CSF) compartment (ventricles). Increased intracranial pressure (ICP), with bulging of the fontanelles, and separation of the sutures are signs of hydrocephalus. Microcephaly (head circumference below the second percentile for age) can be the result of prenatal infection, toxin exposure, malnutrition, or have a genetic cause (see Table 17.3).

Because of the immaturity of the human forebrain at birth, neurological examination of the infant detects mostly reflex responses that require an intact spinal cord and brainstem. As cerebral cortical function matures, some of these reflex patterns decrease and disappear at predictable times during infancy (Table 17.1).

Absence of expected reflexes at the appropriate age indicates depression of central or peripheral motor functions. Asymmetrical responses may indicate lesions in the motor cortex or peripheral nerves. This may also occur with skull fractures after traumatic delivery or postnatal injury. As the infant matures, the neonatal reflexes disappear, and voluntary motor functions follow. If the reflexes of infancy do not disappear, the infant may be experiencing a central motor lesion.

TABLE 17.1 Reflexes of Infancy

Reflex	Age of Appearance of Reflex	Age at Which Reflex Should No Longer Be Obtainable
Moro	Birth	3 months
Stepping	Birth	6 weeks
Sucking	Birth	4 months awake 7 months asleep
Rooting	Birth	4 months awake 7 months asleep
Palmar grasp	Birth	6 months
Plantar grasp	Birth	10 months
Tonic neck	2 months	5 months
Neck righting	4 to 6 months	24 months
Landau	3 months	24 months
Parachute reaction	9 months	Persists indefinitely

STRUCTURAL MALFORMATIONS

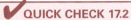

QUICK CHECK 17.2
1. List two defects of neural tube closure.
2. Why do motor and sensory functions worsen with growth in a child with a neural tube defect?
3. What food source or dietary supplement helps to prevent neural tube defects?

Central nervous system (CNS) malformations are responsible for 75% of fetal deaths and 40% of deaths during the first year of life. CNS malformations account for 33% of all apparent congenital malformations, and 90% of CNS malformations are defects of neural tube closure.

Defects of Neural Tube Closure

A stoppage of the normal development of the brain and spinal cord during the first month of embryonic development causes **neural tube defects (NTDs)**. In Canada, one in every 750 children is born with a neural tube defect.[2] Defects of neural tube closure are divided into two categories: (1) anterior midline defects (ventral induction) and (2) posterior defects (dorsal induction). Anterior midline defects may cause brain and face abnormalities with the most extreme form being **cyclopia**. In this condition, the child has one midline orbit and eye with a protruding noselike structure above the orbit. **Spina bifida (split spine)** is the most common NTD and includes anencephaly (*an*, "without"; *enkephalos*, "brain"), encephalocele, meningocele, and myelomeningocele. Vertebrae fail to close in spina bifida. Myelomeningocele is a form of spina bifida with incomplete development of the spine and protrusion of both the spinal cord and the meninges through the skin. Meningocele is a form of spina bifida in which there is protrusion of the meninges, but the spinal cord remains in the spinal canal. Figure 17.2 reviews disorders of embryonic neural development.

Multifactorial (a combination of genes and environment) causes are associated with NTDs. No single gene has been found to cause NTDs, but there can be associated mutations in folate-responsive or folate-dependent pathways.[3] Folic acid deficiency during preconception and early stages of pregnancy increases the risk for NTDs. Supplementation with 400 μg of folic acid per day ensures adequate folate status.[2] The introduction of the mandatory enrichment of flour with folic acid in Canada has resulted in a significant reduction in the incidence of NTDs. Other factors include the increasing use of folic acid supplements and increased prenatal screening and diagnosis leading to pregnancy termination.[3] Other risk factors include a previous NTD pregnancy, maternal diabetes, or obesity, use of anticonvulsant medications, and maternal hyperthermia.[4]

Anencephaly is a defect in which the soft, bony component of the skull and part of the brain are missing.[5] There is a prevalence rate of 1.58 per 10 000 births in Canada each year.[6] These infants are stillborn or die within a few days after birth. The pathological mechanism is unknown. The prenatal use of ultrasound or evaluation of maternal serum alpha fetoprotein (AFP) assists diagnosis.

Encephalocele refers to a herniation or protrusion of the brain and meninges through a defect in the skull, resulting in a saclike structure.[7]

Meningocele is a saclike cyst of meninges filled with spinal fluid and is a mild form of spina bifida (Figure 17.3). It develops during the first 4 weeks of pregnancy when the neural tube fails to close completely. The meninges protrude through the vertebral defect, but there is no involvement of the spinal cord or nerve roots. This condition may produce no neurological deficit or symptoms.

Myelomeningocele (meningomyelocele; spina bifida cystica) is a herniation of a saclike cyst through a defect in the posterior arch of a vertebra. The cysts contain meninges, spinal fluid, and a part of the spinal cord with its nerves. Eighty percent of myelomeningoceles are located in the lumbar and lumbosacral regions, the last regions of the neural tube to close. Myelomeningocele is one of the most common developmental anomalies of the nervous system, affecting about 120 to 150 babies in Canada each year.[8]

Meningocele and myelomeningoceles are present as a skin defect on the infant's back (see Figure 17.3). A transparent membrane that may have neural tissue attached to its inner surface usually covers the defect. This membrane may be intact at birth or may leak CSF, thereby increasing the risks of infection and neuronal damage.

The spinal cord and nerve roots are malformed below the level of the lesion, resulting in loss of motor, sensory, reflex, and autonomic functions. A neurological examination of motor function in the legs, reflexes, and sphincter tone can usually determine the level of spinal cord and nerve root injury (Table 17.2). This examination is useful to predict whether the child will walk, require bladder catheterization, or be at risk of developing scoliosis (see Chapter 40).

Hydrocephalus occurs in 85% of infants with myelomeningocele.[9] Seizures also occur in 30% of those with myelodysplasia. An alteration of motor and sensory functions below the level of the injury occurs. Often these problems worsen as the child grows.[9] This diagnosis occurs with several musculoskeletal and spinal deformities.

Myelomeningoceles are usually associated with the **Chiari II malformation (Arnold-Chiari malformation)**.[9] This defect is a complex malformation of the brainstem and cerebellum. The cerebellar tonsils are displaced downward into the cervical spinal canal. The upper medulla and lower pons are elongated and thin; and the medulla is also displaced downward and sometimes has a "kink" (Figure 17.4). The Chiari II malformation is associated with hydrocephalus; syringomyelia (an abnormality causing cysts at multiple levels within the spinal cord); and cognitive and motor deficits.[10]

Other types of Chiari malformations are not associated with spina bifida. Type I Chiari malformation does not involve the brainstem and may be asymptomatic. In type III, the brainstem or cerebellum extends into a high cervical myelomeningocele. Cerebellar development is lacking with type IV.

Diagnosis of most cases of meningocele and myelomeningocele occurs prenatally, using maternal serological testing (AFP) and prenatal ultrasound. In these cases, delivery of the fetus is by elective Caesarean section to minimize trauma during labour. Surgical repair is critical and may occur in utero or during the first 72 hours of life.[11]

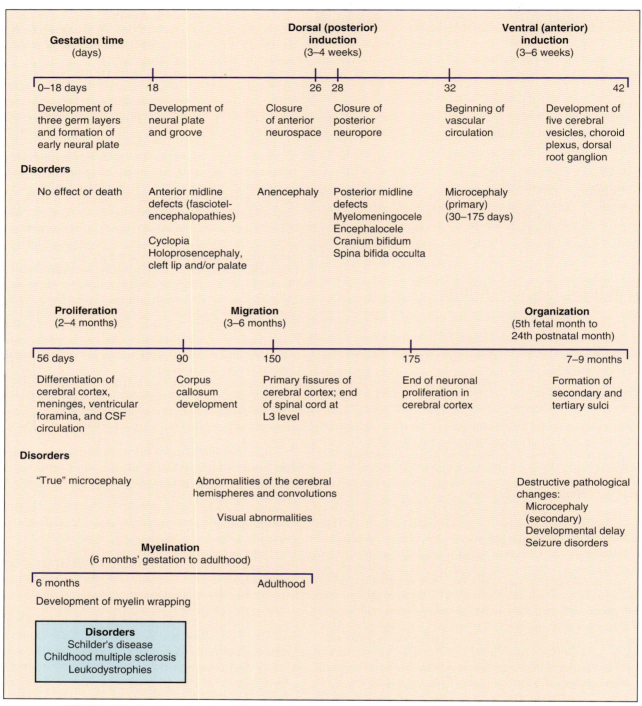

FIGURE 17.2 Disorders Associated With Specific Stages of Embryonic Development. *CSF,* Cerebrospinal fluid.

When a defect occurs without any visible exposure of meninges or neural tissue, the term **spina bifida occulta** is used. The defect is common and occurs to some degree in 10 to 25% of infants.[1] Spina bifida occulta usually causes no neurological dysfunction because the spinal cord and spinal nerves are normal.

Craniostenosis

Skull malformations range from minor defects to major defects that are incompatible with life. **Craniostenosis** (also termed *craniosynostosis*) is the premature closure of one or more of the cranial sutures during the first 18 to 20 months of the infant's life. Males are affected twice as often as females. Fusion of a cranial suture results in an asymmetrical shape of the skull. The general term *plagiocephaly*, meaning "misshapen skull," describes deformities that result from craniostenosis. When a single coronal suture fuses prematurely, the head is flat on that side in front. When the sagittal suture fuses prematurely, head elongation occurs.[1] Single suture craniostenosis is usually only a cosmetic issue. Rarely, when multiple sutures fuse prematurely, brain growth may be

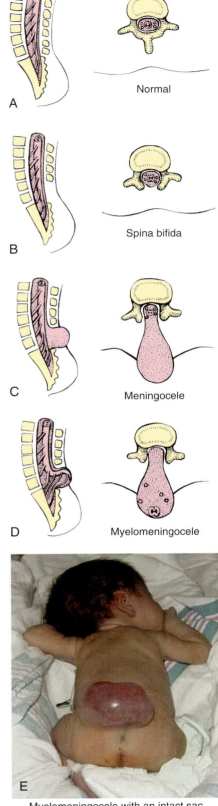

FIGURE 17.3 Normal Spine, Spina Bifida, Meningocele, and Myelomeningocele. (From Hockenberry, M. J., & Wilson, D. [2015]. *Wong's nursing care of infants and children* [10th ed.]. Mosby.)

TABLE 17.2 Functional Alterations in Myelodysplasia Related to Level of Lesion

Level of Lesion	Functional Implications
Thoracic	Flaccid paralysis of lower extremities; variable weakness in abdominal trunk musculature; high thoracic level may mean respiratory compromise; absence of bowel and bladder control
High lumbar	Voluntary hip flexion and adduction; flaccid paralysis of knees, ankles, and feet; may walk with extensive braces and crutches; absence of bowel and bladder control
Mid lumbar	Strong hip flexion and adduction; fair knee extension; flaccid paralysis of ankles and feet; absence of bowel and bladder control
Low lumbar	Strong hip flexion, extension, and adduction and knee extension; weak ankle and toe mobility; may have limited bowel and bladder function
Sacral	Normal function of lower extremities; normal bowel and bladder function

Modified from Sandler, A. D. (2010). Children with spina bifida: Key clinical issues. *Pediatric Clinics of North America, 57*(4), 879–892.

restricted, and surgical repair may prevent neurological dysfunction (Figure 17.5).

Malformations of Brain Development

Reduced growth or accelerated apoptosis causes congenital microcephaly (small brain) (Table 17.3). Increased growth causes megalencephaly (abnormally large brain).

Microcephaly is a defect in generalized brain growth (see Figure 17.5). Cranial size is significantly below average for the infant's age, gender, race, and gestation. The small size of the skull reflects a small brain. *True (primary) microcephaly* commonly occurs because of an autosomal recessive genetic or chromosomal defect. *Secondary (acquired) microcephaly* is associated with various causes including infection, trauma, metabolic disorders, third trimester maternal anorexia, and other genetic syndromes. Developmental delay usually accompanies microcephaly.

Cortical dysplasias are a heterogeneous group of disorders caused by defects in brain development. These disorders may range from a small area of abnormal tissue to an entire brain that is smooth without the normal configuration of gyri and sulci of a developed brain (lissencephaly). The malformation occurs during brain formation. There is a specific genetic defect for some of these disorders. Other disorders are multifactorial or acquired (e.g., intrauterine trauma or infection). Cortical dysplasias increase the risk for seizures that are difficult to control and cause developmental delay and motor dysfunction. Genetic testing assesses risk in other family members.[1]

Congenital hydrocephalus is present at birth and characterized by increased CSF pressure. Blockage within the ventricular system where the CSF flows, an imbalance in the production of CSF, or a reduced reabsorption of CSF may cause this condition.[1] The increased pressure within the ventricular system dilates the ventricles and pushes and compresses the brain tissue against the skull (Figure 17.6). When hydrocephalus develops before fusion of the cranial sutures, the skull can expand to accommodate this additional volume and preserve neuronal function (see photo in Figure 17.6C). The overall incidence of hydrocephalus is approximately 6.07 per 10 000 live births.[10] (Types of hydrocephalus are discussed in Chapter 15.)

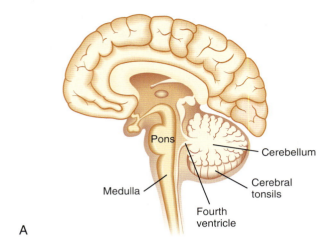
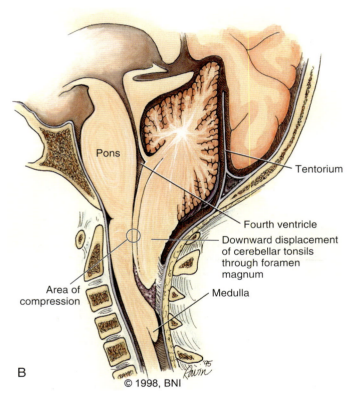

FIGURE 17.4 Normal Brain and Chiari II Malformation. **A,** Diagram of normal brain. **B,** Diagram of Chiari II malformation with downward displacement of cerebellar tonsils and medulla through foramen magnum causing compression and obstruction to flow of cerebrospinal fluid. ([B] Used with permission from Barrow Neurological Institute, Phoenix, Arizona.)

Congenital hydrocephalus may cause fetal death in utero, or the increased head circumference may require Caesarean delivery. When there is separation of the cranial sutures, a tapping of the skull results in a resonant sound. This result is called the Macewen sign ("cracked pot" sign). The eyes may assume a staring expression, with sclera visible above the cornea, called *sunsetting*. Brain malformations, episodes of shunt failure or infection are the usual cause of cognitive impairment in children with hydrocephalus. When treated successfully by shunting or other methods, approximately 30 to 40% of children with uncomplicated congenital hydrocephalus complete schooling and find employment.[12]

The Dandy-Walker malformation (DWM) is a congenital defect of the cerebellum characterized by a large posterior fossa cyst that communicates with the fourth ventricle and an atrophic, upwardly rotated cerebellar vermis.[1] DWM is commonly associated with hydrocephalus caused by compression of the aqueduct of Sylvius. Other causes of blockages within the ventricular system that can result in hydrocephalus include brain tumours, cysts, trauma, arteriovenous malformations, blood clots, infections, and the Chiari malformations.

ALTERATIONS IN FUNCTION: ENCEPHALOPATHIES

> **QUICK CHECK 17.3**
> 1. List three types of cerebral palsy.
> 2. Why does failure to metabolize phenylalanine produce such widespread and devastating effects on development?

Encephalopathy, which means brain pathology, is a general category that includes many syndromes and diseases (see Chapter 16). These disorders may be acute or chronic, as well as static or progressive.

Static Encephalopathies

Static or nonprogressive encephalopathy describes a neurological condition caused by a fixed lesion without active and ongoing disease. Causes include brain malformations or brain injury that may occur during gestation or birth, or at any time during childhood. The extent of the injury or malformation relates directly to the degree of neurological impairment. Anoxia, trauma, and infections are the most common factors that cause injury to the nervous system in the perinatal period. Infections, metabolic disturbances (acquired or genetic), trauma, toxins, and vascular disease may injure the nervous system in the postnatal period.[1]

Cerebral palsy is a disorder of movement, muscle tone, or posture. Injury or abnormal development in the immature brain before, during, or after birth up to 1 year of age is the cause of this disorder. Approximately 1 in 400 persons in Canada are diagnosed with cerebral palsy.[13]

Risk factors include prenatal or perinatal cerebral hypoxia, hemorrhage, infection, genetic abnormalities, or low birth weight. The major types involve spasticity, dystonia, ataxia, or a combination of these symptoms (mixed). Diplegia, hemiplegia, or tetraplegia may be present.

Pyramidal/spastic cerebral palsy results from damage to corticospinal pathways (upper motor neurons). It is associated with increased muscle tone, persistent primitive reflexes, hyperactive deep tendon reflexes, clonus, rigidity of the extremities, scoliosis, and contractures. This form of cerebral palsy accounts for approximately 77 to 93% of cases. Damage to cells in the basal ganglia, thalamus, or cerebellum causes extrapyramidal/nonspastic cerebral palsy. This form of cerebral palsy accounts for approximately 2 to 15% of cases.[14] It includes two subtypes: dystonic and ataxic. Dystonic cerebral palsy is associated with extreme difficulty in fine motor coordination and purposeful movements. Movements are stiff, uncontrolled, and abrupt, resulting from injury to the basal ganglia or extrapyramidal tracts. Damage to the cerebellum causes ataxic cerebral palsy. Alterations in coordination and movement occur with this disorder. There is a broad-based gait and tremor is common with intentional movements. A child may have symptoms of each of these cerebral palsy types.

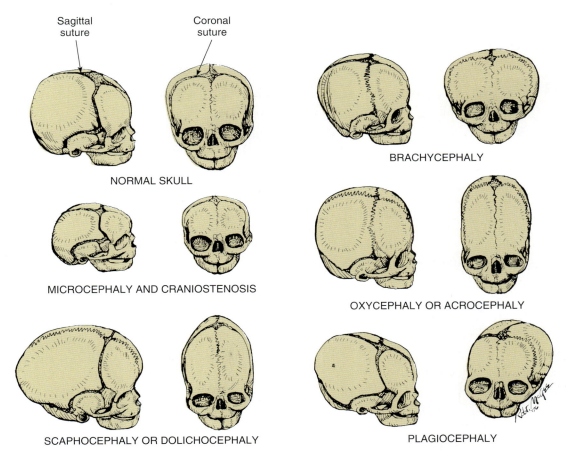

FIGURE 17.5 Normal and Abnormal Head Configurations. *Normal skull:* Bones separated by membranous seams until sutures gradually close. *Microcephaly and craniostenosis:* Microcephaly is head circumference more than 2 standard deviations below the mean for age, gender, race, and gestation and reflects a small brain; craniostenosis is premature closure of sutures. *Scaphocephaly or dolichocephaly* (frequency 56%): Premature closure of sagittal suture, resulting in restricted lateral growth. *Brachycephaly:* Premature closure of coronal suture, resulting in excessive lateral growth. *Oxycephaly or acrocephaly* (frequency 5.8 to 12%): Premature closure of all coronal and sagittal sutures, resulting in accelerated upward growth and small head circumference. *Plagiocephaly* (frequency 13%): Unilateral premature closure of coronal suture, resulting in asymmetrical growth. (From Hockenberry, M. J., & Wilson, D. [2015]. *Wong's nursing care of infants and children* [10th ed.]. Mosby.)

TABLE 17.3 Causes of Microcephaly

Defects in Brain Development	Intrauterine Infections	Perinatal and Postnatal Disorders
Hereditary (recessive) microcephaly	Congenital rubella	Intrauterine or neonatal anoxia
Down syndrome and other trisomy syndromes	Cytomegalovirus infection	Severe malnutrition in early infancy
Fetal ionizing radiation exposure	Congenital toxoplasmosis	Neonatal herpesvirus infection
Maternal phenylketonuria	Zika virus infection	
Cornelia de Lange's syndrome		
Rubinstein-Taybi syndrome		
Smith-Lemli-Opitz syndrome		
Fetal alcohol spectrum disorder		
Angelman syndrome		
Seckel's syndrome		

Children with cerebral palsy often have associated neurological disorders, such as seizures, and intellectual impairment ranging from mild to severe. Other complications include visual impairment, communication disorders, respiratory problems, bowel and bladder problems, and orthopedic disabilities.[15]

Inherited Metabolic Disorders of the Central Nervous System

Many inherited metabolic disorders exist. These disorders typically lead to diffuse brain dysfunction. Early diagnosis and treatment are vital if these infants are to survive without severe neurological problems. Newborn screening in Canada for specific metabolic conditions varies by province or territory. This testing has led to the identification of children at risk of developing metabolic conditions before symptoms develop. Table 17.4 lists some of these inherited metabolic disorders. Inborn errors of metabolism are present at birth, and most cause disturbances of the nervous system. Some disorders may not manifest until childhood or adulthood. Defects in amino acid and lipid metabolism are among the most common.

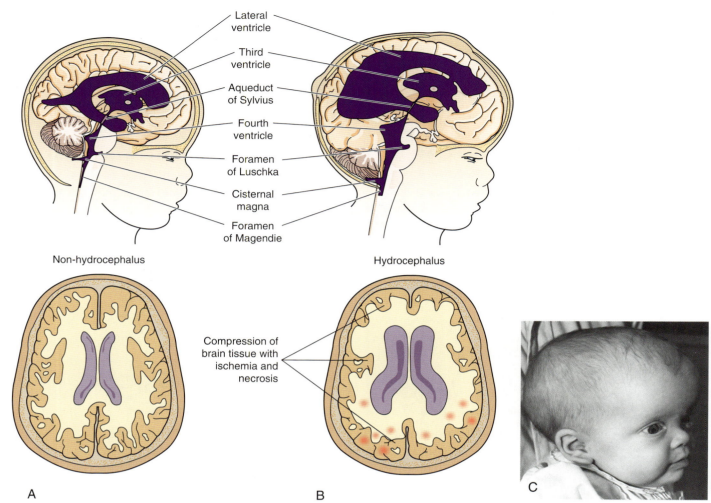

FIGURE 17.6 Hydrocephalus. A block in the flow of cerebrospinal fluid (CSF). **A,** Patent CSF circulation. **B,** Enlarged lateral and third ventricles caused by obstruction of circulation (e.g., stenosis of aqueduct of Sylvius). **C,** Infant born with hydrocephalus. ([C] from McCance, K. L., & Huether, S. E. [2014]. *Pathophysiology: the biological basis for disease in adults and children* [7th ed., p. 668]. Elsevier.)

TABLE 17.4 Inherited Metabolic Disorders of the Central Nervous System

Age of Onset	Disorder
Neonatal period	Pyridoxine dependency, galactosemia, urea cycle defects, maple syrup urine disease and its variant, phenylketonuria (PKU), Menkes' kinky hair syndrome
Early infancy	Tay-Sachs disease and its variants, infantile Gaucher's disease, infantile Niemann-Pick disease, Krabbe disease (leukodystrophy), Farber lipogranulomatosis, Pelizaeus-Merzbacher disease and other sudanophilic leukodystrophies, spongy degeneration of central nervous system (Canavan disease), Alexander's disease, Alpers disease, Leigh disease (subacute necrotizing encephalomyelopathy), congenital lactic acidosis, Zellweger encephalopathy, Lowe syndrome (oculocerebrorenal syndrome)
Late infancy and early childhood	Disorders of amino acid metabolism, metachromatic leukodystrophy, adrenoleukodystrophy, late infantile GM_1 gangliosidosis, late infantile Gaucher's and Niemann-Pick diseases, neuroaxonal dystrophy, mucopolysaccharidosis, mucolipidosis, fucosidosis, mannosidosis, aspartylglycosaminuria, neuronal ceroid lipofuscinoses (Jansky-Bielschowsky disease, Batten's disease, Vogt-Spielmeyer disease (neuronal ceroid lipofuscinosis), Cockayne's syndrome, ataxia telangiectasia
Later childhood and adolescence	Progressive cerebellar ataxias of childhood and adolescence, hepatolenticular degeneration (Wilson's disease), Hallervorden-Spatz disease, Lesch-Nyhan syndrome, Aicardi-Goutieres syndrome, progressive myoclonus epilepsies, homocystinuria, Fabry's disease

Data from Volpe, J. J. (2008). *Neurology of the newborn* (5th ed.). Saunders. For information regarding screening and parent education, see Medical Home Portal at https://www.medicalhomeportal.org.

CHAPTER 17 Developmental Alterations of Neurological Function

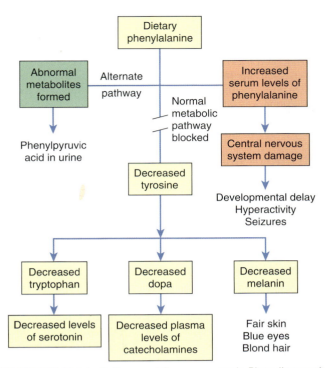

FIGURE 17.7 Metabolic Error and Consequences in Phenylketonuria. (From Hockenberry, M. J., & Wilson, D. [2015]. *Wong's nursing care of infants and children* [10th ed.]. Mosby.)

TABLE 17.5	Common Poisons	
Pharmacological Agents	**Heavy Metals**	**Miscellaneous Agents**
Acetaminophen	Lead	Botulinum toxin
Amphetamines	Acute exposure	Alcohols
Anticonvulsants	Chronic exposure	Ethyl
Antidepressants	Mercury	Isopropyl
Antihistamines	Thallium	Methyl
Atropine	Arsenic	Pesticides
Barbiturates	Iron supplements	Organophosphates
Methadone		Chlorinated hydrocarbons
Phencyclidine		
Salicylates		Mushrooms
Tranquilizers		Venoms
		Snakebite
		Tick paralysis
		Ethylene glycol
		Furniture polish
		Paint solvents

Data from Shannon, M. W., Borron, S. W., & Burns, M. (2007). *Haddad and Winchester's clinical management of poisoning and drug overdose* (4th ed.). Saunders; Swaiman, K. F., Ashwal, S., Ferriero, D. M., et al. (2012). *Pediatric neurology: principles and practice* (5th ed., Vol 2). Mosby.

Defects in Amino Acid Metabolism

Biochemical defects in amino acid metabolism include (1) those in which the transport of an amino acid is impaired, (2) those involving an enzyme or cofactor deficiency, and (3) those encompassing certain chemical components, such as branched-chain or sulphur-containing amino acids. Genetic defects cause most of these disorders.

Phenylketonuria. **Phenylketonuria (PKU)** is an example of an inborn error of metabolism characterized by phenylalanine hydroxylase deficiency. There is an inability of the body to convert the essential amino acid phenylalanine to tyrosine (Figure 17.7). PKU is an autosomal recessive inborn error of metabolism. PKU has an incidence of 1 per 12 000 live births in North America.[16]

Most natural food proteins contain about 15% phenylalanine, an essential amino acid. Phenylalanine hydroxylase controls the conversion of this amino acid to tyrosine in the liver. The body uses tyrosine in the biosynthesis of proteins, melanin, thyroxine, and the catecholamines in the brain and adrenal medulla. Phenylalanine hydroxylase deficiency causes a buildup of phenylalanine in the serum. Increased phenylalanine levels result in abnormalities of the cerebral cortical layers, defective myelination, and cystic degeneration of the grey and white matter. Brain damage occurs prior to detection of the metabolites in the urine and continues as long as phenylalanine levels remain high. Canada and more than 30 other countries use nonselective newborn screening to detect PKU. Treatment of reducing dietary phenylalanine (PKU diet) is effective and allows for normal development. Supplementation with other essential amino acids and nutrients is required to promote adequate growth and development. Mutations in the *PAH* gene are by far the most common cause of PKU.

Storage Diseases

Disorders of lipid metabolism are termed **lysosomal storage diseases**. All disorders in this group have a missing lysosomal enzyme group. Lysosomal storage disorders are rare and include more than 50 known genetic disorders.[1] These disorders cause an excessive accumulation of a particular cell product, occurring in the brain, liver, spleen, bone, and lung. Generally, these disorders are not included in newborn screening. Some of these disorders may be treated with enzyme replacement therapy.[17] The best known of the lysosomal storage disorders is **Tay-Sachs disease (GM2 gangliosidosis)**, an autosomal recessive disorder (*HexA* gene on chromosome 15) caused by deficiency of the lysosomal enzyme hexosaminidase A (HexA). Approximately 80% of individuals diagnosed are of Jewish ancestry. Onset of this disease usually occurs when the infant is 4 to 6 months old. Symptoms of Tay-Sachs include an exaggerated startle response to loud noise, seizures, developmental regression, dementia, and blindness. Death from this disease almost always occurs by 5 years of age. Screening for carriers of the gene defect, along with counselling to prevent disease transmission, is possible.[18]

Acute Encephalopathies
Intoxications of the Central Nervous System

The consideration of a medication-induced encephalopathy should occur in the child with unexplained neurological changes. Such encephalopathies may result from accidental ingestion, therapeutic overdose, intentional overdose, or ingestion of environmental toxins. Table 17.5 lists the most commonly ingested poisons. In Canada 4 392 deaths related to unintentional poisoning were reported in 2017.[19]

Lead poisoning results in high blood levels of lead. If lead poisoning is untreated, lead encephalopathy results and is responsible for serious and irreversible neurological damage. Those at greatest risk are children ages 2 to 3 years and children prone to the practice of **pica**—the habitual, purposeful, and compulsive ingestion of non-food substances, such as clay, soil, and paint chips or paint dust. Lead intoxication also may occur from chronic exposure to lead in cosmetics, inhalation of gasoline vapors, and ingestion of airborne lead.[20]

The occurrence of lead toxicity requiring treatment is rare in Canada.[20] The *Canadian Paediatric Association* has published recommendations for the assessment and treatment of lead poisoning.[20]

Infections of the Central Nervous System

Meningitis is an infection of the meninges and subarachnoid space of the brain and spinal cord. **Encephalitis** is an inflammation within the brain. In many infections of the meninges, encephalitis also is present, and the term *meningoencephalitis* is used. Bacteria, viruses, or other microorganisms can cause inflammation and acute encephalopathy. **Aseptic meningitis** has no evidence of bacterial infection but may be associated with viral infection, systemic disease, or medications.

Bacterial Meningitis

Acute bacterial meningitis is one of the most serious infections to which infants and children are susceptible. In Canada, the 2017 meningitis death rate was 0.2 per 100 000 population.[21] The highest incidence rates are among infants aged less than 1 year. The introduction of conjugate vaccines against *Haemophilus influenzae* type B, *Streptococcus pneumoniae*, and *Neisseria meningitidis* (meningococcus) has decreased the incidence of bacterial meningitis.[1] A vaccine for serogroup B *N. meningitidis* is available in Canada but is not recommended for routine immunization programs for infants, children, adolescents, or adults.[21]

Group B *Streptococcus* causes lethal meningitis and sepsis in neonates. Transmission occurs to the child from the mother's birth canal. *S. pneumoniae* is the most common microorganism in children 1 to 23 months of age. Staphylococcal or streptococcal meningitis can occur in children of any age but takes place more often in children who have had neurosurgery, skull fracture, or a complication of systemic bacterial infection. Infections that begin in the middle ear, sinuses, or mastoid cells also may lead to *S. pneumoniae* infection.

Escherichia coli and group B beta-hemolytic streptococci are the most common causes of meningitis in the newborn period. The second most common microorganism causing bacterial meningitis, particularly in children younger than 4 years, is *Neisseria meningitidis* (meningococcus). This infection has the potential to occur in epidemics. Approximately 2 to 5% of healthy children are carriers of *N. meningitidis*. The incidence of *N. meningitidis* infection increases in adolescence and with crowded environments, such as in student residences. As a result, all persons 11 to 18 years of age should receive immunization against this pathogen.[21]

Pathogens enter the nervous system by direct extension from a contiguous source (e.g., paranasal sinuses or mastoid cells) or, more commonly, by spread through the blood (e.g., infective endocarditis, pneumonia, neurosurgical procedures, and severe burns). Pathogens then cross the blood–brain barrier, enter the CSF, and multiply. Bacterial toxins increase cerebrovascular permeability, causing changes in blood flow and edema. Increased cranial pressure may worsen further by blockage to the CSF circulation. Herniation of the brainstem causes death.

An upper respiratory tract or a gastrointestinal infection often occurs before the onset of acute bacterial meningitis. Inflammation leads to symptoms of fever, headache, vomiting, and irritability and the CNS symptoms of photophobia, nuchal and spinal rigidity, decreased level of consciousness, and seizures. Irritation of the meninges and spinal roots causes pain and resistance to neck flexion (nuchal rigidity), a positive Kernig sign (resistance to knee extension in the supine position with the hips and knees flexed against the body), and a positive Brudzinski sign (flexion of the knees and hips when the neck is flexed forward rapidly). With severe meningeal irritation, the child may show opisthotonic posturing (rigid arching of the back with the head extended). Infants may have bulging fontanelles. Meningococcal meningitis can produce a characteristic petechial rash.

Viral meningitis (aseptic or nonpurulent meningitis) may result from a direct infection of a virus. It may also be secondary to disease, such as measles, mumps, herpes, or leukemia. The key signs of viral meningitis are a mononuclear response in the CSF and the presence of normal glucose levels. The symptoms are similar to those in bacterial meningitis, although usually milder.

Viral encephalitis in children is similar to viral encephalitis in adults (see Chapter 16, Figure 16.13) and can be difficult to distinguish from viral meningitis. Viruses can directly invade the brain, causing inflammation. Postinfectious encephalitis can also develop because of an autoimmune response.[22] Chapter 8 and Chapter 16 discuss encephalopathy resulting from human immunodeficiency virus (HIV).

CEREBROVASCULAR DISEASE IN CHILDREN

Perinatal Stroke

Perinatal arterial ischemic stroke is estimated at 1 in 4 000 live births. It is a leading cause of perinatal brain injury, cerebral palsy, and lifelong disability. Although a cause for perinatal stroke is usually not found, clotting abnormalities may make the child prone to further vascular events.

Childhood Stroke

Childhood stroke occurs in 1 to 13 per 100 000 children per year and may be divided into two categories: ischemic and hemorrhagic.[23]

Ischemic (occlusive) stroke is rare in children. It may result from embolism, sinovenous thrombosis, or congenital or iatrogenic narrowing of vessels leading to decreased flow of blood and oxygen to areas of the brain. Children with arterial ischemic stroke do not have the typical adult risk factors of atherosclerosis and hypertension. Risk factors include cardiac diseases, hematological and vascular disorders, and infection. Approximately 40% of children with acute ischemic stroke have no identifiable risk factors.[1] Sickle cell disease, cerebral arteriopathies, and cardiac anomalies are the common disorders associated with arterial ischemic stroke.[24]

Bleeding from congenital cerebral arteriovenous malformations is the most common cause of **hemorrhagic stroke (intracranial hemorrhage)**. This condition is rare in children younger than 19 years. Immature blood vessels and unstable blood pressure are the usual cause of intraventricular hemorrhage associated with premature birth. There is a high risk of developing posthemorrhagic hydrocephalus.[25]

Epilepsy and Seizure Disorders in Children

The incidence of epilepsy varies greatly with age, and geographical location. In Canada, the incidence of epilepsy in children and youth is higher than in adults. From the ages 1 to 19 years, 60 per 100 000 are affected. From ages 20 years and older, 53 per 100 000 are affected. Approximately 20 000 people in Canada are newly diagnosed each year.[26]

Seizures are the abnormal discharge of electrical activity within the brain. When a sufficient number of neurons become overexcited, they discharge abnormally. This action sometimes results in symptoms (seizures) with alterations in motor function, sensation, autonomic function, behaviour, and consciousness. The symptoms depend on the site and spread of abnormal electrical activity. If a child has more than one unprovoked seizure, that child is said to have **epilepsy**. There are a few exceptions including febrile seizures. Seizures may result from diseases that are primarily neurological (CNS) or are systemic and affect CNS function secondarily (such as diabetes). Structural abnormalities of the brain, hypoxia, intracranial hemorrhage, CNS infection, traumatic injury, electrolyte imbalance, or inborn metabolic disturbances may cause seizures. Febrile seizures occur in about 2 to 5% of children between ages 6 months and 5 years; they are benign and the most common type of childhood seizure. Seizures are sometimes clearly familial. Often the cause of epilepsy is unknown. Table 17.6 reviews the major types of seizure disorders found in children (see also Chapter 15 and Table 15.14).

TABLE 17.6 Major Types of Seizure Disorders Found in Children

Disorder	Manifestations
Generalized Seizure	First symptoms indicate that seizure activity starts in or involves both cerebral hemispheres; consciousness may be impaired; bilateral; an aura may occur before the symptoms
Tonic-clonic	Musculature stiffens, then intense jerking as trunk and extremities undergo rhythmic contraction and relaxation
Atonic	Sudden, momentary loss of muscle tone; drop attacks
Myoclonic	Sudden, brief contractures of a muscle or group of muscles
Absence seizure	Brief loss of consciousness with little or no loss of muscle tone; may experience 20 or more episodes a day lasting about 5 to 10 s each; may have minor movement, such as lip smacking, twitching of eyelids
Partial (Focal) Seizure	Seizure activity that begins with and usually is limited to one part of left or right hemisphere; an aura is common
Simple	Seizure activity that occurs without loss of consciousness
Complex	Seizure activity that occurs with impairment of consciousness
Epilepsy Syndromes	Seizure disorders that display a group of signs and symptoms that occur collectively and characterize or indicate a particular condition
Infantile spasms (West's syndrome)	Form of epilepsy with episodes of sudden flexion or extension involving neck, trunk, and extremities; symptoms range from subtle head nods to violent body contractions (jackknife seizures); onset between 3 and 12 months of age; may be idiopathic, genetic, result of metabolic disease, or in response to central nervous system injury; spasms occur in clusters of 5 to 150 times per day; EEG shows large-amplitude, chaotic, and disorganized pattern called *hypsarrhythmia*
Lennox-Gastaut syndrome	Epileptic syndrome with onset in early childhood, 1 to 5 years of age; includes various generalized seizures—tonic-clonic, atonic (drop attacks), akinetic, absence, and myoclonic; EEG has characteristic "slow spike and wave" pattern; results in delayed cognitive ability, psychomotor developments
Juvenile myoclonic epilepsy	Onset in adolescence; multifocal myoclonus; seizures often occur early in morning, made worse by lack of sleep or after excessive alcohol intake; occasional generalized convulsions; require long-term medication treatment
Benign rolandic epilepsy	Epileptic syndrome typically occurring in the preadolescent age (6 to 12 years); strong association with sleep (seizures typically occur a few hours after sleep onset or just before waking in morning); complex partial seizures with orofacial signs (drooling, distortion of facial muscles); characteristic EEG with centrotemporal (rolandic fissure) spikes
Status Epilepticus	Continuing or recurring seizure activity in which recovery from seizure activity is incomplete; seizure activity can last 30 min or more; medical emergency that requires immediate intervention
Febrile Seizure	Seizure activity associated with a high body temperature but without any serious underlying health issue, occurring most often in children between the ages of 6 months and 5 years

EEG, Electroencephalogram.

CHILDHOOD TUMOURS

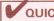 **QUICK CHECK 17.4**
1. Explain the relationship between brainstem function and the principal symptoms of brain tumours in children.

Brain Tumours

Brain tumours are the most common solid tumour and second most common primary neoplasm in children. In Canada, CNS tumours account for 18% of all childhood cancers under the age of 14 years, and 40% of all deaths.[27] Five-year survival for childhood brain tumours is about 73%, varying significantly by tumour type.

Primary brain tumours arise from brain tissue and do not metastasize outside the brain. The cause of brain tumours is unknown. Genetic, environmental, and immune factors may be involved. Exposure to radiation therapy has been the only environmental factor consistently related to the development of brain tumours.[28]

Brain tumours can arise from any CNS cell. Tumours are classified by cell type. Table 17.7 reviews the types and characteristics of childhood brain tumours. Medulloblastoma, ependymoma, astrocytoma, brainstem glioma, craniopharyngioma, and optic nerve glioma constitute approximately 75 to 80% of all pediatric brain tumours. Germ cell tumours are rare. Two thirds of all pediatric brain tumours in children are located in the posterior fossa (Figure 17.8). Treatment strategies and prognoses vary, depending on diagnosis.

Signs and symptoms of brain tumours in children vary from generalized and vague to localized and related specifically to the area of the brain affected. Signs of increased ICP may occur, including headache, vomiting, lethargy, and irritability. If a young child complains of repeated and worsening headache, a thorough investigation should take place because headache is an uncommon complaint in young children. Headache caused by increased ICP usually is worse in the morning. Due to the increased venous drainage when upright, the symptoms gradually improve during the day. The frequency of headache and other symptoms increase as the tumour grows. Irritability or possible apathy and increased sleepiness also may result. Like headache, vomiting occurs more commonly in the morning. Often nausea does *not* precede vomiting, which may become projectile. Unlike with vomiting related to a gastro-intestinal disturbance, the child may be ready to eat immediately after vomiting. Other signs and symptoms include increased head circumference with bulging fontanelles in the child younger than 2 years, cranial nerve palsies, and papilledema (Box 17.1).

Localized findings relate to the degree of disturbance in physiological functioning in the area where the tumour is located. Children with infratentorial tumours exhibit localized signs of impaired coordination and balance, including ataxia, gait difficulties, truncal ataxia, and loss of balance. **Medulloblastoma** occurs as an invasive malignant tumour that develops in the vermis of the cerebellum and may extend into the fourth ventricle. **Ependymoma** develops in the fourth ventricle and arises from the ependymal cells that line the ventricular system. Because both tumours are located in the posterior fossa region along the midline, presenting signs and symptoms are similar. The presence of hydrocephalus and increased ICP is the usual cause of these symptoms. **Cerebellar astrocytomas** are located on the surface of the right or left cerebellar hemisphere and cause unilateral symptoms (occurring on the same side as the tumour), such as head tilt, limb ataxia, and nystagmus.

TABLE 17.7 Brain Tumours in Children

Type	Characteristics
Astrocytoma	Arises from astrocytes, often in cerebellum or lateral hemisphere Slow growing, solid or cystic Often very large before diagnosed Varies in degree of malignancy
Optic nerve glioma	Arises from optic chiasm or optic nerve (association with neurofibromatosis type 1) Slow-growing, low-grade astrocytoma
Medulloblastoma (infiltrating glioma)	Often located in cerebellum, extending into fourth ventricle and spinal fluid pathway Rapidly growing malignant tumour Can extend outside central nervous system
Brainstem glioma	Arises from pons Numerous cell types Compresses cranial nerves V through X
Ependymoma	Arises from ependymal cells lining ventricles Circumscribed, solid, nodular tumours
Craniopharyngioma	Arises near pituitary gland, optic chiasm, and hypothalamus Cystic and solid tumours that affect vision, pituitary, and hypothalamic functions
Germ cell tumour	Arises from germ cells and is most common in pineal and suprasellar region, usually occurring during adolescence

Brainstem gliomas often cause cranial nerve involvement (facial weakness, limitation of horizontal eye movement), cerebellar signs of ataxia, and corticospinal tract dysfunction. Increased ICP generally does not occur.

The area of the sella turcica, the structure containing the pituitary gland, is the site of several childhood brain tumours. The most common of this group is the **craniopharyngioma**. This tumour originates from the pituitary gland or hypothalamus. Usually slow growing, it may be quite large by the time of diagnosis. Symptoms include headache, seizures, diabetes insipidus, early onset of puberty, and growth delay. Other tumours located in this region of the brain include **optic gliomas**. Optic nerve gliomas are associated with neurofibromatosis type 1. This neurocutaneous condition is characterized by café-au-lait macules on the skin and benign tumours of the skin. Tumours that involve the optic tract may cause complete unilateral blindness and hemianopia of the other eye. Optic atrophy is another common finding. Supratentorial tumours of the cerebral hemispheres are more common in neonates and adolescents.[29]

Embryonal Tumours
Neuroblastoma

Neuroblastoma is an embryonal tumour originating outside the CNS in the developing sympathetic nervous system (sympathetic ganglia and the adrenal medulla). Neuroblastoma involves a defect of embryonic tissue and is the most common cancer in infants less than 1 year of age. Approximately 75% of neuroblastomas are found before the child is 5 years old and are rare after 10 years of age. With metastasis apparent in the placenta, diagnosis of these tumours may occur at birth. In Canada, neuroblastoma and other peripheral nervous cell cancers account for 7% of all cancers under the age of 14 years; although it accounts for only about 7% of pediatric malignancies, neuroblastoma causes about 15% of cancer deaths in children.[27,30]

Neuroblastoma is the most common and immature form of the sympathetic nervous system tumours. More than with any other cancer, neuroblastoma has been associated with spontaneous remission, commonly in infants. Prognosis is worse for children older than 2 years of age with spreading disease.[1]

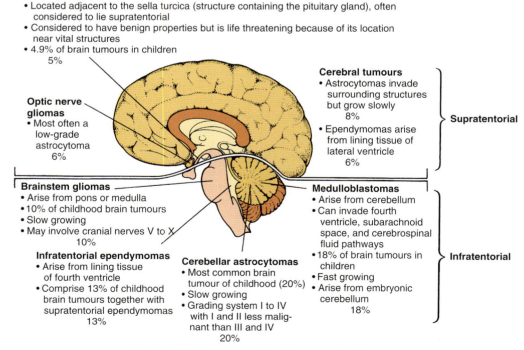

FIGURE 17.8 Location of Brain Tumours in Children.

BOX 17.1 Clinical Manifestations of Brain Tumours

Headache
Recurrent and progressive
In frontal or occipital area
Worse on waking; pain lessens during the day
Worsens by lowering head and straining, such as when defecating, coughing, sneezing

Vomiting
With or without nausea or feeding
Progressively more projectile
More severe in morning
Relieved by moving and changing position

Neuromuscular Changes
Incoordination or clumsiness
Loss of balance (use of wide-based stance, falling, tripping, banging into object)
Poor fine motor control
Weakness
Hyporeflexia or hyperreflexia
Positive Babinski sign
Spasticity
Paralysis

Behavioural Changes
Irritability
Decreased appetite

Failure to thrive
Fatigue (frequent naps)
Lethargy
Coma
Bizarre behaviour (staring, automatic movements)

Cranial Nerve Neuropathy
Cranial nerve involvement varies according to tumour location
Most common signs:
   Head tilt
   Visual defects (nystagmus, diplopia, strabismus, episodic "greying out" of vision, and visual field defects)

Vital Sign Disturbances
Decreased pulse and respiratory rates
Increased blood pressure
Decreased pulse pressure
Hypothermia or hyperthermia

Other Signs
Seizures
Cranial enlargement
Tense, bulging fontanelle at rest*
Separating suture*
Nuchal rigidity
Papilledema (edema of optic nerve)

*Present only in infants and young children.
From Hockenberry, M. N., Rodger, C. C., & Wilson, D. (2020). *Wong's essentials of pediatric nursing* (11th ed.). Mosby.

Although familial tendency has been noted in some cases, a sporadic pattern is found in most children with neuroblastoma. Familial cases of neuroblastoma have an autosomal dominant pattern of inheritance (Chapter 2 discusses mechanisms of inheritance).

The most common location of neuroblastoma is in the retroperitoneal region (65% of cases), most often the adrenal medulla. The tumour is evident as an abdominal mass and may cause anorexia, bowel and bladder alteration, and sometimes spinal cord compression. The second most common location is the mediastinum (15% of cases), where the tumour may cause dyspnea or infection related to airway obstruction. Less often, neuroblastoma may arise from the cervical sympathetic ganglion (3 to 4% of cases). Cervical neuroblastoma often causes Horner's syndrome. This syndrome consists of miosis (pupil contraction), ptosis (drooping eyelid), enophthalmos (backward displacement of the eyeball), and anhidrosis (sweat deficiency).

A number of systemic signs and symptoms are characteristic of neuroblastoma. This includes weight loss, irritability, fatigue, and fever. Severe diarrhea occurs in 7 to 9% of children. Tumour secretion of a hormone called *vasoactive intestinal polypeptide* causes these symptoms.

More than 90% of children with neuroblastoma have increased amounts of catecholamines and associated metabolites in their urine. High levels of urinary catecholamines and serum ferritin are associated with a poor prognosis.

Retinoblastoma

Retinoblastoma is a rare congenital eye tumour of young children that originates in the retina of one or both eyes (Figure 17.9). There are two forms of retinoblastoma: inherited and acquired. The diagnosis of the inherited form of the disease generally occurs during the first year of

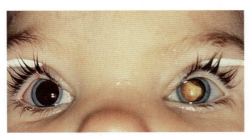

FIGURE 17.9 Retinoblastoma. The tumour occupies a large portion of the inside of the eye globe. (From Damjanov, I. [2006]. *Pathology for the health professions* [3rd ed.]. Saunders. Courtesy Dr. Walter Richardson and Dr. Jamsheed Khan, Kansas City, KS.)

life. The acquired disease most commonly is diagnosed in children 2 to 3 years of age and involves unilateral disease.[31]

Approximately 40% of retinoblastomas are inherited as an autosomal dominant trait with incomplete penetrance (see Figure 2.22). The remaining 60% are acquired. In the early 1970s, Knudson proposed the "two-hit" hypothesis to explain the occurrence of both hereditary and acquired forms of the disease.[1] This hypothesis predicts that two separate events or "hits" must occur in a normal retinoblast cell to cause the cancer. Further, it proposes that in the inherited form, the first hit or mutation occurs in the germ cell (inherited from either parent), and the mutation is contained in every cell of the child's body. In order to transform that cell into cancer, a second, random mutation in a retinoblast cell must occur. Multiple tumours occur in the inherited form because these second mutations are likely to occur in several of the approximately 1 to 2 million retinoblast cells. In contrast, the acquired

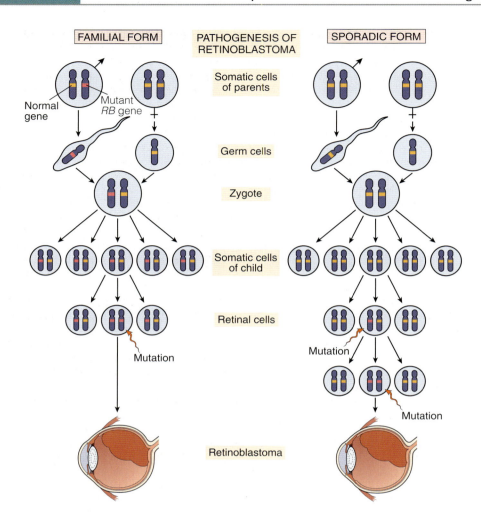

FIGURE 17.10 **The Two-Mutation Model of Retinoblastoma Development.** In inherited retinoblastoma, the transmission of the first mutation occurs through the germline of an affected parent. The second mutation occurs somatically in a retinal cell, leading to development of the tumour. In sporadic retinoblastoma, development of a tumour requires two somatic mutations.

form of retinoblastoma requires two independent hits or mutations to occur in the same somatic cell (after egg fertilization) for the transformation to cancer. As a result, the acquired form of retinoblastoma is much less likely to occur. Figure 17.10 reviews the two-mutation model for these two patterns of mutation.

The primary sign of retinoblastoma is leukocoria, a white pupillary reflex (white reflex) also called *cat's eye reflex*. This finding is caused by the mass behind the lens (see Figure 17.9). It is easy to miss this sign. Other signs and symptoms include strabismus; a red, painful eye; and limited vision.

Because retinoblastoma is a treatable tumour, priorities include saving the child's life and restoring useful vision. The prognosis for most children with retinoblastoma is excellent, with a greater than 90% long-term survival.

DID YOU UNDERSTAND?

Development of the Nervous System in Children
1. The growth and development of the brain occur most rapidly from the third month of gestation through the first year of life.
2. The bones of the skull are separated at the suture lines. The wide junctions of the suture lines (known as *fontanelles*) allow for brain growth. The fontanelles close by 18 months of age.

Structural Malformations
1. Spina bifida (split spine) is the most common disorder of neural tube closure. This disorder includes anencephaly (absence of part of the skull and brain), encephalocele (herniation of the meninges and brain through a skull defect), meningocele (a saclike meningeal cyst that protrudes through a vertebral defect), and myelomeningocele.

2. Premature closure of one or more of the cranial sutures causes craniostenosis and prevents normal skull expansion, resulting in compression of growing brain tissue.
3. Microcephaly is lack of brain growth with delayed mental and motor development.
4. Congenital hydrocephalus results from overproduction, impaired absorption, or blockage of circulation of cerebrospinal fluid.

Alterations in Function: Encephalopathies
1. Static encephalopathies are nonprogressive disorders of the brain that can occur during gestation, birth, or at any time during childhood. Endogenous or exogenous factors can cause these disorders.

2. Prenatal cerebral hypoxia or perinatal traumas are causes of cerebral palsy. Symptoms may include motor dysfunction (including increased muscle tone, increased reflexes, and loss of fine motor coordination), intellectual disability, seizure disorders, or developmental delays.
3. Inherited metabolic disorders that damage the nervous system include defects in amino acid metabolism (phenylketonuria) and lipid metabolism (Tay-Sachs disease) and result in abnormal behaviour, seizures, and deficient psychomotor development.
4. Accidental poisonings from a variety of toxins can cause serious neurological damage.
5. *Neisseria meningitidis* or *Streptococcus pneumoniae* are the common causes of bacterial meningitis. Infection may result from respiratory tract or gastro-intestinal infections. Symptoms include fever, headaches, photophobia, seizures, rigidity, and stupor.
6. Viral meningitis may result from direct infection or be secondary to a systemic viral infection.

Cerebrovascular Disease in Children
1. Ischemic (occlusive) stroke is rare in children but can occur from embolism, sickle cell disease, cerebral arteriopathies, and cardiac anomalies.
2. Hemorrhagic stroke can occur in association with immature blood vessels associated with prematurity or congenital cerebral arteriovenous malformations.
3. Seizure disorders involve abnormal discharges of electrical activity within the brain. They are associated with numerous nervous system disorders and more often are a generalized rather than a partial type of seizure.
4. Generalized seizures include tonic-clonic, atonic, myoclonic, and absence seizures.
5. Partial seizures suggest more localized brain dysfunction.
6. Febrile seizures are provoked and usually limited to children between the ages of 6 months and 5 years. They are benign in nature and the most common type of childhood seizure.

Childhood Tumours
1. Brain tumours are the most common tumours of the nervous system and the second most common type of childhood cancer.
2. Tumours in children most often are located below the tentorial plate (infratentorial tumours).
3. Symptoms of brain tumours may be generalized or localized. The most common general symptoms are the result of increased intracranial pressure and include headache, irritability, vomiting, somnolence, and bulging of fontanelles.
4. Localized signs of infratentorial tumours in the cerebellum include impaired coordination and balance. Cranial nerve signs occur with tumours in or near the brainstem.
5. Signs and symptoms associated with brain tumours and the degree of physiological functioning disturbance depend on the specific location of the tumour.
6. Neuroblastoma is an embryonal tumour of the sympathetic nervous system and can be located anywhere there is sympathetic nervous tissue. Tumour location and size of metastasis influence the person's symptoms.
7. Retinoblastoma is a congenital eye tumour that has two forms: inherited and acquired.

18

Mechanisms of Hormonal Regulation

Kelly Power-Kean, with originating chapter contributions by Valentina L. Brashers and Sue E. Huether

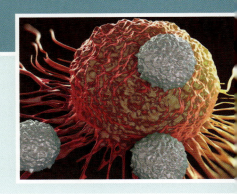

Additional resources are available online at https://evolve.elsevier.com/Canada/Huether/pathophysiology

CHAPTER OUTLINE

Mechanisms of Hormonal Regulation, 427
    Regulation of Hormone Release, 428
    Hormone Transport, 428
    Mechanisms of Hormone Action, 429
Structure and Function of the Endocrine Glands, 431
    Hypothalamic–Pituitary System, 431

Pineal Gland, 436
Thyroid and Parathyroid Glands, 436
Endocrine Pancreas, 438
Adrenal Glands, 439
GERIATRIC CONSIDERATIONS: Aging and Its Effects on Specific Endocrine Glands, 444

LEARNING OBJECTIVES

1. Name the functions of the endocrine system.
2. Discuss the regulation of hormone secretion by positive and negative feedback loops.
3. Discuss the cellular processes of hormone transport and hormone receptors.
4. Compare and contrast upregulation and downregulation of hormone receptors.
5. Discuss hormone receptor binding.
6. Name the hormones of the anterior pituitary and their releasing factor, stimulating hormones, target hormones, and target tissues, including normal outcomes.
7. List the hormones of the posterior pituitary and their actions.
8. Discuss the effects of thyroid hormone (T_3, T_4) and the processes of thyroid hormone regulation.
9. Discuss the effects and processes of the parathyroid hormone.
10. Name and discuss the major functions of the hormones secreted by the alpha, beta, and delta cells.
11. Name and discuss the structure, function, and regulation of secretion of the adrenocortical and medullary hormones.
12. Describe and discuss the neuroendocrine response to stress.

KEY TERMS

1,25-Dihydroxy-vitamin D_3, 437
Adrenal cortex, 440
Adrenal gland, 439
Adrenal medulla, 443
Adrenocorticotropic hormone (ACTH), 431
Aldosterone, 442
Alpha cell, 438
Amylin, 439
Anterior pituitary, 431
Antidiuretic hormone (ADH), 431
Beta cell, 438
C cell, 436
Calcitonin, 436
Chromophil, 431
Chromophobe, 431
Corticotropin-releasing hormone (CRH), 442
Cortisol, 442
Delta cell, 438
Direct effect, 429
Downregulation, 429
F (or PP) cell, 438
First messenger, 430
Follicle, 436
Follicle-stimulating hormone (FSH), 431
Gastrin, 439
Ghrelin, 439
Glucagon, 439
Glucocorticoid, 440
Growth hormone (GH), 431
Hormone, 427
Hormone receptor, 429
Hypothalamus, 431
Insulin, 438
Islet of Langerhans, 438
Isthmus, 436
Luteinizing hormone (LH), 431
Median eminence, 435
Melanocyte-stimulating hormone (MSH), 431
Melatonin, 436
Mineralocorticoid, 442
Negative feedback, 428
Oxytocin, 431
Pancreas, 438
Pancreatic polypeptide, 439
Parathyroid hormone (PTH), 437
Pars distalis, 431
Pars intermedia, 431
Pars nervosa, 435
Pars tuberalis, 431
Permissive effect, 429
Pituitary gland, 431
Pituitary stalk, 435
Positive feedback, 428
Posterior pituitary, 435
Prolactin, 431
Second messenger, 430
Somatostatin, 439
Target cell, 429
Thyroid gland, 436
Thyroid hormone (TH), 436
Thyroid-stimulating hormone (TSH), 428
Thyrotropin-releasing hormone (TRH), 428
Thyroxine-binding globulin, 437
Tropic hormone, 431
Upregulation, 429
Zona fasciculate, 440
Zona glomerulosa, 440
Zona reticularis, 427

CHAPTER 18 Mechanisms of Hormonal Regulation

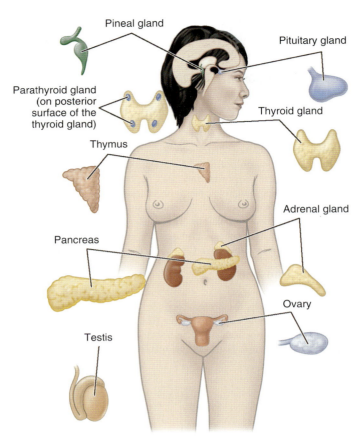

FIGURE 18.1 Major Endocrine Glands. (From Applegate, E. [2011]. *The anatomy and physiology learning system* [4th ed.]. Saunders.)

TABLE 18.1 Structural Categories of Hormones

Structural Category	Examples
Water Soluble	
Peptides	Growth hormone
	Insulin
	Leptin
	Parathyroid hormone
	Prolactin
Glycoproteins	Follicle-stimulating hormone
	Luteinizing hormone
	Thyroid-stimulating hormone
Polypeptides	Adrenocorticotropic hormone
	Antidiuretic hormone
	Calcitonin
	Endorphins
	Glucagon
	Hypothalamic hormones
	Lipotropins
	Melanocyte-stimulating hormone
	Oxytocin
	Somatostatin
	Thymosin
	Thyrotropin-releasing hormone
Amines	Epinephrine
	Norepinephrine
Lipid Soluble	
Thyroxine (an amine, but lipid soluble)	Both thyroxine and tri-iodothyronine
Steroids (cholesterol is a precursor for all steroids)	Estrogens
	Glucocorticoids (cortisol)
	Mineralocorticoids (aldosterone)
	Progestins (progesterone)
	Testosterone
Derivatives of arachidonic acid (autocrine or paracrine action)	Leukotrienes
	Prostacyclins
	Prostaglandins
	Thromboxanes

The endocrine system is composed of various glands throughout the body (Figure 18.1). These glands can create and release special chemical messengers called *hormones*. The endocrine system has five general functions: (1) differentiation of the reproductive and central nervous systems in the developing fetus; (2) stimulation of growth and development during childhood and adolescence; (3) coordination of the male and female reproductive systems, (4) providing an optimal internal environment throughout life; and (5) beginning of corrective and adaptive responses when emergencies occur. The endocrine, nervous, and immune systems work together to regulate responses to the internal and external environments. Hormones send specific regulatory information among cells and organs. Their integration with the nervous system allows them to support communication and control. The mechanisms of communication and control occur within a cell (*autocrine*), between local cells (*paracrine*), and between cells found remotely from each other (*endocrine*). See the *Geriatric Considerations* box at the end of the chapter for a summary of the changes in the structure and function of the endocrine glands that occur with aging.

MECHANISMS OF HORMONAL REGULATION

> ✓ **QUICK CHECK 18.1**
> 1. What are hormones? How do they function?
> 2. What is meant by negative-feedback regulation of hormone release?
> 3. How do first messengers differ from second messengers?
> 4. Where are the receptors found for lipid-soluble hormones?

Endocrine glands respond to specific signals by creating and releasing **hormones** into the circulation. This release then triggers intracellular responses. All hormones share general features:
1. Hormones have specific rates and patterns of **secretion**. Three basic patterns of secretion are (a) diurnal patterns, (b) pulsatile and cyclic patterns, and (c) patterns that depend on levels of circulating substrates (e.g., calcium, sodium, potassium, or the hormones themselves).
2. Hormones work within feedback systems, either negative or positive. These systems support the best internal environment.
3. Hormones affect only target cells with specific receptors for the hormone. They act on these cells to start specific cell functions or activities.
4. Steroid hormones are either excreted by the kidneys or metabolized by the liver. These actions inactivate the hormones and make them more water soluble for renal excretion. Circulating enzymes deactivate peptide hormones. They are then eliminated in the feces or urine.

Hormones are classified according to structure, gland of origin, effects, or chemical makeup. (Table 18.1 categorizes known hormones based on structure.) The secretion and mechanisms of action of hormones are a complex system of combined responses. The endocrine and nervous systems work together to control responses to the internal and external environments.

Regulation of Hormone Release

The release of hormones occurs either to respond to a changed cellular environment or to support the level of another hormone or substance. One or more of the following mechanisms regulates hormone release: (1) chemical factors (such as blood glucose or calcium levels), (2) endocrine factors (a hormone from one endocrine gland controlling another endocrine gland), and (3) neural control. For example, insulin is secreted by the chemical stimulation of increased plasma glucose levels. Cortisol from the adrenal cortex is an endocrine factor that controls and stimulates insulin secretion. Lastly, stimulation of the insulin-secreting cells of the pancreas by the autonomic nervous system is a form of neural control.

Feedback systems supply precise monitoring and control of the cellular environment. Both negative- and positive-feedback systems are important for supporting hormone levels within proper ranges. **Negative feedback** is the most common. This occurs when a changing chemical, neural, or endocrine response to a stimulus decreases the creation and secretion of a hormone. **Positive feedback** occurs when a neural, chemical, or endocrine response increases the creation and secretion of a hormone. For example, Figure 18.2A shows negative feedback within the hypothalamic–pituitary axis and the thyroid gland. Decreased serum levels of the thyroid hormones thyroxine (T_4) and tri-iodothyronine (T_3) stimulate secretion of **thyrotropin-releasing hormone (TRH)** from the hypothalamus. This then stimulates the secretion of **thyroid-stimulating hormone (TSH)**. Secretion of TSH stimulates the creation and secretion of T_3 and T_4. Increasing levels of T_4 and T_3 then generate negative feedback on the pituitary and hypothalamus. This inhibits TSH and TRH creation and decreases the creation and production of thyroid hormones. The lack of negative-feedback inhibition on hormonal release often results in disease-causing excessive hormone production (see Chapter 19).

The female reproductive cycle is an example of positive feedback. The cyclic rise of estradiol levels supplies positive feedback on the anterior pituitary and hypothalamus. This causes an increase in gonadotropin-releasing hormone and follicle-stimulating hormone. These changes result in ovulation (see Chapter 32).

Hormone Transport

Hormones are released into the circulatory system and spread throughout the body. The protein (peptide) hormones (see Table 18.1) are water soluble and circulate in free (unbound) forms. Circulating enzymes break down water-soluble hormones which have a half-life of seconds to minutes. For example, insulinases break down insulin,

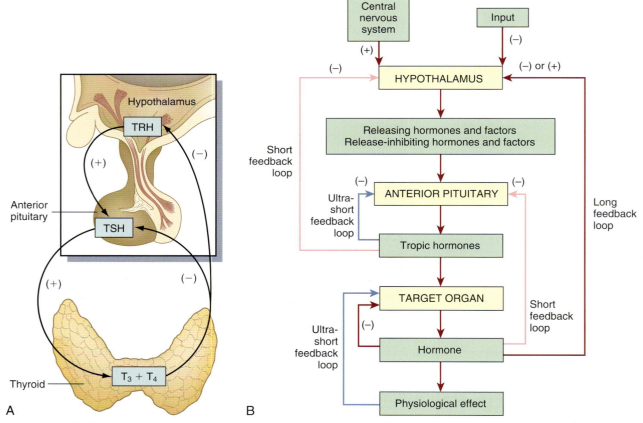

FIGURE 18.2 Feedback Loops. A, An illustration of an endocrine feedback loop involving the hypothalamus and pituitary gland, and end organs; an illustration of the thyroid gland (endocrine regulation). **B,** General model for control and negative feedback (–) to hypothalamic–pituitary target organ systems. Negative-feedback regulation is possible at three levels: target organ (ultra-short feedback), anterior pituitary (short feedback), and hypothalamus (long feedback). (+), Positive feedback; T_3, tri-iodothyronine T_4, thyroxine (tetraiodothyronine); *TRH,* thyroid-releasing hormone; *TSH,* thyroid-stimulating hormone.

TABLE 18.2 Binding Proteins, Their Hormones, and Variables That Affect Their Circulating Levels

Binding Protein	Hormone	Factors That Increase Binding Protein Levels	Factors That Decrease Binding Protein Levels
Corticosteroid-binding globulin	Cortisol Progesterone	Estrogen	Liver disease
Sex hormone–binding globulin	Dihydrotestosterone Testosterone Estradiol	— Hypothyroidism Liver disease	Androgens
Thyroid-binding globulin	Thyroxine Tri-iodothyronine	Estrogen Hyperthyroidism	Testosterone Glucocorticoids Liver disease
Albumin	All lipid-soluble hormones	Estrogen	Liver disease Malnutrition Renal disease

which has a half-life of 3 to 5 minutes. Lipid-soluble hormones (see Table 18.1), such as cortisol and adrenal androgens, are transported bound to a water-soluble carrier or transport protein. These hormones can remain in the blood for hours to days. Only free hormones (those not bound to a carrier protein) can signal a target cell. Because there is balance between the concentrations of free hormones and hormones bound to plasma proteins, a major change in the concentration of binding proteins can affect the concentration of free hormones (Table 18.2). (See Chapter 1 for review of the mechanisms of hormone binding.)

Mechanisms of Hormone Action

Although a hormone is spread throughout the body, only those cells with proper receptors, termed **target cells**, for that hormone are affected. *Hormone receptors* of the target cell have two main functions: (1) to recognize and bind specifically and with high affinity to their hormones and (2) to start a signal to appropriate intracellular effectors.

The sensitivity of the target cell to a hormone is related to the total number of receptors per cell or the affinity (binding) for the receptors to the hormone. The more receptors or the higher the affinity of the receptors, the more sensitive the cell is to the stimulating effects of the hormone. The term **upregulation** describes how low concentrations of hormones increase the number or affinity of receptors per cell. The term **downregulation** describes how high concentrations of hormone decrease the number or affinity of receptors (Figure 18.3). Thus, the cell can adjust its sensitivity to the concentration of the signalling hormone. The receptors on the plasma membrane are constantly created and degraded. As a result, changes in receptor concentration or affinity may occur within hours. The regulation of hormone receptors is important in type 2 diabetes, where there is a decrease in insulin receptor sensitivity that results in hyperglycemia (see Chapter 19). Many physiochemical conditions can affect both the receptor number and the affinity of the hormone for its receptor. Some of these conditions are the fluidity and structure of the plasma membrane, pH, temperature, ion concentration, diet, and the presence of other chemicals (e.g., medications).

Hormones affect target cells directly or permissively. **Direct effects** are the obvious changes in cell function that result from stimulation by a hormone. **Permissive effects** are less obvious hormone-induced changes that help the maximal response or functioning of a cell. For example, insulin via insulin receptors has a direct effect on skeletal muscle cells. Insulin causes increased glucose transport into these cells. Insulin also has a permissive effect on mammary cells, helping the response of these cells to the direct effects of prolactin.

Some hormones have biphasic effects that are dependent on the concentration or secretion pattern of the hormone. For example, in primary hyperparathyroidism, continuous hypersecretion of parathyroid hormone (PTH) leads to bone destruction by osteoclasts. Conversely, stimulation of bone formation occurs with the administration of recombinant PTH in low intermittent doses. Box 18.1 reviews methods of hormone measurement.

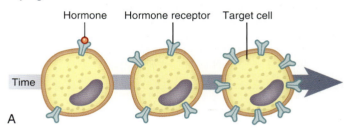

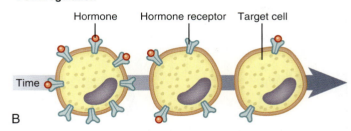

FIGURE 18.3 Regulation of Target Cell Sensitivity. **A,** Low hormone level and upregulation, or an increase in the number of receptors. **B,** High hormone level and downregulation, or a decrease in the number of receptors.

Hormone Receptors

Hormone receptors are found in the plasma membrane or in the intracellular compartment of the target cell (Figure 18.4). Water-soluble (peptide) hormones, which include the protein hormones and the catecholamines, have a high molecular weight and cannot diffuse across the cell membrane. They interact or bind with receptors found in or on the cell membrane. Fat-soluble steroids, vitamin D, retinoic acid, and thyroid hormones move freely across the plasma and nuclear membranes. They then bind with cytosolic or nuclear receptors. Some fat-soluble hormones (e.g., estrogen [see Chapter 32]) may also bind with plasma membrane receptors and can have rapid cellular effects.[1]

BOX 18.1 Methods of Hormone Measurement

Radioimmunoassay (RIA)
In this immunological technique, known amounts of antibody and radio-labelled hormone are placed in an assay tube with the unlabelled hormone. The radio-labelled hormone competes chemically with the unlabelled hormone molecules for binding sites on the antibodies. When increasing amounts of unlabelled hormones are added to the assay, the limited binding sites of the antibody can bind less of the radio-labelled hormone. Therefore, the higher the concentration of the unlabelled hormone, the fewer the number of radioactive *counts*, or labelled hormone, which bind with the fixed concentration of antibody. A quantitative value is obtained using standard reference curves.

Enzyme-Linked Immunosorbent Assay (ELISA)
This assay is used to determine circulating hormone levels. The method is like that of RIA, but is less expensive and easier to conduct. Instead of radio-labelled hormones, an enzyme-labelled hormone is used. The enzyme activity in either the bound or the unbound fraction is determined and related to the concentration of the unlabelled hormone.

Bioassay
This assay uses graded doses of hormone in a reference preparation and then compares the results with an unknown sample. The use of bioassays is more common in investigative endocrinology than in clinical laboratories.

TABLE 18.3 Second Messengers Identified for Specific Hormones

Second Messenger	Associated Hormones
Cyclic adenosine monophosphate (cAMP)	Adrenocorticotropic hormone (ACTH)
	Luteinizing hormone (LH)
	Human chorionic gonadotropin (hCG)
	Follicle-stimulating hormone (FSH)
	Thyroid-stimulating hormone (TSH)
	Antidiuretic hormone (ADH)
	Thyrotropin-releasing hormone (TRH)
	Parathyroid hormone (PTH)
	Glucagon
Cyclic guanosine monophosphate (cGMP)	Atrial natriuretic peptide
Calcium (Ca^{++}) and inositol triphosphate (IP_3)	Angiotensin II
	Gonadotropin-releasing hormone (GnRH)
	Antidiuretic hormone (ADH)
	Luteinizing hormone–releasing hormone (LHRH)
Tyrosine kinases	Insulin
	Growth hormone (GH)
	Leptin
	Prolactin

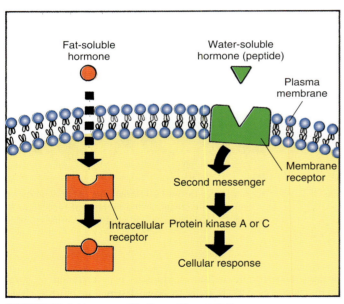

FIGURE 18.4 Hormone Binding at Target Cell.

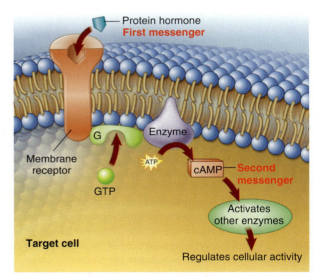

FIGURE 18.5 Mechanism of First and Second Messenger Action. The hormone acts as a "first messenger," delivering its message via the bloodstream to a membrane receptor in the target cell. This function is much like a key fits into a lock. The "second messenger" causes the cell to respond and perform its specialized function. *ATP*, Adenosine triphosphate; *cAMP*, cyclic adenosine monophosphate; *G*, G protein; *GTP*, guanosine triphosphate. (From Patton, K. T., & Thibodeau, G. A. [2018]. *The human body in health and disease* [7th ed.]. Elsevier.)

First and Second Messengers

All water-soluble hormones and some steroid hormones have hormone-specific receptors found in the plasma membranes of cells. Hormone binding with the plasma membrane receptor starts a complex cascade of intracellular effects. In this cascade, the hormone is called the **first messenger**. The hormone–receptor interaction starts a signal that creates a small molecule inside the cell, called the **second messenger**. Second messengers include cyclic adenosine monophosphate (cAMP), cyclic guanosine monophosphate (cGMP), calcium, inositol triphosphate, and the tyrosine kinase system (Table 18.3). The second messenger sends the signal from the receptor to the cytoplasm and nucleus of the cell. This action mediates the effect of the hormone on the target cell (e.g., membrane permeability changes, protein synthesis, inhibition of specific metabolic pathways, enzyme activation, or cellular growth).

When first messengers from the anterior pituitary gland (i.e., adrenocorticotropic hormone (ACTH) and TSH) bind to a cell membrane receptor, intracellular levels of cAMP increase. Second-messenger cAMP activates protein kinases, leading to phosphorylation of cellular proteins. This either activates or deactivates intracellular enzymes, thus directing the actions or products of specific cells (Figure 18.5).

cGMP functions as a second messenger following receptor binding of first messengers (e.g., atrial natriuretic peptide and nitric oxide). These hormones play key roles in cardiovascular and pulmonary health and disease. Research is ongoing related to the use of medications, such as phosphodiesterase inhibitors that target cGMP, for treatment of various diseases.[2,3]

Hormone-receptor binding of first-messenger angiotensin II and antidiuretic hormone (ADH) results in the creation of the second messenger, inositol triphosphate. Inositol triphosphate triggers a release of intracellular calcium, another second messenger. Increased intracellular calcium levels can lead to the formation of the calcium–calmodulin complex. This complex mediates the effects of calcium on intracellular activities that are key for cell metabolism and growth. For example, calmodulin-dependent protein kinases: (1) control intracellular contractile components (myosin and actin, which cause muscle contraction); (2) alter plasma membrane permeability to calcium; and (3) regulate the intracellular enzyme activity that promotes hormone secretion.

Some hormone first messengers, such as insulin, growth hormone (GH), and prolactin, bind to surface receptors that directly activate second messengers of the tyrosine kinase family. These tyrosine kinases include the Janus family of tyrosine kinases (JAK) and signal transducers and activators of transcription (STAT). They regulate a wide range of intracellular processes that contribute to cellular metabolism and growth. Research is currently underway on the use of these first messengers as emerging treatments for diabetes, systemic lupus erythematosus, and cancer.[1,4–6]

Lipid-Soluble (Steroid) Hormone-Receptor Binding

Except for thyroid hormones, the lipid-soluble hormones are created from cholesterol (giving rise to the term *steroid*). These include androgens, estrogens, progestins, glucocorticoids, mineralocorticoids, vitamin D, and retinoid. Because lipid-soluble hormones are relatively small, lipophilic, hydrophobic molecules, they can cross the lipid plasma membrane by simple diffusion (see Chapter 1). Receptors for lipid-soluble hormones are in the cytosol and nucleus and direct gene expression (Figure 18.6). Alteration of gene expression can take hours to days. Studies also reveal that receptors for lipid-soluble hormones are in the plasma membrane and are associated with rapid responses (seconds to minutes) as shown in Figure 18.6.[7,8]

STRUCTURE AND FUNCTION OF THE ENDOCRINE GLANDS

> ✓ **QUICK CHECK 18.2**
> 1. What is the relationship between the hypothalamus and the pituitary?
> 2. What is the action of antidiuretic hormone (ADH)?

Hypothalamic–Pituitary System

The hypothalamic–pituitary axis (HPA) forms the structural and functional basis for the integration of the neurological and endocrine systems. This is referred to as the neuroendocrine system. The HPA produces

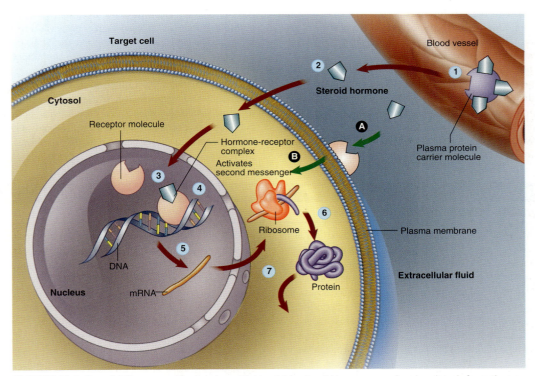

FIGURE 18.6 Steroid Hormone Mechanism. Lipid-soluble steroid hormone molecules detach from the carrier protein (1) and pass through the plasma membrane (2). Hormone molecules then diffuse into the nucleus, where they bind to a receptor to form a hormone-receptor complex (3). This complex then binds to a specific site on a DNA molecule (4), triggering transcription of the genetic information encoded there (5). The resulting messenger RNA *(mRNA)* molecule moves to the cytosol, where it associates with a ribosome, starting the creation of a new protein (6). This new protein—usually an enzyme or channel protein—produces specific effects on the target cell (7). The classic genomic action is typically slow *(red arrows)*. Steroids also may exact rapid effects *(green arrows)* by binding to receptors on the plasma membrane (A) and activating an intercellular second messenger (B). (From Patton, K. T., & Thibodeau, G. A. [2018]. *The human body in health & disease* [7th ed.]. Elsevier.)

several hormones that affect many body functions (Figure 18.7). These functions include those of the thyroid, adrenal gland, and reproductive system.

The hypothalamus is found at the base of the brain. The pituitary gland connects to the hypothalamus by the pituitary stalk, also known as the hypophyseal stalk (Figure 18.8). The anterior pituitary connects to the hypothalamus through hypophysial portal blood vessels (Figure 18.9). The posterior pituitary connects to the hypothalamus via a nerve tract referred to as the *hypothalamohypophysial tract* (Figure 18.10). These connections are key to the functioning of the hypothalamic–pituitary system. The hypothalamus has special neurosecretory cells. These cells are like other neurons in that they have similar electrical properties, organelles, membranes, and synapses. Hypothalamic neurosecretory cells, however, can create and secrete the hypothalamic-releasing hormones that regulate the release of hormones from the anterior pituitary. In addition, these cells create the hormones antidiuretic hormone (ADH) and oxytocin. The posterior pituitary gland releases these hormones. Table 18.4 reviews these hormones.

The pituitary gland is found in the sella turcica (a saddle-shaped depression of the sphenoid bone at the base of the skull). It weighs approximately 0.5 g, except during pregnancy when its weight increases by about 30%. It is composed of two different lobes: (1) the anterior pituitary, or adenohypophysis, and (2) the posterior pituitary, or neurohypophysis (see Figure 18.8). These two lobes differ in their embryonic origins, cell types, and functional relationship to the hypothalamus.

The Anterior Pituitary

The anterior pituitary accounts for 75% of the total weight of the pituitary gland. It is composed of three regions: (1) the pars distalis, (2) the pars tuberalis, and (3) the pars intermedia. The pars distalis is the major part of the anterior pituitary and is the source of the anterior pituitary hormones. The pars tuberalis is a thin layer of cells on the anterior and lateral portions of the pituitary stalk. The pars intermedia lies between the two and secretes melanocyte-stimulating hormone (MSH) in the fetus. In the adult, the distinct pars intermedia disappears, and the individual cells spread throughout the pars distalis and pars nervosa (neural lobe) of the posterior pituitary.

The anterior pituitary is composed of two main cell types: (1) the chromophobes, which appear to be nonsecretory, and (2) the chromophils, which are secretory cells. The chromophils are broken down into seven secretory cell types, and each cell type secretes a specific hormone or hormones. In general, regulation of the anterior pituitary hormones occurs by (1) secretion of hypothalamic peptide hormones or releasing factors, (2) feedback effects of the hormones secreted by target glands, and (3) direct effects of other mediating neurotransmitters. (Figure 18.2 reviews feedback loops.)

The anterior pituitary secretes tropic hormones that affect the physiological function of specific target organs (see Figure 18.7 and Table 18.5). MSH promotes the pituitary secretion of melanin, which darkens skin colour. The glycoprotein hormones follicle-stimulating hormone (FSH) and luteinizing hormone (LH) influence reproductive function. See Chapter 32 for further discussion on these hormones. Adrenocorticotropic hormone (ACTH) regulates the release of cortisol from the adrenal cortex. TSH regulates the activity of the thyroid gland. Growth hormone (GH) and prolactin are *somatotropic hormones* and they have diverse effects on body tissues. Two hormones from the hypothalamus control GH secretion. Growth hormone–releasing hormone (GHRH) increases GH secretion and somatostatin inhibits GH secretion. GH is essential to normal tissue growth and maturation. GH affects aging, sleep, nutritional status, stress, and reproductive hormones. Insulin-like growth factors (IGFs), which are also known as the *somatomedins*, mediate many of the anabolic functions of GH.[1]

There are two primary forms of IGF: IGF-1 and IGF-2, of which IGF-1 is the most biologically active. They both circulate bound to a group of IGF-binding proteins (IGFBPs) that control their availability. IGF-1 binds to IGF-1 receptors mediating the anabolic effects of GH. IGF-1 also binds to insulin receptors, supplying an insulin-like effect on skeletal muscle. IGF-2 has important effects on fetal growth but suppresses GH in the adult. Because of the anabolic effects of GH and IGF-1, they can be used to treat growth disorders, increase muscle mass, and possibly slow the aging process. Their use has been linked to increased rates of cancer[9,10] (see *Health Promotion:* Growth Hormone Supplementation in Aging).

Prolactin primarily functions to cause milk production during pregnancy and lactation. It has immune stimulatory effects and alters immune and inflammatory responses with both physiological and pathological reactions.[11] Vasoactive intestinal polypeptide, serotonin, and growth factors stimulate prolactin's synthesis. Dopamine inhibits the release of prolactin.

HEALTH PROMOTION

Growth Hormone Supplementation in Aging

Genetic and environmental factors influence the process of aging. The aging process is associated with many hormonal and metabolic changes. The term "somatopause" describes the decline of the amounts of GH and IGF with aging. Clinical findings for aging-related somatotropic hormone changes include increased visceral fat, decreased lean body mass, decreased bone density, and changes in reproductive and cognitive function. The underlying mechanisms of aging and its relationship to GH and IGF are complex. For example, GH and IGF promote bone and muscle growth. A recent study suggests that the brain receptor for IGF-1 (an IGF ligand) may be a significant factor in determining overall lifespan and ability to respond to physiological stress. GH and IGF effects on inflammation and immunity also are important in the aging process. Unfortunately, there is still much confusion and controversy over the role of these hormones. Even so, thousands of Canadians self-medicate with a synthetic formulation of GH as an antiaging remedy. The goal of using this hormone is to improve strength, energy, and immunity, as well as use for treatment of heart disease, cancer, impotence, and Alzheimer's disease.

Despite interest in the use of therapeutic doses of recombinant human growth hormone (rhGH) to slow the aging process, all studies have not been positive. Evidence shows that rhGH supplementation can be harmful. Lower lifetime levels of these hormones may provide longevity by supplying protection from cancer and other age-related diseases. Health Canada warns consumers not to self-medicate with human growth hormone GHR-15 due to risks associated with unconfirmed health claims and other potentially harmful effects.

Data from Anisimov, V. N., & Bartke, A. (2013). *Critical Reviews in Oncology/Hematology, 87*(3), 201–223; Ashpole, N. M., Sanders, J. E., Hodges, E. L., et al. (2015). *Experimental Gerontology, 68*, 76–81; Government of Canada. (2005). *Healthy Canadians: Health Canada warns consumers not to use human growth hormone drug called GHR-15*. http://www.healthycanadians.gc.ca/recall-alert-rappel-avis/hc-sc/2005/13695a-eng.php; Haber, D. (2016). *Health promotion and aging: practical application for health professionals* (7th ed.). Springer; Junnila, R. K., List, E. O., Berryman, D. E., et al. (2013). *Nature Reviews Endocrinology, 9*(6), 366–376; Nass, R. (2013). *Endocrinology & Metabolism Clinics of North America, 42*(2), 187–199; Sattler, F. R. (2013). *Best Practice & Research: Clinical Endocrinology & Metabolism, 27*(4), 541–555.

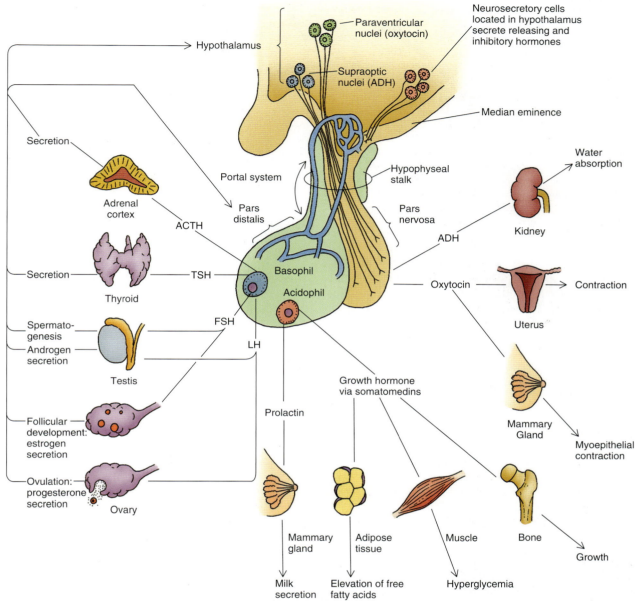

FIGURE 18.7 Pituitary Gland and Its Target Organs. *ACTH,* Adrenocorticotropic hormone; *ADH,* antidiuretic hormone; *FSH,* follicle-stimulating hormone; *LH,* luteinizing hormone; *TSH,* thyroid-stimulating hormone. (From Gartner, L. P., & Hiatt, J. L. [2007]. *Color textbook of histology* [3rd ed.]. Saunders.)

The Posterior Pituitary

The embryonic **posterior pituitary** (neurohypophysis) is derived from the hypothalamus. The posterior pituitary is composed of three parts: (1) the median eminence, located at the base of the hypothalamus; (2) the pituitary stalk; and (3) the infundibular process, also known as the *pars nervosa* or *neural lobe*. The **median eminence** is made largely of the nerve endings of axons from the ventral hypothalamus. It is often considered a part of the posterior pituitary but has at least 10 biologically active hypothalamic-releasing hormones. It also has the neurotransmitters dopamine, norepinephrine, serotonin, acetylcholine, and histamine. The **pituitary stalk** has the axons of neurons that originate in the supraoptic and paraventricular nuclei of the hypothalamus. The pituitary stalk connects the pituitary gland to the brain. Axons originating in the hypothalamus end in the **pars nervosa**. The pars nervosa secretes the hormones of the posterior pituitary (see Figure 18.10).

The posterior pituitary secretes two polypeptide hormones: (1) ADH, also called *arginine vasopressin*, and (2) oxytocin. These hormones differ by only two amino acids. They are created—along with their binding proteins, the neurophysins—in the supraoptic and paraventricular nuclei of the hypothalamus (see Figure 18.10). They are contained in secretory vesicles and move down the axons of the pituitary stalk to the pars nervosa for storage. The posterior pituitary thus is a storage and releasing site for hormones created in the hypothalamus. Cholinergic and adrenergic neurotransmitters mediate the release of ADH and oxytocin. The major stimulus to both ADH and oxytocin release is glutamate. The major inhibitory input is through gamma

434 CHAPTER 18 Mechanisms of Hormonal Regulation

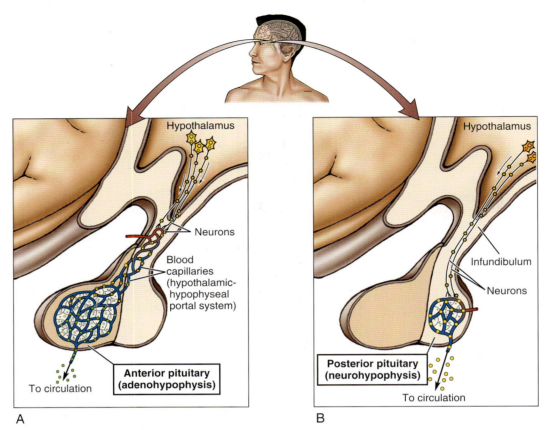

FIGURE 18.8 Pituitary Gland. The pituitary gland sits within the sella turcica of the sphenoid bone of the skull. **A,** Relationship of the hypothalamus to the anterior pituitary gland. **B,** Relationship of the hypothalamus to the posterior pituitary gland. (From Herlihy, B. [2015]. *The human body in health and illness* [5th ed.]. Saunders.)

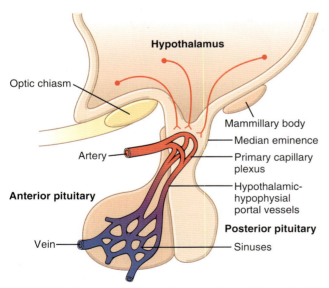

FIGURE 18.9 Hypophysial Portal System. (From Hall, J. E. [2016]. *Guyton and Hall textbook of medical physiology* [13th ed.]. Saunders.)

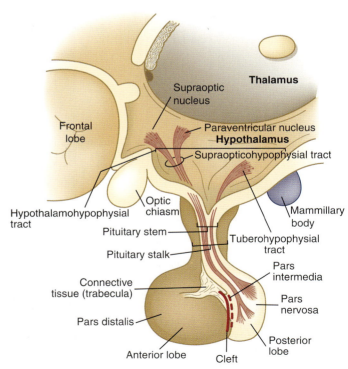

FIGURE 18.10 Nerve Tracts From Hypothalamus to Posterior Lobe of Pituitary Gland.

TABLE 18.4 Hypothalamic Hormones (Hypophysiotropic Hormones)

Hormone	Target Tissue	Action
Thyrotropin-releasing hormone (TRH)	Anterior pituitary	Stimulates release of thyroid-stimulating hormone (TSH); modulates prolactin secretion
Gonadotropin-releasing hormone (GnRH)	Anterior pituitary	Stimulates release of follicle-stimulating hormone (FSH) and luteinizing hormone (LH)
Somatostatin	Anterior pituitary	Inhibits release of growth hormone (GH) and TSH
Growth hormone–releasing hormone (GHRH)	Anterior pituitary	Stimulates release of GH
Corticotropin-releasing hormone (CRH)	Anterior pituitary	Stimulates release of adrenocorticotropic hormone (ACTH) and β-endorphin
Substance P	Anterior pituitary	Inhibits creation and release of ACTH; stimulates secretion of GH, FSH, LH, and prolactin
Prolactin-inhibiting factor (PIF, dopamine)	Anterior pituitary	Inhibits creation and secretion of prolactin
Prolactin-releasing factor (PRF)	Anterior pituitary	Stimulates secretion of prolactin

TABLE 18.5 Tropic Hormones of the Anterior Pituitary and Their Functions

Hormone	Secretory Cell Type	Target Organs	Functions
Adrenocorticotropic hormone (ACTH)	Corticotropic	Adrenal gland (cortex)	Increases steroidogenesis (cortisol and androgenic hormones); creation of adrenal proteins contributing to maintenance of adrenal gland
Melanocyte-stimulating hormone (MSH)	Melanotropic	Anterior pituitary	Promotes secretion of melanin and lipotropin by anterior pituitary; makes skin darker
Somatotropic Hormones			
Growth hormone (GH)	Somatotropic	Muscle, bone, liver	Regulates metabolic processes related to growth and adaptation to physical and emotional stressors, muscle growth, increased protein synthesis, increased liver glycogenolysis, increased fat mobilization
		Liver	Induces formation of somatomedins, or growth factors (IGFs) that have actions like insulin
Prolactin	Lactotropic	Breast	Induces milk production
Glycoprotein Hormones			
Thyroid-stimulating hormone (TSH)	Thyrotropic	Thyroid gland	Increases production and secretion of thyroid hormone
			Increases iodide uptake; promotes hypertrophy and hyperplasia of thymocytes
Luteinizing hormone (LH)	Gonadotropic	In women: granulosa cells	Stimulates ovulation, progesterone production
		In men: Leydig cells	Stimulates testicular growth, testosterone production
Follicle-stimulating hormone (FSH)	Gonadotropic	In women: granulosa cells	Stimulates follicle maturation, estrogen production
		In men: Sertoli cells	Stimulates spermatogenesis
β-Lipotropin	Corticotropic	Adipose cells	Promotes fat breakdown and release of fatty acids
β-Endorphins	Corticotropic	Adipose cells; brain opioid receptors	Produces analgesia; may regulate body temperature, food, and water intake

aminobutyric acid (GABA).[1] Before release into the circulatory system, ADH and oxytocin are split from the neurophysins and are secreted in unbound form.

Antidiuretic hormone. The major homeostatic function of the posterior pituitary is the control of plasma osmolality. This function is regulated by ADH (see Chapter 5). At physiological levels, ADH increases the permeability of the distal renal tubules and collecting ducts (see Chapter 29). This increased permeability leads to increased water reabsorption into the blood. This reabsorption results in concentrated urine and reduced serum osmolality. Hypercalcemia, prostaglandin E, and hypokalemia can inhibit this water reabsorption.

The osmoreceptors of the hypothalamus, found near or in the supraoptic nuclei, primarily regulate the secretion of ADH. The stimulation of these osmoreceptors occurs as plasma osmolality increases. As the rate of ADH secretion increases, more water is reabsorbed by the kidney, and the plasma is diluted back to its set-point osmolality. ADH has no direct effect on electrolyte levels. However, the increased water reabsorption may decrease serum electrolyte concentrations because of a dilutional effect.

Changes in intravascular volume, as detected by baroreceptors in the left atrium, in the carotid arteries, and in the aortic arches, increase ADH secretion. A volume loss of 7 to 25% acts on these receptors to stimulate ADH secretion. Stress, trauma, pain, exercise, nausea, nicotine, exposure to heat, and some medications also increase ADH secretion. ADH secretion decreases with decreased plasma osmolality, increased intravascular volume, hypertension, alcohol ingestion, and an increase in estrogen, progesterone, or angiotensin II levels.

Physiological levels of ADH do not significantly affect vessel tone. However, ADH was originally named *vasopressin* because, at extremely high levels, it causes vasoconstriction and a resulting increase in arterial blood pressure. For example, the administration of high doses of ADH (given as the medication vasopressin [Pitressin]) are given to achieve hemostasis during hemorrhage and to raise blood pressure in shock states.[12,13]

Oxytocin. Oxytocin controls contraction of the uterus and milk ejection in lactating women. It may also affect sperm motility. In both sexes, oxytocin has an antidiuretic effect like that of ADH. The secretion of oxytocin occurs in response to suckling and mechanical distension of the female reproductive tract. Oxytocin binds to its receptors on myoepithelial cells in the mammary tissues and causes contraction of those cells. This contraction increases intramammary pressure and milk expression ("let-down" reflex). Oxytocin also acts on the uterus to stimulate contractions. Oxytocin functions near the end of labour to improve the effectiveness of contractions, promote delivery of the placenta, and stimulate postpartum uterine contractions. Chapter 32 provides a detailed description of the function of this hormone.

Pineal Gland

> ✓ **QUICK CHECK 18.3**
> 1. How does the anterior pituitary regulate the thyroid gland?
> 2. What form of thyroid hormone is biologically active?
> 3. What two organs are the sites of action of parathyroid hormone (PTH)?

The pineal gland is found near the centre of the brain. It is composed of photoreceptive cells that secrete **melatonin**. Noradrenergic sympathetic nerve terminals, controlled by pathways within the hypothalamus, innervate this gland. Tryptophan creates serotonin, which then converts to melatonin. Exposure to dark stimulates the release of melatonin. Light exposure inhibits melatonin release. Melatonin regulates circadian rhythms and reproductive systems. This regulation includes the secretion of the gonadotropin-releasing hormones and the onset of puberty. It also plays an important role in immune regulation and is thought to affect the aging process. Further effects of melatonin include increasing nitric oxide release from blood vessels, removing toxic oxygen free radicals, and decreasing insulin secretion.[1] Melatonin is used in humans to help with sleep disturbances, jet lag, and psychological and inflammatory disorders. Exploration of its utility for many other disorders continues.[14]

Thyroid and Parathyroid Glands

The thyroid gland, found in the neck just below the larynx, produces hormones that control the rates of metabolic processes throughout the body. The four parathyroid glands are near the posterior side of the thyroid and function to control serum calcium levels (Figure 18.11).

Thyroid Gland

Two lobes of the **thyroid gland** lie on either side of the trachea. They are found inferior to the thyroid cartilage and joined by a small band of tissue termed the **isthmus**. The pyramidal lobe is superior to the isthmus (see Figure 18.11). The normal thyroid gland is not visible on inspection, but it may be felt on swallowing.

The thyroid gland consists of **follicles** that hold follicular cells surrounding a viscous substance called *colloid* (Figure 18.12). The follicular cells create and secrete the thyroid hormones. Neurons end on blood vessels within the thyroid gland and on the follicular cells themselves. As a result, neurotransmitters (acetylcholine, catecholamines) may directly affect the secretory activity of follicular cells and thyroid blood flow. The gland stores about a 2-month supply of thyroid hormones.

Also found in the thyroid are parafollicular cells, or C cells (see Figure 18.12). **C cells** secrete various polypeptides, including calcitonin. At high levels, **calcitonin**, also called *thyrocalcitonin*, lowers serum calcium levels by inhibiting bone-resorbing osteoclasts (Table 18.6) (Chapter 38 explains bone resorption). The therapeutic use of calcitonin includes treatment of several bone disorders, including osteogenesis imperfecta, osteoporosis, and Paget's disease. Parafollicular cells can give rise to medullary thyroid carcinoma.

Regulation of thyroid hormone secretion. A negative-feedback loop involving the hypothalamus, the anterior pituitary, and the thyroid gland regulates the **thyroid hormone (TH)** (see Figure 18.2). The creation and storage of TRH occurs within the hypothalamus. The feedback

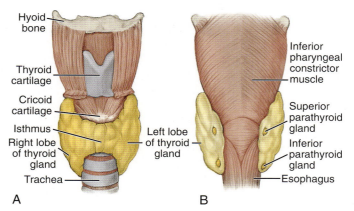

FIGURE 18.11 Thyroid and Parathyroid Glands. *A,* Anterior view. *B,* Posterior view. (From Fehrenbach, M. J., & Herring, S. W. [2012]. *Illustrated anatomy of the head and neck* [4th ed.]. Saunders.)

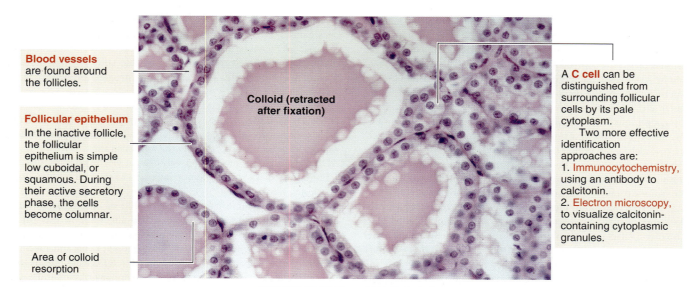

FIGURE 18.12 Thyroid Follicle Cells.

TABLE 18.6 Thyroid Gland Hormones and Their Regulation and Functions

Hormone	Regulation	Functions
Thyroxine (T_4) and tri-iodothyronine (T_3)	T_4 and T_3 levels are controlled by thyroid-stimulating hormone; released in response to metabolic demand Influences on amount secreted: Gender Pregnancy Gonadal- and adrenocortical-increased steroids = ↑ levels Exposure to extreme cold = ↑ levels Nutritional state Chemicals Growth hormone–inhibiting hormone = ↓ levels Dopamine = ↓ levels Catecholamines = ↑ levels	Regulate protein, fat, and carbohydrate catabolism in all cells Regulate metabolic rate of all cells Regulate body heat production Serve as insulin antagonists Maintain growth hormone secretion, skeletal maturation Affect central nervous system development Are necessary for muscle tone and vigour Maintain cardiac rate, force, and output Maintain secretion of gastro-intestinal (GI) tract Affect respiratory rate and oxygen utilization Maintain calcium mobilization Affect red blood cell production Stimulate lipid turnover, free fatty acid release, and cholesterol synthesis
Calcitonin	Elevated serum calcium level—major stimulant for calcitonin Other stimulants: Gastrin Calcium-rich foods (regardless of serum calcium levels) Pregnancy Lowered serum calcium level—suppresses calcitonin release	Lowers serum calcium level by opposing bone-resorbing effects of parathyroid hormone, prostaglandins, and calciferols by inhibiting osteoclastic activity Lowers serum phosphate levels Decreases calcium and phosphorous absorption in GI tract

From Monahan, F. D., Sands, J., Neighbors, M., et al. (2007). *Phipps' medical-surgical nursing: health and illness perspectives* (8th ed.). Mosby.

loop begins with the release of TRH into the hypothalamic–pituitary portal system and circulates to the anterior pituitary. From the interior pituitary it stimulates the release of TSH. The levels of TRH increase with exposure to cold or stress and from decreased levels of thyroxine.

TSH is a glycoprotein created and stored within the anterior pituitary. When the anterior pituitary secretes TSH, it circulates to bind with receptors on the plasma membrane of the thyroid follicular cells. The primary effect of TSH on the thyroid gland is to cause an immediate release of stored TH and an increase in TH creation. TSH also increases growth of the thyroid gland by stimulating thymocyte hyperplasia and hypertrophy. As TH levels rise, there is a negative-feedback effect on the HPA to inhibit TRH and TSH release. This release then results in decreased TH creation and secretion. Serum iodide levels and circulating selenium-dependent enzymes, called deiodinases, also control TH creation. They also inactivate the precursor molecule thyroxine.[15] Table 18.6 details the thyroid gland hormones and their regulation and function.

Creation of thyroid hormone.
The following steps summarize TH creation:
1. The endoplasmic reticulum of the thyroid follicular cells produce uniodinated thyroglobulin.
2. As it is created, thyroglobulin incorporates tyrosine.
3. Carrier proteins found in the outer membrane of the follicular cells actively transfer iodide (the inorganic form of iodine) from the blood into the colloid. The term *iodide trap* describes this active transport system. It is very efficient at accumulating the trace amounts of iodide from the blood.
4. Oxidization of iodide occurs, and it quickly attaches to tyrosine within the thyroglobulin molecule.
5. Coupling of iodinated tyrosine forms thyroid hormones. The coupling of monoiodotyrosine (one iodine atom and tyrosine) and di-iodotyrosine (two iodine atoms and tyrosine) forms tri-iodothyronine (T_3). The coupling of two di-iodotyrosines forms tetraiodothyronine, commonly known as thyroxine (T_4).
6. The storage of thyroid hormones, attached to thyroglobulin, occurs within the colloid.

The thyroid gland normally produces 90% T_4 and 10% T_3. Once released into the circulation, T_3 and T_4 are transported bound to **thyroxine-binding globulin**. Some TH is also transported by thyroxine-binding prealbumin (transthyretin), albumin, or lipoproteins. The bound form serves as a reservoir, while the unbound form is active. In the body tissues, most of the T_4 converts to T_3, which acts on the target cell.[1]

Actions of thyroid hormone. TH has a major effect on the growth, maturation, and function of cells and tissues throughout the body. TH is vital for normal growth and neurological development in the fetus and infant. TH affects metabolic, neurological, cardiovascular, and respiratory functioning across the lifespan. In addition, TH is needed for the metabolism and function of blood cells. It is also needed for normal muscle functioning and the integrity of skin, nails, and hair. Like some steroid hormones, TH binds to intracellular receptor complexes and then influences the genetic expression of specific proteins. TH also affects cell metabolism by changing protein, fat, and glucose metabolism. As a result, there is an increase in heat production and oxygen consumption. Additionally, TH has permissive effects throughout the body by optimizing the actions of other hormones and neurotransmitters (see Table 18.6).

Parathyroid Glands

Normally two pairs of parathyroid glands are present behind the upper and lower poles of the thyroid gland (see Figure 18.11). However, their number may range from two to six.

The parathyroid glands produce **parathyroid hormone (PTH)**, which is the single most important factor in the regulation of serum calcium concentration. The overall effect of PTH secretion is to increase serum calcium concentration and decrease the level of serum phosphate. A decrease in serum-ionized calcium level stimulates PTH secretion. PTH acts directly on the bone to release calcium by stimulating osteoclast activity. PTH also acts on the kidney to increase calcium reabsorption and decrease phosphate reabsorption. The increase in serum calcium concentration inhibits PTH secretion. Surprisingly, intermittent administration of a low dose of PTH stimulates bone formation. This observation led to the use of PTH for treatment of osteoporosis. **1,25-Dihydroxy-vitamin D3** (the active form of vitamin D) works as a cofactor with PTH to promote calcium and phosphate absorption in the gut and enhance bone mineralization. Vitamin D also plays an important role in metabolic processes and controlling inflammation. Approximately one third (32%) of Canadians had concentrations of vitamin D below the recommended level[16] (see *Health Promotion:* Vitamin D).

HEALTH PROMOTION
Vitamin D

Vitamin D is essential for bone health. The prevention and treatment of postmenopausal osteoporosis and renal osteodystrophy includes the use of vitamin D. Vitamin D deficiency affects 32% of all Canadians. About 38% of those affected are between the ages of 12 and 39 years. A study conducted to determine the prevalence of healthy vitamin D status in lactating Inuit women who live in remote regions of the Canadian arctic revealed that only 16 % of participants achieved the minimum vitamin D requirement.

Infections, cancer, heart disease, dementia, diabetes, pain syndromes, and autoimmune disorders have been linked to inadequate serum levels of vitamin D. Controversies continue as to whether these associations indicate a direct cause and effect between low levels of vitamin D and the pathophysiology of these diseases. Debate also exists as to whether vitamin D supplementation reduces risk or improves outcomes of these diseases. Many health organizations recommend increased intake of vitamin D–containing foods (fatty fish, egg yolks, vitamin D–fortified juices, and milk products), increased exposure to sunlight, and supplementation with vitamin D. Health Canada recommends that all Canadians over the age of 2, including pregnant and lactating women, consume 500 mL of milk or fortified soy beverages every day. Adults over the age of 50 years should take a daily vitamin D supplement of 400 units with a goal of achieving a minimum serum level of 50 nmol/L. Lastly, all healthy breastfed term babies should receive a daily vitamin D supplement of 400 units starting at birth and continuing until 1 year of age. Infants who are formula fed receive adequate vitamin D from fortified formula.

Data from Balvers, M. G., Brouwer-Brolsma, E. M., Endenburg, S., et al. (2015). *Journal of Nutritional Science, 4,* e23; Berridge, M. J. (2015). *Biochemical and Biophysical Research Communications, 460*(1), 53–71; Guessous, I. (2015). *BioMed Research International, 2015,* 563403; Hayek Fares, J., & Weiler, H. A. (2018). Vitamin D status and intake of women living in the Canadian Arctic. *Public Health Nutrition, 21*(11), 1988–1994; Health Canada. (2019). *Vitamin D and calcium:* Upda*ted dietary reference intakes.* http://www.hc-sc.gc.ca/fn-an/nutrition/vitamin/vita-d-eng.php; Janz, T., & Pearson, C. (2015). *Health at a glance: vitamin D blood levels of Canadians* (Statistics Canada Catalogue no. 82-624-X), http://www.statcan.gc.ca/pub/82-624-x/2013001/article/11727-eng.htm; Mozos, I., & Marginean, O. (2015). *BioMed Research International, 2015,* 109275; Schöttker, B., & Brenner, H. (2015). *Nutrients, 7*(5), 3264–3278; Statistics Canada. (2019). *Canadian Health Measures Survey: non-environmental laboratory and medication data, 2016 and 2017.* Component of Statistics Canada catalogue no. 11-001-X. https://www150.statcan.gc.ca/n1/en/daily-quotidien/190206/dq190206c-eng.pdf?st=SO-KVKrl.

Phosphate and magnesium concentrations also affect PTH secretion. An increase in serum phosphate level decreases serum calcium level by causing calcium-phosphate precipitation into soft tissue and bone. This action indirectly stimulates PTH secretion. Hypomagnesemia in persons with normal calcium levels acts as a mild stimulant to PTH secretion. However, in persons with hypocalcemia, hypomagnesemia decreases PTH secretion.[1]

Endocrine Pancreas

> ✓ **QUICK CHECK 18.4**
> 1. What are the islets of Langerhans? Where are they found?
> 2. Compare and contrast the actions of alpha, beta, delta, and F cells.
> 3. What is the most potent naturally occurring glucocorticoid? How is its secretion related to that of adrenocorticotropic hormone (ACTH)?
> 4. How does aldosterone influence fluid and electrolyte balance?
> 5. What are catecholamines?

The **pancreas** is both an endocrine gland that produces hormones and an exocrine gland that produces digestive enzymes. (Chapter 35 discusses the exocrine function of the pancreas.) The pancreas is found behind the stomach, between the spleen and the duodenum. The pancreas houses the **islets of Langerhans**. The islets of Langerhans have four types of hormone-secreting cells: (1) **alpha cells**, which secrete glucagon; (2) **beta cells**, which secrete insulin and amylin; (3) **delta cells**, which secrete gastrin and somatostatin; and (4) **F (or PP) cells**, which secrete pancreatic polypeptide. These hormones regulate carbohydrate, fat, and protein metabolism. (The pancreas is illustrated in Figure 18.13.) Nerves from both the sympathetic and the parasympathetic autonomic nervous system innervate the islets.

Insulin

The beta cells of the pancreas create **insulin** from the precursor proinsulin. The creation of proinsulin originates from a larger precursor molecule, preproinsulin. Proinsulin is made of A peptide and B peptide connected by a C peptide and two disulphide bonds. Proteolytic enzymes split C peptide, leaving the bonded A and B peptides as the insulin molecule. Insulin circulates freely in the plasma and is not bound to a carrier. The measurement of serum C peptide level allows for an indirect measurement of serum insulin creation.

Chemical, hormonal, and neural control regulate the secretion of insulin. Insulin secretion is pulsatile. The parasympathetic nervous system stimulates the beta cells, usually before eating a meal, and increases insulin secretion. Other factors stimulating insulin secretion include increased blood levels of glucose, amino acids (leucine, arginine, and lysine), and gastro-intestinal hormones (glucagon, gastrin, cholecystokinin, and secretin). Insulin secretion lessens in response to low blood levels of glucose (hypoglycemia), high levels of insulin (through negative feedback to the beta cells), and sympathetic stimulation of the beta cells in the islets. Prostaglandins also reduce insulin secretion.

At the target cell, insulin signalling is started when insulin binds and activates its cell surface receptor. Cells throughout the body have these receptors. Insulin promotes cellular glucose uptake through glucose transporters (GLUTs). An intracellular cascade of phosphorylation events, protein–protein interactions, and second-messenger generation then occurs. These actions result in diverse metabolic events throughout the body (see details in Figure 18.14).

The sensitivity of the insulin receptor is a key part in supporting normal cellular function. Age, weight, abdominal fat, and physical activity affect insulin sensitivity. Insulin resistance has been linked to many diseases including hypertension, heart disease, and type 2 diabetes mellitus. In obesity, adipocytes release several altered hormones and cytokines that have an important impact on insulin sensitivity. The most effective measures to improve insulin sensitivity in humans are weight loss and exercise.[17]

Insulin is an anabolic hormone that promotes glucose uptake primarily in liver, muscle, and adipose tissue. It also increases the creation of proteins, carbohydrates, lipids, and nucleic acids. It functions mainly in the liver, muscle, and adipose tissue. Table 18.7 reviews the actions of

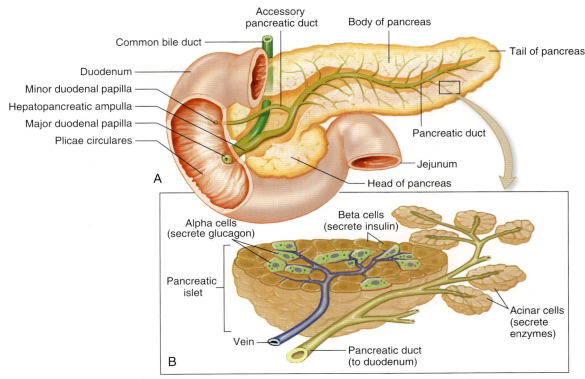

FIGURE 18.13 The Pancreas. **A,** Pancreas dissected to show main and accessory ducts. The main duct may join the common bile duct, as shown here, to enter the duodenum by a single opening at the major duodenal papilla, or the two ducts may have separate openings. The accessory pancreatic duct is usually present and has a separate opening into the duodenum. **B,** Exocrine glandular cells (around small pancreatic ducts) and endocrine glandular cells of the pancreatic islets (next to blood capillaries). Exocrine pancreatic cells secrete pancreatic juice, alpha endocrine cells secrete glucagon, and beta cells secrete insulin and amylin. (From Patton, K. T., & Thibodeau, G. A. [2018]. *The human body in health and disease* [7th ed.]. Elsevier.)

insulin. The net effect of insulin in these tissues is to stimulate protein and fat synthesis and decrease blood glucose level. The brain, red blood cells, kidney, and lens of the eye do not require insulin for glucose transport. Insulin also helps the intracellular transport of potassium, phosphate, and magnesium.

Amylin
Amylin (or islet amyloid polypeptide) is a peptide hormone cosecreted with insulin by beta cells in response to nutrient stimuli. It regulates blood glucose concentration by delaying gastric emptying and suppressing glucagon secretion after meals. Amylin also has a satiety effect, which reduces food intake. Through these mechanisms, amylin has an antihyperglycemic effect.[18]

Glucagon
The alpha cells of the pancreas and cells lining the gastrointestinal tract produce **glucagon**. Glucagon acts primarily in the liver and increases blood glucose concentration by stimulating glycogenolysis and gluconeogenesis in muscle and lipolysis in adipose tissue. Amino acids, such as alanine, glycine, and asparagine, stimulate glucagon secretion. High glucose levels inhibit glucagon release. Low glucose levels stimulate glucagon release. Their processes occur by sympathetic stimulation; thus, it is antagonistic to insulin.[19]

Pancreatic Somatostatin
Delta cells of the pancreas produce **somatostatin** in response to food intake. Somatostatin is essential in carbohydrate, fat, and protein metabolism. It is different from hypothalamic somatostatin, which inhibits the release of GH and TSH. Pancreatic somatostatin is involved in regulating alpha-cell and beta-cell function within the islets. This regulation occurs by reducing secretion of insulin, glucagon, and pancreatic polypeptide.[1]

Gastrin, Ghrelin, and Pancreatic Polypeptide
Pancreatic **gastrin** stimulates the secretion of gastric acid. It is thought that fetal pancreatic gastrin secretion is necessary for adequate islet cell development. **Ghrelin** stimulates GH secretion, controls appetite, and plays a role in obesity and the regulation of insulin sensitivity. F cells release **pancreatic polypeptide** in response to hypoglycemia and protein-rich meals. It reduces gallbladder contraction and exocrine pancreas secretion. Individuals with pancreatic tumours or diabetes mellitus often experience increased amounts of this polypeptide.[20]

Adrenal Glands
The **adrenal glands** are paired, pyramid-shaped organs behind the peritoneum and close to the upper pole of each kidney. A capsule surrounds each gland, which is surrounded by fat, and well supplied with blood. Venous return from the left adrenal gland is to the renal vein and from the right adrenal gland is to the inferior vena cava.

Each adrenal gland consists of two separate portions: an outer cortex and an inner medulla. These two portions have different embryonic origins, structures, and hormonal functions. The adrenal cortex and medulla function like two separate but interrelated glands (Figure 18.15).

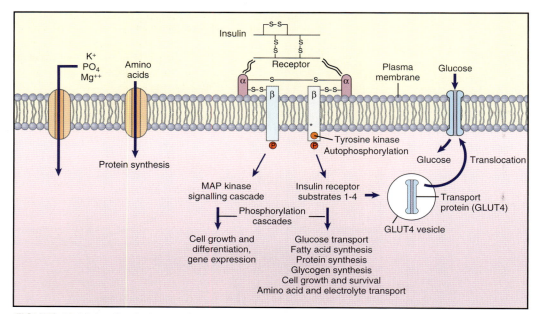

FIGURE 18.14 Insulin Action on Cells. Binding of insulin to its receptor causes autophosphorylation of the receptor, which then itself acts as a tyrosine kinase that phosphorylates insulin receptor substrates 1–4. Activation of numerous target enzymes, such as protein kinase B and mitogen-activated protein (MAP) kinase occurs and these enzymes have a multitude of effects on cell function. The glucose transporter (GLUT4) travels to the plasma membrane, where it helps glucose entry into the cell. Facilitation of the transport of amino acids, potassium (K^+), magnesium (Mg^{++}), and phosphate (PO_4) into the cell also occurs. The induction or suppression of creation of various enzymes, and the regulation of cell growth by signal molecules that modulate gene expression occurs. (Redrawn from Levy, M. N., Koeppen, B. M., & Stanton, B. A. [Eds.]. [2006]. *Berne & Levy principles of physiology* [4th ed.]. Mosby.)

TABLE 18.7 Insulin Actions

	SITES OF INSULIN ACTION		
Actions	**Liver Cells**	**Muscle Cells**	**Adipose Cells**
Glucose uptake	Increased	Increased	Increased
Glucose use	—	—	Increased glycerol phosphate
Glycogenesis	Increased	Increased	—
Glycogenolysis	Decreased	Decreased	—
Glycolysis	Increased	Increased	Increased
Gluconeogenesis	Increased	—	—
Other	Increased fatty acid creation	Increased amino acid uptake	Increased fat esterification
	Decreased ketogenesis	Increased protein synthesis	Decreased lipolysis
	Decreased urea cycle activity	Decreased proteolysis	Increased fat storage

Adrenal Cortex

The **adrenal cortex** accounts for 80% of the weight of the adult gland. The cortex is divided into three zones:[1]
1. The **zona glomerulosa**, the outer layer, constitutes about 15% of the cortex. It primarily produces the mineralocorticoid aldosterone.
2. The **zona fasciculata**, the middle layer, constitutes 78% of the cortex. It secretes the glucocorticoids cortisol, cortisone, and corticosterone.
3. The **zona reticularis**, the inner layer, constitutes 7% of the cortex. It secretes mineralocorticoids (aldosterone), adrenal androgens and estrogens, and glucocorticoids.

ACTH from the pituitary gland stimulates the cells of the adrenal cortex. All hormones of the adrenal cortex are created from cholesterol. The best-known pathway of steroidogenesis involves the conversion of cholesterol to pregnenolone. The final step includes the conversion of pregnenolone to major corticosteroids.

Glucocorticoids

Functions of the glucocorticoids. The **glucocorticoids** are steroid hormones that have metabolic, neurological, anti-inflammatory, and growth-suppressing effects. These functions (Figure 18.16) have direct effects on carbohydrate metabolism. These hormones increase blood glucose concentration. This is achieved by promoting gluconeogenesis in the liver and by decreasing uptake of glucose into muscle cells, adipose cells, and lymphatic cells. In tissues outside the liver, the glucocorticoids stimulate protein catabolism and inhibit amino acid uptake and protein synthesis. The ultimate effect on the body is protein catabolism.

The glucocorticoids act at several sites to suppress immune and inflammatory reactions. One major immunosuppressant effect is the glucocorticoid-mediated decrease in the increase of T lymphocytes (T cells), primarily T-helper cells (Th cells). There is a greater effect on T-helper 1 (Th1) cytokine production (including antiviral interferons)

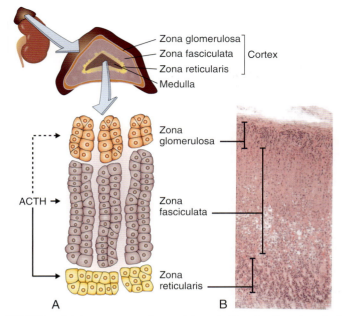

FIGURE 18.15 Structure of the Adrenal Glands Showing Cell Layers (Zonae) of the Cortex. A, Adrenal glands. Each gland consists of cortex and medulla. The cortex has three layers: zona glomerulosa, zona fasciculata, and zona reticularis. B, A part of the medulla is visible at the lower right in the photomicrograph (×35) and at the bottom of the drawing. ([A], from Damjanov, I. [2008]. *Pathophysiology*. Saunders; [B], from Kierszenbaum, A. [2002]. *Histology and cell biology*. Mosby.)

than there is on T-helper 2 (Th2) cytokine production. As such, there is a greater depression of cellular immunity than humoral immunity (see Chapter 7). Glucocorticoids affect innate immunity through several pathways. This includes decreasing the activity of pattern receptors on the surface of macrophages (see Chapter 6). Anti-inflammatory effects of glucocorticoids also include decreased function of natural killer cells, suppression of inflammatory cytokines, and stabilization of lysosomal membranes. These effects decrease the release of proteolytic enzymes. Psychological and physiological stress increases glucocorticoid production. This increase supplies a pathway for the well-described decrease in immunity seen in both acute and chronic stress (see Chapter 9). Use of glucocorticoids for the treatment of disease also leads to suppression of innate and adaptive immunity. This results in the challenging complications of infection and poor wound healing (see Chapter 8).

Other effects of glucocorticoids include inhibition of bone formation and ADH secretion, and stimulation of gastric acid secretion. Glucocorticoids appear to increase the effects of catecholamines. This includes sensitizing the arterioles to the vasoconstrictive effects of norepinephrine. Glucocorticoids also increase TH and GH effects on adipose tissue. A metabolite of cortisol may act like a barbiturate and depress nerve cell function in the brain. This depressed function accounts for the noted effects on mood, such as anxiety and depression, associated with steroid level fluctuation in disease or stress.

Pathologically high levels of glucocorticoids increase the number of circulating erythrocytes. These high levels also increase the appetite, promote fat deposition in the face and cervical areas, and increase uric acid excretion. Decreased serum calcium levels (possibly by inhibiting gastro-intestinal absorption of calcium), suppressed secretion

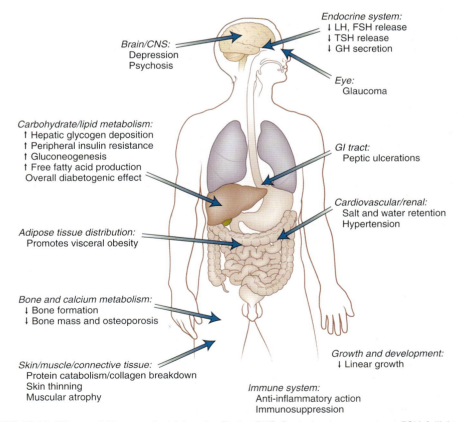

FIGURE 18.16 Effects of Glucocorticoids on the Body. *CNS*, Central nervous system; *FSH*, follicle-stimulating hormone; *GH*, growth hormone; *GI*, gastro-intestinal; *LH*, luteinizing hormone; *TSH*, thyroid-stimulating hormone. (From Stewart, P. M., & Krone, N. P. [2011]. The adrenal cortex. In S. Melmed, K. S. Polonsky, P. R. Larsen, et al. [Eds.], *Williams textbook of endocrinology* [12th ed.]. Saunders.)

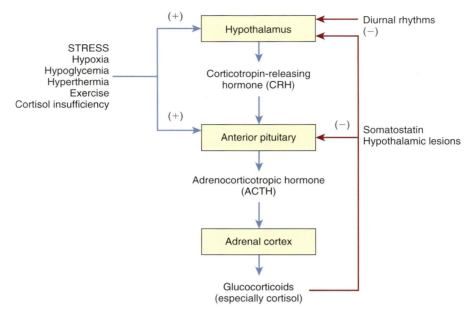

FIGURE 18.17 Feedback Control of Glucocorticoid Creation and Secretion.

and creation of ACTH and interference with the action of GH so that somatic growth is inhibited are also present (see Chapter 19).

Cortisol. The most potent naturally occurring glucocorticoid is cortisol. Cortisol is the main secretory product of the adrenal cortex. A main function of cortisol is to support life and protect the body from stress (see Figure 9.2). The liver is mainly responsible for the deactivation of cortisol.

The hypothalamus and anterior pituitary gland mainly regulate cortisol secretion (Figure 18.17). Several nuclei in the hypothalamus produce corticotropin-releasing hormone (CRH). CRH is stored in the median eminence. Once released, CRH travels through the portal vessels to stimulate the production of ACTH, β-lipotropin, γ-lipotropin, endorphins, and enkephalins by the anterior pituitary. ACTH is the main regulator of cortisol secretion and adrenocortical growth.

ACTH is created as part of a precursor called proopiomelanocortin (POMC). Three factors appear to be mainly involved in regulating the secretion of ACTH: (1) Negative-feedback effects of high circulating levels of cortisol and synthetic glucocorticoids suppress both CRH and ACTH. Low cortisol levels stimulate their secretion. (2) Diurnal rhythms affect ACTH and cortisol levels. In persons with regular sleep–wake patterns, ACTH peaks 3 to 5 hours after sleep begins and declines throughout the day. Cortisol levels follow a similar pattern. (3) Psychological and physiological (e.g., hypoxia, hypoglycemia, hyperthermia, exercise) stress increases ACTH secretion. This leads to increased cortisol levels. (Chapter 14 discusses the neurological mechanisms regulating sleep.) The cells of the immune system produce a form of immunoreactive ACTH (irACTH). This production accounts, in part, for integration of the immune and endocrine systems.

Following secretion, ACTH binds to specific plasma membrane receptors on the cells of the adrenal cortex and on other extra-adrenal tissues. Because both adrenal and extra-adrenal tissues have ACTH receptors, several effects result from stimulation by ACTH. In addition to increasing adrenocortical secretion of cortisol, ACTH supports the size and functions of the adrenal cortex. This support occurs through activation of crucial enzymes and storage of cholesterol for metabolism into steroid hormones. Extra-adrenal effects of ACTH include stimulation of melanocytes and activation of tissue lipase.

Once ACTH stimulates the cells of the adrenal cortex, cortisol creation and secretion immediately occur. In a healthy person, the secretory patterns of ACTH and cortisol are nearly identical. After secretion, some cortisol circulates in bound form attached to albumin but primarily it is bound to the plasma protein transcortin. A smaller amount circulates in the free form and diffuses into cells with specific intracellular receptors for cortisol. Rapid inactivation of ACTH occurs in the circulation, and the liver and kidneys remove the deactivated hormone.

Mineralocorticoids: aldosterone. Mineralocorticoid steroids directly affect ion transport by renal tubular epithelial cells. The transport causes sodium retention and potassium and hydrogen loss. Aldosterone is the most potent naturally occurring mineralocorticoid. Aldosterone conserves sodium by increasing the activity of the sodium–potassium pump of epithelial cells. (Chapter 1 describes the sodium–potassium pump.)

The first stages of aldosterone creation occur in the zona fasciculata and zona reticularis. The final conversion of corticosterone to aldosterone occurs in the zona glomerulosa. The renin-angiotensin-aldosterone (RAA) system (described in Chapter 29) mainly regulates aldosterone creation and secretion. Sodium and water depletion, increased potassium levels, and a diminished effective blood volume activate the RAA system (Figure 18.18). Angiotensin II is the primary stimulant of aldosterone creation and secretion. However, sodium and potassium levels also may directly affect aldosterone secretion. ACTH may transiently stimulate aldosterone creation but does not appear to be a major regulator of secretion.

The daily secretion of approximately 50 to 250 mg of aldosterone occurs when sodium and potassium levels are within normal limits. Of the secreted aldosterone, 50 to 75% binds to plasma proteins. The large proportion of unbound aldosterone adds to its rapid metabolic turnover in the liver, its low plasma concentration, and its short half-life (about 15 minutes). The breakdown of aldosterone occurs in the liver and is excreted by the kidney.

Aldosterone supports extracellular volume by acting on distal nephron epithelial cells to increase reabsorption of sodium and excretion of potassium and hydrogen. This renal effect takes 90 minutes to 6 hours. Chapter 5 describes fluid and electrolyte regulation in more detail. Other effects of aldosterone include enhancement of cardiac muscle contraction, stimulation of ectopic ventricular activity through secondary cardiac pacemakers in the ventricles, stiffening of blood vessels with increased vascular resistance, and decrease in fibrinolysis. Myocardial changes associated with heart failure, resistant hypertension, insulin resistance, and systemic inflammation are associated with pathologically increased levels of aldosterone.[21]

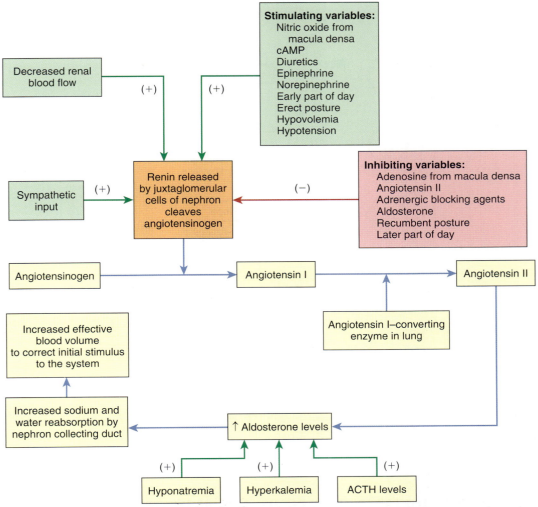

FIGURE 18.18 The Feedback Mechanisms Regulating Aldosterone Secretion. *ACTH*, Adrenocorticotropic hormone; *cAMP*, cyclic adenosine monophosphate.

Adrenal estrogens and androgens. The adrenal cortex secretes minimal amounts of estrogen and androgens. ACTH appears to be the major regulator. Some of the weakly androgenic substances secreted by the cortex (dehydroepiandrosterone [DHEA], androstenedione) are converted by peripheral tissues to stronger androgens, such as testosterone. This conversion accounts for some androgenic effects started by the adrenal cortex. Peripheral conversion of adrenal androgens to estrogens is higher in persons who are aging, obese, or experiencing liver disease or hyperthyroidism.[1] The biological effects and metabolism of the adrenal sex steroids do not vary from those produced by the gonads (see Chapter 32).

Adrenal Medulla

The chromaffin cells (pheochromocytes) of the adrenal medulla secrete and store the catecholamines epinephrine (adrenaline) and norepinephrine (noradrenaline). Creation of both is from the amino acid phenylalanine (Figure 18.19). The adrenal medulla, together with the sympathetic autonomic nervous system, originate from neural crest cells. Only 30% of circulating nonepinephrine comes from the adrenal medulla. The other 70% of norepinephrine comes from nerve terminals. The medulla is only a minor source of norepinephrine. The adrenal medulla functions as a sympathetic ganglion without postganglionic processes. Sympathetic cholinergic preganglion fibres end on the chromaffin cells and secrete catecholamines into the bloodstream. The catecholamines acting in the blood are therefore hormones and not neurotransmitters.

Physiological stress to the body (e.g., traumatic injury, hypoxia, hypoglycemia) triggers release of adrenal catecholamines through acetylcholine (from the preganglionic sympathetic fibres). This release causes the depolarization of the chromaffin cells (see Chapter 9). Depolarization causes exocytosis of the storage granules from the chromaffin cells. Epinephrine and norepinephrine are also released into the bloodstream. ACTH and the glucocorticoids increase the secretion of adrenal catecholamines.[1]

Once released, the catecholamines remain in the plasma for only seconds to minutes. The catecholamines apply their biological effects after binding to plasma membrane receptors (α_1, α_2, β_1, β_2, and β_3) in target cells. This binding activates the adenylyl cyclase system.

Rapid removal of catecholamines from the plasma occurs by being absorbed by neurons for storage in new cytoplasmic granules. They also may be metabolically inactivated and excreted in the urine. The catecholamines directly inhibit their own secretion by decreasing the formation of the enzyme tyrosine hydroxylase.

Catecholamines have diverse effects on the entire body. The *fight-or-flight response* (stress response) characterizes their release and the body's response (see Figures 9.2 and 9.3 and Tables 9.3 and 9.4). Metabolic effects of catecholamines promote hyperglycemia through a variety of mechanisms including interfering with the usual glucose regulatory feedback mechanisms.

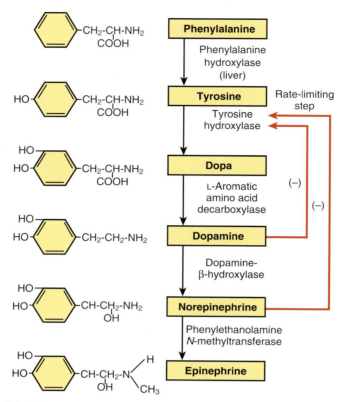

FIGURE 18.19 Creation of Catecholamines.

GERIATRIC CONSIDERATIONS

Aging and Its Effects on Specific Endocrine Glands

General Endocrine Changes With Aging
Aging has many effects on the neuroendocrine system. There are complex changes within the hypothalamic–pituitary axis. Other findings include altered biological activity and circulating levels of hormones, altered secretory response of the endocrine glands, altered metabolism of hormones, and loss of circadian control of hormone secretion.

Pituitary
Posterior: Decrease in size; reduced antidiuretic hormone secretion.
Anterior: Increased fibrosis and moderate increase in size of gland; decline in growth hormone (GH) release.

Thyroid
Glandular atrophy, fibrosis, nodularity, and increased inflammatory infiltrates; decreased thyroxine secretion and turnover, decline in tri-iodothyronine (especially in men), decreased thyroid-stimulating hormone (TSH) secretion; reduced response of plasma TSH concentration to thyroid-releasing hormone (TRH) administration (especially in men).

Growth Hormone and Insulin-Like Growth Factors
The amounts of GH and insulin-like growth factor decline with aging. This decline contributes to decreases in muscle size and function, reduced fat and bone mass, and changes in reproductive and cognitive function. Increased visceral fat and decreased lean body mass and bone density are common in older persons.

Pancreas
It is common for older persons to have glucose intolerance or diabetes. These disorders often are undiagnosed in aging adults. Mechanisms include decreased insulin receptor activity and decreased beta-cell secretion of insulin.

Adrenal
Decreased dehydroepiandrosterone levels lead to decreased creation of androgen-derived estrogen and testosterone. Decreased metabolic clearance of glucocorticoids and cortisol causes decreased cortisol secretion. Decreased levels of aldosterone also occurs. Circadian patterns of adrenocorticotropic hormone and cortisol secretion may change with aging.

Gonads
Postmenopausal women have decreased estrogen and progesterone, increased follicle-stimulating hormone, and increased androgen levels. These changes have many physiological and pathophysiological consequences (see Chapter 32). In men there is a gradual decrease in serum testosterone levels, leading to decreased sexual activity, muscle strength, and bone mineralization.

CHAPTER 18 Mechanisms of Hormonal Regulation

DID YOU UNDERSTAND?

Overview
1. The endocrine system has diverse functions. These functions include sexual differentiation, growth and development, and continuous maintenance of the body's internal environment and responses to stress.
2. Hormones are chemical messengers created by endocrine glands. When released, hormones trigger intracellular responses.

Mechanisms of Hormonal Regulation
1. Hormones have specific negative- and positive-feedback mechanisms. Negative feedback mechanisms are more common. With negative feedback, hormone secretion raises the level of a specific hormone, ultimately causing secretion to subside. This mechanism supports the hormone within a normal physiological range.
2. Endocrine feedback occurs in short, long, and ultra-short feedback loops.
3. Water-soluble hormones circulate throughout the body in unbound form. Lipid-soluble hormones (e.g., steroid, and thyroid hormones) circulate throughout the body bound to carrier proteins. Only unbound hormones can signal a target cell.
4. Hormones affect only target cells with proper receptors. They act on these cells to start specific cell functions or activities.
5. Hormones have two general types of effects on cells: (a) direct effects, or obvious changes in cell function, and (b) permissive effects, or less obvious changes that help cell function.
6. Receptors for hormones may be found on the plasma membrane or in the intracellular compartment of the target cell.
7. Water-soluble hormones act as first messengers, binding to receptors in the cell's plasma membrane. The signals started by hormone-receptor binding are transmitted into the cell by the action of second messengers (i.e., cAMP, cGMP or tyrosine kinase). Second messengers mediate the action of the hormone on the target cell (i.e., protein synthesis or cellular growth).
8. Lipid-soluble hormones (including steroid and thyroid hormones) cross the plasma membrane by diffusion. These hormones diffuse directly into the cell nucleus and bind to nuclear receptors. Plasma membrane receptors may mediate rapid responses of steroid hormones.

Structure and Function of the Endocrine Glands
1. The hypothalamic–pituitary axis (HPA) forms the structural and functional basis for the neuroendocrine system.
2. The hypothalamus regulates anterior pituitary function by secreting, releasing, or inhibiting hormones into the portal circulation.
3. Hypothalamic hormones include prolactin-releasing factor. This factor stimulates secretion of prolactin; prolactin-inhibiting factor (dopamine). Prolactin-inhibiting factor inhibits (1) prolactin secretion; (2) thyrotropin-releasing hormone, which affects release of thyroid hormones; (3) growth hormone–releasing hormone, which stimulates the release of growth hormone (GH); (4) somatostatin, which inhibits the release of GH; (5) gonadotropin-releasing hormone, which facilitates the release of follicle-stimulating hormone (FSH) and luteinizing hormone (LH); (6) corticotropin-releasing hormone (CRH), which facilitates the release of adrenocorticotropic hormone (ACTH) and endorphins; and (7) substance P, which inhibits ACTH release and stimulates the release of many other hormones.
4. The pituitary gland consists of anterior and posterior portions that have different functional relationships to the hypothalamus.
5. The regulation of the hormones of the anterior pituitary occurs by (a) secretion of hypothalamic peptide hormones or releasing factors, (b) feedback effects of the hormones secreted by target glands, and (c) direct effects of other mediating neurotransmitters.
6. Hormones of the anterior pituitary include ACTH, melanocyte-stimulating hormone, somatotropic hormones (GH, prolactin), and glycoprotein hormones (FSH, LH, and thyroid-stimulating hormone [TSH]).
7. The posterior pituitary secretes antidiuretic hormone (ADH), which also is called *vasopressin*, and oxytocin.
8. ADH controls serum osmolality, increases permeability of the renal tubules to water, and causes vasoconstriction when administered in high doses.
9. Oxytocin causes uterine contraction and lactation in women. It may have a role in sperm motility. In both men and women, oxytocin has an antidiuretic effect like that of ADH.
10. The pineal gland secretes melatonin and regulates circadian rhythms and reproduction.
11. The two-lobed thyroid gland has follicles, which secrete some of the thyroid hormones, and C cells, which secrete calcitonin and somatostatin.
12. Regulation of thyroid hormone (TH) is complex and involves the hypothalamus, anterior pituitary, thyroid gland, and many biochemical variables.
13. TSH regulates the secretion of TH through a negative-feedback loop involving the anterior pituitary and hypothalamus.
14. Creation and storage of TSH occurs in the anterior pituitary. The anterior pituitary stimulates secretion of TH by activating intracellular processes. This includes the uptake of iodine necessary for the creation of TH.
15. Once secreted, TH acts on the thyroid gland, the anterior pituitary, and the median eminence to regulate further TH production.
16. Creation of TH depends on the glycoprotein thyroglobulin, which holds tyrosine, a precursor of TH. Tyrosine then combines with iodine to form precursor molecules of the thyroid hormones thyroxine (T_4) and tri-iodothyronine (T_3). These hormones are stored within thyroid colloid until released into the circulation.
17. When released into the circulation, T_3 and T_4 are bound by carrier proteins in the plasma. These proteins store these hormones and supply a buffer for rapid changes in hormone levels. The free form is the active form.
18. Thyroid hormones alter protein synthesis and have a wide range of metabolic effects on proteins, carbohydrates, lipids, vitamins, and other hormones and neurotransmitters. TH also affect heat production and cardiac function.
19. The parathyroid glands normally are found behind the upper and lower poles of the thyroid. These glands secrete parathyroid hormone (PTH), an important regulator of serum calcium and phosphate levels.
20. PTH secretion increases levels of ionized calcium and decreases levels of phosphate in the plasma. In the kidney, PTH increases reabsorption of calcium and decreases reabsorption of phosphorus.
21. The pancreas holds the islets of Langerhans which consist of alpha cells, beta cells, delta cells, and F cells. These cells secrete hormones responsible for much of the carbohydrate metabolism in the body.
22. Alpha cells produce glucagon. Secretion of glucagon is inverse to blood glucose concentrations.
23. Beta cells secrete insulin and amylin. These hormones suppress glucagon secretion and have a satiety effect.

24. Delta cells secrete gastrin and somatostatin. These hormones inhibit glucagon and insulin secretion.
25. F cells secrete pancreatic polypeptide. This hormone inhibits gallbladder contraction and exocrine pancreatic secretion.
26. Insulin is a hormone that regulates blood glucose concentrations and metabolism of fat, protein, and carbohydrates.
27. The paired adrenal glands are found above the kidneys. Each gland consists of an adrenal medulla, which secretes catecholamines, and an adrenal cortex, which secretes steroid hormones.
28. The adrenal cortex secretes steroid hormones. These hormones include glucocorticoids, mineralocorticoids, and adrenal androgens and estrogens.
29. Glucocorticoids directly affect carbohydrate metabolism. This occurs by increasing blood glucose concentration through gluconeogenesis in the liver and by decreasing use of glucose. Glucocorticoids also inhibit immune and inflammatory responses, suppress growth, and promote protein breakdown.
30. The most potent naturally occurring glucocorticoid is cortisol. Cortisol is necessary for the maintenance of life and for protection from stress. The hypothalamus and anterior pituitary regulate the secretion of cortisol.
31. Cortisol secretion is related to secretion of ACTH. CRH stimulates ACTH secretion. ACTH binds with receptors of the adrenal cortex, which activates intracellular mechanisms and leads to cortisol release.
32. Mineralocorticoids are steroid hormones that directly affect ion transport by renal tubular epithelial cells.
33. Aldosterone is the most potent naturally occurring mineralocorticoid. Its primary role is renal reabsorption of sodium and excretion of potassium and hydrogen.
34. The renin-angiotensin-aldosterone (RAA) system regulates aldosterone secretion and is activated by sodium and potassium levels.
35. The principal site of aldosterone action is the kidney, where it causes sodium reabsorption and potassium and hydrogen excretion.
36. Androgens and estrogens secreted by the adrenal cortex act in the same way as those secreted by the gonads.
37. Stimulation of the sympathetic nervous system, ACTH, and glucocorticoids causes the adrenal medulla to secrete the catecholamines epinephrine and norepinephrine.
38. Catecholamines bind with various target cells. They are absorbed by neurons or excreted in the urine. They cause a range of metabolic effects (i.e., hyperglycemia) characterized as the "fight-or-flight response".

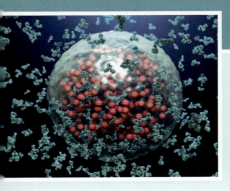

19

Alterations of Hormonal Regulation

Kelly Power-Kean, with originating chapter contributions by Valentina L. Brashers and Sue E. Huether

Additional resources are available online at https://evolve.elsevier.com/Canada/Huether/pathophysiology

CHAPTER OUTLINE

Mechanisms of Hormonal Alterations, 448
Alterations of the Hypothalamic-Pituitary System, 449
    Diseases of the Posterior Pituitary, 449
    Diseases of the Anterior Pituitary, 450
Alterations of Thyroid Function, 453
    Thyrotoxicosis/Hyperthyroidism, 453
    Hypothyroidism, 455
    Thyroid Carcinoma, 457
Alterations of Parathyroid Function, 457
    Hyperparathyroidism, 457
    Hypoparathyroidism, 458

Dysfunction of the Endocrine Pancreas: Diabetes Mellitus, 458
    Types of Diabetes Mellitus, 460
    Acute Complications of Diabetes Mellitus, 465
    Chronic Complications of Diabetes Mellitus, 466
Alterations of Adrenal Function, 470
    Disorders of the Adrenal Cortex, 470
    Tumours of the Adrenal Medulla, 473
CASE STUDY: Type 2 Diabetes Mellitus, 474

LEARNING OBJECTIVES

1. Name three ways target cells fail to respond to hormones, creating dysfunction.
2. Compare the syndrome of inappropriate antidiuretic hormone secretion (SIADH) and diabetes insipidus. Include causes, pathophysiology, manifestations, treatment, and prognosis.
3. Describe the causes of hyper- and hypopituitarism. Name the populations that are at highest risk for developing these disorders.
4. Describe the signs, symptoms, and outcomes of pituitary adenomas and prolactinomas.
5. Explain the development of Graves' disease and thyroid storm. Include the cellular changes, manifestations, treatments, and complications.
6. Describe the causes, treatment, and outcomes for disorders that produce hypothyroidism.
7. Identify the differences between primary and secondary hyperparathyroidism.
8. Describe the similarities and differences in the onset, cause, and pathophysiology of type 1 and type 2 diabetes mellitus.
9. Describe the acute complications of diabetes mellitus. Focus on detection and treatment.
10. List the chronic complications of diabetes mellitus. Discuss how good blood glucose control limits the cellular degeneration for each complication.
11. Describe the function, uses, and mechanisms of the polyol pathway.
12. Compare hypercortical and hypocortical function. Include the causes, pathophysiology, manifestations, treatment, and prognosis.
13. Identify the differences between primary and secondary hyperaldosteronism.
14. Describe pathophysiology, evaluation, and treatment of Addison's disease.
15. Describe tumours of the adrenal medulla.

KEY TERMS

Acromegaly, 452
Addison's disease (primary adrenal insufficiency), 472
Amylin, 460
Autoimmune thyroiditis (Hashimoto's disease, chronic lymphocyte thyroiditis), 455
Beta-cell dysfunction, 464
Central (secondary) thyroid disorders, 453
Congenital adrenal hyperplasia, 472
Cushing's disease, 470
Cushing's syndrome, 470
Cushing's-like syndrome, 470
Dawn phenomenon, 465
Diabetes insipidus (DI), 450
Diabetes mellitus, 458
Diabetic ketoacidosis (DKA), 461
Diabetic neuropathy, 468
Diabetic retinopathy, 467
Feminization, 472
Gestational diabetes mellitus (GDM), 465
Ghrelin, 464
Giantism, 452
Glucagon, 460
Glycosylated hemoglobin (A1C), 459
Graves' disease, 455
Hyperaldosteronism, 472
Hypercortisolism, 470
Hyperosmolar hyperglycemic syndrome (HHS), 465
Hyperparathyroidism, 457
Hyperthyroidism, 453
Hypocortisolism, 472
Hypoglycemia, 465
Hypoparathyroidism, 458
Hypopituitarism, 450
Hypothyroidism, 455

447

Idiopathic Addison's disease (organ-specific autoimmune adrenalitis), 473
Incretin, 464
Insulin resistance, 462
Macular edema, 467
Maturity-onset diabetes of youth (MODY), 464
Metabolic syndrome, 461
Myxedema, 456
Myxedema coma, 456
Nephropathy, 466
Neuropathy, 466
Painless (silent) thyroiditis, 456
Panhypopituitarism, 451
Pheochromocytoma (chromaffin cell tumour), 473
Pituitary adenoma, 451
Postpartum thyroiditis, 456
Pretibial myxedema (Graves' dermopathy), 455
Primary hyperaldosteronism (Conn's syndrome, primary aldosteronism), 472
Primary hyperparathyroidism, 457
Primary thyroid disorder, 453
Prolactinoma, 453
Retinopathy, 466
Secondary hyperaldosteronism, 472
Secondary hyperparathyroidism, 457
Secondary hypocortisolism, 473
Somogyi effect, 465
Subacute thyroiditis (de Quervain's thyroiditis), 456
Subclinical hypothyroidism, 456
Subclinical thyroid disease, 453
Syndrome of inappropriate antidiuretic hormone (SIADH), 449
Tertiary hyperparathyroidism, 457
Thyroid carcinoma, 457
Thyrotoxic crisis (thyroid storm), 455
Thyrotoxicosis, 453
Toxic adenoma, 455
Toxic multinodular goitre, 455
Type 1 diabetes mellitus, 460
Type 2 diabetes mellitus, 461
Virilization, 472

Functions of the endocrine system involve complex interactions between hormones and body systems that support steady states and influence tissue growth and reproductive capabilities. Hypersecretion or hyposecretion of various hormones usually cause endocrine system dysfunction. This dysfunction leads to abnormal hormone concentrations in the blood. Dysfunction also may result from abnormal cell receptor function or an altered intracellular response to the hormone-receptor complex.

MECHANISMS OF HORMONAL ALTERATIONS

QUICK CHECK 19.1
1. What is the mechanism of cell surface receptor–associated disorders?
2. Why do persons with the syndrome of inappropriate antidiuretic hormone (SIADH) produce concentrated urine?
3. Why may individuals with a pituitary adenoma develop visual disturbances?

Notably elevated or notably deceased hormone levels may result from many causes (Table 19.1). Dysfunction of an endocrine gland may involve its failure to produce adequate amounts of biologically free or active hormone (hyposecretion). A gland may also create or release too much hormone (hypersecretion). Feedback systems that recognize the need for a hormone may fail to function properly or may respond to incorrect signals. Breakdown of hormones may occur once they are released into the circulation, or they may be inactivated before reaching the target cell by antibodies that function as circulating hormone inhibitors (e.g., thyroid disease). There are other causes of decreased hormone delivery to target cells. These causes include an inadequate blood supply to the gland or target tissues or an insufficient amount of the proper carrier proteins in the serum. Ectopic sources of hormones are hormones produced by nonendocrine tissues. These hormones may cause abnormally elevated hormone levels without the benefit of the normal feedback system for hormone control (e.g., hormone-producing tumours).

Target cells may not respond correctly to hormonal stimulation for several reasons. There are two general types of target cell insensitivity to hormones:
1. *Cell surface receptor–associated disorders.* These disorders are found mainly in water-soluble hormones, such as insulin. They may present in several ways. They may involve a decrease in the number of receptors, leading to decreased or defective hormone-receptor binding. An impairment of receptor function, resulting in insensitivity to the hormone may occur. The presence of antibodies against specific receptors that either reduce available binding sites or mimic hormone action, suppressing or exaggerating, respectively, the target cell response may

TABLE 19.1 Mechanisms of Hormone Alterations

Inappropriate Amounts of Hormone Delivered to Target Cell	Inappropriate Response by Target Cell
Inadequate Hormone Creation	**Cell Surface Receptor–Associated Disorders**
1. Inadequate quantity of hormone precursors	1. Decrease in the number of receptors
2. Secretory cell unable to convert precursors to active hormone	2. Impaired receptor function (altered affinity for hormones)
Failure of Feedback Systems	3. Presence of antibodies against certain receptors
1. Do not recognize positive feedback, leading to inadequate hormone creation	4. Unusual expression of receptor function
2. Do not recognize negative feedback, leading to excessive hormone creation	
Inactive Hormones	**Intracellular Disorders**
1. Inadequate biologically free hormone	1. Acquired defects in postreceptor signalling cascades
2. Hormone broken down at an altered rate	2. Inadequate creation of a second messenger
3. Circulating hormone inhibitors	3. Altered intracellular enzymes or proteins
Dysfunctional Delivery System	4. Alterations in nuclear coregulators
1. Inadequate blood supply	5. Altered protein synthesis
2. Inadequate carrier proteins	
3. Ectopic production of hormones	

exist. Lastly, an unusual expression of receptor function, as occurs in some tumour cells, may occur.
2. *Intracellular disorders.* These disorders involve defects in postreceptor signalling cascades or inadequate creation of a second messenger. An example is inadequacy of the needed cyclic adenosine monophosphate (cAMP) to transduce the hormonal signal into intracellular events. The target cell for water-soluble hormones may have a faulty response to hormone-receptor binding. This faulty response does not allow for the generation of the required second messenger. Alternatively, the cell may respond abnormally to the second messenger if levels of intracellular enzymes or proteins are altered. (Table 18.3 lists second messengers for various hormones.) As a result, the target cell does not express the usual hormonal effect (e.g., pseudohypoparathyroidism).

Disease-causing mechanisms that affect target cell response for lipid-soluble hormones occur less often than those affecting water-soluble hormones. When they do occur, the mechanisms are like those for water-soluble hormones. This includes changes in the number and binding affinity of intracellular receptors or altered creation of new messenger RNA (mRNA) and substrates for new protein synthesis. In other cases, hormone responsiveness may be linked to alterations in nuclear co-regulators. Nuclear co-regulators are proteins (such as cAMP response element–binding protein) that help or prevent the transcription of the target gene.[1]

ALTERATIONS OF THE HYPOTHALAMIC-PITUITARY SYSTEM

The most common cause of hypothalamic dysfunction is interruption of the pituitary stalk. Causes of this interruption include destructive lesions, rupture after head injury, surgical injury, or tumour. In these cases, an altered connection between the hypothalamus and the pituitary gland causes pituitary disease. For example, without hypothalamic hormones (Figure 19.1), women cease to menstruate, and men experience hypogonadism and impaired spermatogenesis. A decrease in the adrenocorticotropic hormone (ACTH) response to low serum cortisol levels occurs because of the absence of corticotropin-releasing hormone (CRH). The absence of thyrotropin-releasing hormone (TRH) causes hypothalamic hypothyroidism. Low levels of growth hormone–releasing hormone (GHRH) result in growth hormone (GH) deficiency and growth failure in children. An absence of the usual inhibitory control of prolactin secretion (dopamine) causes hyperprolactinemia.

Diseases of the Posterior Pituitary

Diseases of the posterior pituitary cause abnormal secretion of antidiuretic hormone (ADH, also called *arginine vasopressin*). An excess amount of this hormone results in water retention and a hypo-osmolar state. Deficiencies in the amount or response to ADH result in serum hyperosmolarity (see Chapter 5). These complex pathophysiological states have major clinical effects on the modulation of body fluids and electrolytes. They also affect cognitive and emotional responses to stress.

Syndrome of Inappropriate Antidiuretic Hormone

Syndrome of inappropriate antidiuretic hormone (SIADH) occurs when high levels of ADH are present in the absence of normal physiological stimuli for its release. A common cause of SIADH is the ectopic production of ADH by tumours. Examples include small cell carcinoma of the duodenum, stomach, and pancreas; cancers of the bladder, prostate, and endometrium; lymphomas; and sarcomas. Pulmonary disorders associated with SIADH include bronchogenic carcinoma, pneumonia, asthma, cystic fibrosis, and respiratory failure. Central nervous system disorders that may cause SIADH include encephalitis, meningitis, intracranial hemorrhage, tumours, and trauma.

Another important cause of SIADH is surgery. Any surgery can result in increased ADH secretion for as long as 5 to 7 days after surgery. The precise mechanism is uncertain but is likely related to fluid and volume changes following surgery, the amount and type of intravenous fluids given, and the use of opioid analgesics. Following pituitary surgery, stored ADH is released in an unregulated manner. This unregulated release may cause transient SIADH.[2]

Medications are an important cause of SIADH, especially in older persons. These include hypoglycemic medications (e.g., glyburide [Glycron]), opioids, general anaesthetics, antidepressants, antipsychotics, chemotherapeutic agents, nonsteroidal anti-inflammatory medications, and synthetic ADH analogues.[3]

PATHOPHYSIOLOGY The key features of SIADH are the result of increased renal water retention. ADH increases renal collecting duct permeability to water by causing the insertion of aquaporin-2, a water channel protein, into the tubular luminal membrane. This action increases water reabsorption by the kidneys.[3] (Chapter 29 reviews renal function.) This water reabsorption results in an increase of extracellular fluid volume. The increase leads to dilutional hyponatremia (low serum sodium concentration) and hypo-osmolarity. It also produces inappropriately concentrated urine, with respect to serum osmolarity, because water is reabsorbed that normally would be excreted.

CLINICAL MANIFESTATIONS The symptoms of SIADH result from hyponatremia (see Chapter 5). The symptoms are also determined by the severity and rapidity of onset. Thirst, impaired taste, anorexia, dyspnea on exertion, fatigue, and dulled perception occur when the serum sodium level decreases rapidly from 140 to 130 mmol/L. Peripheral edema is absent. Gastro-intestinal (GI) symptoms, including vomiting and abdominal cramps, occur with a drop in sodium concentration from 130 to 120 mmol/L. There is weight gain from water retention, even with nausea and vomiting. Even if hyponatremia develops slowly, serum sodium levels below 110 to 115 mmol/L cause confusion, lethargy, muscle twitching, and convulsions. Severe and sometimes irreversible neurological damage may occur. Symptoms usually resolve with correction of hyponatremia (see Chapter 5).

EVALUATION AND TREATMENT A diagnosis of SIADH requires several manifestations: (1) serum hypo-osmolality and hyponatremia; (2) urine hyperosmolarity (i.e., urine osmolality is greater than expected for the related serum osmolarity); (3) urine sodium excretion that matches sodium intake (i.e., sodium excretion is normal in spite of excessive water reabsorption); (4) normal adrenal and thyroid function; and (5) absence of conditions that can change volume status (e.g., heart failure, hypovolemia, or renal insufficiency).

The treatment of SIADH involves the correction of any underlying causal problems. Fluid restriction with careful monitoring of sodium status and neurological symptoms is also necessary. In severe SIADH, emergency correction of severe hyponatremia by careful administration of hypertonic saline may be needed. Resolution usually occurs within 3 days, with a 2- to 3-kg weight loss and correction of

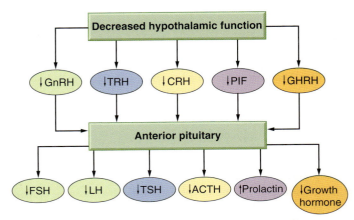

FIGURE 19.1 Loss of Hypothalamic Hormones. *ACTH,* Adrenocorticotropic hormone; *CRH,* corticotropin-releasing hormone; *FSH,* follicle-stimulating hormone; *GHRH,* growth hormone–releasing hormone; *GnRH,* gonadotropin-releasing hormone; *LH,* luteinizing hormone; *PIF,* prolactin-inhibiting factor (probably dopamine); *TRH,* thyrotropin-releasing hormone; *TSH,* thyroid-stimulating hormone.

hyponatremia and salt wasting. If the correction of hyponatremia is too rapid, a severe neurological syndrome called *central pontine myelinolysis* can occur. Demeclocycline (Declomycin) is used to treat resistant or chronic SIADH. This medication causes the renal tubules to develop resistance to ADH. Vasopressin (ADH) receptor antagonists, known as *vaptans*, are also an effective treatment.[3]

Diabetes Insipidus

Diabetes insipidus (DI) is an insufficiency of ADH activity, leading to polyuria (frequent urination) and polydipsia (frequent drinking). There are two forms of DI:

1. *Neurogenic or central DI.* Caused by the insufficient secretion of ADH. It occurs when any organic lesion of the hypothalamus, pituitary stalk, or posterior pituitary interferes with ADH creation, transport, or release. Causative lesions include primary brain tumours, hypophysectomy, aneurysms, thrombosis, infections, and immunological disorders. Central DI is a well-recognized complication of traumatic brain injury. Hereditary disorders that affect ADH genes or result in structural changes in the pituitary gland may also cause central DI.
2. *Nephrogenic DI.* Can be either acquired or genetic and is caused by inadequate response of the renal tubules to ADH. Acquired nephrogenic DI is generally related to disorders and medications that damage the renal tubules or inhibit the generation of cAMP in the tubules. These disorders include pyelonephritis, amyloidosis, destructive uropathies, and polycystic kidney disease. All of these disorders lead to irreversible DI. Medications that may induce a reversible form of nephrogenic DI include lithium carbonate, colchicines, amphotericin B, loop diuretics, general anaesthetics, and demeclocycline (Declomycin). Several genetic causes of nephrogenic DI have also been found. One of the best described is a mutation in the gene that codes for aquaporin-2, which is one of the four water transport channels in the renal tubule.[4]

There is a rare form of DI associated with pregnancy. In gestational DI there is an increase in the level of the vasopressin-degrading enzyme vasopressinase. Clinical signs are usually mild and do not require treatment.[5]

Dipsogenic or *primary polydipsia* may be confused with DI. The cause of primary polydipsia is the chronic ingestion of extremely large quantities of fluid. The fluid washes out the renal medullary concentration gradient, which results in a partial resistance to ADH. This condition resolves with decreased fluid ingestion. It is important to differentiate the psychogenic causes of polydipsia from true DI. Administering an ADH analogue to an individual with psychogenic DI will result in severe hypo-osmolality.

PATHOPHYSIOLOGY Individuals with DI have a partial to total inability to concentrate urine. Insufficient ADH activity causes excretion of large volumes of dilute urine. This leads to increased plasma osmolality. In conscious individuals, the stimulation of the thirst mechanism causes polydipsia—usually a craving for cold drinks. Dehydration develops rapidly without ongoing fluid replacement. Serum hypernatremia and hyperosmolality occurs if the individual with DI cannot conserve as much water as is lost in the urine. There is generally no effect on the concentrations of other serum electrolytes.

CLINICAL MANIFESTATIONS The clinical signs of DI include polyuria, nocturia, continuous thirst, and polydipsia. The urine output is varied but can increase from the normal output of 1 to 2 L/day to 8 to 12 L/day and can be higher than daily fluid intake. Persons with long-standing DI develop a large bladder capacity and hydronephrosis (see Chapter 30). Neurogenic DI usually has a sudden onset. Many persons can recall the exact date of onset of their symptoms. Nephrogenic DI usually has a more gradual onset. Table 19.2 compares the signs and symptoms of DI and SIADH.

EVALUATION AND TREATMENT It is important to distinguish DI from other polyuric states, including diabetes mellitus, osmotically induced diuresis, and psychogenic polydipsia. The criteria for the diagnosis of DI include low urine specific gravity and osmolality, hypernatremia, high serum osmolality, and continued diuresis despite a serum sodium concentration of 145 mmol/L or greater. Confirmation of the diagnosis of DI is generally through water deprivation testing. Distinguishing psychogenic polydipsia from nephrogenic DI is based on plasma ADH levels. ADH levels are low in psychogenic polydipsia and normal or high in nephrogenic DI.

Treatment of neurogenic DI is based on the extent of the ADH deficiency and on the patient's age, endocrine and cardiovascular status, and lifestyle. Some require ADH replacement, but oral or intravenous fluid replacement is usually adequate. ADH replacement therapy for symptomatic central or neurogenic DI includes intravascular, oral, or intranasal administration of the synthetic vasopressin analogue desmopressin (DDAVP).[4] Management of nephrogenic DI requires treatment of any reversible underlying disorders, stopping any causative medications, and correction of associated electrolyte disorders. New treatments aimed at reversing aquaporin-2 dysfunction are being developed.[6] Medications that increase the action of insufficient amounts of endogenous ADH, such as chlorpropamide, carbamazepine (Tegretol), and clofibrate (Atromid), may be used in individuals with incomplete ADH deficiency.

Diseases of the Anterior Pituitary
Hypopituitarism

Characteristics of **hypopituitarism** include the absence of one or more anterior pituitary hormones or the complete failure of all anterior pituitary hormone functions. Hypopituitarism results from an inadequate supply of hypothalamic-releasing hormones, because of damage to the pituitary stalk, or an inability of the gland to produce hormones. The most common causes of hypopituitarism are pituitary infarction or space-occupying lesions, such as pituitary adenomas or aneurysms. Pituitary infarction may occur in women during the postpartum period

TABLE 19.2 Signs and Symptoms of Diabetes Insipidus and Syndrome of Inappropriate Antidiuretic Hormone

Signs and Symptoms	Diabetes Insipidus	Syndrome of Inappropriate Antidiuretic Hormone
Urine output	High	Low (no hypovolemia)
Urine osmolality	Low (<100–200 mmol/kg H_2O)	High (>800 mmol/kg H_2O)
Urine specific gravity	Low (<1.010)	High (>1.020)
Serum sodium	Hypernatremia (>145 mmol/L)	Hyponatremia (<135 mmol/L)
Serum osmolality	Hyperosmolar (>300 mmol/kg)	Hypo-osmolar (<285 mmol/kg)
Symptoms	Polyuria, thirst, high urine output, signs of dehydration	Water retention, low urine output, nausea, vomiting, mental changes

(Sheehan's syndrome) because of blood loss and hypovolemic shock.[7] Traumatic brain injury is increasingly recognized as an important cause of hypopituitarism and can have a significant impact on acute and long-term recovery.[8] Other causes of hypopituitarism include removal or destruction of the gland, infections (e.g., meningitis, syphilis, tuberculosis), autoimmune hypophysitis, and certain medications (e.g., carbamazepine). Mutation of the prophet of pituitary transcription factor (PROP-1) gene involved in early embryonic pituitary development may also be the cause.[9]

PATHOPHYSIOLOGY The pituitary gland is highly vascular and relies heavily upon portal blood flow from the hypothalamus. It is, therefore, at risk of ischemia and infarction. Infarction results in tissue necrosis and edema with swelling of the gland. Expansion of the pituitary within the fixed compartment of the sella turcica further impedes blood supply to the pituitary. Over time, fibrosis of pituitary tissue occurs, and the symptoms of hypopituitarism develop. Adenomas and aneurysms may compress otherwise normal secreting pituitary cells and lead to altered hormonal output.

CLINICAL MANIFESTATIONS The signs and symptoms of hypofunction of the anterior pituitary are variable and depend on the hormones involved. In **panhypopituitarism**, all hormones are deficient, and the individual suffers from many complications. These include cortisol deficiency from lack of ACTH, thyroid deficiency from lack of thyroid-stimulating hormone (TSH), and loss of secondary sex characteristics because of the lack of follicle-stimulating hormone (FSH) and luteinizing hormone (LH). Low levels of GH and insulin-like growth factor 1 (IGF-1) affect growth in children. This can cause physiological and psychological symptoms in adults. Finally, postpartum women cannot lactate because of decreased or absent prolactin.

ACTH deficiency with associated loss of cortisol is a potentially life-threatening disorder. ACTH deficiency usually occurs with generalized pituitary hypofunction. Within 2 weeks of the complete absence of ACTH, symptoms of cortisol insufficiency develop. Symptoms include nausea, vomiting, anorexia, fatigue, and weakness. Hypoglycemia results from increased insulin sensitivity, decreased glycogen reserves, and decreased gluconeogenesis associated with hypocortisolism. ACTH deficiency also limits maximal aldosterone secretion. However, the renin-angiotensin system can stimulate some aldosterone secretion. The glomerular filtration rate decreases, causing decreased urine output.

It is rare to see TSH deficiency alone. It often occurs with other pituitary hormone deficiencies. Symptoms develop 4 to 8 weeks after hypothyrotropinemia occurs. Symptoms include cold intolerance, skin dryness, mild myxedema, lethargy, and decreased metabolic rate. The symptoms often are less severe than those of primary hypothyroidism.

The onset of FSH and LH deficiencies in women of reproductive age is associated with amenorrhea and atrophy of the vagina, uterus, and breasts. In postpubertal males, testicular atrophy and diminished facial hair growth occurs. Both genders experience decreased body hair and decreased libido.

GH deficiency occurs in both children and adults. Several genetic defects have been found in the GH axis in children. One defect is a recessive mutation in the GH gene, resulting in a failure of GH secretion. Mutations also may involve the GH receptor, IGF-1 biosynthesis, IGF-1 receptors, or defects in GH signal transduction.[10] In adults, structural or functional defects of the pituitary are usually a result of GH deficiency. In both children and adults, acute GH and IGF-1 deficiency has been linked to significant metabolic problems seen with critical illness.

In children, growth failure and hypopituitary dwarfism is associated with GH deficiency (Figure 19.2). However, not all children with

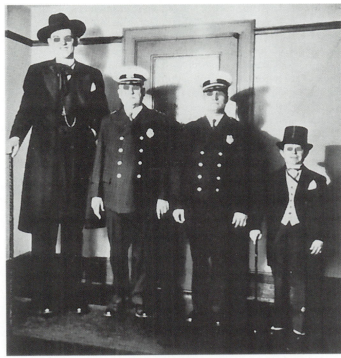

FIGURE 19.2 Hypopituitary Dwarfism and Pituitary Giantism. A pituitary giant and dwarf contrasted with normal-size men. Excessive secretion of growth hormone by the anterior lobe of the pituitary gland during the early years of life produces giants of this type. Deficient secretion of this substance produces well-formed dwarfs. (From Patton, K. T., & Thibodeau, G. A. [2013]. *Anatomy & physiology* [8th ed.]. Mosby.)

short stature have GH deficiency. Symptoms of chronic adult GH deficiency syndrome include increased body fat, decreased strength and lean body mass, osteoporosis, reduced sweating, and dry skin. Psychological problems, including depression, social withdrawal, fatigue, loss of motivation, and a diminished feeling of well-being are also associated with this condition. Without adequate GH replacement, increased mortality can occur. The increased mortality is related to myocardial infarction and stroke associated with dyslipidemias and atherosclerosis.[11]

EVALUATION AND TREATMENT The diagnostic evaluation of suspected pituitary disease is often challenging. Careful interpretation of diagnostic tests together with the individual's signs and symptoms is essential. Simultaneous measurements of the levels of tropic hormones from the pituitary and target endocrine glands are crucial. The more complicated dynamic testing of insulin, TRH, and gonadotropin-releasing hormone (GnRH) may be required. Imaging of the pituitary (magnetic resonance imaging [MRI] or computed tomography [CT] scans) is vital to assess for lesions, such as tumours.

Management of hypopituitarism requires quick correction of the underlying disorder. Replacement of target gland hormones that are deficient because of lack of tropic anterior pituitary hormones is vital. This may include replacement of cortisol, thyroid hormone, GH, and gender-specific steroid hormones.[12] In cases of circulatory collapse, immediate treatment with glucocorticoids and intravenous fluids is critical.

Hyperpituitarism: Primary Adenoma

Pituitary adenomas usually are benign, slow-growing tumours that start from cells of the anterior pituitary. The cause of pituitary adenomas is not known and most occur sporadically. Detection of an altered gene expression is common. Familial pituitary adenomas occur as part of syndromes affecting other organs, such as multiple endocrine neoplasia.[13] Most are microscopic (microadenomas) and are found only on autopsy or incidentally discovered with MRI. Most pituitary microadenomas are hormonally silent and do not pose significant hazards to the individual. Larger adenomas (macroadenomas) are associated with morbidity and mortality caused by alterations in hormone secretion or invasion or impact on surrounding structures.

PATHOPHYSIOLOGY Local growth of the adenoma may influence the optic chiasma and cause various visual disturbances. If the tumour is aggressive, invasion of the cavernous sinuses may occur. This invasion may affect the function of the oculomotor, trochlear, abducens, and trigeminal nerves (see Table 13.6 for review of cranial nerves). Extension to the hypothalamus alters control of wakefulness, thirst, appetite, and temperature.

Hormonal effects of adenomas include hypersecretion from the adenoma itself and hyposecretion from surrounding pituitary cells. The adenomatous tissue secretes the hormone of the cell type from which it arose. This secretion occurs without regard to the needs of the body and without benefit of regulatory feedback mechanisms (autonomous function). Pressure exerted by the tumour in the unexpandable bony sella turcica commonly results in hyposecretion from those cells that are most sensitive to pressure (GH-, FSH-, and LH-secreting cells).[14]

CLINICAL MANIFESTATIONS The clinical manifestations of pituitary adenomas are related to tumour growth and hormone hypersecretion or hyposecretion. Increased tumour size causes headache, fatigue, neck pain or stiffness, and seizures. Visual changes include visual field impairments (often beginning in one eye and progressing to the other) and temporary blindness. Alteration of neuromuscular function occurs if the tumour effects other cranial nerves.

Pituitary adenomas are most often associated with increased secretion of GH and prolactin (see "Hypersecretion of Growth Hormone: Acromegaly" and "Prolactinoma"). Gonadotropic hyposecretion results in menstrual irregularity in women. A decreased libido and receding secondary sex characteristics occur in both genders. If the tumour exerts enough pressure, thyroid and adrenal hypofunction may occur. A lack of TSH and ACTH results in the symptoms of hypothyroidism and hypocortisolism, respectively.

EVALUATION AND TREATMENT Diagnosis of pituitary adenoma involves physical and laboratory evaluations. This includes related hormone assays and radiographic examination of the skull (MRI [preferred] or contrast-enhanced CT). The goal of treatment is to protect the individual from the effects of tumour growth and to control hormone hypersecretion while minimizing damage to appropriately secreting portions of the pituitary. Depending on tumour size and type, treatment may include administration of specific medications to suppress tumour growth, trans-sphenoidal tumour resection, or radiation therapy.[12]

Hypersecretion of Growth Hormone: Acromegaly

Acromegaly results from constant exposure to high levels of GH and IGF-1. Its cause is almost always a GH-secreting pituitary adenoma.[15]

Acromegaly usually occurs in adults in the 40- to 59-year-old age group, although it is often present for years before diagnosis. It is a slowly progressive disease. If untreated, it is associated with a decreased life expectancy. The cause of death from acromegaly is heart disease secondary to hypertension and coronary artery disease, stroke, diabetes mellitus, or colon or lung cancer.

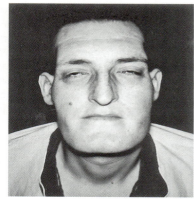

FIGURE 19.3 Acromegaly. (From McCance, K. L., & Huether, S. E. [2019]. *Pathophysiology: the biological basis for disease in adults and children* [8th ed.]. Elsevier, Figure 22.5.)

PATHOPHYSIOLOGY With a GH-secreting adenoma, there is a loss of the GH baseline secretion pattern and sleep-related GH peaks. An irregular secretory pattern takes place. However, suppression of GH levels in acromegalics never fully occurs. Only slight increases of GH and IGF-1 can stimulate growth. In children and adolescents whose epiphyseal plates have not closed, the effect of increased GH levels is called giantism (see Figure 19.2). Skeletal growth is extreme, with some individuals becoming 2.4 to 2.7 metres tall. In the adult, epiphyseal closure has occurred, and increased amounts of GH and IGF-1 cause connective tissue and cytoplasmic matrix increase, as well as excess bony growth. These events result in the typical appearance of acromegaly (Figure 19.3).

GH has significant effects on glucose, lipid, and protein metabolism. Hyperglycemia results from adipocyte inflammation and GH inhibition of peripheral glucose uptake and increased hepatic glucose production. This results in hyperinsulinism and, finally, insulin resistance.[16] Diabetes mellitus occurs when the pancreas cannot secrete enough insulin to balance the effects of GH. Excessive levels of GH and IGF-1 also affect the cardiovascular system. Although there is not a clear understanding of the associated pathophysiological mechanism, hypertension and left ventricular heart failure are seen in one-third to one-half of individuals with acromegaly. Cardiomyopathy associated with progressive and uncontrolled myocardial growth is a significant factor.[17] GH also acts on the renal tubules to increase phosphate reabsorption. This leads to mild hyperphosphatemia. Because the adenoma becomes a space-occupying lesion, hypopituitarism may occur because of compression of surrounding hormone-secreting cells.

CLINICAL MANIFESTATIONS With connective tissue excess, individuals with acromegaly have an enlarged tongue, interstitial edema, enlarged and overactive sebaceous and sweat glands (leading to increased body odour), and coarse skin and body hair. Increased periosteal vertebral bone growth and enlargement of the bones of the face (see Figure 19.3), hands, and feet occurs. The lower jaw and forehead also protrude. Skeletal abnormalities are irreversible.

Increased IGF-1 levels cause ribs to get longer at the bone-cartilage junction. This leads to a barrel-chested appearance, and increased growth of cartilage in joints, which causes backache and arthralgias. With bony and soft tissue overgrowth, nerve entrapment occurs. The entrapment leads to peripheral nerve damage causing weakness, muscular atrophy, footdrop, and sensory changes in the hands.

Symptoms of diabetes mellitus, such as polyuria and polydipsia, may occur because of decreased insulin sensitivity. Acromegaly-associated hypertension usually has no symptoms until heart failure develops. Increased tumour size results in central nervous system symptoms of headache, seizure activity, visual disturbances, and papilledema. Disruption of gonadotropin secretion may occur if there is compression hypopituitarism. This causes amenorrhea in women and sexual dysfunction in men. About 20% of GH-secreting tumours also secrete prolactin, resulting in hypogonadism. Cardiovascular, metabolic, and tumour compression symptoms often improve with treatment.

EVALUATION AND TREATMENT The clinical features of the disease, MRI scans, and elevated levels of IGF-1 confirm diagnosis.[15] GH level is normally elevated and not suppressed with oral glucose tolerance testing. The goals of treatment are to normalize or reduce GH secretion and relieve or prevent complications related to tumour growth. The treatment of choice in acromegaly is trans-sphenoidal surgical removal of the GH-secreting adenoma. Radiation therapy may be effective when rapid control of GH levels is not essential, when the individual is not a good surgical candidate, or when hyperfunction continues after subtotal resection. Somatostatin analogues, such as octreotide (SandoSTATIN), octreotide LAR (SandoSTATIN LAR), and lanreotide (Somatuline), normalize IGF-1 levels and lower GH levels. Pegvisomant (Somavert) can be used to supplement somatostatin analogues. It is an effective medication that causes tissue insensitivity to GH by blocking the GH receptor.[18] Dopaminergic agonists, such as cabergoline (Dostinex), also may be helpful, especially if the tumour also secretes prolactin.

Prolactinoma

Pituitary tumours that secrete prolactin, **prolactinomas**, are the most common hormonally active pituitary tumours. Other conditions or medications can elevate prolactin levels in the absence of a pituitary pathological condition. For example, renal failure, polycystic ovarian disease, primary hypothyroidism, breast stimulation, or even the stress of venipuncture can increase prolactin levels. Prolactin is under tight inhibitory hypothalamic control through the secretion of dopamine. Thus, medications that block the effects of dopamine can increase prolactin level and stimulate growth of prolactin-secreting cells (lactotrophs). These include antipsychotics (risperidone [Risperdal], chlorpromazine [Largactil]), metoclopramide (Reglan), tricyclic antidepressants, and methyldopa (Aldomet). Estrogens increase prolactin concentration by stimulating hyperplasia of prolactin-secreting cells. Any process that interferes with the delivery of dopamine from the hypothalamus to the lactotrophs (pituitary stalk tumour, pituitary stalk transection, or compressive pituitary tumour) also results in hyperprolactinemia. Because TRH stimulates prolactin secretion, in addition to enhancing TSH release, elevation of prolactin concentration may occur in individuals with primary hypothyroidism.

PATHOPHYSIOLOGY The main feature of a prolactinoma is sustained increases in the levels of serum prolactin. The physiological actions of prolactin include breast development during pregnancy, postpartum milk production, and suppression of ovarian function in nursing women. Pathological elevation of prolactin levels in women results in amenorrhea, nonpuerperal milk production (galactorrhea), hirsutism, and osteopenia or osteoporosis resulting from estrogen deficiency. Hyperprolactinemia in men causes hypogonadism and erectile dysfunction.

Because the adenoma becomes an increasingly space-occupying lesion, hypopituitarism may occur because of the compression of surrounding hormone-secreting cells. Central nervous system symptoms may develop because of growth and pressure of the adenoma within the sella turcica. Persons with macro (greater than 1 cm in diameter) or giant (greater than 4 cm in diameter) prolactinomas more commonly experience these complications. These patients are often more difficult to treat.[19]

CLINICAL MANIFESTATIONS Women with hyperprolactinemia generally present with galactorrhea (nonpuerperal milk production) and menstrual disturbances including amenorrhea. In susceptible women, hirsutism develops because of estrogen deficiency. If not detected until after many years, this estrogen deficiency also may result in osteopenia or osteoporosis. Men often develop hypogonadism, gynecomastia, and erectile dysfunction. These conditions may present late when symptoms related to the increasing size of the adenoma occur (i.e., headache or visual impairment).

EVALUATION AND TREATMENT The diagnostic evaluation of hyperprolactinemia includes a careful history to exclude medications that may cause elevations in prolactin concentration. Confirmation of symptoms of hypothyroidism and screening with a serum TSH level is mandatory. To determine the size and location of an adenoma, MRI scanning of the pituitary is indicated. The careful search for a nonpituitary cause should occur if serum prolactin level is less than 50 μg/L.

Dopaminergic agonists (cabergoline) are the treatment of choice for prolactinomas. Restoration of fertility in previously anovulatory women is common. In individuals resistant or intolerant to these medications, trans-sphenoidal surgery and radiotherapy are options.[20] Exploration of new chemotherapeutic and targeted molecular therapies are underway in selected cases.[21]

ALTERATIONS OF THYROID FUNCTION

> **QUICK CHECK 19.2**
> 1. Compare the clinical manifestations of hyperthyroidism and hypothyroidism.
> 2. What is Graves' disease?
> 3. What is myxedema?
> 4. What is the most common cause of thyroid carcinoma?

Disorders of thyroid function develop because of primary dysfunction or disease of the thyroid gland. Secondary dysfunction occurs because of pituitary or hypothalamic alterations. **Primary thyroid disorders** result in alterations of thyroid hormone (TH) levels with secondary feedback effects on pituitary TSH. For example, when there are primary elevations in TH level, TSH level will secondarily decrease because of negative feedback. With a decreased TH level because of a condition affecting the thyroid gland, an elevation of the TSH level will occur. Thyroid disease also can present with minimal or no symptoms but with abnormal laboratory values. This is known as **subclinical thyroid disease**. **Central (secondary) thyroid disorders** are related to disorders of pituitary gland TSH production. When there is excessive TSH production, the TH level elevation is secondary to the primary elevation of TSH concentration. The reverse is true with inadequate TSH production.

Thyrotoxicosis/Hyperthyroidism

PATHOPHYSIOLOGY **Thyrotoxicosis** is a condition that results from any cause of increased TH levels. **Hyperthyroidism** is a form of thyrotoxicosis that occurs when there is excess secretion of TH from the thyroid gland (Figure 19.4). The terms *thyrotoxicosis* and *hyperthyroidism* are often used interchangeably. Common diseases that cause primary hyperthyroidism include Graves' disease, toxic multinodular goitre, and solitary toxic adenoma. TSH-secreting pituitary adenomas less

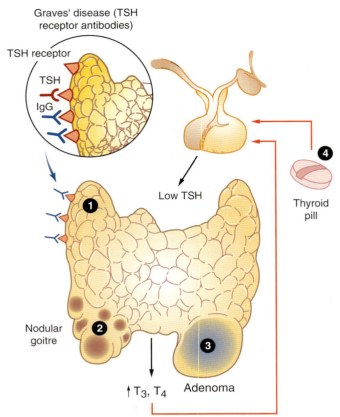

FIGURE 19.4 Common Causes of Hyperthyroidism. Hyperthyroidism may have several causes, among them: **1**, Graves' disease; **2**, toxic multinodular goitre; **3**, follicular adenoma; **4**, thyroid medication. *IgG*, Immunoglobulin G; *TSH*, thyroid-stimulating hormone; T_4, thyroxine; T_3, tri-iodothyronine. (Adapted from Damjanov, I. [2012]. *Pathology for the health professions* [4th ed.]. Saunders.)

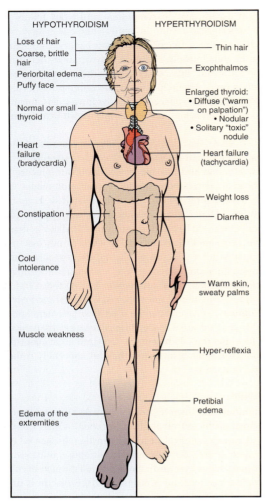

FIGURE 19.5 Clinical Manifestations of Hyperthyroidism and Hypothyroidism. (From Damjanov, I. [2012]. *Pathology for the health professions* [4th ed.]. Saunders.)

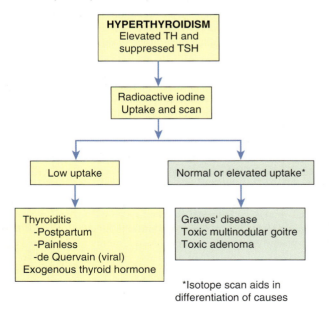

FIGURE 19.6 Evaluation of Hyperthyroidism. The differential diagnosis of hyperthyroidism uses radioactive iodine. *TH*, Thyroid hormone; *TSH*, thyroid-stimulating hormone.

commonly cause *central (secondary) hyperthyroidism*. Thyrotoxicosis not associated with hyperthyroidism includes ectopic thyroid tissue and intake of excessive TH. Each condition is associated with a specific pathophysiology and manifestations. All forms of thyrotoxicosis share some common characteristics.

CLINICAL MANIFESTATIONS The clinical features of thyrotoxicosis are caused by the metabolic effects of increased circulating levels of thyroid hormones. This usually results in an increased metabolic rate. The increase causes heat intolerance and increased tissue sensitivity to stimulation by the sympathetic nervous system. Figure 19.5 summarizes the major manifestations. Enlargement of the thyroid gland (goitre) is common in hyperthyroid conditions caused by stimulation of TSH receptors.

Elevated serum thyroxine (T_4) and tri-iodothyronine (T_3) levels and suppressed serum TSH levels are diagnostic for primary hyperthyroidism. Characteristics of central (secondary) hyperthyroidism caused by TSH-secreting pituitary tumours are normal to increased TSH levels despite elevated TH concentrations. Radioactive iodine is used to test for increased uptake in primary hyperthyroidism (Figure 19.6). The goal of treatment is to control excessive TH production, secretion, or action. Treatment includes antithyroid medication therapy, radioactive iodine therapy (absorbed only by thyroid tissue, causing death of cells), and surgery.[12] A major complication of all treatments for hyperthyroidism is excessive removal of the gland leading to hypothyroidism.

Graves' Disease

Graves' disease is the underlying cause of 50 to 80% of cases of hyperthyroidism. There is a prevalence of approximately 1% of Graves' disease in the Canadian population. It occurs more commonly in women. Although the exact cause of Graves' disease is not known, genetic factors interacting with environmental triggers play an important role in the pathogenesis. Graves' disease is an autoimmune disease and results from a type II hypersensitivity (see Chapter 8). There is stimulation of the thyroid by autoantibodies directed against the TSH receptor. These autoantibodies, called thyroid-stimulating immunoglobulins (TSIs), override the normal regulatory mechanisms. The TSI stimulation of TSH receptors in the gland results in hyperplasia of the gland (goitre) and increased creation of TH, especially of T_3. Increased levels of TH result in the classic signs and symptoms of hyperthyroidism illustrated in Figure 19.5. Inhibition of TSH production by the pituitary is through the usual negative feedback loop.[12]

TSI also contributes to the two major distinguishing clinical manifestations of Graves' disease (ophthalmopathy and dermopathy [pretibial myxedema]). Two categories of ophthalmopathy associated with Graves' disease (Figure 19.7) are (1) functional abnormalities resulting from hyperactivity of the sympathetic division of the autonomic nervous system (lag of the globe on upward gaze and of the upper lid on downward gaze) and (2) infiltrative changes involving the orbital contents with enlargement of the ocular muscles. These changes affect more than half of individuals with Graves' disease. Orbital connective tissue accumulation, inflammation, and edema of the orbital contents result in visual problems. These include exophthalmos (protrusion of the eyeball), periorbital edema, and extraocular muscle weakness, leading to diplopia (double vision).[12] The individual may experience irritation, pain, lacrimation, photophobia, blurred vision, decreased visual acuity, papilledema, visual field impairment, exposure keratosis, and corneal ulceration.

A small number of individuals with Graves' disease and very high levels of TSI experience pretibial myxedema (Graves' dermopathy). This condition is characterized by subcutaneous swelling on the anterior portions of the legs and by indurated and erythematous skin.

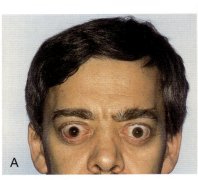
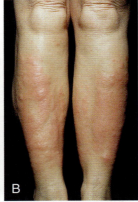

FIGURE 19.7 Thyrotoxicosis (Graves' Disease). **A,** Exophthalmos (large and protruding eyeballs often in association with a large goitre). **B,** Pretibial myxedema associated with Graves' disease; note lumpy and swollen appearance from accumulation of connective tissue and pinkish purple discoloration. ([A], from Belchetz, P., & Hammond, P. [2003]. *Mosby's color atlas and text of diabetes and endocrinology.* Mosby; [B], from Habif, T. [2009]. *Clinical dermatology* [5th ed.]. Mosby.)

Graves' dermopathy is associated with thyrotropin receptor antigens on fibroblasts and recruited T lymphocytes (T cells) that stimulate excessive amounts of hyaluronic acid production in the dermis and subcutaneous tissue.[12] These manifestations occasionally appear on the hands, giving the appearance of clubbing of the fingers (thyroid acropachy).

Hyperthyroidism resulting from nodular thyroid disease. The thyroid gland normally enlarges in response to the increased demand for TH. This demand occurs in puberty, pregnancy, and iodine-deficient states as well as in individuals with immunological, viral, or genetic disorders. When the condition resulting in increased TH resolves, TSH secretion normally subsides and the thyroid gland returns to its original size.

Irreversible changes can occur in some follicular cells. These cells function autonomously and produce excessive amounts of TH. Some follicular cells may cease to function. The balance between the amount of TH produced by hyperfunctioning nodules and that produced by the rest of the gland determines whether an individual develops hyperthyroidism. Toxic multinodular goitre occurs when there are several hyperfunctioning nodules leading to hyperthyroidism. Unlike Graves' disease, there is absence of an autoimmune stimulus. The term toxic adenoma is used if only one nodule is hyperfunctioning. The classic clinical manifestations of hyperthyroidism (see Figure 19.5) usually develop slowly, and exophthalmos and pretibial myxedema do not occur. Nodules may be felt on physical examination and there is increased uptake of radioactive iodine. The incidence of malignancy in toxic nodular goitre is approximately 9%. Most individuals should undergo a fine needle aspiration biopsy of suspicious nodules before treatment. Treatment includes of a combination of radioactive iodine, surgery, and antithyroid medications.[12]

Thyrotoxic crisis. Thyrotoxic crisis (thyroid storm) is a rare but dangerous worsening of the thyrotoxic state in which death can occur within 48 hours without treatment. The condition may develop spontaneously, but it usually occurs in individuals who have undiagnosed or partially treated Graves' disease and are subjected to excessive stress, such as infection, pulmonary or cardiovascular disorders, trauma, seizures, surgery (especially thyroid surgery), obstetrical complications, emotional distress, or dialysis. The increased action of T_4 and T_3 exceeding metabolic demands cause the symptoms of a thyroid crisis.[22]

The systemic symptoms of thyrotoxic crisis include hyperthermia; tachycardia; high-output heart failure; agitation or delirium; and nausea, vomiting, or diarrhea contributing to fluid volume depletion. Treatment includes (1) the use of medications that block TH synthesis (i.e., propylthiouracil or methimazole), (2) the use of beta-blockers for control of cardiovascular symptoms, the administration of (3) steroids or (4) iodine, and (5) supportive care.

Hypothyroidism

Hypothyroidism results from deficient production of TH by the thyroid gland. Hypothyroidism is the most common disorder of thyroid function. This affects 2% of the Canadian population and occurs more commonly in women.[23] It may be primary or central. Primary hypothyroidism accounts for most cases. Central (secondary) hypothyroidism is less common and is related to either pituitary or hypothalamic failure.

The most common cause of primary hypothyroidism in Canada is autoimmune thyroiditis (Hashimoto's disease, chronic lymphocytic thyroiditis). This results in gradual inflammatory destruction of thyroid tissue by infiltration of autoreactive T cells and circulating thyroid autoantibodies (antithyroid peroxidase and antithyroglobulin antibodies). There are several genetic risk factors associated with this disorder. It is also commonly associated with other autoimmune conditions.

Infiltration of thyroid autoantibodies, autoreactive T cells, natural killer cells, and inflammatory cytokines and induction of apoptosis are involved in the tissue destruction seen in Hashimoto's thyroiditis.[24] Radioactive iodine uptake is normal or elevated.

Three conditions experience spontaneous recovery of thyroid function: subacute thyroiditis, painless thyroiditis, and postpartum thyroiditis. **Subacute thyroiditis (de Quervain's thyroiditis)** is a rare nonbacterial inflammation of the thyroid gland often preceded by a viral infection. Fever, tenderness, and enlargement of the thyroid gland go with this condition. The inflammatory process initially results in elevated levels of TH through the release of stored thyroglobulin. This elevated level is then associated with transient hypothyroidism before the gland recovers normal activity. Thyroid antibodies are not present in the blood. Symptoms may last for 2 to 4 months, and nonsteroidal anti-inflammatory medications or corticosteroids usually resolve symptoms. **Painless (silent) thyroiditis** has a course like that of subacute thyroiditis but is pathologically identical to Hashimoto's disease. **Postpartum thyroiditis** is pathologically related to Hashimoto's disease and generally occurs up to 6 months after delivery with a course like that seen in subacute thyroiditis. Thus, a hyperthyroid phase (with a low thyroid radioiodine uptake) precedes the hypothyroid phase in typical cases of subacute, painless, or postpartum thyroiditis. Spontaneous recovery occurs in 95% of these conditions.

Congenital Hypothyroidism

Hypothyroidism in infants occurs when thyroid tissue is absent (thyroid dysgenesis) or with hereditary defects in TH synthesis. Thyroid dysgenesis occurs more often in female infants, with permanent abnormalities in 1 of every 4000 live births. Because TH is essential for embryonic growth, particularly of brain tissue, the infant will be cognitively disabled if there is no T_4 during fetal life.[12] The fetus is dependent on maternal T_4 for the first 20 weeks of gestation.[12] Hypothyroidism may not be evident at birth. Symptoms may include high birth weight, hypothermia, delay in passing meconium, and neonatal jaundice. Examination of cord blood in the first days of life can provide T_4 and TSH levels. Normal growth and intellectual function can occur if treatment with levothyroxine takes place before the child is 3 or 4 months old. The earlier TH replacement is started, the better the child's outcome.[25]

Without early screening, hypothyroidism may not be clear until after 4 months of age. Symptoms include difficulty eating, hoarse cry, and protruding tongue caused by myxedema of oral tissues and vocal cords. Hypotonic muscles of the abdomen with constipation, abdominal protrusion, and umbilical hernia may also occur. Subnormal temperature; lethargy; excessive sleeping; slow pulse rate; and cold, mottled skin may be present. Decreased skeletal growth occurs because of impaired protein synthesis, poor absorption of nutrients, and lack of bone mineralization. The untreated child will be dwarfed with short limbs. A delay in dentition often occurs. Cognitive disability varies with the severity of hypothyroidism and the length of delay before treatment is started.

PATHOPHYSIOLOGY In *primary hypothyroidism*, loss of thyroid function leads to decreased production of TH and increased secretion of TSH and TRH (Figure 19.8). The most common causes of primary hypothyroidism in adults include autoimmune thyroiditis (Hashimoto's disease), loss of thyroid tissue after surgical or radioactive treatment for hyperthyroidism or after head and neck radiation therapy, medications (e.g., lithium and amiodarone [Cordarone]), and geographic iodine deficiency. Infants and children may present with hypothyroidism because of congenital defects. The cause of central

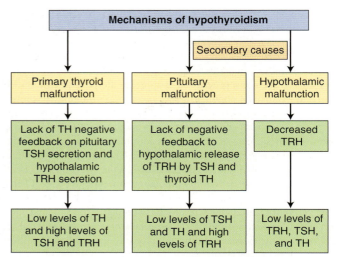

FIGURE 19.8 Mechanisms of Primary and Secondary Hypothyroidism. *TH*, Thyroid hormone; *TRH*, thyrotropin-releasing hormone; *TSH*, thyroid-stimulating hormone.

(secondary) hypothyroidism is the pituitary does not synthesize adequate amounts of TSH or there is a lack of TRH. Pituitary tumours that compress surrounding pituitary cells, or the results of their treatment are the most common causes of central hypothyroidism. Other causes include traumatic brain injury, subarachnoid hemorrhage, or pituitary infarction. Hypothalamic dysfunction results in low levels of TH, TSH, and TRH.[12] **Subclinical hypothyroidism** is a mild thyroid failure estimated to occur in 4 to 8% of adults. An elevation in TSH levels with normal levels of circulating TH represents this condition.[26]

CLINICAL MANIFESTATIONS Hypothyroidism generally affects all body systems and occurs gradually over months or years. The decrease in TH level lowers energy metabolism and heat production. The individual develops a low basal metabolic rate, cold intolerance, lethargy, and slightly lowered basal body temperature (see Figure 19.5). The decrease in the level of TH can lead to too much TSH production, which stimulates thyroid tissue and causes goitre.

The characteristic sign of severe or longstanding hypothyroidism is **myxedema**. This results from the altered makeup of the dermis and other tissues. Large amounts of protein and mucopolysaccharide separate the connective tissue fibres. This complex binds water, producing nonpitting, boggy edema. The edema occurs especially around the eyes, hands, and feet and in the supraclavicular fossae (Figure 19.9). The tongue and laryngeal and pharyngeal mucous membranes thicken, producing thick, slurred speech and hoarseness. **Myxedema coma**, a medical emergency, is a decreased level of consciousness associated with severe hypothyroidism. Signs and symptoms include hypothermia without shivering, hypoventilation, hypotension, hypoglycemia, and lactic acidosis. Older persons with comorbid conditions, such as pulmonary or urinary infections, heart failure, or cerebrovascular accident, and with moderate or untreated hypothyroidism are particularly at risk of developing myxedema coma. It also may occur after overuse of opioids or sedatives or after an acute illness in hypothyroid individuals. Symptoms of hypothyroidism in older persons should not be considered normal aging changes.[27]

EVALUATION AND TREATMENT The documentation of the clinical symptoms of hypothyroidism, and measurement of increased levels of TSH and decreased levels of TH (total T_3 and both total and free T_4)

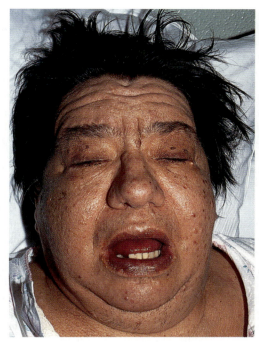

FIGURE 19.9 Myxedema. Note edema around eyes and facial puffiness. The hair is dry. (From Bolognia, J. L., Jorizzo, J., & Schaffer, J. [2012]. *Dermatology* [3rd ed.]. Mosby.)

help in the diagnosis of primary hypothyroidism. When pituitary deficiencies are the cause of hypothyroidism, serum TSH levels and basal metabolic rate (BMR) decrease. Hormone replacement therapy with the hormone levothyroxine (Synthroid) is the treatment of choice. The return of normal TH levels should be timed appropriately. A regimen of hormonal therapy depends on the individual's age, the duration and severity of the hypothyroidism, and the presence of other disorders, particularly cardiovascular disorders.[12] Pregnant women need to be tested for thyroid function.[28]

Thyroid Carcinoma

Thyroid carcinoma is the seventh most common cancer in Canada. It is estimated that 8 600 persons will have been diagnosed with this disease in 2020. The incidence rates of thyroid cancer have been increasing significantly worldwide. The reasons for this trend are unclear. Researchers are examining the role of suspected lifestyle and reproductive factors related to this increased incidence.[29] Exposure to ionizing radiation, especially during childhood, is the most consistent causal factor. Papillary and follicular thyroid carcinomas are the most common types. Medullary and anaplastic thyroid carcinomas are less common. Most tumours are well differentiated.

Most individuals with thyroid carcinoma have normal T_3 and T_4 levels and are therefore euthyroid. Discovery of this cancer is typically in the form of a small thyroid nodule or metastatic tumour in the lungs, brain, or bone. Changes in voice and swallowing and difficulty breathing are related to tumour growth affecting the trachea or esophagus. Ultrasonographic characteristics may be suggestive of malignancy but are neither sensitive nor specific.[12] Fine-needle aspiration of a thyroid nodule usually confirms the diagnosis of thyroid cancer.

Treatment may include partial or total thyroidectomy, TSH suppression therapy (levothyroxine), radioactive iodine therapy (in iodine-concentrating tumours), postoperative radiation therapy, and chemotherapy (especially in anaplastic carcinoma). New research into the molecular pathogenesis of thyroid carcinoma is leading to new therapies.[30]

ALTERATIONS OF PARATHYROID FUNCTION

 QUICK CHECK 19.3
1. How does excessive parathyroid hormone (PTH) affect bones?
2. What are the results of a lack of circulating PTH?

Hyperparathyroidism

Greater-than-normal secretion of parathyroid hormone (PTH) and hypercalcemia characterizes hyperparathyroidism. Classification of hyperparathyroidism is as primary, secondary, or tertiary.[12]

PATHOPHYSIOLOGY Inappropriate excess secretion of PTH by one or more of the parathyroid glands characterizes primary hyperparathyroidism. It is one of the most common endocrine disorders. Parathyroid adenomas account for approximately 80 to 85% of cases. Parathyroid hyperplasia account for another 10 to 15%, and parathyroid carcinoma for about 1% of cases. A variety of genetic causes may result in primary hyperparathyroidism, especially the genes that cause multiple endocrine neoplasia.[31]

Primary hyperparathyroidism presents with an increase in PTH secretion. The usual feedback control mechanisms with this condition are impaired. The calcium level in the blood increases because of increased bone resorption and GI absorption of calcium. However, this increase does not inhibit PTH secretion by the parathyroid gland.

Secondary hyperparathyroidism is a compensatory response of the parathyroid glands to chronic hypocalcemia. This condition can be associated with decreased renal activation of vitamin D (renal failure) (see Chapter 30). There is an increased secretion of PTH, but PTH cannot achieve normal calcium levels because of insufficient levels of activated vitamin D. Other causes of secondary hyperparathyroidism include dietary deficiency in vitamin D or calcium and decreased intestinal absorption of vitamin D or calcium. The ingestion of medications, such as phenytoin (Dilantin), phenobarbital, and laxatives, which either accelerate the metabolism of vitamin D or decrease intestinal absorption of calcium can also be a cause.

Tertiary hyperparathyroidism is excessive secretion of PTH and hypercalcemia that occurs after longstanding secondary hyperparathyroidism. The etiology is unknown but is autonomous secretion of PTH from persistent parathyroid stimulation even after withdrawal of calcium and calcitriol therapy.[12] Treatment is surgical removal of one of the parathyroid glands.

CLINICAL MANIFESTATIONS Hypercalcemia and hypophosphatemia are the hallmarks of primary hyperparathyroidism. The discovery of these conditions may be incidental. Hypercalcemia and hypophosphatemia may be asymptomatic. Affected individuals may also present with symptoms related to the muscular, nervous, and GI systems. These symptoms can include fatigue, headache, depression, anorexia, and nausea and vomiting. Excessive osteoclastic and osteocytic activity resulting in bone resorption may cause pathological fractures, kyphosis of the dorsal spine, and compression fractures of the vertebral bodies. (Chapter 39 discusses bone resorption.)

The increased renal filtration load of calcium leads to increased calcium in the urine. Hypercalcemia also affects proximal renal tubular function. This dysfunction causes metabolic acidosis and production of an abnormally alkaline urine.[12] PTH hypersecretion increases renal phosphate excretion and results in hypophosphatemia (see Chapter 5) and increased phosphate in the urine. The combination of these three variables—hypercalciuria, alkaline urine, and hyperphosphaturia—predisposes the individual to the formation of calcium stones. These stones occur more often in the renal pelvis or renal collecting ducts. These may be associated with infections. Both kidney stones and renal infection can lead to impaired renal function. Hypercalcemia also impairs the concentrating ability of the renal tubule by decreasing its response to ADH. Chronic hypercalcemia of hyperparathyroidism is associated with mild insulin resistance, causing increased insulin secretion to support normal glucose levels.

Secondary hyperparathyroidism caused by renal disease presents clinically with bone resorption and symptoms of hypocalcemia and hyperphosphatemia. Hypocalcemia can cause many significant clinical problems (see Chapter 5). Hyperphosphatemia can cause harmful effects on the cardiovascular system.

EVALUATION AND TREATMENT The findings of increased ionized calcium concentration despite elevated PTH concentration are suggestive of primary hyperparathyroidism. PTH levels also may be inappropriately within the normal range because hypercalcemia should completely suppress PTH production. Treatment suggestion for asymptomatic individuals with mild hypercalcemia includes observation. These individuals are recommended to avoid dehydration and limit their dietary calcium intake. The best treatment of severe primary hyperparathyroidism involves surgical removal of the solitary adenoma. In the case of hyperplasia, complete removal of three and partial removal of the fourth hyperplastic parathyroid glands should occur. In those individuals for whom surgery is not an option, other treatments such as bisphosphonates and calcimimetics (e.g., cinacalcet [Sensipar]) may be considered.

Secondary hyperparathyroidism is likely if serum calcium concentration is low, but PTH level is high. Evaluation for renal function may show chronic renal disease. Treatment for secondary hyperparathyroidism in chronic renal disease is threefold. It requires calcium replacement, dietary phosphate restriction and phosphate binders, and vitamin D replacement. Treatment also may include calcimimetics, which work to increase parathyroid calcium receptor sensitivity, thus lowering PTH levels.[32]

Hypoparathyroidism

Hypoparathyroidism (abnormally low PTH levels) is usually caused by damage to the parathyroid glands during thyroid surgery. This occurs because of the closeness of the parathyroid glands to the thyroid (see Figure 18.11). Hypoparathyroidism also is associated with genetic syndromes, including familial hypoparathyroidism and DiGeorge syndrome (see Chapter 8). Hypomagnesemia also can cause a decrease in PTH secretion and PTH function. An idiopathic or autoimmune form of hypoparathyroidism also exists.[33]

There is an inherited condition associated with hypocalcemia but with normal to elevated levels of PTH called *pseudohypoparathyroidism*. A postreceptor defect in PTH action causes this condition.

PATHOPHYSIOLOGY A lack of circulating PTH causes depressed serum calcium levels and increased serum phosphate levels. In the absence of PTH, resorption of calcium from bone and regulation of calcium reabsorption from the renal tubules are impaired. As a result, phosphate reabsorption by the renal tubules is increased. This increase causes decreased renal phosphate excretion and hyperphosphatemia.

Hypomagnesemia inhibits PTH secretion. When serum magnesium levels return to normal, however, PTH secretion returns to normal. The responsiveness of peripheral tissues to PTH also returns.

Hypomagnesemia may be related to chronic alcoholism, malnutrition, and malabsorption. Other causes include increased renal clearance of magnesium caused by using aminoglycoside antibiotics or certain chemotherapeutic agents, or prolonged magnesium-deficient parenteral nutritional therapy.

CLINICAL MANIFESTATIONS Symptoms associated with hypoparathyroidism are primarily those of hypocalcemia (see Table 5.7). Hypocalcemia causes a lowered threshold for nerve and muscle excitation. Therefore, a slight stimulus may initiate a nerve impulse anywhere along the length of a nerve or muscle fibre. This creates tetany, a condition characterized by muscle spasms, hyper-reflexia, clonic-tonic convulsions, laryngeal spasms, and, in severe cases, death by asphyxiation. Neuromuscular irritability may be evaluated using Trousseau's and Chvostek's signs. Elicitation of Chvostek's sign occurs by tapping the patient's cheek, resulting in twitching of the upper lip. Elicitation of Trousseau's sign occurs by sustained inflation of a sphygmomanometer placed on the patient's upper arm to a level above the systolic blood pressure. A positive result is a painful carpal spasm. Other symptoms of hypocalcemia include dry skin, loss of body and scalp hair, hypoplasia of developing teeth, horizontal ridges on the nails, cataracts, and basal ganglia calcifications (which may be associated with a parkinsonian syndrome). Bone deformities, including brachydactyly and bowing of the long bones, may also occur.

Hypoparathyroidism is also associated with phosphate retention caused by increased renal reabsorption of phosphate. Hyperphosphatemia results from PTH deficiency. Hyperphosphatemia further lowers calcium concentration by inhibiting the activation of vitamin D, thereby lowering the GI absorption of calcium.

EVALUATION AND TREATMENT Hypoparathyroidism is suggested with a low serum calcium concentration and a high phosphorous level in the absence of renal failure, intestinal disorders, or nutritional deficiencies. PTH levels are low in hypoparathyroidism. The measurement of serum magnesium level and urinary calcium excretion also can help in diagnosis. Alleviation of the hypocalcemia is the treatment of choice. In acute states, this treatment involves parenteral administration of calcium. This treatment corrects serum calcium concentration within minutes. Maintenance of serum calcium level is achieved with pharmacological doses of cholecalciferol (vitamin D_3) and oral calcium.[12] Hypoplastic dentition, cataracts, bone deformities, and basal ganglia calcifications do not respond to the correction of hypocalcemia. The other symptoms of hypocalcemia are reversible.

DYSFUNCTION OF THE ENDOCRINE PANCREAS: DIABETES MELLITUS

QUICK CHECK 19.4
1. What are the major differences between type 1 and type 2 diabetes mellitus in relation to insulin?
2. How does obesity contribute to the development of type 2 diabetes?
3. What are three metabolic changes related to hyperglycemia that contribute to diabetic complications?
4. What is the single most important factor to address in the management of diabetes mellitus?

Diabetes mellitus is a group of metabolic diseases characterized by hyperglycemia. The hyperglycemia results from defects in insulin secretion, insulin action, or both. Diabetes Canada estimates that in 2020 Canada had a 10% prevalence rate of diabetes. By 2030, it is

TABLE 19.3 Epidemiology and Etiology of Diabetes Mellitus in Canada

	Type 1 Diabetes: Primary Beta-Cell Defect or Failure	Type 2 Diabetes: Insulin Resistance With Inadequate Insulin Secretion
Incidence		
Frequency	10% of all cases of diabetes mellitus. In 2019, about 11 million Canadians were living with diabetes or prediabetes.	Accounts for most cases (90%). Incidence rate for all diabetes in adults over the age of 20 is 6.3 per 100 000 population. Estimated prevalence of diabetes: 4.2% in 2000, 7.6% in 2010, 10.8% in 2018, 11.9% in 2023, and 13.1% in 2028
Change in incidences	Rates among children and youth have been increasing globally. Canada has one of the highest incidence rates of type 1 diabetes for children under 14 years of age.	Between 2000 and 2016, the number of Canadians living with diabetes increased by an average of 3.3% per year. Diabetes Canada predicts a 39% increase in diabetes (type 1 and type 2 diagnosed) between 2019–2029. Currently 29% of Canadians live with diabetes, undiagnosed diabetes, or prediabetes.
Characteristics		
Age at onset	Peak onset at age 11–13 years (slightly earlier for girls than for boys); rare in children younger than 1 year and adults older than 30 years	Risk of developing diabetes increases after age 40 years. Incidence is increasing among youth.
Gender	Similar in males and females	More males than females
Racial distribution	Rate for White people is 1.5–2 times higher than for visible minorities.	Diabetes diagnosed among Indigenous people is described as an epidemic, with a prevalence three times or higher than that of the general population. In addition, people of South and Southeast Asian, African, and Latin American descent have higher rates of childhood type 2 diabetes, gestational diabetes mellitus, and type 2 diabetes.
Obesity	Generally normal or underweight	Frequent contributing factor to precipitate type 2 diabetes among those susceptible
Etiology		
Common theory	*Autoimmune:* genetic and environmental factors, resulting in gradual process of autoimmune destruction in genetically susceptible individuals. *Nonautoimmune:* Unknown	Genetic susceptibility (polygenic) combined with environmental determinants; defects in beta-cell function combined with insulin resistance. Associated with long-duration obesity
Presence of antibody	Autoantibodies to insulin and to glutamic acid decarboxylase (GAD_{65})	Autoantibodies not present
Insulin resistance	Insulin resistance at diagnosis is unusual, but may occur as individual ages and gains weight.	Insulin resistance is virtually universal and multifactorial in origin.
Insulin secretion	Severe insulin deficiency or no insulin secretion at all	Typically increased at time of diagnosis, but progressively declines over course of illness

Data from Diabetes Canada. (n.d.). *Diabetes: Canada at the tipping point: charting a new path.* https://www.diabetes.ca/CDA/media/documents/publications-and-newsletters/advocacy-reports/canada-at-the-tipping-point-english.pdf; Public Health Agency of Canada. (2011). *Diabetes in Canada: facts and figures from a public health perspective.* https://www.phac-aspc.gc.ca/cd-mc/publications/diabetes-diabete/facts-figures-faits-chiffres-2011/index-eng.php; Public Health Agency of Canada. (2019). *Twenty years of diabetes surveillance using the Canadian Chronic Disease Surveillance System.* https://www.canada.ca/en/public-health/services/publications/diseases-conditions/20-years-diabetes-surveillance.html; Diabetes Canada. (2019). *Diabetes in Canada: backgrounder.* https://www.diabetes.ca/DiabetesCanadaWebsite/media/About-Diabetes/Diabetes%20Charter/2019-Backgrounder-Canada.pdf.

estimated that the prevalence will have increased to 12%.[34] Diabetes rates are three to five times higher in Indigenous populations than in the general population.[34]

Diabetes Canada classifies four categories of diabetes mellitus[35] (Table 19.3), as follows:

1. Type 1 (beta-cell destruction, usually leading to total insulin deficiency).
2. Type 2 (ranging from predominantly insulin resistance with relative insulin deficiency to predominantly an insulin secretory defect with insulin resistance).
3. Other specific types.
4. Gestational diabetes.

The diagnosis of diabetes mellitus is made using various laboratory tests. These tests include **glycosylated hemoglobin (A1C)** levels; fasting plasma glucose (FPG) levels; 2-hour plasma glucose levels during oral glucose tolerance testing (OGTT) using a 75-g oral glucose load; or random glucose levels in an individual with symptoms (Box 19.1).[35] Glycosylated hemoglobin refers to the permanent attachment of glucose to hemoglobin molecules. The test results reflect the average plasma glucose exposure over the life of a red blood cell (about 120 days). The A_{1C} test gives a more exact measure of long-term control of blood glucose levels. This test is critically dependent on the method of measurement and must be related to established standards.

Diabetes Canada classification "prediabetes" describes nondiabetic elevations of A_{1C}, FPG, or 2-hour plasma glucose value during OGTT (see Box 19.1).[35] Diabetes Canada estimates that nearly 6 million Canadians currently have prediabetes.[36] Prediabetes includes impaired glucose tolerance (IGT), which results from decreased insulin secretion,

BOX 19.1 Diagnostic Criteria for Diabetes Mellitus

1. $A_{1C} \geq 6.5\%$ in adults using a standardized, validated assay in the absence of factors that affect the accuracy of the A_{1C} and not for suspected type 1 diabetes
   OR
2. FPG ≥ 7.0 mmol/L (fasting is defined as no caloric intake for at least 8 hours)*
   OR
3. 2-hr PG in a 75 g OGTT ≥ 11.1 mmol/L*
   OR
4. Random PG ≥ 11.1 mmol/L

Diagnosis of Prediabetes
1. FPG 6.1–6.9 mmol/L
   OR
2. 2-hr PG in a 75 g OGTT 7.8–11.0 mmol/L
   OR
3. A_{1C} 6.0–6.4%

*In the absence of symptomatic hyperglycemia, if a single laboratory test result is in the diabetes range, a repeat confirmatory laboratory test (FPG, A_{1C}, 2-hr PG in a 75 g OGTT) must be done on another day. It is preferable that the same test be repeated (in a timely fashion) for confirmation, but a random PG in the diabetes range in an asymptomatic individual should be confirmed with an alternate test. In the case of symptomatic hyperglycemia, the diagnosis has been made and a confirmatory test is not required before treatment is initiated. If results of 2 different tests are available and both are above the diagnostic thresholds, the diagnosis of diabetes is confirmed. To avoid rapid metabolic deterioration in individuals in whom type 1 diabetes is likely (younger or lean or symptomatic hyperglycemia, especially with ketonuria or ketonemia), the initiation of treatment should not be delayed to complete confirmatory testing.

A_{1C}, Hemoglobin A_{1C} or glycosylated hemoglobin; *FPG*, fasting plasma glucose; *OGTT*, oral glucose tolerance testing; *PG*, plasma glucose.

Data from Diabetes Canada Clinical Practice Guidelines Expert Committee. (2018). *Canadian Journal of Diabetes, 42*(Suppl. 1), S1–S325. http://guidelines.diabetes.ca/docs/CPG-2018-full-EN.pdf.

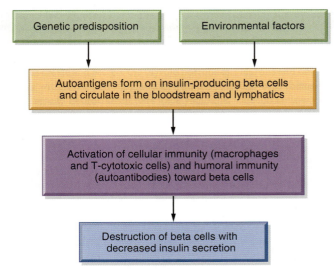

FIGURE 19.10 Pathophysiology of Type 1 Diabetes Mellitus.

Autoimmune type 1 diabetes mellitus is a slowly progressive autoimmune T-cell–mediated disease that destroys beta cells of the pancreas. There is a deficient immune tolerance linked to abnormalities in immune cells and changes in beta-cell antigens. Destruction of beta cells is related to genetic and environmental factors. The strongest genetic association is with human leukocyte antigen (HLA) class II alleles *HLA-DQ* and *HLA-DR*. The *HLA-DR* marker is associated with other autoimmune disorders, such as celiac, Graves', Hashimoto's, and Addison's diseases. Linked environmental factors include exposure to certain medications, foods, and viruses. These gene–environment interactions result in the formation of autoantigens that are expressed on the surface of pancreatic beta cells. These autoantigens circulate in the bloodstream and lymphatics (Figure 19.10). Stimulation of cellular immunity (T-cytotoxic cells and macrophages) and humoral immunity (autoantibodies) occurs, resulting in beta-cell destruction and apoptosis. The destruction of beta cells results from lymphocyte and macrophage infiltration of the islets. This process results in release of inflammatory cytokines, activation of T-helper and T-cytotoxic lymphocytes, and death of islet beta cells. The production of autoantibodies against islet cells, insulin, glutamic acid decarboxylase (GAD), and other cytoplasmic proteins also mediates beta-cell destruction.[38] Insulin synthesis declines and hyperglycemia develops over time.

For insulin synthesis to decline enough such that hyperglycemia occurs, destruction of 80 to 90% of the insulin-secreting beta cells of the islets of Langerhans must occur. Insulin normally suppresses secretion of glucagon. The resulting hypoinsulinemia leads to a marked increase in glucagon secretion. Glucagon, a hormone produced by the alpha cells of the islets, acts in the liver to increase blood glucose level. This is done by stimulating glycogenolysis and gluconeogenesis. In addition to the decline in insulin secretion, there is also a decrease in the secretion of amylin, another beta-cell hormone. One of the key actions of amylin is to suppress glucagon release from the alpha cells. Thus, both alpha-cell and beta-cell functions are abnormal. Both a lack of insulin and a relative excess of glucagon contribute to hyperglycemia in type 1 diabetes.

CLINICAL MANIFESTATIONS In the past, type 1 diabetes was thought to have an abrupt onset. It is now known, however, that the natural history involves a long preclinical period with gradual destruction of beta cells. This destruction eventually leads to insulin deficiency and hyperglycemia. This latent period is longer in adults with onset of type

and impaired fasting glucose (IFG), which is caused by enhanced hepatic glucose output. Individuals with IGT and IFG are at increased risk for cardiovascular disease and premature death and carry a 15 to 50% 5-year risk of developing diabetes, particularly type 2 diabetes.[35] Thus, prevention of diabetes with lifestyle interventions is essential.[36]

Types of Diabetes Mellitus

Type 1 Diabetes Mellitus

Type 1 diabetes mellitus is the most common pediatric chronic disease, with about 10% of Canadians having this form of diabetes. The Canadian prevalence rate of diabetes in children aged 19 years and under is 0.3%, and the incidence is increasing.[37] Between 10 and 13% of individuals with newly diagnosed type 1 diabetes have a first-degree relative (parent or sibling) with type 1 diabetes. There is a 50% concordance rate in twins. Diagnosis is rare during the first 9 months of life and peaks at 12 years of age. Two distinct types of type 1 diabetes have been identified: idiopathic and autoimmune.

PATHOPHYSIOLOGY Idiopathic type 1 diabetes is far less common than autoimmune diabetes. This type of diabetes has a strong genetic link and occurs mostly in people of Asian or African descent. Affected individuals have varying degrees of insulin deficiency.

TABLE 19.4 Clinical Manifestations and Mechanisms for Type 1 Diabetes Mellitus

Manifestation	Rationale
Polydipsia	Because of elevated blood glucose levels, water is osmotically attracted from body cells. This results in intracellular dehydration and stimulation of thirst in hypothalamus.
Polyuria	Hyperglycemia acts as an osmotic diuretic. The amount of glucose filtered by glomeruli of kidney exceeds that which can be reabsorbed by renal tubules. Glycosuria results, accompanied by large amounts of water lost in urine.
Polyphagia	Depletion of cellular stores of carbohydrates, fats, and protein results in cellular starvation and a corresponding increase in hunger.
Weight loss	Weight loss occurs because of fluid loss in osmotic diuresis and loss of body tissue as fats and proteins are used for energy.
Fatigue	Metabolic changes result in poor use of food products, leading to lethargy and fatigue.
Recurrent infections (e.g., boils, carbuncles, and bladder infection)	The increased glucose levels stimulate growth of microorganisms. Diabetes is associated with some immunocompromised individuals.
Prolonged wound healing	Impaired blood supply hinders healing.
Genital pruritus	Hyperglycemia and glycosuria favour fungal growth. Candidal infections, resulting in pruritus, are a common presenting symptom in women.
Visual changes	Blurred vision occurs as water balance in eye fluctuates because of elevated blood glucose levels. Diabetic retinopathy may follow.
Paresthesias	Paresthesias are common manifestations of diabetic neuropathies.
Cardiovascular symptoms (e.g., chest pain, extremity pain, and neurological deficits)	Diabetes contributes to formation of atherosclerotic plaques that involve coronary, peripheral, and cerebrovascular circulations and alterations in microvessels.

1 diabetes and often results in misclassification of those affected as having type 2 diabetes.

Type 1 diabetes affects the metabolism of fat, protein, and carbohydrates. Glucose builds up in the blood and appears in the urine as the renal threshold for glucose is exceeded. This accumulation produces an osmotic diuresis and symptoms of polyuria and thirst (Table 19.4). Wide ranges in blood glucose levels occur. In addition, protein and fat breakdown occurs because of the lack of insulin, resulting in weight loss. Increased metabolism of fats and proteins leads to high levels of circulating ketones, causing a condition known as diabetic ketoacidosis (DKA).

Currently half of individuals with type 1 diabetes are obese. As a result, an increasing number of individuals have both type 1 diabetes and the clinical manifestations of metabolic syndrome, including obesity, dyslipidemia, and hypertension[12] (see Box 19.1). These individuals are at high risk for chronic complications of diabetes, including heart disease and stroke.

EVALUATION AND TREATMENT The criteria for diagnosis of type 1 diabetes are the same as those for type 2 diabetes[35] (see Box 19.1). Many children are diagnosed when they present with the signs and symptoms of DKA. In DKA, exhalation of acetone (a volatile form of ketones) by hyperventilation occurs and gives the breath a sweet or "fruity" odour. Occasionally, diabetic coma is the first symptom of the disease. The diagnosis of diabetes is not difficult when the symptoms of polydipsia, polyuria, polyphagia, weight loss, and hyperglycemia are present in fasting and postprandial states. Measurement of serum C-peptide, a part of proinsulin released during insulin production, is used as a substitute for insulin levels. This measurement is indicative of residual beta-cell mass and function. For diagnosis of type 1 diabetes, the zinc transporter 8 autoantibody (ZnT8Ab) is used. Other important aspects of evaluation include looking for evidence of the chronic complications of type 1 diabetes. These complications include renal, nervous system, cardiac, peripheral vascular, retinal, and bony tissue damage.

Currently, treatment regimens are designed to achieve optimal glucose level control (as measured by the A_{1C} value) without causing significant hypoglycemia events.[35] Management requires individual planning according to type of disease, age, and activity level. All individuals require some combination of insulin therapy, meal planning, and exercise. Several different types of insulin preparations are available. There are new technologies for more physiological insulin delivery systems (e.g., insulin pump therapy).[35] Many different kinds of therapies are being tested to prevent the autoimmune destruction of beta cells. One therapy includes immunosuppression with antirejection medications (see *Health Promotion: Type 1 Diabetes Mellitus*). Finally, islet cell, stem cell, and whole pancreas transplantation has been successful in some individuals.[12]

Type 2 Diabetes Mellitus

Type 2 diabetes mellitus accounts for 90% of all diabetes in Canada.[34] There is an increased prevalence among Indigenous people, as well as people of South and Southeast Asian, African, and Latin American descent. In Canada, the prevalence of diabetes was 17.2% among First Nations individuals living on-reserve, 10.3% among First Nations individuals living off-reserve, and 7.3% among Métis individuals, compared to 5.0% in the non-Indigenous population.[35] There also is an increased prevalence of type 2 diabetes in children, especially those who are obese (see Table 19.3).

A genetic and environmental interaction appears to be responsible for type 2 diabetes.[36] The most well-recognized risk factors are age, obesity, hypertension, physical inactivity, and family history. Researchers have linked more than 60 genes to type 2 diabetes. These genes include those that code for beta-cell mass and beta-cell function (ability to sense blood glucose levels, insulin synthesis, and insulin secretion). Other links include proinsulin and insulin molecular structures, insulin receptors, hepatic synthesis of glucose, glucagon synthesis, and cellular responsiveness to insulin stimulation.[39] These genetic abnormalities, combined with environmental impacts such as obesity, result in the basic pathophysiological mechanisms of type 2 diabetes. These two mechanisms are insulin resistance and decreased insulin secretion by beta cells (Figure 19.11).

There is increasing evidence that diet, including diet during pregnancy, influences the long-term risk of developing type 2 diabetes in children and adults.[40] Metabolic syndrome is a group of disorders (central obesity, dyslipidemia, prehypertension, and an elevated fasting

> **HEALTH PROMOTION**
> *Type 1 Diabetes Mellitus*
>
> An understanding of the exact causes of type 1 diabetes mellitus is not clear. Researchers believe that behavioural patterns, paired with environmental factors, often speed up the disease in genetically disposed people. Studies have shown that the interaction between genetic and environmental factors varies among populations and ethnic groups. Type 1 diabetes is most often associated with the White population, particularly those of northern European descent.
>
> Unfortunately, preventive measures for type 1 diabetes remain unclear. Genetic and environmental risk factors have been found related to type 1 diabetes. By targeting environmental risk factors, increasing awareness of diabetes, and finding people at risk, people may be able to reduce or delay the development of type 1 diabetes.
>
> A person who has a first-degree relative with type 1 diabetes has a 10% chance of developing the disease. Researchers have named several genes they suspect are linked with type 1 diabetes. One specific gene that can accurately predict the development of diabetes has not been found.
>
> Viral infections, especially enteroviruses and dietary microbial toxins, are suspected as factors that may lead to the development of type 1 diabetes. Studies have also revealed possible risk factors, which may include exposure to autoantibodies and cow's milk protein in infancy. When considering the global increased incidence of type 1 diabetes, studies have shown possible contributing factors. These include changes in early feeding patterns, early growth in the first year of life, and the use of antibacterial disinfectants.
>
> When considering the prevention of type 1 diabetes, researchers have become aware of factors that may reduce the risk of developing the disease. These factors include breastfeeding and ensuring optimal vitamin D levels. Researchers feel that breastfeeding has a protective effect from developing type 1 diabetes. A short duration of breastfeeding, however, has been found to be a predisposing factor, especially for those at an increased genetic risk. Researchers also suggest that obesity may promote the development of insulin resistance. This resistance in turn triggers an autoimmune response resulting in the destruction of pancreatic beta cells.

Data from Public Health Agency of Canada. (2011). *Diabetes in Canada: facts and figures from a public health perspective.* http://www.phac-aspc.gc.ca/cd-mc/publications/diabetes-diabete/facts-figures-faits-chiffres-2011/index-eng.php.

blood glucose level) that together give a high risk of developing type 2 diabetes and associated cardiovascular complications (Box 19.2). Estimates show that 19% of Canadian adults have metabolic syndrome, and in those over the age of 65 years, 40% have metabolic syndrome.[41] Metabolic syndrome often develops during childhood and is prevalent among overweight children and adolescents. Many of the same genetic and environmental risks as type 2 diabetes are present in metabolic syndrome. Screening of individuals at risk should take place regularly (see Box 19.2). Early recognition and treatment are critical to reducing cardiovascular events and improving clinical outcomes for individuals with prediabetes and metabolic syndrome. This treatment includes rigorous lifestyle changes.[42]

PATHOPHYSIOLOGY Many organs contribute to insulin resistance, chronic hyperglycemia, and the effects of type 2 diabetes (Figure 19.12). A suboptimal response of insulin-sensitive tissues (especially liver, muscle, and adipose tissue) to insulin defines the term **insulin resistance**. It is associated with obesity. Several mechanisms are involved in abnormalities of the insulin signalling pathway and contribute to insulin resistance. These mechanisms include an abnormality of the insulin molecule, high amounts of insulin antagonists, downregulation of the insulin receptor, and alteration of glucose transporter (GLUT) proteins.

Obesity is one of the most important contributors to insulin resistance and diabetes. Obesity acts through several important mechanisms:

1. Adipokines (leptin and adiponectin) are hormones produced in adipose tissue. Obesity results in increased serum levels of leptin and decreased levels of adiponectin. These changes are associated with inflammation and decreased insulin sensitivity.[43]
2. Elevated levels of serum free fatty acids (FFAs) and intracellular deposits of triglycerides and cholesterol are found in obese individuals. These changes interfere with intracellular insulin signalling, decrease tissue responses to insulin, alter incretin actions, and promote inflammation.
3. Intra-abdominal adipocytes or adipocyte-associated mononuclear cells release inflammatory cytokines and induce insulin resistance. These cytokines are also cytotoxic to beta cells.[43]
4. Obesity is linked with hyperinsulinemia and decreased insulin receptor density.

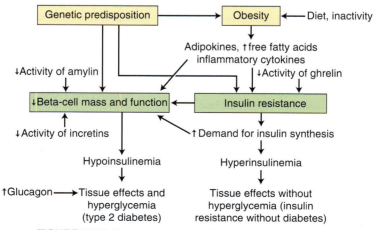

FIGURE 19.11 Pathophysiology of Type 2 Diabetes Mellitus.

CHAPTER 19 Alterations of Hormonal Regulation

BOX 19.2 Criteria for the Diagnosis of Metabolic Syndrome

Three or more of the following five traits:
1. Increased waist circumference (≥102 centimetres in men; ≥88 centimetres in women) for those of North American descent—ranges vary according to ethnicity
2. Plasma triglycerides ≥1.7 mmol/L, or receiving medication for elevated triglycerides
3. Plasma high-density lipoprotein (HDL) cholesterol <1.0 mmol/L (men) or <1.3 mmol/L (women), or medication treatment for decreased HDL
4. Blood pressure systolic ≥130 mm Hg and/or diastolic ≥ 85 mm Hg, or receiving medication for elevated blood pressure
5. Fasting plasma glucose ≥5.6 mmol/L, or receiving medication for elevated glucose

Data from Diabetes Canada Clinical Practice Guidelines Expert Committee. (2018). *Canadian Journal of Diabetes, 42*(Suppl. 1), S1–S325. http://guidelines.diabetes.ca/cpg/chapter3.

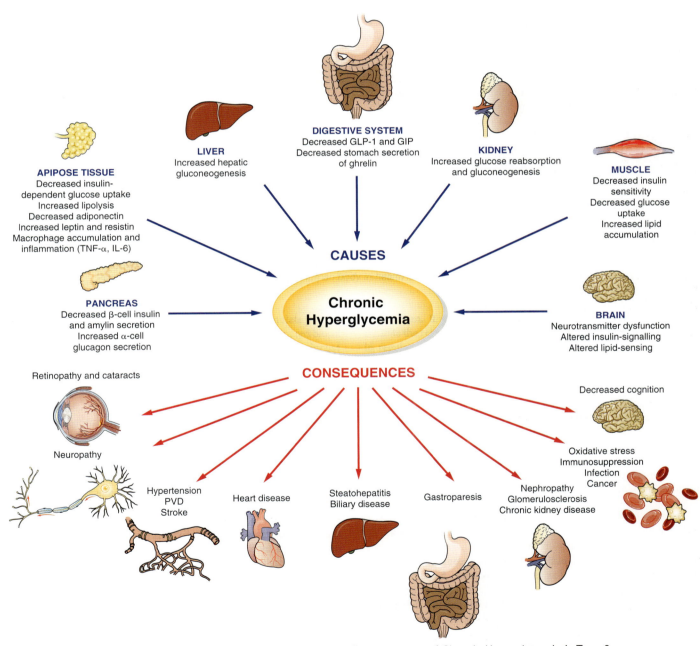

FIGURE 19.12 Multiorgan Causes and Common Consequences of Chronic Hyperglycemia in Type 2 Diabetes Mellitus. *GIP*, Gastric inhibitory polypeptide; *GLP-1*, glucagonlike peptide 1; *IL-6*, interleukin-6; *PVD*, peripheral vascular disease; *TNF-α*, tumour necrosis factor-alpha.

The resulting hyperinsulinemia prevents the clinical appearance of diabetes for many years. Eventually, however, beta-cell dysfunction develops and leads to a deficiency of insulin activity. The islet dysfunction is caused by a combination of a decrease in beta-cell mass and a reduction in normal beta-cell function.[43] A ongoing decrease in the weight and number of beta cells occurs. Many of the remaining cells develop "exhaustion" from increased demand for insulin biosynthesis.

Type 2 diabetes results in an increased glucagon concentration because pancreatic alpha cells become less responsive to glucose inhibition. This lack of responsiveness results in an increase in glucagon secretion. These abnormally high levels of glucagon increase blood glucose level by stimulating glycogenolysis and gluconeogenesis. Like type 1 diabetes, type 2 diabetes also is associated with a deficiency in amylin, further increasing glucagon levels.

A decrease of amylin (islet amyloid polypeptide), another beta-cell hormone, is seen in both type 1 and type 2 diabetes. Amylin increases satiety and suppresses glucagon release from the alpha cells. It also plays a part in islet cell destruction through the deposition of abnormal amyloid polypeptide in the pancreas.[44] Pramlintide, a synthetic analogue of amylin, is used for treatment in type 1 and 2 diabetes in the United States but has not been approved for use in Canada.

Hormones released from the GI tract play a role in insulin resistance, beta-cell function, and diabetes. Ghrelin is a peptide produced in the stomach and pancreatic islets that regulates food intake, energy balance, and hormonal secretion.[45] Decreased levels of circulating ghrelin have been associated with insulin resistance and increased fasting insulin levels. The incretins are a class of peptides that are released from the GI tract in response to food intake. Incretins function to increase the secretion of insulin and have many other positive effects on metabolism. The most studied incretin is called glucagonlike peptide 1 (GLP-1). Studies have shown that beta-cell responsiveness to GLP-1 is reduced both in prediabetes and in type 2 diabetes.[46]

The kidneys also influence the pathophysiology of type 2 diabetes. Renal reabsorption of glucose through the sodium-glucose cotransporter 2 (SGLT2) is an important controller of serum glucose levels. Medications aimed at blocking SGLT2 have resulted in decreased blood glucose level, weight, and blood pressure.[47]

CLINICAL MANIFESTATIONS The clinical manifestations of type 2 diabetes are nonspecific. The affected individual is often overweight, dyslipidemic, hyperinsulinemic, and hypertensive. The individual with type 2 diabetes may show some classic symptoms of diabetes, such as polyuria and polydipsia. More often, persons experiencing type 2 diabetes will have nonspecific symptoms such as fatigue, recurrent infections, visual changes, or symptoms of neuropathy (paresthesias or weakness). In those whose diabetes has progressed without treatment, symptoms related to coronary artery, peripheral artery, and cerebrovascular disease may develop.

EVALUATION AND TREATMENT The diagnostic criteria for type 2 diabetes are the same as those for type 1 (see Box 19.1). Prevention of type 2 diabetes, especially in those individuals with prediabetes, depends on diet and exercise. There is also increasing support for the use of some diabetes medications in high-risk individuals. (See Health Promotion: Type 2 Diabetes Mellitus.)

As with type 1 diabetes, the goal of treatment for individuals with type 2 diabetes is the restoration of a normal blood glucose level and correction of related metabolic disorders. The first approach to treatment of the individual with type 2 diabetes is maintaining an appropriate diet and exercise program.[12] Diet should match activity levels and include more complex carbohydrates, foods low in fats, adequate protein, and

HEALTH PROMOTION
Type 2 Diabetes Mellitus

The incidence of diabetes is increasing worldwide. Estimates show that in 2019, 463 million adults had diabetes and that by 2045, the number will increase to 700 million adults. Approximately 90% of those affected have type 2 diabetes mellitus. The International Diabetes Federation lists Canada among the worst OECD (Organisation for Economic Co-operation and Development) countries for diabetes prevalence. Canadians over 20 years of age face a 50% chance of developing diabetes, and up to 80% of some subgroups among Indigenous peoples face the same risk.

Health promotion interventions play an important role in the prevention and management of type 2 diabetes. Diabetes Canada has suggested three strategies to use as the best prevention for diabetes and its complications:

1. Changing risk factors and conditions by promoting healthy eating, physical activity, and emotional well-being
2. Early identification and effective management of the disease
3. Rehabilitation

Although changing lifestyle factors (e.g., increasing physical activity, eating healthy, and achieving and supporting a healthy weight) can decrease the occurrence of diabetes, successfully carrying out these modifications can be a challenging endeavour. Therefore, it is essential that a comprehensive approach to preventing type 2 diabetes incorporates both population-based strategies and high-risk individual strategies. Health promotion strategies also require leadership from government, local communities, nongovernmental organizations, the business sector, and committed individuals.

In 2018, Diabetes Canada proposed a framework to the government of Canada for a diabetes strategy called *Diabetes 360°*. This comprehensive strategy addressed key needs for Canadians with or at risk of developing diabetes. The primary goal is to dramatically reduce diabetes in Canada and save the health care system billions of dollars. Included in the strategy are recommendations to address the specific needs of the Indigenous peoples in Canada. These recommendations include addressing Truth and Reconciliation's *Calls to Action*, developing an Indigenous diabetes strategy created by Indigenous peoples, prioritizing health and wellness and the determinants of health, addressing the discrepancies in care and health outcomes, ensuring cultural safety and responsiveness, resolving issues of jurisdiction over health affairs, and ensuring stable and sustainable program capital funding.

Data from Diabetes Canada. (2018). *Diabetes 360°: a framework for a diabetes strategy for Canada.* https://www.diabetes.ca/DiabetesCanadaWebsite/media/Advocacy-and-Policy/Diabetes-360-Recommendations.pdf.

fibre. Weight loss results in improved glucose tolerance. Bariatric surgery improves glycemic control, decreases the risk for cardiovascular disease, and promotes weight loss in those morbidly obese. The use of oral hypoglycemic agents are indicated for individuals who require further intervention. Currently, metformin (Glucophage) is considered the primary pharmacological choice for the treatment of type 2 diabetes. A second oral agent, a GLP-1 receptor agonist, or insulin is added if the A_{1C} target is not achieved over 3 months. The use of incretins has increased to treat persons with type 2 diabetes. A combination of medications may be needed. In the later stage of type 2 diabetes, insulin therapy may be necessary because of the progressive loss of beta-cell function.

Other Specific Types of Diabetes Mellitus and Gestational Diabetes Mellitus

Diabetes Canada's classification of diabetes mellitus includes not only the most common forms of diabetes (type 1 and type 2) (see Table 19.3) but also "other specific types" of diabetes mellitus and "gestational diabetes mellitus." Other specific types of diabetes include genetic defects in beta-cell function or insulin action, diseases of the exocrine pancreas, endocrinopathies, medication- or chemical-induced beta-cell dysfunction, infections, and other uncommon autoimmune and inherited disorders. **Maturity-onset diabetes of youth (MODY)** is the best described of these other specific types of diabetes. MODY includes six specific autosomal dominant mutations that affect critical enzymes involved in beta-cell function or insulin action. Approximately 1% of cases of diabetes are monogenic and termed as MODY.[48] Diagnosis and management are like those techniques used for type 2 diabetes.

Any degree of glucose intolerance with onset or first recognition during pregnancy defines **gestational diabetes mellitus (GDM)**. This definition meant that many women with undiagnosed type 1 or type 2 diabetes were diagnosed with GDM. Many of them had progressive disease after delivery. Therefore, Diabetes Canada recommends that women found to have diabetes at their first prenatal visit receive a 75 g OGTT between 6 weeks and 6 months postpartum. Screening for GDM is recommended in asymptomatic, pregnant women between 24 and 28 weeks of gestation.[34] Diabetes Canada's preferred approach for diagnosis of GDM includes screening with a 50 g glucose challenge test (GCT), followed by a 75 g OGTT using the glucose thresholds of fasting 5.3 mmol/L (1 hour: 10.6 mmol/L, and 2 hours: 9.0 mmol/L).[34] Women who are diagnosed with GDM requiring medication for glycemic control should be managed with insulin therapy. Women with type 2 diabetes who are planning a pregnancy should switch from noninsulin antihyperglycemic agents to insulin for glycemic control.[34] Tight glucose control prenatally, during pregnancy, and after delivery is essential to the short- and long-term health of both mother and baby. Women who have GDM have a greatly increased diabetes risk, making consistent follow-up important.

Acute Complications of Diabetes Mellitus

The major acute complications of diabetes mellitus are hypoglycemia, DKA, and **hyperosmolar hyperglycemic syndrome (HHS)** (see comparison in Table 19.5). The **Somogyi effect** (low blood glucose level during the night that may lead to a morning rise in blood glucose level) and **dawn phenomenon** (an early morning rise in blood glucose level related to release of GH, cortisol, and catecholamines without preceding hypoglycemia) also may be seen.

Hypoglycemia in diabetes is also known as *insulin shock* or *insulin reaction*. Individuals with type 2 diabetes are at less risk for hypoglycemia than those with type 1 diabetes because they retain relatively intact glucose counter-regulatory mechanisms. However, hypoglycemia does occur in type 2 diabetes when treatment involves insulin secretagogues (e.g., sulfonylureas) or exogenous insulin. Symptoms include pallor, tremor, anxiety, tachycardia, palpitations, diaphoresis, headache, dizziness, irritability, fatigue, poor judgement, confusion, visual disturbances, hunger, seizures, and coma. Treatment requires immediate replacement of glucose either orally or intravenously. Individuals who are at high risk can be prescribed glucagon for home use. Prevention strategies include individualized management of medications and diet, checking of blood glucose levels, and education.

DKA is a serious complication related to a deficiency of insulin and an increase in the levels of insulin counter-regulatory hormones (catecholamines, cortisol, glucagon, GH) (Figure 19.13). DKA occurs in approximately 30% of children with type 1 diabetes at diagnosis.[49] DKA is much more common in type 1 diabetes because insulin is more deficient (see Table 19.5). Characteristics include hyperglycemia, acidosis, and ketonuria. Insulin normally stimulates lipogenesis and inhibits lipolysis, thus preventing fat catabolism. With insulin deficiency, enhancement of lipolysis occurs and there is an increase for nonesterified fatty acids delivered to the liver. The consequence is increased glyconeogenesis. This increase contributes to hyperglycemia and production of ketone bodies (acetoacetate, hydroxybutyrate, and acetone) by the mitochondria of the liver at a rate that exceeds peripheral use. Accumulation of ketone bodies causes a drop in pH, resulting in metabolic acidosis. Symptoms of DKA include Kussmaul respirations (hyperventilation to compensate for the acidosis), postural dizziness, central nervous system depression, ketonuria, anorexia, nausea, abdominal pain, thirst, and polyuria. Treatment for DKA includes a combination of fluids, insulin, and electrolyte replacement. Patients with type 2 diabetes typically present with a subacute HHS. Characteristics include symptoms like DKA followed by altered

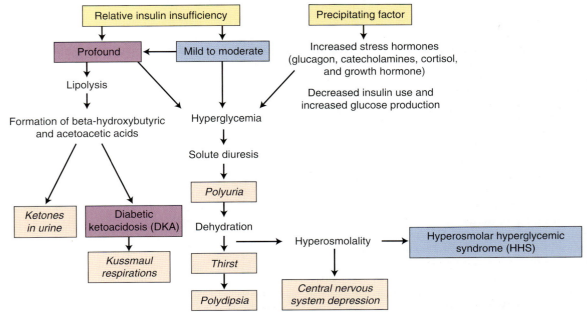

FIGURE 19.13 Pathophysiology of Diabetic Ketoacidosis and Hyperosmolar Hyperglycemia Syndrome in Diabetes Mellitus.

TABLE 19.5 Common Acute Complications of Diabetes Mellitus

	Hypoglycemia in Persons With Diabetes Mellitus	Diabetic Ketoacidosis	Hyperosmolar Hyperglycemic Syndrome
Synonyms	Insulin shock, insulin reaction	Diabetic coma syndrome	Hyperosmolar hyperglycemia nonketotic syndrome
Persons at Risk	Individuals taking insulin; Individuals with rapidly fluctuating blood glucose levels; Individuals with type 2 diabetes taking sulfonylurea agents	Individuals with type 1 diabetes; Individuals with nondiagnosed diabetes	Older persons or very young individuals with type 2 diabetes, nondiabetic persons with predisposing factors, such as pancreatitis; individuals with undiagnosed diabetes
Predisposing Factors	Excessive insulin or sulfonylurea agent intake, lack of sufficient food intake, excessive physical exercise, abrupt decline in insulin needs (e.g., renal failure, immediately postpartum), simultaneous use of insulin-potentiating agents or beta-blocking agents that mask symptoms	Stressful situation such as infection, accident, trauma, emotional stress; omission of insulin; medications that antagonize insulin	Infection, medications that antagonize insulin, comorbid condition
Typical Onset	Rapid	Slow	Slowest
Presenting Symptoms	Adrenergic reaction: pallor, sweating, tachycardia, palpitations, hunger, restlessness, anxiety, tremors. Neurogenic reaction: fatigue, irritability, headache, loss of concentration, visual disturbances, dizziness, hunger, confusion, transient sensory or motor defects, convulsions, coma, death	Malaise, dry mouth, headache, polyuria, polydipsia, weight loss, nausea, vomiting, pruritus, abdominal pain, lethargy, shortness of breath, Kussmaul respirations, fruity or acetone odour to breath	Polyuria, polydipsia, hypovolemia, dehydration (parched lips, poor skin turgor), hypotension, tachycardia, hypoperfusion, weight loss, weakness, nausea, vomiting, abdominal pain, hypothermia, stupor, coma, seizures
Laboratory Analysis	Serum glucose <1.7 mmol/L in newborn (first 2–3 days) and <3.0–3.4 mmol/L in adults	Glucose levels >14 mmol/L, reduction in bicarbonate concentration, increased anion gap, increased plasma levels of β-hydroxybutyrate, acetoacetate, and acetone	Glucose levels >33.6 mmol/L, lack of ketosis, serum osmolarity >320 mmol/L, elevated blood urea nitrogen and creatinine levels

mental status and very high blood glucose levels with high plasma osmolarity.[50]

HHS is an uncommon but significant complication of type 2 diabetes with a high overall mortality. It occurs more often in older persons who have other comorbidities, including infections or cardiovascular or renal disease. HHS differs from DKA in the degree of insulin deficiency (which is more profound in DKA) and the degree of fluid deficiency (which is more marked in HHS). The clinical features of HHS include a very high serum glucose concentration and osmolarity and a near-normal serum bicarbonate level and pH. Glucose levels are considerably higher in HHS than in DKA because of volume depletion. Because the amount of insulin required to inhibit fat breakdown is less than that needed for effective glucose transport, insulin levels are sufficient to prevent excessive lipolysis and ketosis (see Figure 19.13). Clinical manifestations include severe dehydration; loss of electrolytes; and neurological changes, such as stupor. Management includes fluid, insulin, and electrolyte replacement.

Chronic Complications of Diabetes Mellitus

Several serious complications are associated with any type of poorly controlled diabetes mellitus. Most complications are associated with insulin resistance or deficit, chronic hyperglycemia (also known as *glucose toxicity*), and accumulation of advanced glycation end products. In addition, activation of metabolic pathways that cause tissue damage is associated with the chronic complications of diabetes mellitus. These complications include microvascular and macrovascular disease. Microvascular disease occurs with damage to capillaries; **retinopathy**, **nephropathy**, and **neuropathy**. Macrovascular disease occurs with damage to larger vessels; coronary artery, peripheral vascular, and cerebrovascular disease (Table 19.6). Strict control of blood glucose level reduces some complications, particularly nonfatal myocardial infarction, but increases 5-year mortality. Strict control is not recommended for high-risk individuals with type 2 diabetes, but the individual risk–benefit profile should be considered.[51]

Microvascular Disease

Diabetic microvascular complications (disease in capillaries) are a leading cause of blindness, end-stage kidney failure, and various neuropathies. Blockage of capillaries is characteristic of diabetic microvascular disease. The frequency and severity of lesions appear to be related to the length of the disease and the status of glycemic control. Hypoxia and ischemia accompany microvascular disease, especially in the eye,

TABLE 19.6 Chronic Complications of Diabetes Mellitus

Complications	Pathological Mechanisms	Associated Symptoms
Microvascular		
Retinopathy		
Nonproliferative	Microaneurysms, capillary dilation, soft and hard exudates, dot and flame hemorrhages, arteriovenous shunts	May have no visual changes
Proliferative	Formation of new blood vessels, vitreal hemorrhage, scarring, retinal detachment	Loss of visual acuity
Maculopathy	Macular edema	Loss of central vision
Hyperglycemic lens edema	Shunting of glucose to polyol pathway: hyperosmolar fluid in lens	Blurring of vision
Cataract formation	Chronic hyperglycemia	Decreasing visual acuity
Nephropathy	Glomerular basement membrane thickening, mesangial expansion, glomerulosclerosis, focal tubular atrophy; hyperperfusion and hyperfiltration	Microalbuminuria and hypertension slowly progressing to end-stage kidney failure
Neuropathy	Oxidative stress, poor perfusion and ischemia, loss of nerve growth factor	Nerve dysfunction and degeneration
Peripheral neuropathy	Oxidative stress, poor perfusion and ischemia, loss of nerve growth factor	Distal symmetrical sensorimotor polyneuropathy with glove and stocking loss of sensation (pain, vibration, temperature, proprioception); loss of motor nerve function with clawed toes and small muscle wasting in hands and flexor muscles; Charcot joints (loss of sensation results in joint and ligament degeneration, particularly of foot) Acute painful neuropathy with burning pain in legs and feet
Autonomic neuropathy	Oxidative stress, poor perfusion and ischemia, loss of nerve growth factor	Heart rate variability and postural hypotension Gastroparesis (delayed gastric emptying) and diarrhea Loss of bladder tone, urinary retention, and risk for bladder infection Erectile dysfunction and impotence in men
Skin and foot lesions	Loss of sensation, poor perfusion, suppressed immunity, and increased risk for infection	High risk for pressure ulcers and delayed wound healing; abscess formation; development of necrosis and gangrene, particularly of toes and foot; infection and osteomyelitis
Macrovascular		
Cardiovascular	Endothelial dysfunction, dyslipidemia, accelerated atherosclerosis, coagulopathies	Hypertension, coronary artery disease, cardiomyopathy, and heart failure
Cerebrovascular	Endothelial dysfunction, dyslipidemia, accelerated atherosclerosis, coagulopathies	Increased risk for ischemic and thrombotic stroke
Peripheral vascular	Endothelial dysfunction, dyslipidemia, accelerated atherosclerosis, coagulopathies	Claudication, nonhealing ulcers, gangrene
Infection	Impaired immunity, decreased perfusion, recurrent trauma, delayed wound healing, urinary retention	Wound infections, urinary tract infections, increased risk for sepsis

kidney, and nerves. Many individuals with type 2 diabetes will present with microvascular complications. The presence of these complications is related to the long duration of asymptomatic hyperglycemia that generally precedes diagnosis. This evidence stresses the need to screen for diabetes.

Diabetic retinopathy. Diabetic retinopathy is a leading cause of blindness worldwide. Compared with that in type 1 diabetes, retinopathy seems to develop more rapidly in individuals with type 2 diabetes. This is because of the likelihood of longstanding hyperglycemia before diagnosis. Most individuals with diabetes will eventually develop retinopathy. They are also more likely to develop cataracts and glaucoma (see Chapter 14).

Diabetic retinopathy results from relative hypoxemia, damage to retinal blood vessels, red blood cell aggregation, and hypertension (Figure 19.14). There are three stages of retinopathy that lead to loss of vision. In stage I, or the *nonproliferative* stage, there is an increase in retinal capillary permeability, vein dilation, microaneurysm formation, and superficial (flame-shaped) and deep (blot) hemorrhages. In stage II, or the *preproliferative*, a progression of retinal ischemia with areas of poor perfusion that culminate in infarcts occurs. In stage III, or the *proliferative*, the result of neovascularization (angiogenesis) and fibrous tissue formation within the retina or optic disc occurs. Traction of the new vessels on the vitreous humor may cause retinal detachment or hemorrhage into the vitreous humor. As a result, severe blurring or loss of vision may occur. Macular edema is the leading cause of blurred vision among persons with diabetes. Blurring of vision also can be a consequence of hyperglycemia and sorbitol accumulation in the lens. Dehydration of the lens, aqueous humor, and vitreous humor also reduces visual acuity.

Diabetic nephropathy. Diabetes is the most common cause of chronic kidney disease and end-stage kidney disease. Approximately 50% of individuals with diabetes mellitus develop diabetic kidney disease.[52]

Hyperglycemia, advanced glycation end products (AGEs), activation of metabolic pathways, and inflammation all contribute to kidney tissue injury. However, the exact process responsible for destruction of

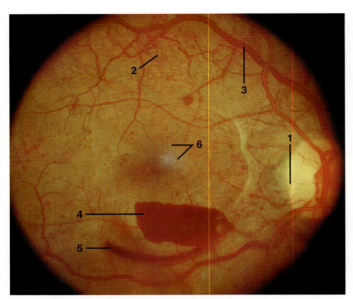

FIGURE 19.14 Diabetic Retinopathy. Neovascularization is present at the optic nerve **1**, and along vascular pathways **2**. Retinal veins are engorged **3**, and a preretinal boat-shaped hemorrhage **4**, is present below the fovea. A more diffuse mild vitreous hemorrhage **5**, is present below the preretinal hemorrhage. A few small, hard exudates are visible in the fovea **6**. (From Palay, D. A., & Krachmer, J. H. [2006]. *Primary care ophthalmology* [2nd ed.]. Mosby.)

kidneys in diabetes is unknown. Renal glomerular changes occur early in diabetes mellitus, occasionally preceding the obvious manifestation of the disease. Hyperglycemia with high renal blood flow (hyperfiltration) causes injury to the glomeruli. This occurs through increases in proximal tubular reabsorption, and by intraglomerular hypertension worsened by systemic hypertension. There is progressive glomerulosclerosis and decreased glomerular blood flow and glomerular filtration. Alterations in glomerular membrane permeability occur with loss of negative charge and albuminuria. Ultimately, there can be tubular and interstitial fibrosis contributing to loss of function.[53]

Microalbuminuria is the first manifestation of diabetic kidney dysfunction. Before proteinuria, no clinical signs or symptoms of progressive glomerulosclerosis are likely to be evident. Later, hypoproteinemia, reduction in plasma oncotic pressure, fluid overload, anasarca (generalized body edema), and hypertension may occur. As renal function continues to deteriorate, individuals with type 1 diabetes may experience hypoglycemia (because of loss of renal insulin metabolism). This process may require a decrease in insulin therapy. As the glomerular filtration rate drops below 10 mL/min, uremic signs occur. These signs include nausea, lethargy, acidosis, anemia, and uncontrolled hypertension (see Chapter 30 for a discussion of renal failure). Proteinuria is strongly correlated with morbidity and mortality from cardiovascular disease.[12] Early diagnosis and control of hypertension and hyperglycemia decreases the severity of nephropathy and delays the onset of end-stage kidney disease.[54]

Diabetic neuropathies. **Diabetic neuropathy** is the most common cause of neuropathy in the Western world. It is the most common complication of diabetes. The underlying pathological mechanism includes both metabolic and vascular factors related to chronic hyperglycemia with ischemia. Demyelination contributing to neural changes and delayed conduction also occurs. Both somatic and peripheral nerve cells show diffuse or focal damage, resulting in polyneuropathy. Sensory neuropathies include distal symmetrical polyneuropathy, focal neuropathy (wristdrop, footdrop), and diabetic amyotrophy (muscle atrophy; weakness; and pain in the muscles of the hip, thigh, and buttocks). Loss of pain, temperature, and vibration sensation is more common than motor involvement. This loss of sensation often involves the extremities first in the hands and feet. Motor neuropathies can affect muscle groups, particularly of the feet. This neuropathy contributes to deformity and unstable balance. Peripheral neuropathy can cause Charcot arthropathy, a progressive deterioration of weight-bearing joints, typically in the foot and ankle. Distal neuropathies combined with vascular complications, infection, or injury can lead to amputation[12] (Figures. 19.15 and 19.16).

Autonomic neuropathies include delayed gastric emptying, diabetic diarrhea, altered bladder function (e.g., decreased sensation of bladder fullness, urge or overflow incontinence), impotence, orthostatic hypotension, and heart rate variability with both tachycardia and bradycardia.[55] Neuropathy may occur during periods of "good" glucose control and may be the initial clinical manifestation of type 2 diabetes. Chronic hyperglycemia also can cause cognitive dysfunction with changes in learning and memory.[56]

Macrovascular Disease

Macrovascular disease is lesions in large- and medium-sized arteries. These lesions increase morbidity and mortality. They also increase the risk for hypertension, accelerated atherosclerosis (Figure 19.17), cardiovascular disease, stroke, and peripheral vascular disease, particularly among individuals with type 2 diabetes. (Chapter 24 discusses atherosclerosis in greater detail.) Children with poorly controlled diabetes have higher risk for developing macrovascular complications earlier in life.[57] The process tends to be more severe and faster in the presence of other risk factors, including obesity, dyslipidemia, and smoking.[57]

Cardiovascular disease. Diabetes increases the risk of cardiovascular disease occurring up to 15 years earlier than in individuals without diabetes.[58] Women with diabetes have a higher risk of developing cardiovascular disease.[59] Hypertension often coexists with diabetes mellitus. It is more prevalent than in the nondiabetic population and can have many causes. In type 1 diabetes, hypertension is associated with the development of microalbuminuria. In type 2 diabetes, hypertension is associated with metabolic syndrome. Hypertension increases the risk for coronary artery disease and stroke. Coronary artery disease is the most common cause of morbidity and mortality in individuals with diabetes mellitus. Mechanisms of disease include (1) vessel injury related to insulin resistance and hyperglycemia oxidative stress; (2) accelerated atherosclerosis associated with high levels of triglycerides, high levels of small low-density lipoproteins (LDLs), and low levels of high-density lipoproteins (HDLs); (3) platelet activation and prothrombosis; and (4) endothelial cell dysfunction.[60] In general, the prevalence of coronary artery disease increases with the duration but not the severity of diabetes. The onset of coronary artery disease can be silent.

The incidence of *heart failure* is higher in individuals with diabetes, even without myocardial infarction. This may be related to cardiomyopathy and the presence of increased amounts of collagen in the ventricular wall and ventricular hypertrophy. There is reduced mechanical adherence of the heart during filling with diastolic and, eventually, systolic failure.[61] (Chapter 24 describes heart disease.) Canadian guidelines exist to reduce the risk and improve treatment of cardiovascular and coronary artery disease in individuals with diabetes.[34]

Stroke. Stroke is twice as common in those with diabetes as in the nondiabetic population.[34] The survival rate for individuals with diabetes after a massive stroke is typically shorter than that for nondiabetic individuals. Hypertension, hyperglycemia, dyslipidemia, and thrombosis are definite risk factors.

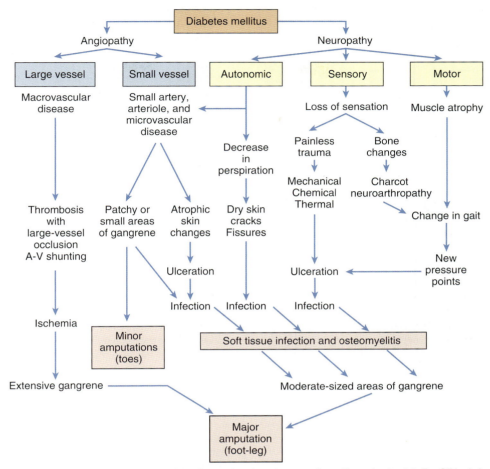

FIGURE 19.15 How Foot Lesions of Diabetes Lead to Amputation. (From Levin, M. E., O'Neal, L., & Bowker, J. [Eds.]. [1993]. *The diabetic foot* [5th ed.]. Mosby.)

Peripheral vascular disease. Diabetes mellitus increases the incidence of peripheral vascular disease (PVD). Symptoms include claudication (pain from reduced blood flow during exercise), ulcers, gangrene, and amputation.[62] Age, duration of diabetes, genetics, and additional risk factors (smoking, dyslipidemia, hypertension) influence the development and management of PVD. In those with diabetes, PVD is more diffuse and often involves arteries below the knee. Blockages of the small arteries and arterioles cause most of the gangrenous changes of the lower extremities and occur in patchy areas of the feet and toes. The lesions begin as ulcers and progress to osteomyelitis or gangrene requiring amputation. Peripheral neuropathies and increased risk for infection advance the disease[12] (see Figure 19.15). Significant morbidity and mortality are associated with major amputation.

Infection

The individual with diabetes is at an increased risk for infection throughout the body for several reasons[12]:

- *The senses.* Impaired vision caused by retinal changes and impaired touch caused by neuropathy. The neuropathy leads to loss of protection with injury and repeated trauma, open wounds, and soft tissue or osseous infection, particularly in the legs and feet (see Figure 19.16).
- *Hypoxia.* Once skin integrity is compromised, susceptibility to infection increases because of hypoxia. In addition, the glycosylated hemoglobin in the red blood cells impedes the release of oxygen to tissues.

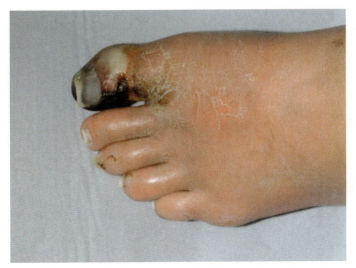

FIGURE 19.16 A Diabetic Foot. (Reprinted with permission from Jeffcoate, W. J., & Harding, K. G. (2003). Diabetic foot ulcers. *The Lancet, 361*(9368), 1545–1551.)

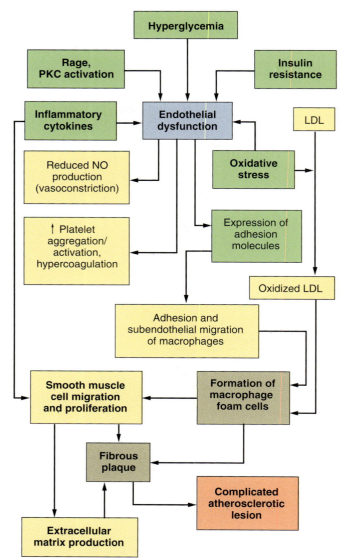

FIGURE 19.17 Diabetes Mellitus and Atherosclerosis. Diabetes with its associated hyperglycemia, relative hypoinsulinemia, oxidative stress, and proinflammatory state contributes to atherogenesis by causing arterial endothelial dysfunction (impaired vasodilation and adhesion of inflammatory cells), dyslipidemia, and smooth muscle proliferation. *LDL,* Low-density lipoprotein; *NO,* nitric oxide; *PKC,* protein kinase C; *RAGE,* receptor advanced glycation end product. (Data from Plutzky, K., Zafrir, B., & Brown, J. D. [2015]. *Vascular biology of atherosclerosis in patients with diabetes, diabetes in cardiovascular disease: a companion to Braunwald's heart disease* [pp. 10, 111–126]. Saunders; Zeadin, M. G., Petlura, C. I., & Werstuck, G. H. [2013]. *Canadian Journal of Diabetes,* 37[5], 345–350.)

- *Pathogens.* Some pathogens multiply rapidly because of increased glucose in body fluids, which supplies an excellent source of energy.
- *Blood supply.* Decreased blood supply results from vascular changes and reduces the supply of white blood cells to the affected area.
- *Suppressed immune response.* Chronic hyperglycemia impairs both innate and adaptive immune responses. This includes abnormal chemotaxis and vasoactive responses, and defective phagocytosis. Clinical signs of infection may be absent.

ALTERATIONS OF ADRENAL FUNCTION

 QUICK CHECK 19.5
1. What are the symptoms of hyperaldosteronism?
2. Hypocortisolism is associated with which major diseases?
3. What are pheochromocytomas?

Disorders of the Adrenal Cortex

Disorders of the adrenal cortex are related to hyperfunction or hypofunction. Hyperfunction that causes increased secretion of cortisol (**hypercortisolism**) leads to Cushing's disease or Cushing's syndrome. Hyperfunction that causes increased secretion of adrenal androgens or estrogens leads to virilization or feminization. Hyperfunction that causes increased levels of aldosterone leads to primary or secondary hyperaldosteronism. These syndromes often have overlapping features. Hypofunction of the adrenal cortex leads to Addison's disease.

Hypercortical Function (Cushing's Syndrome, Cushing's Disease)

Cushing's syndrome refers to the clinical manifestations resulting from chronic exposure to excess cortisol regardless of cause. **Cushing's disease** refers to excess endogenous secretion of ACTH. It is more common in women, but men may have more severe symptoms.[12] *ACTH-dependent hypercortisolism* results from overproduction of pituitary ACTH by a pituitary adenoma (which can occur at any age) or by an ectopic-secreting nonpituitary tumour, such as a small cell carcinoma of the lung (more common in older persons). Cortisol secretion from a rare benign or malignant tumour of one or both adrenal glands (more common in children) causes *ACTH-independent hypercortisolism.* A **Cushing's-like syndrome** may develop as a side effect of long-term glucocorticoid use.[12]

PATHOPHYSIOLOGY Whatever the cause, two observations consistently apply to individuals with hypercortisolism: (1) the normal diurnal or circadian secretion patterns of ACTH and cortisol are lost, and (2) there is no increase in ACTH and cortisol secretion in response to a stressor.[63] With ACTH-dependent hypercortisolism, the excess ACTH stimulates excess production of cortisol and there is loss of feedback control of ACTH secretion. Individuals with ACTH-dependent hypercortisolism experience increased secretion of both cortisol and adrenal androgens, and inhibition of cortisol-releasing hormone. ACTH-independent secreting tumours of the adrenal cortex, however, generally secrete only cortisol. When the secretion of cortisol by the tumour exceeds normal cortisol levels, symptoms of hypercortisolism develop.

CLINICAL MANIFESTATIONS Weight gain is the most common feature. The excess weight results from the accumulation of adipose tissue in the trunk, facial, and cervical areas. These characteristic patterns of fat deposition have been respectively described as "truncal obesity," "moon face," and "buffalo hump" (Figures 19.18 and 19.19).

Glucose intolerance occurs because of cortisol-induced insulin resistance and increased gluconeogenesis and glycogen storage by the liver. Overt diabetes mellitus develops in approximately 20% of individuals with hypercortisolism. Polyuria is a manifestation of hyperglycemia and resultant glycosuria.

The catabolic effects of cortisol on peripheral tissues cause protein wasting. Muscle wasting leads to muscle weakness. In bone, loss of the protein matrix leads to osteoporosis, pathological and vertebral compression fractures, bone and back pain, kyphosis, and reduced height.

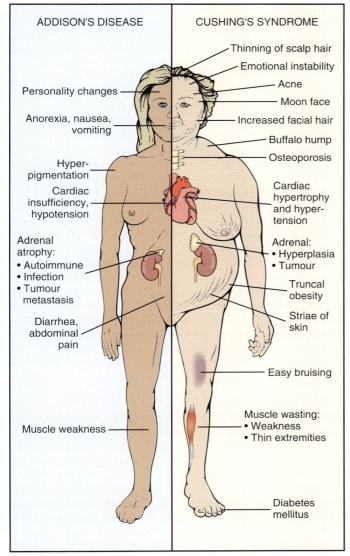

FIGURE 19.18 Symptoms of Addison's Disease and Cushing's Syndrome. (From Goodman, C. C., & Kelly Snyder, T. E. [2013]. *Differential diagnosis for physical therapists* [5th ed.]. Saunders.)

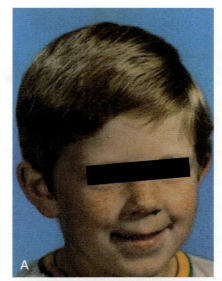
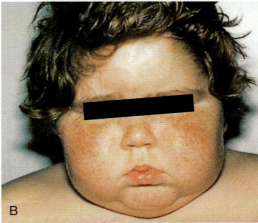

FIGURE 19.19 Cushing's Syndrome. **A**, Patient before onset of Cushing's syndrome. **B**, Patient 4 months later; the demonstration of moon facies is clear. (From Zitelli, B. J., McIntire, S. C., & Nowalk, A. J. [2012]. *Zitelli and Davis' atlas of pediatric physical diagnosis* [6th ed.]. Saunders.)

Cortisol interferes with the action of GH in long bones. As a result, children who present with short stature may be experiencing growth delays related to Cushing's syndrome rather than GH deficiency. Bone disease may contribute to hypercalciuria and resulting renal stones.

In the skin, loss of collagen leads to thin, weakened integumentary tissues. As a result, capillaries are more visible and are easily stretched by adipose deposits. Together, these changes account for the characteristic purple striae seen in the trunk area. Loss of collagenous support around small vessels makes them susceptible to rupture. This leads to easy bruising, even with minor trauma. Thin, atrophied skin is also easily damaged, leading to skin breaks and ulcerations. Bronze or brownish hyperpigmentation of the skin, mucous membranes, and hair occurs when there are very high levels of ACTH.

With elevated cortisol levels, vascular sensitivity to catecholamines increases significantly. This increase leads to vasoconstriction and hypertension. Mineralocorticoid effects promote hypokalemia and sodium and water retention with transient weight gain. Suppression of the immune system and increased susceptibility to infections also occur. Approximately 50% of individuals with Cushing's syndrome experience irritability and depression, disturbed sleep, difficulty concentrating, memory loss, and schizophrenia-like psychosis.[63] Females with ACTH-dependent hypercortisolism may experience symptoms of increased adrenal androgen levels (virilism). These symptoms include increased hair growth (especially facial hair), acne, and oligomenorrhea. Rarely do androgen levels become high enough to cause changes of the voice, recession of the hairline, and hypertrophy of the clitoris.

EVALUATION AND TREATMENT Routine laboratory examinations may reveal hyperglycemia, glycosuria, hypokalemia, and metabolic alkalosis. The use of a variety of laboratory tests confirms the diagnosis of hypercortisolism and determines the underlying disorder. These include urinary free cortisol level higher than 138 nmol/day, abnormal dexamethasone suppressibility of either urinary or serum cortisol, and simultaneous measurement of ACTH and cortisol levels. Late-evening salivary cortisol levels are used as a screening test and to document alterations in the diurnal variation of cortisol level.[63] Imaging procedures are used to diagnose tumours.

Treatment is specific for the cause of hypercorticoadrenalism. Treatments include surgery, medication, and radiation. Differentiation between pituitary ectopic and adrenal causes is essential for effective treatment. Without treatment, approximately 50% of individuals with Cushing's syndrome die within 5 years of onset. Causes of death include overwhelming infection, suicide, complications from generalized arteriosclerosis, and hypertensive disease.

Congenital Adrenal Hyperplasia

Congenital adrenal hyperplasia results from an inherited deficiency of an enzyme that is critical in cortisol biosynthesis. The inefficient production of cortisol causes the concentration of ACTH to increase and causes adrenal hyperplasia. This results in the overproduction of mineralocorticoids or androgens, or both. The most common form is a 21-hydroxylase deficiency, which involves both mineralocorticoid and cortisol synthesis. Affected female children are virilized and may have genital ambiguity. Infants of both genders exhibit salt wasting. Prenatal diagnosis is available and treatment guidelines exist. Disease management requires lifelong treatment with glucocorticoids and mineralocorticoids.[64]

Hyperaldosteronism

Excessive adrenal secretion of aldosterone characterizes hyperaldosteronism. Both primary and secondary forms of hyperaldosteronism can occur. Excessive secretion of aldosterone from an abnormality of the adrenal cortex, usually a single benign aldosterone-producing adrenal adenoma, causes primary hyperaldosteronism (Conn's syndrome, primary aldosteronism). Bilateral adrenal nodular hyperplasia and adrenal carcinomas account for the remainder of cases. The incidence is about 10% of all hypertensive individuals. However, up to 33% of people with resistant hypertension will have evidence of primary hyperaldosteronism.[65]

Secondary hyperaldosteronism results from an extra-adrenal stimulus of aldosterone secretion, most often by angiotensin II through a renin-dependent mechanism. Examples include decreased circulating blood volume (e.g., in dehydration, shock, or hypoalbuminemia) and decreased delivery of blood to the kidneys (e.g., renal artery stenosis, heart failure, or hepatic cirrhosis). Here, the activation of the renin-angiotensin system and later aldosterone secretion may be compensatory. However, in some instances (e.g., heart failure) the increased circulating volume further worsens the condition. Other causes of secondary hyperaldosteronism are Bartter syndrome, a renal tubular defect causing hypokalemia, and renin-secreting tumours of the kidney.

PATHOPHYSIOLOGY Excessive aldosterone secretion and the fluid and electrolyte imbalances that follow cause the pathophysiological alterations in *primary hyperaldosteronism*. Hyperaldosteronism promotes (1) increased renal sodium and water reabsorption with resulting hypervolemia (see Chapter 5) and hypertension and (2) renal excretion of hydrogen and potassium (see Chapter 5). The extracellular fluid volume overload, hypertension, and suppression of renin secretion are characteristic of primary disorders. Edema may not occur with primary aldosteronism because hypervolemia-induced atrial natriuretic factor release results in loss of sodium and water.[66] Hypokalemic alkalosis, changes in myocardial conduction, and skeletal muscle weakness may occur, particularly with severe potassium depletion.

In *secondary hyperaldosteronism*, the effect of increased extracellular volume on renin secretion may vary. If variables stimulate renin secretion, other than pressure-initiated cellular changes at the juxtaglomerular apparatus (see Chapter 29), increased circulating blood volume may not decrease renin secretion through feedback mechanisms. This process occurs in states of increased estrogen levels.

CLINICAL MANIFESTATIONS Hypertension, hypokalemia, and neuromuscular manifestations are the distinctive characteristics of primary hyperaldosteronism. Hypertension is resistant to treatment and can lead to the development of left ventricular dilation and hypertrophy, vascular disease, and kidney disease.[67]

EVALUATION AND TREATMENT Various clinical and laboratory tests are useful in assessing hyperaldosteronism and include:

- Measurement of blood pressure: hypertension is usually present
- Measurement of serum and urinary electrolyte levels: serum sodium level is normal or elevated and serum potassium level is depressed, but urinary potassium level is elevated; metabolic alkalosis may be present
- Evaluation of the plasma aldosterone-to-renin ratio: an increased ratio may indicate hyperaldosteronism
- Aldosterone suppression testing: it is performed using either salt loading or fludrocortisone acetate (Florinef) if the aldosterone-to-renin ratio has increased
- Imaging techniques: they are used to localize an aldosterone-secreting adenoma.

Treatment includes management of hypertension and hypokalemia, as well as correction of any underlying causal abnormalities. If an aldosterone-secreting adenoma is present, surgical removal is needed. Medical management with aldosterone receptor antagonists, such as spironolactone (Aldactone) or eplerenone (Inspra; a medication without the adverse effects of spironolactone) is a good choice in selected cases.

Hypersecretion of Adrenal Androgens and Estrogens

Adrenal tumours—either adenomas or carcinomas, Cushing's syndrome, or defects in steroid synthesis—may cause hypersecretion of adrenal androgens and estrogens. The hormone secreted, the gender of the individual, and the age at which the hypersecretion is started all determine the clinical syndrome that is presented. Hypersecretion of estrogens causes feminization, the development of female secondary sex characteristics. Hypersecretion of androgens causes virilization, the development of male secondary sex characteristics (Figure 19.20).

The effects of an estrogen-secreting tumour are most obvious in males. Results include gynecomastia (98% of cases), testicular atrophy, and decreased libido. In female children, such tumours may lead to early development of secondary sex characteristics. The changes caused by an androgen-secreting tumour are more easily seen in females. They include excessive face and body hair growth (hirsutism), clitoral enlargement, deepening of the voice, amenorrhea, acne, and breast atrophy. In children, virilizing tumours promote early sexual development and bone aging. Treatment of androgen-secreting tumours usually involves surgical removal.

Adrenocortical Hypofunction

Hypocortisolism (low levels of cortisol secretion) develops either because of inadequate stimulation of the adrenal glands by ACTH or because of a primary inability of the adrenals to produce and secrete the adrenocortical hormones. Sometimes there is partial dysfunction of the adrenal cortex, so only synthesis of cortisol and aldosterone or the adrenal androgens is affected. Hypofunction of the adrenal cortex may affect glucocorticoid or mineralocorticoid secretion, or both.

Addison's disease. Primary adrenal insufficiency is termed Addison's disease. It is relatively rare, occurring most often in adults aged 30 to 60 years. Autoimmune mechanisms that destroy adrenal cortical cells cause Addison's disease. It is more common in women. Chronic infections, such as tuberculosis, account for most cases of primary adrenal insufficiency in underdeveloped countries.

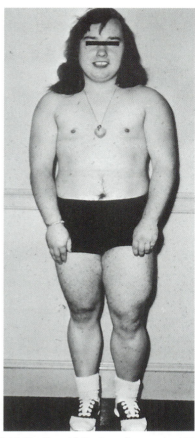

FIGURE 19.20 Virilization. Virilization of a young girl by an androgen-secreting tumour of the adrenal cortex. Masculine features include lack of breast development, increased muscle bulk, and hirsutism (excessive hair). (From Thibodeau, G. A., & Patton, K. T. [2010]. *The human body in health & disease* [4th ed.]. Mosby.)

PATHOPHYSIOLOGY Inadequate corticosteroid and mineralocorticoid synthesis and elevated levels of serum ACTH (loss of negative feedback) characterize Addison's disease. Before clinical manifestations of hypocortisolism are clear, destruction of more than 90% of total adrenocortical tissue must have occurred.

Idiopathic Addison's disease (organ-specific autoimmune adrenalitis) causes adrenal atrophy and hypofunction and is an organ-specific autoimmune disease. It may occur in childhood (type 1) or adulthood (type 2). 21-Hydroxylase autoantibodies and autoreactive T cells specific to adrenal cortical cells are present in 50 to 70% of individuals with idiopathic Addison's disease. This percentage increases in younger persons and in those with other autoimmune diseases. This deficiency allows the increase of immunocytes directed against specific antigens within the adrenocortical cells.[12]

The adrenal glands in idiopathic Addison's disease are smaller than normal and may be misshapen. Idiopathic Addison's disease is often associated with other autoimmune diseases, especially Hashimoto's thyroiditis, pernicious anemia, and idiopathic hypoparathyroidism. In these cases, Addison's disease may be inherited as an autosomal recessive trait. (Chapter 2 describes the mechanisms of inheritance.)

CLINICAL MANIFESTATIONS The symptoms of Addison's disease are primarily a result of hypocortisolism and hypoaldosteronism and are often nonspecific. With mild to moderate hypocortisolism, symptoms begin with weakness and easy fatigability. Skin changes, including hyperpigmentation and vitiligo, may occur. As the condition progresses, anorexia, nausea, vomiting, and diarrhea may develop. Of greatest concern is the development of hypotension that can progress to complete vascular collapse and shock. This is known as *adrenal crisis*, or Addisonian crisis. This crisis develops with undiagnosed disease or acute withdrawal of glucocorticoid therapy.

EVALUATION AND TREATMENT A decrease in serum and urine levels of cortisol and an increase in ACTH levels occurs with primary hypocortisolism. Because of dehydration, blood urea nitrogen levels may increase. Serum glucose level is low. Eosinophil and lymphocyte counts often are elevated. Hyperkalemia occurs in Addison's disease and may cause mild alkalosis (see Chapter 5). The ACTH stimulation test is used to evaluate serum cortisol levels.

The treatment of Addison's disease involves lifetime glucocorticoid and possibly mineralocorticoid replacement therapy. In addition, dietary modifications and correction of any underlying disorders needs to be addressed.[12] With acute stressors (e.g., infection, surgery, or trauma), additional cortisol must be administered to approximate the amount of cortisol that might be expected if normal adrenal function were present (approximately 100 to 300 mg/day). The individual's diet should include at least 150 mmol of sodium per day. If the individual experiences excessive sweating or diarrhea, an increase in sodium intake should occur.

Secondary hypocortisolism. Secondary hypocortisolism commonly results from prolonged administration of exogenous glucocorticoids. This administration suppresses ACTH secretion and causes adrenal atrophy. With removal of the exogenous glucocorticoids, the result is inadequate corticosteroidogenesis. Decreased ACTH secretion also can result from pituitary infarction or tumours that compress ACTH-secreting cells, or hypophysectomy. In all instances of low ACTH levels, adrenal atrophy occurs, and endogenous adrenal steroidogenesis is depressed. Clinical manifestations of secondary hypocortisolism are like those of Addison's disease, although hyperpigmentation usually does not occur. The renin-angiotensin system usually is normal, so aldosterone and potassium levels tend to be normal.

Tumours of the Adrenal Medulla

Pheochromocytomas (chromaffin cell tumours) or sympathetic paragangliomas of the adrenal medulla cause the hyperfunction of the adrenal medulla. They are rare, and about 10% are malignant and metastasize to the lungs, liver, bones, or para-aortic lymph nodes. The tumours are usually random, although up to 40% of them can be inherited.[12]

PATHOPHYSIOLOGY Pheochromocytomas and sympathetic paragangliomas cause excessive production of norepinephrine. Large tumours secrete epinephrine and norepinephrine because of autonomous secretion of the tumour. Approximately 5% of people with these tumours have no symptoms, apparently because the tumour is nonfunctioning. Such tumours can release catecholamines, especially in response to a stressor, such as surgery.

CLINICAL MANIFESTATIONS The clinical manifestations of a pheochromocytoma and sympathetic paragangliomas are related to the chronic effects of catecholamine secretion. The symptoms include persistent hypertension, headache, pallor, diaphoresis, tachycardia, and palpitations. Sustained or paroxysmal hypertension results from increased peripheral vascular resistance. An acute episode of hypertension related to hypersecretion of catecholamines may follow specific events. These events may include exercise, excessive ingestion of tyrosine-containing foods (aged cheese, red wine, beer, yogurt), ingestion of caffeine-containing foods, external pressure on the tumour, and induction of anaesthesia. Hypertension unresponsive to medication therapy is often the first sign of a pheochromocytoma. Headaches appear because of sudden changes in catecholamine levels in the blood, affecting cerebral blood flow. Hypermetabolism and sweating are related to chronic activation of sympathetic receptors in adipocytes, hepatocytes, and other tissues. Glucose intolerance may occur because of catecholamine-induced inhibition of insulin release by the pancreas. These tumours tend to be extremely vascular and can rupture. Rupture may cause massive and potentially fatal hemorrhage.

EVALUATION AND TREATMENT Symptoms of pheochromocytoma can be insidious or intermittent and difficult to diagnose. An increase catecholamine production in the blood or urine confirms the diagnosis. The site of the tumour is then determined using abdominal imaging techniques. Whole-body scanning will evaluate the presence of metastasis.

Management of catecholamine excess is essential to prevent hypertensive emergencies. Treatment requires the use of α- and β-adrenergic blockers. The usual treatment of pheochromocytoma is laparoscopic removal of the tumour. Open resection is completed for large tumours, or with metastasis present. Continuation of medical therapy stabilizes blood pressure before, during, or after surgery.[12] Malignant pheochromocytoma is rarely curable. It is usually managed by a combination of surgical reduction of the tumour and chemotherapy.[68]

CASE STUDY

The patient (preferred pronouns: she/her) is a 42-year-old Inuit resident of a small community in northern Canada. She attended a community well-woman clinic and, through random glucose screening, was informed that her blood glucose reading was high. She was advised to follow up with the community health centre regarding this finding.

- **History of Present Illness**: The patient states she is feeling "pretty good." She does report that she has been very thirsty lately and gets up at least once at night to void. She feels that she has been thirstier because the summer months have been unusually hot, and she has been drinking a lot to keep hydrated. She has also been more tired lately, but attributes that to gaining a lot of weight over the winter. She believes that she has gained at least 15 kg over the winter months, related to inactivity and a poor diet.
- **Past Medical Hx**: Gestational diabetes with third child 10 years ago, hypertension × 6 years, multiple vaginal candida over the past 3 years that she has self-treated with OTC antifungal vaginal suppositories and cream.
- **Obstetrical Gynecological Hx**: G3P3A0, first child at age 21, last child at age 32. All infants were healthy, 3rd child's birthweight was 5 kg. Last Pap test at recent well-woman clinic.
- **Family Hx**: Type 2 diabetes mellitus (DM2) older sister, mother, and maternal grandmother, all diagnosed in their 40 s. Mother and father both have hypertension (HTN). Mother has chronic kidney disease treated with home peritoneal dialysis.
- **Medications**: No prescription, occasional OTC ibuprofen, no vitamin, or herbal supplements
- **Social history**: Married 22 years with 3 children; husband is a mechanic; nonsmoker, nondrinker, no recreational drugs; works full time at local co-op; minimal exercise; eats a diet high in fats and refined sugars
- **Review of Systems**: Recent onset of fatigue, occasional headache and blurred vision, no cardiovascular symptoms, no respiratory symptoms, no nausea or vomiting, occasional constipation, +ve polyuria, +ve polydipsia, +ve nocturia, no hematuria, no dysuria, frequent vaginal candida, no leg cramps or intermittent claudication, no heat/cold intolerance, no rashes
- **Physical Exam**: Overweight Inuit woman in no distress, mucous membranes dry, skin dry and cool with poor skin turgor, +ve acanthosis nigricans, mild arteriolar narrowing of right and left ophthalmic fundus, abdomen soft with central obesity, pedal pulses 1+ bilaterally, no peripheral ulceration, feet cold to touch, sensation to bilateral feet decreased to light touch, vibration and microfilament, remaining exam unremarkable
- **Vital signs**: BP 155/92 LA sitting; pulse 85 regular; RR 16 unlaboured; Temperature 36.8°C oral; BMI 31

Critical Thinking and Clinical Judgement Questions

1. The primary care provider suspects a diagnosis of type 2 diabetes mellitus (DM2). Based on the information provided, identify eight possible risk factors that predispose this patient to that diagnosis.
2. When considering the subjective data provided, identify the clinical symptoms that are consistent with the diagnosis of DM2.
3. When considering the objective data provided, identify 8 clinical signs that are consistent with the diagnosis of DM2.
4. Name the laboratory tests the primary care provider could order to confirm the diagnosis of DM2. Indicate what each test is assessing and provide the expected results to confirm the diagnosis of DM2.
5. What possible treatments might the primary care provider discuss with this patient when considering a diagnosis of DM2?

DID YOU UNDERSTAND?

Mechanisms of Hormonal Alterations

1. Abnormalities in endocrine function may be caused by elevated or depressed hormone levels. These abnormalities result from (a) faulty feedback systems, (b) dysfunction of the gland, (c) altered metabolism of hormones, (d) dysfunction of carrier proteins, or (e) production of hormones from nonendocrine tissues.
2. Target cells may fail to respond to hormonal stimulation because of (a) cell surface receptor–associated disorders, (b) intracellular disorders, or (c) circulating hormone inhibitors.

Alterations of the Hypothalamic–Pituitary System

1. Dysfunction in the action of hypothalamic hormones is most related to interruption of the connection between the hypothalamus and pituitary—the pituitary stalk.
2. Disorders of the posterior pituitary include syndrome of inappropriate antidiuretic hormone (SIADH) and diabetes insipidus (DI). Abnormally high ADH secretion characterizes SIADH; abnormally low ADH secretion characterizes DI.

3. In SIADH, high ADH levels interfere with renal free water clearance. This leads to hyponatremia and hypo-osmolality.
4. DI may be neurogenic (caused by insufficient amounts of ADH) or nephrogenic (caused by an inadequate response to ADH). Its main clinical features are polyuria and polydipsia.
5. Hypopituitarism can be primary (dysfunction of the pituitary) or secondary (dysfunction of the hypothalamus). Primary hypopituitarism can result from a pituitary tumour, trauma, infections, stroke, or surgical removal.
6. Hypopituitarism can affect any or all the pituitary hormones. Symptoms range from mild to life-threatening.
7. Pituitary adenomas cause hyperpituitarism. These tumours are usually benign, and slow growing that arise from cells of the anterior pituitary.
8. Growth of a pituitary adenoma causes neurological and secretory effects. Pressure from the expanding tumour causes hyposecretion of cells, dysfunction of the optic chiasma (leading to visual disturbances), and dysfunction of the hypothalamus and some cranial nerves.
9. Growth hormone (GH) deficiency causes increased body fat, decreased muscle mass, and psychological problems in adults, and hypopituitary dwarfism in children.
10. Hypersecretion of GH in adults causes acromegaly. Pituitary adenoma is the most common cause of acromegaly. Excessive GH secretion in children with open epiphyseal plates causes giantism.
11. Prolonged abnormally high levels of GH lead to excess body and connective tissue and slowly developing renal, thyroid, and reproductive dysfunction.
12. Prolactinomas result in galactorrhea, hirsutism, amenorrhea, hypogonadism, and osteopenia.

Alterations of Thyroid Function
1. Thyrotoxicosis is a general condition in which elevated thyroid hormone (TH) levels cause greater than normal physiological responses. A variety of diseases can cause the condition, each of which has its own pathophysiology and treatment.
2. Hyperthyroidism has a range of endocrine, reproductive, gastrointestinal, integumentary, and ocular manifestations. Increased circulating levels of TH and stimulation of the sympathetic division of the autonomic nervous system cause these manifestations.
3. An autoimmune mechanism that overrides normal mechanisms for control of TH secretion is the cause of Graves' disease. Manifestations include thyrotoxicosis, ophthalmopathy, and circulating thyroid-stimulating immunoglobulins.
4. Toxic nodular goitre and toxic multinodular goitre occur when TH-regulating mechanisms and abnormal hypertrophy of the thyroid gland cause hyperthyroidism.
5. Thyrotoxic crisis is a severe form of hyperthyroidism that is often associated with physiological or psychological stress. Without treatment, death occurs quickly.
6. A deficient production of TH by the thyroid gland causes primary hypothyroidism. Hypothalamic or pituitary dysfunction causes secondary hypothyroidism. Symptoms depend on the degree of TH deficiency. Manifestations include decreased energy metabolism, decreased heat production, and myxedema.
7. An increased level of TSH, which stimulates goitre formation, characterizes primary hypothyroidism.
8. Autoimmune thyroiditis (Hashimoto's disease) is associated with humoral (antibodies) and cellular autoimmune destruction of the thyroid gland and gradual loss of thyroid function. Autoimmune thyroiditis occurs in individuals with genetic susceptibility to an autoimmune mechanism.
9. Subacute thyroiditis is a self-limiting nonbacterial inflammation of the thyroid gland. The inflammation damages follicular cells, causing leakage of tri-iodothyronine (T_3) and thyroxine (T_4). Transient hypothyroidism follows hyperthyroidism. Correction occurs by cellular repair and a return to normal levels in the thyroid.
10. Congenital hypothyroidism is the absence of thyroid tissue during fetal development or defects in hormone synthesis.
11. Myxedema is a sign of hypothyroidism caused by alterations in connective tissue with water-binding proteins. Symptoms include edema and thickened mucous membranes.
12. Myxedema coma is a severe form of hypothyroidism. It may be life-threatening without emergency medical treatment.
13. Thyroid carcinoma is associated with exposure to ionizing radiation, especially in childhood.

Alterations of Parathyroid Function
1. Manifestations of primary or secondary hyperparathyroidism includes greater than normal secretion of parathyroid hormone (PTH).
2. An interruption of the normal mechanisms that regulate calcium and PTH levels causes primary hyperparathyroidism. Manifestations include chronic hypercalcemia, increased bone resorption, and hypercalciuria.
3. Secondary hyperparathyroidism is a compensatory response to hypocalcemia. It often occurs with chronic renal failure and vitamin D deficiency.
4. Tertiary hyperparathyroidism is persistent secretion of PTH after treatment of secondary hyperparathyroidism.
5. Thyroid surgery, autoimmunity, or genetic mechanisms cause hypoparathyroidism.
6. The lack of circulating PTH in hypoparathyroidism causes hypocalcemia, hyperphosphatemia, decreased bone resorption, and hypocalciuria.

Dysfunction of the Endocrine Pancreas: Diabetes Mellitus
1. Diabetes mellitus is a group of metabolic disorders characterized by glucose intolerance, chronic hyperglycemia, and disturbances of carbohydrate, protein, and fat metabolism.
2. A diagnosis of diabetes mellitus is based on elevated plasma glucose concentrations and measurement of glycosylated hemoglobin. Classic signs and symptoms are often present.
3. The two most common types of diabetes mellitus are type 1 and type 2.
4. Characteristics of type 1 diabetes mellitus include loss of beta cells, presence of islet cell antibody, lack of insulin, excess of glucagon, and altered metabolism of fat, protein, and carbohydrates.
5. The cause of type 1 diabetes mellitus is a gradual autoimmune destruction of beta cells in genetically susceptible individuals.
6. In type 1 diabetes, hyperglycemia causes polyuria and polydipsia resulting from osmotic diuresis.
7. The cause of diabetic ketoacidosis (DKA) is an increase in levels of circulating ketones without the inhibiting effects of insulin. Increased levels of circulating fatty acids and weight loss are manifestations of uncontrolled type 1 diabetes mellitus.
8. The cause of type 2 diabetes is the triggering of genetic susceptibility by environmental factors. The most compelling environmental risk factor is obesity.
9. In the obese, many factors contribute to the development of insulin resistance and hyperglycemia. They include metabolic syndrome, altered adipokines, increased fatty acids, inflammation, and hyperinsulinemia,

10. Some insulin production continues in type 2 diabetes, but the weight and number of beta cells decrease. There is a decrease of insulin, amylin, ghrelin, and incretins, and glucagon concentration. All contribute to chronic hyperglycemia.
11. Maturity-onset diabetes of youth (MODY) is a rare monogenetic form of diabetes.
12. Gestational diabetes mellitus is glucose intolerance during pregnancy.
13. Acute complications of diabetes mellitus include hypoglycemia, DKA, and hyperosmolar hyperglycemic syndrome (HHS).
14. Hypoglycemia in diabetes is a complication related to insulin treatment.
15. DKA develops when there is an absolute or relative deficiency of insulin and an increase in the insulin counter-regulatory hormones of catecholamines—cortisol, glucagon, and GH. DKA presents with hyperglycemia, acidosis, and ketonuria.
16. HHS is pathophysiologically like DKA, although levels of free fatty acids are lower in hyperosmolar nonacidotic diabetes. A lack of ketosis shows some level of insulin action. Severe dehydration and electrolyte imbalance are present.
17. Chronic complications of diabetes mellitus include microvascular disease (e.g., neuropathy, retinopathy, nephropathy), macrovascular disease (e.g., coronary artery disease, stroke, peripheral vascular disease), and infection.
18. Microvascular disease associated with diabetes mellitus includes a thickening of the capillary basement membrane, disruption of microcirculation, and a decrease in tissue perfusion.
19. Macrovascular disease associated with diabetes mellitus is most often related to the creation of atherosclerotic plaques in the arterial wall and coagulation defects.
20. The incidence of coronary heart disease, peripheral vascular disease, and stroke is greater in those with diabetes than in nondiabetic individuals.
21. Individuals with diabetes are at risk for a variety of infections. Infection may be related to sensory impairment and resulting injury, hypoxia, increased growth of pathogens in elevated concentrations of glucose, decreased blood supply associated with vascular damage, and impaired immune protection.

Alterations of Adrenal Function

1. Disorders of the adrenal cortex are related to hyperfunction or hypofunction. No known disorders are associated with hypofunction of the adrenal medulla. Medullary hyperfunction causes clinically defined syndromes.
2. Hypercortisol function, or hypercortisolism, causes Cushing's syndrome, which does not involve the pituitary gland, and Cushing's disease, which is hypercortisolism with pituitary involvement. Congenital adrenal hyperplasia is a genetic disorder with deficient steroidogenesis and excess androgen synthesis.
3. Cushing's disease (pituitary-dependent) usually causes hypercortisolism. In rare situations ectopic production of ACTH may be the cause. Complications include obesity, diabetes, protein wasting, immune suppression, and mental status changes.
4. Excessive aldosterone secretion causes primary or secondary hyperaldosteronism. The cause of primary hyperaldosteronism is an abnormality of the adrenal cortex. Secondary hyperaldosteronism involves an extra-adrenal stimulus, often angiotensin.
5. Hyperaldosteronism promotes increased renal sodium and water reabsorption. This results in hypervolemia, increased extracellular fluid volume (which is variable), hypokalemia related to renal reabsorption of sodium, and excretion of potassium.
6. Hypersecretion of adrenal androgens and estrogens can be the result of adrenal tumours. Hypersecretion of estrogens causes feminization. Hypersecretion of androgens causes virilization.
7. Hypofunction of the adrenal cortex can affect glucocorticoid and mineralocorticoid secretion. The cause of hypofunction can be a deficiency of ACTH or by a primary deficiency in the gland itself.
8. The cause of hypocortisolism, or low levels of cortisol, is inadequate adrenal stimulation by ACTH or by primary cortisol hyposecretion. Primary adrenal insufficiency is termed *Addison's disease*.
9. Characteristics of Addison's disease are elevated ACTH levels with inadequate corticosteroid synthesis and output.
10. Manifestations of Addison's disease are related to hypocortisolism and hypoaldosteronism. Signs and symptoms include weakness, fatigability, hypoglycemia and related metabolic problems, lowered response to stressors, hyperpigmentation, vitiligo, and hypovolemia and hyperkalemia.
11. The usual cause of hyperfunction of the adrenal medulla is a pheochromocytoma, a catecholamine-producing tumour. Symptoms of catecholamine excess are related to their sympathetic nervous system effects. They include hypertension, palpitations, tachycardia, glucose intolerance, excessive sweating, and constipation.

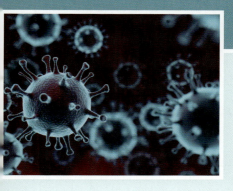

20

Structure and Function of the Hematological System

Kelly Power-Kean, with originating chapter contributions by Sue E. Huether

Additional resources are available online at https://evolve.elsevier.com/Canada/Huether/pathophysiology

CHAPTER OUTLINE

Components of the Hematological System, 478
    Composition of Blood, 478
    Lymphoid Organs, 482
    The Mononuclear Phagocyte System, 484
Development of Blood Cells, 485
    Hematopoiesis, 485
    Development of Erythrocytes, 487
    Development of Leukocytes, 490
    Development of Platelets, 491

Mechanisms of Hemostasis, 491
    Function of Platelets and Blood Vessels, 491
    Function of Clotting Factors, 494
    Retraction and Lysis of Blood Clots, 495
PEDIATRIC CONSIDERATIONS: Hematological Value Changes, 497
GERIATRIC CONSIDERATIONS: Hematological Value Changes, 498

LEARNING OBJECTIVES

1. Describe the components of blood.
2. Discuss the function of plasma and plasma proteins.
3. Discuss the structure and function of the cellular components of blood.
4. Describe the structure and function of the spleen and the lymph nodes.
5. Explain the role of the mononuclear phagocyte system.
6. Describe the process of hematopoiesis.
7. Explain cellular differentiation.
8. Discuss the role of the colony-stimulating factors (CSFs) in the making of blood cells.
9. Explain erythropoiesis and the role of erythropoietin.
10. Explain the function of hemoglobin.
11. List the nutrients required for erythropoiesis to take place. Explain the function of each nutrient.
12. Explain how iron is used in the production of hemoglobin.
13. List several situations that lead to increased leukocyte production.
14. Describe the role of platelets in hemostasis.
15. Explain the difference between the intrinsic and extrinsic clotting pathways.
16. Describe the process of clot breakdown.

KEY TERMS

Agranulocyte, 480
Albumin, 479
Antithrombin III (AT-III), 494
Apoferritin, 489
Apotransferrin, 490
Basophil, 482
Blood clot, 494
Bone marrow, 485
Clotting (coagulation) system, 494
Clotting factor, 480
Collagen, 492
Colony-stimulating factor (CSF, hematopoietic growth factor), 486
Cyclo-oxygenase-1 (COX-1), 493
D-dimer, 494
Deoxyhemoglobin, 488
Endomitosis, 491

Eosinophil, 481
Erythroblast (normoblast), 487
Erythrocyte, 480
Erythropoiesis, 487
Erythropoietin, 486
Extramedullary hematopoiesis, 485
Fibrin degradation product (FDP), 494
Fibrinolysis, 494
Fibrinolytic system, 494
Globin, 487
Globulin, 479
Granulocyte, 480
Hematopoiesis, 485
Hematopoietic stem cell (HSC), 485
Heme, 488
Hemoglobin (Hb), 487
Hemosiderin, 489

Hemostasis, 491
Hepcidin, 490
Immunocyte, 480
Integrin $\alpha_{IIb}\beta_3$ (GPIIb/IIIa), 492
Leukocyte, 480
Lipoprotein, 480
Lymph node, 484
Lymphocyte, 482
Macrophage, 482
Marginating storage pool, 486
Megakaryocytes, 482
Mesenchymal stem cells (MSCs), 485
Methemoglobin, 488
Monocyte, 482
Mononuclear phagocyte system (MPS), 484
Myeloid tissue, 485

Myoglobin, 489
Natural killer (NK) cells, 482
Neutrophil (polymorphonuclear neutrophil [PMN]), 481
Niche, 485
Nitric oxide (NO), 488
Osteoblastic niche, 485
Oxyhemoglobin, 488
Phagocyte, 480
Plasma, 478
Plasma protein, 479
Plasmin, 494
Platelet (thrombocyte), 482
Platelet-release reaction, 492
Primary lymphoid organs, 483
Proerythroblast, 487
Prostacyclin (PGI_2), 491
Protein C, 494
Protein S, 494
Protoporphyrin, 488

478 CHAPTER 20 Structure and Function of the Hematological System

Reticulocyte, 487
Secondary lymphoid organs, 483
Serum, 479
Spleen, 484
Stromal cell, 485
Thrombomodulin, 494
Thrombopoietin (TPO), 491
Thromboxane A$_2$ (TXA$_2$), 494
Tissue factor pathway inhibitor (TFPI), 494
Tissue plasminogen activator (t-PA), 494
Tissue thromboplastin, 494
Transferrin, 490
Urokinaselike plasminogen activator (u-PA), 494
Vascular niche, 485
von Willebrand factor (vWF), 492

All the body's tissues and organs require oxygen and nutrients to survive. The blood that flows through kilometres of vessels throughout the human body supplies these essential nutrients. The red blood cells supply oxygen, and the fluid part of the blood carries nutrients. The blood also cleans waste from the tissues and transports white blood cells and other substances that are needed for protecting the body from injury and infection.

COMPONENTS OF THE HEMATOLOGICAL SYSTEM

> ✓ **QUICK CHECK 20.1**
> 1. What are the unique properties of the erythrocyte's shape?
> 2. Why are plasma proteins important to blood volume?
> 3. Which leukocytes are granulocytes?
> 4. Compare and contrast granulocytes, agranulocytes, phagocytes, and immunocytes.

Composition of Blood

Blood is made up of various cells that circulate suspended in a solution of protein and inorganic materials (plasma). This solution is approximately 92% water and 8% dissolved substances (solutes). The blood volume amounts to about 5.5 L in adults. The constant movement of blood guarantees that critical components are available to all parts of the body to carry out their chief functions. These functions include (1) delivery of substances needed for cellular metabolism in the tissues, (2) removal of the wastes of cellular metabolism, (3) defence against invading microorganisms and injury, and (4) maintenance of acid–base balance.

Plasma and Plasma Proteins

In adults, plasma accounts for 50 to 55% of blood volume (Figure 20.1). **Plasma** is a complex liquid containing a variety of organic and inorganic parts (Table 20.1). The concentration of these elements varies depending on diet, metabolic demand, hormones, and vitamins. Plasma differs from serum. **Serum** is plasma that has been allowed to

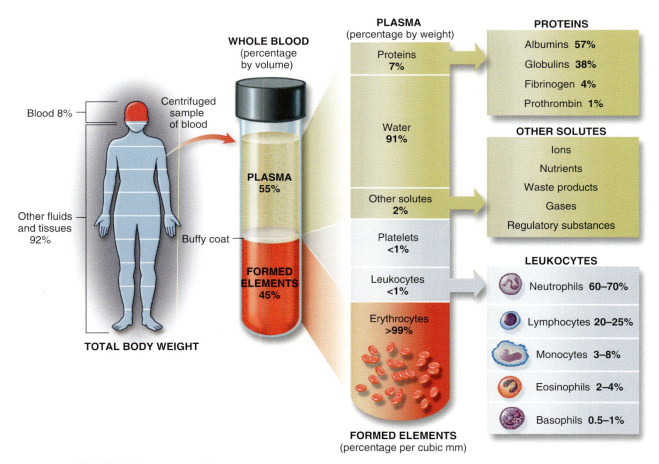

FIGURE 20.1 Make-up of Whole Blood. Approximate values for the components of blood in a normal adult. (From Patton, K. T., & Thibodeau, G. A. [2016]. *Structure & function of the body* [15th ed.]. Mosby.)

TABLE 20.1 Organic and Inorganic Components of Plasma

Constituent	Amount/Concentration	Major Functions
Water (H_2O)	91% of plasma weight	A medium for carrying all other constituents
Electrolytes	Total >1% of plasma	Maintenance of H_2O in extracellular compartment; they act as buffers and function in membrane excitability
Sodium (Na^+)	136–145 mmol/L	
Potassium (K^+)	3.5–5.0 mmol/L	
Calcium (Ca^{++})	2.25–2.75 mmol/L	
Magnesium (Mg^{++})	0.74–1.07 mmol/L	
Chloride (Cl^-)	98–106 mmol/L	
Bicarbonate (HCO_3^-)	21–28 mmol/L	
Phosphate (PO_4^{3+})	0.97–1.45 mmol/L	
Proteins	64–83 g/L	Provision of colloid osmotic pressure of plasma; act as buffers (see text for other functions)
Albumins	35–50 g/L	
Globulins	23–34 g/L	
Fibrinogen	5.8–11.8 µmol/L	
Transferrin	Adult male: 2–5.0 g/L Adult female: 1.9–4.4 g/L	
Ferritin	Male: 12–300 µg/L Female: 10–150 µg/L	
Gases		
Carbon dioxide (CO_2) content	35–45 mm Hg	By-product of oxygenation; most CO_2 content is from HCO_3^- and acts as a buffer
Oxygen (O_2)	Pao_2 80–100 mm Hg (arterial); Pvo_2 40–50 mm Hg (venous)	Oxygenation
Nitrogen gas (N_2)	0.64 mmol/L	By-product of protein catabolism
Nutrients		Supply nutrition and substances for tissue repair
Glucose and other carbohydrates	5.6 mmol/L	
Total amino acids	2.2 mmol/L	
Total lipids	7.5 mmol/L	
Cholesterol	<5.0 mmol/L	
Individual vitamins	0.000 07–1.79 mmol/L	
Individual trace elements	0.000 7–0.2 mmol/L	
Iron	11–32 µmol/L	
Waste Products		
Urea (BUN)	3.6–7.1 mmol/L	End product of protein catabolism
Creatinine (from creatine)	44–106 µmol/L	End product of energy metabolism
Uric acid (from nucleic acids)	160–501 µmol/L	End product of protein metabolism
Indirect bilirubin (from heme)	3.4–12.0 µmol/L	End product of red blood cell destruction
Individual hormones	0.000 01–0.5 g/L	Functions specific to target tissue

PaO_2, Partial pressure of oxygen in arterial blood; *PvO_2*, mixed venous oxygen tension.
Data from Pagana, K. D., Pagana, T. J., Pike-MacDonald, S. A., et al. (2013). *Mosby's Canadian manual of diagnostic and laboratory tests.* Elsevier; Vander, A. J., Luciano, D., & Sherman, J. (2001). *Human physiology: the mechanisms of body function* (8th ed.). McGraw-Hill.

---

clot in the laboratory to remove fibrinogen and other clotting factors that may interfere with diagnostic tests.

The plasma has many proteins (**plasma proteins**). These vary in structure and function. They are classified into two major groups: albumin and globulins. The liver produces most plasma proteins. Plasma cells in the lymph nodes and other lymphoid tissues, however, produce antibodies (see Chapter 7).

Albumin (about 60% of total plasma protein) acts as a carrier molecule for the components of blood and medications. Its key role is regulation of the passage of water and solutes through the capillaries. Albumin molecules are large and do not diffuse freely through the vascular endothelium. They maintain the critical colloidal osmotic pressure (or oncotic pressure) that regulates the passage of fluids and electrolytes into the surrounding tissues (see Chapters 1 and 5). Water and solute particles tend to diffuse out of the arterial portions of the capillaries because blood pressure is greater in arterial than in venous blood vessels. Water and solutes move from tissues into the venous portions of the capillaries where oncotic pressure is greater than intravascular pressure or hydrostatic pressure. In the case of decreased production (e.g., cirrhosis, other diffuse liver diseases, protein malnutrition) or excessive loss of albumin (e.g., certain kidney diseases), the reduced oncotic pressure leads to excessive movement of fluid and solutes into the tissue and decreased blood volume.

The remaining plasma proteins, or **globulins**, are often classified by their properties in an electric field (serum electrophoresis). Under the normal conditions used to perform serum electrophoresis, albumin is the most rapidly moving protein. The globulins are classified by their movement compared to albumin. They include alpha globulins (those moving most closely to albumin), beta globulins, and gamma globulins (those with the least movement). The alpha and beta globulins may be subdivided into subregions (alpha-1, alpha-2, beta-1, or beta-2 globulins). Fibrinogen is a major plasma protein (about 4% of total plasma protein) that would move between the beta and gamma regions but is removed during the formation of serum. The gamma-globulin region consists mainly of antibodies (see Chapter 7).

Plasma proteins can also be classified by function. The functions include clotting, defence, transport, or regulation. The **clotting factors** promote coagulation and stop bleeding from damaged blood vessels. Fibrinogen is the most plentiful of the clotting factors and is the precursor of the fibrin clot (see Figure 20.18). Proteins involved in defence, or protection, against infection include antibodies and complement proteins (see Chapters 6 and 7). Transport proteins bind and carry a variety of inorganic and organic molecules. These include iron (transferrin), copper (ceruloplasmin), lipids and steroid hormones (**lipoproteins**) (see the discussion on membrane transport in Chapter 1), and vitamins (e.g., retinol-binding protein). Regulatory proteins include a variety of enzymatic inhibitors (e.g., α_1-antitrypsin) that protect the tissues from damage, precursor molecules (e.g., kininogen) that are converted into active biological molecules when needed, and protein hormones (e.g., cytokines) that communicate between cells.

Plasma also has other solutes including nutrients, waste products, gases, regulatory substances, and electrolytes. Several inorganic ions regulate cell function, osmotic pressure, and blood pH. These ions include electrolytes, sodium, potassium, calcium, chloride, and phosphate. (Chapters 1 and 5 describe electrolytes.)

Cellular Components of the Blood

The cellular components of the blood are classified as red blood cells (i.e., erythrocytes), white blood cells (i.e., leukocytes), and platelets.

Table 20.2 lists the components of the blood. Figure 20.2 shows the pathways of blood differentiation or maturation.

Erythrocytes. Erythrocytes are the most abundant cells of the blood. They occupy about 48% of the blood volume in men and about 42% in women. Erythrocytes are mostly responsible for tissue oxygenation. Hemoglobin (Hb) carries the gases, and electrolytes regulate gas diffusion through the cell's plasma membrane. The mature erythrocyte lacks a nucleus and cytoplasmic organelles (e.g., mitochondria). As a result, it cannot create protein or carry out oxidative reactions. Because it cannot undergo mitotic division, the erythrocyte has a limited lifespan (approximately 80 to 120 days).

The erythrocyte's size and shape are ideally suited to its function as a gas carrier. It is a small disc with two unique properties: (1) a *biconcave* shape and (2) the capacity to be *reversibly deformed*. The flattened, biconcave shape supplies a surface area:volume ratio that is best for gas diffusion into and out of the cell and for deformity. During its lifespan, the erythrocyte, which is 6 to 8 μm in diameter, repeatedly circulates through splenic sinusoids (Figure 20.3) and capillaries that are only 2 μm in diameter. Reversible deformity allows the erythrocyte to become a more compact torpedolike shape. It can then squeeze through the microcirculation and return to normal.

Leukocytes. Leukocytes defend the body against organisms that cause infection. They also remove debris, including dead or injured host cells (Figure 20.4). Transportation of leukocytes occurs in the circulation, but they act mainly in the tissues. The average adult has approximately 5 to 10×10^9/L of blood.

Leukocytes are classified according to structure as **granulocytes** or **agranulocytes** and according to function as **phagocytes** or **immunocytes**. The granulocytes, which include neutrophils, basophils, and eosinophils, are all phagocytes. (Chapter 6 describes phagocytosis.) Of the agranulocytes, the monocytes and macrophages are phagocytes,

TABLE 20.2 Cellular Components of the Blood

Cell	Structural Characteristics	Normal Amounts of Circulating Blood	Function	Lifespan
Erythrocyte (red blood cell [RBC])	Non-nucleated cytoplasmic disc containing hemoglobin	$4.2–6.1 \times 10^{12}$/L	Gas transport to and from tissue cells and lungs	80–120 days
Reticulocyte index	1.0			
Absolute reticulocyte count	0.5–2.0% of total number of RBCs	Immature erythrocyte		
Leukocyte (white blood cell)	Nucleated cell	$5–10 \times 10^9$/L	Body defence mechanisms	See below
Lymphocyte	Mononuclear immunocyte	20–40% of leukocyte count (leukocyte differential)	Humoral and cell-mediated immunity (see Chapter 7)	Days or years, depending on type
Natural killer cell	Large granular lymphocyte	5–10% circulatory pool (some in spleen)	Defence against some tumours and viruses (see Chapters 6 and 7)	Unknown
Monocyte and macrophage	Large mononuclear phagocyte	2–8% of leukocyte differential	Phagocytosis; mononuclear phagocyte system	Months or years
Eosinophil	Segmented polymorphonuclear granulocyte	1–4% of leukocyte differential	Control of inflammation, phagocytosis, defence against parasites, allergic reactions	Unknown
Neutrophil	Segmented polymorphonuclear granulocyte	55–70% of leukocyte differential	Phagocytosis, particularly during early phase of inflammation	4 days
Basophil	Segmented polymorphonuclear granulocyte	0.5–1.0% of leukocyte differential	Mast cell–like functions, associated with allergic reactions and mechanical irritation	Unknown
Platelet	Irregularly shaped cytoplasmic fragment (not a cell)	$150–400 \times 10^9$/L	Hemostasis after vascular injury; normal coagulation and clot formation/retraction	8–11 days

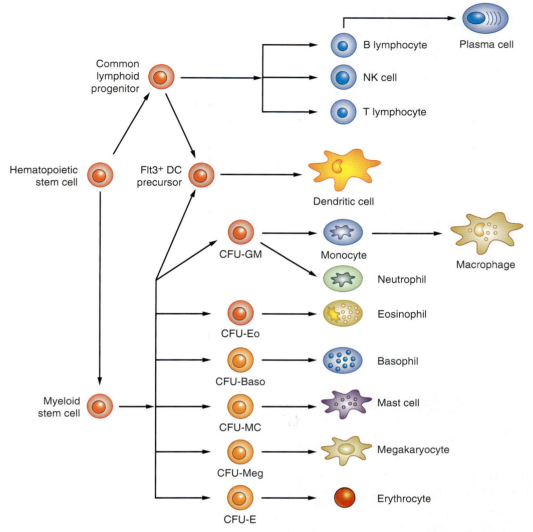

FIGURE 20.2 Differentiation of Hematopoietic Cells. *Arrows* show proliferation and expansion of prehematopoietic stem cell populations. *CFU*, Colony-forming unit; *CFU-GM*, colony-forming unit–granulocyte-macrophage; *Flt3+ DC*, receptor-type tyrosine-protein kinase (Flt3+) dendritic cells (DC); *NK*, natural killer cell. (Chapter 6 discusses mast cells.)

while the lymphocytes are immunocytes (cells that create immunity; see Chapter 7).

Granulocytes. The granulocytes have many membrane-bound granules in their cytoplasm. These granules hold enzymes capable of killing microorganisms and catabolizing debris ingested during phagocytosis. The granules also hold powerful biochemical mediators with inflammatory and immune functions. Granulocytes release these mediators, along with the digestive enzymes, in response to specific stimuli and affect other cells in the circulation. Granulocytes are capable of movement through vessel walls (diapedesis) to get to sites where their action is needed.

The **neutrophil (polymorphonuclear neutrophil [PMN])** is the most numerous granulocyte (Figure 20.5). Neutrophils make up 60 to 70% of the total leukocyte count in adults.

Neutrophils are the chief phagocytes of early inflammation. Soon after bacterial invasion or tissue injury, neutrophils migrate out of the capillaries and into the damaged tissue. It is here that they ingest and destroy contaminating microorganisms and debris. Neutrophils are sensitive to the environment in damaged tissue (e.g., low pH, enzymes released from damaged cells) and die in 1 or 2 days. The breakdown of dead neutrophils releases digestive enzymes from their cytoplasmic granules. These enzymes dissolve cellular debris and prepare the site for healing.

Eosinophils have large, coarse granules and make up 2 to 4% of the normal leukocyte count in adults. Using pattern-recognition receptors, eosinophils are capable of amoeboid movement and phagocytosis. Eosinophils ingest antigen–antibody complexes and are induced by immunoglobulin E (IgE)–mediated hypersensitivity reactions to attack parasites (see Chapters 7 and 8). Eosinophil secondary granules contain toxic chemicals that are highly destructive to parasites and viruses.[1] Eosinophil granules also contain a variety of enzymes (e.g., histaminase) that help to control inflammatory processes. Eosinophils also release leukotrienes, prostaglandins, platelet-activating factor (PAF), and cytokines (e.g., interleukin-1 [IL-1], IL-6, tumour necrosis factor-alpha [TNF-α], granulocyte-macrophage colony–stimulating factor [GM-CSF]) and chemokines (e.g., IL-8) that boost the inflammatory response. During type I hypersensitivity, allergic reactions and asthma are characterized by high eosinophil counts. This increase may be involved in the regulation of inflammation and contribute to the destructive inflammatory processes seen in the lungs of persons who have asthma.

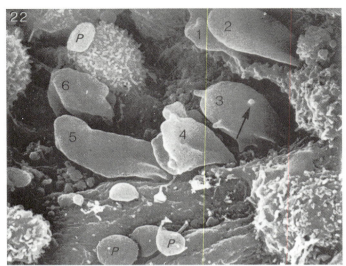

FIGURE 20.3 Red Blood Cells in the Spleen. Scanning electron micrograph of spleen, showing erythrocytes (numbered *1* through *6*) squeezing through the wall in transit from the splenic cord to the sinus. The view shows the endothelial lining of the sinus wall, to which platelets *(P)* adhere, along with "hairy" white blood cells, probably macrophages. The *arrow* shows a protrusion on a red blood cell (×5000). (From Weiss, L. [1974]. A scanning electron microscopic study of the spleen. *Blood, 43*[5], 665–691; reprinted with permission.)

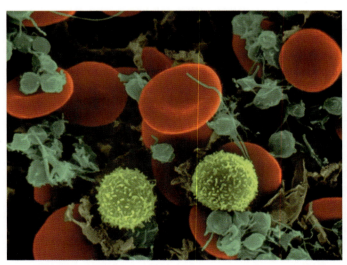

FIGURE 20.4 Blood Cells. Leukocytes are spherical and have irregular surfaces with many extending pili. Leukocytes are the cotton candy–like cells *(yellow)*. Erythrocytes are flattened spheres with a depressed centre *(red)*. (Dennis Kunkel Microscopy/Science Source.)

Basophils make up less than 1% of leukocytes. They are structurally like mast cells (see Figure 20.5). Basophils hold cytoplasmic granules with histamine, chemotactic factors, proteolytic enzymes, and an anticoagulant. Stimulation of basophils also induces creation of vasoactive lipid molecules (e.g., leukotrienes) and cytokines, including IL-6, which affects differentiation of T-helper (Th) 1 and Th2 cells. Basophils also are a rich source of the cytokine IL-4. This cytokine guides B-lymphocyte (B-cell) differentiation toward plasma cells that secrete IgE (see Chapter 7).

Agranulocytes. The agranulocytes include monocytes, macrophages, and lymphocytes. These cells have fewer granules than granulocytes. Monocytes and macrophages make up the mononuclear phagocyte system (MPS) (see "The Mononuclear Phagocyte System" later in this chapter, and Chapter 6). Monocytes and macrophages are powerful

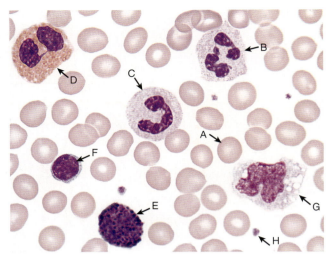

FIGURE 20.5 Leukocytes. Normal cells in peripheral blood: **A**, Erythrocyte (red blood cell); **B**, Neutrophil (segmented); **C**, Neutrophil (banded); **D**, Eosinophil; **E**, Basophil; **F**, Lymphocyte; **G**, Monocyte; **H**, Platelet. (From Keohane, E., Smith, L., & Walenga, J. [2016]. *Rodak's hematology* [5th ed.]. Saunders.)

phagocytes and take part in the immune and inflammatory response. They also ingest dead or defective host cells, particularly blood cells.

Monocytes are immature macrophages (see Figure 20.5). Monocytes are formed and released by the bone marrow into the bloodstream. As they mature, monocytes move into a variety of tissues (e.g., liver, spleen, lymph nodes, peritoneum, gastro-intestinal tract). It is in these tissues that they mature into tissue **macrophages**. Other monocytes may mature into macrophages and move out of the vessels in response to infection or inflammation.

Lymphocytes make up 20 to 25% of the total leukocyte count. They are the primary cells of the immune response (see Figure 20.5 and Chapter 7). Most lymphocytes briefly circulate in the blood and eventually live in lymphoid tissues as mature T lymphocytes (T cells), B lymphocytes (B cells), or plasma cells. (Unit 2 describes lymphocyte function and dysfunction.)

Natural killer (NK) cells resemble lymphocytes. They kill some types of tumour cells (in vitro) and some virus-infected cells without prior exposure (see Chapters 6 and 7). They develop in the bone marrow and circulate in the blood.

Platelets. **Platelets (thrombocytes)** are not true cells but plate-like or disc-shaped anuclear cytoplasmic fragments. They are essential for blood coagulation and control of bleeding. When blood vessel injury stimulates platelets, they can change shape to conform to the need of the injured site. They are formed by the breaking up of large (40 to 100 μm in diameter) cells known as **megakaryocytes**. Platelets hold cytoplasmic granules capable of releasing strong mediators when stimulated by injury to a blood vessel (Figure 20.6).

The normal platelet concentration is approximately 150 to 400×10^9/L of circulating blood. The normal ranges may vary slightly from laboratory to laboratory. An added one-third of the body's available platelets are in a reserve pool in the spleen. A platelet circulates for approximately 8 to 11 days, and ages. It is removed by macrophages, mostly in the spleen.

Lymphoid Organs

> **QUICK CHECK 20.2**
> 1. Why is the spleen considered a hematological organ? Why can humans live without it?
> 2. Why are lymph nodes considered part of the hematological system?
> 3. What is the mononuclear phagocyte system?

CHAPTER 20 Structure and Function of the Hematological System

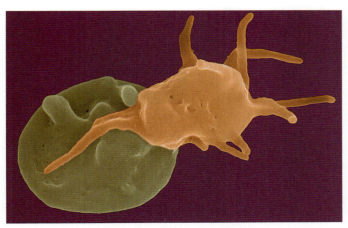

FIGURE 20.6 Coloured Micrograph of Platelets. The platelet on the left is moderately activated, with a generally round shape and the beginning of formation of pseudopodia (footlike extensions from the membrane). The platelet on the right is fully activated, with extensive pseudopodia. (Dennis Kunkel Microscopy/Science Source.)

The lymphoid system is joined with the circulatory system. The lymphoid organs, some of which are merely clusters of lymphoid tissue, are classified as primary or secondary. The **primary lymphoid organs** are the thymus and the bone marrow. The **secondary lymphoid organs** consist of the spleen, lymph nodes, tonsils, and Peyer patches of the small intestine. All the lymphoid organs link the hematological and immune systems. These organs are sites of residence, proliferation, differentiation, or function of lymphocytes and mononuclear phagocytes (monocytes and macrophages). (Chapter 35 describes the liver, which also has hematological functions and is primarily a digestive organ.)

Spleen

The **spleen** is the largest lymphoid organ. It serves as a site of fetal hematopoiesis, filters and cleanses the blood by mononuclear phagocytes, and starts an immune response to bloodborne microorganisms. It is also a reservoir for blood.

The spleen is a concave, encapsulated organ that is about the size of a fist. Strands of connective tissue (trabeculae) extend throughout the spleen from the splenic capsule. These strands divide the spleen into compartments that hold masses of lymphoid tissue called *splenic pulp*.

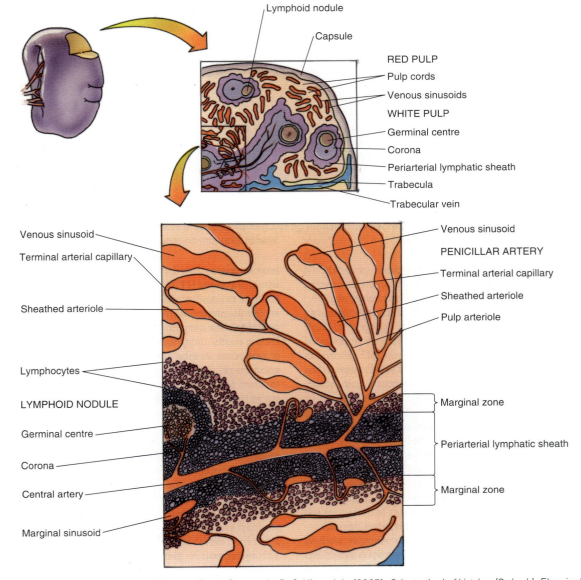

FIGURE 20.7 Diagram of the Spleen. (From Gartner, L. P., & Hiatt, J. L. [2007]. *Color textbook of histology* [3rd ed.]. Elsevier.)

The spleen has many blood vessels, some of which can expand to store blood.

Arterial blood that enters the spleen first meets the white splenic pulp. This pulp is made up of masses of lymphoid tissue holding macrophages and lymphocytes, primarily T cells in proximity to the arterioles (Figure 20.7). Cellular clumps (lymphoid follicles) are formed in the white pulp around the splenic arterioles. The lymphoid follicles are made up of primarily of B cells. These follicles are the chief sites of immune function within the spleen. Here bloodborne antigens meet lymphocytes, starting the immune response and the conversion of lymphoid follicles into germinal centres (see Chapter 7).

Some of the blood continues through the microcirculation and enters highly distensible storage areas, called *venous sinuses*. These sinuses are found in the red pulp of the spleen. The venous sinuses (and the red pulp) can store more than 300 mL of blood. Sudden decreases in blood pressure cause the sympathetic nervous system to stimulate constriction of the sinuses and expel as much as 200 mL of blood into the venous circulation. This mechanism helps to restore blood volume or pressure in the circulation and increases the hematocrit by as much as 4%.

The endothelial lining of the venous sinuses is discontinuous (having gaps between endothelial cells). It is therefore very permeable so that blood cells are allowed to exit the circulation.[2] The red pulp contains a system of loosely interconnected resident macrophages that provide the main site of splenic filtration. Because of the slow circulation in the sinuses, the macrophages easily phagocytose old, damaged, or dead blood cells (mainly erythrocytes), microorganisms, macromolecules, and particles of debris. Hb from phagocytosed erythrocytes is catabolized, and heme (iron) is stored in the cytoplasm of the macrophages or released back into the blood. Blood that filters through the red pulp then moves through the venous sinuses and into the portal circulation.

The spleen is not necessary for life or for adequate hematological function. However, splenic absence from any cause (atrophy, traumatic injury, or removal because of disease) has several secondary effects on the body. For example, leukocytosis (high levels of circulating leukocytes) often occurs after splenectomy. This finding suggests that the spleen has some control over the rate of proliferation of leukocyte stem cells in the bone marrow or their release into the bloodstream. Circulating levels of iron also may decrease, reflecting the spleen's role in the iron cycle. The immune response to encapsulated bacteria, which is primarily an immunoglobulin M (IgM) response, may be severely decreased. This decrease results in increased susceptibility to disseminated infections. Loss of the spleen results in an increase in morphologically defective blood cells in the circulation. This finding confirms the spleen's role in removing old or damaged cells.

Lymph Nodes

Lymph nodes are part of the lymphatic system. Lymphatic vessels collect interstitial fluid from the tissues and transport it, as lymph, through vessels of increasing size to the thoracic duct. From here the lymph drains into the superior vena cava, returning the lymph to the circulation. Lymph nodes are found throughout the body. They filter the lymph during its journey through the lymphatics. A fibrous capsule encloses each lymph node, branches of which (trabeculae) extend inward to divide the node into several sections (Figure 20.8). Reticular fibres of connective tissue divide the sections into a meshwork throughout the lymph node. The node consists of outer (cortex) and inner (paracortex) cortical areas and an inner medulla. Lymph enters through many small afferent lymphatic vessels into the subcapsular sinus, just beneath the capsule. It then drains into the cortical sinuses and then to the medullary sinuses. From there the lymph leaves the node by way of the efferent lymphatic vessel. Blood flows into the lymph nodes through the lymphatic artery, which ends in groups of

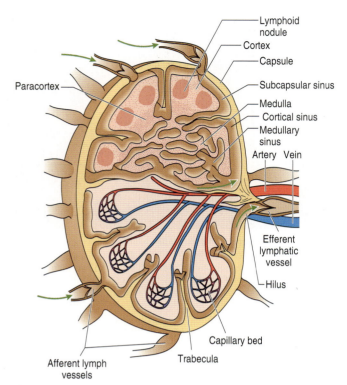

FIGURE 20.8 Cross-section of Lymph Node. Several afferent valved lymphatics bring lymph to node. A single efferent lymphatic leaves the node at the hilus. Note that the artery and vein also enter and leave at the hilus. *Arrows* show direction of lymph flow. (Adapted from Gartner, L. P., & Hiatt, J. L. [2007]. *Color textbook of histology* [3rd ed.]. Saunders.)

postcapillary venules distributed throughout the outer cortex. The lymphatic vein drains the blood.

Lymph nodes are part of the hematological and immune systems. They are the primary site for the first encounter between antigen and lymphocytes. Lymphocytes enter the lymph node from the blood through the postcapillary venules by diapedesis across the endothelial lining. B cells tend to migrate to the cortex and medulla of the nodes, while T cells migrate to the paracortex. Macrophages live in the lymph node. They help filter the lymph of debris, foreign substances, and microorganisms; and supply antigen-processing functions. The dendritic cells meet and process antigens and microorganisms in other tissues, enter the lymph node through the afferent lymph vessels, and migrate throughout the nodes (see Chapter 6). The reticular network supplies adhesive surfaces for trapping large numbers of phagocytes and lymphocytes and helps their organization into follicles or primary nodules. The presence of antigen, either removed from the lymph by macrophages or presented on the surface of dendritic cells, results in the production of secondary nodules having germinal centres. In the germinal centres, lymphocytes, particularly B cells, respond to antigenic stimulation by undergoing proliferation and further differentiation into memory cells and plasma cells (see Chapter 7). Plasma cells travel to the medullary cords. The B-cell proliferation in response to a great deal of antigen (e.g., during infection) may result in lymph node enlargement and tenderness (reactive lymph node).

The Mononuclear Phagocyte System

The **mononuclear phagocyte system (MPS)** (formerly called the *reticuloendothelial system*) is made up of monocytes that differentiate without dividing and live in the tissues for months or perhaps years.[3]

TABLE 20.3 Mononuclear Phagocyte System

Name of Cell	Location
Monocytes/macrophages	Bone marrow and peripheral blood
Kupffer cells (inflammatory macrophages)	Liver
Alveolar macrophages	Lung
Histiocytes	Connective tissue
Macrophages	Bone marrow
Fixed and free macrophages	Spleen and lymph nodes
Pleural and peritoneal macrophages	Serous cavities
Microglial cells	Nervous system
Mesangial cells	Kidney
Osteoclasts	Bone
Langerhans cells	Skin
Dendritic cells	Lymphoid tissue

Table 20.3 lists the various names given to macrophages localized in specific tissues.

Cells of the MPS play an important role in defence. These cells ingest and destroy (by phagocytosis) unwanted materials. These materials include foreign protein particles, circulating immune complexes, microorganisms, debris from dead or injured cells, defective or injured erythrocytes, and dead neutrophils. The osteoclast is a member of the MPS. *Osteoclasts* are multinucleated cells that originate from the monocyte cell lineage (see Figure 20.2). They are specialized for the function of bone resorption; however, they are also known to have phagocytic abilities.

DEVELOPMENT OF BLOOD CELLS

> ✓ **QUICK CHECK 20.3**
> 1. Why is the stem cell system important to hematopoiesis?
> 2. What role do stromal cells play in hematopoiesis?
> 3. Why are some stem cells called pluripotent?

Hematopoiesis

The human requires about 100 billion new blood cells per day. Blood cell production, termed **hematopoiesis**, is constantly ongoing. It occurs in the liver and spleen of the fetus and only in bone marrow (*medullary hematopoiesis*) after birth. This process involves the biochemical stimulation of populations of relatively undifferentiated cells to undergo mitotic division (i.e., proliferation) and maturation (i.e., differentiation) into mature hematological cells. Although proliferation is usually followed by differentiation, certain blood cells proliferate and differentiate at the same time. Erythrocytes and neutrophils generally differentiate fully before entering the blood. Monocytes and lymphocytes continue to mature in the blood and in secondary lymphatic organs.

Hematopoiesis continues throughout life. It increases in response to a need to replenish destroyed circulating cells (e.g., during hemorrhage, hemolytic anemia, consumptive thrombocytopenia) or in response to infection.[2] In general, long-term stimuli, such as chronic diseases, cause a greater increase in hematopoiesis than acute conditions, such as hemorrhage.

Chapter 21 discusses various abnormalities in medullary hematopoiesis. **Extramedullary hematopoiesis** (blood cell production in tissues other than bone marrow) of apparently normal blood cells has been reported in the spleen, liver, and, less often, lymph nodes, adrenal glands, cartilage, adipose tissue, intrathoracic areas, and kidneys. Extramedullary hematopoiesis, however, is usually a sign of disease. It occurs in pernicious anemia, sickle cell anemia, thalassemia, hemolytic disease of the newborn (erythroblastosis fetalis), hereditary spherocytosis, and certain leukemias.

Bone Marrow

Bone marrow is found in the cavities of bone. It is the primary residence of hematopoietic stem cells. It consists of blood vessels, nerves, mononuclear phagocytes, stromal cells, and blood cells in various stages of differentiation. Adults have two kinds of bone marrow: red, or active (hematopoietic) marrow (also called **myeloid tissue**); and yellow, or inactive marrow. The large quantities of fat in inactive marrow make it yellow. Not all bones have active marrow. In adults, active marrow is found in the flat bones of the pelvis (36%), vertebrae (29%), cranium and mandible (13%), sternum and ribs (10%), upper limb girdle (8%), and in the extreme proximal portions of the femur (4%). Inactive marrow is found in the cavities of other bones. (Chapter 38 discusses bones.)

Hematopoietic marrow is vascularized by the primary arteries of the bones, which end in a capillary network forming large venous sinuses. Hematopoietic marrow and fat fill the spaces surrounding the network of venous sinuses. Newly produced blood cells pass through narrow openings between endothelial cells in the venous sinus walls where they enter the circulation. Normally, cells do not enter the circulation until they have differentiated (e.g., developed surface receptors to interact with the endothelium and enter the circulation). Premature release, however, occurs in certain diseases.

The hematological compartment of the bone marrow is made of cellular microenvironments or **niches**. The niches control differentiation of hematopoietic progenitor cells. The cellular make-up of niches includes osteoblasts, osteoclasts, sinusoidal endothelial cells, fibroblasts, megakaryocytes, macrophages, and nerve cells. *Osteoblasts* come from fibroblasts and handle construction of bone. *Osteoclasts* are multinucleate cells of monocytic origin that remodel bone by resorption. Both cells produce cytokines that affect proliferation of hematopoietic cells.[2] At least two populations of stem cells are found in bone marrow niches. **Mesenchymal stem cells (MSCs)** are **stromal cells** that can differentiate into a variety of cells. These cells include osteoblasts, adipocytes, and chondrocytes (produce cartilage). **Hematopoietic stem cells (HSCs)** are originators of all hematological cells. Each type of blood cell originates from a parent stem cell. Both populations of stem cells undergo self-renewal in the bone marrow. This allows added MSCs and HSCs to be produced to replace those undergoing differentiation.[4]

Two types of niches have been found—the osteoblastic (also called *endosteal*) niche and the vascular niche (Figure 20.9). The **osteoblastic niche** is centralized around osteoblasts, which line the surface of bone. The **vascular niche** is organized around sinusoidal endothelial cells. In both niches, HSCs are affected by direct cell-to-cell signalling and soluble mediators produced by cells within each niche. Each niche also has two specialized cells derived from MSCs: CXCL12-abundant reticular (CAR) cells and nestin-expressing cells.[5]

CAR cells look like reticular cells. They have long cellular processes and closely interact with HSCs to provide important intercellular signalling through HSC regulatory molecules. These molecules include chemokine ligand 12 (CXCL12), stem cell factor (SCF, also called *steel factor*), vascular cell adhesion molecule 1 (VCAM-1), and angiopoietin 1 (ANG1). CXCL12 is a chemokine that reacts with a chemokine receptor on HSCs. SCF is expressed as a cell-surface transmembrane protein or a soluble protein and reacts with the HSC KIT receptor (also called *stem cell growth factor receptor, proto-oncogene c-Kit,* or *CD117*). VCAM-1 mediates intercellular adhesion through its receptor, integrin $\alpha_4\beta_1$. ANG1 is secreted and reacts with a tyrosine kinase receptor.

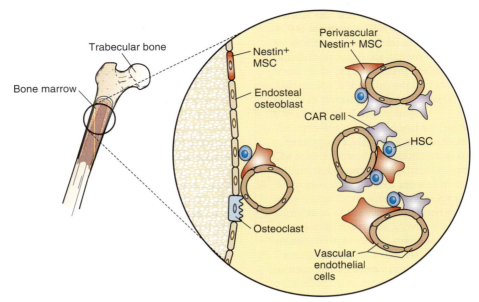

FIGURE 20.9 Bone Marrow Stem Cell Niches. Stem cell niches are microenvironments where stem cells undergo hematopoiesis into all forms of blood cells. Stem cell niches keep and support adult resting hematopoietic stem cells *(HSCs)*. They are activated after cell injury to promote cell renewal or differentiation to form new tissues. The fate of individual HSCs is determined by interactions (intercellular adherence, cytokines, chemokines) with specialized cells within the niches. Within osteoblastic niches the HSC interacts primarily with the osteoblasts and specialized mesenchymal stem cells *(MSCs)* that include nestin-expressing *(Nestin+)* MSCs and CXCL12-abundant reticular *(CAR)* cells. Within the vascular niches, the HSC interacts with vascular endothelial cells, Nestin+ MSC, and a more abundant population of CAR cells.

Nestin-expressing cells express large amounts of the intermediate filament protein, nestin, and particularly SCF and VCAM-1. Although both MSC-derived cells are present in the osteoblastic niche and vascular niche, the CAR cell is the predominant cell in the vascular niche.

Each bone marrow niche affects HSCs differently. In the osteoblastic niche, HSCs are in direct contact with osteoblasts, CAR cells, and nestin-expressing cells. The effect is retention of HSCs in the bone marrow in a quiescent (dormant) state. HSCs that move to the vascular niche directly contact endothelial cells, as well as nestin-expressing cells and larger numbers of perivascular CAR cells. The cumulative signalling events cause HSC proliferation and hematopoietic differentiation.

Cellular Differentiation

All humans originate from a single cell (the fertilized egg) that has the ability to proliferate and differentiate into the huge diversity of cells of the human body. After fertilization, the egg divides over a 5-day period to form a hollow ball (blastocyst) that implants on the uterus. Until about 3 days after fertilization, each cell (blastomere) is undifferentiated and keeps the capacity to differentiate into any cell type. In the 5-day blastocyst, the outer layer of cells has undergone differentiation and commitment to become the placenta. Cells of the inner cell mass, however, continue to have unlimited differentiation potential (currently referred to as being *pluripotent*) and can grow into different kinds of tissue (e.g., blood, nerves, heart, bone). After implantation, cells of the inner cell mass begin differentiation into other cell types. Differentiation is a multistep process. It results in intermediate groups of stem cells with more limited, but still impressive, abilities to differentiate into many different types of cells.

Within the bone marrow niches, each type of blood cell originates from HSCs that proliferate and differentiate under control of a variety of cytokines and growth factors[2] (see Figure 20.2). As with all stem cells, the HSCs are self-renewing (they can proliferate without further differentiation). As a result, a constant population of stem cells is available. Some HSCs will continue differentiation into hematopoietic progenitor cells. Progenitor cells keep proliferative ability but are committed to possible further differentiation into particular types of hematological cells. These cells include lymphoid (lymphocytes, NK cells), granulocyte/monocyte (granulocytes, monocytes, macrophages), and megakaryocyte/erythroid (platelets, erythrocytes) progenitor cells.

Several cytokines take part in hematopoiesis, particularly **colony-stimulating factors (CSFs** or **hematopoietic growth factors)**. CSFs stimulate the proliferation of progenitor cells and their progeny and start the maturation events necessary to produce fully mature cells. Multiple cell types in hematopoietic organs, including endothelial cells, fibroblasts, and lymphocytes, produce the necessary CSFs.

Hematopoiesis in the bone marrow occurs in two separate pools. This includes the stem cell pool and the bone marrow pool. Eventually, mature cells are released into the peripheral circulation (Figure 20.10). The stem cell pool holds pluripotent stem cells and partially committed progenitor cells. The bone marrow pool holds cells that are proliferating and maturing in preparation for release into the circulation and mature cells that are stored for later release into the peripheral blood. The peripheral blood also holds two pools of cells. These pools include those circulating and those stored around the walls of the blood vessels (often called the **marginating storage pool**). The marginating storage pool mainly consists of neutrophils that adhere to the endothelium in vessels where the blood flow is relatively slow. These cells can quickly move into tissues and mucous membranes when needed.

Under certain conditions, the levels of circulating hematological cells need to be rapidly replaced. Medullary hematopoiesis can be increased by any or all of three mechanisms: (1) conversion of yellow

CHAPTER 20 Structure and Function of the Hematological System

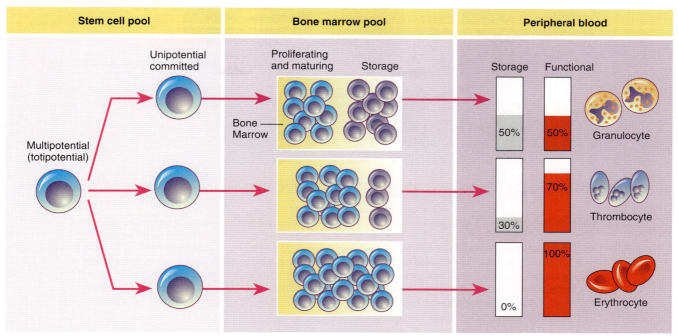

FIGURE 20.10 Hematopoiesis. Hematopoiesis from the stem cell pool; activity is mainly in the bone marrow and in the peripheral blood.

bone marrow, which does not produce blood cells, to red marrow, which does, by the actions of **erythropoietin** (a hormone that stimulates erythrocyte production); (2) faster differentiation of daughter cells; and, presumably, (3) faster proliferation of stem cells.

Development of Erythrocytes

> ✓ **QUICK CHECK 20.4**
> 1. Why is the reticulocyte count important?
> 2. Why is iron important to erythropoiesis?
> 3. What happens to aging erythrocytes?

For almost 100 years it was thought that erythrocytes developed in the spleen. It was not until the 1950s that the bone marrow was named as the site of **erythropoiesis**, or development of red blood cells.

Erythropoiesis
In the bone marrow, erythroid progenitor cells proliferate and differentiate into large, nucleated **proerythroblasts**, which in turn produce cells of the erythroid series. The proerythroblast differentiates through several intermediate forms of **erythroblast** (sometimes called **normoblast**). A progressive elimination of most intracellular structures (including the nucleus), synthesis of Hb, and the process of becoming more compact occurs. Eventually the erythroblast assumes the shape and characteristics of an erythrocyte.

The last immature form is the **reticulocyte**. This form has a mesh-like (reticular) network of ribosomal RNA that is visible microscopically after staining with certain dyes. Reticulocytes stay in the marrow for about 1 day and are released into the venous sinuses. They continue to mature in the bloodstream and may travel to the spleen for several days of added maturation. The normal reticulocyte count is 1% of the total red blood cell count. About 1% of the body's circulating erythrocyte mass normally is made every 24 hours. Therefore, the reticulocyte count is a useful clinical index of erythropoietic activity. It shows whether new red blood cells are being produced.

Most steps of erythropoiesis are primarily under the control of a feedback loop involving the glycoprotein erythropoietin. In healthy humans, the total volume of circulating erythrocytes stays constant. In conditions of tissue hypoxia, erythropoietin is secreted primarily by the peritubular cells of the kidney (Figure 20.11). Rising levels of erythropoietin cause a compensatory increase in erythrocyte production if the oxygen content of blood decreases. This occurs because of anemia, high altitude, or pulmonary disease. The normal steady-state rate of production can increase under anemic or low-oxygen states. Thus, the body responds to reduced oxygenation of blood in two ways: (1) by increasing the intake of oxygen through increased respiration and (2) by increasing the oxygen-carrying capacity of the blood through increased erythropoiesis.

Recombinant human erythropoietin (r-HuEPO) is used in individuals with anemia secondary to decreased erythropoietin from chronic renal failure. An immediate effect of erythropoietin administration is an increase in the blood reticulocyte count, followed by increasing levels of erythrocytes. The most significant side effect is increased blood pressure.

Hemoglobin Synthesis
Hemoglobin (Hb), the oxygen-carrying protein of the erythrocyte, constitutes about 90% of the cell's dry weight. Hb-packed blood cells take up oxygen in the lungs and exchange it for carbon dioxide in the tissues. Hb increases the oxygen-carrying capacity of blood by 100-fold. Each Hb molecule is composed of two pairs of polypeptide chains (the **globins**) and four colourful complexes of iron plus protoporphyrin (the hemes). The hemes are responsible for the blood's ruby-red colour (Figure 20.12).

Several variants of Hb exist. However, they differ only slightly in primary structure based on the use of different polypeptide chains: alpha, beta, gamma, delta, epsilon, or zeta (α, β, γ, δ, ϵ, or ζ).[2] Hemoglobin A (Hb A), the most common type in adults, is composed of two α- and two β-polypeptide chains ($\alpha_2\beta_2$). A normal variant, fetal hemoglobin (Hb F), is a complex of two α- and two γ-polypeptide chains ($\alpha_2\gamma_2$) that binds oxygen with a much greater affinity than adult Hb.

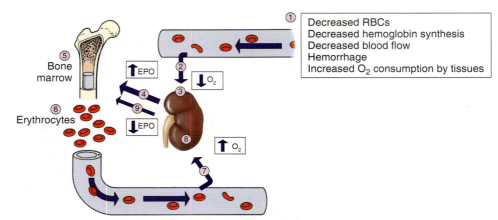

FIGURE 20.11 Role of Erythropoietin in Regulation of Erythropoiesis. (1) Decreased arterial oxygen levels result in (2) decreased tissue oxygen (hypoxia) that (3) stimulates the kidney to increase (4) production of erythropoietin. Erythropoietin is carried to the bone marrow (5) and binds to erythropoietin receptors on proerythroblasts, resulting in increased red blood cell production and maturation and expansion of the erythron (6). The increased release of red blood cells into the circulation often corrects tissue hypoxia (7). (8) Perception of normal oxygen levels by the kidney causes (9) decreased production of erythropoietin (negative feedback) and return to normal levels of erythrocyte production. *EPO*, Erythropoietin; O_2, oxygen (in the blood and tissue); *RBCs*, red blood cells.

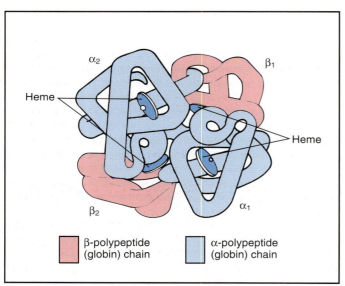

FIGURE 20.12 Molecular Structure of Hemoglobin. The molecule is a spherical tetramer weighing approximately 64 500 daltons. It has a pair of α-polypeptide chains and a pair of β-polypeptide chains and several heme groups.

Heme is a large, flat, iron-protoporphyrin disc. It is synthesized in the mitochondria and can carry one molecule of oxygen.[2] Thus, an individual Hb molecule with its four hemes can carry four oxygen molecules. If all four oxygen-binding sites are occupied by oxygen, the molecule is said to be saturated. Through a series of biochemical reactions, protoporphyrin, a complex four-ringed molecule, is produced and bound with ferrous iron (Fe^{2+}). It is crucial that the iron be correctly charged; reduced Fe^{2+} can bind oxygen, while ferric iron (Fe^{3+}) cannot. Binding of oxygen to Fe^{2+} temporarily oxidizes Fe^{2+} to Fe^{3+} (oxyhemoglobin). However, after the release of oxygen the body reduces the iron to Fe^{2+} and reactivates the Hb (deoxyhemoglobin [reduced Hb]). Without reactivation, the Fe^{3+}-containing Hb (methemoglobin) cannot bind oxygen. An excess of Fe^{3+} occurs with certain medications and chemicals, such as nitrates and sulphonamides.

Several other molecules can competitively bind to deoxyhemoglobin. Carbon monoxide directly competes with oxygen for binding to ferrous ion with an affinity that is about 200-fold greater than that of oxygen. Thus, even a small amount of carbon monoxide can dramatically decrease the ability of Hb to bind and transport oxygen. Hb also binds carbon dioxide, but at a binding site separate from where oxygen binds. In the lungs, carbon dioxide is released, allowing Hb to bind oxygen.

Erythrocytes may play a role in the maintenance of vascular relaxation. Nitric oxide (NO) produced by blood vessels is a major mediator of relaxation and dilation of the vessel walls. In the lungs, Hb can bind oxygen to the ferrous ion and NO to cysteine residues in the globins at the same time (Figure 20.13). As Hb transfers its oxygen to tissue, it may also shed small amounts of NO, contributing to dilation of the blood vessels. This process helps the transfer of oxygen into tissues.

Nutritional Requirements for Erythropoiesis

Normal development of erythrocytes and creation of Hb depend on an optimal biochemical state. An adequate supply of the necessary building blocks including protein, vitamins, and minerals is also needed (Table 20.4). If these components are lacking for a prolonged time, erythrocyte production slows, and anemia (insufficient numbers of functional erythrocytes) may result (see Chapter 21).

Erythropoiesis cannot proceed in the absence of vitamins, especially vitamin B_{12}, folate (folic acid), vitamin B_6, riboflavin, pantothenic acid, niacin, ascorbic acid, and vitamin E. Dietary vitamin B_{12} is a large molecule that requires a protein secreted by parietal cells into the stomach (intrinsic factor) for transport across the ileum. Vitamin B_{12} is stored in the liver and used as needed in erythropoiesis. Decreased B_{12} absorption may lead to pernicious anemia. Folate is necessary for DNA and RNA synthesis. Folate absorption occurs mainly in the upper small intestine and is stored in the liver. Folate deficiency is more common than vitamin B_{12} deficiency and occurs more rapidly. Folate supplements are prescribed for pregnant women because pregnancy increases the demand for folate. Supplements can protect against neural tube defects and may prevent anemia.

Normal Destruction of Senescent Erythrocytes

Mature erythrocytes have cytoplasmic enzymes capable of glycolysis (anaerobic glucose metabolism) and production of small quantities of adenosine triphosphate (ATP). ATP supplies the energy needed to support cell function and keep its plasma membrane pliable[2] (see Figure 1.1). Metabolic processes decrease as the erythrocyte ages. As a result, less ATP is available to support plasma membrane function. The aged red blood cell becomes increasingly fragile and loses its reversible deformability. This process makes it susceptible to rupture while passing through narrowed regions of the microcirculation.

The plasma membrane of the senescent (or aged) red blood cells undergoes phospholipid rearrangement. This causes enrichment of surface phosphatidylserine that is recognized by receptors on macrophages (primarily in the spleen), which selectively remove and sequester the red blood cells. If the spleen is dysfunctional or absent, macrophages in the liver (Kupffer cells) assume control. During digestion of Hb in the macrophage, porphyrin reduces to bilirubin. The bilirubin is then transported to the liver, conjugated, and excreted in the bile as glucuronide (Figure 20.14). Bacteria in the intestinal lumen change conjugated bilirubin into urobilinogen. Although a small part is reabsorbed, most urobilinogen is excreted in feces. Conditions causing increased erythrocyte destruction increase the load of bilirubin for hepatic clearance. This increase leads to increased serum levels of unconjugated bilirubin and increased urinary excretion of urobilinogen. Gallstones (cholelithiasis) can result from a chronically elevated rate of bilirubin excretion.

Iron cycle. About 67% of total body iron is bound to heme in erythrocytes (Hb) and muscle cells (**myoglobin**). About 30% is stored in mononuclear phagocytes (i.e., macrophages) and hepatic parenchymal cells as either ferritin or hemosiderin.[2] The remaining 3% is lost daily in urine, sweat, bile, sloughing of epithelial cells from the skin and intestinal mucosa, and minor bleeding. About 25 mg of iron is needed daily for erythropoiesis. Only 1 to 2 mg of iron is dietary, and the rest is obtained from continual recycling of iron from erythrocytes.

The methemoglobin released from the breakdown of aged or damaged erythrocytes is dissociated by the enzyme heme oxygenase. The iron is released into the bloodstream where it is free to bind again to transferrin or be stored in the macrophage's cytoplasm as ferritin or hemosiderin (Figure 20.15). A minute amount of iron is stored in muscle cells by the heme-containing protein myoglobin. Unavailable stores of iron are present in cytochromes, catalases, and peroxidase enzymes.

The protein ferritin is the major intracellular iron storage protein. **Apoferritin**, which is ferritin without attached iron, can store thousands of atoms of iron. Several apoferritin complexes combine to form the micelle ferritin. Large groups of micelles (if a large amount of iron is present) produce large iron storage complexes, known as **hemosiderin**.

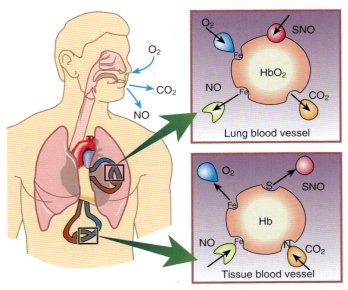

FIGURE 20.13 Hemoglobin Binding to Nitric Oxide. In the lungs, hemoglobin *(Hb)* binds to nitric oxide *(NO)* as S-nitrosothiol *(SNO)*. In tissue, this SNO is released, and free, circulating NO is bound to a different site for exhalation. CO_2, Carbon dioxide; *Fe*, iron; *N*, nitrogen; O_2, oxygen; *S*, sulphur.

TABLE 20.4 Nutritional Requirements for Erythropoiesis

Nutrient	Role in Erythropoiesis	Consequence of Deficiency (see Chapter 21)
Protein (amino acids)	Structural part of plasma membrane	Decreased strength, elasticity, and flexibility of membrane; hemolytic anemia
	Synthesis of hemoglobin	Decreased erythropoiesis and lifespan of erythrocytes
Intrinsic factor	Gastro-intestinal absorption of vitamin B_{12}	Pernicious anemia
Cobalamin (vitamin B_{12})	Synthesis of DNA, maturation of erythrocytes, facilitator of folate metabolism	Macrocytic (megaloblastic) anemia
Folate (folic acid)	Synthesis of DNA and RNA, maturation of erythrocytes	Macrocytic (megaloblastic) anemia
Vitamin B_6 (pyridoxine)	Heme synthesis, possibly increases folate metabolism	Hypochromic-microcytic anemia
Vitamin B_2 (riboflavin)	Oxidative reactions	Normochromic-normocytic anemia
Vitamin C (ascorbic acid)	Iron metabolism, acts as reducing agent to support iron in its ferrous (Fe^{++}) form	Normochromic-normocytic anemia
Pantothenic acid	Heme synthesis	Unknown in humans[a]
Niacin	None, but needed for respiration in mature erythrocytes	Unknown in humans
Vitamin E	Synthesis of heme; possible protection against oxidative damage in mature erythrocytes	Hemolytic anemia with increased cell membrane fragility; shortens lifespan of erythrocytes in individual with cystic fibrosis
Iron	Hemoglobin synthesis	Iron deficiency anemia
Copper	Structural part of plasma membrane	Hypochromic-microcytic anemia

[a]Although pantothenic acid is important for optimal synthesis of heme, experimentally induced deficiency did not produce anemia or other hematopoietic disturbances.
Data from Harmening, D. M. (Ed.). (1997). *Clinical hematology and fundamentals of hemostasis* (3rd ed.). F. A. Davis; Lee, G. R., Bithell, T. C., Foerster, J., et al. (1993). *Wintrobe's clinical hematology* (9th ed.). Lee & Febiger.

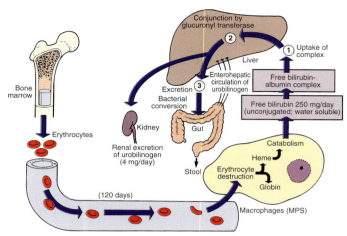

FIGURE 20.14 Metabolism of Bilirubin Released by Heme Breakdown. *MPS*, Mononuclear phagocyte system.

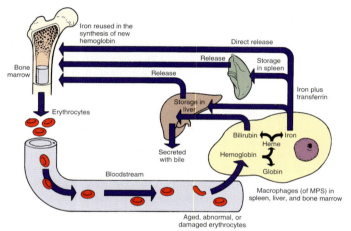

FIGURE 20.15 Iron Cycle. Iron released from gastro-intestinal epithelial cells circulates in the bloodstream associated with its plasma carrier, transferrin. It is delivered to erythroblasts in bone marrow, where most of it is incorporated into hemoglobin. Mature erythrocytes circulate for approximately 120 days, after which they become senescent and are removed by the mononuclear phagocyte system *(MPS)*. Macrophages of MPS (mostly in the spleen) break down ingested erythrocytes and return iron to the bloodstream directly or after storing it as ferritin or hemosiderin.

The iron within deposits of hemosiderin is poorly available to supply iron when needed. The most common cause of hemosiderin deposition is simple bruising. Hemosiderin in small amounts within iron-rich tissues (i.e., spleen, liver, bone marrow) is considered normal. Large groups or its presence in tissue, such as the lungs or subcutaneous tissue, suggest a pathological condition.

Iron from any dietary source, release of iron stores, or erythrocyte catabolism is transported in the blood bound to apotransferrin, thus becoming transferrin. Apotransferrin is a glycoprotein synthesized primarily by hepatocytes in the liver. It is also produced in small amounts by tissue macrophages, submaxillary and mammary glands, and ovaries or testes (see Figure 20.15). Transferrin is transported to the bone marrow, where it binds to transferrin receptors on erythroblasts. Transferrin receptors are on the plasma membrane of all nucleated cells, but at particularly high levels on erythroid precursors and rapidly proliferating cells (e.g., lymphocytes). They are thought to be the only route of cellular entry for transferrin-attached iron. Transferrin is recycled (transferrin cycle) by intracellular dissociation of the iron and secretion of the resulting apotransferrin to the bloodstream.

The iron is transported to the erythroblast's mitochondria (the site of Hb production), where the enzyme heme synthetase inserts ferrous iron into protoporphyrin to form heme. Heme then is bound to globin to form Hb. Iron not used in erythropoiesis is stored temporarily as ferritin or hemosiderin and later excreted.

The body's iron homeostasis is mainly controlled by the hormone hepcidin. Hepcidin is a 25–amino acid peptide made in the liver and released into the plasma. In the plasma it is bound with high affinity to α_2-macroglobulin and with relatively lower affinity to albumin.[6] Hepatocellular hepcidin production is regulated physiologically by the levels of iron in the body, rate of erythropoiesis, and percentage of oxygen saturation. Hepatocytes (liver cells) sense levels of circulating iron by receptors for transferrin. Excess iron is stored in hepatocytes and macrophages, and hepatocytes sense these levels with receptors for bone morphogenetic protein (BMP). Hepcidin production also can be induced by inflammation via IL-6.

Hepcidin regulates iron levels through its binding capacity to ferroportin. Ferroportin is a transmembrane iron exporter found in the plasma membrane of cells that transport or store iron. It is found in macrophages, hepatocytes, and enterocytes (intestinal cells).[2] The body's total iron balance is supported through controlled absorption rather than excretion. Dietary iron (primarily as Fe^{2+}) is transported directly across the membranes of enterocytes in the duodenum and proximal jejunum. (Chapter 1 describes transport mechanisms.) Hepcidin causes internalization and degradation of ferroportin. This process leads to increased intracellular iron stores, decreased dietary iron absorption, and decreased levels of circulating iron. Decreased production of hepcidin leads to release of stored iron and increased dietary absorption. Thus, if the body's iron stores are low or the demand for erythropoiesis increases, dietary iron is transported rapidly through the epithelial cell and into the plasma. If body stores are high and erythropoiesis is not increased, iron transport is stopped, although iron can cross the epithelial cells' plasma membrane passively and is stored as ferritin.

Development of Leukocytes

Leukocytes consist of lymphocytes, granulocytes, and monocytes. Most leukocytes come from HSCs in the bone marrow that differentiate into common lymphoid progenitors and common myeloid progenitors (Figure 20.2 shows the pathways of differentiation). Lymphoid progenitor cells develop into lymphocytes. The lymphocytes enter the bloodstream to undergo further maturation in the primary and secondary lymphoid organs (see Chapter 7). Common myeloid progenitors further differentiate into progenitors for erythrocytes, megakaryocytes, and mast cells, and into granulocyte/monocyte progenitors. The granulocyte/monocyte progenitors further differentiate into monocyte progenitors and granulocyte progenitors. These progenitors then develop into monocytes/macrophages and granulocytes (neutrophils, basophils, eosinophils), respectively. Development from HSC to common granulocyte/monocyte progenitor primarily is under the control of SCF, IL-3, and GM-CSF. Further differentiation into granulocytic and monocytic progenitors is controlled by granulocyte colony-stimulating factor (G-CSF) and macrophage colony-stimulating factor (M-CSF), respectively. The ultimate granulocytic phenotype is determined in the bone marrow by relative local concentrations of early and late-acting cytokines, including GM-CSF, G-CSF, IL-3, IL-5, SCF, and others. Granulocytes are released into the blood within 14 days of development. The bone marrow selectively keeps immature granulocytes as a reserve pool that can be rapidly released in response to the body's needs.

Monocytic progenitors differentiate into monocytes within 24 hours and are released into the circulation. Monocytes mature into various forms of macrophages. This process is usually complete within 1 or 2 days after release.

Most leukocytes exist in the body from days to years, depending on type. Maintenance of optimal levels of granulocytes and monocytes in the blood depends on several factors. These factors include the availability of pluripotent stem cells in the marrow, induction of these into committed stem cells, timely release of new cells from the marrow, and mobilization of the granulocyte reserve pool. Leukocyte production increases in response to infection, to the presence of steroids, and to reduction or depletion of reserves in the marrow. It also is associated with strenuous exercise, convulsive seizures, heat, intense radiation, paroxysmal tachycardias (outbursts of rapid heart rate), pain, nausea and vomiting, and anxiety.

Development of Platelets

Platelets (thrombocytes) are derived from stem cells and progenitor cells that differentiate into megakaryocytes. During thrombopoiesis, the megakaryocyte progenitor is programmed to undergo an endomitotic cell cycle (**endomitosis**). During this cycle DNA replication occurs, but anaphase and cytokinesis are blocked[2] (see Figures 20.2 and 20.6, and Chapter 1). Thus, the megakaryocyte nucleus enlarges and becomes extremely polyploidy (up to 100-fold or more of the normal amount of DNA) without cellular division. At the same time, the numbers of cytoplasmic organelles (e.g., internal membranes, granules) increase, and the cell develops cellular surface elongations and branches that progressively fragment into platelets. A single large megakaryocyte (up to 100 μm) may produce thousands of smaller platelets (2 to 3 μm). Like erythrocytes, platelets released from the bone marrow lack nuclei.

About two-thirds of platelets enter the circulation, and the rest exist in the splenic pool. Platelets circulate in the bloodstream for about 10 days before beginning to lose their ability to carry out biochemical reactions. The spleen sequesters and destroys aging platelets by mononuclear cell phagocytosis. **Thrombopoietin (TPO)**, a hormone growth factor, is the main regulator of the circulating platelet numbers. TPO is mainly produced by the liver and induces platelet production in the bone marrow.[2,7] Platelets express receptors for TPO. When circulating platelet levels are normal, TPO is adsorbed onto the platelet surface and prevented from accessing the bone marrow and initiating further platelet production.[7] When platelet levels are low, the amount of TPO exceeds the number of available platelet TPO receptors, and free TPO can enter the bone marrow. During inflammation, IL-6 induces increased production of TPO. This increased production increases the formation of platelets, which are more thrombogenic.

MECHANISMS OF HEMOSTASIS

✓ **QUICK CHECK 20.5**
1. What specific cells are involved in development of leukocytes?
2. Why are platelets necessary to stop bleeding?
3. Describe the steps of platelet adhesion and aggregation.
4. How does plasminogen start fibrinolysis?

Hemostasis means arrest of bleeding. As a result of hemostasis, damaged blood vessels may support a relatively steady state of blood volume, pressure, and flow. Three equally important components of hemostasis are platelets, clotting factors, and the vasculature (endothelial cells and subendothelial matrix). The following list is the general sequence of events in hemostasis:

1. Vascular injury leads to a transient arteriolar vasoconstriction to limit blood flow to the affected site;
2. Damage to the endothelial cell lining of the vessel exposes the prothrombogenic subendothelial connective tissue matrix, leading to platelet adherence and activation and formation of a *hemostatic plug*, also referred to as a *platelet plug*, to prevent further bleeding (primary hemostasis);
3. Tissue factor, produced by the endothelium, collaborates with secreted platelet factors and activated platelets to activate the clotting (coagulation) system to form fibrin clots and further prevent bleeding (secondary hemostasis);
4. The fibrin/platelet clot contracts to form a more permanent plug; and
5. Regulatory pathways are activated (fibrinolysis) to limit the size of the plug and begin the healing process.

The relative importance of the hemostatic mechanisms clearly varies with vessel size. Damage to large vessels cannot easily be controlled by hemostasis. Instead, these vessels require vascular contraction and dramatically decreased blood flow into the damaged vessels (Table 20.5).

Function of Platelets and Blood Vessels

Platelets normally circulate freely, suspended in plasma, in an inactivated state. Endothelial cells lining the vessels produce NO and the prostaglandin derivative **prostacyclin (PGI2)**. These two substances help support blood flow, blood pressure, and inhibit platelet adhesion and aggregation. NO and PGI_2 are highly synergistic. PGI_2 production varies a great deal in response to stimuli, while NO is released continually to regulate vascular tone. Endothelium also produces adenosine diphosphatase, which degrades adenosine diphosphate (ADP; a potent activator of platelets).

The endothelial cell surface has antithrombotic molecules, such as glycosaminoglycans (e.g., heparan sulphate), thrombomodulin, and plasminogen activators. These limit platelet activation and fibrin deposition. Although thrombomodulin and plasminogen activators help

TABLE 20.5	Types of Bleeding: Sources, Vessel Size, and Sealing Requirements		
Types and Sources of Bleeding	**Involved Vessel**	**Size**	**Sealing Requirements**
Pinpoint petechial hemorrhage (blood leakage from small vessels)	Capillary	Smallest ↓	Generally direct-sealing
	Venule		Mostly fused platelets
	Arteriole		Mostly fused platelets
Ecchymosis (large, soft tissue bleeding)	Vein		Vascular contraction, fused platelets, perivascular and intravascular hemostatic factor activation (see Figure 20-16)
Rapidly expanding "blowout" hemorrhage	Artery	Largest	Greater vascular contraction, more fused platelets, greater perivascular and intravascular hemostatic factor activation

Modified from Harmening, D. M. (Ed.). (1997). *Clinical hematology and fundamentals of hemostasis* (3rd ed.). F. A. Davis.

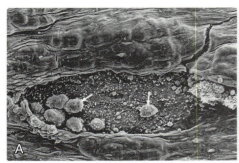 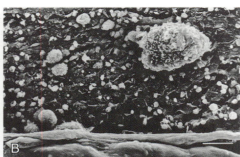 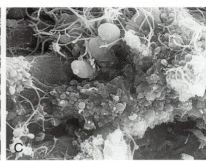

FIGURE 20.16 Platelet Activation. A, After endothelial denudation, platelets and leukocytes adhere to the subendothelium in a monolayer fashion. *Arrows* show adhesion of leukocytes. **B,** Higher-power view showing leukocytes and platelets adherent to the subendothelium. **C,** High magnification of a thrombus showing a mixture of red blood cells and platelets incorporated into the fibrin meshwork. (**A** and **B**, from Libby, P., Bonow R., Mann D. L., et al. [Eds.]. [2007]. *Braunwald's heart disease: a textbook of cardiovascular medicine* [8th ed.]. Saunders; as reproduced from Faggiotto, A., & Ross, R. [1984]. *Arteriosclerosis, 4*[4], 341–356; **C,** from Damjanov, I., & Linder, J. [Eds.]. [1996]. *Anderson's pathology* [10th ed.]. Mosby.)

control hemostasis in normal vessels, their effects are increased during vascular damage and clot formation. Further information is provided on these molecules in the following text describing control of hemostatic mechanisms.

When a vessel is damaged, platelet activation may be started. The role of platelet activation is to (1) contribute to regulation of blood flow into a damaged site through induction of vasoconstriction (vasospasm); (2) initiate platelet-to-platelet interactions resulting in formation of a platelet plug to stop further bleeding; (3) activate the coagulation (or clotting) cascade to stabilize the platelet plug; and (4) initiate repair processes, including clot retraction and clot dissolution. The normal platelet count ranges from 150 to 400×10^9/L. A count below 150 000/mm^3 is defined as thrombocytopenia. However, thrombocytopenia is usually asymptomatic unless the count drops below 100×10^9/L. When the number of platelets is inadequate, abnormal bleeding may occur in response to trauma. Spontaneous major bleeding episodes do not generally occur unless the platelet count falls below 20×10^9/L. However, these values are not absolute, and their clinical significance will vary among individuals.

Platelet activation proceeds through a process of (1) increased adhesion to the damaged vascular wall; (2) platelet degranulation, which stimulates changes in platelet shape; (3) aggregation as platelet–vascular wall and platelet-platelet adherence increases; and (4) activation of the clotting system and development of an immobilizing meshwork of platelets and fibrin (Figure 20.16; and see *Health Promotion:* Sticky Platelets).

The platelet activation process can begin in several ways. If the vessel lining is still intact in an area of inflammation, the endothelial cells may become activated by cytokines and express new proteins on their surface. Several of these, particularly P-selectin, bind specifically yet weakly with receptors on the surface of inactive platelets (e.g., glycoprotein Ib [GPIb]) (Figure 20.17). As inflammation progresses, the platelets adhere more avidly through added receptors that bind through a fibrinogen bridge with the endothelial cell surface. The principal fibrinogen receptor on platelets is the **integrin αIIbβ3** (also known as *glycoprotein PIIb/IIIa* **[GPIIb/IIIa]**).

During vessel damage, the endothelial layer is often compromised. This results in exposure of the underlying matrix that holds **collagen**, fibronectin, and other components. The matrix also holds **von Willebrand factor (vWF)**, and the exposed collagen can bind more vWF from the circulation (see Figure 20.17). Platelets adhere strongly to collagen through the action of several glycoprotein hormones that act as receptors (i.e., glycoprotein VI [GPVI] and integrin $α_2β_1$). They also adhere to vWF through the receptor complex of platelet receptor GPIb and clotting factors IX and V. Progressively the platelets undergo further aggregation through platelet-to-platelet adhesion involving further fibrinogen bridging between receptors (particularly GPIIb/IIIa) on adjacent platelets.

As a result of interactions with the endothelium or the subendothelial matrix, as well as exposure to inflammatory mediators produced by the endothelium and other cells, the platelets are activated. Activation causes reorganization of the platelet cytoskeleton. This process leads to dynamic changes in platelet shape. The platelets go from smooth spheres to those with spiny projections and degranulation (also called the **platelet-release reaction**). The degranulation results in the release of various potent biochemicals.

Platelets have three types of granules—lysosomes, dense bodies, and alpha granules. The contents of the dense bodies and alpha granules are particularly important in hemostasis. Dense bodies are generally proinflammatory (e.g., ADP, calcium, and serotonin). ADP recruits and activates other platelets through specific receptors. ADP also induces the platelet plasma membrane to undergo three important changes. The first change includes becoming ruffled and sticky. They also undergo cellular spreading to make tight contacts between neighbouring platelets,

> ### HEALTH PROMOTION
> #### Sticky Platelets
>
> Investigators report that a genetic trait induces some people to make sticky platelets. People with platelets that tend to stick together have an increased risk of forming deep arterial and venous thromboses. These thromboses can lead to myocardial infarction and cerebrovascular attacks. In pregnant women, sticky blood can result in the blockage of small blood vessels in the placenta. This increases the risk for miscarriage and late-term death of the fetus. People with this condition may also experience complications following cardiac procedures such as angioplasty.
>
> It has been determined that testing for platelet stickiness could determine which people require anticlotting medications to prevent these complications. Treatment for persons who have not experienced significant blood clotting problems may include the administration of a daily baby Aspirin. Those persons with a history of venous thrombosis may require prescription anticoagulant medications such as warfarin (Coumadin). This treatment requires regular blood testing to ensure the blood is at the required consistency to prevent the development of clots or excessive thinning of the blood and the risk of bleeding.

Data from Movva, S., Diamond, H. S., Carsons, S., et al. (2016). *Antiphospholipid syndrome.* https://emedicine.medscape.com/article/333221-overview#a5.

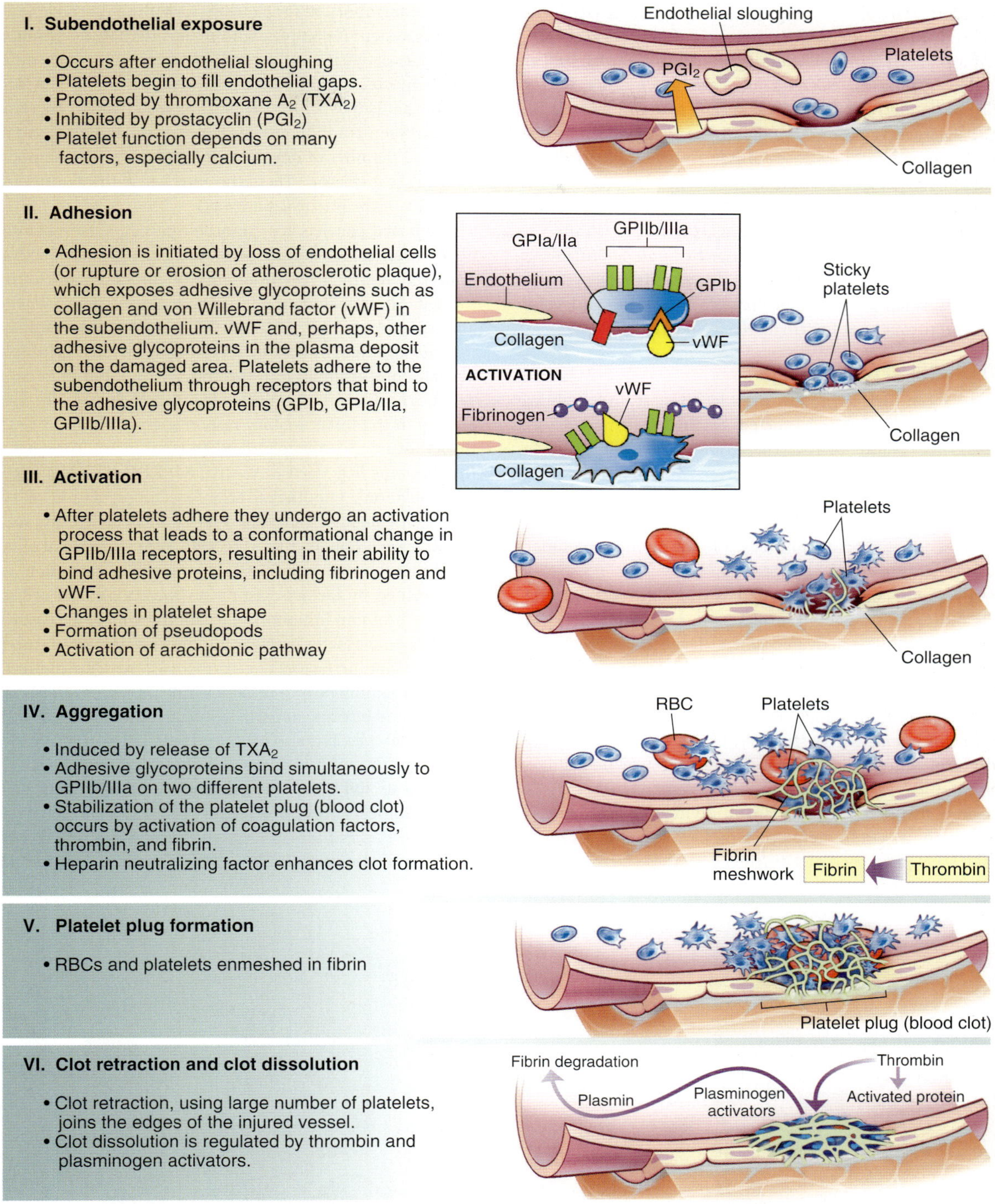
I. Subendothelial exposure
• Occurs after endothelial sloughing
• Platelets begin to fill endothelial gaps.
• Promoted by thromboxane A_2 (TXA_2)
• Inhibited by prostacyclin (PGI_2)
• Platelet function depends on many factors, especially calcium.
Endothelial sloughing
PGI_2
Platelets
Collagen
II. Adhesion
• Adhesion is initiated by loss of endothelial cells (or rupture or erosion of atherosclerotic plaque), which exposes adhesive glycoproteins such as collagen and von Willebrand factor (vWF) in the subendothelium. vWF and, perhaps, other adhesive glycoproteins in the plasma deposit on the damaged area. Platelets adhere to the subendothelium through receptors that bind to the adhesive glycoproteins (GPIb, GPIa/IIa, GPIIb/IIIa).
GPIIb/IIIa
GPIa/IIa
Endothelium
GPIb
Collagen
vWF
ACTIVATION
vWF
Fibrinogen
Collagen
Sticky platelets
Collagen
III. Activation
• After platelets adhere they undergo an activation process that leads to a conformational change in GPIIb/IIIa receptors, resulting in their ability to bind adhesive proteins, including fibrinogen and vWF.
• Changes in platelet shape
• Formation of pseudopods
• Activation of arachidonic pathway
Platelets
Collagen
IV. Aggregation
• Induced by release of TXA_2
• Adhesive glycoproteins bind simultaneously to GPIIb/IIIa on two different platelets.
• Stabilization of the platelet plug (blood clot) occurs by activation of coagulation factors, thrombin, and fibrin.
• Heparin neutralizing factor enhances clot formation.
RBC
Platelets
Fibrin meshwork
Fibrin
Thrombin
V. Platelet plug formation
• RBCs and platelets enmeshed in fibrin
Platelet plug (blood clot)
VI. Clot retraction and clot dissolution
• Clot retraction, using large number of platelets, joins the edges of the injured vessel.
• Clot dissolution is regulated by thrombin and plasminogen activators.
Fibrin degradation
Plasmin
Plasminogen activators
Thrombin
Activated protein

FIGURE 20.17 Blood Vessel Damage, Blood Clot, and Clot Dissolution. *RBC*, Red blood cell.

causing the platelet plug to seal the injured endothelium. Lastly, they undergo externalization of the phospholipid phosphatidylserine, which provides a matrix for activation of clotting factors. Serotonin is a vasoactive amine with histamine-like properties to increase vasodilation and vascular permeability (see Chapter 6). Calcium is necessary for many of the intracellular signalling mechanisms that control platelet activation.

Alpha granules hold a mixture of various factors. This includes clotting factors (fibrinogen, factor V), growth and angiogenic factors (e.g., platelet-derived growth factor [PDGF], vascular endothelial growth factor [VEGF], basic fibroblast growth factor [bFGF]), and angiogenesis inhibitors (e.g., platelet factor 4, thrombospondin, inhibitors of metalloproteinases). Platelet factor 4 also is a heparin-binding protein. Depending on the stimulus, platelets may selectively release promoters or inhibitors of angiogenesis. Many of these mediators also either promote or inhibit platelet activity and the eventual process of clot formation (see Figure 20.17). PDGF stimulates smooth muscle cells and promotes tissue repair. Heparin-binding proteins enhance clot formation at the site of injury.

Platelets also begin producing the prostaglandin derivative **thromboxane A2 (TXA2)**. This substance counters the effects of PGI_2, produced by endothelial cells (see Figure 20.17). TXA_2 causes vasoconstriction and promotes the degranulation of platelets. PGI_2 promotes vasodilation and inhibits platelet degranulation. In platelets, an isoform of cyclo-oxygenase-1 (COX-1) converts arachidonic acid to TXA_2. Aspirin, particularly at low doses, specifically and irreversibly inhibits COX-1, decreasing production of TXA_2 and decreasing platelet activation. Daily intake of low doses of Aspirin leads to more than 95% inhibition of TXA_2 in just a few days.

If blood vessel injury is minor, hemostasis is achieved temporarily by formation of the platelet plug. The plug usually forms within 3 to 5 minutes of injury. Platelet plugs seal the many minute ruptures that occur daily in the microcirculation, particularly in capillaries. With too few platelets, many small hemorrhagic areas called *purpuras* develop under the skin and throughout the tissues (see Chapter 21).

Function of Clotting Factors

A blood clot is a meshwork of protein strands. These strands stabilize the platelet plug and trap other cells, such as erythrocytes, phagocytes, and microorganisms (Figure 20.18). The strands are made of fibrin, which is produced by the clotting (coagulation) system. The clotting system was described in Chapter 6. This system consists of a family of proteins that circulate in the blood in inactive forms. Initiation of the system results in sequential activation (cascade) of multiple members of the system until a fibrin clot is created.

The clotting system is usually presented as two pathways of initiation (intrinsic and extrinsic pathways) that join in a common pathway. The intrinsic pathway is activated when Hageman factor (factor XII) in plasma contacts negatively charged subendothelial substances exposed by vascular injury. The extrinsic pathway is activated when tissue thromboplastin, a substance released by damaged endothelial cells, reacts with clotting factors, particularly factor VII. Both pathways lead to the common pathway and activation of factor X, which continues to clot formation.

The extrinsic pathway is predominant. Individuals with deficiencies in intrinsic pathway components (i.e., factor XI, factor XII), surprisingly, do not have prolonged bleeding because these factors do not seem to be important for clotting. As with the complement cascade, the clotting system is complex with many alternative activators and inhibitors. The relative importance of particular factors may differ between in vivo hemostasis and in vitro testing of clotting. It may also depend on the mechanism by which the pathway is activated. There also is interaction between components of the intrinsic and extrinsic pathways. An activated member of one pathway may activate a member of the other pathway (e.g., factor VIIa of the extrinsic pathway can directly activate factor IX of the intrinsic pathway).

Activated platelets are important participants in clotting. The phosphatidylserine-rich surface produced during platelet activation supplies a matrix on which several important complexes of clotting factors are formed. These include the intrinsic pathway's *tenase complex* (factor X and activated factors VIII and IX) that activates factor X and the *prothrombinase complex* (prothrombin and activated factors X and V) that activates prothrombin into thrombin. Thrombin then converts fibrinogen into fibrin, which polymerizes into a fibrin clot. Thrombin has broad activity in the inflammatory response. In addition to producing fibrin, thrombin is an activator of other substances. This includes coagulation proteins (e.g., factors V, VIII, XI, XIII), platelets (e.g., aggregation, degranulation), endothelial cells (e.g., upregulation of adhesion molecules for leukocytes, increased NO, PGI_2, PDGF), and monocytes (e.g., cytokine secretion, increased receptors for endothelial cells).

Under normal conditions, spontaneous activation of hemostasis is prevented by factors existing on the endothelial cell surface. These include thrombin inhibitors (e.g., antithrombin III), tissue factor inhibitors (e.g., tissue factor pathway inhibitor), and mechanisms for degrading activated clotting factors (e.g., protein C). Antithrombin III (AT-III) is a circulating inhibitor of plasma serine proteases. AT-III is produced by the liver and binds to heparin sulphate found naturally on the surface of endothelial cells. It is also produced with heparin administered clinically to prevent thrombosis. Heparin induces a change in AT-III that greatly improves its ability to inhibit thrombin and other activated clotting factors. Endothelial cells and platelets produce tissue factor pathway inhibitor (TFPI). TFPI works with and reversibly inhibits factor Xa in the prothrombinase complex. It also inhibits other activated clotting factors.

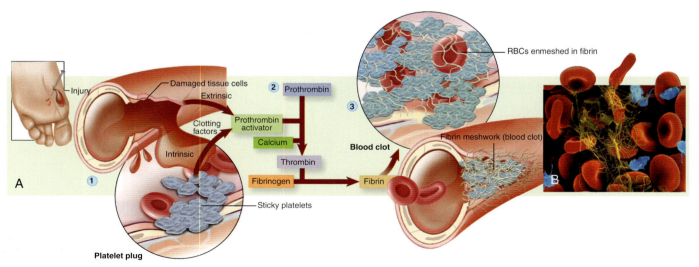

FIGURE 20.18 Blood Clotting Mechanism. A, The complex clotting mechanism can be summarized into three basic steps: **(1)** release of clotting factors from both injured tissue cells and sticky platelets at the injury site (which form a temporary platelet plug); **(2)** series of chemical reactions that eventually result in the formation of thrombin; and **(3)** formation of fibrin and trapping of blood cells to form a clot. **B,** An electron micrograph showing entrapped red blood cells *(RBCs)* in a fibrin clot. (**A,** from Patton, K. T., & Thibodeau, G. A. [2012]. *Structure & function of the body* [14th ed.]. Mosby; **B,** Dennis Kunkel Microscopy/Science Source.)

Thrombomodulin is a thrombin-binding protein on the surface of endothelial cells. Protein C in the circulation binds to thrombomodulin in a thrombin-dependent manner and is converted to activated protein C.[8] Activated protein C, in association with a cofactor (protein S), degrades factors Va and VIIIa. Deficiencies of AT-III, protein C, or protein S are important causes of hypercoagulation (increased clotting). Expression of thrombomodulin and the endothelial cell protein C receptor is downregulated by cytokines and other products of inflammation (e.g., IL-1α, TNF-α, endotoxin). This process enhances clot formation.

Retraction and Lysis of Blood Clots

After a clot is formed, it retracts, or "solidifies." Fibrin strands shorten, becoming denser and stronger. This process approximates the edges of the injured vessel wall and seals the site of injury. Retraction is helped by the large numbers of platelets trapped within the fibrin meshwork. The platelets contract and "pull" the fibrin threads closer together while releasing a factor that stabilizes the fibrin. Contraction expels serum from the fibrin meshwork (see Figure 20.18). This process usually begins within a few minutes after a clot has formed. Expulsion of most of the serum occurs within 20 to 60 minutes.

Lysis (breakdown) of blood clots is carried out by the fibrinolytic system (Figure 20.19). Another plasma protein, plasminogen, is converted to plasmin by several products of coagulation and inflammation, especially by the enzymatic action of tissue plasminogen activator (t-PA). Endothelial cells express t-PA, which is activated maximally after binding to fibrin. Another activator of plasminogen is urokinaselike plasminogen activator (u-PA). The u-PA binds to a specific cellular urokinaselike plasminogen activator receptor (u-PAR), causing activation of plasminogen. This urokinase is the major activator of fibrinolysis in the *extravascular* or tissue compartment, while t-PA is largely involved in *intravascular* fibrinolysis. Several cancers appear to use membrane-bound u-PA to digest intercellular matrix and greatly help tumour invasion and metastasis. Both t-PA and u-PA have been used clinically to treat diseases associated with a blood clot (e.g., pulmonary embolism, myocardial infarction, stroke).[2]

Plasmin is an enzyme that dissolves clots (fibrinolysis). This occurs by degrading fibrin and fibrinogen into fibrin degradation products (FDPs). A major FDP is D-dimer. D-dimer is two D domains from adjacent fibrin monomers that are cross-linked by factor XIIIa and released because of enzymatic cleavage by plasmin. Measurement of levels of circulating D-dimer has been used for diagnosis of deep venous thrombosis or pulmonary embolism.[2] Blood tests for assessing the hematological system are listed in Table 20.6.

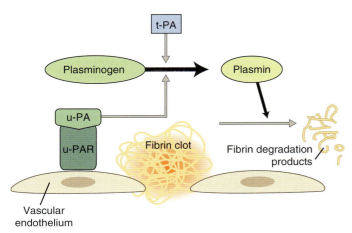

FIGURE 20.19 The Fibrinolytic System. Fibrinolysis is started by the binding of plasminogen to fibrin. Although tissue plasminogen activator (t-PA) starts intravascular fibrinolysis, urokinaselike plasminogen activator (u-PA) is the major activator of fibrinolysis in tissue (extravascular). Plasmin digests the fibrin into smaller soluble pieces (fibrin degradation products). *u-PAR*, Urokinaselike plasminogen activator receptor.

TABLE 20.6 Common Blood Tests for Hematological Disorders

Cell Type and Test	Property Evaluated by Test	Possible Hematological Cause of Abnormal Findings
Erythrocyte		
Red cell count	Number of erythrocytes in 1 mm^3 of peripheral blood	Altered erythropoiesis, anemias, hemorrhage, Hodgkin's disease, leukemia
Mean corpuscular volume (MCV)	Size of erythrocytes	Anemias, thalassemias
Mean corpuscular hemoglobin (MCH)	Amount of hemoglobin (Hb) in each erythrocyte (by weight)	Anemias, hemoglobinopathy
Mean corpuscular hemoglobin concentration (MCHC)	Concentration of Hb in each erythrocyte (percentage of erythrocyte occupied by Hb)	Anemias, hereditary spherocytosis
Hb determination	Amount of Hb (by weight)/L of blood	Anemias
Hematocrit determination	Percentage of a given volume of blood that is occupied by erythrocytes	Hemorrhage, polycythemia, erythrocytosis, anemias, leukemia
Reticulocyte count	Expressed as percentage of reticulocytes in total red blood cell count	Hyperactive or hypoactive bone marrow function
Erythrocyte osmotic fragility test	Cellular shape (biconcavity), structure of plasma membrane	Anemias, hemolytic disease caused by ABO or Rh incompatibility, Hodgkin's disease, polycythemia vera, thalassemia major
Hb electrophoresis	Relative percentage of different types of Hb in erythrocytes	Sickle cell disease, sickle cell trait, hemoglobin C (Hb C) disease, Hb C trait, thalassemias
Sickle cell test	Presence of hemoglobin S (Hb S) in erythrocytes	Sickle cell trait, sickle cell anemia
Glucose-6-phosphate dehydrogenase (G6PD) deficiency test	Deficiency of G6PD in erythrocytes	Hemolytic anemia

Continued

TABLE 20.6 Common Blood Tests for Hematological Disorders—cont'd

Cell Type and Test	Property Evaluated by Test	Possible Hematological Cause of Abnormal Findings
Hemoglobin Metabolism		
Serum ferritin determination	Depletion of body iron (potential deficiency of heme synthesis)	Iron deficiency anemias
Total iron-binding capacity (TIBC)	Amount of iron in serum plus amount of transferrin available in serum	Hemorrhage, iron deficiency anemia, hemochromatosis, hemosiderosis, iron overload, anemias, thalassemia
Transferrin saturation	Percentage of transferrin that is saturated with iron	Acute hemorrhage, hemochromatosis, hemosiderosis, sideroblastic anemia, iron deficiency anemia, iron overload, thalassemia
Porphyrin analysis (protoporphyrin analysis)	Concentration of protoporphyrin in erythrocytes, an indicator of iron-deficient erythropoiesis	Megaloblastic anemia, congenital erythropoietic porphyria
Direct antiglobulin test (DAT)	Antibody binding to erythrocytes	Hemolytic disease of newborn, autoimmune hemolytic anemia, medication-induced hemolytic anemia, transfusion reaction
Antibody screen test (indirect Coombs test)	Detection of antibodies to erythrocyte antigens (other than ABO antigens)	Same as for DAT
Leukocytes: Differential White Cell Count (Absolute Number of Leukocytes×10^9/L of Blood)		
Neutrophil count	Neutrophils×10^9/L	Myeloproliferative disorders, hematopoietic disorders, hemolysis, infection
Lymphocyte count	Lymphocytes×10^9/L	Infectious lymphocytosis, infectious mononucleosis, hematopoietic disorders, anemias, leukemia, lymphosarcoma, Hodgkin's disease
Plasma cell count	Plasma cells×10^9/L	Infectious mononucleosis, lymphocytosis, plasma cell leukemia
Monocyte count	Monocytes×10^9/L	Hodgkin's disease, infectious mononucleosis, monocytic leukemia, non-Hodgkin's lymphoma, polycythemia vera
Eosinophil count	Eosinophils×10^9/L	Hematopoietic disorders, parasitic infections, allergic reactions
Basophil count	Basophils×10^9/L	Chronic myelogenous leukemia, hemolytic anemias, Hodgkin's disease, polycythemia vera
Platelets and Clotting Factors		
Platelet count	Number of circulating platelets per mm^3 of blood	Anemias, multiple myeloma, myelofibrosis, polycythemia vera, leukemia, disseminated intravascular coagulation (DIC), hemolytic disease of the newborn, transfusion reaction, lymphoproliferative disorders
Bleeding time	Duration of bleeding following a standardized superficial puncture wound of skin, integrity of platelet plug, measured in minutes following puncture	Leukemia, anemias, DIC, fibrinolytic activity, purpuras, hemorrhagic disease of the newborn, infectious mononucleosis, multiple myeloma, clotting factor deficiencies, thrombasthenia, thrombocytopenia, von Willebrand's disease
Clot retraction test	Platelet number and function, fibrinogen quantity and use, measured in hours required for expression of serum from a clot incubated in a test tube	Acute leukemia, aplastic anemia, factor XIII deficiency, increased fibrinolytic activity, Hodgkin's disease, hyperfibrinogenemia or hypofibrinogenemia, idiopathic thrombocytopenic purpura, multiple myeloma, polycythemia vera, secondary thrombocytopenia, thrombasthenia
Platelet adhesion studies	Ability of platelets to adhere to foreign surfaces	Anemia, macroglobulinemia, Bernard-Soulier syndrome, multiple myeloma, myeloid metaplasia, plasma cell dyscrasias, thrombasthenia, thrombocytopathy, von Willebrand's disease
Platelet aggregation tests	Ability of platelets to adhere to one another	Afibrinogenemia, Bernard-Soulier syndrome, thrombasthenia, hemorrhagic thrombocythemia, myeloid metaplasia, plasma cell dyscrasias, platelet-release defects, polycythemia vera, preleukemia, sideroblastic anemia, von Willebrand's disease, Waldenström macroglobulinemia, hypercoagulability
Whole blood clotting time (Lee-White coagulation time)	Overall ability of blood to clot, as measured in minutes in a test tube	Afibrinogenemia, clotting factor deficiencies, excessive fibrinolysis, hemorrhagic disease of the newborn, hypofibrinogenemia, hypoprothrombinemia, leukemia

Continued

TABLE 20.6 Common Blood Tests for Hematological Disorders—cont'd

Cell Type and Test	Property Evaluated by Test	Possible Hematological Cause of Abnormal Findings
Circulating anticoagulants (immunoglobulin G antibodies that inhibit coagulation)	Presence of antibodies that neutralize clotting factors and inhibit coagulation, as shown by prolonged clotting time, prothrombin time, or partial thromboplastin time	Afibrinogenemia, presence of fibrin-fibrinogen degradation products, macroglobulinemia, multiple myeloma, DIC, plasma cell dyscrasias
Partial thromboplastin time (PTT)	Effectiveness of clotting factors (except factors VII and VIII), effectiveness of intrinsic pathway of coagulation cascade, as measured in a test tube (in seconds)	Presence of circulating anticoagulants, DIC, clotting factor deficiencies, excessive fibrinolysis, hemorrhagic disease of the newborn, hypofibrinogenemia and afibrinogenemia, prothrombin deficiency, von Willebrand's disease, acute hemorrhage
Prothrombin time	Effectiveness of activity of prothrombin, fibrinogen, and factors V, VII, and X; effectiveness of vitamin K–dependent coagulation factors of extrinsic and common pathways of coagulation cascade as measured in a test tube (in seconds)	Hypofibrinogenemia, dysfibrinogenemia, and afibrinogenemia; presence of circulating anticoagulants; DIC; deficiency of factors V, VII, or X; presence of fibrin degradation products, increased fibrinolytic activity, hemolytic jaundice, hemorrhagic disease of the newborn; acute leukemia, polycythemia vera, prothrombin deficiency, multiple myeloma
Thrombin time	Quantity and activity of fibrinogen as measured in a test tube (in seconds)	Hypofibrinogenemia, dysfibrinogenemia, and afibrinogenemia; presence of circulating anticoagulants; hemorrhagic disease of the newborn, polycythemia vera; increase in fibrinogen-fibrin degradation products; increased fibrinolytic activity
Fibrinogen assay	Amount of fibrinogen available for fibrin formation	Acute leukemia, congenital hypofibrinogenemia or afibrinogenemia, DIC, increased fibrinolytic activity, severe hemorrhage
Fibrin-fibrinogen degradation products (fibrin-fibrinogen split products)	Fibrinogenic activity as measured by levels of fibrin-fibrinogen degradation products (in μmol/L of blood)	Transfusion reactions, DIC, internal hemorrhage in the newborn, deep venous thrombosis, pulmonary embolism

Data from Bick, R. L., Bennett, J. M., & Byrnes, R. K. (Eds.). (1993). *Hematology: clinical and laboratory practice.* Mosby; Byrne, C. J., Saxton, D. F., Pelikan, P. K., et al. (1986). *Laboratory tests: implications for nursing care.* Addison-Wesley; Pagana, K. D., Pagana, T. J., Pike-MacDonald, S. A., et al. (2013). *Mosby's Canadian manual of diagnostic and laboratory tests.* Elsevier.

PEDIATRIC CONSIDERATIONS

Hematological Value Changes

Blood cell counts tend to rise above adult levels at birth and then decrease gradually throughout childhood. Table 20.7 lists normal ranges during infancy and childhood. The immediate rise in values is the result of increased hematopoiesis during fetal life and the increased numbers of cells that result from the trauma of birth and cutting of the umbilical cord.

Average blood volume in the full-term neonate is 85 mL/kg of body weight. The premature infant has a slightly larger blood volume of 90 mL/kg of body weight. In full-term and premature infants, blood volume decreases during the first few months. The average blood volume is 75 to 77 mL/kg, which is like that of older children and adults.

The hypoxic intrauterine environment stimulates erythropoietin production in the fetus and accelerates fetal erythropoiesis. This process produces polycythemia (excessive proliferation of erythrocyte precursors) in the newborn. After birth, the oxygen from the lungs saturates arterial blood, and more oxygen is delivered to the tissues. In response to the change from a placental to a pulmonary oxygen supply during the first few days of life, levels of erythropoietin and the rate of blood cell formation decrease. The active rate of fetal erythropoiesis is reflected by the large numbers of immature erythrocytes (reticulocytes) in the peripheral blood of full-term neonates. After birth, the number of reticulocytes decreases by 50% every 12 hours. As a result, it is rare to find an elevated reticulocyte count after the first week of life. During this period of rapid growth, the rate of erythrocyte destruction is greater than that in later childhood and adulthood. In full-term infants, the normal erythrocyte lifespan is 60 to 80 days. In premature infants, it may be as short as 20 to 30 days. In children and adolescents, it is the same as that in adults—120 days.

The postnatal fall in hemoglobin and hematocrit values is more marked in premature infants than it is in full-term infants. In preschool and school-aged children, hemoglobin, hematocrit, and red blood cell counts gradually rise. Metabolic processes within the erythrocytes of neonates differ a lot from those found in erythrocytes of normal adults. The relatively young population of erythrocytes in newborns uses greater quantities of glucose than do erythrocytes in adults.

The lymphocytes of children tend to have more cytoplasm and less compact nuclear chromatin than do the lymphocytes of adults. A possible explanation is that children tend to have more frequent viral infections, which are associated with atypical lymphocytes. Minor infections, in which the child does not show clinical signs of illness, and the administration of immunizations also may account for the lymphocyte changes.

At birth, the lymphocyte count is high. It continues to rise during the first year of life. Then it steadily declines until the lower value seen in adults is reached. It is unknown whether these developmental differences are physiological or a response to frequent viral infection and immunizations in children.

The neutrophil count, like the lymphocyte count, is high at birth and rises during the first days of life. After 2 weeks, the neutrophil count falls to within or below the normal adult range. Although the exact age can vary by about 7 years of age, the neutrophil count is the same as that of an adult.

The eosinophil count is higher in the first year of life and higher in children than in teenagers or adults. Monocyte counts also are high in the first year of life but then decrease to adult levels. Platelet counts in full-term neonates are comparable to those in adults and remain so throughout infancy and childhood.

TABLE 20.7 Mean Hematological Differential Counts From Birth to Adulthood

Hematological Differential	Newborn (Cord Blood)	2 Weeks of Age	3 Months of Age	6 Months to 6 Years of Age	7–12 Years of Age	Adult
Hemoglobin (g/L)	168	165	120	120	130	130
Hematocrit (%)	55	50	36	37	38	40
Reticulocytes (%)	5	1	1	1	1	1
Leukocytes WBC ($\times 10^9$/L)	9–30	5–20	5.0–19.5	6.0–17.5	4.5–13.5	5–10
Neutrophils (%)	61	40	30	45	55	55
Lymphocytes (%)	31	48	63	48	38	35
Eosinophils (%)	2	3	2	2	2	2
Monocytes (%)	6	9	5	5	5	5
Platelets ($\times 10^9$/L)	140–450	140–450	140–450	140–450	140–450	140–450

WBC, White blood cell.

GERIATRIC CONSIDERATIONS

Hematological Value Changes

Blood make-up changes little with age. An iron deficiency may alter some components. Total serum iron level, total iron-binding capacity, and intestinal iron absorption are all decreased slightly in older persons. The erythrocyte lifespan is normal, although the erythrocytes are replenished more slowly after bleeding. Hemoglobin levels may be low, and the plasma membranes of erythrocytes become increasingly fragile and structurally altered.

Lymphocyte function appears to decrease with age (see Chapters 7 and 8). This decrease causes changes in cellular immunity and some decline in T-cell function. The humoral immune system is less able to respond to antigenic challenge.

No changes in platelet numbers or structure have been seen in older persons, yet platelet adhesiveness probably increases. Although fibrinogen levels and levels of factors V, VII, and IX tend to be increased, no major hypercoagulability has been confirmed.

DID YOU UNDERSTAND?

Components of the Hematological System

1. Blood consists of a variety of components, about 92% water and 8% solutes. In adults, the total blood volume is about 5.5 L.
2. Plasma, a complex aqueous liquid, holds two major groups of plasma proteins: albumins and globulins.
3. The cellular components of the blood are red blood cells (erythrocytes), white blood cells (leukocytes), and platelets.
4. Erythrocytes are the most abundant cells of the blood. They occupy about 48% of the blood volume in men and about 42% in women. Erythrocytes are mainly responsible for tissue oxygenation.
5. Leukocytes are fewer in number than erythrocytes. They constitute about 5 to 10×10^9/L of blood. Leukocytes defend the body against infection and remove dead or injured host cells.
6. Leukocytes are classified as either granulocytes (neutrophils, eosinophils, basophils) or agranulocytes (monocytes/macrophages, lymphocytes).
7. Platelets are anuclear disc-shaped cytoplasmic fragments. Platelets are essential for blood coagulation and control of bleeding.
8. The lymphoid organs are sites of residence, proliferation, differentiation, or function of lymphocytes and mononuclear phagocytes.
9. The spleen is the largest lymphoid organ. It functions as the site of fetal hematopoiesis, filters and cleanses the blood, and acts as a reservoir for lymphocytes and other blood cells.
10. The lymph nodes are the site of development or activity of large numbers of lymphocytes, monocytes, and macrophages.
11. The mononuclear phagocyte system (MPS) is made up of monocytes in bone marrow and peripheral blood and macrophages in tissue.
12. The MPS is an important line of defence against bacteria and other microorganisms in the bloodstream. It cleanses the blood by removing old, injured, or dead blood cells; antigen–antibody complexes; and macromolecules.

Development of Blood Cells

1. Hematopoiesis, or blood cell production, occurs in the liver and spleen of the fetus and in the bone marrow after birth.
2. Hematopoiesis involves two stages: proliferation and differentiation (i.e., maturation). Each type of blood cell has parent cells called *stem cells*.
3. Hematopoiesis continues throughout life to replace blood cells that grow old and die, are killed by disease, or are lost through bleeding.
4. Bone marrow consists of red (hematopoietic) marrow and yellow marrow (fatty tissue). Red marrow is made up of blood vessels, mononuclear phagocytes, stem cells, blood cells in various stages of differentiation, and stromal cells.
5. The bone marrow has many populations of stem cells. Mesenchymal stem cells develop into fibroblasts, osteoclasts, and adipocytes. Hematopoietic stem cells (HSCs) develop into blood cells.
6. Regulation of hematopoiesis occurs in bone marrow niches in which HSCs differentiate. This process is controlled by multiple cytokines and chemokines and through direct contact with osteoblasts (osteoblastic niche) or vascular endothelial cells (vascular niche). In addition, several other specialized cells, including CXCL12-abundant reticular cells and nestin-expressing cells, are involved.
7. Specific hematopoietic growth factors (e.g., colony-stimulating factors) are necessary for the adequate production of myeloid, erythroid, lymphoid, and megakaryocytic lineages.

8. Hemoglobin, the oxygen-carrying protein of the erythrocyte, allows the blood to transport 100 times more oxygen than could be transported dissolved in plasma alone.
9. Regulation of erythropoiesis is mediated by erythropoietin. Erythropoietin is secreted by the kidneys in response to tissue hypoxia. It causes a compensatory increase in erythrocyte production if the oxygen content of the blood decreases because of anemia, high altitude, or pulmonary disease.
10. Erythropoiesis depends on the presence of vitamins. Key vitamins include vitamin B_{12}, folate, vitamin B_6, riboflavin, pantothenic acid, niacin, ascorbic acid, and vitamin E.
11. The iron cycle reuses iron released from old or damaged erythrocytes. Iron binds to transferrin in the blood, is transported to macrophages of the mononuclear phagocyte system, and is stored in the cytoplasm as ferritin.
12. A small hormone called hepcidin, produced by hepatocytes, controls iron homeostasis. This hormone regulates ferroportin. Ferroportin is the principal transporter of iron from stores in hepatocytes and macrophages and from intestinal cells that absorb dietary iron.
13. Maintenance of optimal levels of granulocytes and monocytes in the blood depends on several factors. These factors include the availability of pluripotent stem cells in the marrow, induction of these into committed stem cells, and timely release of new cells from the marrow.
14. Granulocytes and monocytes in the blood develop from common myeloid progenitor cells in the bone marrow. These cells are under the direction of several growth factors, including stem cell factor, interleukin-3, and granulocyte-macrophage colony–stimulating factor.
15. Specific humoral colony-stimulating factors are necessary for the adequate growth of myeloid, erythroid, lymphoid, and megakaryocytic lineages.
16. Platelets develop from megakaryocytes by a process called *endomitosis*. Thrombopoietin controls this process. During endomitosis the megakaryocytes undergo mitosis but not cell division and the cytoplasm and plasma membrane fragment into platelets.

Mechanisms of Hemostasis

1. Hemostasis, or arrest of bleeding, involves (a) vasoconstriction (vasospasm), (b) formation of a platelet plug, (c) activation of the clotting cascade, (d) formation of a blood clot, and (e) clot retraction and clot dissolution.
2. The normal vascular endothelium prevents spontaneous clotting by producing factors. These factors include nitric oxide and prostacyclin that relax the vessels and prevent platelet activation.
3. Lysis of blood clots is the function of the fibrinolytic system. Plasmin, a proteolytic enzyme, splits fibrin and fibrinogen into fibrin degradation products. These products dissolve the clot.

Pediatric Considerations: Hematological Value Changes

1. Blood cell counts tend to rise above adult levels at birth. The levels decline gradually throughout childhood.
2. The lymphocytes of children tend to have more cytoplasm and less compact nuclear chromatin than do the lymphocytes of adults.

Geriatric Considerations: Hematological Value Changes

1. Blood composition changes little with age. Erythrocyte renewal may be delayed after bleeding, most likely because of iron deficiency.
2. Lymphocyte function appears to decrease with age. Most affected is a decrease in cellular immunity.
3. Platelet adhesiveness probably increases with age.

21

Alterations of Hematological Function

Kelly Power-Kean, with originating chapter contributions by Kathryn L. McCance

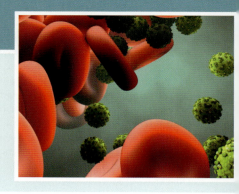

Additional resources are available online at https://evolve.elsevier.com/Canada/Huether/pathophysiology.

CHAPTER OUTLINE

Alterations of Erythrocyte Function, 501
    Classification of Anemias, 501
    Macrocytic-Normochromic Anemias, 503
    Microcytic-Hypochromic Anemias, 505
    Normocytic-Normochromic Anemias, 507
Myeloproliferative Red Blood Cell Disorders, 507
    Polycythemia Vera, 508
    Iron Overload, 509
Alterations of Leukocyte Function, 510
    Quantitative Alterations of Leukocytes, 510

Alterations of Lymphoid Function, 518
    Lymphadenopathy, 518
    Malignant Lymphomas, 518
Alterations of Splenic Function, 524
Hemorrhagic Disorders and Alterations of Platelets and Coagulation, 526
    Disorders of Platelets, 526
    Alterations of Platelet Function, 529
    Disorders of Coagulation, 529
CASE STUDY: Iron Deficiency Anemia, 534

LEARNING OBJECTIVES

1. Define anemia.
2. List the various methods of classifying the anemias.
3. Describe the manifestations of anemia.
4. Describe the pathophysiology of anemia.
5. Compare and contrast the pathophysiology of iron deficiency, pernicious, and folate deficiency anemias.
6. Describe the normocytic-normochromic anemias.
7. Define polycythemia vera and describe its causes.
8. Describe the manifestations of polycythemia vera related to the increased viscosity and volume of blood.
9. Describe the different types of alterations in leukocyte function.
10. Define agranulocytosis and list its clinical manifestations.
11. Describe the manifestations of infectious mononucleosis, including the complications it creates for systems other than the immune system.
12. Classify leukemia as it relates to the maturity of the cells and appearance of the total leukocyte count and differential.
13. Differentiate the leukemias by manifestations, treatment options, and prognosis.
14. Describe Hodgkin's and non-Hodgkin's lymphomas, focusing on differential diagnosis, manifestations, treatment, and prognosis.
15. Describe the pathophysiology, clinical manifestations, and treatment of multiple myeloma.
16. Identify the causes of splenomegaly.
17. Identify the causes of thrombocytopenia.
18. List the causes of impaired hemostasis.
19. Describe the pathophysiology and manifestations of disseminated intravascular coagulation.
20. Describe the conditions that predispose an individual to the development of thrombi.

KEY TERMS

Absolute lymphocytosis, 512
Absolute polycythemia, 508
Acquired sideroblastic anemia (ASA), 506
Acute idiopathic TTP, 528
Acute leukemia, 513
Acute lymphocytic leukemia (ALL), 514
Acute myeloid (or myelogenous) leukemia (AML), 514
Agranulocytosis, 510
Amyloidosis, 523
Anemia, 501

Anisocytosis, 501
Arterial thrombi (pl. *thrombi*), 533
Basopenia, 511
Basophilia, 511
B-cell neoplasm, 521
Bence Jones protein, 523
β_2-Microglobulin, 524
Blast cell, 513
Burkitt lymphoma, 522
Chronic leukemia, 513
Chronic lymphocytic leukemia (CLL), 517

Chronic myeloid (or myelogenous) leukemia (CML), 517
Chronic relapsing TTP, 528
Congestive splenomegaly, 524
Consumptive thrombohemorrhagic disorder, 530
D-dimer, 532
Disseminated intravascular coagulation (DIC), 530
Ecchymoses, 526

Embolus, 533
Eosinopenia, 511
Eosinophilia, 510
Epistaxis, 526
Eryptosis, 503
Erythromelalgia, 529
Essential (primary) thrombocythemia (ET), 528
Fibrin degradation product (FDP), 531
Fibrin split product (FSP), 531

CHAPTER 21 Alterations of Hematological Function

Folate (folic acid), 504
Granulocytopenia, 510
Granulocytosis 510
Hematoma, 526
Hemochromatosis, 509
Hemolysis, 503
Hemostasis 526
Heparin-induced thrombocytopenia (HIT), 527
Hereditary (congenital) sideroblastic anemia, 506
Hereditary hemochromatosis (HH), 509
Heterophilic antibodies, 512
Hodgkin's lymphoma (HL), 519
Hypercoagulability (thrombophilia), 526
Hypersplenism, 524
Hypoplastic anemia, 506
Hypoxemia, 503
Immune thrombocytopenic purpura (ITP) 527
Impaired hemostasis, 529
Infectious mononucleosis (IM), 512
Infiltrative splenomegaly, 525
Intrinsic factor (IF), 504
Iron deficiency anemia (IDA), 505
Janus kinase 2 gene (*JAK2* gene), 508
Koilonychia, 505
Leukemia, 513
Leukocytosis 510
Leukopenia, 510
Lymphadenopathy 518
Lymphoblastic lymphoma (LL), 522
Lymphocytopenia, 512
Lymphocytosis, 512
M protein, 523
Macrocytic (megaloblastic) anemia, 503
Microcytic-hypochromic anemia, 505
Microvasculature thrombosis, 529
Monoclonal gammopathy of undetermined significance (MGUS), 524
Monocytopenia, 511
Monocytosis, 511
Multiple myeloma (MM), 523
Myelodysplastic syndrome (MDS), 506
Myeloproliferative disorder, 517
Neutropenia, 510
Neutrophilia, 510
NK-cell neoplasm, 521
Non-Hodgkin's lymphoma (NHL), 521
Normocytic-normochromic anemia (NNA), 507
Palpable purpura, 526
Pancytopenia, 514
Pernicious anemia (PA), 503
Petechia, 526
Philadelphia chromosome, 514
Phlebotomy, 506
Poikilocytosis, 501
Polycythemia, 507
Polycythemia vera (PV; also, *primary polycythemia*), 508
Purpura, 526
Reed-Sternberg (RS) cell, 519
Relative polycythemia, 507
Reversible sideroblastic anemia (reversible SA), 506
Ringed sideroblast, 506
Secondary thrombocythemia, 528
Shift to the left (leukemoid reaction), 510
Shift to the right, 510
Sideroblastic anemia (SA), 506
Small lymphocytic lymphoma (SLL; also, *CLL/SLL*), 517
Smouldering myeloma, 524
Splenomegaly, 524
T-cell neoplasm, 521
Thrombocythemia (thrombocytosis), 528
Thrombocytopenia, 526
Thromboembolic disease, 526
Thrombosis, 526
Thrombotic thrombocytopenic purpura (TTP), 528
Thrombus, 533
Vasculitis 529
Venous thrombi (pl. *thrombi*), 533
Virchow triad, 533

Alterations of erythrocyte function involve either insufficient or excessive numbers of erythrocytes in the circulation or normal numbers of cells with abnormal components. Anemias are conditions in which there are too few erythrocytes or an insufficient volume of erythrocytes in the blood. Polycythemias are conditions in which erythrocyte numbers or volume is excessive. All of these conditions have many causes and are pathophysiological manifestations of many disease states.

Many disorders involving leukocytes exist. They involve increased numbers of leukocytes (i.e., leukocytosis) in response to infections and proliferative disorders (such as leukemia). Many hematological disorders are malignancies. Many nonhematological malignancies metastasize to bone marrow, affecting leukocyte production. Thus, a large part of this chapter discusses malignant disease.

The primary role of clotting (hemostasis) is to stop bleeding. This happens through an interaction of endothelium lining the vessels, platelets, and clotting factors. A large number of disease states may be associated with a clinically significant increase or decrease in clotting. These clotting disorders result from alterations in any of the three main components of the clotting process.

ALTERATIONS OF ERYTHROCYTE FUNCTION

> ✓ **QUICK CHECK 21.1**
> 1. How do cell size and content determine classification of anemia?
> 2. Why is iron important to hemoglobin synthesis? Why is iron deficiency related to anemia?
> 3. Describe the pathophysiology of iron deficiency anemia.
> 4. How is anemia diagnosed?

Classification of Anemias

Anemia is a reduction in the total number of erythrocytes in the circulating blood or a decrease in the quality or quantity of hemoglobin. Anemias commonly result from (1) impaired erythrocyte production, (2) blood loss (acute or chronic), (3) increased erythrocyte destruction, or (4) a combination of these three factors. Anemias are classified by their causes (e.g., anemia of chronic disease) or by the changes that affect the size, shape, or substance of the erythrocyte. The most common classification of anemias is based on the changes that affect the cell's size and hemoglobin content (Table 21.1). Terms used to identify anemias reflect these characteristics. Terms that end with -*cytic* refer to cell size. Terms that end with -*chromic* refer to hemoglobin content. Other terms describing erythrocytes found in some anemias are **anisocytosis** (assuming various sizes) and **poikilocytosis** (assuming various shapes).

CLINICAL MANIFESTATIONS The main alteration of anemia is a reduced oxygen-carrying capacity of the blood. This alteration results in tissue hypoxia. Symptoms of anemia vary, depending on the body's ability to compensate for the reduced oxygen-carrying capacity. Anemia that is mild and starts gradually is usually easier to compensate. As a result, problems for the individual may only occur during physical exertion. As red blood cell reduction continues, symptoms become more noticeable. Alterations in specific organs and compensation effects are clearer. Compensation usually involves the cardiovascular, respiratory, and hematological systems (Figure 21.1).

A reduction in the number of red blood cells in the blood causes a reduction in the consistency and volume of blood. Initial compensation for cellular loss is movement of interstitial fluid into the blood. This movement causes an increase in plasma volume and supports an adequate blood volume. However, the viscosity (thickness) of the blood decreases.

TABLE 21.1 Morphological Classification of Anemias

Structure of Erythrocytes	Name and Mechanism of Anemia	Primary Cause
Macrocytic-normochromic anemia: large, abnormally shaped erythrocytes, normal hemoglobin concentrations	Pernicious anemia: lack of vitamin B_{12}; abnormal DNA and RNA synthesis in erythroblast; premature cell death	Congenital or acquired deficiency of intrinsic factor; genetic disorder of DNA synthesis
	Folate deficiency anemia: lack of folate; premature cell death	Dietary folate deficiency
Microcytic-hypochromic anemia: small, abnormally shaped erythrocytes and reduced hemoglobin concentration	Iron deficiency anemia: lack of iron for hemoglobin; insufficient hemoglobin	Chronic blood loss, dietary iron deficiency, disruption of iron metabolism or iron cycle
	Sideroblastic anemia: dysfunctional iron uptake by erythroblasts and defective porphyrin and heme synthesis	Congenital dysfunction of iron metabolism in erythroblasts, acquired dysfunction of iron metabolism as result of medications or toxins
	Thalassemia: impaired synthesis of α- or β-chain of hemoglobin A; phagocytosis of abnormal erythroblasts in marrow	Congenital genetic defect of globin synthesis
Normocytic-normochromic anemia: normal size, normal hemoglobin concentration	Aplastic anemia: insufficient erythropoiesis	Depressed stem cell proliferation
	Posthemorrhagic anemia: blood loss	Increased erythropoiesis; iron depletion
	Hemolytic anemia: premature destruction (lysis) of mature erythrocytes in circulation	Increased fragility of erythrocytes
	Sickle cell anemia: abnormal hemoglobin synthesis, abnormal cell shape with susceptibility to damage, lysis, and phagocytosis	Congenital dysfunction of hemoglobin synthesis
	Anemia of chronic disease; abnormally increased demand for new erythrocytes	Chronic infection or inflammation; malignancy

DNA, Deoxyribonucleic acid; *RNA*, ribonucleic acid.

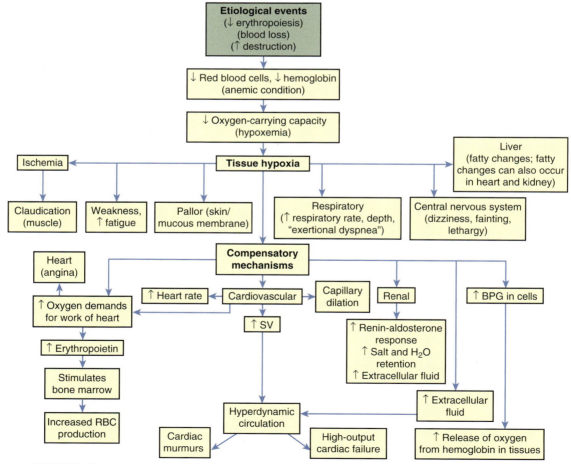

FIGURE 21.1 Progression and Manifestations of Anemia. *BPG*, Bisphosphoglycerate; *RBC*, red blood cell; *SV*, stroke volume.

The "thinner" blood flows faster and more turbulently than normal blood, causing a hyperdynamic circulatory state. This hyperdynamic state creates cardiovascular changes. The changes include increased stroke volume and heart rate. These changes may lead to cardiac dilation and heart valve insufficiency if the underlying anemic condition is not corrected.

Hypoxemia is a reduced oxygen level in the blood. This condition further contributes to cardiovascular dysfunction by causing dilation of arterioles, capillaries, and venules; this dilation increases blood flow through them. Increased peripheral blood flow and venous return further contributes to an increase in heart rate and stroke volume. These symptoms occur in order to meet normal oxygen demand and prevent cardiopulmonary congestion. These compensatory mechanisms may lead to heart failure.

Tissue hypoxia creates added demands and effects on the pulmonary and hematological systems. The rate and depth of breathing increase in an effort to increase oxygen availability. There is also an increase in the release of oxygen from hemoglobin. All of these compensatory mechanisms may cause individuals to experience shortness of breath (dyspnea), a rapid and pounding heartbeat, dizziness, and fatigue. In mild chronic cases, these symptoms may be present only when there is an increased demand for oxygen (e.g., during physical exertion). In severe cases, symptoms may occur at rest.

Manifestations of anemia may be seen in other parts of the body. The skin, mucous membranes, lips, nail beds, and conjunctivae become pale because of reduced hemoglobin concentration. They may also become yellowish (jaundiced) because of build-up of end products of red blood cell destruction (hemolysis) if that is the cause of the anemia. Tissue hypoxia of the skin results in impaired healing and loss of elasticity, as well as thinning and early greying of the hair. Nervous system manifestations may occur where the cause of anemia is a deficiency of vitamin B_{12}. Myelin degeneration occurs, causing a loss of nerve fibres in the spinal cord. This process results in paresthesias (numbness), gait disturbances, extreme weakness, spasticity, and reflex abnormalities. Decreased oxygen supply to the gastro-intestinal (GI) tract often produces abdominal pain, nausea, vomiting, and anorexia. Low-grade fever (less than 38.3°C [100.9°F]) occurs in some anemic individuals. This fever may result from the release of leukocyte pyrogens from ischemic tissues.

When the anemia is severe or acute in onset (e.g., hemorrhage), the first compensatory mechanism is peripheral blood vessel constriction. The constriction diverts blood flow to essential vital organs. Decreased blood flow detected by the kidneys activates the renin-angiotensin response. This causes salt and water retention in an attempt to increase blood volume. These situations are considered to be emergencies and require immediate intervention to correct the underlying problem that caused the acute blood loss.

Therapeutic interventions for slowly developing anemic conditions require treatment of the underlying condition and relief of associated symptoms.[1] Therapies include transfusion, dietary correction, and administration of supplemental vitamins or iron.

Macrocytic-Normochromic Anemias

The macrocytic (megaloblastic) anemias are characterized by unusually large stem cells (megaloblasts) in the marrow. These cells mature into erythrocytes that are unusually large in size (macrocytic), thickness, and volume.[2] These anemias are classified as normochromic because the hemoglobin content is normal. They are the result of ineffective erythrocyte DNA synthesis, commonly caused by deficiencies of vitamin B_{12} (cobalamin) or folate (folic acid). These defective erythrocytes die prematurely, which decreases their numbers in the circulation, causing anemia. Premature death of damaged erythrocytes, eryptosis, is a common mechanism of cellular loss in individuals with anemia secondary to deficiencies of iron, infections (e.g., malaria, mycoplasma), chronic diseases (e.g., diabetes, renal disease), genetic diseases (e.g., beta-thalassemia, glucose-6-phosphate dehydrogenase [G6PD] deficiency, sickle cell trait), and myelodysplastic syndrome.[3]

Defective DNA synthesis in megaloblastic anemias causes red blood cell growth and development to continue at unequal rates. DNA synthesis and cell division are blocked or delayed. However, RNA replication and protein (hemoglobin) synthesis continue normally. Asynchronous development leads to an overproduction of hemoglobin during prolonged cellular division. This process creates a larger-than-normal erythrocyte with a disproportionately small nucleus. With each cell division, the disproportion between RNA and DNA becomes clearer.

Pernicious Anemia

Pernicious anemia (PA), the most common type of macrocytic anemia, is caused by vitamin B_{12} deficiency. It is often associated with the end stage of type A chronic atrophic (autoimmune) gastritis (Figure 21.2C).[4]

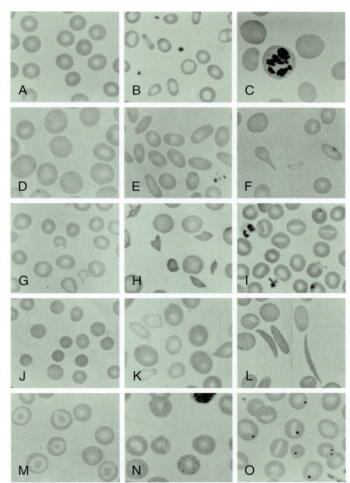

FIGURE 21.2 Appearance of Red Blood Cells in Various Disorders. **A,** Normal blood smear. **B,** Microcytic-hypochromic anemia (iron deficiency). **C,** Macrocytic anemia (pernicious anemia). **D,** Macrocytic anemia in pregnancy. **E,** Hereditary elliptocytosis. **F,** Myelofibrosis (teardrop). **G,** Hemolytic anemia associated with prosthetic heart valve. **H,** Microangiopathic anemia. **I,** Stomatocytes. **J,** Spherocytes (hereditary spherocytosis). **K,** Sideroblastic anemia; note the double population of red blood cells. **L,** Sickle cell anemia. **M,** Target cells (after splenectomy). **N,** Basophil stippling in case of unexplained anemia. **O,** Howell-Jolly bodies (after splenectomy). (From Wintrobe, M.M., et al. (1981). *Clinical hematology* (8th ed.). Lea & Febiger.)

Pernicious means highly injurious or destructive and reflects the fact that this condition was once fatal. It most often affects individuals older than age 30 who are of Northern European descent. However, it has now been recognized in all populations and ethnic groups.

PATHOPHYSIOLOGY The underlying problem in PA is the absence of intrinsic factor (IF). IF is a transporter required for gastric absorption of dietary vitamin B_{12}, a vitamin needed for nuclear maturation and DNA synthesis in red blood cells. Deficiency of IF may be congenital or, more often, an autoimmune process directed against gastric parietal cells. Congenital IF deficiency is a genetic disorder with an autosomal recessive inheritance pattern.[5] The autoimmune form of the disease also has a genetic component. Family clusters have been found. About 20 to 30% of individuals related to persons with PA also have PA. These relatives, particularly first-degree female relatives, also show a higher frequency of the presence of gastric autoantibodies. PA also is often a component of autoimmune polyendocrinopathy. This disorder includes a cluster of autoimmune diseases of endocrine organs (e.g., chronic autoimmune thyroiditis, type 1 diabetes mellitus, Addison's disease, primary hypoparathyroidism, Graves' disease, and myasthenia gravis) that frequently present as comorbidities. Autoimmune thyroiditis and type 1 diabetes mellitus, in particular, are associated with PA.

Most cases of PA result from an autoimmune gastritis (type A chronic gastritis) in which gastric atrophy results from destruction of parietal and zymogenic (relating to an enzyme) cells. Individuals with PA commonly have autoantibodies against the gastric H^+–K^+ ATPase, which is the major protein constituent of parietal cell membranes. Destruction of gastric parietal cells causes gastric mucosal atrophy and results in a deficiency of all secretions of the stomach. This includes hydrochloric acid, pepsin, and IF. Autoantibodies against IF prevent the formation of the B_{12}–IF complex. Thus, PA is secondary to autoimmune destruction of parietal cells, diminishing the production of IF and the presence of autoantibodies that neutralize the ability of remaining IF to transport vitamin B_{12}.

Initiation of the autoimmune process may be secondary to a past infection with *Helicobacter pylori*.[4] Although active infection with *H. pylori* is rare in individuals with PA, more than half of these individuals have circulating antibodies against this microorganism. This finding suggests a history of infection. The current opinion is that in genetically prone individuals, antigens expressed by *H. pylori* mimic the parietal cell H^+–K^+ ATPase. This results in production of an antibody that binds and damages the parietal cell (see Chapter 8 for a discussion of antigenic mimicry and autoimmune disease).

Environmental factors that may contribute to chronic gastritis include excessive alcohol or hot tea ingestion and smoking. Complete or partial removal of the stomach (gastrectomy) causes IF deficiency. Medications known as proton pump inhibitors (PPIs) are used to decrease gastric acidity and may decrease vitamin B_{12} absorption, but it is not thought that they actually cause PA. Although PA is a benign disorder, people with type A chronic gastritis also are at risk of developing gastric adenocarcinoma and gastric carcinoid type I. The incidence rate of carcinoma in these individuals is 2 to 3%.

CLINICAL MANIFESTATIONS PA develops slowly (over 20 to 30 years). By the time an individual seeks treatment, it is usually severe. Early symptoms are often ignored because they are nonspecific and vague. These symptoms include infections, mood swings, and GI, cardiac, or kidney diseases. When the hemoglobin level has decreased to 70 to 80 g/L, the individual experiences classic symptoms of PA, which include weakness, fatigue, paresthesias of feet and fingers, difficulty walking, loss of appetite, abdominal pain, weight loss, and a sore, smooth, beefy red tongue. The skin may become "lemon yellow" (sallow), caused by a combination of pallor and jaundice. Hepatomegaly, a sign of right-sided heart failure, may be present in the older person along with nonpalpable splenomegaly.

Neurological manifestations result from nerve demyelination that may produce neuronal death. The posterior and lateral columns of the spinal cord also may be affected. Damage to these nerves causes a loss of position and vibration sense, ataxia, and spasticity. These complications pose a serious threat because they are not reversible, even with treatment. The cerebrum also may be involved with manifestations of affective disorders, most commonly of the depressive types. Low levels of vitamin B_{12} have been associated with neurocognitive disorders. An increased prevalence of serum vitamin B_{12} deficiency has been reported among individuals with Alzheimer's disease.

EVALUATION AND TREATMENT Diagnosis of PA is based on clinical manifestations and several test results. These tests include blood tests, bone marrow aspiration, serological studies, and gastric biopsy. The presence of circulating antibodies against parietal cells and IF is also useful in diagnosis. Gastric biopsy reveals total achlorhydria (absence of hydrochloric acid), which is diagnostic for PA.

Oral replacement of vitamin B_{12} (cobalamin) is the treatment of choice. Dosing for PA or food-bound cobalamin malabsorption is 1 000 μg/day. Individuals whose deficiency is not corrected by the oral administration receive monthly vitamin B_{12} injections. The effectiveness of cobalamin replacement therapy is determined by a rising reticulocyte count. Blood counts return to normal within 5 to 6 weeks. PA cannot be cured, so maintenance therapy is lifelong.

Untreated PA is fatal, usually because of heart failure. With replacement therapy of vitamin B_{12}, mortality decreases significantly. Death from PA is now rare, and relapses are often the result of nonadherence to therapy.

Folate Deficiency Anemias

Folate (folic acid) is an essential vitamin required for RNA and DNA synthesis within the maturing erythrocyte. Folates are coenzymes required for the synthesis of thymine and purines (adenine and guanine) and the conversion of homocysteine to methionine. Deficient production of thymine, in particular, affects cells undergoing rapid division (e.g., bone marrow cells undergoing erythropoiesis). Humans are totally dependent on dietary intake to meet the daily requirement of 50 to 200 mg/day. Increased amounts are needed for lactating and pregnant females. Folate is absorbed from the upper small intestine and does not require any other element (i.e., IF) to help absorption. After absorption, folate circulates through the liver, where it is stored. Folate deficiency occurs more often than B_{12} deficiency, particularly in alcoholics and individuals with chronic malnourishment. About 10% of North Americans are folate deficient. The incidence of this deficiency has been decreasing in Canada since the fortification of foods with folate and the increased use of folate supplements.

Clinical manifestations are similar to the malnourished appearance of individuals with PA. Other manifestations include cheilosis (scales and fissures of the mouth), stomatitis (inflammation of the mouth), and painful ulcerations of the buccal mucosa and tongue characteristic of *burning mouth syndrome*. Burning mouth syndrome may be secondary to a large number of disorders. These disorders include extremely dry mouth, infection, autoimmune disease, nutritional deficiencies, and other conditions. Dysphagia, flatulence, and watery diarrhea also may be present, as well as histological changes in the GI tract suggestive of sprue (chronic absorption disorder). Undiagnosed inflammatory bowel disease (e.g., Crohn's disease, ulcerative colitis) may be the underlying cause of folate malabsorption in some individuals. Folate deficiency may suppress proliferation of the intestinal mucosa, leading to an increase of GI damage. A thiamine deficiency, which often occurs with folate deficiency, may cause neurological manifestations.

Evaluation of folate deficiency is based on blood tests, measurement of serum folate levels, and clinical manifestations. Treatment requires administration of oral folate preparations until adequate blood levels are obtained and manifestations are reduced or eliminated. Long-term therapy is not necessary if the proper dietary adjustments are made to support adequate intake. After administration of folate, the manifestations of anemia disappear within 1 to 2 weeks.

Microcytic-Hypochromic Anemias

The microcytic-hypochromic anemias are characterized by abnormally small erythrocytes that have abnormally reduced amounts of hemoglobin (Figure 21.2B). Microcytic-hypochromic anemias can result from (1) disorders of iron metabolism, (2) disorders of porphyrin and heme synthesis, or (3) disorders of globin synthesis. Specific conditions include iron deficiency anemia, sideroblastic anemia, and thalassemia.

Iron Deficiency Anemia

Iron deficiency anemia (IDA) is the most common type of anemia worldwide, occurring in both developing and developed countries.[1] Certain populations are at high risk of developing hypoferremia and IDA. This includes individuals living in poverty, women of childbearing age, and children. Iron deficiency in children is associated with many adverse health-related manifestations, especially cognitive impairment, which may be irreversible. Children in developing countries often are affected by chronic parasite infestations that result in blood and iron loss greater than dietary intake.[6] Treatment of these infections results in improvement in appetite, growth, and in the anemia. IDA also occurs in individuals with lead poisoning, and treatment is associated with a decrease in lead levels. An increased prevalence of iron deficiency has been seen in overweight children.

Females in Canada have a higher incidence than males for both hypoferremia and IDA. A peak incidence occurs in the reproductive years and decreases at menopause. Males have a higher incidence during childhood.

PATHOPHYSIOLOGY IDA can occur from one of two different aetiologies or a combination of both inadequate dietary intake of iron and chronic blood loss. In both instances there is no intrinsic dysfunction in iron metabolism. Both aetiologies deplete iron stores and reduce hemoglobin synthesis. A second category is a metabolic or functional iron deficiency. This occurs with various metabolic disorders leading to insufficient iron delivery to bone marrow or impaired iron use (or absorption) within the marrow. Surprisingly, iron stores may be sufficient, but delivery is inadequate to support heme synthesis. This produces a functional or relative iron deficiency.

In developed countries, pregnancy and a continuous loss of blood are the most common causes of IDA. A blood loss of 2 to 4 mL/day (1 to 2 mg of iron) is enough to cause IDA. Menorrhagia (excessive menstrual bleeding) causes primary IDA in females. Males may experience bleeding as a result of ulcers, hiatal hernia, esophageal varices, cirrhosis, hemorrhoids, ulcerative colitis, or cancer. Other causes of blood loss for both genders include the following: (1) use of medications that cause GI bleeding (such as Aspirin or nonsteroidal anti-inflammatory drugs [NSAIDs]); (2) surgical procedures that decrease stomach acidity, intestinal transit time, and absorption (e.g., gastric bypass); (3) insufficient dietary intake of iron; and (4) eating disorders such as pica (the craving and eating of non-nutritional substances, such as dirt, chalk, and paper). *H. pylori* infections also have been found to cause IDA of unknown origin.

Iron in the form of hemoglobin is in constant demand by the body. An important feature of iron is that it can be recycled. The body maintains a balance between iron that is in use as hemoglobin and iron that is stored and available for future hemoglobin synthesis (see Figure 21.2B). Blood loss disrupts this balance by depleting the iron stores more rapidly. Iron contributes to immune function by regulating immune effector mechanisms (such as cytokine activities).

IDA develops slowly through three overlapping stages. In stage I, the body's iron stores for red blood cell production and hemoglobin synthesis are depleted. Red blood cell production proceeds normally with the hemoglobin content of red blood cells also staying normal. In stage II, insufficient amounts of iron are transported to the marrow, and iron-deficient red blood cell production begins. Stage III begins when the hemoglobin-deficient red blood cells enter the circulation to replace normal, aged erythrocytes that have been destroyed. The manifestations of IDA appear in stage III when there is an insufficient iron supply and diminished hemoglobin synthesis.

CLINICAL MANIFESTATIONS The onset of symptoms is gradual. Individuals usually do not seek medical attention until hemoglobin levels drop to 70 or 80 g/L. Early symptoms include fatigue, weakness, shortness of breath, and pale earlobes, palms, and conjunctivae (Figure 21.3).

As the condition progresses and becomes more severe, structural and functional changes occur in epithelial tissue. The fingernails become brittle and "spoon shaped" or concave (koilonychia) (Figure 21.4). Tongue papillae atrophy can cause soreness along with redness and burning (Figure 21.5). These changes can be reversed within 1 to 2 weeks of iron replacement therapy. The corners of the mouth become dry and sore (angular stomatitis). An individual may also experience difficulty with swallowing because of a "web" that develops from mucus and inflammatory cells at the opening of the esophagus. These lesions have the potential to become cancerous.

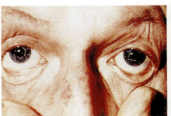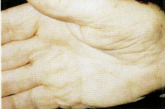

FIGURE 21.3 Pallor and Iron Deficiency. Pallor of the skin, mucous membranes, and palmar creases in an individual with a hemoglobin level of 90 g/L. Palmar creases become as pale as the surrounding skin when the hemoglobin level approaches 70 g/L. (From Hoffbrand, A. V., Pettit, J. E., & Vyas, P. [2009]. *Color atlas of clinical hematology* [4th ed.]. Mosby.)

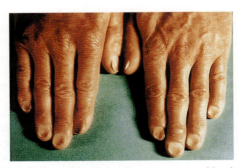

FIGURE 21.4 Koilonychia. The nails are concave, ridged, and brittle. (Courtesy Dr. S. M. Knowles. From Hoffbrand, A. V., Pettit, J. E., & Vyas, P. [2009]. *Color atlas of clinical hematology* [4th ed.]. Mosby.)

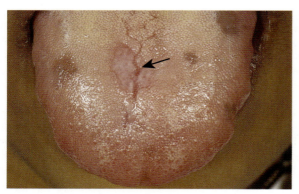

FIGURE 21.5 Glossitis. Tongue of individual with iron deficiency anemia has bald, fissured appearance (*arrow*) caused by loss of papillae and flattening. (From Hoffbrand, A. V., Pettit, J. E., & Vyas, P. [2009]. *Color atlas of clinical hematology* [4th ed.]. Mosby.)

Nonheme iron is a part of many enzymes in the body. A lack of iron may alter other physiological processes and contribute to the clinical manifestations. Individuals with IDA exhibit gastritis, neuromuscular changes, irritability, headache, numbness, tingling, and vasomotor disturbances. The incorrect perception is often made that in older persons, mental confusion, memory loss, and disorientation are "normal" events associated with aging.

EVALUATION AND TREATMENT Evaluation is based on clinical manifestations and laboratory tests. Iron stores are measured directly, by bone marrow biopsy, or indirectly, by tests that measure serum ferritin level, transferrin saturation, or total iron-binding capacity. A sensitive indicator of heme synthesis is the amount of free erythrocyte protoporphyrin (FEP) within erythrocytes.

The first step in treatment of IDA is to find and eliminate, or rule out, sources of blood loss. If this is not done, replacement therapy is ineffective. Iron replacement therapy is needed and is very effective. The use of parenteral iron replacement occurs in cases of uncontrolled blood loss, intolerance to oral iron replacement, intestinal malabsorption, or poor adherence to oral therapy.

Initial doses are continued until the serum ferritin level reaches 50 µg/L, showing that adequate replacement has occurred. A rapid decrease in fatigue, lethargy, and other associated symptoms is generally seen within the first month of therapy. Replacement therapy usually continues for 6 to 12 months after the bleeding has stopped. Menstruating females may need daily oral iron replacement therapy until menopause.

Sideroblastic Anemia

Sideroblastic anemia (SA) makes up a heterogeneous group of inherited and acquired disorders. SA is characterized by anemia of varying severity and the presence of ringed sideroblasts in the bone marrow (Figure 21.2K). **Ringed sideroblasts** are erythroblasts that have iron-laden mitochondria arranged in a circle around one-third or more of the nucleus. More simply, these are red blood cells that have iron granules that have not been synthesized into hemoglobin. Individuals with SA also have increased tissue levels of iron.

PATHOPHYSIOLOGY SAs have various causes, but all have altered heme synthesis in the erythroid cells in bone marrow. **Acquired sideroblastic anemias (ASAs)**, which are the most common, occur as a primary disorder with no known cause (idiopathic). ASAs are also associated with other myeloproliferative or myeloplastic disorders such as myeloma, polycythemia vera, and leukemias. Another form, referred to as **reversible sideroblastic anemias (reversible SAs)**, is secondary to conditions such as alcoholism, medication reactions, copper deficiency, and hypothermia. Reversible SA associated with alcoholism results from nutritional deficiencies of folate. Some medications and copper deficiency also cause reversible SA. Hypothermia causes decreased heme synthesis and incorporation into hemoglobin.

Hereditary (congenital) sideroblastic anemias are rare and occur almost exclusively in males, supporting a recessive X-linked transmission. Other genetic, chromosomal, or enzyme dysfunctions also have been associated with hereditary SA. In all instances, SA anemia is present in infancy or childhood but may remain undetected until mid-life when other conditions, such as diabetes or cardiac failure from iron overload, cause its manifestation.

The leading cause of primary ASA, **myelodysplastic syndrome (MDS)**, is a group of disorders of hematopoietic stem cells demonstrating abnormal growth or cell characteristics.[7] MDS, characterized by abnormalities of multiple cell lineages, may include alterations of neutrophils and platelets. Bleeding from thrombocytopenia and platelet dysfunction is prevalent. Of those who survive, 40% develop acute (myeloblastic) leukemia.

CLINICAL MANIFESTATIONS The anemias of SA are generally moderate to severe, with hemoglobin levels varying from 40 to 100 g/L. In addition to the cardiovascular and respiratory manifestations common to all anemias, individuals with SA may show signs of iron overload (hemochromatosis) and mild to moderate enlargement of the liver (hepatomegaly) and spleen (splenomegaly). Liver function is normal or only mildly affected. Occasionally, the skin may become abnormally coloured (bronze-tinted). Severely affected infants and young children may have growth and development impairment.

EVALUATION AND TREATMENT Initially, SA may be mistaken for deficiency of stem cells in the marrow (**hypoplastic anemia**) or IDA. The diagnosis of SA is made by bone marrow biopsy. The severity of the anemia is variable.

Identification of a causative agent (i.e., medications or toxins) is the initial step in the treatment of SA.[7] Treatment is supportive, with transfusions being the main intervention. Trial administration of oral pyridoxine may occur. Acquired SA related to alcohol abuse and pyridoxine antagonists often shows a complete response to pyridoxine. SA caused by other aetiologies does not show the same improvement.

Initial treatment of individuals with hereditary SA is with pyridoxine therapy. This therapy is effective in approximately one-third of individuals. Structural abnormalities of cells (microcytosis), however, do not disappear. Hemoglobin levels may increase in response to therapy but stabilize at less than normal levels. A therapeutic response to pyridoxine may be supported with lifelong administration of a reduced dosage. Nonresponse to pyridoxine requires blood transfusions.

Evidence of iron overload requires iron depletion therapy to prevent or minimize organ damage. **Phlebotomy**, or removal of blood from the circulation, is used in individuals with mild to moderate anemia without other complications. After iron removal, maintenance phlebotomies are continued. Severely anemic individuals who require transfusions become extremely iron overloaded. With these individuals, the use of deferoxamine, an iron-chelating agent, reduces excess iron levels.

Individuals with acquired SA are less likely to respond to pyridoxine, but SA rarely incapacitates them. When SA is secondary to an identifiable cause, treatment or removal of the cause is essential. In the absence of blood cell abnormalities and iron overload, progression takes place over years. Transfusion and chelation therapy are the same as for hereditary SA when indicated.

Recent advances in treatment for SAs include prolonged administration of erythropoietin and stem cell transplant. Successful treatment of congenital SA with stem cell transplants has occurred. However, this treatment is in the early stages of use and long-term efficacy has not yet been proven. Death from SA is rare and often secondary to complications, such as infection, bone marrow failure, liver failure, cardiac failure, or arrhythmias.

Thalassemia

Thalassemias are inherited blood disorders. They are characterized by abnormal hemoglobin production. The two main types of thalassemia are α-thalassemia and β-thalassemia. See Chapter 22 for detailed information about this disorder.

Normocytic-Normochromic Anemias

Normocytic-normochromic anemias (NNAs) are characterized by erythrocytes that are normal in size and hemoglobin content but insufficient in number.[8] These types of anemia do not share any common etiology, pathological mechanism, or morphological characteristics. They are less common than the macrocytic-normochromic and the microcytic-hypochromic anemias. The four distinct anemias are (1) aplastic (damage to bone marrow erythropoiesis); (2) posthemorrhagic (acute blood loss); (3) hemolytic, which includes acquired (immune destruction of erythrocytes), heredity (e.g., sickle cell, see Figure 21.2L), and hemolysis (destruction by eryptosis); and (4) anemia of chronic inflammation (e.g., chronic kidney disease). The diversity of the NNAs is summarized in Table 21.2. (Sickle cell anemia is discussed in Chapter 22.)

MYELOPROLIFERATIVE RED BLOOD CELL DISORDERS

Hematological dysfunction results from an overproduction of cells, as well as a deficiency. One or more hematopoietic lines may be overproduced in the marrow in response to exogenous (e.g., exposure to radiation, medications) or endogenous (e.g., physiological compensatory response, immune disorder) signals. Excessive red blood cell production is classified as polycythemia (Table 21.3). The two types of polycythemia are relative polycythemia and absolute polycythemia.

Relative polycythemia results from hemoconcentration of the blood. Causes of this condition are associated with dehydration including decreased water intake, diarrhea, excessive vomiting, or increased use of diuretics. Its development is usually of minor concern and resolves with fluid administration or treatment of underlying conditions.

TABLE 21.2 Normocytic-Normochromic Anemias

Anemia	Pathophysiology	Clinical Manifestations	Evaluation and Treatment
Aplastic	Rare; may result from infiltrative disorders of bone marrow, autoimmune diseases, renal failure, splenic dysfunction, vitamin B_{12} or folate deficiency, parvovirus infection, or exposure to radiation, medications, and toxins; also may be congenital Common stem cell population may be altered so it cannot proliferate or differentiate, or stem cell environment is altered to inhibit erythropoiesis Outcome ranges from death to minimal manifestations	Classic cardiovascular and respiratory manifestations with thrombocytopenia, hemorrhage into tissues, leukopenia, and infection	Bone marrow biopsy determines whether anemia is caused by pure RBC aplasia or hypoplasia Treatment of underlying disorder or prevent further exposure to causative agent Blood transfusions, marrow transplant, and pharmacological stimulation of bone marrow function
Posthemorrhagic	Cause is sudden blood loss with normal iron stores	Often obscured by cardiovascular manifestations of acute hemorrhage Severe shock, lactic acidosis, and death can occur if blood loss exceeds 40–50% of plasma volume	Restoration of blood volume by intravenous administration of saline, dextran, albumin, or plasma Transfusion of whole blood also required occasionally
Hemolytic	Acquired: caused by infection, systemic disease, medications or toxins, liver disease, kidney disease, abnormal immune responses Hereditary: caused by abnormalities of RBC membrane or cytoplasmic contents; present at birth Hemolysis: in blood vessels or lymphoid tissues that filter blood (e.g., spleen, liver) Erythrocytes: rigid, slowing their passage and making them vulnerable to phagocytosis Types: warm antibody disease (mediated by IgG antibody specific for erythrocyte antigens), cold antibody disease (mediated by IgM), and medication-induced	Splenomegaly, jaundice, aplastic hemolytic, or megaloblastic crises can develop with viral infection With severe disease, bones become deformed and pathological fractures occur Cardiovascular and respiratory manifestations correspond with severity of anemia	Blood and bone marrow studies Erythroid hyperplasia is found in marrow and blood smears Treatment of acquired disease involves removing cause or treating underlying disorder Other forms of treatment are transfusions, splenectomy, and steroids or folate
Anemia of chronic inflammation	Associated with chronic infections (e.g., AIDS), chronic inflammatory diseases (e.g., rheumatoid arthritis, SLE), and malignancies Causes are decreased erythrocyte lifespan, failure of mechanisms of compensatory erythropoiesis, or disturbance of iron cycle	Manifestations fewer and milder than most other anemias General disability caused by chronic disease limits physical activity so hemoglobin levels adequate; if they drop, signs of iron deficiency anemia develop	Blood tests show iron deficiency in marrow despite normal or increased iron stores elsewhere No treatment is needed unless anemia becomes symptomatic Erythropoietin may be used

AIDS, Acquired immunodeficiency syndrome; *IgG*, immunoglobulin G; *IgM*, immunoglobulin M; *RBC*, red blood cell; *SLE*, systemic lupus erythematosus.

TABLE 21.3 Disorders Classified as Polycythemia

Type of Polycythemia	Mechanism of Increased Erythropoiesis	Cause of Associated Disorder
Primary polycythemia (polycythemia vera)	Excessive proliferation of erythroid precursors in marrow; JAK2 mutation, increased sensitivity of stem cell to erythropoietin	Possible mutation in erythropoietin receptor
Secondary polycythemia	Physiological increase in erythropoietin secretion by kidneys in response to underlying systemic disorder	Tissue hypoxia caused by cardiopulmonary disorders (chronic obstructive pulmonary disease, heart failure), decreased barometric pressure, cardiovascular malformations causing mixing of arterial and venous blood, methemoglobinemia, carboxyhemoglobinemia, smoking, obesity
	"Nonphysiological"[a] increase in erythropoietin secretion	Renal disorders, cerebellar hemangioblastomas, hepatoma (liver tumour), ovarian carcinoma, uterine leiomyoma, pheochromocytoma, adrenocortical hypersecretion
Familial polycythemia	Genetically induced increase in erythroid precursors of marrow Abnormal Hb with increased oxygen affinity Decreased 2,3-DPG Increased sensitivity of stem cells to erythropoietin Increased erythropoietin secretion	Genetic defect

[a]*Nonphysiological* means that there is no obvious physiological explanation for hypersecretion of erythropoietin.
2,3-DPG, 2,3-Diphosphoglycerate; *Hb*, hemoglobin; *JAK2*, Janus kinase 2 gene.

Absolute polycythemia consists of two forms: primary (vera) and secondary. *Secondary polycythemia*, the most common, is a physiological response resulting from erythropoietin secretion caused by hypoxia. Hypoxia occurs in individuals living at higher altitudes (greater than 3000 m), smokers with increased blood levels of carbon monoxide, and individuals with chronic obstructive pulmonary disease or heart failure. Other causes of secondary polycythemia include abnormal types of hemoglobin (e.g., San Diego, Chesapeake), which have a greater affinity for oxygen, and inappropriate secretion of erythropoietin by certain tumours (e.g., renal cell carcinoma, hepatoma, and cerebellar hemangioblastomas).

Polycythemia Vera

Polycythemia vera (PV) (also known as **primary polycythemia**) is a stem cell disorder. Hyperplastic and neoplastic bone marrow alterations occur with PV. These alterations include an abnormal uncontrolled proliferation of red blood cells (often with increased levels of white blood cells [leukocytosis] and platelets [thrombocytosis]). The increase in red blood cells (polycythemia) is responsible for most of the clinical symptoms, including an increase in blood volume and viscosity. PV is one of several disorders collectively known as *myeloproliferative neoplasms* (MPNs). These disorders include certain leukemias, essential thrombocytosis, and chronic bone marrow fibrosis. The disorders all result from abnormal regulation of the hematopoietic stem cells. The common pathogenic feature is the presence of a mutation in the **Janus kinase 2 gene (JAK2 gene)** resulting in an overproduction of blood cells. Because of many characteristics (e.g., overproduction of different blood cells, marrow hypercellularity, or fibrosis) shared by these disorders and a lack of specific molecular markers, the diagnosis can be challenging. The common features include (1) increased proliferative drive in the bone marrow, (2) hematopoiesis of neoplastic stem cells to secondary hematopoietic organs, (3) marrow fibrosis and peripheral deficiencies in blood cells (cytopenias), and (4) variable transformation to acute leukemia.

PV is quite rare, with a peak incidence between the ages of 60 and 80 years and a median incidence of 55 to 60. PV has been seen in individuals younger than the age of 40. Males are twice as likely as females to develop PV. It is more common in Whites of Eastern European Jewish ancestry. PV is rarely seen in children or in multiple members of a single family; however, an autosomal dominant form exists that causes increased secretion of erythropoietin.

PATHOPHYSIOLOGY Erythrocytosis is the essential part of PV. Proliferation of erythroid progenitors occurs in the bone marrow independent of the hormone erythropoietin, but the cells express a normal erythropoietin receptor. Most individuals with PV have an acquired mutation in the tyrosine kinase, Janus kinase 2 (JAK2).[9] Normal JAK2 increases the activity of the erythropoietin receptor and is self-regulatory so that JAK2 activity decreases over time. The mutation associated with PV removes the self-regulatory activity of JAK2. As a result, the erythropoietin receptor is constantly active, regardless of the level of erythropoietin. Overall, the mutated tyrosine kinases bypass normal controls. This causes growth factor–independent proliferation and survival of marrow progenitors or precursor cells. The cause of the mutation is unknown.

CLINICAL MANIFESTATIONS PV is uncommon and occurs insidiously. Clinical manifestations of PV are a result of the increased red blood cell mass and hematocrit. Usually there is an increase in blood volume. Together, all of these factors cause abnormal blood flow that increases blood viscosity. The increased viscosity creates a hypercoagulable state that results in clogging and occlusion of blood vessels. Tissue injury (ischemia) and death (infarction) are the outcome of blood vessel blockage. These outcomes are directly correlated with hematocrit levels. Increases in numbers of thrombocytes, as well as production of dysfunctional platelets, also contribute to this hypercoagulable condition.

Circulatory alterations caused by the thick, sticky blood give rise to other manifestations. This includes plethora (ruddy, red colour of the face, hands, feet, ears, and mucous membranes) and engorgement of retinal and cerebral veins. Other symptoms may include headache, drowsiness, delirium, mania, psychotic depression, chorea, and visual disturbances. Individuals often have an enlarged spleen with abdominal pain and discomfort. Death from cerebral thrombosis is approximately five times greater in individuals with PV.[1]

Cardiovascular function, despite the vascular alterations, is still relatively normal. Cardiac workload and output remain constant. An increased blood volume, however, does increase blood pressure. Blood flow may be affected, causing angina, although cardiovascular infarctions are uncommon. Other cardiovascular manifestations include Raynaud phenomenon and thromboangiitis obliterans.

A unique feature of PV, which is helpful in diagnosis, is the development of intense, painful itching. The itching appears to be increased by heat or exposure to water (aquagenic pruritus). As a result, individuals avoid exposure to water, particularly warm water when bathing or showering. The intensity of itching is related to the concentration of mast cells in the skin and is generally not responsive to antihistamines or topical lotions.

EVALUATION AND TREATMENT PV is often suspected because of clinical features, such as a thrombotic event, splenomegaly, or aquagenic pruritus. Blood and laboratory findings, including an absolute increase in red blood cells and in total blood volume, confirm the diagnosis. Hematocrit levels increasing by one-third of normal levels, and a corresponding increase in hemoglobin and red blood cells, are used for diagnostic purposes. Erythrocytes appear normal, but anisocytosis may be present. There also may be moderate increases in white blood cells and platelets. A bone marrow examination may be done but is not very valuable unless performed in association with cytogenetic and molecular studies for relevant mutations in *JAK2*.[10] The presence of a *JAK2* mutation confirms the diagnosis.[10] Treatment of PV consists of reducing red blood cell proliferation and blood volume, controlling symptoms, and preventing clogging and clotting of the blood vessels. In low-risk individuals (e.g., those younger than age 60 or with no history of thrombosis and without risk factors for cardiovascular disease), the recommended therapy is phlebotomy (300 to 500 mL at a time) and low-dose Aspirin. Frequent phlebotomies also reduce iron levels, a condition that impedes erythropoiesis.

Hydroxyurea (Droxia), a nonalkylating myelosuppressive, is the medication of choice for myelosuppression because of a reduced incidence to cause leukemia and thrombosis. Radioactive phosphorus (^{32}P) also is used as an effective and easily tolerated intervention to suppress erythropoiesis. Its effects may last up to 18 months. Side effects of ^{32}P include suppression of hematopoiesis resulting in anemia, leukopenia, and thrombocytopenia. Acute leukemia is also a side effect, although most often it occurs after 7 or more years of treatment. Interferon-alpha has been used when other forms of treatment have failed.

Survival for 10 to 15 years is common. However, without proper treatment, 50% of individuals with PV die within 18 months of the onset of first symptoms because of thrombosis or hemorrhage. A significant potential outcome of PV is the conversion to acute myeloid (or myelogenous) leukemia (AML). This occurs spontaneously in 10% of individuals and generally is resistant to conventional therapy. Conversion to AML is most likely related to treatment methods associated with cytotoxic myelosuppressive agents. Although PV is a chronic disorder, proper therapy results in remissions and prevention of pathological outcomes.

Iron Overload

Iron overload can be primary, as in hereditary hemochromatosis, or secondary. The secondary causes of iron overload include anemias with inefficient erythropoiesis (e.g., SA, aplastic anemia), dietary iron overload, or conditions that require repeated blood transfusions or iron dextran injections. Iron absorption is regulated by erythropoietin, tissue oxygenation, and iron stores (see Chapter 20).

Hereditary Hemochromatosis

Hemochromatosis is caused by excessive iron absorption. Hereditary hemochromatosis (HH) is a common inherited, autosomal recessive disorder of iron metabolism.[1] It is characterized by increased GI iron absorption with tissue iron deposition. Excess iron is deposited first in the liver and pancreas, followed by the heart, joints, and endocrine glands. Excess iron causes tissue damage that can lead to diseases such as cirrhosis, diabetes, heart failure, arthropathies, and impotence. HH affects more males than females.

HH is caused by two genetic base-pair alterations, C282Y and H63D. These are mutations in the *HFE* gene on chromosome 6. Homozygosity of C282Y is the most common genotype and accounts for 82 to 90% of HH cases. The remaining cases appear to be caused by environmental factors or other genotypes. *HFE* mutations are common in Canada, affecting an estimated 1 in 300 Canadians, primarily of Northern European descent.[11] Current research estimates that 1 in 9 Canadians are heterozygotes or carriers of HH.[11]

PATHOPHYSIOLOGY In HH, regulation of intestinal absorption of dietary iron is abnormal, causing iron accumulation. The *HFE* gene directs intestinal absorption of dietary iron by regulating the liver-derived protein hepcidin. Hepcidin lowers plasma iron level; a deficiency in hepcidin, caused by genetic mutations, causes iron overload. The gene mutations in HH reduce hepcidin synthesis. This reduces the level of circulating plasma hepcidin. The decreased hepcidin-ferroportin (iron transporter) interaction leads to more iron outward flow (efflux) from cells in the small intestinal mucosa. This outward flow causes a rise in iron concentration and a systemic overload. The iron overload leads to excess iron tissue deposits. These deposits can eventually result in liver fibrosis, cirrhosis, hepatocellular carcinoma, diabetes, hypothyroidism, arthritis, cardiomyopathies, and skin hyperpigmentation.

With HH there appears to be a long latent period with individual variation in biochemical expression. Variation depends on environmental factors such as blood loss from menstruation or donation, alcohol intake, and diet. Cirrhosis is a late-stage development of HH that can shorten life expectancy. Cirrhosis also is a risk factor for hepatocellular carcinoma that occurs between 40 and 60 years of age. Cirrhosis prevention is a major goal of HH screening and treatment.

CLINICAL MANIFESTATIONS Clinical manifestations of HH include fatigue, malaise, abdominal pain, arthralgias, and impotence. Clinical findings include hepatomegaly, abnormal liver enzymes, bronzed skin, diabetes, and cardiomegaly. Many individuals are diagnosed as a result of serum iron studies as part of a health screening panel. Most affected individuals (greater than 75%) are asymptomatic and have a low frequency (less than 25%) of cirrhosis, diabetes, or skin pigmentation.

EVALUATION AND TREATMENT Laboratory findings in individuals with HH show elevations in serum iron levels, transferrin saturation, and ferritin levels. Documentation of iron overload relies on quantitative phlebotomy with calculation of the amount of iron removed. Alternatively, a liver biopsy can determine the amount of hepatic iron. With the use of genetic testing, individuals who are C282Y homozygous or compound heterozygous, less than 40 years old, and have normal liver functions, no further workup is necessary.

Treatment of HH is simple and consists of phlebotomy of 550 mL of whole blood, which is equivalent to 200 to 250 mg of iron. Frequency of phlebotomy depends on ferritin levels and should continue until the ferritin level is between 20 and 50 μg/L. Initially, phlebotomy may be needed weekly but once therapeutic ferritin levels are reached, phlebotomy may only be needed every 2 to 3 months. Blood banks now accept blood donations from persons with documented HH. Iron-chelating agents are sometimes used in addition to phlebotomy. Individuals with HH should be instructed to refrain from taking iron and vitamin C supplements and consuming raw shellfish. In addition, alcohol should be used in moderation. Family screening is recommended for all first-degree relatives of a person with HH.

ALTERATIONS OF LEUKOCYTE FUNCTION

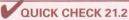
QUICK CHECK 21.2
1. What condition is manifested by an increase in the numbers of circulating granulocytes and monocytes?
2. What is the cause of infectious mononucleosis (IM)?
3. What are the classic symptoms of IM?

Leukocyte function is affected if too many or too few white blood cells are present in the blood or if the cells that are present are structurally or functionally defective. Phagocytic cells (granulocytes, monocytes, macrophages) may lose their ability to act as phagocytes, and the lymphocytes may lose their ability to respond to antigens. (Chapter 6 describes disruptions of inflammatory and immune processes caused by leukocyte disorders.) Other leukocyte alterations include infectious mononucleosis (IM) and cancers of the blood including leukemia and multiple myeloma (MM).

Quantitative Alterations of Leukocytes

Quantitative alterations are increases or decreases in numbers and functions of leukocytes in the blood. **Leukocytosis** is present when the count is higher than normal. **Leukopenia** is present when the count is lower than normal. Leukocytosis and leukopenia may affect a specific type of white blood cell and may result from a variety of physiological conditions and alterations.

Leukocytosis occurs as a normal protective response to physiological stressors. These stressors include invading microorganisms, strenuous exercise, emotional changes, temperature changes, anaesthesia, surgery, pregnancy, and some medications, hormones, and toxins. It also is caused by pathological conditions, such as malignancies and hematological disorders. Unlike leukocytosis, leukopenia is never normal and is defined as an absolute blood cell count less than 4×10^9/L. Leukopenia is associated with a decrease in neutrophils, which increases risk for infection. When the neutrophil count falls below 1×10^9/L, the risk for infection increases drastically. With counts below 0.5×10^9/L, the possibility for life-threatening infections is high. Leukopenia may be caused by radiation, anaphylactic shock, autoimmune disease (e.g., systemic lupus erythematosus), immune deficiencies (see Chapter 8), and certain chemotherapeutic agents.

Granulocyte and Monocyte Alterations

Increased numbers of circulating granulocytes (neutrophils, eosinophils, basophils) and monocytes are mainly a physiological response to infection. Increased numbers also occur as a result of myeloproliferative disorders that increase stem cell proliferation in the bone marrow.[1]

Decreased numbers occur when infectious processes deplete the supply of circulating granulocytes and monocytes, drawing them out of the circulation and into infected tissues faster than they can be replaced. Decreases also can be caused by disorders that suppress marrow function, such as severe congenital neutropenia, or immune-related neutropenia.[1]

Granulocytosis is an increase in granulocytes (neutrophils, eosinophils, or basophils) and begins with the release of stored blood cells. **Neutrophilia** is another term that is used to describe *granulocytosis* because neutrophils are the most numerous of the granulocytes (Table 21.4). Neutrophilia is seen in the early stages of infection or inflammation and is confirmed when the absolute count exceeds 7.5×10^9/L. Release and depletion of stored neutrophils stimulates granulopoiesis to replenish neutrophil reserves. Specific conditions associated with neutrophilia and other white blood cells are found in Table 21.4.

When the demand for circulating mature neutrophils exceeds the supply, immature neutrophils are released from the bone marrow. Premature release of the immature cells is responsible for the phenomenon known as a **shift to the left**, or **leukemoid reaction**. This refers to the microscopic detection of disproportionate numbers of immature leukocytes in peripheral blood smears. To understand this phenomenon, visualize cellular differentiation, maturation, and release (see Figure 20.2) as progressing from left to right. The early release of immature white blood cells prevents the completion of the sequence and shifts the distribution of leukocytes in the blood toward those on the left side of the diagram. This phenomenon is also seen in the blood smear of individuals with leukemia, hence the term *leukemoid reaction*. As infection or inflammation decreases, granulopoiesis replaces circulating granulocytes. As such, a **shift to the right** (return to normal) occurs.

Neutropenia is a condition associated with a decrease in circulating neutrophils. It exists clinically when the neutrophil count is less than 2×10^9/L. Decrease in neutrophils occurs in severe prolonged infections when production of granulocytes cannot keep up with demand.[1]

Other causes of neutropenia, in the absence of infection, may be (1) decreased neutrophil production or ineffective granulopoiesis, (2) reduced neutrophil survival, and (3) abnormal neutrophil distribution and sequestration. Neutropenia also is classified as primary or secondary. Primary disorders are further named as congenital or acquired. Primary acquired neutropenia is associated with multiple conditions. These conditions include hypoplastic anemia or aplastic anemia, leukemia (AML/chronic lymphocytic leukemia [CLL]), lymphomas (Hodgkin's, non-Hodgkin's), and MDS. The megaloblastic anemias (vitamin B_{12} and folate deficiency) as well as starvation and anorexia nervosa cause neutropenia. This occurs because of an inadequate supply of vitamins and nutrients for protein production.

Congenital defects in neutrophil production include cyclic neutropenia, neutropenia with congenital immunodeficiencies, and multiple syndromes. Syndromes include Kostmann, Shwachman-Diamond, Diamond-Blackfan, and Barth. Reduced neutrophil survival and abnormal distribution and sequestration are usually secondary to other disorders. Neutropenia occurs in a variety of immunological disorders. These disorders include systemic lupus erythematosus, rheumatoid arthritis, Felty's and Sjögren's syndromes, splenomegaly, and medication-related causes.

Severe neutropenia, **granulocytopenia** (less than 0.5×10^9/L), or **agranulocytosis** (complete absence of granulocytes in blood) is usually secondary to arrested hematopoiesis in the bone marrow or massive cell destruction in the circulation. Chemotherapeutic agents used to treat hematological and other malignancies cause bone marrow suppression. Several other medications cause agranulocytosis. This condition occurs rarely but carries a high mortality of 10 to 50%. Clinical manifestations of agranulocytosis include severe infection (particularly of the respiratory system) leading to septicemia, general malaise, fever, tachycardia, and ulcers in the mouth and colon. If this condition is untreated, sepsis caused by agranulocytosis results in death within 3 to 6 days. Table 21.4 details other conditions associated with neutropenia.

Eosinophilia is an absolute increase (greater than 4.5×10^9/L) in the total number of circulating eosinophils. Allergic disorders (type 1) associated with asthma, hay fever, parasitic infections, and medication reactions often cause eosinophilia. Hypersensitivity reactions trigger the release of eosinophil chemotactic factor of anaphylaxis (ECF-A). The release of histamine from mast cells attracts eosinophils to the area. Mast cells release interleukin-5 (IL-5), which stimulates the bone marrow to produce more eosinophils into the blood. Areas with a lot of mast cells, such as the respiratory and GI tracts, are commonly affected. Eosinophilia also may occur in dermatological disorders, eosinophilia-myalgia syndrome, and parasitic invasion. Other conditions associated with eosinophilia are detailed in Table 21.4.

CHAPTER 21 Alterations of Hematological Function

TABLE 21.4 Other Conditions Associated with Neutrophils, Eosinophils, Basophils, Monocytes, and Lymphocytes

Condition	Cause	Example
Neutrophil		
Neutrophilia (granulocytosis)	Inflammation or tissue necrosis	Surgery, burns, MI, pneumonitis, rheumatic fever, rheumatoid arthritis
	Infection	Bacterial: Gram-positive (staphylococci, streptococci, pneumococci), Gram-negative (*Escherichia coli*, *Pseudomonas* species)
	Physiological	Exercise, extreme heat or cold, third-trimester pregnancy, emotional distress
	Hematological	Acute hemorrhage, hemolysis, myeloproliferative disorder, chronic granulocytic leukemia
	Medications or chemicals	Epinephrine, steroids, heparin, histamine, endotoxin
	Metabolic	Diabetes (acidosis), eclampsia, gout, thyroid storm
	Neoplasm	Liver, GI tract, bone marrow
Neutropenia	Decreased marrow production	Radiation, chemotherapy, leukemia, aplastic anemia, abnormal granulopoiesis
	Increased destruction	Splenomegaly, hemodialysis, autoimmune disease
	Prolonged infection	Gram-negative (typhoid), viral (influenza, hepatitis B, measles, mumps, rubella), severe infections, protozoal infections (malaria)
Eosinophil		
Eosinophilia	Allergy	Asthma, hay fever, medication sensitivity
	Infection	Parasites (trichinosis, hookworm), chronic (fungal, leprosy, TB)
	Malignancy	CML, lung, stomach, ovary, Hodgkin's lymphoma
	Dermatosis	Pemphigus, exfoliative dermatitis (medication-induced)
	Medications	Digitalis, heparin, streptomycin, tryptophan (eosinophilia-myalgia syndrome), penicillins, propranolol
Eosinopenia	Stress response	Trauma, shock, burns, surgery, mental distress
	Medications	Steroids (Cushing's syndrome)
Basophil		
Basophilia	Inflammation	Infection (measles, chickenpox), hypersensitivity reaction (immediate)
	Hematological	Myeloproliferative disorders (CML, polycythemia vera, Hodgkin's lymphoma, hemolytic anemia)
	Endocrine	Myxedema, antithyroid therapy
Basopenia	Physiological	Pregnancy, ovulation, stress
	Endocrine	Graves' disease
Monocyte		
Monocytosis	Infection	Bacterial (subacute bacterial endocarditis, TB), recovery phase of infection
	Hematological	Myeloproliferative disorders, Hodgkin's lymphoma, agranulocytosis
	Physiological	Normal newborn
Monocytopenia	Rare	
Lymphocyte		
Lymphocytosis	Physiological	4 months to 4 years
	Acute infection	Infectious mononucleosis, CMV infection, pertussis, hepatitis, mycoplasma pneumonia, typhoid
	Chronic infection	Congenital syphilis, tertiary syphilis
	Endocrine	Thyrotoxicosis, adrenal insufficiency
	Malignancy	ALL, CLL, lymphosarcoma cell leukemia
Lymphocytopenia	Immunodeficiency syndrome	AIDS, agammaglobulinemia
	Lymphocyte destruction	Steroids (Cushing's syndrome), radiation, chemotherapy
		Hodgkin's lymphoma
		Heart failure, renal failure, TB, SLE, aplastic anemia

AIDS, Acquired immunodeficiency syndrome; *ALL*, acute lymphocytic leukemia; *CLL*, chronic lymphocytic leukemia; *CML*, chronic myeloid (or myelogenous) leukemia; *CMV*, cytomegalovirus; *GI*, gastro-intestinal; *MI*, myocardial infarction; *SLE*, systemic lupus erythematosus; *TB*, tuberculosis.

Eosinopenia is a decrease in the number of circulating eosinophils. It is generally caused by movement of eosinophils into inflammatory sites. It may be seen in Cushing's syndrome and as a result of stress caused by surgery, shock, trauma, burns, or mental distress. Other conditions associated with eosinopenia are detailed in Table 21.4.

Basophilia is an increase in the number of circulating basophils. It is rare and generally is a response to inflammation and immediate hypersensitivity reactions. Basophils hold histamine that is released during an allergic reaction. Increased numbers of basophils are seen in myeloproliferative disorders, such as chronic myeloid leukemia and myeloid metaplasia. Other conditions associated with basophilia are detailed in Table 21.4.

Basopenia (also known as *basophilic leukopenia*) is a decrease in circulating numbers of basophils. It is seen in hyperthyroidism, acute infection, ovulation and pregnancy, and long-term therapy with steroids. Other conditions associated with basopenia are detailed in Table 21.4.

Monocytosis is an increase in the number of circulating monocytes. It is often transient and not related to a dysfunction of monocyte production. If present, it is usually associated with neutropenia during bacterial infections. This occurs mainly in the late stages or recovery stage when monocytes are needed to phagocytize surviving microorganisms and debris. Increased monocytes also may show marrow recovery from agranulocytosis. Monocytosis is often seen in chronic infections such as tuberculosis (TB), brucellosis, listeriosis, and subacute bacterial endocarditis. Monocytosis has been found to correlate with the extent of myocardial damage following myocardial infarctions. Other conditions associated with monocytosis are detailed in Table 21.4. Monocytopenia, a decrease in the number of circulating monocytes, is rare but has been found with hairy cell leukemia and prednisone therapy.

Lymphocyte Alterations

Quantitative alterations of lymphocytes occur when lymphocytes are activated by antigenic stimuli, usually microorganisms (see Chapter 7). Lymphocytosis is an increase in the number (absolute lymphocytosis) or proportion of lymphocytes in the blood. It is rare in acute bacterial infections and is seen most commonly in acute viral infections, particularly those caused by the Epstein-Barr virus (EBV). Other disorders associated with lymphocytosis are detailed in Table 21.4.

Lymphocytopenia is a decrease in the number of circulating lymphocytes in the blood. It may be attributed to (1) abnormalities of lymphocyte production associated with neoplasias and immune deficiencies and (2) destruction by medications, viruses, or radiation. It is also known to occur without any detectable cause. Conditions associated with lymphocytopenia are detailed in Table 21.4. The lymphocytopenia associated with heart failure and other acute illnesses may be caused by elevated cortisol levels. Lymphocytopenia is a major problem in acquired immune deficiency syndrome (AIDS). AIDS-related lymphocytopenia is caused by human immunodeficiency virus (HIV), which destroys T-helper lymphocytes. (For a detailed discussion of AIDS, see Chapter 8.)

Infectious Mononucleosis

Infectious mononucleosis (IM) is a benign, acute, self-limiting, lymphoproliferative clinical syndrome characterized by acute infection of B lymphocytes (B cells). The most common cause is EBV.[1] EBV is a global lymphotropic herpesvirus and accounts for approximately 85% of IM cases. Other viruses that cause symptoms resembling IM include cytomegalovirus (CMV), adenovirus, HIV, hepatitis A, influenza A and B, and rubella. Bacteria that cause similar symptoms include *Toxoplasma gondii*, *Corynebacterium diphtheriae*, and *Coxiella burnetii*. The classic symptoms are pharyngitis, lymphadenopathy, and fever.

It is estimated that 90 to 95% of all humans are infected with EBV, with infection occurring most often during early childhood.[1,2] These early infections are usually asymptomatic and supply immunity to EBV; thus, early EBV infections rarely develop into IM. IM may arise when the first infection occurs during adolescence or later. Symptomatic IM usually affects young adults between ages 15 and 35 years of age. Peak incidence occurs between ages 1 to 6 and 14 to 20 years. The overall incidence rate for this age group is 2 to 3 cases per 1000 persons per year. Children from low socioeconomic environments are particularly susceptible to infections with EBV. IM is uncommon in individuals older than age 40; however, if it does occur, it is commonly caused by CMV.[3]

Transmission of EBV is usually through saliva from close personal contact (e.g., kissing, hence the term *kissing disease*). The virus also may be secreted in other mucosal secretions of the genital, rectal, and respiratory tracts, as well as blood. The infection begins with widespread invasion of the B cells, which have receptors for EBV. The virus initially infects the oropharynx, nasopharynx, and salivary epithelial cells with later spread into lymphoid tissues and B cells.

In the immunocompetent individual, unaffected B cells produce antibodies (immunoglobulins IgG, IgA, IgM) against the virus. At the same time, there is a massive proliferation of T-cytotoxic cells (CD8) that are directed against EBV-infected cells (see Chapter 7). The immune response against EBV-infected cells is largely responsible for the cellular proliferation in the lymphoid tissue (lymph nodes, spleen, tonsils, and, occasionally, liver). Once the virus enters the bloodstream, the infection spreads throughout the body. Inflammation at the site of first viral entry (the mouth and throat) causes sore throat and fever.

CLINICAL MANIFESTATIONS The incubation period for IM is approximately 30 to 50 days. Early flulike symptoms, such as headache, malaise, joint pain, and fatigue, may appear during the first 3 to 5 days, although some individuals are without symptoms. At the time of diagnosis, the individual commonly presents with the classic group of symptoms: fever, sore throat (pharyngitis), cervical lymph node enlargement, and fatigue. The pharyngitis is usually diffuse with a whitish or greyish green, thick exudate. It can be painful, causing the individual to seek treatment. Characteristics with progression may include a generalized lymphadenopathy, enlarged spleen, and appearance in the blood of atypical activated T lymphocytes (mononucleosis cells). IM is usually self-limiting, and recovery occurs in a few weeks. Fatigue, however, may last for 1 to 2 months after resolution of the infection.

Severe clinical complications are rare. With progression of IM, general lymph node enlargement may develop with enlargement of the spleen and liver. Splenomegaly is clinically clear 50% of the time and is proven radiologically 100% of the time. Difficulty in detecting splenomegaly with physical examination contributes to the underestimation of actual enlargement. Splenic rupture is rare and can occur spontaneously as a result of mild trauma. This complication occurs primarily in men younger than 25 years of age and between days 4 and 21 after the onset of symptoms. It is the most common cause of death related to IM. Other causes of fatalities are hepatic failure, extensive bacterial infection, and viral myocarditis. Other organ systems are rarely involved, but such involvement may be present with characteristic manifestations, such as hepatitis with jaundice and anemia, encephalitis, meningitis, Guillain-Barré syndrome, and Bell's palsy. Eye manifestations may include eyelid and periorbital edema, dry eyes, keratitis, uveitis, and conjunctivitis. Reye syndrome has been known to develop in children with EBV infection. Pulmonary and respiratory failure has been documented, but it is more likely to occur in immunocompromised individuals. Approximately 3 to 10% of adults older than 40 years of age have never been infected with EBV and are susceptible to IM later in life. In these individuals, the classic symptoms are not generally present, making diagnosis more difficult.

EVALUATION AND TREATMENT The blood of affected individuals has an increased number of white blood cells with many atypical forms. The diagnosis of IM depends on the following findings: (1) an increase in the number of lymphocytes, commonly based on Hoagland criteria of at least 50% lymphocytes and at least 10% atypical lymphocytes in the blood; (2) a positive heterophile antibody reaction (monospot test); and (3) a rising titer of specific antibodies for EBV antigens. Heterophilic antibodies are a heterogeneous group of IgM antibodies that are agglutinins against nonhuman red blood cells (e.g., horse, sheep). They are detected by qualitative (monospot test) or quantitative (heterophile antibody test) methods. Use of the monospot test is limited because other infections (e.g., CMV, adenovirus) and toxoplasmosis also produce heterophilic antibodies. Thus 5 to 15% of monospot tests return false-positive results. Heterophilic antibodies in the blood increase as the condition progresses. However, some individuals and children younger than 4 years of age do not produce these antibodies. Diagnosis of EBV infection may be increased with newer viral-specific tests that show EBV-specific antibodies.

Treatment is supportive and consists of rest and relief of symptoms with analgesics and antipyretics. Aspirin is avoided with children because of its association with Reye syndrome. *Streptococcal pharyngitis*, which occurs in 20 to 30% of cases, is treated with penicillin or erythromycin (Erythrocin). The use of ampicillin (Principen) or amoxicillin (Amoxil) is known to cause a rash. Bed rest with avoidance of strenuous activity and contact sports is indicated. Steroids are used when severe complications, such as impending airway obstruction, or other organ involvement (central nervous system manifestations, thrombocytopenic purpura, myocarditis, pericarditis) are present. Acyclovir (Zovirax) has been used in immunocompromised individuals but is not considered standard therapy. In the rare event of splenic rupture, the treatment has been removal of the spleen and continues to be the choice in hemodynamically unstable individuals. Current research, however, is suggesting that it may be better to repair the spleen to avoid overwhelming postsplenectomy infection.

Leukemias

> **QUICK CHECK 21.3**
> 1. How are leukemias classified?
> 2. What is the pathogenesis of acute lymphocytic leukemia (ALL)?
> 3. What is the significance of the Philadelphia chromosome, and how is it related to leukemia?

Leukemia is a clonal malignant disorder of the bone marrow and usually, but not always, of the blood. The common pathological feature of all forms of leukemia is an uncontrolled proliferation of malignant leukocytes. This uncontrolled proliferation causes an overcrowding of bone marrow and decreased production and function of normal hematopoietic cells. Chromosomal abnormalities and translocations are common in most leukemias. When genes become mutated, they create genomic anomalies that block cell maturation and activate pro-growth signalling pathways that prevent apoptotic cell death.

Over time, the classification of leukemia has become increasingly complex, with many changes. These changes have created a blurring between the once discrete categories *lymphoma* and *leukemia*. Some cancers known as *lymphoma* have *leukemic* presentations, and evolution to leukemia is not unusual during the progression of incurable lymphoma. The World Health Organization (WHO) currently groups the lymphoid neoplasms into five broad categories, which are defined by the cell of origin:
1. Precursor B-cell neoplasms (immature B cells)
2. Peripheral B-cell neoplasms (mature B cells)
3. Precursor T-cell neoplasms (immature T cells)
4. Peripheral T-cell and NK (natural killer)-cell neoplasms (mature T cells and NK cells)
5. Hodgkin's lymphoma (Reed-Sternberg [RS] cell and variants)

Most lymphoid neoplasm classifications relate to stages of cell differentiation of B-cell or T-cell differentiation (Figure 21.6A). Figure 21.6B shows a simple schematic overview of the main types of leukemia.

Acute leukemia is characterized by undifferentiated or immature cells, usually a **blast cell**. The onset of disease is abrupt and rapid. Without treatment, disease progression results in a short survival time. In **chronic leukemia**, the predominant cell is more differentiated but does not function normally, with a relatively slow progression. There are four major types of leukemia: acute lymphocytic (ALL), acute myelogenous (AML), chronic lymphocytic (CLL), and chronic myelogenous (CML).

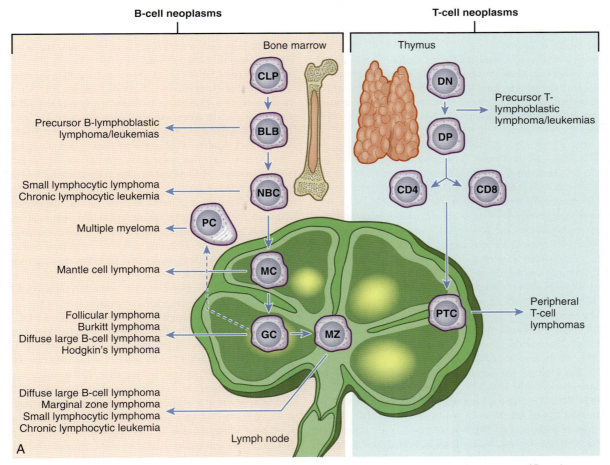

FIGURE 21.6 Origin of Lymphoid Neoplasms. **A**, Specific lymphoid tumours emerge from stages of B- and T-cell differentiation. **B**, Overview of main types of leukemia. Acute myeloid lymphoma (*AML*) may arise *de novo* or be preceded by myelodysplastic phase.

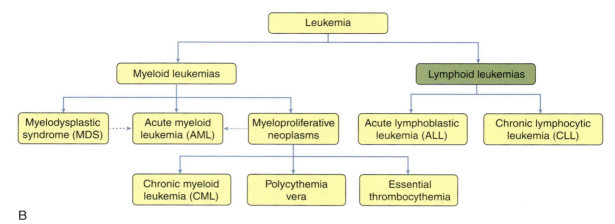

FIGURE 21-6, cont'd Not all cases of myelodysplastic syndrome (MDS) evolve to AML (*dashed line*). Some myelodysplastic neoplasms can transform into AML, although very rarely (*dotted line*). *BLB*, Pre-B lymphoblast; *CLP*, common lymphoid precursor; *DN*, CD4/CD8 double-negative pro-T cell; *DP*, CD4/CD8 double-positive pre-T cell; *GC*, germinal centre B cell; *MC*, mantle B cell; *MZ*, marginal zone B cell; *NBC*, naïve B cell; *PTC*, peripheral T cell. ([A] From Kumar, V., Abbas, A., & Aster, J. C. [2016]. *Robbins & Cotran pathologic basis of disease* [9th ed.]. Saunders; [B] from Khwaja, A., Bjorkholm, M., Gale, R. E., et al. [2016]. Acute myeloid leukaemia. *Nature Reviews Disease Primers, 2*, 16010. https://doi.org/10.1038/nrdp.2016.10.)

Leukemia occurs with varying frequencies at different ages and is more common in adults than in children. In 2020, it was estimated that 6 900 Canadians would be diagnosed with leukemia, with males having a slightly higher incidence than females. Estimated deaths for 2020 were 3 000 individuals.[14] Leukemia accounts for about 32% of all childhood cancers.[15] CLL and AML are the most common types in adults. CML is found mostly in adults.

Over the past 2 decades, the rates of induced remission and survival in most forms of leukemia have increased. This progress is a result of more effective treatments, improved blood product and antimicrobial support, and specialized nursing care. Chemotherapy and bone marrow transplant have increased the survival rates of individuals with acute leukemia.[1]

PATHOPHYSIOLOGY All leukemias have certain pathophysiological features in common. Most lymphoid neoplasms arise from B-cell and T-cell differentiation pathways. The leukemias are clonal disorders driven by genetically abnormal stem-like cancer cells (SLCCs).[16] Abnormal immature white blood cells, called *leukemic blasts*, fill the bone marrow and spill into the blood. The leukemic blasts literally "crowd out" the marrow and cause cellular proliferation of the other cell lines to cease. Normal granulocytic-monocytic, lymphocytic, erythrocytic, and megakaryocytic progenitor cells cease to function, resulting in **pancytopenia** (a reduction in all cellular components of the blood). Almost 90% of ALLs have chromosomal changes that correlate with immunophenotyping and sometimes confer prognostic significance. Genetic translocations (mitotic errors) are seen in leukemic cells. One of these translocations, the **Philadelphia chromosome**, is seen in 95% of those with CML and 30% of adults with ALL (Figure 21.7). The Philadelphia chromosome results from a reciprocal translocation between the long arms of chromosomes 9 and 22. A unique protein (BCR-ABL protein) is encoded from two genes (*BCR* from chromosome 22 and *ABL* from chromosome 9) artificially linked at the junction of translocation. BCR-ABL1 appears to excessively activate intracellular pathways, leading to increased proliferation, decreased sensitivity to apoptosis, and premature release of immature cells into the circulation. In most leukemias and lymphomas, a single major genetic abnormality does not lead to an aggressive malignancy.

The first event is usually followed by a series of secondary genetic changes. Therefore, the original tumour becomes genetically unstable and diverse. In most cases, leukemic cells are ejected into the blood, where they accumulate. These cells also may infiltrate and accumulate in the liver, spleen, lymph nodes, and other organs. The presentation of large numbers of leukemic cells in the blood may be one of the most dramatic indicators of leukemia. Leukemia, however, is still a primary disruption of the bone marrow.

Risk factors for the onset of leukemia include environmental factors as well as other diseases. Increased risk for ALL has been linked to exposure to X-rays before birth, being exposed to ionizing radiation (postnatally), past treatment with chemotherapy, and certain genetic conditions including Down syndrome, neurofibromatosis type 1(NF1), Shwachman syndrome, Bloom's syndrome, and ataxia telangiectasia. There is growing concern about the effect of low-dose radiation on later risk for leukemia.[17] There is a significant tendency for leukemia to reappear in families. A unique characteristic of ALL, unlike other forms, is that ALL develops at different rates in different geographic locations, although the reason for this is unclear. Individuals in developed countries and in higher socioeconomic categories have an increased incidence of ALL. Acute leukemia also may develop secondary to certain acquired disorders, including CML, CLL, PV, myelofibrosis, HL, MM, ovarian cancer, and SA.

Potential risk factors for AML include smoking, earlier chemotherapy, and exposure to ionizing radiation. AML is the most reported secondary cancer after high doses of chemotherapy for HL, non-Hodgkin's lymphoma (NHL), MM, ovarian cancer, and breast cancer.

Acute leukemias. Acute leukemias consist of two types: **acute lymphocytic leukemia (ALL)** and **acute myeloid (or myelogenous) leukemia (AML)**.[1] ALL is an aggressive, fast-growing leukemia with too many lymphoblasts, or immature white blood cells found in blood and bone marrow. It also is called *acute lymphoblastic leukemia*. AML is an aggressive fast-growing leukemia with too many myeloblasts or immature white blood cells that are not lymphoblasts found in the bone marrow and blood. It also is called *acute myeloblastic leukemia* and *acute nonlymphocytic leukemia* (ANLL). AML is the more common acute leukemia occurring in adults, with the median age at diagnosis being around 70 years. There is a rise in the age-related incidence

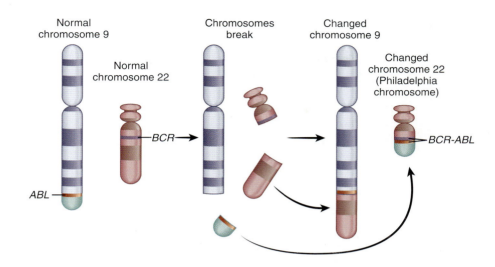

FIGURE 21.7 Philadelphia Chromosome. A piece of chromosome 9 and a piece of chromosome 22 break off and trade places. The *BCR-ABL* gene is formed on chromosome 22 where the piece of chromosome 9 attaches. The changed chromosome 22 is called *Philadelphia chromosome*. (Adapted from National Cancer Institute. [2014]. *Childhood acute lymphoblastic leukemia treatment.* National Institutes of Health.)

of AML around 40 to 50 years of age, and a steep increase from 60 to 64 years of age. Individuals of both genders and all ages experience acute leukemias with the incidence increasing dramatically in individuals older than 50 years. North American and Scandinavian countries have the highest mortality. Eastern European countries, Asia (except Japan), and Central America have the lowest mortality. Japan's higher mortality is the result of the atomic bombs dropped in World War II. Blacks have consistently shown a lower mortality than Whites. In 2016, 385 Canadians were diagnosed with ALL and 1 090 were diagnosed with AML. In 2017, 144 Canadians died from ALL and 1 184 died from AML.[18,19] The risk factors for ALL include being exposed to X-rays before birth, exposure to ionizing radiation (postnatal), and past treatment with chemotherapy.

PATHOPHYSIOLOGY ALL presumably progresses from malignant transformation of B- or C-cell progenitor cells (like a stem cell) (Figure 21.8). Most cases of ALL occur in children and often in the first decade. Although adults account for about 20% of all cases, their mortality rate is significantly higher. The significant difference between the incidence of ALL in adults and children may be because of differences in the biology of the disease. B-cell ALL occurs mainly in children and is strongly associated with chromosomal aneuploidy of various types. Adult ALL is a mixture of cancers of precursor B- and T-cell origin. The identification of mutations found in ALL is ongoing and includes mutations that drive cell growth and mutations that increase tyrosine kinase activity.

Genetic alterations in AML alter genes that encode the transcription factors needed for normal myeloid differentiation. As a result, differentiation becomes arrested. These mutations affect the epigenome, suggesting that epigenetic alterations are key in AML. Mutations may lead to proliferation by activating growth factor signalling, as well as a decreased rate of apoptosis. Therefore, the bone marrow and peripheral blood are characterized by leukocytosis and a predominance of blast cells. With an increase in the immature blast cells, they replace normal myelocytic cells, megakaryocytes, and erythrocytes. This displacement can lead to complications of bleeding, anemia, and infection. Several hereditary conditions are known to increase the risk for AML (e.g., Down syndrome, Fanconi anemia, Bloom's syndrome, and others).

CLINICAL MANIFESTATIONS Within days to a few weeks of the first symptoms is an abrupt stormy onset, which is more prevalent in ALL. The clinical manifestations of all varieties of acute leukemia are generally similar. Table 21.5 reviews the mechanisms associated with common manifestations. Signs and symptoms related to bone marrow depression include fatigue caused by anemia, bleeding resulting from thrombocytopenia, and fever caused by infection. Bleeding may occur in the skin, gums, mucous membranes, and GI tract. Visible signs include petechiae and ecchymosis, as well as discoloration of the skin, gingival bleeding, hematuria, and mid-cycle or heavy menstrual bleeding.

Infection sites include the mouth, throat, respiratory tract, lower colon, urinary tract, and skin. Gram-negative bacilli (*Escherichia coli, Pseudomonas aeruginosa*, and *Klebsiella pneumoniae*) may cause these infections. Fever, often accompanied by chills, is an early sign.

Anorexia is accompanied by weight loss, diminished sensitivity to sour and sweet tastes, wasting of muscle, and difficulty swallowing. Liver, spleen, and lymph node enlargement occur more commonly in ALL than in AML. Liver and spleen enlargement commonly occur together. The leukemic individual often experiences abdominal pain and tenderness. Pain in the bones and joints is thought to result from leukemia infiltration with secondary stretching of the periosteum.

Neurological manifestations are common and may be caused by either leukemic infiltration or cerebral bleeding. Headache, vomiting, papilledema, facial palsy, blurred vision, auditory disturbances, and meningeal irritation can occur if leukemic cells infiltrate the cerebral or spinal meninges.

EVALUATION AND TREATMENT Blood tests and examination of bone marrow confirms diagnosis. For ALL, diagnostic confusion with AML, hairy cell leukemia, and malignant lymphoma is not uncommon.[20] It is critical to obtain an accurate diagnosis because of the differences in treatment and prognosis of ALL and AML.[20] Also critical is that bone

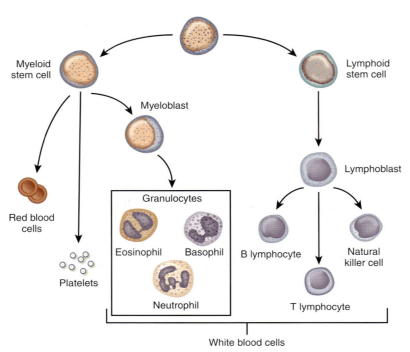

FIGURE 21.8 **Leukemia Arises From Stemlike Cells.** A blood stem cell undergoes multiple steps to finally become a red blood cell, platelet, or white blood cell. (Modified from National Cancer Institute. [2014]. *Adult acute lymphoblastic leukemia treatment (PDQ)*. Author. https://www.cancer.gov/cancertopics/pdq/treatment/adultALL/HealthProfessional.)

TABLE 21.5 Clinical Manifestations and Related Pathophysiology in Leukemia

Clinical Manifestations	Laboratory Abnormalities	Cause	Comments
Anemia	Relative *proportion* of erythroblasts to total count (decreased in anemia) is key	Decreased stem cell input or ineffective erythropoiesis, or both	In acute leukemia, anemia is usually present from beginning, often first symptom noticed, and severe; mild form without symptoms is common in CML and CLL; hemorrhage common in acute forms, occasional in CML, but rare in CLL
Bleeding (purpura, petechiae, ecchymosis, hemorrhage)	Decreased and possibly abnormal platelets	Reduction in megakaryocytes leading to thrombocytopenia	Bleeding more common in acute than in chronic leukemia
Infection	Increased multisegmented neutrophils	Opportunistic organisms; decreased protection resulting from granulocytopenia or immune deficiency secondary to chemotherapy, corticosteroids, and disease process	Major sites of infection: oral cavity, throat, lower colon, urinary tract, lungs, and skin; prevention of infection focuses on restoring host defences, decreasing invasive procedures, and reducing colonization of organisms
Weight loss	Decreased 24-hr urinary creatinine excretion; hypoalbuminemia	Condition can be attributed to pain, depression, chemotherapy, radiation therapy, loss of appetite, and alterations in taste	Severe weight loss may be related to excess production of TNF-α
Bone pain	Often no radiographic evidence of bone problems	Result of bone infiltration by leukemic cells or intramedullary infection	If combination medication regimens are ineffective, radiation therapy is used
Liver, spleen, and lymph node enlargement	Biopsy abnormal for liver and spleen	Leukemic cell infiltration	Lymph nodes also undergo leukemia proliferation in CLL
Elevated uric acid level	Normal excretion of uric acid is 300–500 mg/day; leukemic individual can excrete 50 times more	Increased catabolism of protein and nucleic acid; urate precipitation increased from dehydration caused by anorexia or fever and medication therapy	Hyperuricemia is present in both acute leukemia and CML; treatment focuses on increasing urine pH or decreasing acid production with medication allopurinol

CLL, Chronic lymphocytic leukemia; *CML*, chronic myeloid (or myelogenous) leukemia; *TNF-α*, tumour necrosis factor-alpha.

marrow aspirates be done by an oncologist, hematologist, hematopathologist, or general pathologist who is experienced in interpreting specimens.[20]

Chemotherapy, used in various combinations, is the treatment of choice for leukemia. Other treatments include radiation therapy, chemotherapy with stem cell transplant, and other medication therapy. Supportive measures include blood transfusions, antibiotics, antifungals, and antivirals. It is critical that stem cell transplants be done in hospitals with very experienced staff for both the procedure and the recovery phase.

Attainment of complete remission (CR) requires fairly aggressive treatment. Treatment is divided into two phases: *remission induction* (to attain remission) and *post remission* (to maintain remission). Factors influencing increased survival rate include the use of combined and multimodality treatment methods; improved supportive services, such as blood banking and nutritional support; and antimicrobial treatment. The presence of the Philadelphia chromosome (seen in about 5% of children with ALL, in 30% of adults with ALL, and occasionally in AML) is a poor prognostic indicator.

Myelosuppression is both a consequence of leukemia and a treatment for the disease. Hematological support with blood products and granulocyte colony-stimulating factor (G-CSF) or granulocyte-macrophage colony–stimulating factor (GM-CSF) has effectively shortened the time of neutropenia and improved survival by reducing the risk for infection.

Chronic leukemias. The two main types of chronic leukemia are (1) **chronic myelogenous leukemia (CML)** and (2) **chronic lymphocytic leukemia (CLL)**. CML is also called *chronic granulocytic leukemia* and *chronic myeloid leukemia*. CML can occur, depending on the lineage of the malignant cells (e.g., chronic neutrophilic leukemia [CNL] or chronic eosinophilic leukemia [CEL]). CML is a slowly progressing disease with too many blood cells (not lymphocytes) made in the bone marrow. In adults, CLL is the most common leukemia in the Western world. CLL is a slow-growing cancer in which too many immature lymphocytes (white blood cells) are found mostly in the blood and bone marrow. CLL and **small lymphocytic lymphoma (SLL**; also, **CLL/SLL)** differ only in the amount of proliferation of peripheral blood lymphocytes. Unlike cells in acute leukemia, chronic leukemic cells are well differentiated and can be readily named. CML is mostly a disease of adults but can occur in children or adolescents. The peak incidence is the fifth to sixth decades. Individuals with chronic leukemia have a longer life expectancy, usually extending several years from the time of diagnosis.

The chronic leukemias account for the majority of cases in adults. In Canada, it is estimated there were 1 745 new cases of CLL in 2016 and 611 deaths in 2017. There were about 600 new cases of CML in 2016, and 140 deaths in 2017.[21,22] The incidences of CLL and CML increase significantly in individuals over 40 years of age, with prevalence in the sixth through eighth decades. CML is one of a group of diseases called **myeloproliferative disorders**—acquired abnormalities in signalling pathways that lead to growth factor–independent proliferation.

PATHOPHYSIOLOGY CML is clonal and is thought to arise from a hematopoietic stem cell. The cells seen in CML are heterogeneous in differentiation, depending on the stage of the disease. During the chronic phase, the predominant cell is a long-lasting hematopoietic stem cell. The Philadelphia chromosome (see Figure 21.7) is present in more than 95% of persons diagnosed with CML, and the presence of the BCR-ABL1 protein is responsible for initiation of CML (Figure 21.9). The only known cause of CML is exposure to ionizing radiation.

CLL cells that accumulate in the bone marrow do not interfere with normal blood cell production to the extent found in acute leukemias. This significant feature may explain the reduced severity in the beginning stage of disease. The major pathophysiologic deficit in CLL is the

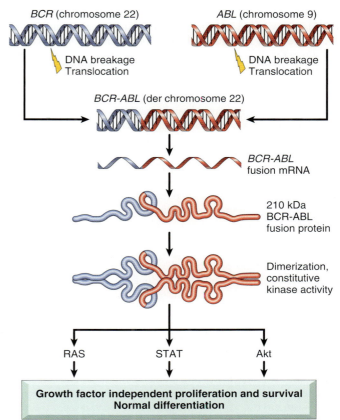

FIGURE 21.9 Pathogenesis of Chronic Myeloid Leukemia. The breakage and joining of *BCR* and *ABL* creates the chimeric fusion gene *BCR-ABL*. *BCR-ABL* genetically encodes an active BCR-ABL intracellular tyrosine kinase (an enzyme that controls intracellular "on–off" switches). The ABL kinase in turn induces signalling through the same pro-growth and pro-survival pathways that are activated by normal hematological growth factors. Altogether the activation of many downstream pathways drives growth factor–independent proliferation and survival of bone marrow progenitors. *Akt*, Protein kinase B; *RAS*, renin-angiotensin system; *STAT*, signal transducer and activator of transcription. (From Kumar, V., Abbas, A. K., & Aster, J. C. [Eds.]. [2021]. *Robbins and Cotran pathologic basis of disease* [10th ed.]. Elsevier.)

failure of B cells to mature into plasma cells that synthesize immunoglobulins, resulting in hypogammaglobulinemia (60% of individuals). The cause of CLL is unknown.

CLINICAL MANIFESTATIONS Chronic leukemia advances slowly and insidiously. About 70% of individuals with CLL are asymptomatic at the time of diagnosis. When symptoms do appear, the most common finding is lymphadenopathy. The most significant effect of CLL is suppression of humoral immunity and increased infection with encapsulated bacteria. Often, the level of neutrophils is depressed. This depression adds to the risk for infection. Invasion of most organ cells is uncommon. Infiltration does occur in lymph nodes, liver, spleen, and salivary glands. CNS involvement is rare. About 10% of individuals develop a more aggressive malignancy, usually a diffuse large B-cell lymphoma. In these individuals, extreme fatigue, weight loss, night sweats, low-grade fever, elevated levels of the enzyme lactic dehydrogenase, hypercalcemia, anemia, and thrombocytopenia are common.

Individuals with CML may progress through three phases of the disease. These phases include a chronic phase lasting 2 to 5 years, during which symptoms may not be apparent; an accelerated phase of 6 to

18 months, during which the primary symptoms develop; and a terminal blast phase ("blast crisis") with a survival of only 3 to 6 months. The accelerated phase is characterized by excessive proliferation and accumulation of malignant cells. Splenomegaly is prominent and becomes painful. Lymphadenopathy generally is not present. Liver enlargement also occurs, but liver function is rarely altered. Hyperuricemia is common and produces gouty arthritis. Infections, fever, and weight loss also are seen often. The terminal blast phase is characterized by rapid and progressive leukocytosis with an increase in basophils. In the later stages of the terminal phase, which then resembles AML, blast cells or promyelocytes predominate, and the individual experiences a "blast crisis."

The acute effects of CML resemble those of acute leukemia but with more prominent and painful splenomegaly. Lymphadenopathy generally is found only in the acute phase of the disease. Hyperuricemia is usually present and produces gouty arthritis. Infections, fever, and weight loss are common findings in individuals with CML.

EVALUATION AND TREATMENT Diagnosis of chronic leukemia depends on laboratory analyses of peripheral blood and bone marrow. Diagnosis of CLL is based on detection of a monoclonal B-cell lymphocytosis in the blood. The cells must have the characteristic immunophenotype (CD5+, CD19+, CD20 [weak], CD23+) at levels in excess of 5 000 cells/mm^3 over a sustained period of time (usually 4 weeks). Confusion with other diseases may be avoided by determination of cell-surface markers.

Treatment of CLL includes periodic observation with treatment of infection, hemorrhage, or immunological complications. Because the disease mostly occurs in the elderly and the rate of progression is slow, it is often simply observed until the disease progresses. Randomized trials show no survival advantage for immediate versus delayed treatment of those individuals with early-stage disease.[23] For individuals with progressing CLL, treatment with conventional doses of chemotherapy is not curative. Individuals treated with allogeneic stem cell transplantation have achieved prolonged disease-free survival.[24] Antileukemic therapy is frequently unnecessary in uncomplicated early disease.[24] A large variation in survival exists, ranging from several months to a normal life expectancy. Treatment must be individualized on the basis of clinical behaviour of the disease.[24] Complications of pancytopenia, including hemorrhage and infection, are a major cause of death for these individuals. Typically, individuals with CLL survive 10 years or more. Those with certain risk factors, however, have a more aggressive disease, shortening their survival to less than 3 years.

Current treatment modalities for CML do not cure the disease or prevent blastic transformation. Standard treatment consists of combined chemotherapy, biological response modifiers, and allogenic stem cell transplantation. Stem cell transplantation use is limited by donor availability and by high toxicity in older persons (older than 65 years). Imatinib mesylate (Gleevec), a tyrosine kinase inhibitor, led to changes in the management of CML. Other tyrosine kinase inhibitors have been developed; however, concerns about disease persistence and resistance still exist.[24] Gleevec produces a complete cytogenic response in more than 80% of newly diagnosed persons; however, it does not cure CML because it does not kill leukemia stem cells.

ALTERATIONS OF LYMPHOID FUNCTION

> ✓ **QUICK CHECK 21.4**
> 1. Contrast the main features of Hodgkin's lymphoma with those of non-Hodgkin's lymphoma.
> 2. What is Burkitt lymphoma?
> 3. Explain the statement: Multiple myeloma (MM) is heterogeneous.
> 4. What are the main pathological features of MM?

Lymphadenopathy

Lymphadenopathy is characterized by enlarged lymph nodes (Figure 21.10). Lymph node enlargement occurs because of an increase in the size and number of its germinal centres. The proliferation of lymphocytes and monocytes (immature phagocytes) or invasion by malignant cells causes these increases. Normally, lymph nodes are not palpable or are barely palpable. Enlarged lymph nodes are characterized by being palpable and often also may be tender or painful to touch.

Localized lymphadenopathy usually indicates drainage of an area associated with an inflammatory process or infection (reactive lymph node). *Generalized lymphadenopathy* occurs less often and is generally seen in the presence of infections, autoimmune diseases, or disseminated malignancy. Palpable nodes, however, do not always show serious disease and may indicate a minor trauma or infection. The location and size of the enlarged nodes are important factors in diagnosing the cause of the lymphadenopathy. Other important factors include the individual's age, gender, and geographic location. Generalized lymphadenopathy occurs with NHL, CLL, histiocytosis, and disorders that produce lymphocytosis. In general, lymphadenopathy results from four types of conditions: (1) neoplastic disease, (2) immunological or inflammatory conditions, (3) endocrine disorders, or (4) lipid storage diseases. Diseases of unknown cause, including autoimmune diseases and reactions to medications, also may lead to generalized lymphadenopathy.

Malignant Lymphomas

Lymphomas consist of a diverse group of neoplasms that develop from the proliferation of malignant lymphocytes in the lymphoid system.

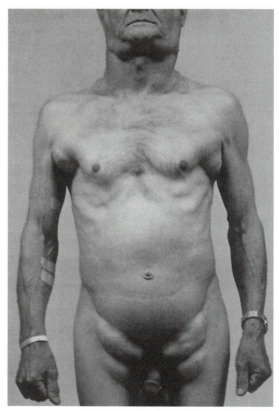

FIGURE 21.10 Lymphadenopathy. Individual with lymphocyte leukemia with extreme but symmetrical lymphadenopathy. (Courtesy Dr. A. R. Kagan, Los Angeles. From Ackerman, L. V., del Regato, J. A., Spjut, H. J., et al. [1985]. *Cancer: diagnosis, treatment, and prognosis* [6th ed.]. Mosby.)

The WHO publishes the Revised European American Lymphoma (REAL) classification, which is based on the cell type from which the lymphoma probably originated. The basic groups include HL and NHL. Three major groups of lymphoid malignancies based on morphology and cell lineage include (1) B-cell neoplasms; (2) T-cell neoplasms, and (3) NK-cell neoplasms. MM, which was previously classified independently, is now included as a B-cell lymphoma. NHL can be further divided into cancers that have an *indolent* (slow-growing) course or an *aggressive* (fast-growing) course. Both HL and NHL occur in children and adults. The overall treatment and prognosis depend on the stage and type of lymphoma.

Lymphoma is the most common blood cancer in Canada. Incidence rates of lymphoma differ with respect to age, gender, geographic location, and socioeconomic class. It was estimated that in 2020, 10 400 Canadians would be diagnosed with NHL and 1 000 would be diagnosed with HL.[25,26] Since the early 1970s, the incidence of NHL has nearly doubled. The exact reason for this increase is still a mystery. However, a part of the increase has been attributed to lymphomas developing in association with immune deficiencies, including AIDS and organ transplants. The incidence of HL has declined over the same time period, especially among older persons.

In general, lymphomas are the result of genetic mutations or viral infection. Globally, however, the incidence of lymphoma (except for BL) has increased in more developed countries. As a result, researchers are studying many potential risk factors. These factors include diet, obesity, metabolic syndrome, sedentary lifestyle, stress, advances in medical care and access, increases in longevity, and exposure to compounds from industrialization. Malignant transformation produces a cell with uncontrolled and excessive growth that accumulates in the lymph nodes and other sites, producing tumour masses. Lymphomas usually start in the lymph nodes or lymphoid tissues of the stomach or intestines.

Hodgkin's Lymphoma

Hodgkin's lymphoma (HL) is a malignant lymphoma that progresses from one group of lymph nodes to another. HL includes the development of systemic symptoms, and the presence of B cells called **Reed-Sternberg (RS) cells**[1] (see Pathophysiology section). In about 70% of cases, RS cells are infected with EBV. In Canada, estimates of new cases of HL include 1 000 in 2020 and 100 deaths.[26] The incidence of HL is higher in males, and the median age of diagnosis is 64 years. The incidence is greater in White individuals than in Black individuals. Denmark, the Netherlands, and the United States have the highest incidence of HL and Japan and Australia have the lowest.

HL peaks at two different ages: early in life, during the second and third decades, and later in life, during the sixth and seventh decades.

PATHOPHYSIOLOGY It is widely accepted that the RS cell is the malignant transformed lymphocyte (Figure 21.11). RS cells are often large and binucleate with occasional mononuclear variants. RS cells are necessary for the diagnosis of HL. In rare instances, cells resembling RS cells can be found in benign illnesses, as well as in other forms of cancer, including NHL and solid tissue cancers and in IM.

The triggering mechanism for the malignant transformation of cells is still unknown. Classic HL appears to be derived from a B cell in the germinal centre that has not undergone successful immunoglobulin gene rearrangement (see Chapter 7) and would normally be induced to undergo apoptosis. Survival of this cell may be linked to infection with EBV. Laboratory and epidemiological studies have linked HL with EBV infections. RS cells secrete and release cytokines (e.g., IL-10, transforming growth factor-beta [TGF-β]) that result in the accumulation of inflammatory cells, producing local and systemic effects. HL

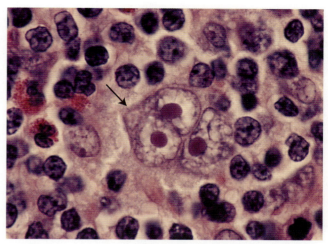

FIGURE 21.11 Lymph Nodes. Diagnostic Reed-Sternberg cell (*arrow*). A large multinucleated or multilobed cell with inclusion body–like nucleoli surrounded by a halo of clear nucleoplasm. (From Damjanov, I., & Linder, J. [Eds.]. [1996]. *Anderson's pathology* [10th ed.]. Mosby.)

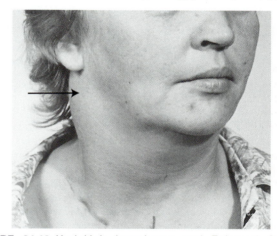

FIGURE 21.12 Hodgkin's Lymphoma and Enlarged Cervical Lymph Node. Typical enlarged cervical lymph node in the neck (*arrow*) of a 35-year-old woman with Hodgkin's lymphoma. (From Ackerman, L. V., del Regato, J. A., Spjut, H. J., et al. [1985]. *Cancer: diagnosis, treatment, and prognosis* [6th ed.]. Mosby.)

is subcategorized into two main types: classic Hodgkin's and nodular lymphocyte–predominant Hodgkin's. Classic HL is subclassified into four types: (1) nodular sclerosis Hodgkin's lymphoma (grades 1 and 2), (2) lymphocyte rich classical Hodgkin's lymphoma, (3) mixed cellularity Hodgkin's lymphoma, and (4) lymphocyte depletion Hodgkin's lymphoma. These types are based on the morphology of RS cells and the characteristics of the inflammatory cell infiltrate in the tumour. Lymphocyte-predominant disease presents with earlier-stage disease, longer survival, and fewer treatment failures than classic HL.[27] However, despite a more favourable prognosis, lymphocyte-predominant HL has a tendency to histologically transform into diffuse large B-cell lymphoma by 10 years in approximately 10% of people.[28]

CLINICAL MANIFESTATIONS The complex action of cytokines and other growth factors that are secreted and released by the malignant cells explain the many clinical features of HL. These substances induce infiltration and proliferation of inflammatory cells. These actions result in an enlarged, painless lymph node in the neck (often the first sign of HL) (Figure 21.12). The discovery of an asymptomatic mediastinal

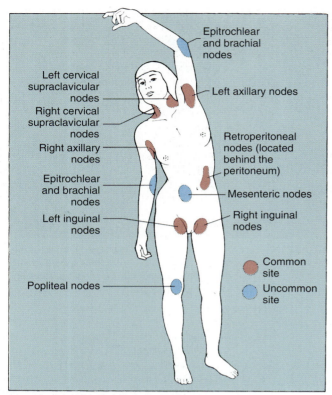

FIGURE 21.13 Common and Uncommon Involved Lymph Node Sites for Hodgkin's Lymphoma.

TABLE 21.6 Definitions of Stages of Hodgkin's Lymphoma

Stage	Criteria
I	Involvement of a single lymph node region (I) or localized involvement of a single extralymphatic organ or site (I_E)[a]
II	Involvement of two or more lymph node regions on same side of diaphragm (II) or localized involvement of a single associated extralymphatic organ or site and its regional lymph node(s), with or without involvement of other lymph node regions on same side of diaphragm (II_E)
III	Involvement of lymph node regions on both sides of diaphragm (III), which may also be accompanied by localized involvement of an associated extralymphatic organ or site (III_E), by involvement of the spleen (III_S), or by both (III_{E+S})
IV	Disseminated (multifocal) involvement of one or more extralymphatic organs, with or without associated lymph node involvement, or isolated extralymphatic organ involvement with distant (nonregional) nodal involvement
A: No systemic symptoms present	
B: Unexplained fevers >38°C [100.4°F], drenching night sweats, or weight loss >10% of body weight	

[a]The number of lymph node regions involved may be shown by a subscript (e.g., II_3).
From National Comprehensive Cancer Network. (2014). Hodgkin lymphoma. In *NCCN practice guidelines, Version 2. 2014: Hodgkin lymphoma* (originally adapted from Carbono, P. P., Kaplan, H. S., Musshoff, K., et al. [1971]. *Cancer Research, 31*[11], 1860–1861).

mass on routine chest X-ray is common. The cervical, axillary, inguinal, and retroperitoneal lymph nodes are commonly affected in HL (Figure 21.13). Local symptoms caused by pressure and obstruction of the lymph nodes are the result of the lymphadenopathy.

About one-third of individuals will have some common systemic symptoms. These symptoms include intermittent fever without other symptoms of infection, drenching night sweats, itchy skin (pruritus), and fatigue. These constitutional symptoms accompanied by weight loss are associated with a poor prognosis.

Although HL rarely arises in the lung, mediastinal and hilar node adenopathy can cause secondary involvement of the trachea, bronchi, pleura, or lungs. Retroperitoneal nodes can involve vertebral bodies and nerves and also can cause displacement of ureters. Spinal cord involvement is more common in the dorsal and lumbar regions. Skin lesions, although uncommon, include psoriasis and eczematoid lesions, causing itching and scratching.

As a result of direct invasion from mediastinal lymph nodes, pericardial involvement can cause pericardial friction rub, pericardial effusion, and engorgement of neck veins. The GI tract and urinary tract are rarely involved. Anemia is often found in individuals with HL accompanied by a low serum iron level and reduced iron-binding capacity. Other laboratory findings include elevated sedimentation rate, leukocytosis, and eosinophilia. Leukopenia occurs in advanced stages of HL.

Splenic involvement in HL depends on histological type. In mixed cellularity and lymphocytic deletion types of HL, the spleen is involved in 60% of cases. With lymphocyte and nodular sclerosis types, 34% of cases involve the spleen.

EVALUATION AND TREATMENT Because of the variability in symptoms, early definitive detection may be challenging. Asymptomatic lymphadenopathy can progress undetected for several years. Diagnosis is made from physical examination and history, complete blood count (CBC), blood chemistry studies including sedimentation rate, lymph node biopsy, pathology review for RS cells, and immunophenotyping for disease markers.[29] Highly indicative of HL is a lymph node biopsy with scattered RS cells and cellular infiltrate. The current staging system for HL is the Ann Arbor staging system with Cotswolds modifications.[30] Clinical staging includes personal history; physical examination; laboratory studies, including sedimentation rate; and thoracic and abdominal/pelvic computed tomography (CT) scans[27] (Table 21.6). Positron emission tomography (PET) scans, usually combined with CT scans, have replaced gallium scans and lymphangiography for clinical staging.[31] Staging laparotomy should be considered only when the results will allow substantial reduction in treatment. It should not be done in individuals who require chemotherapy. If the laparotomy is needed for treatment decisions, the risks of potential morbidity should be considered.[31] For those at high risk of relapse, conventional CT scans are employed for screening to avoid the increased false-positive test results and increased radiation exposure of serial PET-CT scans.[29] Prognostic indicators include clinical stage, histological type, tumour cell concentration and tumour burden, constitutional symptoms, and age of the individual.

The effectiveness of treatment is related to many factors. This includes age, gender, and general health of the individual; signs and symptoms; stage of the disease; blood test results; type of HL; and classification of the disease as recurrent or progressive. Adult HL can usually be cured with early diagnosis and treatment.[29,31] Three types of treatment are used: chemotherapy, radiation therapy, and surgery. Treatment for pregnant women includes watchful waiting and steroid therapy. Newer treatments undergoing testing include chemotherapy and radiation therapy with stem cell transplant and monoclonal antibody therapy.[29,31] Treatment with chemotherapy or radiation therapy, or both, may increase the risk for secondary cancers, cardiovascular disease, and other health problems.

Non-Hodgkin's Lymphoma

Non-Hodgkin's lymphomas (NHLs) are a heterogeneous group of lymphoid tissue neoplasms with differing biologic and clinical patterns of activity and responses to treatment. For unknown reasons, NHL incidence rates increased worldwide from 1950 to 2000, tripling in adults older than 65 years of age. The WHO/REAL classification of NHL includes (1) **B-cell neoplasms**, which include of a variety of lymphomas including myelomas that originate from B cells at various stages of differentiation; and (2) **T-cell neoplasms** and **NK-cell neoplasms**, which include lymphomas that originate from either T or NK cells. These cancers are differentiated from HL by a lack of RS cells and other cellular changes not characteristic of HL.

In 2020, it was estimated that 10 400 Canadians would be diagnosed with NHL, and 2 900 Canadians would die from the disease.[29] The median age of diagnosis is 67 years with a higher occurrence in men. The highest incidences are in North America, Europe, Oceania, and several African countries.[32] Part of the increased incidence has been attributed to diagnostic improvements as well as AIDS-related cancers following the HIV epidemic.[32] Conversely, the mortality has risen at a slower rate. It is thought that newer treatment modalities are improving survival rates.

PATHOPHYSIOLOGY NHL is a progressive clonal expansion of B cells, T cells, or NK cells. B cells account for 85 to 90% of NHLs, with most of the rest being T cells and rarely NK cells. A small percentage originates from macrophages. Oncogenes may be activated by chromosomal translocations, or the tumour-suppressor loci may be inactivated by deletion or mutation of chromosomes. Certain subtypes may have altered genomes by oncogenic viruses. The various subtypes of NHL may be named by specific diagnostic markers related to various cytogenetic lesions. The most common type of chromosomal alteration in NHL is translocation, which disrupts the genes encoded at the breakpoints. Unlike HL, NHL spreads in a less predictable way and spreads widely early.[29] Diffuse large B-cell lymphoma (DLBCL) is the most common form of NHL.

Risk factors for adult NHL include being older, male, or White. Other risk factors include being afflicted by certain inherited immune disorders, an autoimmune disease, or HIV/AIDS; exposure to a variety of mutagenic chemicals or certain pesticides; infection with certain cancer-related viruses (e.g., EBV, HIV, HTLV-1, hepatitis C, and human herpesvirus-8); and immune suppression related to organ transplant. Gastric infection with *H. pylori* increases the risk for gastric lymphomas. NHL is a disease of middle age, usually found in persons more than 50 years old.

CLINICAL MANIFESTATIONS Clinical manifestations of NHL usually begin as localized or generalized lymphadenopathy, similar to HL. Differences in clinical features are noted in Table 21.7. The cervical, axillary, inguinal, and femoral lymph node chains are the most commonly affected sites. Generally, the swelling is painless, and the nodes have enlarged and transformed over a period of months or years. Other sites of involvement are the nasopharynx, GI tract, bone, thyroid, testes, and soft tissue. Some individuals have retroperitoneal and abdominal masses with symptoms of abdominal fullness, back pain, ascites (fluid in the peritoneal cavity), skin rash or itchy skin, fatigue, fever of unknown origin, drenching night sweats, and leg swelling.

Lymphomas are classified as low, intermediate, or high grade. A low-grade lymphoma, which also may be termed *indolent*, has a slow progression. Individuals with low-grade lymphoma commonly present

TABLE 21.7 Clinical Differences Between Non-Hodgkin's Lymphoma and Hodgkin's Lymphoma

Characteristics	Non-Hodgkin's Lymphoma	Hodgkin's Lymphoma
Nodal involvement	Multiple peripheral nodes	Localized to single axial group of nodes (i.e., cervical, mediastinal, para-aortic)
	Mesenteric nodes and Waldeyer's tonsillar ring commonly involved	Mesenteric nodes and Waldeyer's tonsillar ring rarely involved
Spread	Noncontiguous	Orderly spread by contiguity
B symptoms[a]	Uncommon	Common
Extranodal involvement	Common	Rare
Extent of disease	Rarely localized	Often localized

[a]Fever, weight loss, night sweats.

with a painless, peripheral adenopathy. Spontaneous regression of these nodes may occur, mimicking the presence of an infection. Night sweats with an elevated temperature (more than 38°C [100.4°F]) and weight loss, as well as extranodular involvement, are not commonly present in the early stages but are common in advanced or end-stage disease. Cytopenia, or reduction in the number of blood cells, reflective of bone marrow involvement is often seen. Hepatomegaly is common. Splenomegaly is present in approximately 40% of individuals. Fatigue and weakness are more prevalent with advanced stages.

Intermediate- and high-grade lymphomas, which are more aggressive, have a more varied clinical presentation. A high-grade lymphoma also may be termed *aggressive*.

EVALUATION AND TREATMENT The primary means for diagnosis of NHL is biopsy. A common finding in NHL is noncontiguous lymph node involvement, which is not common in HL. Staging is determined from radiological studies, biopsy, and examination of bone marrow aspirate.

Treatment for NHL is quite diverse and depends on type (B cell or T cell), tumour stage, histological status (low, intermediate, or high grade), symptoms, age, and presence of comorbidities.[33,34] Depending on the type (B cell or T cell) of the tumour, stage of disease, and aggressiveness of the tumour, treatment is usually initiated at the time of diagnosis. However, because treatment is not curative for some low-grade indolent lymphomas that are widely disseminated, observation without treatment may be the best choice. These indolent tumours are often not symptomatic for the individual and this approach improves quality of life. In some cases, the disease may be so slow growing that treatment is not needed for an extended period of time.

Treatment with chemotherapy alone may be adequate for many individuals, although radiation therapy is often included. Low-dose chemotherapy has been followed by autologous stem cell transplantation in some NHLs or for recurrent disease. Treatment using monoclonal antibody alone or in combination with radiation therapy (radioimmunotherapy) also is being used.

Individuals with NHL can survive for extended periods. A partial remission may be achieved in some cases in which evidence of the disease remains, but the disease does not progress. Survival with nodular lymphoma ranges up to 15 years, but those with diffuse disease

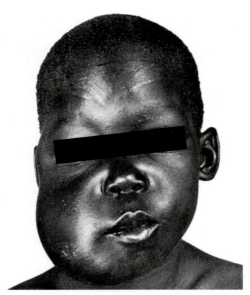

FIGURE 21.14 Burkitt Lymphoma. Burkitt lymphoma involving the jaw in a young African boy. (Courtesy I. Magrath, MD, Bethesda, MD. From Zitelli, B. J., McIntire, S. C., & Nowalk, A. J. [2012]. *Zitelli and Davis' atlas of pediatric physical diagnosis* [6th ed.]. Saunders.)

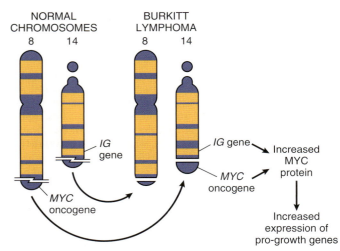

FIGURE 21.15 Burkitt Lymphoma Cells. The 8,14 chromosomal translocation and associated oncogenes in Burkitt lymphoma. *IG*, Immunoglobulin; *MYC*, myelocytomatosis viral oncogene homologue.

generally do not survive as long. Overall, the survival rates of NHL are less than those for HL. Survival rates for NHL are 77% at 1 year, 59% at 5 years, and 42% at 10 years.

Burkitt lymphoma. Burkitt lymphoma (BL) is a B-cell NHL with unique clinical and epidemiological features. It is aggressive and is the fastest growing human tumor. There are three main types of BL: endemic, sporadic, and immunodeficiency-related. *Endemic* BL commonly occurs in Africa and is linked to the EBV, and *sporadic* BL occurs worldwide. *Immunodeficiency-related* BL is most often seen in individuals with AIDS. BL occurs most often in children and young adults. Endemic cases, usually from Africa, involve a rapidly growing tumor of the jaw and facial bones (Figure 21.14). It is now understood that Burkitt lymphoma is heterogeneous, and pathological confirmation is sometimes challenging. In Canada, BL is rare. It is characterized by extensive bone marrow invasion and replacement, and usually involves the abdomen.[35]

PATHOPHYSIOLOGY Almost all cases of BL are associated with EBV. It is suspected that suppression of the immune system by other illnesses (e.g., HIV infection, chronic malaria) increases the individual's susceptibility to EBV. B cells are particularly sensitive because of specific surface receptors for EBV. As a result, the B cell undergoes chromosomal translocations that result in overexpression of the *c-MYC* proto-oncogene and loss of control of cell growth (Figure 21.15). The most common translocation (75% of individuals) is between chromosomes 8 (having the *c-MYC* gene) and 14 (having the immunoglobulin heavy chain genes). Other translocations have been reported between chromosome 8 and chromosomes 2 or 22, which have genes for immunoglobulin light chains.

CLINICAL MANIFESTATIONS In non-African BL, the most common presentation is abdominal swelling. Most tumours manifest at extranodal locations. More advanced disease may involve the eyes, ovaries, kidneys, or glandular tissue (breast, thyroid, tonsil). It presents with type B symptoms (night sweats, fever, weight loss). Common manifestations may include nausea and vomiting; loss of appetite or change in bowel habits, or both; GI bleeding; symptoms of an acute abdominal condition; intestinal perforation; and renal failure.

EVALUATION AND TREATMENT Usually indicative of BL is the presence of tumours in the jaw and facial bones, enlarged lymph nodes, and bone marrow having malignant B cells. Laboratory studies include CBC, electrolytes, liver and renal function tests, lactate dehydrogenase, hepatitis B, HIV, and uric acid.[33,34] Treatment involves aggressive multi-drug regimens, such as combination chemotherapy. There is no role for radiation therapy in people with BL.[33,34]

Lymphoblastic lymphoma. Lymphoblastic lymphoma (LL) is a rare variant of NHL overall (2 to 4%) but accounts for almost one-third of cases of NHL in children and adolescents, with a male predominance. The majority of LL (90%) is of T-cell origin; the rest arises from B cells. LL is similar to acute lymphoblastic leukemia and may be considered a variant of that disease.

PATHOPHYSIOLOGY The disease arises from a clone of relatively immature T cells that becomes malignant in the thymus. As with most lymphoid tumours, LL is often associated with translocations, primarily of the chromosomes that encode for the T-cell receptor (chromosomes 7 and 14). These aberrations result in increased expression of a variety of transcription factors and loss of growth control.

CLINICAL MANIFESTATIONS The first sign of LL is usually a painless lymphadenopathy in the neck. Peripheral lymph nodes in the chest become involved in about 70% of individuals. Involved nodes are found mostly above the diaphragm. LL is an aggressive tumour that presents as stage IV in most people. T-cell LL is associated with a unique mediastinal mass (up to 75%) because of the clear origin of the tumour in the thymus. The mass results in dyspnea and chest pain and may cause compression of bronchi or the superior vena cava. The tumour may infiltrate the bone marrow in about half of those affected. Suppression of bone marrow hematopoiesis leads to increased susceptibility to infections. Other organs, including the liver, kidney, spleen, and brain, also may be affected. Many individuals express type B symptoms: fever, night sweats, and significant weight loss.

EVALUATION AND TREATMENT The most common therapeutic approach is combined chemotherapy (intensive therapy). In early stages of the disease, the response rate is high with increased survival.

The 5-year survival in children is 80 to 90% and 45 to 55% in adults. Although LL is easily treated, there is a high relapse rate: 40 to 60% of adults.

Multiple myeloma. Multiple myeloma (MM) is a clonal plasma cell cancer characterized by the slow proliferation of tumour cell masses in the bone marrow. (Figure 21.16).[36] These masses are associated with lytic bone lesions (round, punched-out regions of bone). Uncommon variants include *solitary myeloma (plasmacytoma)* with a single mass in bone or soft tissue and *smoldering myeloma*, which is defined by a lack of symptoms and a high plasma abnormal antibody called the M protein.

Myeloma cells live in the bone marrow and are usually not found in the peripheral blood. As the number of myeloma cells increases, fewer red blood cells, white blood cells, and platelets are produced. Myeloma may spread to other tissues, especially in very advanced stages of the disease. The reported incidence of MM has doubled in the past two decades, possibly as a result of more sensitive testing used for diagnosis. The annual incidence rate in Western industrialized countries is 4 per 100 000, and it was estimated that 2 900 new cases would be diagnosed in Canada in 2017.[37] MM occurs in all races, but in the United States the incidence in Black individuals is about twice that of White individuals. It rarely occurs before the age of 40 years—the peak age of incidence is between 65 and 70 years. It is slightly more common in men than in women. Other risk factors include exposure to radiation or certain chemicals, including pesticides, and a history of monoclonal gammopathy of undetermined significance (MGUS; see "Clinical Manifestations") or plasmacytoma.

PATHOPHYSIOLOGY MM is a plasma cell neoplasia that causes lytic bone lesions (bony disease; radiologically appears as punched-out defects), hypercalcemia, renal failure, anemia, and immune abnormalities.[35] Multiple mutations in different pathways alter the intrinsic biology of the plasma cell, generating the features of myeloma.[36] MM tumours are highly heterogeneous.[38] Defining driver mutations and heterogeneity is essential for treatment decisions. Many myelomas are aneuploidy and, in most individuals with myeloma, chromosomal translocations are the most common. Development of further secondary genetic alterations causes progression to an aggressive MM. Investigators are studying various epigenetic alterations and interactions with extracellular matrix proteins. For example, myeloma cells interact and secrete peptides that adhere to stromal cells, inducing cytokines that possibly promote inflammation. Myeloma cells are prone to the accumulation of misfolded protein, such as unpaired immunoglobulin chains. Misfolded proteins activate apoptosis.

Malignant plasma cells arise from one clone of B cells that produce abnormally large amounts of one class of immunoglobulin (usually IgG, occasionally IgA, and rarely IgM, IgD, or IgE). The malignant transformation may begin early in B-cell development, possibly before meeting antigens in the secondary lymphoid organs. The myeloma cells return either to the bone marrow or to other soft tissue sites. Cytokines, particularly IL-6, have been named as essential factors that promote the growth and survival of MM cells. (Lymphocytes and cytokines are described in Chapter 6.) IL-6 acts as an osteoclast-activating factor and stimulates osteoclasts to reabsorb bone. This process results in bone lesions and hypercalcemia (high calcium levels in the blood) attributable to the release of calcium from the breakdown of bone.

The antibody produced by the transformed plasma cell is often defective, having truncations, deletions, and other abnormalities, and is often referred to as a *paraprotein* (abnormal protein in the blood). Because of the large number of malignant plasma cells, the abnormal antibody, called the **M protein**, becomes the most prominent protein in the blood (as Figure 21.18 shows). Suppression of normal plasma cells by the myeloma results in diminished or absent normal antibodies. The excessive amount of M protein also may contribute to many of the clinical manifestations of the disease. Frequently, the myeloma produces free immunoglobulin light chain (Bence Jones protein) that is present in the blood and urine and contributes to damage of renal tubular cells.

CLINICAL MANIFESTATIONS MM is characterized by elevated levels of calcium in the blood (hypercalcemia), renal failure, anemia, and bone lesions. The hypercalcemia and bone lesions result from infiltration of the bone by malignant plasma cells and stimulation of osteoclasts to reabsorb bone. This process results in the release of calcium (hypercalcemia) and the development of lytic lesions of bone (Figure 21.17). Destruction of bone tissue causes pain, the most

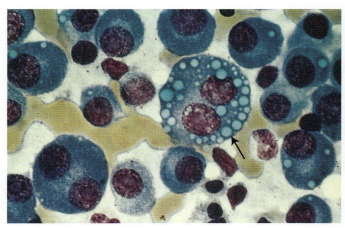

FIGURE 21.16 Multiple Myeloma, Bone Marrow Aspirate. Normal marrow cells are largely replaced by plasma cells, including atypical forms with multiple nuclei (*arrow*), and cytoplasmic droplets holding immunoglobulin. (From Kumar, V., Abbas, A. K., & Aster, J. C. [Eds.]. [2021]. *Robbins and Cotran pathologic basis of disease* [10th ed.]. Elsevier.)

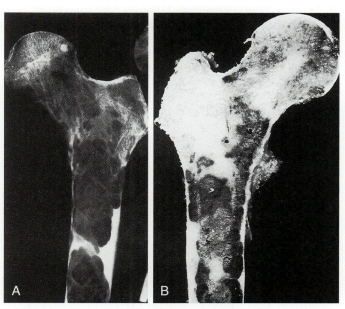

FIGURE 21.17 Multiple (Plasma Cell) Myeloma. **A**, Roentgenogram of femur showing extensive bone destruction caused by tumour. Note the absence of reactive bone formation. **B**, Gross specimen from the same individual; myelomatous sections appear as dark granular sections. (From Kissane, J. M. [Ed.]. [1990]. *Anderson's pathology* [9th ed.]. Mosby.)

common presenting symptom, and pathological fractures. The bones most commonly involved, in decreasing order of frequency, are the vertebrae, ribs, skull, pelvis, femur, clavicle, and scapula. Spinal cord compression, because of the weakened vertebrae, occurs in about 10% of individuals. A condition called **amyloidosis** may occur, in which antibody proteins increase and stick together in peripheral nerves and organs, such as the kidney and heart. Signs and symptoms of amyloidosis include fatigue, purple spots on the skin, enlarged tongue, diarrhea, edema, and numbness or tingling in the legs and feet.

Proteinuria is seen in 90% of individuals. Renal failure may be either acute or chronic and is usually secondary to the hypercalcemia. Bence Jones protein may lead to damage of the proximal tubules. Anemia is usually normocytic and normochromic and results from inhibited erythropoiesis caused by tumour cell infiltration of the bone marrow.

The high concentration of paraprotein in the blood may lead to hyperviscosity syndrome. The increased viscosity interferes with blood circulation to various sites (brain, kidneys, extremities). Hyperviscosity syndrome is seen in up to 20% of persons. Added neurological symptoms (e.g., confusion, headaches, blurred vision) may occur secondary to hypercalcemia or hyperviscosity.

Suppression of the humoral (antibody-mediated) immune response results in repeated infections, primarily pneumonias and pyelonephritis. The most commonly involved microorganisms are encapsulated bacteria that are particularly sensitive to the effects of antibody; pneumonia caused by *Streptococcus pneumoniae*, *Staphylococcus aureus*, or *K. pneumoniae*; or pyelonephritis caused by *E. coli* or other Gram-negative organisms. Cell-mediated (T-cell) function is relatively normal. Overwhelming infection is the leading cause of death from MM.

MM is a progressive disorder and is often preceded by a condition known as **monoclonal gammopathy of undetermined significance (MGUS)**. MGUS is diagnosed by the presence of an M protein in the blood or urine without other evidence of MM.[39,40] MGUS is present in approximately 1% of the general population and in 3% of individuals older than 70 years. Although MGUS is considered nonpathological and requires no treatment, about 2% of individuals with MGUS progress to malignant plasma cell disorders. Progression of MM following MGUS advances to asymptomatic MM and finally symptomatic MM. Asymptomatic MM also may be referred to as **smouldering myeloma** and indolent myeloma.[39,40] Smouldering myeloma is usually characterized by the presence of an M protein and clonal bone marrow plasma cells, but with no indication of end-organ damage.

EVALUATION AND TREATMENT Diagnosis of MM is made by symptoms and radiographic and laboratory studies. A definitive diagnosis requires a bone marrow biopsy. The International Myeloma Working Group's criteria[41] for the diagnosis of MM include biomarkers (monoclonal components in serum and urine; quantification of immunoglobulins IgG, IgA, and IgM; and characterization of the heavy and light chains by immunofixation) and the presence of hypercalcemia, renal failure, anemia, and bone lesions (CRAB). Several types of radiological studies document the presence of bone lesions and areas of destruction. Quantitative measurements of immunoglobulins (IgG, IgM, IgA) are usually done, and serum electrophoretic analysis reveals increased levels of M protein (see Figure 21.18). Bence Jones protein may be observed in the urine or serum by immunoelectrophoresis, or in the serum using available enzyme-linked immunosorbent assays (ELISAs). However, variants of MM include individuals in which free light chain only is produced and a rare variant that produces only free heavy chain; about 1% of cases are nonsecretory so that neither M protein nor Bence Jones protein is produced. Measurement of another protein, free **β2-microglobulin**, is used as an indicator of prognosis or effectiveness of therapy.

Treatment options include combinations of chemotherapy; other medication therapy; targeted therapy; high-dose chemotherapy with stem cell transplant; biological therapy; radiation therapy (bone lesions of the spine); and—sometimes—surgery. New therapies, called *proteasome inhibitors*, are emerging. Dose intensification improves outcomes in younger persons; however, long-term remissions occur in a minority of people. Gene expression profiling (GEP) helps improve the treatment of MM because it identifies prognostic subgroups and defines the molecular pathways associated with these subgroups. Newer agents (e.g., bortezomib, lenalidomide) have expanded therapeutic regimens for end-stage myeloma. The median survival for all stages of MM is 3 years. Approval of new drugs has changed the management of MM, and research for survival improvement is ongoing.

ALTERATIONS OF SPLENIC FUNCTION

> **QUICK CHECK 21.5**
> 1. Name the major causes of splenomegaly.
> 2. How does splenomegaly differ from hypersplenism?

The complexities of splenic function are not totally understood, and its mysteries are still being studied. The normal functions of the spleen that may impact disease states include (1) phagocytosis of blood cells and particulate matter (e.g., bacteria), (2) antibody production, (3) hematopoiesis, and (4) sequestration of formed blood elements. The spleen is part of the mononuclear phagocyte system and is involved in all systemic inflammations, hematopoietic disorders, and many metabolic disorders.

In the past, **splenomegaly** (enlargement of the spleen) has been associated with various disease states. It is now recognized that splenomegaly is not necessarily pathologic; an enlarged spleen may be present in certain individuals without any evidence of disease. Splenomegaly may be, however, one of the first physical signs of underlying conditions, and its presence should not be ignored. In conditions where splenomegaly is present, the normal functions of the spleen may become overactive, producing a syndrome known as **hypersplenism**.

Current criteria showing the presence of hypersplenism include (1) cytopenias (anemia, leukopenia, thrombocytopenia, or combinations of these), (2) cellular bone marrow, (3) splenomegaly, and (4) improvement after splenectomy. Some individuals may seek treatment for problems even though they have not met all of these clinical criteria. Therefore, the relevance and significance of hypersplenism are still uncertain. Primary hypersplenism is recognized when no etiological factor has been found. Secondary hypersplenism occurs in the presence of another condition.

PATHOPHYSIOLOGY Specific conditions causing splenomegaly and resulting hypersplenism are many (Box 21.1). Different pathological processes that produce splenomegaly are described briefly.

Acute inflammatory or infectious processes cause splenomegaly because of an increased demand for defensive activities. Acutely enlarged spleens secondary to infection may become so filled with erythrocytes that their natural rubbery resilience is lost. As a result, they become fragile and vulnerable to blunt trauma. Splenic rupture is a complication associated with IM. Rupture occurs mostly in males between days 4 and 21 of acute illness.

Congestive splenomegaly is accompanied by ascites, portal hypertension, and esophageal varices. It is most commonly seen in those with hepatic cirrhosis. Splenic hyperplasia develops in disorders that increase splenic workload. It is associated most commonly with various types of anemia (e.g., hemolytic) and chronic myeloproliferative disorders (i.e., PV).

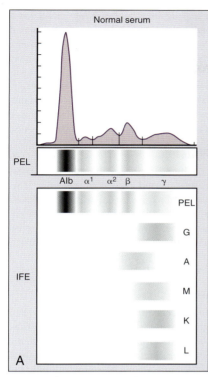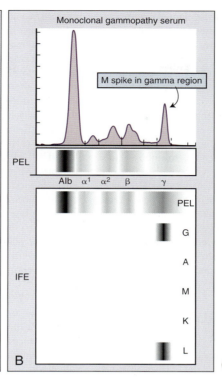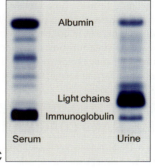

FIGURE 21.18 **M Protein.** Serum protein electrophoresis (*PEL*) is used to screen for M proteins in multiple myeloma. **A**, In normal serum the proteins separate into several regions between albumin (*Alb*) and a broad band in the gamma (γ) region, where most antibodies (gamma globulins) are found. Immunofixation (*IFE*) can show the location of IgG (*G*), IgA (*A*), IgM (*M*), and kappa (κ) and lambda (*L*) light chains. **B**, Serum from an individual with multiple myeloma holds a sharp M protein (*M spike*). The M protein is monoclonal and has only one heavy chain and one light chain. In this instance, the IFE identifies the M protein as an IgG having a lambda light chain. **C**, Serum, and urine protein electrophoretic patterns in an individual with multiple myeloma. Serum shows an M protein (*Immunoglobulin*) in the gamma region, and the urine has a large amount of the smaller-sized light chains with only a small amount of the intact immunoglobulin. *Ig*, Immunoglobulin. ([A and B], from Abeloff, M., Armitage, J., Niederhuber, J., et al. [2008]. *Abeloff's clinical oncology* [4th ed.]. Churchill Livingstone. [C], from McPherson, R., & Pincus, M. [2012]. *Henry's clinical diagnosis and management by laboratory methods* [22nd ed.]. Saunders.)

BOX 21.1 Diseases Related to Classification of Splenomegaly

Inflammation or Infection
Acute: viral (hepatitis, infectious mononucleosis, cytomegalovirus), bacterial (salmonella, Gram-negative), parasitic (typhoid)
Subacute or chronic: bacterial (subacute bacterial endocarditis, tuberculosis), parasitic (malaria), fungal (histoplasmosis), Felty's syndrome, systemic lupus erythematosus, rheumatoid arthritis, thrombocytopenia

Congestive
Cirrhosis, heart failure, portal vein obstruction (portal hypertension), splenic vein obstruction

Infiltrative
Gaucher's disease, amyloidosis, diabetic lipemia

Tumours or Cysts
Malignant: polycythemia rubra vera, chronic or acute leukemias, Hodgkin's lymphoma, metastatic solid tumours

Nonmalignant: Hamartoma
Cysts: true cysts (lymphangiomas, hemangiomas, epithelial, endothelial); false cysts (hemorrhagic, serous, inflammatory)

Infiltrative splenomegaly is the result of engorgement of the macrophages with indigestible materials associated with various "storage diseases." Tumours and cysts cause actual growth of the spleen. Metastatic tumours in the spleen are rare and may result from primary tumours of the skin, lung, breast, and cervix.

CLINICAL MANIFESTATIONS Overactivity of the spleen results in hematological alterations that affect all blood components. Sequestering of red blood cells, granulocytes, and platelets results in a reduction of all circulating blood cells. The spleen may sequester up to 50% of the red blood cell population, thereby upsetting the normal physiological concentration of red blood cells in the circulation. The rate of splenic pooling is related to spleen size and the degree of increased blood flow through it. Sequestering exposes the red blood cells to splenic conditions that speed up destruction, further contributing to the decreased red blood cell concentration. Anemia is the result of these joint activities. An increase in blood volume may potentiate anemia. This increase produces a dilutional effect on the already reduced concentration of red blood cells. The dilutional effect, as well as the removal and destruction of red blood cells, depends primarily on the degree of splenomegaly.

White blood cells and platelets also are affected by sequestering, although not to the same degree as the red blood cell. The size of the spleen is the determining factor in the number of cells sequestered.

EVALUATION AND TREATMENT Treatment for hypersplenism is splenectomy; however, it may not always be indicated. A splenectomy is considered necessary to alleviate the destructive effects on red blood cells. Clinical indicators should determine the need for splenectomy, not necessarily specific conditions. Splenectomy for splenic rupture is no longer considered mandatory because of the possibility of overwhelming sepsis after removal. Repair and preservation are now considered before the decision to remove the spleen. Splenectomy also may be performed as treatment for hairy cell leukemia, Felty's syndrome, agnogenic myeloid metaplasia, thalassemia major, Gaucher's disease, hemodialysis, splenomegaly, splenic venous thrombosis, and thrombotic thrombocytopenic purpura (TTP).

Individuals are able to lead normal lives after splenectomy. However, blood cell abnormalities often exist after removal of the spleen (i.e., red blood cells become thinner, broader, and wrinkled; white blood cell counts initially increase and then plateau; platelet counts rise after surgery and then stabilize). A major postoperative complication following splenectomy is overwhelming postsplenectomy infection (OPI). Unless treated in time, OPI may rapidly progress to septic shock and possibly disseminated intravascular coagulation (DIC).

HEMORRHAGIC DISORDERS AND ALTERATIONS OF PLATELETS AND COAGULATION

> **QUICK CHECK 21.6**
> 1. Compare and contrast thrombocytopenia with thrombocytosis.
> 2. Why does vitamin K deficiency predispose an individual to a coagulation disorder?
> 3. Name three pathological causes of disseminated intravascular coagulation (DIC). Describe the manifestations associated with DIC.
> 4. Compare and contrast a thrombus with an embolus.

The arrest of bleeding, or **hemostasis**, depends on adequate numbers of platelets, normal levels of coagulation factors, and absence of defects in vessels walls. The range of abnormal bleeding varies widely from massive bleeds, such as rupture of large vessels like the aorta, to small bleeds in skin or mucosal membranes. Diminished or excessive levels of coagulation factors can lead to defective hemostasis or spontaneous and unnecessary clotting. (Chapter 20 discusses hemostasis.) Diminished hemostasis results in either internal or external **hemorrhage**, defined as copious or heavy discharge of blood from blood vessels. A classification of hemorrhagic disorders is included in Table 21.8.

Purpuric disorders, red or purple discolored spots on skin, occur when there is a deficiency of normal platelets necessary to plug damaged vessels or prevent leakage from the tiny tears that occur daily in capillaries. More serious internal bleeding occurs from events that simply overwhelm hemostatic mechanisms. These events include rupture of large blood vessels, trauma, and diseases associated with massive hemorrhage including abdominal aneurysm. Between these smaller bleeds and massive bleeds are deficiencies of coagulation factors found with the hemophilias (see Chapter 22). Disorders that result in spontaneous clotting can develop from genetic disorders of the clotting system components or from acquired diseases that activate clotting. These disorders are known collectively as **thromboembolic disease**. Additionally, any disorder of the blood that predisposes to clotting of blood or **thrombosis** is called **hypercoagulability** (thrombophilia).

Disorders of Platelets

Quantitative or qualitative abnormalities of platelets can interrupt normal blood coagulation and prevent hemostasis.[42] The quantitative abnormalities are thrombocytopenia, a decrease in the number of circulating platelets, and thrombocythemia, an increase in the number of platelets. Qualitative disorders affect the structure or function of individual platelets and can coexist with the quantitative disorders. Qualitative disorders usually prevent platelet adherence and aggregation, preventing formation of a platelet plug.

Thrombocytopenia

Thrombocytopenia is defined as a platelet count less than 150×10^9/L of blood, although most individuals do not consider the decrease significant unless it falls below 100×10^9/L of blood.[43,44] Hemorrhage associated with minor trauma does not appreciably increase until the count falls below 50×10^9/L. Spontaneous bleeding without trauma can occur with counts ranging from 10 to 15×10^9/L, resulting in skin manifestations (i.e., petechiae, ecchymoses, and larger purpuric spots) or frank bleeding from mucous membranes. Severe spontaneous bleeding may result if the count is less than 10×10^9/L and can be fatal if it occurs in the GI tract, respiratory tract, or CNS.

Before the diagnosis of thrombocytopenia is made, pseudothrombocytopenia must be ruled out. This phenomenon occurs in approximately 1 in 1000 to 1 in 10000 laboratory samples and results from an error in platelet counting when a blood sample is analyzed by an automated cell counter. Platelets in the blood sample may become nonspecifically agglutinated by immunoglobulins in the presence of ethylenediaminetetraacetic acid (EDTA), a preservative in banked blood. The agglutinated platelets are not counted, thus giving a clear, but false, thrombocytopenia. Thrombocytopenia also may be falsely diagnosed because of a dilutional effect seen after massive transfusion of platelet-poor packed cells to treat a hemorrhage. This occurs when more than 10 units of blood have been transfused within a 24-hour period. The hemorrhage that necessitated the transfusion also accelerates the loss of platelets, contributing to the pseudothrombocytopenic state. Splenic sequestering of platelets in hypersplenism (congestive) also induces an apparent thrombocytopenia, as does hypothermia (less than 25°C [77°F]), which is reversed when temperatures return to normal. These events suggest an increased platelet sequestration in response to chilling.

TABLE 21.8 Classification of Hemorrhagic Disorders

Type of Defect	Example	Manifestation
Defects of primary hemostasis	Platelet defects or von Willebrand's disease	Usually present with small bleeds in skin or mucosal membrane; bleeds are usually petechiae (<3-mm minute hemorrhages) or purpuras (>3-mm red-purple discolorations); common in capillaries; also includes epistaxis (nose bleeds), gastro-intestinal bleeds, or excessive menstruation
Defects of secondary hemostasis	Coagulation factor defects	Bleeds into soft tissue, muscle, or joints; intracranial bleeds may occur
Generalized defects of small vessels	Palpable purpura and ecchymoses	Extravasated blood creates a palpable mass (or palpable purpura), ecchymoses (simply called a *bruise*), or a larger palpable lesion (or hematoma); systemic disorders disrupt small blood vessels, called *vasculitis*

PATHOPHYSIOLOGY Thrombocytopenia results from decreased platelet production, increased consumption, or both. The condition may be either congenital or acquired and may be either primary or secondary to other acquired or congenital conditions.[45] Thrombocytopenia secondary to congenital conditions occurs in a large number of diseases, although each is relatively rare.[45]

Acquired thrombocytopenia is more common and may occur as a result of decreased platelet production secondary to viral infections (e.g., EBV, rubella, CMV, HIV), medications (e.g., thiazides, estrogens, quinine-containing medications, chemotherapeutic agents, ethanol), nutritional deficiencies (vitamin B_{12} or folic acid in particular), chronic renal failure, bone marrow hypoplasia (e.g., aplastic anemia), radiation therapy, or bone marrow infiltration by cancer. Most common forms of thrombocytopenia are the result of increased platelet consumption. Examples include heparin-induced thrombocytopenia, idiopathic (immune) thrombocytopenia purpura, TTP, and DIC.

Heparin-induced thrombocytopenia. Heparin is a common cause of medication-induced thrombocytopenia.[45] Approximately 4% of individuals treated with unfractionated heparin develop **heparin-induced thrombocytopenia (HIT)**. The incidence is lower (about 0.1%) with the use of low-molecular-weight heparin. HIT is an immune-mediated, adverse drug reaction caused by IgG antibodies against the heparin–platelet factor 4 complex leading to platelet activation through platelet Fc γIIa receptors.[45] The release of additional platelet factor 4 from activated platelets and activation of thrombin lead to increased platelet consumption and a decrease in platelet counts beginning 5 to 10 days after administration of heparin.

CLINICAL MANIFESTATIONS The hallmark of HIT is thrombocytopenia. A decrease of approximately 50% in the platelet count is seen in more than 95% of individuals. However, 30% or more of those with thrombocytopenia are also at risk for venous or arterial thrombosis. This risk occurs because a *prothrombotic state* is caused by antibody binding to platelets, inducing activation, aggregation, and consumption (thus the term *thrombocytopenia* in the syndrome name) of platelets. Venous thrombosis is more common and results in deep venous thrombosis (DVT) and pulmonary emboli. Arterial thrombosis affects the lower extremities, causing limb ischemia. Arterial thrombosis may lead to cerebrovascular accidents and myocardial infarctions. Other major arteries also may be affected (e.g., renal, mesenteric, upper limb). Although platelet counts are low, bleeding is uncommon.

EVALUATION AND TREATMENT Diagnosis is primarily based on clinical observations. The individual presents with dropping platelet counts after 5 days or longer of heparin treatment. On average, platelet counts may fall to 60×10^9/L. Because most individuals have undergone surgery and the onset of symptoms, including thrombosis, may be delayed until after release from the hospital, other possible causes of thrombocytopenia (e.g., infection, other medication reactions) must be considered. Tests are available to measure antiheparin-platelet factor 4 antibodies. The sensitivity of this test is extremely high (> 90%), but the specificity is less because of false-positive reactions (e.g., those receiving dialysis). Treatment is the withdrawal of heparin and use of alternative anticoagulants.

Immune thrombocytopenia purpura. The most common cause of thrombocytopenia, secondary to increased platelet destruction is **immune thrombocytopenic purpura (ITP)**. The incidence of ITP is estimated to range from 5.8 to 6.6 per 100 000 in the general population and tends to increase with age. ITP may be acute or chronic. The acute form is often seen in children and typically lasts 1 to 2 months with a CR. In some cases, it may last for up to 6 months, and some children (7 to 28%) may progress to the chronic condition (see Chapter 22). Acute ITP is usually secondary to infections (particularly viral) or other conditions that lead to large amounts of antigen in the blood, such as medication allergies or systemic lupus erythematosus. Under these conditions, the antigen usually forms immune complexes with circulating antibody. It is thought that the immune complexes bind to Fc receptors on platelets, leading to their destruction in the spleen. The acute form of ITP usually resolves as the source of antigen is resolved (infection) or removed (medications).

Chronic ITP is caused by autoantibody-mediated destruction against platelet-specific antigens. This form is more commonly seen in adults, being most prevalent in women between 20 and 40 years old, although it can be found in all ages. The chronic form tends to get progressively worse. It can occur from a variety of predisposing conditions or exposures (secondary) or have no known risk factors (primary). The autoantibodies are generally of the IgG class and are against one or more of several platelet glycoproteins (e.g., GPIIb/IIIa, GPIIb/IX, GPIa/IIa). The antibodies bind directly to the platelet antigens, after which the antibody-coated platelets are recognized and removed from the circulation by macrophages in the spleen.

CLINICAL MANIFESTATIONS Initial manifestations range from minor bleeding problems (development of petechiae and purpura) over the course of several days to major hemorrhage from mucosal sites (epistaxis, hematuria, menorrhagia, bleeding gums). Rarely will an individual present with intracranial bleeding or other sites of internal bleeding.

During pregnancy, a woman with ITP may have a newborn that is also thrombocytopenic. If the fetal platelets express the same antigen as the mother, the maternal antibody will coat the platelets, potentially resulting in thrombocytopenia in utero. A variant of neonatal thrombocytopenia (*neonatal alloimmune thrombocytopenia*) occurs when the mother does not have ITP but makes IgG antibodies against an antigen inherited from the father found on fetal platelets but not on maternal platelets.[46]

EVALUATION AND TREATMENT Diagnosis of ITP is based on a history of bleeding and associated symptoms (weight loss, fever, headache). Physical examination includes notations on the type, location, and severity of bleeding. Evidence of infections (bacterial, HIV and other viral), medication history, family history, and evidence of thrombosis are assessed. Other diagnostic tests include CBC and peripheral blood smear. Unlike some other forms of thrombocytopenia, there is usually no evidence of splenectomy. Testing for antiplatelet antibodies is usually not helpful. Although most cases of ITP are associated with elevated levels of IgG on platelets, other forms of thrombocytopenia also have a high incidence of platelet-associated antibodies; thus, the specificity is low.[47] In addition, some cases of ITP will not present with elevated platelet-associated antibodies. The sensitivity is 75 to 94%; therefore, a negative test does not rule out ITP.

The acute form of ITP usually resolves without major clinical consequences. The chronic form (like many autoimmune diseases) is variable with multiple remissions and exacerbations. Treatment is palliative, not curative, and focuses on prevention of platelet destruction. Initial therapy for ITP is glucocorticoids (e.g., prednisone). This therapy suppresses the immune response and prevents sequestering and further destruction of platelets. If steroid therapy is ineffective, other reagents may be used. Treatment with intravenous immune globulin (IVIg) is used to prevent major bleeding. The response rate is 80%, but the effects are transient, lasting only days to a few weeks. Anti-Rh_o(D) (RhoGAM) has been used with limited success to treat individuals who are Rh-positive. Newer medications are now available.

If other therapies are ineffective, splenectomy is considered to remove the site of platelet destruction. However, splenectomy is not without risks. Approximately 10 to 20% of individuals who undergo a splenectomy suffer a relapse and require further treatment. In that situation, it is thought that the liver has become the site for platelet destruction. If splenectomy is unsuccessful and life-threatening thrombocytopenia persists, more aggressive immunosuppressive medications (e.g., azathioprine [Nu-azathioprine], cyclophosphamide) are usually recommended. Because of potential complications, these medications are reserved for individuals who are severely thrombocytopenic and refractive to other therapies.

Thrombotic thrombocytopenic purpura. **Thrombotic thrombocytopenic purpura (TTP)** is a multisystem disorder characterized by thrombotic microangiopathy (TMA) (small or microvessel disease) in which platelets aggregate and cause occlusion of arterioles and capillaries within the microcirculation.[48] Aggregation may lead to increased platelet consumption and organ ischemia. TTP is uncommon, occurring in about five per million individuals per year. The incidence is increasing and does appear to be an actual increase and not just the result of improved recognition. One suspected etiological factor for TMA, TTP, and hemolytic uremic syndrome (HUS) is medication induced. A recent report categorizes multiple medications that have been associated with drug-induced TMA (DITMA). The results of this study emphasize the importance of assessing medications as a possible etiology of TTP.[49]

There are two types of TTP: familial and acquired idiopathic. The familial type is rarer and is usually chronic, relapsing, and typically seen in children. When the disease is recognized and treated early, the child experiences predictable recurring episodes at approximately 3-week intervals that are responsive to treatment. Acquired TTP is more common and more acute and severe. It occurs mostly in females in their 30s and is rarely seen in infants and older persons.

Platelet aggregation and microthrombi formation is found throughout the entire vascular system, causing damage to multiple organs. The most susceptible organs for damage include the kidney, brain, and heart. Also affected are the pancreas, spleen, and adrenal glands. The thrombi are composed of platelets with minimal fibrin and red blood cells, differentiating them from thrombi secondary to intravascular coagulation.

CLINICAL MANIFESTATIONS Chronic relapsing TTP is a rare familial form of TTP observed in children and usually recognized and successfully treated. The acquired **acute idiopathic TTP** is much more common and more severe.[48] TTP is clinically related to and must be distinguished from other thrombotic microangiopathic conditions, including HUS, malignant hypertension, pre-eclampsia, and pregnancy-induced HELLP (*h*emolysis, *e*levated *l*iver enzymes, *l*ow *p*latelet count) syndrome. Early diagnosis and treatment are essential because TTP may prove fatal within 90 days.

Acute idiopathic TTP is characterized by a "pentad" of symptoms. Only 20 to 30% of those with acute idiopathic TTP present with the classic pentad. These symptoms include (1) extreme thrombocytopenia (less than 20×10^9/L), (2) intravascular hemolytic anemia, (3) ischemic signs and symptoms most often involving the CNS (about 65% present with memory disturbances, behavioural irregularities, headaches, or coma), (4) kidney failure (present in about 65%), and (5) fever (present in about 33%).

EVALUATION AND TREATMENT A routine blood smear usually shows fragmented red blood cells *(schizocytes)* produced by shear forces when red blood cells are in contact with the fibrin mesh in clots that form in the vessels. As a result of tissue injury, serum levels of lactate dehydrogenase (LDH) may be very high, and low-density lipoprotein (LDL) levels may be elevated. Tests for antibody on red blood cells are negative, excluding immune hemolytic anemia.

Prompt treatment can significantly reduce the death rate. Plasma exchange with fresh frozen plasma is the treatment of choice, achieving a 70 to 85% response rate. Additionally, steroids (glucocorticoids) are administered. In the absence of major organ damage, this approach may lead to complete recovery with no long-term complications. The anti-CD20 monoclonal antibody rituximab (Rituxan) has shown some success in people who are refractory to plasma exchange.[50] Relapses do occur at a rate of 13 to 36%. Recurrences have been reported, sometimes delayed until 9 years after treatment. Individuals who do not respond to conventional treatment may be candidates for splenectomy; however, postoperative hemorrhage still is a dangerous complication. Immunosuppression therapy has been successful in some individuals.

Thrombocythemia

Thrombocythemia (also called **thrombocytosis**) is characterized by a platelet count greater than 400×10^9/L of blood.[43,44] Thrombocythemia may be primary or secondary (reactive) and is usually asymptomatic until the count exceeds 1000×10^9/L. Then intravascular clot formation (thrombosis), hemorrhage, or other abnormalities can occur.

PATHOPHYSIOLOGY Essential (primary) thrombocythemia (ET) is a chronic myeloproliferative neoplasm characterized by an increase in platelet production (or thrombocytosis) resulting from a defect in the bone marrow megakaryocyte progenitor cells. Abnormal blood clotting commonly occurs in individuals with essential thrombocythemia causing many clinical manifestations. Other disease features include leukocytosis, splenomegaly, thrombosis, bleeding, microcirculatory symptoms, itching (or pruritus), and risk for leukemic or bone marrow fibrotic transformation.[51] The most common mutated genes in ET are the Janus kinase 2 *(JAK2)* and calreticulin *(CALR)* genes. Other mutated genes also can occur and contribute to ET. The *JAK2* mutation causes overactivity in cell signaling from JAK2 protein. JAK2, a tyrosine kinase, is an essential player downstream of cytokine receptors, such as the thrombopoietin (affects platelet proliferation) and erythropoietin (affects erythrocyte proliferation) receptors. More simply, both erythropoietin and thrombopoietin send their signals and resulting proliferation through JAK2. Along with increased platelets, there may be an increase in the number of red blood cells, showing a myeloproliferative disorder. However, the increase in red blood cells is not to the extent seen in PV. Red blood cells in ET tend to aggregate and adhere to the endothelium and contribute to the blockage of flow in the microvasculature and altered interactions between platelets and the vascular endothelium.[52] The *JAK2* (V617F) mutation is present in 50 to 60% of persons with ET. It is more common in middle-aged individuals, with the majority of cases occurring between ages 50 and 60 years. There is no known gender preference. There also is a rare hereditary type of ET called *familial essential thrombocythemia* (FET) that is inherited in an autosomal dominant pattern.

Secondary thrombocythemia may occur after splenectomy because platelets that normally would be stored in the spleen remain in circulating blood. The increase in platelets may be gradual, with thrombocythemia not occurring for up to 3 weeks after splenectomy. Reactive thrombocythemia may occur during some inflammatory conditions, such as rheumatoid arthritis and cancers. In these conditions, excessive production of some cytokines (e.g., IL-6, IL-11) may induce increased production of thrombopoietin in the liver, resulting in increased megakaryocyte proliferation. Reactive thrombocythemia also may occur during a variety of physiological conditions, such as after exercise.

CLINICAL MANIFESTATIONS Clinical manifestations vary among individuals. Those with ET are at risk for large-vessel arterial or venous thrombosis. The most common complication is **microvasculature thrombosis** leading to ischemia in the fingers, toes, or cerebrovascular regions.[53] The primary presenting symptoms of microvasculature thrombosis are erythromelalgia, headache, and paresthesias. **Erythromelalgia** is unilateral or bilateral warm, congested, red hands and feet with painful burning sensations, particularly in the forefoot sole and one or more toes. The lower extremities are affected more often and only one side may be involved. The pain is started by standing, exercise, or warmth and relieved by elevation and cooling. In extreme situations, acrocyanosis (bluish or purple colouring of hands or feet) and gangrene may result.

Arterial thrombosis is more common than venous thrombosis and may involve the coronary and renal arteries. Deep venous thrombosis of the lower extremities and pulmonary embolism are the major sites for venous involvement. Other common venous sites include intraabdominal venous thrombosis (portal and hepatic). People older than 60 years of age or those with prior history of thrombotic events have as much as a 25% chance of developing a cerebral, cardiac, or peripheral arterial thrombus and, less often, developing a pulmonary embolism or deep venous thrombosis. Conversion to acute leukemia is found in less than 10%.[54] Symptoms related to microvascular thrombosis in the CNS include headache, dizziness with paresthesias, transient ischemic attacks, strokes, visual disturbances, and seizures. Major thrombotic events, not related to the platelet count, occur in about 20 to 30% of individuals with ET. Prior history of thrombotic events, advanced age, and duration of thrombocytosis are predictors of future thrombotic complications. Individuals older than age 60 are at greatest risk.

Although thrombosis is the more common symptom, hemorrhage can also occur. Sites for bleeding include the GI tract, skin, mucous membranes, urinary tract, gums, teeth sockets after extraction, joints, eyes, and brain. GI bleeding may be mistaken for a duodenal ulcer. Hemorrhage is not severe and generally occurs in the presence of very high platelet counts. Transfusions are needed only occasionally. Bleeding and clotting may occur simultaneously, and individuals will not necessarily be "bleeders" or "clotters."

EVALUATION AND TREATMENT Initial diagnosis is not difficult; as many as two-thirds of cases are diagnosed from a routine CBC. Secondary thrombocytosis also may occur as a moderate rise in the platelet count that resolves with treatment or resolution of the underlying condition. The World Health Organization requires that the following four criteria be met for a diagnosis of ET: (1) sustained platelet count of at least $450 \times 10^9/L$; (2) bone marrow biopsy showing proliferation of enlarged mature megakaryocytes and no increase of granulocyte or erythrocyte precursors; (3) failure to meet the criteria of PV, myelofibrosis, CML, or other myelodysplastic syndrome; and (4) presence of JAK2 617F or another clonal marker or evidence of reactive thrombocytosis.[54] Since ET can be mistaken for CML, careful differentiation is necessary because treatment varies significantly.

Treatment of ET is directed toward preventing thrombosis or hemorrhage.[54] Reducing the platelet count is still a significant treatment issue. Hydroxyurea (Hydrea), a nonalkylating myelosuppressive agent, has been the medication of choice to suppress platelet production. Long-term use, however, may cause progression to other myeloplastic disorders, particularly AML or myelofibrosis.[54] Another medication used to treat ET is interferon (IFN). IFN has a response rate of 80% but may not be effective for everyone because of side effects. Anagrelide interferes with platelet maturation rather than production, thus not interfering with red and white blood cell growth and development. Low-dose Aspirin may be effective to alleviate erthromyalgia and transient neurological manifestations. ET is not necessarily considered life-threatening, but in those older than age 60 and who have had earlier incidences of thrombosis, complications are more common and associated with a higher risk of mortality.

Alterations of Platelet Function

Qualitative alterations in platelet function are characterized by an increased bleeding time in the presence of a normal platelet count. Associated clinical manifestations include spontaneous petechiae and purpura, and bleeding from the GI tract, genito-urinary tract, pulmonary mucosa, and gums. Congenital alterations in platelet function (thrombocytopathies) are quite rare.[55]

Acquired disorders of platelet function are more common than congenital disorders and may be categorized into three principal causes: (1) medications, (2) systemic inflammatory conditions, and (3) hematological alterations.

Multiple medications are known to interfere with platelet function in several ways: inhibition of platelet membrane receptors, inhibition of prostaglandin pathways, and inhibition of phosphodiesterase activity. Aspirin is the most commonly used medication that affects platelets. It irreversibly inhibits cyclo-oxygenase function for several days after administration. NSAIDs also affect cyclo-oxygenase, although in a reversible fashion.

Systemic disorders that affect platelet function are chronic renal disease, liver disease, cardiopulmonary bypass surgery, and severe deficiencies of iron or folate and antiplatelet antibodies associated with autoimmune disorders. Hematological disorders associated with platelet dysfunction include chronic myeloproliferative disorders, MM, leukemias, and myelodysplastic syndromes and dysproteinemias.

Disorders of Coagulation

Disorders of coagulation are usually caused by defects or deficiencies in one or more of the clotting factors. (Chapter 20 describes the normal function of clotting factors.) Qualitative or quantitative abnormalities interfere with or prevent the enzymatic reactions that transform clotting factors, circulating as plasma proteins, into a stable fibrin clot (see Figure 20.17). Some clotting factor defects are inherited and involve a single factor, such as the hemophilias and von Willebrand's disease. Other coagulation defects are acquired and tend to result from deficient synthesis of clotting factors by the liver. Causes include liver disease and dietary deficiency of vitamin K.

Other coagulation disorders are attributed to pathological conditions that trigger coagulation inappropriately, engaging the clotting factors and causing detrimental clotting within blood vessels. For example, any cardiovascular abnormality that alters normal blood flow by acceleration, deceleration, or obstruction can create conditions in which coagulation proceeds within the vessels. An example of this is thromboembolic disease, in which blood clots obstruct blood vessels. Coagulation is also stimulated by the presence of tissue factor (TF) that is released by damaged or dead tissues. **Vasculitis**, or inflammation of the blood vessels, along with vessel damage activates platelets, which in turn activates the coagulation cascade. In extensive or prolonged vasculitis, blood clot formation can suppress mechanisms that normally control clot formation and dissolution, leading to clogging of the vessels. In each of these acquired conditions, normal hemostatic function proves harmful to the body by consuming coagulation factors excessively or by overwhelming normal control of clot formation and breakdown (fibrinolysis) (see Figure 20.19).

Impaired Hemostasis

Impaired hemostasis, or the inability to promote coagulation and the development of a stable fibrin clot, is commonly associated with liver

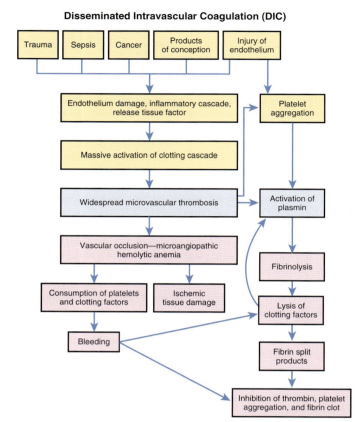

FIGURE 21.19 Pathophysiology of Disseminated Intravascular Coagulation.

dysfunction. The dysfunction may be caused by either specific liver disorders or lack of vitamin K.

Vitamin K deficiency. Vitamin K, a fat-soluble vitamin, is required for the synthesis and regulation of prothrombin; the procoagulant factors (VII, IX, X); and the anticoagulant factors within the liver (proteins C and S).[56] Unknown is the contribution of vitamin K to the overall supply by the intestinal flora. The primary source of vitamin K is found in green leafy vegetables. The most common cause of vitamin deficiency is parenteral nutrition in combination with antibiotics that destroy normal gut flora. Rarely is the deficiency caused by a lack of dietary intake. Bulimia, however, can suppress vitamin K–dependent activity. Parenteral administration of vitamin K is the treatment of choice and usually results in correction of the deficiency within 8 to 12 hours. Fresh frozen plasma also may be administered but is usually reserved for individuals with life-threatening hemorrhages or those who require emergency surgery.

Liver disease. Liver disease (e.g., acute or chronic hepatocellular diseases, cirrhosis), vitamin K deficiency, or liver surgery includes hemostatic derangements with defects in the clotting or fibrinolytic systems and platelet function. The hepatic parenchyma cells produce most of the factors involved in hemostasis. As a result, damage to the liver often results in decreased production of factors involved in clotting. The level of factor VII is the first to decline after liver damage because of its rapid turnover. Factor IX levels are less affected and do not decline until the liver destruction is well advanced. The liver also is a major site for production of plasminogen and α_2-antiplasmin of the fibrinolytic system, as well as thrombopoietin and the metalloprotease ADAMTS13. Diminished thrombopoietin may lead to thrombocytopenia from decreased platelet production. Decreased production of ADAMTS13 results in increased levels of large precursor molecules of von Willebrand's factor. This leads to the formation of large aggregates of platelets.

With severe liver disease, such as cirrhosis, most clotting factors are significantly depressed. Levels of clotting system regulators, such as antithrombin, protein C, protein S, and fibrinogen, also are decreased. The fibrolytic system is commonly active because of plasmin inhibitor and other activators that are unaffected. Thrombocytopenia occurs in affected individuals because of diminished thrombopoietin and ADAMTS13, as well as increased sequestration (pooling) of platelets in the spleen. As a result, the spleen is often enlarged in cirrhosis and is associated with portal hypertension. These individuals may appear to have a condition similar to DIC (see "Consumptive Thrombohemorrhagic Disorders", below).

Treatment of hemostasis alterations in liver disease must be comprehensive to cover all aspects of dysfunctions. Fresh frozen plasma administration is the treatment of choice. All individuals, however, do not tolerate the volume needed to adequately replace all deficient factors. Alternative modalities include the addition of exchange transfusions and platelet concentration to plasma administration.

Consumptive Thrombohemorrhagic Disorders

Consumptive thrombohemorrhagic disorders are a heterogeneous group of conditions that show the entire spectrum of hemorrhagic and thrombotic pathological findings. Symptoms range from the subtle to the devastating. They generally are considered to be intermediary disease processes that complicate a vast number of primary disease states. These disorders are also characterized by confusion and controversy related to their diagnosis, treatment, and management. No one definition can cover all possible varieties of these disorders. DIC, however, is most commonly used in the clinical setting to describe a pathological condition associated with hemorrhage and thrombosis.

Disseminated intravascular coagulation. **Disseminated intravascular coagulation (DIC)** is an acquired clinical syndrome characterized by widespread activation of coagulation resulting in formation of fibrin clots in medium and small vessels or microvasculature throughout the body.[56] Widespread clotting may lead to blockage of blood flow to organs, resulting in multiple organ failure. The excess clotting may result in consumption of platelets and clotting factors, leading to a tendency to bleed despite widespread clots.

The clinical course of DIC is largely determined by the stimulus intensity, host response, and comorbidities. It ranges from an acute, severe, life-threatening process that is characterized by massive hemorrhage and thrombosis to a chronic, low-grade condition. The chronic condition includes subacute hemorrhage and diffuse microcirculatory thrombosis. DIC may be localized to one specific organ or generalized, involving multiple organs.

The diagnosis of DIC has been challenging because of the complexity and wide variations in clinical manifestations. Diagnostic criteria have been established and include a systemic thrombohemorrhagic disorder with laboratory evidence of (1) clotting activation, (2) fibrinolytic activation, (3) coagulation inhibitor consumption, and (4) biochemical evidence of end-organ damage or failure.

DIC is secondary to a wide variety of well-defined clinical conditions, specifically those capable of activating the clotting cascade.

Sepsis is the most common condition associated with DIC. Gram-negative microorganisms, as well as some Gram-positive microorganisms, fungi, protozoa (malaria), and viruses (influenza, herpes), are capable of precipitating DIC by causing damage to the vascular endothelium. Gram-negative endotoxins are the primary cause of endothelial damage. DIC may occur in up to 50% of individuals with Gram-negative sepsis. DIC occurs in approximately 10 to 20% of individuals with metastatic cancer or acute leukemia. The adenocarcinomas most frequently associated with DIC include the lung, pancreas, colon, and stomach.[57] Direct tissue damage (e.g., massive trauma, extensive surgery, severe burns) also results in release of TF, an initiator of DIC, by the endothelium. Severe trauma, especially to the brain, can induce DIC. DIC occurs in about two-thirds of individuals with a systemic inflammatory response to trauma. Some complications of pregnancy also are associated with DIC. Incidences range from 50% for women with placental abruptions to less than 10% for severe pre-eclampsia. Other causes of DIC have been found, most notably blood transfusion. Transfused blood dilutes the clotting factors, as well as circulating naturally occurring antithrombins. In hemolytic transfusion reactions, the endothelium is damaged by complement-mediated reactions.

PATHOPHYSIOLOGY DIC results from abnormally widespread and ongoing activation of clotting—coagulopathy—in small and mid-size vessels that alters the microcirculation, leading to ischemic necrosis in various organs, particularly the kidney and lung. Concomitantly, DIC can be caused by the imbalance between the coagulant system and the fibrinolytic system (which generates plasmin) to support normal circulation. DIC can cause widespread deposition of fibrin in the microcirculation that leads to ischemia, microvascular thrombotic obstruction, and organ failure (Figure 21.19).

Seemingly paradoxical, DIC involves both widespread clotting and bleeding because of simultaneous procoagulant activation, fibrinolytic activation, and consumption of platelets and coagulation factors, which results directly in serious bleeding (see Figure 21.19).

DIC is not a disease but is secondary to a variety of conditions (Box 21.2) because of activation of the clotting cascade. The common pathway for DIC appears to be excessive and widespread exposure to TF. This may occur by several mechanisms: (1) damage to the vascular endothelium results in exposure to TF; (2) when stimulated by inflammatory cytokines, endothelial cells and monocytes express surface TF; (3) endotoxin triggers the release of many cytokines that can both promote and cause progression of DIC; (4) sepsis is associated with many cytokines, interleukins, and platelet-activating factor that promote DIC as well as activate endothelial cells that stimulate thrombi development; and (5) TF may be released directly into the bloodstream from circulating white blood cells.

> **BOX 21.2 Conditions Associated With Disseminated Intravascular Coagulation (DIC)**
>
> *Malignancy:* acute myelocytic leukemia, metastatic solid tumours (pancreas, prostate)
> *Infections:* bacterial (Gram-negative endotoxin, Gram-positive mucopolysaccharides), viral (hepatitis, CMV, dengue, HIV), fungal, parasitic, rickettsial
> *Pregnancy complications:* eclampsia/pre-eclampsia, placental abruption, amniotic fluid embolism, dead fetus syndrome
> *Severe trauma:* head injury, burns, crush injuries, tissue necrosis, severe hypo- or hyperthermia
> *Liver disease:* obstructive jaundice, acute liver failure, fatty liver of pregnancy
> *Intravascular hemolysis:* transfusion reactions, medication-induced hemolysis, viper snake bites, graft versus host disease
> *Medical devices:* aortic balloon, prosthetic devices
> *Hypoxia and low blood flow states:* arterial hypotension secondary to shock, cardiopulmonary arrest
> *Vascular disorders:* Giant hemangiomas (Kasabach-Merritt syndrome), aortic aneurysms

CMV, Cytomegalovirus; *HIV,* human immunodeficiency virus.

TF binds clotting factor VII, which leads to conversion of prothrombin to thrombin and formation of fibrin clots (see Figure 20.19). This pathway appears to be the primary route by which DIC is started.

Not only is the clotting system extensively activated in DIC, but also the activities of the predominant natural anticoagulants (TF pathway inhibitor, antithrombin III, protein C) are greatly diminished. During DIC, the activation of clotting is prolonged and is a result of certain conditions (e.g., bacteremia or endotoxemia). Thrombin generation is increased and is insufficiently balanced by impaired anticoagulant systems, such as antithrombin and protein C.[58] The overall result is fibrin generation and deposition in the vascular system. In early DIC, plasmin (naturally occurring clot busting or fibrinolytic agent) produced from endothelial cells causes fibrinolysis to support circulation. Bleeding can occur with excess fibrinolytic activity. However, fibrinolysis becomes blunted by high levels of plasminogen activator inhibitor-1 (PAI-1), a fibrinolytic inhibitor.[58] Over time the activity of plasmin is diminished by PAI-1. Although some fibrinolytic activity stays, the level is inadequate to control the systemic deposition of fibrin. The slow breakdown of fibrin by plasmin produces **fibrin split products (FSPs)** (also known as **fibrin degradation products [FDPs]**). These products are powerful anticoagulants that are normally removed from blood by fibronectin and macrophages. FSPs, along with thrombin, induce further cytokine release from monocytes, contributing to endothelial damage and TF release. During DIC, the presence of FSPs is prolonged. Low levels of fibronectin suggest a poor prognosis.

Although thrombosis is generalized and widespread, individuals with DIC are at risk for hemorrhage. Hemorrhage is secondary to the abnormally high consumption of clotting factors and platelets, as well as the anticoagulant properties of FSPs, which interfere with fibrin mesh formation or polymerization. Both thrombin and FSPs have a high affinity for platelets and cause platelet activation and aggregation—an event that occurs early in the development of DIC—which helps microcirculatory coagulation and obstruction in the initial phase. However, platelet consumption exceeds production, resulting in a thrombocytopenia that increases bleeding.

Activation of clotting also leads to activation of other inflammatory pathways, including the kallikrein–kinin and complement systems (see Chapter 6). Activation of these systems contributes to increased vascular permeability, hypotension, and shock. Activated complement components also induce platelet destruction, which initially contributes to the thrombosis and later to the thrombocytopenia.

The deposition of fibrin clots in the circulation interferes with blood flow, causing widespread organ hypoperfusion. This condition may lead to ischemia, infarction, and necrosis. This process further potentiates and complicates the existing DIC process by causing further release of TF and eventually organ failure. Manifestations of multisystem organ dysfunction and failure ultimately result.

In addition to initiation of clotting by TF, DIC may be precipitated by direct proteolytic activation of factor X. The proteolytic activation of factor X has been described as "thrombin mimicry" and is the result of proteases directly converting fibrinogen to fibrin. These proteases may come from snake venom, some tumour cells, or the pancreas and liver, where they are released during episodes of pancreatitis and various stages of liver disease. Direct proteolytic activity appears to be independent of any type of damage to the endothelium or tissue.

Whatever starts the process of DIC, the cycle of thrombosis and hemorrhage persists until the underlying cause of the DIC is removed or proper therapeutic interventions are used.

CLINICAL MANIFESTATIONS Clinical signs and symptoms of DIC present a wide spectrum of possibilities, depending on the underlying disease process that initiates DIC and whether the DIC is acute or

> **BOX 21.3 Clinical Manifestations Associated With Disseminated Intravascular Coagulation (DIC)**
>
> **Integumentary System**
> Widespread hemorrhage and vascular lesions
> Oozing from puncture sites, incisions, mucous membranes
> Acrocyanosis (irregular-shaped cyanotic patches)
> Gangrene
>
> **Central Nervous System**
> Subarachnoid hemorrhage
> Altered state of consciousness (slight confusion to convulsions and coma)
>
> **Gastro-Intestinal System**
> Occult bleeding to massive gastro-intestinal bleeding
> Abdominal distension
> Malaise
> Weakness
>
> **Pulmonary System**
> Pulmonary infarctions
> ARDS
> Cyanosis
> Tachypnea
> Hypoxemia
>
> **Renal System**
> Hematuria
> Oliguria
> Renal failure

ARDS, Acute respiratory distress syndrome.

chronic (Box 21.3). Most symptoms are the result of either bleeding or thrombosis. Acute DIC presents with rapid development of hemorrhaging (oozing) from venipuncture sites, arterial lines, or surgical wounds or development of ecchymotic lesions (purpura, petechiae) and hematomas. Other sites of bleeding include the eyes (sclera, conjunctiva), the nose, and the gums. Most individuals with DIC have bleeding at three or more unrelated sites, and any combination may be seen. Shock of variable intensity, out of proportion to the amount of blood loss, also may be seen. Hemorrhaging into closed compartments of the body also can occur and may precede the development of shock.

Manifestations of thrombosis are not always as clear, even though it is often the first pathological alteration to occur. The first observations may be bleeding and sometimes very extensive hemorrhage. Several organ systems are susceptible to microvascular thrombosis associated with dysfunction: cardiovascular, pulmonary, central nervous, renal, and hepatic systems. Acute and correct clinical interpretations are critical to preventing progression of DIC that may lead to multisystem organ dysfunction and failure. (Chapter 24 discusses multiple organ dysfunction syndrome.) Indicators of multisystem dysfunction include changes in level of consciousness or behaviour, confusion, seizure activity, oliguria, hematuria, hypoxia, hypotension, hemoptysis, chest pain, and tachycardia. Symmetrical cyanosis of fingers and toes (blue finger/toe syndrome), nose, and breast may be seen and shows macrovascular thrombosis. This may lead to infarction and gangrene that may require amputation. Jaundice also is seen and most likely results from red blood cell destruction rather than liver dysfunction.

Individuals with chronic or low-grade DIC do not present with the overt manifestations of hemorrhaging and thrombosis but instead have subacute bleeding and diffuse thrombosis. These individuals are described as having *compensated DIC*, or *nonovert DIC*. The major characteristic of this state is an increased turnover and decreased survival time of the components of hemostasis: platelets and clotting factors. Occasionally, diffuse or localized thrombosis develops, but this outcome is infrequent.

EVALUATION AND TREATMENT No single laboratory test can be used to effectively diagnose DIC. Diagnosis is based primarily on clinical symptoms and confirmed by a combination of laboratory tests. The person must present with a clinical condition that is known to be associated with DIC. The most commonly used combination of laboratory tests usually confirms thrombocytopenia or a rapidly decreasing platelet count on repeated testing, prolongation of clotting times, the presence of FSPs, and decreased levels of coagulation inhibitors. Platelet counts below $100 \times 10^9/L$ or a progressive decrease in platelet counts is sensitive for DIC, although not highly specific. These changes usually show consumption of platelets.

The standard coagulation tests (e.g., prothrombin time [PT], activated partial thromboplastin time [aPTT]) also have a high degree of sensitivity, but they are not highly specific for DIC. As a result of consumption of circulating clotting factors, these tests are usually abnormal, ranging from shortened to prolonged times. However, conditions other than DIC may prolong clotting times.

Detection of FSPs is more specific for DIC. Detection of D-dimers is a widely used test for DIC. A **D-dimer** is a molecule produced by plasmin degradation of cross-linked fibrin in clots. D-dimers in the blood can be quantified using ELISA tests that include commercially available and highly specific monoclonal antibody against the D-dimer. Agglutination tests for other FSPs are available. Levels of FSPs are elevated in the plasma in 95 to 100% of cases; however, they are less specific and only document the presence of plasmin and its action on fibrin. ELISAs for markers of thrombin activity are sometimes used.

Levels of coagulation inhibitors (e.g., antithrombin III [AT-III], protein C) can be measured by assays that rely on function or by ELISAs that quantify the amount of the specific inhibitor. AT-III levels can supply key information for diagnosing and monitoring therapy of DIC. Initial levels of functional AT-III are low in DIC because thrombin is irreversibly complexed with activated clotting factors and AT-III.

Treatment of DIC is directed toward (1) ending the underlying pathological condition, (2) controlling ongoing thrombosis, and (3) supporting organ function. Elimination of the underlying pathological condition is the first intervention in the treatment phase to remove the trigger for activation of clotting. Once the stimulus is gone, production of coagulation factors in the liver leads to restoration of normal plasma levels within 24 to 48 hours.

Control of thrombosis is more difficult to reach. Heparin is used for this treatment. Its use, however, is controversial because its mechanism of action is binding to and activating AT-III, which is deficient in many types of DIC. Currently, heparin is only indicated in certain types of situations related to DIC. For instance, heparin seems to be effective in DIC caused by a retained dead fetus or associated with acute promyelocytic leukemia. Organ function is compromised by microthrombi, and there is a risk of losing an extremity because of vascular occlusion; thus, heparin is also indicated in these conditions. However, heparin's usefulness for DIC that is precipitated by septic shock has not been proven and so is contraindicated in that instance. Heparin is also contraindicated when there is evidence of postoperative bleeding, peptic ulcer, or CNS bleeding.

Replacement of deficient coagulation factors, platelets, and other coagulation elements is gaining recognition as an effective treatment modality. Their use is not without controversy, however, because a major concern with replacement therapy is the possible risk of adding components that will increase the rate of thrombosis. Clinical judgement is the key factor in determining whether replacement is to be used as a treatment modality. Several clinical trials are evaluating replacement of anticoagulants (i.e., AT-III, protein C). Antifibrinolytic medications also are used in treatment but are limited to instances of life-threatening bleeding that have not been controlled by blood part replacement therapy.

Maintenance of organ function is achieved by fluid replacement to sustain adequate circulating blood volume and support best tissue and organ perfusion. Fluids may be needed to restore blood pressure, cardiac output, and urine output to normal parameters.

Thromboembolic Disorders

Certain conditions within the blood vessels predispose an individual to develop clots spontaneously. A stationary clot attached to the vessel wall is called a **thrombus** (Figure 21.20). A thrombus is composed of fibrin and blood cells and can develop in either the arterial or the venous system. **Arterial thrombi** form under conditions of high blood flow and are composed mostly of platelet aggregates held together by fibrin strands. **Venous thrombi** form under conditions of low flow and are composed mostly of red blood cells with larger amounts of fibrin and few platelets.

A thrombus eventually reduces or obstructs blood flow to tissues or organs, such as the heart, brain, or lungs, depriving them of essential nutrients critical to survival. A thrombus also has the potential of detaching from the vessel wall and circulating within the bloodstream (referred to as an **embolus**). The embolus may become lodged in smaller blood vessels, blocking blood flow into the local tissue or organ, and leading to ischemia. Whether episodes of thromboembolism are life-threatening depends on the site of vessel occlusion.

Therapy consists of removal or dissolution of the clot and supportive measures. Anticoagulant therapy is effective in treating or preventing venous thrombosis. It is not as useful in treating or preventing arterial thrombosis. Parenteral heparin is the major anticoagulant used to treat thromboembolism. Oral warfarin (Coumadin) medications are also often used, including a newer direct factor Xa inhibitor (rivaroxaban [Xarelto]). More aggressive therapy may be indicated for such conditions as pulmonary embolism, coronary thrombosis, or thrombophlebitis. Streptokinase (Kabikinase), tissue plasminogen activator (Alteplase) (t-PA), and urokinase (Kinlytic) activate the fibrinolytic system and are administered to speed up the lysis of known thrombi. These medications are known as fibrinolytic or thrombolytic therapy and are prescribed cautiously because they can cause hemorrhagic complications.

The risk of developing spontaneous thrombi is related to several factors, referred to as the **Virchow triad**: (1) injury to the blood vessel endothelium, (2) abnormalities of blood flow, and (3) hypercoagulability of the blood.

Endothelial injury to blood vessels can result from atherosclerosis (plaque deposits on arterial walls) (see Chapter 24). Atherosclerosis initiates platelet adhesion and aggregation, promoting the development of atherosclerotic plaques that enlarge, causing further damage and occlusion. Other causes of vessel endothelial injury may be related to hemodynamic alterations associated with hypertension and turbulent blood flow. Injury also is caused by radiation injury, exogenous chemical agents (e.g., toxins from cigarette smoke), endogenous agents (e.g., cholesterol), bacterial toxins or endotoxins, or immunological mechanisms.

Sites of turbulent blood flow in the arteries and stasis of blood flow in the veins increase the risk for thrombus formation. In areas of turbulence, platelets and endothelial cells may be activated, leading to thrombosis. In sites of stasis, platelets may remain in contact with the endothelium for prolonged lengths of time, and clotting factors that would normally be diluted with fresh flowing blood are not diluted and may become activated. The most common clinical conditions that predispose to venous stasis and subsequent thromboembolic phenomena are major surgery (e.g., orthopedic surgery), acute myocardial infarction, heart failure, limb paralysis, spinal injury, malignancy, advanced age, the postpartum period, and bed rest longer than 1 week. Turbulence and stasis occur with ulcerated atherosclerotic plaques (myocardial infarction), hyperviscosity (polycythemia), and conditions with deformed red blood cells (sickle cell anemia).

Hypercoagulability, or thrombophilia, increases the risk for venous thrombosis. Hypercoagulability is differentiated according to whether it results from primary (hereditary) or secondary (acquired) causes.

Hereditary thrombophilias. Thrombophilias can result from both inherited conditions and, more commonly, acquired conditions.[59] Several inherited conditions increase the risk of developing thrombosis, and most are autosomal dominant. Thus, individuals who are homozygous for the mutation are at greatest risk for thrombosis. These include mutations in platelet receptors, coagulation proteins, fibrinolytic proteins, and other factors. The particular mutations that have been most strongly linked as risk factors for venous thrombosis or for arterial thrombosis leading to coronary artery disease or stroke include those that affect fibrinogen, prothrombin (G20210A variant), factor V (factor V Leiden) of the coagulation system. Other inherited thrombophilias are risk factors mostly for venous thrombosis and include deficiencies in protein C, protein S, and AT-III.[59] Other hereditary thrombophilias are less common.

Tests to diagnose inherited thrombophilias include PT; PTT; and levels of protein C, protein S, and AT-III. More elaborate tests to detect precise mutations in factor V, prothrombin, or methylenetetrahydrofolate reductase may be indicated.

Acquired hypercoagulability. Deficiencies in proteins S and C and AT-III may be acquired and contribute to a hypercoagulable state.[60] Conditions associated with an acquired protein deficiency include DIC, liver disease, infection, deep venous thrombosis, acute respiratory distress syndrome, L-asparaginase therapy, HUS, and TTP. The

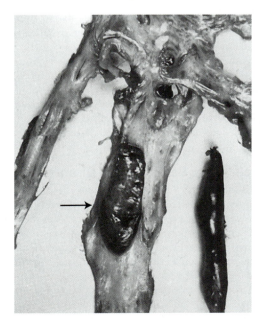

FIGURE 21.20 Thrombus. Thrombus arising in valve pocket at upper end of superficial femoral vein (*arrow*). Postmortem clot on the right is shown for comparison. (From McLachlin, J., & Paterson, J. C. [1951]. *Surgery, Gynecology & Obstetrics, 93*[1], 1–8.)

postoperative state also predisposes an individual to protein C or S deficiency; however, its role in contributing to deep venous thrombosis is still unclear.

Acquired hypercoagulable states include antiphospholipid syndrome (APS).[60] APS is an autoimmune syndrome characterized by autoantibodies against plasma membrane phospholipids and phospholipid-binding proteins. As with most autoimmune diseases, the predominantly affected individual is female and of reproductive age. Those with APS are at risk for both arterial and venous thrombosis and a variety of obstetrical complications, including pregnancy loss and pre-eclampsia/eclampsia. In severe cases the individual may die from recurrent major thrombus formation.[61] The pathophysiology is related to autoantibodies directly reacting with platelets or endothelial cells (increasing the risk for thrombosis) or the placental surface (resulting in damage to the placenta). The predominant diagnostic tests measure prolongation of laboratory blood coagulation tests related to an antibody inhibitor (lupus anticoagulant) and specific ELISAs for antibodies against phospholipids (e.g., anticardiolipin antibody) or proteins that bind to phospholipids (e.g., β_2-glycoprotein I). Highly effective therapy (i.e., unfractionated, or low-molecular-weight heparin with low-dose Aspirin) is available to prevent the obstetric complications.[61]

CASE STUDY

Jana Silva is a 25-year-old college student who presents to her primary care provider for an annual checkup. When asked by the primary care provider how she has been feeling, Ms. Silva states, "I have been feeling really tired for the past 4 months and I don't seem to have any energy".

History of Present Illness: 1-year history of menorrhagia; gradual onset of extreme fatigue and decreased energy, menstrual cycle every 28 days, 5 days of heavy flow and intense cramping.

Past Medical Hx: unremarkable, G0P0A0

Medications: ibuprofen 200 mg 6 times daily during menses and PRN for headaches, no herbal, no vitamins

Social history: nonsmoker, nondrinker, no recreational drugs, strict vegetarian for 6 years

Review of Systems: negative history of hematuria, hematemesis, hemoptysis, or melena, 2-month history of intense cravings for crushed ice, frequent headaches

Physical Exam: tachycardia, pale cool skin with normal turgor, pale conjunctiva and palmar creases, and pale moist oral mucosa. Remaining exam unremarkable.

Vital signs: BP 110/60 left arm sitting; RR 20 unlaboured; Pulse: 130 regular; Temperature 37°C oral; BMI 28

Critical Thinking and Clinical Judgement Questions

1. The primary care provider suspects a diagnosis of iron deficiency anemia. Based on the information provided, identify three possible contributing factors for this diagnosis.
2. When considering the subjective data provided, identify the clinical symptoms that are consistent with the diagnosis of iron deficiency anemia.
3. When considering the objective data provided, identify the clinical signs that are consistent with the diagnosis of iron deficiency anemia.
4. Name the laboratory tests that the primary care provider could order to confirm the diagnosis of iron deficiency anemia. Indicate what each test is assessing and provide the expected results that would confirm a diagnosis of iron deficiency anemia.
5. What possible treatments might the primary care provider discuss with this patient?

DID YOU UNDERSTAND?

Alterations of Erythrocyte Function

1. *Anemia* is defined as a reduction in the number or volume of circulating red blood cells or a decrease in the quality or quantity of hemoglobin.
2. The most common classification of anemias is based on changes in the cell size—represented by the cell suffix -*cytic*—and changes in the cell's hemoglobin content—represented by the suffix -*chromic*.
3. Clinical manifestations of anemia can be found in all organs and tissues. Decreased oxygen delivery to tissues causes fatigue, dyspnea, syncope, angina, compensatory tachycardia, and organ dysfunction.
4. Macrocytic (megaloblastic) anemias are characterized by unusually large stem cells in the marrow that mature into very large erythrocytes. Macrocytic anemias are caused most commonly by deficiencies of vitamin B_{12} or folate. Pernicious anemia, the most common type of macrocytic anemia, can be fatal unless vitamin B_{12} replacement is given.
5. Microcytic-hypochromic anemias are characterized by abnormally small red blood cells with insufficient hemoglobin content. The most common cause is iron deficiency.
6. Iron deficiency anemia (IDA) is the most common type of anemia worldwide. It usually develops slowly, with a gradual, insidious onset of symptoms, including fatigue, weakness, dyspnea, alteration of various epithelial tissues, and vague neuromuscular complaints.
7. IDA is usually a result of a chronic blood loss or decreased iron intake. Once the source of blood loss is found and corrected, iron replacement therapy can be started.
8. Sideroblastic anemias (SAs) are a heterogeneous group of inherited and acquired disorders. SAs have various causes, but all share altered heme synthesis.
9. Normocytic-normochromic anemias are characterized by insufficient numbers of normal erythrocytes. Included in this category are aplastic, posthemorrhagic, hemolytic, and anemia of chronic inflammation.

Myeloproliferative Red Blood Cell Disorders

1. Polycythemia vera (PV) is a stem cell disorder with hyperplastic and neoplastic bone marrow changes. It is characterized by excessive proliferation of erythrocyte precursors in the bone marrow. Polycythemia is responsible for most of the clinical symptoms, including increased blood volume and viscosity. Frequent phlebotomies reduce iron levels, and hydroxyurea is the medication of choice for myelosuppression.
2. PV may spontaneously convert to acute myeloid (or myelogenous) leukemia.

Alterations of Leukocyte Function

1. Quantitative alterations of leukocytes (too many or too few) can be caused by bone marrow dysfunction or premature destruction

of cells in the circulation. Many quantitative changes in leukocytes occur in response to invasion by microorganisms.
2. Leukocytosis is a condition in which the leukocyte count is higher than normal. It is usually a response to physiological stressors and invasion of microorganisms.
3. Leukopenia is present when the leukocyte count is lower than normal. It is caused by pathological conditions, such as malignancies and hematological disorders.
4. Granulocytosis occurs in response to infection and inflammation.
5. Granulocytopenia, a significant decrease in the number of neutrophils, can be a life-threatening condition if sepsis occurs. It is often caused by chemotherapeutic agents, severe infection, and radiation.
6. Eosinophilia results most commonly from allergic disorders, parasitic invasion, and ingestion or inhalation of toxic foreign particles.
7. Basophilia is rare and generally is a response to inflammation and immediate hypersensitivity reactions. Basopenia is a decrease in circulating numbers of basophils.
8. Monocytosis is an increase in the number of circulating monocytes and is often transient. It occurs during the late or recuperative phase of infection. Monocytopenia is a decrease in the number of circulating monocytes.
9. Lymphocytopenia is a decrease in the number of circulating lymphocytes in the blood. It is associated with neoplasias, immune deficiencies, and destruction by medications, viruses, or radiation.
10. Infectious mononucleosis (IM) is an acute infection of B cells most commonly associated with the Epstein-Barr virus (EBV). The classic symptoms are pharyngitis, lymphadenopathy, and fever. The proliferation of infected B cells may be uncontrolled and lead to B-cell lymphomas.
11. Transmission of EBV is usually through saliva from close personal contact. IM is self-limiting, and treatment consists of rest and symptomatic treatment.
12. The common pathological feature of all forms of leukemia is an uncontrolled proliferation of malignant leukocytes. This causes an overcrowding of bone marrow and decreased production and function of normal hematopoietic cells.
13. The classification of leukemias is based on the cell type involved—myeloid or lymphoid—and the rate of progression—acute or chronic. There are four major types of leukemia: (a) acute lymphocytic leukemia (ALL), (b) acute myeloid (or myelogenous) leukemia (AML), (c) chronic lymphocytic leukemia (CLL), and (d) chronic myeloid (or myelogenous) leukemia (CML).
14. The exact cause of leukemia is unknown. Several risk factors and related genetic aberrations are associated with the onset of malignancy. The leukemias are clonal disorders driven by genetically abnormal stem-like cancer cells.
15. Abnormal immature white blood cells, called *blasts*, fill the bone marrow and spill into the blood. The blasts overcrowd the marrow and cause cellular proliferation of the other cell lines to cease.
16. The major clinical manifestations of leukemia include fatigue caused by anemia, bleeding caused by thrombocytopenia, fever secondary to infection, anorexia, and weight loss.
17. Treatment depends on the type of leukemia and includes observation, steroids, chemotherapy, monoclonal antibodies, and transplant options.
18. Chronic leukemias progress slowly and insidiously. Acute leukemias can have an abrupt stormy onset.

Alterations of Lymphoid Function

1. Lymphadenopathy is characterized by enlarged lymph nodes.
2. Lymphomas consist of a diverse group of neoplasms that develop from the proliferation of malignant lymphocytes in the lymphoid system. There are three major categories of lymphomas: (a) B-cell neoplasms, (b) T-cell and natural killer (NK)–cell neoplasms, and (c) the two general categories of Hodgkin's lymphoma (HL) and non-Hodgkin's lymphoma (NHL).
3. Lymphomas are the result of genetic mutations or viral infection. Malignant transformation produces a cell with uncontrolled and excessive growth that accumulates in the lymph nodes and other sites, producing tumour masses.
4. HL is characterized by the presence of B cells called the Reed-Sternberg cells.
5. The pathogenesis of HL may be linked to infection with EBV.
6. An enlarged, painless mass or swelling, most commonly in the neck, is a first sign of HL. Asymptomatic lymphadenopathy, however, can progress undetected for years.
7. Treatment of HL includes chemotherapy, radiation therapy, and surgery. Treatment with chemotherapy or radiation therapy, or both, may increase the risk for secondary cancers, cardiovascular disease, and other health problems.
8. NHL is not a single disease, but a heterogeneous group of proliferative lymphoid tissue neoplasms. Clonal expansion of B cells accounts for the majority of NHLs. Oncogenes may be activated by chromosomal translocation or by deletion of tumour-suppressor genes. Certain subtypes may have altered genomes by oncogenic viruses.
9. With NHL, the swelling of lymph nodes is painless, and the nodes enlarge and transform over a period of months or years.
10. Standard treatment for NHL includes radiation therapy, chemotherapy, target therapy (monoclonal antibody therapy, proteasome inhibitor therapy), plasmapheresis, biological therapy, and watchful waiting.
11. Burkitt lymphoma is a B-cell tumour and involves the jaw and facial bones and sometimes the abdomen. Burkitt lymphoma is heterogeneous and may involve infection with EBV and suppression of the immune system by other illnesses.
12. Treatment for Burkitt lymphoma is intensive chemotherapy.
13. Multiple myeloma (MM) is a neoplasm of plasma cells in the bone marrow and usually not found in the peripheral blood. It is characterized by multiple malignant tumour masses of plasma cells scattered throughout the skeletal system and sometimes found in soft tissue.
14. MM tumours are highly heterogeneous and involve mutations in different signalling pathways. Chromosomal translocations are common. The exact cause of MM is unknown, but risk factors include radiation, certain chemicals, and a history of monoclonal gammopathy of undetermined significance (MGUS).
15. The common presentation of MM is characterized by elevated levels of calcium in the blood, renal failure, anemia, and bone lesions.
16. Treatment includes chemotherapy, radiation therapy, plasmapheresis, and stem cell transplant.

Alterations of Splenic Function

1. Splenomegaly may be considered normal in certain individuals, but its presence is associated with various diseases.
2. Splenomegaly results from (a) acute inflammatory or infectious processes, (b) congestive disorders, (c) infiltrative processes, and (d) tumours or cysts.
3. Hypersplenism results from splenomegaly. Hypersplenism results in sequestering of the blood cells, causing increased destruction of red blood cells, leukopenia, and thrombocytopenia.

Hemorrhagic Disorders and Alterations of Platelets and Coagulation

1. The arrest of bleeding is called *hemostasis*.

2. Thrombocytopenia is characterized by a platelet count below 150×10^9/L of blood. The most significant count is less than 100×10^9/L, and a count less than 50×10^9/L increases the potential for hemorrhage associated with minor trauma.
3. Thrombocytopenia exists in primary or secondary forms. It is associated with autoimmune diseases, viral infections, medications, nutritional deficiencies, chronic renal failure, cancer, radiation therapy, bone marrow hypoplasia, and disseminated intravascular coagulation (DIC).
4. Immune thrombocytopenic purpura (ITP) is the most common cause of thrombocytopenia, secondary to increased platelet destruction.
5. Thrombocythemia is characterized by a platelet count greater than 400×10^9/L of blood. It is symptomatic when the count exceeds $1\,000 \times 10^9$/L, at which time the risk for intravascular clot formation (thrombosis), hemorrhage, or other abnormalities can occur.
6. Essential (primary) thrombocythemia is a myeloproliferative neoplasm characterized by an increase in platelet production and often an increase in red blood cell production.
7. Qualitative alterations in normal platelet function prevent platelet plug formation and may result in prolonged bleeding times. Acquired disorders of platelet function are more common than congenital disorders.
8. Disorders of coagulation are usually caused by defects or deficiencies in one or more of the clotting factors. Coagulation is stimulated by the presence of tissue factor that is released by damaged or dead tissues.
9. Coagulation is impaired when there is a deficiency of vitamin K because of insufficient production of prothrombin and synthesis of clotting factors VII, IX, and X, often associated with liver diseases.
10. DIC is an acquired clinical syndrome characterized by widespread activation of coagulation, resulting in formation of fibrin clots in medium and small vessels or microvasculature throughout the body. Widespread clotting may lead to blockage of blood flow to organs, resulting in multiple organ failure. The size of clotting may result in consumption of platelets and clotting factors, leading to a tendency to bleed despite widespread clots.
11. DIC is secondary to a wide variety of clinical conditions; sepsis is the most common condition associated with DIC.
12. For a diagnosis of DIC, the person must present with a clinical condition that is known to be associated with DIC.
13. Treatment of DIC is directed toward (a) ending the underlying pathological condition, (b) controlling ongoing thrombosis, and (c) supporting organ function.
14. Thromboembolic disorders result from a fixed (thrombus) or moving (embolus) clot that blocks flow within a vessel, denying nutrients to tissues distal to the occlusion. Death can result when clots obstruct blood flow to the heart, brain, or lungs.
15. The term *Virchow triad* refers to three factors that can cause thrombus formation: (a) injury to the blood vessel endothelium, (b) abnormalities of blood flow, and (c) hypercoagulability of the blood.
16. Hypercoagulability, or thrombophilia, is a condition in which an individual is at risk for thrombosis.

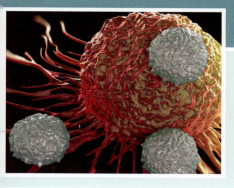

22

Developmental Alterations of Hematological Function

Kelly Power-Kean, with originating chapter contributions by Laura A. Linder and Kathryn L. McCance

Additional resources are available online at https://evolve.elsevier.com/Canada/Huether/pathophysiology.

CHAPTER OUTLINE

Disorders of Erythrocytes, 537
　Acquired Disorders, 538
　Inherited Disorders, 540
Disorders of Coagulation and Platelets, 545
　Inherited Hemorrhagic Disease, 545
　Antibody-Mediated Hemorrhagic Disease, 546

Neoplastic Disorders, 547
　Leukemia, 547
　Lymphomas, 548

LEARNING OBJECTIVES

1. Name the causes and symptoms that are unique to childhood iron deficiency anemia.
2. Describe the maternal–newborn blood incompatibilities that cause hemolytic diseases in newborns.
3. Describe the genetic abnormalities that produce sickle cell anemia and the thalassemias.
4. Describe the four types of sickle cell crisis.
5. Compare and contrast the types of thalassemia.
6. Differentiate between the inherited hemophilias. Discuss treatment options and complications of the disorders.
7. Describe the acquired antibody-mediated hemorrhagic diseases of childhood.
8. Name the childhood leukemias and discuss the causes.
9. Describe the etiology, morbidity, and mortality of Hodgkin's and non-Hodgkin's lymphomas in childhood.

KEY TERMS

α-Thalassemia major, 544
α-Thalassemia minor, 544
α-Thalassemia trait, 544
Aplastic crisis, 542
β-Thalassemia major (Cooley's anemia), 544
β-Thalassemia minor, 544
Blast cell, 547
Glucose-6-phosphate dehydrogenase (G6PD) deficiency, 538
Hemoglobin H disease, 544
Hemoglobin S (Hb S), 540
Hemolytic anemia, 538
Hemolytic disease of the fetus and newborn (HDFN) (erythroblastosis fetalis), 538
Hemophilia A, 545
Hemophilia B, 545
Hodgkin's lymphoma (HL), 548
Hydrops fetalis, 539
Hyperbilirubinemia, 539
Hyperhemolytic crisis, 542
Icterus gravis neonatorum, 539
Icterus neonatorum (neonatal jaundice), 539
Immune thrombocytopenic purpura (ITP), 546
Kernicterus, 539
Leukemia, 547
Leukemic cell, 547
Lymphoblast, 547
Lymphoma, 548
Non-Hodgkin's lymphoma (NHL), 548
Sequestration crisis, 542
Sickle cell anemia, 540
Sickle cell disease, 540
Sickle cell–hemoglobin C disease, 541
Sickle cell–thalassemia disease, 540
Sickle cell trait, 540
Thalassemia, 538
Vaso-occlusive crisis (thrombotic crisis), 542

This chapter includes conditions in children that affect red blood cells, the coagulation process and platelets, and disorders involving white blood cells. Discussions of both acquired conditions and inherited conditions are also presented.

DISORDERS OF ERYTHROCYTES

✓ QUICK CHECK 22.1
1. Why is Rh incompatibility rare today?
2. Why do clinical manifestations of sickle cell disease not appear until the infant is at least 6 months old?
3. Why do children with thalassemia major develop cardiovascular complications?

TABLE 22.1 Anemias of Childhood

Cause	Anemic Condition
Deficient Erythropoiesis or Hemoglobin Synthesis	
Decreased stem cell population in marrow (congenital or acquired pure red cell aplasia)	Normocytic-normochromic anemia
Decreased erythropoiesis despite normal stem cell population in marrow (infection, inflammation, cancer, chronic renal disease, congenital dyserythropoiesis)	Normocytic-normochromic anemia
Deficiency of a factor or nutrient needed for erythropoiesis	
Cobalamin (vitamin B_{12}), folate	Megaloblastic anemia
Iron	Microcytic-hypochromic anemia
Increased or Premature Hemolysis	
Alloimmune disease (maternal–fetal Rh, ABO, or minor blood group incompatibility)	Autoimmune hemolytic anemia
Autoimmune disease (idiopathic autoimmune hemolytic anemia, symptomatic systemic lupus erythematosus, lymphoma, medication-induced autoimmune processes)	Autoimmune hemolytic anemia
Inherited defects of plasma membrane structure (spherocytosis, elliptocytosis, stomatocytosis) or cellular size or both (pyknocytosis)	Hemolytic anemia
Infection (bacterial sepsis, congenital syphilis, malaria, cytomegalovirus infection, rubella, toxoplasmosis, disseminated herpes)	Hemolytic anemia
Intrinsic and inherited enzymatic defects (deficiencies) of glucose-6-phosphate dehydrogenase, pyruvate kinase, 5′-nucleotidase, glucose phosphate isomerase	Hemolytic anemia
Inherited defects of hemoglobin synthesis	Sickle cell anemia Thalassemia
Disseminated intravascular coagulation (see Chapter 21)	Hemolytic anemia
Galactosemia	Hemolytic anemia
Prolonged or recurrent respiratory or metabolic acidosis	Hemolytic anemia
Blood vessel disorders (cavernous hemangiomas, large vessel thrombus, renal artery stenosis, severe coarctation of aorta)	Hemolytic anemia

Anemia is the most common blood disorder in children. As with adult anemias, anemias occurring in children result from inadequate erythropoiesis or early destruction of erythrocytes. Iron deficiency is the most common cause of insufficient erythropoiesis. Iron deficiency can result from insufficient dietary intake or chronic loss of iron caused by bleeding. The hemolytic anemias of childhood are either inherited or acquired. They may be divided into disorders that result from destruction caused by (1) intrinsic abnormalities of the erythrocytes and (2) damaging factors external to the erythrocytes.

The most dramatic form of acquired congenital hemolytic anemia is hemolytic disease of the fetus and newborn (HDFN), also termed *erythroblastosis fetalis*. HDFN results when maternal blood and fetal blood are incompatible. This causes the mother's immune system to produce antibodies against fetal erythrocytes.

Intracellular defects in red blood cells include enzyme deficiencies and defects of hemoglobin synthesis. The most common deficiency is glucose-6-phosphate dehydrogenase (G6PD) deficiency. The defects of hemoglobin synthesis, which manifest as sickle cell disease or thalassemia, depends on which component of hemoglobin is defective. Table 22.1 lists these and other causes of childhood anemia.

Acquired Disorders

Iron Deficiency Anemia

IDA is the most common nutritional disorder worldwide, with the highest incidence occurring between 6 months and 2 years of age. IDA is common in Canada with prevalence higher in toddlers, adolescent girls, and women of childbearing age.[1] There are certain Indigenous populations in Canada in whom the prevalence is very high. IDA causes clinical manifestations mostly related to inadequate hemoglobin synthesis.[2] Iron is *critical* to the developing child, especially for normal brain development. Without it, the damage from the periods of IDA is irreversible.

IDA can result from (1) dietary lack of iron, (2) problems with iron absorption, (3) blood loss, and (4) increased requirement for iron. Inadequate intake of iron is the most common cause of IDA during the first few years of life. Blood loss is the most common cause during childhood and adolescence.

Dietary lack of iron is not common in developed countries, where iron is readily absorbed from heme found in meat. In developing countries, food may be less available. Although iron is found in plants, it is a more poorly absorbed form.[2] Infants are at increased risk for IDA because of very small amounts of iron in milk. Availability of iron from breast milk is higher than that from cow's milk. Chronic diarrhea, fat malabsorption, and sprue have impaired absorption.

Blood loss may not always be obvious. For example, blood loss caused by a gastro-intestinal lesion, parasitic infestation, or hemorrhagic disease can be occult (hidden) and result in chronic IDA. Chronic parasite infestations, which result in blood and iron loss greater than dietary intake, often occur in children in developing countries. Treatment of parasitic infections results in improvement in appetite and growth, as well as reduction of anemia. Infants and young children who drink excessive amounts of cow's milk may also develop IDA because of chronic intestinal blood loss. A protein in cow's milk may induce inflammation that damages the intestinal mucosa, causing diffuse, chronic microhemorrhage. Cellular components of both innate and adaptive immunity may play significant roles in the development of cow's milk allergy.

The association between IDA and lead poisoning is controversial. New areas of investigation include iron deficiency in overweight children and the association of *Helicobacter pylori* infection with IDA.[3,4]

PATHOPHYSIOLOGY No matter the cause, iron deficiency produces a hypochromic-microcytic anemia.[2] In the early stages, the body may respond by increasing red blood cell activity in the bone marrow. This may temporarily prevent the development of anemia. As the body's iron stores are decreased, anemia develops. Low serum levels of ferritin and transferrin saturation lead to lowered hemoglobin and hematocrit levels.

CLINICAL MANIFESTATIONS The symptoms of mild anemia—listlessness and fatigue—may go unnoticed in infants and young children, who are unable to describe these symptoms. Clinical indicators of anemia also are nonspecific, such as irritability, decreased activity tolerance, weakness, and lack of interest in play, and may be attributed to other causes. As a result, parents may not note persistent changes in the child's behaviour until moderate anemia has developed. Other clinical manifestations, such as pallor, anorexia, tachycardia, and systolic murmurs, are often not present until hemoglobin levels fall below 50 mmol/L.

Other symptoms and signs of chronic IDA include splenomegaly, widened skull sutures, decreased physical growth, developmental delays, pica (a behaviour in which nonfood substances, such as clay, are eaten), and altered neurological and intellectual functions. The child's attention span, alertness, and learning ability are most affected.

EVALUATION AND TREATMENT Laboratory tests confirm the diagnosis of IDA. These tests include hemoglobin, hematocrit, serum iron, and ferritin levels and the total iron binding capacity. Obtaining a thorough account of the child's present illness and dietary history and performing a complete physical examination are essential to the evaluation and treatment of IDA. Treatment is similar for both children and adults (see Chapter 21). Oral administration of a simple ferrous salt is usually sufficient. Taking iron supplements with a vitamin C source helps promote absorption.[2] The administration of iron in a liquid form should be through a straw or a dropper placed back on the tongue to prevent staining the teeth. To prevent recurrences of IDA, dietary modification must occur. This includes increasing the intake of iron-rich foods and limiting the intake of cow's milk to the recommended daily allowance for age.

Hemolytic Disease of the Fetus and Newborn

The most common cause of hemolytic anemia in newborns is alloimmune disease. **Hemolytic disease of the fetus and newborn (HDFN) (erythroblastosis fetalis)** can occur only if antigens on fetal erythrocytes differ from antigens on maternal erythrocytes. Most cases are caused by ABO incompatibility. This occurs if the mother and fetus have different ABO blood types. About 1 in 3 cases of HDFN is caused by Rh incompatibility, which occurs when the fetus is Rh-positive, and the mother is Rh-negative. Some minor blood antigens also may be involved (see Chapter 7).

ABO incompatibility occurs in about 20 to 25% of all pregnancies. Only 1 in 10 of these cases results in HDFN. Rh incompatibility occurs in less than 10% of pregnancies. It rarely causes HDFN in the first incompatible fetus. During the first pregnancy, erythrocytes from the fetus cause the mother's immune system to produce antibodies. These antibodies can then affect fetuses in subsequent incompatible pregnancies.

PATHOPHYSIOLOGY Three conditions need to be met for HDFN to occur: (1) the mother's blood contains preformed antibodies against fetal erythrocytes or produces them on exposure to fetal erythrocytes; (2) sufficient amounts of antibody (usually immunoglobulin G [IgG]) cross the placenta and enter fetal blood; and (3) IgG binds with sufficient numbers of fetal erythrocytes to cause widespread antibody-mediated hemolysis or splenic removal. (Chapter 8 describes antibody-mediated cellular destruction.)

In most cases of HDFN, the mother has blood type O and the fetus has blood type A or B. Maternal antibodies may be formed against type B erythrocytes if the mother is type A or against type A erythrocytes if the mother is type B.

ABO incompatibility can cause HDFN even if fetal erythrocytes do not escape into the maternal circulation during pregnancy. HDFN occurs because the blood of most adults already contains anti-A or anti-B antibodies. The production of these antibodies occurs on exposure to certain foods or infection by Gram-negative bacteria. As a result, IgG against type A or B erythrocytes are created in maternal blood. This IgG can enter the fetal circulation throughout the first incompatible pregnancy. Anti-O antibodies do not exist because type O erythrocytes are not antigenic. Anti-Rh antibodies form only in response to the presence of Rh-positive erythrocytes from the fetus in the blood of a Rh-negative mother. The mixing of fetal blood with the mother's blood occurs at the time of delivery. Exposure may also occur through transfused blood, and, rarely, previous sensitization of the mother by her own mother's incompatible blood (Figure 22.1).

The first Rh-incompatible pregnancy generally presents no difficulties for the fetus. This is because few fetal erythrocytes cross the placental barrier during the pregnancy. When the placenta detaches at birth, many fetal erythrocytes often enter the mother's bloodstream. If the mother is Rh-negative and the fetus is Rh-positive, the mother produces anti-Rh antibodies. These anti-Rh antibodies persist in the bloodstream for a long time. If the next offspring is Rh-positive, the mother's anti-Rh antibodies can enter the bloodstream of the fetus and destroy the erythrocytes.

The destruction of IgG-coated fetal erythrocytes usually occurs in the spleen. As hemolysis proceeds, the fetus becomes anemic. Erythropoiesis increases, especially in the liver and spleen. The release of immature nucleated cells (erythroblasts) into the bloodstream (hence the name *erythroblastosis fetalis*) then occurs. The degree of anemia depends on several factors: (1) the length of time the antibody has been in the fetal circulation; (2) the concentration of the antibody; and (3) the ability of the fetus to compensate for increased hemolysis. The formation of unconjugated (indirect) bilirubin occurs during breakdown of hemoglobin. The bilirubin is then transported across the placental barrier into the maternal circulation and is excreted by the mother. Hyperbilirubinemia occurs in the neonate after birth because excretion of lipid-soluble unconjugated bilirubin through the placenta is no longer possible.

HDFN is typically more severe in Rh incompatibility than in ABO incompatibility. Rh incompatibility is more likely to result in severe or even life-threatening anemia, death *in utero*, or damage to the central nervous system. Severe anemia alone can cause death because of cardiovascular complications. Extensive hemolysis also results in increased levels of unconjugated bilirubin in the neonate's circulation. If bilirubin levels exceed the liver's ability to conjugate and excrete bilirubin, it can be deposited in the brain, a condition known as **kernicterus**.

Fetuses that do not survive anemia *in utero* usually are stillborn, with gross edema in the entire body, a condition called **hydrops fetalis**. Death can occur as early as 17 weeks' gestation and results in spontaneous abortion.

CLINICAL MANIFESTATIONS Neonates with mild HDFN may appear healthy or slightly pale, with slight enlargement of the liver or spleen. Extreme pallor, splenomegaly, and hepatomegaly indicate severe anemia, which predisposes the neonate to cardiovascular failure and shock. Life-threatening Rh incompatibility is rare largely because of the routine use of Rh immunoglobulin.

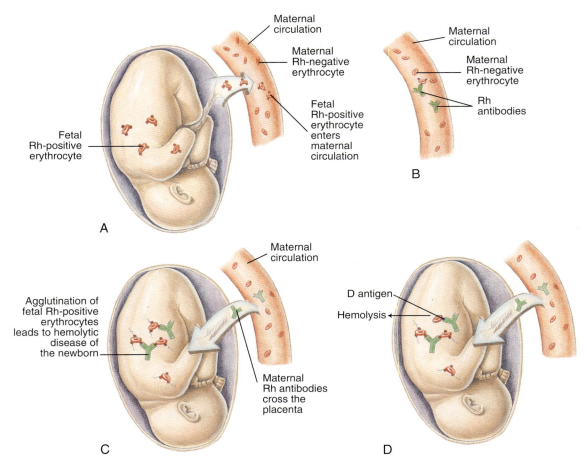

FIGURE 22.1 Hemolytic Disease of the Newborn. **A**, Before or during delivery, Rh-positive erythrocytes from the fetus enter the blood of a Rh-negative woman through a tear in the placenta. **B**, The mother is sensitized to the Rh antigen and produces Rh antibodies. Because this sensitization usually happens after delivery, there is no effect on the fetus in the first pregnancy. **C**, During a subsequent pregnancy with a Rh-positive fetus, Rh-positive erythrocytes cross the placenta, enter the maternal circulation, and **D**, stimulate the mother to produce antibodies against the Rh antigen. (Modified from Seeley, R. R., Stephens, T. D., Tate, P., et al. [1995]. *Anatomy and physiology* [3rd ed.]. Mosby.)

Because the maternal antibodies remain in the neonate's circulatory system after birth, erythrocyte destruction can continue. Without replacement transfusions, in which the neonate receives Rh-negative red blood cells, severe **hyperbilirubinemia** and **icterus neonatorum (neonatal jaundice)** can develop shortly after birth. If kernicterus develops, it can cause cerebral damage including intellectual disabilities, cerebral palsy, or high-frequency deafness. It may even cause death (**icterus gravis neonatorum**).

EVALUATION AND TREATMENT Fetuses and neonates with ABO incompatibility usually do not need additional monitoring or treatment. Fetuses and infants at risk for HDFN because of Rh incompatibility may require additional monitoring and treatment. Routine evaluation of fetuses at risk for HDFN includes the Coombs' test. The indirect Coombs' test measures antibodies in the mother's circulation and indicates whether the fetus is at risk for HDFN. The direct Coombs' test measures antibody already bound to the surfaces of fetal erythrocytes. It is used primarily to confirm the diagnosis of antibody mediated HDFN. If a prior history of fetal hemolytic disease is present, additional diagnostic tests are done to assess risk with the current pregnancy. These include maternal antibody titres, fetal blood sampling, amniotic fluid spectrophotometry, and ultrasound fetal assessment.

Prevention is the key to managing HDFN that results from Rh incompatibility. Immunoprophylaxis using Rh immune globulin (RhoGAM), a preparation of antibodies against Rh antigen D (anti-D Ig), prevents a Rh-negative woman from producing antibodies. If the administration of Rh immune globulin to a Rh-negative woman occurs within 72 hours of exposure to Rh-positive erythrocytes, she will not produce antibodies against the D antigen. As a result, the next Rh-positive baby she conceives will be protected. Updated guidelines also state that if anti-D Ig is not given within 72 hours, every effort should still be made to administer it within 10 days.[5]

Inherited Disorders
Sickle Cell Disease

Sickle cell disease is a group of autosomal recessive disorders characterized by the production of **hemoglobin S (Hb S; sickle hemoglobin)** within the erythrocytes. A genetic mutation in which one amino acid (valine) replaces another (glutamic acid) causes the formation of Hb S (Figure 22.2). Under conditions of decreased oxygen tension and dehydration, Hb S stretches and becomes longer. This process causes the erythrocyte to assume a characteristic sickle shape (see Figure 22.2). These sickled cells also die prematurely, resulting in hemolytic anemia.

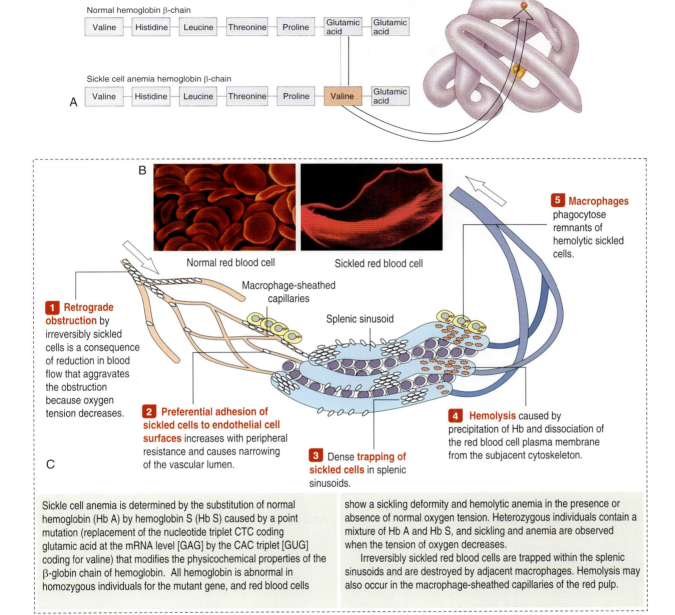

FIGURE 22.2 Sickle Cell Hemoglobin. A, Sickle cell hemoglobin is produced by a recessive allele of the gene encoding the β-chain of the protein hemoglobin. It represents a single amino acid change—from glutamic acid to valine at the sixth position of the chain. In this model of a hemoglobin molecule, the position of the mutation can be seen near the end of the upper arm. **B,** Colour-enhanced electron micrograph shows normal erythrocytes and sickled blood cell. **C,** Summary of sickle cell. ([A], from Raven, P. H., & Johnson, G. B. [1992]. *Biology* [3rd ed.]. Mosby; [B], Dennis Kunkel Microscopy/Science Source; [C], from Kierszenbaum, A., & Tres, L. [2012]. *Histology and cell biology: An introduction to pathology* [3rd ed.]. Mosby.)

The most prevalent types of sickle cell disease are sickle cell anemia, sickle cell–thalassemia, and sickle cell–Hb C (Table 22.2). (See Chapter 2 for a discussion of genetic inheritance of disease.) Sickle cell anemia, a homozygous form, is the most severe. It results when the individual inherits two copies of Hb S. Sickle cell–thalassemia and sickle cell–Hb C disease are heterozygous forms in which the child inherits Hb S from one parent and another type of abnormal hemoglobin from the other parent. Sickle cell trait occurs when the child inherits Hb S from one parent and normal hemoglobin (Hb A) from the other. This heterozygous carrier state rarely has clinical manifestations. All forms of sickle cell disease are lifelong conditions.

Sickle cell disease is most common among persons with ancestry from sub-Saharan Africa. Although less common, it also is present among individuals with ancestry from Mediterranean countries, the Arabian Peninsula, parts of India, and Spanish-speaking areas of South America. Estimates are that 5 000 people have been diagnosed with the disease in Canada.[6] The number of Canadian patients with sickle cell disease will continue to increase, related to high rates of immigration

TABLE 22.2 Inheritance of Sickle Cell Disease

Hemoglobin Inherited From First Parent	Hemoglobin Inherited From Second Parent	Form of Sickle Cell Disease in Child
Hemoglobin (Hb) S (an abnormal hemoglobin)	Hb S	Sickle cell anemia: homozygous inheritance in which child's hemoglobin is mostly Hb S, with remainder Hb F (fetal hemoglobin)
Hb S	Defective or insufficient α- or β-chains of Hb A (α- or β-thalassemia)	Sickle cell–thalassemia disease (heterozygous inheritance of Hb S and α- or β-thalassemia)
Hb S	Hb C or D (both abnormal hemoglobins)	Sickle cell–hemoglobin C (or D) disease (heterozygous inheritance of hemoglobin S and either C or D)
Hb S	Normal hemoglobins (mostly Hb A)	Sickle cell trait, carrier state (heterozygous inheritance of Hb S and normal hemoglobin)

from countries with high prevalence. Expectations are of improved outcomes for those affected by sickle cell disease with advances in medical care. Sickle cell–hemoglobin C disease is less common (1 in 800 births), and sickle cell–thalassemia disease occurs in 1 in 1 700 births.

Sickle cell trait occurs in 7 to 13% of African Americans. Its prevalence in African countries, such as Nigeria and the Democratic Republic of Congo, may be as high as 30%.[7] The sickle cell trait may provide protection against lethal forms of malaria. This results in a genetic advantage for carriers who reside in endemic regions for malaria (e.g., sub-Saharan Africa and some Mediterranean countries).

PATHOPHYSIOLOGY Hb S is soluble and usually causes no problem when properly oxygenated. When oxygen tension decreases, the abnormal β-globin chain of Hb S polymerizes, forming abnormal fluid polymers. As these polymers realign, they cause the red blood cell to form into the sickle shape. Decreased oxygenation, pH, and dehydration of the individual trigger the sickling process. Acute illness, stress, temperature changes, and living at higher altitude can cause decreased oxygen tension, leading to sickling.

Sickled erythrocytes tend to plug the blood vessels. This increases the viscosity of the blood, which slows circulation and causes vascular occlusion, pain, and organ infarction. Viscosity increases the time of exposure to less oxygenation, promoting further sickling. Sickled cells undergo hemolysis in the spleen or become sequestered there, causing blood pooling and infarction of splenic vessels. The anemia that follows triggers erythropoiesis in the marrow and, in extreme cases, in the liver (Figure 22.3).

Sickling usually is not permanent. Most sickled erythrocytes regain a normal shape after reoxygenation and rehydration. Sickling causes irreversible plasma membrane damage. In persons with sickle cell anemia, in which the erythrocytes contain a high percentage of Hb S (75 to 95%), up to 30% of the erythrocytes can become irreversibly sickled.

CLINICAL MANIFESTATIONS The clinical manifestations of sickle cell disease can vary. Some individuals have mild symptoms, and others suffer from repeated vaso-occlusive crises.[8] When sickling occurs, the general manifestations of hemolytic anemia include pallor, fatigue, jaundice, and irritability. Extensive sickling can cause four types of crises:

1. **Vaso-occlusive crisis (thrombotic crisis).** This crisis begins with sickling in the microcirculation. As blood flow is obstructed by sickled cells, vasospasm occurs, and a "logjam" effect blocks all blood flow through the vessel. Unless the process is reversed, thrombosis and infarction of local tissue follow. Vaso-occlusive crisis is extremely painful and may last for days or even weeks. An average duration is 4 to 6 days. The frequency of this type of crisis is variable and unpredictable. Vaso-occlusion in vessels to the brain can result in stroke. Chronic vaso-occlusion in vessels to the kidneys results in end-stage renal disease.

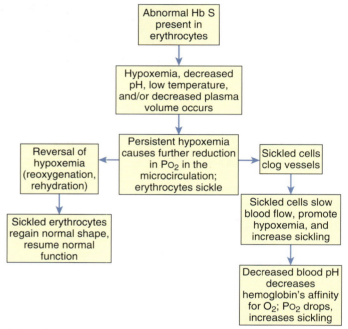

FIGURE 22.3 Sickling of Erythrocytes. *Hb S*, Hemoglobin S; O_2, oxygen; Po_2, partial pressure of oxygen.

2. **Sequestration crisis.** This type of crisis is usually seen in children less than 5 years of age. Large amounts of blood become acutely pooled in the liver and spleen. Because the spleen can hold as much as one-fifth of the body's blood supply at one time, the risk of mortality is high. About half of children who experience sequestration crises will have recurrent episodes.

3. **Aplastic crisis.** The cause of profound anemia is decreased erythropoiesis despite an increased need for new erythrocytes. In sickle cell anemia, erythrocyte survival is only 10 to 20 days. Normally the bone marrow is able to compensate to replace the cells lost through premature hemolysis. If this compensatory response does not occur, aplastic crisis develops. This type of crisis typically lasts 7 to 10 days.

4. **Hyperhemolytic crisis.** Although unusual, this crisis may occur in association with certain medications or infections. It has also been reported as an acute or chronic reaction following a blood transfusion.

The clinical manifestations of sickle cell disease usually do not appear until the infant is at least 6 months old. At that time postnatal concentrations of Hb F decrease causing concentrations of Hb S to rise (Figure 22.4). Infection is the most common cause of death related to sickle cell disease. Sepsis and meningitis develop in as many as 10% of children with sickle cell anemia during the first 5 years of life.

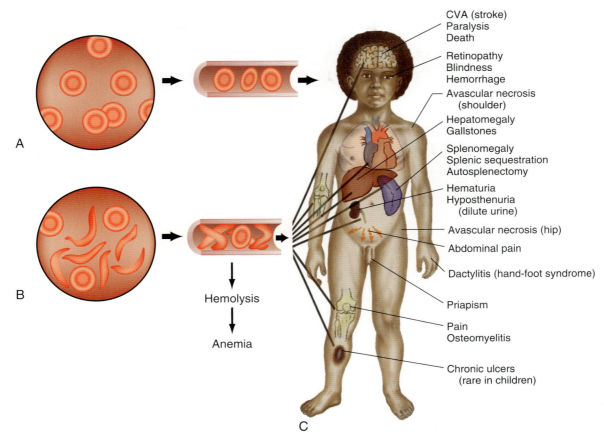

FIGURE 22.4 Differences Between Effects of A, Normal and B, Sickled Red Blood Cells on Blood Circulation, and Selected Consequences in a Child. C, Tissue Effects of Sickle Cell Anemia. *CVA,* Cerebrovascular accident. ([A and B], adapted from Hockenberry, M. J., & Wilson, D. [Eds.]. [2015]. *Wong's nursing care of infants and children* [10th ed.]. Mosby.)

Sickle cell–Hb C disease is usually milder than sickle cell anemia. The main clinical problems are related to vaso-occlusive crises. These events are thought to result from higher hematocrit and viscosity. In older children, sickle cell retinopathy, renal necrosis, and aseptic necrosis of the femoral heads occur along with obstructive crises.

Sickle cell–thalassemia has the mildest clinical manifestations of all the sickle cell diseases. The normal hemoglobins, particularly Hb F, inhibit sickling. The erythrocytes tend to be small (microcytic) and to contain less hemoglobin (hypochromic), making them less likely to occlude the microcirculation, even when in a sickled state.

EVALUATION AND TREATMENT The sickle cell trait does not affect life expectancy or interfere with daily activities. On rare occasions, severe hypoxia caused by shock, vigorous exercising at high altitudes, flying at high altitudes in unpressurized aircraft, or undergoing anaesthesia is associated with vaso-occlusive episodes in persons with sickle cell trait. These cells form an ivy shape instead of a sickle shape.

The parents' hematological history and clinical manifestations may suggest that a child has sickle cell disease, but hematological tests are necessary for diagnosis. If the sickle solubility test confirms the presence of Hb S in peripheral blood, hemoglobin electrophoresis provides information about the amount of Hb S in erythrocytes. Prenatal diagnosis can be made after chorionic villus sampling as early as 8 to 10 weeks' gestation or by amniotic fluid analysis at 15 weeks' gestation (Figure 22.5). Newborn screening for sickle cell disease should be performed according to provincial recommendations.

Advances in identification of the disease and supportive care have improved survival of children with sickle cell disease. Supportive care emphasizes preventing consequences of anemia and avoiding crises, which includes ensuring adequate hydration, infection prevention, and pain management. Genetic counselling and psychological support are important for the child and family.

A common treatment for sickle cell disease is hydroxyurea. Hydroxyurea inhibits DNA synthesis and causes an increase in Hb F concentration. It also provides an anti-inflammatory effect by decreasing leukocyte production. These outcomes are thought to decrease crises. Transfusion therapy can decrease morbidity and mortality associated with sickle cell disease, particularly in those at increased risk for stroke.[9] Despite these benefits, transfusion can result in iron overload, which can cause liver damage and fibrosis, delayed physical and sexual development, and heart disease. Chelation therapy to remove excess iron is often required.[10]

Hematopoietic stem cell transplantation offers the only cure for sickle cell disease. This treatment, however, does have risks. Current research is seeking to reduce the toxicities associated with transplantation while optimizing long-term outcomes.

Thalassemias

The α- and β-thalassemias are inherited autosomal recessive disorders that cause an impaired rate of synthesis of one of the two chains—α or β—of adult hemoglobin (Hb A). Beta-thalassemia is most prevalent among Greek, Italian, some Arab, and Sephardic Jewish people. Alpha-thalassemia is most common among Chinese, Vietnamese, Cambodians, and Laotians. Both α- and β-thalassemias are common among Black people. Beta-thalassemias are more common than alpha-thalassemias. Both types are further classified as major or minor. The

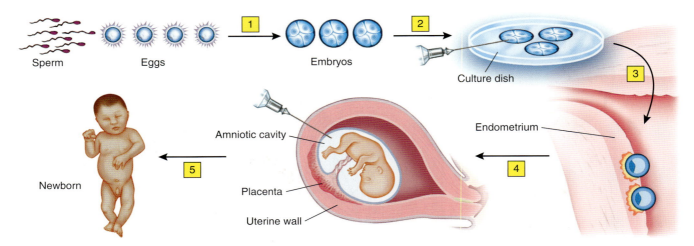

FIGURE 22.5 Prepregnancy Sickle Cell Test. This technique has potential for detection of other inherited diseases. (1) Fertilization produces several embryos. (2) The embryos are tested for the presence of the gene. (3) The embryos without the gene are implanted. (4) Amniocentesis confirms whether the fetus (or fetuses) has the sickle cell gene. (5) Child is born without being affected by sickle cell.

classification is based on the number of genes that control α- or β-chain synthesis. It is also based on the combination of mutations and whether they are homozygous (thalassemia major) or heterozygous (thalassemia minor). The anemic manifestation of thalassemia is microcytic-hypochromic hemolytic anemia.

PATHOPHYSIOLOGY Mutations that decrease the synthesis of β-globin chains cause the β-thalassemias. These conditions lead to anemia, tissue hypoxia, and red blood cell hemolysis. β-Chain production is depressed moderately in the heterozygous form, **β-thalassemia minor**, and severely in the homozygous form, **β-thalassemia major** (also called **Cooley's anemia**). As a result, erythrocytes have a reduced amount of hemoglobin and an accumulation of free α-chains (Figure 22.6). Free α-chains are unstable and easily precipitate in the cell. Mononuclear phagocytes in the marrow destroy most erythroblasts that contain precipitates. Destruction results in ineffective erythropoiesis and anemia. Some of the precipitate-carrying cells mature and enter the bloodstream. These cells are destroyed prematurely in the spleen, resulting in mild hemolytic anemia.

There are four forms of α-thalassemia: (1) **α-thalassemia trait** (the carrier state), in which a single α-chain–forming gene is defective; (2) **α-thalassemia minor**, in which two genes are defective; (3) **hemoglobin H disease**, in which three genes are defective; and (4) **α-thalassemia major**, a fatal condition in which all four α-forming genes are defective. Death is inevitable because α-chains are absent, and oxygen cannot be released to the tissues.

CLINICAL MANIFESTATIONS β-Thalassemia minor causes mild to moderate microcytic-hypochromic anemia. The degree of reticulocytosis depends on the severity of the anemia and results in skeletal changes. Hemolysis of immature (and therefore fragile) erythrocytes may cause a slight elevation in serum iron and indirect bilirubin levels. Persons with β-thalassemia minor may experience mild splenomegaly, bronze colouring of the skin, and hyperplasia of the bone marrow, but they are less likely to experience life-threatening complications.

Persons with β-thalassemia major may become quite ill and show impaired physical growth and development. Anemia is severe and results in a significant cardiovascular burden with high-output heart failure. In the past, death resulted from heart failure. Today, blood transfusions can increase lifespan by one to two decades. Death usually is caused by hemochromatosis (from transfusions). Liver enlargement occurs because of progressive hemosiderosis. Extramedullary hemopoiesis and increased destruction of red blood cells causes spleen enlargement. Skeletal changes begin in infancy and include spinal impairment that slows linear growth and subsequent upper and lower limb-length discrepancy. Deformity of the facial bones in response to hyperplastic marrow results in a characteristic chipmunk-like facial appearance.

Persons who inherit the mildest form of α-thalassemia (the α-thalassemia trait) usually are symptom-free or have mild microcytosis. α-Thalassemia minor has clinical manifestations that are virtually identical to those of β-thalassemia minor. This includes mild microcytic-hypochromic reticulocytosis, bone marrow hyperplasia, increased serum iron concentrations, and moderate splenomegaly.

Signs and symptoms of α-thalassemia major are like those of β-thalassemia major, but milder. Moderate microcytic-hypochromic anemia, enlargement of the liver and spleen, and bone marrow hyperplasia are evident.

α-Thalassemia major causes hydrops fetalis. This is the most severe form of α-thalassemia, caused by deletion of all four α-globin genes. The infant suffers from severe tissue anoxia and may develop fulminant intrauterine heart failure. Signs of fetal distress became evident by the third trimester of pregnancy. In the past, severe tissue anoxia led to death in utero. Intrauterine transfusions now prevent many of these deaths.

EVALUATION AND TREATMENT Evaluation of thalassemia is based on familial disease history, clinical manifestations, and blood tests. Peripheral blood smears that show microcytosis, and hemoglobin electrophoresis that demonstrates diminished amounts of α- or β-chains confirm the diagnosis. Prenatal diagnosis is sometimes made, and families are referred for genetic counselling. The analysis of fetal DNA from withdrawn amniotic fluid is a screening test to detect hydrops fetalis (α-thalassemia major). Newborn screening for thalassemia should follow provincial recommendations. Offering molecular genetic testing of at-risk siblings allows for early diagnosis and treatment.

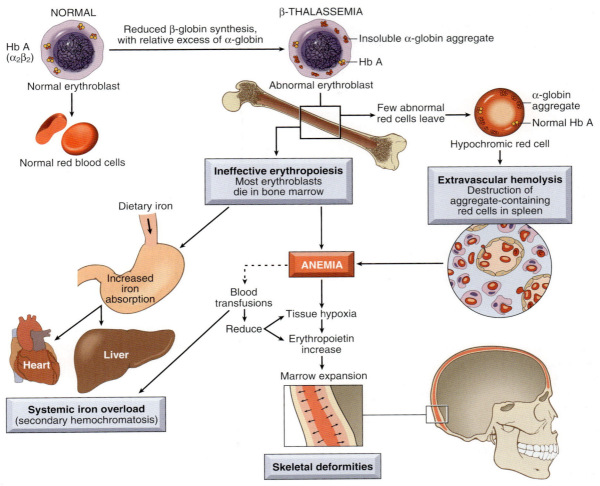

FIGURE 22.6 Pathogenesis of β-Thalassemia Major. The aggregates of unpaired α-globin chains are a hallmark of the disease. Blood transfusions can diminish the anemia, but they add to the systemic iron overload. *Hb A*, Hemoglobin A. (From Kumar, V., Abbas, A. K., & Aster, J. C. [Eds.]. [2021]. *Robbins and Cotran pathologic basis of disease* [10th ed.]. Elsevier.)

Treatment is largely supportive and involves a regular transfusion program and chelation therapy to reduce transfusion iron overload (see Figure 22.6). Milder forms of thalassemia rarely require transfusion. Allogeneic hematopoietic stem cell transplantation is the only cure. Optimal clinical management may decrease the need for splenectomy.

DISORDERS OF COAGULATION AND PLATELETS

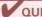 **QUICK CHECK 22.2**
1. List the major disorders of coagulation and platelets found in children.
2. Why are persons with hemophilia at risk of developing degenerative joint changes?
3. What is the major abnormality in immune thrombocytopenic purpura?

Inherited Hemorrhagic Disease
Hemophilias

The hemophilias are a group of inherited bleeding disorders resulting from mutations in coagulation factors. The focus of this section will be hemophilia A and hemophilia B. Both are X-linked recessive conditions, thus affecting mainly males and homozygous females.[11] A third type, hemophilia C, is an autosomal recessive condition that results from a deficiency of factor XI. Table 22.3 lists the coagulation factors and deficiencies associated with clinical bleeding.

Hemophilia A is defined as factor VIII deficiency and is the most common hereditary disease associated with life-threatening bleeding. A mutation in factor VIII, an essential cofactor for factor IX in the coagulation cascade, is the cause.

Hemophilia B results from a mutation in the *F9* gene, which codes for factor IX. Because both factors VIII and IX function together to activate factor X, hemophilia A and B are clinically indistinguishable. The incidence of hemophilia A is about 1 in 5000 male births. Hemophilia B is five times less common, with an incidence of about 1 in 30 000 male births. Hemophilia affects about 1 in 10 000 male births worldwide.[12] All ethnic groups are equally affected.

PATHOPHYSIOLOGY As X-linked recessive conditions, hemophilia A and B are most frequently inherited from a mother who is heterozygous for a mutation in either the *F8* or *F9* gene. Approximately 30% of cases, however, result from a new mutation. This new mutation can

TABLE 22.3 The Coagulation Factors and Associated Disorders

Clotting Factors	Synonym	Disorder
I	Fibrinogen	Congenital deficiency (afibrinogenemia) and dysfunction (dysfibrinogenemia)
II	Prothrombin	Congenital deficiency or dysfunction
V	Labile factor or proaccelerin	Congenital deficiency (parahemophilia)
VII	Stable factor or proconvertin	Congenital deficiency
VIII	Antihemophilic factor	Congenital deficiency is hemophilia A (classic hemophilia)
IX	Christmas factor	Congenital deficiency is hemophilia B
X	Stuart-Prower factor	Congenital deficiency
XI	Plasma thromboplastin antecedent	Congenital deficiency, sometimes referred to as *hemophilia C*
XII	Hageman factor	Congenital deficiency is *not* associated with clinical symptoms
XIII	Fibrin-stabilizing factor	Congenital deficiency

occur in either a carrier female or in an affected male. More than 1 300 mutations have been associated with factor VIII and IX deficiency. Affected individuals within the same family will have the same mutation; however, the mutation causing hemophilia may be different across families.[11]

The clinical manifestation of deficiencies of factor VIII and factor IX occurs almost exclusively in males. The *F8* and *F9* genes are located on the long arm of the X chromosome. A mutation in either of these genes typically results in either deficient or abnormal function of the corresponding clotting factor. Because a male's DNA contains only one X chromosome, hemophilia affects mostly males. In females, who have the second copy of the X chromosome, the mutation results in the clinical manifestations of hemophilia. The other X chromosome usually produces a sufficient quantity of normal functioning clotting factors. Females who are heterozygous carriers typically do not experience excessive bleeding. Because X-inactivation or lyonization (see Chapter 2) is a random process, phenotypes of women who are heterozygous carriers can vary. Fifty percent of female carriers have low clotting factor levels. Although very uncommon, it is possible for a female to be homozygous for mutations in the *F8* or *F9* gene and, therefore, have hemophilia.[11]

CLINICAL MANIFESTATIONS The clinical manifestations and severity of hemophilia depend largely on the level of factor VIII and IX activity. Joint bleeding is the most characteristic type of bleeding in hemophilia. The joints most often affected are the knees, ankles, and elbows. Bleeding into muscles, usually from trauma, also can occur. Oral bleeding is common in the setting of dental surgery. Spontaneous painless hematuria is relatively common in hemophilia. It does not result in significant blood loss but requires evaluation. Hematuria accompanied by pain requires quick evaluation and treatment.

Intracranial bleeds, bleeding of internal organs, and bleeding into the tissues of the neck, chest, or abdomen are all life-threatening. Delayed or suboptimal treatment of these bleeds may lead to permanent brain injury, loss of organ function, or death.

EVALUATION AND TREATMENT A positive family history may expedite a diagnosis of hemophilia. When a mother who is a known or suspected carrier is pregnant, genetic testing in utero through amniocentesis or chorionic villus sampling (CVS) may reveal a hemophilia diagnosis before childbirth. In the absence of a positive family history, a personal bleed history, laboratory testing, family history, and physical assessment contribute to a thorough evaluation and accurate diagnosis. In general, those with hemophilia A or B will have a prolonged partial thromboplastin time (PTT), and the prothrombin time (PT) will be normal. Measurement of factor VIII (hemophilia A) and factor IX (hemophilia B) levels is necessary for diagnosis.

Most children with hemophilia A (factor VIII deficiency) can be treated with recombinant factor VIII. Most children with hemophilia B (factor IX deficiency) can be treated with recombinant factor IX. The reconstitution of recombinant factor in a small volume of diluent, then administered by slow intravenous push, raises the factor level almost immediately. Emerging therapies for hemophilia include the use of PEGylated factor. Adding a polyethylene glycol (PEG) molecule results in an extended half-life of the involved factor.[12]

Antibody-Mediated Hemorrhagic Disease

The antibody-mediated hemorrhagic diseases are caused by the immune response. Antibody-mediated destruction of platelets or antibody-mediated inflammatory reactions to allergens damage blood vessels and cause seepage into tissues. The thrombocytopenic purpuras may be intrinsic or idiopathic. They also may be transient phenomena transmitted from mother to fetus. The inflammatory, or "allergic," purpuras, although rare, occur in response to allergens in the blood. All these disorders first appear during infancy or childhood.

Immune Thrombocytopenic Purpura

Primary **immune thrombocytopenic purpura (ITP)** (previously referred to as **idiopathic thrombocytopenic purpura**) is the most common disorder of platelet consumption. Autoantibodies bind to the plasma membranes of platelets. This causes platelet sequestration and destruction by mononuclear phagocytes in the spleen and other lymphoid tissues at a rate that exceeds the ability of the bone marrow to produce them. Medications, infections, lymphomas, or an unknown cause trigger the destruction of platelets.

PATHOPHYSIOLOGY The autoantibodies that produce the destruction are often of the IgG class and are usually against the platelet membrane glycoproteins (IIb-IIIa or Ib-IX). Approximately 70% of cases of ITP are preceded by a viral illness (e.g., cytomegalovirus [CMV], Epstein-Barr virus [EBV], parvovirus, or respiratory tract infection) prior to the eruption of petechiae or purpura by 1 to 3 weeks.

CLINICAL MANIFESTATIONS Bruising and a generalized petechial rash often occur with acute onset. Petechiae can develop into ecchymoses. Asymmetrical bruising is typical and is often on the legs and trunk. Hemorrhagic bullae of the gums, lips, and other mucous membranes may be prominent. Epistaxis (nose bleeding) may be severe and difficult to control. Except for signs of bleeding, the child appears well. The spleen, bone marrow, and blood are the sites of principal changes.[13] The acute phase lasts 1 to 2 weeks, but thrombocytopenia often persists. Intracranial hemorrhage is the most serious complication of ITP; however, the incidence is less than 1%. In some cases, the onset is more gradual, and manifestations consist of moderate bruising and a few petechiae.

EVALUATION AND TREATMENT Laboratory tests reveal an isolated low platelet count, and the few platelets observed on a smear are large, reflecting increased bone marrow production. The Ivy test (a bleeding time test) is prolonged. Children with typical features of ITP should not undergo bone marrow aspiration. The primary treatment for children with ITP is observation, regardless of platelet count. When bleeding is present, treatment is with an infusion of intravenous immune globulin (IVIg) or a short course of corticosteroids.

Even without treatment, the prognosis for children with ITP is excellent; 75% recover completely within 3 months. After the initial acute phase, spontaneous clinical manifestations subside. By 6 months after onset, 70 to 80% of affected children have regained normal platelet counts.[14] Persistent ITP in children is considered chronic, and immunosuppressive therapies are used.[15]

NEOPLASTIC DISORDERS

> ✓ **QUICK CHECK 22.3**
> 1. List the childhood leukemias in order of rate of incidence.
> 2. Why do children with leukemia experience bone or joint pain?
> 3. What are the common types of non-Hodgkin's lymphomas in children?

Leukemia

Leukemia is cancer of the blood-forming tissues, such as the bone marrow, that most often produces abnormal white blood cells called **leukemic cells**. Once in the blood, leukemic cells can spread to other organs, such as the lymph nodes, spleen, and brain. Leukemia is the most common malignancy in children and teens. The four most common types of leukemia are (1) acute lymphoblastic leukemia (ALL), (2) acute myeloid leukemia (AML), (3) chronic lymphocytic leukemia (CLL), and (4) chronic myeloid leukemia (CML).[16]

About 75% of leukemias among children and teens are ALLs. The remaining cases are AMLs and related neoplasms. Chronic leukemias are rare in children and account for fewer than 5% of cases.

ALL is most common in early childhood, peaking between 2 and 4 years of age.[17] AML is slightly more common during the first 2 years of life and during the teenage years. It occurs equally among boys and girls of all races. ALL is more common in boys than girls and among White children.[18]

The cause of most childhood cancer is unknown. Inherited mutations cause about 5% of all childhood cancers. Genetic mutations can occur during fetal development. Genetic conditions associated with leukemia include Down syndrome, neurofibromatosis, Shwachman-Diamond syndrome, Bloom's syndrome, and ataxia-telangiectasia. Epigenetic modifications, including DNA methylation, have been proposed as mediating events between environmental exposures and subsequent disease development.[17]

Many studies have shown that exposure to ionizing radiation can lead to the development of childhood leukemia and possibly other cancers.[19] There is recent concern for performing computed tomography (CT) scans in children. The increased use of these scans combined with wide variability in radiation doses has resulted in many children receiving a high dose of radiation.[20] Studies of other possible risk factors, including parental exposure to cancer-causing chemicals, prenatal exposure to pesticides, childhood exposure to common infectious agents, and living near a nuclear power plant, have produced inconsistent results. Higher risks of cancer have not been seen in children of individuals treated for cancer not caused by an inherited mutation.[21,22]

PATHOPHYSIOLOGY ALL is composed of immature B (pre-B) or T (pre-T) cells called **lymphoblasts**. The bone marrow is dense with lymphoblasts that replace the normal marrow and disrupt normal function. Many of the chromosomal abnormalities documented in ALL cause dysregulation of the expression and function of transcription factors required for normal B-cell and T-cell development.[23] The mutations can include both a gain or loss of function that are required for normal development.

AML is caused by acquired oncogenic mutations that impair differentiation. This results in the accumulation of immature myeloid blasts in the marrow and other organs. Epigenetic alterations are frequent in AML and have a central role. The bone marrow crowding by blasts produces marrow failure and complications, including anemia, thrombocytopenia, and neutropenia. AML is very heterogeneous because myeloid cell differentiation is complex. Leukemia—ALL or AML—is typically distinguished from lymphoma by the presence of less than 20% leukemic blasts.

CLINICAL MANIFESTATIONS The onset of leukemia may be abrupt or insidious. Children with leukemia may present with symptoms only 1 week before diagnosis. The most common symptoms reflect the consequences of bone marrow failure. These include decreased levels of red blood cells and platelets and changes in white blood cells. Pallor, fatigue, petechiae, purpura, bleeding, and fever generally are present. Approximately 45% of children have a hemoglobin level below 70 mmol/L. Epistaxis often occurs in children with severe thrombocytopenia.

Fever is usually present because of (1) infection associated with the decrease in functional neutrophils and (2) hypermetabolism associated with the ongoing rapid growth and destruction of leukemic cells. White blood cell counts greater than 200×10^9/L can cause leukostasis, an intravascular clumping of cells that results in infarction and hemorrhage, usually in the brain and lung.

Renal failure because of hyperuremia (high uric acid levels) can be associated with ALL, particularly at diagnosis or during the first phase of treatment. Extramedullary invasion with leukemic cells can occur in almost all body tissue. The central nervous system (CNS) is a common site of infiltration of extramedullary leukemias. Less than 10% of children with ALL will have CNS involvement at diagnosis. The most common symptoms of CNS involvement relate to increased intracranial pressure. This increased pressure causes early morning headaches, nausea, vomiting, irritability, and lethargy. Gonadal involvement with testicular infiltration also may occur.

Leukemic infiltration into bones and joints is common. Reports of joint pain may lead to the diagnosis of leukemia in some children. In most children, bone pain is characterized as migratory, vague, and without areas of swelling or inflammation. However, if joint pain is the primary symptom and some swelling is associated with the pain, misdiagnoses of rheumatoid arthritis and rheumatic fever have occurred. Other organs reported to be sites of leukemic invasion include the kidneys, heart, lungs, thymus, eyes, skin, and gastro-intestinal tract.

EVALUATION AND TREATMENT Leukemia is diagnosed through blood tests and examination of peripheral blood smears. Completion of a bone marrow aspiration usually occurs to further characterize the leukemia. The **blast cell** is the hallmark of acute leukemia (Figure 22.7). Healthy children have less than 5% blast cells in the bone marrow and none in the peripheral blood. In ALL, the bone marrow often is replaced by 80 to 100% blast cells. Counts of normally developing red blood cells, platelets and granulocytes are usually decreased. Occasionally, the marrow appears hypocellular, making the diagnosis difficult to differentiate from aplastic anemia. When this difficulty occurs, bone marrow biopsy or biopsy of extramedullary sites is necessary to confirm the diagnosis.

Approximately 85% of children with ALL will become 5-year survivors of their illness. Chemotherapy is the treatment of choice for

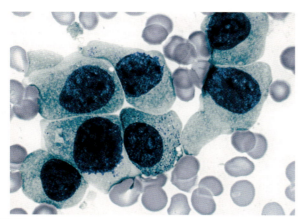

FIGURE 22.7 Monoblasts From Acute Monoblastic Leukemia. Monoblasts in a marrow smear from an individual with acute monoblastic leukemia. The monoblasts are larger than myeloblasts and usually have abundant cytoplasm, often with delicate scattered azurophilic granules (an element that stains well with blue aniline dyes). (From Damjanov, I., & Linder, J. [Eds.]. [1996]. *Anderson's pathology* [10th ed.]. Mosby.)

acute leukemia. Radiation of the CNS is used only in selected cases. Identification of various risk groups among children with ALL has led to the development of different intensities of medication protocols. As a result, treatment is targeted specifically for a particular risk group. For children who experience relapses of ALL, treatment with chimeric antigen receptor T cells (CAR-T cells) is showing promise.[24,25]

AML is more difficult to treat than ALL. Combination chemotherapy is the most common approach to treatment. Those children with unfavourable cytogenetic markers and those who experience a relapse of their disease will often undergo hematopoietic stem cell transplantation.[19]

CML accounts for less than 5% of childhood leukemias. Biologically targeted medications, known as tyrosine kinase inhibitors (TKIs), are becoming the mainstay of treatment, specifically for individuals whose disease has the *BCR/ABL* translocation.[26] Several TKIs are approved for use in children and are administered orally. Treatment requires continued adherence the medication regimen. The health impact of long-term TKI therapy is not yet known.[26]

Lymphomas

Lymphoma (HL and NHL) develops from the proliferation of malignant lymphocytes (immune cells) in the lymphoid system (see Chapters 12 and 21). Lymphomas are malignant growths that arise from discrete tissue masses.[27] Lymphoid neoplasms involve some recognizable stage of lymphocyte B- or T-cell differentiation.

Some lymphomas occasionally have leukemic presentations, and evolution to "leukemia" is not unusual during the progression of incurable "lymphomas." The terms merely reflect the usual tissue distribution.[28] The World Health Organization provides a classification scheme for lymphoma that was updated in 2016.[29]

In Canada, NHL and HL represent about 11% of all cases of childhood cancer. About 100 children younger than 14 years of age are diagnosed with lymphoma in Canada each year.[30] NHL (including Burkitt lymphoma) occurs more often than HL. Either group of diseases is rare before the age of 5 years, and the relative incidence increases throughout childhood. Boys are more likely to be diagnosed with a malignant lymphoma. Children with inherited or acquired immune deficiency syndrome, such as Wiskott-Aldrich syndrome, ataxia-telangiectasia, and Bloom's syndrome are at particular risk for developing NHL.

Non-Hodgkin's Lymphoma

Non-Hodgkin's lymphomas (NHLs) are cancers of immune cells. NHLs are a large and diverse group of tumours. Some tumours develop more slowly, and others develop more quickly and aggressively. Childhood NHL usually becomes evident as a diffuse disease. It can be further subdivided into four major types: (1) B-cell NHL (Burkitt and Burkitt-like lymphoma, and Burkitt leukemia); (2) diffuse large B-cell lymphoma; (3) lymphoblastic lymphoma; and (4) anaplastic large cell lymphoma.[31] The common types of NHL in children are different than those in adults. The most common types of NHL in children are Burkitt lymphoma (40%), lymphoblastic lymphoma (25 to 30%), and large cell lymphoma (10%).

PATHOPHYSIOLOGY Burkitt lymphoma will be discussed as an example of pathogenesis of NHL in children. All forms of Burkitt lymphoma are associated with translocations of the *MYC* gene on chromosome 8 that lead to increased MYC protein levels.[32] MYC is a transcriptional regulator that increases the expression of genes required for aerobic glycolysis, called the *Warburg effect* (see Chapter 10). Most Burkitt lymphomas are latently infected with EBV.[33] EBV is also present in about 25% of HIV-associated tumours and 15 to 20% of sporadic cases.[34]

CLINICAL MANIFESTATIONS NHL can arise from any lymphoid tissue. Signs and symptoms therefore are specific for the site involved. Associated signs of NHL include swelling of the lymph nodes in the neck, underarm, stomach, or groin; trouble swallowing; painless lump or swelling in a testicle; weight loss for unknown reason; night sweats; and trouble breathing. Involvement of facial bones, particularly the jaw, is common in African Burkitt lymphoma.

EVALUATION AND TREATMENT Physical examination and health history confirms the diagnosis, followed by biopsy of disease sites. Usual sites include the involved lymph nodes, tonsils, spleen, liver, bowel, or skin. Burkitt lymphoma is aggressive and responds well to treatment. With intensive chemotherapy, a cure may occur in most children and young adults.

Hodgkin's Lymphoma

Hodgkin's lymphoma (HL) is a group of lymphoid cancers. Unlike NHL, HL arises in a single chain of lymph nodes and spreads first in a contiguous way to lymphoid tissue. HL is characterized by the presence of Reed-Sternberg cells, which are large cells derived from the germinal centre of B cells (Figure 22.8). The World Health Organization has identified five types of HL: (1) nodular sclerosis, (2) mixed cellularity, (3) lymphocyte rich, (4) lymphocyte depletion, and (5) lymphocyte predominance. The first four types are considered the *classic* types of HL with similar expression of Reed-Sternberg cells. In the lymphocyte predominance type, the Reed-Sternberg cell is distinctive but different than the others. HL is a common type of cancer in young adults and adolescents but rare in childhood.

PATHOPHYSIOLOGY The Reed-Sternberg cells fail to express most of the normal B-cell genes, as well as those of T-cells. The causes of the genetic rearrangements or reprogramming are not fully known. They are thought to be the result of widespread epigenetic changes. Activation of the transcription factor NF-κB, which controls transcription of DNA, is a common event in classic HL.[34] EBV infection may activate NF-κB. Lymph nodes in individuals with infectious mononucleosis hold EBV-infected B cells, resembling Reed-Sternberg cells. This suggests that the EBV proteins may have a role in changes of the B cells into Reed-Sternberg cells.[34] NF-κB is involved in many biological processes, including inflammation, immunity, cell growth, differentiation, and apoptosis. Loss-of-function mutations in major histocompatibility

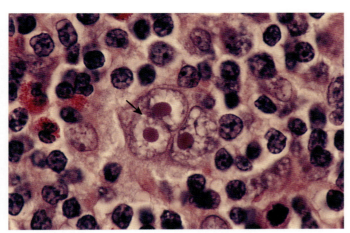

FIGURE 22.8 Diagnostic Reed-Sternberg Cell. A large multinucleated or multilobated cell with inclusion body–like nucleoli *(arrow)* surrounded by a halo of clear nucleoplasm. (From Damjanov, I., & Linder, J. [2000]. *Pathology: A color atlas.* Mosby.)

class I antigens may allow Reed-Sternberg cells to avoid the normal host immune response.[35]

CLINICAL MANIFESTATIONS Painless lymphadenopathy in the lower cervical chain, with or without fever, is the most common symptom in children. Other lymph nodes and organs also may be involved (Figure 22.9). Mediastinal involvement can cause pressure on the trachea or bronchi, leading to airway obstruction. Extranodal primary sites in HL are rare. Initial symptoms consist of anorexia, malaise, and fatigue. Intermittent fever is present in 30% of children, and weight loss also may be present. HL has a well-defined staging system that considers the extent and location of disease and the presence of fever, weight loss, or night sweats at diagnosis.

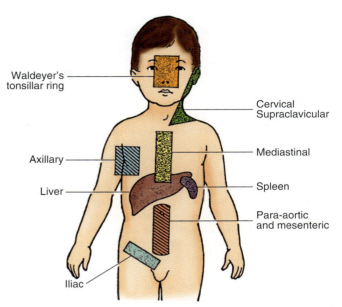

FIGURE 22.9 Main Areas of Lymphadenopathy and Organ Involvement in Hodgkin's Lymphoma. (From Hockenberry, M. J., & Wilson, D. [Eds.]. [2015]. *Wong's nursing care of infants and children* [10th ed.]. Mosby.)

EVALUATION AND TREATMENT Treatment for HL includes chemotherapy and radiation therapy. Historically, survivors had a much greater risk of developing a secondary cancer, such as lung cancer, melanoma, and breast cancer. Treatment protocols suggest minimizing the use of radiotherapy and using less toxic chemotherapy. Targeted therapies, including monoclonal antibodies such as brentuximab vedotin (Adcetris) and immune checkpoint inhibitors, may have a greater role in treating HL.

> ### DID YOU UNDERSTAND?

Disorders of Erythrocytes
1. Anemia is the most common blood disorder in children. Ineffective erythropoiesis or premature destruction of erythrocytes are the cause of childhood anemias.
2. Iron deficiency anemia (IDA) is the most common nutritional disorder worldwide. IDA has the highest incidence occurring between 6 months and 2 years of age. Iron is critical for the developing child.
3. No matter the cause of IDA, it produces a hypochromic-microcytic anemia, eventually lowering hemoglobin and hematocrit.
4. Hemolytic disease of the fetus and newborn (HDFN) results from incompatibility between the maternal and the fetal blood. It may involve differences in Rh factors or blood type (ABO). Maternal antibodies form in response to the presence of fetal incompatible erythrocytes in the blood of a Rh-negative mother. The maternal antibodies then enter the fetal circulation and cause hemolysis of fetal erythrocytes.
5. The key to treatment of HDFN resulting from Rh incompatibilities lies in prevention or immunoprophylaxis.
6. Sickle cell disease is a group of disorders characterized by the production of abnormal hemoglobin S (Hb S).
7. Sickle cell disease is an inherited, autosomal recessive disorder expressed as sickle cell anemia, sickle cell–thalassemia disease, or sickle cell–hemoglobin C disease. Sickle cell anemia, a homozygous form, is the most severe.
8. Sickle cell–thalassemia disease and sickle cell–hemoglobin C disease are heterozygous forms in which the child inherits another type of abnormal hemoglobin from one parent. Sickle cell trait, in which the child inherits Hb S from one parent and normal hemoglobin (Hb A) from the other, is a heterozygous carrier state that rarely has clinical manifestations.
9. Sickle cell disease causes a change in the shape of red blood cells, resulting in deoxygenation or dehydration.
10. The α- and β-thalassemias are inherited autosomal recessive disorders that cause an impaired rate of synthesis of one of the α or β chains of adult hemoglobin.

Disorders of Coagulation and Platelets
1. Hemophilia A is defined as factor VIII deficiency. It is the most common hereditary disease associated with life-threatening bleeding. It is caused by a mutation in factor VIII, an essential cofactor in the coagulation cascade. Factor IX deficiency is most often called *hemophilia B*.
2. Hemophilia may be inherited or caused by a spontaneous mutation of the factor gene.
3. The antibody-mediated hemorrhagic diseases are a group of disorders caused by the immune response. Antibody-mediated destruction of platelets or antibody-mediated inflammatory reactions to allergens damage blood vessels and cause seepage into tissues.

4. Immune thrombocytopenic purpura is a disorder of platelet consumption in which antiplatelet antibodies bind to the plasma membranes of platelets. This binding results in platelet sequestration and destruction by mononuclear phagocytes at a rate that exceeds the ability of the bone marrow to produce them.

Neoplastic Disorders

1. Leukemia is cancer of the blood-forming tissues that most often produces abnormal white blood cells called *leukemic cells*.
2. Among children and teens, about 75% of leukemias are acute lymphoblastic leukemia (ALL). The remaining cases are acute myeloid leukemia (AML). Chronic leukemias are rare in children.
3. The cause of childhood leukemia is unknown. About 5% of all childhood cancers are caused by inherited mutations.
4. Studies have shown that exposure to ionizing radiation can lead to the development of childhood leukemia and other cancers.
5. ALL causes dysregulation of the expression and function of transcription factors required for normal B-cell and T-cell development.
6. Epigenetic alterations are frequent in AML and have a key role.
7. The onset of leukemia may be abrupt or insidious. The most common symptoms reflect the consequences of bone marrow failure. These changes include decreased levels of red blood cells and platelets and changes in white blood cells.
8. Lymphomas are malignant proliferations that arise from discrete tissue masses. Lymphoid neoplasms involve some recognizable stage of lymphocyte B- or T-cell differentiation.
9. Some lymphomas occasionally have leukemic presentations.
10. The lymphomas of childhood are Hodgkin's lymphoma (HL) and non-Hodgkin's lymphoma (NHL).
11. NHL are neoplasms of immune cells. The most common types of NHL in children are Burkitt lymphoma (40%), lymphoblastic lymphoma (25 to 30%), and large cell lymphoma (10%).
12. Most Burkitt lymphomas are infected with the Epstein-Barr virus (EBV). There is increased evidence of NHL in children with congenital immunodeficiency syndromes.
13. Unlike NHL, HL arises in a single chain of lymph nodes and spreads first in a contiguous way to lymphoid tissue.
14. HL is characterized by the presence of Reed-Sternberg cells. These are large cells derived from the germinal centre of B cells.

23

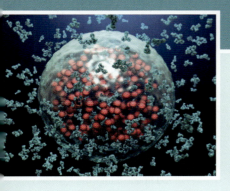

Structure and Function of the Cardiovascular and Lymphatic Systems

Mohamed Toufic El-Hussein, with originating chapter contributions by Kathryn L. McCance

Additional resources are available online at https://evolve.elsevier.com/Canada/Huether/pathophysiology.

CHAPTER OUTLINE

The Circulatory System, 552
The Heart, 552
    Structures That Direct Circulation Through the Heart, 553
    Structures That Support Cardiac Metabolism: The Coronary Vessels, 555
    Structures That Control Heart Action, 556
    Factors Affecting Cardiac Output, 563

The Systemic Circulation, 566
    Structure of Blood Vessels, 566
    Factors Affecting Blood Flow, 568
    Regulation of Blood Pressure, 571
    Regulation of the Coronary Circulation, 575
The Lymphatic System, 575

LEARNING OBJECTIVES

1. Describe the functions of the heart and the pulmonary system.
2. Describe the cardiac cycle.
3. Describe the structures of the heart and the location of the great vessels.
4. Describe the function and location of the cardiac conduction system.
5. Identify the components of an electrocardiogram.
6. Discuss the four unique characteristics of the myocardial cells and conduction system.
7. Discuss how factors influencing cardiac output reflect cardiac performance.
8. Use Starling's law and Laplace's law to demonstrate the interrelationship between preload, afterload, and contractility.
9. Discuss how various reflexes and biochemicals affect heart function.
10. Compare and contrast the structure and function of arteries, veins, and capillaries.
11. Describe the critical role of the endothelium for vascular function.
12. Discuss factors influencing the systemic blood pressure and blood flow.
13. Identify the factors that regulate blood pressure.
14. Discuss the function of the renin-angiotensin-aldosterone system in regulating blood pressure.
15. Discuss factors that regulate the flow of blood in the coronary circulation.
16. Discuss the normal structure and function of the lymphatic system.

KEY TERMS

Actin, 563
Adrenomedullin (ADM), 574
Afferent lymphatic vessel, 577
Afterload, 565
Angiogenesis, 557
Anisotropic band (A band), 563
Aorta, 555
Aortic semilunar valve, 555
Arteriogenesis, 557
Arteriole, 566
Arteries, 566
Artery, 566
Atrioventricular node (AV node), 559
Atrioventricular valve (AV valve), 555
Automatic cell, 560
Automaticity, 560
Autoregulation, 576
Bainbridge reflex, 566
Baroreceptor reflex, 566
Blood flow, 571
Blood velocity, 571
Bundle of His (atrioventricular bundle [AV bundle]), 560
Capillaries, 566
Capillary, 566
Cardiac action potential, 557
Cardiac cycle, 555
Cardiac output, 564
Cardiac vein, 557
Cardiomyocyte, 554
Cardiovascular vasomotor control centre, 566
Chordae tendineae, 555
Collateral artery, 557
Conduction system, 556
Coronary artery, 557
Coronary ostium (*pl.*, ostia), 557
Coronary perfusion pressure, 575
Coronary sinus, 557
Cross-bridge theory of muscle contraction, 563
Depolarization, 560
Diastole, 555
Diastolic blood pressure, 573
Diastolic depolarization, 560
Efferent lymphatic vessel, 577
Ejection fraction, 564
Elastic artery, 567
Endocardium, 554
Endothelial cell, 570
Endothelium, 570
Epinephrine, 566
Excitation–contraction coupling, 563
Fenestration, 570
Great cardiac vein, 557
Heart rate, 554
Inferior vena cava, 555
Inotropic agent, 566
Intercalated disc, 563
Isotropic band (I band), 562
Laminar flow, 571
Laplace's law, 565
Left atrium, 554
Left bundle branch (LBB), 560

551

Left coronary artery (LCA), 557
Left heart, 553
Left ventricle, 554
Lumen, 568
Lymph, 577
Lymph node, 577
Lymphatic vein, 577
Lymphatic venule, 577
M line, 563
Mean arterial pressure (MAP), 573
Mediastinum, 553
Metarteriole, 568
Mitral and tricuspid complex, 555
Mitral valve (left atrioventricular valve, bicuspid valve), 555
Muscle pump, 571
Muscular artery, 568
Myocardial contractility, 563
Myocardial oxygen consumption (MVO_2), 563
Myocardium, 554
Myoglobin, 575
Myosin, 563
Natriuretic peptide (NP), 574
Nitric oxide (NO), 575
P wave, 560
Papillary muscle, 555
Perfusion, 574
Pericardial cavity, 554
Pericardial fluid, 554
Pericardial sac, 554
Pericardium, 554
Peripheral vascular system, 566
Poiseuille's law, 571
PR interval, 560
Precapillary sphincter, 568
Preload, 565
Pressure, 571
Prolapse, 555
Pulmonary artery, 555
Pulmonary circulation, 553
Pulmonary vein, 555
Pulmonic semilunar valve, 555
Pulse pressure, 573
Purkinje fibre, 560
QRS complex, 560
QT interval, 560
Radius (diameter), 571
Refractory period, 560
Repolarization, 560
Resistance, 571
Rhythmicity, 560
Right atrium, 554
Right bundle branch (RBB), 560
Right coronary artery (RCA), 557
Right heart, 553
Right lymphatic duct, 577
Right ventricle, 554
Semilunar valve, 555
Shear stress, 557
Sinoatrial node (SA node, sinus node), 559
ST interval, 560
Starling's law of the heart, 565
Stenosis, 557
Stroke volume, 564
Superior vena cava, 555
Systemic circulation, 553
Systemic vascular resistance (SVR), 565
Systole, 555
Systolic blood pressure, 573
Systolic compressive effect, 575
T wave, 560
Thoracic duct, 577
Titin, 563
Total peripheral resistance (TPR), 565
Total resistance, 571
Tricuspid valve, 555
Tropomyosin, 563
Troponin C, 563
Troponin I, 563
Troponin T, 563
Troponin–tropomyosin complex, 563
Tunica externa (adventitia), 567
Tunica intima, 567
Tunica media, 567
Turbulent (flow), 571
Vasa vasorum, 567
Vascular compliance, 571
Vasoconstriction, 568
Vasodilation, 568
Vein, 571
Ventricular end-diastolic pressure (VEDP), 565
Ventricular end-diastolic volume (VEDV), 565
Venule, 566
Z line, 563

The functions of the circulatory system are delivery of oxygen, nutrients, hormones, and immune system components, to body tissues. The circulatory system is also responsible for removing metabolism waste products. The blood vessels connected to the heart, along with the lymphatic vessels, achieve delivery and removal of waste products. The nervous and endocrine systems regulate the heart and blood vessels. Immune system components, nutrients, and oxygen are supplied by the immune, digestive, and respiratory systems, respectively. Gaseous wastes of metabolism are expired through the lungs, whereas the kidneys and digestive tract remove other wastes.

The vascular endothelium is a multifunctional tissue that is essential to normal vascular, immune, and hemostatic system function. Endothelial dysfunction is a critical factor in the development of vascular and other diseases.[1]

THE CIRCULATORY SYSTEM

QUICK CHECK 23.1
1. What are the functions of the pericardial sac?
2. Why is the thickness of the myocardium different in the right and left ventricles?
3. Trace the flow of blood through the heart during one cardiac cycle.

The heart is composed of two conjoined pumps. The right side pump, or **right heart**, which pumps blood through the lungs, is also known as the **pulmonary circulation** and is described in Chapter 26. The left side pump, or **left heart**, which sends blood throughout the **systemic circulation**, supplies all the body except the lungs (Figure 23.1). These two systems are serially connected, thus the output of one becomes the input of the other.

Arteries carry blood from the heart to all parts of the body, where they branch into arterioles and even smaller vessels, ultimately becoming a fine meshwork of capillaries. Capillaries allow the closest contact and exchange between the blood and the interstitial space, or interstitium—the environment in which cells live. Venules, and eventually veins, carry blood from the capillaries back to the heart. Some of the plasma or liquid part of the blood passes through the walls of the capillaries into the interstitial space. The lymphatic system returns fluid and lymph to the cardiovascular system. The lymphatic system is a critical component of the immune system as described in Chapters 6 and 7.

THE HEART

Adult hearts weigh between 200 and 350 grams and are about fist sized. The heart lies obliquely (diagonally) in the **mediastinum**, the area above the diaphragm and between the lungs. Heart structures can be categorized by three functions:

1. *Structural support of heart tissues and circulation of pulmonary and systemic blood through the heart.* This category includes the heart wall and fibrous skeleton that enclose and support the heart, dividing it into four chambers; the valves directing flow through the chambers; and the great vessels conducting blood to and from the heart.
2. *Maintenance of heart cells.* This category includes all the vessels of the coronary circulation—the arteries and veins that serve the metabolic needs of all the heart cells—and the heart's lymphatic vessels.
3. *Stimulation and control of heart action.* Among these structures are the nerves and specialized muscle cells that direct the rhythmic contraction and relaxation of the heart muscles, propelling blood throughout the pulmonary and systemic circulatory systems.

CHAPTER 23 Structure and Function of the Cardiovascular and Lymphatic Systems

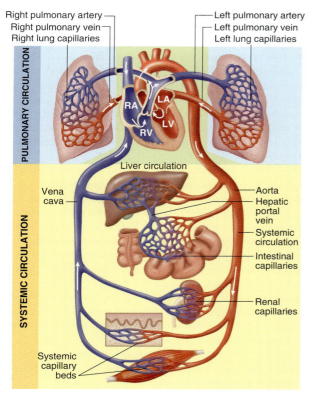

FIGURE 23.1 Diagram of the Pulmonary and Systemic Circulatory Systems. The right heart pumps unoxygenated blood *(blue)* through the pulmonary circulation, where oxygen enters the blood and carbon dioxide is exhaled, and the left heart pumps oxygenated blood *(red)* to and from all the other organ systems in the body. *LA,* Left atrium; *LV,* left ventricle; *RA,* right atrium; *RV,* right ventricle. (From Patton, K. T., Thibodeau, G. A., & Douglas, M. M. [2012]. *Essentials of anatomy & physiology.* Elsevier.)

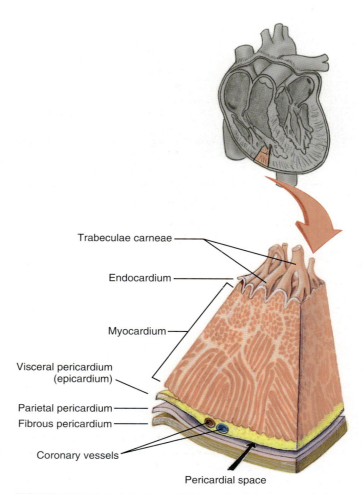

FIGURE 23.2 Wall of the Heart. This section of the heart wall shows the fibrous pericardium, the parietal and visceral layers of the serous pericardium (with the pericardial space between them), the myocardium, and the endocardium. Note the fatty connective tissue between the visceral layer of the serous pericardium (epicardium) and the myocardium. Note also that the endocardium covers tubular projections of myocardial muscle tissue called *trabeculae.* (Revised from Applegate, E. [2011]. *The anatomy and physiology learning system* [4th ed.]. Saunders.)

Structures That Direct Circulation Through the Heart
The Heart Wall

The three layers of the heart wall—the epicardium, myocardium, and endocardium—are enclosed in a double-walled membranous sac, the **pericardium** (Figure 23.2). The **pericardial sac** has three main functions: (1) it prevents displacement of the heart during gravitational acceleration or deceleration, (2) it serves as a physical barrier to protect the heart against infection and inflammation coming from the lungs and pleural space, and (3) it contains pain receptors and mechanoreceptors that can cause reflex changes in blood pressure and **heart rate**. The **pericardial cavity** is a fluid-containing space (also referred to as *pericardial space*) that separates the two layers of the pericardium: the parietal and the visceral pericardia (see Figure 23.2). The mesothelial layer of the pericardium secretes the **pericardial fluid** (about 20 mL) that lubricates the membranes that line the pericardial cavity, enabling them to slide smoothly over one another with minimal friction as the heart beats. The amount and character of the pericardial fluid are altered if the pericardium is inflamed (see Chapter 24).

The smoothness of the outer layer of the heart, the epicardium, also minimizes the friction between the heart wall and the pericardial sac. The thickest layer of the heart wall, the **myocardium**, is composed of cardiac muscle and is anchored to the heart's fibrous skeleton. The heart muscle cells, **cardiomyocytes**, provide the contractile force needed for blood to flow through the heart and into the pulmonary and systemic circulations. About 0.5 to 1% of the cardiomyocytes are replaced annually. Over a lifetime, about half of these muscle cells are replaced.[2]

The internal lining of the myocardium, the **endocardium**, is composed of connective tissue and squamous cells (see Figure 23.2). This lining is continuous with the endothelium that lines all the arteries, veins, and capillaries of the body, creating a continuous, closed circulatory system.

Chambers of the Heart

The heart has four chambers: the **left atrium**, the **right atrium**, the **right ventricle**, and the **left ventricle**. These chambers form two pumps in series: the right heart is a low-pressure system pumping blood through the lungs, and the left heart is a high-pressure system pumping blood to the rest of the body (Figure 23.3). The atria are smaller than the ventricles and have thinner walls. The ventricles have a thicker myocardial layer and constitute much of the bulk of the heart. A continuum of muscle fibres that originate from the fibrous skeleton at the base of the heart form the ventricles.

The wall thickness of each cardiac chamber depends on the amount of pressure or resistance it must overcome to eject blood. The two atria have the thinnest walls because they are low-pressure chambers that

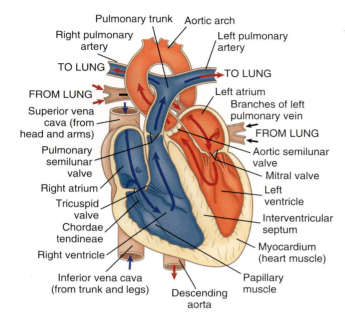

FIGURE 23.3 Structures That Direct Blood Flow Through the Heart. The blue and red arrows indicate the pathways of unoxygenated and oxygenated blood flow through chambers, valves, and major vessels.

serve as storage units and channels for blood that is emptied into the ventricles. Normally, there is little resistance to flow from the atria to the ventricles. The ventricles, on the other hand, must propel the blood all the way through the pulmonary or systemic vessels. The mean pulmonary artery pressure, the force the right ventricle must overcome, is only 15 mm Hg, whereas the mean arterial pressure the left ventricle must pump against is about 92 mm Hg. Because the pressure is markedly higher in the systemic circulation, the wall of the left ventricle is about three times thicker than that of the right ventricle.

The right ventricle is shaped like a crescent or triangle, which enables a bellowslike action that efficiently ejects large volumes of blood through the pulmonary semilunar valve into the low-pressure pulmonary system. The larger left ventricle is bullet shaped, which allows it to generate enough pressure to eject blood through a relatively larger aortic semilunar valve into the high-pressure systemic circulation.

The septal membrane separates the right and left sides of the heart and prevents blood from crossing between the two circulatory systems. The interatrial septum separates the atria, and the interventricular septum separates the ventricles. Because the fetus does not depend on the lungs for oxygenation, there is an opening before birth between the right and left atria called the *foramen ovale* that facilitates circulation. This opening closes functionally at the time of birth as the higher pressure in the left atrium pushes a flap, the septum primum, over the hole. In 75 to 80% of infants, these septa are permanently fused within the first year of life[3,4] (see Chapter 25).

Fibrous Skeleton of the Heart

Four rings of dense fibrous connective tissue provide a firm anchorage for the attachments of the atrial and ventricular musculature, as well as the valvular tissue (Figure 23.4). The fibrous rings are adjacent and form a central, fibrous supporting structure collectively termed the *annuli fibrosi cordis*.

Valves of the Heart

The four heart valves ensure that blood only flows one way through the heart. When the ventricles are relaxed, the two atrioventricular valves (AV valves) open and blood flows from the relatively higher pressure in the atria to the lower pressure in the ventricles. As the ventricles contract, ventricular pressure increases and causes these valves to close and prevent backflow into the atria. The semilunar valves of the heart open when intraventricular pressure exceeds aortic and pulmonary pressures, and blood flows out of the ventricles and into the pulmonary and systemic circulations. After ventricular contraction and ejection, intraventricular pressure falls and the pulmonic semilunar valve and aortic semilunar valve close when the pressure in the vessels is greater than the pressure in the ventricles, thus preventing backflow into the right and left ventricles, respectively. The actions of the heart valves are shown in Figures 23.3 and 23.4.

The AV (tricuspid and mitral) valve openings are composed of tissue flaps called *leaflets* or *cusps*, which are attached at the upper margin to a ring in the heart's fibrous skeleton. Chordae tendineae attach the end of the lower margin of the valve leaflets to the papillary muscles (see Figure 23.3). The papillary muscles, extensions of the myocardium, help hold the cusps together and downward at the onset of ventricular contraction, thus preventing their backward expulsion or prolapse into the atria.

The AV valve in the right heart is called the tricuspid valve because it has three cusps. The left AV valve is a bicuspid (two-cusp) valve called the mitral valve (left atrioventricular valve, bicuspid valve). The tricuspid and mitral valves function as a unit because the atria, fibrous rings, valvular tissue, chordae tendineae, papillary muscles, and ventricular walls are connected. Collectively, these six structures are known as the mitral and tricuspid complex.

Blood leaves the right ventricle through the pulmonic semilunar valve, and it leaves the left ventricle through the aortic semilunar valve (see Figures 23.3 and 23.4). Both the pulmonic and aortic semilunar valves have three cup-shaped cusps that arise from the fibrous skeleton.

The Great Vessels

Blood moves in and out of the heart through several large veins and arteries (see Figure 23.3). The right heart receives venous blood from the systemic circulation through the superior vena cava and inferior vena cava, which join and then enter the right atrium. Blood leaving the right ventricle enters the pulmonary circulation through the pulmonary artery, which divides into right and left branches to transport unoxygenated blood from the right heart to the lungs. The pulmonary arteries branch further into the pulmonary capillary beds, where oxygen and carbon dioxide exchange occurs.

Four pulmonary veins, two from the right lung and two from the left lung, carry oxygenated blood from the lungs to the left side of the heart. The oxygenated blood moves through the left atrium and ventricle, out into the aorta that subsequently branches into the systemic arteries that supply the body.

Blood Flow During the Cardiac Cycle

The pumping action of the heart consists of contraction and relaxation of the heart muscle, or myocardium. Each ventricular contraction and the relaxation that follows it constitute one cardiac cycle. (Blood flow through the heart during a single cardiac cycle is illustrated in Figure 23.5.) During the period of relaxation, termed diastole, blood fills the ventricles. The ventricular contraction that follows, termed systole, propels the blood out of the ventricles and into the pulmonary and systemic circulations. Contraction of the left ventricle occurs slightly earlier than contraction of the right ventricle.

The five phases of the cardiac cycle are said to begin with the opening of the mitral and tricuspid valves and atrial contraction (see Figures 23.6 and 23.7). Closing of the mitral and tricuspid valves as passive ventricular filling begins marks the end of one cardiac cycle.

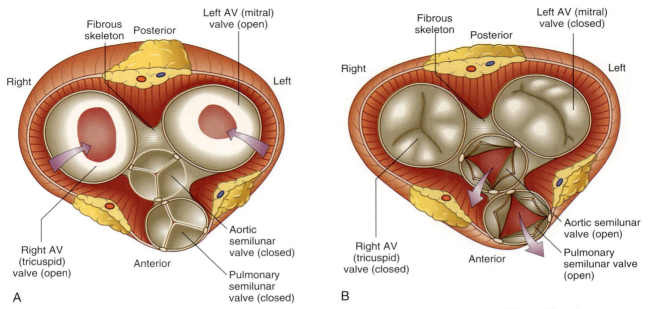

FIGURE 23.4 Transverse Section of the Heart Showing the Atrioventricular (Mitral and Tricuspid) and Semilunar (Aortic and Pulmonary) Valves. Superior view with the atria and vessels removed. *Arrows* indicate direction of blood flow. **A,** When the heart is filling with blood, the AV valves are open and the semilunar valves are closed. **B,** When blood is leaving the heart, the semilunar valves are open and the AV valves are closed. *AV,* Atrioventricular. (From Naish, J. [2015]. *Medical sciences* [2nd ed.]. Saunders.)

Normal Intracardiac Pressures

Normal intracardiac pressures are shown in Table 23.1.

Structures That Support Cardiac Metabolism: The Coronary Vessels

> ✓ **QUICK CHECK 23.2**
> 1. Draw a diagram of the conduction system of the heart.
> 2. Why are the left and right coronary vessels considered the major coronary vessels?

TABLE 23.1	Normal Intracardiac Pressures	
	Mean (mm Hg)	Range (mm Hg)
Right atrium	4	0–8
Right ventricle		
Systolic	24	15–28
End-diastolic	4	0–8
Left atrium	7	4–12
Left ventricle		
Systolic	130	90–140
End-diastolic	7	4–12

The coronary circulation, which is part of the systemic circulation, supplies the myocardium and other heart structures with oxygen and nutrients. The **coronary arteries** originate at the upper edge of the aortic semilunar valve cusps (Figure 23.8B) and receive blood through openings in the aorta called the **coronary ostia**. The **cardiac veins** empty into the right atrium through another ostium, the opening of a large vein called the **coronary sinus** (Figure 23.8C). (Regulation of the coronary circulation, which is similar to regulation of flow through systemic and pulmonary vessels, is described in "Regulation of the Coronary Circulation")

Coronary Arteries

The major coronary arteries, the **right coronary artery (RCA)** and the **left coronary artery (LCA)** (Figure 23.8A), traverse the epicardium, myocardium, and endocardium and branch to become arterioles and then capillaries. Their main branches are outlined in Box 23.1. The coronary arteries are smaller in women than in men because women's hearts weigh proportionately less than men's hearts.

Collateral Arteries

Collateral arteries are anastomoses or connections between branches of the same coronary artery or connections of branches of the RCA with branches of the left. The epicardium contains more collateral vessels than the endocardium. New collateral vessels are formed through two processes: **arteriogenesis** (new artery growth branching from preexisting arteries) and **angiogenesis** (growth of new capillaries within a tissue).[5] **Shear stress**, which results from increased blood flow speed within and just beyond areas of stenosis, as well as the production of growth factors and cytokines, including monocyte chemoattractant protein-1 (MCP-1) and vascular endothelial growth factor (VEGF), stimulates collateral circulation growth.[6] The collateral circulation assists in supplying blood and oxygen to myocardium that has become ischemic following gradual narrowing, or **stenosis**, of one or more major coronary arteries (coronary artery disease). Unfortunately, diabetes, which predisposes to coronary artery disease, also impedes collateral formation because of increased production of antiangiogenic factors, such as endostatin and angiostatin.

Coronary Capillaries

The heart requires an extensive capillary network to function. Blood travels from the arteries to the arterioles and then into the capillaries, where oxygen and other nutrients enter the myocardium, whereas waste products enter the blood. At rest, the heart extracts 50 to 80%

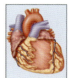
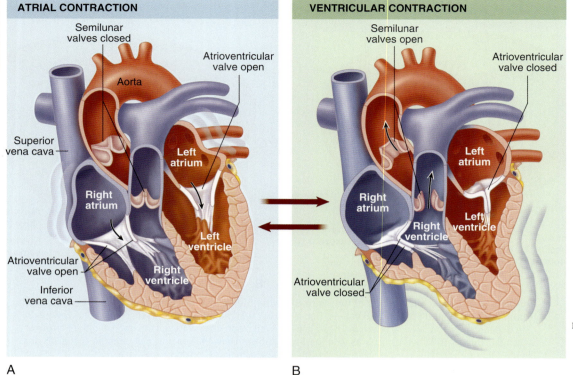

FIGURE 23.5 Blood Flow Through the Heart During a Single Cardiac Cycle. **A,** During diastole, blood flows into the atria, atrioventricular valves are pushed open, and blood begins to fill the ventricles. Atrial systole squeezes blood remaining in the atria into the ventricles. **B,** During ventricular systole, the ventricles contract, pushing blood out through semilunar valves into the pulmonary artery (right ventricle) and the aorta (left ventricle). (Adapted from Patton, K. T., & Thibodeau, G. A. [2018]. *The human body in health and disease* [7th ed.]. Elsevier Inc.)

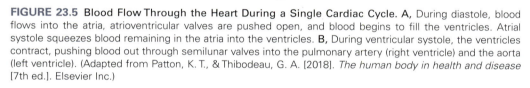

Left coronary artery. Arises from single ostium behind left cusp of aortic semilunar valve. It ranges from a few millimetres to a few centimetres long and passes between left arterial appendage and pulmonary artery. Generally, it divides into two branches: the left anterior descending artery and the circumflex artery. Other branches are distributed diagonally across the free wall of the left ventricle.

Left anterior descending artery (or anterior interventricular artery). Delivers blood to portions of left and right ventricles and much of interventricular septum. It travels down the anterior surface of the interventricular septum toward apex of the heart.

Circumflex artery. Travels in a groove (*coronary sulcus*) that separates left atrium from left ventricle and extends to left border of heart. It supplies blood to left atrium and lateral wall of left ventricle and often branches to posterior surfaces of left atrium and left ventricle.

Right coronary artery. Originates from an ostium behind the right aortic cusp, travels from behind the pulmonary artery, and extends around the right heart to the heart's posterior surface, where it branches to atrium and ventricle. The *right coronary artery* has three major branches: the conus (supplies blood to upper right ventricle), the right marginal branch (supplies right ventricle to the apex), and the posterior descending branch (lies in posterior interventricular sulcus and supplies smaller branches to both ventricles).

of the oxygen delivered to it, and coronary blood flow is directly correlated with myocardial oxygen consumption.[7] Any alteration of the cardiac muscles dramatically affects blood flow in the capillaries.

Coronary Veins and Lymphatic Vessels

After passing through the capillary network, blood from the coronary arteries drains into the cardiac veins located alongside the arteries. Most of the venous drainage of the heart occurs through veins in the visceral pericardium. The veins then feed into the **great cardiac vein** (see Figure 23.8C) and coronary sinus on the posterior surface of the heart, between the atria and ventricles, in the coronary sulcus.

The myocardium has an extensive system of lymphatic capillaries and collecting vessels within the layers of the myocardium and the valves. With cardiac contraction, the lymphatic vessels drain fluid to lymph nodes in the anterior mediastinum that empty into the superior vena cava. The lymphatics are important for protecting the myocardium against infection and injury.

Structures That Control Heart Action

Life depends on continuous repetition of the cardiac cycle (systole and diastole), which requires the transmission of electrical impulses, termed **cardiac action potentials**, through the myocardium.[7] (Action potentials are described in Chapters 1 and 5.) The muscle fibres of the myocardium are electrically coupled so that action potentials pass from cell to cell rapidly and efficiently.

The myocardium contains its own pacemakers and **conduction system**—specialized cells that enable it to generate and transmit action potentials without input from the nervous system (Figure 23.9). The pacemaker cells are concentrated at two sites, or nodes, in the myocardium. Nodes of specialized cells stimulate the cardiac cycle. Although the autonomic nervous system (both sympathetic and parasympathetic fibres) innervates the heart, neural impulses are not needed to

CHAPTER 23 Structure and Function of the Cardiovascular and Lymphatic Systems

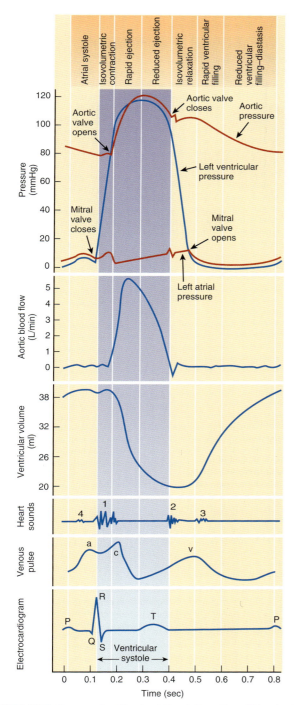

FIGURE 23.6 Composite Chart of Heart Function. This chart is a composite of several diagrams of heart function (cardiac pumping cycle, blood pressure, blood flow, volume, heart sounds, venous pulse, and electrocardiogram), all on the same time scale.

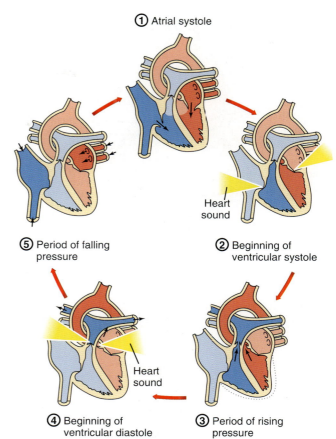

FIGURE 23.7 The Five Phases of the Cardiac Cycle. (1) Atrial systole: Atria contract, pushing blood through the open tricuspid and mitral valves into the ventricles. Semilunar valves are closed. (2) Beginning of ventricular systole. Ventricles contract, increasing pressure within the ventricles. The tricuspid and mitral valves close, causing the first heart sound. (3) Period of rising pressure: semilunar valves open when pressure in the ventricle exceeds that in the arteries. Blood spurts into the aorta and pulmonary arteries. (4) Beginning of ventricular diastole: pressure in the relaxing ventricles drops below that in the arteries. Semilunar valves snap shut, causing the second heart sound. (5) Period of falling pressure: blood flows from veins into the relaxed atria. Tricuspid and mitral valves open when pressure in the ventricles falls below that in the atria. (Adapted from Solomon, E. [2016]. *Introduction to human anatomy and physiology* [4th ed.]. Saunders.)

contraction and the degree and duration of myocardial relaxation. Normal or appropriate function depends on the supply of these substances, which is why coronary artery disease can seriously disrupt heart function.

The Conduction System

> **QUICK CHECK 23.3**
> 1. What are the pathways of conduction through the heart?
> 2. What does each of the electrocardiogram waves (P, Q, R, S, T) represent?
> 3. Define *automaticity* and *rhythmicity*.

Normally, electrical impulses arise in the **sinoatrial node (SA node, sinus node)**, the usual pacemaker of the heart. The SA node is located at the junction of the right atrium and superior vena cava, just superior to the tricuspid valve. Both sympathetic and parasympathetic nerve fibres heavily innervate the SA node.[8] In the resting adult, the SA node

maintain the cardiac cycle. Thus, the heart will beat in the absence of any innervation, one of the many factors that allow heart transplantation to be successful.

Substances delivered to the myocardium in coronary blood influence heart action. Nutrients and oxygen are needed for cellular survival and normal function. Hormones and biochemical substances, including medications, can affect the strength and duration of myocardial

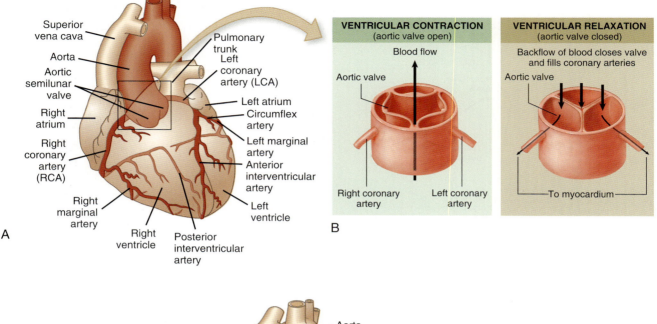
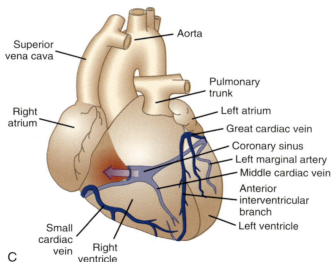

FIGURE 23.8 Coronary Circulation. A, Arteries. B, Coronary artery openings from the aorta. C, Veins. Both (A) and (C) are anterior views of the heart. Vessels near the anterior surface are more darkly coloured than vessels of the posterior surface seen through the heart. (B) Placement of the coronary artery opening behind the leaflets of the aortic valve allows the coronary arteries to fill during ventricular relaxation. ([A–C], from Patton, K. T., & Thibodeau, G. A. [2018]. *The human body in health & disease* [7th ed.]. Elsevier.)

generates about 60 to 100 action potentials per minute, depending on age and physical condition. Each action potential travels rapidly from cell to cell and through the atrial myocardium, carrying the action potential onward to the **atrioventricular node (AV node)**, as well as causing both atria to contract, beginning systole.[8]

The AV node, located in the right atrial wall superior to the tricuspid valve and anterior to the ostium of the coronary sinus, conducts the action potentials onward to the ventricles. The autonomic parasympathetic ganglia that serve as receptors for the vagus nerve innervate the AV node, causing slowing of impulse conduction.

Conducting fibres from the AV node converge to form the **bundle of His (atrioventricular bundle [AV bundle])**, within the posterior border of the interventricular septum. The bundle of His then gives rise to the right and left bundle branches. The **right bundle branch (RBB)** is thin and travels without much branching to the right ventricular apex. Damage to the endocardium increases the RBB's susceptibility to interruption of impulse conduction because of its thinness and relative lack of branches. The **left bundle branch (LBB)** in some hearts divides into two branches, or fascicles. The left anterior bundle branch (LABB) passes the left anterior papillary muscle and the base of the left ventricle and crosses the aortic outflow tract. Damage to the aortic valve or the left ventricle can interrupt this branch. The left posterior bundle branch (LPBB) travels posteriorly, crossing the left ventricular inflow tract to the base of the left posterior papillary muscle. This branch spreads diffusely through the posterior inferior left ventricular wall. Blood flow through this portion of the left ventricle is relatively nonturbulent, so the LBB is somewhat protected from injury caused by wear and tear.

The **Purkinje fibres** are the terminal branches of the RBB and LBB. They extend from the ventricular apexes to the fibrous rings and penetrate the heart wall to the outer myocardium. The first areas of the

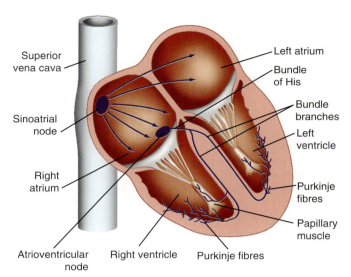

FIGURE 23.9 **The Cardiac Conduction System.** Specialized cardiac muscle cells in the heart wall rapidly conduct an electrical impulse throughout the myocardium. The sinoatrial node (pacemaker) initiates the signal that spreads through the atrial myocardium to the atrioventricular node. The atrioventricular node then initiates a signal that is conducted through the atrioventricular bundle (of His) and Purkinje fibres to reach the ventricular myocardium. (From Koeppen, B. M. [Ed.]. [2010]. *Berne & Levy physiology* [6th ed.]. Mosby.)

TABLE 23.2 **Intracellular and Extracellular Ion Concentrations in the Myocardium**

	Intracellular Concentration (mmol/L)	Extracellular Concentration (mmol/L)
Sodium (Na^+)	5	135–145
Potassium (K^+)	150	3.5–5.0
Chloride (Cl^-)	5	98–106
Calcium (Ca^{++})	10^{-7}	Total Ca: 2.25–2.75 Ionized: 1.05–1.30

ventricles to be excited are portions of the interventricular septum. The septum is activated from both the RBB and the LBB. The extensive network of Purkinje fibres promotes the rapid spread of the impulse to the ventricular apexes. The basal and posterior portions of the ventricles are the last to be activated.

Propagation of cardiac action potentials. The movement of ions—including sodium, potassium, calcium, and chloride—across cardiac cell membranes causes electrical activation of the muscle cells; this is called **depolarization**. Deactivation of muscle cells, also called **repolarization**, occurs the same way. (Movement of ions across cell membranes is described in Chapter 1; electrical activation of muscle cells is described in Chapter 38.)

Movement of ions into and out of the cell creates an electrical (voltage) difference across the cell membrane, called the *membrane potential*. The resting membrane potential of myocardial cells is between −80 and −90 mV, whereas that of the SA node is between −50 and −60 mV and that of the AV node is between −60 and −70 mV.[8] During depolarization, the inside of the cell becomes less negatively charged. In cardiac cells, as in other excitable cells, when the resting membrane potential (in millivolts) becomes more negative with depolarization and reaches the threshold potential for cardiac cells, a cardiac action potential is fired. Table 23.2 summarizes the intracellular and extracellular ionic concentrations of cardiac muscle. Medications that alter the movement of these ions (e.g., calcium) have profound effects on the action potential and can alter heart rate. The various phases of the cardiac action potential are related to changes in the permeability of the cell membrane to sodium, potassium, chloride, and calcium. Threshold is the point at which the cell membrane's selective permeability to these ions is temporarily disrupted, leading to an "all or nothing" depolarization. If the resting membrane potential becomes more negative because of a decrease in extracellular potassium concentration (hypokalemia), it is termed *hyperpolarization*.

A **refractory period**, during which no new cardiac action potential can be initiated regardless of the stimulus, follows depolarization. This effective or absolute refractory period corresponds to the time needed for the reopening of channels that permit sodium and calcium influx into the cells. A relative refractory period occurs near the end of repolarization, following the effective refractory period. During this time, the membrane can be depolarized again but only if a greater-than-normal stimulus is initiated. Abnormal refractory periods as a result of disease can cause abnormal heart rhythms or dysrhythmias, including ventricular fibrillation and cardiac arrest (see Chapter 24).

The electrocardiogram. Skin electrodes record an electrocardiogram, which is the summation of all the cardiac action potentials that originate from myocardial cell electrical activity (Figure 23.10). The **P wave** represents atrial depolarization. The **PR interval** is a measure of time from the onset of atrial activation to the onset of ventricular activation (normally 0.12 to 0.20 second). The PR interval represents the time necessary for electrical activity to travel from the sinus node through the atrium, AV node, and His–Purkinje system to activate ventricular myocardial cells. The **QRS complex** represents the sum of all ventricular muscle cell depolarization. The configuration and amplitude of the QRS complex may vary considerably among individuals. The duration is normally between 0.06 and 0.10 second. During the **ST interval**, the entire ventricular myocardium is depolarized. The **QT interval** is sometimes called the "electrical systole" of the ventricles. It lasts about 0.4 second but varies inversely with the heart rate. The **T wave** represents ventricular repolarization.

Automaticity. Automaticity, or the property of generating spontaneous depolarization to threshold, enables the SA and AV nodes to generate cardiac action potentials without any external stimulus. Cells capable of spontaneous depolarization are called **automatic cells**. The automatic cells of the cardiac conduction system can stimulate the heart to beat even when it is transplanted and thus has no innervation. Spontaneous depolarization is possible in automatic cells because the membrane potential of these special cells does not actually "rest" during return to the resting membrane potential. Instead, it slowly depolarizes toward threshold during the diastolic phase of the cardiac cycle. Because threshold is approached during diastole, return to the resting membrane potential in automatic cells is called **diastolic depolarization**. The electrical impulse normally begins in the SA node because its cells depolarize more rapidly than other automatic cells.

Rhythmicity. Rhythmicity is the regular generation of an action potential by the heart's conduction system. The SA node sets the pace because normally it has the fastest rate. The SA node depolarizes spontaneously 60 to 100 times per minute. If the SA node is damaged, the AV node can become the heart's pacemaker at a rate of about 40 to 60 spontaneous depolarizations per minute. Eventually, however, conduction cells in the atria usually take over from the AV node. Purkinje fibres are capable of spontaneous depolarization but at an even slower rate than the AV node.

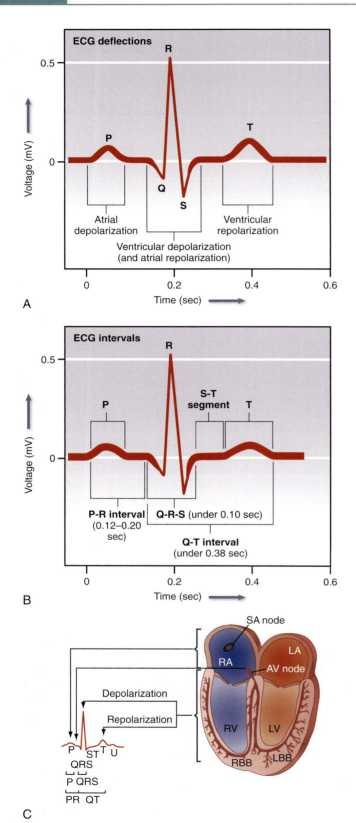

FIGURE 23.10 Electrocardiogram and Cardiac Electrical Activity. **A,** Normal ECG. Depolarization and repolarization. **B,** ECG intervals among P, QRS, and T waves. **C,** Schematic representation of ECG and its relationship to cardiac electrical activity. *AV,* Atrioventricular; *ECG,* electrocardiogram; *LA,* left atrium; *LBB,* left bundle branch; *LV,* left ventricle; *RA,* right atrium; *RBB,* right bundle branch; *RV,* right ventricle.

Cardiac Innervation

✓ **QUICK CHECK 23.4**
1. Describe the interactions of actin, myosin, and the troponin–tropomyosin complex in controlling heart function.
2. Define *excitation–contraction coupling*.

Although the heart's nodes and conduction system are able to generate action potentials independently, the autonomic nervous system influences both the rate of impulse generation (firing), depolarization, and repolarization of the myocardium, and the strength of atrial and ventricular contraction. Autonomic neural transmission produces changes in the heart and circulatory system faster than metabolic or humoral agents. Speed is important, for example, in stimulating the heart to increase its pumping action during times of stress and fear—the so-called fight-or-flight response—or with increased physical activity. Although increased delivery of oxygen, glucose, hormones, and other bloodborne factors sustains increased cardiac activity, the rapid initiation of increased activity depends on the sympathetic and parasympathetic fibres of the autonomic nervous system.

Sympathetic and parasympathetic nerves. Sympathetic and parasympathetic nerve fibres innervate all parts of the atria and ventricles and the SA and AV nodes. In general, sympathetic stimulation increases electrical conductivity and the strength of myocardial contraction, and vagal parasympathetic nerve activity does the opposite, slowing the conduction of action potentials through the heart and reducing the strength of contraction. Thus, the sympathetic and parasympathetic nerves affect the speed of the cardiac cycle (heart rate, or beats per minute), and the sympathetic nerves also influence the diameter of the coronary vessels (Figure 23.11). Sympathetic nervous activity enhances myocardial performance. The sympathetic nervous system stimulation of the SA node therefore rapidly increases heart rate. Furthermore, neurally released norepinephrine or circulating catecholamines interact with β-adrenergic receptors on the cardiac cell membranes. The overall effect is an increased influx of calcium (Ca^{++}), which increases the contractile strength of the heart and increases the speed of electrical impulses through the heart muscle and the nodes.[8] The release of vasodilating metabolites resulting from increased myocardial contraction causes increased sympathetic discharge, which dilates the coronary vessels.[7]

The parasympathetic nervous system affects the heart through the vagus nerve, which releases acetylcholine. Acetylcholine causes decreased heart rate and slows conduction through the AV node.

Myocardial Cells

Cardiomyocytes are composed of long, narrow fibres that contain bundles of longitudinally arranged myofibrils; a nucleus (cardiac muscle); mitochondria; an internal membrane system (the sarcoplasmic reticulum); cytoplasm (sarcoplasm); and a plasma membrane (the sarcolemma), which encloses the cell. Cardiac and skeletal muscle cells also have an "external" membrane system made up of transverse tubules (T tubules) formed by inward pouching of the sarcolemma. The sarcoplasmic reticulum forms a network of channels that surrounds the muscle fibre.

Because the myofibrils in both cardiac and skeletal fibres consist of alternating light and dark bands of protein, the fibres look striped, or striated. The dark and light bands of the myofibrils create repeating longitudinal units, called *sarcomeres*, which are between 1.6 and 2.2 μm long (Figures 23.12 and 23.13). The length of these sarcomeres determines the limits of myocardial stretch at the end of diastole and subsequently the force of contraction during systole. Alterations in

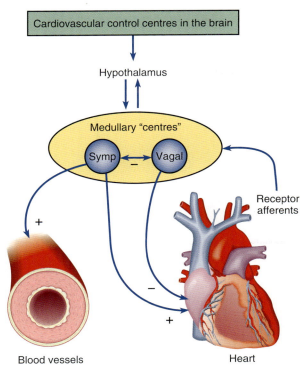

FIGURE 23.11 Autonomic Innervation of Cardiovascular System. (+), Activation; (−), inhibition.

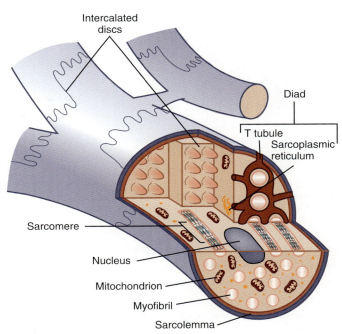

FIGURE 23.12 Cardiac Muscle Fibre. Unlike other types of muscle fibres, cardiac muscle fibres are typically branched with junctions, called *intercalated discs*, between adjacent myocytes. Like skeletal muscle cells, cardiac muscle cells contain sarcoplasmic reticula and T tubules, although these structures are not as highly organized as in skeletal muscle fibres.

sarcomere size are seen in both physiological and pathological myocardial hypertrophy.

Hypertrophy, or enlargement, of the heart may occur through growth in either the length or the width of the sarcomeres in both normal and disease conditions. When normal stimuli, such as physical activity or pregnancy, cause hypertrophy, myocardial contractility is increased and when the stimulus is removed, regression of the hypertrophy occurs. Conversely, hypertension or myocardial infarction lead to disease-related hypertrophy, resulting in reduced contractility and often heart failure. It has long been thought that this pathological hypertrophy was not reversible, but new research has shown that reversal may be possible.

Placement of a left ventricular assist device in patients with hypertrophic heart failure awaiting a heart transplant has resulted in regression of the ventricular hypertrophy, occasionally to the point that heart transplant was not required. Research on the mechanisms involved in regression has shown that gene activation, several signalling pathways, angiogenesis, and autophagy are all involved. The hope is that identification of these mechanisms will lead to new and more effective pharmaceutical treatments for heart failure that currently is associated with a poor long-term prognosis.[9–11]

Differences between cardiac and skeletal muscle reflect heart function. Cardiac cells are arranged in branching networks throughout the myocardium, whereas skeletal muscle cells tend to be arranged in parallel units throughout the length of the muscle. Cardiac fibres have only one nucleus, whereas skeletal muscle cells have many nuclei. Other differences enable cardiac fibres to do the following:
- *Transmit action potentials quickly from cell to cell.* Electrical impulses are transmitted rapidly from cardiac fibre to cardiac fibre because the network of fibres connects at **intercalated discs**, which are thickened portions of the sarcolemma. The intercalated discs contain three junctions: desmosomes or macula adherens; fascia adherens, which mechanically attach one cell to another; and gap junctions, also known as *tight junctions*, which allow the electrical impulse to spread from cell to cell through a low-resistance pathway (see Chapter 1). Changes in the function of these junctional elements may cause an increased risk for arrhythmias.[8]
- *Maintain high levels of energy synthesis.* Molecules such as adenosine triphosphate (ATP) supply the heart, which cannot rest and is in constant need of energy, unlike skeletal muscles. Therefore, the cytoplasm surrounding the bundles of myofibrils in each cardiomyocyte contains a large number of mitochondria (25 to 33% of cell volume). Cardiac muscle cells have more mitochondria than do skeletal muscle cells to provide the necessary respiratory enzymes for aerobic metabolism and supply quantities of ATP sufficient for the constant action of the myocardium.[12]
- *Gain access to more ions, particularly sodium and potassium, in the extracellular environment.* Cardiac fibres contain more T tubules than do skeletal muscle fibres (see Figure 23.12). This increased closeness to the T tubules gives each myofibril in the myocardium faster access to molecules needed for the transmission of action potentials, a process that involves transport of sodium and potassium through the walls of the T tubules. Because the T tubule system is continuous with the extracellular space and the interstitial fluid, it facilitates the rapid transmission of the electrical impulses from the surface of the sarcolemma to the myofibrils inside the fibre. This rapid transmission activates all the myofibrils of one fibre at the same time. The sarcoplasmic reticulum is located around the myofibrils. As an action potential is transmitted through the T tubules, it induces the sarcoplasmic reticulum to release its stored calcium, thus activating the contractile proteins **actin** and **myosin**.

Actin, myosin, and the troponin–tropomyosin complex. Within each myocardial sarcomere are myosin molecules that resemble golf

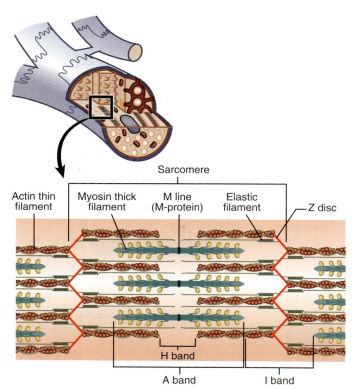

FIGURE 23.13 Structure of a Sarcomere. The sarcomere is the basic contractile unit of a muscle cell. The Z disc is the anchor for the contractile elements actin and myosin. Actin attaches directly to the Z disc, whereas myosin is attached to it by elastic titin filaments. The myosin filaments are connected to each other by M-protein at the M line. The A, H, and I bands refer to parts of the sarcomere as they were originally seen by light microscopy.

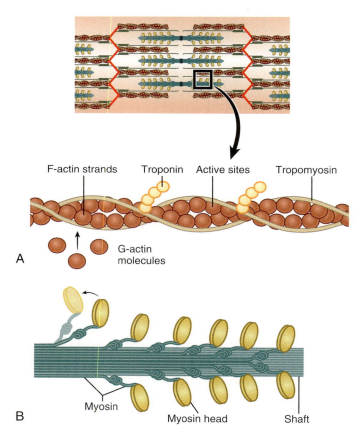

FIGURE 23.14 Structure of Myofilaments. A, Thin myofilament. B, Thick myofilament.

clubs with two large, ovoid heads at one end of the shaft (Figure 23.14B). The two heads contain an actin binding site and a site of adenosine-triphosphatase (ATPase) activity. Thick filaments of myosin overlapping with thinner actin molecules form the central dark band of the sarcomere called the **anisotropic band**, or **A band** (see Figures 23.13 and 23.14). A thick filament has about 200 myosin molecules bundled together with their outward-facing heads named *cross-bridges* because they can form force-generating bridges by binding with exposed actin molecules, resulting in contraction (Figure 23.14A). Actin molecules are part of the thin filaments (see Figures 23.13 and 23.14). The light bands, called **isotropic bands** (or **I bands**), of the sarcomere contain only actin molecules and no myosin (see Figure 23.13). Thin filaments of actin extend from each side of the **Z line**, a dense fibrous structure at the centre of each I band. The area from one dark Z line to the next Z line defines one sarcomere. The centre of the sarcomere is the H zone, a less dense region with a central thin, dark **M line**.[12]

A single **tropomyosin** molecule (a relaxing protein) lies alongside seven actin molecules. Troponin, another relaxing protein, associates with the tropomyosin molecule, forming the **troponin–tropomyosin complex** (see Figures 23.14A, and 23.15). The troponin complex itself has three components. **Troponin T** aids in the binding of the troponin complex to actin and tropomyosin, **troponin I** inhibits the ATPase of actomyosin, and **troponin C** contains binding sites for the calcium ions involved in contraction. Troponin T and I molecules are released into the bloodstream during myocardial injury and are measured to evaluate if a myocardial infarction or other damage has occurred. When troponin and tropomyosin cover the myosin binding sites on actin, the cross-bridges release calcium and the myocardium relaxes. The sarcomere also contains a giant elastic protein, **titin**, which attaches myosin to the Z line, acts as a spring, and influences myocardial stiffness.[12] Titin structure impacts myocardial diastolic filling and has been found to play a role in heart failure.[13]

Myocardial metabolism. Cardiomyocytes depend on the constant production of ATP, which is synthesized within the mitochondria mainly from glucose, fatty acids, and lactate. If the myocardium is underperfused because of coronary artery disease, anaerobic metabolism must be used for energy (see Chapter 1). The metabolic processes provide energy that fuels muscle contraction and relaxation, electrical excitation, membrane transport, and synthesis of large molecules. Normally, the amount of ATP produced supplies sufficient energy to pump blood throughout the system.

Cardiac work is expressed as **myocardial oxygen consumption (MV̇O2)**, which is closely correlated with total cardiac energy requirements. Three major factors determine the MV̇O$_2$: (1) amount of wall stress during systole, estimated by measuring the systolic blood pressure; (2) duration of systolic wall tension, measured indirectly by the heart rate; and (3) contractile state of the myocardium, which is not measured clinically.

The coronary arteries deliver oxygen to the myocardium. The cardiac muscle immediately uses approximately 70 to 75% of this oxygen, leaving little oxygen in reserve. Since the oxygen content of the blood and the amount of oxygen extracted from the blood cannot be increased under normal circumstances, increasing coronary blood flow is the only way to meet any increased energy needs. MV̇O$_2$ increases with exercise and decreases with hypotension and hypothermia. As

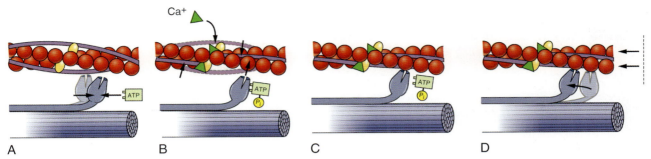

FIGURE 23.15 Cross-bridge Theory of Muscle Contraction. **A,** Each myosin cross-bridge in the thick filament moves into a resting position after an adenosine triphosphate *(ATP)* molecule binds and transfers its energy. **B,** Calcium ions *(Ca+)* released from the sarcoplasmic reticulum bind to troponin in the thin filament, allowing tropomyosin to shift from its position blocking the active sites of actin molecules. **C,** Each myosin cross-bridge then binds to an active site on a thin filament, displacing the remnants of ATP hydrolysis— adenosine diphosphate and inorganic phosphate *(Pi)*. **D,** The release of stored energy from step (A) provides the force needed for each cross-bridge to move back to its original position, pulling actin along with it. Each cross-bridge will remain bound to actin until another ATP molecule binds to it and pulls it back into its resting position (A). (Adapted from Thibodeau, G. A., & Patton, K. T. [1999]. *Anatomy & physiology* [4th ed.]. Mosby.)

myocardial metabolism and consumption of oxygen increase, the local concentration of local vasoactive metabolic factors increases. Some of these factors—such as adenosine, nitric oxide, and prostaglandins— dilate coronary arterioles, thus increasing coronary blood flow.[14]

Myocardial Contraction and Relaxation

Myocardial contractility is a change in developed tension at a given resting fibre length, which basically is the ability of the heart muscle to shorten. At the molecular level, thin filaments of actin slide over thick filaments of myosin, called the **cross-bridge theory of muscle contraction**. Anatomically, contraction occurs when the sarcomere shortens, so adjacent Z lines move closer together (see Figure 23.13). The degree of shortening depends on the amount of overlap between the thick and thin filaments.

Calcium and excitation–contraction coupling. Excitation–contraction coupling is the process by which an action potential arriving at the muscle fibre plasma membrane triggers the cycle, leading to cross-bridge formation and contraction. Cycle activation depends on calcium availability; thus, the concentration of calcium ions within the cardiomyocytes regulates the amount of force it develops. Calcium enters the myocardial cell from the interstitial fluid after electrical excitation that increases membrane calcium permeability. Two types of calcium channels (L-type, T-type) are found in cardiac tissues.[12] The L-type, or long-lasting, channels predominate and are the channels blocked by calcium channel–blocking medications (verapamil [Isoptin], nifedipine [Adalat], diltiazem [Cardizem]).[12] The T-type, or transient, channels are much less abundant in the heart. Current available calcium channel–blocking medications do not block the T-type channels; therefore, T-type channel blockers are being investigated.[15] Calcium entering the cell triggers the release of additional calcium from the two storage sites within the sarcomere: the sarcoplasmic reticulum and tubule system. Calcium ions then diffuse toward the myofibrils, where they bind with troponin (see Figure 23.15).

The calcium–troponin complex interaction facilitates the contraction process. In the resting state, troponin I is bound to actin and the tropomyosin molecule covers the sites where the myosin heads bind to actin, thereby preventing interaction between actin and myosin (see Figure 23.15). Calcium binds to troponin C, which ultimately results in tropomyosin moving troponin I, thus uncovering the binding sites on the myosin heads. Myosin and actin can now form cross-bridges, and ATP can be dephosphorylated to adenosine diphosphate (ADP). Under these circumstances, sliding of the thick and thin filaments can occur, and the muscle contracts (see Figure 23.15).[12]

Myocardial relaxation. Relaxation is as vital to optimal cardiac function as contraction, and calcium, troponin, and tropomyosin also facilitate relaxation. After contraction, free calcium ions are actively pumped out of the cell back into the interstitial fluid or stored back in the sarcoplasmic reticulum and tubule system. As the concentration of calcium within the sarcomere decreases, troponin releases its bound calcium. The tropomyosin complex moves and blocks the active sites on the actin molecule, preventing cross-bridge formation with the myosin heads. If the ability of the myocardium to relax is impaired, it can lead to increased diastolic filling pressures and eventually heart failure.[16]

Factors Affecting Cardiac Output

 QUICK CHECK 23.5
1. Explain four ways that aging impacts the cardiovascular system.
2. Why is Starling's law of the heart important to the understanding of heart failure?
3. Discuss the baroreceptor reflex and explain its influence on blood pressure and heart rate.

Measuring the cardiac output evaluates cardiac performance. **Cardiac output** is calculated by multiplying heart rate in beats per minute (beats/min) by **stroke volume** in litres per beat. Normal adult cardiac output is about 5 L/min at rest given a heart rate of about 70 beats/min and a normal stroke volume of about 70 mL.[7]

With each heartbeat, the ventricles eject much of their blood volume, and the amount ejected per beat is called the **ejection fraction**. Echocardiography, computed tomography (CT) scan, nuclear medicine scan, or cardiac catheterization estimate the ejection fraction, which is calculated by dividing stroke volume by end-diastolic volume. The end-diastolic volume of the normal ventricle is about 70 to 80 mL/m^2, and the normal ejection fraction of the resting heart measured with gated myocardial perfusion imaging is 66%±8% for women and 58%±8% for men.[17]

Factors that increase contractility, such as increased sympathetic nervous system activity, also increase ejection fraction. A decrease in

TABLE 23.3	Cardiovascular Function in Older Persons	
Determinant	Resting Cardiac Performance	Exercise Cardiac Performance[a]
Cardiac output	Unchanged	Decreases because of a decrease in maximum heart rate
Heart rate	Slight decrease	Increases less than in younger people
Stroke volume	Slight increase	No change
Ejection fraction	Unchanged	Decreased
Afterload	Increased	Increased
End-diastolic volume	Unchanged	Increased
End-systolic volume	Unchanged	Increased
Contraction	Decreased velocity	Decreased
Myocardial wall stiffness	Increased	Increased
Maximum oxygen consumption	Not applicable	Decreased
Plasma catecholamines	—	Increased

[a]Changes in healthy men and women up to age 80 years as compared with those who are 20 years of age.
Data from Lakatta, E. G., Najjar, S. S., Schulman, S. P., et al. (2011). Aging and cardiovascular disease in the elderly. In V. Fuster, R. A. Walsh, R. A. Harrington, et al. (Eds.), *Hurst's the heart* (13th ed., pp. 2196–2225). McGraw-Hill.

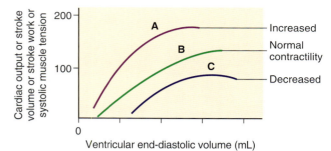

FIGURE 23.16 Starling's Law of the Heart. The relationship between length and tension in the heart. End-diastolic volume determines end-diastolic length of ventricular muscle fibres and is proportional to tension generated during systole, as well as to cardiac output, stroke volume, and stroke work. A change in myocardial contractility causes the heart to perform on a different length-tension curve. *A*, Increased contractility; *B*, normal contractility; *C*, heart failure or decreased contractility. (See text for further explanation.)

ejection fraction may indicate ventricular failure. The effects of aging on cardiovascular function are summarized in Table 23.3.

The factors that determine cardiac output are (1) preload, (2) afterload, (3) myocardial contractility, and (4) heart rate. Preload, afterload, and contractility all affect stroke volume.

Preload

Preload is the volume and pressure inside the ventricle at the end of diastole (**ventricular end-diastolic volume [VEDV]** and **ventricular end-diastolic pressure [VEDP]**). Two primary factors determine the preload: (1) the amount of venous blood returning to the ventricle during diastole and (2) the amount of blood left in the ventricle after systole (end-systolic volume). Venous return is dependent on blood volume and flow through the venous system and the AV valves. End-systolic volume is dependent on the strength of ventricular contraction and the resistance to ventricular emptying. Clinically, measuring the central venous pressure (CVP) for the right side of the heart and the pulmonary artery wedge pressure for the left side estimates the preload. Normal values for these two estimates are 1 to 5 mm Hg and 4 to 12 mm Hg, respectively.[18]

Laplace's law states that wall tension generated in the wall of the ventricle (or any chamber or vessel) to produce a given intraventricular pressure depends directly on ventricular size or internal radius and inversely on ventricular wall thickness. VEDV, which determines the size of the ventricle and the stretch of the cardiac muscle fibres, therefore affects the tension (or force) for contraction. **Starling's law of the heart** indicates that the volume of blood in the heart at the end of diastole determines the length of its muscle fibres and is directly related to the force of contraction during the next systole. Muscle fibres have an optimal resting length from which to generate the maximum amount of contractile strength. Within a physiological range of muscle stretching, increased preload increases stroke volume (and therefore cardiac output and stroke work) (Figure 23.16, curve B). Excessive ventricular filling and preload (increased VEDV) stretches the heart muscle beyond optimal length and stroke volume begins to fall. Factors that increase contractility cause the heart to operate on a higher length-tension curve (see Figure 23.16, curve A). Factors that decrease contractility (see Figure 23.16, curve C) cause the heart to operate at a lower length-tension curve. Figure 23.17 illustrates the relationship between VEDV and stroke volume, cardiac output, and stroke work.

Increases in preload (VEDV) may not only cause a decline in stroke volume but also result in increases in VEDP. These changes can lead to heart failure (see Chapter 24). Increased VEDP causes pressures to increase or "back up" into the pulmonary or systemic venous circulation, thus increasing the movement of plasma out through vessel walls, causing fluid to accumulate in lung tissues (pulmonary edema; see Chapter 27) or in peripheral tissues (peripheral edema).

Afterload

Left ventricular **afterload** is the resistance to ejection of blood from the left ventricle. It is the load that the muscle must move during contraction (see Figure 23.17). Aortic systolic pressure is an index of afterload. Pressure in the ventricle must exceed aortic pressure before blood can be pumped out during systole. Low aortic pressures (decreased afterload) enable the heart to contract more rapidly and efficiently, whereas high aortic pressures (increased afterload) slow contraction and cause higher workloads against which the heart must function to eject blood. Increased aortic pressure is usually the result of increased **systemic vascular resistance (SVR)**, sometimes referred to as **total peripheral resistance (TPR)**. In individuals with hypertension, increased TPR means that afterload is chronically elevated, resulting in increased ventricular workload and hypertrophy of the myocardium. In some individuals, changes in afterload are the result of aortic valvular disease. SVR is calculated by dividing mean arterial pressure by cardiac output. The normal range is 700 dyne/sec/cm^{-5}.[7,18]

Myocardial Contractility

Stroke volume, or the volume of blood ejected per beat during systole, also depends on the *force* of contraction, myocardial contractility, or the degree of myocardial fibre shortening. Three major factors determine the force of contraction (see Figure 23.17):

1. *Changes in the stretching of the ventricular myocardium caused by changes in VEDV (preload).* As discussed previously, increased venous return to the heart distends the ventricle, thus increasing

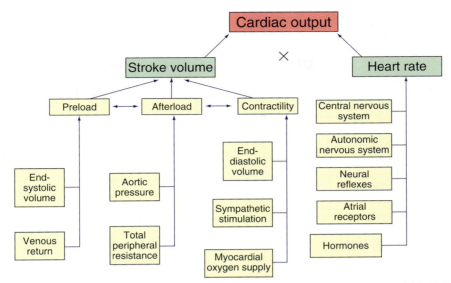

FIGURE 23.17 Factors Affecting Cardiac Performance. Cardiac output, the amount of blood (in litres) ejected by the heart per minute, depends on heart rate (beats per minute) and stroke volume (millilitres of blood ejected during ventricular systole).

preload, which increases the stroke volume and, subsequently, cardiac output, up to a certain point. However, an excessive increase in preload leads to decreased stroke volume.

2. *Alterations in the inotropic stimuli of the ventricles.* Hormones, neurotransmitters, or medications that affect contractility are called **inotropic agents**. The most important endogenous positive inotropic agents are **epinephrine** and norepinephrine released from the sympathetic nervous system. Other positive inotropes include thyroid hormone and dopamine. The most important negative inotropic agent is acetylcholine released from the vagus nerve. Many medications have positive or negative inotropic properties that can have profound effects on cardiac function. In sepsis, a variety of cytokines, including tumour necrosis factor-alpha (TNF-α) and interleukin-1β, have been shown to impair myocardial contractility.[19]

3. *Adequacy of myocardial oxygen supply.* Oxygen and carbon dioxide levels (tensions) in the coronary blood also influence contractility. With severe hypoxemia (arterial oxygen saturation of less than 50%), contractility is decreased. With less severe hypoxemia (arterial oxygen saturation of more than 50%), contractility is stimulated. The myocardial response to circulating catecholamines and contractility is enhanced in response to moderate degrees of hypoxemia.[20]

Preload, afterload, and contractility all interact with one another to determine stroke volume and cardiac output. Changes in any one of these factors can result in deleterious effects on the others, resulting in heart failure (see Chapter 24).

Heart Rate

As described previously, SA node activity is the primary determinant of the heart rate. The average heart rate in healthy adults is about 70 beats/min. This rate diminishes by 10 to 20 beats/min during sleep and can accelerate to more than 100 beats/min during muscular activity or emotional excitement. In well-conditioned athletes, resting heart rate is normally about 50 to 60 beats/min. In highly trained or elite athletes, the resting heart rate can be below 50 beats/min. Athletes also have a greater stroke volume and lower peripheral resistance in active muscles than they had before training. The control of heart rate includes activity of the central nervous system, autonomic nervous system, neural reflexes, atrial receptors, and hormones (see Figure 23.17).

Cardiovascular control centres in the brain. The **cardiovascular vasomotor control centre** is in the medulla and pons areas of the brainstem, with additional areas in the hypothalamus, cerebral cortex, and thalamus.[21] The hypothalamic centres regulate cardiovascular responses to changes in temperature, the cerebral cortex centres adjust cardiac reaction to a variety of emotional states, and the brainstem control centre regulates heart rate and blood pressure (see Figure 23.11).

The nerve fibres from the cardiovascular control centre synapse with autonomic neurons that influence the rate of firing of the SA node. As previously discussed, increased heart rate occurs with sympathetic (adrenergic) stimulation. When the parasympathetic nerves to the heart are stimulated (primarily via the vagus nerve), heart rate slows and the sympathetic nerves to the heart, arterioles, and veins are inhibited.[8] At rest, the heart rate in healthy individuals is primarily under the control of parasympathetic stimulation. Administration of medications that block parasympathetic function (anticholinergic) or physical interruption of the vagus nerve causes significant tachycardia (abnormally fast heart rate) because this inhibitory parasympathetic influence is lost.

Neural reflexes. Output from the **baroreceptor reflexes** influences short-term regulation of the vascular smooth muscle of resistance arteries, myocardial contractility, and heart rate, all components of blood pressure control. The baroreceptors or pressoreceptors are located in the aortic arch and carotid arteries. If blood pressure decreases, the baroreceptor reflex accelerates heart rate, increases myocardial contractility, and increases vascular smooth muscle contraction in the arterioles, thus raising blood pressure. This reflex is critical to maintaining adequate tissue perfusion. When blood pressure increases, the baroreceptors increase their rate of discharge, sending neural impulses over a branch of the glossopharyngeal nerve (cranial nerve IX) and through the vagus nerve to the cardiovascular control centres in the medulla. These reflexes increase parasympathetic activity and decrease sympathetic activity, causing the resistance arteries to dilate, decreasing myocardial contractility and heart rate. The role of baroreceptors in influencing blood pressure is discussed in more detail in "Baroreceptors" later in this chapter.

Atrial receptors. Mechanoreceptors that influence heart rate exist in both atria.[21] They are located where the veins, venae cavae, and pulmonary veins enter their respective atria. Bainbridge reflex is the name for the changes in the heart rate that may occur after intravenous infusions of blood or other fluid. The change in heart rate is thought to be caused by a reflex mediated by these atrial volume receptors that are innervated by the vagus nerve (volume receptors are thought to respond to increased plasma volume). Although this reflex can be elicited in humans, its relevance is uncertain at this time.[22]

Stimulation of these atrial receptors also increases urine volume, presumably because of a neurally mediated reduction in antidiuretic hormone. In addition, peptides of the atrial natriuretic family are released from atrial tissue in response to the increases in blood volume. These peptides have diuretic and natriuretic (salt excretion) properties, resulting in decreased blood volume and pressure. The atrial natriuretic peptides also have been shown to relax vascular smooth muscle and oppose myocardial hypertrophy, leading to measurement of blood levels to evaluate clinical status and raising interest in their use as therapeutic agents.[23]

Hormones and biochemicals. Hormones and other biochemically active substances affect the arteries, arterioles, venules, capillaries, and contractility of the myocardium. Norepinephrine, mainly released as a neurotransmitter from the adrenal medulla, dilates vessels of the liver and skeletal muscle and causes an increase in myocardial contractility. Some adrenocortical hormones, such as hydrocortisone, potentiate the effects of the catecholamines, norepinephrine and epinephrine.

Thyroid hormones enhance sympathetic activity and increase cardiac output. Growth hormone, working together with insulinlike growth factor 1 (IGF-1), also has been shown to increase myocardial contractility.[24] Decreases in levels of growth hormone or thyroid hormone may result in bradycardia (heart rate below 60 beats/min), reduced cardiac output, and low blood pressure. (Other hormones are discussed in "Regulation of Blood Pressure," later in this chapter.)

THE SYSTEMIC CIRCULATION

> ✓ **QUICK CHECK 23.6**
> 1. What is the function of the arterioles?
> 2. Identify the functions of the endothelium.
> 3. Why does the total cross-sectional area in the capillary system lower the resistance to flow?

The arteries and veins of the systemic circulation are illustrated in Figure 23.18. Oxygenated blood leaves the left side of the heart through the aorta and flows into the systemic arteries. These arteries branch into small arterioles, which branch into the smallest vessels, the capillaries, where nutrient and waste product exchange between the blood and tissues occurs. Blood from the capillaries then enters tiny venules that join to form the larger veins, which return venous blood to the right heart. Peripheral vascular system is the term used to describe the part of the systemic circulation that supplies the skin and the extremities, particularly the legs and feet.

Structure of Blood Vessels

Blood vessel walls are composed of three layers: (1) the tunica intima (innermost, or intimal, layer), (2) tunica media (middle, or medial, layer) and (3) the tunica externa or adventitia (outermost, or external, layer), which also contains nerves and lymphatic vessels. These layers are illustrated in Figure 23.19. Blood vessel walls vary in thickness depending on the thickness or absence of one or more of these three layers. The vasa vasorum, small vessels located in the tunica externa, nourish cells of the larger vessel walls.

Arterial Vessels

An artery is a thick-walled pulsating blood vessel that transports blood away from the heart. In the systemic circulation, arteries carry oxygenated blood. Arterial walls are composed of elastic connective tissue, fibrous connective tissue, and smooth muscle. Elastic arteries, such as the aorta, the branches of the aorta, and the trunk of the pulmonary artery, have a thick tunica media with more elastic fibres than smooth muscle fibres. Elasticity allows the vessel to absorb energy and stretch as blood is ejected from the heart during systole. During diastole, elasticity promotes recoil of the arteries, maintaining blood pressure within the vessels.

Muscular arteries, medium- and small-sized arteries, are farther from the heart than the elastic arteries. They contain more muscle fibres and fewer elastic fibres than the elastic arteries and they function to distribute blood to arterioles throughout the body. Because their smooth muscle can contract or relax, they play a role in blood flow control and in directing flow to body parts with the highest need at any point in time. Contraction narrows the vessel lumen (the internal cavity of the vessel), which diminishes flow through the vessel (vasoconstriction). When the smooth muscle layer relaxes, more blood flows through the vessel lumen (vasodilation).

An artery becomes an arteriole where the diameter of its lumen narrows to less than 0.5 mm. Arterioles are mainly composed of smooth muscle. Constriction or dilation of these smooth muscles regulates the flow of blood into the capillaries to either slow or increase the flow (Figure 23.20). The thick smooth muscle layer of the arterioles is a major determinant of the resistance blood encounters as it flows through the systemic circulation.

The capillary network is composed of connective channels called metarterioles, and "true" capillaries (see Figure 23.20). Metarterioles have discontinuous smooth muscle cells in their tunica media, whereas capillaries have no smooth muscle cells. There is a ring of smooth muscle called the precapillary sphincter at the point where capillaries branch from metarterioles. As the sphincters contract and relax, they regulate blood flow through the capillary beds. The precapillary sphincters help to maintain arterial pressure and regulate selective flow to vascular beds.

Capillaries are composed solely of a layer of endothelial cells surrounded by a basement membrane. Their thin walls and unique structure make possible the rapid exchange of water and small (low molecular weight) soluble molecules. Some larger molecules, such as albumin and cells of the innate and adaptive components of the immune system, may also be exchanged between the blood and the interstitial fluid. In some capillaries, the endothelial cells contain oval windows or pores termed fenestrations covered by a thin diaphragm.

Substances pass between the capillary lumen and the interstitial fluid (1) through junctions between endothelial cells, (2) through fenestrations in endothelial cells, (3) in vesicles moved by active transport across the endothelial cell membrane, or (4) by diffusion through the endothelial cell membrane. A single capillary may be only 0.5 to 1 mm in length and 0.01 mm in diameter, but the capillaries are so numerous their total surface area may be more than 600 m^2 (about 100 football fields).

Endothelium

The vascular endothelium is important to several body functions and is sometimes considered a separate endocrine organ. All tissues depend on a blood supply, and the blood supply depends on endothelial cells, which form the lining (or endothelium) of the blood vessel (Figure 23.21). The vascular endothelium has important roles in coagulation, antithrombogenesis, and fibrinolysis. In addition, it plays a role in immune system function, tissue and vessel growth, wound

CHAPTER 23 Structure and Function of the Cardiovascular and Lymphatic Systems

healing, and the contraction and relaxation of vessels (vasomotion).[25] Table 23.4 summarizes some of the more important endothelial functions. Endothelial injury and dysfunction are central processes in many of the most common and serious cardiovascular disorders, including hypertension and atherosclerosis (see Chapter 24).

Veins

Compared with arteries, **veins** are thin walled with more fibrous connective tissue and have a larger diameter (see Figure 23.19). Veins also are more numerous than arteries. The smallest venules downstream from the capillaries have an endothelial lining and are surrounded by connective tissue. The largest venules have some smooth muscle fibres in their thin tunica media. The venous tunica externa has less elastic tissue than that in arteries, so veins do not recoil as much or as rapidly after distension. Like arteries, veins receive nourishment from tiny vasa vasorum.

Veins contain valves to facilitate the one-way flow of blood toward the heart (Figure 23.22). These valves are folds of the tunica intima and resemble the semilunar valves of the heart. When a person stands up, contraction of the skeletal muscles of the legs compresses the deep veins of the legs and assists the flow of blood toward the heart. This important mechanism of venous return is called the **muscle pump** (Figure 23.22B).

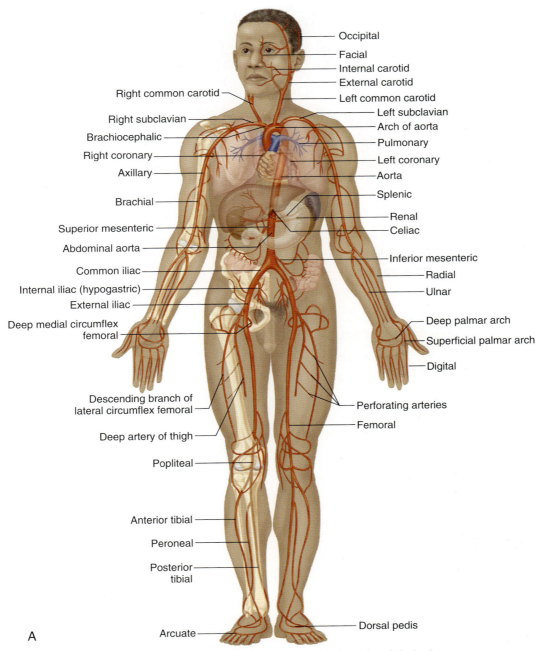

FIGURE 23.18 Circulatory System. **A,** Principal arteries of the body.

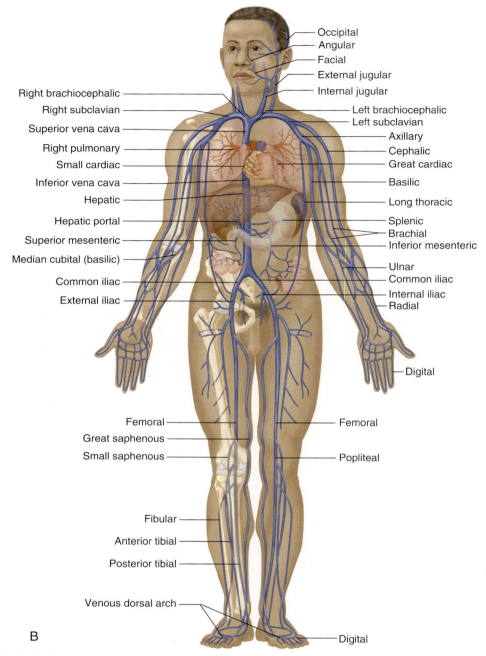

FIGURE 23.18, cont'd B, Principal veins of the body. (From Patton, K. T., Thibodeau, G. A., & Douglas, M. M. [2012]. *Essentials of anatomy & physiology*. Elsevier.)

Factors Affecting Blood Flow

Blood flow, the amount of fluid moved per unit of time, is usually expressed as litres or millilitres per minute (L/min or mL/min). Factors that influence blood flow include pressure, resistance, velocity, turbulent versus laminar flow, and compliance, with the most important of these being pressure and resistance.

Pressure and Resistance

Pressure in a liquid system is the force exerted on the liquid per unit area and is expressed clinically as millimetres of mercury (mm Hg), or torr (1 torr = 1 mm Hg). Blood flow to an organ depends partly on the pressure difference between the arterial and venous vessels supplying that organ. Fluid moves from the arterial "side" of the capillaries where the pressure is higher to the venous side where the pressure is lower.

Resistance is the opposition to blood flow. Most opposition to blood flow results from the diameter and length of the vessels. Changes in blood flow through an organ result from changes in the vascular resistance within the organ because of increases or decreases in vessel diameter and the opening or closing of vascular channels. Resistance in a vessel is inversely related to blood flow—that is, increased resistance leads to decreased blood flow. **Poiseuille's law** indicates that resistance is directly related to tube length and blood viscosity and inversely related to the radius of the tube to the fourth power (r^4). Because blood

CHAPTER 23 Structure and Function of the Cardiovascular and Lymphatic Systems

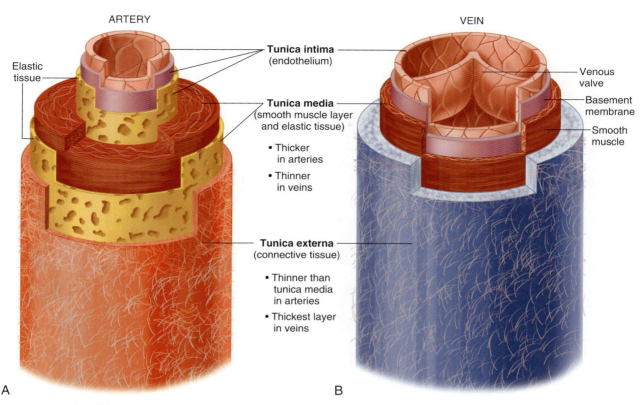

FIGURE 23.19 Structure of the Blood Vessels. The tunica externa of the veins is colour-coded *blue* and the arteries *red*. (From Patton, K. T., & Thibodeau, G. A. [2016]. *Structure & function of the body* [15th ed.]. Elsevier.)

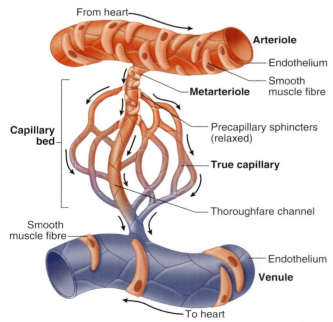

FIGURE 23.20 Microcirculation. Altering the tone of precapillary sphincters surrounding arterioles and metarterioles controls the local blood flow through a capillary network. In the diagram, the sphincters are relaxed, permitting blood flow to enter the capillary bed. (From Patton, K. T., Thibodeau, G. A., & Douglas, M. M. [2012]. *Essentials of anatomy & physiology*. Elsevier.)

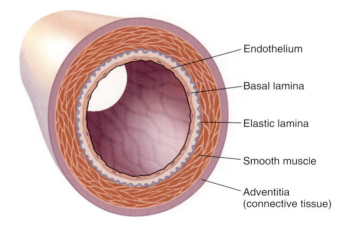

FIGURE 23.21 Vascular Endothelium. The endothelial cells arrange themselves as a single-layer lining that has numerous critical functions (see Table 23.4).

flow is inversely related to resistance, the greater the resistance, the lower the blood flow will be. Resistance to flow cannot be measured directly, but it can be calculated if the pressure difference and flow volumes are known. The radius and length of the blood vessel, as well as the blood viscosity, determine the resistance to blood flow in a single vessel. The most important factor determining resistance *in a single vessel* is the radius or diameter of the vessel's lumen. Small changes in the lumen's radius or diameter lead to large changes in vascular

TABLE 23.4 Functions of the Endothelium

Function	Actions Involved
Filtration and permeability	Facilitates transport of large molecules via vesicular transport movement through intercellular junctions
	Facilitates transport of small molecules via movement of vesicles, through opening of tight junctions, and across cytoplasm
Vasomotion	Stimulates vascular relaxation through production of nitric oxide, prostacyclin, and other vasodilators
	Stimulates vascular constriction through production of endothelin-1 and of angiotensin II by the action of endothelial angiotensin-converting enzyme on angiotensin I
Hemostatic balance	Maintains a balance between procoagulant and anticoagulant factors, as well as profibrinolytic and antifibrinolytic factors; endothelial surface is normally antithrombotic
	Counteracts coagulation through anticoagulant factors, including prostacyclin, nitric oxide, antithrombin, thrombomodulin, tissue factor pathway inhibitor, and heparins
	Activates coagulation through procoagulant factors, including tissue factor (factor VII), factor VIII, factor V, and plasminogen activator inhibitor-1 (PAI-1)
	Controls coagulation through profibrinolytic factors: tissue- and urokinase-type plasminogen activating factor and plasminogen activator inhibitor-1 (PAI-1)
	Breaks down blood clots through antifibrinolytic factor: tissue plasminogen activator
Inflammation/immunity	Expresses chemotactic agents and adhesion molecules that support white blood cells (including monocytes, neutrophils, and lymphocytes) moving into tissues
	Expresses receptors for oxidized lipoproteins, allowing them to enter vascular intima
Angiogenesis/vessel growth	Releases growth factors such as endothelin-1 and heparins for vascular smooth muscle cells
Lipid metabolism	Expresses receptors for lipoprotein lipase and low-density lipoproteins

From Griendling, K. K., Harrison, D. G., & Alexander, R. W. (2011). Biology of the vessel wall. In V. Fuster, R. A. Walsh, R. A. Harrington, et al. (Eds.), *Hurst's the heart* (13th ed., pp. 153–171). McGraw-Hill; Rajendran, P., Rengarajan, T., Thangavel, J., et al. (2013). The vascular endothelium and human diseases. *International Journal of Biological Sciences, 9*(10), 1057–1069.

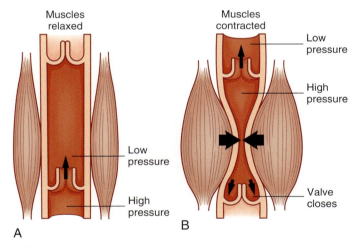

FIGURE 23.22 Venous Valves and the Muscle Pump. In veins, one-way valves aid circulation by preventing backflow of venous blood when pressure in a local area is low. **A,** Blood is moved toward the heart as valves in the veins are forced open by pressure from volume of blood downstream and the neighbouring muscles are relaxed. **B,** When pressure below the valve drops, blood begins to flow backward but fills the "pockets" formed by the valve flaps, pushing the flaps together and thus blocking further backward flow. Contraction in the adjacent muscles and the valves of the systemic veins assist in the return of unoxygenated blood to the right heart.

resistance. Clinically, vasoconstriction will contribute to an increase in resistance whereas vasodilation will cause a decrease in resistance that may be reflected by a fall in blood pressure. Because vessel length is relatively constant, whereas lumen size is quite variable, length is not as important as lumen size in determining flow through a single vessel. Because viscosity is relatively constant, blood vessel radius is usually the key factor in determining TPR. An exception to this rule is when red blood cell volume, measured as hematocrit, is elevated, which is relatively rare. Conditions with elevated hematocrits include a lack of body water, cyanotic congenital heart disease (see Chapter 25), or polycythemia (see Chapter 21), and can lead to increased cardiac work because of increased vascular resistance.

Resistance to flow through a *system of vessels*, or **total resistance**, depends not only on characteristics of individual vessels but also on whether the vessels are arranged in series or in parallel and on the total cross-sectional area of the system. Vessels arranged in parallel provide less resistance than vessels arranged in series. Blood flowing through the distributing arteries, beginning with branches off the aorta and ending at arterioles in the capillary bed, encounters more resistance than blood flowing through the capillary bed itself, where flow is distributed among many short, tiny branches arranged in parallel (Figure 23.23). The total cross-sectional area of the arteriolar system is greater than that of the arterial system, yet the greater number of arterioles arranged in series leads to great resistance to flow in the arteriolar system. In contrast, the capillary system has a larger number of vessels arranged in parallel and the total cross-sectional area is much greater; thus, there is lower resistance overall through the capillary system. The resulting slow velocity of flow in each capillary is optimal for capillary–tissue exchange.

Velocity

Blood velocity or speed is the *distance* blood travels in a unit of time, usually centimetres per second. It is directly related to blood flow (*amount* of blood moved per unit of time) and inversely related to the cross-sectional area of the vessel in which the blood is flowing (see Figure 23.23). As blood moves from the aorta to the capillaries, the total cross-sectional area of the vessels increases and the velocity decreases.

Laminar Versus Turbulent Flow

Flow through a tubular system can be either laminar or turbulent. Blood flow through the vessels, except where vessels split or branch, is usually laminar. In **laminar flow**, concentric layers of molecules move "straight ahead," with each layer flowing at a slightly different velocity (Figure 23.24). The cohesive attraction between the fluid and the vessel wall prevents the molecules of blood that are in contact with the wall from moving at all. The next thin layer of blood is able to slide slowly past the stationary layer and so on until, at the centre, the blood velocity is greatest. Large vessels have

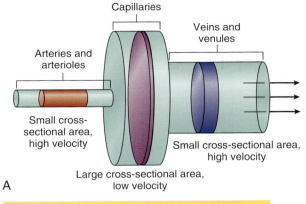

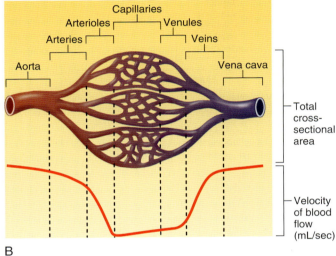

FIGURE 23.23 Relationship Between Cross-sectional Area and Velocity of Blood Flow. Blood flows with great speed in the large arteries. However, branching of arterial vessels increases the total cross-sectional area of the arterioles and capillaries, reducing the flow rate. When capillaries merge into venules and venules merge into veins, the total cross-sectional area decreases, causing the flow rate to increase. (From Patton, K. T. [2019]. *Anatomy & physiology* [10th ed.]. Elsevier.)

room for a large centre layer, therefore, they have less resistance to flow and greater flow and velocity than smaller vessels.

Where flow is obstructed, the vessel turns, or blood flows over rough surfaces, the flow becomes **turbulent** with whorls or eddy currents that produce noise, causing a murmur to be heard on auscultation. Resistance increases with turbulence, which frequently occurs in areas with atherosclerotic plaque (see Chapter 24).

Vascular Compliance

Vascular compliance is the increase in volume a vessel can accommodate for a given increase in pressure. Compliance depends on factors related to the nature of a vessel wall, such as the ratio of elastic fibres to muscle fibres in the wall. Elastic arteries are more compliant than muscular arteries. The veins are more compliant than either type of artery, and they can serve as storage areas for the circulatory system.

Compliance determines a vessel's response to pressure changes. For example, the venous system can accommodate a large volume of blood with only a small increase in pressure. In the less compliant arterial system, where smaller volumes and higher pressures are normal, even small changes in blood volume can cause significant changes in arterial pressure.

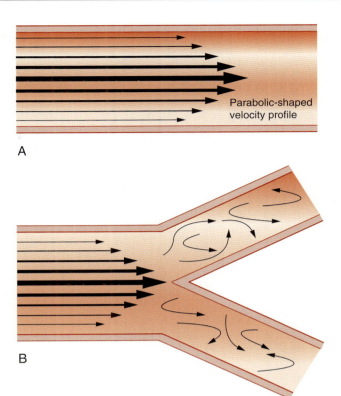

FIGURE 23.24 Laminar and Turbulent Blood Flow. A, Laminar flow. Fluid flows in long, smooth-walled tubes as if it were composed of a large number of concentric layers. **B,** Turbulent flow. Turbulent flow is caused by numerous small currents flowing cross-wise or oblique to the long axis of the vessel, resulting in flowing whorls and eddying currents.

Stiffness is the opposite of compliance. Several conditions and disorders can cause stiffness, with the most common being aging and atherosclerosis (see Chapter 24).

Regulation of Blood Pressure

> ✓ **QUICK CHECK 23.7**
> 1. Identify the factors and relationships regulating blood pressure.
> 2. Why is capillary flow increased with increased mean arterial pressure?
> 3. Why is angiotensin significant in blood flow?
> 4. Define *natriuretic peptides* and *adrenomedullin*.

Arterial Pressure

Arterial blood pressure is determined by the cardiac output multiplied by the peripheral resistance (Figure 23.25). The **systolic blood pressure** is the highest arterial blood pressure following ventricular contraction or systole. The **diastolic blood pressure** is the lowest arterial blood pressure that occurs during ventricular filling or diastole. The **mean arterial pressure (MAP)**, which is the average pressure in the arteries throughout the cardiac cycle, depends on the elastic properties of the arterial walls and the mean volume of blood in the arterial system. MAP can be approximated from the measured values of the systolic (P_s) and diastolic (P_d) pressures as follows:

$$MAP = P_d + \frac{1}{3}(P_s - P_d)$$

The normal range for MAP is 70 to 110 mm Hg.[26] The difference between the systolic pressure and diastolic pressure ($P_s - P_d$) is called

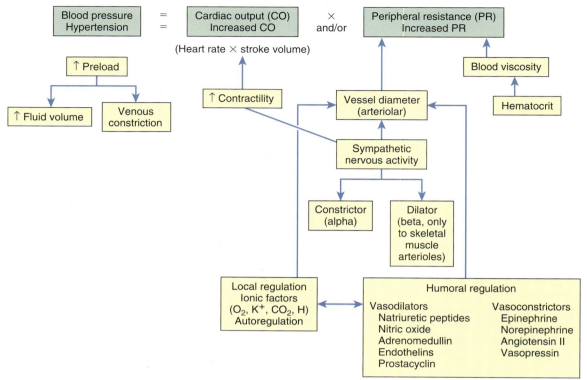

FIGURE 23.25 Factors and Relationships Regulating Blood Pressure. CO_2, Carbon dioxide; H, hydrogen; K^+, potassium; O_2, oxygen.

the **pulse pressure** and typically is between 40 and 50 mm Hg.[7] Pulse pressure is directly related to arterial wall stiffness and stroke volume.

During a wide range of physiological conditions, including changes in body position, muscular activity, and circulating blood volume, arterial pressure is regulated within a fairly narrow range to maintain tissue **perfusion**, or blood supply to the capillary beds. The major factors and relationships that regulate arterial blood pressure are summarized in Figure 23.25.

Effects of Cardiac Output

Alterations in heart rate, stroke volume (volume of blood ejected during each ventricular contraction), or both can change the cardiac output (minute volume) of the heart. An increase in cardiac output without a decrease in peripheral resistance will cause MAP and flow rate to increase. The higher arterial pressure increases blood flow through the arterioles. On the other hand, a decrease in the cardiac output causes a drop in the mean arterial blood pressure and arteriolar flow if peripheral resistance stays constant.

Effects of Total Peripheral Resistance

Total resistance in the systemic circulation, known as either *SVR* or *TPR*, is primarily a function of arteriolar diameter. If cardiac output remains constant, arteriolar constriction raises MAP by reducing the flow of blood into the capillaries, whereas arteriolar dilation has the opposite effect. Reflex control of total cardiac output and peripheral resistance includes (1) sympathetic stimulation of heart, arterioles, and veins; and (2) parasympathetic stimulation of the heart (Figure 23.26). The cardiovascular centre in the medulla receives input from arterial baroreceptors and chemoreceptors throughout the vascular system and then modifies vagal and sympathetic output to control heart rate and contractility, plus vascular diameter. Vasoconstriction is regulated by an area of the brainstem that maintains a constant (tonic) output of norepinephrine from sympathetic fibres in the peripheral arterioles. This tonic activity is essential for maintenance of blood pressure.

Baroreceptors. As discussed previously, baroreceptors are stretch receptors located predominantly in the aorta and in the carotid sinus (Figure 23.26A). They respond to changes in smooth muscle fibre length by altering their rate of discharge and supplying sensory information to the cardiovascular centre in the brainstem. When activated (stretched), the baroreceptors decrease cardiac output (by lowering heart rate and stroke volume) and peripheral resistance, and thus lower blood pressure. (Postural changes and the baroreceptor reflex are discussed in Chapter 24.)

Arterial chemoreceptors. Specialized areas within the aortic arch and carotid arteries are sensitive to concentrations of oxygen, carbon dioxide, and hydrogen ions (pH) in the blood (Figure 23.26B). Although these chemoreceptors are most important for respiratory control, they also transmit impulses to the medullary cardiovascular centres that regulate blood pressure. A decrease in arterial oxygen concentration or an increase in carbon dioxide concentration contributes to an increase in heart rate, stroke volume, and blood pressure, whereas an increase in carbon dioxide concentration causes decreases in these variables. Alteration in arterial oxygen concentration is the major chemoreceptive reflex. The effects of altered pH or carbon dioxide levels are minor.[21]

Effect of Hormones

Hormones influence blood pressure regulation through their effects on vascular smooth muscle and blood volume. By constricting or dilating the arterioles in organs, hormones can (1) increase or decrease the flow in response to the body's needs, (2) redistribute blood volume during hemorrhage or shock, and (3) regulate heat loss. The key

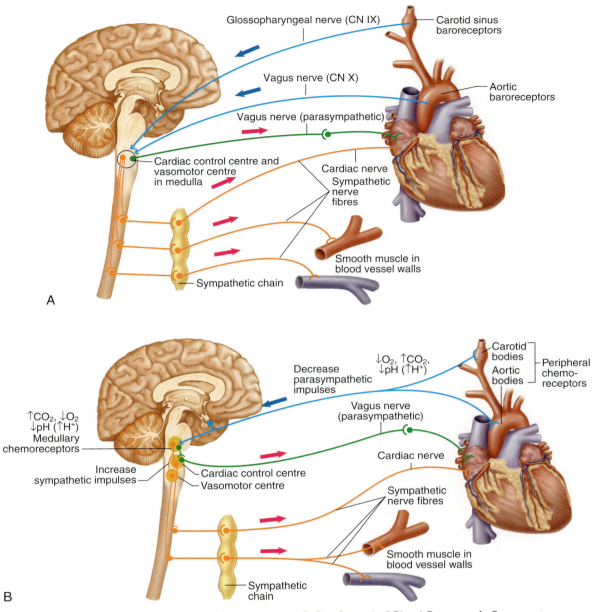

FIGURE 23.26 Baroreceptors and Chemoreceptor Reflex Control of Blood Pressure. **A,** Baroreceptor reflexes. **B,** Vasomotor chemoreflexes. *CN,* Cranial nerve; CO_2, carbon dioxide; H^+, hydrogen; O_2, oxygen. (Modified from Patton, K. T. [2019]. *Anatomy & physiology* [10th ed.]. Elsevier.)

vasoconstrictor hormones include angiotensin II, vasopressin (or antidiuretic hormone), epinephrine, and norepinephrine. The main vasodilator hormones are the atrial natriuretic hormones. By causing fluid retention or loss, aldosterone, vasopressin, and the natriuretic hormones can influence stroke volume and thus blood pressure.

A variety of other factors, including adipokines and insulin, may be related to the hypertension that occurs with chronic conditions, such as adiposity and diabetes mellitus. These factors have not been clearly demonstrated to play a role in blood pressure regulation in healthy individuals.[27] Research has suggested that the risk for cardiovascular disease and hypertension that often co-occurs with diabetes mellitus is more closely related to insulin resistance than to insulin levels.[28] **Adrenomedullin (ADM)** is a vasodilating peptide present in cardiovascular, pulmonary, renal, and other tissues. Because increases in ADM levels are associated with heart failure and myocardial infarction, ADM levels may be useful for risk categorization in people with these conditions.[29]

Vasoconstrictor hormones. The vasoconstrictor hormones include epinephrine, norepinephrine, and angiotensin II, which is part of the renin-angiotensin-aldosterone system. Vasopressin (also known as *antidiuretic hormone*) is also considered a vasoconstrictor hormone. Epinephrine, the catecholamine hormone released from the adrenal medulla, causes vasoconstriction in most vascular beds except the coronary, liver, and skeletal muscle circulations. Norepinephrine mainly acts as a neurotransmitter; however, some norepinephrine is also released from the adrenal medulla. When released into the circulation, it is a more potent vasoconstrictor than epinephrine. Although angiotensin II and vasopressin are vasoconstrictors, they are not thought to have a major role in blood pressure control in normal circumstances.

Vasopressin and aldosterone also affect blood pressure by increasing fluid reabsorption in the kidneys and stimulating thirst in the hypothalamus, which in turn results in excessive fluid intake. Eventually these mechanisms lead to increase in blood volume. Vasopressin causes the reabsorption of water from tubular fluid in the distal tubule and collecting duct of the nephron. Aldosterone, the end product of the renin-angiotensin-aldosterone system, stimulates the reabsorption of sodium, chloride, and water from the same locations in the kidney (Figure 23.27; also see Chapters 5 and 18).

Vasodilator hormones. The natriuretic peptides (NPs) or hormones (see Figure 23.27), including atrial natriuretic peptide (ANP), B-type natriuretic peptide (BNP), C-type natriuretic peptide (CNP), and urodilatin, function as both vasodilators and regulators of sodium and water excretion (natriuresis and diuresis). Increased pressure or diastolic volume in the heart stimulates the release of these peptide hormones. Increased levels of BNP predict increased risk for a poor outcome in heart failure (see *Health Promotion:* B-type Natriuretic Peptide and Heart Failure), pulmonary embolism, valvular heart disease, and chronic coronary artery disease.[30]

Effects of Other Mediators

A variety of other mediators have been demonstrated to cause arteriolar vasodilation or vasoconstriction. Some of the vasodilating mediators include nitric oxide, ADM, the endothelins, and prostacyclin. These mediators are being investigated to determine whether they or their inhibitors might be useful medications for the treatment of cardiovascular diseases or whether their levels might be useful in determining the prognosis of persons with known disease.

Nitric oxide (NO), an intercellular and intracellular signalling molecule produced in endothelial cells, has a variety of roles in vascular function, including acting as a vasodilator and inhibitor of smooth muscle proliferation. Nitric oxide also has been referred to as *endothelium-derived relaxing factor* (EDRF). One way that diabetes may contribute to hypertension is through inhibition of nitric oxide production by impeding a family of enzymes—the nitric oxide synthases.[31] Understanding the role of nitric oxide in producing vasodilation explains why sublingual nitroglycerine has been a useful treatment for coronary artery spasm.[32]

ADM, a peptide with powerful vasodilatory activity, is present in numerous tissues. It is a member of the calcitonin gene–related peptide family. Although it has been found to have numerous cardiovascular effects, including a role in fetal cardiovascular system development and vasodilation, its exact role in adult human cardiovascular function and disease is unclear. Some research indicates that elevated ADM levels may be useful disease indicators.[33]

The endothelins are a family of three peptides (ET-1, ET-2, and ET-3) and four receptors produced in cells in the vascular smooth muscle, the endothelium, the kidneys, and other organs. Understanding the physiological and pathological roles of these peptides has been complicated by the fact that endothelin binding to the type-A receptor causes vasodilation and natriuresis, whereas binding to the type-B receptor causes the opposite response—vasoconstriction plus sodium and water retention.[34] Inhibitors to ET-1 have been approved for the treatment of pulmonary hypertension.[35]

Prostacyclin is a vasodilator that is produced by the actions of cyclo-oxygenases (COX-1 and COX-2) on arachidonic acid. It also has the additional properties of opposing clot formation (antithrombotic), decreasing platelet activity, and inhibiting the release of growth factors from macrophages and the endothelial cells.[32] Nonsteroidal anti-inflammatory drugs (NSAIDs) that inhibit these cyclo-oxygenases have been associated with cardiovascular disease risk in healthy people and in those with a known cardiovascular disease.[36,37]

Venous Pressure

The main determinants of venous blood pressure are (1) the volume of fluid within the veins and (2) the compliance (distensibility) of the vessel walls. The venous system typically accommodates about 66% of the total blood volume at any time, with venous pressure averaging less than 10 mm Hg. The systemic arteries accommodate about 11% of the total blood volume, with an average arterial pressure (blood pressure) of about 100 mm Hg. The remainder of the blood volume is within the heart, capillaries, and pulmonary circulation.[26]

The sympathetic nervous system controls venous compliance. The walls of the veins are highly innervated by sympathetic fibres that control venous smooth muscle. Rather than constriction that would occur in the arteries, smooth muscle contraction in the veins results in stiffening of the vessel walls. This stiffening reduces venous distensibility and increases venous blood pressure, forcing more blood through the veins and into the right heart.

Two other mechanisms that increase venous pressure and venous return to the heart are (1) the skeletal muscle pump and (2) the respiratory pump. During skeletal muscle contraction, the veins within the muscles are partially compressed, causing decreased venous capacity and increased return to the heart (see Figure 23.26). The respiratory pump acts during inspiration, when the veins of the abdomen are partially compressed by the downward movement of the diaphragm. Increased abdominal pressure moves blood toward the heart.

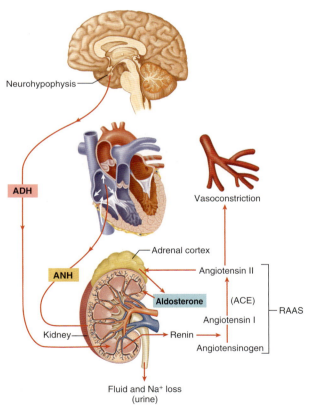

FIGURE 23.27 Three Mechanisms That Influence Total Plasma Volume. The antidiuretic hormone *(ADH)* mechanism and renin-angiotensin-aldosterone system *(RAAS)* tend to increase water, sodium, and chloride retention and thus increase total plasma volume. The atrial natriuretic hormone *(ANH)* mechanism antagonizes these mechanisms by promoting water, sodium, and chloride loss, thus promoting a decrease in total plasma volume. *ACE,* Angiotensin-converting enzyme. (Modified from Patton, K. T. [2019]. *Anatomy & physiology* [10th ed.]. Elsevier.)

> **HEALTH PROMOTION**
>
> ### B-type Natriuretic Peptide and Heart Failure
>
> Heart failure occurs because of chronic and progressive loss of functioning cardiac myocytes and a disruption of the ability of the myocardium to contract normally, which triggers a variety of compensatory mechanisms. Compensatory mechanisms, such as an increase in adrenergic nervous system activity and excessive activation of the renin-angiotensin-aldosterone system, will initially restore cardiovascular contractility. However, over time, continual activation of these systems can lead to detrimental dysfunction in myocardial pumping ability, left ventricular remodelling, and subsequent cardiac decompensation.
>
> BNP is a hormone that was initially identified in the brain but is now recognized as being released primarily from the heart, particularly the ventricles. The normal reference range for BNP is less than 100 ng/L. Values increase with age and weight and are higher in women than men. The production of BNP increases in response to ventricular volume expansion and pressure overload. It also increases to counteract the possible deleterious effects of the compensatory mechanisms. BNP has diuretic, natriuretic, and vasodilator actions. It also inhibits the renin-angiotensin-aldosterone system, the secretion of endothelin, and systemic and renal sympathetic activity. BNP may protect against collagen formation and accumulation, and the pathological cardiac remodelling that contributes to the worsening of heart failure. As such, an elevated BNP serum level is a marker of ventricular distress and useful in diagnosing and monitoring the severity of heart failure. BNP levels higher than 400 correlate with heart failure. The severity of heart failure is directly correlated with the level of BNP. That is, the higher the BNP level, the greater the severity of heart failure.
>
> In 2015, Lourenço, Ribeiro, Pintalhão, and colleagues established that BNP is the gold standard for heart failure prognostic prediction. They also concluded that a decrease in BNP levels independently predicts better survival and lower mortality. For example, patients in whom BNP decreased by greater than 30% had a hazard ratio of death of 0.57 (0.37 to 0.89). Also in 2015, Egom suggested that a linear relationship exists between plasma BNP levels and cardiovascular mortality. It should be noted that elevated BNP does not differentiate between ventricular systolic or ventricular diastolic dysfunction.
>
> Studies reveal that BNP is a marker that is highly sensitive and specific. The greater value of BNP is in repeated measurement to monitor the progression of disease and in evaluating the response to medical therapy. As a marker, BNP is particularly useful in the emergency department setting for patients who present with acute dyspnea. BNP measurement is also a valuable tool in differentiating cardiac from noncardiac causes of respiratory distress. Several studies have shown that concentrations of BNP are substantially higher in patients with acute heart failure when compared with those with dyspnea due to other causes.

Data from Egom, E. E. (2015). BNP and heart failure: preclinical and clinical trial data. *Journal of Cardiovascular Translational Research, 8*(3), 149–157. doi:10.1007/s12265-015-9619-3; Kessenich, C.R. (2011). BNP and heart failure: what is the connection? *Nurse Practitioner, 36*(1), 13–14. doi:10.1097/01.npr.0000391180.55502.18; Lourenço, P., Ribeiro, A., Pintalhão, M., et al. (2015). Predictors of six-month mortality in BNP-matched acute heart failure patients. *American Journal of Cardiology, 116*(5), 744–748. doi:10.1016/j.amjcard.2015.05.046.

Regulation of the Coronary Circulation

Coronary blood flow is directly proportional to the perfusion pressure and inversely proportional to the vascular resistance of the coronary bed. **Coronary perfusion pressure** is the difference between pressure in the aorta and pressure in the coronary vessels. Thus, aortic pressure is the driving pressure for the arteries and arterioles that perfuse the myocardium. Vasodilation and vasoconstriction maintain coronary blood flow despite stresses imposed by the constant contraction and relaxation of the heart muscle and despite shifts (within a physiological range) of coronary perfusion pressure.

Several unique anatomical factors influence coronary blood flow. Because of their anatomical location, the aortic valve cusps can obstruct coronary blood flow by occluding the openings of the coronary arteries during systole. Also, during systole, the coronary arteries are compressed by ventricular contraction. The resulting **systolic compressive effect** is particularly evident in the subendocardial layers of the left ventricular wall and can greatly increase resistance to coronary blood flow with the result that most left ventricular coronary blood flow occurs during diastole. During the period of systolic compression, when flow is slowed or stopped, **myoglobin**, a protein in heart muscle that binds oxygen, provides the supply of oxygen to the myocardium. Myoglobin's oxygen levels are replenished during diastole.

Autoregulation

Autoregulation (automatic self-regulation) of organs alters the resistance (diameter) in their arterioles and thereby enables organs to regulate blood flow. Autoregulation in the coronary circulation maintains the blood flow at a nearly constant rate at perfusion pressures (MAP) between 60 and 140 mm Hg when other influencing factors are held constant.[21] Thus autoregulation helps to ensure constant coronary blood flow despite shifts in the perfusion pressure within the stated range.

Given that blood flow is directly related to pressure and inversely related to resistance, for flow to stay constant as pressure decreases resistance also has to decrease. Therefore, the mechanisms underlying autoregulation must be related to control of smooth muscle contraction in the arteriolar walls. Although the exact mechanisms underlying autoregulation are unknown, research has indicated that factors influencing calcium release with the myocardium are involved and perhaps also the accumulation of vasodilatory products of metabolism, such as adenosine.[21,38]

Autonomic Regulation

Although the coronary vessels, themselves, contain sympathetic (α- and β-adrenergic) and parasympathetic neural receptors, coronary blood flow during regular activity is regulated locally by the factors that cause autoregulation. During exercise, however, the vasodilating effects of β_2-receptors on the smaller coronary resistance arteries are responsible for about 25% of any increase in blood flow. At the same time, α-adrenergic receptors in larger arteries cause vasoconstriction to direct the blood flow to the inner layers of the myocardium.[21]

THE LYMPHATIC SYSTEM

> ✓ **QUICK CHECK 23.8**
> 1. Why is the lymphatic system considered a circulatory system?
> 2. What happens to lymph in lymph nodes?

The lymphatic system is a one-way network of lymphatic vessels and the lymph nodes (Figures 23.28 and 23.29) that is important for immune function, fluid balance, and transport of lipids, hormones, and cytokines. Every day about 3 L of fluid filters out of venous capillaries

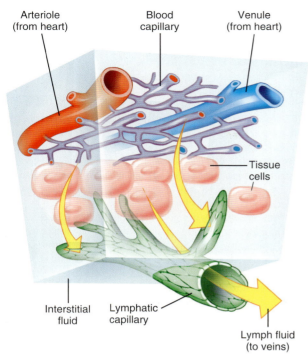

FIGURE 23.28 Role of the Lymphatic System in Fluid Balance. Fluid from plasma flowing through the capillaries moves into interstitial spaces. Although most of this interstitial fluid is either absorbed by tissue cells or reabsorbed by blood capillaries, some of the fluid tends to accumulate in the interstitial spaces. This lymph then diffuses into the lymphatic vessels that carry it to the lymph nodes and then into the systemic venous blood. *Green* is used to diagram the lymphatic vessels, although the lymphatic vessels, particularly the smaller ones, are almost transparent. (Modified from Patton, K. T. [2019]. *Anatomy and physiology* [10th ed.]. Elsevier.)

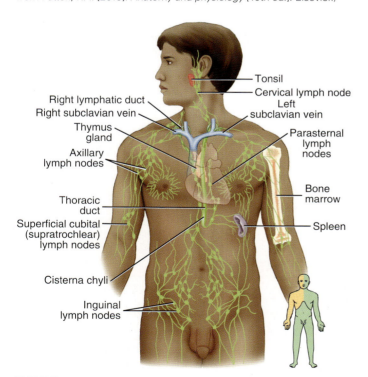

FIGURE 23.29 Principal Organs of the Lymphatic System. (From VanMeter, K. C., & Hubert, R. J. [2010]. *Microbiology for the healthcare professional.* Mosby.)

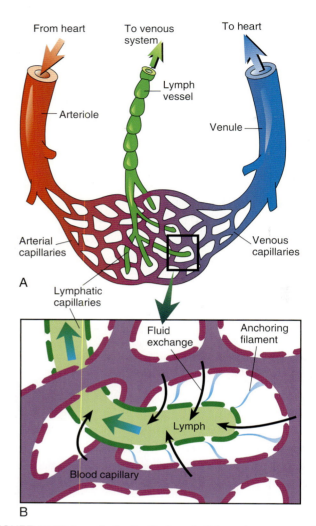

FIGURE 23.30 Lymphatic Capillaries. **A,** Schematic representation of lymphatic capillaries. **B,** Anatomical components of microcirculation.

in body tissues and is not reabsorbed. This fluid becomes the lymph that is carried by the lymphatic vessels to the chest, where it enters the venous circulation. The lymphatic vessels run in the same sheaths with the arteries and veins. (Lymph nodes and lymphoid tissues are described in Chapters 6 and 8.) In this pumpless system, a series of valves ensures one-way flow of the excess interstitial fluid (now called *lymph*) toward the heart. The lymphatic capillaries are closed at the distal ends, as shown in Figure 23.30.

Lymph consists primarily of water and small amounts of dissolved proteins, mostly albumin, that are too large to be reabsorbed into the less permeable blood capillaries. Lymph also carries two types of immune system cells: lymphocytes and antigen-presenting cells. The antigen-presenting cells are carried to the next lymph node in the system while lymphocytes traffic between lymph nodes. Once within the lymphatic system, lymph travels through **lymphatic venules** and **lymphatic veins** that drain into one of two large ducts in the thorax: the right lymphatic duct and the thoracic duct. The **right lymphatic duct** drains lymph from the right arm and the right side of the head and thorax, whereas the larger **thoracic duct** receives lymph from the rest of the body (see Figure 23.29). The right lymphatic duct and the thoracic duct drain lymph into the right and left subclavian veins, respectively.

Lymphatic veins are thin walled like the veins of the cardiovascular system. In larger lymphatic veins, endothelial flaps form valves similar to those in blood-carrying veins (see Figure 23.30). The valves allow lymph to flow in only one direction as lymphatic vessels are compressed intermittently by skeletal muscle contraction, pulsatile expansion of the artery in the same sheath, and contraction of the smooth muscles in the walls of the lymphatic vessels (see Figure 23.28).

As lymph is transported toward the heart, it is filtered through thousands of bean-shaped **lymph nodes** clustered along the lymphatic vessels (see Figure 23.29). Lymph enters the nodes through **afferent lymphatic vessels**, filters through the sinuses in the node, and leaves by way of **efferent lymphatic vessels** (see Figure 23.28). Lymph flows slowly through a node, allowing phagocytosis of foreign substances within the node and delivery of lymphocytes. (Phagocytosis is described in Chapter 7.)

DID YOU UNDERSTAND?

Overview
1. The circulatory system is part of the body's transport and communication systems. It delivers oxygen, nutrients, metabolites, hormones, neurochemicals, proteins, and blood cells including lymphocytes and leukocytes throughout the body and carries metabolic wastes to the kidneys, lungs, and liver for excretion.

The Circulatory System
1. The circulatory system consists of the heart and the blood and lymphatic vessels and is made up of two separate but serially conjoined connected pump systems: the pulmonary circulation and the systemic circulation. The lymphatic system is a one-way network consisting of lymphatic vessels and lymph nodes.
2. The low-pressure pulmonary circulation is driven by the right side of the heart; its function is to deliver blood to the lungs for oxygenation.
3. The higher-pressure systemic circulation is driven by the left side of the heart and functions to provide oxygenated blood, nutrients, and other key substances to body tissues and transport waste products to the lungs, kidneys, and liver for excretion.
4. The lymphatic vessels collect fluids from the interstitium and return the fluids to the circulatory system. The lymphatic vessels also deliver antigens, microorganisms, and cells to the lymph nodes.

The Heart
1. The heart consists of two atria and two ventricles separated by valves (two atrioventricular valves [AV valves].
2. The heart wall is made up of three layers: the epicardium (outer layer), the myocardium (muscular layer), and the endocardium (inner lining). The myocardial layer of the two atria is thinner than the myocardial layer of the ventricles
3. The right and left sides of the heart are separated by portions of the heart wall called the *interatrial septum* and the *interventricular septum*.
4. Deoxygenated (venous) blood from the systemic circulation enters the right atrium through the superior and inferior venae cavae. From the right atrium, the blood passes through the right AV (tricuspid) valve into the right ventricle. In the ventricle, the blood flows from the inflow tract to the outflow tract and then through the pulmonary semilunar valve (pulmonary valve) into the pulmonary artery, which delivers it to the lungs for oxygenation.
5. Oxygenated blood from the lungs enters the left atrium through the four pulmonary veins (two from the left lung and two from the right lung). From the left atrium, the blood passes through the left AV valve (mitral valve) into the left ventricle. In the ventricle, the blood flows from the inflow tract to the outflow tract and then through the aortic semilunar valve (aortic valve) into the aorta, which delivers it to systemic arteries of the entire body.
6. The pumping action of the heart consists of two phases: diastole, during which the myocardium relaxes, and the ventricles fill with blood; and systole, during which the myocardium contracts, forcing blood out of the ventricles. A cardiac cycle includes one systolic contraction and the diastolic relaxation that follows it. Each cardiac cycle represents one heartbeat.
7. The conduction system of the heart generates and transmits electrical impulses (cardiac action potentials) that stimulate systolic contractions. The autonomic nerves (sympathetic and parasympathetic fibres) can adjust heart rate and force of contraction, but they do not originate the heartbeat.
8. Each cardiac action potential travels from the SA node to the AV node to the bundle of His (atrioventricular bundle [AV bundle]), through the bundle branches, and finally to the Purkinje fibres and ventricular myocardium, where the impulse stops. It is prevented from reversing its path by the refractory period of cells that have just been polarized. The refractory period ensures that diastole (relaxation) will occur, thereby completing the cardiac cycle.
9. The normal electrocardiogram is the sum of all cardiac action potentials. The P wave represents atrial depolarization. The QRS complex is the sum of all ventricular cell depolarizations. The ST interval occurs when the entire ventricular myocardium is depolarized.
10. Cardiac action potentials are generated by the SA node at a rate of 60 to 100 impulses per minute. The impulses can travel through the conduction system of the heart, stimulating myocardial contraction as they go.
11. Adrenergic receptor number, type, and function govern autonomic (sympathetic) regulation of heart rate, contractile strength, and the dilation or constriction of coronary arteries. The presence of specific receptors on the myocardium and coronary vessels determines the effects of the neurotransmitters norepinephrine and epinephrine.
12. Unique features that distinguish myocardial cells from skeletal cells enable myocardial cells to transmit action potentials faster (through intercalated discs), synthesize more adenosine triphosphate (because of a large number of mitochondria), and have readier access to ions in the interstitium (because of an abundance of transverse tubules). These combined differences enable the myocardium to work constantly, which is not required by skeletal muscle.
13. Cross-bridges between actin and myosin enable contraction. Calcium ions interacting with the troponin complex help initiate the contraction process. Subsequently, myocardial relaxation begins as troponin releases calcium ions.
14. Cardiac performance is affected by preload, afterload, myocardial contractility, and heart rate.
15. Preload, or pressure generated in the ventricles at the end of diastole, depends on the amount of blood in the ventricle. Afterload is

the resistance to ejection of the blood from the ventricle. Afterload depends on pressure in the aorta.

16. Myocardial stretch determines the force of myocardial contraction. The greater the stretch, the stronger the contraction, up to a certain point. This relationship is known as Starling's law of the heart.
17. Contractility is the potential for myocardial fibre shortening during systole. It is determined by the amount of stretch during diastole (i.e., preload) and by sympathetic stimulation of the ventricles.
18. Heart rate is determined by the SA node and by components of the autonomic nervous system, including cardiovascular control centres in the brain, receptors in the aorta and carotid arteries, and hormones, including catecholamines (epinephrine, norepinephrine).

The Systemic Circulation

1. Blood flows from the left ventricle into the aorta and from the aorta into arteries that eventually branch into arterioles and capillaries, the smallest of the arterial vessels. Oxygen, nutrients, and other substances needed for cellular metabolism pass from the capillaries into the interstitium, where they are taken up by the cells. Capillaries also absorb metabolic waste products from the interstitium.
2. Venules, the smallest veins, receive capillary blood. From the venules, the venous blood flows into larger and larger veins until it reaches the venae cavae, through which it enters the right atrium.
3. Blood vessel walls have three layers: (1) the tunica intima (inner layer), (2) the tunica media (middle layer), and (3) the tunica externa (the outer layer).
4. Layers of the blood vessel wall differ in thickness and composition from vessel to vessel, depending on the vessel's size and location within the circulatory system. In general, the tunica media of arteries close to the heart has more elastic fibres because these arteries must be able to distend during systole and recoil during diastole. Distributing arteries farther from the heart contain more smooth muscle fibres because they constrict and dilate to control blood pressure and volume within specific capillary beds.
5. Blood flow into the capillary beds is controlled by the contraction and relaxation of smooth muscle bands (precapillary sphincters) at junctions between metarterioles and capillaries.
6. Endothelial cells line the blood vessels. The endothelium is a life-support tissue. It functions as a filter (altering permeability), changes in vasomotion (constriction and dilation), and is involved in clotting and inflammation.
7. Blood flow through the veins is assisted by the contraction of skeletal muscles (the muscle pump), and backward flow is prevented by one-way valves, which are particularly important in the deep veins of the legs.
8. Blood flow is affected by blood pressure, resistance to flow within the vessels, blood consistency (which affects velocity), anatomical features that may cause turbulent or laminar flow, and compliance (distensibility) of the vessels.
9. The greater a vessel's length and the blood's viscosity and the narrower the radius of the vessel's lumen, the greater the resistance within the vessel.
10. Total peripheral resistance, or the resistance to flow within the entire systemic circulatory system, depends on the combined lengths and radii of all the vessels within the system and on whether the vessels are arranged in series (greater resistance) or in parallel (lesser resistance).
11. Blood flow is also influenced by neural stimulation (vasoconstriction or vasodilation) and by autonomic features that cause turbulence within the vascular lumen (e.g., protrusions from the vessel wall, twists and turns, vessel branching).
12. Arterial blood pressure is influenced and regulated by factors that affect cardiac output (heart rate, stroke volume), total resistance within the system, and blood volume.
13. Antidiuretic hormone, the renin-angiotensin-aldosterone system, and natriuretic peptides can all alter blood volume and thus blood pressure.
14. Venous blood pressure is influenced by blood volume within the venous system and compliance of the venous walls.
15. Blood flow through the coronary circulation is governed by the same principles as flow through other vascular beds plus two adaptations dictated by cardiac dynamics. First, blood flows into the coronary arteries during diastole rather than systole, because during systole the cusps of the aortic semilunar valve block the openings of the coronary arteries. Second, systolic contraction inhibits coronary artery flow by compressing the coronary arteries.
16. Myoglobin in heart muscle stores oxygen for use during the systolic phase of the cardiac cycle.
17. Autoregulation enables the coronary vessels to maintain optimal perfusion pressure despite systolic compression.

The Lymphatic System

1. The vessels of the lymphatic system run in the same sheaths as the arteries and veins.
2. Lymph (interstitial fluid) is absorbed by lymphatic venules in the capillary beds and travels through ever larger lymphatic veins until it empties through the right lymphatic duct or thoracic duct into the right or left subclavian veins, respectively.
3. As lymph travels toward the thoracic ducts, it passes through thousands of lymph nodes clustered around the lymphatic veins. The lymph nodes are sites of immune function and are ideally placed to sample antigens and cells carried by the lymph from the periphery of the body into the central circulation.

24

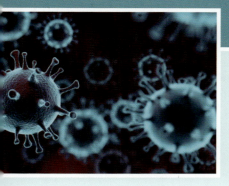

Alterations of Cardiovascular Function

Mohamed Toufic El-Hussein, with originating chapter contributions by Valentina L. Brashers

Additional resources are available online at https://evolve.elsevier.com/Canada/Huether/pathophysiology.

CHAPTER OUTLINE

Diseases of the Veins, 580
  Varicose Veins and Chronic Venous Insufficiency, 580
  Thrombus Formation in Veins, 580
  Superior Vena Cava Syndrome, 581
Diseases of the Arteries, 581
  Hypertension, 581
  Orthostatic (Postural) Hypotension, 588
  Aneurysm, 589
  Thrombus Formation, 590
  Embolism, 590
  Peripheral Vascular Disease, 590
  Atherosclerosis, 591
  Peripheral Artery Disease, 592
  Coronary Artery Disease, Myocardial Ischemia, and Acute Coronary Syndromes, 595
Disorders of the Heart Wall, 606
  Disorders of the Pericardium, 606
  Pericardial Effusion, 607
  Disorders of the Myocardium: The Cardiomyopathies, 608
  Disorders of the Endocardium, 609
  Cardiac Complications in AIDS, 616
Manifestations of Heart Disease, 616
  Heart Failure, 616
  Dysrhythmias, 620
Shock, 621
  Impairment of Cellular Metabolism, 621
  Impairment of Oxygen Use, 621
  Clinical Manifestations of Shock, 625
  Treatment for Shock, 625
  Types of Shock, 625
  Multiple Organ Dysfunction Syndrome, 630
COMORBIDITIES: Cardiovascular Comorbidities, 633
GERIATRIC CONSIDERATIONS: Aging and Cardiovascular Function, 634
CASE STUDY, 634

LEARNING OBJECTIVES

1. Describe the alterations in vascular flow that result in deep venous thrombosis (DVT), stasis ulcers, chronic insufficiencies, and superior vena cava syndrome.
2. Describe the differences between primary, secondary, and complicated hypertension.
3. Describe malignant hypertension.
4. Describe the clinical symptoms and pathophysiology of postural and idiopathic hypotension.
5. Compare the differences between true and false aneurysms.
6. Compare the differences between a thrombus and an embolus.
7. Describe the pathophysiology of Buerger's and Raynaud's disease.
8. Identify the risk factors for atherosclerosis.
9. Identify the characteristics of peripheral arterial disease.
10. Describe the development of coronary artery disease.
11. Describe the progression of coronary artery disease from ischemia to infarction.
12. Describe the diagnostic evaluation of myocardial infarction, and the significance of timely intervention.
13. Compare the differences between acute coronary syndromes.
14. Describe the pathophysiology and symptoms of pericardial disorders.
15. Compare the differences between dilated, hypertrophic, and restrictive cardiomyopathies.
16. Describe the types of valvular dysfunctions.
17. Describe acute rheumatic fever and how it leads to rheumatic heart disease and valvular injury.
18. Describe infective endocarditis.
19. Explain the significance of dysrhythmias.
20. Compare left and right heart failure
21. Describe the different types of shock.
22. Identify the relationship between sepsis, septic shock, and multiple organ dysfunction syndrome.

KEY TERMS

Acute coronary syndrome, 595
Acute pericarditis, 606
Anaphylactic shock, 627
Anaphylaxis, 627
Aneurysm, 589
Aortic regurgitation, 611
Aortic stenosis, 610
Arteriolar remodelling, 584
Arteriosclerosis, 591
Atherosclerosis, 591
Cardiogenic shock, 626
Cardiomyopathy, 608
Chronic orthostatic hypotension, 589
Chronic venous insufficiency (CVI), 580
Chylomicron, 595
Complicated plaque, 592
Constrictive pericarditis (restrictive pericarditis [chronic pericarditis]), 607
Coronary artery disease (CAD), 595
Deep venous thrombosis (DVT), 580
Diastolic heart failure, 619
Dilated cardiomyopathy, 608

Dyslipidemia (dyslipoproteinemia), 595
Dysrhythmia (arrhythmia), 620
Electrocardiogram (ECG), 588
Embolism, 590
Embolus, 590
Endothelial injury, 592
False aneurysm, 589
Fatty streak, 592
Fibrous plaque, 592
Foam cell, 592
Heart failure (HF), 616
Heart failure with preserved ejection fraction (HfpEF), 619
Heart failure with reduced ejection fraction (HfrEF), 616
Hibernating myocardium, 603
High-output failure, 620
High-sensitivity C-reactive protein (hs-CRP), 592
Hypertension, 581
Hypertensive crisis (malignant hypertension), 587
Hypertensive hypertrophic cardiomyopathy, 608
Hypertrophic cardiomyopathy, 608
Hypertrophic obstructive cardiomyopathy, 608
Hypovolemic shock, 626
Infarction, 595
Infective endocarditis, 614
Intermittent claudication, 592
Ischemia, 595
Left ventricular failure, 616
Lipoprotein, 595
Lipoprotein(a) (Lp[a]), 597
Mental stress–induced ischemia, 599
Metabolic syndrome (MetS), 597
Microvascular angina (MVA), 599
Mitral regurgitation, 612
Mitral stenosis, 611
Mitral valve prolapse syndrome (MVPS), 612
Multiple organ dysfunction syndrome (MODS), 630
Myocardial infarction (MI), 601
Myocardial remodelling, 603
Myocardial stunning, 603
Neurogenic shock (vasogenic shock), 626
Nonbacterial thrombotic endocarditis, 615
Non-ST elevation myocardial infarction (non-STEMI), 601
Orthostatic (postural) hypotension (OH), 588
Percutaneous coronary intervention (PCI), 601
Pericardial effusion, 607
Peripheral artery disease (PAD), 592
Plaque, 591
Pressure–natriuresis relationship, 584
Primary hypertension, 582
Prinzmetal's angina, 599
Raynaud's phenomenon, 591
Restrictive cardiomyopathy, 609
Rheumatic fever, 612
Rheumatic heart disease, 612
Right ventricular failure, 620
Secondary hypertension, 582
Septic shock, 627
Shock, 621
Silent ischemia, 599
ST elevation myocardial infarction (STEMI), 601
Stable angina pectoris, 598
Superior vena cava syndrome (SVCS), 581
Supply-dependent oxygen consumption, 632
Systemic inflammatory response syndrome (SIRS), 627
Systolic heart failure, 616
Tamponade, 607
Thromboangiitis obliterans (Buerger's disease), 590
Thromboembolus, 580
Thrombus, 580
Transmural myocardial infarction, 602
Tricuspid regurgitation, 612
True aneurysm, 589
Unstable angina, 601
Valvular hypertrophic cardiomyopathy, 608
Valvular regurgitation (valvular insufficiency or valvular incompetence), 609
Valvular stenosis, 609
Varicose vein, 580
Venous stasis ulcer, 580
Ventricular remodelling, 616

DISEASES OF THE VEINS

QUICK CHECK 24.1
1. What is chronic venous insufficiency?
2. What are the risk factors for deep venous thrombosis?
3. Name three causes of superior vena cava syndrome.

Varicose Veins and Chronic Venous Insufficiency

A **varicose vein** is a distended, tortuous, and palpable vessel that results from pooling of blood (Figure 24.1; see Figure 23.26). Varicose veins typically involve the saphenous veins of the leg. Trauma that damages valves in the saphenous vein with the action of gravity on blood in the legs leads to gradual venous distension, resulting in varicose veins.

If a valve is damaged, a section of the vein is subjected to the pressure of a larger volume of blood under the influence of gravity.[1] The vein swells as it becomes engorged and surrounding tissue becomes edematous. Edema of surrounding tissue is due to the increased hydrostatic pressure that pushes plasma through the vessel wall. Venous distension develops over time in individuals who stand for long periods, wear constricting garments, or cross the legs at the knees (see Figure 23.27). Risk factors also include age, female gender, a family history of varicose veins, obesity, pregnancy, deep venous thrombosis (DVT), and previous leg injury. Prolonged increased pressure in the vein damages venous valves, rendering them incompetent and unable to maintain normal venous pressure.

Varicose veins and valvular incompetence can progress to chronic venous insufficiency, especially in obese individuals. **Chronic venous insufficiency (CVI)** is inadequate venous return over a long period.

Venous hypertension, circulatory stasis, and tissue hypoxia cause an inflammatory reaction in vessels and skin ulcerations. Symptoms include edema of the lower extremities and hyperpigmentation of the skin of the feet and ankles. Edema may extend to the knees. Circulation to the extremities can become so sluggish that the metabolic demands of the cells to obtain oxygen and nutrients and to remove wastes are barely met. Any trauma or pressure can therefore lower the oxygen supply and cause cell death and necrosis (**venous stasis ulcers**) (Figure 24.2). Infection can occur because poor circulation impairs the delivery of the cells and biochemicals necessary for the immune and inflammatory responses.

Treatment of varicose veins and CVI begins conservatively, and excellent wound healing results have followed noninvasive treatments such as elevating the legs, wearing compression stockings, and performing physical exercise.[2] Invasive management includes endovenous ablation, sclerotherapy or surgical ligation, conservative vein resection, and vein stripping.[3]

Thrombus Formation in Veins

A **thrombus** is a blood clot that remains attached to a vessel wall (see Figure 21.20). A detached thrombus is a **thromboembolus**. Venous thrombi are more common than arterial thrombi because flow and pressure are lower in the veins than in the arteries. **Deep venous thrombosis (DVT)** occurs primarily in the lower extremity. Three factors (Virchow triad) promote venous thrombosis: (1) venous stasis (e.g., immobility, age, heart failure), (2) venous endothelial damage (e.g., trauma, intravenous medications), and (3) hypercoagulable states (e.g., inherited disorders, malignancy, pregnancy, use of oral contraceptives or hormone replacement therapy). Orthopedic trauma or surgery, spinal cord injury, and obstetric/gynecological conditions can be

CHAPTER 24 Alterations of Cardiovascular Function

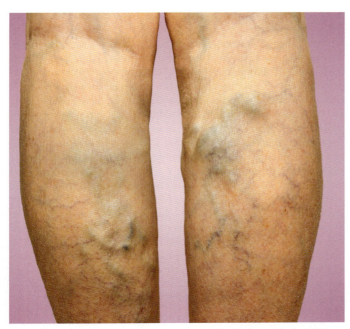

FIGURE 24.1 Varicose Veins of the Leg. (iStockphoto/Marina113)

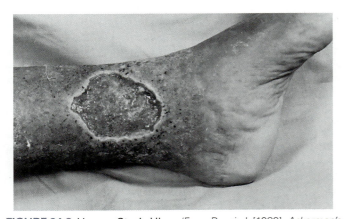

FIGURE 24.2 Venous Stasis Ulcer. (From Rosai, J. [1989]. *Ackerman's surgical pathology* [7th ed., vol. 2]. Mosby.)

associated with up to a 100% likelihood of DVT. Genetic abnormalities related to states of hypercoagulability, such as factor V Leiden mutation, prothrombin mutations, and deficiencies of protein C, protein S, and antithrombin, increase the risk of venous thrombosis.[4]

Accumulation of clotting factors and platelets leads to thrombus formation in the vein, near a venous valve. Inflammation around the thrombus promotes further platelet aggregation, causing pain and redness in the deep veins of the legs. If the thrombus creates significant obstruction to venous blood flow, increased pressure in the vein leads to edema of the extremity. Most thrombi will dissolve without treatment. Untreated DVT increases the risk of embolization, where a part of the blood clot breaks off and travels to the lungs, causing a blockage in one of the arteries (e.g., pulmonary embolism) (see Chapter 27). Persistent venous obstruction leads to CVI and post-thrombotic syndrome, which is characterized by pain, edema, and ulceration of the affected limb.[5]

Because DVT is usually asymptomatic and difficult to detect clinically, prevention is important in at-risk individuals. Prevention may include early ambulation, pneumatic devices, and prophylactic anticoagulation. If thrombosis does occur, a combination of serum D-dimer measurement and Doppler ultrasonography are used to confirm the diagnosis. Management most often consists of anticoagulation therapy using heparin (low-molecular-weight heparin) and warfarin (Coumadin).[6] New oral anticoagulant therapies, such as factor Xa inhibitors and direct thrombin inhibitors, have been shown to have a more favourable benefit-to-risk ratio and are rapidly becoming the treatments of choice.[7] Thrombolytic therapy or placement of an inferior vena cava filter may be indicated in select individuals.[4,6]

Superior Vena Cava Syndrome

Superior vena cava syndrome (SVCS) is a progressive occlusion of the superior vena cava (SVC) that leads to venous distension in the upper extremities and head. Causes include bronchogenic cancer (75% of cases), lymphomas, and metastasis of other cancers.[8] Other less common causes include tuberculosis, mediastinal fibrosis, and cystic fibrosis. Pacemaker wires, central venous catheters, and pulmonary artery catheters with associated thrombosis account for nearly 40% of cases.[9] The SVC is a relatively low-pressure vessel that lies in the closed thoracic compartment, therefore, tissue expansion can easily compress the SVC. The right mainstem bronchus abuts the SVC so that cancers occurring in this bronchus may exert pressure on the SVC. Additionally, the SVC is surrounded by lymph nodes and lymph chains that commonly become involved in thoracic cancers and compress the SVC during tumour growth. The onset of SVCS is most often slow to develop, because of collateral venous drainage to the azygos vein.

Clinical manifestations of SVCS are edema and venous distension in the upper extremities and face, including the ocular beds. Affected persons complain of a feeling of fullness in the head or tightness of shirt collars, necklaces, and rings. Cerebral edema may cause headache, visual disturbance, and impaired consciousness. The skin of the face and arms may become purple and taut, and capillary refill time is prolonged. Respiratory distress may be present because of edema of bronchial structures or compression of the bronchus by a carcinoma.

Chest X-ray, Doppler studies, computed tomography (CT), magnetic resonance imaging (MRI), and ultrasound are used to make the diagnosis. Because of its slow onset and the development of collateral venous drainage, SVCS is generally not a vascular emergency, but it is an oncological emergency. Treatment for malignant disorders can include radiation therapy, surgery, chemotherapy, and the administration of diuretics, steroids, and anticoagulants, as necessary. Treatment for nonmalignant causes may include bypass surgery using various grafts, thrombolysis (both locally and systemically), balloon angioplasty, and placement of intravascular stents.[8]

DISEASES OF THE ARTERIES

> **QUICK CHECK 24.2**
> 1. What are the major risk factors for hypertension?
> 2. Summarize the pathophysiology of primary hypertension.
> 3. What is malignant hypertension?
> 4. What are the causes of orthostatic hypotension?

Hypertension

Hypertension is consistent elevation of systemic arterial blood pressure.[10] Approximately 7.5 million Canadians have hypertension. Hypertension is considered to be the main factor contributing to mortality, disability-adjusted life years (DALYs), and years of life lost (YLL) in Canada. About 90% of Canadians are expected to develop hypertension if they live an average lifespan.[11]

The chance of developing primary hypertension increases with age. According to Hypertension Canada's *2020 Comprehensive Guidelines for the Prevention, Diagnosis, Risk Assessment, and Treatment of Hypertension in Adults and Children*, hypertension continues to be the main risk factor for cardiovascular disease (CVD) in Canada. The main risk factors for hypertension are diabetes mellitus, chronic kidney disease, inadequate of consumption of fresh fruits and vegetables, and sedentary behaviour. The aforementioned risk factors determine the timing and frequency of screening. The prevalence of hypertension is higher in those of African descent and in those with diabetes.

Hypertension Canada defines **hypertension** as a mean systolic blood pressure (SBP) greater than or equal to 140 mm Hg or diastolic blood pressure (DBP) greater than or equal to 90 mm Hg when a *non-automated* office blood pressure measurement is used (Table 24.1). Alternately, hypertension is also defined as a mean SBP greater than or equal to 135 mm Hg or DBP greater than or equal to 85 mm Hg when an *automated* office blood pressure measurement is used.[12] Figure 24.3 presents a hypertension diagnostic algorithm for adults.

The 2020 guidelines add that a patient is diagnosed with hypertension if the mean awake SBP is ≥135 mm Hg or DBP is ≥85 mm Hg, or if the mean 24-hour SBP is ≥130 mm Hg or DBP is ≥80 mm Hg. White coat hypertension should be diagnosed if the out-of-office ambulatory blood pressure measurement (ABPM) or home blood pressure measurement (HBPM) average is not elevated and, as such, pharmacological treatment should not be initiated. Prior to diagnosing white coat hypertension, it is recommended that the ABPM be recorded to confirm that the mean awake blood pressure (BP) is < 135/85 mm Hg and that the mean 24-hour BP is < 130/80 mm Hg. If the out-of-office measurement is not documented after the first visit, then patients can be diagnosed as hypertensive using serial office blood pressure measurement (OBPM) visits if during the second visit the mean OBPM (averaged across all visits) is ≥140 mm Hg SBP and/or ≥90 mm Hg DBP in patients with macrovascular target organ damage, diabetes mellitus, or chronic kidney disease (glomerular filtration rate [GFR] < 60 mL/min/1.73 m². If during the third visit the mean OBPM (averaged across all visits) is ≥160 mm Hg SBP or ≥100 mm Hg DBP, and during the fourth and fifth visits the mean OBPM (averaged across all visits) is ≥140 mm Hg SBP or ≥90 mm Hg DBP, then the patient is diagnosed with hypertension. If during the last visit the patient is not diagnosed as hypertensive and does not show evidence of macrovascular target organ damage, the patient's BP should be assessed at annual intervals.[13]

Patients who are prescribed antihypertensive drugs should be followed up every month or every 2 months depending on their BP, until the BP recorded on two successive visits is less than the target. Symptomatic patients should be seen urgently, especially if they experience severe hypertension, intolerance to antihypertensive drugs, or target organ damage. Standard OBPM should be used for follow-up. Measurement using electronic (oscillometric) upper arm devices is preferred over auscultation. ABPM or HBPM is recommended for follow-up of patients with demonstrated white coat effect.[13]

According to Hypertension Canada, all Canadian adults should have their blood pressure checked each time they visit a clinic, regardless of the reason. It is recommended that health care providers use automated measurement of blood pressure rather than manual measurement. It is also recommended that these measurements be done multiple times and be unattended. In 2020, Hypertension Canada released the updated guidelines recommending that the measurement frequency for ABPM (24-hour ambulatory BP monitoring) is at 20- to 30-minute intervals throughout the day and night, adding that the minimum number of readings should be 20 daytime and 7 night-time readings. The greater the number of readings, the more precise the average BP. Despite varied measurement protocols, HBPM has been shown to predict health outcomes better than OBPMs. Out-of-office BP measurements are recommended to rule out white coat hypertension and to assess for masked hypertension. White coat hypertension patients tend to be overtreated, however. Studies have shown that treated and untreated individuals have similar long-term cardiovascular risk to that of treated and untreated normotensive individuals. In individuals with diabetes, diagnosis of hypertension is probable when OBPM is 130/80 for 3 or more measurements on different days.[13]

Patients are also encouraged to record and report out-of-office blood pressure measurements to confirm the initial diagnosis of hypertension. Optimum management of the hypertensive patient requires thorough assessment and evaluation. Patients should be reminded that modification of health behaviour is effective in preventing hypertension, treating hypertension, and reducing cardiovascular risk. However, a combination of both health behaviour changes and medications is often necessary to achieve target blood pressures. Patients should be taught how to measure blood pressure at home to be involved in self-monitoring and self-management, and to promote adherence to medications and a healthy diet.[14]

Normal blood pressure is associated with the lowest cardiovascular risk, whereas those who fall into the prehypertension category are at risk of developing hypertension and many associated cardiovascular complications unless lifestyle modification and treatment are instituted. All stages of hypertension are associated with increased risk for target organ disease events, such as myocardial infarction (MI), kidney disease, and stroke. Both stage I and stage II hypertension need effective long-term therapy.

Most cases (92 to 95%) of hypertension are diagnosed as **primary hypertension** (also called *essential hypertension* or *idiopathic hypertension*). **Secondary hypertension** accounts for 5 to 8% of cases, and is caused by an underlying disorder such as renal disease.

Factors Associated With Primary Hypertension

The Indigenous population in Canada and primary hypertension. In Canada, the rate of developing and dying of heart disease and stroke among Indigenous people is twice that in the rest of the population. Moreover, Indigenous people are three to four times more likely to experience type 2 diabetes mellitus than non-Indigenous people, and they are 10.5 times more likely to die from coronary heart disease. About 40% of the Indigenous population in Canada lives on reserves, thus they do not have prompt access to health care facilities and their standard of living is often lower than that of the average Canadian.[15] A lower standard of living is linked to unhealthy behaviours such as smoking, eating mostly processed, high-salt, and high-cholesterol diets.[16] Indigenous people typically have heart attacks earlier in life than non-Indigenous people. The Indigenous population has a higher prevalence of physical inactivity, smoking, overweight, obesity, high blood pressure, and diabetes—all of which are risk factors for CVD and

TABLE 24.1 Classification of Blood Pressure for Adults Age 18 Years and Older

Category	Systolic (mm Hg)		Diastolic (mm Hg)
Normal	<120	AND	<80
Prehypertension	120–139	OR	80–89
Stage 1 hypertension	140–159	OR	90–99
Stage 2 hypertension	≥160	OR	≥100

Data from James, P. A., Oparil, S., Carter, B., et al. (2014). *JAMA, 311*(5), 507–520.

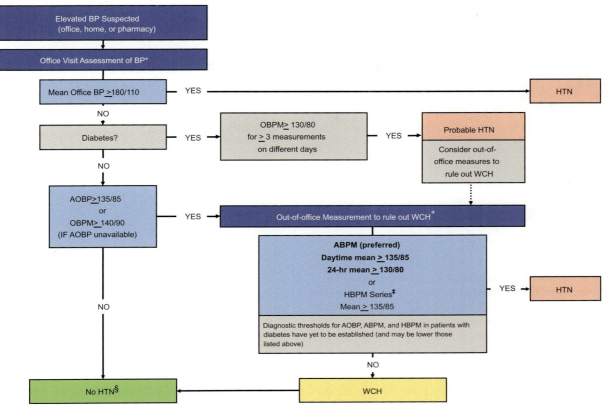

FIGURE 24.3 Hypertension Diagnostic Algorithm For Adults. The diagnostic algorithm has been revised for the 2020 Guidelines. In 2017 and 2018, diabetes was included in the diagnostic algorithm to provide a comprehensive overview of the diagnosis of hypertension. However, this created several challenges: the OBPM diagnostic threshold is different in patients with diabetes; evidence for defining AOBP and out-of-office (ABPM and HBPM) diagnostic thresholds is lacking; and the potential prognostic value of out-of-office measurements in patients with diabetes, including the identification of white coat hypertension or masked hypertension, exists, but definitions are not established. The committee elected to revise the 2018 algorithm to include the recommendation that a series of 3 to 5 office measurements can be used to establish a diagnosis of hypertension in diabetes. Although it is plausible that an AOBP threshold could be lower, there is currently no published evidence to guide a specific AOBP threshold. There are no studies to date that have established ABPM or HBPM thresholds in patients with diabetes. Other guideline bodies have elected to estimate corresponding values for HBPM and ABPM on the basis of the established thresholds for the general population; however, the evidence is not clear and these are not validated for diabetes. With respect to identifying white coat hypertension in patients with diabetes, there are currently no evidence-based definitions. However, a comprehensive review of the published evidence is required to establish thresholds upon which diagnostic and treatment decisions can be based. *ABPM*, Ambulatory blood pressure measurement; *AOBP*, automated office blood pressure (performed with the patient unattended in a private room); *BP*, blood pressure; *HBPM*, home blood pressure measurement; *HTN*, hypertension; *OBPM*, office blood pressure measurement (measurements are performed in the office using an electronic upper arm device with a provider in the room); *WCH*, white coat hypertension. * If AOBP is used, use the mean calculated and displayed by the device. If OBPM is used, take at least three readings, discard the first and calculate the mean of the remaining measurements. A history and physical exam should be performed, and diagnostic tests ordered. †Serial office measurements over 3 to 5 visits can be used if ABPM or HBPM are not available. ‡Home BP Series: Two readings taken each morning and evening for 7 days (28 total). Discard first day readings and average the last 6 days. §In a patient with suspected masked hypertension, ABPM or HBPM could be considered to rule out masked hypertension. (Reprinted from Rabi, D., McBrien, K., Woo, V., et al. [2020]. Hypertension Canada's 2020 comprehensive guidelines for prevention, diagnosis, risk assessment, and treatment for hypertension in adults and children. *Canadian Journal of Cardiology, 36*[5], 596–624. https://www.onlinecjc.ca/action/showPdf?pii=S0828-282X%2820%2930191-4.)

hypertension. Indigenous people are more likely to have high blood pressure than the non-Indigenous population. As well, smoking rates among Indigenous people are, on average, twice as high as those of non-Indigenous people (39% versus 20.5%).[17]

New immigrants and primary hypertension. New immigrants to Canada often have fewer chronic conditions upon arrival compared with the native-born population. This trend is referred to as the *healthy immigrant effect* and reflects that fact that when immigrants first arrive in their new homeland, they tend to be healthier than the native-born population. However, new immigrants to Canada tend to experience a rapid deterioration in their general health status after living in Canada for several years due to lifestyle changes that impact their physical

RISK FACTORS
Primary Hypertension

Family history
Advancing age
Cigarette smoking
Obesity
Heavy alcohol consumption
Gender (men greater than women before age 55; women greater than men after 55)
Being of African descent
Being of Indigenous descent
Immigration-related change in socioeconomic status
High dietary sodium intake
Low dietary intake of potassium, calcium, magnesium
Glucose intolerance

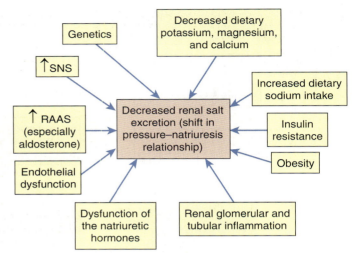

FIGURE 24.4 Factors That Cause a Shift in the Pressure–Natriuresis Relationship. Numerous factors have been implicated in the pathogenesis of sodium retention in individuals with hypertension. These factors cause less renal excretion of salt than would normally occur with increased blood pressure. This is called a shift in the pressure–natriuresis relationship and is thought to be a central process in the pathogenesis of primary hypertension. *RAAS*, Renin-angiotensin-aldosterone system; *SNS*, sympathetic nervous system.

activity and dietary habits.[18] Dietary acculturation, which is the process by which immigrants adopt the dietary practices of the host country, has been associated with obesity, diabetes, and hypertension.[19] Dietary acculturation for immigrant groups has largely been attributed to the "Westernization" of immigrant diets, as characterized by an increased consumption of unhealthy north American foods (e.g., fast food, junk food).[19] In addition, immigrants may also be eating the foods of their festivals ("festival foods") more regularly. Festival foods are calorically rich foods that are typically consumed only a few times a year, during festivals or special occasions in the home country, and usually in limited amounts. After immigration, immigrants tend to prepare these festival foods more frequently and eat them in larger quantities. As such, in the process of acculturation, festival foods become "traditional foods" that are eaten on a more regular basis.[19] Immigration-related cultural changes have been found to be independently associated with high blood pressure.[18]

PATHOPHYSIOLOGY Hypertension results from a sustained increase in peripheral resistance (arteriolar vasoconstriction), an increase in circulating blood volume, or both.

Primary Hypertension

The cause of primary hypertension has not been identified. A combination of epigenetic changes and environmental factors such as diet and lifestyle is thought to be responsible for its development.[20] Multiple pathophysiological mechanisms mediated by a host of neurohumoral effects are involved in the maintenance of elevated blood pressure. Inflammation, endothelial dysfunction, obesity-related hormones, and insulin resistance also contribute to both increased peripheral resistance and increased blood volume. Increased vascular volume is related to a decrease in renal excretion of salt, often referred to as a shift in the pressure–natriuresis relationship (Figure 24.4). This shift means that for a given blood pressure, individuals with hypertension tend to secrete less salt in their urine.

The sympathetic nervous system (SNS) has been implicated in both the development and the maintenance of elevated blood pressure and plays a role in hypertensive end-organ damage.[21] Increased SNS activity causes increased heart rate and systemic vasoconstriction, thus raising the blood pressure. Additional mechanisms of SNS-induced hypertension include structural changes in blood vessels (vascular remodelling), renal sodium retention (shift in the pressure–natriuresis curve), insulin resistance, increased renin and angiotensin levels, and procoagulant effects.[22]

The renin-angiotensin-aldosterone system and cardiovascular disease. In hypertensive individuals, overactivity of the renin-angiotensin-aldosterone system (RAAS) contributes to salt and water retention and increased vascular resistance (see Figure 23.27). There are two primary renin-angiotensin-aldosterone systems. The first RAAS leads to the release of renin, the synthesis of angiotensin II (Ang II) through angiotensin-converting enzyme (ACE), stimulation of the angiotensin II type 1 receptor (AT1R), and secretion of aldosterone. The RAAS has multiple effects on the cardiovascular system and plays an important role in the complications associated with metabolic syndrome (MetS). Ang II and aldosterone contribute to hypertensive hypertrophy and fibrosis of heart muscle, decreased contractility, and an increased susceptibility to arrhythmias and heart failure (HF). Further, Ang II causes systemic vasoconstriction, renal salt and water retention, and stimulates tissue growth and inflammation.[23-34] High levels of Ang II contribute to endothelial dysfunction, thus decreasing the release of endothelial vasodilators and anticoagulants. Ang II elevation in the blood is also associated with insulin resistance, remodelling of blood vessels, atherogenesis, and platelet aggregation.[29] In the kidney, Ang II causes a shift in the pressure–natriuresis curve, inflammation, and glomerular remodelling and is a major contributor to renal failure in individuals with hypertension and diabetes.

Further, Ang II mediates **arteriolar remodelling**, which is structural change in the vessel wall that results in permanent increases in peripheral resistance and contributes to atherogenesis[28] (see Figure 23.33). Ang II is associated with end-organ effects of hypertension, including atherosclerosis, renal disease, cardiac hypertrophy, and HF.[23,34] Finally, aldosterone not only contributes to sodium retention by the kidney but also has other deleterious effects on the cardiovascular system and contributes to insulin resistance.[35]

In contrast, the second RAAS serves a counter-regulatory system. Activation of a second ACE pathway (ACE2) leads to the synthesis of angiotensin (1–7) (Ang [1–7]) from Ang II. Ang (1–7) stimulates Mas receptors in the brain, blood vessels, heart, kidney, gut, pancreas, and inflammatory cells and has vasodilatory, antiproliferative, antifibrotic, and antithrombotic effects. These protective effects lead to lower blood

HEALTH PROMOTION

Hypertension

According to the 2020 Hypertension Guidelines, adjusting modifiable risk factors such as excess body fat, low dietary potassium (low fruit and vegetable intake), physical inactivity, and high alcohol intake can help prevent and control hypertension for most individuals.

Hypertension is related to eating an unhealthy diet, specifically one that is high in sodium. It is estimated that high sodium intake causes 32% of all cases of hypertension in Canada. Current national guidelines recommend consuming less than 2 000 mg of sodium per day. Reducing sodium intake at a population level has been shown repeatedly to be cost saving, effective, and efficient in preventing early CVD.

Canada has the highest rate of hypertension awareness, treatment, and control worldwide. However, Hypertension Prevention and Control and Hypertension Canada recommend public policies for the prevention and control of hypertension. For example, they recommend screening for high blood pressure and providing education about healthy behaviours. Following are some individual health behaviours that are also recommended to help prevent and control hypertension:

- **Physical exercise**

   To decrease the odds of developing hypertension in individuals with normal blood pressure and to help patients with reducing their BP, it is recommended that the individual accumulates 30 to 60 minutes of moderate-intensity dynamic exercise, such as walking, jogging, cycling, or swimming) on 4 to 7 days per week in addition to the routine activities of daily living. It is worth noting that higher intensities of exercise are not more effective. The use of resistance or weight training exercise (such as free-weight lifting, fixed-weight lifting, or handgrip exercise) does not adversely influence BP in normotensive or hypertensive individuals with SBP/DBP of 140 to 159/90 to 99 mm Hg.

- **Weight reduction**
1. All adults should ensure that their height, weight, and waist circumference are measured and their body mass index calculated.
2. Body mass index should be maintained and waist circumference is best kept less than 102 cm for men and less than 88 cm for women in normotensive individuals to prevent hypertension and for hypertensive patients to reduce BP. All overweight hypertensive individuals should be advised to lose weight.
3. Weight loss strategies should use a multidisciplinary approach that includes dietary education, increased physical activity, and behavioural intervention.

- **Alcohol consumption**

   It is recommended that healthy adults abstain from alcohol or reduce alcohol intake to 2 drinks per day or less to prevent hypertension. In adults with hypertension who drink more than 2 drinks per day, a reduction in alcohol intake is associated with decreased BP and is recommended. Adults diagnosed with hypertension and who consume 6 or more drinks of alcohol per day must cut down their alcohol intake to 2 or fewer drinks per day to reduce their BP.

   A safe limit for alcohol consumption has not been identified. The incidence of hypertension increases with any amount of alcohol consumption in men, and with more than 2 drinks per day in women. There is positive linear association between alcohol consumption and mortality.

- **Diet**

   Hypertensive patients at increased risk of hypertension are encouraged to consume a diet that emphasizes fruits, vegetables, low-fat dairy products, whole grain foods rich in dietary fibre, and protein from plant sources that is reduced in saturated fat and cholesterol (Dietary Approaches to Stop Hypertension [DASH]) diet.

- **Sodium intake**

   Sodium intake should be reduced to 2 000 mg (5 g of salt or 87 mmol of sodium) per day in patients diagnosed with hypertension or patients prone to develop hypertension.

   Supplementation of calcium and magnesium is not recommended for the prevention or treatment of hypertension.

- **Potassium intake**

   Dietary potassium intake should be increased in patients with hypertension to reduce BP unless they are at risk of hyperkalemia.

- **Stress management**

   Stress management in hypertensive patients in whom stress might be contributing to high BP should be considered. Cognitive-behavioural interventions and relaxation techniques should be individualized for maximum benefits in patients with hypertension.

Adapted from Rabi, D. M., McBrien, K. A., Sapir-Pichhadze, R., et al. (2020). Hypertension Canada's 2020 comprehensive guidelines for the prevention, diagnosis, risk assessment, and treatment of hypertension in adults and children. *Canadian Journal of Cardiology, 36*(5), 596–624. https://www.onlinecjc.ca/article/S0828-282X(20)30191-4/fulltext.

---

pressure, less vascular inflammation and clotting, and decrease in tissue remodelling and damage to target organ tissues. This pathway appears to be especially important in protecting renal tissue and improving insulin sensitivity in those with diabetes and hypertension. Research is under way to develop pharmacological interventions, such as synthetic Mas agonists, Ang (1-7) formulations, and ACE2 activators that will stimulate these protective RAAS pathways. More recently, additional RAAS pathways have been identified that play a role in proto-oncogene stimulation, hypothalamic function, and central nervous system function.[23–34]

Medications, such as ACE inhibitors and angiotensin receptor blockers (ARBs), oppose the activity of the RAAS and are effective in reducing blood pressure and protecting against target organ damage.[32] Also, the use of ACE2 to create Ang (1–7), which has cardiovascular, cerebrovascular, and metabolic protective effects,[31] may lead to new and more effective medications.[26] *Health Promotion: Hypertension* provides information on how individuals can help prevent and control hypertension.

Populations with high dietary sodium intake have long been shown to have an increased incidence of hypertension.[36] Low dietary potassium, calcium, and magnesium intakes also are risk factors because without their intake, sodium is retained. The natriuretic hormones modulate renal sodium (Na^+) excretion and require adequate potassium, calcium, and magnesium to function properly. The natriuretic hormones include atrial natriuretic peptide (ANP), B-type natriuretic peptide (BNP), C-type natriuretic peptide (CNP), and urodilatin. Dysfunction of these hormones, along with alterations in the RAAS and the SNS, causes an increase in vascular tone and a shift in the pressure–natriuresis relationship. In hypertension, increased ANP and BNP levels are linked to an increased risk for ventricular hypertrophy, atherosclerosis, and HF.[37] Salt retention leads to water retention and increased blood volume, which contributes to an increase in blood pressure and results in subtle renal injury, renal vasoconstriction, and ischemia. Renal tissue ischemia causes inflammation of the kidney and contributes to dysfunction of the glomeruli and tubules, which promotes additional sodium retention.[38]

HEALTH PROMOTION
Obesity and Hypertension

The Obesity Population Risk Tool (OPoRT)[a] was developed and validated in Canada as a means to estimate population trajectories of obesity based on the distribution of risk factors collected in population surveys.[b] The OPoRT was applied to the 2013/14 Canadian Community Health Survey (CCHS) to estimate the future burden of obesity, identify subgroups at an elevated risk, and demonstrate the use of a tool that can be used to inform obesity prevention. A total of 121 486 people responded to the CCHS. Analysis was restricted to individuals ≥ 18 years of age at baseline ($n = 111\ 772$). Pregnant women were excluded from the sample because their body weight measurements were not accurate ($n = 110\ 825$). Individuals with missing BMI were also excluded and, as such, the final sample size was 105 297.

According to the OPoRT, the 10-year burden of obesity in Canada is estimated at 326 cases per 1 000, or a total of 8.54 million obese individuals by 2023/24, which amounts to an increase of 1.70 million cases from 2013/14. Other findings were:

- More men will be affected by obesity than women (347 cases per 1 000 compared with 305 cases per 1 000).
- Individuals between the ages 35 to 49 (374 cases per 1 000 or $n = 2.52$ million of the total predicted number of cases) are the age group with the highest predicted burden of obesity.
- Respondents who identified as White and Canadian-born are expected to experience a greater burden of obesity than visible minorities and immigrants (338 cases per 1 000 compared with 286 cases per 1 000; 349 cases per 1 000 compared with 262 cases per 1 000, respectively).
- Participants who reported being food insecure were predicted to have approximately 40% more burden of obesity than respondents who were food secure (324 cases per 1 000 compared with 452 cases per 1 000).
- Former heavy smokers were predicted to have the greatest burden of obesity (419 cases per 1 000) compared with non-smokers (304 cases per 1 000), amounting to an over 25% relative difference between the two categories.
- Respondents who reported being physically inactive have an increased burden of obesity compared with those who were physically active (364 cases per 1 000 compared with 294 cases per 1 000).
- Light alcohol drinkers will have a higher predicted burden of obesity (364 cases per 1 000) compared to respondents who never drank (321 cases per 1 000). The heavy drinker category ($n = 3.56$ million) will amount to the greatest total number of persons with obesity with a burden of 345 cases per 1 000.
- A dose-response increase in burden of obesity was noticed as the number of health risk behaviours (smoking, alcohol consumption, and physical inactivity) increased from zero (281 cases per 1 000) to three (372 cases per 1 000).
- Northwest Territories (445 cases per 1 000), Nunavut (444 cases per 1 000), Nova Scotia and New Brunswick (401 cases per 1 000 for each province) were predicted to have the highest burden of obesity. British Columbia (271 cases per 1 000), followed by Quebec (315 cases per 1 000), and Ontario (322 cases per 1 000) were predicted to have the lowest burden of obesity due to the large population of immigrants who live in these provinces and often have healthier behaviours than their Canadian-born counterparts.[c,d]

Predicting rates of obesity across Canada over 10 years will help researchers and public health decision makers determine how to direct investments to the regions where the incidence of obesity is trending high. Population-level strategies to raise awareness and guide individuals on making good food choices through clear package labeling, reducing prices as an incentive, while working with industry to improve the nutritional quality of foods by reducing fat, sugar, and salt have proven to be effective strategies to combat obesity. Developing national benchmarks to eliminate excess nutrients and reducing calorie or portion sizes are also recommended strategies. In addition, policies aimed at improving the environment and infrastructure, promoting physical activity, and improving the acceptability and safety of active transport can also help reach many individuals in the population. There is consensus, on the basis of research and practice, that public health strategies designed to tackle risk factors for obesity have been demonstrated to be cost-effective.

[a] O'Neill, M., Kornas, K., & Rosella, L. (2019). The future burden of obesity in Canada: a modelling study. *Canadian Journal of Public Health, 110*(6), 768–778. doi:10.17269/s41997-019-00251-y. https://www.ncbi.nlm.nih.gov/pmc/articles/PMC6900264/.
[b] Lebenbaum, M., Espin-Garcia, O., Li, Y., et al. (2018). Development and validation of a population based risk algorithm for obesity: the Obesity Population Risk Tool (OPoRT). *PLoS One, 13*(1), e0191169. https://doi.org/10.1371/journal.pone.0191169.
[c] De Maio, F., & Kemp, E. (2010). The deterioration of health status among immigrants to Canada. *Global Public Health, 5*(5), 462–478. https://doi.org/10.1080/17441690902942480.
[d] Lu, Y., Kaushal, N., Denier, N., et al. (2017). Health of newly arrived immigrants in Canada and the United States: differential selection on health. *Health & Place, 48*, 1–10. https://doi.org/10.1016/j.healthplace.2017.08.001.

Inflammation plays a role in the pathogenesis of hypertension.[39] Activation of innate and adaptive immunity results in damage to endothelial cells.[40] Endothelial injury and tissue ischemia result in the release of vasoactive inflammatory cytokines. Although many of these cytokines (e.g., histamine, prostaglandins) have vasodilatory actions in acute inflammatory injury, chronic inflammation leads to decreased production of vasodilators (such as nitric oxide), vascular remodelling, and smooth muscle contraction. Inflammation also contributes to insulin resistance, decreased natriuresis, and autonomic dysfunction (increased SNS activity).[41–43]

Obesity is recognized as an important risk factor for hypertension in both adults and children and contributes to many of the neurohumoral, metabolic, renal, and cardiovascular processes that cause hypertension (see *Health Promotion: Obesity and Hypertension*).[44] Obesity causes changes in the adipokines (i.e., leptin and adiponectin) and also is associated with increased activity of the SNS and the RAAS.[45] Obesity is linked to inflammation, endothelial dysfunction, and insulin resistance and an increased risk for cardiovascular complications from hypertension.[44]

Finally, insulin resistance is common in hypertension, even in individuals without clinical diabetes. Insulin resistance is associated with decreased endothelial release of nitric oxide and other vasodilators.[46] It also affects renal function and causes renal salt and water retention. Insulin resistance is associated with overactivity of the SNS and the RAAS. It is interesting to note that in many individuals with diabetes who are treated with medications that increase insulin sensitivity, blood pressure often declines, even in the absence of antihypertensive medications. The interactions between obesity, hypertension, insulin resistance, and lipid disorders in MetS result in a high risk for CVD.[46]

It is likely that primary hypertension is an interaction between many of these factors leading to sustained increases in blood volume and peripheral resistance. The pathophysiology of primary hypertension is summarized in Figure 24.5.

Secondary Hypertension

An underlying disease process or medication that raises peripheral vascular resistance or cardiac output can cause secondary hypertension. Examples include renal vascular or parenchymal disease,

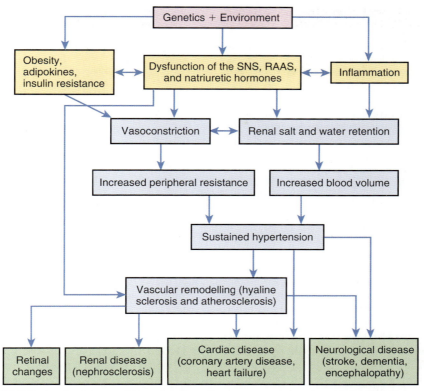

FIGURE 24.5 Pathophysiology of Hypertension. Numerous genetic vulnerabilities have been linked to hypertension and these, in combination with environmental risks, cause neurohumoral dysfunction (sympathetic nervous system *[SNS]*, renin-angiotensin-aldosterone system *[RAAS]*, and natriuretic hormones) and promote inflammation and insulin resistance. Insulin resistance and neurohumoral dysfunction contribute to sustained systemic vasoconstriction and increased peripheral resistance. Inflammation contributes to renal dysfunction, which, in combination with the neurohumoral alterations, results in renal salt and water retention and increased blood volume. Increased peripheral resistance and increased blood volume are two primary causes of sustained hypertension.

adrenocortical tumours, adrenomedullary tumours (pheochromocytoma), and medications (oral contraceptives, corticosteroids, antihistamines). If the cause is identified and removed before permanent structural changes occur, blood pressure returns to normal.

Complicated Hypertension

As hypertension becomes more severe and chronic, tissue damage can occur in the blood vessels and tissues leading to target-organ damage in the heart, kidney, brain, and eyes. Cardiovascular complications of sustained hypertension include left ventricular hypertrophy, angina pectoris, HF, coronary artery disease (CAD), MI, and sudden death. In response to hypertension, several neurohormonal substances, including catecholamines from the SNS and Ang II, lead to myocardial hypertrophy. Hypertrophy is characterized by changes in the myocyte proteins, apoptosis of myocytes, and deposition of collagen in heart muscle, which causes it to become thickened, scarred, and less able to relax during diastole, leading to HF with preserved ejection fraction.[47] In addition, the increased size of the heart muscle increases demand for oxygen delivery over time, the contractility of the heart is impaired, and the individual is at increased risk for MI and HF with reduced ejection fraction. Vascular complications include the formation, dissection,[48] and rupture of aneurysms (outpouchings in vessel walls) and atherosclerosis leading to vessel occlusion.

Renal complications of complicated hypertension include parenchymal damage, nephrosclerosis, renal arteriosclerosis, and renal insufficiency or failure. Microalbuminuria (small amounts of protein in the urine) occurs in 10 to 25% of individuals with primary hypertension and is now recognized as an early sign of impending renal dysfunction and a significantly increased risk for cardiovascular events, especially in those who also have diabetes.[49] Complications specific to the retina include retinal vascular sclerosis, exudation, and hemorrhage. Cerebrovascular complications include transient ischemia, stroke, cerebral thrombosis, aneurysm, hemorrhage, and dementia.[50] The pathological effects of complicated hypertension are summarized in Table 24.2.

Hypertensive crisis (or **malignant hypertension**) is rapidly progressive hypertension in which diastolic pressure is usually greater than 140 mm Hg. It can occur in those with primary hypertension, but the reason why some people develop this complication and others do not is unknown. Other causes include complications of pregnancy, cocaine or amphetamine use, reaction to certain medications, adrenal tumours, and alcohol withdrawal. High arterial pressure renders the cerebral arterioles incapable of regulating blood flow to the cerebral capillary beds. High hydrostatic pressures in the capillaries cause vascular fluid to exude into the interstitial space. If blood pressure is not reduced, cerebral edema and cerebral dysfunction (encephalopathy) increase until death occurs. Organ damage resulting from malignant hypertension is life-threatening. Besides encephalopathy, hypertensive crisis can cause papilledema, cardiac failure, uremia, retinopathy, and cerebrovascular accident and is considered a medical emergency.[51]

CLINICAL MANIFESTATIONS Hypertension is called a silent disease because the early stages of hypertension have no clinical manifestations

TABLE 24.2 Pathological Effects of Sustained, Complicated Primary Hypertension

Site of Injury	Mechanism of Injury	Potential Pathological Effect
Heart		
Myocardium	Increased workload combined with diminished blood flow through coronary arteries	Left ventricular hypertrophy, myocardial ischemia, heart failure
Coronary arteries	Accelerated atherosclerosis (coronary artery disease)	Myocardial ischemia, myocardial infarction, sudden death
Kidneys	Reduced blood flow, increased arteriolar pressure, RAAS and SNS stimulation, and inflammation	Glomerulosclerosis and decreased glomerular filtration, end-stage renal disease
Brain	Reduced blood flow and oxygen supply; weakened vessel walls, accelerated atherosclerosis	Transient ischemic attacks, cerebral thrombosis, aneurysm, hemorrhage, acute brain infarction
Eyes (retinas)	Retinal vascular sclerosis, increased retinal artery pressures	Hypertensive retinopathy, retinal exudates and hemorrhages
Aorta	Weakened vessel wall	Dissecting aneurysm
Arteries of lower extremities	Reduced blood flow and high pressures in arterioles, accelerated atherosclerosis	Intermittent claudication, gangrene

RAAS, Renin-angiotensin-aldosterone system; *SNS*, sympathetic nervous system.

other than elevated blood pressure. Some hypertensive individuals never have signs, symptoms, or complications, whereas others become very ill and may die because of hypertension. Other individuals may develop anatomical and physiological damage caused by past hypertensive disease, despite current blood pressure measurements being within normal ranges. If elevated blood pressure is not detected and treated, it becomes established and may begin to accelerate its effects on tissues when the individual is 30 to 50 years of age. This sets the stage for the complications of hypertension that begin to appear during the fourth, fifth, and sixth decades of life.

Most clinical manifestations of hypertensive disease are caused by complications that damage organs and tissues outside the vascular system. Besides elevated blood pressure, the signs and symptoms, therefore, tend to be specific to the organs or tissues affected. Evidence of heart disease, renal insufficiency, central nervous system dysfunction, impaired vision, impaired mobility, vascular occlusion, or edema can all be caused by sustained hypertension.

EVALUATION AND TREATMENT A single elevated blood pressure reading does not mean that a person has hypertension. At initial presentation, patients who exhibit features of a hypertensive urgency or emergency should be diagnosed as hypertensive and require immediate management. In all other patients, at least 2 more readings should be taken during the same visit.[13] Diagnosis requires the measurement of blood pressure on at least two separate occasions, averaging two readings at least 2 minutes apart, with the following conditions: the person is seated, the arm is supported at heart level, the person must be at rest for at least 5 minutes, and the person should not have smoked or ingested any caffeine in the previous 30 minutes.[12] Diagnostic tests for further evaluation of hypertension include 24-hour blood pressure monitoring in select individuals, complete blood count, urinalysis, biochemical blood profile (measures levels of plasma glucose, sodium, potassium, calcium, magnesium, creatinine, cholesterol, and triglycerides), and an **electrocardiogram (ECG)**. Individuals who have elevated blood pressure are assumed to have primary hypertension unless their history, physical examination, or initial diagnostic screening indicates secondary hypertension. Once the diagnosis is made, a careful evaluation for other cardiovascular risk factors and for end-organ damage should be done.

Treatment of primary hypertension depends on its severity. Hypertension Canada recommends beginning with lifestyle modification in preventing and treating hypertension.[12] Important lifestyle modifications include following an exercise program, making dietary modifications, stopping smoking, and losing weight. Reducing salt intake is an important dietary modification and has been shown to significantly reduce blood pressure in both hypertensive and normotensive individuals.[36,52] Pharmacological treatment of hypertension reduces the risk for end-organ damage and prevents major diseases, such as MI and stroke. Hypertension Canada recommends that treatment begin with thiazide diuretics alone or in combination with Ang II blockers (ACE inhibitors or ARBs) or calcium channel blockers.[53] Beta-blockers were found to have a higher rate of stroke than Ang II blockers and are no longer recommended as first-line medications. Individuals with HF, chronic kidney disease, or a history of MI or stroke should begin antihypertensive treatment with an ACE inhibitor or ARB. Some individuals require two or more medications for blood pressure control.

Hypertension Canada also recommends that antihypertensive therapy be prescribed for average DBP measurements of greater than or equal to 100 mm Hg or average SBP measurements of greater than or equal to 160 mm Hg in patients without macrovascular target-organ damage or other cardiovascular risk factors. It also strongly recommends that antihypertensive therapy be considered for average DBP readings greater than or equal to 90 mm Hg or for average systolic blood pressure readings greater than or equal to 140 mm Hg in the presence of macrovascular target-organ damage or other independent cardiovascular risk factors.[53]

Careful follow-up to support continued adherence, determine response, and monitor for potential adverse effects of these medications is important.

Orthostatic (Postural) Hypotension

> **QUICK CHECK 24.3**
> 1. How does Laplace's law function in aneurysms?
> 2. What is a thrombus?
> 3. Why are emboli dangerous?

The term **orthostatic (postural) hypotension (OH)** refers to a decrease in systolic blood pressure of at least 20 mm Hg or a decrease in diastolic blood pressure of at least 10 mm Hg within 3 minutes of moving to a standing position.[54] *Idiopathic*, or primary, OH implies no known initial cause. This kind of OH is often called *neurogenic* and is usually the result of primary neurological disorders or secondary to conditions that affect autonomic function.[55] It affects men more often than women and usually occurs between the ages of 40 and 70 years. Primary OH affects up to 18% of older persons, and it is a significant risk factor for falls and associated injury, with increased mortality.[56]

Recently, OH has been implicated in contributing to depression and dementia.[57]

Normally when an individual stands, baroreceptor-mediated reflex arteriolar and venous constriction and increased heart rate compensate for the gravitational changes on the circulation. Other compensatory mechanisms include mechanical factors, such as the closure of valves in the venous system, contraction of the leg muscles, and a decrease in intrathoracic pressure.[57] The normally increased sympathetic activity during upright posture is mediated through a stretch receptor (baroreceptor) reflex that responds to shifts in volume caused by postural changes. This reflex promptly increases heart rate and constricts the systemic arterioles. Thus, arterial blood pressure is maintained. These mechanisms are dysfunctional or inadequate in individuals with OH, consequently, upon standing, blood pools and normal arterial pressure cannot be maintained.

OH may be acute or chronic. Acute OH is caused when the normal regulatory mechanisms are sluggish as a result of (1) altered body chemistry, (2) medication action (e.g., antihypertensives, antidepressants), (3) prolonged immobility caused by illness, (4) starvation, (5) physical exhaustion, (6) any condition that produces volume depletion (e.g., dehydration, diuresis, potassium or sodium depletion), or (7) any condition that results in venous pooling (e.g., pregnancy, extensive varicosities of the lower extremities). Older persons are particularly susceptible to this type of OH.

Chronic orthostatic hypotension may be (1) secondary to a specific disease or (2) idiopathic or primary. The diseases that cause secondary OH are endocrine disorders (e.g., adrenal insufficiency, diabetes), metabolic disorders (e.g., porphyria), or diseases of the central or peripheral nervous systems (e.g., Parkinson's disease, multiple system atrophy, intracranial tumours, cerebral infarcts, Wernicke encephalopathy, peripheral neuropathies). Cardiovascular autonomic neuropathy is a common cause of OH in persons with diabetes and is a serious and often overlooked complication. In addition to cardiovascular symptoms, associated impotence and bowel and bladder dysfunction are common.

Dizziness, blurring or loss of vision, and syncope or fainting occur in OH because of insufficient vasomotor compensation and reduction of blood flow through the brain. Although no curative treatment is available for idiopathic OH, often it can be managed adequately with a combination of nondrug and medication therapies—increasing fluid and salt intake, wearing thigh-high stockings, and taking mineralocorticoids and vasoconstrictors.[55,57]

Aneurysm

An aneurysm is a localized dilation or outpouching of a vessel wall or cardiac chamber (Figure 24.6). True aneurysms involve all three layers of the arterial wall and are best described as a weakening of the vessel wall (Figure 24.7A). Most are fusiform and circumferential, whereas *saccular aneurysms* are basically spherical in shape. A false aneurysm is an extravascular hematoma that communicates with the intravascular space. A common cause of this type of lesion is a leak between a vascular graft and a natural artery.

Aneurysms most commonly occur in the thoracic or abdominal aorta. The aorta is particularly susceptible to aneurysm formation because of constant stress on the vessel wall and the absence of penetrating vasa vasorum in the media layer. Genetic and environmental risk factors (such as smoking and diet) are implicated in the pathogenesis of aortic aneurysms.[58] Atherosclerosis is the most common cause of arterial aneurysms because plaque formation erodes the vessel wall and contributes to inflammation. Inflammation eventually leads to the release of proteinases that can further weaken the vessel. In hypertension, increasing wall stress also contributes to aneurysm formation.

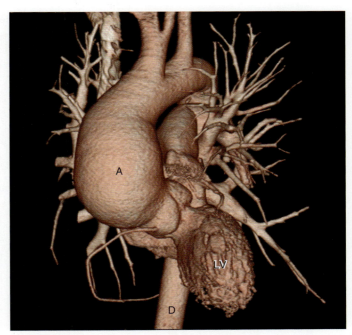

FIGURE 24.6 Aneurysm. A three-dimensional CT scan shows the aneurysm *(A)* involving the ascending thoracic aorta. *D*, Descending aorta; *LV*, left ventricle.

Collagen vascular disorders (e.g., Marfan's syndrome), syphilis, and other infections that affect arterial walls also can cause aneurysms.

Cardiac aneurysms most commonly form after MI when intraventricular tension stretches the noncontracting infarcted muscle. The stretching produces infarct expansion, a weak and thin layer of necrotic muscle, and fibrous tissue that bulges with each systole.

Clinical manifestations depend on where the aneurysm is located. Aortic aneurysms often are asymptomatic until they rupture, and then cause severe pain and hypotension. Thoracic aortic aneurysms can cause dysphagia (difficulty swallowing) and dyspnea (breathlessness). An aneurysm that impairs flow to an extremity causes symptoms of ischemia. Cerebral aneurysms, which often occur in the circle of Willis, are associated with signs and symptoms of increased intracranial pressure. Signs and symptoms of stroke occur when cerebral aneurysms leak. (Cerebral aneurysms are described in Chapter 16.) Aneurysms in the heart present with dysrhythmias, HF, and embolism of clots to the brain or other vital organs.

Aortic aneurysms can be complicated by acute aortic syndromes, which include aortic dissection, hemorrhage into the vessel wall, or vessel rupture. Dissection of the layers of the arterial wall occurs when there is a tear in the intima and blood enters the wall of the artery (Figure 24.7B). Dissections can involve any part of the aorta (ascending, arch, or descending) and can disrupt flow through arterial branches, thus creating a surgical emergency.

Ultrasonography, CT, MRI, or angiography are used to confirm the diagnosis of an aneurysm. Medical treatment is indicated for slow-growing aortic aneurysms, particularly in early stages, and includes cessation of smoking, reduction of blood pressure and blood volume, and implementation of β-adrenergic blockade. For those aneurysms that are dilating rapidly or have become large, surgical treatment is indicated and usually includes replacement with a prosthetic graft. Endovascular surgical techniques are commonly used for aneurysm repair and management of acute aortic rupture.[59]

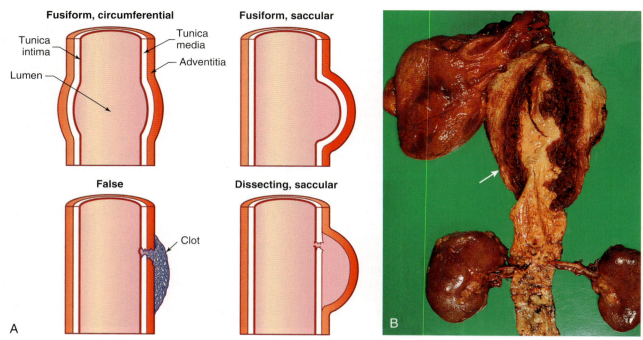

FIGURE 24.7 Longitudinal Sections Showing Types of Aneurysms. A, Weakening of the vessel wall causes the formation of true aneurysms, the fusiform circumferential and fusiform saccular aneurysms. Trauma leading to break in the vessel wall causes false and saccular aneurysms. **B,** Dissecting aneurysm of thoracic aorta *(arrow)*. ([B], from Damjanov, I., & Linder, J. [Eds.]. [1996]. *Anderson's pathology* [10th ed.]. Mosby.)

Thrombus Formation

As in venous thrombosis, arterial thrombi tend to develop when intravascular conditions promote activation of coagulation, or when there is stasis of blood flow. These conditions include those in which there is intimal irritation or roughening (such as in surgical procedures), inflammation, traumatic injury, infection, low blood pressures, or obstructions that cause blood stasis and pooling within the vessels. (Mechanisms of coagulation are described in Chapter 20.) Inflammation of the endothelium leads to activation of the clotting cascade, causing platelets to adhere readily. An anatomical change in an artery (such as an aneurysm) can contribute to thrombus formation, particularly if the change results in a pooling of arterial blood. Thrombi also form on heart valves altered by calcification or bacterial vegetation. Valvular thrombi are most commonly associated with inflammation of the endocardium (endocarditis) and rheumatic heart disease. Widespread arterial thrombus formation can occur in shock, particularly shock resulting from septicemia. In septic shock, systemic inflammation activates the intrinsic and extrinsic pathways of coagulation, resulting in microvascular thrombosis throughout the systemic arterial circulation.

Arterial thrombi pose two potential threats to the circulation. First, the thrombus may grow large enough to occlude the artery, causing ischemia in tissues supplied by the artery. Second, the thrombus may dislodge, becoming a thromboembolus that travels through the vascular system until it occludes flow into a distal systemic vascular bed.

Diagnosis of arterial thrombi is usually accomplished through the use of Doppler ultrasonography and angiography. Pharmacological treatment involves the administration of heparin, warfarin derivatives, thrombin inhibitors, or thrombolytics.[60] A balloon-tipped catheter also can be used to remove or compress an arterial thrombus. Various combinations of medication and catheter therapies are sometimes used concurrently.

Embolism

An **embolus** is a bolus of matter circulating in the bloodstream (**embolism**) that can lead to an obstruction of a vessel. The embolus may consist of a dislodged thrombus, air bubble, aggregate of amniotic fluid, fat, bacteria, cancer cells, or a foreign substance. An embolus travels in the bloodstream until it reaches a vessel through which it cannot pass. No matter how tiny it is, an embolus will eventually lodge in a systemic or pulmonary vessel determined by its source. Pulmonary emboli originate on the venous side (mostly from the deep veins of the legs) of the systemic circulation or in the right heart. Arterial emboli most commonly originate in the left heart and are associated with thrombi after MI, valvular disease, left ventricular failure, endocarditis, and dysrhythmias.

Embolism causes ischemia or infarction in tissues distal to the obstruction, producing organ dysfunction and pain. Infarction and subsequent necrosis of a central organ are life-threatening. For example, occlusion of a coronary artery will cause an MI, whereas occlusion of a cerebral artery causes a stroke (see Chapter 16). The types of emboli are summarized in Table 24.3.

Peripheral Vascular Disease
Thromboangiitis Obliterans (Buerger's Disease)

 QUICK CHECK 24.4
1. What is Buerger's disease?
2. Compare the differences between the manifestations of Buerger's disease and Raynaud's phenomenon.

Thromboangiitis obliterans (Buerger's disease) is an inflammatory disease of the periph.eral arteries and is associated with smoking. Buerger's disease is an autoimmune condition characterized by the formation of thrombi filled with inflammatory and immune cells.[61]

TABLE 24.3	Types of Emboli
Type	**Characteristics**
Arteries	
Arterial thromboembolism	Dislodged thrombus; source is usually from heart; most common sites of obstruction are lower extremities (femoral and popliteal arteries), coronary arteries, and cerebral vasculature
Veins	
Venous thromboembolism	Dislodged thrombus; source is usually from lower extremities; obstructs branches of pulmonary artery
Air embolism	Bolus of air displaces blood in vasculature; source usually room air entering circulation through intravenous (IV) lines; trauma to chest also may allow air from lungs to enter vascular space
Amniotic fluid embolism	Bolus of amniotic fluid; extensive intra-abdominal pressure attending labour and delivery can force amniotic fluid into bloodstream of mother; introduces antigens, cells, and protein aggregates that trigger inflammation, coagulation, and immune responses
Bacterial embolism	Aggregates of bacteria in bloodstream; source is subacute bacterial endocarditis or abscess
Fat embolism	Globules of fat floating in bloodstream associated with trauma to long bones; lungs in particular are affected
Foreign matter	Small particles or fibres introduced during trauma or through an IV or intra-arterial line; coagulation cascade is initiated and thromboemboli form around particles

Inflammatory cytokines and toxic oxygen free radicals contribute to accompanying vasospasm.[62] Over time, these thrombi become organized and fibrotic and result in permanent occlusion and obliteration of portions of small- and medium-sized arteries in the feet and sometimes in the hands. Although collateral vessels develop in Buerger's disease, they are inadequate to supply the extremities with blood. These collateral vessels have a characteristic corkscrew shape, thought to be a result of dilated vasa vasorum in the affected artery.

The chief symptom of Buerger's disease is pain and tenderness of the affected part, usually affecting more than one extremity. Clinical manifestations resulting from sluggish blood flow include rubor (redness of the skin) and cyanosis. Dilated capillaries under the skin cause rubor and tissue ischemia causes cyanosis. Chronic ischemia causes the skin to thin and become shiny and the nails to become thickened and malformed. In advanced disease, profound ischemia of the extremities resulting from vessel obliteration can cause gangrene necessitating amputation. Buerger's disease has also been associated with cerebrovascular disease (stroke), mesenteric disease, and rheumatic symptoms (joint pain).

Diagnosis of Buerger's disease is made by identification of the following common features—age less than 45 years, smoking history, evidence of peripheral ischemia—and by exclusion of other causes of arterial insufficiency. The most important part of treatment is cessation of cigarette smoking. If the person continues to smoke, the likelihood of recurrence of the disease and gangrene requiring amputation is high. Vasodilators are prescribed to alleviate vasospasm, and the individual receives instruction in exercises that use gravity to improve blood flow.

Raynaud's Phenomenon

Raynaud's phenomenon is characterized by attacks of vasospasm in the small arteries and arterioles of the fingers and, less commonly, the toes. Primary Raynaud's phenomenon is a common primary vasospastic disorder of unknown origin. Secondary Raynaud's phenomenon is associated with systemic diseases, particularly collagen vascular disease (scleroderma), vasculitis, malignancy, pulmonary hypertension, chemotherapy, cocaine use, hypothyroidism, thoracic outlet syndrome, trauma, serum sickness, or long-term exposure to environmental conditions such as cold temperatures or vibrating machinery in the workplace. Blood vessels in affected individuals demonstrate endothelial dysfunction with an imbalance in endothelium-derived vasodilators (e.g., nitric oxide) and vasoconstrictors (e.g., endothelin-1).[63] Platelet activation also may play a role, and autoantibodies have been identified in some individuals. Brief exposure to cold, vibration, or emotional stress can trigger vasospastic attacks, especially in young women, leading to secondary Raynaud's phenomenon. Genetic predisposition may play a role in its development.

Vasospastic attacks as a result of ischemia lead to changes in skin colour and sensation in either disorder. Vasospasm occurs with varying frequency and severity and causes pallor, numbness, and the sensation of coldness in the digits. Attacks tend to be bilateral, and manifestations usually begin at the tips of the digits and progress to the proximal phalanges. Sluggish blood flow resulting from ischemia may cause the skin to appear cyanotic. Rubor, throbbing pain, and paresthesias follow as blood flow returns. Skin colour returns to normal after the attack, but frequent, prolonged attacks interfere with cellular metabolism, causing the skin of the fingertips to thicken and the nails to become brittle. In severe, chronic Raynaud's phenomenon, ischemia can eventually cause ulceration and gangrene.

Once evident, the clinical manifestations confirm the diagnosis of Raynaud's phenomenon. Nailfold capillaroscopy is a sensitive method of diagnosis and can improve management and follow-up of individuals with associated collagen vascular disorders.[64] Treatment for Raynaud's phenomenon consists of removing the stimulus or treating the primary disease process. Treatment of Raynaud's phenomenon begins with avoidance of stimuli that trigger attacks (e.g., cold temperatures, emotional stress) and cessation of cigarette smoking to eliminate the vasoconstricting effects of nicotine. If attacks of vasospasm become frequent or prolonged, vasodilators, such as calcium channel blockers, nitric oxide agonists, alpha-blockers, prostaglandin analogues, or endothelin antagonists, are administered.[63] Sympathectomy may be indicated in severe cases, but may not be effective. If ischemia leads to ulceration and gangrene, amputation may be necessary.

Atherosclerosis

> **QUICK CHECK 24.5**
> 1. Discuss the development of *atherosclerosis*.
> 2. Describe how hypertension and dyslipidemia increase the likelihood of developing coronary artery disease.
> 3. Compare the differences between myocardial ischemia, angina, and silent ischemia.

Arteriosclerosis is a condition characterized by thickening and hardening of the vessel wall. **Atherosclerosis** is a form of arteriosclerosis that is caused by the accumulation of lipid-laden macrophages within the arterial wall, which leads to the formation of a lesion called a **plaque**. Atherosclerosis is not a single disease entity but rather a pathological process that can affect vascular systems throughout the body, resulting in ischemic syndromes that can vary widely in their severity and clinical manifestations. It is the leading cause of CAD and cerebrovascular disease. (Atherosclerosis of the coronary arteries is described in "Coronary Artery Disease, Myocardial Ischemia, and Acute Coronary Syndromes," later in this chapter, and atherosclerosis of the cerebral arteries is described in Chapter 16.)

PATHOPHYSIOLOGY Atherosclerosis begins with injury to the endothelial cells that line artery walls. Pathologically, the lesions progress from endothelial injury and dysfunction to fatty streak to fibrotic plaque to complicated lesion (Figure 24.8). Possible causes of endothelial injury include the common risk factors for atherosclerosis, such as smoking, hypertension, diabetes, increased levels of low-density lipoprotein (LDL), decreased levels of high-density lipoprotein (HDL), and autoimmunity. Other "nontraditional" risk factors include increased serum markers for inflammation and thrombosis (such as high-sensitivity C-reactive protein [hs-CRP], troponin I, adipokines, infection, and air pollution). These risk factors are discussed in more detail in "Coronary Artery Disease, Myocardial Ischemia, and Acute Coronary Syndromes," later in this chapter.

Injured endothelial cells become inflamed. Inflammation plays a fundamental role in mediating the steps in the initiation and progression of atherogenesis.[65] Inflamed endothelial cells cannot make normal amounts of antithrombic and vasodilating cytokines.[66]

The next step in atherogenesis occurs when inflamed endothelial cells express adhesion molecules that bind macrophages and other inflammatory and immune cells (Figure 24.9). Binding to damage-associated molecular patterns (DAMPs) released from injured cells, and release of numerous inflammatory cytokines (e.g., tumour necrosis factor-alpha [TNF-α], interferons, interleukins, and C-reactive protein [CRP]) and enzymes that further injure the vessel wall activate macrophages.[65,67]

The inflammatory process that generates toxic oxygen free radicals causes oxidation (i.e., addition of oxygen) of LDL that has accumulated in the vessel intima. Dyslipidemia, diabetes, smoking, and hypertension contribute to LDL oxidation and its accumulation in the vessel wall.[68] Oxidized LDL causes additional adhesion molecule expression with the recruitment of monocytes that differentiate into macrophages. These macrophages penetrate into the intima, where they engulf oxidized LDL. These lipid-laden macrophages are now called foam cells, and when they accumulate in significant amounts, they form a lesion called a fatty streak (see Figures 24.8 and 24.9). These lesions can be found in the walls of arteries of most people, even young children. Once formed, fatty streaks produce more toxic oxygen free radicals, recruit T lymphocytes (T cells) leading to autoimmunity, and secrete additional inflammatory mediators, resulting in progressive damage to the vessel wall.[65]

Macrophages also release growth factors that stimulate smooth muscle cell proliferation.[67] Smooth muscle cells in the region of endothelial injury proliferate, produce collagen, and migrate over the fatty streak, forming a fibrous plaque (see Figure 24.10). The fibrous plaque may calcify, protrude into the vessel lumen, and obstruct blood flow to distal tissues (especially during exercise), which may cause symptoms (e.g., angina or intermittent claudication).

Many plaques, however, are "unstable," meaning they are prone to rupture even before they affect blood flow significantly and are clinically silent until they rupture. Plaque rupture occurs because of innate and adaptive immune responses to tissue injury, including activation of proteinases (matrix metalloproteinases and cathepsins) and bleeding within the lesion (plaque hemorrhage), which accelerates apoptosis of cells within the plaque.[65] Plaques that have ruptured are called complicated plaques. Once rupture occurs, exposure of underlying tissue results in platelet adhesion, initiation of the clotting cascade, and rapid thrombus formation. The thrombus may suddenly occlude the affected vessel, resulting in ischemia and infarction. Aspirin or other antithrombotic agents are used to prevent this complication of atherosclerotic disease.

CLINICAL MANIFESTATIONS Atherosclerosis presents with symptoms and signs that result from inadequate perfusion of tissues because of obstruction of the vessels that supply them. Partial vessel obstruction may lead to transient ischemic events, often associated with exercise or stress. As the lesion becomes complicated, increasing obstruction with superimposed thrombosis may result in tissue infarction. Obstruction of peripheral arteries can cause significant pain and disability. Atherosclerosis leading to CAD is the major cause of myocardial ischemia. Atherosclerotic obstruction of the vessels supplying the brain is the major cause of stroke. Similarly, atherosclerotic lesions can compromise blood supply to any part of the body, causing ischemia.

EVALUATION AND TREATMENT In evaluating individuals for the presence of atherosclerosis, obtaining a complete health history (including risk factors and symptoms of ischemia) is essential. Physical examination may reveal arterial bruits and evidence of decreased blood flow to tissues. Laboratory data that include measurement of levels of lipids, blood glucose, and hs-CRP are also indicated. Judicious use of X-ray films, electrocardiography, ultrasonography, nuclear scanning, CT, MRI, and angiography may be necessary to identify affected vessels, particularly coronary vessels.[69]

Current management of atherosclerosis is focused on detection and treatment of preclinical lesions with medications aimed at stabilizing and reversing plaques before they rupture. Once a lesion obstructs blood flow, the primary goal in the management of atherosclerosis is to restore adequate blood flow to the affected tissues. If an individual has presented with acute ischemia (e.g., MI, stroke), interventions are specific to the diseased area (discussed further under those topics). In situations in which the disease process does not require immediate intervention, management focuses on reduction of risk factors and prevention of plaque progression. Management strategies include implementation of an exercise program, cessation of smoking, and control of hypertension and diabetes where appropriate while reducing LDL cholesterol level by diet or medications, or both. Management of atherosclerotic risk factors is discussed further in Chapter 24.

Peripheral Artery Disease

Peripheral artery disease (PAD) refers to atherosclerotic disease of arteries that perfuse the limbs, especially the lower extremities. PAD affects an estimated 800 000 Canadians over 40 years of age.[70] The risk factors for PAD are the same as those previously described for atherosclerosis, but it is especially prevalent in older persons with diabetes and has a very strong link with smoking.[71]

Lower extremity ischemia resulting from arterial obstruction in PAD can be gradual or acute. In most individuals, atherosclerosis in the iliofemoral vessels gradually increase obstruction to arterial blood flow to the legs, resulting in pain with ambulation called intermittent claudication. If a thrombus forms over the atherosclerotic lesion, complete obstruction of blood flow can occur acutely, causing severe pain, loss of pulses, and skin colour changes in the affected extremity.

Evaluation for PAD requires a careful history and physical examination that focuses on finding evidence of atherosclerotic disease (e.g., bruits), determining a difference in blood pressure measured at the ankle versus the arm (ankle-brachial index), and measuring blood flow using noninvasive Doppler.[72] Treatment includes risk factor reduction (smoking cessation and treatment of diabetes, hypertension, and dyslipidemia) and antiplatelet therapy. Symptomatic PAD should be managed with vasodilators in combination with antiplatelet or

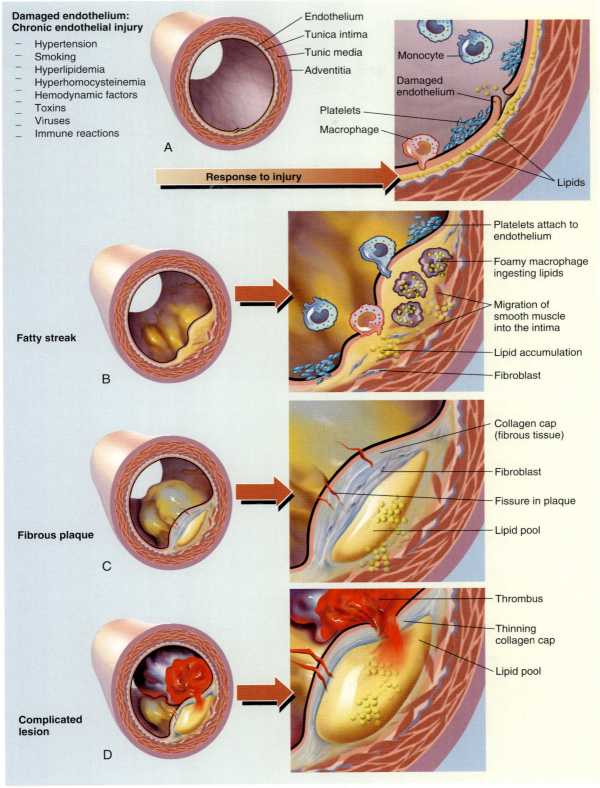

FIGURE 24.8 Progression of Atherosclerosis. A, Damaged endothelium. **B,** Diagram of fatty streak and lipid core formation (see Figure 24.9 for a diagram of oxidized low-density lipoprotein [LDL]). **C,** Diagram of fibrous plaque. Raised plaques are visible: some are yellow; others are white. **D,** Diagram of complicated lesion; thrombus is red; collagen is blue. Plaque is complicated by red thrombus deposition.

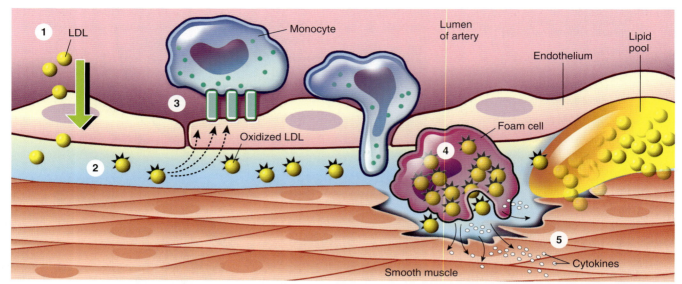

FIGURE 24.9 Low-density Lipoprotein Oxidation. 1, Low-density lipoprotein *(LDL)* enters the arterial tunica intima through an intact endothelium. In hypercholesterolemia, the influx of LDL exceeds the eliminating capacity and an extracellular pool of LDL is formed. Association of LDL with the extracellular matrix enhances this process. 2, Enzymatic or nonenzymatic reactions generate oxygen free radicals, which oxidize intimal LDL. 3, This generates proinflammatory lipids that induce endothelial expression of the adhesion molecule. Vascular cell adhesion molecule-1 activates complement and stimulates chemokine secretion. All of these factors cause adhesion and entry of mononuclear leukocytes, particularly monocytes and T cells. 4, Monocytes differentiate into macrophages. Macrophages upregulate and internalize oxidized LDL and transform into foam cells. Macrophage update of oxidized LDL also leads to presentation of its fragments to antigen-specific T cells. 5, This process induces an autoimmune reaction that leads to production of proinflammatory cytokines. Such cytokines include interferon-gamma, tumour necrosis factor-alpha, and interleukin-1, which act on endothelial cells to stimulate expression of adhesion molecules and procoagulant activity. Cytokines also act on macrophages to activate proteases, endocytosis, nitric oxide (NO), and cytokines in addition to acting on smooth muscle cells to induce NO production and inhibit growth, collagen, and actin expression. (Modified from Crawford, M. H., DiMarco, J. P., & Paulus, W. J. [2010]. *Cardiology* [3rd ed.]. Mosby.)

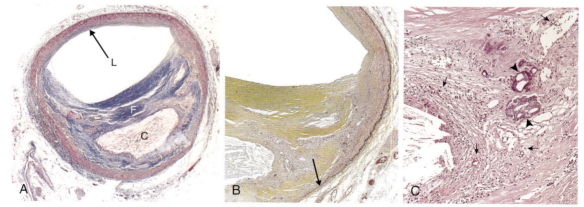

FIGURE 24.10 Histological Features of Atheromatous Plaque in the Coronary Artery. A, Overall architecture demonstrating fibrous cap *(F)* and a central necrotic (largely lipid) core *(C)*. The lumen *(L)* has been moderately narrowed. Note that a segment of the wall is plaque free *(arrow)*, so that there is an eccentric lesion. In this section, collagen has been stained blue (Masson's trichrome stain). B, Higher power photograph of a section of the plaque shown in (A) stained for elastin *(black)*, demonstrating that the internal and external elastic membranes are destroyed and the media of the artery is thinned under the most advanced plaque *(arrow)*. C, Higher magnification photomicrograph at the junction of the fibrous cap and core, showing scattered inflammatory cells, calcification *(arrowhead)*, and neovascularization *(small arrows)*. (From Kumar, V., Abbas, A., & Aster J. [2007]. *Robbins basic pathology* [9th ed.]. Saunders.)

antithrombotic medications (Aspirin, ticlopidine [Ticlid], or clopidogrel [Plavix]), and cholesterol-lowering medications.[73] Aerobic exercise is a crucial part of therapy.[10] If acute or refractory symptoms occur, emergent percutaneous or surgical revascularization may be indicated. Newer treatment modalities that are being explored include autologous stem cell therapies and angiogenesis.[74]

Coronary Artery Disease, Myocardial Ischemia, and Acute Coronary Syndromes

Coronary artery disease (CAD), myocardial ischemia, and MI form a pathophysiological continuum that deprives the heart muscle of blood-borne oxygen and nutrients and impairs the pumping ability of the heart. The earliest lesions of the continuum are those of CAD, which is usually caused by atherosclerosis (see Figure 24.10). CAD can diminish the myocardial blood supply until deprivation impairs myocardial metabolism enough to cause ischemia, a local state in which the cells are temporarily deprived of blood supply. The cells remain alive but cannot function normally. Persistent ischemia or the complete occlusion of a coronary artery causes the acute coronary syndromes including infarction, or irreversible myocardial damage.

Development of Coronary Artery Disease

A systematic review demonstrated that 90% of Canadians have suboptimal cardiovascular health status secondary to multiple cardiovascular risk factors; increased rates of obesity and diabetes; and lack of control of hypertension, dyslipidemia, and blood glucose.[75]

More than 1.4 million Canadians have heart disease. It is also one of the leading causes of death in Canada, claiming more than 33 600 lives per year.[76] Fortunately, the incidence and mortality statistics for CAD have been decreasing over the past 15 years because of more aggressive recognition, prevention, and treatment. Risk factors for CAD are the same as those for atherosclerosis and can be categorized as conventional (major) versus nontraditional (novel), and as modifiable versus nonmodifiable. The plethora of new information obtained about the conventional risk factors has markedly improved prevention and management of CAD. In addition, nontraditional risk factors have been identified that have provided insight into the pathogenesis of CAD and may lead to more effective interventions in the future.

Conventional or major risk factors for CAD that are nonmodifiable include (1) advanced age, (2) male gender or women after menopause, and (3) family history. Aging and menopause are associated with increased exposure to risk factors and poor endothelial healing. Family history may contribute to CAD through genetics and shared environmental exposures. Modifiable major risks include (1) dyslipidemia, (2) hypertension, (3) cigarette smoking, (4) diabetes mellitus (insulin resistance), (5) obesity, (6) sedentary lifestyle, and (7) atherogenic diet. Fortunately, modification of these factors can dramatically reduce the risk for CAD.[77]

Dyslipidemia. The link between CAD and abnormal levels of lipoproteins is well documented. The term lipoprotein refers to lipids, phospholipids, cholesterol, and triglycerides bound to carrier proteins. Most cells require lipids (cholesterol in particular) for the manufacture and repair of plasma membranes. Cholesterol is also a necessary component for the manufacture of such essential substances as bile acids and steroid hormones.

The cycle of lipid metabolism is complex. Dietary fat is packaged into particles known as *chylomicrons* in the small intestine. Chylomicrons transport exogenous lipids from the intestine to the liver and peripheral cells, thus playing an important role in the absorption of fat. Chylomicrons are the least dense of the lipoproteins and primarily contain triglyceride. Some of the triglyceride may be removed and either stored by adipose tissue or used by muscle as an energy source. The liver takes up the chylomicron remnants, which are composed mainly of cholesterol. A series of chemical reactions in the liver results in the production of several lipoproteins that vary in density and function. These include very-low-density lipoproteins (VLDLs), which contain primarily triglyceride; LDLs, which carry mostly cholesterol; and HDL molecules with protein as the main components.

Dyslipidemia (or dyslipoproteinemia) refers to abnormal concentrations of serum lipoproteins. It has been defined by the Third Report of the National Cholesterol Education Program in the United States[78] (Table 24.4), although more recent Canadian guidelines place less emphasis on specific serum lipoprotein levels.[79] These abnormalities are the result of a combination of genetic and dietary factors. Primary or familial dyslipoproteinemias result from genetic defects that cause abnormalities in lipid-metabolizing enzymes and abnormal cellular lipid receptors. Secondary causes of dyslipidemia include the existence of several common systemic disorders, such as diabetes, hypothyroidism, pancreatitis, and renal nephrosis, as well as the use of certain medications, such as some diuretics, glucocorticoids, interferons, and antiretrovirals.

LDL is responsible for the delivery of cholesterol to the tissues, and an increased serum concentration of LDL is a strong indicator of coronary risk. The hepatic receptors that bind LDL and limit liver synthesis of this lipoprotein control serum levels of LDL. High dietary intake of cholesterol and saturated fats, in combination with a genetic predisposition to accumulations of LDL in the serum (e.g., dysfunction of the hepatic LDL receptor), results in high levels of LDL in the bloodstream. LDL migration into the vessel wall, oxidation, and phagocytosis by macrophages are key steps in the pathogenesis of atherosclerosis (see Figure 24.9). LDL also plays a role in endothelial injury, inflammation, and immune responses that have been identified as being important in atherogenesis.[68] The term *LDL* actually describes several types of LDL molecules. Measurement of LDL subfractions allows for a better prediction of coronary risk. For example, LDL cholesterol measurements enable the detection of the small, dense LDL particles that are the most atherogenic, and apolipoprotein B (structural protein found in both LDL and VLDL) levels are a very strong predictor of future coronary events. Recent guidelines from the Canadian Cardiovascular Society focus on treating dyslipidemia in the context of other risk factors.[79] (See *Health Promotion*: Recommendations for Managing Cholesterol.)

TABLE 24.4 Criteria for Dyslipidemia

	Optimal	Near-Optimal	Desirable	Low	Borderline	High	Very High
Total cholesterol			<5 mmol/L	4.15–5.19 mmol/L	5.2–6.19 mmol/L	≥6.2–7.2 mmol/L	>7.21 mmol/L
LDL	<2.59 mmol/L	2.59–3.34 mmol/L			3.37–4.11 mmol/L	4.14–4.90 mmol/L	≥4.92 mmol/L
Triglycerides			<0.45–1.81 mmol/L		150–199	200–499	≥5.6 mmol/L
HDL				<1.036 mmol/L		≥1.55 mmol/L	

HDL, High-density lipoprotein; LDL, low-density lipoprotein.
Data from Expert Panel on Detection, Evaluation, and Treatment of High Blood Cholesterol in Adults. (2001). *JAMA, 285*(19), 2486–2497.

HEALTH PROMOTION

Recommendations for Managing Cholesterol

The Heart and Stroke Foundation of Canada recommends that cholesterol be tested in the following individuals:
- Men over 40 years of age
- Women who are over 50 years of age, postmenopausal, or both
- Individuals with heart disease, diabetes, or high blood pressure
- Individuals with a waist circumference greater than 94 cm (37 in.) for men and 80 cm (31.5 in.) for women
- Individuals who smoke or have smoked within the last year
- Men with erectile dysfunction
- Individuals with family history of heart disease or stroke

It also recommends that individuals prevent or manage cholesterol levels by doing the following:

1. **Eat a healthy balanced diet**.
   - Choose a variety of whole and minimally processed foods at every meal. This means foods that are not packaged or that have few ingredients.
   - Fill half your plate with vegetables and fruit at every meal. Choose vegetables and fruit for snacks. Select fresh, frozen, or canned vegetables and fruit. You want them to be plain, without sauce, sugar, or salt added.
   - Choose whole grains. Look for whole-grain breads, barley, oats (including oatmeal), quinoa, brown rice, bulgur, farro, etc.
   - Mix up your protein foods. Choose more vegetarian options such as beans, lentils, tofu, and nuts. Include vegetarian options as often as possible in your weekly meal plan. Make sure your meat is lean and poultry is without the skin, and include fish a couple of times per week. Limit your portion sizes.
   - Choose lower fat dairy products or alternatives with no added sugar. Select 1% or skim milk, plain yogurt, and lower fat cheeses.
   - Plan healthy snacks with at least two different types of food. For example, try hummus and baby carrots, apple wedges and lower fat cheese, or plain yogurt with berries.
   - Drink water or lower fat plain milk to satisfy thirst. Avoid sugary drinks, including soft drinks, sports drinks, sweetened milk or alternatives, fruit drinks, 100% fruit juice, and ready-to-drink sweetened coffees and teas.

2. **Cook and eat more meals at home**. Cooking at home allows you to select whole and minimally processed foods.
   - Develop and share skills in food preparation and cooking with your family.
   - Buy a healthy cookbook or use the healthy recipes at http://www.heartandstroke.ca/recipes. Select the top 10 recipes your family loves and get everyone involved in the meal preparation.
   - Reduce the amount of sugar, salt, and solid fats used in your favourite recipes.

3. **Make eating out a special occasion**. Eating out usually results in you consuming large amounts of food and more fat, salt, and sugar.
   - Try to limit the number of times you eat in a restaurant per month.
   - When you do eat out, choose restaurants that serve freshly made dishes using whole and minimally processed foods and provide nutrition information.
   - Share meals or ask for half the meal to be packed up to eat the next day.

4. **Achieve and maintain a healthy weight**. Being overweight or obese increases your LDL or bad cholesterol level, lowers your HDL or good cholesterol level, and raises your triglyceride levels. Reducing your weight is a positive way to reduce your blood cholesterol levels. Help is available at https://www.heartandstroke.ca/healthy-living/healthy-weight.

5. **Physical activity**. Being physically active will help improve your cholesterol levels and general heart health. Aim for 150 minutes a week. That is less than 25 minutes per day! Choose activities you like. Cycling, swimming, gardening, and walking are great ways to keep active.

6. **Be smoke-free**. Smoking is a risk factor for heart disease. It reduces the level of your HDL "good" cholesterol. Once you quit, within a few weeks your HDL levels will start to rise.

From Heart & Stroke Foundation of Canada. (2017). *How to Manage Your Cholesterol*. https://www.heartandstroke.ca/heart-disease/risk-and-prevention/condition-risk-factors/managing-cholesterol. Reproduced with the permission of the Heart and Stroke Foundation of Canada. www.heartandstroke.ca.

The Canadian Cardiovascular Harmonized National Guidelines Endeavour (C-CHANGE) *Guideline for the Prevention and Management of Cardiovascular Disease in Primary Care: 2018 Update*[80] recommends the following:

- A target LDL-C below < 2.0 mmol/L or > 50% reduction of LDL-C in individuals for whom treatment is begun, to decrease the risk of cardiovascular disease (CVD) events. Alternative target variables are apolipoprotein B (apoB) < 0.8 g/L or non–HDL-C < 2.6 mmol/L. Recommendations include:
  - A > 50% reduction of LDL-C for patients with LDL-C > 5.0 mmol/L in individuals for whom treatment is begun, to decrease the risk of CVD events and mortality.
  - Management that includes statin therapy in high-risk conditions including clinical atherosclerosis, abdominal aortic aneurysm, most diabetes mellitus (DM), chronic kidney disease (age > 50 years), and those with LDL-C ≥ 5.0 mmol/L to decrease the risk of CVD events and mortality.
- For individuals not at LDL-C goal despite statin therapy as described above, a combination of statin therapy with second-line agents may be used to achieve the goal; the agent used should be selected based upon the size of the existing gap to LDL-C goal. Recommendations include:
  - Management that includes statin therapy for individuals at high risk (modified Framingham Risk Score [FRS] ≥ 20%) to decrease the risk of CVD events.
  - Management that includes statin therapy for individuals at intermediate risk (modified FRS 10%–19%) with LDL-C ≥ 3.5 mmol/L to decrease the risk of CVD events.
  - Statin therapy should also be considered for persons at intermediate risk with LDL-C < 3.5 mmol/L but with apoB ≥ 1.2 g/L or non–HDL-C ≥ 4.3 mmol/L, or in men aged ≥ 50 years and women aged ≥ 60 years with ≥ 1 CV risk factor.[80]

Low levels of HDL cholesterol also are a strong indicator of coronary risk. HDL is responsible for "reverse cholesterol transport," which returns excess cholesterol from the tissues to the liver for processing or elimination in the bile. HDL also participates in endothelial repair and decreases thrombosis. It can be fractionated into several particle densities (HDL-2 and HDL-3) that have different effects on vascular function. Exercise, weight loss, fish oil consumption, and moderate alcohol use result in modest increases in HDL level. Despite the wealth of evidence that HDL plays an important role in preventing atherosclerotic coronary disease, studies have suggested that raising overall levels of HDL is not adequate to prevent CVD. Niacin and fibrates are medications that can cause modest increases in HDL levels that are not correlated with an improvement in cardiovascular risk in individuals without documented coronary disease (primary prevention). Medications that are aimed specifically at increasing HDL levels include recombinant apolipoprotein A-I (ApoA-I) mimetics, thiazolidinediones (used to treat diabetes), and cholesteryl ester transfer protein inhibitors, but they have not been shown to be effective in preventing heart disease. Recent studies suggest that it is not the serum levels of HDL that are key to determining CAD risk, but rather HDL functionality, which is harder to measure.[81,82]

Other lipoproteins associated with increased cardiovascular risk include elevated levels of serum VLDLs (triglycerides) and increased **lipoprotein(a) (Lp[a])** levels. Triglycerides are associated with an increased risk for CAD, especially in combination with other risk factors such as diabetes. Lp(a) is a genetically determined molecular complex between LDL and a serum glycoprotein called *apolipoprotein A* and has been shown to be an important risk factor for atherosclerosis, especially in women.

Hypertension. Hypertension is responsible for a twofold to threefold increased risk for atherosclerotic CVD. It contributes to endothelial injury, a key step in atherogenesis. It also can cause myocardial hypertrophy, which increases myocardial demand for coronary flow. Overactivity of the SNS and RAAS commonly found in hypertension also contributes to the genesis of CAD.

The Canadian Cardiovascular Harmonized National Guidelines Endeavour (C-CHANGE) *Guideline for the Prevention and Management of Cardiovascular Disease in Primary Care: 2018 Update* recommends that initial therapy should be with either monotherapy or single-pill combination. The recommended monotherapy choices are a thiazide or thiazide-like diuretic, with longer-acting diuretics preferred. Another recommended monotherapy is a beta-blocker in patients who are less than 60 years of age. An ACE inhibitor (in patients who are not Black) or an ARB is also an appropriate monotherapy. A long-acting calcium channel blocker (CCB) has also proven to be an effective monotherapy. A single-pill combination of an ACE inhibitor combined with a CCB is also available when monotherapy is not effective. ARB with a CCB, or ACE inhibitor or ARB with a diuretic are also available as combination therapy. It is worth noting that alpha-blockers are not recommended as first-line agents for uncomplicated hypertension and beta-blockers are not recommended as first-line therapy for uncomplicated hypertension in patients aged ≥ 60 yr. Moreover, ACE inhibitors are not recommended as first-line therapy for uncomplicated hypertension in Black patients.[80]

Cigarette smoking. Both direct and passive (environmental) smoking increase the risk for CAD. Smoking has a direct effect on endothelial cells and the generation of oxygen free radicals that contribute to atherogenesis.[83] Nicotine stimulates the release of catecholamines (epinephrine and norepinephrine), which increase heart rate and peripheral vascular constriction. As a result, blood pressure increases, as do cardiac workload and oxygen demand. Cigarette smoking is associated with an increase in LDL levels and a decrease in HDL levels. The risk for CAD increases with heavy smoking and decreases when smoking is stopped.

Diabetes mellitus (insulin resistance). Insulin resistance and diabetes mellitus are extremely important risk factors for CAD. Insulin resistance and diabetes have multiple effects on the cardiovascular system, including damage to the endothelium, thickening of the vessel wall, increased inflammation, increased thrombosis, glycation of vascular proteins, and decreased production of endothelial-derived vasodilators, such as nitric oxide.[84] Diabetes also is associated with dyslipidemia (see Chapter 19). Good diabetic control is linked to reduced risk for CAD.

The Canadian Cardiovascular Harmonized National Guidelines Endeavour (C-CHANGE) *Guideline for the Prevention and Management of Cardiovascular Disease in Primary Care: 2018 Update* recommends that all patients with diabetes should follow a comprehensive, multifaceted approach to reduce CV risk, including:

- A1C ≤ 7.0% implemented early in the course of diabetes.
- Patients with DM must maintain SBP of < 130 mm Hg and DBP of < 80 mm Hg, in addition to receiving additional vascular-protective medications and achievement of healthy weight goals through healthy eating, regular physical activity, and smoking cessation.
- To reduce the risk of chronic kidney disease and retinopathy in patients with type 2 diabetes, an A1C ≤ 6.5% must be achieved especially if patients are at low risk of hypoglycemia.[80]

Obesity or a sedentary lifestyle. In Canada, 14.9% of adults have a combination of obesity, dyslipidemia, hypertension, and insulin resistance, called **metabolic syndrome (MetS)**, which is associated with an even higher risk for CAD events. The importance of MetS for public health is demonstrated by its significant association with chronic disease relative to the general population. The 10-year incidence estimate for diabetes and mean percent risk for a fatal CVD event were higher in those with MetS compared to those without (18.0% versus 7.1% for diabetes, and 4.1% versus 0.8% for CVD). MetS is prevalent in Canadian adults, and a high proportion of individuals with MetS have diagnosed or undiagnosed chronic conditions. Projection estimates for the incidence of chronic disease associated with MetS demonstrate higher rates in individuals with this condition. Thus, MetS may be a relevant risk factor in the development of chronic disease.[85]

Abdominal obesity has the strongest link with increased CAD risk and is related to inflammation, insulin resistance, decreased HDL level, increased blood pressure, and fewer changes in hormones called adipokines (leptin and adiponectin).[86] A sedentary lifestyle not only increases the risk for obesity but also has an independent effect on increasing CAD risk. Physical activity and weight loss offer substantial reductions in risk factors for CAD.[87]

Atherogenic diet. Diet plays a complex role in atherogenic risk. Diets high in salt, fats, trans fats, and carbohydrates have all been implicated. There are many recommendations regarding diet modification to reduce coronary risk; following a Mediterranean diet is one of the most effective.

Nontraditional risk factors. Nontraditional, or novel, risk factors for CAD include increased serum markers for inflammation and thrombosis (troponin I, adipokines, infection, and air pollution). The amount of risk conferred by these relatively newly identified factors is still being explored.

Markers of inflammation and thrombosis. Of the numerous markers of inflammation that have been linked to an increase in CAD risk (hs-CRP, fibrinogen, protein C, plasminogen activator inhibitor), the relationship between serum levels of hs-CRP and CAD has been explored in the greatest depth. hs-CRP is a protein mostly synthesized in the liver and used as an indirect measure of atherosclerotic plaque–related inflammation. An elevated serum level of hs-CRP is strongly correlated with an increased risk for coronary events,[88] but it is a nonspecific measure of inflammation and may indicate the presence of other inflammatory conditions. The primary use of hs-CRP is as an aid to decision making about pharmacological interventions for individuals with other risk factors for coronary disease.[89] Other markers of inflammation associated with CAD include the erythrocyte sedimentation rate and concentrations of von Willebrand factor, interleukin-6 (IL-6), IL-18, tumour necrosis factor, fibrinogen, and cluster of differentiation (CD) 40 ligand. Interestingly, the long-term use of some anti-inflammatories, such as ibuprofen (Advil), has been linked to increased (rather than decreased) risk for CAD because of their potentiation of clotting in certain tissues.[90]

Troponin I. Troponin I (TnI) is a serum protein whose measurement is used as a sensitive and specific diagnostic test to help identify myocardial injury during acute coronary syndromes. Highly sensitive TnI assays are used in individuals without a history of CAD to assess risk for future coronary heart disease events, mortality, and HF.

Adipokines. Adipokines are a group of hormones released from adipose cells. Obesity causes increased levels of leptin, which is implicated in hypertension and diabetes, and decreased levels of adiponectin, which is a hormone that functions to protect the vascular endothelium and is anti-inflammatory.[91,92] Other adipokines also have been linked to inflammation in endothelial cells.[93] Weight loss, exercise, and healthy diet improve adipokine levels.

Infection. Infections with various microorganisms, including *Chlamydia pneumoniae*, *Helicobacter pylori*, and cytomegalovirus, have been linked to an increased risk for CAD, although cause and effect have not been proven. Periodontal disease also has been linked to an increased risk for CAD. One hypothesis is that systemic infection results in increased inflammation of vessels and, therefore, contributes to vascular disease. Unfortunately, the use of antibiotics for the prevention and treatment of CAD has not yielded consistently positive results.

Air pollution. Exposure to air pollution, especially roadway exposures, is strongly correlated with coronary risk. It is postulated that toxins in pollution contribute to macrophage activation, oxidation of LDL, thrombosis, and inflammation of vessel walls.[94]

Myocardial Ischemia

PATHOPHYSIOLOGY The coronary arteries normally supply blood flow sufficient to meet the demands of the myocardium as it labours under varying workloads. Oxygen is extracted from these vessels with maximal efficiency. If demand increases, healthy coronary arteries can dilate to increase the flow of oxygenated blood to the myocardium. Narrowing of a major coronary artery by more than 50% impairs blood flow enough to hamper cellular metabolism when myocardial demand increases.

Myocardial ischemia develops if the flow or oxygen content of coronary blood is insufficient to meet the metabolic demands of myocardial cells (Figure 24.11). Imbalances between coronary blood supply and myocardial demand can result from a number of conditions. The most common cause of decreased coronary blood flow and resultant myocardial ischemia is the formation of atherosclerotic plaques in the coronary circulation. As the plaque increases in size, it may partially occlude the vessel lumina, thus limiting coronary flow and causing ischemia, especially during exercise. As discussed earlier in this chapter, some plaques are "unstable," meaning they are prone to ulceration or rupture. When this ulceration or rupture occurs, underlying tissues of the vessel wall are exposed, resulting in platelet adhesion and thrombus formation (see Figures 24.7 and 24.15). Thrombus formation can suddenly stop blood supply to the heart muscle, resulting in acute myocardial ischemia, and if the vessel obstruction cannot be reversed rapidly, ischemia will progress to infarction. Myocardial ischemia also can result from other causes of decreased blood and oxygen delivery to the myocardium, such as coronary spasm, hypotension, dysrhythmias, and decreased oxygen-carrying capacity of the blood (e.g., anemia, hypoxemia). Common causes of increased myocardial demand for blood include tachycardia, exercise, hypertension (hypertrophy), and valvular disease.

Myocardial cells become ischemic within 10 seconds of coronary occlusion, thus hampering pump function and depriving the myocardium of a glucose source necessary for aerobic metabolism. Anaerobic processes take over, and lactic acid accumulates. After several minutes, the heart cells lose the ability to contract and cardiac output decreases. Cardiac cells remain viable for approximately 20 minutes under ischemic conditions. If blood flow is restored, aerobic metabolism resumes, contractility is restored, and cellular repair begins. If perfusion is not restored, then MI occurs (see Figure 24.11).

CLINICAL MANIFESTATIONS Individuals with reversible myocardial ischemia present clinically in several ways. Chronic coronary obstruction results in recurrent predictable chest pain called *stable angina*. Abnormal vasospasm of coronary vessels results in unpredictable chest pain called *Prinzmetal's angina*. Myocardial ischemia that does not cause detectable symptoms is called *silent ischemia*.

1. **Stable angina pectoris.** Angina is chest pain caused by myocardial ischemia. The gradual luminal narrowing and hardening of the arterial walls, with associated inflammation, endothelial cell dysfunction, and a decrease in endogenous vasodilators cause stable angina. These changes are more prevalent in individuals with obesity, diabetes, and dyslipidemia.[95] Affected vessels cannot dilate in response to increased myocardial demand associated with physical exertion or emotional stress. With rest, blood flow is restored and necrosis of myocardial cells does not occur. Angina pectoris is typically experienced as transient substernal chest discomfort, ranging from a sensation of heaviness or pressure to moderately severe pain. Individuals often describe the sensation by clenching a fist over the left sternal border. The discomfort may be mistaken for indigestion. The buildup of lactic acid or abnormal stretching of the ischemic myocardium that irritates myocardial nerve fibres causes pain. These afferent sympathetic fibres enter the spinal cord from levels C3 to T4, accounting for a variety of locations and radiation patterns of anginal pain. Discomfort may radiate to the neck, lower jaw, left arm, and left shoulder, or occasionally to the back or down the right arm. Pallor, diaphoresis, and dyspnea may be associated with the pain. Rest and nitrates usually relieve the pain. However, myocardial ischemia in women may not present with typical anginal pain. Common symptoms in women include atypical chest pain, palpitations, sense of unease, and severe fatigue. In addition, it is estimated that half of women with stable angina do not have obstructive CAD,

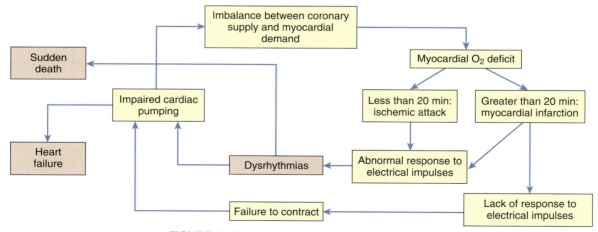

FIGURE 24.11 Cycle of Ischemic Events. O_2, Oxygen.

but rather have "microvascular angina" that results from vasoconstriction of small coronary arterioles deep in the myocardium[96] (see *Health Promotion: Women and Microvascular Angina*).

2. **Prinzmetal's angina.** Prinzmetal's angina (also called *variant angina*) is chest pain attributable to transient ischemia of the myocardium that occurs unpredictably and often at rest. Vasospasm of one or more major coronary arteries with or without associated atherosclerosis causes pain. The pain often occurs at night during rapid eye movement sleep and may have a cyclic pattern of occurrence. The angina may result from decreased vagal activity, hyperactivity of the SNS, or decreased nitric oxide activity. Other causes include altered calcium channel function in arterial smooth muscle or impaired production or release of inflammatory mediators, such as serotonin, histamine, endothelin, or thromboxane.[97] Serum markers of inflammation, such as CRP and IL-6, are elevated in individuals with this form of angina. Prinzmetal's angina is usually a benign condition, but it can occasionally cause serious dysrhythmias, especially if treatment is withdrawn. Therefore, calcium channel blockers or long-acting nitrates should be continued even if clinical remission is achieved.[98]

3. **Silent ischemia** and **mental stress–induced ischemia.** Myocardial ischemia may not cause detectable symptoms such as angina. Ischemia can be totally asymptomatic (and referred to as *silent ischemia*), or individuals may complain of fatigue, dyspnea, or a feeling of unease. Some individuals only have silent ischemia, and episodes of silent ischemia are common in individuals who also experience angina. One proposed mechanism for the absence of angina in silent myocardial ischemia is the presence of a global or regional abnormality in left ventricular sympathetic afferent innervation. The most common cause of autonomic dysfunction leading to silent ischemia is diabetes mellitus. Other causes include surgical denervation during coronary artery bypass grafting (CABG) or cardiac transplantation, or following ischemic local nerve injury by MI. Also of interest is silent ischemia occurring in some individuals during mental stress (Figures 24.12 and 24.13). Chronic stress has been linked to an increase in the number of inflammatory cytokines and a hypercoagulable state that may contribute to acute ischemic events.[99,100] Stress radionucleotide imaging detects silent ischemia. Detection and management of silent ischemia caused by coronary disease is important because it is an indicator of increased risk for serious cardiovascular events.[101]

EVALUATION AND TREATMENT Many individuals with reversible myocardial ischemia will have a normal physical examination between events. Physical examination of those experiencing myocardial ischemia may disclose rapid pulse rate or extra heart sounds (gallops or murmurs), and pulmonary congestion indicating impaired left ventricular function. The presence of xanthelasmas (small fat deposits) around the eyelids or arcus senilis of the eyes (a yellow lipid ring around the cornea) suggests severe dyslipidemia and possible atherosclerosis. The presence of peripheral or carotid artery bruits suggests probable atherosclerotic disease and increases the likelihood that CAD is present.

Electrocardiography is a critical tool for the diagnosis of myocardial ischemia. Ischemic cells distort the electrical impulses that are measured across the myocardium during an ECG. Because many individuals have normal ECGs when there is no pain, diagnosis requires that

HEALTH PROMOTION

Women and Microvascular Angina

Heart disease and stroke are the leading cause of death among Canadian women, with more women dying from heart disease than from all cancers combined. Heart disease and stroke kill seven times as many women as does breast cancer.

Overall, 42% of women suffering a heart attack do not experience chest pain. Women with myocardial ischemia often have either no symptoms or atypical symptoms, such as palpitations, anxiety, weakness, and fatigue. Additionally, many women with angina are found to have cardiac ischemia yet no evidence of obstructive CAD on cardiac catheterization, a condition sometimes called *cardiac syndrome x*. Evidence is accumulating that nearly half of women with myocardial ischemia suffer from coronary microvascular disease, a condition often called **microvascular angina (MVA)**. Small intramyocardial arterioles constrict in MVA, causing ischemic pain that is less predictable than with typical epicardial CAD. The pathophysiology is complex and still being elucidated, but there is strong evidence that endothelial dysfunction, decreased endogenous vasodilators, inflammation, changes in adipokines, and platelet activation are contributing factors. Managing MVA can be challenging because women with this condition have less coronary microvascular dilation in response to nitrates than do those without MVA. Aggressive interventions to reduce modifiable risk factors for CAD are an important component of management, especially smoking cessation, exercise, and diabetes management. The combination of non-nitrate vasodilators, such as calcium channel blockers with HMG-CoA reductase inhibitors (statins), also has been shown to be effective in many women, and new medications, such as ranolazine (Ranexa) and ivabradine (Lancora), have shown promise in the treatment of MVA.

Data from: Arthur, H. M., Campbell, P., Harvey, P. J., et al. (2012). *Canadian Journal of Cardiology, 28*(2, Suppl.), S42–S49; Ashley, K. E., & Geraci, S. A. (2013). *Southern Medical Journal, 106*(7), 427–433; Heart Research Institute (CAN). (n.d.). *Women and heart disease.* http://www.hricanada.org/about-heart-disease/women-and-heart-disease; Luo, C., Long, M., Hu, X., et al. (2014). *Circulation, 7*(1), 43–48; Recio-Mayoral, A., Rimoldi, O. E., Camici, P. G., et al. (2013). *JACC Cardiovascular Imaging, 6*(6), 660–667; Russo, G., Di Franco, A., Lamendola, P., et al. (2013). *Cardiovascular Drugs and Therapy, 27*(3), 229–234; Taqueti, V. R., & Ridker, P. M. (2013). *JACC Cardiovasc Imaging, 6*(6), 668–671; Zhang, X., Li, Q., Zhao, J., et al. (2014). *Coronary Artery Disease, 25*(1), 40–44; Zuchi, C., Tritto, I., Ambrosio, G., et al. (2013). *International Journal of Cardiology, 163*(2), 132–140.

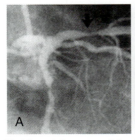 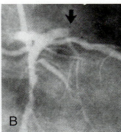 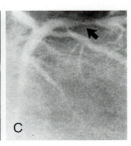

FIGURE 24.12 Mental Stress and Angiogram of Coronary Arteries. **A,** Baseline. **B,** Transient total occlusion of left anterior descending branch of the left coronary artery after mental stress. **C,** After nitrates and nifedipine, artery reopened to same diameter as baseline. (Modified from Stern, S. [Ed.]. [1998]. *Silent myocardial ischemia.* Mosby.)

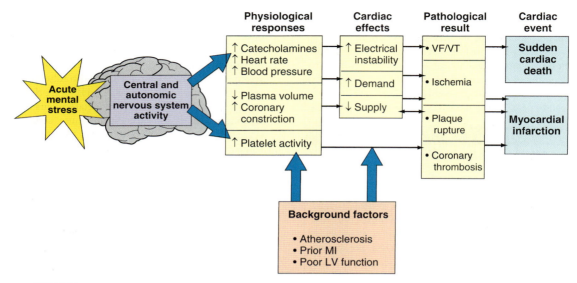

FIGURE 24.13 Pathophysiological Model of the Effects of Acute Stress as a Trigger of Cardiac Clinical Events. Acting via the central and autonomic nervous systems, stress can produce a cascade of physiological responses that may lead to myocardial ischemia, especially in persons with coronary artery disease, potentially fatal dysrhythmia, plaque rupture, or coronary thrombosis. *LV,* Left ventricular; *MI,* myocardial infarction; *VF,* ventricular fibrillation; *VT,* ventricular tachycardia. (From Krantz, D. S., Kop, W. J., Santiago, H. T., et al. [1996]. Mental stress as a trigger of myocardial ischemia and infarction. In P. C. Deedwania, & G. H. Tofler, [Eds.], *Triggers and timing of cardiac events* [2nd ed.]. Saunders.)

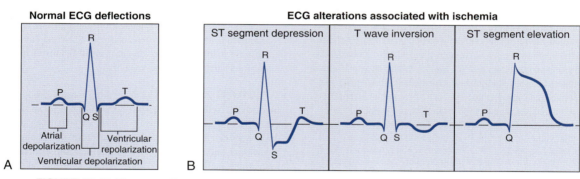

FIGURE 24.14 Electrocardiogram and Ischemia. A, Normal electrocardiogram *(ECG).* **B,** Electrocardiographic alterations associated with ischemia.

an ECG be performed during an attack of angina or during exercise stress testing. The ST segment and the T wave segments of the ECG respectively correlate with ventricular contraction and relaxation (see Figure 23.10). Transient ST segment depression and T wave inversion are characteristic signs of ischemia that involves only the inner wall of the myocardium (subendocardial ischemia). ST elevation is indicative of ischemia involving the full myocardial wall (transmural ischemia) (Figure 24.14). The ECG tracings correlate with different parts of the myocardium and, therefore, can give some indication of which coronary artery is involved.

Stress radionucleotide imaging is indicated to detect ischemic changes in asymptomatic individuals with multiple risk factors for coronary disease, such as diabetes and dyslipidemia, and for older individuals who plan to start vigorous exercise. Currently, the diagnostic modality of choice for the diagnosis of myocardial ischemia is single-photon emission computed tomography (SPECT), which is effective at identifying ischemia and estimating coronary risk.[102] Stress echocardiography is another technique used to diagnose CAD. Unfortunately, these tests cannot detect the presence of vulnerable plaques that are the cause of the majority of acute coronary syndromes.[103] CT, noninvasive coronary angiography using electron beam CT, protein-weighted MRI, and intravascular ultrasound are noninvasive tests for evaluating coronary atherosclerotic lesions and measuring coronary artery calcium concentration. The sensitivity and specificity of these tests vary widely.[102] Coronary angiography helps determine the anatomical extent of CAD, but the procedure is expensive and carries some risk. It is used primarily to determine whether possible percutaneous coronary intervention (PCI) or CABG surgery is warranted for individuals whose noninvasive studies suggest severe disease.

The primary aims of therapy for myocardial ischemia and stable angina are to increase coronary blood flow and to reduce myocardial oxygen consumption. Recommendations for appropriate diet, exercise, and risk reduction strategies have been widely distributed, and the use of lipid-lowering statins has been shown to be effective for both primary and secondary prevention of CAD.[79,104] Reversing vasoconstriction, reducing plaque growth and rupture, and preventing clotting improve coronary blood flow. Manipulation of blood pressure, heart rate, contractility, and left ventricular volume reduce myocardial oxygen demand. Several classes of medications are useful for increasing coronary flow and decreasing myocardial demand, especially nitrates, beta-blockers, and calcium channel blockers.[102,105,106]

Percutaneous coronary intervention (PCI) is a procedure whereby stenotic (narrowed) coronary vessels are dilated with a catheter. Indications for PCI in stable angina include persistent symptoms despite optimal medical therapy or severe disease that indicates a high risk for infarction.[102] Restenosis of the artery is the major complication of the procedure. Placement of a coronary stent can reduce this risk. Pharmacological treatment with antithrombotics, such as Aspirin, clopidogrel, or glycoprotein IIb/IIIa receptor antagonists, after stenting also can improve outcomes.

Severe CAD can be surgically treated by a CABG, usually using the saphenous vein from the lower leg.

Acute Coronary Syndromes

> **QUICK CHECK 24.6**
> 1. Describe the processes of coronary artery disease.
> 2. Describe the pathophysiology of myocardial infarction.
> 3. Describe the complications associated with myocardial infarction.

The process of atherosclerotic plaque progression can be gradual. Thrombus formation over a ruptured or ulcerated atherosclerotic plaque leads to sudden coronary obstruction, causing acute coronary syndromes (Figure 24.15). **Unstable angina** is the result of reversible myocardial ischemia and is a harbinger of impending infarction. **Myocardial infarction (MI)** results when there is prolonged ischemia causing irreversible damage to the heart muscle. MI can be further subdivided into **non-ST elevation myocardial infarction (non-STEMI)** and **ST elevation myocardial infarction (STEMI)**. Sudden cardiac death can occur as a result of any of the acute coronary syndromes.

An atherosclerotic plaque that is prone to rupture is called "unstable" and has a core that is especially rich in deposited oxidized LDL and a thin fibrous cap (Figure 24.16). These unstable plaques may not extend into the lumen of the vessel and may be clinically silent until they rupture. Plaque disruption (ulceration or rupture) occurs because of the effects of shear forces, inflammation with release of multiple inflammatory mediators, secretion of macrophage-derived degradative enzymes, and apoptosis of cells at the edges of the lesions. Exposure of the plaque substrate activates the clotting cascade. In addition, platelet activation results in the release of coagulants and exposure of platelet glycoprotein IIb/IIIa surface receptors, resulting in further platelet aggregation and adherence. The resulting thrombus can form very quickly (Figure 24.17A). The release of vasoconstrictors, such as thromboxane A_2 and endothelin, further exacerbates vessel obstruction. The thrombus may shatter before permanent myocyte damage has occurred (unstable angina) or it may cause prolonged ischemia with infarction of the heart muscle (MI) (Figure 24.17B).

Unstable angina. Unstable angina is a form of acute coronary syndrome that results from reversible myocardial ischemia. It is important to recognize this syndrome because it signals that the atherosclerotic plaque has become complicated, and infarction may soon follow. Unstable angina occurs when a fairly small fissuring or superficial erosion of the plaque leads to transient episodes of thrombotic vessel occlusion and vasoconstriction at the site of plaque damage. This thrombus is labile and occludes the vessel for no more than 10 to 20 minutes, with return of perfusion before significant myocardial necrosis occurs. Unstable angina presents as new-onset angina, angina that is occurring at rest, or angina that is increasing in severity or frequency (Box 24.1).

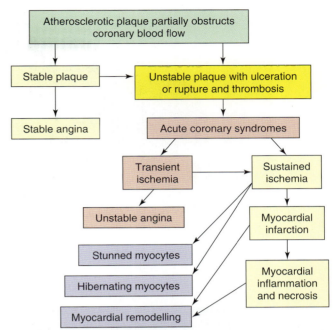

FIGURE 24.15 Pathophysiology of Acute Coronary Syndromes. The atherosclerotic process can lead to stable plaque formation and stable angina or can result in unstable plaques that are prone to rupture and thrombus. Thrombus formation on a ruptured plaque that disperses in less than 20 minutes leads to transient ischemia and unstable angina. If the vessel obstruction is sustained, myocardial infarction with inflammation and necrosis of the myocardium results. In addition, myocardial infarction is associated with other structural and functional changes, including myocyte stunning and hibernation and myocardial remodelling (see Figure 24.34).

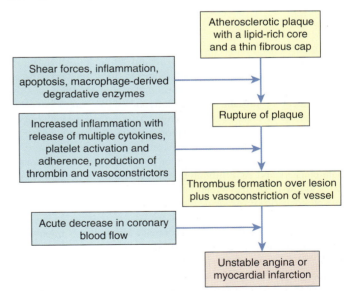

FIGURE 24.16 Pathogenesis of Unstable Plaques and Thrombus Formation.

Individuals may experience increased dyspnea, diaphoresis, and anxiety as the angina worsens. Physical examination may reveal evidence of ischemic myocardial dysfunction such as pulmonary congestion. The ECG most commonly shows ST segment depression and T wave inversion during pain that resolve as the pain is relieved. ECG changes without serum cardiac isoenzyme evidence of myocyte necrosis was traditionally used to diagnose unstable angina. However, the advent of

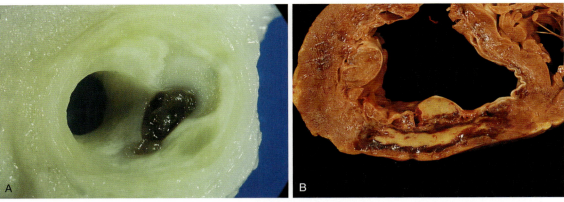

FIGURE 24.17 Plaque Disruption and Myocardial Infarction. **A,** Plaque disruption. The cap of the lipid-rich plaque has become torn with the formation of a thrombus, mostly inside the plaque. **B,** Myocardial infarction. This infarct is 6 days old. The centre is yellow and necrotic with a hemorrhagic red rim. The responsible arterial occlusion is probably in the right coronary artery. The infarct is on the posterior wall. (From Damjanov, I., & Linder, J. [Eds.]. [1996]. *Anderson's pathology* [10th ed.]. Mosby.)

> **BOX 24.1 Three Principal Presentations of Unstable Angina**
>
> 1. Rest angina: Angina occurring at rest and prolonged, usually >20 minutes
> 2. New-onset angina: New-onset angina of at least CCS Class III severity
> 3. Increasing angina: Previously diagnosed angina that has become distinctly more frequent, longer in duration, or lower in threshold (i.e., increased by ≥1 CCS class to at least CCS Class III severity)

CCS, Canadian Cardiovascular Society.
From Anderson, J., Adams, C. D., Antman, E. M., et al. (2007). *Journal of the American College of Cardiology, 50,* e1–e157; originally adapted from Braunwald, E. (1989). *Circulation, 80,* 410–414.

---

highly sensitive measurements of myocardial damage (high-sensitivity cardiac troponin T [hs-cTnT]) that can identify tiny amounts of enzymes released from damaged myocytes has blurred the distinction between unstable angina and MI.[107] Therefore, the current guidelines for the management of unstable angina and non-STEMI are identical.[108] Management of unstable angina requires immediate hospitalization with administration of oxygen, Aspirin, nitrates, and morphine if pain is still present. Additional antithrombotic therapy with clopidogrel or glycoprotein IIb/IIIa platelet receptor antagonists may be indicated. Beta-blockers and ACE inhibitors also may be used. Anticoagulants (such as low-molecular-weight heparin) or direct thrombin inhibitors (e.g., fondaparinux [Arixtra]) also can be given. Rapid intervention with PCI also may be indicated.[108]

Myocardial infarction. When coronary blood flow is interrupted for an extended period of time, myocyte necrosis occurs. This results in MI. Plaque progression, disruption, and subsequent clot formation are the same for MI as they are for unstable angina (see Figures 24.14, 24.15, and 24.16). In this case, however, the thrombus is less labile and occludes the vessel for a prolonged period, such that myocardial ischemia progresses to myocyte necrosis and death. Pathologically, there are two major types of MI: subendocardial infarction and transmural infarction. Clinically, however, MI is categorized as non-STEMI or STEMI.[109]

If the thrombus disintegrates before complete distal tissue necrosis has occurred, the infarction will involve only the myocardium directly beneath the endocardium (subendocardial MI) (Figure 24.18). This infarction will usually present with ST segment depression and T wave inversion without Q waves. Therefore, it is termed *non-STEMI.* It is especially important to recognize this form of acute coronary syndrome because recurrent clot formation on the disrupted atherosclerotic plaque is likely. If the thrombus lodges permanently in the vessel, the infarction will extend through the myocardium all the way from endocardium to epicardium, resulting in severe cardiac dysfunction (**transmural myocardial infarction**) (see Figure 24.18). Transmural MI will usually result in marked elevations in the ST segments on ECG, and these individuals are categorized as having STEMI. Clinically, it is important to identify those individuals with STEMI because they are at highest risk for serious complications and should receive definitive intervention without delay.

PATHOPHYSIOLOGY After 8 to 10 seconds of decreased blood flow, the affected myocardium becomes cyanotic and cooler. Myocardial oxygen reserves are used quickly (within about 8 seconds) after complete cessation of coronary flow. Glycogen stores decrease as anaerobic metabolism begins. Unfortunately, glycolysis can supply only 65 to 70% of the total myocardial energy requirement and produces much less adenosine triphosphate (ATP) than aerobic processes. Hydrogen ions and lactic acid accumulate. Because myocardial tissues have poor buffering capabilities and myocardial cells are sensitive to low cellular pH, accumulation of these products further compromises the myocardium. Acidosis may make the myocardium more vulnerable to the damaging effects of lysosomal enzymes and may suppress impulse conduction and contractile function, thereby leading to HF.

Oxygen deprivation also is accompanied by electrolyte disturbances, specifically the loss of potassium, calcium, and magnesium from cells. Myocardial cells deprived of necessary oxygen and nutrients lose contractility, thereby diminishing the pumping ability of the heart. Ischemia causes the myocardial cells to release catecholamines, predisposing the individual to serious imbalances of sympathetic and parasympathetic function, irregular heartbeats (dysrhythmia), and HF. Catecholamines mediate the release of glycogen, glucose, and stored fat from body cells. Therefore, plasma concentrations of free fatty acids and glycerol rise within 1 hour after the onset of acute MI. Excessive levels of free fatty acids can have a harmful detergent effect on cell membranes. Norepinephrine elevates blood glucose levels through stimulation of liver and skeletal muscle cells and suppresses pancreatic beta-cell activity, which reduces insulin secretion and elevates blood glucose concentration further. Infiltration of inflammatory cells contributes to tissue

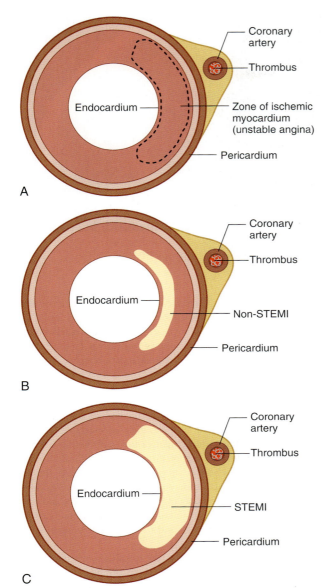

FIGURE 24.18 Unstable Angina, Non-STEMI, and STEMI. **A,** Unstable angina. Coronary thrombosis leads to myocardial ischemia. **B,** Non-STEMI. Persistent coronary occlusion leads to infarction of the myocardium closest to the endocardium. **C,** STEMI. Continued coronary occlusion leads to transmural infarction extending from endocardium to pericardium. *Non-STEMI,* Non-ST elevation myocardial infarction; *STEMI,* ST elevation myocardial infarction.

injury.[110] Ang II is released during myocardial ischemia and contributes to the pathogenesis of MI in several ways. First, it results in the systemic effects of peripheral vasoconstriction and fluid retention, which increase myocardial workload. Second, it is a growth factor for vascular smooth muscle cells, myocytes, and cardiac fibroblasts, resulting in structural changes in the myocardium called *remodelling*. Finally, Ang II promotes catecholamine release and causes coronary artery spasm.

Reperfusion injury once blood flow is restored can exacerbate ischemic injury. This process involves the release of toxic oxygen free radicals, calcium flux, and pH changes that cause a sustained opening of mitochondrial permeability transition pores (mPTPs) and contribute to resultant cellular death. Many innovative therapies are being explored to reduce reperfusion injury.[110]

Cardiac cells can withstand ischemic conditions for about 20 minutes before irreversible hypoxic injury causes cellular death (apoptosis) and tissue necrosis. This results in the release of intracellular enzymes such as creatine phosphokinase-myocardial bound (CPK-MB) and myocyte proteins such as the troponins through the damaged cell membranes into the interstitial spaces. The lymphatics absorb the enzymes and transport them into the bloodstream, where serological tests detect them.

MI results in both structural and functional changes of cardiac tissues (Figure 24.19). Gross tissue changes at the area of infarction may not become apparent for several hours, despite almost immediate onset (within 30 to 60 seconds) of electrocardiographic changes. Cardiac tissue surrounding the area of infarction also undergoes changes. **Myocardial stunning** is a temporary loss of contractile function that persists for hours to days after perfusion has been restored. This pathophysiological state can occur both with MI and in individuals who suffer ischemia during cardiovascular procedures or during central nervous system trauma. Alterations in electrolyte pumps and calcium homeostasis and the release of toxic oxygen free radicals cause stunning of the myocardium. Stunning can contribute to HF, shock, and dysrhythmias. Recurrent episodes of transient myocardial ischemia (angina) before MI can result in myocyte adaptation to oxygen deprivation with reduced stunning and preservation of myocardium.[111] This process, termed *ischemic preconditioning*, is being studied to determine whether it has potential prophylactic or therapeutic uses.[112] **Hibernating myocardium** describes tissue that is persistently ischemic and undergoes metabolic adaptation to prolong myocyte survival until perfusion can be restored. PCI or surgery aimed at reperfusion of hibernating myocardium can restore significant cardiac function.[113] **Myocardial remodelling** is a process mediated by Ang II, aldosterone, catecholamines, adenosine, and inflammatory cytokines that causes myocyte hypertrophy and loss of contractile function in the areas of the heart distant from the site of infarction. Remodelling can be limited through rapid restoration of coronary flow and the use of renin-angiotensin-aldosterone blockers and beta-blockers after MI.[114]

The severity of functional impairment depends on the size of the lesion and the site of infarction. Functional changes can include (1) decreased cardiac contractility with abnormal wall motion, (2) altered left ventricular compliance, (3) decreased stroke volume, (4) decreased ejection fraction, (5) increased left ventricular end-diastolic pressure (LVEDP), and (6) sinoatrial node malfunction. Life-threatening dysrhythmias and HF often follow MI.

With infarction, ventricular function is abnormal and the ejection fraction falls, resulting in increases in ventricular end-diastolic volume (VEDV). If the coronary obstruction involves the perfusion to the left ventricle, pulmonary venous congestion ensues. If the right ventricle becomes ischemic, increases in systemic venous pressures occur.

MI causes a severe inflammatory response that ends with wound repair (see Chapter 6). Damaged cells undergo degradation, fibroblasts proliferate, and scar tissue is synthesized. Many cell types, hormones, and nutrient substrates must be available for optimal healing to proceed. Within 24 hours, leukocytes infiltrate the necrotic area, and proteolytic enzymes from scavenger neutrophils degrade necrotic tissue. The collagen matrix that is deposited is initially weak, mushy, and vulnerable to reinjury. Unfortunately, it is at this time in the recovery period (10 to 14 days after infarction) that individuals feel more like increasing activities and may stress the newly formed scar tissue. The scar tissue, which is strong but cannot contract and relax like healthy myocardial tissue completely replaces the necrotic area after 6 weeks.

CLINICAL MANIFESTATIONS The first symptom of acute MI is usually sudden, severe chest pain. The pain is similar to that of angina pectoris but more severe and prolonged. It may be described as heavy

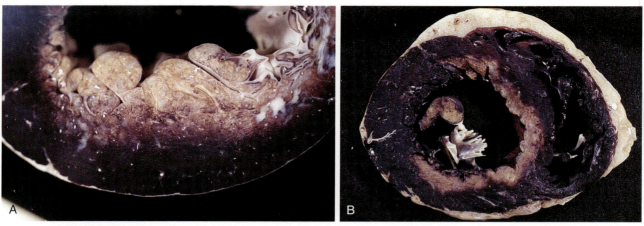

FIGURE 24.19 Myocardial Infarction. **A,** Local infarct confined to one region. **B,** Massive large infarct caused by occlusion of three coronary arteries. (From Damjanov, I., & Linder, J. [Eds.]. [1996]. *Anderson's pathology* [10th ed.]. Mosby.)

and crushing, such as a "truck sitting on my chest." Radiation to the neck, jaw, back, shoulder, or left arm is common. Some individuals, especially those who are older persons or have diabetes, experience no pain, thereby having a "silent" infarction. Infarction often simulates a sensation of unrelenting indigestion. Nausea and vomiting may occur because of reflex stimulation of vomiting centres by pain fibres. Vasovagal reflexes from the area of the infarcted myocardium also may affect the gastro-intestinal tract.

Various cardiovascular changes are found on physical examination:
- The SNS is reflexively activated to compensate, resulting in a temporary increase in heart rate and blood pressure.
- Abnormal extra heart sounds reflect left ventricular dysfunction.
- Pulmonary findings of congestion including dullness to percussion and inspiratory crackles at the lung bases can occur if the individual develops HF.
- Peripheral vasoconstriction may cause the skin to become cool and clammy.

The number and severity of postinfarction complications depend on the location and extent of necrosis, the individual's physiological condition before the infarction, and the availability of swift therapeutic intervention. Sudden cardiac death can occur in individuals with myocardial ischemia even if infarction is absent or minimal, and is a multifactorial problem. Risk factors for sudden death are related to three factors: ischemia, left ventricular dysfunction, and electrical instability. These factors interact with each other (Figure 24.20). Table 24.5 lists the most common complications.

EVALUATION AND TREATMENT The diagnosis of acute MI is made on the basis of history, physical examination, ECG results, and serial cardiac troponin elevations (Box 24.2). The cardiac troponins (troponin I and troponin T) are the most specific indicators of MI. A transient rise in these plasma enzyme levels can confirm the occurrence of MI and indicate its severity. Blood is drawn for troponin level determination as soon as possible after the onset of symptoms, and serial serum levels are assessed for several days. If serological tests show abnormally high levels of troponin, acute MI has occurred. Elevation of troponin level may not occur immediately after infarction and laboratory confirmation that an infarction has occurred may be delayed up to 12 hours.

MI can occur in various regions of the heart wall and may be described as anterior, inferior, posterior, lateral, subendocardial, or transmural, depending on the anatomical location and extent of tissue damage from infarction. Twelve-lead ECGs help localize the affected area through identification of changes in ST segments and T waves (Figure 24.21). The infarcted myocardium is surrounded by a zone of hypoxic injury, which may progress to necrosis or return to normal, and adjacent to this zone of hypoxic injury is a zone of reversible ischemia (see Figure 24.21). A characteristic Q wave often develops on ECG some hours later in STEMI.

Cardiac troponin I (cTnI) is the most specific indicator of MI, and measurement of its level should be performed on admission to the emergency department. cTnI level elevation is detectable 2 to 4 hours after onset of symptoms. Additional measurements within 6 to 9 hours and again at 12 to 24 hours are recommended if clinical suspicion is high and previous samples were negative. Troponin levels also can be used to estimate infarct size and, therefore, the likelihood of complications. Additional laboratory data may reveal leukocytosis and elevated CRP, both of which indicate inflammation. The individual's blood glucose level is usually elevated, and the glucose tolerance level may remain abnormal for several weeks.

Acute MI requires admission to the hospital, often directly into a coronary care unit. While most guidelines continue to recommend the use of oxygen in acute MI, a recent review did not demonstrate a clear benefit of oxygen therapy.[115] The individual should be given an Aspirin immediately (ticlopidine if allergic to Aspirin). Pain relief is of utmost importance and involves the use of sublingual nitroglycerine and morphine sulphate. Continuous monitoring of cardiac rhythms and enzymatic changes is essential, because the first 24 hours after onset of symptoms is the time of highest risk for sudden death. Non-STEMI is treated in the same way as unstable angina, including antithrombotics, anticoagulation or PCI, or both.[108] STEMI is best managed with emergent PCI and antithrombotics.[116] Thrombolytics may be used if PCI is not readily available. Hyperglycemia is treated with insulin. Once the person is stabilized, further management includes ACE inhibitors, beta-blockers, and statins.[116] Individuals who are in shock require aggressive fluid resuscitation, ionotropic medications, and possible emergent invasive procedures.

Bed rest, followed by gradual return to activities of daily living, reduces the myocardial oxygen demands of the compromised heart. Individuals not receiving thrombolytic or heparin infusion must receive DVT prophylaxis as long as their activity is significantly limited. Stool softeners are given to eliminate the need for straining, which can precipitate bradycardia and can be followed by increased venous return to the heart, causing possible cardiac overload. Education regarding

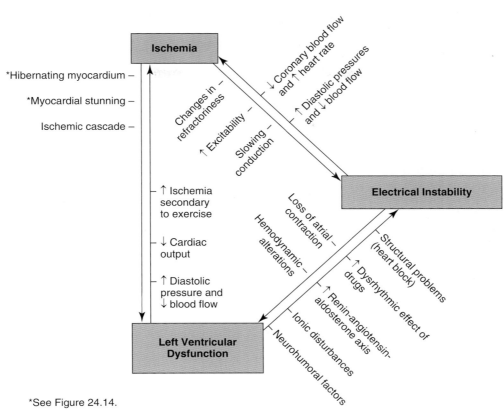

*See Figure 24.14.

FIGURE 24.20 Three Interacting Factors Related to Sudden Cardiac Death. The three factors are ischemia, left ventricular dysfunction, and electrical instability.

TABLE 24.5 Complications With Myocardial Infarctions

Type	Characteristics
Dysrhythmias	• Disturbances of cardiac rhythm that affect 90% of persons with cardiac infarction • Causes are ischemia, hypoxia, autonomic nervous system imbalances, lactic acidosis, electrolyte abnormalities, alterations of impulse conduction pathways or conduction abnormalities, medication toxicity, or hemodynamic abnormalities
Left ventricular failure (heart failure)	• Characterized by pulmonary congestion, reduced myocardial contractility, and abnormal heart wall motion • Cardiogenic shock can develop
Inflammation of pericardium (pericarditis)	• Pericardial friction rubs • Often noted 2 to 3 days later and associated with anterior chest pain that worsens with respiratory effort
Dressler postinfarction syndrome	• Essentially a delayed form of pericarditis that occurs 1 week to several months after acute myocardial infarction (MI) syndrome • Thought to be immunological response to necrotic myocardium marked by pain, fever, friction rub, pleural effusion, and arthralgias
Organic brain syndrome	• Occurs if blood flow to brain is impaired secondary to MI
Transient ischemic attacks or cerebrovascular accident	• Occur if thromboemboli detach from clots that form in cardiac chambers or on cardiac valves
Rupture of heart structures	• Cause is necrosis of tissue in or around papillary muscles • Papillary muscles of chordae tendineae cordis affected • Predisposing factors include thinning of wall, poor collateral flow, shearing effect of muscular contraction against stiffened necrotic area, marked necrosis at terminal end of blood supply, and aging of myocardium with laceration of myocardial microstructure
Rupture of wall of infarcted ventricle	• Can be caused by aneurysm formation when pressure becomes too great
Left ventricular aneurysm	• Late (month to years) complication of MI that can contribute to heart failure and thromboemboli
Infarctions around septal structures	• Occur in those structures that separate heart chambers and lead to septal rupture • Associated with audible, harsh cardiac murmurs; increased left ventricular end-diastolic pressure; and decreased systemic blood pressure
Systemic thromboembolism	• May disseminate from debris and clots that collect inside dilated aneurysmal sacs or from infarcted endocardium
Pulmonary thromboembolism	• Usually from deep venous thrombi of legs • Reduced incidence associated with early mobilization and prophylactic anticoagulation therapy
Sudden death	• Dysrhythmias frequently causative, particularly ventricular fibrillation • Risk for death increased by age more than 65 years, previous angina pectoris, hypotension or cardiogenic shock, acute systolic hypertension at time of admission, diabetes mellitus, dysrhythmias, and previous MI

BOX 24.2 Universal Definition of Myocardial Infarction

The term *myocardial infarction* should be used when there is evidence of myocardial necrosis in a clinical setting with myocardial ischemia. Under these conditions any one of the following criteria meets the diagnosis for myocardial infarction:
- Detection of rise and/or fall of cardiac biomarkers (preferably troponin) with at least one value above the 99th percentile of the upper reference limit (URL) together with evidence of myocardial ischemia with at least one of the following:
- Symptoms of ischemia
- Electrocardiogram (ECG) changes indicative of new ischemia (new ST–T changes or new left bundle branch block [LBBB])
- Development of pathological Q waves in the ECG
- Imaging evidence of new loss of viable myocardium or new regional wall motion abnormality
- Sudden, unexpected cardiac death, involving cardiac arrest, often with symptoms suggestive of myocardial ischemia, and accompanied by presumably new ST elevation, or new LBBB, and/or evidence of fresh thrombus by coronary angiography and/or at autopsy
- Cardiac death occurring before blood samples could be obtained, or at a time before the appearance of cardiac biomarkers in the blood
- For percutaneous coronary interventions (PCIs) in persons with normal baseline troponin values, elevations of cardiac biomarkers greater than the 99th percentile URL are indicative of periprocedural myocardial necrosis. By convention, increases of biomarkers greater than 3 × 99th percentile URL have been designated as defining PCI-related myocardial infarction. A subtype related to a documented stent thrombosis is recognized.
- For coronary artery bypass grafting (CABG) in persons with normal baseline troponin values, elevations of cardiac biomarkers greater than the 99th percentile URL are indicative of periprocedural myocardial necrosis. By convention, increases of biomarkers greater than 5 × 99th percentile URL plus either new pathological Q waves or new LBBB, or angiographically documented new graft or native coronary artery occlusion, or imaging evidence of new loss of viable myocardium have been designated as defining CABG-related myocardial infarction.
- Pathological findings of an acute myocardial infarction

Data from Linden, B. (2013). *BJCN, 8*(1), 8–9. doi:10.12968/bjca.2013.8.1.8; Thygesen, K., Alpert, J. S., Jaffe, A. S., et al. (2012). *Circulation, 126*(16), 2020–2035; Thygesen, K., Alpert, J. S., Jaffe, A. S., et al. (2015). The universal definition of myocardial infarction. In M. Tubaro, P. Vranckx, S. Price, et al. (Eds.), *The ESC textbook of intensive and acute cardiovascular care* (2nd ed., pp. 356–364). Oxford: Oxford University Press; Thygesen, K., Alpert, J. S., White, H. D., et al. (2007). *Journal of the American College of Cardiology, 50*, 2173–2195.

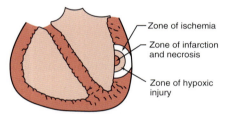
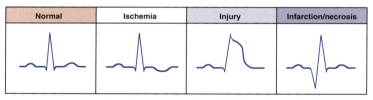

FIGURE 24.21 Electrocardiographic Alterations Associated With the Three Zones of Myocardial Infarction.

appropriate diet and caffeine intake, smoking cessation, exercise, and other aspects of risk factor reduction is crucial for secondary prevention of recurrent myocardial ischemia.

DISORDERS OF THE HEART WALL

 QUICK CHECK 24.7
1. Why does pericarditis develop?
2. What are cardiomyopathies? List the major disorders.
3. Briefly describe the pathophysiological effects of the cardiomyopathies.

Disorders of the Pericardium

Pericardial disease is a localized manifestation of another disorder, such as infection (bacterial, viral, fungal, rickettsial, or parasitic), trauma, surgery, neoplasm, metabolic, immunological, or vascular disorder (uremia, rheumatoid arthritis, systemic lupus erythematosus, periarteritis nodosa). The pericardial response to injury from these diverse causes may consist of acute pericarditis, pericardial effusion, or constrictive pericarditis.

Acute Pericarditis

Acute pericarditis is acute inflammation of the pericardium. The etiology of acute pericarditis is most often idiopathic. Viral infections with coxsackie, influenza, hepatitis, measles, mumps, or varicella viruses can also cause acute pericarditis. It also is the most common cardiovascular complication of human immunodeficiency virus (HIV) infection.

Other causes include MI, trauma, neoplasm, surgery, uremia, bacterial infection (especially tuberculosis), connective tissue disease (especially systemic lupus erythematosus and rheumatoid arthritis), or radiation therapy.[117] The pericardial membranes become inflamed and roughened, and a pericardial effusion may develop that can be serous, purulent, or fibrinous (Figure 24.22). Possible sequelae of pericarditis include recurrent pericarditis, pericardial constriction, and cardiac tamponade.

Symptoms may follow several days of fever and usually begin with the sudden onset of severe retrosternal chest pain that worsens with respiratory movements and when assuming a recumbent position. The pain may radiate to the back as a result of irritation of the phrenic nerve (innervates the trapezius muscles) as it traverses the pericardium. Individuals with acute pericarditis also report dysphagia, restlessness, irritability, anxiety, weakness, and malaise.

Physical examination often discloses low-grade fever (less than 38°C [100.4°F]) and sinus tachycardia. A friction rub—a scratchy, grating sound—may be heard at the cardiac apex and left sternal border and is highly suggestive of pericarditis. The roughened pericardial membranes rubbing against each other cause this sound. Friction rubs are not always present and may be intermittently heard and transient. Hypotension or the presence of a pulsus paradoxus (a decrease in systolic blood pressure of greater than 10 mm Hg with inspiration) is suggestive of cardiac tamponade, which can be life-threatening. Electrocardiographic changes may reflect inflammatory processes through PR segment depression and diffuse ST segment elevation without Q waves, and they may remain abnormal for days or even

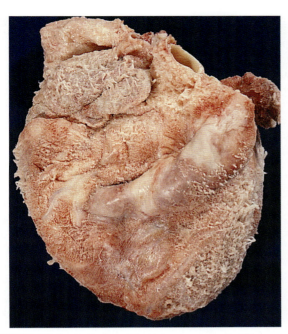

FIGURE 24.22 Acute Pericarditis. Note shaggy coat of fibres covering the surface of heart. (From Damjanov, I., & Linder, J. [2000]. *Pathology: a color atlas*. Mosby.)

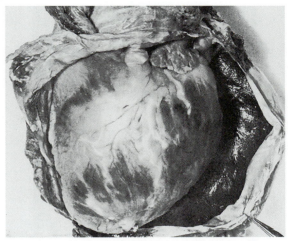

FIGURE 24.23 Exudate of Blood in the Pericardial Sac From Rupture of Aneurysm. (From Damjanov, I., & Linder, J. [2000]. *Pathology: a color atlas*. Mosby.)

weeks.[117] Ultrasound, CT scanning, and MRI may be used as diagnostic modalities. Acute pericarditis requires at least two of the following four criteria for diagnosis: (1) chest pain characteristics of pericarditis, (2) pericardial rub, (3) characteristic electrocardiographic changes, and (4) new or worsening pericardial effusion.[117]

Treatment for uncomplicated acute pericarditis consists of relieving symptoms and includes administration of anti-inflammatory agents, such as salicylates and nonsteroidal anti-inflammatory drugs (NSAIDs), and colchicine. Approximately one-third of cases will be complicated by the development of idiopathic recurrent pericarditis.[118] Exploration of the underlying cause is important. If pericardial effusion develops, aspiration of the excessive fluid may be necessary.

Pericardial Effusion

Pericardial effusion is the accumulation of fluid in the pericardial cavity and can occur in all forms of pericarditis. Most are idiopathic (20%), but other causes (such as neoplasm and infection) must be considered.[117] Analysis of the fluid obtained through pericardiocentesis allows for identification of the likely source of the fluid.[119] The fluid may be a transudate, such as the serous effusion that develops with left ventricular failure, overhydration, or hypoproteinemia. More often, however, the fluid is an exudate, which reflects pericardial inflammation like that seen with acute pericarditis, heart surgery, some chemotherapeutic agents, infections, and autoimmune disorders such as systemic lupus erythematosus. (Types of exudate are described in Chapter 6.) Exudative effusions also are found in up to 12% of individuals with STEMI.[120] If the fluid is serosanguineous, the underlying cause is likely to be tuberculosis, neoplasm, uremia, or radiation. Idiopathic serosanguineous (cause unknown) effusion is possible, however. Effusions of frank blood are generally related to aneurysms, trauma, or coagulation defects (Figure 24.23). If chyle leaks from the thoracic duct, it may enter the pericardium and lead to cholesterol pericarditis.

Pericardial effusion, even in large amounts, is not necessarily clinically significant, except that it indicates an underlying disorder. If an effusion develops gradually, the pericardium can stretch to accommodate large quantities of fluid without compressing the heart. If the fluid accumulates rapidly, however, even a small amount (50 to 100 mL) may create sufficient pressure to cause cardiac compression, a serious condition known as tamponade. The danger is that pressure exerted by the pericardial fluid eventually will equal diastolic pressure within the heart chambers, which will interfere with right atrial filling during diastole. The decrease in right atrial filling causes increased venous pressure, systemic venous congestion, and signs and symptoms of right ventricular failure (distension of the jugular veins, edema, hepatomegaly). Decreased atrial filling leads to decreased ventricular filling, decreased stroke volume, and reduced cardiac output. Life-threatening circulatory collapse may occur.

Findings during physical examination are included in Beck's triad (sinus tachycardia, elevated jugular venous pressure, low blood pressure) and pulsus paradoxus. Cardiac tamponade is a clinical diagnosis, but assessment of the patient's condition and diagnosis of the underlying cause of the tamponade can be obtained through lab studies, electrocardiography, echocardiography, or other imaging techniques. The treatment of cardiac tamponade is the removal of pericardial fluid to help relieve the pressure surrounding the heart. An important clinical finding is pulsus paradoxus, in which arterial blood pressure during expiration exceeds arterial pressure during inspiration by more than 10 mm Hg. Pulsus paradoxus in patients with pericardial effusion is an ominous sign for cardiac tamponade and indicates impairment of diastolic filling of the left ventricle. The presence of a large pericardial effusion or tamponade magnifies the normally insignificant effect of inspiration on intracardiac flow and volume. Other clinical manifestations of pericardial effusion are distant or muffled heart sounds, poorly palpable apical pulse, dyspnea on exertion, and dull chest pain. A chest X-ray film may disclose a "water-bottle configuration" of the cardiac silhouette. An echocardiogram can detect an effusion as small as 20 mL and is a reliable and accurate diagnostic test, although CT scans also may be done.[117]

Treatment of pericardial effusion or tamponade generally consists of pericardiocentesis (aspiration of excessive pericardial fluid) and treatment of the underlying condition. Persistent pain may be treated with analgesics, anti-inflammatory medications, or steroids. Surgery may be required if the underlying cause of tamponade is trauma or aneurysm. A pericardial "window" may be surgically created to prevent tamponade.[121]

Constrictive Pericarditis

Constrictive pericarditis, or restrictive pericarditis (chronic pericarditis), was synonymous with tuberculosis years ago, and tuberculosis

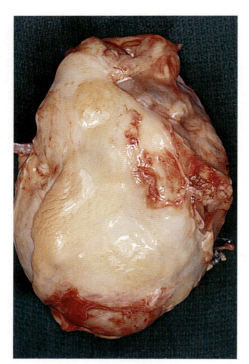

FIGURE 24.24 Constrictive Pericarditis. The fibrotic pericardium encases the heart in a rigid shell. (From Damjanov, I., & Linder, J. [2000]. *Pathology: a color atlas*. Mosby.)

continues to be an important cause of pericarditis in immunocompromised individuals. Currently, this form of pericardial disease is more commonly idiopathic or associated with viral infection, radiation exposure, collagen vascular disorders, sarcoidosis, neoplasm, uremia, or cardiac surgery.[117] In constrictive pericarditis, fibrous scarring with occasional calcification of the pericardium causes the visceral and parietal pericardial layers to adhere, obliterating the pericardial cavity. The fibrotic lesions encase the heart in a rigid shell (Figure 24.24). Like tamponade, constrictive pericarditis compresses the heart and eventually reduces cardiac output. Unlike tamponade, however, constrictive pericarditis always develops gradually.

Symptoms tend to be exercise intolerance, dyspnea on exertion, fatigue, and anorexia. Clinical assessment shows edema, distension of the jugular vein, hepatic congestion, and systemic hypotension. Restricted ventricular filling may cause a pericardial knock (early diastolic sound).

ECG findings include nonspecific ST and T wave abnormalities and atrial fibrillation (AF). Chest X-ray films often disclose prominent pulmonary vessels and calcification of the pericardium. CT, MRI, and transesophageal echocardiography are used to detect pericardial thickening and constriction and to distinguish constrictive pericarditis from restrictive cardiomyopathy. Pericardial biopsy may be needed to determine the etiology.

Initial treatment for constrictive pericarditis consists of restriction of dietary sodium intake and administration of diuretics to improve cardiac output. Management also may include use of anti-inflammatory medications and treatment of any underlying disorder. If these modalities are unsuccessful, surgical excision of the restrictive pericardium is indicated (pericardial decortication).[117]

Disorders of the Myocardium: The Cardiomyopathies

The **cardiomyopathies** are a diverse group of diseases that primarily affect the myocardium itself. They may, however, be secondary to

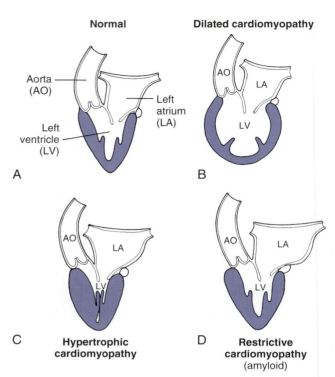

FIGURE 24.25 Diagram Showing Major Distinguishing Pathophysiological Features of the Three Types of Cardiomyopathy. **A,** The normal heart. **B,** In the dilated type of cardiomyopathy, the heart has a globular shape and the largest circumference of the left ventricle is not at its base but midway between apex and base. **C,** In the hypertrophic type, the wall of the left ventricle is greatly thickened, the left ventricular cavity is small, but the left atrium may be dilated because of poor diastolic relaxation of the ventricle. **D,** In the restrictive (constrictive) type, the left ventricular cavity is normal size, but, again, the left atrium is dilated because of the reduced diastolic compliance of the ventricle. (From Kissane, J. M. [Ed.]. [1990]. *Anderson's pathology* [9th ed.]. Mosby.)

infectious disease, toxin exposure, systemic connective tissue disease, infiltrative and proliferative disorders, or nutritional deficiencies. Many cases are idiopathic; others are caused by ischemia, hypertension, inherited disorders, infections, toxins, or systemic inflammatory disorders. Some are preceded by myocarditis, however, most individuals with acute myocarditis recover without sequelae.[117] The cardiomyopathies are categorized as dilated (formerly, congestive), hypertrophic, or restrictive, depending on their physiological effects on the heart (Figure 24.25).

Dilated cardiomyopathy is usually the result of ischemic heart disease, valvular disease, diabetes, renal failure, alcohol or medication toxicity, peripartum complications, or infection.[117] There is a strong genetic basis for dilated cardiomyopathy, and it can be associated with inherited disorders, such as muscular dystrophy. It is characterized by impaired systolic function leading to increases in intracardiac volume, ventricular dilation, and HF with reduced ejection fraction (Figure 24.26). Individuals complain of dyspnea, fatigue, and pedal edema. Findings on examination include a displaced apical pulse, S_3 gallop, peripheral edema, jugular venous distension, and pulmonary congestion. Chest X-ray and echocardiogram are used to confirm the diagnosis, and management is focused on reducing blood volume, increasing contractility, and reversing the underlying disorder if possible.[117] Heart transplant is required in severe cases.

Hypertrophic cardiomyopathy refers to two major categories of thickening of the myocardium: (1) hypertrophic obstructive

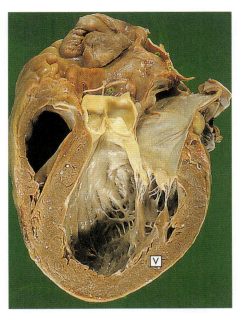

FIGURE 24.26 Dilated Cardiomyopathy. The dilated left ventricle has a thin wall *(V)*. (From Stevens, A., Lowe, J. S., & Scott, I. [2009]. *Core pathology* [3rd ed.]. Mosby.)

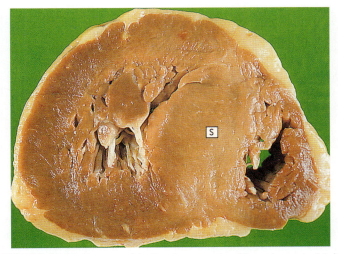

FIGURE 24.27 Hypertrophic Cardiomyopathy. There is marked left ventricular hypertrophy, which often affects the septum *(S)*. (From Stevens, A., Lowe, J. S., & Scott, I. [2009]. *Core pathology* [3rd ed.]. Mosby.)

cardiomyopathy (asymmetric septal hypertrophic cardiomyopathy or subaortic stenosis) and (2) hypertensive or valvular hypertrophic cardiomyopathy. **Hypertrophic obstructive cardiomyopathy** is the most commonly inherited cardiac disorder. It is characterized by thickening of the septal wall (Figure 24.27), which may cause outflow obstruction to the left ventricle outflow tract.[117] Obstruction of left ventricular outflow can occur when the heart rate is increased and the intravascular volume is decreased. This type of hypertrophic cardiomyopathy is a significant risk factor for serious ventricular dysrhythmias and sudden death.[117,122] There are other conditions that cause hypertrophic changes in the ventricles. **Hypertensive hypertrophic cardiomyopathy** and **valvular hypertrophic cardiomyopathy** are the most common.[123] These conditions occur because of increased resistance to ventricular ejection, which is commonly seen in individuals with hypertension or valvular stenosis (usually aortic). In this case, hypertrophy of the myocytes is an attempt to compensate for increased myocardial workload. Long-term dysfunction of the myocytes develops over time, with diastolic dysfunction appearing first and leading eventually to systolic dysfunction of the ventricle. Individuals with hypertrophic cardiomyopathy may be asymptomatic or may complain of angina, syncope,[48] dyspnea on exertion, and palpitations. Examination may reveal extra heart sounds and murmurs. Echocardiography and cardiac catheterization can confirm the diagnosis.

Restrictive cardiomyopathy is characterized by restrictive filling and increased diastolic pressure of either or both ventricles with normal or near-normal systolic function and wall thickness. It may occur idiopathically or as a cardiac manifestation of systemic diseases, such as amyloidosis, scleroderma, sarcoidosis, lymphoma, and hemochromatosis, or a number of inherited storage diseases.[117] The myocardium becomes rigid and noncompliant, impeding ventricular filling and raising filling pressures during diastole. The most common clinical manifestation of restrictive cardiomyopathy is right ventricular failure with systemic venous congestion. Cardiomegaly and dysrhythmias are common. A thorough evaluation for the underlying cause should be initiated (and may include myocardial biopsy). Treatment is aimed at the underlying cause. Death occurs as a result of HF or dysrhythmias.

Disorders of the Endocardium

> ✓ **QUICK CHECK 24.8**
> 1. Compare the effect of aortic stenosis with mitral stenosis on the left ventricle and atrium.
> 2. Describe aortic regurgitation, mitral regurgitation, and tricuspid regurgitation.
> 3. What are the common symptoms of mitral valve prolapse?
> 4. What is the cause of rheumatic heart disease?

Valvular Dysfunction

Disorders of the endocardium (the innermost lining of the heart wall) damage the heart valves, which are composed of endocardial tissue. Endocardial damage can be either congenital or acquired. The acquired forms result from inflammatory, ischemic, traumatic, degenerative, or infectious alterations of valvular structure and function. One of the most common causes of acquired valvular dysfunction is degeneration or inflammation of the endocardium secondary to rheumatic heart disease (Table 24.6). Structural alterations of the heart valves are caused by remodelling changes in the valvular extracellular matrix and lead to stenosis, incompetence, or both.

In **valvular stenosis**, the valve orifice is constricted and narrowed, so blood cannot flow forward and the workload of the cardiac chamber proximal to the diseased valve increases (Figure 24.28). Pressure (intraventricular or atrial) rises in the chamber to overcome resistance to flow through the valve, necessitating greater exertion by the myocardium and producing myocardial hypertrophy.

Although all four heart valves may be affected, in adults those of the left heart (mitral and aortic valves) are far more commonly affected than those of the right heart (tricuspid and pulmonic valves). In **valvular regurgitation** (also called **valvular insufficiency** or **valvular incompetence**), the valve leaflets, or cusps, fail to shut completely, permitting blood flow to continue even when the valve is presumably closed (see Figure 24.28). During systole or diastole, some blood leaks back into the chamber proximal to the diseased valve, which increases the volume of blood the heart must pump and increases the workload of both the atrium and the ventricle. Increased volume leads to chamber dilation, and increased workload leads to hypertrophy, both of which are compensatory mechanisms intended to increase the

TABLE 24.6 Clinical Manifestations of Valvular Stenosis and Regurgitation

Manifestation	Aortic Stenosis	Mitral Stenosis	Aortic Regurgitation	Mitral Regurgitation	Tricuspid Regurgitation
Most common cause	Congenital bicuspid valve, degenerative (calcific) changes with aging, rheumatic heart disease	Rheumatic heart disease	Infective endocarditis; aortic root disease (connective tissue diseases, Marfan's syndrome); dilation of aortic root from hypertension and aging	Myxomatous degeneration (mitral valve prolapse)	Congenital
Cardiovascular outcome (untreated)	Left ventricular hypertrophy followed by left ventricular failure; decreased coronary blood flow with myocardial ischemia	Left atrial hypertrophy and dilation with fibrillation, followed by right ventricular failure	Left ventricular hypertrophy and dilation, followed by left ventricular failure	Left atrial hypertrophy and dilation, followed by left ventricular failure	Right ventricular failure
Pulmonary effects	Pulmonary edema: dyspnea on exertion	Pulmonary edema: dyspnea on exertion, orthopnea, paroxysmal nocturnal dyspnea, predisposition to respiratory tract infections, hemoptysis, pulmonary hypertension	Pulmonary edema with dyspnea on exertion	Pulmonary edema with dyspnea on exertion	Dyspnea
Central nervous system effects	Syncope, especially on exertion	Neural deficits only associated with emboli (e.g., hemiparesis)	Syncope	None	None
Pain	Angina pectoris	Atypical chest pain	Angina pectoris	Atypical chest pain	Palpitations
Heart sounds	Systolic murmur heard best at right parasternal second intercostal space and radiating to neck	Low, rumbling diastolic murmur heard best at apex and radiating to axilla; accentuated first heart sound, opening snap	Diastolic murmur heard best at right parasternal second intercostal space and radiating to neck	Murmur throughout systole heard best at apex and radiating to axilla	Murmur throughout systole heard best at left lower sternal border

Data from Mann, D. L., Zipes, D. P., Libby, P., et al. (Eds.). (2014). *Braunwald's heart disease: a textbook of cardiovascular medicine* (10th ed.). Saunders.

pumping capability of the heart but that lead to cardiac dysfunction over time. Eventually, myocardial contractility diminishes, ejection fraction drops, and diastolic pressure increases, and the ventricles fail from being overworked. Depending on the severity of the valvular dysfunction and the capacity of the heart to compensate, valvular alterations cause a range of symptoms and some degree of incapacitation (see Table 24.6).

In general, the transthoracic echocardiography (TTE) is used to diagnose valvular disease and assess the severity of valvular obstruction or regurgitation before the onset of symptoms. CT or MRI may be indicated in certain settings. Valvular lesions are staged and appropriate management is determined by using four general categories: (1) at risk, (2) progressive, (3) asymptomatic severe, and (4) symptomatic severe.[124] Management almost always includes careful medical management, valvular repair, or valve replacement followed by long-term anticoagulation therapy and prophylaxis for endocarditis as needed. The purpose of valvular intervention is to improve symptoms and prolong survival, as well as to minimize complications, such as asymptomatic irreversible ventricular dysfunction, pulmonary hypertension, stroke, and AF.[124]

Stenosis.

Aortic stenosis. **Aortic stenosis** is the most common valvular abnormality, affecting nearly 2% of adults older than 65 years of age.[125] It has three common causes: (1) congenital bicuspid valve, (2) degeneration with aging, and (3) inflammatory damage caused by rheumatic heart disease. Aortic stenosis also is associated with many risk factors for CAD, including hypertension, smoking, and dyslipidemia. Aortic valve degeneration with aging is associated with chronic inflammation, lipoprotein deposition in the tissue, and leaflet calcification. The orifice of the aortic valve narrows, causing resistance to blood flow from the left ventricle into the aorta (Figure 24.29). Outflow obstruction increases pressure within the left ventricle as it tries to eject blood through the narrowed opening. Left ventricular hypertrophy develops to compensate for the increased workload. Eventually, hypertrophy increases myocardial oxygen demand, which the coronary arteries may not be able to supply, leading to attacks of angina. In addition, aortic stenosis is frequently accompanied by atherosclerotic coronary disease, further contributing to inadequate coronary perfusion. Untreated aortic stenosis can lead to hypertrophic cardiomyopathy, dysrhythmias, MI, and HF.[125]

Aortic stenosis usually develops gradually. Classic symptoms include angina, syncope, and dyspnea. Clinical manifestations include decreased stroke volume and narrowed pulse pressure (the difference between systolic and diastolic pressures). Heart rate is often slow, and pulses are delayed. Resistance to flow leads to a crescendo-decrescendo systolic heart murmur heard best at the right parasternal second intercostal space, and may radiate to the neck. Echocardiography can be used to assess the severity of valvular obstruction before the onset of

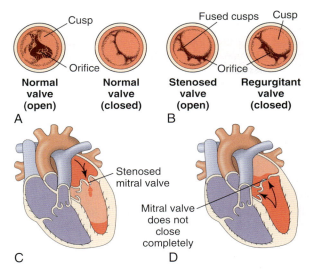

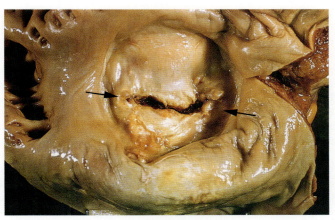

FIGURE 24.30 Mitral Stenosis With Classic "Fish Mouth" Orifice. (From Kumar, V., Abbas, A. K., & Aster, J. C. [Eds.]. [2021]. *Robbins and Cotran pathologic basis of disease* [10th ed.]. Elsevier.)

FIGURE 24.28 Valvular Stenosis and Regurgitation. **A,** Normal position of the valve leaflets, or cusps, when the valve is open and closed. **B,** Open position of a stenosed valve *(left)* and open position of a closed regurgitant valve *(right)*. **C,** Hemodynamic effect of mitral stenosis. The stenosed valve is unable to open sufficiently during left atrial systole, inhibiting left ventricular filling. **D,** Hemodynamic effect of mitral regurgitation. The mitral valve does not close completely during left ventricular systole, permitting blood to re-enter the left atrium.

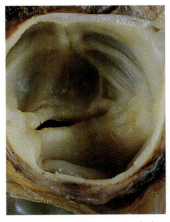

FIGURE 24.29 Aortic Stenosis. Mild stenosis in valve leaflets of a young adult. (From Damjanov, I., & Linder, J. [2000]. *Pathophysiology: a color atlas*. Mosby.)

symptoms. Medical management includes vasodilator therapy. Surgical valve replacement with either a mechanical or a bioprosthetic valve is indicated for both symptomatic and asymptomatic individuals with severe stenosis.[124] Percutaneous placement of a prosthetic valve avoids major heart surgery in selected individuals.[124,126] Once individuals become symptomatic from aortic stenosis, the prognosis is poor.

Mitral stenosis. Mitral stenosis impairs the flow of blood from the left atrium to the left ventricle. Mitral stenosis is the most common form of rheumatic heart disease. Autoimmunity in response to group A β-hemolytic streptococcal M protein antigens leads to inflammation and scarring of the valvular leaflets. Scarring causes the leaflets to become fibrous and fused, and the chordae tendineae cordis become shortened (Figure 24.30).

Impedance to blood flow results in incomplete emptying of the left atrium and elevated atrial pressure as the chamber tries to force blood through the stenotic valve. Continued increases in left atrial volume and pressure cause atrial dilation and hypertrophy. The risk of developing AF and dysrhythmia-induced thrombi is high. As mitral stenosis progresses, symptoms of decreased cardiac output occur, especially during exertion. Continued elevation of left atrial pressure and volume causes pressure to rise in the pulmonary circulation. If untreated, chronic mitral stenosis develops into pulmonary hypertension, pulmonary edema, and right ventricular failure.

Blood flow through the stenotic valve results in a rumbling decrescendo diastolic murmur heard best over the cardiac apex and radiating to the left axilla. If the mitral valve is forced open during diastole, it may make a sharp noise called an opening snap. The first heart sound (S_1) is often accentuated and somewhat delayed because of increased left atrial pressure. Other signs and symptoms are generally those of pulmonary congestion and right ventricular failure. Chest X-ray films, electrocardiography, and echocardiography are used to evaluate atrial enlargement and valvular obstruction. Management includes use of anticoagulation therapy and control of heart rate. Mitral stenosis can often be repaired with percutaneous balloon commissurotomy, but may require valve replacement in advanced cases.[124]

Regurgitation.

Aortic regurgitation. Aortic regurgitation results from an inability of the aortic valve leaflets to close properly during diastole because of abnormalities of the leaflets, the aortic root and annulus, or both. It can be primary, caused by congenital bicuspid valve or degeneration in older persons. Aortic regurgitation can also be secondary to chronic hypertension, rheumatic heart disease, bacterial endocarditis, syphilis, connective tissue disorders (e.g., Marfan's syndrome and ankylosing spondylitis), appetite-suppressing medications, trauma, or atherosclerosis.[125] During systole, blood is ejected from the left ventricle into the aorta. During diastole, some of the ejected blood flows back into the left ventricle through the leaking valve. Volume overload occurs in the ventricle because it receives blood both from the left atrium and from the aorta during diastole. The hemodynamic abnormalities depend on the amount of regurgitation. As the end-diastolic volume of the left ventricle increases, myocardial fibres stretch to accommodate the extra fluid. Compensatory dilation permits the left ventricle to increase its stroke volume and maintain cardiac output. Ventricular hypertrophy also occurs as an adaptation to the increased volume and because of increased afterload created by the high stroke volume and resultant systolic hypertension. Over time, ventricular dilation and hypertrophy eventually cannot compensate for aortic incompetence, and HF develops.

Clinical manifestations include widened pulse pressure resulting from increased stroke volume and diastolic backflow. Turbulence across the aortic valve during diastole produces a decrescendo murmur in the second, third, or fourth intercostal spaces parasternally and may radiate to the neck. Large stroke volume and rapid runoff of blood from the aorta cause prominent carotid pulsations and bounding peripheral pulses (Corrigan's pulse). Other symptoms are usually associated with HF that occurs when the ventricle can no longer pump adequately. Dysrhythmias are a common complication of aortic regurgitation. Echocardiography is used to estimate the severity of regurgitation, and valve replacement surgery may be delayed for many years through careful use of vasodilators and inotropic agents.[124]

Mitral regurgitation. **Mitral regurgitation** can be primary because of mitral valve prolapse, rheumatic heart disease, infective endocarditis, MI, connective tissue diseases (Marfan's syndrome), and dilated cardiomyopathy. It can also be secondary because of ischemic or nonischemic myocardial disease, which damages the chordae tendineae or the mitral annulus.[124] Mitral regurgitation permits backflow of blood from the left ventricle into the left atrium during ventricular systole, producing a holosystolic (throughout systole) murmur heard best at the apex, which radiates into the back and axilla. Because of increased volume from the left atrium, the left ventricle becomes dilated and hypertrophied to maintain adequate cardiac output. The volume of backflow re-entering the left atrium gradually increases, causing atrial dilation and associated AF. As the left atrium enlarges, the valve structures stretch and become deformed, leading to further backflow. As mitral valve regurgitation progresses, left ventricular function may become impaired to the point of failure. Eventually, increased atrial pressure leads to pulmonary hypertension and failure of the right ventricle. Mitral incompetence is usually well tolerated—often for years—until ventricular failure occurs. HF is the cause of most clinical manifestations. Echocardiography is used to estimate the severity of regurgitation, and transcatheter or surgical repair or valve replacement may become necessary.[127] Surgical repair must be done emergently if MI causes acute mitral regurgitation.

Tricuspid regurgitation. **Tricuspid regurgitation** is more common than tricuspid stenosis. Congenital defects, rheumatic heart disease, endocarditis, or trauma can cause primary tricuspid regurgitation.[125] However, 80% of the cases of tricuspid regurgitation are functional because of annular dilatation and leaflet tethering abnormalities related to dilation of the right ventricle secondary to pulmonary hypertension.[124] Tricuspid valve incompetence leads to volume overload in the right atrium and ventricle, increased systemic venous blood pressure, and right ventricular failure. Pulmonic valve dysfunction can have the same consequences as tricuspid valve dysfunction.

Mitral Valve Prolapse Syndrome

In **mitral valve prolapse syndrome (MVPS)**, one or both of the cusps of the mitral valve billow upward (prolapse) into the left atrium during systole (Figure 24.31). The most common cause of MVPS is myxomatous degeneration of the leaflets in which the cusps are redundant, thickened, and scalloped because of changes in tissue proteoglycans, increased levels of proteinases, and infiltration by myofibroblasts. Mitral regurgitation occurs if the ballooning valve permits blood to leak into the atrium.

Because mitral valve prolapse can be associated with other inherited connective tissue disorders (Marfan's syndrome, Ehlers-Danlos syndrome, osteogenesis imperfecta), it has been suggested that it results from a genetic or environmental disruption of valvular development during the fifth or sixth week of gestation. There also may be a relationship between symptomatic mitral valve prolapse and hyperthyroidism.

Many cases of mitral valve prolapse are completely asymptomatic. Cardiac auscultation on routine physical examination may disclose a regurgitant murmur or midsystolic click in an otherwise healthy individual, or echocardiography may demonstrate the condition in the absence of auscultatory findings. Symptomatic mitral valve prolapse can cause palpitations related to dysrhythmias, tachycardia, lightheadedness, syncope, fatigue (especially in the morning), lethargy, weakness, dyspnea, chest tightness, hyperventilation, anxiety, depression, panic attacks, and atypical chest pain. Many symptoms are vague and puzzling and are unrelated to the degree of prolapse. Most individuals with mitral valve prolapse have an excellent prognosis, do not develop symptoms, and do not require any restriction in activity or medical management. Occasionally, beta-blockers are needed to alleviate syncope, severe chest pain, or palpitations.

Acute Rheumatic Fever and Rheumatic Heart Disease

Acute rheumatic fever is a systemic febrile illness associated with inflammation of the joints, skin, nervous system, and heart.[128] Delayed exaggerated immune response to infection by group A β-hemolytic streptococcus in genetically predisposed individuals can cause **rheumatic fever**. If untreated, rheumatic fever can cause scarring and deformity of cardiac structures, resulting in **rheumatic heart disease**. While acute rheumatic fever (ARF) is now considered to be a disease of the past in Canada, its incidence in Indigenous communities is 21.3 per 100 000, which is 75 times greater than the overall Canadian estimated incidence.[129]

PATHOPHYSIOLOGY ARF can develop only as a sequel to pharyngeal infection by group A β-hemolytic streptococcus. Streptococcal skin infections do not progress to ARF because the strains of the microorganism that affect the skin do not have the same antigenic molecules in their cell membranes as those that cause pharyngitis and, therefore, do not elicit the same kind of immune response. However, both skin and pharyngeal infections can cause acute glomerulonephritis.

ARF is the result of an abnormal humoral and cell-mediated immune response to group A streptococcal cell membrane antigens called M proteins (Figure 24.32).[130,131] This immune response cross-reacts with molecularly similar self-antigens in heart, muscle, brain, and joints, causing an autoimmune response that results in diffuse, proliferative, and exudative inflammatory lesions in these tissues. The inflammation may subside before treatment, leaving behind damage to the heart valves. Repeated attacks of ARF cause chronic proliferative changes in the previously mentioned organs with resultant tissue scarring, granuloma formation, and thrombosis.

Approximately 10% of individuals with rheumatic fever develop rheumatic heart disease. In developed countries, the peak incidence of the development of rheumatic heart disease occurs in adults between the ages of 25 and 34. Although rheumatic fever can cause carditis in all three layers of the heart wall, the primary lesion usually involves the endocardium. Endocardial inflammation causes swelling of the valve leaflets, with secondary erosion along the lines of leaflet contact. Small, beadlike clumps of vegetation containing platelets and fibrin are deposited on eroded valvular tissue and on the chordae tendineae cordis. These lesions can become progressively adherent. Scarring and shortening of the involved structures occur over time. The valves lose their elasticity, and the leaflets may adhere to each other.

If inflammation penetrates the myocardium, called *myocarditis*, localized fibrin deposits develop that are surrounded by areas of necrosis. These fibrinoid necrotic deposits are called *Aschoff bodies*. Pericardial inflammation is usually characterized by serofibrinous effusion within the pericardial cavity. Cardiomegaly and left ventricular failure may occur during episodes of untreated acute or recurrent rheumatic fever. Conduction defects and AF often are associated with rheumatic heart disease.

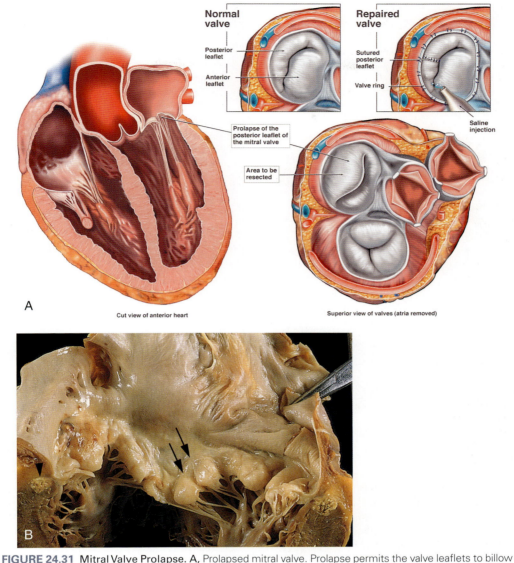

FIGURE 24.31 Mitral Valve Prolapse. A, Prolapsed mitral valve. Prolapse permits the valve leaflets to billow back *(arrows)* into the atrium during left ventricular systole. The billowing causes the leaflets to part slightly, permitting regurgitation into the atrium. **B,** Looking down into the mitral valve, the ballooning *(arrows)* of the leaflets is seen. (From Kumar, V., Abbas, A. K., & Aster, J. C. [Eds.]. [2015]. *Robbins and Cotran pathologic basis of disease* [9th ed.]. Philadelphia: Saunders. [A], Nucleus Medical Media Inc.)

CLINICAL MANIFESTATIONS The common symptoms of ARF are fever, lymphadenopathy, arthralgia, nausea, vomiting, epistaxis (nosebleed), abdominal pain, and tachycardia. The major clinical manifestations of ARF usually occur singly or in combination 1 to 5 weeks after streptococcal infection of the pharynx. They are carditis, acute migratory polyarthritis, chorea, erythema marginatum, and subcutaneous nodules.

ARF is a clinical diagnosis and has no single confirmatory test. The most common approach to diagnosis is to use the Jones criteria (Table 24.7). The Jones criteria were first proposed in 1944 and modified in 2015. The main modifications were the inclusion of echocardiography for the diagnosis of carditis, risk stratification based on two sets of criteria, and the establishment of specific recommendations for diagnosis of recurrent ARF.[132] The diagnosis of the initial episode of ARF requires documentation of a recent streptococcal infection and at least two major or one major and two minor criteria (see Table 24.7).

EVALUATION AND TREATMENT Supportive evidence for group A β-hemolytic streptococci includes positive throat cultures and measurement of serum antibodies against the hemolytic factor streptolysin O. Cultures may be negative when the rheumatic attack begins, however. Several other antibody tests are sensitive prognosticators of streptococcal infection, including antideoxyribonuclease B (anti-DNase B), antihyaluronidase, and antistreptozyme (ASTZ). Elevated measurements of white blood cell count, erythrocyte sedimentation rate, and C-reactive protein indicate inflammation. All three are usually increased at the time cardiac or joint symptoms begin to appear. Echocardiographic screening for rheumatic heart disease in children with a history of rheumatic fever is controversial because not all detectable abnormalities are clinically relevant.[133]

Therapy for ARF is aimed at eradicating the streptococcal infection and involves a 10-day regimen of oral penicillin or erythromycin administration. NSAIDs are used as anti-inflammatory agents for

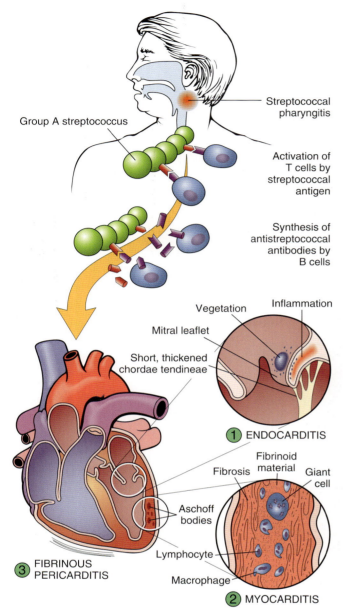

FIGURE 24.32 **Pathogenesis and Structural Alterations of Acute Rheumatic Heart Disease.** Beginning usually with a sore throat, rheumatic fever can develop only as a sequel to pharyngeal infection by group A β-hemolytic streptococcus. Suspected as a hypersensitivity reaction, it is proposed that antibodies directed against the M proteins of certain strains of streptococci cross-react with tissue glycoproteins in the heart, joints, and other tissues. The exact nature of cross-reacting antigens has been difficult to define, but it appears that the streptococcal infection causes an autoimmune response against self-antigens. Inflammatory lesions are found in various sites. Aschoff bodies are the most distinctive within the heart. The chronic sequelae result from progressive fibrosis because of healing of the inflammatory lesions and the changes induced by valvular deformities. (From Damjanov, I. [2012]. *Pathology for the health professions* [4th ed.]. Saunders.)

TABLE 24.7 Summary of the 2015 Jones Criteria

Evidence of Preceding GAS Infection (at Least One of the Following)
1. Increased or rising antistreptolysin O titer or other streptococcal antibodies (anti-DNase B). A rise in titre is better evidence than a single titre result
2. A positive throat culture for group A β-hemolytic streptococci
3. A positive rapid group A streptococcal carbohydrate antigen test in a child whose clinical presentation suggests a high pretest probability of streptococcal pharyngitis

Risk Stratification

Low-Risk Population	Moderate/High Risk Population
ARF incidence ≤2 per 100 000 school-aged children or all-age RHD prevalence of ≤2 per 1 000 population year	Children not clearly from a low-risk population

Major Criteria

Clinical and/or subclinical carditis	Clinical and/or subclinical carditis
Polyarthritis	Monoarthritis, polyarthritis, and/or polyarthralgia
Chorea	Chorea
Erythema marginatum	Erythema marginatum
Subcutaneous nodules	Subcutaneous nodules

Minor Criteria

Prolonged PR interval	Prolonged PR interval
Polyarthralgia	Monoarthralgia
≥38.5°C	≥38°C
Peak ESR ≥60 mm in 1 hour and/or CRP ≥3.0 mg/dL	Peak ESR ≥30 mm in 1 hour and/or CRP ≥3.0 mg/dL

ARF, Acute rheumatic fever; *CRP*, C-reactive protein; *ESR*, erythrocyte sedimentation rate; *GAS*, group A streptococcal; *RHD*, rheumatic heart disease.
From Zühlke, L., Beaton, A., Engel, M. A., et al. (2017). *Current Treatment Options in Cardiovascular Medicine*, *19*(2), 15.

both rheumatic carditis and arthritis. Serious carditis may require corticosteroids and diuretics. Because recurrent rheumatic fever occurs in more than half of affected children, continuous prophylactic antibiotic therapy may be necessary for as long as 5 years. Several potential group A β-hemolytic streptococcus vaccines are being developed. Rheumatic heart disease may require surgical repair of damaged valves.

Infective Endocarditis

> ✓ **QUICK CHECK 24.9**
> 1. What three critical elements are required for the pathogenesis of infective endocarditis?
> 2. Why does infective endocarditis involve several organ systems?
> 3. What effect does AIDS have on the heart?

Infective endocarditis is a general term used to describe infection and inflammation of the endocardium—especially the cardiac valves. Bacteria are the most common cause of infective endocarditis, especially streptococci, staphylococci, and enterococci, which account for more than 80% of cases.[124] Other causes include viruses, fungi, rickettsia, and parasites. Infective endocarditis was once a lethal disease, but morbidity and mortality diminished significantly with the advent of antibiotics and improved diagnostic techniques (see *Risk Factors: Infective Endocarditis*).

RISK FACTORS
Infective Endocarditis

- Acquired valvular heart disease
- Implantation of prosthetic heart valves
- Congenital lesions associated with highly turbulent flow (e.g., ventricular septal defect)
- Previous attack of infective endocarditis
- Intravenous medication use
- Long-term indwelling intravenous catheterization (e.g., for pressure monitoring, feeding, hemodialysis)
- Implantable cardiac pacemakers
- Heart transplant with defective valve

PATHOPHYSIOLOGY The pathogenesis of infective endocarditis requires at least three critical elements (Figure 24.33):

1. *Endocardial damage.* Trauma, congenital heart disease, valvular heart disease, and the presence of prosthetic valves are the most common risk factors for endocardial damage that lead to infective endocarditis. Turbulent blood flow caused by these abnormalities usually affects the atrial surface of atrioventricular valves or the ventricular surface of semilunar valves. Endocardial damage exposes the endothelial basement membrane, which contains a type of collagen that attracts platelets, triggers the inflammatory process, and stimulates sterile thrombus formation on the membranes (**nonbacterial thrombotic endocarditis**).
2. *Adherence of bloodborne microorganisms to the damaged endocardial surface.* Bacteria may enter the bloodstream during injection drug use, trauma, dental procedures that involve manipulation of the gingiva, cardiac surgery, genitourinary procedures and indwelling catheters in the presence of infection, or gastro-intestinal instrumentation, or they may spread from uncomplicated upper respiratory tract or skin infections. Bacteria adhere to the damaged endocardium using adhesins.[134]
3. *Formation of infective endocardial vegetations* (Figure 24.34). Bacteria infiltrate the sterile thrombi and accelerate fibrin formation by activating the clotting cascade. These vegetative lesions can form anywhere on the endocardium but usually occur on heart valves and surrounding structures. Although endocardial tissue is constantly bathed in antibody-containing blood and is surrounded by scavenging monocytes and polymorphonuclear leukocytes, bacterial colonies are inaccessible to host defences because they are embedded in the protective fibrin clots. Embolization from these vegetations can lead to abscesses and characteristic skin changes, such as petechiae, splinter hemorrhages, Osler nodes, and Janeway lesions.

CLINICAL MANIFESTATIONS Fever occurs in 80% of cases.[134] Infective endocarditis causes varying degrees of valvular dysfunction and may be associated with manifestations involving several organ systems (respiratory [lungs], sensory [eyes], genitourinary [kidneys], musculoskeletal [bones, joints], and central nervous systems), making diagnosis exceedingly difficult. Signs and symptoms of infective endocarditis are caused by infection and inflammation, systemic spread of microemboli, and immune complex deposition. The "classic" findings are fever, new, or changed cardiac murmur and petechial lesions of the skin, conjunctiva, and oral mucosa. Characteristic physical findings include Osler nodes (painful erythematous nodules on the pads of the fingers and toes) and Janeway lesions (nonpainful hemorrhagic lesions on the palms and soles). Central nervous system complications

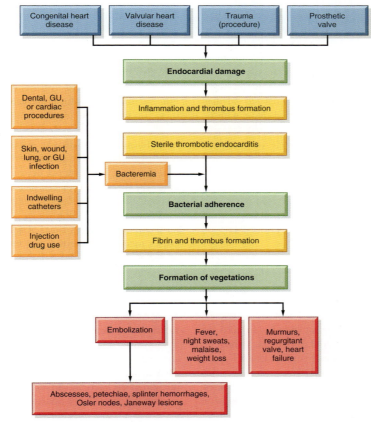

FIGURE 24.33 Pathogenesis of Infective Endocarditis. *GU,* Genitourinary.

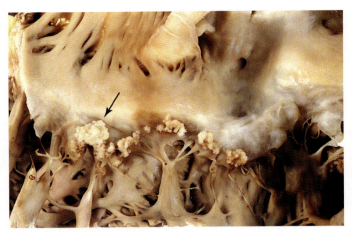

FIGURE 24.34 Bacterial Endocarditis of Mitral Valve. The valve is covered with large, irregular vegetations (arrow). (From Damjanov, I., & Linder, J. [2000]. *Pathology: a color atlas.* Mosby.)

are the most frequent and the most severe extracardiac complications and include stroke, abscess, and meningitis.[134,135] Other manifestations include weight loss, back pain, night sweats, and HF. Splenic, renal, pulmonary, peripheral arterial, coronary, and ocular emboli may lead to a wide variety of signs and symptoms.

EVALUATION AND TREATMENT The criteria for the diagnosis of infective endocarditis are called the *Duke criteria* and include repetitive blood cultures positive for bacteria and evidence for endocardial involvement (murmurs or documented regurgitation) along with recognized risk factors, fever, and vascular complications.[134] Serum measures, such as C-reactive protein, also are elevated. Echocardiography should be performed immediately. Antimicrobial therapy is generally given for several weeks, beginning with intravenous and ending with oral administration. In some cases, two different antibiotics are given simultaneously to eliminate the offending microorganism and prevent the development of medication resistance.[124,134] Other medications may be necessary to treat left ventricular failure secondary to valvular dysfunction. Surgery that involves excision of infected tissue with or without valve replacement improves outcomes in many persons with infective endocarditis, especially those with severe HF or persistent bacteremia despite antibiotic therapy.

Antibiotic prophylaxis to prevent infective endocarditis is indicated for those with prosthetic valves, a history of infective endocarditis, unrepaired cyanotic congenital heart disease, and heart transplant with valvular defect in the setting of gingival procedures or in the presence of documented acute gastro-intestinal or genitourinary infection.[124]

Cardiac Complications in AIDS

Individuals with HIV infection and acquired immune deficiency syndrome (AIDS) are at risk for cardiac complications including dilated cardiomyopathy, myocarditis, pericardial effusion, endocarditis, pulmonary hypertension, and nonantiretroviral medication–related cardiotoxicity. In addition, cardiac involvement may be induced by various bacterial, viral, protozoal, mycobacterial, and fungal pathogens that complicate AIDS. Malignancies, such as lymphoma and Kaposi sarcoma, are seen often in individuals with AIDS and can affect the heart. HIV has been found to cause immune activation that increases the risk for coronary atherosclerosis.[136,137] Furthermore, treatment with antiretroviral therapy can cause dyslipidemia and atherosclerotic disease.

Left ventricular failure is the most common complication of HIV infection and is related to left ventricular dilation and dysfunction and sudden death.[138] Pericardial effusion, ventricular dysrhythmias, electrocardiographic changes, and right ventricular dilation and hypertrophy are other less common findings.

MANIFESTATIONS OF HEART DISEASE

> ✓ **QUICK CHECK 24.10**
> 1. What is ventricular remodelling?
> 2. Why are changes in left ventricular end-diastolic volume important for left ventricular failure?
> 3. What is the vicious cycle of heart failure with preserved ejection fraction?

Heart Failure

Heart failure (HF) is when the heart is unable to generate an adequate cardiac output, causing inadequate perfusion of tissues or increased diastolic filling pressure of the left ventricle, or both, so that pulmonary capillary pressures are increased. It affects nearly 10% of individuals older than age 65 and is the most common reason for admission to the hospital in that age group. Ischemic heart disease and hypertension are the most important predisposing risk factors.[10] Other risk factors include age, obesity, diabetes, renal failure, valvular heart disease, cardiomyopathies, myocarditis, congenital heart disease, and excessive alcohol use. Numerous genetic polymorphisms have been linked to an increased risk for HF, including genes for cardiomyopathies, myocyte contractility, and neurohumoral receptors. Most causes of HF result from dysfunction of the left ventricle (HF with reduced ejection fraction and HF with preserved ejection fraction). The right ventricle also may be dysfunctional, especially in pulmonary disease (right ventricular failure). Finally, some conditions cause inadequate perfusion despite normal or elevated cardiac output (high-output failure). (See *Health Promotion*: Canadian Heart Failure Statistics.)

Left Ventricular Failure

Left ventricular failure is further categorized as HF with reduced ejection fraction or HF with preserved ejection fraction. It is possible for these two types of HF to occur simultaneously in one individual.

Heart failure with reduced ejection fraction (HFrEF), or **systolic heart failure**, is defined as an ejection fraction of less than 40% and an inability of the heart to generate an adequate cardiac output to perfuse vital tissues. Cardiac output depends on the heart rate and stroke volume. The three major determinants of stroke volume are contractility, preload, and afterload[139] (see Chapter 23).

Diseases that disrupt myocyte activity reduce contractility. MI is the most common primary cause of decreased contractility. Other primary causes include myocarditis and cardiomyopathies. Secondary causes of decreased contractility, such as recurrent myocardial ischemia and increased myocardial workload, contribute to inflammatory, immune, and neurohumoral changes (activation of the SNS and RAAS) that mediate a process called ventricular remodelling.[34] **Ventricular remodelling** results in disruption of the normal myocardial extracellular structure with resultant dilation of the myocardium and causes progressive myocyte contractile dysfunction over time (Figure 24.35). When contractility is decreased, stroke volume falls and left ventricular end-diastolic volume (LVEDV) increases. This decreased contractility causes dilation of the heart and an increase in preload.

Preload, or LVEDV, increases with decreased contractility or an excess of plasma volume (intravenous fluid administration, renal failure, mitral valvular disease). Increases in LVEDV can actually

HEALTH PROMOTION
Canadian Heart Failure Statistics

In Canada, the annual direct costs of heart failure (HF) are estimated to be more than $2.8 billion, due to hospitalizations and the associated costs. According to data from the Canadian Institute for Health Information (CIHI), 60 000 patients were hospitalized between 2013 and 2014 as a consequence of HF. Unfortunately, the number of visits due to HF has been increasing over the last couple of years, reaching a 13% increase in the last 6 years. Currently, 600 000 Canadians are living with HF, and these numbers are expected to increase as the Canadian population gets older, placing an increased burden on the Canadian health care system.

Living conditions play an important role in the longevity of Canadians and their cardiovascular health. Studies have shown that low-income Canadians tend to experience more heart attacks than Canadians with better incomes. Job insecurity plays a significant role in contributing to undue stress, increasing the physiological and psychological load, eventually overwhelming the body, and leading to sleep deprivation, high blood pressure, and heart disease. Job insecurity also has a negative impact on personal relationships, parenting effectiveness, and children's behaviour.

The following health care interventions can help patients prevent and manage HF:

- Promoting healthy lifestyle behaviours that preserve and maintain the current capacity and potentially improve cardiovascular fitness and future health status
- Promoting activities that strengthen mind–body interactions
- Empowering patients and families to understand HF symptoms and collaborating with them to manage those symptoms using health-promoting behaviours
- Promoting opportunities for social networking and interaction to overcome patients' barriers to socialization to enhance quality of life
- Promoting an atmosphere that focuses on wellness rather than illness, eventually creating hope for people living with HF
- Encouraging and rewarding health-promoting behaviours and lifestyle changes that emphasize health

Although health-promoting behaviours may not change the course of the disease, they can influence the patient's response to the illness condition, thereby mitigating its effect on quality of life.

Data from Clark, A. P., Stuifbergen, A., Gottlieb, N. H., et al. (2006). *Holistic Nursing Practice, 20*(2), 73–79; Heart and Stroke Foundation. (2016). *Canada is failing our heart failure patients* [Press release]. https://www.heartandstroke.ca/-/media/pdf-files/canada/2017-heart-month/heartandstroke-reportonhealth-2016.ashx?rev=87b86c6911fa441ca3f9bf4de5a02d32; Mikkonen, J., & Raphael, D. (2010). *Social determinants of health: the Canadian facts*. York University School of Health Policy and Management. http://www.thecanadianfacts.org/the_canadian_facts.pdf.

improve cardiac output up to a certain point, but as preload continues to rise, it causes a stretching of the myocardium that eventually can lead to dysfunction of the sarcomeres and decreased contractility. This relationship is described by Starling's law of the heart (see Figure 23.16). Decreased contractility leads to further increases in preload (Figure 24.36).

Increased afterload is most commonly a result of increased peripheral vascular resistance, such as that seen with hypertension. Nearly 75% of cases of HF have antecedent hypertension.[10] Although much less common, it also can be the result of aortic valvular disease. With increased afterload, there is resistance to ventricular emptying and more workload for the ventricle. The ventricle responds with hypertrophy, which is a form of myocardial remodelling. This process differs from the physiological myocyte response to increased workload (exercise) in which the workload is intermittent rather than sustained, resulting in an increase in muscle mass but no distortion of the cardiac architecture. Sustained afterload leads to pathological hypertrophy mediated by Ang II and catecholamines and results in an increase in oxygen demand by the thickened myocardium.[140] A state of relative ischemia develops that further contributes to changes in the myocytes themselves and ventricular remodelling (Figure 24.37). In addition, hypertrophic remodelling results in alteration of the cardiac extracellular matrix and deposition of collagen between the myocytes, which can disrupt the integrity of the muscle, decrease contractility, and increase the likelihood that the ventricle will dilate and fail.[141] These changes in ventricular structure and function are referred to as *hypertensive hypertrophic cardiomyopathy*.

As cardiac output falls, renal perfusion diminishes with activation of the RAAS, which acts to increase peripheral vascular resistance and plasma volume, thus further increasing afterload and preload. In addition, baroreceptors in the central circulation detect the decrease in perfusion and stimulate the SNS to cause yet more vasoconstriction and the hypothalamus to produce antidiuretic hormone (ADH). This vicious cycle of decreasing contractility, increasing preload, and increasing afterload causes progressive worsening of left ventricular failure.

In addition to these hemodynamic interactions, HFrEF is characterized by a complex constellation of neurohumoral, inflammatory, and metabolic processes. Ang II and aldosterone have direct toxicity to the myocardium, contributing to remodelling, myocyte death, and fibrosis. Catecholamines released by the SNS also are toxic to the myocardium and contribute to remodelling.[34] Natriuretic peptides are released in an effort to improve renal salt and water excretion but are inadequate to compensate for these neurohumoral perturbations.[141] Insulin resistance and diabetes not only contribute to HF but also are a complication of HF with changes in myocyte metabolism. Inflammatory cytokines, such as TNF-α, are released in HF, contributing to myocardial damage as well as systemic weight loss (cardiac cachexia). Finally, changes in the metabolic processes within the myocardium also are affected with a decreased ability of the heart to produce energy and an increase in release of toxic metabolites.[142] These neurohumoral, inflammatory, and metabolic aspects of left HFrEF have led to the routine use of combinations of medications that inhibit angiotensin, aldosterone, and catecholamines and increase salt excretion in an effort to prevent long-term damage to the myocardium, as well as the exploration of new treatment modalities focused on reducing inflammation and improving myocardial metabolic function.[142,143]

The interaction of these hemodynamic, neurohumoral, inflammatory, and metabolic processes results in a steady decline in myocardial function. Pathologically, the heart muscle exhibits gradual changes in myocyte structure and function, with apoptosis of cells, deposition of fibrin, and remodelling of the myocardium such that contractility and cardiac output decline. A vicious cycle of decreasing contractility, increasing preload, and increasing afterload develops, causing the progressive worsening of symptoms associated with left ventricular failure (Figure 24.38).

The clinical manifestations of left ventricular failure are the result of pulmonary vascular congestion and inadequate perfusion of the systemic circulation. Individuals experience dyspnea, orthopnea, cough of frothy sputum, fatigue, decreased urine output, and edema. Physical examination often reveals pulmonary edema (cyanosis, inspiratory crackles, pleural effusions), hypotension or hypertension, an S_3 gallop, and evidence of underlying CAD or hypertension. The diagnosis can be further confirmed with echocardiography showing decreased cardiac output and cardiomegaly. The level of serum BNP can also help make the diagnosis of HF and give some insight into its severity.[144]

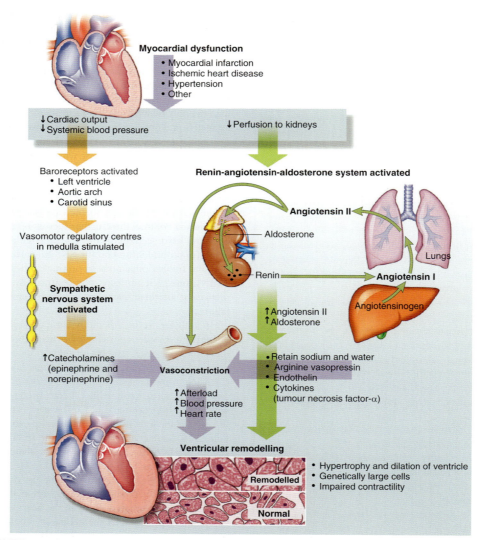

FIGURE 24.35 Pathophysiology of Ventricular Remodelling. Myocardial dysfunction activates the renin-angiotensin-aldosterone and sympathetic nervous systems, releasing neurohormones (angiotensin II, aldosterone, catecholamines, and cytokines). These neurohormones contribute to ventricular remodelling. (Redrawn from Carelock, J., & Clark, A. P. Heart failure: pathophysiologic mechanisms: the same neurohormonal actions that initially preserve cardiac output subsequently cause functional deterioration. New drug breakthroughs may provide a solution. *American Journal of Nursing, 101*[12], 26–33. https://journals.lww.com/ajnonline/Citation/2001/12000/Heart_Failure__Pathophysiologic_Mechanisms__The.17.aspx?trendmd-shared=0.)

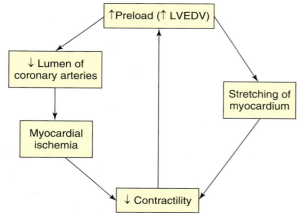

FIGURE 24.36 Effect of Elevated Preload on Myocardial Oxygen Supply and Demand. *LVEDV*, Left ventricular end-diastolic volume.

Management of HFrEF is aimed at interrupting the worsening cycle of decreasing contractility, increasing preload, and increasing afterload. The acute onset of left ventricular failure is most often the result of acute myocardial ischemia and must be managed in conjunction with management of the underlying coronary disease. Oxygen, nitrate, and morphine administration improves myocardial oxygenation and helps relieve coronary spasm while lowering preload through systemic venodilation. Inotropic medications, such as dopamine, dobutamine (Dobutrex), and milrinone, increase contractility and can help raise the blood pressure in hypotensive individuals but must be monitored carefully.[145] Diuretics reduce preload. ACE inhibitors, ARBs, and aldosterone blockers reduce both preload and afterload by decreasing aldosterone levels and reducing peripheral vascular resistance. Finally, individuals with severe HFrEF failure may benefit from acute coronary bypass or PCI. These people often are supported with the intra-aortic balloon pump (IABP) or left ventricular assist devices (LVADs) until surgery can be performed.

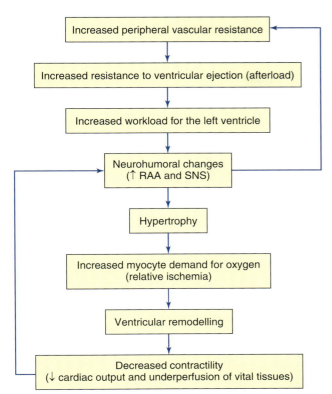

FIGURE 24.37 Role of Increased Afterload in the Pathogenesis of Heart Failure. *RAAS*, Renin-angiotensin-aldosterone system; *SNS*, sympathetic nervous system.

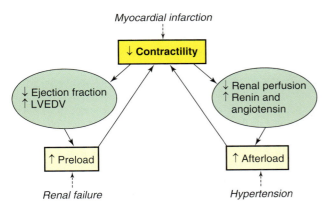

FIGURE 24.38 Vicious Cycle of Heart Failure With Reduced Ejection Fraction. Although the initial insult may be one of primary decreased contractility (e.g., myocardial infarction), increased preload (e.g., renal failure), or increased afterload (e.g., hypertension), all three factors play a role in the progression of left ventricular failure. *LVEDV*, Left ventricular end-diastolic volume.

Management of chronic left ventricular failure is based on current clinical guidelines and clinical severity.[146] The overall goals are to reduce preload and afterload. Salt restriction and diuretics (loop diuretics) are effective in reducing preload. ACE inhibitors (or Ang II receptor blockers) reduce preload and afterload and have been shown to significantly reduce mortality in individuals with chronic left ventricular failure. Aldosterone blockers, such as spironolactone, also are associated with improved outcomes.[147] Beta-blockers improve symptoms and increase survival but must be used carefully to avoid hypotension. The inotropic medication digoxin may be considered in selected individuals, especially those with refractory HF or AF.[146]

Although many individuals with left ventricular failure die suddenly from dysrhythmias, prophylactic administration of antidysrhythmics has not been shown to improve survival. In individuals with sustained ventricular tachycardia, implantable cardioverter-defibrillators should be considered. Cardiac resynchronization therapy is proving to be an important modality in selected individuals.[148] For those individuals with CAD, coronary bypass surgery or PCI may improve perfusion to ischemic myocardium (hibernating myocardium) and improve cardiac output. Surgical interventions may be performed (including improving ventricular geometry, implanting assist devices) or heart transplantation may need to be considered. Experimental therapies, including natriuretic peptide analogues, gene transfer, and stem cell therapies, are being explored.[149] Gene therapy offers some exciting new hope for severe HF.

Heart failure with preserved ejection fraction (HFpEF), or *diastolic heart failure*, can occur singly or along with HFrEF.[150] Isolated HFpEF is defined as pulmonary congestion despite a normal stroke volume and cardiac output. Accurate estimation of the prevalence of HFpEF in Canada is challenging due to lack of standardization in diagnostic criteria and inherent difficulties in its diagnosis. However, a recent study estimated that the overall prevalence of HFpEF in the general population ranges between 1.1 and 5.5%.[151]

HFpEF is preceded by a condition called *preclinical diastolic dysfunction* (PDD) in which affected individuals do not have symptoms, but have early changes in ventricular relaxation and a high untreated risk of developing HF.[152] HFpHF results from decreased compliance of the left ventricle and abnormal diastolic relaxation such that a normal LVEDV results in an increased LVEDP. This pressure is reflected back into the pulmonary circulation and results in pulmonary edema, pulmonary hypertension, and right ventricular hypertrophy.[153] The amount of left ventricle stiffness and right ventricular hypertrophy are the strongest pathophysiological predictors of complications from HFpEF.[154] The major causes of diastolic dysfunction include hypertension-induced myocardial hypertrophy and myocardial ischemia–induced ventricular remodelling. Hypertrophy and ischemia cause a decreased ability of the myocytes to actively pump calcium from the cytosol, resulting in impaired relaxation. Other causes include aortic valvular disease, mitral valve disease, pericardial diseases, and cardiomyopathies. Diabetes also increases the risk for diastolic dysfunction. Like HFrEF, HFpEF is characterized by sustained activation of the RAAS and the SNS.

Individuals with diastolic dysfunction present with dyspnea on exertion and fatigue. Evidence of pulmonary edema (inspiratory crackles on auscultation, pleural effusions) is usually not present in resting individuals without tachycardia. Late in diastole, atrial contraction with rapid ejection of blood into the noncompliant ventricle may give rise to an S_4 gallop. Electrocardiography often reveals evidence of left ventricular hypertrophy, and chest X-ray may show pulmonary congestion without cardiomegaly (Table 24.8). There also may be evidence of underlying coronary disease, hypertension, or valvular disease. Diagnosis is based on three factors: signs and symptoms of HF, normal left ventricular ejection fraction, and evidence of diastolic dysfunction. Clinical Doppler echocardiography is used to confirm the diagnosis, which demonstrates poor ventricular filling with normal ejection fractions.[155]

Management is aimed at improving ventricular relaxation and prolonging diastolic filling times to reduce diastolic pressure. No therapy has been shown to improve survival, and calcium channel blockers, beta-blockers, ACE inhibitors, and ARBs have been used with varying success.[156] Treatment with the 3-hydroxy-3-methyl-glutaryl-coenzyme A (HMG-CoA) reductase inhibitors (statins) has consistently resulted in improvements in left ventricle diastolic function.[156,157] Inotropic

TABLE 24.8 Comparison of HFrEF and HFpEF

Characteristic	HFrEF	HFpEF
Gender	Males greater than females	Females greater than males
Left ventricular ejection fraction	Decreased	Normal
Left ventricular chamber size	Increased	Decreased
Left ventricular hypertrophy on electrocardiogram	Possible	Probable
Chest radiography	Pulmonary congestion with cardiomegaly	Pulmonary congestion without cardiomegaly
Gallop	S_3	S_4

HFpEF, Heart failure with preserved ejection fraction; *HFrEF*, heart failure with reduced ejection fraction.
Adapted from Jessup, M., & Brozena, S. (2003). *New England Journal of Medicine, 348*(20), 2007–2018.

medications are not indicated in isolated HFpEF because contractility and ejection fraction are not affected. Digoxin may be used to slow the heart rate in individuals with HFpEF and AF. Outcomes for individuals with HFpEF are as poor as those with HFrEF, and there has been no improvement in prognosis despite numerous new treatment trials.[158]

Right Ventricular Failure

Right ventricular failure is defined as the inability of the right ventricle to provide adequate blood flow into the pulmonary circulation at a normal central venous pressure. It can result from left ventricular failure when an increase in left ventricular filling pressure is reflected back into the pulmonary circulation. As pressure in the pulmonary circulation rises, the resistance to right ventricular emptying increases (Figure 24.39). The right ventricle is poorly prepared to compensate for this increased afterload and will dilate and fail. As a result, pressure will rise in the systemic venous circulation, leading to peripheral edema and hepatosplenomegaly. Treatment relies on management of the left ventricular dysfunction as just outlined. When right ventricular failure occurs in the absence of left ventricular failure, it is typically attributable to diffuse hypoxic pulmonary disease such as chronic obstructive pulmonary disease (COPD), cystic fibrosis, and acute respiratory distress syndrome (ARDS). These disorders result in an increase in right ventricular afterload. The mechanisms for this type of right ventricular failure (cor pulmonale) are discussed in Chapter 27. Finally, MI, cardiomyopathies, and pulmonic valvular disease interfere with right ventricular contractility and can lead to right ventricular failure.

High-Output Failure

High-output failure is the inability of the heart to adequately supply the body with bloodborne nutrients, despite adequate blood volume and normal or elevated myocardial contractility. In high-output failure, the heart increases its output but the body's metabolic needs are still not met. Common causes of high-output failure are anemia, septicemia, hyperthyroidism, and beriberi (Figure 24.40).

Anemia decreases the oxygen-carrying capacity of the blood. Metabolic acidosis occurs as the body's cells switch to anaerobic metabolism (see Chapter 5). In response to metabolic acidosis, heart rate and stroke volume increase in an attempt to improve tissue perfusion. If anemia is severe, however, even maximum cardiac output does not supply the cells with enough oxygen for metabolism.

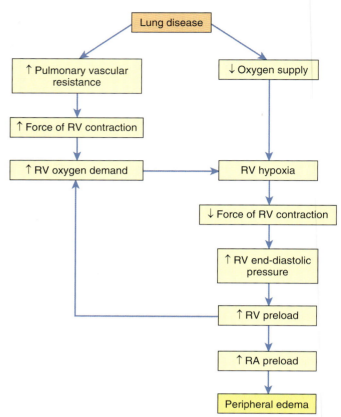

FIGURE 24.39 Right Ventricular Failure. *RA*, Right atrial; *RV*, right ventricular.

In septicemia, disturbed metabolism, bacterial toxins, and the inflammatory process cause systemic vasodilation and fever. Faced with a lowered systemic vascular resistance (SVR) and an elevated metabolic rate, cardiac output increases to maintain blood pressure and prevent metabolic acidosis. In overwhelming septicemia, however, the heart may not be able to raise its output enough to compensate for vasodilation. Body tissues show signs of inadequate blood supply despite a high cardiac output.

Hyperthyroidism accelerates cellular metabolism through the actions of elevated levels of thyroxine from the thyroid gland. This may occur chronically (thyrotoxicosis) or acutely (thyroid storm). Because the body's increased demand for oxygen threatens to cause metabolic acidosis, cardiac output increases. If blood levels of thyroxine are high and the metabolic response to thyroxine is vigorous, even an abnormally elevated cardiac output may be inadequate.

In North America, malnutrition secondary to chronic alcoholism causes beriberi (thiamine deficiency). Beriberi causes a mixed type of HF. Thiamine deficiency impairs cellular metabolism in all tissues, including the myocardium. In the heart, impaired cardiac metabolism leads to insufficient contractile strength. In blood vessels, thiamine deficiency leads to peripheral vasodilation, which decreases SVR. HF ensues as decreased SVR triggers increased cardiac output, which the impaired myocardium is unable to deliver. The strain of demands for increased output in the face of impaired metabolism may deplete cardiac reserves until low-output failure begins.

Dysrhythmias

A **dysrhythmia**, or **arrhythmia**, is a disturbance of heart rhythm. Normal heart rhythms are generated by the sinoatrial node and travel through the heart's conduction system, causing the atrial and

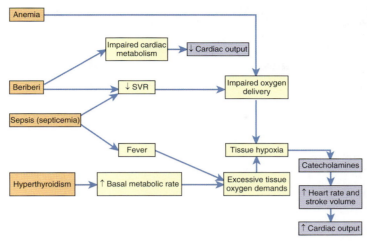

FIGURE 24.40 High-output Failure. *SVR,* Systemic vascular resistance.

ventricular myocardium to contract and relax at a regular rate that is appropriate to maintain circulation at various levels of physical activity (see Chapter 23). Dysrhythmias range in severity from occasional "missed" or rapid beats to serious disturbances that impair the pumping ability of the heart, contributing to HF and death. An abnormal rate of impulse generation (Table 24.9) from the sinoatrial node or other pacemaker or an abnormal conduction of impulses (Table 24.10) through the heart's conduction system, including the myocardial cells themselves, can cause dysrhythmias.

SHOCK

> ✓ **QUICK CHECK 24.11**
> 1. Describe the mechanisms operative in shock.
> 2. Why does myocardial infarction often cause cardiogenic shock?
> 3. How is hypovolemic shock manifested?
> 4. Why is anaphylactic shock considered a medical emergency?

In **shock** the cardiovascular system fails to perfuse the tissues adequately, resulting in widespread impairment of cellular metabolism. Because tissue perfusion can be disrupted by any factor that alters heart function, blood volume, or blood pressure, shock has many causes and various clinical manifestations. Ultimately, however, shock progresses to organ failure and death, unless compensatory mechanisms reverse the process or clinical intervention succeeds. Untreated severe shock overwhelms the body's compensatory mechanisms through positive feedback loops that initiate and maintain a downward physiological spiral.

The term *multiple organ dysfunction syndrome* (MODS) describes the failure of two or more organ systems after severe illness and injury and is a frequent complication of severe shock. The disease process is initiated and perpetuated by uncontrolled inflammatory and stress responses. It is progressive and is associated with significant mortality.

Impairment of Cellular Metabolism

The final common pathway in shock of any type is impairment of cellular metabolism. Figure 24.41 illustrates the pathophysiology of shock at the cellular level.

Impairment of Oxygen Use

In all types of shock, the cell either is not receiving an adequate amount of oxygen or is unable to use oxygen. Without oxygen, the cell shifts from aerobic to anaerobic metabolism. Anaerobic metabolism is a less efficient method of extracting energy from carbon bonds, and the cell begins to use its stores of ATP faster than stores can be replaced. Without ATP, the cell cannot maintain an electrochemical gradient across its selectively permeable membrane. Specifically, the cell cannot operate the sodium–potassium pump. Sodium and chloride accumulate inside the cell, and potassium exits the cell. Cells of the nervous system and myocardium are profoundly and immediately affected. The resting potentials of these cells are reduced, and action potentials decrease in amplitude. Various clinical manifestations of impaired central nervous system and myocardial function result.

As sodium moves into the cell, water follows. Throughout the body, the water drawn from the interstitium into the cells is "replaced" by water that is, in turn, drawn out of the vascular space. This decreases circulatory volume. Within the cells, water causes cellular edema that disrupts cellular membranes, releasing lysosomal enzymes that injure the cells internally and then leak into the interstitium. Compensatory mechanisms, including inflammation and activation of the clotting cascade, further impair oxygen use and contribute to the complications of shock, such as acute tubular necrosis (ATN), ARDS, and disseminated intravascular coagulation (DIC).

In addition to decreasing ATP stores, anaerobic metabolism affects the pH of the cell, and metabolic acidosis develops. A compensatory mechanism enables cardiac and skeletal muscles to use lactic acid as a fuel source, but only for a limited time. The decreasing pH of the cell that is functioning anaerobically has serious consequences. Enzymes necessary for cellular function dissociate under acid conditions. Enzyme dissociation stops cell function, repair, and division. As lactic acid is released systemically, blood pH drops, reducing the oxygen-carrying capacity of the blood (see Chapter 4). Therefore, less oxygen is delivered to the cells. Further acidosis triggers the release of more lysosomal enzymes because the low pH disrupts lysosomal membrane integrity.

Impairment of Glucose Use

Impaired glucose delivery or impaired glucose uptake by the cells (see Figure 24.41) can cause impaired glucose use. The reasons for inadequate glucose delivery are the same as those enumerated for inadequate oxygen delivery. In addition, in septic and anaphylactic shock, glucose metabolism may be increased or disrupted because of fever or bacteria; moreover, the presence of vasoactive toxins, endotoxins, histamine, and kinins can prevent glucose uptake.

TABLE 24.9 Disorders of Impulse Formation

Type	Electrocardiogram	Effect	Pathophysiology	Treatment
Sinus bradycardia	P rate 60 or less PR interval normal QRS for each P	Increased preload Decreased mean arterial pressure	Hyperkalemia: slows depolarization Vagal hyperactivity: unknown Digoxin toxicity common Late hypoxia: lack of adenosine triphosphate (ATP)	If hypotensive, treat cause Sympathomimetics, anticholinergics Pacemaker placement
Simple sinus tachycardia	P rate 100–150 PR interval normal QRS for each P	Decreased filling times Decreased mean arterial pressure Increased myocardial demand	Catecholamines: rise in resting potential and calcium influx Fever: unknown Early heart failure: compensatory response to decreased stroke volume Lung disease: hypoxic cell metabolism Hypercalcemia	Oxygen, bed rest Calcium blockers
Premature atrial contractions (PACs) or beats[a]	Early P waves that may have morphological changes PR interval normal QRS for each P	Occasional decreased filling time and mean arterial pressure	Electrolyte disturbances (especially hypercalcemia): alter action potentials Hypoxia and elevated preload: cell membrane disturbances	Treat underlying cause Digoxin
Sinus dysrhythmias	Rate varies P–P regularly irregular, short with inspiration, long with exhalation PR interval normal QRS for each P	Variable filling times Variable mean arterial pressure Variable oxygen demand	Unknown Common in young children and young adults	None
Atrial tachycardia (includes premature atrial tachycardia if onset is abrupt)	P rate 151–250 P morphology may differ from sinus P PR interval normal P/QRS ratio variable	Decreased filling time Decreased mean arterial pressure Increased myocardial demand	Same as PACs: leads to increased atrial automaticity, atrial re-entry Digoxin toxicity: common Aging	Control ventricular rate Digoxin, calcium channel blockers, vagus stimulation Pacemaker to override atrial conduction Cardioversion
Atrial flutter[a]	P rate 251–300, morphology may vary from sinus P PR interval usually not observable P/QRS ratio variable	Decreased filling time Decreased mean arterial pressure	Same as atrial tachycardia	Same as atrial tachycardia
Atrial fibrillation[a,*]	P rate >300 and usually not observable No PR interval QRS rate variable and rhythm irregular	Same as atrial flutter	Same as atrial tachycardia	Same as atrial tachycardia
Idiojunctional rhythm	P absent or independent QRS normal, rate 41–59, regular	Decreased cardiac output from loss of atrial contribution to ventricular preload	Atrial and sinus bradycardia, standstill, or block	Same as sinus bradycardia
Junctional bradycardia	P absent or independent QRS normal, rate 40 or less	Same as idiojunctional rhythm	Same as idiojunctional rhythm Vagal hyperactivity	Same as sinus bradycardia
Premature junctional contractions (PJCs) or beats	Early beats without P waves QRS morphology normal	Decreased cardiac output from loss of atrial contribution to ventricular preload for that beat	Hyperkalemia (5.4–6 mmol/L) Hypercalcemia, hypoxia, and elevated preload (see PACs)	Same as PAC
Accelerated junctional rhythm	P absent or independent QRS morphology normal, rate 60–99	Decreased cardiac output from loss of atrial contribution to ventricular preload	Same as PJCs	Same as PAC

Continued

TABLE 24.9 Disorders of Impulse Formation—cont'd

Type	Electrocardiogram	Effect	Pathophysiology	Treatment
Junctional tachycardia	P absent or independent QRS morphology normal, rate 100 or more	Decreased cardiac output from loss of atrial contribution to ventricular preload Increased myocardial demand because of tachycardia	Same as PJCs	Same as PAC
Idioventricular rhythm[b]	P absent or independent QRS >0.11 and rate 20–39	Same as idiojunctional rhythm	Sinus, atrial, and junctional bradycardia, standstill, or block	Same as sinus bradycardia
Ventricular bradycardia[b]	P absent or independent QRS >0.11 and rate 60 or less	Same as idiojunctional rhythm	Same as idiojunctional rhythm	Same as sinus bradycardia
Agonal rhythm/ electromechanical dissociation[b]	P absent or independent QRS >0.11 and rate 20 or less	Absent or barely present cardiac output and pulse Not compatible with life	Depolarization and contraction not coupled: electrical activity present with little or no mechanical activity Usually caused by profound hypoxia	Vigorous pharmacological treatment aimed at restoring rate and force Usually ineffective May attempt to use pacemaker
Ventricular standstill or asystole[b]	P absent or independent QRS absent	No cardiac output Not compatible with life	Profound ischemia, hyperkalemia, acidosis	Same as agonal rhythm, plus electrical defibrillation
Premature ventricular contractions (PVCs) or depolarizations[a]	Early beats with P waves QRS occasionally opposite in deflection from usual QRS	Same as premature junctional contractions	Same as PJCs, aging and induction of anaesthesia Impulse originates in cell outside normal conduction system and spreads through intercalated disks	Pharmacological interventions to change thresholds, refractory periods; reduce myocardial demand, increase supply
Accelerated ventricular rhythm	P absent or independent QRS >0.11 and rate of 41–99	Same as accelerated junctional rhythm	Same as PVCs	Removal of cause Same as PVCs
Ventricular tachycardia[b]	P absent or independent QRS >0.11 and rate 100 or more	Same as junctional tachycardia	Same as PVCs	Same as PVCs, plus electrical cardioversion
Ventricular fibrillation[b]	P absent QRS >300 and usually not observable	Same as ventricular standstill	Same as PVCs Rapid infusion of potassium	Same as PVCs, plus electrical cardioversion

[a]Most common in adults.
[b]Life-threatening in adults.
*El Hussein, M. T., & Kilfoil, L. (2020). The ABCs of atrial fibrillation. *Nurse Practitioner*, 45(8), 28–33. doi:10.1097/01.NPR.0000681780.47800.a3.

TABLE 24.10 Disorders of Impulse Conduction

Type	Electrocardiogram	Effect	Pathophysiology	Treatment
Sinus block	Occasionally absent P, with loss of QRS for that beat	Occasional decrease in cardiac output Increase in preload for following beat	Local hypoxia, scarring of intra-atrial conduction pathways, electrolyte imbalances Increased atrial preload	Conservative Usually does not progress in severity Pharmacological treatment includes vagolytics, sympathomimetics, pacing
First-degree block[a]	PRI >0.2 sec	None	Same as sinus block Hyperkalemia (>7 mmol/L) Hypokalemia (<3.5 mmol/L) Formation of myocardial abscess in endocarditis	Conservative Discovery and correction of cause
Second-degree block, Mobitz I, or Wenckebach[a]	Progressive prolongation of PRI until one QRS is dropped Pattern of prolongation resumes	Same as sinus block	Hypokalemia (<3.5 mmol/L) Faulty cell metabolism in AV node Severity increases as heart rate increases Supports theory that AV node is fatiguing Digoxin toxicity, beta blockade CAD, MI, hypoxia, increased preload, valvular surgery and disease, diabetes	Same as sinus block

Continued

TABLE 24.10 Disorders of Impulse Conduction—cont'd

Type	Electrocardiogram	Effect	Pathophysiology	Treatment
Second-degree block or Mobitz II	Same as sinus block	Same as sinus block	Hypokalemia (<3.5 mmol/L) Faulty cell metabolism below AV node Antidysrhythmics, tricyclic antidepressants CAD, MI, hypoxia, increased preload, valvular surgery and disease, diabetes	More aggressively than Mobitz I, because can progress to type III Pacemaker after pharmacological treatment
Third-degree block[b]	P waves present and independent of QRS No observed relationship between P and QRS Always AV dissociation	Same as idiojunctional rhythm	Hypokalemia (<3.5 mmol/L) Faulty cell metabolism low in bundle of His MI, especially inferior wall, as nodal artery interrupted; results in ischemia of AV node	Pacemaker after pharmacological treatment Temporary pacing if caused by inferior MI, because ischemia usually resolves
Atrioventricular dissociation	P waves present and independent of QRS, but not always because of block (e.g., ventricular tachycardia) AV dissociation not always third-degree block	Decreased cardiac output from loss of atrial contribution to ventricular preload Variable effect on myocardial demand, depending on ventricular rate	May result from third-degree block or accelerated junctional or ventricular rhythm or be caused by sinus, atrial, and junctional bradycardias	Treat according to cause Pacemaker or reducing rate of AV or ventricular discharge, or increasing rate of sinus or AV node discharge
Ventricular block	QRS >0.11 sec R-S-R'' in V_1, V_2, V_5, V_6	None	Faulty cell metabolism in right and left bundle branches RBBB more common than LBBB because of dual blood supply to left bundle branch HF, MR, especially anterior MI, because of infarct of fascicles Left anterior hemiblock more common than left posterior hemiblock because posterior fascicles have dual blood supply	Isolated RBBB or LBBB or hemiblock not treated If acute and/or associated with acute anterior MI, treated with permanent pacer and vigorous pharmacological therapy
Aberrant conduction	QRS >0.11 sec	None, unless ventricular rate abnormalities present	Conduction of impulse through intercalated disks because conduction system transiently blocked as a result of hypoxia, electrolyte imbalances, digoxin toxicity, excessively rapid rate of discharge	Correct underlying cause
Pre-excitation syndromes (Wolff-Parkinson-White and Lown-Ganong-Levine)	P present with QRS for each PPRI <0.12 sec and QRS <0.11 sec because of delta wave in PRI	None	Congenital presence of accessory pathways (bundle of Kent and fibre of Mahaim) that conduct very rapidly and bypass AV node, causing early ventricular depolarization in relation to atrial depolarization Prone to tachycardias and atrial fibrillation that can result in very rapid ventricular rates (reason unknown)	Aimed at aligning refractory periods of accessory pathway and AV node to prevent re-entry May slow rate with medication therapy May surgically cut pathways

[a]Most common in adults.
[b]Life-threatening in adults.
AV, Atrioventricular; *CAD*, coronary artery disease; *HF*, heart failure; *LBBB*, left bundle branch block; *MI*, myocardial infarction; *MR*, mitral regurgitation; *PRI*, PR interval; *RBBB*, right bundle branch block.

Some compensatory mechanisms activated by shock contribute to decreased glucose uptake by the cells. High serum levels of cortisol, thyroid hormone, and catecholamines account for hyperglycemia and insulin resistance, tachycardia, increased SVR, and increased cardiac contractility. Cells shift to glycogenolysis, gluconeogenesis, and lipolysis to generate fuel for survival (see Chapter 1). Except in the liver, kidneys, and muscles, the body's cells have extremely limited stores of glycogen. In fact, total body stores can fuel the metabolism for only about 10 hours. The depletion of fat and glycogen stores is not itself a cause of organ failure, but the energy costs of glycogenolysis and lipolysis are considerable and contribute to cell failure.

The depletion of protein also is a cause of organ failure. When gluconeogenesis causes proteins to be used for fuel, these proteins are no longer available to maintain cellular structure, function, repair,

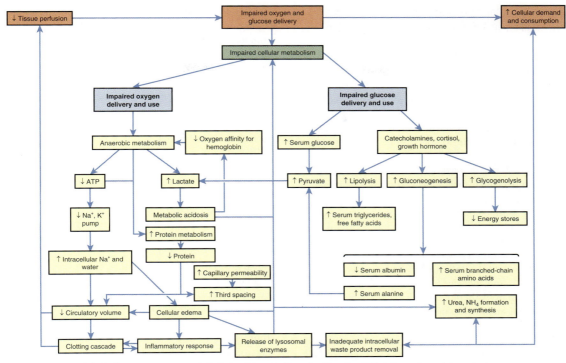

FIGURE 24.41 Impaired Cellular Metabolism in Shock. *ATP,* Adenosine triphosphate.

and replication. The breakdown of protein occurs in starvation states, hyperdynamic metabolic states, and septic shock. During anaerobic metabolism, protein metabolism liberates alanine, which is converted to pyruvate. In sepsis, pyruvic acid is changed into lactic acid, and a positive feedback loop is formed. As proteins are broken down anaerobically, ammonia and urea are produced. Ammonia is toxic to living cells. Uremia develops, and uric acid further disrupts cellular metabolism. Serum albumin and other plasma proteins are consumed for fuel first. Serum protein consumption decreases capillary osmotic pressure and contributes to the development of interstitial edema, creating another positive feedback loop that decreases circulatory volume. In septic shock, plasma protein breakdown includes metabolism of immunoglobulins, thereby impairing immune system function when it is most needed.

Protein breakdown weakens skeletal and cardiac muscle, causing muscle wasting. Skeletal muscle wasting impairs the muscles that facilitate breathing. Muscle wasting therefore alters the actions of both the heart and the lungs. The delivery of oxygen and glucose to the cells is directly reduced, as is the removal of waste products, forming another positive feedback loop.

A final outcome of impaired cellular metabolism is the buildup of metabolic end products in the cell and interstitial spaces. Waste products are toxic to the cells and further disrupt cellular function and membrane integrity. Once a sufficiently large number of cells from vital organs have damage to cellular membranes, leakage of lysosomal enzymes, and depletion of ATP, shock can be irreversible.

Clinical Manifestations of Shock

The clinical manifestations of shock are variable depending on the type of shock, and observable and measurable signs and symptoms are often conflicting in nature. Subjective complaints in shock are usually nonspecific. The individual may report feeling sick, weak, cold, hot, nauseated, dizzy, confused, afraid, thirsty, and short of breath. Hypotension, characterized by a mean arterial pressure below 60 mm Hg, is common to almost all shock states. It is considered a late sign of decreased tissue perfusion. Cardiac output and urinary output are usually variable early in shock states but generally become decreased as the shock syndrome progresses. Respiratory rate is usually increased, and respiratory alkalosis may be an important early indicator of impending shock. Other variable indicators of shock include alterations of heart rate, core body temperature, skin temperature, SVR, and skin colour. Altered sensorium may be another indicator of poor tissue perfusion. Decreased mixed venous oxygen saturation indicates poor tissue oxygenation and an alteration in cellular oxygen extraction and can be used to monitor response to therapy.

Treatment for Shock

The first treatment for shock is to discover and correct or remove the underlying cause. Simultaneously, management should be directed at improvement in microcirculatory tissue perfusion. General supportive treatment includes administration of intravenous fluids to expand intravascular volume, use of vasopressors and supplemental oxygen, and control of glucose levels. Further treatment depends on the cause and severity of the shock syndrome, which is discussed with each type of shock. Once positive feedback loops are established, intervention in shock is difficult. Prevention and very early treatment offer the best prognosis.

Types of Shock

Shock is classified by cause as cardiogenic (caused by HF), hypovolemic (caused by insufficient intravascular fluid volume), neurogenic (caused by neural alterations of vascular smooth muscle tone), anaphylactic (caused by immunological processes), or septic (caused by infection). As described previously, each of these share similar effects on tissues and cells but can vary in their clinical manifestations and severity.

Cardiogenic Shock

Cardiogenic shock is defined as decreased cardiac output and evidence of tissue hypoxia in the presence of adequate intravascular volume. Most cases of cardiogenic shock follow MI, but shock also can follow left ventricular failure, dysrhythmias, acute valvular dysfunction, ventricular or septal rupture, myocardial or pericardial infections, massive pulmonary embolism, cardiac tamponade, and medication toxicity. Microcirculation changes within the myocardium contribute to decreased contractility and worsening cardiac output.[159] Compensatory neurohumoral responses contribute to the overall pathophysiology (Figure 24.42).

The clinical manifestations of cardiogenic shock are caused by widespread impairment of cellular metabolism. They include impaired thought process, dyspnea and tachypnea, systemic venous and pulmonary edema, dusky skin colour, marked hypotension, oliguria, and ileus. Management of cardiogenic shock includes careful fluid and vasopressor administration followed by early angiography, IABP counterpulsation, ventricular assist devices, extracorporeal membrane oxygenation, and early revascularization (PCI or bypass surgery).[160] Cardiogenic shock is often unresponsive to treatment, with a mortality of more than 70% reported. New therapies being explored include anti-inflammatory medications and nitric oxide synthase inhibitors.

Hypovolemic Shock

Hypovolemic shock is caused by loss of whole blood (hemorrhage), plasma (burns), or interstitial fluid (diaphoresis, diabetes mellitus, diabetes insipidus, emesis, diarrhea, or diuresis) in large amounts. Hypovolemic shock begins to develop when intravascular volume has decreased by about 15%.

Hypovolemia is offset initially by compensatory mechanisms (Figure 24.43). Heart rate and SVR increase, boosting both cardiac output and tissue perfusion pressures. Interstitial fluid moves into the vascular compartment. The liver and spleen add to blood volume by disgorging stored red blood cells and plasma. In the kidneys, renin stimulates aldosterone release and the retention of sodium (and hence water), whereas ADH from the posterior pituitary gland increases water retention. However, if the initial fluid or blood loss is great or if loss continues, compensation fails, resulting in decreased tissue perfusion. As in cardiogenic shock, oxygen and nutrient delivery to the cells is impaired and cellular metabolism fails. Anaerobic metabolism and lactate production result in lactic acidosis and serum and cellular electrolyte abnormalities.

The clinical manifestations of hypovolemic shock include high SVR, poor skin turgor, thirst, oliguria, low systemic and pulmonary preloads, rapid heart rate, thready pulse, and mental status deterioration. The differences between the signs and symptoms of hypovolemic shock and those of cardiogenic shock are mainly caused by differences in fluid volume and cardiac muscle health. Management begins with rapid fluid replacement with crystalloids and blood products.[161] For hemorrhagic hypovolemic shock, the administration of pharmacological doses of ADH can improve blood pressure. Hypothermia and coagulopathies frequently complicate treatment.[161] If adequate tissue perfusion cannot be restored promptly, systemic inflammation and multiple organ dysfunction are likely.

Neurogenic Shock

Neurogenic shock (sometimes called **vasogenic shock**) is the result of widespread and massive vasodilation that results from parasympathetic overstimulation and sympathetic understimulation (Figure 24.44) (see Chapter 23). This type of shock can be caused by any factor that stimulates parasympathetic or inhibits sympathetic stimulation of vascular smooth muscle. Trauma to the spinal cord or medulla and conditions that interrupt the supply of oxygen or glucose to the medulla can cause neurogenic shock by interrupting sympathetic

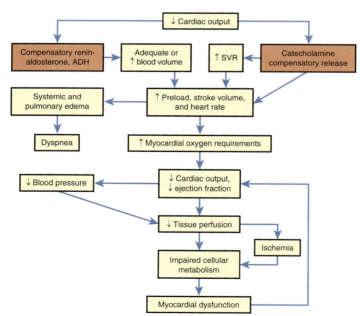

FIGURE 24.42 Cardiogenic Shock. Shock becomes life-threatening when compensatory mechanisms (in *orange boxes*) cause increased myocardial oxygen requirements. Renal and hypothalamic adaptive responses (i.e., renin-angiotensin-aldosterone and antidiuretic hormone *[ADH]*) maintain or increase blood volume. The adrenal gland releases catecholamines (e.g., mostly epinephrine, some norepinephrine), causing vasoconstriction and increases in contractility and heart rate. These adaptive mechanisms, however, increase myocardial demands for oxygen and nutrients. These demands further strain the heart, which can no longer pump an adequate volume, resulting in shock and impaired metabolism. *SVR*, Systemic vascular resistance.

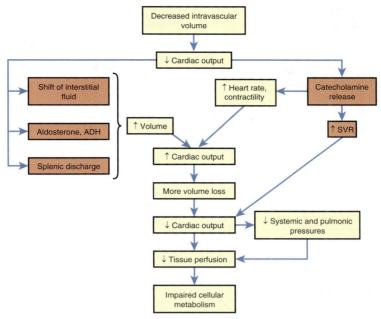

FIGURE 24.43 Hypovolemic Shock. This type of shock becomes life-threatening when compensatory mechanisms (in *orange boxes*) are overwhelmed by continued loss of intravascular volume. *ADH*, Antidiuretic hormone; *SVR*, systemic vascular resistance.

activity. Depressive medications, anaesthetic agents, and severe emotional stress and pain are other causes. The loss of vascular tone results in "relative hypovolemia," in which blood volume has not changed but SVR decreases drastically so that the amount of space containing the blood has increased.[162] The pressure in the vessels falls below that which is needed to drive nutrients across capillary membranes to the cells. In addition, neurological insult may cause bradycardia, which decreases cardiac output and further contributes to hypotension and underperfusion of tissues. As with other types of shock, neurogenic shock leads to impaired cellular metabolism. Management includes the careful use of fluids and vasopressors until blood pressure stabilizes.

Anaphylactic Shock

Anaphylactic shock results from a widespread hypersensitivity reaction known as anaphylaxis. The lifetime prevalence of anaphylaxis is 0.5 to 2%.[163] The basic physiological alteration is the same as that of neurogenic shock: vasodilation and relative hypovolemia, leading to decreased tissue perfusion and impaired cellular metabolism (Figure 24.45). Anaphylactic shock is characterized by other effects that rapidly involve the entire body.

Anaphylactic shock begins with exposure of a sensitized individual to an allergen. Common allergens known to cause these reactions are insect venoms, shellfish, peanuts, latex, and medications such as penicillin. In genetically predisposed individuals, these allergens initiate a vigorous humoral immune response (type I hypersensitivity reaction) that results in the production of large quantities of immunoglobulin E (IgE) antibody (see Chapter 8). Allergen bound to IgE causes degranulation of mast cells. Mast cells release a large number of vasoactive and inflammatory cytokines. The released substances mediate an extensive immune and inflammatory response, including vasodilation and increased vascular permeability, resulting in peripheral pooling and tissue edema. Extravascular effects include constriction of extravascular smooth muscle, often causing laryngospasm and bronchospasm (see Chapter 27) and cramping abdominal pain with diarrhea.

The onset of anaphylactic shock is usually sudden, and progression to death can occur within minutes unless emergency treatment is given. The primary clinical manifestations of anaphylaxis include anxiety, dizziness, difficulty breathing, stridor, wheezing, pruritus with hives (urticaria), swollen lips and tongue, and abdominal cramping. A precipitous fall in blood pressure occurs, followed by impaired mentation. Other signs include decreased SVR, with high or normal cardiac output, and oliguria. The diagnosis can be confirmed by a number of serum markers, such as plasma histamine and tryptase.[164] Treatment begins with removal of the antigen (if possible). Epinephrine is administered intramuscularly to cause vasoconstriction and reverse airway constriction.[165] Fluids are given intravenously to reverse the relative hypovolemia, and antihistamines and corticosteroids are administered to stop the inflammatory reaction. Vasopressors and inhaled β-adrenergic agonist bronchodilators may also be necessary.

Septic Shock

> **✓ QUICK CHECK 24.12**
> 1. What are some of the important causes of septic shock?
> 2. What is the systemic inflammatory response syndrome?
> 3. Why is correction of the underlying problem the most important treatment for all kinds of shock?

Septic shock begins with an infection that progresses to bacteremia, then systemic inflammatory response syndrome (SIRS) with sepsis, then severe sepsis, then septic shock, and finally MODS. Causes and definitions of each component of septic shock are presented in Table 24.11.[166]

In 2011, 1 in 18 deaths in Canada involved sepsis, a serious medical condition caused by an overwhelming immune response to an infection. Deaths involving sepsis increased significantly between 2000 and 2007 and then remained stable between 2007 and 2011. Between 2000 and 2007, deaths involving sepsis were higher among males than

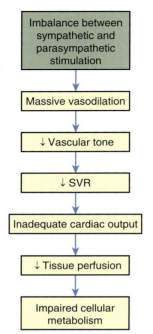

FIGURE 24.44 Neurogenic Shock. *SVR,* Systemic vascular resistance.

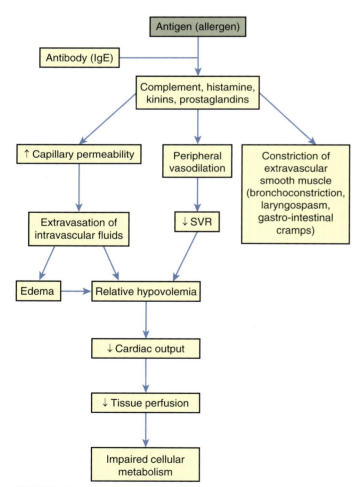

FIGURE 24.45 Anaphylactic Shock. *IgE,* Immunoglobulin E; *SVR,* systemic vascular resistance.

TABLE 24.11	Causes and Definitions of Septic Shock
Cause	**Definition**
Infection	Microbial phenomenon characterized by inflammatory response to presence of microorganisms or invasion of normally sterile host tissue by those microorganisms
Bacteremia	Presence of viable bacteria in blood
Systemic inflammatory response syndrome (SIRS)	Systemic inflammatory response to a variety of severe clinical insults manifested by two or more of the following signs: Temperature >38°C (100.4°F) or <36°C (96.8°F) Heart rate >90 beats/min Respiratory rate >20 breaths/min or arterial blood carbon dioxide level <32 mm Hg White blood cell count >12 000 cells/mm³, <4 000 cells/mm³, or containing <10% immature forms (bands)
Sepsis	Systemic response to infection characterized by two or more of SIRS criteria
Severe sepsis	Sepsis associated with organ dysfunction
Septic shock	Severe sepsis complicated by persistent hypotension refractory to early fluid therapy
Multiple organ dysfunction syndrome	Presence of altered organ function in an acutely ill individual such that homeostasis cannot be maintained without intervention

Data adapted from American College of Chest Physicians/Society of Critical Care Medicine Consensus Conference. (1992). *Critical Care Medicine, 20*(6), 864–874; Levy, M. M., Fink, M. P., Marshall, J. C., et al. (2003). *Critical Care Medicine, 31*(4), 1250–1256.

females, although between 2007 and 2011 the difference between the sexes narrowed. From 2009 to 2011, sepsis contributed to 53.4% of all deaths from infectious diseases and 5.5% of all deaths in Canada.[167]

Although death rates from septic shock have been declining, septic shock remains a highly lethal condition.[168] Septic shock can be caused by community-acquired or health care–associated infections, especially pneumonia and intra-abdominal and urinary tract infections. Indwelling arterial and central venous catheters also are an important source of infection (see *Health Promotion:* Sepsis Prevention: Central Line–Associated Bloodstream Infection).[156] Most often, sepsis is caused by bacteria, with *Staphylococcus aureus* and *Streptococcus pneumoniae* being the most common Gram-positive causes. *Escherichia coli, Klebsiella* species, and *Pseudomonas aeruginosa* are the most common Gram-negative causes.[169] Septic shock also can be caused by fungi and viruses, and in almost one-third of cases, the infectious organism is never identified. The source and virulence of the infectious microorganism, as well as the underlying health of the affected individual, significantly affect prognosis. Risk factors for septic shock include the individual's genetic composition, underlying chronic diseases, immune deficiency states, and timeliness of therapeutic interventions for infection.

Systemic inflammatory response syndrome (SIRS) reportedly has a low performance for distinguishing infection from non-infection.[170] A study of patients diagnosed by SIRS (SIRS patients) or a quick sequential organ failure assessment (qSOFA) (qSOFA patients) confirmed the ability of both for predicting infection after hospital admission. The study retrospectively analyzed the data from a multicenter prospective study. When emergency physicians suspected infection, SIRS or the qSOFA were applied. A total of 1 045 patients was eligible for this study. The

HEALTH PROMOTION

Sepsis Prevention: Central Line–Associated Bloodstream Infection

Central line–associated bloodstream infection (CLABSI) is an important cause of sepsis and septic shock. Central lines are most commonly placed in the central venous circulation for administering medications, performing hemodialysis, and monitoring hemodynamics. Catheters can be placed in several ways, including surgical and percutaneous access methods, depending on the purpose of the catheter. Risk factors for CLABSI include extremes of age, underlying systemic and immunocompromising conditions, and catheter-related factors, such as number of catheters, site of catheter insertion, and length of time the catheter has been in place. Over 40 acute-care hospitals across Canada submitted data between 2009 and 2018 for hip and knee surgical site infections (SSIs), cerebrospinal fluid shunt SSIs, paediatric cardiac SSIs and/or central line associated bloodstream infections (CLABSIs). Between 2009 and 2018, there were 2 973 reported CLABSIs, the majority of which occurred in adult mixed critical care units (ICUs) (n = 1 331; 44.8%) and NICUs (n = 1 102; 37.1%). Among CLABSIs identified in adult ICUs, the median age was 63 years (IQR[a] = 52–73 years). Males represented 62% of adult CLABSIs. One-third of adult CLABSI patients died within 30 days following the first positive culture (32.3%, n = 482/1 492). Among CLABSIs identified in paediatric intensive care units (PICUs), the median age was six months (IQR = 2–22 months). Males represented 51% of PICU cases and within 30 days of positive culture, 11% of infected patients had died (n = 37/342). Among CLABSIs identified in the neonatal intensive care unit (NICU), the median age at first positive culture was 20 days (IQR = 10–45 days). Males represented 57% of NICU cases and within 30 days of positive culture, 8% of infected patients had died (n = 88/1 077). Overall, NICUs had higher rates of CLABSIs (2.7 cases per 1 000 line-days, on average) than PICUs (1.9/1 000 line-days), adult mixed ICUs (1.1/1 000 line-days) and adult cardiovascular surgery ICUs (0.7/1 000 line-days). While rates remained relatively constant for adult ICUs and PICUs, a 54.8% decrease was observed among NICUs (from 4.2 to 1.9/1 000 line-days, 2009 to 2018, p<0.0001).

Data from Canadian Nosocomial Infection Surveillance Program. (2020). Device-associated infections in Canadian acute-care hospitals from 2009 to 2018. *Canada Communicable Disease Report, 46*(11/12), 387–387. https://doi.org/10.14745/ccdr.v46i1112a05.
[a]*IQU*, Interquartile range.

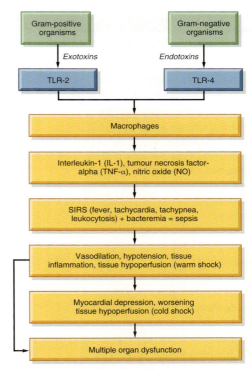

FIGURE 24.46 Septic Shock. *SIRS*, Systemic inflammatory response syndrome; *TLR*, Toll-like receptor.

SIRS patients accounted for 91.6% of qSOFA patients and they showed a higher rate of final infection than that of non-SIRS patients irrespective of the qSOFA diagnosis. The SIRS significantly predicted an ultimate infection (p=0.018) in patients who met the SIRS and qSOFA simultaneously. The study concluded that the SIRS patients included almost all qSOFA patients and SIRS showed a better performance for predicting infection for qSOFA in patients who met both definitions.[170]

Most septic shock begins when bacteria enter the bloodstream to produce bacteremia. These bacteria and their associated toxins initiate an innate immune response. Gram-negative microorganisms release endotoxins, and Gram-positive microorganisms release exotoxins, lipoteichoic acids, and peptidoglycans. These pathogen-associated molecular patterns (PAMPs), as well as molecules released from injured cells (damage-associated molecular patters), trigger the septic syndrome by interacting with pattern-associated receptors on macrophages, such as Toll-like receptor 2 (TLR-2) for Gram-positive PAMPs and Toll-like receptor 4 (TLR-4) for Gram-negative PAMPs (Figure 24.46).[169,171] These microbial molecules also activate complement, coagulation, kinins, and inflammatory cells.

The release of inflammatory mediators triggers intense cellular responses and the subsequent release of secondary mediators, including cytokines, complement fragments, prostaglandins, platelet-activating factor, oxygen free radicals, nitric oxide, and proteolytic enzymes (see *Risk Factors*: Proinflammatory Mediators Contributing to Septic Shock). Chemotaxis, activation of granulocytes, and reactivation of the phagocytic cells and inflammatory cascades result. This systemic inflammation, especially through the action of nitric oxide, leads to widespread vasodilation with compensatory tachycardia and increased cardiac output in the early stages of septic shock (hyperdynamic phase).[171] Later in the course of disease, inflammatory mediators, such as complement and interleukins, depress myocardial contractility such that cardiac output falls and tissue perfusion decreases. Tissue perfusion and cellular oxygen extraction also are affected by activation of the clotting cascade through the action of platelet-activating factor and depletion of the endogenous anticoagulant protein C.[169,171] Furthermore, unresponsiveness to or depletion of vasoactive factors such as vasopressin contributes to hypotension and tissue hypoperfusion. The inflammatory response can become overwhelming, leading to SIRS.[172] SIRS can progress to widespread tissue hypoxia, necrosis, and apoptosis, which leads to septic shock and MODS. It has been determined that there is a parallel release of anti-inflammatory mediators and impairment of phagocytic and adaptive immune cell function that accompanies SIRS, causing a depression in the immune response to infection that contributes to the overall shock syndrome.[169,172]

Clinical manifestations of septic shock are the result of inflammation, decreased perfusion of vital tissues, and an alteration in oxygen extraction by all cells. In early shock, tachycardia causes cardiac output to remain normal or become elevated, although myocardial contractility is reduced. Temperature instability is present, ranging from hyperthermia to hypothermia. Effects on other organ systems may result in deranged renal function, jaundice, clotting abnormalities with DIC, deterioration of mental status, and ARDS. Gastro-intestinal mucosa changes cause the translocation of bacteria from the gut into the bloodstream. Increased permeability of the gut also can lead to increased

RISK FACTORS
Proinflammatory Mediators Contributing to Septic Shock

More than 100 inflammatory mediators have been implicated in the pathogenesis of septic shock. The following are some of the most important contributors:

Tumour Necrosis Factor-Alpha (TNF-α)
Produced from macrophages, natural killer cells, and mast cells in response to endotoxin and interleukins
Net effect: generates same symptoms of septic shock as those seen with interleukins; thus is redundant

Interleukin-1β (IL-1β)
Released by macrophages and lymphocytes in septic shock in response to bacterial toxins
Net effect: produces fever, vasodilation and hypotension, edema, myocardial depression, and elevated white blood count

Interleukin-6 (IL-6)
Released by macrophages and lymphocytes during infection
Net effect: fever, elevated white blood count

Nitric Oxide (NO)
Released by activated macrophages and neutrophils
Net effect: damages tissues and causes systemic vasodilation and hypotension

Platelet-Activating Factor (PAF)
Released from mononuclear phagocytes, platelets, and some endothelial cells in response to endotoxin
Net effect: contributes to widespread clotting, generates same symptoms of shock as those seen with interleukins and TNF-α, and may initiate multiple organ failure

Complement
Activated by bacterial products and antigen/antibody complexes
Net effect: damages tissues and amplifies the inflammatory process by cellular chemotaxis and promotion of phagocytosis

inflammation and immune reactions attributable to toxins carried by the intestinal lymphatics.

The diagnosis of septic shock rests on the recognition of the systemic manifestations of overwhelming inflammation (SIRS) in individuals with suspected or documented infection. Determining the cause and severity of septic shock can be aided by measurement of levels of serum lactate, troponin,[173] C-reactive protein, and procalcitonin.[174] The management of septic shock has shown improved outcomes[171] by following the Surviving Sepsis Guidelines (see *Health Promotion:* The Surviving Sepsis Guidelines). These guidelines include rapid goal-directed resuscitation with fluids and vasopressors, antibiotic administration, and respiratory support.[175] Control of hyperglycemia with insulin, treatment of complications associated with MODS, careful nutritional support, and prevention of stress ulcers and DVT are also essential. Despite improvements in septic shock–related mortality in recent years, mortality remains high and new treatments are being explored.[176]

Multiple Organ Dysfunction Syndrome

 QUICK CHECK 24.13
1. Why can multiple organ dysfunction syndrome be initiated by either a septic or a nonseptic insult?
2. Why are inflammation and clotting triggered when the vascular endothelium is injured?
3. Describe the mechanisms that result in decreased oxygen delivery to the tissues in MODS.

HEALTH PROMOTION
The Surviving Sepsis Guidelines

The Surviving Sepsis Campaign: International Guidelines for Management of Sepsis and Septic Shock: 2016 focused on five clinical variables: hemodynamics, infection, adjunctive therapies, metabolic, and ventilation. In terms of resuscitation, goal-directed therapy that was the intention of previous guidelines had been challenged by more recent trials, and is no longer recommended. The guidelines recommend assessment of hemodynamic status after the initial fluid bolus, before further fluid is administered. In addition to hemodynamic evaluation of physiological variables, assessment should include invasive hemodynamic monitoring to determine the type of shock if the clinical diagnosis does not lead to accurate diagnosis. The new guidelines recommend the use of pulse or stroke volume variations induced by mechanical ventilation or passive leg raise test over static variables such as intravascular pressures or volumes to predict the patient's responsiveness to fluid.

Contrary to previous guidelines that recommended specific target values of central venous pressure, recent data have shown that central venous pressure has limited value for the prediction of the response to fluids. The 2016 guidelines recommend that when fluid administration is initiated, the fluid challenge technique should be used to evaluate the effect and safety of fluid administration. If hemodynamic factors continue to improve in response to fluids, further fluid should be administered. Fluid administration should be withheld when the response to fluids is no longer beneficial, a step often overlooked in clinical practice. Several studies have demonstrated that excessive fluid administration is associated with an increase in mortality. Recent guidelines transitioned from a quantitative resuscitation strategy to a more patient-centered resuscitation approach guided by hemodynamic assessment of dynamic variables, such as fluid responsiveness.

Infection control, for example removal of a catheter or device, and early antibiotic therapy is the cornerstone of treatment. Source control should always be obtained as soon as possible. The new guidelines recommend that antibiotics should be given within 1 hour maximum. Several studies demonstrated that delaying antibiotic administration is associated with an increased risk of mortality.

In addition to the timely administration of antibiotics, it is essential to ascertain that the clinician selects the most appropriate antibiotic with the right dosage and indication. The dosing strategies should be based on the drug's pharmacokinetics/pharmacodynamics principles in treating patients with sepsis. For example, due to the tendency to have increase in volume of distribution of drugs in septic patients, some clinicians argue that the recommended initial doses of antibiotics are often insufficient. A recommendation was made for the use of empirical combination therapy in patients with septic shock where two different classes of antibiotics are used to cover a single pathogen that is susceptible to both agents. This recommendation in the new guidelines is related to the increasing frequency of resistant bacteria to antibiotics and as such, multidrug combinations of classes of antibiotics decrease the odds of inadequate coverage.

Unlike previous editions, the 2016 SSC guidelines do not include recommendations for pediatric patients with sepsis, because the specific aspects could not be covered in a few paragraphs in the adult guidelines.

From Rhodes, A., Evans, L. E., Alhazzani, W., et al. (2017). Surviving sepsis campaign: international guidelines for management of sepsis and septic shock: 2016. *Intensive Care Medicine, 43*(3), 304–377. https://link.springer.com/article/10.1007/s00134-017-4683-6.

Multiple organ dysfunction syndrome (MODS) is the progressive dysfunction of two or more organ systems resulting from an uncontrolled inflammatory response to a severe illness or injury. The organ dysfunction can progress to organ failure and death (Figure 24.47).

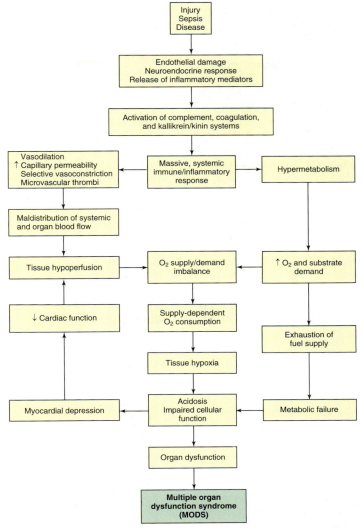

FIGURE 24.47 Pathogenesis of Multiple Organ Dysfunction Syndrome. O_2, Oxygen.

Although sepsis and septic shock are the most common causes, any severe injury or disease process that activates a massive systemic inflammatory response in the host can initiate MODS. These triggers include severe trauma, burns, acute pancreatitis, obstetrical complications, major surgery, circulatory shock, some medications, and gangrenous or necrotic tissue.

MODS is a common cause of mortality in Critical Care Units. Mortality for individuals ranges from 36 to 100% if there is failure of five or more organs, with liver and kidney failure being the most common.[177] People at greatest risk of developing MODS are older persons and persons with significant tissue injury or pre-existing disease (Box 24.3).

PATHOPHYSIOLOGY As a result of the initiating insult (sepsis, injury, or disease), the neuroendocrine system is activated with the release of the stress hormones cortisol, epinephrine, and norepinephrine into the bloodstream (see Chapter 8). Vascular endothelial damage occurs as a direct result of injury or from damage by bacterial toxins and inflammatory mediators, such as nitric oxide, tumour necrosis factor, and IL-1, which are released into the circulation. The vascular endothelium becomes permeable, allowing fluid and protein to leak into the interstitial spaces, contributing to hypotension and hypoperfusion. Leakage of fluid into the lungs causes ARDS. When the endothelium is damaged, platelets and tissue thromboplastin are activated, resulting in systemic microvascular coagulation that may lead to DIC (see Chapter 21).[178]

Because of the release of inflammatory mediators, four major plasma enzyme cascades are activated: complement, coagulation, fibrinolytic, and kallikrein/kinin. The overall effect of the activation of these cascades is a hyperinflammatory and hypercoagulant state that maintains the interstitial edema formation, cardiovascular instability, endothelial damage, and clotting abnormalities characteristic of MODS.[179] A massive systemic immune and inflammatory response then develops involving neutrophils, macrophages, and mast cells (Table 24.12). The inflammatory process initiated is the same as that described in septic shock and SIRS and sets the stage for MODS.

The numerous inflammatory and clotting processes operating in MODS cause maldistribution of blood flow and hypermetabolism. Oxygen delivery to the tissues decreases despite the supranormal systemic blood flow for several reasons:
- Shunting of blood past selected regional capillary beds is caused when inflammatory mediators override the normal vascular tone.

- Interstitial edema, resulting from microvascular changes in permeability, contributes to decreased oxygen delivery by creating a relative hypovolemia and by increasing the distance oxygen must travel to reach the cells.
- Capillary obstruction occurs because of formation of microvascular thrombi and the aggregation of white blood cells.

Hypermetabolism in MODS with accompanying alterations in carbohydrate, fat, and lipid metabolism is initially a compensatory measure to meet the body's increased demands for energy. The alterations in metabolism affect all aspects of substrate utilization. The net result of hypermetabolism is depletion of oxygen and fuel supplies.

Myocardial depression also accompanies MODS. The cause is unclear but inflammatory cytokines, bacterial products, and ischemia have been implicated. Decreased cardiac output contributes to poor perfusion of tissues and exacerbation of MODS.

Maldistribution of blood flow, coagulation, myocardial depression, ARDS, and the hypermetabolic state combine to create an imbalance in oxygen supply and demand. This imbalance is critical in the pathogenesis of MODS because it results in a pathological condition known as **supply-dependent oxygen consumption**. Ordinarily, the amount of oxygen consumed by the cells depends only on the demands of the cells, because there is an adequate reserve of oxygen that can be delivered if needed. The reserve, however, has been exhausted in MODS, and the amount of oxygen consumed becomes dependent on the amount the circulation is able to deliver. The amount of oxygen delivered is often inadequate in MODS. Therefore, tissue hypoxia with cellular acidosis and impaired cellular function ensue and result in multiple organ failure.

CLINICAL MANIFESTATIONS There may be a lag time between the inciting event and the onset of symptoms that may last for as long as 24 hours. The individual develops a low-grade fever, tachycardia, dyspnea, altered mental status, and hyperdynamic and hypermetabolic states. ARDS is often an early manifestation of MODS (see Chapter 27) and is characterized by tachypnea, pulmonary edema with crackles and diminished breath sounds, use of accessory muscles, and hypoxemia.

As the syndrome continues, hypermetabolic and hyperdynamic states intensify and signs of liver and kidney failure appear. Liver failure presents with jaundice, abdominal distension, liver tenderness, muscle wasting, and hepatic encephalopathy. All facets of metabolism, substance detoxification, and immune response are impaired. Albumin and clotting factor synthesis decreases, protein wastes accumulate, and liver tissue macrophages (Kupffer cells) no longer function effectively. Progressive oliguria, azotemia, and edema mark the development of renal failure. Anuria, hyperkalemia, and metabolic acidosis may occur if renal shutdown is severe.

The gastro-intestinal system also shows evidence of dysfunction. The gastro-intestinal system is sensitive to ischemic and inflammatory injury. Clinical manifestations of bowel involvement are hemorrhage, ileus, malabsorption, diarrhea or constipation, vomiting, anorexia, and abdominal pain. Stress ulceration of the stomach lining is a common complication of shock and MODS and, although usually painless, can result in massive blood loss and death. Compounding the damage caused by injury to the bowel is the phenomenon of bacterial translocation. When mediators and severe ischemia injure the mucosal epithelium, bacteria and toxins pass from the gut into the portal circulation. The overwhelmed liver is unable to clear these products and they move into the systemic circulation. Thus, whether infection or some other injury was the precipitating cause of MODS, sepsis occurs once the gut barrier is damaged.

Hematological failure and myocardial failure are usually later manifestations. The signs and symptoms of cardiac failure in the hypermetabolic, hyperdynamic phase of MODS are similar to those of septic shock: tachycardia, bounding pulse, increased cardiac output, decreased SVR, and hypotension. In the terminal stages, hypodynamic circulation with bradycardia, profound hypotension, and ventricular

---

BOX 24.3 Other Common Triggers of MODS

Severe trauma	Heat stroke
Major surgery	Liver failure
Burns	Mesenteric ischemia
Circulatory shock	Propofol infusion syndrome
Acute pancreatitis	Persistent inflammatory foci
Acute renal failure	Necrotic tissue
Acute respiratory distress syndrome	Disseminated intravascular coagulation
Blood transfusion	

MODS, Multiple organ dysfunction syndrome.
Data from Abboud, B., Daher, R., & Boujaoude, J. (2008). *World Journal of Gastroenterology, 14*(35), 5361–5370; Adukauskiené, D., Dockiene, I., Naginiene, R., et al. (2008). *Medicina (Kaunas), 44*(7): 536–540; Beger, H. G., & Rau, B. M. (2007). *World Journal of Gastroenterology, 13*(38), 5043–5051; Bouchama, A., & Knochel, J. P. (2002). *New England Journal of Medicine, 346*, 1978–1988; Broessner, G., Beer, R., Franz, G., et al. (2005). *Critical Care, 9*(5), R498–R501; Carnovale, A., Rabitti, P. G., Manes, G., et al. (2005). *Journal of the Pancreas (Online), 6*(5), 438–444; Ciesla, D. J., Moore, E. E., Johnson, J. L., et al. (2005). *Archives of Surgery, 140*(5): 432–440; Gando, S. (2010). *Critical Care Medicine, 38*(2), S35–S42; Kam, P. C. A., & Cardone, D. (2007). *Anesthesia, 62*(1), 690–701; Oeckler, R. A., & Hubmayr, R. D. (2007). *European Respiratory Journal, 30*(6), 1216–1226; Shaheem, M. A., & Akhtar, A. J. (2007). *Journal of the National Medical Association, 99*(12), 1402–1406; Varghese, G. M., John, G., Thomas, K., et al. (2005). *Emergency Medicine J, 22*, 185–187; Vincent, J. L., Nelson, D. R., & Williams, M. D. (2011). *Critical Care Medicine, 39*(5), 1050–1055; Zaccheo, M. M., & Bucher, D. H. (2008). *Critical Care Nurse, 28*(3), 18–26.

TABLE 24.12 Cells of Inflammation and Multiple Organ Dysfunction

Cell	Activators	Contribution to Multiple Organ Dysfunction
Neutrophils	Complement, kinins, endotoxin, clotting factors	Release of phagocytic products: toxic oxygen free radicals, superoxide ion, hydrogen peroxide, hydroxyl radicals, proteases, platelet-activating factor (PAF), arachidonic acid metabolites (prostaglandins, thromboxane, leukotrienes)
		Endothelial damage, vasodilation, vasopermeability, microvascular coagulation, selective vasoconstriction, hypotension, shock
Macrophages	Complement, endotoxin, chemotactic factors	Release of same phagocytic products as neutrophils
		Release of monokines: tumour necrosis factor (TNF), interleukin-1 (IL-1)
		TNF produces fever, anorexia, hyperglycemia, weight loss
Mast cells	Direct injury, endotoxin, complement	Release of histamine, PAF, arachidonic acid metabolites
		Vasodilation, vasopermeability, hypotension, shock

dysrhythmias may develop. Encephalopathy, characterized by mental status changes ranging from confusion to deep coma, may occur at any time. Ischemia and inflammation are responsible for the central nervous system manifestations, which include apprehension, confusion, disorientation, restlessness, agitation, headache, decreased cognitive ability and memory, and decreased level of consciousness. When ischemia is severe, seizures and coma can occur. Death may occur as early as 14 days or after a period of several weeks.

EVALUATION AND TREATMENT Early detection of organ failure is extremely important so that supportive measures can be initiated immediately. Frequent assessment of the clinical status of individuals at known risk is essential. The Acute Physiology and Chronic Health Evaluation (APACHE) II and III systems are used to assess for severity and progression of MODS. Once organ failure develops, monitoring of laboratory values and hemodynamic parameters also can be used to assess the degree of impairment.

There is no specific treatment for MODS, and therapeutic management consists of prevention and support. Prevention consists of controlling the initial insult, treating infections quickly, and supporting healing. Management goals include controlling infection, restoring oxygenation and perfusion, and supporting organ function. Sources of infection are removed and antimicrobials are administered. Ventilatory support is initiated to maintain adequate oxygen saturation, and fluids are administered to maintain vascular volume. Nutritional support must be provided to meet metabolic demand. Dialysis also may be required.

COMORBIDITIES

Cardiovascular Comorbidities

Chronic Obstructive Pulmonary Disease

Patients with chronic obstructive pulmonary disease (COPD) have higher odds of developing ischemic heart disease and myocardial infarction (MI) in comparison to patients without COPD. Thus, there is a strong correlation between COPD, heart failure, and ischemic heart disease.

The correlation between COPD and CVDs varies according to different COPD phenotypes. Patients with chronic bronchitis and recurrent exacerbations experience more cardiovascular events (arrhythmias, MI, and heart failure) than those without exacerbations, because of an underlying inflammatory–hypoxic state, and the difficulty lies in differentiating between COPD exacerbations and both ischemia and heart failure. On the other hand, the emphysematous phenotype has stronger association with diastolic dysfunction because of lung hyperinflation, which adversely influences ventricular filling and cardiac output.[a]

Type 2 diabetes mellitus is a major risk factor for angina, heart failure, MI, and atherosclerosis. Individuals with diabetes have a two- to threefold increased risk of heart attack and stroke. One study established that adults with diabetes had the same risk for future MI as adults with previous MI and without diabetes.[b] Unfortunately, CVD remains a leading cause of morbidity and mortality in people with types 1 or 2 diabetes mellitus.[c]

COVID-19

Another recent cardiovascular comorbidity is coronavirus disease 2019 (COVID-19). Angiotensin-converting enzyme 2 (ACE2), an enzyme used by severe acute respiratory syndrome coronavirus 2 (SARS-CoV-2) to enter epithelial cells, is often upregulated in patients treated with angiotensin-converting enzyme inhibitors (ACEIs) and angiotensin receptor blockers (ARBs) for CVD. It is hypothesized that the increase in ACE2 expression is associated with a greater COVID-19 severity in patients receiving ACEI or ARBs.

It is well established that ACE2 is targeted by SARS-CoV-2 to gain entrance into cells. It is also established that ACE2 plays a major anti-inflammatory role in RAS signalling by converting Ang II, an essential promotor of inflammation, to Ang (1–7), which carries anti-inflammatory properties.

There is an age-associated decline in ACE2 expression (anti-inflammatory), with simultaneous age-associated increase in RAS signalling throughout the body (proinflammatory). Exaggerated forms of this proinflammatory profile are common pathophysiological sequalae of hypertension and diabetes, and are highly prevalent in older people. In order to restore the cellular physiological function of patients with hypertension or DM who are receiving ACEIs/ARBs, they will have upregulation of their ACE2 receptors. Based on these hypotheses, the following question was posed: Knowing that ACE2 receptors are the "gateway of SARS-CoV-2 entry" into cells, how can the decrease in ACE2 receptors in older people and those with CVD predispose for greater COVID-19 severity?[d]

It is logical that greater expression of ACE2 leads to higher predisposition to COVID-19. However, when it comes to COVID-19 severity, reduction in ACE2 levels with aging and the associated upregulation of Ang II proinflammatory pathway likely predispose older individuals with cardiovascular comorbidities to severe forms of COVID-19. The direct binding of SARS-CoV-2 to ACE2 gives the virus additional power to control the receptor and reduce the surface expression of ACE2 since the virus is now attached to it. Eventually, this leads to upregulation of Ang II inflammatory signaling in the lungs, resulting in acute lung injury. Therefore, older persons who already have reduced ACE2 levels are more likely to be subjected to exaggerated inflammation due to the further reduction in ACE2 receptors expression after COVID-19 attaches to them.

Tuberculosis

Another comorbidity that accelerates the development of coronary artery disease is tuberculosis (TB). The greatest number of TB cases in Canada exists among foreign-born nationals. Unfortunately over the last 10 years, Canada reported that the incidence rate of TB has consistently been highest among Canadian-born Indigenous individuals.[e] In 2017, the rate of active tuberculosis in Canada was 4.9 per 100 000 population, whereas the rate in Canadian-born Indigenous peoples was 21.5 per 100 000 population.[f]

A systematic review and meta-analysis compared the risk of coronary heart disease among patients with TB versus individuals without TB. A total of four cohort studies (83 500 cases of TB) met the eligibility criteria and were included into the meta-analysis. The pooled analysis found that patients with TB have an increased risk of developing coronary heart disease with the pooled risk ratio of 1.76 (95% CI, 1.05–2.95; I^2 of 97%).[g]

---

[a]Corrao, S., Brunori, G., Lupo, U., et al. (2017). Effectiveness and safety of concurrent beta-blockers and inhaled bronchodilators in COPD with cardiovascular comorbidities. *European Respiratory Review, 26*(145), 160123. https://doi.org/10.1183/16000617.0123-2016.

[b]Haffner, S. M., Lehto, S., Rönnemaa, T., et al. (1998). Mortality from coronary heart disease in subjects with type 2 diabetes and in nondiabetic subjects with and without prior myocardial infarction. *New England Journal of Medicine, 339*, 229–34.

[c]Schmidt, A. M. (2019). Diabetes mellitus and cardiovascular disease: emerging therapeutic approaches. *Arteriosclerosis, Thrombosis, and Vascular Biology, 39*(4), 558–568.

[d]AlGhatrif, M., Cingolani, O., & Lakatta, E. (2020). The dilemma of coronavirus disease 2019, aging, and cardiovascular disease: insights from cardiovascular aging science. *JAMA Cardiology, 5*(7), 747–748. https://doi:10.1001/jamacardio.2020.1329. https://jamanetwork.com/journals/jamacardiology/article-abstract/2764300.

[e]Government of Canada. (2014). Chapter 1: Epidemiology of tuberculosis in Canada. *Canadian Tuberculosis Standards* (7th ed.). https://www.canada.ca/en/public-health/services/infectious-diseases/canadian-tuberculosis-standards-7th-edition/edition-13.html#a6_0.

[f]Government of Canada. (2019). *Tuberculosis: monitoring.* https://www.canada.ca/en/public-health/services/diseases/tuberculosis/surveillance.html.

[g]Wongtrakul, W., Charoenngam, N., & Ungprasert, P. (2020). Tuberculosis and risk of coronary heart disease: a systematic review and meta-analysis. *Indian Journal of Tuberculosis, 67*(2), 182–188. https://doi.org/10.1016/j.ijtb.2020.01.008.

CI, Confidence interval; I^2, heterogeneity.

GERIATRIC CONSIDERATIONS
Aging and Cardiovascular Function

Older persons make up the majority of patients in current cardiovascular clinical practice. Pharmacokinetics is impacted, leading to alteration in drug distribution. Older persons have a lower total body water content, thus lipophilic drugs have increased volume of distribution with a prolonged half-life, whereas hydrophilic drugs tend to have a smaller distribution volume in the elderly. This leads to increased concentrations of water-soluble drugs that can lead to toxicity.

Lower serum protein levels in older persons can lead to increased free (non-protein bound) concentrations of drugs, which increases the risk of drug toxicity for a given dose.

Older persons also experience platelet dysfunction, decreased coagulation factors synthesis, and increased fragility of blood vessels.

The physical and medical changes associated with aging increase the risk of mechanical and nonmechanical falls in older persons, which increases their risk for bleeding. The process of starting older persons on anticoagulation is associated with risk, because aging is also associated with a simultaneous increase in thrombosis and bleeding risks. Older persons are at higher risk of experiencing cardiac arrhythmias, including atrial fibrillation, ventricular arrhythmia, and sudden cardiac death resulting from degenerative changes and fibrous infiltration of cardiac tissue and conduction system. Electrophysiological changes in cardiac ion channels as a result of aging can increase the risk to the side effects of antiarrhythmic medications.

Older persons experience alterations in the rate of absorption, distribution, metabolism and elimination of antiarrhythmic drugs which increases the risk of toxicity. The rhythm control choices in older persons are very limited. Flecainide and propafenone (class Ic agents) should not be used frequently in older persons, because they increase the risk of proarrhythmia, especially in patients with structural heart disease. Atherosclerotic vascular disease, left ventricular hypertrophy, and myocardial dysfunction in older persons makes them poor candidates for class Ic agents. Sotalol is excreted by the kidneys and has restricted use in the elderly because of poor renal clearance. Amiodarone has extensive side effect profile but is considered the antiarrhythmic choice in older persons with AF. The use of amiodarone in older persons is a clinical challenge because it is a potent inhibitor to a number of drug metabolizing enzymes and drug transporters, including CYP3A4, CYP2C9, and P-glycoprotein. In addition, the expected hepatic, thyroid, and pulmonary side effects of amiodarone are much more pronounced in older persons.

Hypertension is a very common problem in older persons. Older persons have sluggish baroreceptor and sympathetic neural responses; as such, caution must be exercised when reducing blood pressure in older persons to avoid adverse effects, particularly postural hypotension, which can increase the risk of falls and major fractures. Reducing blood pressure in older persons has been shown to lead to impaired mental function, confusion, sleepiness, dizziness, and syncope with postural hypotension, thus significantly impairing the quality of life.[a]

[a]Ayan, M., Pothineni, N. V., Siraj, A., et al. (2016). Cardiac drug therapy—considerations in the elderly. *Journal of Geriatric Cardiology, 13*(12), 992–997. https://www.ncbi.nlm.nih.gov/pmc/articles/PMC5351831/.

CASE STUDY

A 66-year-old female Indigenous truck driver presented to the emergency department with a 20-minute episode of diaphoresis and chest pain. The chest pain was described as central, radiating to the left arm and neck, and crushing in nature. The pain settled promptly following 2 tablets (325 mg) of ASA given orally (crushed) and 3 sprays of nitroglycerin sublingually administered by paramedics on the way to the emergency department. The patient's father died of heart attack at age 54, and the patient herself has smoked 20 cigarettes daily (38 pack-year history). The patient contracted TB at the age of 12 while living on reserve, and does not remember receiving treatment.

On examination she appeared restless and was unable to complete sentences fully. While there were no heart murmurs present on cardiac auscultation, an extra heart sound was heard at the apex with the patient in the left lateral decubitus position interpreted as S3. Blood pressure was 180/105 mm Hg, heart rate was 101 bpm and regular, oxygen saturation was 97%.

Critical Thinking and Clinical Judgement Questions

1. What are the risk factors that predisposed the patient to the development of CAD?
2. What is the most likely diagnosis for this patient? (Provide justification for your answer.)
3. An ECG was requested and showed ST-segment elevation in V1–V4 with ST depression on leads I, AVL, V5 and V6. How would the nurse expect this patient to be managed?
4. The patient was taken to the catheterization lab where the left anterior ventricular coronary artery was shown to be completely occluded. Following successful percutaneous intervention and one drug eluding stent implantation in the left anterior ventricular coronary artery, normal flow was restored (thrombosis in myocardial infarction, TIMI = 3); 72 hours later, she was ready to be discharged home.

The patient was keen to return to work and asked when she could do so; however the cardiologist recommended that she take some time off. Prior to discharge, the patient looked upset and asked the nurse why she could not immediately go back to work. How would the nurse justify to the patient the rationale for not immediately going back to work?

DID YOU UNDERSTAND?

Diseases of the Veins

1. Chronic venous insufficiency (CVI) is inadequate venous return over a long period that causes pathological ischemic changes in the vasculature, skin, and supporting tissues.
2. Venous stasis ulcers follow the development of CVI and probably develop as a result of the borderline metabolic state of the cells in the affected extremities.
3. Deep venous thrombosis (DVT) results from stasis of blood flow, endothelial damage, or hypercoagulability. The most serious complication of DVT is pulmonary embolism.
4. Superior vena cava syndrome is a progressive occlusion of the superior vena cava that leads to venous distension in the upper extremities and head.

Diseases of the Arteries

1. Hypertension can be primary (without a known cause) or secondary (caused by an underlying disease).
2. The exact cause of primary hypertension is unknown, although several hypotheses are proposed, including overactivity of the sympathetic nervous system (SNS), and overactivity of the renin-angiotensin-aldosterone system (RAAS). Sodium and water retention by the kidneys, hormonal inhibition of sodium–potassium transport across cell walls, and complex interactions involving insulin resistance, inflammation, and endothelial function have also been implicated as possible causes of primary hypertension.
3. Hypertension is managed with both pharmacological and nonpharmacological methods that lower the blood volume and the total peripheral resistance.
4. A thrombus is a clot that remains attached to a vascular wall. An embolus is a mobile aggregate of a variety of substances that occludes the vasculature. Sources of emboli include clots, air, amniotic fluid, bacteria, fat, and foreign matter. These emboli cause ischemia and necrosis when a vessel is totally blocked.
5. The most common source of arterial emboli is the heart as a result of mitral and aortic valvular disease and atrial fibrillation, followed by myxomas. Tissues affected include the lower extremities, the brain, and the heart.
6. Emboli to the central organs cause tissue death in lungs, kidneys, and mesentery.
7. Peripheral vascular diseases include Buerger's disease and Raynaud's phenomenon, involving arterioles of the extremities.
8. Atherosclerosis is a form of arteriosclerosis and is the leading contributor to coronary artery disease (CAD) and cerebrovascular disease.
9. Atherosclerosis is an inflammatory disease that begins with endothelial injury.
10. Important steps in atherogenesis include vasoconstriction, adherence of macrophages, release of inflammatory mediators, oxidation of low-density lipoprotein, formation of foam cells and fatty streaks, and development of fibrous plaque.
11. Once a plaque has formed, it can rupture, resulting in clot formation and instability and vasoconstriction, which lead to obstruction of the lumen and inadequate oxygen delivery to tissues.
12. Ischemic heart disease is most commonly the result of CAD and the ensuing decrease in myocardial blood supply.
13. Peripheral artery disease is the result of atherosclerotic plaque formation in the arteries that supply the extremities, and it causes pain and ischemic changes in the nerves, muscles, and skin of the affected limb.
14. CAD is the result of an atherosclerotic plaque that gradually narrows the coronary arteries or that ruptures and causes sudden thrombus formation.
15. Many risk factors contribute to the onset and escalation of CAD, including traditional risk factors such as dyslipidemia, cigarette smoking, hypertension, diabetes mellitus (insulin resistance), obesity, and sedentary lifestyle, and nontraditional risk factors such as elevated C-reactive protein levels, hyperhomocysteinemia, and changes in adipokines.
16. Atherosclerotic plaque progression can be gradual and cause stable angina pectoris, which is predictable chest pain caused by myocardial ischemia in response to increased demand (e.g., exercise) without infarction.
17. Prinzmetal's angina results from coronary artery vasospasm.
18. Myocardial ischemia may be asymptomatic, which is called *silent ischemia*, and is a risk factor for the development of the acute coronary syndromes.
19. Sudden coronary obstruction because of thrombus formation causes the acute coronary syndromes. These syndromes include unstable angina, non-ST elevation myocardial infarction (non-STEMI), and ST elevation myocardial infarction (STEMI).
20. Unstable angina results in reversible myocardial ischemia.
21. Myocardial infarction (MI) is caused by prolonged, unrelieved ischemia that interrupts blood supply to the myocardium. After about 20 minutes of myocardial ischemia, irreversible hypoxic injury causes cellular death and tissue necrosis.
22. Dysrhythmias and cardiac failure are the most common complications of acute MI.
23. An increase in plasma enzyme levels is used to diagnose the occurrence of MI as well as indicate its severity. Elevations of the isoenzymes creatine kinase-myocardial bound, troponins, and lactate dehydrogenase 1 (LDH-1) are most predictive of an MI.
24. Treatment of an MI includes revascularization (thrombolytics or PCI) and administration of antithrombotics, angiotensin-converting enzyme (ACE) inhibitors, and beta-blockers. Pain relief and fluid management also are key components of care.

Disorders of the Heart Wall

1. Inflammation of the pericardium, or *pericarditis*, may result from several sources (e.g., infection, trauma or surgery, neoplasm).
2. Fluid may collect within the pericardial sac (pericardial effusion). Cardiac function may be severely impaired if the accumulation of fluid occurs rapidly and involves a large volume.
3. Cardiomyopathies are a diverse group of primary myocardial disorders that are usually the result of remodelling, neurohumoral responses, and hypertension. The size of the cardiac muscle walls and chambers may increase or decrease depending on the type of cardiomyopathy, thereby altering contractile activity.
4. The hemodynamic integrity of the cardiovascular system depends to a great extent on properly functioning cardiac valves. Congenital or acquired disorders that result in stenosis, regurgitation, or both can structurally alter the valves.
5. Mitral valve prolapse syndrome (MVPS) describes the condition in which the mitral valve leaflets do not position themselves properly during systole. MVPS may be a completely asymptomatic condition or can result in unpredictable symptoms.
6. Rheumatic fever is an inflammatory disease that results from a delayed immune response to a streptococcal infection in genetically predisposed individuals. Severe or untreated cases of rheumatic fever may progress to rheumatic heart disease, a potentially disabling cardiovascular disorder.
7. Infective endocarditis is a general term for infection and inflammation of the endocardium, especially the cardiac valves. If left unchecked, severe valve abnormalities, chronic bacteremia, and systemic emboli may occur as vegetations detach from the valve surface and travel through the bloodstream. Antibiotic therapy can limit the extension of this disease.

Manifestations of Heart Disease

1. Heart failure (HF) can be divided into HF with reduced ejection fraction (systolic) and HF with preserved ejection fraction (diastolic).
2. The most common causes of left ventricular failure are MI and hypertension.
3. HF with reduced ejection fraction (systolic) is caused by increased preload, decreased contractility, or increased afterload. These processes result in an increased left ventricular end-diastolic volume and an increased left ventricular end-diastolic pressure that cause increased pulmonary venous pressures and pulmonary edema.

4. In addition to the hemodynamic changes of left ventricular failure, there is a neuroendocrine response that tends to exacerbate and perpetuate the condition.
5. The neuroendocrine mediators of HF include the SNS and the RAAS, thus diuretics, beta-blockers, and ACE inhibitors are important components of pharmacological therapy.
6. HF with preserved ejection fraction (diastolic HF) is a clinical syndrome characterized by the symptoms and signs of HF, a preserved ejection fraction, and abnormal diastolic function.
7. Diastolic dysfunction means that the LVEDP is increased, even if volume and cardiac output are normal.
8. Right ventricular failure can result from left ventricular failure or pulmonary disease.
9. A dysrhythmia (arrhythmia) is a disturbance of heart rhythm. Dysrhythmias range in severity from occasional missed beats or rapid beats to disturbances that impair myocardial contractility and are life-threatening.
10. Dysrhythmias can occur because of an abnormal rate of impulse generation or an abnormal conduction of impulses.

Shock

1. Shock is a widespread impairment of cellular metabolism involving positive feedback loops that places the individual on a downward physiological spiral leading to multiple organ dysfunction syndrome (MODS).
2. Types of shock are cardiogenic, hypovolemic, neurogenic, anaphylactic, and septic. MODS can develop from all types of shock.
3. The final common pathway in all types of shock is impaired cellular metabolism—cells switch from aerobic to anaerobic metabolism. Energy stores drop, and cellular mechanisms relative to membrane permeability, action potentials, and lysozyme release fail.
4. Anaerobic metabolism results in activation of the inflammatory response, decreased circulatory volume, and decreasing pH.
5. Impaired cellular metabolism results in cellular inability to use glucose because of impaired glucose delivery or impaired glucose intake, resulting in a shift to glycogenolysis, gluconeogenesis, and lipolysis for fuel generation.
6. Glycogenolysis is effective for only about 10 hours. Gluconeogenesis results in the use of proteins necessary for structure, function, repair, and replication that leads to more impaired cellular metabolism.
7. Gluconeogenesis contributes to lactic acid, uric acid, and ammonia buildup, interstitial edema, and impairment of the immune system, as well as general muscle weakness, leading to decreased respiratory function and cardiac output.
8. Anaphylactic shock is caused by physiological recognition of a foreign substance. The inflammatory response is triggered, and a massive vasodilation with fluid shift into the interstitium follows. The relative hypovolemia leads to impaired cellular metabolism.
9. Septic shock begins with impaired cellular metabolism caused by uncontrolled septicemia. The infecting agent triggers the inflammatory and immune responses. This inflammatory response is accompanied by widespread changes in tissue and cellular function.
10. MODS is the progressive failure of two or more organ systems after a severe illness or injury. It can be triggered by chronic inflammation, necrotic tissue, severe trauma, burns, adult respiratory distress syndrome, acute pancreatitis, and other severe injuries.
11. MODS involves the stress response; changes in the vascular endothelium resulting in microvascular coagulation; release of complement, coagulation, and kinin proteins; and numerous inflammatory processes. Consequences of all these mediators are a maldistribution of blood flow, hypermetabolism, hypoxic injury, and myocardial depression.
12. Clinical manifestations of MODS include inflammation, tissue hypoxia, and hypermetabolism. All organs can be affected including the kidney, lung, liver, gastro-intestinal tract, and central nervous system.

25

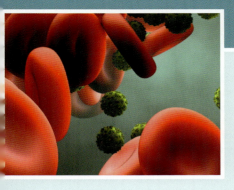

Developmental Alterations of Cardiovascular Function

Mohamed Toufic El-Hussein, with originating chapter contributions by Nancy Pike and Jennifer Peterson

Additional resources are available online at https://evolve.elsevier.com/Canada/Huether/pathophysiology.

CHAPTER OUTLINE

Congenital Heart Disease, 637
- Obstructive Defects, 639
- Defects With Increased Pulmonary Blood Flow, 641
- Defects With Decreased Pulmonary Blood Flow, 643
- Mixing Defects, 644
- Heart Failure, 646

Acquired Cardiovascular Disorders, 647
- Kawasaki Disease, 648
- Systemic Hypertension, 649

LEARNING OBJECTIVES

1. Identify risk factors for congenital cardiac defects.
2. Describe anatomical (shunt) defects and cyanotic and acyanotic congenital heart defects.
3. Differentiate between congenital heart defects that increase, decrease, or do not change pulmonary blood flow.
4. Discuss the pathophysiology, manifestations, and treatment for coarctation of the aorta.
5. Describe the clinical manifestations and potential treatments for aortic and pulmonary stenosis.
6. Describe the pathophysiology and manifestations of a patent ductus arteriosus.
7. Describe the clinical manifestations and potential treatments for atrial and ventricular septal defects.
8. Discuss the pathophysiology of tetralogy of Fallot.
9. Identify how heart failure in childhood differs from adulthood.
10. Discuss the pathophysiology of Kawasaki disease in childhood.
11. Compare childhood systemic hypertension to adulthood primary hypertension.

KEY TERMS

Acyanotic heart defect, 638
Aortic stenosis (AS), 639
Atrial septal defect (ASD), 642
Atrioventricular canal (AVC) defect (atrioventricular septal defect [AVSD], endocardial cushion defect [ECD]), 642
Coarctation of the aorta (COA), 639
Congenital heart disease (CHD), 637
Cyanosis, 638
Cyanotic heart defect, 638
Foramen ovale, 642
Heart failure (HF), 647
Hypoplastic left heart syndrome (HLHS), 646
Kawasaki disease (KD), 648
Left-to-right shunt, 638
Patent ductus arteriosus (PDA), 641
Patent foramen ovale (PFO), 642
Pulmonary atresia, 640
Pulmonary stenosis (PS), 640
Right-to-left shunt, 638
Shunt, 638
Subvalvular aortic stenosis, 640
Supravalvular aortic stenosis, 640
Systemic hypertension, 649
Tetralogy of Fallot (TOF), 643
Total anomalous pulmonary venous connection (TAPVC), 645
Transposition of the great arteries (TGA; transposition of the great vessels [TGV]), 644
Tricuspid atresia, 644
Truncus arteriosus (TA), 646
Valvular aortic stenosis, 639
Ventricular septal defect (VSD), 642

Cardiovascular disorders in children are classified as congenital or acquired. **Congenital heart disease (CHD)** is the most common. The diagnosis and management of congenital heart disease continue to improve with the use of fetal echocardiography and early interventional catheterization or surgical repair. Acquired heart disease in children continues to present challenges to the practitioner. Although guidelines for diagnosing acquired diseases are available, work is still needed in developing standards of treatment and long-term follow-up protocols.

CONGENITAL HEART DISEASE

 QUICK CHECK 25.1
1. What are the three principal classifications of congenital heart disease?
2. Describe the different characteristics that determine whether the defects are cyanotic or acyanotic.
3. What is the most common type of congenital heart defect?

Several environmental and genetic risk factors are associated with the incidence of different types of CHD. Among the environmental risk factors are (1) maternal conditions, such as intrauterine viral infections (especially rubella), diabetes mellitus, phenylketonuria, alcoholism, hypercalcemia, medications (e.g., thalidomide, phenytoin [Dilantin]), and complications of advanced maternal age; (2) antepartal bleeding; and (3) prematurity (Table 25.1).[1,2]

Genetic risk factors also have been implicated in the incidence of CHD (Table 25.2). Only a small percentage of cases of CHD are clearly linked solely to genetic or environmental factors. However, the cause of most defects is multifactorial.[1,2]

In Canada, 1 in 80 to 100 children are born with CHD. Sixty years ago only about 20% of these children survived to adulthood. The survival rate has improved over the years, reaching 90%, and resulting in a growing population of young adults who require lifelong cardiac care.[3]

There are approximately 257 000 Canadians living with CHD; two-thirds are adults and at least half face the prospect of complications, multiple surgeries, and/or premature or sudden death.

A congenital heart defect can be categorized according to (1) whether the defect causes cyanosis, (2) whether the defect causes increased or decreased blood flow into the pulmonary circulation, and (3) whether the defect causes obstruction of blood flow from the ventricles (Figure 25.1). The normal movement of blood through the right side of the heart and into the pulmonary system is separate from the blood flow through the left side of the heart into the systemic circulation (Figure 25.2A). Abnormal movement from one side of the heart to the other is termed a *shunt*. Shunting of blood flow from the left heart into the right heart is called a *left-to-right shunt* and occurs in conditions such as atrial septal defect (ASD) and ventricular septal defect (Figure 25.2B). This left-to-right shunt increases blood flow into the

TABLE 25.1 Maternal Conditions and Environmental Exposures and the Associated Congenital Heart Defects

Cause	Type of Congenital Heart Defect
Infection	
Intrauterine	Patent ductus arteriosus (PDA), pulmonary stenosis (PS), coarctation of the aorta (COA)
Systemic viral	PDA, PS, COA
Rubella	PDA, PS, COA
Coxsackie B5	Endocardial fibroelastosis
Radiation	Specific cardiovascular effect not known
Metabolic Disorders	
Diabetes	Ventricular septal defect (VSD), cardiomegaly, transposition of the great vessels
Phenylketonuria	COA, PDA
Hypercalcemia	Supravalvular aortic stenosis, PS; aortic hyperplasia
Medications	
Thalidomide (Thalomid)	No specific lesion
Dextroamphetamine (Dexedrine)	One case of reported transposition
Alcohol	Tetralogy of Fallot (TOF), atrial septal defect (ASD), VSD
Peripheral Conditions	
Increased maternal age	VSD, TOF (relationship unclear)
Antepartal bleeding	Various defects (relationship unclear)
Prematurity	PDA, VSD
High altitude	PDA, ASD (increased incidence)

TABLE 25.2 Congenital Heart Disease in Selected Fetal Chromosomal Aberrations

Conditions	Incidence of CHD (%)	Common Defects (in Decreasing Order of Frequency)
Chromosome 5p deletion syndrome (cri du chat syndrome)	25	VSD, PDA, ASD
Trisomy 13 syndrome	90	VSD, PDA, dextrocardia
Trisomy 18 syndrome	99	VSD, PDA, PS
Trisomy 21 (Down syndrome)	50	AVSD, VSD
Turner's syndrome (XO)	35	COA, AS, ASD
Klinefelter's variant (XXXXY)	15	PDA, ASD

AS, Aortic stenosis; *ASD*, atrial septal defect; *AVSD*, atrioventricular septal defect; *CHD*, congenital heart disease; *COA*, coarctation of the aorta; *PDA*, patent ductus arteriosus; *PS*, pulmonary stenosis; *VSD*, ventricular septal defect.
From Park, M. K. (2014). *Pediatric cardiology for practitioners* (6th ed.). Mosby.

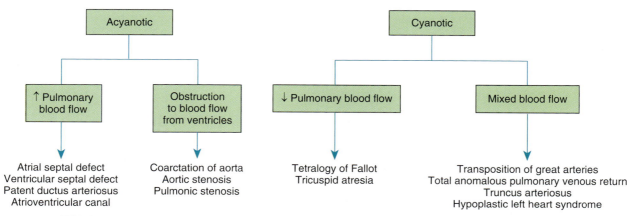

FIGURE 25.1 Comparison of Acyanotic–Cyanotic and Hemodynamic Classification Systems of Congenital Heart Disease. (From Hockenberry, M. J., & Wilson, D. [2015]. *Wong's nursing care of infants and children* [10th ed.]. Mosby.)

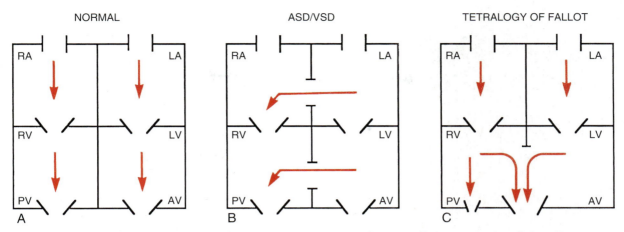

FIGURE 25.2 Shunting of Blood in Congenital Heart Disease. **A**, Normal. **B**, Acyanotic defect. **C**, Cyanotic defect. *ASD*, Atrial septal defect; *AV*, aortic valve; *LA*, left atrium; *LV*, left ventricle; *PV*, pulmonic valve; *RA*, right atrium; *RV*, right ventricle; *VSD*, ventricular septal defect. (From Hockenberry, M. J., & Wilson, D. [2015]. *Wong's nursing care of infants and children* [10th ed.]. Mosby.)

pulmonary circulation. Because blood continues to flow through the lungs before passing into the systemic circulation, there is no decrease in tissue oxygenation or cyanosis. Thus defects that cause left-to-right shunt are termed **acyanotic heart defects**. Other types of acyanotic heart defects obstruct blood flow from the ventricles but do not cause shunting. **Cyanotic heart defects** frequently cause shunting of blood from the right side of the heart directly into the left side of the heart (**right-to-left shunt**). This type of shunt decreases blood flow through the pulmonary system, causing less than normal oxygen delivery to the tissues and resultant cyanosis (see Chapter 27). Tetralogy of Fallot (TOF) occurs in 5 to 10% of all CHD and is the most common cyanotic heart defect.[2] In this condition, narrowing of the pulmonary outflow tract increases right heart pressures, thus forcing blood through a defect in the ventricular septum into the left heart (Figure 25.2C). **Cyanosis**, a bluish discoloration of the skin indicating that tissues are not receiving normal amounts of oxygen, also can be caused by other types of heart defects that result in the mixing of venous and arterial blood that enter the systemic circulation.

Most congenital heart defects are named to describe the underlying defect (e.g., valvular abnormalities; abnormal openings in the septa, including persistence of the foramen ovale; continued patency of the ductus arteriosus; and malformation or abnormal placement of the great vessels). Descriptions of the most common defects follow.

Obstructive Defects

Coarctation of the Aorta

PATHOPHYSIOLOGY **Coarctation of the aorta (COA)** is an abnormal localized narrowing of the aorta just proximal to the insertion of the ductus arteriosus. Before birth, the ductus arteriosus bypasses this obstruction and allows blood to flow from the pulmonary artery into the distal aorta. However, once the ductus functionally closes within 15 hours after birth, blood flow to the lower extremities is then restricted by the coarctation. Clinically, there is increased blood pressure proximal to the defect (head and upper extremities, right greater than left) and decreased blood pressure distal to the obstruction (torso and lower extremities) (Figure 25.3).

CLINICAL MANIFESTATIONS The location and severity of the COA determine whether an infant will become symptomatic after the ductus arteriosus closes. If the COA is severe, infants will present with low cardiac output, poor tissue perfusion, acidosis, and hypotension. Physical examination of the infant will reveal weak or absent femoral pulses. Children with undiagnosed COA will present with unexplained upper extremity hypertension.[1,2]

EVALUATION AND TREATMENT Physical examination and measurement of upper and lower extremity blood pressures will often suggest the diagnosis. Echocardiography, magnetic resonance imaging (MRI), and cardiac catheterization may be needed to confirm the diagnosis. Initial treatment in the symptomatic newborn consists of continuous intravenous infusion of prostaglandin E_1 to maintain the patency of the ductus arteriosus. Once the symptomatic newborn is stabilized, surgical correction is indicated.[4]

Surgical correction consists of either resection of the narrowed portion of the aorta with an end-to-end anastomosis or enlargement of the constricted section using a graft taken from a portion of the left subclavian artery. Because this defect is outside the heart and pericardium, cardiopulmonary bypass usually is not required and a thoracotomy incision is used. However, coarctation repair may be part of a more complex operation, which might require a sternotomy incision and cardiopulmonary bypass.

Studies have shown percutaneous balloon angioplasty with or without the use of a stent to be an effective, less invasive option for treating native COA or for reducing residual postoperative coarctation in most children.[1,2,5] Other complications include aneurysm formation and blood vessel injury from arterial access.

Aortic Stenosis

PATHOPHYSIOLOGY **Aortic stenosis (AS)** is a narrowing or stricture of the left ventricular outlet, causing resistance of blood flow from the left ventricle into the aorta (Figure 25.4). The physiological consequence of severe AS is hypertrophy of the left ventricular wall, which eventually leads to increased end-diastolic pressure, resulting in pulmonary venous and pulmonary arterial hypertension. If severe, there may be decreased cardiac output and pulmonary vascular congestion. Left ventricular hypertrophy impedes coronary artery perfusion and may result in subendocardial ischemia and associated papillary muscle dysfunction that cause mitral insufficiency.

There are three types of AS. **Valvular aortic stenosis** occurs as a consequence of malformed or fused cusps, resulting in a unicuspid or

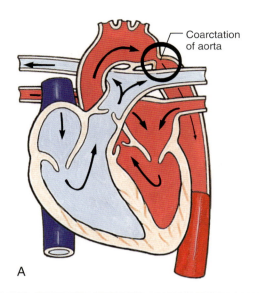

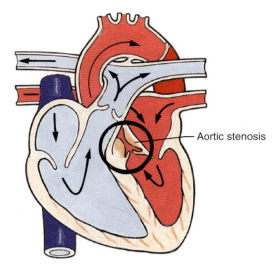

FIGURE 25.4 Aortic Stenosis. Narrowing of the aortic valve causing resistance to blood flow in the left ventricle, decreased cardiac output, left ventricular hypertrophy, and pulmonary congestion. (From Hockenberry, M. J., & Wilson, D. [Eds.]. [2013]. *Wong's essentials of pediatric nursing* [9th ed.]. Mosby.)

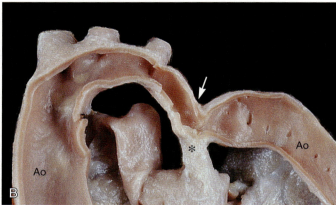

FIGURE 25.3 Postductal and Preductal Coarctation of the Aorta. A, Postductal coarctation occurs distal to ("after") the insertion of the closed ductus arteriosus into the aortic arch. Preductal coarctation occurs proximal to ("before") the insertion of the patent ductus arteriosus. The coarctation consists of a flap of tissue that protrudes from the tunica media of the aortic wall. **B,** Coarctation of the aorta with typical indentation of the aortic wall *(arrow)* opposite the ductal arterial ligament *(asterisk). Ao,* Aorta. ([A], from Hockenberry, M. J., & Wilson, D. [2013]. *Wong's essentials of pediatric nursing* [9th ed.]. Mosby; [B], from Damjanov, I., & Linder, J. [Eds.]. [1996]. *Anderson's pathology* [10th ed.]. Mosby.)

bicuspid valve. Valvular AS is a serious defect because (1) the obstruction tends to be progressive; (2) there may be sudden episodes of myocardial ischemia or low cardiac output that, on rare occasions, can result in sudden death in late childhood or adolescence; and (3) surgical repair will not result in a normal valve.[1,2]

Subvalvular aortic stenosis is a stricture caused by a fibrous ring below a normal valve. It can also be caused by a narrowed left ventricular outflow tract in combination with a small aortic valve annulus. **Supravalvular aortic stenosis**, a narrowing of the aorta just above the valve, occurs infrequently.[6]

CLINICAL MANIFESTATIONS Infants with significant AS demonstrate signs of decreased cardiac output with faint pulses, hypotension, tachycardia, and poor feeding. A loud, harsh systolic ejection murmur is expected. Older children also may have complaints of exercise intolerance and, rarely, chest pain. Children are at risk for bacterial endocarditis, although prophylaxis with antibiotics is no longer routinely recommended (see *Health Promotion:* Endocarditis Risk).

EVALUATION AND TREATMENT Valvular AS diagnosis is confirmed by echocardiography. Mild to moderate valvular AS does not usually require intervention or restriction of activity. Treatment of severe valvular AS varies, with nonsurgical palliation the initial treatment of choice by many interventional cardiologists. Dilation of the stenotic valve with balloon angioplasty, which is performed in the cardiac catheterization laboratory, still carries a high morbidity and mortality in the critically ill neonate; however, in older infants and children it compares favourably with surgical valvotomy.[5] Balloon angioplasty is, however, associated with the risk for aortic regurgitation (insufficiency). Children undergoing this procedure almost always require surgical intervention at some time to relieve recurrent narrowing or worsening regurgitation.[5]

Surgical treatment for valvular AS depends on the severity of the stenosis, previous interventions, and age of the child. Aortic valve commissurotomy or valvotomy may be used as an early intervention. Aortic valve replacement may be required if the valve is severely dysplastic. Mechanical valve replacement is usually deferred as long as possible to minimize the number of valve replacements related to growth. AS requires lifelong evaluation and treatment. Multiple surgical or catheterization interventions are expected.

Pulmonary Stenosis

PATHOPHYSIOLOGY **Pulmonary stenosis (PS)** is a narrowing or stricture of the pulmonary valve that causes resistance to blood flow from the right ventricle to the pulmonary artery (Figure 25.5). Generally, moderate to severe stenosis causes right ventricular hypertrophy. **Pulmonary atresia** is an extreme form of PS with total fusion of the valve leaflets (blood cannot flow to the lungs); the right ventricle may be hypoplastic. In some cases of right ventricular outflow obstruction, the narrowing is below the valve (infundibular or subvalve PS).

CLINICAL MANIFESTATIONS Most infants are asymptomatic if the PS is mild to moderate. Newborns with severe PS or pulmonary atresia

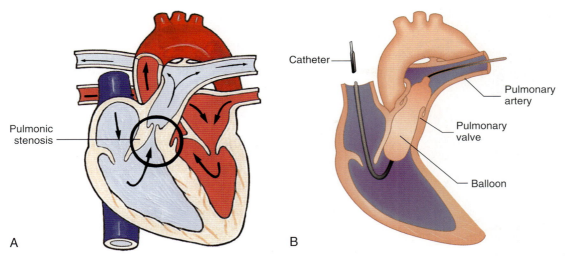

FIGURE 25.5 Pulmonary Stenosis. A, The pulmonary valve narrows at the entrance of the pulmonary artery. **B,** Balloon angioplasty is used to dilate the valve. A catheter is inserted across the stenotic pulmonic valve into the pulmonary artery, and a balloon at the end of the catheter is inflated while it is positioned across the narrowed valve opening. ([A], from Hockenberry, M. J., & Wilson, D. [Eds.]. [2013]. *Wong's essentials of pediatric nursing* [9th ed.]. Mosby.)

HEALTH PROMOTION
Endocarditis Risk

Children with CHD are at risk of developing endocarditis. According to the Canadian Dental Association (CDA), only those patients at greatest risk of developing infective endocarditis must receive short-term prophylactic antibiotics before common, routine dental and surgical procedures, because the risks of taking prophylactic antibiotics outweigh the benefits for most patients. The CDA supports the growing body of evidence that promotes dental hygiene and care rather than prophylactic antibiotics and emphasizes the importance of achieving and maintaining excellent oral health and practising daily oral hygiene.

In Canada, dental plans are available to only 26% of low-income workers. Among the 74% of these lower-income workers without plans, only 39% are seen by a dentist on a yearly basis.

The CDA recommends that people with the following should take prophylactic antibiotics before routine dental and surgical procedures:
- Prosthetic cardiac valve
- History of infective endocarditis
- Serious congenital heart conditions
- Repaired congenital heart defect with prosthetic material or device
- Repaired congenital heart defect with residual defect at the site or adjacent to the site of a prosthetic patch or a prosthetic device
- A cardiac transplant that develops a problem in a heart valve

The CDA suggests that prophylactic antibiotics are no longer needed for patients with the following conditions:
- Mitral valve prolapse
- Rheumatic heart disease
- Bicuspid valve disease
- Calcified aortic stenosis
- Congenital heart conditions such as ventricular septal defect, atrial septal defect, and hypertrophic cardiomyopathy

Data from American Heart Association. (2017). *What is infective endocarditis?* https://www.heart.org/-/media/files/health-topics/answers-by-heart/what-is-infective-endocarditis.pdf?la=en; Canadian Dental Association. (2014). *CDA position on prevention of infective endocarditis.* https://www.cda-adc.ca/_files/position_statements/infectiousEndocarditis.pdf; Mikkonen, J., & Raphael, D. (2010). *Social determinants of health: the Canadian facts* (p. 39). York University School of Health Policy and Management. http://www.thecanadianfacts.org/the_canadian_facts.pdf.

---

will be cyanotic (from a right-to-left shunt through an ASD) and may have signs of decreased cardiac output. A harsh systolic murmur is expected with PS. Pulmonary atresia produces a continuous murmur.

EVALUATION AND TREATMENT Echocardiography confirms the diagnosis and determines the severity of the PS. The treatment of choice for infants with moderate-to-severe PS is balloon angioplasty (Figure 25.5B). A catheter with a special balloon device is used to dilate the area of narrowing. Multiple studies have proven the effectiveness and safety of balloon angioplasty in reducing the pressure gradient across the pulmonic valve.[5] In rare cases, surgical valvotomy may be required. Pulmonary blood flow is supported with prostaglandin E_1 infusion to maintain the patency of the ductus arteriosus in cases of pulmonary atresia with right ventricle–dependent coronary circulation in the neonatal period until surgery is performed to supply pulmonary blood flow.[5]

Both balloon dilation and surgical valvotomy leave the pulmonary valve incompetent (insufficient); however, most children are usually able to tolerate pulmonary valve incompetence and are asymptomatic. Long-term problems with restenosis are rare for uncomplicated PS.[1,2,5]

Defects With Increased Pulmonary Blood Flow
Patent Ductus Arteriosus

PATHOPHYSIOLOGY Patent ductus arteriosus (PDA) is failure of the fetal ductus arteriosus (artery connecting the aorta and pulmonary artery) to functionally close within the first 15 hours after birth. However, several weeks after birth (Figure 25.6) may be needed for attainment of true anatomical closure, in which the ductus loses the ability to reopen. The continued patency of this vessel allows blood to flow from the higher-pressure aorta to the lower-pressure pulmonary artery, causing a left-to-right shunt.

shunt from the left atrium to the right atrium.[7] Left-to-right shunting of blood can occur with a large ASD.

Another opening in the atrial septal wall that is part of normal fetal communication, which usually closes after birth, is the foramen ovale. When the lungs become functional at birth, the pulmonary pressure decreases and the left atrial pressure exceeds that of the right. The pressure change forces the septum to functionally close the foramen ovale. If it does not close, it is called a patent foramen ovale (PFO). About one out of four adults has a PFO without CHD; however, in children with CHD, the foramen ovale often remains open.

CLINICAL MANIFESTATIONS Infants with a large ASD may develop pulmonary overcirculation and slow growth. Some older children and adults will experience shortness of breath with activity as the right ventricle becomes less compliant with age. A systolic ejection murmur and a widely split second heart sound are the expected findings on physical examination.

EVALUATION AND TREATMENT Diagnosis is confirmed by echocardiography. The ASD may be closed surgically with primary repair (sutured closed) or with a patch (pericardium or Dacron). Surgical repair involves open-heart surgery with cardiopulmonary bypass. Catheterization device closure offers a less invasive alternative for children with an ASD that meets anatomical and size criteria.[8] All options have low morbidity and mortality.

Ventricular Septal Defect

PATHOPHYSIOLOGY A ventricular septal defect (VSD) is an opening of the septal wall between the ventricles. VSDs are the most common type of congenital heart defect and account for 15 to 20% of all such defects.[2] VSDs are similar to ASDs in that blood will shunt from left to right. Left-to-right shunting of blood can occur with a large VSD. Depending on the size and location, many VSDs close spontaneously, most often within the first 2 years of life.

CLINICAL MANIFESTATIONS Depending on the size and degree of shunting and pulmonary vascular resistance (PVR), children may have no symptoms or have clinical effects from excessive pulmonary blood flow. In the infant, excessive pulmonary blood flow from left-to-right shunting causes dyspnea and tachypnea symptoms, commonly referred to as *heart failure* (HF), even though the heart muscle functions well with a VSD. A holosystolic (pansystolic) murmur is expected.

If the degree of shunting is significant and not corrected, the child is at risk of developing pulmonary hypertension.

EVALUATION AND TREATMENT Diagnosis is confirmed by echocardiography. Cardiac catheterization may be needed to calculate the degree of shunting and to directly measure the pressures in the heart. Smaller VSDs require minimal treatment and may close completely or become small enough that surgical closure is not required. If the infant has severe HF or failure to thrive that is unmanageable with medical therapy, early surgical repair is performed. Surgical repair involves open-heart surgery with cardiopulmonary bypass. The opening is either sutured closed (primary) or covered with a patch (pericardium or Dacron). Nonsurgical device closure is available but only under restricted conditions.[5,9] Endocarditis prophylaxis is only recommended for 6 months after surgical or device closure and indefinitely with a residual VSD after patch closure.[9]

Atrioventricular Canal Defect

PATHOPHYSIOLOGY Atrioventricular canal (AVC) defect, also known as atrioventricular septal defect (AVSD) or by the traditional term endocardial cushion defect (ECD), is the result of incomplete

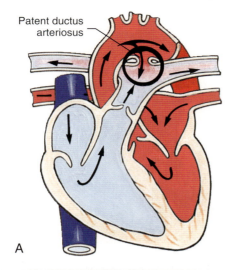

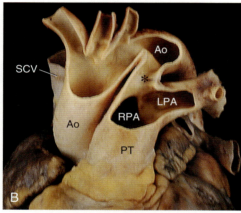

FIGURE 25.6 Patent Ductus Arteriosus. A, Patent ductus arteriosus (PDA) with left-to-right shunt. **B,** PDA in an adult with pulmonary hypertension. *Ao,* Aorta; *LPA,* left pulmonary artery; *PT,* pulmonary trunk; *RPA,* right pulmonary artery; *SCV,* subclavian vein. ([A], from Hockenberry, M. J., & Wilson, D. [2013]. *Wong's essentials of pediatric nursing* [9th ed.]. St. Louis: Mosby; [B], from Damjanov, I., & Linder, J. [Eds.]. [1996]. *Anderson's pathology* [10th ed.]. Mosby.)

CLINICAL MANIFESTATIONS Infants may be asymptomatic or show signs of pulmonary overcirculation, such as dyspnea, fatigue, and poor feeding. There is a characteristic machinery like murmur in both systole and diastole. Aortic flow (run-off) into the lower pressure pulmonary circulation produces low diastolic blood pressure, widened pulse pressure, and bounding pulses. Children are at risk for bacterial endocarditis and may develop pulmonary hypertension in later life from chronic excessive pulmonary blood flow.

EVALUATION AND TREATMENT Diagnosis is confirmed with echocardiography. Administration of indomethacin (Indocin, a prostaglandin inhibitor) has proved successful in closing a PDA in premature infants and some newborns. Surgical division of the PDA through a left thoracotomy also may be done; in some cases the procedure can be performed with thoracoscopy. Closure with an occlusion device during cardiac catheterization is performed in select children older than 6 months of age. Both surgical and nonsurgical procedures are considered low risk.[2,5]

Atrial Septal Defect

PATHOPHYSIOLOGY An atrial septal defect (ASD) is an opening in the septal wall between the two atria. This opening allows blood to

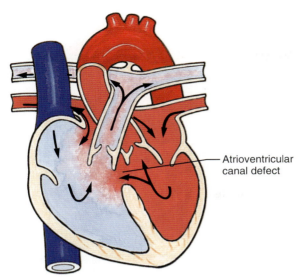

FIGURE 25.7 Atrioventricular Canal Defect. (From Hockenberry, M. J., & Wilson, D. [2013]. *Wong's essentials of pediatric nursing* [9th ed.]. Mosby.)

fusion of endocardial cushions (Figure 25.7). AVC defect consists of an ostium primum ASD and inlet VSD with associated abnormalities of the atrioventricular valve tissue. These valve abnormalities range from a cleft in the mitral valve to a common mitral and tricuspid valve. The directions and pathways of flow are determined by pulmonary and systemic resistance, left and right ventricular pressures, and the compliance of each chamber. Flow is generally from left to right. AVC defect is a common cardiac defect in children with Down syndrome. However, children with this defect can have a normal karyotype.

CLINICAL MANIFESTATIONS Infants with this defect often display moderate to severe HF attributable to left-to-right shunting and pulmonary overcirculation. Infants with pulmonary hypertension and high pulmonary resistance have less shunting and therefore minimal signs of HF. There may be mild cyanosis that increases with crying. Those with a large left-to-right shunt will have a murmur, and those with minimal shunt may not have a murmur. Children with AVC defect are at risk of developing irreversible pulmonary hypertension if left surgically untreated.

EVALUATION AND TREATMENT AVC defect is one of the most frequent diagnoses made with fetal echocardiography. Cardiac catheterization usually is not needed. Initial treatment goals include aggressive medical management of HF and nutritional supplementation. Complete surgical repair is most common and typically performed between 3 and 6 months of age to prevent irreversible pulmonary hypertension. This procedure consists of patch closure of the septal defects and reconstruction of the atrioventricular (AV) valve tissue (either repair of the mitral valve cleft or fashioning of two AV valves). If the mitral valve defect is severe, valve replacement may be needed.

Defects With Decreased Pulmonary Blood Flow
Tetralogy of Fallot
PATHOPHYSIOLOGY The classic form of **tetralogy of Fallot (TOF)** includes four defects: (1) VSD, (2) PS, (3) overriding aorta, and (4) right ventricular hypertrophy (Figure 25.8). The pathophysiology varies widely, depending not only on the degree of PS but also on the pulmonary and systemic vascular resistance to flow. If total resistance to

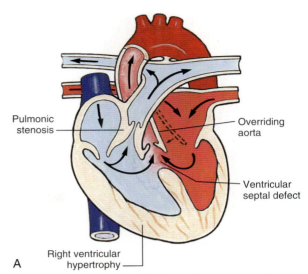

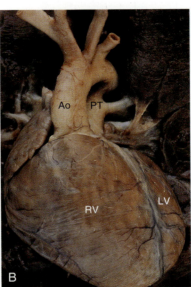

FIGURE 25.8 Tetralogy of Fallot. **A**, Tetralogy of Fallot hemodynamics. **B**, Right ventricular hypertrophy and overriding aorta *(Ao)*. *LV*, Left ventricle; *PT*, pulmonary trunk; *RV*, right ventricle. ([A], from Hockenberry, M. J., & Wilson, D. [2013]. *Wong's essentials of pediatric nursing* [9th ed.]. St. Louis: Mosby; [B], from Damjanov, I., & Linder, J. [Eds.]. [1996]. *Anderson's pathology* [10th ed.]. Mosby.)

pulmonary flow is greater than systemic resistance, the shunt is from right to left. If systemic resistance is more than pulmonary resistance, the shunt is from left to right. PS decreases blood flow to the lungs and, consequently, the amount of oxygenated blood that returns to the left heart. Physiological compensation to chronic, severe hypoxia includes production of more red blood cells (polycythemia), development of collateral bronchial vessels, and enlargement of the nail beds (clubbing).

CLINICAL MANIFESTATIONS Some infants may be acutely cyanotic at birth. In others, progression of hypoxia and cyanosis may be more gradual over the first year of life as the PS worsens. Acute episodes of cyanosis and hypoxia can occur, called *hypercyanotic spells*, *blue spells*, or *"tet" spells*. These spells (increased right-to-left shunt) may occur during crying or after feeding. Oxygen has little effect in improving

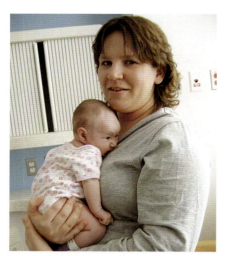

FIGURE 25.9 Infant Held in a Knee–Chest Position. (From Hockenberry, M. J., & Wilson, D. [2013]. *Wong's essentials of pediatric nursing* [9th ed.]. Mosby.)

hypoxemia, but placing the infant in a knee–chest position (Figure 25.9) and administering morphine sulphate subcutaneously or intravenously is most commonly used to treat "tet" spells. If prolonged or frequent, these spells are an indication for emergent evaluation and surgical treatment.

Chronic cyanosis may cause clubbing of the fingers and poor growth in children. Squatting or the knee–chest position can help with cyanosis in these children because it increases peripheral resistance in the systemic circulation, which causes an increase in pressures in the left heart and consequent reduction in right-to-left shunting and improvement in pulmonary perfusion. Children with unrepaired TOF are at risk for emboli, stroke, brain abscess, seizures, and loss of consciousness or sudden death following a "tet" spell.

EVALUATION AND TREATMENT Diagnosis is confirmed with echocardiography. Elective surgical repair is usually performed in the first year of life. Indications for earlier repair include increasing cyanosis or the development of hypercyanotic spells. Complete repair involves closure of the VSD, resection of the infundibular stenosis, and application of a pericardial patch to enlarge the right ventricular outflow tract that can extend across the pulmonary valve annulus (transannular patch).

Tricuspid Atresia

PATHOPHYSIOLOGY Tricuspid atresia is failure of the tricuspid valve to develop; consequently, there is no communication from right atrium to right ventricle (Figure 25.10). Blood flows through an ASD or a PFO to the left atrium and through a VSD to the right ventricle. This condition is often associated with PS or transposition of the great arteries. There is complete mixing of unoxygenated and oxygenated blood in the left side of the heart, resulting in systemic desaturation and mild cyanosis. The physiological process that causes lesion development is variable, depending on the great vessel anatomy and amount of PS.

CLINICAL MANIFESTATIONS A murmur is noted, and cyanosis is usually seen in the newborn period. Tachycardia, dyspnea, fatigue, and poor feeding may be noted with excessive pulmonary blood flow. Older children may have signs of chronic hypoxemia with clubbing. Children are at risk for bacterial endocarditis, brain abscess, and stroke.

EVALUATION AND TREATMENT After diagnosis is confirmed by echocardiography, the neonate with decreased pulmonary blood flow

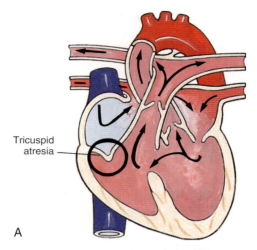

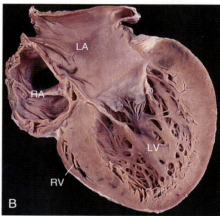

FIGURE 25.10 Tricuspid Atresia. **A**, Tricuspid atresia hemodynamics. **B**, Small right ventricle *(RV)* slit of ventricular septal defect; left ventricle *(LV)* is enlarged. *LA*, Left atrium; *RA*, right atrium. ([A], from Hockenberry, M. J., & Wilson, D. [2013]. *Wong's essentials of pediatric nursing* [9th ed.]. Mosby; [B], from Damjanov, I., & Linder, J. [Eds.]. [1996]. *Anderson's pathology* [10th ed.]. Mosby.)

is treated with a continuous infusion of prostaglandin E_1 to maintain the patency of the ductus arteriosus until surgical intervention. If the ASD is restrictive, an atrial septostomy is performed during cardiac catheterization or under echocardiographic guidance.[10] Treatment is accomplished in staged procedures. Once the infant is stabilized, a Blalock-Taussig shunt (systemic to pulmonary artery anastomosis) is placed to increase blood flow to the lungs.

Further surgery is undertaken between 4 and 8 months of age, depending on the child's growth and degree of cyanosis. Surgical outcomes are best in the child with normal ventricular function and low PVR. For children with borderline PVR, a fenestration (opening) can be created in the baffle or graft to relieve high systemic pulmonary venous pressures if needed.

Postoperative complications that increase hospital stay include pleural and pericardial effusions, elevated PVR, and ventricular dysfunction.

Mixing Defects

Transposition of the Great Arteries or Transposition of the Great Vessels

PATHOPHYSIOLOGY In transposition of the great arteries (TGA) or transposition of the great vessels (TGV), the pulmonary artery

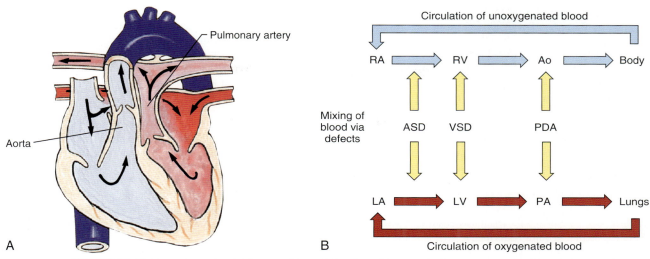

FIGURE 25.11 Hemodynamics in Transposition of the Great Vessels. **A,** Complete transposition of the great vessels with an intact interventricular septum. The aorta arises from the right ventricle and the pulmonary artery from the left ventricle. **B,** Oxygen saturation in the two, parallel circuits. *Ao,* Aorta; *ASD,* atrial septal defect; *LA,* left atrium; *LV,* left ventricle; *PA,* pulmonary artery; *PDA,* patent ductus arteriosus; *RA,* right atrium; *RV,* right ventricle; *VSD,* ventricular septal defect. ([A], from Hockenberry, M. J., & Wilson, D. [2013]. *Wong's essentials of pediatric nursing* [9th ed.]. Mosby.)

leaves the left ventricle and the aorta exits the right ventricle (Figure 25.11). Associated defects, such as ASD, VSD, or PDA, permit mixing of saturated and desaturated blood, which maintains adequate tissue oxygenation for a limited time.

CLINICAL MANIFESTATIONS Clinical manifestations depend on the type and size of the associated defects. Children with limited communication between cardiac chambers are severely cyanotic, acidotic, and ill at birth. Those with large septal defects or a PDA may be less severely cyanotic but may have symptoms of pulmonary overcirculation. Classically, no murmur is heard unless there is an associated VSD.

EVALUATION AND TREATMENT Diagnosis is suspected by physical examination and confirmed with echocardiography. Administration of intravenous prostaglandin E_1 to maintain the patency of the ductus arteriosus may be initiated to temporarily increase oxygen delivery. Enlargement of the PFO by balloon atrial septostomy may be performed during cardiac catheterization or under echocardiographic guidance to increase mixing and maintain cardiac output.[5,10]

The most preferred type of surgical repair for TGA performed in the first weeks of life is the arterial switch procedure. It involves transecting the great arteries and anastomosing the main pulmonary artery to the native proximal aorta (just above the aortic valve) and anastomosing the ascending aorta to the native proximal pulmonary artery. The coronary arteries are moved with a "button" of tissue from the proximal aorta to the proximal pulmonary artery, creating a new aorta. Reimplantation of the coronary arteries is critical to the infant's survival, and the arteries must be reattached without torsion or kinking to provide the heart with its supply of oxygen. The advantage of the arterial switch procedure is the re-establishment of normal circulation with the left ventricle acting as the systemic pump. Potential complications of the arterial switch include narrowing at the great artery anastomoses, neoaortic valve regurgitation, or coronary artery insufficiency.[2] Long-term results for the arterial switch operation are usually good.

Total Anomalous Pulmonary Venous Connection

PATHOPHYSIOLOGY Total anomalous pulmonary venous connection (TAPVC) is a rare defect characterized by failure of the pulmonary veins to join the left atrium during cardiac development. TAPVC is also called *total anomalous pulmonary venous return* (TAPVR) or *total anomalous pulmonary venous drainage* (TAPVD) (Figure 25.12). The pulmonary venous return is connected to the right side of the circulation rather than to the left atrium.

The right atrium receives all the blood that normally would flow into the left atrium. As a result, the right side of the heart is enlarged and the left side, especially the left atrium, is smaller than normal. An associated ASD or PFO allows systemic venous blood to shunt from the right atrium to the left side of the heart. As a result, the oxygen saturation of the blood in both sides of the heart (and, ultimately, in the systemic arterial circulation) is the same. If the pulmonary blood flow is increased, pulmonary venous return is also large, and the amount of saturated blood is relatively high. However, if there is obstruction

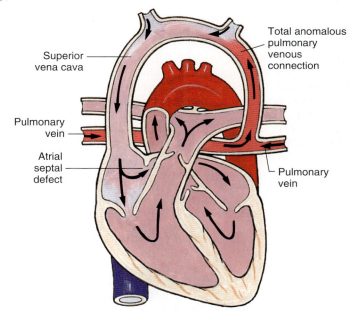

FIGURE 25.12 Total Anomalous Pulmonary Venous Connection.

to pulmonary venous drainage, the infant has severe cyanosis and low cardiac output. Infracardiac TAPVC often is associated with obstruction of pulmonary venous drainage and is a surgical emergency with higher mortality than the unobstructed types.

CLINICAL MANIFESTATIONS Most infants develop cyanosis early in life. The degree of cyanosis is inversely related to the amount of pulmonary blood flow. Children with unobstructed TAPVC may be asymptomatic until PVR decreases during infancy, increasing pulmonary blood flow, with resulting signs of pulmonary overcirculation. Cyanosis becomes worse with pulmonary vein obstruction; once obstruction occurs, the infant's condition usually deteriorates rapidly. Without intervention, cardiac failure will progress to death. Murmur is not a common feature of TAPVC.

EVALUATION AND TREATMENT Diagnosis is suspected with echocardiography but may require confirmative angiography. Corrective repair is usually required in early infancy. The surgical approach varies with the anatomical defect. In general, however, the common pulmonary vein (venous confluence) is sutured to the left atrium, the ASD is closed, and the anomalous pulmonary venous connection or vertical vein may be ligated.

Truncus Arteriosus
PATHOPHYSIOLOGY Truncus arteriosus (TA) is failure of normal septation and division of the embryonic outflow tract into a pulmonary artery and an aorta, resulting in a single vessel that exits the heart. There is always an associated VSD with mixing of the systemic and arterial circulations (Figure 25.13), causing some degree of cyanosis. Blood ejected from the heart flows preferentially to the lower-pressure pulmonary arteries, causing increased pulmonary blood flow.

CLINICAL MANIFESTATIONS Most infants are symptomatic with moderate HF and variable cyanosis, poor growth, and activity intolerance. Children are at risk for brain abscess and bacterial endocarditis.

EVALUATION AND TREATMENT Diagnosis is made by echocardiography. Corrective repair is a modification of the Rastelli procedure and is performed in the first few weeks or months of life. It involves closing the VSD so that the TA receives the outflow from the left ventricle and excising the pulmonary arteries from the aorta and attaching them to the right ventricle by means of a homograft (cadaver) conduit. These children require additional procedures to replace the conduit since its size becomes inadequate in relation to growth or narrows because of calcification over time.

Hypoplastic Left Heart Syndrome
PATHOPHYSIOLOGY Hypoplastic left heart syndrome (HLHS) is underdevelopment of the left side of the heart. Features include small left atrium, small or absent mitral valve, small or absent left ventricle, and small or absent aortic valve. Coarctation also is expected (Figure 25.14). Most blood from the left atrium flows across the PFO to the right atrium, to the right ventricle, and out of the pulmonary artery. The descending aorta receives blood from the PDA supplying systemic blood flow and filling the aorta and coronary arteries as well.

CLINICAL MANIFESTATIONS HLHS presents in the early newborn period as mild cyanosis, tachypnea, and low cardiac output if not already detected by fetal echocardiography. Support of the systemic circulation is accomplished with prostaglandin E_1 infusion. If HLHS is not suspected and the PDA closes, there is progressive deterioration with cyanosis and decreased cardiac output, leading to cardiovascular collapse. If untreated, HLHS is usually fatal in the first months of life.

EVALUATION AND TREATMENT Echocardiography shows all of the features of HLHS. Cardiac catheterization is rarely required. A multistage surgical repair approach is used. Infants successfully treated for HLHS have improved survival rates related to advances in surgical and medical technology. Long-term (10 to 15 years) health problems after the Fontan procedure related to reduced right ventricular function and high central venous pressures have been reported to impact quality of life.[11,12]

Heart Failure

> ✓ **QUICK CHECK 25.2**
> 1. Why is it critical to recognize and treat children during the acute phase of Kawasaki disease?
> 2. Discuss the causes of obesity in children and the cardiovascular effects.

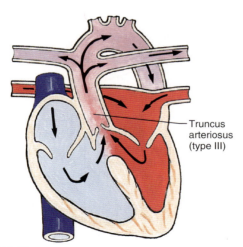

FIGURE 25.13 Truncus Arteriosus. The truncus arteriosus (TA) fails to divide into the pulmonary artery and aorta, and the interventricular septum fails to close at the top. Blood from both ventricles mixes in the TA and then enters the pulmonary and systemic circuits. (From Hockenberry, M. J., & Wilson, D. [2013]. *Wong's essentials of pediatric nursing* [9th ed.]. Mosby.)

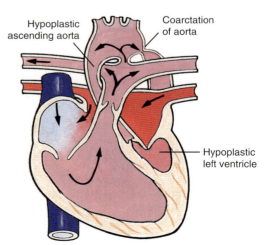

FIGURE 25.14 Hypoplastic Left Heart Syndrome. (From Hockenberry, M. J., & Wilson, D. [Eds.]. [2009]. *Wong's essentials of pediatric nursing* [8th ed.]. Mosby.)

TABLE 25.3 Causes of Heart Failure Resulting From Congenital Heart Disease

Age of Onset	Cause
At birth	HLHS
	Volume overload lesions
	Severe tricuspid or pulmonary insufficiency
	Large systemic AV fistula
First week	TGA
	PDA in small premature infants
	HLHS (with more favourable anatomy)
	TAPVR, particularly those with pulmonary venous obstruction
	Others
	Systemic AV fistula
	Critical AS or PS
1–4 weeks	COA with associated anomalies
	Critical AS
	Large left-to-right shunt lesions (VSD, PDA) in premature infants
	All other lesions previously listed
4–6 weeks	Some left-to-right shunt lesions, such as AVSD
6 weeks to 4 months	Large VSD
	Large PDA
	Others, such as anomalous left coronary artery from PA

AS, Aortic stenosis; *AV*, atrioventricular; *AVSD*, atrioventricular septal defect; *COA*, coarctation of the aorta; *HLHS*, hypoplastic left heart syndrome; *PA*, pulmonary artery; *PDA*, patent ductus arteriosus; *PS*, pulmonary stenosis; *TAPVR*, total anomalous pulmonary venous return; *TGA*, transposition of the great arteries; *VSD*, ventricular septal defect.
Modified from Park, M. K. (2014). *Pediatric cardiology for practitioners* (6th ed.). Mosby.

BOX 25.1 Clinical Manifestations of Heart Failure

Impaired Myocardial Function
Tachycardia
Sweating (inappropriate)
Decreased urinary output
Fatigue
Weakness
Restlessness
Anorexia
Pale, cool extremities
Weak peripheral pulses
Decreased blood pressure
Gallop rhythm
Cardiomegaly

Pulmonary Congestion
Tachypnea
Dyspnea

Retractions (infants)
Flaring nares
Exercise intolerance
Orthopnea
Cough, hoarseness
Cyanosis
Wheezing
Grunting

Systemic Venous Congestion
Weight gain
Hepatomegaly
Peripheral edema, especially periorbital
Ascites
Neck vein distension

From Hockenberry, M. J., & Wilson, D. (Eds.). (2013). *Wong's essentials of pediatric nursing* (9th ed.). Mosby.

Heart failure (HF) is a common complication of many congenital heart defects. HF occurs when the heart is unable to maintain sufficient cardiac output to meet the metabolic demands of the body. The most common congenital causes of HF in infancy and childhood are listed in Table 25.3. Classic HF in children also can be acquired, usually resulting from cardiomyopathies, dysrhythmias, or electrolyte disturbances. Pulmonary overcirculation from a large left-to-right shunt is often called *heart failure* but is not usually associated with decreased ventricular function and failure to meet metabolic demands. However, the clinical manifestations are similar, such as failure to thrive, tachypnea, tachycardia, and exercise intolerance.[2]

In general, the pathophysiological mechanisms of HF in infants and children are similar to those in adults. It is most often a result of decreased left ventricular systolic function and the associated left atrial and pulmonary venous hypertension and pulmonary venous congestion. The same compensatory mechanisms are activated in the face of inadequate cardiac output. Right ventricular failure is rare in childhood.

Left ventricular failure in infants is manifested as poor feeding and sucking, often leading to failure to thrive. In left ventricular failure, dyspnea, tachypnea, and diaphoresis may be accompanied by retractions, grunting, and nasal flaring. Wheezing, coughing, and rales are rare in childhood HF.[1,2,13] Common skin changes, such as pallor or mottling, are often present (Box 25.1). Signs of systemic venous congestion, such as hepatomegaly, weight gain, ascites, and peripheral edema, can be present but could be suggestive of other medical conditions such as renal or nutritional deficiencies.

A thorough physical examination with emphasis on cardiac and pulmonary findings will often reveal the degree of HF. Plotting a child's growth (height, weight, head circumference) is an important method of assessing a child's health. Infants with HF or pulmonary overcirculation usually have low weight with normal length and head circumference measurements. The failure to thrive is usually the result of increased metabolic expenditure relative to caloric intake. An electrocardiogram (ECG) also should be performed to determine the presence of dysrhythmia or hypertrophy. A chest X-ray is useful in assessing the presence of cardiomegaly and signs of increased pulmonary circulation or pulmonary edema with echocardiography to assess impaired function and possible etiology. B-type natriuretic peptide (BNP) has emerged as another diagnostic test of HF in children to confirm or exclude a cardiac cause for the symptoms.[2,14]

Treatment is aimed at decreasing cardiac workload and increasing the efficiency of heart function. Severe CHD is typically managed with surgical repair if applicable. Medical management initially consists of diuretics, such as furosemide (Lasix). Depending on the degree of HF, other diuretics can be used in combination with furosemide to counteract potassium losses. Agents that reduce afterload, such as captopril (Capoten) or enalapril (Vasotec) and beta-blockers, are employed to further manage severe HF.[1,2,13] Children with end-stage HF on maximal medical therapy can be supported on a ventricular assist device (VAD) while awaiting cardiac transplantation in severe cases that meet eligibility.[13]

ACQUIRED CARDIOVASCULAR DISORDERS

Acquired heart diseases refer to disease processes or abnormalities that occur after birth. They result from various causes, such as infection, genetic disorders, autoimmune processes in response to infection, environmental factors, or autoimmune diseases. Examples of acquired heart diseases include Kawasaki disease (KD), myocarditis, rheumatic heart disease, cardiomyopathy, and systemic hypertension. This chapter discusses KD and systemic hypertension. Myocarditis, rheumatic heart disease, and cardiomyopathy are discussed in Chapter 24.

Kawasaki Disease

Kawasaki disease (KD), formerly known as *mucocutaneous lymph node syndrome*, is an acute, usually self-limiting systemic vasculitis that may result in cardiac sequelae without treatment. Although KD occurs throughout the world, the greatest number of cases are seen in Japan.[1,2] KD's high prevalence in Japan reflects the genetic component of KD, with the case rate being highest among Asians and lower among White and Black children.

KD is primarily a condition of young children. Eighty percent of cases are seen in children younger than 5 years of age, with the incidence peaking in the toddler age group. Males are affected slightly more than females. The peak incidence is in the winter and spring.[1,2]

The etiology of KD remains unknown. Current etiological theories centre on an immunological response to an infectious, toxic, or antigenic substance.[2,14]

PATHOPHYSIOLOGY KD progresses pathologically and clinically in the following stages. In the early or acute phase, small capillaries, arterioles, and venules become inflamed, as does the heart itself. In the subacute state, inflammation spreads to larger vessels and aneurysms of the coronary arteries may develop. In the convalescent stage, medium-sized arteries begin the granulation process and may cause coronary artery thickening with increased risk for thrombosis. After the convalescent stage, inflammation wanes with potential scarring, calcification, and stenosis of the affected vessels.

CLINICAL MANIFESTATIONS The clinical course of KD progresses in three stages: acute, subacute, and convalescent. In the acute phase, the child with classic or typical KD has fever, conjunctivitis, oral changes ("strawberry" tongue), rash, erythema of the palms and soles, and lymphadenopathy, and is often irritable. During this phase, myocarditis may develop. The subacute phase begins when the fever ends and continues until the clinical signs have resolved. It is at this time that the child is most at risk for coronary artery aneurysm development. Desquamation of the palms and soles occurs at this time, as well as marked thrombocytosis. The convalescent phase is marked by the elevation of the erythrocyte sedimentation rate and C-reactive protein level, as well as by an increased platelet count. Arthritis or arthralgia of the joints may be present. This phase continues until all laboratory values return to normal—usually about 6 to 8 weeks after onset.[1,2] Atypical or "incomplete" KD can be seen in infants and children who lack the diagnostic criteria (have fewer than four signs) or "classic" physical findings. Recognition can be difficult and often results in delay of treatment with possible cardiovascular sequelae.[2,14]

EVALUATION AND TREATMENT The diagnostic criteria for KD are based on clinical features, which state that the child must exhibit fever for more than 5 days along with four of five criteria (Box 25.2). Children diagnosed with KD usually have leukocytosis, increased erythrocyte sedimentation rates, thrombocytosis, and elevated liver enzymes. An echocardiogram is obtained at the time of diagnosis as a baseline measurement to assess for coronary aneurysms or inflammation. Serial echocardiograms are obtained after treatment to assess for development of coronary aneurysms or regression of those present early in the course of the disease. Treatment includes oral administration of Aspirin and intravenous infusion of gamma globulin (most often only one dose). Aspirin is continued until the manifestations of inflammation are resolved but may be used indefinitely in children with residual coronary artery abnormalities.

Treatment with Aspirin and immunoglobulin during the acute phase has decreased the morbidity of KD and has reduced the incidence of coronary abnormalities from approximately 20% to less than 10% at 6 to 8 weeks after initiation of therapy. Most children recover completely from KD, including regression of aneurysms. The most common cardiovascular sequela is coronary thrombosis.[14]

> **BOX 25.2 Diagnostic Criteria for Kawasaki Disease**
>
> The child must exhibit five of the following six criteria, including fever:
> 1. Fever for 5 or more days (often diagnosed with shorter duration of fever if other symptoms are present)
> 2. Bilateral conjunctival infection without exudation
> 3. Changes in the oral mucous membranes, such as erythema, dryness, and fissuring of the lips; oropharyngeal reddening; or "strawberry tongue"
> 4. Changes in the extremities, such as peripheral edema, peripheral erythema, and desquamation of palms and soles, particularly periungual peeling
> 5. Polymorphous rash, often accentuated in the perineal area
> 6. Cervical lymphadenopathy (one lymph node >1.5 cm)
>
> Modified from Hockenberry, M. J., & Wilson, D. (Eds.). (2013). *Wong's essentials of pediatric nursing* (9th ed.). Mosby.

Multisystem Inflammatory Syndrome (MIS)

Severe acute respiratory syndrome coronavirus-2 (SARS-CoV-2), or COVID-19, was discovered in December 2019 and is caused by a novel coronavirus, a highly infectious pathogen. COVID-19 is structurally related to the virus that causes severe acute respiratory syndrome (SARS). The initial clinical sign of the SARS-CoV-2-related disease is usually pneumonia seen on x-ray. Reports also describe gastrointestinal symptoms and asymptomatic infections, especially among young children. The first known published case of classic KD associated with COVID-19 was reported in Hospital Pediatrics journal in late April 2020.[15]

It is logical, considering the temporal association, that KD-like illness is a post-infectious disease caused by SARS-CoV-2. Despite the temporal association, a causal link with COVID-19 has not been confirmed.[16] While evidence suggests that children are minimally impacted by COVID-19, recently physicians have noted a new syndrome resembling KD (vasculitis) in children. The syndrome was labelled pediatric multisystem inflammatory syndrome (MIS-C),[17] and is manifested by fever, rash, hypotension, gastrointestinal symptoms, and organ dysfunction. Patients eventually develop warm vasoplegic shock that rarely responds to fluid volume resuscitation.[18] Patients are also at risk of developing small pleural pericardial and ascitic effusions, suggestive of a systemic inflammatory process. Typical respiratory symptoms are not common.

While the multisystem inflammatory syndrome (MIS) resembles KD, the classic symptoms of KD (such as bilateral conjunctival injection, strawberry tongue, and rash) are often lacking.[19] Age of children affected with MIS-C appears to be higher than for classic KD which is usually age 3. Moreover, children of African descent are more likely to develop MIS-C, while KD is more common in children of Asian ancestry, reflecting an ethnic predisposition. Another difference is the presence of gastrointestinal symptoms in patients with SARS-COV-2, which has the potential to infect enterocytes via angiotensin converting enzyme 2 (ACE2) receptors being expressed in gastric epithelia, which can lead to diarrhea in approximately one-third of infected adults. The MIS associated with COVID-19 seems to present more gastrointestinal symptoms like vomiting, diarrhea, and abdominal pain compared to classical Kawasaki diseases.

Laboratory values indicate that MIS has more elevated CRP (C-reactive protein), D-dimer ferritin, elevated cardiac enzymes, and low lymphocyte count in complete blood count (CBC) than Kawasaki syndrome does.

In addition to multi-organ failure, the complications of MIS include thrombosis, ischemic events, and coronary aneurysms. ECG in patients with MIS usually is nonspecific, whereas echocardiography can show echo-bright coronary arteries that have the potential to progress to coronary aneurysm. Finally, it has been found that MIS-C presents with low platelet count, while KD presents with increased platelet count. Patients with MIS are treated with intravenous immunoglobulins and Aspirin. Aspirin should be withheld if the patient is at risk of bleeding. Children with MIS should be followed up by a cardiologist to rule out coronary abnormalities caused by the virus.

Systemic Hypertension

Systemic hypertension in children is defined as systolic and diastolic blood pressure levels greater than the 95th percentile for age and gender on at least three occasions (Tables 25.4 and 25.5). The Fourth Task Force on Blood Pressure Control in Children uses height as an additional criterion to the blood pressure guidelines.[1,20]

Hypertension is classified into two categories: primary (or essential) hypertension, in which a specific cause cannot be identified; and secondary hypertension, in which a cause *can* be identified (Box 25.3). Hypertension in children differs from adult hypertension in etiology and presentation. Young children, when diagnosed with hypertension, are often found to have secondary hypertension caused by some underlying disease, such as renal disease or COA (see Box 25.3). An increased prevalence of primary hypertension in older children has been noted. Researchers are now focusing on primary hypertension in older children in relation to morbidity and the presence of early atherosclerotic disease. Certain factors influence blood pressure in children. Children who are overweight are often hypertensive. Smoking also is associated with an increased risk for hypertension.[20-22]

PATHOPHYSIOLOGY In infants and children, a cause of hypertension is almost always found. In general, the younger the child with significant hypertension, the more likely a correctable cause can be determined. Therefore, a thorough evaluation needs to be performed.[2,21]

The pathophysiology of primary hypertension in children is not clearly understood but may result from a complex interaction of a strong predisposing genetic component with disturbances in sympathetic vascular smooth muscle tone, humoral agents (angiotensin, catecholamines), renal sodium excretion, and cardiac output. New studies have shown that an increased level of leptin, a hormone produced by adipose tissue, is associated with hypertension in obese children.[22] Ultimately, these factors impair the ability of the peripheral vascular bed to relax.

CLINICAL MANIFESTATIONS Most children with systemic hypertension are asymptomatic. It is necessary that a thorough history and physical examination be obtained. The examination should include an accurate blood pressure measurement obtained in the right arm with the arm supported at the level of the heart; three separate measurements using an appropriate-size cuff also are needed for an accurate blood pressure reading.[20-22]

EVALUATION AND TREATMENT In children, the history and physical examination should be directed at determining the etiology of hypertension, such as COA or renal disease (Table 25.6). A CBC, serum chemistry levels (including blood urea nitrogen and creatinine), uric acid level, urinalysis, urine culture, lipid profile, and renal ultrasound are part of the routine evaluation for renal disease (Table 25.7). Blood pressure differential between upper and lower extremities and echocardiography can be used to identify COA. If COA is found, surgical correction or balloon angioplasty with or without a stent is initiated, depending on the child's age and the severity of the coarctation. If hypertension is determined to be essential, or primary, in nature, nonpharmacological therapy is used initially. Moderate weight loss and exercise can decrease systolic and diastolic pressures in many children. Appropriate diet, regular physical activity, and avoidance of smoking have been shown to be effective in reducing blood pressure.[1] Ambulatory blood pressure monitoring (ABPM) has the potential to become an important tool in the evaluation and management of childhood hypertension.[23]

TABLE 25.4 Normative Blood Pressure Levels (Systolic/Diastolic [Mean]) by DINAMAP Monitor in Children 5 Years Old and Younger

Age	Mean BP Levels (mm Hg)	90th Percentile	95th Percentile
1–3 days	64/41 (50)	75/49 (50)	78/52 (62)
1 month to 2 years	95/58 (72)	106/68 (83)	110/71 (86)
2–5 years	101/57 (74)	112/66 (82)	115/68 (85)

BP, Blood pressure.
Data from Park, M. K. (2014). *Pediatric cardiology for practitioners* (6th ed.). Mosby; modified from Park, M. K., & Menard, S. M. (1989). *American Journal of Diseases in Children, 143*, 860.

TABLE 25.5 Auscultatory Blood Pressure Values for Boys and Girls Aged 6 to 17 Years (Systolic/Diastolic K5)

Age and Gender	Mean BP Levels (mm Hg)	90th Percentile	95th Percentile
6–7 years			
Boys	95–96 / 53–55	105–107 / 64–66	108–110 / 67–70
Girls	94–94 / 52–54	103–104 / 63–65	106–107 / 66–68
8–9 years			
Boys	97–99 / 56–57	108–109 / 68–68	111–113 / 71–71
Girls	96–98 / 56–56	106–108 / 67–67	109–111 / 70–70
10–11 years			
Boys	100–102 / 57–57	111–113 / 68–68	114–116 / 71–71
Girls	100–102 / 57–57	110–112 / 68–68	113–115 / 71–71
12–13 years			
Boys	105–108 / 56–56	116–118 / 68–68	119–122 / 71–71
Girls	104–105 / 57–57	113–115 / 68–68	116–118 / 71–71
14–15 years			
Boys	110–113 / 57–57	121–124 / 68–69	122–127 / 71–72
Girls	106–107 / 58–58	116–117 / 68–69	119–119 / 72–72
16–17 years			
Boys	114–114 / 59–62	125–125 / 71–73	128–128 / 74–77
Girls	107–108 / 59–59	117–118 / 69–70	120–121 / 73–73

BP, Blood pressure; K5, Korotkoff phase 5.
From Park, M. K. (2014). *Pediatric cardiology for practitioners* (6th ed.). Mosby.

BOX 25.3 Conditions Associated With Secondary Hypertension in Children

Renal
Renal parenchymal disease
    Glomerulonephritis, acute and chronic
    Pyelonephritis, acute and chronic
    Congenital anomalies (polycystic or dysplastic kidneys)
    Obstructive uropathies (hydronephrosis)
    Hemolytic-uremic syndrome
    Collagen disease (periarteritis, lupus)
    Renal damage from nephrotoxic medications, trauma, or radiation
Renovascular disease
    Renal artery disorders (e.g., stenosis, polyarteritis, thrombosis)
    Renal vein thrombosis

Cardiovascular
Coarctation of the aorta
Conditions with large stroke volume (patent ductus arteriosus, aortic insufficiency, systemic arteriovenous fistula, complete heart block) (these conditions cause only systolic hypertension)

Endocrine
Hyperthyroidism (systolic hypertension)
Excessive catecholamine levels
    Pheochromocytoma
    Neuroblastoma
Adrenal dysfunction
    Congenital adrenal hyperplasia
        11-β-Hydroxylase deficiency
        17-Hydroxylase deficiency
    Cushing's syndrome
    Hyperaldosteronism
        Primary
            Conn's syndrome
            Idiopathic nodular hyperplasia
            Dexamethasone-suppressible hyperaldosteronism
        Secondary
            Renovascular hypertension
            Renin-producing tumour (juxtaglomerular cell tumour)
Hyperparathyroidism (and hypercalcemia)

Neurogenic
Increased intracranial pressure (any cause, especially tumours, infections, trauma)
Poliomyelitis
Guillain-Barré syndrome
Dysautonomia (Riley-Day syndrome)

Medications and Chemicals
Sympathomimetic medications (nose drops, cough medications, cold preparations, theophylline [Uniphyl])
Amphetamines
Corticosteroids
Nonsteroidal anti-inflammatory drugs
Oral contraceptives
Heavy-metal poisoning (mercury, lead)
Cocaine, acute or chronic use
Cyclosporine
Thyroxine
Tacrolimus

Miscellaneous
Hypervolemia and hypernatremia
Stevens-Johnson syndrome
Bronchopulmonary dysplasia (newborns)

From Park, M. K. (2014). *Pediatric cardiology for practitioners* (6th ed.). Mosby.

Medication therapy is controversial in children with primary hypertension; however, when nonpharmacological therapy fails, the approach is similar to the treatment of hypertension in adults with the use of angiotensin-converting enzyme inhibitors or angiotensin receptor blocker medications.[2,20] The current emphasis on preventive cardiology, especially for children, is significant because many investigators believe signs of atherosclerosis are present during childhood.[1,20–22]

TABLE 25.6 Most Common Causes of Chronic Sustained Hypertension

Age Group	Causes
Newborn	Renal artery thrombosis, renal artery stenosis, congenital renal malformation, COA, bronchopulmonary dysplasia
<6 years	Renal parenchymal disease, COA, renal artery stenosis
6–10 years	Renal artery stenosis, renal parenchymal disease, primary hypertension
>10 years	Primary hypertension, renal parenchymal disease

COA, Coarctation of the aorta.
From Park, M. K. (2014). *Pediatric cardiology for practitioners* (6th ed.). Mosby.

TABLE 25.7 Routine and Special Laboratory Tests for Hypertension

Laboratory Tests	Significance of Abnormal Results
Urinalysis, urine culture, blood urea nitrogen, and creatinine levels	Renal parenchymal disease
Serum electrolyte levels (hypokalemia)	Hyperaldosteronism, primary or secondary
	Adrenogenital syndrome
	Renin-producing tumours
ECG, chest X-ray studies	Cardiac cause of hypertension, also baseline function
Intravenous pyelography (or ultrasonography, radionuclide studies, computed tomography of kidneys)	Renal parenchymal diseases
	Renovascular hypertension
	Tumours (neuroblastoma, Wilms tumour)
Plasma renin activity, peripheral	High-renin hypertension
	Renovascular hypertension
	Renin-producing tumours
	Some caused by Cushing's syndrome
	Some caused by essential hypertension
	Low-renin hypertension
	Adrenogenital syndrome
	Primary hyperaldosteronism
24-hr urine collection for 17-ketosteroids and 17-hydroxycorticosteroids	Cushing's syndrome
	Adrenogenital syndrome
24-hr urine collection for catecholamine levels and vanillylmandelic acid	Pheochromocytoma
	Neuroblastoma
Aldosterone	Hyperaldosteronism, primary or secondary
	Renovascular hypertension
	Renin-producing tumours
Renal vein plasma renin activity	Unilateral renal parenchymal disease
	Renovascular hypertension
Abdominal aortogram	Renovascular hypertension
	Abdominal COA
	Unilateral renal parenchymal diseases
	Pheochromocytoma
Intra-arterial digit subtraction angiography	Renovascular hypertension

COA, Coarctation of the aorta; *ECG*, electrocardiogram.
From Park, M. K. (2014). *Pediatric cardiology for practitioners* (6th ed.). Mosby.

DID YOU UNDERSTAND?

Congenital Heart Disease

1. Environmental risk factors associated with the incidence of CHD typically are (a) maternal conditions, including intrauterine viral infections, diabetes mellitus, medications, and complications of advanced maternal age; (b) antepartal bleeding; and (c) prematurity.
2. Genetic risk factors associated with CHD include, but are not limited to, Down syndrome, trisomies 13 and 18, cri du chat syndrome, and Turner's syndrome.
3. Classification of a congenital heart defect is based on (a) whether the defect causes cyanosis, (b) whether the defect causes increased or decreased blood flow into the pulmonary circulation, and (c) whether the defect causes obstruction of blood flow from the ventricles.
4. Acyanotic heart defects that increase pulmonary blood flow consist of abnormal openings (atrial septal defect, ventricular septal defect, patent ductus arteriosus, or atrioventricular canal defect) that permit blood to shunt from left (systemic circulation) to right (pulmonary circulation).
5. Obstruction of ventricular outflow is commonly caused by aortic stenosis (left ventricle) or pulmonary stenosis (right ventricle).
6. In less severe obstruction, ventricular outflow remains normal because of compensatory ventricular hypertrophy stimulated by increased afterload and, in postductal coarctation of the aorta (COA), development of collateral circulation around the coarctation.
7. Cyanotic congenital defects in which saturated and desaturated blood mix within the heart or great arteries include tetralogy of Fallot (TOF), transposition of the great arteries, total anomalous pulmonary venous connection, truncus arteriosus, and hypoplastic left heart syndrome.
8. In cyanotic heart defects that decrease pulmonary blood flow (TOF), myocardial hypertrophy cannot compensate for restricted right ventricular outflow. Flow to the lungs decreases, and cyanosis is caused by an insufficient volume of oxygenated blood and right-to-left shunt.

9. Heart failure (HF) is usually the result of congenital heart defects that increase blood volume in the pulmonary circulation. A clinical manifestation of HF unique to children is failure to thrive.

Acquired Cardiovascular Disorders

1. Two examples of acquired heart disease in children are Kawasaki disease (KD) and systemic hypertension.
2. KD is an acute systemic vasculitis that also may result in the development of coronary artery aneurysms and thrombosis if untreated.
3. Systemic hypertension in children differs from hypertension in adults in etiology and presentation. When significant hypertension is found in a young child, the examiner should evaluate for the presence of secondary hypertension, most commonly renal disease or COA.

26

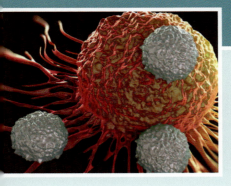

Structure and Function of the Pulmonary System

Mohamed Toufic El-Hussein, with originating chapter contributions by Valentina L. Brashers

Additional resources are available online at https://evolve.elsevier.com/Canada/Huether/pathophysiology.

CHAPTER OUTLINE

Structures of the Pulmonary System, 654
    Conducting Airways, 654
    Gas-Exchange Airways, 655
    Pulmonary and Bronchial Circulation, 655
    Control of the Pulmonary Circulation, 656
    Chest Wall and Pleura, 657
Function of the Pulmonary System, 657
    Ventilation, 658

    Neurochemical Control of Ventilation, 659
    Mechanics of Breathing, 660
    Gas Transport, 662
GERIATRIC CONSIDERATIONS: Aging and the Pulmonary System, 666

LEARNING OBJECTIVES

1. Trace a molecule of air inhaled from the environment as it travels through the pulmonary system.
2. List the conducting airways, their location, and their function.
3. Identify the structures involved in gas exchange.
4. Describe the importance of surfactant.
5. Describe the structures that surround the pulmonary system.
6. Identify the factors essential to successful ventilation, perfusion, and diffusion.
7. Describe mechanical and chemo-receptors, noting the importance of each in respiration.
8. Describe lung compliance and compare it to elastic recoil.
9. Describe the mechanics of breathing.
10. Describe the partial pressure of oxygen and its measurement.
11. Describe how ventilation and perfusion are interrelated.
12. Describe the clinical significance of the oxyhemoglobin dissociation.
13. Describe the mechanisms of carbon dioxide transport from the body tissues to the lungs
14. Describe the factors affecting carbon dioxide diffusion across the alveolar membrane.
15. Describe the causes of pulmonary vasoconstriction.

KEY TERMS

Acinus, 655
Alveolar duct, 655
Alveolar ventilation, 658
Alveolocapillary membrane, 655
Alveolus (*pl.*, alveoli), 655
Bohr effect, 666
Bronchus (*pl.*, bronchi), 654
Carina, 654
Central chemoreceptor, 660
Collectin, 661
Compliance, 661

Elastic recoil, 661
Goblet cell, 655
Haldane effect, 666
Hilum (*pl.*, hila), 654
Hypoxic pulmonary vasoconstriction, 656
Irritant receptor, 659
J-receptor, 659
Larynx, 654
Mediastinum, 654
Minute volume (minute ventilation), 658

Nasopharynx, 654
Oropharynx, 654
Oxygen saturation (SaO_2), 664
Oxyhemoglobin (HbO_2), 665
Oxyhemoglobin dissociation curve, 665
Partial pressure (of a gas), 662
Peripheral chemoreceptor, 659
Pleura (*pl.*, pleurae), 657
Pleural space (pleural cavity), 657
Respiratory bronchiole, 655

Respiratory centre, 659
Stretch receptor, 659
Surface tension, 661
Surfactant, 655
Thoracic cavity, 657
Trachea, 654
Ventilation, 658
Ventilation–perfusion ratio ($\dot{V}/\dot{Q}$), 663

The primary function of the pulmonary system is the exchange of gases between the environmental air and the blood. The three steps in this process are (1) ventilation, the movement of air into and out of the lungs; (2) diffusion, the movement of gases between air spaces in the lungs and the bloodstream; and (3) perfusion, the movement of blood into and out of the capillary beds of the lungs to body organs and tissues. The first two steps are carried out by the pulmonary system and the third by the cardiovascular system (see Chapter 23). Normally the pulmonary system functions efficiently under a variety of conditions and with little energy expenditure.

STRUCTURES OF THE PULMONARY SYSTEM

> ✓ **QUICK CHECK 26.1**
> 1. List the major components of the pulmonary system.
> 2. Which components of the pulmonary system contribute to the body's defence?
> 3. What are conducting airways?
> 4. Describe an alveolus.

The pulmonary system includes two lungs, the upper and lower airways, the blood vessels that serve these structures (Figure 26.1), the diaphragm, and the chest wall or thoracic cage. The lungs are divided into lobes: three in the right lung (upper, middle, lower) and two in the left lung (upper, lower). Each lobe is further divided into segments and lobules. The **mediastinum** is the space between the lungs and contains the heart, great vessels, and esophagus. A set of conducting airways, or bronchi, delivers air to each section of the lung. The lung tissue that surrounds the airways supports them, preventing distortion or collapse of the airways as gas moves in and out during ventilation. The diaphragm is a dome-shaped muscle that separates the thoracic and abdominal cavities and is involved in ventilation.

The lungs are protected from exogenous contaminants by a series of mechanical barriers (Table 26.1). These defence mechanisms are so effective that, in the healthy individual, contamination of the lung tissue itself, particularly by infectious agents, is rare.

Conducting Airways

The conducting airways allow air into and out of the gas-exchange structures of the lung. The **nasopharynx**, **oropharynx**, and related structures are often called the *upper airway* (Figure 26.2). These structures are lined with a ciliated mucosa that warms and humidifies inspired air and removes foreign particles from it. The mouth and oropharynx are used for ventilation when the nose is obstructed or when increased flow is required (e.g., during exercise). Filtering and humidifying are not as efficient with mouth breathing.

The **larynx** connects the upper and lower airways and is made up of the endolarynx and its surrounding triangular-shaped bony and cartilaginous structures. The endolarynx encompasses two pairs of folds: the false vocal cords (supraglottis) and the true vocal cords. The slit-shaped space between the true cords forms the glottis (see Figure 26.2). The vestibule is the space above the false vocal cords. The laryngeal box is formed of three large cartilages (epiglottis, thyroid, cricoid) and three smaller cartilages (arytenoid, corniculate, cuneiform) connected by ligaments. The supporting cartilages prevent collapse of the larynx during inspiration and swallowing. The internal laryngeal muscles control vocal cord length and tension, and the external laryngeal muscles move the larynx as a whole. Both sets of muscles are important to swallowing, ventilation, and vocalization.[1] The internal muscles contract during swallowing to prevent aspiration into the trachea. These muscles also contribute to voice pitch.

The **trachea**, which is supported by U-shaped cartilage, connects the larynx to the bronchi, the conducting airways of the lungs. The trachea branches into two main airways, or **bronchi** (*sing.*, **bronchus**), at the **carina** (see Figure 26.1). The right and left main bronchi enter the

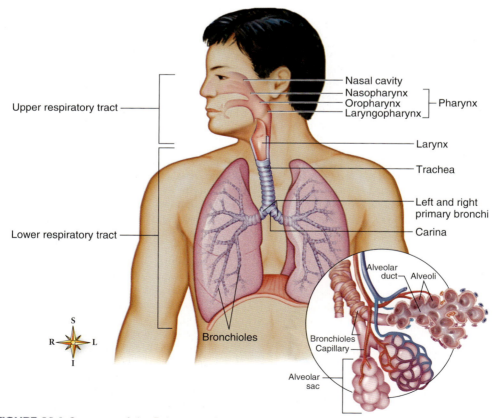

FIGURE 26.1 Structure of the Pulmonary System. The upper and lower respiratory tracts (airways) are illustrated. The enlargement in the circle depicts the acinus, where oxygen and carbon dioxide are exchanged. (From Patton, K. T., & Thibodeau, G. A. [2016]. *Structure & function of the body* [15th ed.]. Mosby.)

TABLE 26.1 Pulmonary Defence Mechanisms

Structure or Substance	Mechanism of Defence
Upper respiratory tract mucosa	Maintains constant temperature and humidification of gas entering lungs; traps and removes foreign particles, some bacteria, and noxious gases from inspired air
Nasal hairs and turbinates	Trap and remove foreign particles, some bacteria, and noxious gases from inspired air
Mucous blanket	Protects trachea and bronchi from injury; traps most foreign particles and bacteria that reach lower airways
Cilia	Propel mucous blanket and entrapped particles toward oropharynx, where they can be swallowed or expectorated
Irritant receptors in nares (nostrils)	Trigger sneeze reflex when stimulated by chemical or mechanical irritants, resulting in the rapid removal of irritants from nasal passages
Irritant receptors in trachea and large airways	Trigger cough reflex when stimulated by chemical or mechanical irritants, resulting in the removal of irritants from lower airways
Alveolar macrophages	Ingest and remove bacteria and other foreign material from alveoli by phagocytosis (see Chapters 6 and 7)

lungs at the **hila** (*sing.*, **hilum**), or "roots" of the lungs, along with the pulmonary blood and lymphatic vessels. From the hila the main bronchi branch further, as shown in Figure 26.3.

The bronchial walls have three layers: an epithelial lining, a smooth muscle layer, and a connective tissue layer. The epithelial lining of the bronchi contains single-celled exocrine glands—the mucous-secreting **goblet cells**—and ciliated cells. The goblet cells produce a mucous blanket that protects the airway epithelium, and the ciliated epithelial cells rhythmically beat this mucous blanket toward the trachea and pharynx where it can be swallowed or expectorated by coughing. The layers of epithelium that line the bronchi become thinner with each successive branching (see Figure 26.3).

Gas-Exchange Airways

The conducting airways terminate in the **respiratory bronchioles**, **alveolar ducts**, and **alveoli** (*sing.*, **alveolus**). These thin-walled structures together are sometimes called the **acinus** (see Figures 26.1 and 26.3), and all of them participate in gas exchange.[2]

The alveoli are the primary gas-exchange units of the lung, where oxygen (O_2) enters the blood and carbon dioxide (CO_2) is removed (Figure 26.4). Tiny passages called *pores of Kohn* permit some air to pass through the septa from alveolus to alveolus, promoting collateral ventilation and even distribution of air among the alveoli. The lungs contain approximately 25 million alveoli at birth and 300 million by adulthood.

Lung epithelial cells provide a protective interface with the environment and are essential for adequate gas exchange, preventing entry of foreign agents, regulating ion and water transport, and maintaining mechanical stability of the alveoli.[3] Two major types of epithelial cells appear in the alveolus. Type I alveolar cells provide structure, and type II alveolar cells secrete **surfactant**, a lipoprotein that coats the inner surface of the alveolus and lowers alveolar surface tension at end-expiration, thereby preventing lung collapse.[1,2,4,5]

Like the bronchi, alveoli contain cellular components of immunity and inflammation, particularly the mononuclear phagocytes (called *alveolar macrophages*). These cells ingest foreign material that reaches the alveolus and prepare it for removal through the lymphatics. (Phagocytosis and the mononuclear phagocyte system are described in Chapters 6 and 7.)

Pulmonary and Bronchial Circulation

> ✓ **QUICK CHECK 26.2**
> 1. What are the functions of the pulmonary circulation and of the bronchial circulation?
> 2. What is the most important factor causing pulmonary artery constriction?
> 3. What are the characteristics of the pleural space?

The pulmonary circulation eases gas exchange, delivers nutrients to lung tissues, acts as a reservoir for the left ventricle, and serves as a filtering system that removes clots, air, and other debris from the circulation.

Although the entire cardiac output from the right ventricle goes into the lungs, the pulmonary circulation has a lower pressure and resistance than the systemic circulation. Pulmonary arteries are exposed to about one-fifth of the pressure of the systemic circulation. Usually about one-third of the pulmonary vessels are filled with blood (perfused) at any given time. More vessels become perfused when right ventricular cardiac output increases. Therefore, increased delivery of blood to the lungs does not normally increase mean pulmonary artery pressure.

The pulmonary artery divides and enters the lung at the hila, branching with each main bronchus and with all bronchi at every division. Thus, every bronchus and bronchiole has an accompanying artery or arteriole. The arterioles divide at the terminal bronchioles to form a network of pulmonary capillaries around the acinus. Capillary walls consist of an endothelial layer and a thin basement membrane, which often fuses with the basement membrane of the alveolar septum. As a result, there is very little separation between blood in the capillary and gas in the alveolus.

The shared alveolar and capillary walls compose the **alveolocapillary membrane** (respiratory membrane) (Figure 26.5). Gas exchange occurs across this membrane. With normal perfusion, approximately 100 mL of blood in the pulmonary capillary bed is spread very thinly over 70 to 100 m^2 of alveolar surface area. Any disorder that thickens the membrane impairs gas exchange.

Each pulmonary vein drains several pulmonary capillaries. Unlike the pulmonary arteries, pulmonary veins are dispersed randomly throughout the lung and then leave the lung at the hila and enter the left atrium. They have no valves.

The bronchial circulation is part of the systemic circulation, and it both moistens inspired air and supplies nutrients to the conducting airways, large pulmonary vessels, and membranes (pleurae) that surround the lungs. Not all of its capillaries drain into its own venous system. Some empty into the pulmonary vein and contribute to the normal venous mixture of oxygenated and deoxygenated blood or right-to-left shunt (right-to-left shunts are described in Chapter 27). The bronchial circulation does not participate in gas exchange.[6]

Lung vasculature also includes deep and superficial pulmonary lymphatic capillaries. Fluid and alveolar macrophages migrate from the alveoli to the terminal bronchioles, where they enter the lymphatic system. Both deep and superficial lymphatic vessels leave the lung at the hilum through a series of mediastinal lymph nodes. The lymphatic system plays an important role in both providing immune defence and keeping the lung free of fluid. (The lymphatic system is described in Chapter 23.)

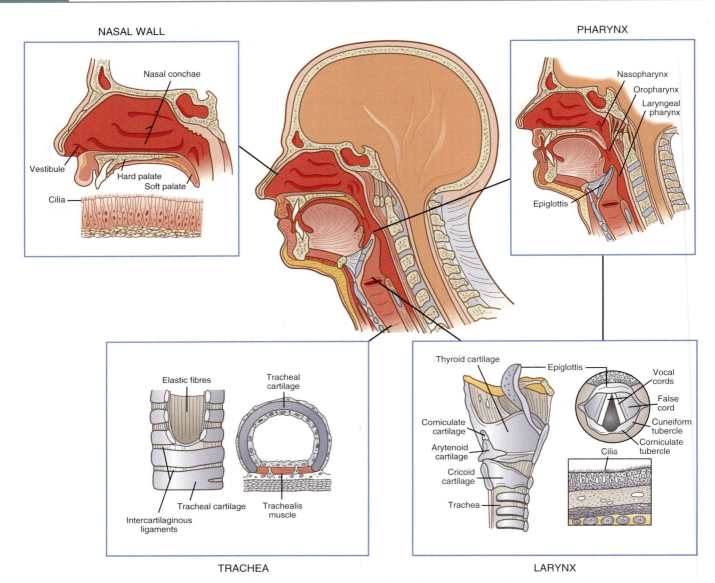

FIGURE 26.2 Structures of the Upper Airway. (Redrawn from Thompson, J. M., McFarland, G. K., Hirsch, J. E., et al. [2002]. *Mosby's clinical nursing* [5th ed.]. Mosby.)

Control of the Pulmonary Circulation

The calibre of pulmonary artery lumina decreases as smooth muscle in the arterial walls contracts. Contraction increases pulmonary artery pressure. Calibre increases as these muscles relax, decreasing blood pressure. Contraction (vasoconstriction) and relaxation (vasodilation) primarily occur in response to local humoral conditions, even though the pulmonary circulation is innervated by the autonomic nervous system (ANS), as is the systemic circulation.

The most important cause of pulmonary artery constriction is a low alveolar partial pressure of oxygen (Po_2). Vasoconstriction is caused by alveolar and pulmonary venous hypoxia, often termed **hypoxic pulmonary vasoconstriction**, and results from an increase in intracellular calcium levels in vascular smooth muscle cells in response to low O_2 concentration and the presence of charged O_2 molecules called *oxygen radicals*.[7] It can affect only one portion of the lung (i.e., one lobe that is obstructed, decreasing its partial pressure of oxygen in alveolar gas [PAO_2]) or the entire lung. If only one segment of the lung is involved, the arterioles to that segment constrict, shunting blood to other, well-ventilated portions of the lung. This reflex improves the lung's efficiency by better matching ventilation and perfusion. If all segments of the lung are affected, however, vasoconstriction occurs throughout the pulmonary vasculature and pulmonary hypertension (elevated pulmonary artery pressure) can result. The pulmonary vasoconstriction caused by low alveolar Po_2 is reversible if the alveolar Po_2 is corrected. Chronic alveolar hypoxia can result in structural changes in pulmonary arterioles causing permanent pulmonary artery hypertension, which eventually leads to right ventricular failure (cor pulmonale).[7]

Acidemia also causes pulmonary artery constriction. If the acidemia is corrected, the vasoconstriction is reversed. (Respiratory acidosis and metabolic acidosis are described in Chapter 5.) An elevated partial pressure of carbon dioxide in arterial blood ($PaCO_2$) value without a drop in pH does not cause pulmonary artery constriction. Other biochemical factors that affect the calibre of vessels in pulmonary

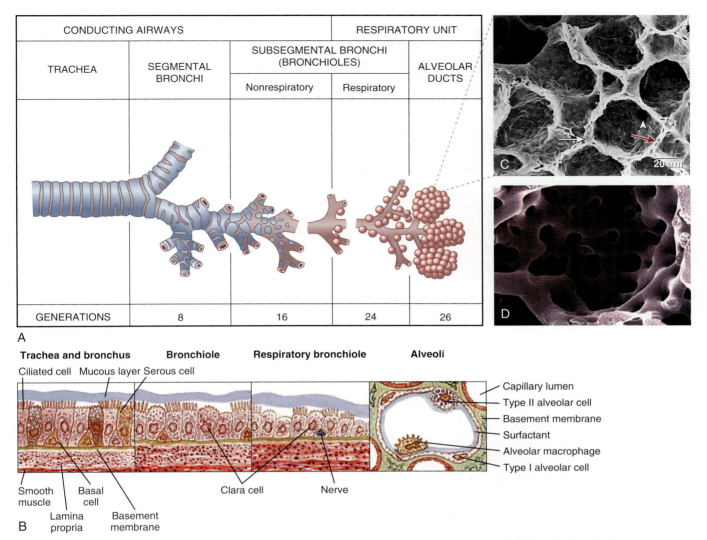

FIGURE 26.3 Structures of the Lower Airway. **A**, Structures of lower respiratory airway. **B**, Changes in bronchial wall with progressive branching. **C**, Electron micrograph of alveoli: *long white arrow* identifies type II pneumocyte (secretes surfactant); *white arrowhead* identifies pores of Kohn; *red arrow* identifies alveolar capillary. **D**, Plastic cast of pulmonary capillaries at high magnification. ([A], Redrawn from Thompson, J. M., McFarland, G. K., Hirsch, J. E., et al. [2002]. *Mosby's clinical nursing* [5th ed.]. Mosby; [B], from Wilson, S. F., & Thompson, J. M. [1990]. *Respiratory disorders*. Mosby; [C], from Mason, R. J., Broaddus, M. D., Martin, T. R., et al. [2010]. *Murray and Nadel's textbook of respiratory medicine* [5th ed.]. Saunders; [D], courtesy A. Churg, MD, and J. Wright, MD, Vancouver, Canada. From Leslie, K. O., & Wick, M. R. [2011]. *Practical pulmonary pathology: a diagnostic approach* [2nd ed.]. Saunders.)

circulation are histamine, prostaglandins, serotonin, nitric oxide, and bradykinin (see the *Geriatric Considerations:* Aging and the Pulmonary System box at the end of the chapter).

Chest Wall and Pleura

The chest wall (skin, ribs, intercostal muscles) protects the lungs from injury. The intercostal muscles of the chest wall, along with the diaphragm, accessory muscles, and abdominal muscles, do the muscular work of breathing. The **thoracic cavity** is contained by the chest wall and encases the lungs (Figure 26.6). A serous membrane called the **pleura** (*pl.*, **pleurae**) adheres firmly to the lungs and then folds over itself and attaches firmly to the chest wall. The membrane covering the lungs is the *visceral pleura*, and lining the thoracic cavity is the *parietal pleura*. The area between the two pleurae is called the **pleural space**, or **pleural cavity**. Normally, only a thin layer of fluid secreted by the pleura (pleural fluid) fills the pleural space, lubricating the pleural surfaces and allowing the two layers to slide over each other without separating. Pressure in the pleural space is usually negative or subatmospheric (−4 to −10 mm Hg).

FUNCTION OF THE PULMONARY SYSTEM

> ✓ **QUICK CHECK 26.3**
> 1. How do ventilation and respiration differ?
> 2. Describe three functions of the respiratory centre in the brainstem.
> 3. What are the three types of lung receptors?
> 4. How do the functions of central and peripheral chemoreceptors differ?

The pulmonary system (1) ventilates the alveoli, (2) diffuses gases into and out of the blood, and (3) perfuses the lungs so that the organs and tissues of the body receive blood that is rich in O_2 and deficient in CO_2.

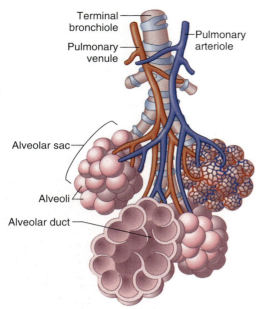

FIGURE 26.4 Alveoli. Bronchioles subdivide to form tiny tubes called *alveolar ducts*, which end in clusters of alveoli called *alveolar sacs*. (From Patton, K. T., & Thibodeau, G. A. [2018]. *The human body in health & disease* [7th ed.]. Elsevier.)

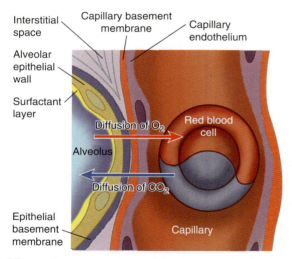

FIGURE 26.5 Cross-section Through an Alveolus Showing Histology of the Alveolar-Capillary Membrane (Respiratory Membrane). The dense network of capillaries forms an almost continuous sheet of blood in the alveolar walls, providing a very efficient arrangement for gas exchange. CO_2, Carbon dioxide; O_2, oxygen. (Adapted from Montague, S. E., Watson, R., & Herbert, R. [2005]. *Physiology for nursing practice* [3rd ed.]. Elsevier.)

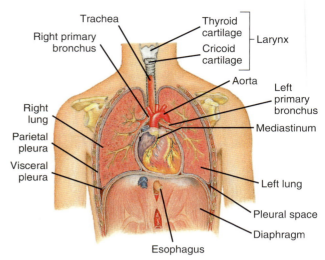

FIGURE 26.6 Thoracic (Chest) Cavity and Related Structures. The thoracic (chest) cavity is divided into three subdivisions (left and right pleural divisions and mediastinum) by a partition formed by a serous membrane called the *pleura*. (From Thibodeau, G. A., & Patton, K. T. [1996]. *Anatomy & physiology* [3rd ed.]. Mosby.)

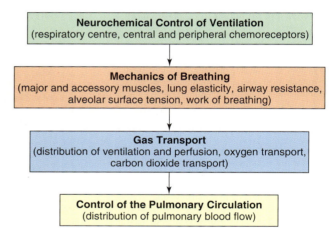

FIGURE 26.7 Functional Components of the Respiratory System. The central nervous system responds to neurochemical stimulation of ventilation and sends signals to the chest wall musculature. The response of the respiratory system to these impulses is influenced by several factors that impact the mechanisms of breathing and, therefore, affect the adequacy of ventilation. Gas transport between the alveoli and pulmonary capillary blood depends on a variety of physical and chemical activities. Finally, the control of the pulmonary circulation plays a role in the appropriate distribution of blood flow.

Each component of the pulmonary system contributes to one or more of these functions (Figure 26.7).

Ventilation

Ventilation is the mechanical movement of gas or air into and out of the lungs. It is often misnamed *respiration*, which is actually the exchange of O_2 and CO_2 during cellular metabolism. "Respiratory rate" is actually the ventilatory rate, or the number of times gas is inspired and expired per minute. The amount of effective ventilation is calculated by multiplying the ventilatory rate (breaths per minute) by the volume or amount of air per breath (litres per breath or tidal volume). This is called the **minute volume** (or **minute ventilation**) and is expressed in litres per minute.

CO_2, the gaseous form of carbonic acid (H_2CO_3), is produced by cellular metabolism. The lung eliminates about 10 000 mmol of carbonic acid per day in the form of CO_2, which is produced at the rate of approximately 200 mL/min. CO_2 is eliminated to maintain a normal arterial CO_2 pressure ($PaCO_2$) of 40 mm Hg and normal acid–base balance (see Chapter 5 for a discussion of acid–base regulation). Adequate ventilation is necessary to maintain normal $PaCO_2$ levels. Diseases that limit ventilation result in CO_2 retention. The adequacy of **alveolar ventilation** cannot be accurately determined by observation of ventilatory rate, pattern, or effort. If a health care provider needs to determine the adequacy of ventilation, an arterial blood gas analysis must be performed to measure $PaCO_2$.

Neurochemical Control of Ventilation

Breathing is usually involuntary, because homeostatic changes in ventilatory rate and volume are adjusted automatically by the nervous system to maintain normal gas exchange. Voluntary breathing is necessary for talking, singing, laughing, and deliberately holding one's breath. The mechanisms that control respiration are complex (Figure 26.8).

The respiratory centre in the brainstem controls respiration by sending impulses to the respiratory muscles, causing them to contract and relax. The respiratory centre is made up of several groups of neurons: the dorsal respiratory group (DRG), the ventral respiratory group (VRG), the pneumotaxic centre, and the apneustic centre.[1,2,4]

The basic automatic rhythm of respiration is set by the DRG, which receives afferent input from peripheral chemoreceptors in the carotid and aortic bodies. It also receives input from mechanical, neural, and chemical stimuli; in addition to receiving input from receptors in the lungs.[8] The VRG contains both inspiratory and expiratory neurons and is almost inactive during normal, quiet respiration, becoming active when increased ventilatory effort is required. The pneumotaxic centre and apneustic centre, situated in the pons, do not generate primary rhythm but, rather, act as modifiers of the rhythm established by the medullary centres. The pattern of breathing can be influenced by emotion, pain, and disease.

Lung Receptors

Three types of lung receptors send impulses from the lungs to the DRG:
1. **Irritant receptors** (C fibres) are found in the epithelium of all conducting airways. They are sensitive to noxious aerosols (vapours), gases, and particulate matter (e.g., inhaled dusts), which cause them to initiate the cough reflex.[9] When stimulated, irritant receptors also cause bronchoconstriction and increased ventilatory rate.
2. **Stretch receptors** are located in the smooth muscles of airways and are sensitive to increases in the size or volume of the lungs. They decrease ventilatory rate and volume when stimulated, an occurrence sometimes referred to as the *Hering-Breuer reflex*. This reflex is active in newborns and assists with ventilation. In adults, this reflex is active only at high tidal volumes (such as with exercise) and may protect against excess lung inflation. Bronchopulmonary C fibres and a subset of stretch-sensitive, acid-sensitive myelinated sensory nerves mediate the cough reflex.[10]
3. **J-receptors** (juxtapulmonary capillary receptors) are located near the capillaries in the alveolar septa. They are sensitive to increased pulmonary capillary pressure, which stimulates them to initiate rapid, shallow breathing; hypotension; and bradycardia.[5]

The lung is innervated by the ANS. Fibres of the sympathetic division in the lung branch from the upper thoracic and cervical ganglia of the spinal cord. Fibres of the parasympathetic division of the ANS travel

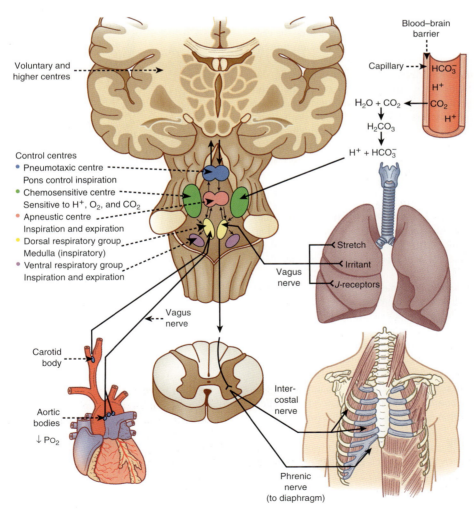

FIGURE 26.8 Neurochemical Respiratory Control System. CO_2, Carbon dioxide; H^+, hydrogen; H_2CO_3, carbonic acid; H_2O, water; HCO_3^-, bicarbonate; O_2, oxygen; Po_2, partial pressure of oxygen.

in the vagus nerve to the lung. (Structures and function of the ANS are discussed in detail in Chapter 13.) The parasympathetic and sympathetic divisions control airway calibre (interior diameter of the airway lumen) by stimulating bronchial smooth muscle to contract or relax. The parasympathetic receptors cause smooth muscle to contract, whereas sympathetic receptors cause it to relax. Bronchial smooth muscle tone depends on equilibrium—that is, equal stimulation of contraction and relaxation. The parasympathetic division of the ANS is the main controller of airway calibre under normal conditions. Constriction occurs if the irritant receptors in the airway epithelium are stimulated by irritants in inspired air, by inflammatory mediators (e.g., histamine, serotonin, prostaglandins, leukotrienes), by many medications, and by humoral substances.

Chemoreceptors

Chemoreceptors monitor the pH, $PaCO_2$, and PaO_2 (partial pressure of oxygen in arterial blood) of arterial blood. **Central chemoreceptors** monitor arterial blood indirectly by sensing changes in the pH of cerebrospinal fluid (CSF) (see Figure 26.8).[11] They are located near the respiratory centre and are sensitive to hydrogen ion concentration in the CSF. (Chapter 5 describes the relationship between ions and the pH, or acid–base status, of body fluids.) The pH of the CSF reflects arterial pH because CO_2 in arterial blood can diffuse across the blood–brain barrier (the capillary wall separating blood from cells of the central nervous system) into the CSF until the partial pressure of carbon dioxide (P_{CO_2}) is equal on both sides. CO_2 that has entered the CSF combines with water (H_2O) to form carbonic acid, which subsequently dissociates into hydrogen ions that are capable of stimulating the central chemoreceptors. In this way, $PaCO_2$ regulates ventilation through its impact on the pH (hydrogen ion content) of the CSF.[1,2,4,11]

If alveolar ventilation is inadequate, $PaCO_2$ increases. CO_2 diffuses across the blood–brain barrier until P_{CO_2} values in the blood and the CSF reach equilibrium. As the central chemoreceptors sense the resulting decrease in pH (increase in hydrogen ion concentration), they stimulate the respiratory centre to increase the depth and rate of ventilation. Increased ventilation causes the P_{CO_2} of arterial blood to decrease below that of the CSF, and CO_2 diffuses out of the CSF, returning its pH to normal.

The central chemoreceptors are sensitive to very small changes in the pH of CSF (equivalent to a 1 to 2 mm Hg change in P_{CO_2}) and can maintain a normal $PaCO_2$ under many different conditions, including strenuous exercise.[11] If inadequate ventilation, or hypoventilation, is long term (e.g., in chronic obstructive pulmonary disease), these receptors become insensitive to small changes in $PaCO_2$ ("reset") and regulate ventilation poorly.[12]

The peripheral chemoreceptors are somewhat sensitive to changes in $PaCO_2$ and pH but are sensitive primarily to O_2 levels in arterial blood (PaO_2). As PaO_2 and pH decrease, peripheral chemoreceptors, particularly in the carotid bodies, send signals to the respiratory centre to increase ventilation. However, the PaO_2 must drop well below normal (to approximately 60 mm Hg) before the peripheral chemoreceptors have much influence on ventilation. If $PaCO_2$ is elevated as well, ventilation increases much more than it would in response to either abnormality alone. The peripheral chemoreceptors become the major stimulus to ventilation when the central chemoreceptors are reset by chronic hypoventilation.[13]

Mechanics of Breathing

> ✓ **QUICK CHECK 26.4**
> 1. Describe the work of the diaphragm in ventilation.
> 2. What is the function of surfactant?
> 3. How is elastic recoil related to compliance?
> 4. What causes changes in airway resistance?

The mechanical aspects of inspiration and expiration are known collectively as the *mechanics of breathing* and involve (1) major and accessory muscles of inspiration and expiration, (2) elastic properties of the lungs and chest wall, and (3) resistance to airflow through the conducting airways. Alterations in any of these properties increase the work of breathing or the metabolic energy needed to achieve adequate ventilation and oxygenation of the blood.

Major and Accessory Muscles

The major muscles of inspiration are the diaphragm and the external intercostal muscles (muscles between the ribs) (Figure 26.9). The diaphragm is a dome-shaped muscle that separates the abdominal and thoracic cavities. When it contracts and flattens downward, it increases the volume of the thoracic cavity, creating a negative pressure that draws gas into the lungs through the upper airways and trachea. Contraction of the external intercostal muscles elevates the anterior portion of the ribs and increases the volume of the thoracic cavity by increasing its front-to-back (anterior–posterior [AP]) diameter. Although the external intercostals may contract during quiet breathing, inspiration at rest is usually assisted by the diaphragm only.

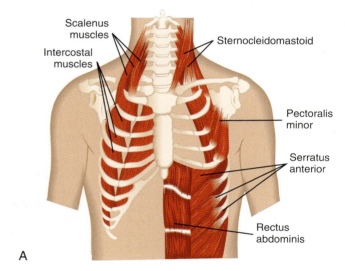

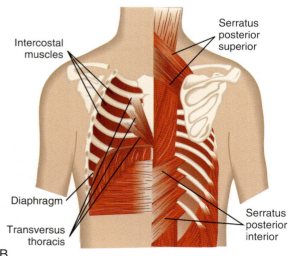

FIGURE 26.9 Muscles of Ventilation. **A**, Anterior view. **B**, Posterior view. (Modified from Thompson, J. M., McFarland, G. K., Hirsch, J. E., et al. [2002]. *Mosby's clinical nursing* [5th ed.]. Mosby.)

The accessory muscles of inspiration are the sternocleidomastoid and scalene muscles. Like the external intercostals, these muscles enlarge the thorax by increasing its AP diameter. The accessory muscles assist inspiration when the minute volume (volume of air inspired and expired per minute) is high, as during strenuous exercise, or when the work of breathing is increased because of disease. The accessory muscles do not increase the volume of the thorax as efficiently as the diaphragm does.

There are no major muscles of expiration because normal, relaxed expiration is passive and requires no muscular effort. The accessory muscles of expiration, the abdominal and internal intercostal muscles, assist expiration when minute volume is high, during coughing, or when airway obstruction is present. When the abdominal muscles contract, intra-abdominal pressure increases, pushing up the diaphragm and decreasing the volume of the thorax. The internal intercostal muscles pull down the anterior ribs, decreasing the AP diameter of the thorax.

Alveolar Surface Tension

Surface tension occurs at any gas–liquid interface and refers to the tendency for liquid molecules that are exposed to air to adhere to one another. This phenomenon can be seen in the way liquids "bead" when splashed on a waterproof surface.

Within a sphere, such as an alveolus, surface tension tends to make expansion difficult. According to Laplace's law, the pressure (P) required to inflate a sphere is equal to two times the surface tension $(2\,T)$ divided by the radius (r) of the sphere, or $P = 2\,T/r$. As the radius of the sphere (or alveolus) decreases, more and more pressure is required to inflate it. If the alveoli were lined only with a waterlike fluid, taking breaths would be extremely difficult.

Alveolar ventilation, or distension, is made possible by surfactant, which lowers surface tension by coating the air–liquid interface in the alveoli. Surfactant, a lipoprotein (90% lipids and 10% protein) produced by type II alveolar cells, includes two groups of *surfactant* proteins. One group consists of small hydrophobic molecules that have a detergent like effect that separates the liquid molecules, thereby decreasing alveolar surface tension.[2,14] The second group of surfactant proteins consists of large hydrophilic molecules called **collectins** that are capable of inhibiting foreign pathogens (see Chapter 6).[15]

As the radius of an alveolus shrinks, the surface tension of the surfactant-lined sphere decreases, and as the radius expands, the surface tension increases. Thus, normal alveoli are much easier to inflate at low lung volumes (i.e., after expiration) than at high volumes (i.e., after inspiration). The decrease in surface tension caused by surfactant also is responsible for keeping the alveoli free of fluid. If surfactant is not produced in adequate quantities, alveolar surface tension increases, causing alveolar collapse, decreased lung expansion, increased work of breathing, and severe gas-exchange abnormalities.

Elastic Properties of the Lung and Chest Wall

The lung and chest wall have elastic properties that permit expansion during inspiration and return to resting volume during expiration. The elasticity of the lung is caused both by elastin fibres in the alveolar walls and surrounding the small airways and pulmonary capillaries, and by surface tension at the alveolar air–liquid interface.[13] The elasticity of the chest wall is the result of the configuration of its bones and musculature.

Elastic recoil is the tendency of the lungs and chest wall to return to the resting state after inspiration. Normal elastic recoil permits passive expiration, eliminating the need for major muscles of expiration. Passive elastic recoil may be insufficient during laboured breathing (high minute volume), when the accessory muscles of expiration may be needed. The accessory muscles are used also if disease compromises elastic recoil (e.g., in emphysema) or blocks the conducting airways.

Normal elastic recoil depends on an equilibrium between opposing forces of recoil in the lungs and chest wall. Under normal conditions, the chest wall tends to recoil by expanding outward. The tendency of the chest wall to recoil by expanding is balanced by the tendency of the lungs to recoil or inward collapse around the hila. The opposing forces of the chest wall and lungs create the small negative intrapleural pressure.

Balance between the outward recoil of the chest wall and inward recoil of the lungs occurs at the resting level, the end of expiration, where the functional residual capacity (FRC) is reached. However, muscular effort is needed to overcome lung resistance to expansion. During inspiration, the diaphragm and intercostal muscles contract, air flows into the lungs, and the chest wall expands. During expiration, the muscles relax and the elastic recoil of the lungs causes the thorax to decrease in volume until, once again, balance between the chest wall and lung recoil forces is reached (Figure 26.10).

Compliance is the measure of lung and chest wall distensibility and is defined as volume change per unit of pressure change. It represents the relative ease with which these structures can be stretched and is, therefore, the opposite of elasticity. Compliance is determined by the alveolar surface tension and the elastic recoil of the lung and chest wall.

Increased compliance indicates that the lungs or chest wall is abnormally easy to inflate and has lost some elastic recoil. A decrease in compliance indicates that the lungs or chest wall is abnormally stiff or difficult to inflate. Compliance increases with normal aging and with disorders such as emphysema. Compliance decreases in individuals with acute respiratory distress syndrome, pneumonia, pulmonary edema, and pulmonary fibrosis. (These disorders are described in Chapter 27.)

Airway Resistance

Airway resistance, which is similar to resistance to blood flow (described in Chapter 23), is determined by the length, radius, and cross-sectional area of the airways and by the density, viscosity, and velocity of the gas (Poiseuille's law). Resistance (R) is computed by dividing change in pressure (P) by rate of flow (F), or $R = P/F$ (Ohm's law). Airway resistance is normally very low. One-half to two-thirds of total airway resistance occurs in the nose. The next highest resistance is in the oropharynx and larynx. There is very little resistance in the conducting airways of the lungs because of their large cross-sectional area. Airway resistance is affected by the diameter of the airways. Bronchodilation, which decreases resistance to airflow, is caused by β_2-adrenergic receptor stimulation. Bronchoconstriction, which increases airway resistance, can be caused by stimulation of parasympathetic receptors in the bronchial smooth muscle and by numerous irritants and inflammatory mediators.[2] Airway resistance can also be increased by edema of the bronchial mucosa and by airway obstructions such as mucus, tumours, or foreign bodies. Pulmonary function tests (PFTs) measure lung volumes and flow rates and can be used to diagnose lung disease.

Work of Breathing

The work of breathing is determined by the muscular effort (and therefore O_2 and energy) required for ventilation. Normally very low, the work of breathing may increase considerably in diseases that disrupt the equilibrium between forces exerted by the lung and chest wall. More muscular effort is required when lung compliance decreases (e.g., in pulmonary edema), chest wall compliance decreases (e.g., in spinal deformity or obesity), or airways are obstructed by bronchospasm or mucous plugging (e.g., in asthma or bronchitis). An increase in the

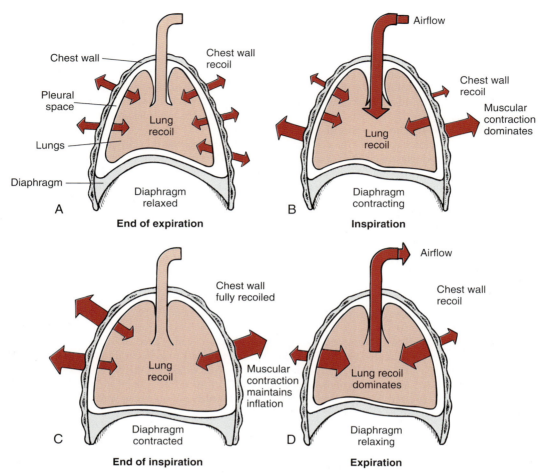

FIGURE 26.10 Interaction of Forces During Inspiration and Expiration. **A,** Outward recoil of the chest wall equals inward recoil of the lungs at the end of expiration. **B,** During inspiration, contraction of respiratory muscles, assisted by chest wall recoil, overcomes the tendency of lungs to recoil. **C,** At the end of inspiration, respiratory muscle contraction maintains lung expansion. **D,** During expiration, respiratory muscles relax, allowing elastic recoil of the lungs to deflate the lungs.

work of breathing can result in a marked increase in O_2 consumption and an inability to maintain adequate ventilation (Figure 26.11).

Gas Transport

> ✓ **QUICK CHECK 26.5**
> 1. What are the eight steps of gas transport?
> 2. What is barometric pressure? How is it related to physiological pressure measurements?
> 3. Describe the relationship between ventilation and pulmonary blood flow.
> 4. How does the alveolocapillary membrane function in ventilation and perfusion?
> 5. Describe the process of oxyhemoglobin association and dissociation.

Gas transport is the delivery of O_2 to the cells of the body and the removal of CO_2. It has four steps: (1) ventilation of the lungs, (2) diffusion of O_2 from the alveoli into the capillary blood, (3) perfusion of systemic capillaries with oxygenated blood, and (4) diffusion of O_2 from systemic capillaries into the cells. Steps in the transport of CO_2 occur in reverse order: (1) diffusion of CO_2 from the cells into the systemic capillaries, (2) perfusion of the pulmonary capillary bed by venous blood, (3) diffusion of CO_2 into the alveoli, and (4) removal of CO_2 from the lung by ventilation. Alterations in the respiratory or cardiovascular system are likely to derange certain steps in gas exchange at the cellular level.

Measurement of Gas Pressure

A gas is composed of millions of molecules moving randomly and colliding with each other and with the wall of the space in which they are contained. These collisions exert pressure. If the same number of gas molecules is contained in a small and a large container, the pressure is greater in the small container because more collisions occur in the smaller space (Figure 26.12).

Barometric pressure (P_B) (atmospheric pressure) is the pressure of gas molecules in air at specific altitudes. At sea level, P_B is 760 mm Hg and is the sum of the pressures of each gas in the air at sea level. The portion of the total pressure of any individual gas is its partial pressure (see Figure 26.12). At sea level, the air consists of O_2 (20.9%), nitrogen (78.1%), and a few other trace gases. The **partial pressure** of O_2 is equal to the percentage of O_2 in the air (20.9%) times the total P_B (760 mm Hg at sea level), or 159 mm Hg (760 × 0.209 = 158.84 mm Hg). (Symbols used in the measurement of gas pressures and pulmonary ventilation are defined in Table 26.2.)

The heart pumps against gravity to perfuse the pulmonary circulation. As blood is pumped into the lung apices of a sitting or standing individual, some blood pressure is dissipated in overcoming gravity. As a result, blood pressure at the apices is lower than that at the bases. Because greater pressure causes greater perfusion, the bases of the lungs are better perfused than the apices (Figure 26.13). Thus, ventilation and perfusion are greatest in the same lung portions—the lower lobes—and depend on body position. If a standing individual assumes a supine or side-lying position, the areas of the lungs that are then most dependent become the best ventilated and perfused.

Alveolar pressure (gas pressure in the alveoli) affects the distribution of perfusion in the pulmonary circulation. Gas-containing alveoli surround the pulmonary capillary bed, unlike the systemic capillary bed. If the gas pressure in the alveoli exceeds the blood pressure in the capillary, the capillary collapses and flow ceases. This outcome is most likely to occur in portions of the lung where blood pressure is lowest and alveolar gas pressure is greatest—that is, at the apex of the lung.

The lungs are divided into three zones on the basis of relationships among all the factors affecting pulmonary blood flow. Alveolar pressure and the forces of gravity, arterial blood pressure, and venous blood pressure affect the distribution of perfusion, as shown in Figure 26.14.

In zone I, alveolar pressure exceeds pulmonary arterial and venous pressures. The capillary bed collapses, and normal blood flow ceases. Normally zone I is a very small part of the lung at the apex. In zone II, alveolar pressure is greater than venous pressure but not arterial pressure. Blood flows through zone II, but alveolar pressure impedes to a certain extent. Zone II is normally above the level of the left atrium. In zone III, both arterial and venous pressures are greater than alveolar pressure; as such, blood flow is not affected. Zone III is in the base of the lung. Blood flow through the pulmonary capillary bed increases in regular increments from the apex to the base.

Although both blood flow and ventilation are greater at the base of the lungs than at the apices, they are not perfectly matched in any zone. Perfusion exceeds ventilation in the bases, and ventilation exceeds perfusion in the apices of the lung. The relationship between ventilation and perfusion is expressed as a ratio called the **ventilation–perfusion ratio ($\dot{V}/\dot{Q}$)**.[1] The normal $\dot{V}/\dot{Q}$ is 0.8, indicating that perfusion exceeds ventilation under normal conditions.

Oxygen Transport

Approximately 1 000 mL (1 L) of O_2 is transported to the body's cells each minute. O_2 is transported in the blood in two forms: a small amount dissolves in plasma, and the remainder binds to hemoglobin molecules. Without hemoglobin, O_2 would not reach the cells in sufficient amounts to maintain normal metabolic function. (Hemoglobin is discussed in detail in Chapter 20, and cellular metabolism is explored in Chapter 1.)

Diffusion across the alveolocapillary membrane. The alveolocapillary membrane is ideal for O_2 diffusion because it has a large total surface area (70 to 100 m^2) and is very thin (0.5 μm). In addition, the partial pressure of oxygen molecules in alveolar gas (P_AO_2) is much greater than that in capillary blood, a condition that promotes rapid diffusion down the concentration gradient from the alveolus into the capillary. The partial pressure of oxygen (oxygen tension) in mixed venous or pulmonary artery blood (PvO_2) is approximately 40 mm Hg as it enters the capillary, and alveolar oxygen tension (P_AO_2) is approximately 100 mm Hg at sea level. Therefore, a pressure gradient of 60 mm Hg eases the diffusion of O_2 from the alveolus into the capillary (Figure 26.15).

Blood remains in the pulmonary capillary for about 0.75 second, but only 0.25 second is required for O_2 concentration to equilibrate (equalize) across the alveolocapillary membrane. Therefore, O_2 has enough time to diffuse into the blood, even during increased cardiac output, which speeds blood flow and shortens the time the blood remains in the capillary.

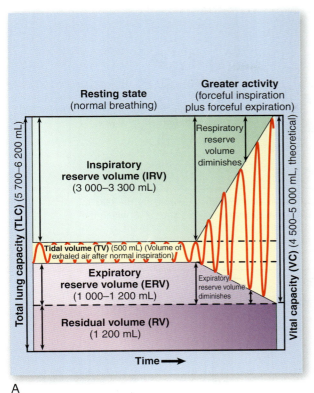
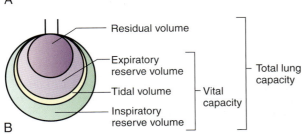

FIGURE 26.11 Pulmonary Ventilation and Lung Volumes. The chart in **A** shows a tracing like that produced with a spirometer. The diagram in **B** shows the pulmonary volumes as relative proportions of an inflated balloon. During normal, quiet breathing, about 500 mL of air is moved into and out of the respiratory tract *(TV)*. During forceful breathing (like that during and after heavy exercise), an extra 3 300 mL can be inspired *(IRV)*, and an extra 1 000 mL or so can be expired *(ERV)*. The largest volume of air that can be moved in and out during ventilation is called the vital capacity *(VC)*. Air that remains in the respiratory tract after a forceful expiration is called the residual volume *(RV)*. (From Patton, K. T., & Thibodeau, G. A. [2018]. *The human body in health & disease* [7th ed.]. Elsevier.)

Distribution of Ventilation and Perfusion

Effective gas exchange depends on an approximately even distribution of gas (ventilation) and blood (perfusion) in all portions of the lungs.[1] The lungs are suspended from the hila in the thoracic cavity. When an individual is in an upright position (sitting or standing), gravity pulls the lungs down toward the diaphragm and compresses their lower portions or bases. The alveoli in the upper portions, or apices, of the lungs contain a greater residual volume of gas and are larger and less numerous than those in the lower portions. Because surface tension increases as the alveoli become larger, the larger alveoli in the upper portions of the lung are more difficult to inflate (less compliant) than the smaller alveoli in the lower portions of the lung. Therefore, during ventilation most of the tidal volume is distributed to the bases of the lungs, where compliance is greater.

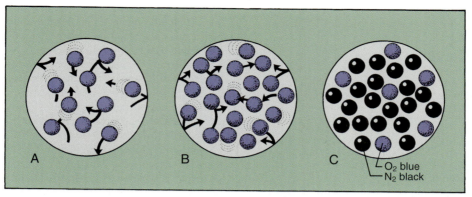

FIGURE 26.12 Relationship Between Number of Gas Molecules and Pressure Exerted by the Gas in an Enclosed Space. **A,** Theoretically, 10 molecules of the same gas exert a total pressure of 10 within the space. **B,** If the number of molecules is increased to 20, total pressure is 20. **C,** If there are different gases in the space, each gas exerts a partial pressure: here the partial pressure of nitrogen (N_2) is 20, that of oxygen (O_2) is 6, and the total pressure is 26.

TABLE 26.2 Common Pulmonary Abbreviations

Symbol	Definition
FEV_1	Forced expiratory volume in 1 second
FiO_2	Fraction of inspired oxygen
FRC	Functional residual capacity
FVC	Forced vital capacity
P	Pressure (usually partial pressure) of a gas
PaO_2	Partial pressure of oxygen in arterial blood
P_AO_2	Partial pressure of oxygen in alveolar gas
$P(A-a)O_2$	Difference between alveolar and arterial partial pressure of oxygen (A–a gradient)
$PaCO_2$	Partial pressure of carbon dioxide in arterial blood
P_B	Barometric or atmospheric pressure
$PvCO_2$	Venous partial pressure of carbon dioxide
PvO_2	Partial pressure of oxygen in mixed venous or pulmonary artery blood
Q	Perfusion or blood flow
SaO_2	Saturation of hemoglobin (in arterial blood) with oxygen
SvO_2	Saturation of hemoglobin (in mixed venous blood) with oxygen
V	Volume or amount of gas
V_A	Alveolar ventilation
V_D	Dead-space ventilation
V_E	Minute capacity
V_T	Tidal volume or average breath
$\dot{V}/\dot{Q}$	Ratio of ventilation to perfusion (the overhead dot means measurement over time, usually 1 minute)

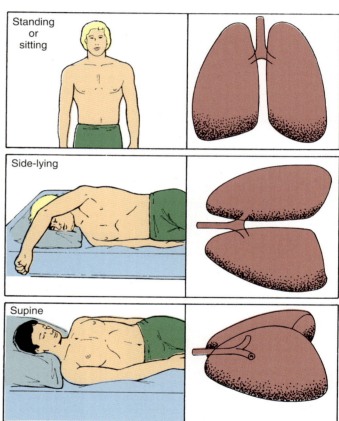

FIGURE 26.13 Pulmonary Blood Flow and Gravity. The greatest volume of pulmonary blood flow normally will occur in the gravity-dependent areas of the lung. Body position has a significant effect on the distribution of pulmonary blood flow. Shaded areas represent gravity-dependent pulmonary blood flow.

Determinants of arterial oxygenation. As O_2 diffuses across the alveolocapillary membrane, it dissolves in the plasma, where it exerts pressure (PaO_2). As the PaO_2 increases, O_2 moves from the plasma into the red blood cells (erythrocytes) and binds with hemoglobin molecules. O_2 continues to bind with hemoglobin until the hemoglobin-binding sites are filled or *saturated*. O_2 then continues to diffuse across the alveolocapillary membrane until the PaO_2 (O_2 dissolved in plasma) and P_AO_2 (O_2 in the alveolus) equilibrate, eliminating the pressure gradient across the alveolocapillary membrane. At this point, diffusion stops (see Figure 26.15).

The majority (97%) of the O_2 that enters the blood is bound to hemoglobin. The remaining 3% stays in the plasma and creates PaO_2.

Arterial blood gas measurement is done to measure the PaO_2. **Oxygen saturation ($SaO2$)** is the percentage of the available hemoglobin that is bound to O_2 and can be measured using a device called an *oximeter*.

Because hemoglobin transports all but a small fraction of the O_2 carried in arterial blood, changes in hemoglobin concentration affect the O_2 content of the blood. Decreases in hemoglobin concentration below the normal value of 150 g/L of blood reduce O_2 content, and increases in hemoglobin concentration may increase O_2 content, minimizing the

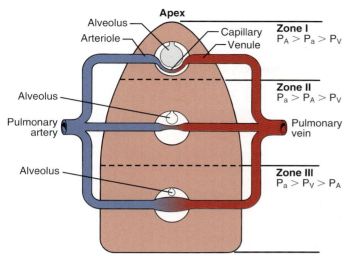

FIGURE 26.14 Gravity and Alveolar Pressure. Effects of gravity and alveolar pressure on pulmonary blood flow in the three lung zones. In zone I, alveolar pressure (P_A) is greater than arterial pressure (P_a) and venous pressure (P_v), and no blood flow occurs. In zone II, arterial pressure exceeds alveolar pressure, but alveolar pressure exceeds venous pressure. Blood flow occurs in this zone, but alveolar pressure compresses the venules (venous ends of the capillaries). In zone III, both arterial and venous pressures are greater than alveolar pressure and blood flow fluctuates depending on the difference between arterial pressure and venous pressure.

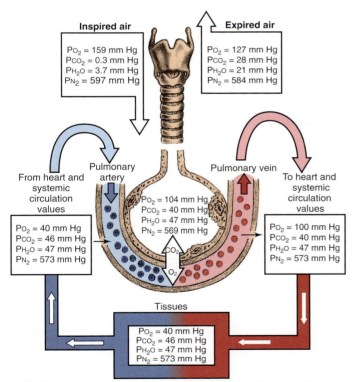

FIGURE 26.15 Partial Pressure of Respiratory Gases in Normal Respiration. The numbers shown are average values near sea level. The values of Po_2, Pco_2, and PN_2 fluctuate from breath to breath. CO_2, Carbon dioxide; O_2, oxygen; Pco_2, partial pressure of carbon dioxide; PH_2O, partial pressure of water; PN_2, partial pressure of nitrogen; Po_2, partial pressure of oxygen. (Modified from Thompson, J. M., McFarland, G. K., Hirsch, J. E., et al. [2002]. *Mosby's clinical nursing* [5th ed.]. Mosby.)

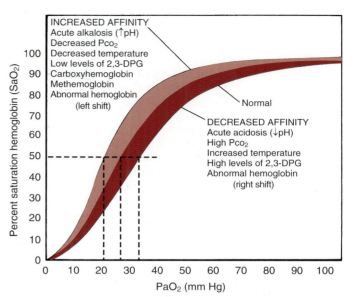

FIGURE 26.16 Oxyhemoglobin Dissociation Curve. The horizontal or flat segment of the curve at the top of the graph is the arterial or association portion, or that part of the curve where oxygen (O_2) is bound to hemoglobin and occurs in the lungs. This portion of the curve is flat because partial pressure changes of O_2 between 60 and 100 mm Hg do not significantly alter the percentage saturation of hemoglobin with O_2 and allow adequate hemoglobin saturation at a variety of altitudes. If the relationship between SaO_2 and PaO_2 were linear (in a downward sloping straight line) instead of flat between 60 and 100 mm Hg, there would be inadequate saturation of hemoglobin with O_2. The steep part of the oxyhemoglobin dissociation curve represents the rapid dissociation of O_2 from hemoglobin that occurs in the tissues. During this phase there is rapid diffusion of O_2 from the blood into tissue cells. The P_{50} is the PaO_2 at which hemoglobin is 50% saturated, normally 26.6 mm Hg. A lower than normal P_{50} represents increased affinity of hemoglobin for O_2, whereas a high P_{50} is seen with decreased affinity. Note that variation from the normal is associated with decreased (low P_{50}) or increased (high P_{50}) availability of O_2 to tissues *(dashed lines)*. The shaded area shows the entire oxyhemoglobin dissociation curve under the same circumstances. *2,3-DPG*, 2,3-Diphosphoglycerate; PaO_2, partial pressure of oxygen in arterial blood; Pco_2, partial pressure of carbon dioxide; SaO_2, saturation of hemoglobin (in arterial blood) with oxygen. (From Lane, E. E., & Walker, J. F. [1987]. *Clinical arterial blood gas analysis*. Mosby.)

impact of impaired gas exchange. In fact, increased hemoglobin concentration is a major compensatory mechanism in pulmonary diseases that impair gas exchange. For this reason, measurement of hemoglobin concentration is important in assessing individuals with pulmonary disease. If cardiovascular function is normal, the body's initial response to low O_2 content is to accelerate cardiac output. In individuals who also have cardiovascular disease, this compensatory mechanism is ineffective, making increased hemoglobin concentration an even more important compensatory mechanism. (Hemoglobin structure and function are described in Chapter 20.)

Oxyhemoglobin association and dissociation. When hemoglobin molecules bind with O_2, **oxyhemoglobin (HbO2)** forms. Binding occurs in the lungs and is called *oxyhemoglobin association* or *hemoglobin saturation with oxygen* (SaO_2). The reverse process, where O_2 is released from hemoglobin, occurs in the body tissues at the cellular level and is called *hemoglobin desaturation*. When hemoglobin saturation and desaturation are plotted on a graph, the result is a distinctive S-shaped curve known as the **oxyhemoglobin dissociation curve** (Figure 26.16).

Several factors can change the relationship between PaO_2 and SaO_2, causing the oxyhemoglobin dissociation curve to shift to the right or left (see Figure 26.16). A shift to the right depicts hemoglobin's decreased affinity for O_2 or an increase in the ease with which oxyhemoglobin dissociates and O_2 moves into the cells. A shift to the left depicts hemoglobin's increased affinity for O_2, which promotes association in the lungs and inhibits dissociation in the tissues.

Acidosis (low pH) and hypercapnia (increased $PaCO_2$) shift the oxyhemoglobin dissociation curve to the right. In the tissues, metabolic activity increases levels of CO_2 and hydrogen ions, thus decreasing the affinity of hemoglobin for O_2. Alkalosis (high pH) and hypocapnia (decreased $PaCO_2$) shift the curve to the left. In the lungs, as CO_2 diffuses from the blood into the alveoli, the blood CO_2 level is reduced and the affinity of hemoglobin for O_2 is increased. Changes in CO_2 and hydrogen ion concentrations in the blood cause shifting in the oxyhemoglobin dissociation curve, known as the **Bohr effect**. Changes in body temperature and increased or decreased levels of 2,3-diphosphoglycerate (2,3-DPG), a substance normally present in erythrocytes, also shift the oxyhemoglobin dissociation curve. Hyperthermia and increased 2,3-DPG levels shift the curve to the right. Hypothermia and decreased 2,3-DPG levels shift the curve to the left.

Carbon Dioxide Transport

CO_2 is carried in the blood in three ways: (1) dissolved in plasma (PCO_2), (2) as bicarbonate (HCO_3^-), and (3) as carbamino compounds. As CO_2 diffuses out of the cells into the blood, it dissolves in the plasma. Approximately 10% of the total CO_2 in venous blood and 5% of the CO_2 in arterial blood are transported dissolved in the plasma (venous partial pressure of carbon dioxide [$PvCO_2$] and $PaCO_2$, respectively). As CO_2 moves into the blood, it diffuses into the red blood cells. Within the red blood cells, CO_2, with the help of the enzyme carbonic anhydrase, combines with water to form carbonic acid and then quickly dissociates into hydrogen and bicarbonate. As carbonic acid dissociates, the hydrogen binds to hemoglobin, where it is buffered, and the bicarbonate moves out of the red blood cell into the plasma. Approximately 60% of the CO_2 in venous blood and 90% of the CO_2 in arterial blood are carried in the form of bicarbonate. The remainder combines with blood proteins, hemoglobin in particular, to form carbamino compounds. Approximately 30% of the CO_2 in venous blood and 5% of the CO_2 in arterial blood are carried as carbamino compounds.

CO_2 is 20 times more soluble than O_2 and diffuses quickly from the tissue cells into the blood. Diffusion of O_2 out of the blood and into the cells enhances the entrance of CO_2 into the blood. Reduced hemoglobin (hemoglobin that is dissociated from O_2) can carry more CO_2 than can hemoglobin saturated with O_2. Therefore, the drop in oxygen saturation (SaO_2) at the tissue level increases the ability of hemoglobin to carry CO_2 back to the lung.

The diffusion gradient for CO_2 in the lung is only approximately 6 mm Hg (venous PCO_2 = 46 mm Hg; alveolar PCO_2 = 40 mm Hg) (see Figure 26.15). Yet CO_2 is so soluble in the alveolocapillary membrane that the CO_2 in the blood quickly diffuses into the alveoli, where it is removed from the lung with each expiration. Diffusion of CO_2 in the lung is so efficient that diffusion defects that cause hypoxemia (low O_2 content of the blood) do not as readily cause hypercapnia (excessive CO_2 in the blood).

The binding of O_2 with hemoglobin in the lung enhances the diffusion of CO_2 out of the blood. As hemoglobin binds with O_2, the amount of CO_2 carried by the blood decreases. Thus, in the tissue capillaries, O_2 dissociation from hemoglobin helps the pickup of CO_2, and the binding of O_2 to hemoglobin in the lungs helps the release of CO_2 from the blood. This effect of O_2 on CO_2 transport is called the **Haldane effect**.

GERIATRIC CONSIDERATIONS
Aging and the Pulmonary System

Elasticity/Chest Wall
- Chest wall compliance decreases because ribs become ossified and joints are stiffer, resulting in increased work of breathing
- Kyphoscoliosis may curve the vertebral column, decreasing lung volumes
- Intercostal muscle strength decreases
- Elastic recoil diminishes, possibly the result of loss of elastic fibres

Result: Lung compliance increases and vital capacity (VC) declines, residual volume (RV) increases, total lung capacity (TLC) is unchanged, ventilatory reserves decline, and ventilation–perfusion ratios fall.

Gas Exchange
- Pulmonary capillary network decreases
- Alveoli dilate, and peripheral airways lose supporting tissues
- Surface area for gas exchange decreases
- pH and PCO_2 do not change much, but PO_2 declines
- Sensitivity of respiratory centres to hypoxia or hypercapnia decreases
- Ability to initiate an immune response against infection decreases

NOTE: Maximum PaO_2 at sea level can be estimated by multiplying the person's age by 0.3 and subtracting the product from 100.

Exercise
- Decreased PaO_2 and diminished ventilatory reserve lead to decreased exercise tolerance
- Early airway closure inhibits expiratory flow
- Changes depend on activity and fitness levels earlier in life
- An active, physically fit individual has fewer changes in function at any age than does a sedentary individual
- Respiratory muscle strength and endurance decrease, but exercise can maintain and enhance it

Lung Immunity
- Alterations in alveolar complement and surfactant and an increase in pro-inflammatory cytokines increase the risk for pulmonary disease and infection

GERIATRIC CONSIDERATIONS—cont'd
Aging and the Pulmonary System

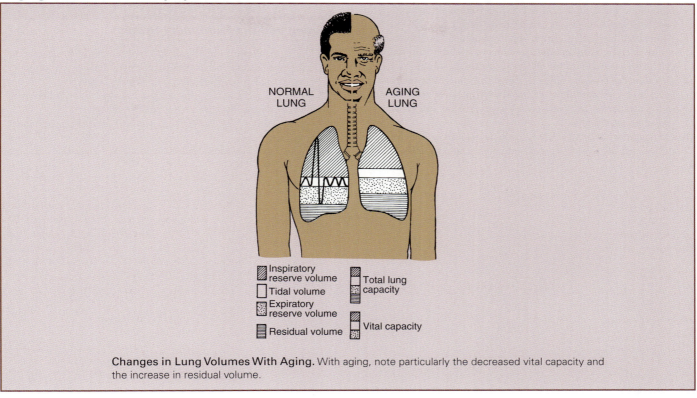

Changes in Lung Volumes With Aging. With aging, note particularly the decreased vital capacity and the increase in residual volume.

Data from Carpagnano, G. E., Turchiarelli, V., Spanevello, A., et al. (2013). *Aging Clinical and Experimental Research, 25*(3), 239–245; Lalley, P. M. (2013). *Respiratory Physiology & Neurobiology, 187*(3), 199–210; Lowery, E. M., Brubaker, A. L., Kuhlmann, E., et al. (2013). *Clinical Interventions in Aging, 8,* 1489–1496; Miller, M. R. (2010). *Seminars in Respiratory and Critical Care Medicine, 31*(5), 521–527; Moliva, J. I., Rajaram, M. V., Sasindran, S. J., et al. (2014). *Age (Dordr), 36*(3), 9633; Ramly, E., Kaafarani, H. M., & Velmahos, G. C. (2015). *Surgery Clinics of North America, 95*(1), 53–69; Weiss, C. O., Hoenig, H. H., Varadhan, R., et al. (2010). *Journals of Gerontology: Series A: Biological Sciences and Medical Sciences, 65*(3), 287–294.

DID YOU UNDERSTAND?

Structures of the Pulmonary System
1. Air is inspired and expired through the conducting airways: nasopharynx, oropharynx, trachea, bronchi, and bronchioles.
2. Gas exchange occurs in structures beyond the respiratory bronchioles: in the alveolar ducts and the alveoli. Together these structures compose the acinus.
3. The primary gas-exchange units of the lungs are the alveoli. The membrane that surrounds each alveolus and contains the pulmonary capillaries is called the *alveolocapillary membrane*.
4. Pulmonary circulation, a separate division of the circulatory system, perfuses the gas-exchange airways. A branch of the systemic circulation called the *bronchial circulation perfuses* the bronchi and other lung structures.
5. The pulmonary circulation is innervated by the autonomic nervous system (ANS), but vasodilation and vasoconstriction are controlled mainly by local and humoral factors, particularly arterial oxygenation and acid–base status.
6. The chest wall is lined by a serous membrane called the *parietal pleura*; the lungs are encased in a separate membrane called the *visceral pleura*. The *pleural space* is the area where these two pleurae contact and slide over one another.

Function of the Pulmonary System
1. The pulmonary system enables oxygen (O_2) to diffuse into the blood and carbon dioxide (CO_2) to diffuse out of the blood.
2. Ventilation is the process by which air flows into and out of the gas-exchange airways.
3. Chemoreceptors in the circulatory system and brainstem sense the effectiveness of ventilation by monitoring the pH status of cerebrospinal fluid and the O_2 content (partial pressure of oxygen) of arterial blood.
4. The type II alveolar cells produce surfactant, a lipoprotein that lines the alveoli. Surfactant reduces alveolar surface tension and permits the alveoli to expand as air enters.
5. Elastic recoil is the tendency of the lungs and chest wall to return to their resting state after inspiration. Compliance is the measure of lung and chest wall distensibility and is defined as volume change per unit of pressure change.
6. Gas transport depends on ventilation of the alveoli, diffusion across the alveolocapillary membrane, perfusion of the pulmonary and systemic capillaries, and diffusion between systemic capillaries and tissue cells.

7. Efficient gas exchange depends on an even distribution of ventilation and perfusion within the lungs. Both ventilation and perfusion are greatest in the bases of the lungs because the alveoli in the bases are more compliant (their resting volume is low) and perfusion is greater in the bases as a result of gravity.
8. Almost all the O_2 that diffuses into pulmonary capillary blood is transported by hemoglobin, a protein contained within red blood cells. The remainder of the O_2 is transported dissolved in plasma.
9. O_2 enters the body by diffusing down the concentration gradient, from high concentrations in the alveoli to lower concentrations in the capillaries. Diffusion ceases when alveolar and capillary O_2 pressures equilibrate.
10. Compared with O_2, CO_2 is more soluble in plasma. Therefore, CO_2 diffuses readily from tissue cells into plasma and from plasma into the alveoli. CO_2 returns to the lungs dissolved in plasma, as bicarbonate, or in carbamino compounds (e.g., bound to hemoglobin).

GERIATRIC CONSIDERATIONS
Aging and the Pulmonary System

1. Aging affects the mechanical aspects of ventilation by decreasing chest wall compliance and elastic recoil of the lungs. Changes in these elastic properties reduce the ventilatory reserve.
2. With aging, the surface area for gas exchange and capillary perfusion may decrease, reducing exercise capacity.
3. Level of fitness and associated systemic disease affect individual lung function.

27

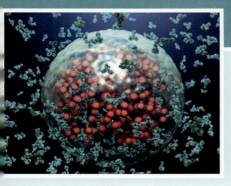

Alterations of Pulmonary Function

Mohamed Toufic El-Hussein, with originating chapter contributions by Valentina L. Brashers and Sue E. Huether

Additional resources are available online at https://evolve.elsevier.com/Canada/Huether/pathophysiology.

CHAPTER OUTLINE

Clinical Manifestations of Pulmonary Alterations, 670
    Signs and Symptoms of Pulmonary Disease, 670
    Conditions Caused by Pulmonary Disease or Injury, 672
Disorders of the Chest Wall and Pleura, 673
    Chest Wall Restriction, 673
    Pleural Abnormalities, 674
Pulmonary Disorders, 675
    Restrictive Lung Diseases, 675
    Obstructive Lung Diseases, 682
    Respiratory Tract Infections, 688

Pulmonary Vascular Disease, 691
Malignancies of the Respiratory Tract, 693
COMORBIDITIES: The Negative Impact of Comorbidities on the Disease Course of COVID-19, 697
COMORBIDITIES: Chronic Obstructive Pulmonary Disease Comorbidities, 698
GERIATRIC CONSIDERATIONS: Chronic Obstructive Pulmonary Disease in Older Persons, 699
CASE STUDY, 699

LEARNING OBJECTIVES

1. Identify the clinical indicators of pulmonary disease.
2. Define hyperventilation and hypoventilation.
3. Discuss alterations in arterial blood gas values that indicate pulmonary disease.
4. Differentiate between hypoxia and hypoxemia.
5. Define acute respiratory failure and identify risk factors.
6. Identify the types of pneumothorax, including manifestations and causes.
7. Compare and contrast pleural effusion and empyema.
8. Discuss how the structure, form, and integrity of the chest wall influence pulmonary function.
9. Discuss the clinical manifestations and underlying mechanisms of atelectasis.
10. Distinguish between the pleural abnormalities of bronchiectasis, bronchiolitis, and bronchiolitis obliterans.
11. Describe how inhaling toxic or allergenic substances causes respiratory dysfunction.
12. Describe the pathophysiology associated with pulmonary edema and acute respiratory distress syndrome.
13. Describe similarities, clinical manifestations, underlying mechanisms, and consequences of obstructive pulmonary diseases.
14. Discuss the role of inflammation in asthma.
15. Compare and contrast the clinical symptoms and underlying mechanisms of bacterial pneumonia, viral pneumonia, and tuberculosis.
16. Describe the cellular changes, clinical manifestations, treatments, outcomes, and complications of pulmonary embolus.
17. Discuss the risk factors and pathological changes associated with pulmonary hypertension.
18. Describe the different types of lung cancer.

KEY TERMS

Abscess, 691
Absorption atelectasis, 676
Acute bronchitis, 688
Acute lung injury (ALI), 678
Acute respiratory distress syndrome (ARDS), 678
Adenocarcinoma, 695
Air trapping, 687
Alveolar dead space, 673
Aspiration, 675
Asthma, 682
Atelectasis, 676

Bronchiectasis, 676
Bronchiolitis, 677
Bronchiolitis obliterans, 677
Bronchiolitis obliterans organizing pneumonia (BOOP), 677
Cavitation, 691
Cheyne-Stokes respiration, 671
Chronic bronchitis, 686
Chronic obstructive pulmonary disease (COPD), 684
Clubbing, 671

Compression atelectasis, 676
Consolidation, 689
Cor pulmonale, 693
Cough, 670
Cyanosis, 671
Dyspnea, 670
Emphysema, 687
Empyema (infected pleural effusion), 675
Extrinsic allergic alveolitis (hypersensitivity pneumonitis), 678

Exudative effusion, 675
Flail chest, 674
Hemoptysis, 670
Hypercapnia, 672
Hypersensitivity pneumonitis (extrinsic allergic alveolitis), 678
Hyperventilation, 671
Hypocapnia, 671
Hypoventilation, 671
Hypoxemia, 672
Hypoxia, 672

Idiopathic pulmonary fibrosis (IPF), 677
Ischemia, 672
Kussmaul respiration (hyperpnea), 671
Large cell carcinoma, 696
Laryngeal cancer, 694
Latent TB infection (LTBI), 691
Lung cancer, 694
Open pneumothorax (communicating pneumothorax), 674
Orthopnea, 670
Oxygen toxicity, 677
Paroxysmal nocturnal dyspnea (PND), 670
Pleural effusion, 675
Pneumoconiosis, 677
Pneumonia, 688
Pneumothorax, 674
Pulmonary artery hypertension (PAH), 692
Pulmonary edema, 678
Pulmonary embolism (PE), 692
Pulmonary fibrosis, 677
Pulsus paradoxus, 683
Respiratory failure, 673
Shunting, 672
Small cell (oat cell) carcinoma, 696
Squamous cell carcinoma, 695
Status asthmaticus, 683
Surfactant impairment, 676
Tension pneumothorax, 674
TNM classification, 696
Transudative effusion, 675
Tuberculosis (TB), 691

Pulmonary disease is often classified as acute or chronic, obstructive or restrictive, or infectious or noninfectious. Symptoms of lung disease are common and associated not only with primary lung disorders but also with diseases of other organ systems, particularly the heart.

CLINICAL MANIFESTATIONS OF PULMONARY ALTERATIONS

QUICK CHECK 27.1
1. List the primary signs and symptoms of pulmonary disease.
2. What abnormal breathing patterns are seen with pulmonary disease?
3. What mechanisms produce hypercapnia?
4. What mechanisms produce hypoxemia?

Signs and Symptoms of Pulmonary Disease

Pulmonary disease is associated with many signs and symptoms, the most common of which are dyspnea and cough. Others include abnormal sputum, hemoptysis, altered breathing patterns, hypoventilation and hyperventilation, cyanosis, clubbing, and chest pain.

Dyspnea

Dyspnea is a subjective experience of breathing discomfort that comprises qualitatively distinct sensations that vary in intensity. Dyspnea is an individual experience and derives from interactions among multiple physiological, psychological, social, and environmental factors, and it may induce secondary physiological and behavioural responses.[1] It is often described as breathlessness, air hunger, shortness of breath, laboured breathing, and preoccupation with breathing. Dyspnea may be the result of pulmonary disease or many other conditions, such as pain, heart disease, trauma, and psychogenic disorders.[2]

The severity of the experience of dyspnea may not directly correlate with the severity of underlying disease. Either diffuse or focal disturbances of ventilation, gas exchange, or ventilation–perfusion relationships can cause dyspnea, as can the increased work of breathing or any disease that damages lung tissue (lung parenchyma). Stimulation of many receptors can contribute to the sensation of dyspnea, including afferent receptors in the cortex and medulla and mechanoreceptors in the chest wall, upper airway receptors, and central and peripheral chemoreceptors.[3]

The more severe signs of dyspnea include flaring of the nostrils and use of accessory muscles of respiration. Retraction (pulling back) of the supercostal or intercostal muscles is predominant in children. Dyspnea is frequently associated with significant anxiety. To quantify dyspnea, both ordinal rating scales and visual analogue scales are used.

Dyspnea may occur transiently or can become chronic. Dyspnea first presents during exercise and is called *dyspnea on exertion*. **Orthopnea** is dyspnea that occurs during heart failure when an individual lies flat, which causes the abdominal contents to exert pressure on the diaphragm, decreasing the efficiency of the respiratory muscles. **Paroxysmal nocturnal dyspnea (PND)** occurs when individuals with pulmonary or cardiac disease awake at night gasping for air and have to sit or stand to relieve the dyspnea. Dyspnea may be unrecognized in mechanically ventilated individuals and is often accompanied by pain and anxiety. A focused assessment and change in ventilator settings may be required.[4]

Cough

Cough is a protective reflex that helps clear the airways by an explosive expiration. Inhaled particles, accumulated mucus, inflammation, or the presence of a foreign body initiates the cough reflex by stimulating the irritant receptors in the airway. There are few such receptors in the most distal bronchi and the alveoli. Therefore, it is possible for significant amounts of secretions to accumulate in the distal respiratory tree without cough being initiated. The cough reflex consists of inspiration, closure of the glottis and vocal cords, contraction of the expiratory muscles, and reopening of the glottis, causing a sudden, forceful expiration that removes the offending matter. The effectiveness of the cough depends on the depth of the inspiration and the degree to which the airways narrow, increasing the velocity of expiratory gas flow. Those with an inability to cough effectively are at greater risk for pneumonia.

Acute cough is cough that resolves within 2 to 3 weeks of the onset of illness or resolves with treatment of the underlying condition. It is most commonly the result of upper respiratory tract infections, allergic rhinitis, acute bronchitis, pneumonia, heart failure, pulmonary embolus, or aspiration. *Chronic cough* is defined as cough that is persistent and in individuals who do not smoke. Postnasal drainage syndrome, asthma, eosinophilic bronchitis, laryngeal hypersensitivity, and gastroesophageal reflux disease can trigger chronic cough.[5] In persons who smoke, chronic bronchitis is the most common cause of chronic cough, although lung cancer must always be considered. Individuals taking angiotensin-converting enzyme inhibitors for cardiovascular disease may develop chronic cough that resolves with discontinuation of the medication.

Abnormal Sputum

Changes in the amount, colour, and consistency of sputum provide information about progression of disease and effectiveness of therapy. The gross and microscopic appearances of sputum enable the clinician to identify cellular debris or microorganisms, which aids in diagnosis and choice of therapy.

Hemoptysis

Hemoptysis is the coughing up of blood or bloody secretions. Hemoptysis is sometimes confused with hematemesis, which is the vomiting of blood. Blood produced with coughing is usually bright red, has an alkaline pH, and is mixed with frothy sputum. Blood that is vomited is dark, has an acidic pH, and is mixed with food particles.

Hemoptysis usually indicates infection or inflammation that damages the bronchi (bronchitis, bronchiectasis) or the lung parenchyma (pneumonia, tuberculosis, lung abscess). Other causes include cancer, pulmonary infarction, or pulmonary venous stenosis. The amount and duration of bleeding provide important clues about its source. Bronchoscopy, combined with chest computed tomography (CT), is used to confirm the site of bleeding.

Abnormal Breathing Patterns

Normal breathing (eupnea) is rhythmic and effortless. The resting ventilatory rate is 8 to 16 breaths per minute, and tidal volume ranges from 400 to 800 mL. A short expiratory pause occurs with each breath, and the individual takes an occasional deeper breath, or sighs. Sigh breaths, which help to maintain normal lung function, are usually 1.5 to 2 times the normal tidal volume and occur approximately 10 to 12 times per hour.

The rate, depth, regularity, and effort of breathing undergo characteristic alterations in response to physiological and pathophysiological conditions. Patterns of breathing automatically adjust to minimize the work of respiratory muscles. Strenuous exercise or metabolic acidosis induces Kussmaul respiration (hyperpnea), which is characterized by a slightly increased ventilatory rate, very large tidal volumes, and no expiratory pause.

Laboured breathing occurs whenever there is an increased work of breathing, especially if the airways are obstructed. In large airway obstruction, a slow ventilatory rate, large tidal volume, increased effort, prolonged inspiration and expiration, and stridor or audible wheezing (depending on the site of obstruction) are typical. In small airway obstruction, such as that seen in asthma and chronic obstructive pulmonary disease (COPD), a rapid ventilatory rate, small tidal volume, increased effort, prolonged expiration, and wheezing are often present. Pulmonary fibrosis, for example, stiffens the lungs and chest wall. This decreases compliance, resulting in small tidal volumes and rapid ventilatory rate (tachypnea), a hallmark of *restricted breathing*.

Shock and severe cerebral hypoxia (insufficient oxygen [O_2] in the brain) contribute to gasping respirations that consist of irregular, quick inspirations with an expiratory pause. Anxiety can cause sighing respirations, which consist of irregular breathing characterized by frequent, deep sighing inspirations. Cheyne-Stokes respiration is characterized by alternating periods of deep and shallow breathing. Apnea lasting from 15 to 60 seconds is followed by ventilations that increase in volume until a peak is reached; then ventilation (tidal volume) decreases again to apnea. Cheyne-Stokes respiration results from any condition that reduces blood flow to the brainstem, which in turn slows impulses sending information to the respiratory centres of the brainstem. Neurological impairment above the brainstem is also a contributing factor (see Figure 15.1).

Hypoventilation and Hyperventilation

Hypoventilation is inadequate alveolar ventilation in relation to metabolic demands. Hypoventilation occurs when minute volume (tidal volume × respiratory rate) is reduced. Alterations in pulmonary mechanics or in the neurological control of breathing cause hypoventilation.[6] When alveolar ventilation is normal, carbon dioxide (CO_2) is removed from the lungs at the same rate as it is produced by cellular metabolism and arterial and alveolar partial pressure of carbon dioxide (PCO_2) values remain at normal levels (40 mm Hg). With hypoventilation, CO_2 removal does not keep up with CO_2 production and partial pressure of carbon dioxide in arterial blood ($PaCO_2$) increases, causing hypercapnia ($PaCO_2$ greater than 44 mm Hg) (see Table 26.2 for a definition of gas partial pressures and other pulmonary abbreviations). This increase in $PaCO_2$ results in respiratory acidosis that can affect the function of many tissues throughout the body. Hypoventilation is often overlooked until it is severe because breathing pattern and ventilatory rate may appear to be normal and changes in tidal volume can be difficult to detect clinically. Blood gas analysis (i.e., measurement of the $PaCO_2$ of arterial blood) reveals the hypoventilation. Pronounced hypoventilation can cause secondary hypoxemia, somnolence, or disorientation.

Hyperventilation is alveolar ventilation exceeding metabolic demands. The lungs remove CO_2 faster than it is produced by cellular metabolism, resulting in decreased $PaCO_2$, or hypocapnia ($PaCO_2$ less than 36 mm Hg). Hypocapnia results in a respiratory alkalosis that also can interfere with tissue function. Like hypoventilation, arterial blood gas analysis is used to determine hyperventilation. Hyperventilation commonly occurs with severe anxiety, acute head injury, pain, and in response to conditions that cause hypoxemia.

Cyanosis

Cyanosis is a bluish discoloration of the skin and mucous membranes. Increasing amounts of desaturated or reduced hemoglobin (which is bluish) in the blood causes cyanosis. It generally develops when 5 g of hemoglobin is desaturated, regardless of hemoglobin concentration.

Poor circulation resulting from intense peripheral vasoconstriction—like that observed in persons who have Raynaud's disease, are in cold environments, or are severely stressed—causes *peripheral cyanosis* (slow blood circulation in fingers and toes). Peripheral cyanosis is best seen in the nail beds. Decreased arterial oxygenation (low PaO_2) from pulmonary diseases or pulmonary or cardiac right-to-left shunts causes *central cyanosis*. Central cyanosis is best detected in buccal mucous membranes and lips.

Lack of cyanosis does not necessarily indicate that oxygenation is normal. In adults, cyanosis is not evident until severe hypoxemia is present and, therefore, is an insensitive indication of respiratory failure. For example, severe anemia (inadequate hemoglobin concentration) and carbon monoxide poisoning (in which hemoglobin binds to carbon monoxide instead of to O_2) can cause inadequate oxygenation of tissues without causing cyanosis. Individuals with polycythemia (an abnormal increase in numbers of red blood cells), however, may have cyanosis when oxygenation is adequate. Therefore, cyanosis must be interpreted in relation to the underlying pathophysiological condition. If cyanosis is suggested, the PaO_2 should be measured.

Clubbing

Clubbing is the selective bulbous enlargement of the end (distal segment) of a digit (finger or toe) (Figure 27.1). Clubbing severity can be graded from 1 to 5 based on the extent of nail bed hypertrophy and the amount of changes in the nails themselves. It is usually painless. Clubbing is commonly associated with diseases that disrupt the normal pulmonary circulation and cause chronic hypoxemia, such as bronchiectasis, cystic fibrosis, pulmonary fibrosis, lung abscess, and congenital heart disease, and is rarely reversible. It is proposed that whole megakaryocytes enter the systemic circulation and become impacted in the fingertip circulation. Megakaryocytes and megakaryocyte fragments are activated to release platelet-derived growth factor (PDGF). PDGF promotes growth, vascular permeability, and monocyte and neutrophil chemotaxis and leads to an increased number of vascular smooth muscle cells and fibroblasts, all of which are seen in the pathology of clubbing.[7] It can sometimes be seen in individuals with lung cancer even without hypoxemia because of the effects of inflammatory cytokines and growth factors (hypertrophic osteoarthropathy).[8]

Pain

Pain caused by pulmonary disorders originates in the pleurae, airways, or chest wall.[9] Infection and inflammation of the parietal pleura cause sharp or stabbing pain (pleurodynia) when the pleura stretches during inspiration. The pain is usually localized to a portion of the chest wall, where a unique breath sound called a *pleural friction rub* may be heard over the

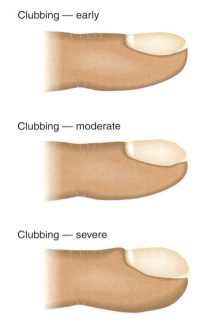

FIGURE 27.1 Clubbing of Fingers Caused by Chronic Hypoxemia. (Modified from Seidel, H. M., Stewart, R. W., Ball, J. W., et al. [2011]. *Mosby's guide to physical examination* [7th ed.]. Mosby.)

painful area. Laughing or coughing makes pleural pain worse. Pleural pain is common with pulmonary infarction (tissue death) caused by pulmonary embolism (PE) and emanates from the area around the infarction.

Infection and inflammation of the trachea or bronchi (tracheitis or tracheobronchitis, respectively) can cause central chest pain that is pronounced after coughing. It can be difficult to differentiate from cardiac pain. High blood pressure in the pulmonary circulation (pulmonary hypertension) can cause pain during exercise that is often mistaken for cardiac pain (angina pectoris).

Pain in the chest wall is muscle pain or rib pain. Excessive coughing (which makes the muscles sore) and rib fractures or thoracic surgery produce such pain. Inflammation of the costochondral junction (costochondritis) also can cause chest wall pain. Chest wall pain can often be reproduced by pressing on the sternum or ribs.

Conditions Caused by Pulmonary Disease or Injury
Hypercapnia

Hypercapnia is associated with hypoventilation of the alveoli, and leads to increased CO_2 concentration in the arterial blood (increased $PaCO_2$). As discussed in Chapter 26, CO_2 is easily diffused from the blood into the alveolar space; as such minute volume (respiratory rate × tidal volume) determines not only alveolar ventilation but also $PaCO_2$. Hypoventilation is often overlooked because the breathing pattern and ventilatory rate may appear to be normal; therefore, it is important to obtain blood gas analysis to determine the severity of hypercapnia and resultant respiratory acidosis (acid–base balance is described in Chapter 5).

There are many causes of hypercapnia. Most are a result of a decreased drive to breathe or an inadequate ability to respond to ventilatory stimulation. Some of these causes include:
- depression of the respiratory centre by medications
- diseases of the medulla, including infections of the central nervous system or trauma
- abnormalities of the spinal conducting pathways, as in spinal cord disruption or poliomyelitis
- diseases of the neuromuscular junction or of the respiratory muscles themselves, as in myasthenia gravis or muscular dystrophy
- thoracic cage abnormalities, as in chest injury or congenital deformity
- large airway obstruction, as in tumours or sleep apnea, and
- increased work of breathing or physiological dead space, as in emphysema.

Hypercapnia and the associated respiratory acidosis result in electrolyte abnormalities that may cause dysrhythmias. Individuals also may present with somnolence and even coma because of changes in intracranial pressure associated with high levels of arterial CO_2, which causes cerebral vasodilation. Alveolar hypoventilation with increased alveolar CO_2 concentration limits the amount of O_2 available for diffusion into the blood, thereby leading to secondary hypoxemia.

Hypoxemia

Hypoxemia, or reduced oxygenation of arterial blood (reduced PaO_2), is caused by respiratory alterations, whereas hypoxia (or ischemia) is reduced oxygenation of cells in tissues. Although hypoxemia can lead to tissue hypoxia, tissue hypoxia can result from other abnormalities unrelated to alterations of pulmonary function, such as low cardiac output or cyanide poisoning.

Hypoxemia results from problems with one or more of the major mechanisms of oxygenation:
1. O_2 delivery to the alveoli
    a. O_2 content of the inspired air (fraction of inspired oxygen [FiO_2])
    b. Ventilation of alveoli
2. Diffusion of O_2 from the alveoli into the blood
    a. Balance between alveolar ventilation and perfusion ($\dot{V}/\dot{Q}$ match)
    b. Diffusion of O_2 across the alveolar capillary barrier
3. Perfusion of pulmonary capillaries

The amount of O_2 in the alveoli is called the PaO_2 and is dependent on two factors. The first factor is the presence of adequate O_2 content of the inspired air. The amount of O_2 in inspired air is expressed as the percentage or fraction of air that is composed of O_2, called the FiO_2. The FiO_2 of air at sea level is approximately 21%, or 0.21. Anything that decreases the FiO_2 (such as high altitude) decreases the PaO_2. A second factor is the amount of alveolar minute volume (tidal volume × respiratory rate). Hypoventilation results in an increase in partial pressure of carbon dioxide in alveolar gas and a decrease in PaO_2 such that there is less O_2 available in the alveoli for diffusion into the blood. This type of hypoxemia can be completely corrected if alveolar ventilation is improved by increases in the rate and depth of breathing. Hypoventilation causes hypoxemia in unconscious persons; in persons with neurological, muscular, or bone diseases that restrict chest expansion; and in individuals who have COPD.

Diffusion of O_2 from the alveoli into the blood is also dependent on two factors. The first is the balance between the amount of air that enters alveoli ($\dot{V}$) and the amount of blood perfusing the capillaries around the alveoli ($\dot{Q}$). An abnormal ventilation–perfusion ratio ($\dot{V}/\dot{Q}$) is the most common cause of hypoxemia (Figure 27.2). The normal $\dot{V}/\dot{Q}$ is 0.8 because perfusion is somewhat greater than ventilation in the lung bases and because some blood is normally shunted to the bronchial circulation. $\dot{V}/\dot{Q}$ *mismatch* refers to an abnormal distribution of ventilation and perfusion. Inadequate ventilation of well-perfused areas of the lung (low $\dot{V}/\dot{Q}$) causes hypoxemia. Mismatching of this type, called shunting, occurs in atelectasis, in asthma as a result of bronchoconstriction, and in pulmonary edema and pneumonia when alveoli are filled with fluid. When blood passes through portions of the pulmonary capillary bed that receive no ventilation, the pulmonary capillaries in that area constrict and a right-to-left shunt occurs, resulting in decreased systemic PaO_2 and hypoxemia. Poor perfusion of well-ventilated portions of the lung (high $\dot{V}/\dot{Q}$), resulting in wasted ventilation, causes hypoxemia. The most common cause of high $\dot{V}/\dot{Q}$ is a pulmonary embolus that impairs blood flow to a segment of the

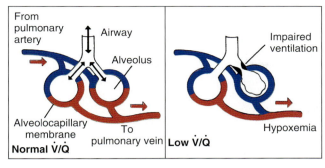
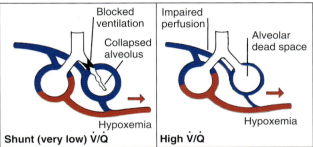

FIGURE 27.2 Ventilation–Perfusion Abnormalities. $\dot{V}/\dot{Q}$, Ventilation–perfusion ratio.

lung. An area where alveoli are ventilated but not perfused is termed **alveolar dead space**.

The second factor affecting diffusion of O_2 from the alveoli into the blood is the alveolocapillary membrane. Diffusion of O_2 through the alveolocapillary membrane is impaired if the membrane is thickened or the surface area available for diffusion is decreased. Thickened alveolocapillary membranes, as occur with edema (tissue swelling) and fibrosis (formation of fibrous lesions), increase the time required for O_2 to diffuse from the alveoli into the capillaries. If diffusion is slowed enough, the P_{O_2} levels of alveolar gas and capillary blood do not have time to equilibrate during the fraction of a second that blood remains in the capillary. Destruction of alveoli, as in emphysema, decreases the alveolocapillary membrane surface area available for diffusion. Hypercapnia is seldom produced by impaired diffusion because CO_2 diffuses so easily from capillary to alveolus that the individual with impaired diffusion would die from hypoxemia before hypercapnia could occur.

Hypoxemia can result from blood flow bypassing the lungs. It can occur because of intracardiac defects that cause right-to-left shunting or because of intrapulmonary arteriovenous malformations.

Hypoxemia is most often associated with a compensatory hyperventilation and the resultant respiratory alkalosis (i.e., decreased $PaCO_2$ and increased pH). However, in individuals with associated ventilatory difficulties, hypoxemia may be complicated by hypercapnia and respiratory acidosis. Hypoxemia results in widespread tissue dysfunction and, when severe, can lead to organ infarction. In addition, hypoxic pulmonary vasoconstriction can contribute to increased pressures in the pulmonary artery (pulmonary artery hypertension [PAH]) and lead to right ventricular failure or cor pulmonale. Clinical manifestations of acute hypoxemia may include cyanosis, confusion, tachycardia, edema, and decreased renal output.

Acute Respiratory Failure

> **✓ QUICK CHECK 27.2**
> 1. How does chest wall restriction affect ventilation?
> 2. How does pneumothorax differ from pleural effusion?
> 3. What causes empyema?

Respiratory failure is defined as inadequate gas exchange such that PaO_2 is less than or equal to 60 mm Hg or $PaCO_2$ is greater than or equal to 50 mm Hg, with pH less than or equal to 7.25.[10] Respiratory failure can result from direct injury to the lungs, airways, or chest wall or indirectly because of disease or injury involving another body system, such as the brain, spinal cord, or heart. It can occur in individuals who have an otherwise normal respiratory system or in those with underlying chronic pulmonary disease. Most pulmonary diseases can cause episodes of acute respiratory failure. If the respiratory failure is primarily hypercapnic, it is the result of inadequate alveolar ventilation and the individual must receive ventilatory support with a bag-valve mask, noninvasive positive pressure ventilation, or intubation and placement on mechanical ventilation. If the respiratory failure is primarily hypoxemic, it is the result of inadequate exchange of O_2 between the alveoli and the capillaries and the individual must receive supplemental O_2 therapy. Many people will have combined hypercapnic and hypoxemic respiratory failure and will require both kinds of support.

Respiratory failure is an important potential complication of any major surgical procedure, especially those that involve the central nervous system, thorax, or upper abdomen. The most common postoperative pulmonary problems are atelectasis, pneumonia, pulmonary edema, and pulmonary emboli. People who smoke are at risk, particularly if they have pre-existing lung disease. Limited cardiac reserve, neurological disease, chronic renal failure, chronic hepatic disease, and infection also increase the tendency to develop postoperative respiratory failure.

Prevention of postoperative respiratory failure includes frequent turning and position changes, deep-breathing exercises, and early ambulation to prevent atelectasis and accumulation of secretions. Humidification of inspired air can help loosen secretions. Incentive spirometry gives individuals immediate feedback about tidal volumes, which encourages them to breathe deeply. Supplemental O_2 is given for hypoxemia, and antibiotics are given as appropriate to treat infection. If respiratory failure develops, the individual may require mechanical ventilation or extracorporeal membrane oxygenation (ECMO).

DISORDERS OF THE CHEST WALL AND PLEURA

There are many conditions that can affect the chest wall or pleura, or both, and influence the function of the respiratory system. Chest wall disorders primarily affect tidal volume and, therefore, result in hypercapnia. Pleural diseases impact both ventilation and oxygenation.

Chest Wall Restriction

If the chest wall is deformed, traumatized, immobilized, or heavy from the accumulation of fat, the work of breathing increases and ventilation may be compromised because of a decrease in tidal volume. The degree of ventilatory impairment depends on the severity of the chest wall abnormality. Grossly obese individuals are often dyspneic on exertion or when recumbent. Individuals with severe kyphoscoliosis (lateral bending and rotation of the spinal column, with distortion of the thoracic cage) often present with dyspnea on exertion that can progress to respiratory failure. Obesity and kyphoscoliosis are risk factors for respiratory failure or infections in individuals admitted to the hospital for other problems, particularly those who require surgery. Other musculoskeletal abnormalities that can impair ventilation are ankylosing spondylitis (see Chapter 39) and pectus excavatum (a deformity characterized by depression of the sternum).

Impairment of respiratory muscle function caused by neuromuscular diseases such as poliomyelitis, muscular dystrophy, myasthenia gravis, and Guillain-Barré syndrome (see Chapter 16) also can restrict the chest wall and impair pulmonary function. Muscle weakness can result in hypoventilation, inability to remove secretions, and hypoxemia.

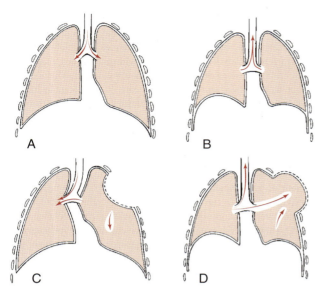

FIGURE 27.3 Flail Chest. Normal respiration: **A**, inspiration; **B**, expiration. Paradoxical motion: **C**, inspiration, area of lung underlying unstable chest wall flattens on inspiration; **D**, expiration, unstable area inflates. Note movement of mediastinum toward opposite lung during inspiration.

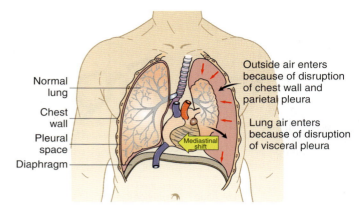

FIGURE 27.4 Pneumothorax. Air in the pleural space causes the lung to collapse around the hilus and may push mediastinal contents (heart and great vessels) toward the other lung.

Pain from chest wall injury, surgery, or disease can cause significant hypoventilation, especially in those with underlying lung disease. Trauma to the thorax can not only restrict chest expansion because of pain but also cause structural and mechanical changes that impair the ability of the chest to expand normally. **Flail chest** results from the fracture of several consecutive ribs in more than one place or fracture of the sternum and several consecutive ribs. These multiple fractures result in instability of a portion of the chest wall, causing paradoxical movement of the chest with breathing. During inspiration, the unstable portion of the chest wall moves inward and during expiration it moves outward, impairing movement of gas in and out of the lungs (Figure 27.3).

Chest wall restriction results in a decrease in tidal volume. An increase in respiratory rate can compensate for small decreases in tidal volume, but many individuals will progress to hypercapnic respiratory failure. Pulmonary function testing (reduction in forced vital capacity [FVC]), arterial blood gas measurement (hypercapnia), and radiographs are used to diagnosis chest wall restriction. Treatment is aimed at any reversible underlying cause but is otherwise supportive. In severe cases, mechanical ventilation may be indicated.

Pleural Abnormalities
Pneumothorax

Pneumothorax is the presence of air or gas in the pleural space caused by a rupture in the visceral pleura (which surrounds the lungs) or the parietal pleura and chest wall. As air separates the visceral and parietal pleurae, it destroys the negative pressure of the pleural space and disrupts the equilibrium between elastic recoil forces of the lung and chest wall. The lung then tends to recoil by collapsing toward the hilum (Figure 27.4).

Primary (spontaneous) pneumothorax occurs unexpectedly in healthy individuals (usually men) between 20 and 40 years of age and is caused by the spontaneous rupture of blebs (blisterlike formations) on the visceral pleura. Bleb rupture can occur during sleep, rest, or exercise. The ruptured blebs are usually located in the apexes of the lungs.

The cause of bleb formation is not known, although more than 80% of these individuals have been found to have emphysema-like changes in their lungs even if they have no history of smoking or no known genetic disorder. Approximately 10% of affected individuals have a significant family history of primary pneumothorax that has been linked to mutations in the folliculin gene.[11] Chest trauma (such as a rib fracture or stab and bullet wounds that tear the pleura; rupture of a bleb or bulla [larger vesicle], as occurs in emphysema; or mechanical ventilation, particularly if it includes positive end-expiratory pressure [PEEP]) can cause *secondary pneumothorax*. Transthoracic needle aspiration is the most common cause of *iatrogenic pneumothorax* by primary pneumothorax, and secondary pneumothorax can present as either open or tension. In **open pneumothorax (communicating pneumothorax)**, air pressure in the pleural space equals barometric pressure because air that is drawn into the pleural space during inspiration (through the damaged chest wall and parietal pleura or through the lungs and damaged visceral pleura) is forced back out during expiration. In **tension pneumothorax**, however, the site of pleural rupture acts as a one-way valve, permitting air to enter on inspiration but preventing its escape by closing during expiration. As more and more air enters the pleural space, air pressure in the pneumothorax begins to exceed barometric pressure. Air pressure in the pleural space pushes against the already recoiled lung, causing compression atelectasis, and against the mediastinum, compressing and displacing the heart, great vessels, and trachea (*mediastinal shift*). The pathophysiological effects of tension pneumothorax are life-threatening (see Figure 27.4).

Clinical manifestations of spontaneous or secondary pneumothorax begin with sudden pleural pain, tachypnea, and dyspnea. Depending on the size of the pneumothorax, physical examination may reveal absent or decreased breath sounds and hyper-resonance to percussion on the affected side. Severe hypoxemia, tracheal deviation away from the affected lung, and hypotension (low blood pressure) complicate tension pneumothorax. Deterioration occurs rapidly and immediate treatment is required. Diagnosis of pneumothorax is made with chest radiographs, ultrasound, and CT. Aspiration, usually with insertion of a chest tube that is attached to a water-seal drainage system with suction or a small-bore catheter with a one-way valve, is used to treat pneumothorax.[12] After the pneumothorax is evacuated and the pleural rupture is healed, the chest tube is removed. For individuals with persistent air leaks, other interventions may be needed including thoracoscopic surgical techniques or pleurodesis (instillation of a caustic substance, such as talc, into the pleural space).

TABLE 27.1 Mechanism of Pleural Effusion[a]

Type of Fluid/Effusion	Source of Accumulation	Primary or Associated Disorder
Transudate (hydrothorax)	Watery fluid that diffuses out of capillaries beneath pleura (i.e., capillaries in lung or chest wall)	Cardiovascular disease that causes high pulmonary capillary pressures; liver or kidney disease that disrupts plasma protein production, causing hypoproteinemia (decreased oncotic pressure in blood vessels)
Exudate	Fluid rich in cells and proteins (leukocytes, plasma proteins of all kinds; see Chapter 5) that migrates out of capillaries	Infection, inflammation, or malignancy of pleura that stimulates mast cells to release biochemical mediators that increase capillary permeability
Pus (empyema)	Microorganisms and debris of infection (leukocytes, cellular debris) accumulate in pleural space	Pulmonary infections, such as pneumonia; lung abscesses; infected wounds
Blood (hemothorax)	Hemorrhage into pleural space	Traumatic injury, surgery, rupture, or malignancy that damages blood vessels
Chyle (chylothorax)	Chyle (milky fluid containing lymph and fat droplets) that moves from lymphatic vessels into pleural space instead of passing from gastro-intestinal tract to thoracic duct	Traumatic injury, infection, or disorder that disrupts lymphatic transport

[a]The principles of diffusion are described in Chapter 1; mechanisms that increase capillary permeability and cause exudation of cells, proteins, and fluid are discussed in Chapter 5.

Pleural Effusion

Pleural effusion is the presence of fluid in the pleural space. The source of the fluid is usually from blood vessels or lymphatic vessels lying beneath the pleural space, but occasionally an abscess or other lesion may drain into the pleural space. Pleural effusions that enter the pleural space from intact blood vessels can be **transudative** (watery) or **exudative** (high concentrations of white blood cells and plasma proteins). Other types of pleural effusion are characterized by the presence of pus (empyema), blood (hemothorax), or chyle (chylothorax). Mechanisms of pleural effusion are summarized in Table 27.1.

Small collections of fluid may not affect lung function and remain undetected. Most will be removed by the lymphatic system once the underlying condition is resolved. In larger effusions, dyspnea, compression atelectasis with impaired ventilation, and pleural pain are common. Mediastinal shift and cardiovascular manifestations occur in a large, rapidly developing effusion. Physical examination shows decreased breath sounds and dullness to percussion on the affected side. A pleural friction rub can be heard over areas of inflamed pleura.

Chest X-ray and thoracentesis (needle aspiration) are used to confirm the diagnosis and determine the type of effusion, in addition to providing symptomatic relief. If the effusion is large, drainage usually requires the placement of a chest tube and surgical interventions may be needed to prevent recurrence of the effusion.

Empyema

Empyema (infected pleural effusion) is the presence of pus in the pleural space and develops when the pulmonary lymphatics become blocked, leading to an outpouring of contaminated lymphatic fluid into the pleural space. Empyema occurs most commonly in older persons and children and usually develops as a complication of pneumonia, surgery, trauma, or bronchial obstruction from a tumour. Commonly documented infectious organisms include *Staphylococcus aureus*, *Escherichia coli*, anaerobic bacteria, and *Klebsiella pneumoniae*.

Individuals with empyema present clinically with cyanosis, fever, tachycardia (rapid heart rate), cough, and pleural pain. Breath sounds are decreased directly over the empyema. Chest radiographs, thoracentesis, and sputum culture are used to make the diagnosis. The treatment for empyema includes the administration of appropriate antimicrobials and drainage of the pleural space with a chest tube. In severe cases, ultrasound-guided pleural drainage, instillation of fibrinolytic agents, or introduction of deoxyribonuclease (DNase) into the pleural space is needed for adequate drainage. Surgical debridement may be required.[13]

PULMONARY DISORDERS

> ✓ **QUICK CHECK 27.3**
> 1. Contrast *aspiration* and *atelectasis*.
> 2. What are some of the causes of pulmonary fibrosis?
> 3. What symptoms are produced by inhalation of toxic gases?
> 4. Describe pneumoconiosis and give two examples.
> 5. Briefly describe the role of neutrophils in acute respiratory distress syndrome.

Restrictive Lung Diseases

Restrictive lung diseases are characterized by decreased compliance of the lung tissue. This decrease in lung compliance means that it takes more effort to expand the lungs during inspiration, which increases the work of breathing. Individuals with lung restriction have dyspnea, an increased respiratory rate, and a decreased tidal volume. Pulmonary function testing reveals a decrease in FVC. Restrictive lung diseases can cause $\dot{V}/\dot{Q}$ mismatch and affect the alveolocapillary membrane, which reduces the diffusion of O_2 from the alveoli into the blood and results in hypoxemia. Some of the most common restrictive lung diseases in adults are aspiration, atelectasis, bronchiectasis, bronchiolitis, pulmonary fibrosis, inhalation disorders (e.g., pneumoconiosis and allergic alveolitis), pulmonary edema, and acute lung injury (ALI)/acute respiratory distress syndrome (ARDS).

Aspiration

Aspiration is the passage of fluid and solid particles into the lung. It tends to occur in individuals whose normal swallowing mechanism and cough reflex are impaired by central or peripheral nervous system abnormalities. Predisposing factors include an altered level of consciousness caused by substance abuse, sedation, or anaesthesia; seizure disorders; stroke; neuromuscular disorders that cause dysphagia; and feeding through a nasogastric tube. The right lung, particularly the right lower lobe, is more susceptible to aspiration than the left lung because the branching angle of the right mainstem bronchus is straighter than the branching angle of the left mainstem bronchus.

Aspiration of large food particles or gastric fluid with pH of less than 2.5 has serious consequences. Solid food particles can obstruct a bronchus, resulting in bronchial inflammation and collapse of airways distal to the obstruction. If the aspirated solid is not identified and removed by bronchoscopy, a chronic, local inflammation develops that may lead to recurrent infection and bronchiectasis (permanent dilation of the bronchus).

Aspiration of oral or pharyngeal secretions can lead to aspiration pneumonia. Intubation of the trachea also can cause aspiration and bacterial pneumonia. Aspiration of acidic gastric fluid may cause severe pneumonitis. Bronchial damage includes inflammation, loss of ciliary function, and bronchospasm. In the alveoli, acidic fluid damages the alveolocapillary membrane. This damage to the alveolocapillary membrane allows plasma and blood cells to move from capillaries into the alveoli, resulting in hemorrhagic pneumonitis. The lung becomes stiff and noncompliant as surfactant production is disrupted, leading to further edema and collapse. Hypoventilation may develop as this process progresses and systematic complications, such as hypotension, may occur.

Clinical manifestations of aspiration include the sudden onset of choking and intractable cough with or without vomiting, fever, dyspnea, and wheezing. Some individuals have no symptoms acutely; instead, they have recurrent lung infections, chronic cough, or persistent wheezing over months and even years.

Preventive measures for individuals at risk are more effective than treatment of known aspiration. The most important preventive measures include use of a semirecumbent position, surveillance of enteral feeding, use of promotility agents, and avoidance of excessive sedation. Nasogastric tubes, which are often used to remove stomach contents, are used to prevent aspiration but also can cause aspiration if fluid and particulate matter are regurgitated as the tube is being placed.

Treatment of aspiration pneumonitis includes use of supplemental O_2 and mechanical ventilation with PEEP and administration of corticosteroids. Fluids are restricted to decrease blood volume and minimize pulmonary edema. Bacterial pneumonia may develop as a complication of aspiration pneumonitis and must be treated with broad-spectrum antimicrobials.

Atelectasis

Atelectasis is the collapse of lung tissue. There are three types of atelectasis:

1. **Compression atelectasis** is caused by external pressure exerted by tumour, fluid, or air in the pleural space or by abdominal distension pressing on a portion of lung, causing alveoli to collapse.
2. **Absorption atelectasis** results from removal of air from obstructed or hypoventilated alveoli or from inhalation of concentrated O_2 or anaesthetic agents.
3. **Surfactant impairment** results from decreased production or inactivation of surfactant, which is necessary to reduce surface tension in the alveoli and thus prevent lung collapse during expiration. Surfactant impairment can occur because of premature birth, ARDS, anaesthesia induction, or mechanical ventilation.

Atelectasis tends to occur after surgery, especially in those who have been administered general anaesthetics.[14] Postoperative individuals are often in pain, breathe shallowly, are reluctant to change position, and produce viscous secretions that tend to pool in dependent portions of the lung, especially following thoracic or upper abdominal surgery. Atelectasis increases shunt, decreases compliance, and may lead to perioperative hypoxemia.

Clinical manifestations of atelectasis are similar to those of pulmonary infection including dyspnea, cough, fever, and leukocytosis. Prevention and treatment of postoperative atelectasis usually include deep-breathing exercises (often with the aid of an incentive spirometer), frequent position changes, and early ambulation. Deep breathing promotes ciliary clearance of secretions, stabilizes the alveoli by redistributing surfactant, and promotes collateral ventilation through the pores of Kohn, promoting expansion of collapsed alveoli (Figure 27.5). Postoperative noninvasive positive-pressure ventilation (NIPPV) has been shown to improve oxygenation and ventilation for high-risk individuals (i.e., individuals who are obese or in respiratory distress).

Bronchiectasis

Bronchiectasis is persistent abnormal dilation of the bronchi. There may be a genetic predisposition or a defect in host defence.[15] It usually occurs in conjunction with other respiratory conditions that are associated with chronic bronchial inflammation, such as obstruction of an airway with mucous plugs, atelectasis, aspiration of a foreign body, infection, cystic fibrosis (see Chapter 28), tuberculosis,

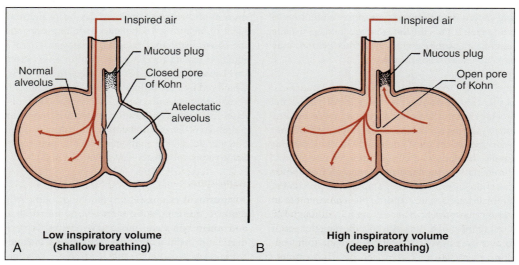

FIGURE 27.5 Pores of Kohn. **A**, Absorption atelectasis caused by lack of collateral ventilation through pores of Kohn. **B**, Restoration of collateral ventilation during deep breathing.

congenital weakness of the bronchial wall, or immunocompromised health status. Chronic inflammation of the bronchi leads to destruction of elastic and muscular components of their walls, obstruction of the bronchial lumen, traction from adjacent fibrosis, and permanent dilation. Bronchiectasis also is associated with a number of systemic disorders, such as rheumatological disease, inflammatory bowel disease, and immunodeficiency syndromes (e.g., acquired immune deficiency syndrome [AIDS]). There may be no known cause.

The primary symptom of bronchiectasis is a chronic productive cough that may date back to a childhood illness or infection. The disease is commonly associated with recurrent lower respiratory tract infections and expectoration of voluminous amounts of foul-smelling purulent sputum (measured in cupfuls). Hemoptysis and clubbing of the fingers (from chronic hypoxemia) are common. Pulmonary function studies show decreases in FVC and expiratory flow rates. Hypoxemia eventually leads to cor pulmonale. High-resolution CT is used to confirm the diagnosis. Bronchiectasis is treated with sputum culture, antibiotics, anti-inflammatory medications, bronchodilators, chest physiotherapy, and supplemental O_2.

Bronchiolitis

Bronchiolitis is a diffuse, inflammatory obstruction of the small airways or bronchioles occurring most commonly in children. In adults it usually occurs with chronic bronchitis but can occur in otherwise healthy individuals in association with an upper or lower respiratory tract viral infection, with inhalation of toxic gases, or be of unknown etiology.[16] Bronchiolitis also is a serious complication of stem cell and lung transplantation and can progress to **bronchiolitis obliterans**, a fibrotic process that occludes airways and causes permanent scarring of the lungs. **Bronchiolitis obliterans organizing pneumonia (BOOP)** is a complication of bronchiolitis obliterans in which the alveoli and bronchioles become filled with plugs of connective tissue.

Clinical manifestations include a rapid ventilatory rate; marked use of accessory muscles; low-grade fever; dry, nonproductive cough; and hyperinflated chest. A decrease in the $\dot{V}/\dot{Q}$ results in hypoxemia. Spirometry and bronchoscopy with biopsy are used to make the diagnosis. Bronchiolitis is treated with appropriate antibiotics, corticosteroids, immunosuppressive agents, and chest physiotherapy (humidified air administration, coughing and deep-breathing exercises, postural drainage).

Pulmonary Fibrosis

Pulmonary fibrosis is an excessive amount of fibrous or connective tissue in the lung. Formation of scar tissue after active pulmonary disease (e.g., ARDS, tuberculosis), in association with a variety of autoimmune disorders (e.g., rheumatoid arthritis, progressive systemic sclerosis, sarcoidosis), can cause pulmonary fibrosis.

Inhalation of harmful substances (e.g., coal dust, asbestos) can also contribute to the development of pulmonary fibrosis. Chronic inflammation leads to fibrosis and causes a marked loss of lung compliance. The lung becomes stiff and difficult to ventilate, and the diffusing capacity of the alveolocapillary membrane may decrease, causing hypoxemia. Diffuse pulmonary fibrosis has a poor prognosis.

Pulmonary fibrosis is known as idiopathic pulmonary fibrosis when there is no specific cause. **Idiopathic pulmonary fibrosis (IPF)** is the most common idiopathic interstitial lung disorder. It is more common in men than in women and most cases occur after age 60. Although IPF is characterized by chronic inflammation, recent studies suggest that it results from multiple injuries at different lung sites with aberrant healing responses to alveolar epithelial cell injury, which probably occurs in response to a combination of environmental insults and genetic predispositions.[17] Fibroproliferation of the interstitial lung tissue around the alveoli causes decreased O_2 diffusion across the alveolocapillary membrane and hypoxemia. As the disease progresses, decreased lung compliance leads to increased work of breathing, decreased tidal volume, and resultant hypoventilation with hypercapnia.

The primary symptom of IPF is increasing dyspnea on exertion. Physical examination reveals diffuse inspiratory crackles. Pulmonary function testing (decreased FVC), high-resolution CT, and lung biopsy are used to confirm the diagnosis. Treatment includes O_2, corticosteroids, and cytotoxic medications, although success rates are low, and toxicities are high. Newer therapies include antifibrotic medications (N-acetylcysteine [Mucomyst], pirfenidone [Esbriet]), nintedanib (Ofev; an angiogenesis inhibitor), interferon alfa-2 (Intron A), and anticoagulation therapy.[18] Selected individuals may benefit from lung transplantation.

Inhalation Disorders

Exposure to toxic gases. Inhalation of gaseous irritants can cause significant respiratory dysfunction. Commonly encountered toxic gases include smoke, ammonia, hydrogen chloride, sulphur dioxide, chlorine, phosgene, and nitrogen dioxide. Inhalation injuries in burns can include toxic gases from household or industrial combustants, heat, and smoke particles. Inhaled toxic particles cause damage to the airway epithelium and promote mucus secretion, inflammation, mucosal edema, ciliary damage, pulmonary edema, and surfactant inactivation. The cellular effects of toxic gases and polluted air are described in Chapter 4. ARDS and pneumonia are common complications of acute toxic inhalation. Initial symptoms include burning of the eyes, nose, and throat; coughing; chest tightness; and dyspnea. Hypoxemia is common. Treatment includes administration of supplemental O_2, mechanical ventilation with PEEP, and support of the cardiovascular system. Corticosteroids are sometimes used, although their effectiveness has not been well documented. Most individuals respond quickly to therapy. Some, however, may improve initially and then deteriorate as a result of bronchiectasis or bronchiolitis.

Prolonged exposure to high concentrations of supplemental O_2 can result in a relatively rare condition known as **oxygen toxicity**. O_2 free radicals mediate the severe inflammatory response leading to the underlying mechanism of injury. Damage to alveolocapillary membranes results in disruption of surfactant production, production of interstitial and alveolar edema, and a reduction in lung compliance. Treatment involves ventilatory support and a reduction of inspired O_2 concentration to less than 60% as soon as tolerated.

Pneumoconiosis. **Pneumoconiosis** represents any change in the lung caused by inhalation of inorganic dust particles, usually occurring in the workplace. As in all cases of environmentally acquired lung disease, the individual's history of exposure is important in determining the diagnosis. Pneumoconiosis often occurs after years of exposure to the offending dust, with progressive fibrosis of lung tissue.

The dusts of silica, asbestos, and coal are the most common causes of pneumoconiosis. Others include talc, fibreglass, clays, mica, slate, cement, cadmium, beryllium, tungsten, cobalt, aluminum, and iron. Deposition of these materials in the lungs causes the release of proinflammatory cytokines. This leads to chronic inflammation with scarring of the alveolocapillary membrane, resulting in pulmonary fibrosis and progressive pulmonary deterioration. Clinical manifestations with advancement of disease include cough, chronic sputum production, dyspnea, decreased lung volumes, and hypoxemia. Chest X-ray or CT and obtaining a complete occupational history are used to confirm the diagnosis. Treatment is usually palliative and focuses on preventing further exposure and improving working conditions, along with pulmonary rehabilitation and management of associated hypoxemia and bronchospasm.

Hypersensitivity pneumonitis. The inhalation of organic particles or fumes can cause **hypersensitivity pneumonitis (extrinsic allergic alveolitis)**, an allergic, inflammatory disease of the lungs. Many allergens can cause this disorder, including grains, silage, bird droppings or feathers, wood dust (particularly redwood and maple), cork dust, animal pelts, coffee beans, fish meal, mushroom compost, and moulds that grow on sugarcane, barley, and straw. The lung inflammation is a hypersensitivity response that occurs after repeated, prolonged exposure to the allergen causing pneumonitis. Lymphocytes and inflammatory cells infiltrate the interstitial lung tissue, releasing a variety of autoimmune and inflammatory cytokines.[19]

Hypersensitivity pneumonitis can be acute, subacute, or chronic. The acute form causes fever, cough, and chills a few hours after exposure. With continued exposure, the disease becomes chronic and pulmonary fibrosis develops. Obtaining a history of allergen exposure, performing serum antibody testing, chest X-ray, bronchoalveolar lavage, CT, and, in some cases, lung biopsy are needed to make the diagnosis. Treatment consists of removal of the offending agent and administration of corticosteroids.[20]

Pulmonary Edema

Pulmonary edema is excess fluid in the lung. The normal lung is kept dry by lymphatic drainage and a balance among capillary hydrostatic pressure, capillary oncotic pressure, and capillary permeability. In addition, surfactant lining the alveoli repels water, keeping fluid from entering the alveoli. Predisposing factors for pulmonary edema include heart disease, ARDS, and inhalation of toxic gases. The pathogenesis of pulmonary edema is shown in Figure 27.6.

The most common cause of pulmonary edema is left-sided heart disease. When the left ventricle fails, filling pressures on the left side of the heart increase and cause a concomitant increase in pulmonary capillary hydrostatic pressure. When the hydrostatic pressure exceeds the oncotic pressure (which holds fluid in the capillary), fluid moves from the capillary into the interstitial space (the space within the alveolar septum between the alveolus and capillary). When the flow of fluid out of the capillaries exceeds the lymphatic system's ability to remove it, pulmonary edema develops.

Another cause of pulmonary edema is capillary injury that increases capillary permeability, as in cases of adult respiratory distress syndrome or inhalation of toxic gases, such as ammonia. Capillary injury and inflammation cause water and plasma proteins to leak out of the capillary and move into the interstitial space, increasing the interstitial oncotic pressure (which is usually very low). As the interstitial oncotic pressure begins to exceed the capillary oncotic pressure, water moves out of the capillary and into the lung. (Mechanisms of edema are discussed in Chapter 5, Figures 5.1 and 5.2). Tumours and fibrotic tissue obstruct the lymphatic system and increase systemic venous pressure, resulting in pulmonary edema.

Clinical manifestations of pulmonary edema include dyspnea, hypoxemia, and increased work of breathing. Physical examination may disclose inspiratory crackles (rales) and dullness to percussion over the lung bases. In severe edema, pink frothy sputum is expectorated, hypoxemia worsens, and hypoventilation with hypercapnia may develop.

The treatment of pulmonary edema depends on its cause. If the edema is caused by increased hydrostatic pressure resulting from heart failure, therapy is directed toward improving cardiac output with diuretics, vasodilators, and medications that improve the contraction of the heart muscle. If edema is the result of increased capillary permeability resulting from injury, the treatment is focused on removing the offending agent and implementing supportive therapy to maintain adequate ventilation and circulation. Individuals with either type of pulmonary edema require supplemental O_2. Mechanical ventilation may be needed if edema significantly impairs ventilation and oxygenation.

Acute Lung Injury/Acute Respiratory Distress Syndrome

Acute lung injury (ALI)/acute respiratory distress syndrome (ARDS) represents a spectrum of acute lung inflammation and diffuse alveolocapillary injury. Both ALI and ARDS are defined as (1) the acute onset of bilateral infiltrates on chest radiograph, (2) a low ratio of PaO_2 to the fraction of inhaled O_2 under positive airway pressure, and (3) not derived from hydrostatic pulmonary edema. Biomarkers that can be used to diagnose ARDS are under investigation.[21] Advances in therapy have decreased overall mortality in people younger than

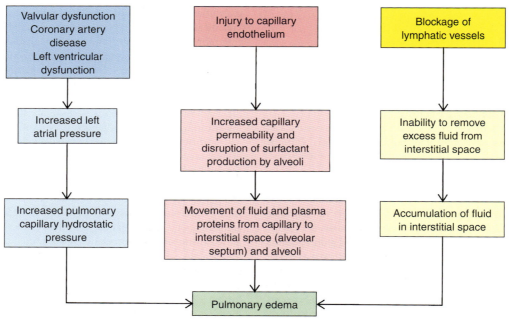

FIGURE 27.6 Pathogenesis of Pulmonary Edema.

60 years to approximately 40%, although mortality in older persons and those with severe infections remains much higher. The most common predisposing factors are genetic factors, sepsis, and multiple trauma. There are many other causes, including pneumonia, burns, aspiration, cardiopulmonary bypass surgery, pancreatitis, blood transfusions, drug overdose, inhalation of smoke or noxious gases, fat emboli, high concentrations of supplemental O_2, radiation therapy, and disseminated intravascular coagulation.

Over 10 000 Canadian patients die each year from ARDS. The mortality rate from ALI/ARDS is close to 50%. Often patients are so sick that they need to be on mechanical ventilation, which itself may result in ventilator-induced lung injury (VILI). Studies have reported that lung stretch due to cyclical stretching can increase the mortality rate by nearly 10%. In Canada, annually, thousands of patients sustain a severe injury to the lung (e.g., severe pneumonia) that results in ARDS. The estimated cost associated with a single patient admission to hospital with ARDS approaches $15 000, putting the national expenditure for this condition at over $2 billion annually.[22]

PATHOPHYSIOLOGY All disorders causing ALI/ARDS cause acute injury to the alveolocapillary membrane, producing massive pulmonary inflammation, increased capillary permeability, severe pulmonary edema, shunting, $\dot{V}/\dot{Q}$ mismatch, and hypoxemia. ARDS can occur directly (from aspiration of highly acidic gastric contents, inhalation of toxic gases) or indirectly (from circulating inflammatory mediators released in response to systemic disorders, such as sepsis and trauma). Lung injury and inflammation damage the alveolocapillary membrane, causing pulmonary edema, often referred to as *noncardiogenic pulmonary edema*. ARDS progresses through three overlapping phases characterized by histological changes in the lung: exudative (inflammatory), proliferative, and fibrotic[23,24] (Figure 27.7). The three phases are described as follows:

1. *Exudative phase (within 72 hours):* Neutrophils and other cells (platelets, macrophages, lung epithelial, and endothelial cells) that release a cascade of inflammatory cytokines are activated, causing damage to the alveolocapillary membrane, and greatly increasing capillary membrane permeability. Fluids, proteins, and blood cells leak from the capillary bed into the pulmonary interstitium and flood the alveoli (hemorrhagic exudate). Surfactant is inactivated. The resulting pulmonary edema and hemorrhage severely reduce lung compliance and impair alveolar ventilation. The inflammatory mediators also cause pulmonary vasoconstriction, contributing to ventilation–perfusion mismatch. The inflammatory mediators causing the alveolocapillary damage of ARDS often cause inflammation, endothelial damage, and capillary permeability throughout the body, resulting in systemic inflammatory response syndrome (SIRS). SIRS then leads to multiple organ dysfunction syndrome (MODS) and may cause death (see Chapter 24 and Figure 24.46).
2. *Proliferative phase (within 4 to 21 days):* Resolution of the pulmonary edema and proliferation of type II pneumocytes, fibroblasts, and myofibroblasts take place. The intra-alveolar hemorrhagic exudate becomes a cellular granulation tissue appearing as hyaline membranes and there is progressive hypoxemia.
3. *Fibrotic phase (within 14 to 21 days):* Remodelling and fibrosis of lung tissue take place. The fibrosis progressively obliterates the alveoli, respiratory bronchioles, and interstitium, leading to a decrease in functional residual capacity (FRC) and continuing $\dot{V}/\dot{Q}$ mismatch with severe right-to-left shunt. The result of this overwhelming inflammatory response by the lungs is acute respiratory failure.

CLINICAL MANIFESTATIONS The clinical manifestations of ARDS are progressive:
1. Dyspnea and hypoxemia with poor response to O_2 supplementation
2. Hyperventilation and respiratory alkalosis
3. Decreased tissue perfusion, metabolic acidosis, and organ dysfunction
4. Increased work of breathing, decreased tidal volume, and hypoventilation
5. Hypercapnia, respiratory acidosis, and worsening hypoxemia
6. Respiratory failure, decreased cardiac output, hypotension, and death

EVALUATION AND TREATMENT Diagnosis is based on a history of the lung injury, physical examination, blood gas analysis, and radiological examination. Measurement of serum biomarkers (i.e., surfactant proteins, mucin-associated antigens, and interleukins) may aid in the diagnosis and prognosis of ARDS.[21] Treatment is based on early detection, supportive therapy, and prevention of complications. Supportive therapy is focused on maintaining adequate oxygenation and ventilation while preventing infection. It often requires various modes of mechanical ventilation. Pharmacological therapy continues to be explored. Low-dose corticosteroids may improve survival in selected individuals but need further investigation.[25]

ARDS and COVID-19. The coronavirus disease 2019 (COVID-19) is responsible for the pathogenesis of severe acute respiratory syndrome-coronavirus-2 (SARS-CoV-2)-induced lung injury. Clinical data indicate that severe COVID-19 is manifested as viral pneumonia-induced acute respiratory distress syndrome (ARDS). The COVID-19 pathogenesis mechanism is extrapolated from our understanding of influenza A virus-induced pneumonia.

Influenza-induced ARDS is triggered by the virus's single-stranded RNA genome in the cytoplasm of respiratory epithelial cells. Cytoplasmic viral RNA stimulates the release of type-I and -III interferons (IFN-I and -III) and the proinflammatory cytokines interleukin (IL)-1ß and IL-18 through the activation of pathways such as Toll-like receptors, and mitochondria-associated antiviral signalling proteins. The induction of these antiviral pathways results in the upregulation of interferon-stimulated genes and the recruitment of effector and regulatory immune cells. Alveolar macrophages respond to these cues by phagocytosing infected and apoptotic epithelial cells, to promote viral clearance. Alveolar macrophages also release proinflammatory and chemotactic cytokines including IL-6 and IL-8. The lung epithelial cell and alveolar macrophage work synergistically to recruit other immune cell types, such as neutrophils and natural killer (NK) cells. Neutrophils cause nonspecific necrosis of epithelial cells via the secretion of effector compounds, such as neutrophil extracellular traps. While these processes exert protective effects against the influenza virus and other pathogens, they also contribute to lung injury when they remain unchecked.[26] NK cells cause pronecrotic and proapoptotic effects by secreting cytotoxic granzymes and perforins. Continuous and unchecked NK cell-mediated cytotoxicity can contribute uncontrolled lung injury.[27]

Infiltrating monocyte-derived macrophages and dendritic cells are also involved in secreting proinflammatory molecules, such as TNF-α and nitric oxide, to promote influenza clearance. Unfortunately, in the process of clearing the influenza virus, alveolar injury through the induction of epithelial cell apoptosis takes place.

Dendritic cells connect the innate with adaptive immune systems by sampling viral antigens from lung alveoli. Afterwards, the dendritic cells migrate to the lymph nodes draining the infected area. Dendritic cells in the lymph nodes act as antigen-presenting cells for naïve CD8+ and CD4+ T-cells. Once activated, the T cells expand and mature in an antigen-specific manner, after which the activated T cells migrate to the lung, where the CD8+ T-cells induce the lysis of cells presenting viral

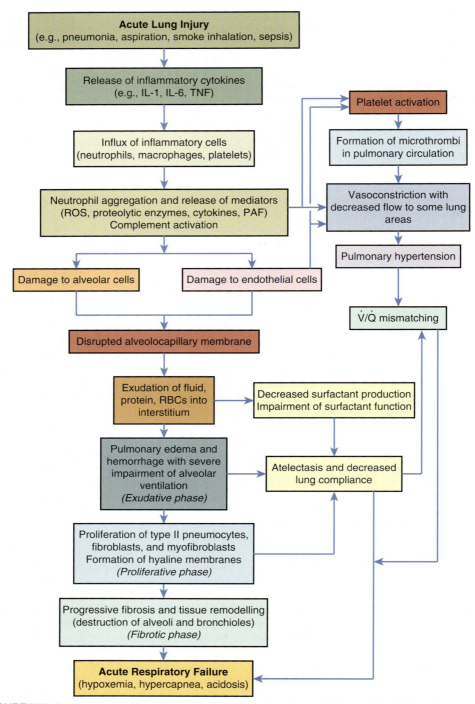

FIGURE 27.7 Pathogenesis of Acute Respiratory Distress Syndrome. *IL*, Interleukin; *PAF*, platelet-activating factor; *RBCs*, red blood cells; *ROS*, reactive oxygen species; *TNF*, tumour necrosis factor; *V̇/Q̇*, ventilation–perfusion ratio.

antigens, and CD4+ T-cells modulate the inflammatory response in a myriad of ways. CD4+ T-cells secrete more cytokines, including IFN-II. The aforementioned complex immune process leads to the active clearance of the influenza virus, but at the expense of severe lung injury from epithelial cell destruction and prolonged inflammation, often seen clinically as ARDS in affected patients. Surprisingly, postmortem studies of patients who died as a result of influenza induced-ARDS demonstrated undetectable viral loads in most patients, suggesting that the direct cytotoxic effects of the virus are not the main causes of death, but rather it is caused by the host's failure to deactivate or modulate inflammation in order to promote repair of damaged lung tissue.

Advanced age is the leading risk factor for developing severe COVID-19. Data from Italy and China reported case-fatality rates of 15 to 20% among patients aged >80 years, compared with <1% in patients aged <50 years.

SARS-CoV-2, an enveloped, single-stranded RNA virus, belongs to the *Betacoronavirus* genus and shares 79% of its RNA sequence with the virus that caused the 2003–2004 SARS epidemic.[28] On their envelope, these viruses contain a spike (S)-protein which mediates viral fusion and endocytosis. The viral fusion occurs after the virus binds to the human ACE2 receptor, which triggers enzymatic activation of the virus by the host proteases. After endocytosis, the transcription of the viral genome is started with the help of viral RNA-dependent RNA polymerase and then translated by host ribosomes to synthesise viral proteins. Afterwards, the mature virions are assembled in the cytoplasm, where they are primed for exocytosis.[29]

SARS-CoV-2 has affinity, mediated by the human ACE2 receptor and the host membrane serine protease TMPRSS2 for S-protein cleavage and activation, to bind to the ciliated airway epithelial cells and type II pneumocytes.[30] In addition to this affinity, the SARS-CoV-2 has a furin cleavage site that expands its affinity and increases its infectivity. The furin cleavage site allows S-protein fusion domain exposure by universal furin proteases. These furin proteases are found on the membranes of numerous cells across the body that also express ACE2, such as vascular endothelial cells.[31]

SARS-CoV-2 transmissibility has a mean incubation period of 5 days, with viral loads peaking before symptom onset, and declines thereafter. Posterior naso/oropharyngeal swabs for COVID-19 viruses will test positive for a minimum of 8 days and a median of 20 days from the appearance of symptoms.[32] The maximum duration of viral shedding is unclear; evidence suggests that in most cases it is likely to wane by day 40 postinfection.

There is variability in the symptoms reported during the early symptomatic phase of infection, ranging from fever, fatigue, dry cough, and diarrhea, to sore throat and loss of taste. Some patients remain asymptomatic in this phase.[33] In many patients, the prodromal symptoms are followed by the pulmonary phase of infection, which is characterized by dyspnea, radiographic pulmonary infiltrates, and hypoxemia.[34]

Morbidity and mortality related to COVID-19 occur in the inflammatory phase, which features a dysregulated immune response and hypercoagulable state that is associated with cardiac and renal failure, cerebrovascular disease, and ARDS.[35,36] The latter is the most commonly occurring symptom, representing a major percentage of COVID-19 patients that require intensive care unit (ICU) admission.[33] Patients who survive follow a recovery phase, in which inflammation resolves and damaged lung tissue is repaired, ultimately restoring organ system allostasis.

Management. Timely intubation is indicated for refractory hypoxaemia or hypercapnia, or with evidence of increased work of breathing on clinical examination.[37] Noninvasive ventilation has been associated with worse outcomes when the PaO_2/FiO_2 ratio is <150 in ARDS.[38] In patients with mild hypoxemia and without high respiratory drive or work of breathing, dire consequences of intubation and invasive ventilation related to sedation, paralysis, and endotracheal (ET) tube complications may outweigh benefits. Lower tidal volume is recommended at 4 mL/kg of the predicted body weight to keep plateau pressure <30 cm H_2O. Low tidal volume ventilation results in improved outcomes in patients with and without ARDS and should be the starting point for ventilatory management of patients with ARDS. Consider higher PEEP in patients with evidence of higher potential for lung recruitment as seen on a CT scan. Higher PEEP might be beneficial in patients with high recruitability, with better gas exchange, and reduced risk of VILI. Higher PEEP can be harmful in patients with low recruitability, who have hypoxemia resulting largely from pulmonary vascular pathology; high PEEP can lead to adverse hemodynamic effects or barotrauma. Improvement in partial pressure of arterial oxygen with increased PEEP can be misleading. In the absence of contraindications, use prone positioning in mechanically ventilated patients, with a PaO_2/FiO_2 ratio <150. Prone positioning is associated with improved outcomes in patients with moderate or severe ARDS, with improved ventilation or perfusion matching, more homogeneous distribution of ventilation, and reduced risk of VILI.[39] Staffing and resource demands can limit feasibility during surges in case volume. Efficacy and safety of prone positioning in awake, non-intubated patients remains unclear and is being evaluated in clinical trials in patients with COVID-19.[40] Consider venovenous ECMO for patients with refractory hypoxaemia or high driving pressures or respiratory acidosis despite conventional lung-protective measures; that is high PEEP or prone positioning.

Refractory hypoxemia is the leading cause of potentially injurious levels of mechanical ventilation. Staffing and resource demands can limit feasibility of using ECMO, especially when the number of cases increases.[41]

Vaping and Lung Injury. Electronic (e-) cigarettes have been introduced as a way of stopping or reducing tobacco smoking in adults, and function by heating liquids to generate aerosols for inhalation.

In 2017, 4.6 million Canadians aged 15 years and older had tried an e-cigarette (an increase from 3.9 million in 2015), whereas 460 000 youths aged 15 to 19 and 704 000 young adults aged 20 to 24, had tried an e-cigarette (unchanged from 2015).[42]

Past-30-day use of e-cigarettes was reported by 863 000 Canadians aged 15 years and older. 127 000 youths aged 15 to 19, 145 000 young adults aged 20 to 24, and 590 000 adults aged 25 years and older had used an e-cigarette in the past 30 days.[42]

Among Canadians who had ever tried an e-cigarette, 64% (3.0 million) reported that the last e-cigarette they used contained nicotine, 24% (1.1 million) reported using an e-cigarette that did not contain nicotine, and 12% (546 000) were uncertain; 1.1 million current or former smokers reported using e-cigarettes as a cessation aid in the past two years. Almost half, or 2.2 million, of those who ever tried an e-cigarette reported that they borrowed, shared, or bought them from a friend or relative. Among past-30-day e-cigarette users, the most commonly reported reasons for using e-cigarettes included the following: because e-cigarettes help people to quit smoking cigarettes; e-cigarettes might be less harmful than smoking cigarettes; and e-cigarettes may be less harmful than cigarettes to people around them. Nearly one in four Canadians were unaware how much a person risked harming themselves by using an e-cigarette.

Electronic cigarette use, also called vaping, needs a battery to produce aerosols from the heated liquids (or e-liquids). The liquids consist of propylene glycol, glycerin, flavourings and in most cases, nicotine. Some users may choose liquids that contain tetrahydrocannabinol (THC), the psychoactive component of cannabis. E-cigarette aerosols contain heavy metals and volatile organic compounds. Many other constituents of e-cigarette aerosols have also been detected, such as acetone, formaldehyde, and N-nitrosonornicotine, a tobacco-specific nitrosamine. The e-cigarette is sometimes also used for illicit drug delivery.

Vaping was promoted as a safer alternative to traditional tobacco cigarettes, but recent evidence suggests that vaping is associated with a myriad of lung injuries. Symptoms may include dyspnea that may be severe and rapidly progressive, leading to severe respiratory failure that often requires intubation, and sometimes ECMO. In some cases, vaping resulted in a fatal outcome in previously healthy adolescents and adults. There have been reports of a large number of adverse outcomes relating to e-cigarette consumption (vaping), which has been referred to as "vaping associated pulmonary illness" (VAPI).[43]

VAPI (and e-cigarette or vaping use-associated lung injury [EVALI]) is a diagnosis of exclusion because there are no specific clinical, laboratory, radiological, or pathological indicators of the disease. It can mimic or be associated with respiratory infections but presents with a great variety of symptoms (e.g., cough, chest pain, or shortness of breath, abdominal pain, nausea, vomiting, or diarrhea). In some patients, the gastro-intestinal symptoms precede the respiratory symptoms. Respiratory or gastro-intestinal symptoms may be associated with constitutional symptoms such as fever, chills, and weight loss in the majority of patients. Sick patients need admission to the ICU for intubation and mechanical ventilation. An emerging association between the use of e-cigarettes and COPD has also been noted in some patients.[43]

Radiological presentations. The radiological patterns depend on the frequency, dose, and chemical characteristics of the inhaled substances, and on the vaping device used. Chest CT scans in general can demonstrate bilateral ground-glass opacities (GGO), with sparing of the lung periphery, and centrilobular ground-glass nodules.

The following interstitial pneumonias have been described in VAPI cases:[43]
- Hypersensitivity pneumonitis
- Acute eosinophilic pneumonia
- Pneumonia with pleural effusions
- Organizing pneumonia
- *Acute lung injury* and *acute respiratory distress syndrome (ARDS)* have also been associated with vaping and VAPI
- *Diffuse alveolar hemorrhage (DAH)* has mainly been associated with cocaine and cannabis use unrelated to vaping practices. *Respiratory bronchiolitis-associated pneumonitis (respiratory bronchiolitis–associated interstitial lung disease [RBILD])* has been clearly linked to e-cigarette use. *Giant-cell interstitial pneumonia* (a pneumoconiosis from exposure to hard metal) is a rare diagnosis made on the basis of findings in a surgical biopsy of the lung. The findings in this patient were attributed to hard metal (cobalt) contamination in her vape pen. The biopsy showed fibrosis characterized by peripheral reticulation, GGO, and mild traction bronchiectasis. The patient's symptoms improved after cessation of vaping. On the chest CT scan, it presented as GGO, architectural distortion, and linear opacities in a peribronchiolar distribution
- *Acute lipoid pneumonia* can be caused by inhaling vaporized oil particles when using e-cigarettes
- *Bronchiolitis*

Treatment. Treatment of VAPI is mainly empirical. There are no trials investigating the state-of-the-art treatment of VAPI. Generally, patients should refrain from vaping and should receive oxygen support as needed, by nasal cannula, an oxygen mask, high-flow nasal cannula, noninvasive ventilation, mechanical ventilation, or even ECMO. High-dose systemic corticosteroids with intravenous methyl-prednisolone, followed by 1 mg/kg prednisolone daily, should be initiated. Early initiation of IV cephalosporines and macrolides PO for community-acquired pneumonia should always be considered for patients with severe symptoms, because VAPI can be associated with concurrent respiratory infections. If clinically or radiologically suspected, monotherapy with macrolides may be a useful treatment option in case of bronchiolitis. Ipratropium/salbutamol inhalations are useful in patients with severe bronchial obstruction. Prognosis is relatively good, even in severe disease, although fatalities have been described. The mean duration of hospitalization overall was 6.7 days; in the age group of ≥51 years, it was 14.8 days.[43]

Obstructive Lung Diseases

> **✓ QUICK CHECK 27.4**
> 1. What mechanisms cause airway obstruction in asthma?
> 2. Define *chronic bronchitis*.
> 3. How does emphysema affect oxygenation and ventilation?

Obstructive lung disease is characterized by airway obstruction that is worse with expiration. More force (i.e., use of accessory muscles of expiration) is required to expire a given volume of air and emptying of the lungs is slowed. The unifying symptom of obstructive lung diseases is dyspnea, and the unifying sign is wheezing. Individuals have an increased work of breathing, ventilation–perfusion mismatching, and a decreased forced expiratory volume in 1 second (FEV_1). The most common obstructive diseases are asthma, chronic bronchitis, and emphysema. Because many individuals have chronic bronchitis with emphysema, these diseases together are often called *chronic obstructive pulmonary disease* (COPD).

Asthma

Asthma is a chronic inflammatory disorder of the bronchial mucosa that causes bronchial hyper-responsiveness, constriction of the airways, and variable airflow obstruction that is reversible. Asthma occurs at all ages and is the third-most common chronic disease in Canada[44] (see *Health Promotion*: Asthma). The prevalence of asthma is increasing.[45]

> ### HEALTH PROMOTION
> #### Asthma
>
> According to Statistics Canada (2017), asthma is the third most common chronic disease[a] and children are the most affected, often needing hospital admission.[b] The Public Health Agency of Canada estimates that over 3.8 million people in Canada currently suffer from asthma;[c] approximately 850 000 of those are children under the age of 14.[b]
>
> Asthma is the most common chronic disease in children.[d] Every day, 317 Canadians are diagnosed with asthma.[e]
>
> Severe asthma impacts between 150 000 and 250 000 Canadians.[f] Severe asthma occurs when symptoms of asthma persist; it is often associated with multiple episodes of worsening attacks, despite being on multiple asthma medicines and practising a high degree of medication adherence and good trigger management.
>
> Some Canadian communities are highly impacted by asthma, for example, asthma is 40% more prevalent among Indigenous communities than in the general Canadian population.[g]
>
> In Canada, many asthma patients do not have control over their asthma; 53% of Canadians with asthma have what doctors call "poorly controlled" asthma. This designation means that the asthma treatment is ineffective. Those who have poorly controlled asthma have poorer health outcomes and quality of life as compared with individuals with well-controlled asthma.
>
> Asthma is a billion-dollar problem in Canada. According to the Conference Board of Canada, the cost of hospitalization, health care professional services, and medication and indirect costs (including decreased productivity) for asthma in 2012 was estimated at $2.1 billion annually. The cost of asthma to the Canadian economy is expected to climb to $4.2 billion annually by 2030.[g]

[a] Statistics Canada. (2017). Chronic conditions, 2016. *Health Fact Sheets* (Catalogue no.82–625-X), September. https://www150.statcan.gc.ca/n1/pub/82–625-x/2017001/article/54858-eng.htm.
[b] Canadian Institute for Health Information (CIHI). (2018). *Asthma hospitalizations among children and youth in Canada: trends and inequalities*. https://www.cihi.ca/sites/default/files/document/asthma-hospitalization-children-2018-chartbook-en-web.pdf.
[c] Public Health Agency of Canada. (2018). *Report from the Canadian Chronic Disease Surveillance System: asthma and chronic obstructive pulmonary disease (COPD) in Canada, 2018*. https://www.canada.ca/content/dam/phac-aspc/documents/services/publications/diseases-conditions/asthma-chronic-obstructive-pulmonary-disease-canada-2018/pub-eng.pdf.
[d] World Health Organization. (2020). *Asthma*. https://www.who.int/en/news-room/fact-sheets/detail/asthma.
[e] The Ontario Asthma Surveillance Information System (OASIS) and the Institute for Clinical Evaluative Sciences (ICES), Ontario. (2014). *Asthma statistics*. https://lab.research.sickkids.ca/oasis/oasis-statistics/.
[f] Statistics Canada. (2020). *Canadian community health survey (CCHS)—annual component*. https://www.statcan.gc.ca/eng/survey/household/3226.
[g] Asthma Canada. (2020). *Asthma facts and statistics*. https://asthma.ca/wp-content/uploads/2020/07/Asthma-101.pdf.

Asthma is a familial disorder, and more than 100 genes have been identified that may play a role in the susceptibility, pathogenesis, and treatment response of asthma. Specific gene expressions may impart associated *phenotypes* with specific inflammatory markers (i.e., cells, cytokines, or exhaled nitric oxide) or *endotypes* including clinical characteristics, biomarkers, lung physiology, genetics, histopathology, epidemiology, and treatment response.[46] Other risk factors include age at onset of disease, levels of allergen exposure, urban residence, exposure to indoor and outdoor air pollution, tobacco smoke, recurrent respiratory tract viral infections, gastroesophageal reflux disease, and obesity (which promotes a proinflammatory state).[47–49] Exposure to inhaled irritants can cause inflammation and damage to airways independent of allergen sensitivity. This exposure leads to irritant (or nonallergic) asthma, as well as increases the hyper-responsiveness of the airways to allergens in those with a history of atopy (allergy).[50] Inhaled irritants affect both the epigenetics of asthma and asthma presentation, including age of onset, symptoms, and gender differences.[51]

Exposure to high levels of certain allergens during childhood increases the risk for asthma. Furthermore, decreased exposure to certain infectious organisms appears to create an immunological imbalance that favours the development of allergy and asthma. This complex relationship has been called the *hygiene hypothesis*.[52] Recently, the relationship between the microbiome and asthma risk is shedding light on these complex interactions.[53]

PATHOPHYSIOLOGY Airway epithelial exposure to antigen initiates both an innate and an adaptive immune response in sensitized individuals[54] (see Chapter 8). Many cells and cellular elements contribute to the persistent inflammation of the bronchial mucosa and hyper-responsiveness of the airways, including dendritic cells (antigen-presenting macrophages), T-helper 2 lymphocytes (Th2 cells), B lymphocytes (B cells), mast cells, neutrophils, eosinophils, and basophils. There are both an immediate (early asthmatic response) and a late (delayed) response.

During the *early asthmatic response*, antigen exposure to the bronchial mucosa activates dendritic cells, which present antigen to T-helper cells. T-helper cells differentiate into Th2 cells, releasing inflammatory cytokines and interleukins that activate B cells (plasma cells) and eosinophils. Plasma cells produce antigen-specific immunoglobulin E (IgE), which binds to the surface of mast cells. Subsequent cross-linking of IgE molecules with the antigen causes mast cell degranulation with the release of inflammatory mediators, including histamine, bradykinins, leukotrienes and prostaglandins, platelet-activating factor, and interleukins[55] (see Figures 8.11 and 8.12 for additional details). These inflammatory mediators cause vasodilation, increased capillary permeability, mucosal edema, bronchial smooth muscle contraction (bronchospasm), and mucus secretion from mucosal goblet cells with narrowing of the airways and obstruction to airflow. Eosinophils cause direct tissue injury and release of toxic neuropeptides that contribute to increased bronchial hyper-responsiveness[56] (Figures 27.8–27.10).

The *late asthmatic response* begins 4 to 8 hours after the early response. Chemotactic recruitment of eosinophils, neutrophils, and lymphocytes during the acute response causes a latent release of inflammatory mediators, again inciting bronchospasm, edema, and mucus secretion with obstruction to airflow. Synthesis of leukotrienes contributes to prolonged smooth muscle contraction. Eosinophils cause direct tissue injury with fibroblast proliferation and airway scarring. Damage to ciliated epithelial cells contributes to impaired mucociliary function, with the accumulation of mucus and cellular debris forming plugs in the airways. Untreated inflammation can lead to long-term airway damage that is irreversible and is known as *airway remodelling* (subepithelial fibrosis, smooth muscle hypertrophy).[57]

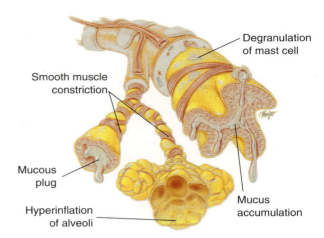

FIGURE 27.8 Bronchial Asthma. Thick mucus, mucosal edema, and smooth muscle spasm cause obstruction of small airways; breathing becomes laboured and expiration is difficult. (Modified from Des Jardins, T., & Burton, G. G. [1995]. *Clinical manifestations and assessment of respiratory disease* [3rd ed.]. Mosby.)

Airway obstruction increases resistance to airflow and decreases flow rates, especially expiratory flow. Impaired expiration causes air trapping, hyperinflation distal to obstructions, and increased work of breathing. Changes in resistance to airflow are not uniform throughout the lungs and the distribution of inspired air is uneven, with more air flowing to the less resistant portions. Continued air trapping increases intrapleural and alveolar gas pressures and causes decreased perfusion of the alveoli. Increased alveolar gas pressure, decreased ventilation, and decreased perfusion lead to variable and uneven ventilation–perfusion relationships within different lung segments. Hyperventilation is triggered by lung receptors responding to increased lung volume and obstruction. The result is early hypoxemia without CO_2 retention. Hypoxemia further increases hyperventilation through stimulation of the respiratory centre, causing $PaCO_2$ to decrease and pH to increase (respiratory alkalosis). With progressive obstruction of expiratory airflow, air trapping becomes more severe, and the lungs and thorax become hyperexpanded, positioning the respiratory muscles at a mechanical disadvantage. This leads to a decrease in tidal volume with increasing CO_2 retention and respiratory acidosis. Respiratory acidosis signals respiratory failure, especially when left ventricular filling, and thus cardiac output, becomes compromised because of severe hyperinflation.

CLINICAL MANIFESTATIONS Individuals are asymptomatic between attacks, and pulmonary function tests are normal. At the beginning of an attack, the individual experiences chest constriction, expiratory wheezing, dyspnea, nonproductive coughing, prolonged expiration, tachycardia, and tachypnea. Severe attacks involve the accessory muscles of respiration, and wheezing is heard during both inspiration and expiration. A **pulsus paradoxus** (decrease in systolic blood pressure during inspiration of more than 10 mm Hg) may be noted. Peak flow measurements should be obtained. Because the severity of blood gas alterations is difficult to evaluate by clinical signs alone, arterial blood gas tensions should be measured if O_2 saturation falls below 90%. Usual findings are hypoxemia with an associated respiratory alkalosis. In the *late asthma response*, symptoms can be even more severe than the initial attack.

If bronchospasm is not reversed by usual treatment measures, the individual is considered to have acute severe bronchospasm or **status asthmaticus**.[58] If status asthmaticus continues, hypoxemia worsens,

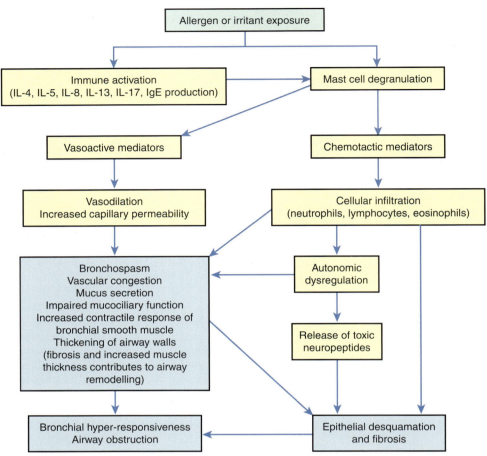

FIGURE 27.9 Pathophysiology of Asthma. Allergen or irritant exposure results in a cascade of inflammatory events leading to acute and chronic airway dysfunction. *IgE,* Immunoglobulin E; *IL,* interleukin.

expiratory flows and volumes decrease further, and effective ventilation decreases. Acidosis develops as the $PaCO_2$ level begins to rise. Asthma becomes life-threatening at this point if treatment does not reverse this process quickly. A silent chest (no audible air movement) and a $PaCO_2$ of greater than 70 mm Hg are ominous signs of impending death.

EVALUATION AND TREATMENT The diagnosis of asthma is supported by a history of allergies and recurrent episodes of wheezing, dyspnea, and cough or exercise intolerance. Further evaluation includes spirometry, which may document reversible decreases in FEV_1 during an induced attack.

The evaluation of an acute asthma attack requires the rapid assessment of arterial blood gases and expiratory flow rates (using a peak flow meter) and a search for underlying triggers, such as infection. Hypoxemia and respiratory alkalosis are expected early in the course of an acute attack. The development of hypercapnia with respiratory acidosis signals the need for mechanical ventilation. Management of the acute asthma attack requires immediate administration of O_2 and inhaled beta-agonist bronchodilators. In addition, oral corticosteroids should be administered early in the course of management.[59] Careful monitoring of gas exchange and airway obstruction in response to therapy provides information necessary to determine whether hospitalization is necessary. Antibiotics are not indicated for acute asthma unless there is a documented bacterial infection.

Management of asthma begins with avoidance of allergens and irritants. Individuals with asthma tend to underestimate the severity of their asthma and extensive education is important, including use of a peak flow meter and adherence to an action plan. In the mildest form of asthma (intermittent), short-acting beta-agonist inhalers are prescribed. For all categories of persistent asthma, anti-inflammatory medications are essential, and inhaled corticosteroids are the mainstay of therapy. In individuals who are not adequately controlled with inhaled corticosteroids, leukotriene antagonists can be considered. In more severe asthma, long-acting beta agonists can be used to control persistent bronchospasm; however, these agonists can actually worsen asthma in some individuals with certain genetic polymorphisms.[60] Immunotherapy has been shown to be an important tool in reducing asthma exacerbations and can now be given sublingually.[61] Monoclonal antibodies to IgE (omalizumab [Xolair]) have been found to be helpful as adjunctive therapy to inhaled steroids.[62] Biomarkers and epigenetic markers are being evaluated to personalize treatment and reduce mortality.[63,64]

Asthma Canada has issued stepwise guidelines for the diagnosis and management of chronic asthma based on clinical severity (see https://asthma.ca/get-help/resources/). The Canadian Paediatric Society and the Canadian Thoracic Society have issued age-specific guidelines for diagnosis and management of asthma in preschoolers (see http://www.cps.ca/en/documents/position/asthma-in-preschoolers).

Chronic Obstructive Pulmonary Disease

Chronic obstructive pulmonary disease (COPD) is defined as a common preventable and treatable disease characterized by persistent airflow limitation that is usually progressive and associated with an enhanced chronic inflammatory response in the airways and the lung

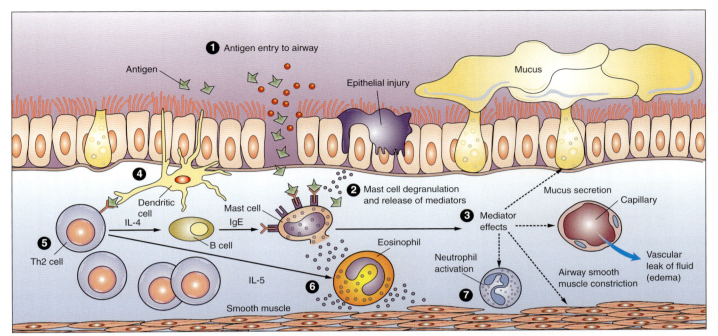

FIGURE 27.10 Acute Asthmatic Responses. Inhaled antigen (1) binds to mast cells covered with preformed immunoglobulin E *(IgE)*. Mast cells degranulate (2) and release inflammatory mediators such as histamine, bradykinins, leukotrienes, prostaglandins, platelet-activating factor, and interleukins. Secreted mediators (3) induce active bronchospasm (airway smooth muscle constriction), edema from increased capillary permeability, and airway mucus secretion from goblet cells. At the same time, antigen is detected by (4) dendritic cells that process and present it to Th2 cells (5), which produce interleukin-4 *(IL-4)* and many other interleukins (see text). IL-4 promotes switching of B cells to favour IgE production. Th2 cells also produce interleukin-5 *(IL-5)* (6), which activates eosinophils. Eosinophil products, such as major basic protein and eosinophilic cationic protein, damage the respiratory epithelium. Many inflammatory cells, including neutrophils (7), also contribute to the inflammatory process and airway obstruction.

to noxious particles or gases. Exacerbations and comorbidities contribute to the overall severity of disease.[65] COPD is the most common chronic lung disease in the world, and the fourth-leading cause of death globally. However, COPD prevalence in women is higher throughout the lifespan. Risk factors for COPD include tobacco smoke (cigarette, pipe, cigar, and environmental tobacco smoke), occupational dusts and chemicals (vapours, irritants, and fumes), indoor air pollution from biomass fuel used for cooking and heating (in poorly vented dwellings), outdoor air pollution (see *Health Promotion*: Tips to Keep Lungs Healthy), and any factor that affects lung growth during gestation and childhood (low birth weight, respiratory tract infections).[66] Genetic and epigenetic susceptibilities have been identified including polymorphisms of genes that code for tumour necrosis factor, surfactant, proteases, and antiproteases and acquired failure of DNA repair.[67] The clinical phenotypes of COPD discussed here are chronic bronchitis and emphysema. An inherited mutation in the α_1-antitrypsin gene results in the development of COPD at an early age, even in individuals who do not smoke.

According to Statistics Canada, 4% of Canadians aged 35 to 79 self-reported being diagnosed with COPD, whereas direct measurements of lung function from the Canadian Health Measures Survey (CHMS) indicate that 13% of Canadians had a lung function score indicative of COPD; that is, a FEV_1/FVC ratio of less than 0.70. The disparity between self-reported and measured COPD in the CHMS suggests that COPD is underdiagnosed in Canada. Further, Canadians aged 60 to 79 (19%) were more likely to have measured COPD than those aged 40 to 59 (11%). Despite the gravity of COPD, 60 to 85% of patients (most with mild to moderately severe COPD) are thought to remain undiagnosed.[68]

HEALTH PROMOTION
Tips to Keep Lungs Healthy

1. **Get help to quit smoking.** Smoke from cigarettes, cigars, and pipes contains over 4 000 harmful chemicals, 50 of which are known to cause cancer. As such, smoking can cause lung cancer and chronic obstructive pulmonary disease (COPD).
2. **Stay away from secondhand smoke.** Second-hand smoke is a mix of chemicals produced by burning tobacco. Two-thirds of the smoke from a cigarette is not inhaled by the smoker. Instead, it enters the air around the smoker and is sometimes inhaled by people sharing the same space, increasing their risk of developing a disease and even dying.
3. **Wash your hands well with soap and water.** Around 80% of common infectious respiratory diseases like colds and flu are spread through touch. Avoid excessive use of antibacterial soaps and cleaners to prevent antibiotic resistance. Also, use an alcohol-based hand sanitizer in cases where you do not have access to soap and water.
4. **Take part in minimizing air pollution.** Avoid idling your car engine and open-air burning. Avoid using pesticides and other chemicals on your lawn and garden. Walk or use public transit. Do not forget to ventilate your house to make sure that you are getting a lot of fresh, clean air. Always open your windows when cleaning, painting, installing new carpet, or doing other household projects.
5. **Wear protective gear if you work around dust and asbestos.** By protecting your lungs from potential health hazards at work, you can decrease the risk of developing lung diseases such as lung cancer, asthma, and COPD.

Adapted and reproduced with permission from the Minister of Health, 2017. Public Health Agency of Canada, 2008. *How do I keep my lungs healthy?* https://www.phac-aspc.gc.ca/cd-mc/crd-mrc/healthy_lungs-poumons_en_sante-eng.php.

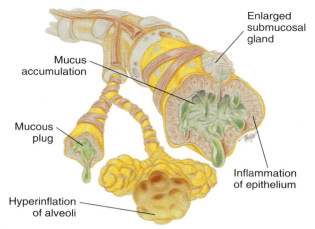

FIGURE 27.11 Chronic Bronchitis. Inflammation and thickening of mucous membrane with accumulation of mucus and pus leading to obstruction characterized by productive cough. (Modified from Des Jardins, T., & Burton, G. G. [1995]. *Clinical manifestations and assessment of respiratory disease* [3rd ed.]. Mosby.)

Chronic Bronchitis

Chronic bronchitis is defined as hypersecretion of mucus and chronic productive cough for at least 3 months of the year (usually the winter months) for at least 2 consecutive years.

PATHOPHYSIOLOGY Inspired irritants result in airway inflammation with infiltration of neutrophils, macrophages, and lymphocytes into the bronchial wall. Continual bronchial inflammation causes bronchial edema, an increase in the size and number of mucous glands and goblet cells in the airway epithelium, smooth muscle hypertrophy with fibrosis, and narrowing of airways. Thick, tenacious mucus is produced and cannot be cleared because of impaired ciliary function (Figure 27.11). The lung's defence mechanisms are, therefore, compromised, increasing susceptibility to pulmonary infection and injury and ineffective repair. Frequent infectious exacerbations from bacterial colonization of damaged airways are complicated by bronchospasm with dyspnea and productive cough.[69,70] The pathogenesis of chronic bronchitis is shown in Figure 27.12.

This process initially affects only the larger bronchi, but eventually all airways are involved. The thick mucus and hypertrophied bronchial smooth muscle constrict the airways and lead to obstruction,

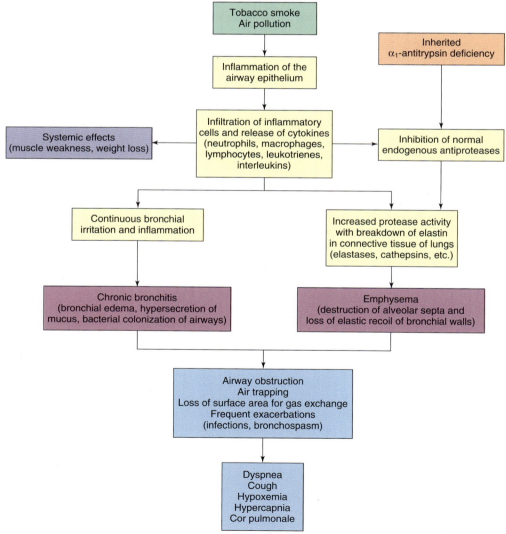

FIGURE 27.12 Pathogenesis of Chronic Bronchitis and Emphysema (Chronic Obstructive Pulmonary Disease).

CHAPTER 27 Alterations of Pulmonary Function

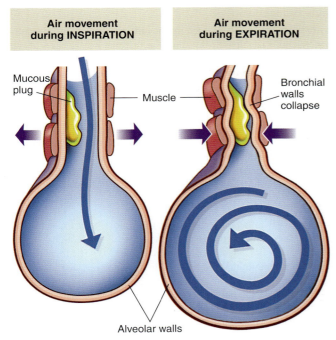

FIGURE 27.13 Mechanisms of Air Trapping in Chronic Obstructive Pulmonary Disease. Mucous plugs and narrowed airways cause air trapping and hyperinflation of alveoli on expiration. During inspiration, the airways are pulled open, allowing gas to flow past the obstruction. During expiration, decreased elastic recoil of the bronchial walls results in collapse of the airways and prevents normal expiratory airflow.

TABLE 27.2 Clinical Manifestations of Chronic Obstructive Lung Disease

Clinical Manifestations	Chronic Bronchitis	Emphysema
Productive cough	Classic sign	With infection
Dyspnea	Late in course	Common
Wheezing	Intermittent	Common
History of smoking	Common	Common
Barrel chest	Occasionally	Classic
Prolonged expiration	Always present	Always present
Cyanosis	Common	Uncommon
Chronic hypoventilation	Common	Late in course
Polycythemia	Common	Late in course
Cor pulmonale	Common	Late in course

particularly during expiration when the airways are narrowed (Figure 27.13). Obstruction eventually leads to ventilation–perfusion mismatch with hypoxemia. The airways collapse early in expiration, trapping gas in the distal portions of the lung (hyperinflation).[71] Air trapping expands the thorax and positions the respiratory muscles at a mechanical disadvantage. This air trapping leads to decreased tidal volume, hypoventilation, and hypercapnia.

CLINICAL MANIFESTATIONS Table 27.2 lists the common clinical manifestations of chronic bronchitis and emphysema.

EVALUATION AND TREATMENT Diagnosis is based on history of symptoms, physical examination, chest imaging, pulmonary function tests (i.e., a FEV_1/FVC ratio less than 0.7), and blood gas analyses. These tests reflect the progressive nature of the disease. Prevention of chronic bronchitis is essential because pathological changes are not reversible. By the time an individual seeks medical care for symptoms, considerable airway damage is present. If the individual stops smoking, disease progression can be halted.[72] Influenza and pneumococcal vaccinations should be up to date.

Bronchodilators, mucolytics, antioxidants, and anti-inflammatory medications are prescribed as needed to control cough and reduce dyspnea. Chest physiotherapy may be helpful and includes deep breathing and postural drainage. During acute exacerbations (infection and bronchospasm), individuals require treatment with antibiotics and steroids and may need mechanical ventilation.[73] Chronic use of oral steroids may be needed late in the course of the disease but should be considered a last resort. Individuals with severe hypoxemia will require home O_2 therapy. O_2 is administered with care to individuals with severe hypoxemia and CO_2 retention. Chronic elevation of $PaCO_2$ diminishes the sensitivity of central chemoreceptors, and they no longer act as the primary stimulus for breathing. Teaching includes nutritional counselling, respiratory hygiene, recognition of the early signs of infection, and techniques that relieve dyspnea, such as pursed-lip breathing. In addition, many comorbidities accompany COPD and require monitoring and therapy, including cardiovascular disorders, metabolic diseases, bone disease, stroke, lung cancer, cachexia, skeletal muscle weakness, anemia, depression, and cognitive decline. Chronic low-grade systemic inflammation may be associated with these conditions.[74]

Emphysema

Emphysema is abnormal permanent enlargement of gas-exchange airways (acini) accompanied by destruction of alveolar walls without obvious fibrosis. Obstruction results from changes in lung tissues rather than mucus production and inflammation, as in chronic bronchitis. The major mechanism of airflow limitation is loss of elastic recoil.

Primary emphysema, which accounts for 1 to 3% of all cases of emphysema, is commonly linked to an inherited deficiency of the enzyme α_1-antitrypsin. Normally α_1-antitrypsin inhibits the action of many proteolytic enzymes (i.e., elastases released by neutrophils); therefore, α_1-antitrypsin deficiency (an autosomal recessive trait) increases the likelihood of developing emphysema because proteolysis in lung tissues is not inhibited.[75] α_1-Antitrypsin deficiency is suggested in individuals who develop emphysema before 40 years of age and in individuals who do not smoke but still develop the disease. The major cause of secondary emphysema is the inhalation of tobacco smoke, although air pollution, occupational exposures, and childhood respiratory tract infections are known to be contributing factors.

PATHOPHYSIOLOGY Emphysema is characterized by destruction of alveoli through the breakdown of elastin within the septa by an imbalance between proteases and antiproteases, oxidative stress, and apoptosis of lung structural cells (see Figure 27.12).[76] Alveolar destruction also produces large air spaces within the lung parenchyma (bullae) and air spaces adjacent to pleurae (blebs) (Figure 27.14). Bullae and blebs are not effective in gas exchange and result in significant ventilation–perfusion mismatching and hypoxemia. Expiration becomes difficult because loss of elastic recoil reduces the volume of air that can be expired passively, and air is trapped in the lungs (see Figure 27.13). **Air trapping** causes hyperexpansion of the chest, placing the muscles of respiration at a mechanical disadvantage. It results in increased workload of breathing, so that late in the course of disease, many individuals will develop hypoventilation and hypercapnia. Persistent inflammation in the airways can result in hyper-reactivity of the

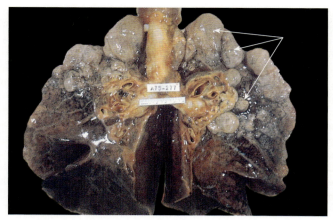

FIGURE 27.14 Bullous Emphysema With Large Apical and Subpleural Bullae *(arrows).* (From Kumar, V., Abbas, A. K., Fausto, N., et al. [Eds.]. [2007]. *Robbins basic pathology* [8th ed.]. Saunders.)

bronchi with bronchoconstriction, which may be partially reversible with bronchodilators. Destruction of alveolar walls and pulmonary capillaries also causes PAH and cor pulmonale. Chronic inflammation also can have significant systemic effects including weight loss, muscle weakness, and increased susceptibility to comorbidities, such as infection.

CLINICAL MANIFESTATIONS The clinical manifestations of emphysema are listed in Table 27.2.

EVALUATION AND TREATMENT Emphysema is usually diagnosed and staged by pulmonary function measures. In COPD, pulmonary function tests indicate obstruction to gas flow during expiration with a marked decrease in FEV_1. Chronic management of emphysema begins with smoking cessation. Pharmacological management is based on clinical severity (mild, moderate, severe, or very severe). Inhaled anticholinergic agents and beta agonists should be prescribed. Inhaled corticosteroids are indicated for severe COPD, although long-term therapy with oral steroids should be avoided if possible. Pulmonary rehabilitation, improved nutrition, and breathing techniques can improve symptoms. Progressive pulmonary dysfunction with hypoxemia and hypercapnia may require long-term O_2 therapy and ventilation, if indicated.[77] A class of medications called *phosphodiesterase E4* (PDE4) inhibitors is proving to be effective in selected individuals with severe COPD.[73] α_1-Antitrypsin augmentation may be indicated for primary emphysema.[78] Selected individuals with severe emphysema can benefit from lung volume reduction surgery.[79]

Respiratory Tract Infections

 QUICK CHECK 27.5
1. Compare pneumococcal and viral pneumonia as to severity of disease.
2. Describe the pathophysiological features of tuberculosis.
3. How does lung abscess present clinically?

Respiratory tract infections are a common cause of short-term disability in Canada and the United States. Most of these infections—the common cold, pharyngitis (sore throat), and laryngitis—involve only the upper airways. Although the lungs have direct contact with the atmosphere, they usually remain sterile. Infections of the lower respiratory tract occur most often in the very young and very old or those with impaired immunity.

Acute Bronchitis

Acute bronchitis is acute infection or inflammation of the airways or bronchi and is usually self-limiting. The vast majority of cases of acute bronchitis are caused by viruses. Many of the clinical manifestations are similar to those of pneumonia (i.e., fever, cough, chills, malaise), but physical examination does not reveal signs of pulmonary consolidation and chest radiographs do not show infiltrates. Individuals with viral bronchitis usually have a nonproductive cough that often occurs in paroxysms and is aggravated by cold, dry, or dusty air. In some cases, purulent sputum is produced. Chest pain often develops from the effort of coughing. Treatment consists of rest, Aspirin, humidity, and a cough suppressant, such as codeine. Bacterial bronchitis is treated with rest, antipyretics, humidity, and antibiotics.

Pneumonia

Pneumonia is infection of the lower respiratory tract caused by bacteria, viruses, fungi, protozoa, or parasites. It is the eighth leading cause of death in Canada and the United States.[80,81] The incidence and mortality of pneumonia are highest in older persons. Risk factors for pneumonia include advanced age, compromised immunity, underlying lung disease, alcoholism, altered consciousness, impaired swallowing, smoking, ET intubation, malnutrition, immobilization, underlying cardiac or liver disease, and residence in a long-term care facility. The causative microorganism influences the clinical presentation of the individual, the treatment plan, and the prognosis.

Pneumonia can be categorized as community-acquired pneumonia (CAP), health care–associated pneumonia (HCAP), hospital-acquired pneumonia (HAP), or ventilator-associated pneumonia (VAP). CAP is a significant cause of morbidity, mortality, and health care costs. As many as 36% of patients with CAP require critical care unit (CCU) admission, and these patients have mortality ranging from 21 to 58%. Moreover, patients with CAP in the CCU have longer durations of stay compared with those who are not in the CCU, which is associated with higher hospital costs.[82] CAP is the eighth leading cause of death in Canada and the United States and the leading cause of infection-related hospitalization.[83]

HCAP is defined as occurring in individuals with recent hospitalization, residence in a long-term care facility or extended care facility, home infusion therapy, chronic dialysis, or home wound care, although more recent studies suggest nonambulatory status, tube feedings, and the use of gastric acid suppressive agents also should be considered as criteria for HCAP.[84] It is estimated that nearly one-third of all hospital admissions for pneumonia are now considered HCAP.

HAP is the second most common health care–associated infection (urinary tract infection [UTI] is the most common) but has the greatest mortality (overall 20 to 50% mortality). VAP is a health care–associated infection that occurs in 9 to 27% of individuals who require intubation and mechanical ventilation.[85-87]

The microorganisms that most commonly cause CAP are different from those that cause HCAP, HAP, and VAP (Box 27.1). The most common CAP is caused by *Streptococcus pneumoniae* (also known as *pneumococcus*), which results in hospitalization in more than half of affected individuals and an overall hospital mortality of about 10%.[88] *Mycoplasma pneumoniae* is a common cause of atypical pneumonia in young people, especially those living in group housing such as dormitories and army barracks. Community-acquired methicillin-resistant *Staphylococcus aureus* (MRSA) is becoming more common.[89,90] Influenza and respiratory syncytial virus are the most common causes of viral CAP in adults.[91] VAP is a frequent complication in the CCU (see *Health Promotion:* Ventilator-Associated Pneumonia). Immunocompromised individuals (e.g., those with human immunodeficiency virus [HIV] or those undergoing organ transplantation) are especially susceptible to *Pneumocystis jirovecii* (formerly called

BOX 27.1 Etiological Microorganisms for Pneumonia in Adults

Cap	HCAP/HAP/VAP	Immunocompromised Individuals
Streptococcus pneumoniae	Pseudomonas aeruginosa	Pneumocystis jirovecii
Moraxella catarrhalis	Staphylococcus aureus	Mycobacterium tuberculosis
Haemophilus influenzae	Klebsiella pneumoniae	Atypical mycobacteria
Oral anaerobic bacteria	Escherichia coli	Fungi
Influenza virus		Respiratory viruses
Respiratory syncytial virus		Protozoa
Staphylococcus aureus		Parasites
Chlamydia pneumoniae		
Legionella pneumophila		
Mycoplasma pneumoniae		

CAP, Community-acquired pneumonia; HAP, hospital-acquired pneumonia; HCAP, health care–associated pneumonia; VAP, ventilator-associated pneumonia.

Pneumocystis carinii), mycobacterial infections, and fungal infections of the respiratory tract. These infections can be difficult to treat and have a high mortality.

PATHOPHYSIOLOGY Aspiration of oropharyngeal secretions is the most common route of lower respiratory tract infection; thus, the nasopharynx and oropharynx constitute the first line of defence for most infectious agents. Another route of infection is through the inhalation of microorganisms that have been released into the air when an infected individual coughs, sneezes, or talks, or from aerosolized water such as that from contaminated respiratory therapy equipment. This route of infection is most important in viral and mycobacterial pneumonias and in *Legionella* outbreaks. ET tubes become colonized with bacteria that form biofilms (i.e., protected colonies of bacteria that are resistant to host defences and treatment with antibiotics) and can seed the lung with microorganisms, especially during ET suctioning. Pneumonia also can occur when bacteria are spread to the lung in the blood from bacteremia that can result from infection elsewhere in the body or from intravenous drug abuse.

In healthy individuals, pathogens that reach the lungs are expelled or controlled by mechanisms of self-defence (see Chapters 6, 7, and 8). If a microorganism evades the upper airway defence mechanisms, such as the cough reflex and mucociliary clearance, the next line of defence is the airway epithelial cell. Airway epithelial cells can recognize some pathogens directly (e.g., *P. aeruginosa* and *S. aureus*). The most important guardian cell of the lower respiratory tract is the alveolar macrophage; it recognizes pathogens through its pattern-recognition receptors (e.g., Toll-like receptors). Macrophages present infectious antigens to the adaptive immune system, activating T cells and B cells with the induction of both cellular and humoral immunity. Release of tumour necrosis factor-alpha (TNF-α) and IL-1 from macrophages and chemokines and chemotactic signals from mast cells and fibroblasts contributes to widespread inflammation in the lung and recruitment of neutrophils from the capillaries of the lungs into the alveoli. The resulting inflammatory mediators and immune complexes can damage bronchial mucous membranes and alveolocapillary membranes,

HEALTH PROMOTION
Ventilator-Associated Pneumonia

Ventilator-associated pneumonia (VAP) is a common complication of mechanical ventilation and is the most serious infection in the critical care unit (CCU). VAP is associated with higher mortality, morbidity, and costs. Although there are many risk factors, including age greater than 65 years, presence of comorbidities, use of sedation, supine posture, poor oral hygiene, and immunocompromised status, the principal determinant of VAP development is the presence of the ET tube. Common etiological microorganisms include *Staphylococcus aureus* and *Pseudomonas aeruginosa*; multidrug-resistant strains are common. Bacterial colonization of the oropharynx occurs soon after placement of the ET tube with subsequent aspiration and pooling of bacteria near the ET tube cuff. Many bacteria are capable of forming a protective coating, called a *biofilm*, on the surface of the ET tube that contributes to bacterial replication and makes microorganisms less vulnerable to antibiotics. Injury to the tracheal mucosa and decreased mucociliary clearance contribute to lower airway infection. Analgesic and sedation agents alter cellular function and reduce the immune response. Implementation of certain treatment protocols has shown improved outcomes regarding VAP prevention and mortality reduction, especially the use of a "bundle" of techniques including raising the head of the bed, improving oral hygiene, providing continuous suction of subglottic secretions by antimicrobial-impregnated ET tubes, using checklists, and encouraging effective team communication. Recent studies have suggested that surveillance cultures could improve the prescribing of appropriate antibiotics and that the addition of aerosolized antibiotics may improve treatment outcomes.

According to the Canadian Patient Safety Institute, VAP is the leading cause of death among hospital-acquired infections in Canada. Hospital mortality of ventilated patients who developed VAP in Canadian hospitals is 46%, compared with 32% for ventilated patients who do not develop VAP.

In Canada, it is estimated that VAP is associated with an increase of 7.6 days of ventilation, an increase of 8.7 days in the CCU, and an increase in total stay of 11.5 days. It also plays a role in 6 to 30% of additional deaths in critically ill patients.

Data from Canadian Patient Safety Institute. (2016). *Measures: ventilator-associated pneumonia (VAP)*. https://www.patientsafetyinstitute.ca/en/toolsResources/psm/Pages/VAP-measurement.aspx; Kallet, R. H. (2015). *Respiratory Care, 60*(10), 1495–1508; Klompas, M., Speck, K., Howell, M. D., et al. (2014). *JAMA Internal Medicine, 174*(5), 751–761; Kollef, M. H., Hamilton, C. W., & Montgomery, A. B. (2013). *Current Opinion in Infectious Disease, 26*(6), 538–544; Luna, C. M., Bledel, I., & Raimondi, A. (2014). *Current Opinion in Infectious Disease, 27*(2), 184–193; Mietto, C., Pinciroli, R., Patel, N., et al. (2013). *Respiratory Care, 58*(6), 990–1007; Rouze, A., & Nseir, S. (2013). *Current Opinion in Critical Care, 19*(5), 440–447; Smith, M. A., Hibino, M., Falcione, B. A., et al. (2014). *Annals of Pharmacotherapy, 48*(1), 77–85.

causing the acini and terminal bronchioles to fill with infectious debris and exudate. Some microorganisms release toxins from their cell walls that can cause further lung damage and consolidation of lung tissue. The accumulation of exudate in the acinus leads to dyspnea and to $\dot{V}/\dot{Q}$ mismatching and hypoxemia.

Pneumococcus (*S. pneumoniae*) is the most common and lethal cause of outpatient and inpatient pneumonias.[92] Pneumococci can infect the lungs through inhalation of aerosolized bacteria or, more commonly, by aspiration of colonized oropharyngeal secretions. These bacteria have several virulence factors; most important, they have capsules that make phagocytosis by alveolar macrophages more difficult, and they have the ability to release a variety of toxins (including pneumolysin, which damages airway and alveolar cells).[93] An intense inflammatory response is initiated with release of TNF-α and IL-1.[94] Neutrophils and inflammatory exudates cause alveolar edema, which leads to the other changes shown in Figure 27.15.

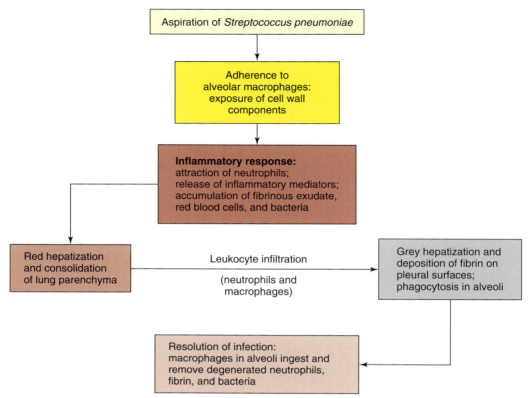

FIGURE 27.15 Pathophysiological Course of Pneumococcal Pneumonia.

Viral pneumonia is a seasonal and usually mild and self-limiting CAP. It can set the stage for a secondary bacterial infection by damaging ciliated epithelial cells, which normally prevent pathogens from reaching the lower airways. Immunocompromised individuals are at risk for very serious viral infections, such as pneumonia caused by cytomegalovirus. Viral pneumonia also can be a complication of another viral illness, such as chickenpox or measles (spread from the blood). New or atypical forms of viral infection, such as swine influenza A (H1N1) virus, avian influenza A (H5N1) virus, and the coronavirus that causes severe acute respiratory syndrome (SARS), are affecting previously healthy populations and pose a considerable threat for pandemics.[95]

Viruses destroy the ciliated epithelial cells and invade the goblet cells and bronchial mucous glands. Sloughing of destroyed bronchial epithelium occurs throughout the respiratory tract, preventing mucociliary clearance. Bronchial walls become edematous and infiltrated with leukocytes. In severe cases, the alveoli are involved with decreased compliance and increased work of breathing.

CLINICAL MANIFESTATIONS Most cases of pneumonia are preceded by a viral upper respiratory tract infection. Individuals then develop fever, chills, productive or dry cough, malaise, pleural pain, and sometimes dyspnea and hemoptysis. Physical examination may show signs of pulmonary consolidation, such as dullness to percussion, inspiratory crackles, increased tactile fremitus, egophony, and whispered pectoriloquy. Individuals also may demonstrate symptoms and signs of underlying systemic disease or sepsis.

EVALUATION AND TREATMENT Diagnosis is made on the basis of history and physical examination (tachypnea, tachycardia, crackles, bronchial breath sounds, findings of pleural effusion), white blood cell count, oxygenation and pH, chest X-rays, stains and cultures of respiratory tract secretions, and blood cultures before starting antibiotics. The white blood cell count is usually elevated, although it may be low if the individual is debilitated or immunocompromised. Serum procalcitonin level can be used to help differentiate bacterial from viral infection and guide therapy. Chest radiographs show infiltrates that may involve a single lobe of the lung or may be more diffuse. Once the diagnosis of pneumonia has been made, the pathogen is identified by means of sputum characteristics (Gram stain, colour, odour) and cultures or, if sputum is absent, blood cultures. Because many pathogens exist in the normal oropharyngeal flora, the specimen may be contaminated with pathogens from oral secretions. If sputum studies fail to identify the pathogen, the individual is immunocompromised, or the individual's condition worsens, further diagnostic studies may include thoracentesis, bronchoscopy, or lung biopsy. Urine antigen testing offers rapid pathogen identification for *Legionella pneumophila*, *S. pneumoniae*, and *Histoplasma capsulatum* but requires culture for microbial specificity.[96]

Prevention of pneumonia includes avoidance of aspiration, respiratory isolation of immunocompromised individuals, and vaccination. The first step in the management of pneumonia is establishing adequate ventilation and oxygenation. Adequate hydration and good pulmonary hygiene (e.g., deep breathing, coughing, chest physiotherapy) also are important. Antibiotics are given within 4 hours to treat bacterial pneumonia; however, resistant strains of microorganisms are becoming more prevalent and require secondary antibiotics.[96] When a specific microorganism is not identified, empirical antibiotics are chosen on the basis of the likely causative microorganism.[84] Viral pneumonia is usually treated with supportive therapy alone; however, antivirals may be needed in severe cases. Infections with opportunistic microorganisms may be polymicrobial and require multiple medications, including antifungals.

Tuberculosis

Tuberculosis (TB) is an infection caused by *Mycobacterium tuberculosis*, an acid-fast bacillus that usually affects the lungs but may invade other body systems. TB is a leading cause of death from a curable infectious disease in the world. TB cases increased greatly during the mid-1990s as a result of AIDS, but incidence of both diseases has decreased since 2000.[97] Emigration of infected individuals from high-prevalence countries, transmission in crowded institutional settings, homelessness, substance abuse, and lack of access to screening and medical care have contributed to the spread of TB.

For most Canadians, the risk of developing TB is very low. However, there are about 1 600 new cases of TB reported in Canada every year.[98] In Canada, 1 640 new active and retreatment TB cases were reported in 2013, and the incidence rate for 2013 was 4.7 per 100 000 population. These figures are comparable to both the number of TB cases reported in 2012 (1 699) and the incidence rate for 2012 (4.9 per 100 000 population).[99]

PATHOPHYSIOLOGY TB is highly contagious and is transmitted from person to person in airborne droplets. In immunocompetent individuals, the microorganism is usually contained by the inflammatory and immune response systems. This results in **latent TB infection (LTBI)** and is associated with no clinical evidence of disease.

Once the bacilli are inspired, they lodge in the lung periphery, usually in the upper lobe, and cause localized nonspecific pneumonitis (lung inflammation). Some bacilli migrate through the lymphatics and become lodged in the lymph nodes, where they encounter lymphocytes and initiate the immune response. Inflammation in the lung causes activation of alveolar macrophages and neutrophils. These phagocytes engulf the bacilli and begin the process by which the body's defence mechanisms isolate the bacilli, preventing them from spreading. However, the bacterium is successful as a pathogen because it can survive and multiply within macrophages and resist lysosomal killing, forming a granulomatous lesion (see Chapter 6) called a *tubercle*. Infected tissues within the tubercle die, forming cheeselike material called *caseation necrosis*. Collagenous scar tissue then grows around the tubercle, completing the isolation of the bacilli. The immune response is complete after about 10 days, preventing further multiplication of the bacilli.

Once the bacilli are isolated in tubercles and immunity develops, TB may remain dormant for life. If the immune system is impaired, reactivation with progressive disease occurs and may spread through the blood and lymphatics to other organs. Infection with HIV is the single greatest risk factor for reactivation of TB infection. Cancer, immunosuppressive medications (e.g., corticosteroids), poor nutritional status, and renal failure can also reactivate disease.

CLINICAL MANIFESTATIONS LTBI is asymptomatic. Symptoms of active disease often develop so gradually that they are not noticed until the disease is advanced. Common clinical manifestations include fatigue, weight loss, lethargy, anorexia (loss of appetite), and a low-grade fever that usually occurs in the afternoon. A cough that produces purulent sputum develops slowly and becomes more frequent over several weeks or months. Night sweats and general anxiety are often present. Dyspnea, chest pain, and hemoptysis may occur as the disease progresses. Extrapulmonary TB disease is common in HIV-infected individuals and may cause neurological deficits, meningitis symptoms, bone pain, and urinary symptoms.

EVALUATION AND TREATMENT TB is diagnosed by a positive tuberculin skin test (TST; purified protein derivative [PPD]), sputum culture, immunoassays, and chest radiographs.[100] A positive skin test indicates the need for yearly chest radiographs to detect active disease. In addition, individuals who have received the TB vaccine with bacille Calmette-Guérin (BCG) will have a positive TST even if they have never had TB. When active pulmonary disease is present, the tubercle bacillus can be cultured from the sputum and may be seen with an acid-fast stain. However, sputum culture can take up to 6 weeks to become positive. Two immunoassays (enzyme-linked ImmunoSpot and quantitative blood interferon-gamma assay) are available. These new tests are more sensitive and specific than TST for the diagnosis of latent TB and are not confounded by previous BCG vaccination.[101]

Treatment consists of combination antibiotic therapy to control active disease or prevent reactivation of LTBI. Adverse effects are common and new medications are being explored.[102] Two worrisome treatment categories of TB have become more prevalent in recent years. "Multidrug-resistant TB" and "extensively resistant TB" now account for approximately 2 to 5% of cases worldwide. Multiple second-line medications are required for treatment success.[103] The BCG vaccine is used in countries where TB is endemic.

In Canada, the BCG vaccine is not recommended for routine use in the population. However, BCG may be recommended for certain populations in Canada; for example, infants in high-incidence communities and travellers who are returning for an extended stay to a high-incidence country where BCG is routinely given. For infants born in Canada who will be moving to and staying for an extended period in a country with high TB incidence and where BCG vaccination is still standard practice, vaccination is recommended soon after arrival in the high-incidence country.[104] New vaccines are in clinical trials.[105] Treatment of TB HIV co-infection requires monitoring of medication interactions and toxicities.[106]

Abscess Formation and Cavitation

An **abscess** is a circumscribed area of suppuration and destruction of lung parenchyma. Abscess formation follows consolidation of lung tissue, in which inflammation causes alveoli to fill with fluid, pus, and microorganisms. Aspiration abscess can occur from aspiration of anaerobes, such as those found in individuals who have pneumonia or who are infected with *Klebsiella* or *Staphylococcus*. Aspiration abscess is usually associated with alcohol misuse, seizure disorders, general anaesthesia, and swallowing disorders. Necrosis (death and decay) of consolidated tissue may progress proximally until it communicates with a bronchus. **Cavitation** is the process of the abscess emptying into a bronchus and cavity formation. Abscess communication with a bronchus causes production of copious amounts of often foul-smelling sputum, and occasionally hemoptysis. Other clinical manifestations include fever, cough, chills, and pleural pain. The diagnosis is made by chest radiography. Treatment includes appropriate antibiotics and chest physiotherapy (chest percussion and postural drainage). Bronchoscopy may be performed to drain the abscess.

Pulmonary Vascular Disease

> ✓ **QUICK CHECK 27.6**
> 1. What factors influence the impact of an embolus?
> 2. List three causes of pulmonary hypertension.
> 3. What is cor pulmonale?

Blood flow through the lungs can be disrupted by disorders that occlude the vessels, increase pulmonary vascular resistance, or destroy the vascular bed. Effects of altered pulmonary blood flow may range from insignificant dysfunction to severe and life-threatening changes in ventilation–perfusion ratios. Major disorders include PE, pulmonary hypertension, and cor pulmonale.

Pulmonary Embolism

Pulmonary embolism (PE) is occlusion of a portion of the pulmonary vascular bed by an embolus. PE most commonly results from embolization of a clot from deep venous thrombosis involving the lower leg (see Chapter 24). Other less common emboli include tissue fragments, lipids (fats), a foreign body, an air bubble, or amniotic fluid. Risk factors for PE include conditions and disorders that promote blood clotting as a result of venous stasis (immobilization, heart failure), hypercoagulability (inherited coagulation disorders, malignancy, hormone replacement therapy, oral contraceptives), and injuries to the endothelial cells that line the vessels (trauma, infection, caustic intravenous infusions). Genetic risks include factor V Leiden, antithrombin II, protein S, protein C, and prothrombin gene mutations. No matter its source, a blood clot becomes an embolus when all or part of it detaches from the site of formation and begins to travel in the bloodstream.

PATHOPHYSIOLOGY The effect of the embolus depends on the extent of pulmonary blood flow obstruction, the size of the affected vessels, the nature of the embolus, and the secondary effects. Pulmonary emboli can result in any of the following:

- *Embolus with infarction:* an embolus that causes infarction (death) of a portion of lung tissue
- *Embolus without infarction:* an embolus that does not cause permanent lung injury (perfusion of the affected lung segment is maintained by the bronchial circulation)
- *Massive occlusion:* an embolus that occludes a major portion of the pulmonary circulation (i.e., main pulmonary artery embolus)
- *Multiple pulmonary emboli:* multiple emboli may be chronic or recurrent

Significant obstruction of the pulmonary vasculature leads to increased pulmonary artery vasoconstriction, pulmonary hypertension, and right ventricular dilation and afterload.[107] The pathogenesis of massive PE caused by a thrombus is summarized in Figure 27.16.

If the embolus does not cause infarction, the clot is dissolved by the fibrinolytic system and pulmonary function returns to normal. If pulmonary infarction occurs, shrinking and scarring develop in the affected area of the lung.

CLINICAL MANIFESTATIONS In most cases, the clinical manifestations of PE are nonspecific; therefore, evaluation of risk factors and predisposing factors is an important aspect of diagnosis. Although most emboli originate from clots in the lower extremities, deep venous thrombosis is often asymptomatic, and clinical examination has low sensitivity for the presence of clot, especially in the thigh and pelvis.

An individual with PE usually presents with the sudden onset of pleuritic chest pain, dyspnea, tachypnea, tachycardia, and unexplained anxiety. Occasionally syncope (fainting) or hemoptysis occurs. With large emboli, a pleural friction rub, pleural effusion, fever, and leukocytosis may be noted. Recurrent small emboli may not be detected until progressive incapacitation, precordial pain, anxiety, dyspnea, and right ventricular enlargement are exhibited. Massive occlusion causes severe pulmonary hypertension and shock.

EVALUATION AND TREATMENT Routine chest radiographs and pulmonary function tests are not definitive for PE in the first 24 hours. Arterial blood gas analyses usually demonstrate hypoxemia and hyperventilation (respiratory alkalosis). The diagnosis is made by measuring elevated levels of D-dimer in the blood (a product of thrombus degradation) in combination with CT scanning or magnetic resonance imaging (MRI). Measurement of the levels of brain natriuretic peptide and troponin is useful in PE associated with right ventricular dysfunction.[108]

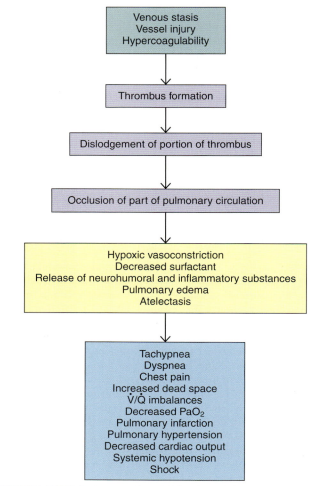

FIGURE 27.16 Pathogenesis of Massive Pulmonary Embolism Caused by a Thrombus (Pulmonary Thromboembolism). PaO_2, Partial pressure of oxygen in arterial blood; $\dot{V}/\dot{Q}$ ventilation–perfusion ratio.

Prevention of PE includes elimination of predisposing factors for individuals at risk. Venous stasis in hospitalized persons is minimized by leg elevation, bed exercises, position changes, early postoperative ambulation, and pneumatic calf compression. Clot formation is also prevented by prophylactic low-dose anticoagulant therapy.

Anticoagulant therapy is the primary treatment for PE. Initial anticoagulant therapy usually includes low-molecular-weight heparins (e.g., enoxaparin [Lovenox]) and factor Xa inhibitors. If a massive life-threatening embolism occurs, a fibrinolytic agent, such as streptokinase (Kabikinase), is sometimes used, and some individuals will require catheter-directed therapies or surgical thrombectomy. A filter in the inferior vena cava can prevent emboli from reaching the lungs. After stabilization, anticoagulation is continued for several months.[109]

Pulmonary Artery Hypertension

Pulmonary artery hypertension (PAH) is defined as a mean pulmonary artery pressure greater than 25 mm Hg at rest. PAH is classified into several groups:[110]

- No known cause or associated with inheritance, medications or toxins, connective tissue disease, or infection
- Pulmonary hypertension attributable to left ventricular disease (see Chapter 24)
- Pulmonary hypertension caused by chronic lung disease or hypoxia, or both

- Chronic thromboembolic pulmonary hypertension
- Pulmonary hypertension caused by other multifactorial mechanisms including blood, metabolic, and systemic disorders.

COPD is the most common lung disease associated with PAH, but any condition that causes chronic hypoxemia can result in pulmonary hypertension.

PATHOPHYSIOLOGY Idiopathic pulmonary arterial hypertension (IPAH) (also called *pulmonary hypertension caused by unclear multifactorial mechanisms*) is characterized by endothelial dysfunction with overproduction of vasoconstrictors, such as thromboxane and endothelin, and decreased production of vasodilators, such as prostacyclin and nitric oxide. Vascular growth factors are released, causing fibrosis and thickening of vessel walls (called *remodelling*) with luminal narrowing and abnormal vasoconstriction.[111] These changes cause resistance to pulmonary artery blood flow, thus increasing the pressure in the pulmonary arteries and right ventricle. Gas exchange is reduced with restriction in lung volumes. As resistance and pressure increase, the workload of the right ventricle increases and subsequent right ventricular hypertrophy, followed by failure, may occur (cor pulmonale). The pathogenesis of PAH and cor pulmonale resulting from disease of the respiratory system or hypoxia is shown in Figure 27.17.

Pulmonary hypertension associated with lung respiratory disease or hypoxia, or both, is a serious complication of many acute and chronic pulmonary disorders, such as COPD and hypoventilation associated with obesity. These conditions are complicated by hypoxic pulmonary vasoconstriction, which further increases pulmonary artery pressure.

CLINICAL MANIFESTATIONS Pulmonary hypertension may not be detected until it is quite severe. The symptoms are often masked by other forms of pulmonary or cardiovascular disease. The first indication of PAH may be an abnormality seen on a chest radiograph (enlarged right heart border) or an electrocardiogram that shows right ventricular hypertrophy. Manifestations of fatigue, chest discomfort, tachypnea, and dyspnea (particularly with exercise) are common. Examination may reveal peripheral edema, jugular venous distension, a precordial heave, and accentuation of the pulmonary component of the second heart sound.

EVALUATION AND TREATMENT Definitive diagnosis of PAH can be made only with right heart catheterization. Common diagnostic modalities used to determine the cause include chest X-ray, echocardiography, and CT. The diagnosis of IPAH is made when all other causes of pulmonary hypertension have been ruled out.

General therapies for PAH include administration of O_2, diuretics, and anticoagulants and avoidance of contributing factors, such as air travel, decongestant medications, nonsteroidal anti-inflammatory drugs, pregnancy, and tobacco use. Medications used in the treatment of PAH include prostacyclin and its analogues, endothelin antagonists, phosphodiesterase-5 inhibitors, and a soluble guanylate cyclase activator. None of these medications are curative, but there is improved morbidity and mortality.[112] Percutaneous catheter-based therapies are under development.[113] Individuals who do not achieve adequate clinical remission may require lung transplantation.

The most effective treatment for pulmonary hypertension associated with lung respiratory disease or hypoxia, or both, is treatment of the primary disorder. Supplemental O_2 may be indicated to reverse hypoxic vasoconstriction.

Cor Pulmonale

Cor pulmonale is defined as right ventricular enlargement (hypertrophy, dilation, or both) caused by PAH (see Figure 27.17).[114]

PATHOPHYSIOLOGY Cor pulmonale develops as PAH exerts chronic pressure overload in the right ventricle. Pressure overload increases the work of the right ventricle and causes hypertrophy of the normally thin-walled heart muscle. This pressure overload eventually progresses to dilation and failure of the ventricle.

CLINICAL MANIFESTATIONS The clinical manifestations of cor pulmonale may be obscured by underlying respiratory or cardiac disease and appear only during exercise testing. The heart may appear normal at rest, but with exercise, cardiac output falls. The electrocardiogram may show right ventricular hypertrophy. The pulmonary component of the second heart sound, which represents closure of the pulmonic valve, may be accentuated, and a pulmonic valve murmur also may be present. Tricuspid valve murmur may accompany the development of right ventricular failure. Increased pressures in the systemic venous circulation cause jugular venous distension, hepatosplenomegaly, and peripheral edema.

EVALUATION AND TREATMENT Diagnosis is based on physical examination, imaging, and electrocardiography or echocardiography, or both. The goal of treatment for cor pulmonale is to decrease the workload of the right ventricle by lowering pulmonary artery pressure. Treatment is the same as that for pulmonary hypertension, and its success depends on reversal of the underlying lung disease.

Malignancies of the Respiratory Tract

> ✓ **QUICK CHECK 27.7**
> 1. Describe squamous cell carcinoma of the vocal cords.
> 2. Differentiate the two types of non–small cell lung cancer.
> 3. What are paraneoplastic syndromes?

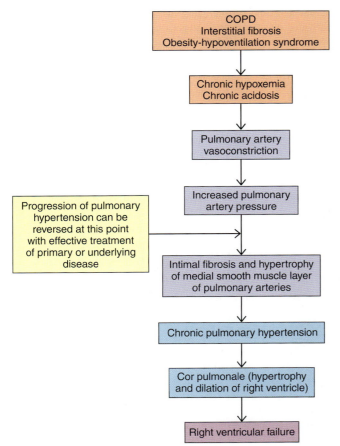

FIGURE 27.17 Pathogenesis of Pulmonary Hypertension and Cor Pulmonale. *COPD,* Chronic obstructive pulmonary disease.

Laryngeal Cancer

According to the Canadian Cancer Society, in 2017 an estimated 1 150 Canadians were diagnosed with laryngeal cancer and 440 would die from it. In 2017, an estimated greater number of men (970) than women (180) were diagnosed with laryngeal cancer. Moreover, an estimated greater number of men (350) than women (95) would die from it.[115] In Canada, the incidence rates of laryngeal cancer decreased significantly from 1992 to 2013 for both males (3.2% per year) and females (3.4% per year).[116]

The primary risk factor for laryngeal cancer is tobacco smoking; risk is further heightened with the combination of smoking and alcohol consumption. The human papillomavirus (HPV 6 and 11) also has been linked to both benign and malignant disease of the larynx.[117] The highest incidence is in men between 50 and 75 years of age.

PATHOPHYSIOLOGY Carcinoma of the true vocal cords (glottis) is more common than that of the supraglottic structures (epiglottis, aryepiglottic folds, arytenoids, false cords). Tumours of the subglottic area are rare. Squamous cell carcinoma is the most common cell type, although small cell carcinomas also occur (Figure 27.18). Metastasis develops by spread to the draining lymph nodes, and distant metastasis is rare.

CLINICAL MANIFESTATIONS The presenting symptoms of laryngeal cancer include hoarseness, dyspnea, and cough. Progressive hoarseness can result in voice loss. Dyspnea is rare with supraglottic tumours but can be severe in subglottic tumours. Cough may follow swallowing. Laryngeal pain is likely with supraglottic lesions.

EVALUATION AND TREATMENT Evaluation of the larynx includes external inspection and palpation of the larynx and the lymph nodes of the neck. Indirect laryngoscopy provides a stereoscopic view of the structure and movement of the larynx. A biopsy also can be obtained during this procedure. Direct laryngoscopy provides more thorough visualization of the tumour. Imaging procedures facilitate the identification of tumour boundaries and the degree of extension to surrounding tissue.

Combined chemotherapy and radiation or surgical resection can result in cure in selected cases; however, sequelae such as swallowing and speech difficulties may result.[118] Total laryngectomy is required when lesions are extensive and involve the cartilage. Swallowing and speech therapy after treatment can significantly improve recovery.

Lung Cancer

The term lung cancer refers to tumours that arise from the epithelium of the respiratory tract (bronchogenic carcinomas). Other pulmonary tumours, such as mesotheliomas (associated with asbestos exposure), occur less commonly (Table 27.3).

Lung cancer is the leading cause of cancer death in Canada; it causes more cancer deaths among Canadians than breast, colorectal, and prostate cancer combined. Despite its prevalence, the lung cancer death rate (especially for men) has dropped substantially over the past 25 years in Canada, which has led to a decline in the overall cancer death rate. In 2010, lung cancer was responsible for 27% of the premature deaths caused by cancer in Canada.[119]

The most common cause of lung cancer is tobacco smoking (see Figure 11.5) (see Health Promotion: Facts on Tobacco Use). Smokers with obstructive lung disease (low FEV_1 measurements) are at a much greater risk of developing lung cancer. Other risk factors for lung cancer include radon gas exposure, secondhand smoke (environmental tobacco smoke), occupational exposures to certain workplace toxins, radiation, and air pollution (see Chapter 11 and Figures 11.1, 11.18, and 11.19). Genetic risks include polymorphisms of the genes responsible for growth factor receptors, angiogenesis, apoptosis, DNA repair, and detoxification of inhaled smoke.[120] Lung cancers are classified by cell type and molecular profiling. The most common types of lung cancer are presented here.

Types of lung cancer. Primary lung cancers arise from cells that line the bronchi within the lungs and are therefore called *bronchogenic carcinomas*. Although there are many types of lung cancer, they can be divided into two major categories: non–small cell lung carcinoma (NSCLC) and neuroendocrine tumours of the lung. The category of non–small cell lung carcinoma accounts for 75 to 85% of all lung cancers and can be subdivided into three types of lung cancer: squamous cell carcinoma, adenocarcinoma, and large cell undifferentiated carcinoma. They are further described by genotyping (i.e., epidermal growth factor receptor *[EGFR]* gene or anaplastic lymphoma kinase *[ALK]* gene mutations and rearrangements), which is important for targeted personalized therapy.[121] Neuroendocrine tumours of the lung arise from the bronchial mucosa and include small cell carcinoma,

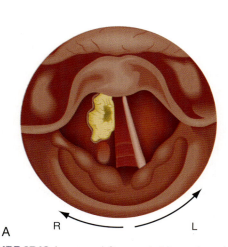
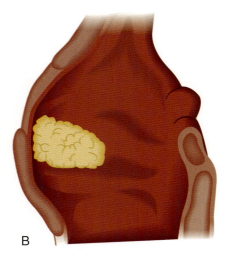

FIGURE 27.18 Laryngeal Cancer. **A,** Mirror view of carcinoma of the right false cord partially hiding the true cord. **B,** Lateral view. (Redrawn from Ackerman, L. V., del Regato, J. A., Spjut, H. J., et al. [1985]. *Ackerman and del Regato's cancer* [2nd ed.]. Mosby.)

TABLE 27.3 Characteristics of Lung Cancers

Tumour Type	Growth Rate	Metastasis	Means of Diagnosis	Clinical Manifestations and Treatment
Non–Small Cell Carcinoma				
Squamous cell carcinoma	Slow	Late; mostly to hilar lymph nodes	Biopsy, sputum analysis, bronchoscopy, electron microscopy, immunohistochemistry	Cough, hemoptysis, sputum production, airway obstruction, hypercalcemia; treated surgically, chemotherapy and radiation as adjunctive therapy
Adenocarcinoma	Moderate	Early; to lymph nodes, pleura, bone, adrenal glands, and brain	Radiography, fibre-optic bronchoscopy, electron microscopy	Pleural effusion; treated surgically, chemotherapy as adjunctive therapy
Large cell carcinoma	Rapid	Early and widespread	Sputum analysis, bronchoscopy, electron microscopy (by exclusion of other cell types)	Chest wall pain, pleural effusion, cough, sputum production, hemoptysis, airway obstruction resulting in pneumonia; treated surgically
Neuroendocrine Tumours of the Lung				
Small cell carcinoma	Very rapid	Very early; to mediastinum, lymph nodes, brain, bone marrow	Radiography, sputum analysis, bronchoscopy, electron microscopy, immunohistochemistry	Cough, chest pain, dyspnea, hemoptysis, localized wheezing, airway obstruction, signs and symptoms of excessive hormone secretion; treated by chemotherapy and ionizing radiation to thorax and central nervous system
Other Pulmonary Tumours				
Malignant pleural mesothelioma (MPM)	Rapid	Early; to lymph nodes, lungs, heart, bone	Radiography, thoracentesis	Chest pain, chronic cough, signs of pleural effusion

HEALTH PROMOTION

Facts on Tobacco Use

According to the Registered Nurses' Association of Ontario (RNAO), smoking cigarettes is mentally and physically addictive. It is estimated that 45 000 Canadians over the age of 35 die every year as a result of smoking. Smoking cigarettes increases the risk for heart disease, cancer, lung disease, pregnancy complications, stomach problems, and gum problems.

Passive or secondhand smoke can cause cancer due to the presence of many chemicals in secondhand smoke, and at least 50 of them are known to be associated with cancer. Passive smoking leads to 1 100 and 7 800 deaths per year in Canada, with at least one-third of them in Ontario. Children are also impacted by secondhand smoke and become more prone to breathing problems and lung infections.

For smokers who want to quit smoking, the RNAO recommends the following tips:

- Using a calendar, pick a "quit date" to stop smoking. This date should make sense to you in your busy life. Stick to this date!
- Prepare yourself for situations that you know will be difficult without smoking.
- Take it one day at a time. When you first stop, try to change the places where you do your daily routine.
- Keep busy, try to increase your level of activity. Congratulate yourself often: think positive.
- Ask at least one friend and some family members to help support you through the process.
- Count or save the money you would have spent on cigarettes and treat yourself to something special.
- Don't try "just one" cigarette, it will take you back to the start.

From Registered Nurses Association of Ontario (RNAO). (2009). *Deciding to Quit Smoking Health Education Fact Sheet.* http://rnao.ca/sites/rnao-ca/files/Deciding_to_Quit_Smoking.pdf.

large cell neuroendocrine carcinoma, and typical carcinoid and atypical carcinoid tumours. Small cell carcinoma is the most common of these neuroendocrine tumours, accounting for 15 to 20% of all lung cancers. Characteristics of these tumours, including clinical manifestations, are listed in Table 27.3. Many cancers that arise in other organs of the body metastasize to the lungs; however, these are not considered lung cancers and are categorized by their primary site of origin.

Non–small cell lung cancer. Squamous cell carcinoma accounts for about 30% of bronchogenic carcinomas and is associated with smoking and COPD. These tumours are typically located near the hila and project into bronchi (Figure 27.19A). Because of this central location, symptoms of nonproductive cough or hemoptysis are common. Pneumonia and atelectasis are often associated with squamous cell carcinoma (see Figure 27.19A). Chest pain is a late symptom associated with large tumours. These tumours are often fairly well localized and tend not to metastasize until late in the course of the disease.

Adenocarcinoma (tumour arising from glands) of the lung constitutes 35 to 40% of all bronchogenic carcinomas (Figure 27.19B). Pulmonary adenocarcinoma develops in a stepwise fashion through atypical adenomatous hyperplasia, adenocarcinoma in situ, and minimally invasive adenocarcinoma to invasive carcinoma.[122] These tumours, which are usually smaller than 4 cm, more commonly arise in the peripheral regions of the pulmonary parenchyma. They may be asymptomatic and discovered by routine chest roentgenogram in the early stages, or the individual may present with pleuritic chest pain and shortness of breath from pleural involvement by the tumour.

Included in the category of adenocarcinoma is bronchioloalveolar cell carcinoma. These tumours arise from terminal bronchioles and alveoli and are now being referred to as *adenocarcinoma in situ* or *minimally invasive adenocarcinoma*.[123] They are slow-growing tumours with an unpredictable pattern of metastasis through the pulmonary arterial system and mediastinal lymph nodes.

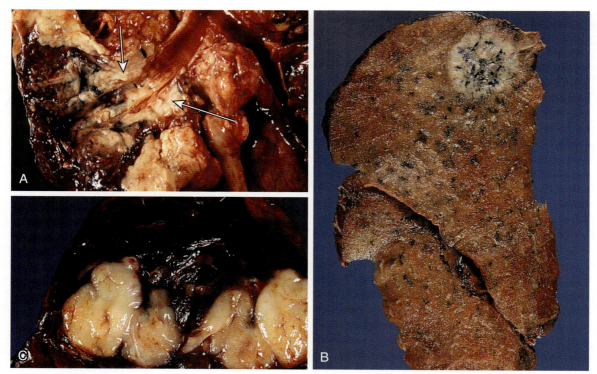

FIGURE 27.19 Lung Cancer. **A,** Squamous cell carcinoma (see *arrows*). This hilar tumour originates from the main bronchus. The *arrows* indicate the main bronchus. **B,** Peripheral adenocarcinoma. The tumour shows prominent black pigmentation, suggestive of having evolved in an anthracotic scar. **C,** Small cell carcinoma. The tumour forms confluent nodules. On cross section, the nodules have an encephaloid appearance. (From Damjanov, I., & Linder, J. [Eds.]. [1996]. *Anderson's pathology* [10th ed.]. Mosby.)

Large cell carcinoma (undifferentiated). Large cell carcinomas constitute approximately 10% of bronchogenic carcinomas. These transformed epithelial cells have lost all evidence of differentiation and are considered an undifferentiated non–small cell carcinoma. Recent studies have confirmed that these tumours arise from squamous, glandular, or neuroendocrine precursor cells, and molecular analyses have made it possible to target some of these aggressive cancers for immunological therapy.[124] These tumours commonly arise centrally, can grow to distort the trachea, and cause widening of the carina.

Neuroendocrine tumours. Small cell (oat cell) carcinomas are the most common type of neuroendocrine lung tumours and have the highest correlation with tobacco smoking. Small cell carcinoma arises from neuroendocrine cells that contain neurosecretory granules. Most of these tumours are central in origin (hilar and mediastinal) (Figure 27.19C). Cell sizes range from 6 to 8 µm, have a rapid rate of growth, and tend to metastasize early and widely.[125] Small cell carcinomas tend to present at tumour, node, metastasis (TNM) stage IV and have the worst prognosis. They are often associated with ectopic hormone production. Ectopic hormone production is important to the clinician because resulting signs and symptoms called *paraneoplastic syndromes* may be the first manifestation of the underlying cancer. Examples include hyponatremia (antidiuretic hormone), Cushing's syndrome (adrenocorticotropic hormone), hypocalcemia (calcitonin), gynecomastia (gonadotropins), carcinoid syndrome (serotonin), and Lambert-Eaton myasthenic syndrome (paraneoplastic cerebellar degeneration).

PATHOPHYSIOLOGY Tobacco smoke contains more than 30 carcinogens and is responsible for causing 80 to 90% of lung cancers. These carcinogens, along with inherited genetic predisposition to cancers, result in tumour development. Once lung cancer is initiated by these carcinogen-induced mutations, further tumour development is promoted by growth factors that alter cell growth and differentiation, such as epidermal growth factor, and by production of inflammatory mediators, such as toxic O_2 free radicals. The bronchial mucosa suffers multiple carcinogenic "hits" because of repetitive exposure to tobacco smoke and, eventually, epithelial cell changes begin to be visible on biopsy. These changes progress from metaplasia to carcinoma in situ and finally to invasive carcinoma. Further tumour progression includes invasion of surrounding tissues and finally metastasis to distant sites including the brain, bone marrow, and liver (see Chapter 10 for details of cancer biology).

CLINICAL MANIFESTATIONS Table 27.3 summarizes the characteristic clinical manifestations of neuroendocrine tumours of the lung. Symptoms are often attributed to side effects of smoking; and when they are severe enough to motivate the individual to seek medical advice, the disease is usually advanced.

EVALUATION AND TREATMENT Screening for lung cancer remains controversial but use of low-dose spiral CT scanning decreases the risk of dying from lung cancer by 20% in heavy smokers.[126] Diagnostic tests for the evaluation of lung cancer include sputum cytological studies, chest imaging, virtual bronchoscopy, radial probe endobronchial ultrasound, electromagnetic navigational bronchoscopy, and biopsy. Biopsy determines the cell type, and the evaluation of lymph nodes and other organ systems is used to determine the stage of the cancer.[127] The histological cell type, the genotype, and the stage of the disease are major factors that influence choice of therapy. The current accepted system for the staging of non–small cell cancer is the TNM classification (*T* indicates the extent of the primary tumour, *N* indicates nodal involvement,

HEALTH PROMOTION

Lung Cancer

In Canada, lung cancer is the most common cancer diagnosis and the leading cause of death from cancer for men and women.[a] The Canadian Cancer society estimated that in 2020:[a]

- 29 800 Canadians would be diagnosed with lung cancer. This represents 13% of all new cancer cases in 2020.
- 21 200 Canadians would die from lung cancer. This represents 25% of all cancer deaths in 2020.
- 15 000 men will be diagnosed with lung cancer and 11 000 will die from it
- 14 800 women will be diagnosed with lung cancer and 10 200 will die from it.
- On average, 81 Canadians will be diagnosed with lung cancer every day and 58 Canadians will die from lung cancer every day.

In Canada, the incidence of lung cancer is currently higher in men than in women (although this gap is beginning to narrow), and more than 85% of cases are related to smoking tobacco. About 44% of Canadians (12.6 million) smoke or have quit smoking.[b]

Lung cancer has a poor prognosis, and the 5-year relative survival ratio is among the lowest for all types of cancer in Canada (17% in 2013).[c]

Cigarette smoking is the main risk factor for developing lung cancer and is associated with over 85% of the cases of this disease in Canada. The 2012 Canadian Tobacco Use Monitoring Survey (CTUMS) reported that 44% of adults (4.6 million Canadians) were current or previous smokers (16% are current smokers). Other factors that increase risk for lung cancer include secondhand exposure to tobacco smoke, exposure to radon and other toxic substances (e.g., asbestos, arsenic, diesel exhaust, silica, and chromium), having a first-degree relative with lung cancer, and undergoing radiation therapy to the chest.[d]

The Canadian Task Force on Preventive Health Care (CTFPHC) recommendations for lung-cancer screening are as follows:[e,f]

- Low-dose computed tomography (LDCT) screening is recommended for adults aged 55 to 74 years with at least a 30 pack-year smoking history who currently smoke or quit less than 15 years ago. Screening should take place every year for up to three consecutive years. Screening should ONLY be carried out in health care settings with expertise in early diagnosis and treatment of lung cancer.
- No screening with LDCT is recommended for all other adults, regardless of age, smoking history, or other risk factors.
- No screening with chest X-ray, with or without sputum cytology, is recommended.

*"Pack-year" is defined as the (average number of cigarette packs smoked daily) × (number of years smoking).

[a]Canadian Cancer Society. (2020). *Lung cancer statistics*. https://www.cancer.ca/en/cancer-information/cancer-type/lung/statistics/?region=pe.
[b]Canadian Task Force on Preventive Health Care. (2016). Recommendations on screening for lung cancer. *Canadian Medical Association Journal*, 188(6), 425–432. https://www.cmaj.ca/content/188/6/425.
[c]Canadian Cancer Society. (2014). *Risk factors for lung cancer 2014*. https://www.cancer.ca/en/cancer-information/cancer-type/lung/risks/?region=on.
[d]Health Canada. (2012). *Canadian Tobacco Use Monitoring Survey (CTUMS) 2012*. https://www.hc-sc.gc.ca/hc-ps/tobac-tabac/research-recherche/stat/ctums-esutc_2012-eng.php.
[e]Canadian Task Force on Preventive Health Care. (2014). *CTFPHC Guidelines: Lung cancer*. https://canadiantaskforce.ca/wp-content/uploads/2016/03/2015-lung-cancer-protocol-en.pdf.
[f]Canadian Task Force on Preventive Health Care. (2014). *CTFPHC guidelines: Lung cancer—protocol*. https://canadiantaskforce.ca/wp-content/uploads/2016/03/2015-lung-cancer-protocol-en.pdf.

COMORBIDITIES

The Negative Impact of Comorbidities on the Disease Course of COVID-19

Coronavirus disease 2019 (COVID-19) is an infection caused by a virus and leads to severe acute respiratory syndrome coronavirus 2 (SARS-CoV-2). The mortality rate ranges between 3 to 7%.[132] Fulminant pneumonia leading to acute respiratory distress syndrome and multiple organ failure is often associated with high mortality results.[133] Recent evidence suggests that comorbidities are often linked to a more severe course of COVID-19 infection and poor clinical outcomes.[134] Given the high rate of infectivity and the high mortality of COVID-19, it is important to understand the impact of comorbidities on the course of the disease's progression.

Researchers performed a systematic search to evaluate the potential role of all reported comorbidities on COVID-19 disease progression.[135] They searched MEDLINE, Embase, Cochrane Central Register of Controlled Trials, Web of Science, and Scopus between 01/01/2020 and 05/11/2020. Outcomes evaluated were mortality, admission to a critical care unit (CCU), and severity of COVID-19, and 61 cohort studies with 31 089 patients were included in the meta-analysis. The overall mortality rate was 10.0% (19.9% of patients admitted to CCU), while the severity was 24.0%. Underlying chronic kidney disease, cardiovascular disease, cerebrovascular disease, chronic obstructive pulmonary disease, hypertension, malignancy, diabetes, and immunodeficiency were associated with increased risk of mortality, and patients with a history of cerebrovascular disease, COPD, cardiovascular disease, hypertension, diabetes, and malignancy needed more frequent admission to intensive care than other patients without these comorbidities.

In summary, cerebrovascular disease, COPD, cardiovascular disease, hypertension, diabetes mellitus, and malignancy are major risk factors for poor prognosis in patients with COVID-19. Findings from this meta-analysis demonstrate the critical role of comorbidities in determining the clinical outcomes of COVID-19. These results have the potential to be used for risk stratification of patients with SARS-CoV-2 and should be factored in when establishing a prognostic tool.

A study in the UK explored the impact of age, hypertension, diabetes, or coronary heart disease on patients hospitalized with COVID-19.[136] Of 269 070 participants aged older than 65, 507 (0.2%) became COVID-19 hospital inpatients, of which 141 (27.8%) died. Common comorbidities in hospitalized inpatients were hypertension (59.6%), history of fall or fragility fractures (29.4%), coronary heart disease (21.5%), type 2 diabetes (type 2, 19.9%), and asthma (17.6%). Age group, sex, ethnicity, and education, pre-existing diagnoses of dementia, type 2 diabetes, chronic obstructive pulmonary disease, pneumonia, depression, atrial fibrillation, and hypertension emerged as independent risk factors for COVID-19 hospitalization. Chronic kidney disease and asthma were risk factors for COVID-19 hospitalization in women, but not men.

and *M* indicates the extent of distant metastasis) (see Chapter 10). In contrast, small cell lung cancers are only staged as either limited (confined to the area of origin in the lung) or extensive.

The only proven way of reducing the risk for lung cancer is the cessation of smoking and avoidance of environmental toxins.[128] For all types of early-stage lung carcinoma, the preferred treatment is surgical resection. Once metastasis has occurred, total surgical resection is more difficult and survival rates dramatically decrease. For individuals with non–small cell carcinoma with metastasis at diagnosis, adjunctive radiation and chemotherapy and treatment based on molecular markers may improve outcomes.[129] Treatment modalities, including dose-intensified radiation, radiofrequency ablation, microwave ablation, cryotherapy, and brachytherapy, may be available as primary or palliative treatment for those for whom surgical removal is not an option. Research is in progress to advance personalized genetic and immunological approaches to treatment[130,131] (see *Health Promotion*: Lung Cancer).

COMORBIDITIES

Chronic Obstructive Pulmonary Disease Comorbidities[137]

Historically, COPD descriptions were centred around its impact on respiratory function. Currently, comorbidities play a significant role in contributing to the severity of symptoms and COPD progression. Some comorbidities are clustered with specific COPD phenotypes. For example, there is a stronger association between airway-predominant disease and cardio-metabolic comorbidities, whereas in emphysema-predominant COPD, sarcopenia, and osteoporosis are common. These patterns suggest different inflammatory pathways acting by COPD phenotype.

Osteoporosis is a major concern in COPD, particularly among men. Although β-blocker use for cardiac indications in COPD remains low, recent evidence suggests that this group of medications could decrease COPD exacerbations. Gastroesophageal reflux disease (GERD) is consistently associated with poor COPD outcomes, but mechanisms and impact of treatment are still unclear. Nontraditional comorbid conditions, such as cognitive impairment, anxiety, and depression, have a significant impact in COPD outcomes.

Obesity, low lung function, advanced age, and tobacco use are risk factors shared by COPD and cardiovascular disease. Epidemiological studies have established that there is a direct association between the presence of COPD and cardiovascular conditions (congestive heart failure, stroke, and cardiac arrhythmia), in addition to an association between worsening spirometry severity and increased odds of cardiovascular disease.

There is evidence that steroids are part of the reason for osteoporosis in COPD. Vertebral fractures (a significant consequence of osteoporosis) have double the incidence among persons with COPD, compared with those without chronic lung disease. Two consistent associations of osteoporosis in COPD are the high prevalence among men and a robust association with emphysema-predominant disease. These associations are aligned with the hypothesis that osteoporosis and emphysema are components of a specific disease phenotype, with specific mechanistic pathways involved. This idea is supported by the findings of increased levels of TNF-α and IL-6, which are enhancers of osteoclast activity, among COPD patients with osteoporosis, compared with those without osteoporosis.

Type 2 diabetes and the presence of metabolic syndrome are more frequent with COPD than the general population, and the risk of developing diabetes is also higher among those with COPD. The increase in incidence of diabetes is because of use of steroids, including inhaled steroids. Presence of diabetes in COPD is associated with a threefold increase in mortality. In contrast with osteoporosis, diabetes, and the metabolic syndrome are more frequent with a nonemphysematous, airway-predominant imaging phenotype of COPD, suggesting that inflammatory pathways could differ among emphysema and chronic bronchitis-predominant phenotypes.

With advanced COPD, there is an increase in the proportion of underweight patients, a phenomenon that is also more frequent among those with emphysematous phenotype. COPD patients not only lose weight, but also have a different body composition, with low fat-free mass index, because of increase or redistribution of fat tissue in addition to the loss of muscle mass. These changes have been explained as primed by the persistent low-level inflammation characteristic of COPD. The impact of changing weight and body composition is multidimensional: whereas low muscle mass is associated with lower exercise capacity, which also affects respiratory muscle function, greater visceral fat in COPD is associated with poor clinical outcomes, in particular with more cardiovascular events.

Experimental evidence suggests that poor physical activity, triggered by cachexia, could accelerate inflammatory lung and muscle damage. Nutritional support and rehabilitation efforts can result in modest weight gain, with no significant changes in spirometry measures, but with beneficial effects on respiratory and systemic muscle function and modest gains in walking distance and quality of life. The frequency of GERD is higher among COPD sufferers than in the general population. The interest in this comorbidity has been growing, because of its consistent association with more frequent COPD exacerbations, higher costs, and decreased quality of life. There are many potential, and unproved, reasons for the association, including chronic micro aspiration, trans diaphragmatic pressure changes, abnormal swallowing patterns, and esophageal motility. In studies of subjects with COPD, GERD treatment was associated with better scores in quality-of-life measures but not with differences in exacerbations.

Depression and anxiety are common in COPD with both conditions being more frequent among younger patients, women, and those with airway disease-predominant symptoms. Clinical outcomes are worse for patients with anxiety or depression, compared with COPD patients without these comorbidities. Specific programs designed to manage anxiety and depression in COPD are limited but must be considered for all patients. Unfortunately, only a minority of persons with COPD have their emotional needs appropriately addressed.

COPD and COVID-19

How does COPD increase the risk of severe COVID-19? The precise mechanisms of how this occurs have not been fully explained; however, there are various hypotheses.

The host engagement for SARS-CoV-2 to the nasal mucosa is the first hypothesis. The nasal mucosa are rich in a protein called angiotensin converting enzyme-2 (ACE-2).[138,139] The virus uses this protein as its receptor to enter the epithelial cells. Once inside, the virus seizes the cellular machinery of the host to produce daughter virions, which are released into the extracellular environment to infect the adjacent cells. The virus also propagates to the distal parts of the respiratory tract. Without ACE-2, infection is aborted. The ACE-2 expression levels in lungs are associated with the degree of severity of COVID-19, such that the high levels of ACE-2 receptors are often linked to severe manifestations of COVID-19. It is now known that patients with COPD have increased expression of ACE-2 in the lower respiratory tract, which is often amplified by active smoking, and increases the risk for development of severe COVID-19.[140,141]

Another hypothesis is that patients with COPD often exhibit increased sensitivity of the renin-angiotensin-aldosterone system as a result of up-regulation of ACE and angiotensin II that may be exacerbated during acute SARS-CoV-2 infection, causing acute pulmonary hypertension and pulmonary edema.[142] Corticosteroids may offer some protection against COVID-19, and during the COVID-19 pandemic, patients with COPD must be encouraged to use their prescribed inhaled corticosteroids. Long-acting bronchodilators are first line therapies for COPD, followed by inhaled corticosteroids for patients with frequent exacerbators. During severe exacerbations, COPD patients are managed with antibiotics and oral corticosteroids.[143] For exacerbations related to SARS-CoV-2 infection, patients should be given systemic dexamethasone in cases where supplemental oxygenation or invasive mechanical ventilation are needed. In these settings, the use of dexamethasone has been shown to reduce mortality by 18 to 36%.[144] COVID-19 is a growing concern in patients with COPD, but with appropriate inhaler therapy, COPD patients can be "protected" from the severe consequences of SARSCoV-2 during this pandemic.[145]

COPD and Tuberculosis

While tuberculosis (TB) was almost completely eliminated in non-Indigenous people born in Canada, Indigenous peoples in Canada continue to be affected by TB.[146] The relationship between TB and COPD is sophisticated, and a substantial number of patients with TB develop post-tubercular airway disease or TB-associated COPD. Several studies have suggested that COPD patients are also at high risk of developing pulmonary TB. Furthermore, COPD is a common comorbidity in patients with TB, second only to diabetes. TB also negatively affects the long-term outcomes of COPD, causing early mortality and increased frequency of COPD exacerbations. COPD also alters the clinical presentation of TB and increases the risk of morbidity and mortality from TB.[147]

COMORBIDITIES—cont'd

Given the prevalence of TB among the Indigenous peoples in Canada, it is worth zeroing in on the relationship between TB and COVID-19. In 2020, researchers conducted a study to determine if latent or active TB increased susceptibility to SARS-COV-19 infection and disease severity, and led to more rapid development of COVID-19 pneumonia. They established that TB infection increases susceptibility to SARS-CoV-2 and increases COVID-19 severity. TB infection status of COVID-19 patients should be checked routinely at hospital admission. Patients with active or latent TB were more susceptible to SARS-CoV-2, and COVID-19 symptom development and progression were more rapid and severe. Tuberculosis status must be suspected in certain at-risk populations and assessed carefully on admission. The management and therapeutic strategies should be adjusted accordingly to prevent rapid development of severe COVID-19 complications.[148]

Functional Comorbidities

The growing burden of COPD among older persons is a major comorbidity, but apart from being a risk factor for the presence of other chronic conditions, the systemic impact of aging threatens the independence and ability to participate in the complex process of self-care required in COPD. Cognitive dysfunction, chronic pain, geriatric conditions, and limitations with activities of daily living are as important in COPD as other classical comorbidities, as they predict the development of disability and future dependencies and nursing care utilization.[137]

GERIATRIC CONSIDERATIONS

Chronic Obstructive Pulmonary Disease in Older Persons

COPD in older persons is a complex disorder with several unique age-related aspects. Underlying changes in pulmonary lung function and poor sensitivity to bronchoconstriction and hypoxia with advancing age can place older persons at greater risk of mortality or other complications from COPD.[149]

Most individuals achieve peak pulmonary function at approximately age 20, after which airflow limitation increases with age, principally because of physiological changes in lung elastic recoil, chest wall stiffness, and respiratory muscle strength. Collagen and elastin influence elastic recoil in the lungs. Although the lung content of collagen may not change with age, collagen tends to become more cross-linked, whereas elastin tends to undergo degeneration, resulting in a loss of elastic recoil with age. Bronchiolar airway size tends to decrease after the age of 40 irrespective of pulmonary disease.

Other pulmonary changes with age include larger diameter of the alveolar ducts, with associated smaller alveolar sacs and increases in alveolar basal laminae. The overall result of these changes is an airway pattern referred to as "senile emphysema" that can occur in nonsmokers and sometimes mimics smoking-induced COPD. These age-related changes are in contrast to airflow limitation caused by COPD, which is largely a consequence of small-airway disease and parenchymal destruction. Loss of muscle mass in older persons as a result of poor nutrition, menopause, or andropause can further undermine respiratory capacity, leading to decreased physical activity level. Older persons have less ability to perceive increases in airway resistance. They also have less peripheral chemosensitivity to CO_2, which can lead to an impaired ventilatory response in the setting of hypercapnia. This may lead to delays in seeking care and may cause a disconnect between reported symptoms and severity of respiratory impairment. Taken together, these factors may contribute to the higher mortality rates in older persons from pulmonary disease than that seen in younger populations.

COPD patients are at higher risk of experiencing respiratory infections because of alterations in their mucociliary clearance mechanisms and increased production of the specific cell adhesion molecules that mediate attachment of bacteria and viruses in the airways. Expression of platelet adhesion factor receptor (a cell adhesion molecule for *Streptococcus pneumoniae* and untypable *Haemophilus influenza*) and ICAM-1 (a cell adhesion molecule for rhinovirus) are significantly elevated in COPD patients and smokers compared with normal controls.[150,151] Elevated levels of these proteins may increase the risk of respiratory infection and bacterial colonization. In addition, certain treatments, such as inhaled corticosteroids, can further increase the risk of pneumonia in COPD patients.

Streptococcus pneumoniae is a bacterium associated with invasive pneumococcal disease (IPD) and community-acquired pneumonia (CAP).[152] Two types of vaccines are used in Canada for the prevention of diseases caused by *S. pneumoniae* in adults: pneumococcal 23-valent polysaccharide (PNEU-P-23) vaccine containing 23 pneumococcal serotypes, and pneumococcal 13-valent conjugate (PNEU-C-13) vaccine containing 13 pneumococcal serotypes. PNEU-P-23 vaccine is recommended for the prevention of IPD in adults who are 65 years of age and older. In July 2015, PNEU-C-13 vaccine was authorized for the prevention of IPD and CAP caused by the serotypes included in the vaccine, for all adults 18 years of age and older. The PNEU-P-23 vaccine is a safe and effective tool in preventing IPD in immunocompetent adults over 65 years of age, while evidence on the effectiveness in preventing CAP remains inconclusive. The available Canadian epidemiological data indicate that the burden of IPD among individuals 65 years of age and over due to PNEU-C-13 serotypes is decreasing, but the burden of IPD caused by unique PNEU-P-23 serotypes and those not included in any currently available vaccine remains substantial.[152] All people with chronic lung disease, including COPD and individuals who required medical care for asthma in the past 12 months, should receive the pneumococcal vaccine.[153]

CASE STUDY

Ms. Taleb, a 59-year-old female who works as an accountant, presents to the clinic with cough, shortness of breath, and increased sputum production. Her past medical history is significant for COPD with chronic bronchitis, hypertension, diabetes, hyperlipidemia, and GERD. She reports that her sputum has increased in consistency and amount over the past few days. Her last exacerbation was about 6 months ago, for which she received oral antibiotics. This is her third exacerbation in the past year. She has a 40-pack-year history of cigarette smoking and quit smoking 3 years ago. She does not take chronic steroids and is not adherent to her medical therapy.

Physical exam reveals rhonchi and expiratory wheezes. Her vital signs are blood pressure 140/83 mm Hg, pulse rate 80 beats/min, respiration rate 20 breaths/min, temperature 37.9°C, and O_2 saturation 92% nasal prongs 1 L/min. She has no known drug allergies. A sputum Gram stain in the office reveals purulent sputum (presence of WBCs). Chest x-ray findings are negative for pneumonia, and a COVID-19 test is pending. The physicians ordered droplet and contact isolation.

Critical Thinking and Clinical Judgement Questions

1. What is the relationship between Ms. Taleb's COPD and cigarette smoking?
2. Is there a relationship between COPD and GERD?
3. Why was Ms. Taleb at higher risk of contracting COVID-19?
4. What are the potential pathophysiological conditions that can lead to increased oxygen demands or desaturation?
5. The physician ordered a short course of dexamethasone. Explain the rationale for starting this medication.

DID YOU UNDERSTAND?

Clinical Manifestations of Pulmonary Alterations

1. Dyspnea is the feeling of breathlessness and increased respiratory effort.
2. Coughing is a protective reflex that expels secretions and irritants from the lower airways.
3. Changes in the sputum volume, consistency, or colour may indicate underlying pulmonary disease.
4. Hemoptysis is expectoration of bloody mucus.
5. Hypoventilation is decreased alveolar ventilation caused by airway obstruction, chest wall restriction, or altered neurological control of breathing and results in increased partial pressure of carbon dioxide in arterial blood ($PaCO_2$), or hypercapnia.
6. Hyperventilation is increased alveolar ventilation produced by anxiety, head injury, or severe hypoxemia and causes decreased $PaCO_2$ (hypocapnia).
7. Cyanosis is a bluish discoloration of the skin caused by desaturation of hemoglobin, polycythemia, or peripheral vasoconstriction.
8. Clubbing of the fingertips is associated with diseases that interfere with oxygenation of the tissues.
9. Chest pain can result from inflamed pleurae, trachea, bronchi, ribs, or respiratory muscles.
10. Hypoxemia is a reduced PaO_2 caused by (a) decreased O_2 content of inspired gas, (b) hypoventilation, (c) O_2 diffusion abnormality, (d) ventilation–perfusion mismatch, or (e) shunting.

Disorders of the Chest Wall and Pleura

1. Chest wall compliance is diminished by obesity and kyphoscoliosis (which compress the lungs), and by neuromuscular diseases that impair chest wall muscle function.
2. Flail chest results from rib or sternal fractures that disrupt the mechanics of breathing.
3. Pneumothorax is the accumulation of air in the pleural space. It can be caused by spontaneous rupture of weakened areas of the pleura or can be secondary to pleural damage caused by disease, trauma, or mechanical ventilation.
4. Tension pneumothorax is a life-threatening condition caused by trapping of air in the pleural space, producing displacement of the great vessels and heart.
5. Pleural effusion is the accumulation of fluid in the pleural space resulting from disorders that promote transudation or exudation from capillaries underlying the pleura or from blockage or injury to lymphatic vessels that drain into the pleural space.
6. Empyema is the presence of pus in the pleural space (infected pleural effusion); it usually occurs because of lymphatic drainage from sites of bacterial pneumonia.

Pulmonary Disorders

1. Pulmonary disorders can be restrictive (limiting lung volumes) or obstructive (limiting airflow) or both.
2. Aspiration of food particles or pharyngeal or gastric secretions can cause obstruction, inflammation, or pneumonitis.
3. Atelectasis is the collapse of alveoli resulting from compression of lung tissue or absorption of gas from obstructed alveoli.
4. Bronchiectasis is abnormal dilation of the bronchi secondary to another pulmonary disorder, usually infection or inflammation.
5. Bronchiolitis is the inflammatory obstruction of small airways. It occurs most commonly in children.
6. Pulmonary fibrosis is excessive connective tissue in the lung that diminishes lung compliance; it may be idiopathic or caused by disease and is associated with chronic inflammation.
7. Inhalation of toxic gases or prolonged exposure to high concentrations of oxygen (O_2) can damage the bronchial mucosa or alveolocapillary membrane and cause inflammation or acute respiratory failure.
8. Pneumoconiosis, which is caused by inhalation of dust particles in the workplace, can cause pulmonary fibrosis, increase susceptibility to lower airway infection, and initiate tumour formation.
9. Hypersensitivity pneumonitis (extrinsic allergic alveolitis) is an allergic or hypersensitivity reaction to many allergens causing lung inflammation.
10. Pulmonary edema is excess water in the lung caused by increased capillary hydrostatic pressure, decreased capillary oncotic pressure, or increased capillary permeability. Obstructive lung disease is characterized by airway obstruction that causes difficult expiration. Asthma is an inflammatory disease of the airways resulting from a type I hypersensitivity immune response involving the activity of antigen, immunoglobulin E, mast cells, eosinophils, and other inflammatory cells and mediators.
11. In asthma, airway obstruction is caused by episodic attacks of bronchospasm, bronchial inflammation, mucosal edema, and increased mucus production.
12. Chronic obstructive pulmonary disease (COPD) is the coexistence of chronic bronchitis and emphysema.
13. Chronic bronchitis causes airway obstruction resulting from inflammation, bronchial smooth muscle hypertrophy, and production of thick, tenacious mucus.
14. In emphysema, destruction of the alveolar septa and loss of passive elastic recoil lead to alveolar enlargement, airway collapse, obstruction of gas flow, and air trapping during expiration.
15. Acute bronchitis is usually a self-limiting viral infection.
16. Pneumococcal pneumonia (*Streptococcus pneumoniae*) is the most common acute lung infection, resulting in an inflammatory response with four phases: (a) consolidation, (b) red hepatization, (c) grey hepatization, and (d) resolution.
17. Viral pneumonia can be severe, but is more often an acute, self-limiting lung infection usually caused by the influenza virus. Atypical forms and new forms can cause severe acute respiratory syndrome (SARS).
18. Tuberculosis (TB) is a lung infection caused by *Mycobacterium tuberculosis* (tubercle bacillus). Pulmonary vascular diseases are caused by embolism or hypertension in the pulmonary circulation.
19. Pulmonary embolism is most often the result of embolism of part of a clot from deep venous thrombosis and causes vascular obstruction, $\dot{V}/\dot{Q}$ mismatch, hypoxemia, and pulmonary hypertension.
20. Pulmonary artery hypertension (pulmonary artery pressure greater than 25 mm Hg at rest) can be idiopathic or associated with left ventricular failure, lung disease, or recurrent pulmonary emboli that increase resistance to blood flow in the pulmonary artery or its branches.
21. Cor pulmonale is right ventricular enlargement or failure caused by pulmonary hypertension.
22. Lung cancer, the most common cause of cancer death in Canada, is commonly caused by tobacco smoking.
23. Lung cancer (bronchogenic carcinoma) cell types include non–small cell carcinoma (squamous cell carcinoma, adenocarcinoma, and large cell undifferentiated carcinoma) and, less commonly, neuroendocrine tumours (small cell carcinoma, large cell neuroendocrine carcinoma, and typical carcinoid and atypical carcinoid tumours).

28

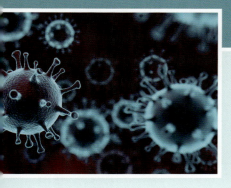

Developmental Alterations of Pulmonary Function

Mohamed Toufic El-Hussein, with originating chapter contributions by Valentina L. Brashers

Additional resources are available online at https://evolve.elsevier.com/Canada/Huether/pathophysiology.

CHAPTER OUTLINE

Disorders of the Upper Airways, 702
  Infections of the Upper Airways, 702
  Aspiration of Foreign Bodies, 703
  Obstructive Sleep Apnea Syndrome, 704
Disorders of the Lower Airways, 704
  Respiratory Distress Syndrome of the Newborn, 704
  Bronchopulmonary Dysplasia, 705

Respiratory Tract Infections, 706
Aspiration Pneumonitis, 709
Asthma, 709
Acute Lung Injury/Acute Respiratory Distress Syndrome, 710
Cystic Fibrosis, 711
Sudden Unexpected Infant Death, 711

LEARNING OBJECTIVES

1. Compare and contrast croup (laryngotracheobronchitis), acute epiglottitis, and aspiration of a foreign body, with reference to the differential diagnosis, treatment, and prognosis.
2. Identify how obstructive sleep apnea in childhood differs from adulthood.
3. Describe the pathology and causes of respiratory distress syndrome of the newborn.
4. Discuss the causes of bronchopulmonary dysplasia in the premature newborn.
5. Discuss the symptoms, causes, and differential diagnosis of bronchiolitis.
6. Describe the differences between viral, bacterial, atypical, and aspiration pneumonia.
7. Identify how an allergic response can trigger childhood asthma attacks.
8. Describe the typical blood gas abnormalities found during an acute asthma attack.
9. Identify how acute respiratory distress syndrome in childhood differs from adulthood.
10. Describe the pathophysiology, clinical manifestations, and treatment for a child with cystic fibrosis.
11. Describe sudden unexpected infant death.

KEY TERMS

Acute epiglottitis, 703
Acute respiratory distress syndrome (ARDS), 710
Aspiration pneumonitis, 709
Asthma, 709
Atypical pneumonia (*Mycoplasma pneumoniae, Chlamydophila pneumoniae*), 708
Bacterial pneumonia, 707
Bacterial tracheitis, 703
Bronchiolitis, 706
Bronchopulmonary dysplasia (BPD), 705
Croup, 702
Cystic fibrosis (CF), 711
Cystic fibrosis transmembrane conductance regulator (CFTR) protein, 711
Obstructive sleep apnea syndrome (OSAS), 704
Peritonsillar abscess, 703
Pneumonia, 707
Respiratory distress syndrome (RDS) of the newborn, 704
Sudden unexpected infant death (SUID), 711
Tonsillar abscess, 703
Tonsillar infections, 703
Upper airway obstruction, 702
Viral pneumonia, 707

Age, genetics, and environmental conditions determine the physiological maturation and alterations of respiratory function in children. Infants, especially premature infants, may present special problems because of incomplete development of the airways, circulation, chest wall, and immune system. A variety of upper and lower airway infections can cause respiratory compromise or play a role in the pathogenesis of more chronic pulmonary disease. Pulmonary dysfunction can be categorized into disorders of either the upper or the lower airways.

DISORDERS OF THE UPPER AIRWAYS

> **QUICK CHECK 28.1**
> 1. Compare between croup and epiglottitis.
> 2. What symptoms indicate aspiration of a foreign body?
> 3. What signs and symptoms suggest obstructive sleep apnea syndrome?

Disorders of the upper airways can cause significant obstruction to airflow. Common causes of **upper airway obstruction** in children are infections, foreign body aspiration, obstructive sleep apnea, and trauma.

Infections of the Upper Airways

Table 28.1 compares some of the more common upper airway infections.

Croup

Croup is an acute laryngotracheitis and almost always occurs in children between 6 months and 5 years of age, with a peak incidence at 2 years of age. Parainfluenza is the most common cause of croup in 85% of cases. Other causes include respiratory syncytial virus (RSV), rhinovirus, adenovirus, rubella virus, or atypical bacteria.

PATHOPHYSIOLOGY Subglottic inflammation and edema from the infection is the main pathogenesis of the viral croup (Figure 28.1). The cricoid cartilage is structurally the narrowest point of the airway, making edema in this area critical. As illustrated in Figure 28.2, increased resistance to airflow leads to increased work of breathing, which generates more negative intrathoracic pressure that, in turn, may exacerbate dynamic collapse of the upper airway.

CLINICAL MANIFESTATIONS Typically, the child experiences rhinorrhea, sore throat, and low-grade fever for a few days, and then develops a harsh (seal-like) barking cough, inspiratory stridor, and hoarse voice. The quality of voice, cough, and stridor may suggest the location of the obstruction (Figure 28.3). Most cases resolve spontaneously within 24 to 48 hours and do not warrant hospital admission. A child with severe croup usually displays deep retractions (Figure 28.4), stridor, agitation, tachycardia, and sometimes pallor or cyanosis.

EVALUATION AND TREATMENT The degree of symptoms determines the level of treatment. Most children with croup require no treatment; however, some cases require outpatient treatment. These children usually have only mild stridor or retractions and appear alert, playful, and able to eat.

Glucocorticoids—either injected, oral (dexamethasone [Dexasone]), or nebulized (budesonide [Pulmicort])—have been shown to improve symptoms.[1] The presence of stridor at rest, moderate or severe retractions of the chest, or agitation suggests more severe disease and does require inpatient observation and treatment. For acute respiratory distress, nebulized epinephrine (Adrenalin) stimulates α- and β-adrenergic receptors and decreases mucosal edema and airway secretions.[2]

Heliox (helium–oxygen mixture) can be used in severe cases, although it is not yet considered a mainstay of routine treatment.

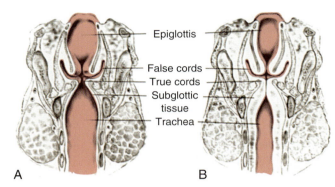

FIGURE 28.1 The Larynx and Subglottic Trachea. **A**, Normal trachea. **B**, Narrowing and obstruction from edema caused by croup. (From Hockenberry, M. J., & Wilson, D. [Eds.]. [2015]. *Wong's nursing care of infants and children* [10th ed.]. Mosby.)

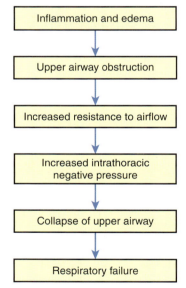

FIGURE 28.2 Upper Airway Obstruction With Croup.

TABLE 28.1 Comparison of Upper Airway Infections

Condition	Age	Onset	Etiology	Pathophysiology	Symptoms
Acute laryngotracheobronchitis	6 months to 3 years	Usually gradual	Viral	Inflammation from larynx to bronchi	Harsh cough; stridor; low-grade fever; may have nasal discharge, conjunctivitis
Acute tracheitis	1 to 12 years	Abrupt or following viral illness	*Staphylococcus aureus*	Inflammation of upper trachea	High fever; toxic appearance; harsh cough; purulent secretions
Acute epiglottitis	2 to 6 years	Abrupt	*Haemophilus influenzae*, group A streptococci	Inflammation of supraglottic structures	Severe sore throat; dysphagia; high fever; toxic appearance; muffled voice; may drool; dyspnea; sits erect and quietly

influenzae, or group A beta-hemolytic *Streptococcus* (GABHS) are the most common causes of bacterial tracheitis. Treatment of viral croup with corticosteroids has increased the risk for bacterial tracheitis. The presence of airway edema and copious purulent secretions leads to airway obstruction. Bacterial tracheitis is treated with immediate administration of antibiotics and endotracheal intubation to prevent total upper airway obstruction.[4]

Acute Epiglottitis

Historically, acute epiglottitis was caused by *Haemophilus influenzae* type b (Hib). Since the advent of the *H. influenzae* vaccine, the overall incidence of acute epiglottitis has been reduced.

PATHOPHYSIOLOGY The epiglottis arises from the posterior tongue base and covers the laryngeal inlet during swallowing. Bacterial invasion of the mucosa with associated inflammation leads to the rapid development of edema, causing severe, life-threatening obstruction of the upper airway.[5]

CLINICAL MANIFESTATIONS In the classic form of the disease, a child between 2 and 7 years of age suddenly develops high fever, irritability, sore throat, inspiratory stridor, and severe respiratory distress. The child appears anxious and has a voice that sounds muffled ("hot potato" voice). Drooling, absence of cough, preference to sit, and dysphagia (inability to swallow) are common.[6] In addition to appearing ill, the child will generally adopt a position of leaning forward (tripoding) to try to improve breathing. Death can occur in a few hours.

EVALUATION AND TREATMENT Acute epiglottitis is a life-threatening emergency. Efforts should be made to keep the child calm and undisturbed. Examination of the throat should not be attempted because it may trigger laryngospasm and cause respiratory collapse. With severe airway obstruction, the airway may be secured with intubation, and antibiotics are administered promptly. Racemic epinephrine and corticosteroids may be given until definitive management of the airway can be achieved.[7]

Tonsillar Infections

Tonsillar infections (tonsillitis) are occasionally severe enough to cause upper airway obstruction. Upper airway obstruction because of tonsillitis is a well-known complication of infectious mononucleosis, especially in a young child. Formation of a tonsillar abscess complicates tonsillitis, which can further contribute to airway obstruction. Peritonsillar abscess is usually unilateral and is most often a complication of acute tonsillitis.[8] The abscess must be drained and the child given antibiotics.[9] Some children with recurrent tonsillitis benefit from adenotonsillectomy.[10]

Aspiration of Foreign Bodies

Aspiration of foreign bodies (FBs) into the airways usually occurs in children 1 to 4 years of age. Cough reflex expels most objects, but some objects may lodge in the larynx, trachea, or bronchi. Large objects (e.g., hard candy, a bite of hotdog, nuts, popcorn, grapes, beans, toy pieces, fragments of popped balloons, or coins) may occlude the airway and become life-threatening. Items of particular concern are batteries and magnets. The aspiration event commonly is not witnessed or is not recognized when it happens because the coughing, choking, or gagging symptoms may resolve quickly. FBs lodged in the larynx or upper trachea cause cough, stridor, hoarseness or inability to speak, respiratory distress, and agitation or panic; the presentation is often dramatic and so frightening that bronchoscopic removal may be necessary.

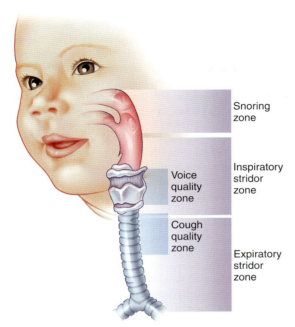

FIGURE 28.3 Listening Can Help Locate the Site of Airway Obstruction. A loud, gasping snore suggests enlarged tonsils or adenoids. In inspiratory stridor, the airway is compromised at the level of the supraglottic larynx, vocal cords, subglottic region, or upper trachea. Expiratory stridor results from a narrowing or collapse in the trachea or bronchi. Airway noise during both inspiration and expiration often represents a fixed obstruction of the vocal cords or subglottic space. Hoarseness or a weak cry is a by-product of obstruction at the vocal cords. If a cough is croupy, suspect constriction below the vocal cords. (Redrawn from Eavey, R. D. [1986]. *Contemporary Pediatrics, 3*[6]: 79; original illustration by Paul Singh-Roy.)

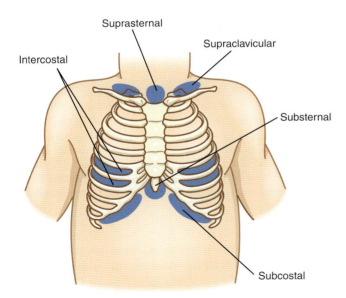

FIGURE 28.4 Areas of Chest Muscle Retraction.

Heliox improves gas flow and decreases the flow resistance of the narrowed airway.[3]

Bacterial tracheitis. Bacterial tracheitis (pseudomembranous croup) is the most common potentially life-threatening upper airway infection in children. *Staphylococcus aureus* (including methicillin-resistant *Staphylococcus aureus* [MRSA] strains), *Haemophilus*

Obstructive Sleep Apnea Syndrome

Obstructive sleep apnea syndrome (OSAS) is defined by partial or intermittent complete upper airway obstruction during sleep with disruption of normal ventilation and sleep patterns.

PATHOPHYSIOLOGY Reduced airway diameter and increased upper airway collapsibility are the common causes of OSAS. Obstruction of the upper airway during sleep results in cyclic episodes of increasing respiratory effort and changes in intrathoracic pressures with oxygen desaturation, hypercapnia, and arousal. The child goes back to sleep and the cycle repeats. Adenotonsillar hypertrophy, obesity, and craniofacial anomalies are associated with decreased airway diameter. Infants are at risk because they have both anatomical and physiological predispositions toward airway obstruction and gas exchange abnormalities.[11]

CLINICAL MANIFESTATIONS Common manifestations of OSAS include snoring and laboured breathing, sweating, and restlessness during sleep, which may be continuous or intermittent. There may be episodes of increased respiratory effort but no audible airflow, often terminated by snorting, gasping, repositioning, or arousal. Daytime sleepiness/napping is occasionally reported, as well as nocturnal enuresis.

EVALUATION AND TREATMENT Careful history and physical examination should be done on all children whose parents present with snoring. Imaging of the upper airway may be used to rule out adenoidal hypertrophy or upper airway narrowing.[12] The most definitive evaluation is the polysomnographic sleep study, which documents obstructed breathing and physiological impairment. If obstructive sleep apnea is documented or strongly suspected clinically, children are most often referred for tonsillectomy and adenoidectomy (T & A) on the basis of described symptoms and physical findings, such as enlarged tonsils, adenoidal facies, and mouth breathing.

DISORDERS OF THE LOWER AIRWAYS

QUICK CHECK 28.2
1. Why are premature infants susceptible to respiratory distress syndrome?
2. Describe the pathological findings of "new bronchopulmonary dysplasia."

Lower airway disease is one of the leading causes of morbidity in the first year of life and continues to be an important component of other illnesses progressing into childhood. Pulmonary disorders commonly observed include neonatal respiratory distress syndrome, bronchopulmonary dysplasia (BPD), infections, asthma, cystic fibrosis (CF), and acute respiratory distress syndrome (ARDS).

Respiratory Distress Syndrome of the Newborn

Respiratory distress syndrome (RDS) of the newborn (previously known as *hyaline membrane disease*) is a significant cause of neonatal morbidity and mortality. It occurs almost exclusively in premature infants.[13] RDS occurs in 50 to 60% of infants born at 29 weeks' gestation and decreases significantly by 36 weeks. Risk factors are summarized in *Risk Factors: Respiratory Distress Syndrome of the Newborn.*

RISK FACTORS
Respiratory Distress Syndrome of the Newborn

- Premature birth or low birth weight
- Male gender
- Caesarean delivery without labour
- Diabetic mother
- Perinatal asphyxia

PATHOPHYSIOLOGY Surfactant deficiency causes RDS, which decreases the alveolar surface area available for gas exchange. Surfactant is a lipoprotein with a detergent-like effect that separates the liquid molecules inside the alveoli, thereby decreasing alveolar surface tension. Without surfactant, alveoli collapse at the end of each exhalation. Usually, alveolar cells do not secrete surfactant normally until approximately 30 weeks' gestation. In addition to surfactant deficiency, premature infants are born with underdeveloped and small alveoli that are difficult to inflate and have thick walls and inadequate capillary blood supply such that gas exchange is significantly impaired. Furthermore, the infant's chest wall is weak and highly compliant, therefore the rib cage tends to collapse inward with respiratory effort. The net effect is atelectasis (collapsed alveoli), resulting in significant hypoxemia. Atelectasis is difficult for the neonate to overcome because it requires a significant negative inspiratory pressure to open the alveoli with each breath. This increased work of breathing may result in hypercapnia. Hypoxia and hypercapnia cause pulmonary vasoconstriction and increase intrapulmonary resistance and shunting. This pulmonary vasoconstriction results in hypoperfusion of the lung and a decrease in effective pulmonary blood flow. Increased pulmonary vascular resistance may even cause a partial return to fetal circulation, with right-to-left shunting of blood through the ductus arteriosus and foramen ovale. Inadequate perfusion of tissues and hypoxemia contribute to metabolic acidosis.

Increased pulmonary capillary permeability results in further worsening of the process of alveolar ventilation. Many premature infants with RDS will require mechanical ventilation, which damages the alveolar epithelium. Together these conditions result in the leakage of plasma proteins into the alveoli. Fibrin deposits in the air spaces create the appearance of "hyaline membranes," for which the disorder was originally named. The plasma proteins leaked into the air space have the additional adverse effect of inactivating any surfactant that may be present. The pathogenesis of RDS is summarized in Figure 28.5.

CLINICAL MANIFESTATIONS Signs of RDS appear within minutes of birth and include tachypnea (respiratory rate greater than 60 breaths/min), expiratory grunting, intercostal and subcostal retractions, nasal flaring, and cyanosis. Severity tends to increase over the first 2 days of life. Apnea and irregular respirations occur as the infant tires. Severity of hypoxemia and difficulty in providing supplemental oxygenation have resulted in the Vermont Oxford Neonatal Network definition of RDS: a partial pressure of oxygen in arterial blood (PaO_2) less than 50 mm Hg in room air, central cyanosis in room air, or a need for supplemental oxygen to maintain PaO_2 greater than 50 mm Hg, as well as classic chest film appearance.[14] The typical chest radiograph shows diffuse, fine granular densities within the first 6 hours of life. This "ground glass" appearance is associated with alveolar flooding. Ventilatory support is often required.

EVALUATION AND TREATMENT Diagnosis is made based on premature birth or other risk factors, chest radiographs, pulse oximetry measurements, and, if needed, analysis of amniotic fluid or tracheal aspirates to estimate lung maturity (lecithin/sphingomyelin ratio [L/S ratio]). Some neonates require immediate resuscitation because of asphyxia or severe respiratory distress. For women who are at risk for preterm birth, antenatal treatment with glucocorticoids induces rapid acceleration of lung maturation and stimulation of surfactant production in the fetus and significantly reduces the incidence of RDS and death.[15,16]

Administration of exogenous surfactant (either synthetic or natural) prophylaxis through nebulizer or nasal continuous positive airway pressure (CPAP) ventilation beginning within 15 to 30 minutes of birth

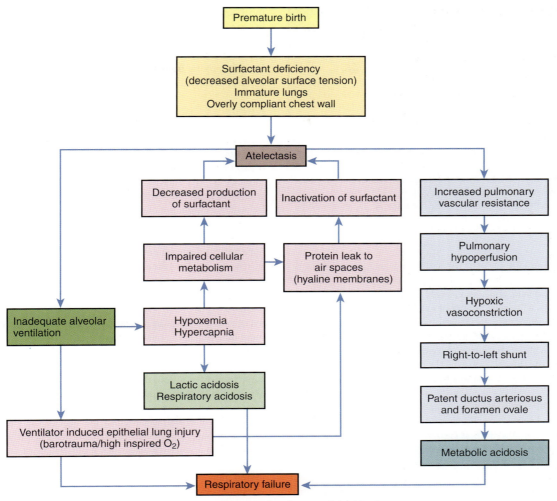

FIGURE 28.5 Pathogenesis of Respiratory Distress Syndrome of the Newborn.

is the current recommendation for infants weighing less than 1000 g. For infants weighing more than 1000 g, surfactant replacement is based on clinical need.

Most infants survive RDS and, in many cases, recovery may be complete within 10 to 14 days.[17]

Bronchopulmonary Dysplasia

Bronchopulmonary dysplasia (BPD), also known as *chronic lung disease of prematurity*, is the major cause of pulmonary disease in infants. It is associated with premature birth (usually before 28 weeks' gestation), prolonged (at least 28 days) perinatal supplemental oxygen, and positive pressure ventilation. Risk factors for BPD[18] are summarized in *Risk Factors:* Bronchopulmonary Dysplasia.

The widespread use of antenatal glucocorticoids and postnatal surfactant has lessened the incidence and severity of RDS, and BPD is occurring primarily in the smallest premature infants (23 to 28 weeks' gestation) who have received mechanical ventilation. The presence of antenatal chorioamnionitis with fetal involvement, postnatal sepsis, a patent ductus arteriosus, and genetic susceptibility confer additional risks of developing BPD.[18]

PATHOPHYSIOLOGY Lung immaturity and inflammation contribute to the development of BPD. Before the widespread use of surfactant therapy, BPD was a disease characterized by airway injury, inflammation, and parenchymal fibrosis (*classic BPD*). With the initiation

> **RISK FACTORS**
> **Bronchopulmonary Dysplasia**
> - Premature birth (especially ≤28 weeks)
> - Positive-pressure ventilation
> - Supplemental oxygen administration
> - Antenatal chorioamnionitis
> - Postnatal sepsis or pneumonia
> - Patent ductus arteriosus
> - Nutritional deficiencies
> - Early adrenal insufficiency
> - Genetic susceptibility

of surfactant therapy, what is called the *new BPD* is most common and is a form of arrested lung development. There is poor formation of the alveolar structure with fewer and larger alveoli and decreased surface area for gas exchange. Persistent inflammation contributes to pulmonary capillary fibrosis, ventilation–perfusion mismatch, pulmonary hypertension, and decreased exercise capacity.[19,20] Table 28.2 and Figure 28.6 illustrate the pathophysiology of BPD.

CLINICAL MANIFESTATIONS The clinical definition of BPD includes need for supplemental oxygen at 36 weeks' postmenstrual age or gestational age (the time elapsed between the first day of the last normal

TABLE 28.2 Comparison of Classic and New Bronchopulmonary Dysplasia	
Classic BPD	**New BPD**
Metaplasia of respiratory epithelium	Less severe squamous metaplasia
Smooth muscle hypertrophy	Less smooth muscle hypertrophy
Significant fibrosis	Less fibrosis
Large vascular modifications	Abnormal pulmonary vascular structure
	Small number and increased diameter of alveoli
	Increase in elastic tissue

BPD, Bronchopulmonary dysplasia.
Adapted from Monte, L. F., Silva Filho, L. V., Miyoshi, M. H., et al. (2005). *Journal of Pediatrics (Rio J), 81*(2), 99–110, Table 3. https://www.scielo.br/scielo.php?pid=s0021-75572005000300004&script=sci_arttext&tlng=en.

menstrual period and the day of birth), and for at least 28 days after birth. It also details a graded severity dependent on required respiratory support at term (mild, moderate, and severe, based on oxygen requirements and ventilatory needs). Clinically, the infant exhibits hypoxemia and hypercapnia caused by ventilation–perfusion mismatch and diffusion defects. The work of breathing increases and the ability to feed may be impaired. Intermittent bronchospasm, mucus plugging, and pulmonary hypertension characterize the clinical course. Of the most severely affected infants, dusky spells may occur with agitation, feeding, or gastroesophageal reflux.

EVALUATION AND TREATMENT Infants with severe BPD require prolonged assisted ventilation. Prevention of lung damage with noninvasive respiratory support, such as early nasal CPAP or nasal intermittent positive-pressure ventilation (IPPV), is used in clinical situations when permitted. When compared with mechanical ventilation, use of CPAP has resulted in fewer days of oxygen and ventilator requirement by reducing the amount of lung injury.[21] Diuretics are used to control pulmonary edema. Bronchodilators reduce airway resistance. Inhaled corticosteroids improve the rate of extubation and reduce the time that mechanical ventilation is required.[22] Prophylactic caffeine citrate administration, vitamin A supplementation, and careful fluid and nutritional support are routinely used and have resulted in improved outcomes.[23] Children with BPD will need to be monitored into adulthood for the development of chronic lung disease.

Respiratory Tract Infections

> **✓ QUICK CHECK 28.3**
> 1. Describe the typical presentation of respiratory syncytial virus bronchiolitis.
> 2. What clinical features distinguish bacterial pneumonia from atypical pneumonia?

Respiratory tract infections are common in children and are a frequent cause for emergency department visits and hospitalizations. Clinical presentation, age of the child, and season of the year can often provide clues to the etiological agent, even when the agent cannot be proved.

Bronchiolitis

Bronchiolitis is a common, viral respiratory tract infection of the small airways that occurs almost exclusively in infants and young toddlers and is a major reason for hospitalization. It has a seasonal, yearly incidence, from approximately November to April, and is the leading cause of hospitalization for infants during the winter season. The most common associated pathogen is RSV, but bronchiolitis also may be associated with human metapneumovirus and human bocavirus. Healthy infants usually make a full recovery from RSV bronchiolitis, but infants who were premature (birth weight less than 2500 g) or who have underlying BPD or heart disease may have a much higher risk for a more severe or even deadly course.

PATHOPHYSIOLOGY Viral infection causes necrosis of the bronchial epithelium and destruction of ciliated epithelial cells. There is infiltration with lymphocytes around the bronchioles and a cell-mediated hypersensitivity to viral antigens with release of lymphokines causing inflammation, as well as activation of eosinophils, neutrophils, and monocytes. The submucosa becomes edematous and cellular debris and fibrin form plugs within the bronchioles. Edema of the bronchiolar wall, accumulation of mucus and cellular debris, and bronchospasm narrow many peripheral airways. Other airways become partially or completely occluded. Atelectasis occurs in some areas of the lung and hyperinflation occurs in others.

The mechanics of breathing are disrupted by bronchiolitis. Airway narrowing causes obstruction of airflow that is worse on expiration. This airway narrowing leads to air trapping, hyperinflation, and increased functional residual capacity (FRC). Airway resistance and hyperinflation result in increased work of breathing and the development of hypercapnia in severe cases.

CLINICAL MANIFESTATIONS Symptoms usually begin with significant rhinorrhea followed by a tight cough over the next several days, along with systemic signs of decreased appetite, lethargy, and fever. Infants typically have tachypnea, variable degrees of respiratory distress, and abnormal auscultatory findings of the chest. Wheezing is most common, but rales or rhonchi also may be present. Chest radiographs often reveal hyperexpanded lungs, patchy or peribronchial infiltrates, and, sometimes, atelectasis of the right upper lobe. Very young infants may present with severe apnea before lower respiratory tract symptoms appear, and these apneas frequently require mechanical ventilation. Many children also may present with conjunctivitis or otitis media.

EVALUATION AND TREATMENT According to the Canadian Paediatric Society, bronchiolitis is a clinical diagnosis. Typically, diagnosis is made by review of history, signs, and symptoms (e.g., rhinitis, cough, wheezing, chest retractions, tachypnea). Laboratory, radiological examination (chest X-ray), blood tests, and viral or bacterial cultures are not routinely performed.

The decision to admit a child with bronchiolitis to the hospital depends on the risk for progression to severe disease, respiratory status, ability to maintain adequate hydration, the family's ability to cope at home, and the age of the child. The use of antibiotics is not recommended, unless there is suspicion of an underlying bacterial infection.[24] Most cases are mild and require no specific treatment and may be monitored as outpatients. Continuous oxygen saturation monitoring may be indicated for high-risk children in the acute phase of illness, and intermittent monitoring or spot checks are appropriate for lower-risk children and patients who are improving clinically. When treatment is indicated, it is primarily supportive in nature, including hydration, minimal handling, gentle nasal suctioning, and oxygen therapy. Preventive treatment with RSV-specific monoclonal antibody (palivizumab [Synagis]), provided as a monthly injection for 5 months through the RSV season, is recommended for high-risk infants younger than 2 years who meet specific criteria (e.g., hemodynamically significant heart disease and chronic lung disease of prematurity). Other preventive measures include use of hand hygiene and alcohol-based

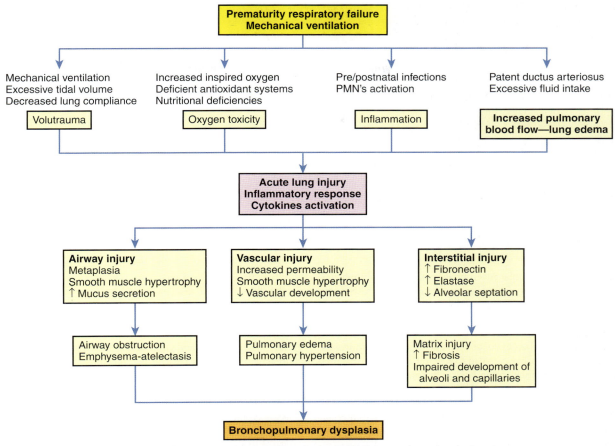

FIGURE 28.6 Pathophysiology of Bronchopulmonary Dysplasia. *PMN*, Polymorphonuclear leukocyte.

decontamination, prevention of exposure to tobacco smoke, and promotion of infant breastfeeding. If intravenous fluids are used for hydration, an isotonic solution (0.9% sodium chloride/5% dextrose) is recommended, together with routine monitoring of serum sodium.

Pneumonia

Pneumonia is infection and inflammation in the terminal airways and alveoli. Community-acquired pneumonia (CAP) is a major cause of morbidity and mortality in children, particularly in developing countries. The most common agents are viruses, followed by bacteria, and atypical microorganisms (e.g., mycoplasma) (Table 28.3), and clinical symptoms often do not differentiate viral from bacterial or atypical pneumonia. Risk factors for developing CAP are age younger than 2 years, overcrowded living conditions, winter season, recent antibiotic treatment, day-care attendance, and passive smoke exposure. Nutritional status, age, and underlying disease process influence morbidity and mortality rates related to CAP.

PATHOPHYSIOLOGY Viral pneumonia is two to three times more likely to occur in children than in adults, and incidence generally follows a seasonal pattern. Bacterial co-infections are common. RSV is the most common viral pneumonia in young children. A number of other viruses are important, including parainfluenza, influenza, human rhinovirus, human metapneumovirus, and adenoviruses.[25] Acquisition of these viruses is by direct contact, droplet transmission, or aerosol exposure. There is initial destruction of the ciliated epithelium of the distal airway with sloughing of cellular material. A mononuclear-predominant inflammatory response occurs, in the interstitium initially, and later may involve the alveoli as well. Early in the course of the disease, it is often difficult to determine whether the pneumonia is viral or bacterial. Viral pneumonia often presents with cough and no fever. Differences in the clinical presentation can help to determine origin, such as degree of elevation of temperature, absolute neutrophil counts, and percentage of bands. Ultimately, diagnosis requires laboratory confirmation using immunofluorescence tests. Development of safe drugs to treat and prevent viral pneumonia continues to be a focus of much research.[26]

Bacterial pneumonia beyond the neonatal period is most commonly the result of infection with streptococci and staphylococci microorganisms. Pneumococcal (*Streptococcus pneumoniae*) pneumonia is the most common cause of community-acquired bacterial pneumonia and presents acutely and with variable severity.[27] Childhood immunization with polyvariant pneumococcal conjugate vaccine appears to decrease the incidence of pneumococcal pneumonia in children younger than 2 years of age.[28] Staphylococcal pneumonia and group A streptococcal pneumonia can be particularly fulminant (sudden, severe) and necrotizing (causing cell death) with a high incidence of accompanying empyema, pneumatocele (a lung lesion filled with air), and sepsis. *H. influenzae* pneumonia has become rare because of widespread immunization.

Bacterial pneumonia usually begins with aspiration of nasopharyngeal bacteria. A preceding viral infection sometimes sets the stage for bacterial infection by causing epithelial damage, reduced mucociliary clearance in the trachea and major bronchi, and a reduced immune response. Once in the alveolar region, bacteria encounter local host defences, such as antibodies, complement, and cytokines, which prepare

TABLE 28.3 Common Types of Pneumonia in Children

Type	Causal Agent	Age	Onset	Signs/Symptoms
Viral pneumonia	Respiratory syncytial virus (RSV), influenza, adenovirus, others	Infants for RSV, all ages for others	Acute or gradual, winter and early spring	Mild to high fever, cough, rhinorrhea, malaise, rales, rhonchi, wheezing, or apnea; variable radiographic pattern
Pneumococcal pneumonia	Pneumococci (*Streptococcus pneumoniae*)	Usually 1 to 4 years	Acute, follows an upper respiratory tract infection, winter and early spring	High fever, productive cough, pleuritic pain, increased respiration rate, decreased breath sounds in area of consolidation; lobar infiltrate or "round pneumonia" on radiograph
Staphylococcal pneumonia	*Staphylococcus aureus* (including methicillin-resistant strains)	1 week to 2 years	Acute, winter	High fever, cough, respiratory distress; empyema or pneumatoceles common
Streptococcal pneumonia	Group A beta-hemolytic streptococci	All ages	Acute, any season	High fever, chills, respiratory distress, sepsis, or shock
Mycoplasmal and chlamydial pneumonia	*Mycoplasma pneumoniae, Chlamydophila pneumoniae*	School-age and adolescents	Gradual	Low-grade fever, cough

bacteria for ingestion by alveolar macrophages. Alveolar macrophages recognize bacteria with their surface receptors and phagocytose them. If these mechanisms fail, macrophages release numerous inflammatory cytokines, and neutrophils will be recruited into the lung.[29] An intense, cytokine-mediated inflammation will ensue. Vascular engorgement, edema, and a fibrinopurulent exudate occur. Alveolar filling prevents gas exchange and, if extensive, can lead to respiratory failure. If sepsis occurs at the same time, shock and end-organ hypoperfusion will cause metabolic acidosis.

The clinical presentation of bacterial pneumonia, particularly pneumococcal, may include a preceding viral illness followed by fever with chills and rigors, shortness of breath, and an increasingly productive cough. Occasionally, there is blood streaking of the sputum. Respiratory rate and oxygen saturation also are important clinical indicators. Auscultation usually shows such abnormalities as crackles or decreased breath sounds. Other, less specific findings may include malaise, emesis, abdominal pain, and chest pain. Chest films will usually present with a lobar pattern in older children and adolescents but may appear patchier with a bronchopneumonic pattern in younger children.

Atypical pneumonia (*Mycoplasma pneumoniae, Chlamydophila pneumoniae*) is the most common cause of CAP for school-age children and young adults. *Chlamydophila* pneumonia is clinically indistinguishable from and is typically grouped with *Mycoplasma* as "atypical pneumonia." Transmission is from person to person with a 2- to 3-week incubation period.

Mycoplasmic microorganisms lack cell walls but have a limiting membrane and a specialized receptor for attaching to ciliated respiratory epithelial cells. Local sloughing of cells occurs. Peribronchial lymphocytic infiltration develops, along with neutrophil recruitment to the airway lumen. The pattern resembles bronchitis or bronchopneumonia. Onset is usually gradual, resembling a typical upper respiratory tract infection but with low-grade fever, cough, and chest pain.[30] *Mycoplasma* can cause a wide spectrum of disease and is more extensive as a cause of complications than previously noted. It also is occurring more frequently in infants and younger children. Most cases are not clinically severe and full recovery should be expected. Complications, when they do occur, can include bronchopneumonia, parapneumonic effusions, and necrotizing pneumonitis.

EVALUATION AND TREATMENT Guidelines have been developed to improve and aid assessment and management of pediatric pneumonia.[31,32] Diagnosis of pneumonia is based on clinical and laboratory findings. The etiological agent can sometimes be inferred from the age of the child and clinical scenario.[33] Chest X-ray in bacterial pneumonia often will initially produce a patchy infiltration and later reveal a segmental or lobar disease. A viral infection is more likely to be associated with an interstitial pattern. Biomarkers (i.e., procalcitonin) facilitate more rapid diagnosis and guide antibiotic therapy. The high-sensitivity C-reactive protein (hs-CRP) is less specific, and its level is elevated in both viral and bacterial infections.[34] Several microbiological tests are available, such as polymerase chain reaction (PCR) and nucleic acid amplification tests (NAATs).

Some pneumonias may be treated on an outpatient basis; however, many children require oxygen supplementation and, occasionally, assisted ventilation. This requirement is particularly true with infants who have a viral interstitial pneumonia, such as RSV. In addition, adequate hydration, proper nutrition, and supportive pulmonary therapy are required to reduce the duration and severity of illness. Many infants are markedly tachypneic and unable to coordinate their breathing with swallowing; they may require enteral feeding. Aspiration is always a risk with infants in respiratory distress.

Appropriate antibiotic administration for bacterial pneumonias is dependent on age and severity assessment. Local patterns of resistance must be considered when choosing appropriate antibiotics. Pneumococcal and mycoplasmal pneumonias present some unique treatment obstacles and may need a multifaceted approach to care including vaccine antigens and immune adjuvant therapies in addition to antibiotics.[35] Children should be vaccinated against influenza and pneumococcus.

Aspiration Pneumonitis

> **QUICK CHECK 28.4**
> 1. What are the key features of the early and late asthmatic responses?
> 2. Explain the full progression of blood gas abnormalities in a severe asthma attack.
> 3. What is air trapping and how is it manifested in children?

Aspiration pneumonitis is caused by a foreign substance, such as food, meconium, secretions (saliva or gastric), or environmental compounds, entering the lung and resulting in inflammation of the lung tissue. The aspiration of meconium from amniotic fluid can occur at birth.[36] Neurologically compromised children or children with chronic lung disease may have chronic pulmonary aspiration (CPA), which can cause progressive lung disease, bronchiectasis, and respiratory failure.[37]

CPA is the leading cause of death in children who are neurologically compromised because of failure of protective reflexes and difficulty swallowing.[37] Children undergoing sedation or anaesthesia also may aspirate oral secretions contaminated with anaerobic bacteria or acidic stomach contents. The severity of lung injury after an aspiration incident is determined by the volume and pH of the material aspirated and the presence of pathogenic bacteria. Very low pH or extremely high pH will cause a significant inflammatory response. With hydrocarbon ingestions, lung injury is determined by the volatility and viscosity of the aspirated substance. A low-viscosity substance, such as gasoline or lighter fluid, is the most toxic, and high-viscosity hydrocarbons, such as petroleum jelly or mineral oil, are much less likely to cause a pneumonitis. Treatment for aspiration pneumonitis depends on the material aspirated but can include broad-spectrum antibiotics with failure to improve after 48 hours. Children with CPA and a large amount of upper respiratory tract secretions may benefit from salivary gland injection with botulinum toxin A (BTX-A) to suppress secretion.[38]

Asthma

Asthma is a chronic inflammatory disease characterized by bronchial hyper-reactivity and reversible airflow obstruction, usually in response to an allergen (see Chapter 27). It is the most prevalent chronic disease in childhood, affecting 490 000 Canadian children between the ages of 4 and 11.[39,40] Populations most affected include those living in an urban setting, and those of low socioeconomic status.[40]

Childhood asthma results from a complex interaction between *genetic* susceptibility and *environmental* factors. Many genotypes are associated with susceptibility and phenotypes of asthma, including early-onset mild allergic asthma, asthma with severe exacerbations, later-onset asthma associated with obesity, severe nonatopic asthma, and corticosteroid-dependent asthma. Important risk factors include early exposure to allergens (e.g., air pollution, dust mites, cockroach antigen, cat exposure, and tobacco smoke), respiratory tract infections, preterm birth, and childhood obesity.[41–44] The *hygiene hypothesis* proposes that infants and children exposed to a highly hygienic environment and who receive vaccinations to prevent certain infections lack adequate exposure to common pathogens and therefore do not achieve balanced immune responses as they mature[45] (see Chapter 27).

About 70 to 80% of acute wheezing episodes in children with asthma are associated with viral respiratory tract infection (i.e., RSV, human rhinoviruses, and parainfluenza viruses). In infants and toddlers less than 2 years old, the most common of these is RSV. In older children and adults, the major viral trigger is rhinovirus (the "common cold" virus). Bacterial respiratory tract infections also can trigger asthma.[46] Vitamin D insufficiency may be a risk factor for airway inflammation and wheezing in children because vitamin D suppresses T-helper 2 (Th2)-mediated allergic disease.[47]

PATHOPHYSIOLOGY The pathophysiology of asthma in children is similar to that for adults and is described in Chapter 27. Asthma is initiated by a type I hypersensitivity reaction primarily mediated by Th2 lymphocytes whose cytokines activate mast cells, eosinophilia, leukocytosis, and enhanced B-lymphocyte immunoglobulin E (IgE) production (see Chapter 8; see also Figures 27.8, 27.9, 27.10). As in adults, inflammation, bronchospasm, and mucus production in the airways lead to ventilation–perfusion mismatch with hypoxemia and expiratory airway obstruction with air trapping and increased work of breathing. In young children, airway obstruction can be more severe because of the smaller diameter of their airways.

CLINICAL MANIFESTATIONS Clinical manifestations of an acute asthma attack include coughing, expiratory wheezing, and shortness of breath. Breath sounds may become faint when air movement is poor. The child may speak in clipped sentences or not at all because of dyspnea. Sometimes hyperinflation (barrel chest) is visible. Respiratory rate and heart rate are elevated. Nasal flaring and use of accessory muscles with retractions in the substernal, subcostal, intercostal, suprasternal, or sternocleidomastoid areas are evident. Infants may appear to be "head bobbing" because of sternocleidomastoid muscle use. Pulsus paradoxus (decrease in systolic blood pressure of more than 10 mm Hg during inspiration) may be present. The child may appear anxious or diaphoretic, important signs of respiratory compromise.

Findings in chronic asthma may include hyperinflation of the thorax or pectus excavatum. Clubbing should not be seen with asthma and, if present, should trigger evaluation for other conditions such as CF. Exercise intolerance may indicate underlying asthma.

EVALUATION AND TREATMENT Asthma is often underdiagnosed and undertreated, especially in preschool-age children because asthma symptoms overlap with other respiratory illnesses, such as bronchitis or upper respiratory tract infections. Diagnosis of asthma is based on episodes of wheezing as well as a variety of risk factors including parental history of asthma, atopic dermatitis, sensitization to aeroallergens or foods, blood eosinophilia, or wheezing not associated with upper respiratory tract illnesses. Confirmation of the diagnosis of asthma relies on pulmonary function testing using spirometry, which can be accomplished only after the child is 5 to 6 years of age. For younger children, an empirical trial of asthma medications is commonly initiated.

The Canadian Thoracic Society and the Canadian Paediatric Society have made several recommendations for diagnosing asthma in children who are 1 to 5 years of age. Diagnosis should be based on observation of signs or symptoms of airflow obstruction and reversibility of airflow obstruction (i.e., improvement in signs or symptoms with asthma therapy). Moreover, there should be no clinical suspicion of an alternative diagnosis (e.g., bronchiolitis, which often presents as wheezing in a child less than 1 year of age).[48] For children with recurrent (two or more) episodes of asthma like symptoms *and wheezing* on presentation, direct observation of improvement with an inhaled bronchodilator should be made by a physician to confirm the diagnosis. An alternative diagnostic method for children with recurrent (two or more) episodes of asthmalike symptoms, *no wheezing* on presentation, *frequent symptoms*, or any *moderate or severe exacerbation* is a 3-month therapeutic trial with a medium daily dose of inhaled corticosteroid (with short-acting β_2-agonists, as needed). Clear and consistent improvement in the frequency and severity of symptoms, exacerbations, or both confirms the diagnosis.[48]

The goal of asthma therapy is to achieve long-term control by reduction in impairment and risk.[48,49] Child and family education and appropriate allergen avoidance techniques should begin immediately. Care providers need to periodically assess asthma control in children. Key features for assessment include nighttime awakenings, interference with normal activities, use of short-acting β_2 agonists, pulmonary function testing, and exacerbations requiring steroids. Peak flow meters are often used to help guide treatment. Before therapy is augmented, care providers need to assess medication administration techniques, environmental controls, and comorbidities. For reduction in therapy, the asthma needs to be under good control for a minimum of 3 months.[49]

The pharmacological treatment of asthma in children is essentially the same as that for adults and is initiated in a stepwise sequence based on asthma severity and response to treatment (see Chapter 27). Management of asthma medications in children is often difficult because fluctuation in severity of symptoms is common.

Acute Lung Injury/Acute Respiratory Distress Syndrome

> **QUICK CHECK 28.5**
> 1. How are the alveoli and capillaries affected by the inflammation of acute respiratory distress syndrome?
> 2. What aspects of lung disease in cystic fibrosis are the focus of current therapies?
> 3. What are the risk factors for sudden unexpected infant death?

Acute respiratory distress syndrome (ARDS) can occur in children and is a dramatic, life-threatening condition resulting from a direct acute lung injury (ALI) such as pneumonia, aspiration, near drowning, or smoke inhalation; or from a systemic insult, such as sepsis or multiple trauma, either of which activates an inflammatory response that causes alveolocapillary injury. Mortality in pediatric ARDS remains high, at approximately 40%.[50]

PATHOPHYSIOLOGY The pathophysiology of ARDS in children is the same as that described for adults in Chapter 27 (see Figure 27.7).

CLINICAL MANIFESTATIONS ARDS develops acutely after ALI, usually within 24 hours, although occasionally it is delayed by up to a few days. ARDS is characterized by progressive respiratory distress, severe hypoxemia, decreased pulmonary compliance, and diffuse densities on chest radiograph. Initially, hyperventilation occurs, but carbon dioxide retention may ultimately occur as well because of inadequate functional air space and respiratory muscle fatigue. The severity of the overall picture is modified by comorbid factors, such as the presence of sepsis or multiorgan failure, and by the presence or absence of complications, such as health care–associated pneumonia. Some children who recover have residual pulmonary abnormalities.

EVALUATION AND TREATMENT Treatment for ARDS remains supportive in nature, and the goals are to maintain adequate tissue oxygenation, minimize ALI, and avoid iatrogenic pulmonary complications. Most individuals with ARDS require mechanical ventilation and often relatively high levels of positive end-expiratory pressure (PEEP) to promote alveolar ventilation and stabilization, and redistribution of alveolar edema fluid into the interstitium. Lung-protective ventilation strategies may include low tidal volume and permissive hypercapnia, permissive hypoxemia to prevent oxygen toxicity, prone positioning, high-frequency oscillatory ventilation, and airway pressure release ventilation. Use of corticosteroids in children with ARDS is controversial and remains at the discretion of the clinician. Extracorporeal membrane oxygenation (ECMO) can provide cardiac or respiratory support, or both, but does not heal the underlying condition.[51]

Cystic Fibrosis

Cystic fibrosis (CF) is an autosomal recessive inherited disease that results from defective epithelial chloride ion transport. The CF gene is located on chromosome 7. There are more than 1 800 known mutations of this gene divided into six classes with varying severity of disease expression. Classes 1 through 3 are associated with more severe disease and 4 through 6 with milder pulmonary disease and pancreatic sufficiency. Mortality correlates respectively with the aforementioned classes.[52] CF primarily affects White individuals (approximately 1 in 3 000). There are approximately 1 000 new cases of CF diagnosed each year, and the median age at diagnosis is 6 months. The projected mean age of survival is the early 40 s.[52]

PATHOPHYSIOLOGY CF is a multiorgan disease that affects the lungs, digestive tract (see Chapter 37), and reproductive organs. The cystic fibrosis transmembrane conductance regulator (CFTR) gene mutation results in the abnormal expression of cystic fibrosis transmembrane conductance regulator (CFTR) protein, which is an activated chloride channel present on the surface of many types of epithelial cells, including those lining airways, bile ducts, pancreas, sweat ducts, and vas deferens. The most important effects are on the lungs, and respiratory failure is almost always the cause of death. The typical features of CF lung disease are mucus plugging, chronic inflammation, and chronic infection of the small airways. The mucus plugging results from both increased production and altered physicochemical properties of the mucus. Mucus-secreting airway cells (goblet cells and submucosal glands) are increased in number and size. CF mucus is dehydrated and viscous because of defective chloride secretion and excess sodium absorption. The periciliary fluid layer is depleted in volume, impairing the mobility of the cilia and thereby allowing mucus to adhere to the airway epithelium, along with bacteria and injurious by-products from neutrophils. Neutrophils are present in great excess in the airways and release damaging oxidants and proteases (i.e., elastase) that cause direct damage to lung structural proteins, induce airway cells to produce interleukin-8 (IL-8) (which attracts more neutrophils and stimulates mucus secretion), and destroy immunoglobulin G (IgG) and complement components important for opsonization and phagocytosis of pathogens[53] (Figure 28.7).

The CF airway microenvironment favours bacterial colonization. *S. aureus* and *H. influenzae* are common in younger children, and *Pseudomonas aeruginosa* ultimately colonizes airways in at least 75% of children with CF.[54] Their biofilm resists β-lactam antibiotics, and rapid mutation of the biofilm makes these children antibiotic

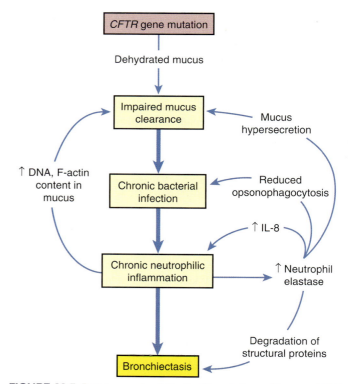

FIGURE 28.7 Pathogenesis of Cystic Fibrosis Lung Disease. *CFTR*, Cystic fibrosis transmembrane conductance regulator; *IL-8*, interleukin-8.

resistant.[55] Persistence of these microorganisms incites chronic local inflammation and airway damage with microabscess formation, bronchiectasis, patchy consolidation and pneumonia, peribronchial fibrosis, and cyst formation (Figure 28.8).[56] Peripheral bullae may develop and pneumothorax may occur. Hemoptysis, sometimes life-threatening, may occur because of the erosion of enlarged bronchial arteries. Over time, pulmonary vascular remodelling occurs because of localized hypoxia and arteriolar vasoconstriction. Pulmonary hypertension and cor pulmonale may develop in the late stages of disease.

CLINICAL MANIFESTATIONS The most common presenting symptoms of CF are respiratory or gastro-intestinal (see Chapter 37). Respiratory symptoms include persistent cough or wheeze, excessive sputum production, and recurrent or severe pneumonia. Physical signs that develop over time include barrel chest and digital clubbing. More subtle presentations include chronic sinusitis and nasal polyps.

EVALUATION AND TREATMENT The standard method of diagnosis (screening) are the immunoreactive trypsinogen (IRT) blood test and the sweat test, which reveal sweat chloride concentration in excess of 60 mmol/L. Alternative or supplemental methods include genotyping for *CFTR* mutations. Every province and territory in Canada, except Quebec, has committed to newborn screening for CF. In 2015, Cystic Fibrosis Canada continued to engage the Quebec government regarding the importance of newborn screening. Canadian researchers used data from the Canadian Cystic Fibrosis Registry to evaluate the impact of newborn screening on long-term health outcomes. They demonstrated that those identified with CF at birth have fewer lung infections, reduced hospitalizations, and better nutritional status.[57] Another health economics study revealed that it is also more cost-effective, from the perspective of the public health system, than not implementing newborn screening.

Treatment is primarily focused on pulmonary health and nutrition (see Chapter 37). Common pulmonary therapies include techniques to promote mucus clearance, such as chest physiotherapy and related mechanical devices; use of bronchodilators; and administration of aerosolized dornase alfa (Pulmozyme) and hypertonic saline, which liquefy mucus.[58,59] Oral, inhaled, or intravenous antibiotics are used to treat exacerbations of pulmonary infection. Different classes of antibiotics are used to treat different pathogens and to overcome antibiotic resistance.[60,61] Recombinant human growth hormone has been shown to improve lung function, height, and weight in children with severe CF.[62] Individuals with end-stage lung disease may consider lung transplantation.[63] Newer approaches to gene therapy are being explored, including mutation-specific targets.[64]

SUDDEN UNEXPECTED INFANT DEATH

Sudden unexpected infant death (SUID) remains a disease of unknown cause and is the most common cause of unexplained infant death in Western countries. It is defined as "sudden death of an infant under 1 year of age which remains unexplained after a thorough case investigation, including performance of a complete autopsy, examination of the death scene, and review of the clinical history."[65]

The incidence of SUID is low during the first month of life, with the peak incidence at 2 to 4 months of age. It is unusual after 6 months of age. SUID almost always occurs during nighttime sleep, when infants are least likely to be observed. A seasonal variation has been noted, with higher frequencies during the winter months. This has been related to a higher rate of respiratory tract infections during those months, and such infections are often reported to have preceded the death. The sleeping room also may be overheated or the infant overwrapped.

In 1993, the Government of Canada, recommended that infants be placed on their backs to sleep, and in 1999 it reinforced this message by launching the Back to Sleep campaign. In Canada, between 1999 and 2004, the rate of SUID decreased by 50%. This decline may be attributable, in part, to changes in parental behaviour such as placing infants on their backs to sleep and decreasing maternal smoking during pregnancy.[66]

According to an American Academy of Pediatrics policy statement, infants should be placed on a separate surface specifically made for infants in the same room with parents until the age of 1. While there is no evidence supporting moving an infant to his or her own room before 1 year of age, keeping the infant in the parents' bedroom during the first 6 months of age is highly recommended because the rates of SUID and other sleep-related deaths, especially those occurring in bed-sharing situations, are highest in the first 6 months. Placing the infant's specially designed bed close to the parents' bed so that the parents can view and reach the infant can facilitate feeding, comforting, and monitoring. Room-sharing reduces SUID risk and removes the possibility of suffocation, strangulation, and entrapment that can occur when the infant is sleeping in the adult bed.[67,68]

Clinical risk groups are summarized in *Risk Factors*: Sudden Unexpected Infant Death. About 75% of all SUID victims have no known predisposing clinical risk factor.[69]

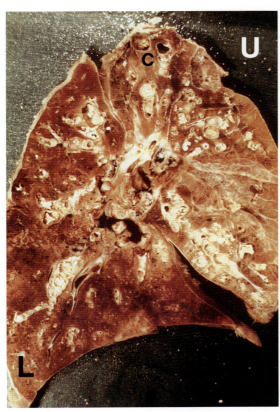

FIGURE 28.8 Pathology of the Lung in End-Stage Cystic Fibrosis. Key features are widespread mucus impaction of airways and bronchiectasis, especially from the upper lobe *(U)*, with hemorrhagic pneumonia in the lower lobe *(L)*. Small cysts *(C)* are present at the apex of the lung. (From Kleinerman, J., & Vauthy, P. [1976]. *Pathology of the lung in cystic fibrosis.* Cystic Fibrosis Foundation.)

> **RISK FACTORS**
> *Sudden Unexpected Infant Death*
>
> - Prone and side-lying sleeping positions
> - Sleeping on soft bedding
> - Overheated sleeping environment
> - Lower socioeconomic status
> - Mothers younger than 20
> - Low birth weight or growth-restricted infants
> - Male infants
> - Preterm birth
> - Multiple gestations
> - Sibling who died of SUID
> - Smoking during pregnancy
> - Exposure to tobacco smoke
> - Lack of prenatal care
> - Parent's illicit drug use or binge drinking
> - Larger family size
>
> Data from Bergman, N. J. (2015). *Pediatric Research, 77*(1–1), 10–19; Blackwell, C., Moscovis, S., Hall, S., et al. (2015). *Frontiers in Immunology, 6*, 44; Hakeem, G. F., Oddy, L., Holcroft, C. A., et al. (2015). *World Journal of Pediatrics, 11*(1), 41–47; Van Nguyen, J. M., & Abenhaim, H. A. (2013). *American Journal of Perinatology, 30*(9), 703–714.

The etiology of SUID remains unknown but probably involves a combination of predisposing factors, including a vulnerable infant and environmental stressors. There has been longstanding interest in hypotheses involving impaired autonomic regulation and failure of cardiovascular, ventilatory, and arousal responses to hypoxemia or hypercapnia. There also is a potential relationship between SUID, auditory function, and central chemosensitivity to carbon dioxide.[70,71]

Alternative theories involve airway obstruction events, such as control of tongue movements related to inspiratory activity, increased vagal tone, sudden intrapulmonary shunting because of abnormalities of surfactant or pulmonary vessels, exaggerated inflammation, or exaggerated inflammation in response to bacterial pathogens from the nasopharynx or viral respiratory tract infections.[72] Genetic factors may predispose certain individuals to SUID. The most important risk factor genes include those involved in the regulation of the immune system, cardiac abnormalities, and brainstem function.[73–75]

Currently, the best strategies for reducing SUID seem to be avoidance of all the controllable risk factors. Parents of infants with clinical risk should be taught cardiopulmonary resuscitation (CPR) as a precaution. Home monitoring has not been demonstrated to decrease the incidence of SUID, and more research is needed.[76] Some at-risk infants may warrant cardiorespiratory monitoring after careful consideration of the individual situation.

DID YOU UNDERSTAND?

Disorders of the Upper Airways

1. Spasmodic croup is characterized by a barking cough but occurs in older children, is of sudden onset at night and without fever, and has unknown etiology.
2. Tonsillar infections are usually caused by GABHS and can be complicated by tonsillar abscesses.

Disorders of the Lower Airways

1. Respiratory distress syndrome (RDS) of the newborn usually occurs in premature infants who are born before surfactant production and alveolocapillary development are complete. Atelectasis and hypoventilation cause shunting, hypoxemia, and hypercapnia.
2. Bronchopulmonary dysplasia (BPD) is the result of tissue injury and repair and disrupted alveolar development in the lungs of infants who required ventilatory support during a time when their lungs were underdeveloped because of their prematurity. Surfactant therapy has improved outcomes.
3. Bronchiolitis is a viral lower respiratory tract infection that presents with runny nose, wheezing, cough, and tachypnea in infants and is usually caused by infection with respiratory syncytial virus (RSV).
4. Viral pneumonia and bacterial pneumonia cause varying degrees of illness in children. Viral pneumonia is the most common type of pneumonia and frequently precedes bacterial pneumonia.
5. Aspiration pneumonitis is caused by inhalation of a foreign substance, such as food, milk, secretions, or environmental compounds, into the lung, and results in inflammation.
6. Asthma is a chronic inflammatory disease characterized by bronchial hyper-reactivity and reversible airflow obstruction and is usually a type I hypersensitivity response to an antigen. Its origins are multifactorial, including genetic, allergic, and viral-triggered mechanisms.
7. Acute respiratory distress syndrome results from acute lung injury and can occur when there is an insult to the lung that activates an inflammatory response causing alveolar capillary injury, usually within 24 hours.
8. Cystic fibrosis (CF) is an autosomal recessive genetic disease that affects the epithelial lining of many organ systems, especially the respiratory and gastro-intestinal systems. Airway secretions are particularly thick and tenacious, and the airways develop chronic bacterial infection with pathogens such as *Pseudomonas aeruginosa* and *Staphylococcus aureus*.

Sudden Unexpected Infant Death

1. Sudden unexpected infant death (SUID) is the leading cause of postnatal death for infants outside of the hospital setting and is associated with low birth weight, prone sleeping position, and other environmental factors.

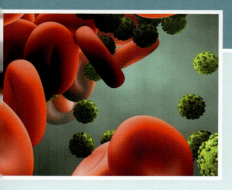

29

Structure and Function of the Renal and Urological Systems

Mohamed Toufic El-Hussein, with originating chapter contributions by and Sue E. Huether

Additional resources are available online at https://evolve.elsevier.com/Canada/Huether/pathophysiology.

CHAPTER OUTLINE

Structures of the Renal System, 714
  Structures of the Kidney, 714
Urinary Structures, 718
  Ureters, 718
Renal Blood Flow, 719
  Autoregulation of Intrarenal Blood Flow, 719
  Neural Regulation of Renal Blood Flow, 720
  Hormones and Other Factors Regulating Renal Blood Flow, 720
Kidney Function, 720
  Nephron Function, 720
  Hormones and Nephron Function, 724
  Aldosterone, 725
  Natriuretic Peptides, 725
  Renal Hormones, 725
Tests of Renal Function, 726
  Renal Clearance, 726
  Plasma Creatinine Concentration, 726
  Blood Urea Nitrogen, 726
PEDIATRIC CONSIDERATIONS: Pediatrics and Renal Function, 728
GERIATRIC CONSIDERATIONS: Aging and Renal Function, 728

LEARNING OBJECTIVES

1. Describe the anatomy of the renal system.
2. Diagram the structures and major functions of the nephron.
3. List the major vessels that supply blood to the kidneys.
4. Explain the relationship between renal blood flow and glomerular filtration rate.
5. Discuss the role of the sympathetic nervous system in the regulation of renal blood flow.
6. Describe the role of the renin-angiotensin system as it relates to renal blood flow.
7. List several factors that affect glomerular filtration rate.
8. Briefly explain the process of urine formation.
9. Identify the electrolytes reabsorbed and secreted by the proximal and distal tubes.
10. Describe the countercurrent exchange system of urine concentration.
11. Identify hormones activated or secreted by the kidney and describe their actions.
12. Discuss the clinical significance of blood urea nitrogen and creatinine measurements.

KEY TERMS

Afferent arteriole, 717
Aldosterone, 725
Antidiuretic hormone (ADH), 724
Arcuate artery, 716
Atrial natriuretic peptide (ANP), 725
Autoregulation of intrarenal blood flow, 719
Bladder, 718
Bowman capsule, 715
Bowman space, 715
Calyx (*pl.*, calyces), 714
Collecting duct, 716
Cortex, 714
Cortical nephron, 715
Countercurrent exchange system, 723
Cystatin C, 726
Detrusor muscle, 718
Distal convoluted tubule, 716
Diuretic, 725
Effective renal blood flow (ERBF), 726
Effective renal plasma flow (ERPF), 726
Efferent arteriole, 717
Erythropoietin (EPO), 726
Excretion, 720
External urethral sphincter, 719
Filtration slit, 715
Glomerular capillary, 717
Glomerular filtration, 720
Glomerular filtration membrane, 715
Glomerular filtration rate (GFR), 719
Glomerulotubular balance, 722
Glomerulus, 715
Hilum, 714
Intercalated cell, 716
Interlobar artery, 716
Internal urethral sphincter, 719
Juxtaglomerular apparatus, 716
Juxtaglomerular cell, 716
Juxtamedullary nephron, 715
Kidney, 714
Lobe, 714
Loop of Henle, 716
Macula densa, 716
Medulla, 714
Mesangial cell, 715
Mesangial matrix, 715
Micturition, 718
Midcortical nephron, 715
Natriuretic peptides, 725
Nephron, 715
Net filtration pressure (NFP), 720
Peritubular capillary, 717
Plasma creatinine (P_{cr}) concentration, 726
Podocyte, 715
Principal cell, 716
Proximal convoluted tubule, 716
Pyramid, 714
Renal artery, 716
Renal capsule, 714
Renal columns, 714
Renal corpuscle, 715

CHAPTER 29 Structure and Function of the Renal and Urological Systems

Renal fascia, 714
Renal papilla (*pl.*, papillae), 718
Renal vein, 717
Renalase, 720
Renin-angiotensin-aldosterone system (RAAS), 720
Tamm-Horsfall protein (THP), 724
Transport maximum (T_m), 721
Trigone, 718
Tubular reabsorption, 720
Tubular secretion, 720
Tubuloglomerular feedback, 719
Urea, 724
Ureter, 718
Urethra, 719
Urinalysis, 727
Urine concentration, 722
Urine dilution, 722
Urodilatin, 720
Uromodulin, 724
Vasa recta, 717
Vitamin D, 725

The primary function of the kidney is to maintain a stable internal environment for optimal cell and tissue metabolism. The kidneys accomplish these life-sustaining tasks by balancing solute and water transport, excreting metabolic waste products, conserving nutrients, and regulating acids and bases. The kidney also has an endocrine function and secretes the hormones renin, erythropoietin (EPO), and 1,25-dihydroxy-vitamin D_3 for regulation of blood pressure, erythrocyte production, and calcium metabolism, respectively. The kidney also can release glucose into the circulation by the processes of glycogenolysis and gluconeogenesis. Urine is formed through the processes of glomerular filtration, tubular reabsorption, and secretion within the kidney. The bladder stores the urine received from the kidney by way of the ureters. Urine is then released from the bladder through the urethra.

STRUCTURES OF THE RENAL SYSTEM

> ✓ **QUICK CHECK 29.1**
> 1. What is the major structural difference between the cortex and medulla of the kidney?
> 2. What is the function of the nephron?
> 3. Why are proteins not filtered at the glomerulus?

Structures of the Kidney

The **kidneys** are paired organs located in the posterior region of the abdominal cavity behind the peritoneum. They lie on either side of the vertebral column, with their upper and lower poles extending from the twelfth thoracic vertebra to the third lumbar vertebra (Figure 29.1). The right kidney is slightly lower and is displaced downward by the overlying liver. Each kidney is approximately 11 cm long, 5 to 6 cm wide, and 3 to 4 cm thick. A tightly adhering capsule (the **renal capsule**) surrounds each kidney, which is embedded in a mass of perirenal fat. The capsule and fatty layer are covered with a double layer of **renal fascia** composed of fibrous tissue. The cushion of adipose tissue (paranephric fat) and the position of the kidney between the abdominal organs and muscles of the back protect it from trauma. The **hilum** is a medial indentation in the kidney and is the location of the entry and exit for the renal blood vessels, nerves, lymphatic vessels, and ureter.

The structures of the kidney are summarized in Figure 29.2. The outer layer of the kidney is called the **cortex** and contains all of the glomeruli, most of the proximal tubules, and some segments of the distal convoluted tubule. The **medulla** forms the inner part of the kidney and consists of regions called **pyramids**. **Renal columns** are an extension of the cortex and extend between the pyramids to the renal pelvis. The pyramids extend into the renal pelvis and contain the loops of Henle and collecting ducts. The minor and major **calyces** are chambers receiving urine from the collecting ducts and form the entry into the renal pelvis, which is an extension of the upper ureter.

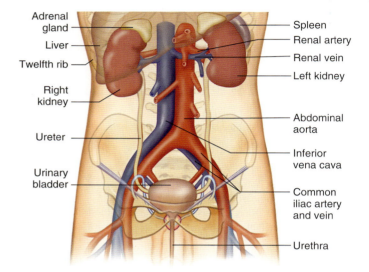

FIGURE 29.1 Organs of the Urinary System. (From Patton, K. T., & Thibodeau, G. A. [2018]. *The human body in health & disease* [7th ed.]. Mosby.)

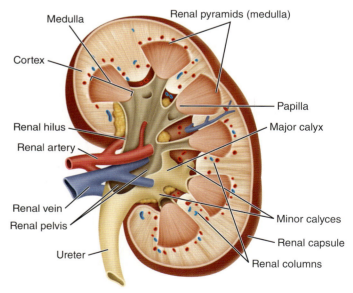

FIGURE 29.2 Internal Structure of the Kidney. (From Solomon, E. [2016]. *Introduction to human anatomy and physiology* [4th ed.]. Saunders.)

The structural unit of the kidney is the lobe. Each **lobe** is composed of a pyramid and the overlying cortex. There are about 14 to 18 lobes in each kidney.

Nephron

The **nephron** is the functional unit of the kidney. Each kidney contains approximately 1.2 million nephrons. The nephron is a tubular structure with subunits that include the renal corpuscle, proximal convoluted tubule, loop of Henle, distal convoluted tubule, and collecting duct, all of which contribute to the formation of final urine (Figure 29.3). The different structures of the epithelial cells lining various segments of the tubule facilitate the special functions of secretion and reabsorption (Figure 29.4).

The kidney has three kinds of nephrons: (1) superficial **cortical nephrons** (85% of all nephrons), which extend partially into the medulla; (2) **midcortical nephrons** with short or long loops; and (3) **juxtamedullary nephrons** (about 12% of nephrons), which lie close to and extend deep into the medulla (about 40 mm) and are important for the concentration of urine (Figure 29.5). The **glomerulus** is a tuft of capillaries that loop into the **Bowman capsule** (**Bowman space**), like fingers pushed into bread dough. **Mesangial cells** (shaped like smooth muscle cells) secrete the **mesangial matrix** (a type of connective tissue) and lie between and support the capillaries (Figure 29.6). Mesangial cells also have phagocytic abilities similar to monocytes, release inflammatory cytokines, and can contract to regulate glomerular capillary blood flow.[1] Together, the glomerulus, the Bowman capsule, and mesangial cells are called the **renal corpuscle**.

The **glomerular filtration membrane** filters blood components through its three layers: (1) an inner capillary endothelium, (2) a middle basement membrane, and (3) an outer layer of capillary epithelium. The capillary endothelium is composed of cells in continuous contact with the basement membrane and contains pores. The middle basement membrane is a selectively permeable network of glycoproteins and mucopolysaccharides. The epithelium has specialized cells called **podocytes** from which pedicles (foot projections) radiate and adhere to the basement membrane. The pedicles interlock with the pedicles of adjacent podocytes, forming an elaborate network of intercellular clefts (**filtration slits**, or slit membranes). The endothelium,

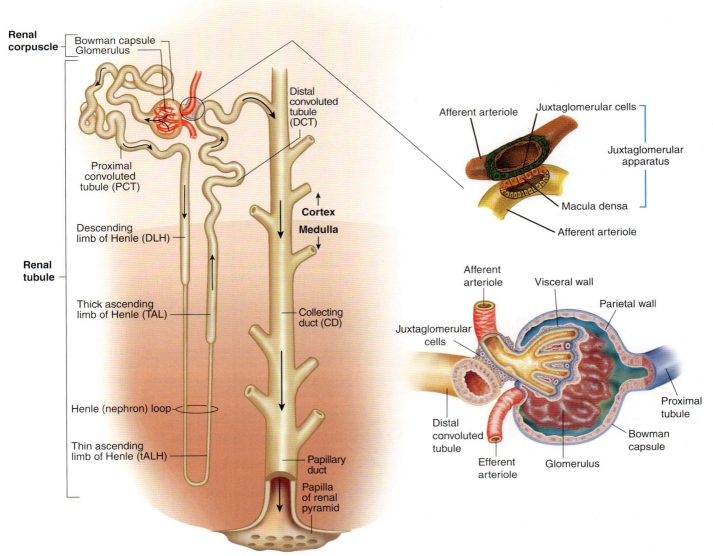

FIGURE 29.3 Components of the Nephron. (From Damjanov, I. [2012]. *Pathology for the health professions* [4th ed.]. Mosby; Patton, K. T., Thibodeau, G. A., & Douglas, M. M. [2012]. *Essentials of anatomy & physiology*. Mosby.)

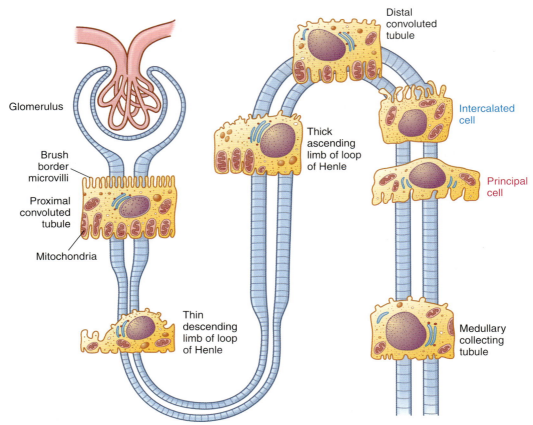

FIGURE 29.4 Epithelial Cells of the Various Segments of Nephron Tubules. The brush border and high number of mitochondria in cells of the proximal tubule promote reabsorption of 50% of the glomerular filtrate. Intercalated cells secrete H^+ (through K^+ exchange) or reabsorb HCO_3^-. Principal cells are influenced by aldosterone and reabsorb Na^+ and water and secrete K^+. H^+, Hydrogen; HCO_3^-, bicarbonate; K^+, potassium; Na^+, sodium.

basement membrane, and podocytes are covered with protein molecules bearing anionic (negative) charges that retard the filtration of anionic proteins and prevent proteinuria. The glomerular filtration membrane separates the blood of the glomerular capillaries from the fluid in the Bowman space and allows all components of the blood to be filtered, with the exception of blood cells and plasma proteins with a molecular weight greater than 70 000. The glomerular filtrate passes through the three layers of the glomerular membrane and forms the primary urine.

The glomerulus is supplied by the afferent arteriole and drained by the efferent arteriole. A group of specialized cells known as **juxtaglomerular cells** (renin-releasing cells) are located around the afferent arteriole where it enters the glomerulus (see Figure 29.3). Between the afferent and efferent arterioles is the **macula densa** (sodium-sensing cells) of the distal convoluted tubule (see Figure 29.6). Together the juxtaglomerular cells and macula densa cells form the **juxtaglomerular apparatus** (see Figure 29.3). Control of renal blood flow (RBF), glomerular filtration, and renin secretion occurs at this site.[2]

The **proximal convoluted tubule** continues from the Bowman space and has an initial convoluted segment (pars convoluta) and then a straight segment (pars recta) that descends toward the medulla (see Figure 29.3). The wall of the proximal tubule consists of one layer of cuboidal epithelial cells with a surface layer of microvilli (a brush border) that increases reabsorptive surface area. This is the only surface inside the nephron where the cells are covered with a brush border of microvilli (see Figure 29.4). The proximal convoluted tubule joins the **loop of Henle**, which extends into the medulla. The cells of the thick segment are cuboidal and actively transport several solutes, but not water. The thin ascending segment of the loop of Henle narrows and is composed of thin squamous cells with no active transport function.

The **distal convoluted tubule** has straight and convoluted segments. It extends from the macula densa to the **collecting duct**, a large tubule that descends down the cortex and through the renal pyramids of the inner and outer medullae, draining urine into the minor calyx. In the distal convoluted tubule, **principal cells** reabsorb sodium and secrete potassium, and **intercalated cells** secrete hydrogen and reabsorb potassium and bicarbonate.

Blood Vessels of the Kidney

The blood vessels of the kidney closely parallel nephron structure. The major vessels are:

1. **Renal arteries** arise as the fifth branches of the abdominal aorta, divide into anterior and posterior branches at the renal hilum, and then subdivide into lobar arteries supplying blood to the lower, middle, and upper thirds of the kidney.
2. **Interlobar artery** subdivisions travel down renal columns and between pyramids and form afferent glomerular arteries.
3. **Arcuate arteries** consist of branches of interlobar arteries at the cortical-medullary junction; they arch over the base of the pyramids and run parallel to the surface.

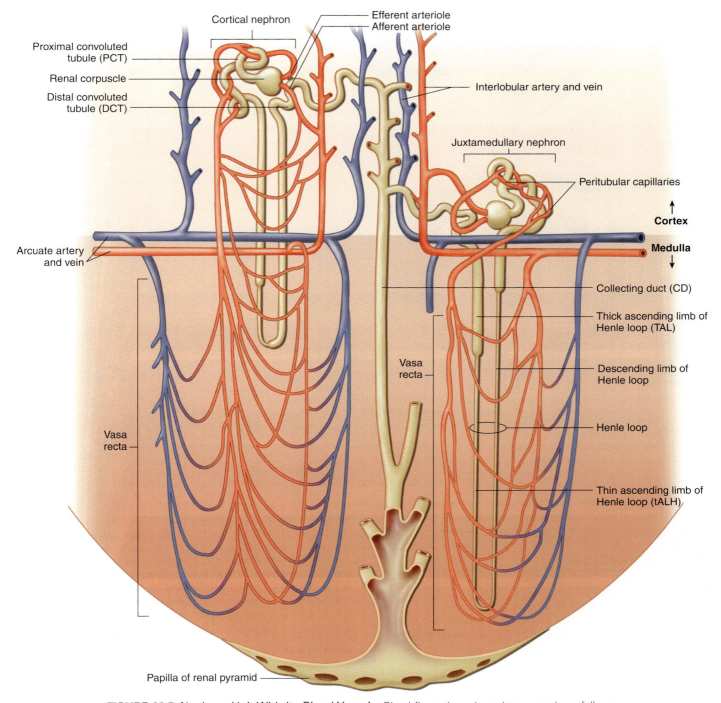

FIGURE 29.5 **Nephron Unit With Its Blood Vessels.** Blood flows through nephron vessels as follows: interlobular artery, afferent arteriole, glomerulus, efferent arteriole, peritubular capillaries (around the tubules), venules, interlobular vein. (From Patton, K. T., Thibodeau, G. A., & Douglas, M. M. [2012]. *Essentials of anatomy & physiology.* Mosby.)

4. **Glomerular capillaries** consist of four to eight vessels and are arranged in a fistlike structure; they arise from the **afferent arteriole** and empty into the **efferent arteriole**, which carries blood to the peritubular capillaries. They are the major resistance vessels for regulating intrarenal blood flow (see "Autoregulation of Intrarenal Blood Flow").
5. **Peritubular capillaries** surround convoluted portions of the proximal and distal convoluted tubules and the loop of Henle; they are adapted for cortical and juxtamedullary nephrons.
6. **Vasa recta** is a network of capillaries that forms loops and closely follows the loop of Henle; it is the only blood supply to the medulla (important for formation of concentrated urine).
7. **Renal veins** follow the arterial path in reverse direction and have the same names as the corresponding arteries; they eventually empty into the inferior vena cava. The lymphatic vessels also tend to follow the distribution of the blood vessels.

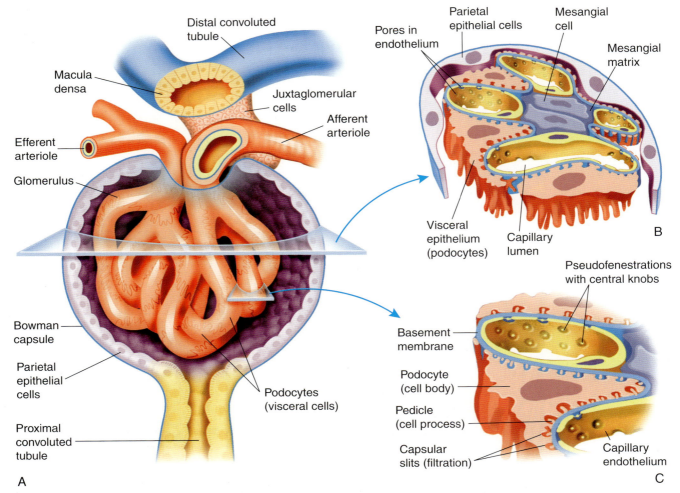

FIGURE 29.6 Anatomy of the Glomerulus and Juxtaglomerular Apparatus. A, Longitudinal cross section of glomerulus and juxtaglomerular apparatus. B, Horizontal cross section of glomerulus. C, Enlargement of glomerular capillary filtration membrane.

URINARY STRUCTURES

✓ **QUICK CHECK 29.2**
1. Where is pain from the ureters referred?
2. How do the bladder and urethra function in urine regulation?
3. What is autoregulation in the kidney? What other regulatory mechanisms are at work in renal function?

Ureters

The urine formed by the nephrons flows from the distal convoluted tubules and collecting ducts through the papillary ducts to the **renal papillae** (projections of the ducts) into the calyces, where it is collected in the renal pelvis (see Figures 29.2 and 29.5), and then funnelled into the **ureters**. Each adult ureter is approximately 30 cm long and is composed of long, intertwining smooth muscle bundles. The lower ends pass obliquely through the posterior aspect of the bladder wall. The close approximation of smooth muscle cells permits the direct transmission of electrical stimulation from one cell to another. The resulting downward peristaltic contraction from intrinsic pacemaker activity propels urine into the bladder. Contraction of the bladder during **micturition** (urination) compresses the lower end of the ureter, preventing reflux. Peristalsis is maintained even when the ureter is denervated, so ureters can be transplanted.

Sensory innervation for the upper part of the ureter arises from sympathetic inputs from the tenth thoracic nerve roots, with referred pain to the umbilicus. The innervation of lower segments arises from the parasympathetic sacral nerves, with referred pain to the vulva or penis. The ureters have a rich blood supply. The primary arteries come from the kidney, with contributions from the lumbar and superior vesical arteries.

Bladder and Urethra

The **bladder** is a bag composed of smooth muscle fibres that forms the **detrusor muscle** and its smooth lining of uroepithelium (also called *transitional epithelium*). As the bladder fills with urine, it distends and the layers of uroepithelium within the lining slide past each other and become thinner as bladder volume increases. The uroepithelium forms the interface between the urinary space and the underlying vasculature and connective, nervous, and muscle tissue. Uroepithelium also lines the urinary tract from the renal pelvis to the urethra. The uroepithelium maintains an important barrier function to prevent movement of water and solutes between the urine and the blood. It communicates information about urine pressure and composition to surrounding nerve and muscle cells.[3] The **trigone** is a smooth triangular area between the openings of the two ureters and the urethra (Figure 29.7). The position of the bladder varies with age and sex. The bladder has a profuse blood supply, accounting for the bleeding that readily occurs with trauma, surgery, or inflammation.

CHAPTER 29 Structure and Function of the Renal and Urological Systems

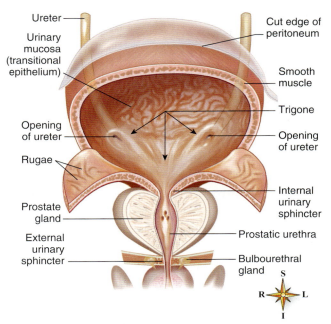

FIGURE 29.7 Structure of the Urinary Bladder. Frontal view of a dissected urinary bladder (male) in a fully distended position. (From Patton, K. T., & Thibodeau, G. A. [2018]. *The human body in health & disease* [7th ed.]. Mosby.)

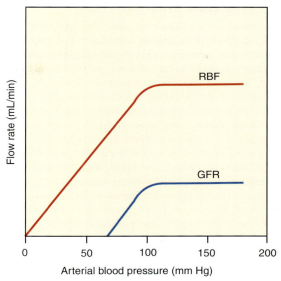

FIGURE 29.8 Renal Autoregulation. Renal blood flow *(RBF)* and glomerular filtration rate *(GFR)* are stabilized in the face of changes in perfusion pressure. (From Koeppen, B. M., & Stanton, B. A. [2010]. *Berne and Levy physiology* [6th ed., updated]. Mosby.)

The **urethra** extends from the inferior side of the bladder to the outside of the body. A ring of smooth muscle forms the **internal urethral sphincter** at the junction of the urethra and bladder. The **external urethral sphincter** is composed of striated skeletal muscle and is under voluntary control. The entire urethra is lined with mucus-secreting glands. The female urethra is short (3 to 4 cm). The male urethra is long (18 to 20 cm) and has three main segments: prostatic, membranous, and penile. The prostatic urethra is closest to the bladder. It passes through the prostate gland and contains the openings of the ejaculatory ducts. The membranous urethra passes through the floor of the pelvis. The penile segment forms the remainder of the tube. It is surrounded by the corpus spongiosum erectile tissue and contains the openings of the bulbourethral mucous glands.

The innervation of the bladder and internal urethral sphincter is supplied by parasympathetic fibres of the autonomic nervous system. The reflex arc required for micturition is stimulated by mechanoreceptors that respond to stretching of tissue, sensing bladder fullness and sending impulses to the sacral level of the cord. When the bladder accumulates 250 to 300 mL of urine, the bladder contracts and the internal urethral sphincter relaxes through activation of the spinal reflex arc (known as the *micturition reflex*). At this time, a person feels the urge to void. The reflex can be inhibited or facilitated by impulses coming from the brain, resulting in voluntary control of micturition by the relaxation or contraction of the external sphincter.

RENAL BLOOD FLOW

The kidneys are highly vascular organs and usually receive 1 000 to 1 200 mL of blood per minute, or about 20 to 25% of the cardiac output. With a normal hematocrit of 45%, about 600 to 700 mL of blood flowing through the kidney per minute is plasma. From the renal plasma flow (RPF), 20% (approximately 120 to 140 mL/min) is filtered at the glomerulus and passes into the Bowman capsule. The filtration of the plasma per unit of time is known as the **glomerular filtration rate (GFR)**, which is directly related to the perfusion pressure of the glomerular capillaries.

The remaining 80% (about 480 mL/min) of plasma flows through the efferent arterioles to the peritubular capillaries. The ratio of glomerular filtrate to RPF per minute (125/600 = 0.20) is called the *filtration fraction*. Normally all but 1 to 2 mL/min of the glomerular filtrate is reabsorbed from nephron tubules and returned to the circulation by the peritubular capillaries.

The GFR is directly related to RBF, which is regulated by intrinsic autoregulatory mechanisms, by neural regulation, and by hormonal regulation. In general, blood flow to any organ is determined by the arteriovenous pressure differences across the vascular bed. If mean arterial pressure decreases or vascular resistance increases, RBF declines and urinary output decreases. Normal urinary output is about 30 mL/hour minimum in adults or 0.5 to 1.0 mL/kg/hr.

Autoregulation of Intrarenal Blood Flow

In the kidney, a local mechanism tends to keep the rate of glomerular perfusion and, therefore, the GFR, fairly constant over a range of arterial pressures between 80 and 180 mm Hg (Figure 29.8). Changes in afferent arteriolar resistance occur in the same direction. Therefore, RBF and GFR are relatively constant, a relationship maintained by an intrinsic autoregulatory myogenic mechanism of contraction when blood vessels are stretched. The purpose of **autoregulation of intrarenal blood flow** is to keep RBF and GFR constant when there are increases or decreases in systemic blood pressure. Solute and water excretion, and thus blood volume, are regulated despite arterial pressure changes.[4]

A second mechanism of autoregulation is **tubuloglomerular feedback**. Because the GFR in an individual nephron increases or decreases, the macula densa cells in the distal convoluted tubule sense the increasing or decreasing amounts of filtered sodium. When GFR and sodium concentration increase, the macula densa cells stimulate afferent arteriolar vasoconstriction and decrease GFR. The opposite occurs with decreases in GFR and sodium concentration at the macula densa. This mechanism prevents large fluctuations in body water and salt.[5]

Neural Regulation of Renal Blood Flow

The blood vessels of the kidney are innervated by sympathetic nerve fibres located primarily on afferent arterioles. When systemic arterial pressure decreases, increased renal sympathetic nerve activity is mediated reflexively through the carotid sinus and the baroreceptors of the aortic arch. The sympathetic nerves release catecholamines. This release stimulates afferent renal arteriolar vasoconstriction and decreases RBF and GFR, increases renal tubular sodium and water reabsorption, and increases blood pressure. Decreased afferent renal sympathetic nerve activity produces the opposite effects. The integrated response regulates water and sodium balance. Renalase is a hormone released by the kidney and heart that promotes the metabolism of catecholamines, and in this way participates in blood pressure regulation.[6] The sympathetic nervous system also participates in hormonal (i.e., angiotensin II) regulation of RBF. There is no significant parasympathetic innervation. The innervation of the kidney arises primarily from the celiac ganglion and greater splanchnic nerve.

Hormones and Other Factors Regulating Renal Blood Flow

Hormones and other mediators can alter the resistance of the renal vasculature by stimulating vasodilation or vasoconstriction. A major hormonal regulator of RBF is the renin-angiotensin-aldosterone system (RAAS), which can increase systemic arterial pressure and change RBF. Renin is an enzyme formed and stored in the cells of the arterioles of the juxtaglomerular apparatus (see Figure 29.3). Renin release is triggered by decreased blood pressure in the afferent arterioles, decreased sodium chloride concentration in the distal convoluted tubule, sympathetic nerve stimulation of β-adrenergic receptors on the juxtaglomerular cells, and the release of prostaglandins.[7] Numerous physiological effects of the RAAS stabilize systemic blood pressure and preserve the extracellular fluid volume during hypotension or hypovolemia. Actions include sodium reabsorption, systemic vasoconstriction, sympathetic nerve stimulation, and thirst stimulation with increased fluid intake. The effects of aldosterone combine with those of antidiuretic hormone (ADH) in regulating blood volume and are summarized in Figure 29.9 (see also Figures 5.4 and 18.18).

Natriuretic peptides are synthesized and released from the heart and are natural antagonists to the RAAS. Natriuretic peptides cause vasodilation and increase sodium and water excretion and decrease blood pressure. They assist in protecting the heart from volume overload. Urodilatin is renal natriuretic peptide produced by cells in the distal convoluted tubule and collecting duct. It increases RBF, causing diuresis.

KIDNEY FUNCTION

> **QUICK CHECK 29.3**
> 1. Outline the process of glomerular filtration.
> 2. What types of absorption/reabsorption take place in the proximal tubule, the loops of Henle, and the distal convoluted tubule?
> 3. What is the countercurrent exchange system? What substances are involved?
> 4. What hormones are activated or synthesized by the kidney?

Nephron Function

The nephron can perform many functions at the same time (Figure 29.10):
1. Filter plasma at glomerulus
2. Reabsorb and secrete different substances along tubular structures
3. Form a filtrate of protein-free fluid (ultrafiltration)
4. Regulate the filtrate to maintain body fluid volume, electrolyte composition, and pH within narrow limits
5. Glomerular filtration, tubular reabsorption, tubular secretion, and excretion

Glomerular filtration is the movement of fluid and solutes across the glomerular capillary membrane into the Bowman space. Tubular reabsorption is the movement of fluids and solutes from the tubular lumen to the peritubular capillary plasma. Tubular secretion is the transfer of substances from the plasma of the peritubular capillary to the tubular lumen. The transport mechanisms are both active and passive (processes that are defined in Chapter 1). Excretion is the elimination of a substance in the final urine (Figure 29.11).

Glomerular Filtration

The fluid filtered by the glomerular capillary filtration membrane and released into the proximal convoluted tubule is protein-free but contains electrolytes (such as sodium, chloride, and potassium) and organic molecules (such as creatinine, urea, and glucose) in the same concentrations as found in plasma. Like other capillary membranes, the glomerulus is freely permeable to water and relatively impermeable to large colloids, such as plasma proteins. The molecule's size and electrical charge and the small size of the filtration slits in the glomerular epithelium affect the permeability of substances crossing the glomerulus and entering the proximal convoluted tubule.

Capillary pressures also affect glomerular filtration. The hydrostatic pressure within the capillary is the major force for moving water and solutes across the filtration membrane and into the Bowman capsule. Two forces oppose the filtration effects of the glomerular capillary hydrostatic pressure (P_{GC}): (1) the Bowman capsule hydrostatic pressure (P_{BC}) and (2) the effective glomerular capillary oncotic pressure (π_{GC}). Because the fluid in the Bowman space normally contains only minute amounts of protein, it does not usually have an oncotic influence on the plasma of the glomerular capillary (Figure 29.12).

The combined effect of forces favouring and forces opposing filtration determines the filtration pressure. The net filtration pressure (NFP) is the sum of forces favouring and opposing filtration. The estimated values contributing to the forces of net filtration are presented in Table 29.1.

As the protein-free fluid is filtered into the Bowman capsule, the plasma oncotic pressure increases and the hydrostatic pressure decreases. The increase in glomerular capillary oncotic pressure is great enough to reduce the NFP to zero at the efferent end of the capillary and to stop the filtration process effectively. The low hydrostatic pressure and the increased oncotic pressure in the efferent arteriole then are transferred to the peritubular capillaries and facilitate reabsorption of fluid from the proximal convoluted tubules.

Filtration rate. The total volume of fluid filtered by the glomeruli averages 180 L/day, or approximately 120 mL/min, which is a phenomenal amount considering the size of the kidneys. Because only 1 to 2 L of urine is excreted per day, 99% of the filtrate is reabsorbed into the peritubular capillaries and returned to the blood. The factors determining the GFR are directly related to the pressures that favour or oppose filtration (see Figure 29.12 and Table 29.1).

Obstruction to the outflow of urine (caused by strictures, stones, or tumours along the urinary tract) can cause a retrograde increase in hydrostatic pressure at the Bowman space and a decrease in GFR. Low levels of plasma protein in the blood can result in a decrease in glomerular capillary oncotic pressure, which increases GFR. Excessive loss of *protein-free fluid* from vomiting, diarrhea, use of diuretics, or excessive sweating can increase glomerular capillary oncotic pressure and decrease the GFR. Renal disease also can cause changes in pressure

CHAPTER 29 Structure and Function of the Renal and Urological Systems

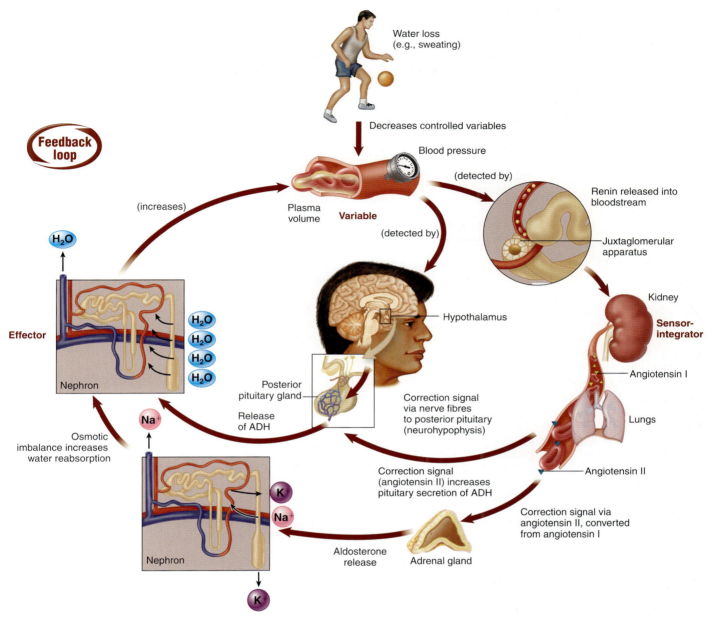

FIGURE 29.9 Cooperative Roles of Antidiuretic Hormone and Aldosterone in Regulating Urine and Plasma Volume. The drop in blood pressure that accompanies loss of fluid from the internal environment triggers the hypothalamus to rapidly release antidiuretic hormone *(ADH)* from the posterior pituitary gland. ADH increases water reabsorption of the kidney by increasing water permeability of the distal convoluted tubules and collecting ducts. The drop in blood pressure also is detected by each nephron's juxtaglomerular apparatus, which responds by secreting renin. Renin triggers the formation of angiotensin II, which stimulates release of aldosterone from the adrenal cortex. Aldosterone then slowly boosts water *(H_2O)* reabsorption by the kidneys by increasing reabsorption of sodium *(Na^+)*. Because angiotensin II also stimulates secretion of ADH, it serves as an additional link between the ADH and aldosterone mechanisms. K^+, Potassium. (From Patton, K. T., & Thibodeau, G. A. [2019]. *Anatomy & physiology* [10th ed.]. Mosby.)

relationships by altering capillary permeability and the surface area available for filtration (see Chapter 30).

Proximal convoluted tubule. By the end of the proximal tubule, approximately 60 to 70% of filtered sodium and water and about 50% of urea have been actively reabsorbed, along with 90% or more of potassium, glucose, bicarbonate, calcium, phosphate, amino acids, and uric acid. Chloride, water, and urea are reabsorbed passively but linked to the active transport of sodium (a cotransport mechanism). For some molecules, active transport in the renal tubules is limited as the carrier molecules become saturated, a phenomenon known as **transport maximum (Tm)**. For example, when the carrier molecules for glucose reabsorption in the proximal convoluted tubule become saturated (i.e., with the development of hyperglycemia), the excess will be excreted in the urine.

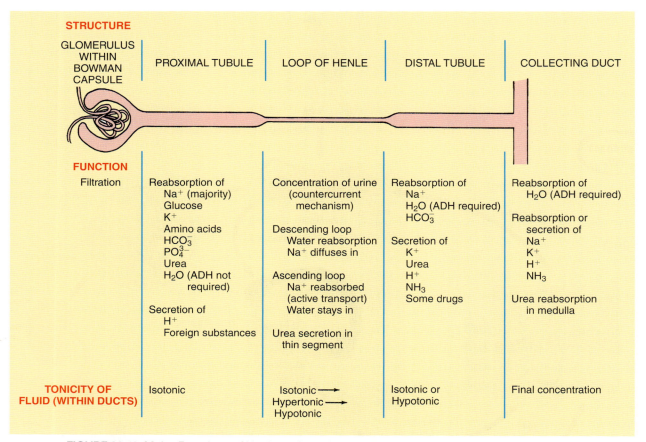

FIGURE 29.10 Major Functions of Nephron Segments. *ADH,* Antidiuretic hormone; *H+,* hydrogen; *H₂O,* water; *HCO⁻₃,* bicarbonate; *K+,* potassium; *Na+,* sodium; *NH₃,* ammonia; *PO4⁻₃,* phosphate. (Modified from Hockenberry, M. J., & Wilson, D. [Eds.]. [2007]. *Wong's nursing care of infants and children* [8th ed.]. Mosby.)

Active reabsorption of sodium is the primary function of the proximal convoluted tubule. Water, most other electrolytes, and organic substances are cotransported with sodium. The osmotic force generated by active sodium transport promotes the passive diffusion of water out of the tubular lumen and into the peritubular capillaries. Passive transport of water is further enhanced by the elevated oncotic pressure of the blood in the peritubular capillaries, which is created by the previous filtration of water at the glomerulus. The reabsorption of water leaves an increased concentration of urea within the tubular lumen, creating a gradient for its passive diffusion to the peritubular plasma. As the positively charged sodium ions leave the tubular lumen, negatively charged chloride ions passively follow to maintain electroneutrality. Because the inner membrane of the proximal tubular cell has a limited permeability to chloride, chloride reabsorption lags behind that of sodium.

Hydrogen ions are actively exchanged for sodium ions in the tubular lumen. The hydrogen ions (H+) then combine with bicarbonate. Bicarbonate is completely filtered at the glomerulus, and approximately 90% is reabsorbed in the proximal tubule. In the tubular lumen, hydrogen and bicarbonate ions form carbonic acid (H_2CO_3), which rapidly breaks down, or dissociates, to carbon dioxide (CO_2) and water (H_2O). These then diffuse into the tubular cell, where carbonic anhydrase again catalyzes the CO_2 and H_2O to form bicarbonate (HCO3−) and H+. The H+ is secreted again, and bicarbonate combines with sodium and is transported to the peritubular capillary blood as $NaHCO_3$ (a sodium bicarbonate buffer). Bicarbonate is thus conserved, and the hydrogen is reabsorbed as water. Therefore, these ions normally do not contribute to the urinary excretion of acid or the addition of acid to the blood.

In addition to the proximal tubular secretion of hydrogen ions, secretory transport mechanisms exist for creatinine, other organic bases, and endogenous and exogenous organic acids including *para-aminohippurate* (PAH) and penicillin (Box 29.1). These secretory mechanisms eliminate medications and other exogenous chemical products from the body, often after first conjugating them with sulphate and glucuronic acid in the liver. Many medications and their metabolites are eliminated from the body in this way. When the renal tubules are damaged, metabolic by-products and medications may accumulate, causing toxic levels in the body.

Normally, 99% of the glomerular filtrate is reabsorbed. When the GFR spontaneously decreases or increases, the renal tubules, primarily the proximal tubules, automatically adjust their rate of reabsorption of sodium and water to balance the change in GFR. This prevents wide fluctuations in the excretion of sodium and water into the urine and is known as **glomerulotubular balance**.

Loop of Henle and distal convoluted tubule. Urine can be hypotonic, isotonic, or hypertonic. **Urine concentration** or **urine dilution** occurs principally in the loop of Henle, distal convoluted tubules, and collecting ducts. The structural features of the medullary hairpin loops allow the kidney to concentrate urine and conserve water for the body. The transition of the filtrate into the final urine reflects the concentrating ability of the loops. Final adjustments in urine composition are

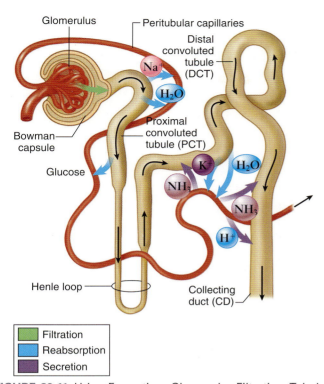

FIGURE 29.11 Urine Formation: Glomerular Filtration, Tubular Reabsorption, and Tubular Secretion. These are the three processes by which the kidneys excrete urine. Water (H_2O), electrolytes, glucose, and organic molecules are filtered at the glomerulus. Sodium (Na^+) and glucose are reabsorbed into peritubular capillaries by active transport from the proximal convoluted tubules, and H_2O reabsorption follows by osmosis. Na^+ is reabsorbed by active transport from distal convoluted tubules; more Na^+ is conserved when aldosterone is secreted. Osmotic reabsorption of H_2O from the distal convoluted tubules occurs when antidiuretic hormone is present. Secretion of ammonia (NH_3), hydrogen (H^+), and potassium (K^+) occurs from peritubular capillaries into distal convoluted tubules by active transport. (From Patton, K. T., & Thibodeau, G. A. [2018]. *The human body in health & disease* [7th ed.]. Mosby.)

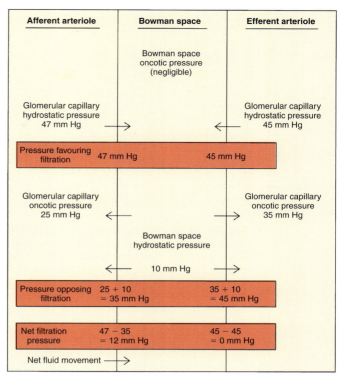

FIGURE 29.12 Glomerular Filtration Pressures.

TABLE 29.1 Glomerular Filtration Pressures

Forces	Pressures	Beginning of Capillary	End of Capillary
Promoting Filtration			
Glomerular capillary hydrostatic pressure	P_{GC}	47	45
Bowman capsule oncotic pressure	π_{BC}	Negligible effect	Negligible effect
Opposing Filtration			
Bowman capsule hydrostatic pressure	P_{BC}	10	10
Glomerular capillary oncotic pressure	π_{GC}	25	35
Net filtration pressure		12	0

BOX 29.1 Substances Transported by Renal Tubules

Reabsorption	Secretion
Albumin	Choline
Ascorbate	Creatinine
Fructose	Histamine
Galactose	Methylguanidine
Glutamate	*para*-aminohippurate
Glucose	Penicillin and many other medications
Phosphate	Steroid glucuronides
Sulphate	Thiamine
Xylose	

made by the distal convoluted tubule and collecting duct according to body needs.

Production of concentrated urine involves a **countercurrent exchange system**, in which fluid flows in opposite directions through the parallel tubes of the loop of Henle. A concentration gradient causes fluid to be exchanged across the parallel pathways. The longer the loop, the greater the concentration gradient; the concentration gradient increases from the cortex to the tip of the medulla. The loops of Henle multiply the concentration gradient, and the vasa recta blood vessels act as a countercurrent exchanger for maintaining the gradient. The process is initiated in the thick ascending limb of the loop of Henle with the active transport of chloride and sodium out of the tubular lumen and into the medullary interstitium (Figure 29.13). Because the lumen of the ascending limb is impermeable to water, water cannot follow the sodium–chloride transport. This impermeability to water causes the ascending tubular fluid to become hypo-osmotic and the medullary interstitium to become hyperosmotic. The descending limb of the loop, which receives fluid from the proximal tubule, is highly permeable to water but it is the only place in the nephron that does not actively transport either sodium or chloride. Sodium and chloride may, however, diffuse into the descending tubule from the interstitium.

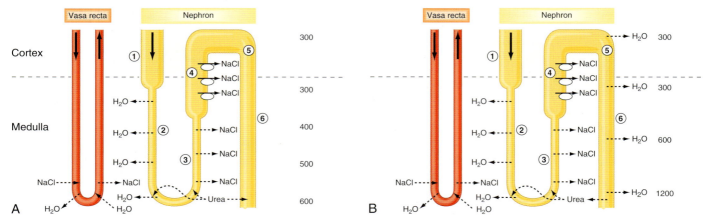

FIGURE 29.13 Countercurrent Mechanism for Concentrating and Diluting Urine. A, Urine dilution; **B,** urine concentration. (1) Filtrate isotonic to plasma. (2) Descending thin limb permeable to water (H_2O). (3) Ascending thin limb impermeable to H_2O; permeable to ions. (4) Ascending thick limb actively transports sodium chloride *(NaCl)*; impermeable to H_2O and urea. (5) Distal convoluted tubule actively resorbs NaCl; resorbs H_2O in presence of antidiuretic hormone. (6) Medullary collecting duct actively resorbs NaCl, and slightly permeable to H_2O and urea. (NOTE: Numbers on illustration represent milliosmoles [mOsm]. See text for details.) (From Koeppen, B. M., & Stanton, B. A. [2010]. *Berne and Levy physiology* [6th ed., updated]. Mosby.)

The hyperosmotic medullary interstitium causes water to move out of the descending limb, and the remaining fluid in the descending tubule becomes increasingly concentrated while it flows toward the tip of the medulla. While the tubular fluid rounds the loop and enters the ascending limb, sodium and chloride are removed and water is retained. The fluid then becomes more and more dilute as it encounters the distal convoluted tubule.

The slow rate of blood flow and the hairpin structure of the vasa recta blood vessels allow blood to flow through the medullary tissue without disturbing the osmotic gradient. When blood flows into the descending limb of the vasa recta, it encounters the increasing osmotic concentration gradient of the medullary interstitium. Water moves out and sodium and chloride diffuse into the descending vasa recta. The plasma becomes increasingly concentrated as it flows toward the tip of the medulla.

As blood flows away from the tip of the medulla and toward the cortex, the surrounding interstitial fluid becomes comparatively more dilute. Water then moves back into the vasa recta, and sodium and chloride diffuse out and the plasma again becomes more dilute. The net result is a preservation of the medullary osmotic gradient. If blood were to flow rapidly through the vasa recta, as occurs in some renal diseases, the medullary concentration gradient would be washed away and the ability to concentrate urine and conserve water would be lost. The efficiency of water conservation is related to the length of the loops of Henle: the longer the loops, the greater the ability to concentrate the urine.

Urea is the major constituent of urine along with water. The glomerulus freely filters urea, and tubular reabsorption depends on urine flow rate, with less reabsorption at higher flow rates. Approximately 50% of urea is excreted in the urine, and 50% is recycled within the kidney. This recycling contributes to the osmotic gradient within the medulla and is necessary for the concentration and dilution of urine (see Figure 29.13). Because urea is an end product of protein metabolism, individuals with protein deprivation cannot maximally concentrate their urine.[8]

Another function of the loop of Henle is the production of uromodulin (also known as Tamm-Horsfall protein [THP]), the most abundant protein in human urine. This protein binds to uropathogens to prevent urinary tract infection, protects the uroepithelium from injury, protects against kidney stone formation, and is associated with progression of kidney disease.[9]

The convoluted portion of the distal convoluted tubule is poorly permeable to water but readily reabsorbs ions and contributes to the dilution of the tubular fluid. The later, straight segment of the distal convoluted tubule and the collecting duct are permeable to water as controlled by ADH released from the posterior pituitary gland. Sodium is readily reabsorbed by the later segment of the distal convoluted tubule and collecting duct under the regulation of the hormone aldosterone (see Chapter 18). Potassium is actively secreted in these segments and is also controlled by aldosterone and other factors related to the concentration of potassium in body fluids (see Chapter 5).

Hydrogen is secreted by the distal convoluted tubule and combines with nonbicarbonate buffers (i.e., ammonium and phosphate) for the elimination of acids in the urine (see Figure 5.11). The distal convoluted tubule thus contributes to the regulation of acid–base balance by excreting hydrogen ions into the urine and by adding new bicarbonate to the plasma. The mechanism is similar to the conservation of bicarbonate by the proximal tubule, except that the hydrogen ion is excreted in the urine and influences acid–base balance (see Figure 5.11). The specific mechanisms of acid–base balance and acid excretion are described in Chapter 5.

Urine Composition

Urine is normally clear yellow or amber in colour. Cloudiness may indicate the presence of bacteria, cells, or high solute concentration. The pH ranges from 4.6 to 8.0, but it is normally acidic, providing protection against bacteria. Specific gravity ranges from 1.001 to 1.035. Normal urine does not contain glucose or blood cells and only occasionally contains traces of protein, usually in association with rigorous exercise.

Hormones and Nephron Function
Antidiuretic Hormone

The distal convoluted tubule in the cortex receives the hypo-osmotic urine from the ascending limb of the loop of Henle. The concentration of the final urine is controlled by **antidiuretic hormone (ADH)**, which is secreted from the posterior pituitary or neurohypophysis. ADH increases water permeability and reabsorption in the last segment of the distal convoluted tubule and along the entire length of the collecting ducts, which pass through the inner and outer zones of the medulla. The water diffuses into the ascending limb of the vasa recta and returns to the systemic circulation. The excreted urine can have a high osmotic concentration, up to 1400 mOsm. The volume is normally reduced to about 1% of the amount filtered at the glomerulus. (The mechanism for the regulation of ADH and plasma osmolality is described in Chapters 5 and 18.)

Aldosterone

Aldosterone is synthesized and secreted by the adrenal cortex under the regulation of the RAAS (see Chapter 18). Aldosterone stimulates the epithelial cells of the distal convoluted tubule and collecting duct to reabsorb sodium (promoting water reabsorption) and increases the excretion of potassium and hydrogen ions.

Natriuretic Peptides

Natriuretic peptides are a group of peptide hormones, including **atrial natriuretic peptide (ANP)**, secreted from myocardial cells in the atria, and B-type natriuretic peptide (BNP), secreted from myocardial cells in the cardiac ventricles.[10] When the heart dilates during volume expansion or heart failure, ANP and BNP inhibit sodium and water absorption by kidney tubules, inhibit secretion of renin and aldosterone, vasodilate the afferent arterioles, and constrict the efferent arterioles. The result is increased urine formation leading to a decrease in blood volume and blood pressure. C-type natriuretic peptide is secreted from the vascular endothelium and causes vasodilation in the nephron.

Urodilatin is secreted by the distal convoluted tubules and collecting ducts and causes vasodilation and natriuretic and diuretic effects.

Diuretics as a Factor in Urine Flow

A **diuretic** is any agent enhancing the flow of urine. Clinically, diuretics interfere with renal sodium reabsorption and reduce extracellular fluid volume. Diuretics are commonly used to treat hypertension and edema caused by heart failure, cirrhosis, and nephrotic syndrome.

Diuretics are divided into five general categories: (1) osmotic diuretics, (2) carbonic anhydrase inhibitors (inhibitors of urinary acidification), (3) inhibitors of loop sodium or chloride transport, (4) aldosterone antagonists (potassium-sparing diuretics), and (5) aquaretics. (The physiological mechanism related to each category is summarized in Table 29.2.)

Renal Hormones

Certain hormones are either activated or synthesized by the kidney. These hormones have significant systemic effects and include urodilatin, the active form of vitamin D, and EPO.

Vitamin D

Vitamin D is a hormone that can be obtained in the diet or synthesized by the action of ultraviolet radiation (sun exposure) on cholesterol in the skin. These forms of vitamin D_3 (cholecalciferol) are inactive and require two hydroxylations to establish a metabolically active form. The first step occurs in the liver and the second in the kidneys.

Vitamin D is necessary for the absorption of calcium and phosphate by the small intestine. The renal hydroxylation step is stimulated by parathyroid hormone (see Chapter 18). A decreased plasma calcium level (less than 2.25 mmol/L) stimulates the secretion of parathyroid

TABLE 29.2 Action of Diuretics

Diuretic	Site of Action	Action	Common Side Effects
Osmotic Diuretics			
Mannitol (Osmitrol) Glycerol Urea (Ureaphil)	Proximal tubule	Freely filtered but not reabsorbed; osmotically attract water and diminish sodium reabsorption	Hypokalemia, dehydration
Carbonic Anhydrase Inhibitors			
Acetazolamide (Diamox)	Proximal tubule	Inhibits carbonic anhydrase; blocks hydrogen ion secretion and reabsorption of sodium and bicarbonate	Hypokalemia, systemic acidosis, alkaline urine
Inhibitors of Sodium or Chloride Reabsorption			
Thiazides Hydrochlorothiazide (HCTZ, Urozide)	Distal convoluted tubules	Inhibit sodium and chloride reabsorption; mildly suppress carbonic anhydrase; reduce calcium excretion	Hypokalemia, metabolic alkalosis
Furosemide (Lasix) Ethacrynic acid (Edecrin)	Thick ascending limb of loop of Henle	Inhibit active transport of chloride, sodium, and potassium	Hypokalemia, uric acid retention
Torsemide (Demadex) Bumetanide (Burinex)	Cortical vasodilation	Increase rate of urine formation	Hypokalemia, uric acid retention
Potassium-Sparing Diuretics			
Spironolactone (Aldactone)	Distal convoluted tubule/collecting duct	Inhibits aldosterone, blocks sodium reabsorption, and results in potassium retention	Hyperkalemia, nausea, confusion, gynecomastia
Triamterene (APO Triazide) and amiloride (Midamor)	Distal convoluted tubule/collecting duct	Inhibit sodium reabsorption and inhibit potassium excretion	Nausea, vomiting, headache, granulocytopenia, skin rash
Aquaretics			
Vasopressin (V_2) blockers (e.g., conivaptan [Vaprisol])	Distal convoluted tubule/collecting ducts	Block action of antidiuretic hormone	Dehydration

hormone. Parathyroid hormone then stimulates a sequence of events to help restore plasma calcium concentration toward normal levels (2.25 to 2.75 mmol/L):

1. Calcium mobilization from bone
2. Synthesis of 1,25-dihydroxy-vitamin D_3
3. Absorption of calcium from the intestine
4. Increased renal calcium reabsorption
5. Decreased renal phosphate reabsorption

Serum phosphate concentration fluctuations also influence the renal hydroxylation of vitamin D. Decreased levels stimulate active 1,25-dihydroxy-vitamin D_3 formation, and increased levels inhibit formation. The formation of 1,25-dihydroxy-vitamin D_3 results in compensatory changes in phosphate absorption from bone and intestine. Individuals with renal disease have a deficiency of 1,25-dihydroxy-vitamin D_3 and show symptoms of disturbed calcium and phosphate balance (see Chapters 5, 18, and 30).

Erythropoietin

Erythropoietin (EPO) stimulates the bone marrow to produce red blood cells in response to tissue hypoxia and may have tissue-protective effects.[11] Erythrocyte production is discussed in Chapter 20. The stimulus for EPO release is decreased oxygen delivery in the kidneys. Oxygen-sensing EPO-producing cells are peritubular fibroblasts located in the juxtamedullary cortex.[12] The anemia of chronic kidney disease, in which kidney cells have become nonfunctional, can be related to the lack of this hormone (see Chapter 30).

Kidney function changes throughout the lifespan, and major changes are summarized in the *Pediatric Considerations:* Pediatrics and Renal Function and *Geriatric Considerations:* Aging and Renal Function boxes at the end of the chapter.

TESTS OF RENAL FUNCTION

QUICK CHECK 29.4
1. Why is creatinine clearance a good estimate of glomerular filtration rate (GFR)?
2. What is the relationship between plasma creatinine concentration and GFR?

Renal Clearance

A number of specific renal functions can be measured by renal clearance. Renal clearance techniques determine how much of a substance can be cleared from the blood by the kidneys per given unit of time. The application of this principle permits an indirect measure of GFR, tubular secretion, tubular reabsorption, and RBF.

Clearance and Renal Blood Flow

A clearance formula also can be used to estimate RPF and RBF using a molecule called *para*-aminohippuric acid (PAH). Some PAH is filtered at the glomerulus, and most of the remainder is secreted into the tubules in one circulation through the kidney. If all the PAH were removed from the plasma during a single pass through the kidney, total RPF could be determined. Because the supporting and nonsecreting structures of the kidney receive 10 to 15% of the **effective renal blood flow (ERBF)**, clearance of PAH measures only what is known as **effective renal plasma flow (ERPF)**, which is 85 to 90% of the true RPF.

Clearance and Glomerular Filtration Rate

The GFR provides the best estimate of functioning renal tissue and is important for assessing or monitoring kidney damage and medication dosing. Damage to the glomerular membrane or loss of nephrons leads to a corresponding decrease in GFR. The measurement of GFR requires the use of a substance that has a stable plasma concentration; is freely filtered at the glomerulus; is not secreted, reabsorbed, or metabolized by the tubules; and is easy to measure. Inulin (a fructose polysaccharide) is one substance that meets the criteria for measurement of GFR.

The accurate determination of inulin clearance requires constant infusion to maintain a stable plasma level. This is time-consuming and inconvenient. Therefore, the clearance of creatinine, a natural substance produced by muscle and released into the blood at a relatively constant rate, is commonly used as an estimate clinically. It is freely filtered at the glomerulus, but a small amount is secreted by the renal tubules. Therefore, creatinine clearance overestimates the GFR, but within tolerable limits. Creatinine clearance provides a good clinical measure of GFR because only one blood sample is required in addition to an accurately collected 24-hour volume of urine. **Cystatin C** is a stable protein in serum filtered at the glomerulus and metabolized in the tubules. Serum levels of cystatin C also are a marker for estimating GFR, particularly for mild to moderate impaired renal function.[13] A combined creatinine and cystatin C estimate of GFR was developed in 2012 and considers age, race, and sex.[14]

Formulas are used to estimate GFR.[15] The Cockcroft–Gault formula is commonly used and considers age, body weight, and plasma creatinine (P_{cr}) values. The U.S. National Kidney Foundation recommends using the Modification of Diet in Renal Disease (MDRD) equation.[16] The Chronic Kidney Disease Epidemiology Collaboration (2009 CKD-EPI) equation has been developed as a more precise estimate of GFR than the MDRD and considers age, sex, and ethnicity.[17] In 2012, cystatin C and combined creatinine and cystatin C equations were developed. Calculators for estimates of GFR using these formulas are readily available on the Internet (e.g., see http://touchcalc.com/ip_epi_gfr/ip_ckd_epi). Normal GFR values are 90 to 120 mL/min.

Plasma Creatinine Concentration

A chronic decline in the GFR over weeks or months is reflected in the **plasma creatinine (P_{cr}) concentration** (normal value = 44 to 97 µmol/L for females; 53 to 106 µmol/L for males). The P_{cr} concentration has a stable value when the GFR is stable because creatinine has a constant rate of production as a product of muscle metabolism. The amount filtered is approximately equal to the amount excreted. When the GFR declines, the P_{cr} increases proportionately. Thus, the GFR and P_{cr} are inversely related. If the GFR were to decrease by 50%, the filtration and excretion of creatinine would be reduced by 50% and creatinine would accumulate in plasma to twice the normal value. Therefore, elevated P_{cr} values represent decreasing GFR. In the new steady state, however, the total amount of creatinine excreted in the urine would remain the same because of the proportionate decrease in GFR and increase in P_{cr}.

The application of this principle is simple and useful for monitoring progressive changes in renal function. The test is most valuable for monitoring the progress of chronic rather than acute renal disease because it takes 7 to 10 days for the plasma creatinine level to stabilize when GFR declines. Serial measures can be obtained over a long time and plotted as a curve of glomerular function. The P_{cr} also becomes elevated during trauma or the breakdown of muscle tissue. In such instances, the value is then not useful for estimating GFR.

Blood Urea Nitrogen

The concentration of urea nitrogen in the blood reflects glomerular filtration and urine-concentrating capacity. Because urea is filtered at the glomerulus, blood urea nitrogen (BUN) levels increase as glomerular filtration drops. Because urea is reabsorbed by the blood through the permeable tubules, the BUN value rises in states of dehydration and with acute and chronic kidney disease when passage of fluid through the tubules slows. BUN values also change as a result of altered protein intake and protein catabolism. The normal range for BUN levels in the adult is 3.6 to 7.1 mmol/L of blood.

Urinalysis

Urinalysis is a noninvasive and relatively inexpensive diagnostic procedure. The best results are obtained from a fresh, cleanly voided specimen because decay permits changes in the composition of urine. Urinalysis includes evaluation of colour, turbidity, protein, pH, specific gravity, sediment, and supernatant. Urine tests are listed in Table 29.3, and bladder function tests are listed in Table 29.4.

TABLE 29.3 Normal Renal Function Tests

Test	Normal Value	Interpretation
Urine		
Colour	Amber-yellow	Medications and foods may change urine colour
Turbidity	Clear	Purulent matter will make urine cloudy
pH	4.6–8.0	Bacteria create an alkaline urine
Specific gravity (density of water = 1.000)		Gravity represents concentrating ability or density of urine in relation to density of water (i.e., higher when contains glucose or protein; lower with dilute urine)
Adults	1.010–1.025	
Infants	1.010–1.018	
Blood	Negative	Blood indicates bleeding along urinary tract
Microscopic Urine		
Bacteria	None	Bacteria indicates infection
Red blood cells	Negative	Red blood cells indicate bleeding along urinary tract
White blood cells	Negative	White blood cells indicate urinary tract infection
Crystals	Negative	Crystals may indicate stones
Fat	Negative	Fat can be associated with nephrosis
Casts	Occasional	A few casts are normal; many may represent renal disease
Urinary Chemistry		
Bilirubin	Negative	An increase may cause dark orange colour
Urobilinogen	0.5–4 mg/24 hours	An increase may indicate red blood cell hemolysis
Ketones	Negative	Ketones represent an increase in fat metabolism
Glucose	Negative	Glucose usually signifies hyperglycemia
Sodium	40–220 mmol/day	Sodium can increase or decrease with renal disease
Potassium	25–120 mmol/day	Potassium can increase or decrease with renal disease, potassium intake, aldosteronism, or diuretic use
Protein	Negative-trace	Protein indicates dysfunction of glomerulus
Normal Serum Values		
BUN	3.6–7.1 mmol/L	Blood urea nitrogen (BUN) is elevated with diseased kidneys
Creatinine	Elevated with decreased GFR	
Male	53–106 µmol/L	
Female	44–97 µmol/L	
Cystatin C	0.0444–0.11667 mmol/L	This test provides early detection of decreased glomerular filtration rate (GFR)
Potassium		Potassium is elevated in kidney failure

TABLE 29.4 Bladder Function Tests

Procedure	Description
Urodynamic Tests	
Cystometry (cystometrogram)	Measures bladder pressure using a pressure-measuring catheter; fluid volume and pressures are measured as bladder is filled with fluid; simultaneous pressures may be measured in rectum; sensations of bladder fullness are also recorded; coughing or straining can lead to involuntary bladder contractions
	Bladder capacity: male, 350–750 mL; female, 350–550 mL
	Intrabladder pressure with empty bladder: 40 cm H_2O
	Detrusor pressure: <10 cm H_2O
	Residual urine: <30 mL
Uroflowmetry	Measures time it takes to empty a full bladder of urine; flow rates may be faster with urge incontinence or slower with prostatic obstruction

(Continued)

TABLE 29.4 Bladder Function Tests—cont'd

Procedure	Description
Postvoid residual urine	Measures residual urine in bladder after voiding; urine can be removed with catheter and measured, or ultrasound imaging can be used to measure urine; postvoid residual of more than 200 mL is abnormal and requires further evaluation
Measurement of leak point pressure	Measures pressure at which bladder fluid will leak from bladder without warning
Pressure flow study	Measures pressure required to empty bladder; pressure flow study identifies bladder outlet obstruction such as that occurring with prostate enlargement
Electromyography	Measures nerve impulses and muscle activity in urethral sphincter by placing sensors on skin near urethra and rectum or by placing sensors on catheter placed in urethra or rectum
Video urodynamics	Takes pictures and videos during filling and emptying of bladder; imaging equipment uses X-rays or ultrasound waves; this test shows size and shape of urinary tract
Direct Visualization Diagnostic Procedures	
Cystoscopy	Cystoscope (a type of endoscope) is inserted through urethra and is used to visualize inside of bladder
Ureteroscopy	Ureteroscope is inserted through urethra and bladder and directly into ureter and upper urinary tract to visualize upper urinary tract

H_2O, Water.

PEDIATRIC CONSIDERATIONS
Pediatrics and Renal Function

Glomerular filtration rate (GFR) in infants does not reach adult levels until 1 to 2 years of age, and newborns have a decreased ability to efficiently remove excess water and solutes. Their shorter loops of Henle also decrease concentrating ability and produce a more dilute urine than that produced by adults. Risks for metabolic acidosis are increased during the first few months of life while the mechanisms for excreting acid and retaining bicarbonate are maturing. These normal developmental processes result in a narrow safety margin for fluid and electrolyte balance when there is any disturbance such as diarrhea, infection, fever, fasting for diagnostic tests, improper feeding, fluid replacement, or medication administration. Newborns diurese 2 to 3 days after birth, which is reflected by a decrease in total body water and body weight. An increased risk of toxicity accompanies medication administration. Low–birth weight infants have a delay in achieving full renal function and may not have full GFR until 8 years of age. They also are at a greater risk for low nephron numbers and chronic kidney disease as adults.

Data from Filler, G., Yasin, A., & Medeiros, M. (2014). *Pediatric Nephrology, 29*(2), 183–192; Hoseini, R., Otukesh, H., Rahimzadeh, et al. (2012). *Iranian Journal of Kidney Diseases, 6*(3), 166–172; Lankadeva, Y. R., Singh, R. R., Tare, M., et al. (2014). *American Journal of Physiology—Renal Physiology, 306*(8), F791–F800; Sulemanji, M., & Vakili, K. (2013). *Seminars in Pediatric Surgery, 22*(4), 195–198.

GERIATIC CONSIDERATIONS
Aging and Renal Function

- Structural changes commonly occur in the kidney with aging, including loss of renal mass, arterial sclerosis, an increased number of sclerotic glomeruli, loss of tubules, and interstitial fibrosis. These changes contribute to a slow decline in glomerular filtration rate (GFR) and a reduction in creatinine clearance in most individuals, but it generally is not significant enough to lead to severe loss of renal function. As the number of nephrons decreases and degenerative changes occur, nephrons are less able to concentrate urine and less able to tolerate dehydration, excessive water loads, or electrolyte imbalances, particularly with physiological stress. Up to 45% of people older than 70 years of age have chronic kidney disease.
- The presence of comorbid conditions, such as hypertension and diabetes mellitus, accelerates the decline of renal function. Response to acid–base changes and reabsorption of glucose may be delayed.
- Medications eliminated by the kidney can accumulate in the plasma, causing toxic reactions; GFR and medication dosage should be carefully evaluated.
- Decreased thirst sensation and diminished water intake may alter water balance.
- Impairment in renal blood flow, hormonal regulatory systems, and metabolism of medications may alter sodium and water balance.
- Older donor kidneys show decreased regenerative capacity.

Data from Baldea, A. J. (2009). *Surgical Clinics of North America, 95*(1), 71–83; Bolignano, D., Mattace-Raso, F., Sijbrands, E. J., et al. (2014). *Ageing Research Reviews, 14*, 65–80; Karam, Z., & Tuazon, J. (2013). *Clinics in Geriatric Medicine, 29*(3), 555–564; Presta, P., Lucisano, G., Fuiano, L., et al. (2012). *International Urology and Nephrology, 44*(2), 625–632; Sands, J. M. (2012). *Journal of Gerontology, Series A: Biological Sciences and Medical Sciences, 67*(12), 1352–1357; Schmitt, R., & Melk, A. (2012). *American Journal of Transplant, 12*(11), 2892–2900; Tonelli, M., & Riella, M. C. (2014). *Nature Reviews Nephrology, 10*(3), 127–128.

CHAPTER 29 Structure and Function of the Renal and Urological Systems

DID YOU UNDERSTAND?

Structures of the Renal System

1. The kidneys are paired structures lying bilaterally between the twelfth thoracic and third lumbar vertebrae and behind the peritoneum of the abdominal cavity.
2. The kidney is composed of an outer cortex and an inner medulla.
3. The calyces receive urine from the distal convoluted tubules and join to form the renal pelvis, which is continuous with the upper end of the ureter.
4. The nephron is the urine-forming unit of the kidney and is composed of the glomerulus, proximal convoluted tubule, hairpin loops of Henle, distal convoluted tubule, and collecting duct.
5. The glomerulus contains loops of capillaries supported by mesangial cells. The capillary walls serve as a filtration membrane for the formation of the primary urine.
6. The proximal tubule is lined with microvilli to increase surface area and enhance reabsorption of water, solutes, and electrolytes.
7. The hairpin loops of Henle transport solutes and water, contributing to the hypertonic state of the medulla, and are important for the concentration and dilution of urine.
8. The distal convoluted tubule adjusts acid–base balance by excreting acid into the urine and forming new bicarbonate ions. It reabsorbs water with the influence of antidiuretic hormone and reabsorbs sodium and excretes potassium with the influence of aldosterone.
9. The ureters extend from the renal pelvis to the posterior wall of the bladder. Urine flows through the ureters and into the bladder by means of peristaltic contraction of the ureteral muscles.
10. The bladder is a bag composed of the detrusor and trigone muscles and innervated by parasympathetic fibres. When accumulation of urine reaches 250 to 300 mL, mechanoreceptors, which respond to stretching of tissue, stimulate the micturition reflex.

Renal Blood Flow

1. Renal blood flows at about 1 000 to 1 200 mL/min, or 20 to 25% of the cardiac output.
2. Blood flow through the glomerular capillaries is maintained at a constant rate in spite of a wide range of arterial pressures by autoregulation of the glomerular capillaries.
3. The glomerular filtration rate (GFR) is the filtration of plasma per unit of time and is directly related to the perfusion pressure of renal blood flow (RBF).
4. Renin is an enzyme secreted from the juxtaglomerular apparatus in response to decreased blood pressure and causes the generation of angiotensin II, a potent vasoconstrictor. The renin-angiotensin-aldosterone system is thus a regulator of RBF.

Kidney Function

1. The major function of the nephron is urine formation, which involves the processes of glomerular filtration, tubular reabsorption, tubular secretion, and excretion.
2. Glomerular filtration is favoured by capillary hydrostatic pressure and opposed by oncotic pressure in the capillary and hydrostatic pressure in the Bowman capsule. The balance of favouring and opposing filtration forces is known as net filtration pressure.
3. The GFR is approximately 120 mL/min, and 99% of the filtrate is reabsorbed.
4. The proximal convoluted tubule reabsorbs about 60 to 70% of the filtered sodium and water and 90% or more of other electrolytes.
5. Because most molecules are reabsorbed by active transport, the carrier mechanism can become saturated at a point known as the transport maximum (T_m). Molecules not reabsorbed are excreted with the urine.
6. The concentration or specific gravity of the final urine is a function of the level of antidiuretic hormone (ADH). This hormone stimulates the distal convoluted tubules and collecting ducts to reabsorb water. The countercurrent exchange system of the long loops of Henle and their accompanying capillaries establishes a concentration gradient within the renal medulla to facilitate the reabsorption of water from the collecting duct.
7. The kidney secretes or activates a number of hormones having systemic effects, including vitamin D, erythropoietin, and the natriuretic hormone urodilatin.

Tests of Renal Function

1. Creatinine, a substance produced by muscle, is measured in both plasma and urine to calculate a commonly used clinical measurement of GFR.
2. Plasma creatinine concentration, cystatin C level, and blood urea nitrogen (BUN) level are estimates of glomerular function. BUN value also is an indicator of hydration status.
3. Formulas for estimating GFR can be helpful clinical indicators of renal function.
4. Urinalysis involves evaluation of colour, turbidity, protein, pH, specific gravity, sediment, and supernatant. Presence of bacteria, red blood cells, white blood cells, casts, or crystals in the urine sediment may indicate a renal or bladder disorder.

Pediatric Considerations: Pediatrics and Renal Function

1. Compared with adults, infants and children have more dilute urine because of higher blood flow and shorter loops of Henle.
2. Children are more affected than adults by fluid imbalances resulting from diarrhea, infection, or improper feeding because of their limited ability to quickly regulate changes in pH or osmotic pressure.

Geriatric Considerations: Aging and Renal Function

1. Older persons have a decreased ability to concentrate urine and are less able to tolerate dehydration or water loads because they have fewer nephrons.
2. Responses to acid–base changes and reabsorption of glucose are delayed in older persons.
3. In older persons, medications eliminated by the kidney can accumulate in the plasma, causing toxic reactions.

30

Alterations of Renal and Urinary Tract Function

Mohamed Toufic El-Hussein, with originating chapter contributions by Sue E. Huether

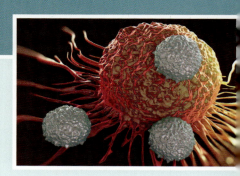

Additional resources are available online at https://evolve.elsevier.com/Canada/Huether/pathophysiology.

CHAPTER OUTLINE

Urinary Tract Obstruction, 731
   Upper Urinary Tract Obstruction, 731
   Lower Urinary Tract Obstruction, 733
   Tumours, 736
Urinary Tract Infection, 736
   Causes of Urinary Tract Infection, 737
   Types of Urinary Tract Infection, 737
Glomerular Disorders, 739
   Glomerulonephritis, 739
   Nephrotic and Nephritic Syndromes, 742
Acute Kidney Injury, 744
   Classification of Kidney Dysfunction, 744
   Classification of Acute Kidney Injury, 744
   COVID-19–Associated Acute Kidney Injury, 746
Chronic Kidney Disease, 748
   Creatinine and Urea Clearance, 750

Fluid and Electrolyte Balance, 750
Calcium, Phosphate, and Bone, 751
Protein, Carbohydrate, and Fat Metabolism, 751
Cardiovascular System, 751
Pulmonary System, 752
Hematological System, 752
Immune System, 752
Neurological System, 752
Gastro-intestinal System, 752
Endocrine and Reproductive Systems, 752
Integumentary System, 752
COMORBIDITIES, 753
GERIATRIC CONSIDERATIONS: Aging and Chronic Kidney Disease, 753
CASE STUDY, 754

LEARNING OBJECTIVES

1. Discuss the causes and effects of obstruction in various locations within the urinary tract.
2. Describe the pathophysiology of kidney stone formation.
3. Compare and contrast the types of stones.
4. Describe what is meant by neurogenic bladder and overactive bladder syndrome.
5. List the anatomical causes of resistance to urine flow and the signs of urinary obstruction.
6. Describe the two most common tumours of the renal and urological systems: renal carcinoma and bladder tumours.
7. Discuss the etiology, infectious agents, manifestations, treatments, and complications of urinary tract infections.
8. Describe acute and chronic pyelonephritis; include the pathophysiology, clinical manifestations, evaluation, and treatments of each.
9. Identify the causes of glomerulonephritis and the resulting changes in glomerular structure and function.
10. Compare and contrast acute, rapidly progressive, and chronic glomerulonephritis.
11. Describe the progression of nephrotic syndrome from causation through complications.
12. Differentiate between prerenal, intrarenal, and postrenal causes of acute kidney injury.
13. Describe the pathophysiology of acute tubular necrosis (ATN).
14. Discuss the clinical manifestations, treatment options, outcomes, and complications of acute kidney injury.
15. Discuss the clinical manifestations of chronic kidney disease and explain what is meant by the term uremia.

KEY TERMS

Acute cystitis, 737
Acute glomerulonephritis, 739
Acute kidney injury (AKI), 744
Acute tubular necrosis (ATN), 744
Anuria, 746
Azotemia, 744
Calcium stone, 733
Calculus (*pl.*, calculi) (urinary stone), 732
Chronic glomerulonephritis, 741
Chronic kidney disease (CKD), 748
Chronic pyelonephritis, 739
Compensatory hypertrophy, 732
Cystinuric (xanthine) stone, 733
Detrusor areflexia, 734
Detrusor hyper-reflexia (overactivity), 734
Detrusor hyper-reflexia with vesico-sphincter dyssynergia, 734
Diabetic nephropathy, 741
Dyssynergia, 734
End-stage kidney disease (ESKD), 744
Hydronephrosis, 731
Hydroureter, 731
Hyperfunction, 732
Intrarenal (intrinsic) acute kidney injury, 745
Kidney failure, 744
Low bladder wall compliance, 735
Lupus nephritis, 741
Nephritic syndrome, 742
Nephrotic syndrome, 742

CHAPTER 30 Alterations of Renal and Urinary Tract Function

Neurogenic bladder, 734
Nonbacterial infectious cystitis, 738
Noninfectious cystitis, 738
Nonoliguric renal failure, 746
Obstructive uropathy, 731
Oliguria, 746
Overactive bladder (OAB) syndrome, 734

Painful bladder syndrome/interstitial cystitis (PBS/IC), 738
Partial obstruction of the bladder outlet or urethra, 734
Pelvic organ prolapse, 734
Postobstructive diuresis, 732
Postrenal acute kidney injury, 746
Prerenal acute kidney injury, 744

Prostate enlargement, 734
Pyelonephritis, 738
Renal adenoma, 736
Renal cell carcinoma (RCC), 736
Renal colic, 733
Renal insufficiency, 744
Renal transitional cell carcinoma (RTCC), 736
Rhabdomyolysis, 746

Staghorn calculus, 733
Struvite stone, 733
Tubulointerstitial fibrosis, 731
Uremia (uremic syndrome), 744
Ureterohydronephrosis, 731
Urethral stricture, 734
Uric acid stone, 733
Urinary tract infection (UTI), 737

Renal and urinary function can be affected by a variety of disorders. The most common type of urinary dysfunction is infection of the bladder. Stones, tumours, or inflammation also can obstruct the urinary tract. Renal function can be impaired by disorders of the kidney itself or by systemic diseases and may ultimately result in acute kidney injury (AKI) or chronic kidney disease (CKD). Because the kidney filters the blood, it is directly linked to every other organ system. Kidney failure, whether acute or chronic, is therefore a life-threatening condition.

URINARY TRACT OBSTRUCTION

> ✓ **QUICK CHECK 30.1**
> 1. List two typical complications of urinary tract obstruction, and briefly describe them.
> 2. How do kidney stones form?
> 3. Which population group is at greatest risk for bladder tumours?

Urinary tract obstruction is an interference with the flow of urine at any site along the urinary tract (Figure 30.1). A blockage may be anatomical or functional. The obstruction impedes flow proximal to the blockage, dilates structures distal to the obstruction, increases the risk for infection, and compromises renal function. Anatomical changes in the urinary system caused by obstruction are referred to as **obstructive uropathy**. The severity of an obstructive uropathy is determined by (1) the location of the obstructive lesion, (2) the involvement of ureters and kidneys, (3) the severity (completeness) of the blockage, (4) the duration of the blockage, and (5) the nature of the obstructive lesion.[1,2] Obstructions may be relieved or partially alleviated by correction of the obstruction, although permanent impairments occur if a complete or partial obstruction persists over a period of weeks to months or longer.

Upper Urinary Tract Obstruction

Common causes of upper urinary tract obstruction include stricture or congenital compression of a calyx at the ureteropelvic–ureterovesical junction (e.g., stones [calculi], or vesicoureteral reflux) (see Chapter 31); compression from an aberrant vessel, tumour, or abdominal inflammation and scarring (retroperitoneal fibrosis); or ureteral blockage from stones or a malignancy of the renal pelvis or ureter.

Obstruction of the upper urinary tract causes dilation of the ureter, renal pelvis, calyces, and renal parenchyma proximal to the site of urinary blockage, resulting from a "backing up" of urine. The increased pressure is transmitted to the glomerulus, which decreases filtration. Dilation of the ureter is referred to as **hydroureter** (accumulation of urine in the ureter), and dilation of the renal pelvis and calyces proximal to a blockage is referred to as **hydronephrosis** or **ureterohydronephrosis** (dilation of both the ureter and the pelvicaliceal system) (Figure 30.2). Dilation of the upper urinary tract is an early response to obstruction and includes smooth muscle hypertrophy

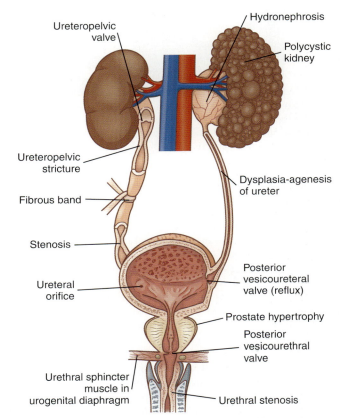

FIGURE 30.1 Major Sites of Urinary Tract Obstruction.

and accumulation of urine above the level of blockage (urinary stasis). Unless the obstruction is relieved, the dilation leads to enlargement and **tubulointerstitial fibrosis** with deposition of excessive amounts of collagen and other proteins. These changes occur in the distal nephrons and affect renal function within approximately 7 days. By 14 days, obstruction has adversely affected both distal and proximal tubular aspects of the nephron units. Within 28 days, the glomeruli of the kidney have been damaged, and the renal cortex and medulla are reduced in size (thinned). Tubular damage initially decreases the kidney's ability to concentrate urine, causing an increase in urine volume despite a decrease in glomerular filtration rate (GFR). The affected kidney is unable to conserve sodium, bicarbonate, and water or to excrete hydrogen or potassium, leading to metabolic acidosis and dehydration. The magnitude of this damage, and the kidney's ability to recover normal regulatory function, is affected by the severity and duration of the obstruction. With complete obstruction and compression of the renal vasculature, damage to the renal tubules occurs in a matter of hours,

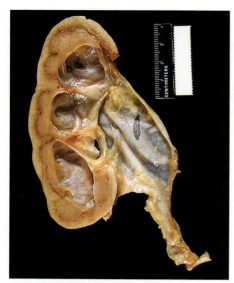

FIGURE 30.2 Hydronephrosis of the Kidney. There is marked dilation of the renal pelvis and calyces with thinning of the overlying cortex and medulla due to compression atrophy. (From Kumar, V., Abbas, A. K., & Aster, J. C. [Eds.]. [2021]. *Robbins and Cotran pathologic basis of disease* [10th ed.]. Elsevier.)

and irreversible damage occurs within 4 weeks. Nevertheless, even in the face of a complete obstruction, the human kidney may recover at least partial function provided that the blockage is removed within 56 to 69 days.[3] This recovery requires a period of approximately 4 months. Partial obstruction (in the absence of renal infection) leads to subtler but ultimately permanent impairments, including loss of the kidney's ability to concentrate urine, reabsorb bicarbonate, excrete ammonia, or regulate metabolic acid–base balance.

The body is able to partially counteract the negative consequences of unilateral obstruction by a process called **compensatory hypertrophy** and **hyperfunction**.[4] Compensatory response is the result of two growth processes: obligatory growth occurs under the influence of somatomedins, and compensatory growth occurs under the influence of still unidentified hormone(s). These processes cause the unobstructed kidney to increase the size of individual glomeruli and tubules but not the total number of functioning nephrons. The ability of the body to engage in compensatory hypertrophy and hyperfunction diminishes with age, and the process is reversible when relief of obstruction results in recovery of function by the obstructed kidney.

Relief of bilateral, partial urinary tract obstruction or complete obstruction of one kidney is usually followed by a brief period of diuresis (commonly called **postobstructive diuresis**).[5] Postobstructive diuresis is a physiological response and is typically mild, representing a restoration of fluid and electrolyte imbalance caused by the obstructive uropathy. Occasionally, relief of obstruction will cause rapid excretion of large volumes of water, sodium, or other electrolytes, resulting in a urine output of 10 L/day or more. Rapid postobstructive diuresis causes dehydration and fluid and electrolyte imbalances that must be promptly corrected. Risk factors for severe postobstructive diuresis include chronic, bilateral obstruction; impairment of one or both kidneys' ability to concentrate urine or reabsorb sodium (acquired nephrogenic diabetes insipidus); hypertension; edema and weight gain; heart failure; and uremic encephalopathy.

Kidney Stones

Calculi, or **urinary stones**, are masses of crystals, protein, or other substances that are a common cause of urinary tract obstruction in adults. Calculi can be located in the kidneys, ureters, and urinary bladder.[6] Most renal stones are unilateral. The risk for urinary calculi formation is influenced by a number of factors, including age, sex, ethnicity, geographical location, seasonal factors, fluid intake, diet, and occupation. Most persons develop their first stone before age 50 years. Geographical location influences the risk for stone formation because of indirect factors, including average temperature, humidity, and rainfall, and their influence on fluid intake and dietary patterns. Persons who regularly consume an adequate volume of water and those who are physically active are at reduced risk when compared with persons who are inactive or consume lower volumes of water.

Urinary calculi can be classified according to the primary minerals (salts) that make up the stones. The most common stone types include calcium oxalate or phosphate (70 to 80%), struvite (magnesium-ammonium-phosphate) (15%), and uric acid (7%). Cystine stones are rare (<1%).[7]

PATHOPHYSIOLOGY Calculus formation is complex and related to (1) supersaturation of one or more salts in the urine, (2) precipitation of the salts from a liquid to a solid state, (3) growth through crystallization or agglomeration (sometimes called *aggregation*), and (4) the presence or absence of stone inhibitors (e.g., uromodulin [Tamm-Horsfall protein]).[8] *Supersaturation* is the presence of a higher concentration of a salt within a fluid (in this case, the urine) than the volume is able to dissolve to maintain equilibrium.

Human urine contains many ions capable of *precipitating* from solution and forming a variety of salts. The salts form crystals that are retained and grow into stones. *Crystallization* is the process by which crystals grow from a small *nidus* or nucleus to larger stones in the presence of supersaturated urine. Although supersaturation is essential for free stone formation, the urine need not remain continuously supersaturated for a calculus to grow once its nidus has precipitated from solution. Intermittent periods of supersaturation after the ingestion of a meal or during times of dehydration from limited oral intake or secondary to continued use of diuretics are sufficient for stone growth in many individuals. In addition, the renal tubules and papillae have many surfaces that may attract a crystalline nidus (Randall plaque) and add biological material (matrix) forming a stone.[9] *Matrix* is an organic material (i.e., mucoprotein) in which the components of a kidney stone are embedded.

The temperature and pH of the urine also influence the risk for precipitation and calculus formation, and pH is most important. An alkaline urinary pH (pH >7.0) significantly increases the risk for calcium phosphate stone formation, whereas acidic urine (pH <5.0) increases the risk for uric acid stone formation. Cystine and xanthine also precipitate more readily in acidic urine.

Stone or *crystal growth-inhibiting substances*, such as potassium citrate, Tamm-Horsfall protein, pyrophosphate, and magnesium, are capable of crystal growth inhibition, thereby reducing the risk for calcium phosphate or calcium oxalate precipitation in the urine and preventing subsequent stone formation.

The size of a stone determines the likelihood that it will pass through the urinary tract and be excreted through micturition.[10] Stones smaller than 5 mm have about a 50% chance of spontaneous (painful) passage, whereas stones that are 1 cm have almost no chance of spontaneous passage.

Retention of crystal particles occurs primarily at the papillary collecting ducts. Although most crystals are flushed from the tract through antegrade urine flow, urinary stasis (i.e., from benign prostatic hyperplasia, neurogenic bladder), anatomical abnormalities (strictures), or inflamed epithelium within the urinary tract may prevent prompt flushing of crystals from the system, thus increasing the risk for calculus formation.

Calcium stones account for 70 to 80% of all stones requiring treatment. Calcium oxalate accounts for about 80% of these stones and calcium phosphate about 15%. Most individuals have idiopathic calcium urolithiasis, a condition whose exact etiology has not yet been defined. Stones can form freely in supersaturated urine or detach from interstitial sites within the tubules (Randall plaque formation) near the tip of the renal papillae. Hypercalciuria, hyperoxaluria, hyperuricosuria, hypocitraturia, mild renal tubular acidosis, or crystal growth inhibitor deficiencies and alkaline urine are associated with calcium stones. Hypercalciuria is attributable to intestinal hyperabsorption of dietary calcium and decreased renal calcium reabsorption. Hyperparathyroidism and bone demineralization associated with prolonged immobilization are also known to cause hypercalciuria. Although oxalate in the diet influences the risk of developing calcium stones, primary hyperoxaluria is a rare, inherited disorder.

Struvite stones primarily contain magnesium-ammonium-phosphate as well as varying levels of matrix. Matrix forms in an alkaline urine and during infection with a urease-producing bacterial pathogen, such as *Proteus*, *Klebsiella*, or *Pseudomonas*. Struvite calculi may grow quite large and branch into a staghorn configuration (**staghorn calculus**) that approximates the pelvicaliceal collecting system.

Uric acid stones occur in persons who excrete excessive uric acid in the urine, such as those with gouty arthritis. Uric acid is primarily a product of biosynthesis of endogenous purines and is secondarily affected by consumption of purines (e.g., meat and beer) in the diet. A consistently acidic urine (pH <5.0) greatly increases this risk. Cystine and xanthine are amino acids that precipitate more readily in acidic urine. Cystinuria and xanthinuria are both genetic disorders of amino acid metabolism, and excess of these amino acids in urine can cause **cystinuric (xanthine) stone** formation in the presence of a low urine pH of 5.5 or less.

CLINICAL MANIFESTATIONS Renal colic, described as moderate to severe pain often originating in the flank and radiating to the groin, usually indicates obstruction of the renal pelvis or proximal ureter.[11] Colic that radiates to the lateral flank or lower abdomen typically indicates obstruction in the midureter, and bothersome lower urinary tract symptoms (urgency, frequent voiding, urge incontinence) indicate obstruction of the lower ureter or ureterovesical junction. The pain can be severe and incapacitating and may be accompanied by nausea and vomiting. Gross or microscopic hematuria may be present.

EVALUATION AND TREATMENT The evaluation and diagnosis of urinary calculi is based on presenting symptoms and history combined with a focused physical assessment. Imaging studies determine the location of the calculi, the severity of obstruction, and associated obstructive uropathy. The history queries dietary habits, the age of the first stone episode, stone analysis, and presence of complicating factors including hyperparathyroidism or recent gastro-intestinal or genito-urinary surgery. Urinalysis (including pH) is obtained, and a 24-hour urine is completed to identify calcium oxalate, calcium citrate, and other significant constituents. In addition, every effort is made to retrieve and analyze calculi that are passed spontaneously or retrieved through aggressive intervention. To diagnose and manage underlying metabolic disorders, additional tests are completed for those with suspected hyperparathyroidism (elevated serum calcium levels) or cystine or uric acid (high purine diet) stones.

The goals of treatment are to manage acute pain, promote stone passage, reduce the size of stones already formed, and prevent new stone formation. The components of treatment include (1) managing pain, (2) reducing the concentration of stone-forming substances by increasing urine flow rate with high fluid intake, (3) adjusting the pH of the urine (e.g., make it more alkaline with potassium citrate administration), (4) decreasing the amount of stone-forming substances in the urine by decreasing dietary intake or endogenous production or by altering urine pH, and (5) removing stones using percutaneous nephrolithotomy, ureteroscopy, or ultrasonic or laser lithotripsy to fragment stones for excretion in the urine. Prevention of recurrent stones includes increasing fluid intake to generate 2.5 L of urine per day, avoiding intake of colas and other soft drinks acidified with phosphoric acid, avoiding dietary oxalate (e.g., chocolate, beets, nuts, rhubarb, spinach, strawberries, tea, wheat bran), eating less animal protein, limiting sodium intake, and, for calcium stone prevention, maintaining a dietary calcium intake of 1 000 to 1 200 mg/day. Potassium citrate may be used to raise urinary pH.[12,13]

Lower Urinary Tract Obstruction

Obstructive disorders of the lower urinary tract are primarily related to storage of urine in the bladder or emptying of urine through the bladder outlet. The causes of obstruction include both neurogenic and anatomical alterations or, in some instances, a combination of both. Incontinence is a common symptom, and types of incontinence are reviewed in Table 30.1.

In Canada, the continence care community generally agrees that incontinence affects about 10% of the population. That translates into approximately 3.5 million Canadians who experience some form of incontinence.[14] Individual research estimates for the prevalence of incontinence in Canada range from 2 to 50% of the population, depending on the study, the research method, and the questions posed. For example, asking the question "Are you incontinent?" will collect a

TABLE 30.1 Types of Incontinence

Type	Description
Urge incontinence (most common in older persons)	• Involuntary loss of urine associated with abrupt and strong desire to void (urgency) • Often associated with involuntary contractions of detrusor • When associated with neurological disorder, this is called detrusor hyper-reflexia; when no neurological disorder exists, this is called detrusor instability • May be associated with decreased bladder wall compliance
Stress incontinence (most common in women <60 years and men who have had prostate surgery)	• Involuntary loss of urine during coughing, sneezing, laughing, or other physical activity associated with increased abdominal pressure
Overflow incontinence	• Involuntary loss of urine with overdistension of bladder • Associated with neurological lesions below S1, polyneuropathies, and urethral obstruction (e.g., enlarged prostate)
Mixed incontinence (most common in older women)	• Combination of both stress and urge incontinence
Functional incontinence	• Involuntary loss of urine attributable to dementia or immobility

Data from Agency for Health Care Policy and Research, National Guideline Clearing House. (2014). *Assessment and diagnosis: guidelines on urinary incontinence.* https://www.ahrq.gov/; Khandelwal, C., & Kistler, C. (2013). *American Family Physician, 87*(8), 543–550.

TABLE 30.2	Neurogenic Bladder	
Site of Lesion	Cause (Symptoms)	Diseases
Lesions above C2 involve pontine micturition centre (UMN disorder)	Detrusor hyper-reflexia (urgency and urine leakage)	Stroke, traumatic brain injury, multiple sclerosis (MS), hydrocephalus, cerebral palsy, Alzheimer's disease, brain tumours
Lesions between C2 and S1 (UMN disorder)	Detrusor hyper-reflexia with vesico-sphincter dyssynergia (functional bladder outlet obstruction)	Spinal cord injury C2–T12, MS, transverse myelitis, Guillain-Barré syndrome, disc problems
Lesions below S1 (cauda equina syndrome) (LMN disorder)	Acontractile detrusor, with or without urethral sphincter incompetence (stress urinary incontinence)	Myelodysplasia, peripheral polyneuropathies, MS, tabes dorsalis, spinal injury T12–S1, cauda equina syndrome, herpes simplex/zoster

LMN, Lower motor neuron; *UMN*, upper motor neuron.

dramatically lower rate of positive responses than the question "Do you suffer from occasional leakage of urine?" There tends to be a greater prevalence of incontinence among women than men. It is assumed that this difference is related to childbearing and other consequences of being female.[14]

Neurogenic Bladder

Neurogenic bladder is a general term for bladder dysfunction caused by neurological disorders (Table 30.2). The types of dysfunction are related to the sites in the nervous system controlling sensory and motor bladder function. Lesions developing in upper motor neurons of the brain and spinal cord result in dyssynergia (loss of coordinated neuromuscular contraction) and overactive or hyper-reflexive bladder function. Lesions in the sacral area of the spinal cord or peripheral nerves result in underactive, hypotonic, or atonic (flaccid) bladder function, often with loss of bladder sensation.

Neurological disorders that develop above the pontine micturition centre result in detrusor hyper-reflexia (overactivity), also known as an uninhibited or reflex bladder. This is an upper motor neuron disorder in which the bladder empties automatically when it becomes full and the external sphincter functions normally. Because the pontine micturition centre remains intact, there is coordination between detrusor muscle contraction and relaxation of the urethral sphincter. Stroke, traumatic brain injury, dementia, and brain tumours are examples of disorders that result in detrusor hyper-reflexia. Symptoms include urine leakage and incontinence.

Neurological lesions that occur below the pontine micturition centre but above the sacral micturition centre (between C2 and S1) are also upper motor neuron lesions and result in detrusor hyper-reflexia with vesico-sphincter dyssynergia. There is loss of pontine coordination of detrusor muscle contraction and external sphincter relaxation, so both the bladder and the sphincter are contracting at the same time, causing a functional obstruction of the bladder outlet.[15] Spinal cord injury, multiple sclerosis, Guillain-Barré syndrome, and vertebral disc problems are causes of this disorder. There is diminished bladder relaxation during storage with small urine volumes and high intravesicular (inside the bladder) pressures. The result is an overactive bladder syndrome with symptoms of frequency, urgency, urge incontinence, and increased risk for urinary tract infection (UTI).

Lesions involving the sacral micturition centre (below S1; may also be termed *cauda equina syndrome*) or peripheral nerve lesions result in detrusor areflexia (acontractile detrusor), a lower motor neuron disorder. The result is an acontractile detrusor or atonic bladder with retention of urine and distension. If the sensory innervation of the bladder is intact, the full bladder will be sensed but the detrusor may not contract. This is an *underactive bladder syndrome* and may have symptoms of stress and overflow incontinence. Myelodysplasia, multiple sclerosis, tabes dorsalis, and peripheral polyneuropathies are associated with this disorder.

Overactive Bladder Syndrome

Overactive bladder (OAB) syndrome is a syndrome of detrusor overactivity characterized by urgency with involuntary detrusor contractions during the bladder filling phase that may be spontaneous or provoked.[16] There is coordination between the contracting bladder and the external sphincter, but the detrusor is too weak to empty the bladder, resulting in urinary retention with overflow or stress incontinence. *Overactive bladder* is defined by the International Continence Society as a symptom syndrome of urgency, with or without urge incontinence and usually associated with frequency and nocturia.[16] OAB syndrome affects millions of adults and children. Adults are often reluctant to discuss this syndrome with their health care provider.

Anatomical Obstructions to Urine Flow

Anatomical causes of resistance to urine flow include urethral stricture, prostatic enlargement in men, pelvic organ prolapse in women, and tumour compression. Symptoms of obstruction are more common in men and include (1) frequent daytime voiding (urination more than every 2 hours while awake); (2) nocturia (awakening more than once each night to urinate for adults younger than 65 years of age or more than twice for older persons); (3) poor force of stream; (4) intermittency of urinary stream; (5) bothersome urinary urgency, often combined with hesitancy; and (6) feelings of incomplete bladder emptying despite micturition.

A urethral stricture is a narrowing of its lumen and occurs when infection, injury, or surgical manipulation produces a scar that reduces the calibre of the urethra. The vast majority of urethral strictures occur in men; they are rare in women. The severity of obstruction is influenced by its location within the urethra, its length, and the minimum calibre of urethral lumen within the stricture. Specifically, proximal urethral strictures cause more severe obstruction than do strictures of the distal urethra, longer strictures tend to be more obstructive, and the magnitude of blockage is inversely proportional to the urethral calibre.[17,18]

Prostate enlargement is caused by acute inflammation, benign prostatic hyperplasia, or prostate cancer (see Chapter 34). Each of these disorders can cause encroachment on the urethra with obstruction to urine flow and the symptoms summarized previously.

Severe pelvic organ prolapse (see Chapter 33) in a woman causes bladder outlet obstruction when a cystocele (the downward protrusion or herniation of the bladder into the vagina) descends below the level of the urethral outlet. A cystocele reaching or protruding beyond the vaginal introitus creates the greatest risk for obstruction, particularly if the bladder neck has been surgically repaired without simultaneous repair of the cystocele. In rare circumstances in men, the bladder may herniate into the scrotum, causing a similar type of obstruction.

Partial obstruction of the bladder outlet or urethra initially causes an increase in the force of detrusor contraction. If the blockage persists, afferent nerves within the bladder wall are adversely affected, leading to urinary urgency and, in some cases, overactive detrusor contractions (a myogenic cause of OAB). When obstruction persists, there is an increased deposition of collagen within the smooth muscle bundles of the detrusor muscle (trabeculation), possibly in an attempt to increase the force of its contraction strength. Ultimately, the bladder wall loses its ability to stretch and accommodate urine, a condition called **low bladder wall compliance**, and the detrusor loses its ability to contract efficiently. Low bladder wall compliance chronically elevates intravesicular pressure, greatly increasing the likelihood of hydroureter, hydronephrosis, and impaired renal function.

EVALUATION AND TREATMENT Although the history and physical examination are critical to the evaluation of lower urinary tract disorders, it must be remembered that no symptom or cluster of symptoms has been identified that accurately differentiates the various causes of these disorders. For example, symptoms such as urgency, urge incontinence, frequent urination, and nocturia may develop because of OAB or either increased or decreased bladder outlet resistance. Reduced resistance is associated with the symptom of stress incontinence (incontinence with coughing or sneezing) and symptoms of increased resistance are similar to bladder outlet obstruction, including poor force of urinary stream, hesitancy, and feelings of incomplete bladder emptying.

Various diagnostic tests assist with evaluation. The *postvoid urine* is measured by catheterization within 5 to 15 minutes of urination or through a bladder ultrasound machine that measures bladder height and width to provide an approximation of urine within the vesicle. This measurement may be combined with *uroflowmetry*, a graphic representation of the force of the urinary stream expressed as millilitres voided per second. A *cystometric test* uses a catheter and manometer to evaluate bladder urine volume and pressure in relation to involuntary bladder contraction (the leak point pressure) and the urge to void. Each of these measurements assesses the lower urinary tract's efficiency in evacuating urine through micturition, but neither differentiates poor detrusor contraction strength from obstruction as a cause of urinary retention. Instead, *multichannel urodynamic testing* is used to identify obstruction, quantify its severity, and measure detrusor contraction strength (Figure 30.3). *Video urodynamic* recordings can also demonstrate OAB and detrusor sphincter dyssynergia. An evaluation of renal function, including functional imaging studies and measurement of serum creatinine level, is completed particularly when obstruction is severe and associated with elevated residuals or UTI.

Because the bladder neck consists of circular smooth muscle with adrenergic innervation, OAB and detrusor sphincter dyssynergia may be managed by α-adrenergic blocking (antimuscarinic) medications. In intractable cases, botulinum toxin type A (Botox) injections or surgery is recommended.[19] Detrusor sphincter dyssynergia may be managed by intermittent catheterization in combination with higher-dose antimuscarinic medications to prevent overactive detrusor contractions and associated dyssynergia while ensuring regular, complete bladder evacuation by catheterization. Alternatively, men with dyssynergia may be managed by condom catheter containment, supplemented by an α-adrenergic-blocking medication or transurethral sphincterotomy (surgical incision of the striated sphincter) to relieve obstruction. Low bladder wall compliance may be managed by antimuscarinic medications and intermittent catheterization; however, more severe cases may require augmentation enterocystoplasty (enlargement of the low compliant bladder wall using a detubularized piece of small bowel), urinary diversion, or long-term in-dwelling catheterization. Untreated OAB impairs health and quality of life, causes depression, leads to social isolation, and causes significant economic burden. In the older person, OAB may cause risk for falls and UTI.[20]

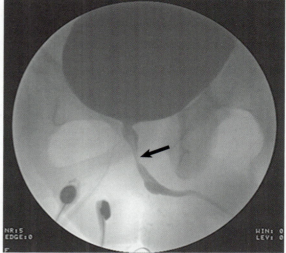
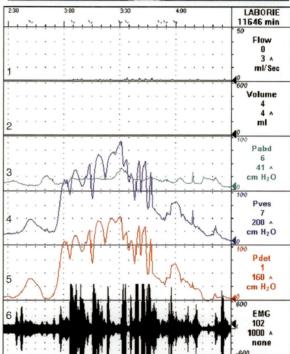

FIGURE 30.3 Neurogenic Detrusor Overactivity With Detrusor Sphincter Dyssynergia. The *arrow* indicates narrowing of the striated sphincter consistent with electromyographic activity *(line 6)* noted on the urodynamic tracing. Note the characteristic poor flow pattern *(line 1)* with elevated voiding pressures *(lines 4 and 5)* indicating obstruction. Line 1, Urine flow rate; line 2, urine volume; line 3, abdominal pressure *(Pabd)*; line 4, intravesicular (inside bladder) pressure *(Pves)*; line 5, detrusor muscle pressure *(Pdet)*; line 6, bladder electromyelogram *(EMG)*.

Prostate enlargement is managed by treating the underlying cause of the prostate enlargement with medication or surgery. Urinary retention may require transient placement of a suprapubic catheter. Urethral stricture is treated with urethral dilation accomplished by using a steel instrument shaped like a catheter (urethral sound) or a series of incrementally increasing catheterlike tubes (filiforms and followers). Long, dense strictures typically require surgical repair to prevent recurrence.

Tumours

Renal Tumours

There are a number of different types of kidney tumours. **Renal adenomas** (benign tumours) are uncommon but are increasing in number. The tumours are encapsulated and are usually located near the cortex of the kidney. Because the tumours can become malignant, they are usually surgically removed. **Renal cell carcinoma (RCC)** is the most common renal neoplasm. **Renal transitional cell carcinoma (RTCC)** is rare and primarily arises in the renal parenchyma and renal pelvis. Risk factors include cigarette smoking, obesity, and uncontrolled hypertension. With surgical resection, 5-year survival is about 90% for stage I (encapsulated) cancer.[21]

The Canadian Cancer Society estimated that in 2020, 7 500 Canadians (4 900 men and 2 600 women) were diagnosed with kidney and renal pelvis cancer. It also estimated that close to 1 950 Canadians (1 300 men and 680 women) died from this disease in 2020. RCC usually occurs in men (two times more often than in women) between 50 and 60 years of age.[22]

PATHOGENESIS RCCs are adenocarcinomas that usually arise from the tubular epithelium, commonly in the renal cortex. The etiology is unknown. They are classified according to cell type and extent of metastasis. *Clear cell tumours*, the most common, present a better prognosis than granular cell or spindle tumours. Confinement within the renal capsule, together with treatment, is associated with a better survival rate. The tumours usually occur unilaterally (Figure 30.4). About 25% of individuals with RCC present with metastasis.[23]

CLINICAL MANIFESTATIONS The classic clinical manifestations of renal tumours are hematuria, dull and aching flank pain, palpable flank mass, and weight loss, but all of these symptoms occur in fewer than 10% of cases. Further, they represent an advanced stage of disease, whereas earlier stages are often silent (painless hematuria). The most common sites of distant metastasis are the lung, lymph nodes, liver, bone, thyroid gland, and central nervous system.

EVALUATION AND TREATMENT Diagnosis is based on the clinical symptoms, plain X-ray films of the abdomen, intravenous pyelography, renal angiography, computed tomography (CT) or positron emission tomography using [124]I-girentuximab, and a radiolabelled monoclonal antibody that binds to clear cell cancer cells. The tumour, node, metastasis (TNM) classification is used to stage RCC.[24] Staging systems using molecular tumour markers are rapidly improving.[25] Treatment for localized disease is surgical removal of the affected kidney (radical nephrectomy) or partial nephrectomy for smaller tumours, with combined use of chemotherapeutic agents. Radiofrequency ablation also may be used for early-stage tumours when surgery is not an option. Metastatic disease is treated with immunotherapy (i.e., bevacizumab [angiogenesis inhibitor such as sunitinib (Sutent) or sorafenib (Nexavar)], T-cell activators, interferon-alpha, and interleukin-2) and target therapies including vascular endothelial growth factor or the mammalian target of rapamycin pathways, or both. Cell-based vaccines are showing promise.[26,27] Survival is related to tumour grade, tumour cell type, and extent of metastasis.

Bladder Tumours

The development of bladder cancer is most common in men older than 60 years. *Transitional cell (urothelial) carcinoma* is the most common bladder malignancy, and tumours are usually superficial. More advanced tumours are muscle invasive. Less common forms are squamous cell and adenocarcinoma (cells that produce mucus). The Canadian Cancer Society estimated that in 2020, 12 200 Canadians (9 400 men and 2 800 women) were diagnosed with bladder cancer. It also estimated that 2 600 Canadians (1 850 men and 720 women) died from this disease in 2017.[28]

PATHOGENESIS The risk for primary bladder cancer is greater among people who smoke or are exposed to metabolites of aniline dyes, high levels of arsenic in drinking water, heavy consumption of phenacetin, or have uroepithelial schistosomiasis infection. Bladder cancer results from a genetic alteration in normal bladder epithelium.[29] Metastasis is usually to lymph nodes, liver, bones, or lungs. The TNM classification is used for staging bladder carcinoma.[30] Secondary bladder cancer develops by invasion of cancer from bordering organs, such as cervical carcinoma in women or prostatic carcinoma in men.

CLINICAL MANIFESTATIONS Gross painless hematuria is the archetypal clinical manifestation of bladder cancer. Episodes of hematuria tend to recur, and they are often accompanied by bothersome lower urinary tract symptoms including daytime voiding frequency, nocturia, urgency, and urge urinary incontinence, particularly for carcinoma in situ. Flank pain may occur if tumour growth obstructs one or both ureterovesical junctions.

EVALUATION AND TREATMENT Cystoscopy with tissue biopsy confirms the diagnosis of bladder cancer. Urine cytological study (pathological analysis of sloughed cells within the urine) is used for screening high-risk individuals. Use of biological markers for bladder cancer diagnosis and treatment prognosis are under investigation.[31] Transurethral resection or laser ablation, combined with intravesical chemotherapy or biological therapy, is effective for superficial tumours. Radical cystectomy with urinary diversion and adjuvant chemotherapy is required for locally invasive tumours.[32]

URINARY TRACT INFECTION

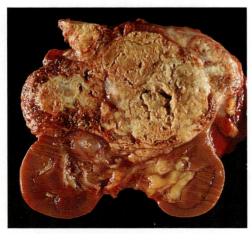

FIGURE 30.4 Renal Cell Carcinoma. Renal cell carcinomas usually are spheroidal masses composed of yellow tissue mottled with hemorrhage, necrosis, and fibrosis. (From Damjanov, I., & Linder, J. [Eds.]. [1996]. *Anderson's pathology* [10th ed.]. Mosby.)

> ✓ **QUICK CHECK 30.2**
> 1. Why is cystitis more common in women?
> 2. What is interstitial cystitis?
> 3. How does pyelonephritis differ from cystitis?

CHAPTER 30 Alterations of Renal and Urinary Tract Function

Causes of Urinary Tract Infection

A **urinary tract infection (UTI)** is an inflammation of the urinary epithelium usually caused by bacteria from gut flora. A UTI can occur anywhere along the urinary tract, including the urethra, prostate, bladder, ureter, or kidney. At risk are premature newborns; prepubertal children; sexually active and pregnant women; women treated with antibiotics that disrupt vaginal flora; spermicide users; estrogen-deficient postmenopausal women; individuals with in-dwelling catheters; and persons with diabetes mellitus, neurogenic bladder, or urinary tract obstruction. Cystitis is more common in women because of the shorter urethra and the closeness of the urethra to the anus (increasing the possibility of bacterial contamination). Up to 50% of women may have a lower UTI at some time in their life.[33] Canadian women make about 500 000 visits to doctors per year due to UTIs.[34] Generally, UTIs are mild and without complications, and they occur in individuals with a normal urinary tract; these infections are termed *uncomplicated UTIs*. A *complicated UTI* develops when there is an abnormality in the urinary system or a health problem that compromises host defences, such as human immunodeficiency virus (HIV), kidney transplant, diabetes mellitus, or spinal cord injury. UTI may occur alone or in association with pyelonephritis, prostatitis, or kidney stones.[35] Up to 40% of cases of septic shock are caused by urosepsis.[36] Factors associated with UTI are summarized in Figure 30.5.

Several factors normally combine to protect against UTIs. Most bacteria are washed out of the urethra during micturition. The low pH and high osmolality of urea, the presence of Tamm-Horsfall protein or uromodulin (secreted by renal tubular cells in the distal loop of Henle), and secretions from the uroepithelium provide a bactericidal effect. The ureterovesical junction closes during bladder contraction, preventing reflux of urine to the ureters and kidneys. Both the longer urethra and the presence of prostatic secretions decrease the risk for infection in men. A UTI occurs when a pathogen circumvents or overwhelms the host's defence mechanisms and rapidly reproduces.

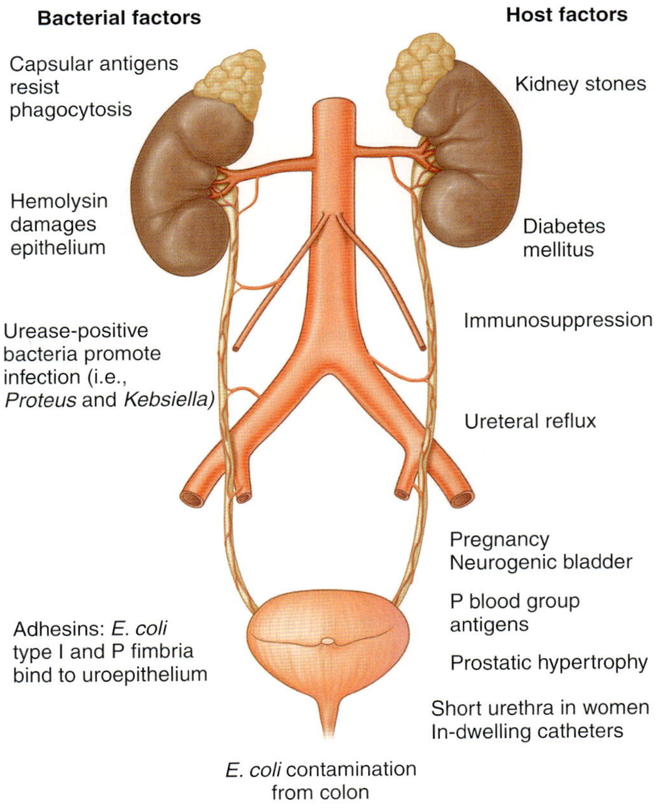

Types of Urinary Tract Infection
Acute Cystitis

Acute cystitis is an inflammation of the bladder and is the most common site of UTI. The morphological appearance of the bladder through cystoscopy describes different types of cystitis. With mild inflammation, the mucosa is hyperemic (red). More advanced cases may show diffuse hemorrhage (termed *hemorrhagic cystitis*), pus formation, or suppurative exudates (termed *suppurative cystitis*) on the epithelial surface of the bladder. Prolonged infection may lead to sloughing of the bladder mucosa with ulcer formation (termed *ulcerative cystitis*). The most severe infections may cause necrosis of the bladder wall (termed *gangrenous cystitis*).

PATHOPHYSIOLOGY The most common infecting microorganisms are uropathic strains of *Escherichia coli* and the second most common is *Staphylococcus saprophyticus*. Less common microorganisms include *Klebsiella*, *Proteus*, *Pseudomonas*, fungi, viruses, parasites, or tubercular bacilli. Schistosomiasis is the most common cause of parasitic invasion of the urinary tract on a global basis; it infects more than 200 million people and has a strong association with bladder cancer.[37]

Bacterial contamination of the normally sterile urine usually occurs by retrograde movement of Gram-negative bacilli into the urethra and bladder and then to the ureter and kidney. Uropathic strains of *E. coli* have type-1 fimbriae that bind to latex catheters and receptors on the uroepithelium. They resist flushing during normal micturition. These strains also have P fimbriae (pyelonephritis-associated fimbriae) that bind to the uroepithelium of individuals with P blood group antigen and readily ascend the urinary tract (see Figure 30.5). Some women may be genetically susceptible to certain strains of *E. coli* attachment.[38] Hematogenous infections are uncommon and often preceded by septicemia. Infection initiates an inflammatory response and the symptoms of cystitis. The inflammatory edema in the bladder wall stimulates discharge of stretch receptors, initiating symptoms of bladder fullness with small volumes of urine and producing the urgency and frequency of urination associated with cystitis.

CLINICAL MANIFESTATIONS Many individuals with bacteriuria are asymptomatic, and older persons have the highest risk. Clinical manifestations of cystitis are related to the inflammatory response and usually include frequency, urgency, dysuria (painful urination), and suprapubic and low back pain. Hematuria, cloudy urine, and flank pain are more serious symptoms. Approximately 10% of individuals with bacteriuria have no symptoms, and 30% of individuals with symptoms are abacteriuric. Older persons with cystitis may be asymptomatic or demonstrate confusion or vague abdominal discomfort. Older persons who have recurrent UTIs and other concurrent illness have a higher risk for mortality.[39]

EVALUATION AND TREATMENT Infections in symptomatic individuals are diagnosed by urine culture of specific microorganisms with counts of 10 000/mL or more from freshly voided urine. Urine dipstick testing that is positive for leukocyte esterase or nitrite reductase can be used for the diagnosis of uncomplicated UTI. Risk factors, such as urinary tract obstruction, should be identified and treated. Evidence of bacteria from urine culture and antibiotic sensitivity warrants treatment with a microorganism-specific antibiotic. Acute uncomplicated cystitis in nonpregnant women can be diagnosed without an office visit or urine culture. If a urine culture and sensitivity are ordered, the

Bacterial factors
- Capsular antigens resist phagocytosis
- Hemolysin damages epithelium
- Urease-positive bacteria promote infection (i.e., *Proteus* and *Kebsiella*)
- Adhesins: *E. coli* type I and P fimbria bind to uroepithelium

Host factors
- Kidney stones
- Diabetes mellitus
- Immunosuppression
- Ureteral reflux
- Pregnancy
- Neurogenic bladder
- P blood group antigens
- Prostatic hypertrophy
- Short urethra in women
- In-dwelling catheters
- *E. coli* contamination from colon

FIGURE 30.5 Mechanisms of Urinary Tract Infection. *E. coli*, *Escherichia coli*.

urine specimen must be obtained before the initiation of any antibiotic therapy; 3 to 7 days of treatment is most common.[40] Complicated UTI requires 7 to 14 days of treatment. From 20 to 25% of women have relapsing infection within 7 to 10 days, requiring prolonged antibiotic treatment. Follow-up urine cultures should be obtained 1 week after initiation of treatment and at monthly intervals for 3 months. Clinical symptoms are frequently relieved, but bacteriuria may still be present. Repeat cultures should be obtained every 3 to 4 months until 1 year after treatment for evaluation and treatment of recurrent infection[41] (see *Health Promotion*: Urinary Tract Infection and Antibiotic Resistance).

Painful Bladder Syndrome/Interstitial Cystitis

Painful bladder syndrome/interstitial cystitis (PBS/IC) is a condition that includes nonbacterial infectious cystitis (viral, mycobacterial, chlamydial, fungal), noninfectious cystitis (radiation injury, chemical, autoimmune, hypersensitivity), and interstitial cystitis. It occurs most commonly in women ages 20 to 30 years who have symptoms of cystitis, such as frequency, urgency, dysuria, and nocturia, but with negative urine cultures and no other known etiology. Nonbacterial infectious cystitis is most common among those who are immunocompromised. Noninfectious cystitis is associated with radiation or chemotherapy treatment for pelvic and urogenital cancers.

The cause of PBS/IC is unknown. An autoimmune reaction may be responsible for the inflammatory response, which includes mast cell activation, altered uroepithelial permeability, and increased sensory nerve sensitivity. Inflammation and fibrosis of the bladder wall are accompanied by the presence of hemorrhagic ulcers (Hunner's ulcers), and bladder volume may decrease as a result of fibrosis. Alteration of the bladder uroepithelial proteoglycan layer makes it more susceptible to penetration by bacteria. Characteristic symptoms of PBS/IC include bladder fullness, urinary frequency (including nocturia), small urine volume, and chronic pelvic pain with symptoms lasting longer than 9 months. Diagnosis of PBS/IC requires the exclusion of other diagnoses, and extensive evaluations are completed. No single treatment is effective. Oral and intravesical therapies, sacral nerve stimulation, and botulinum toxin type A are used for symptom relief. Surgery is used in refractory cases.[42,43]

Acute Pyelonephritis

Pyelonephritis is an infection of one or both upper urinary tracts (ureter, renal pelvis, and interstitium). Common causes are summarized in Table 30.3. Urinary obstruction and reflux of urine from the bladder (vesicoureteral reflux) are the most common underlying risk factors. One or both kidneys may be involved. Most cases occur in women.

PATHOPHYSIOLOGY Microorganisms usually associated with acute pyelonephritis include *E. coli*, *Proteus*, or *Pseudomonas*. The latter two microorganisms are more commonly associated with infections after urethral instrumentation or urinary tract surgery. These microorganisms also split urea into ammonia, making alkaline urine that increases the risk for stone formation. The infection is probably spread by ascending uropathic microorganisms along the ureters, but dissemination also may occur by way of the bloodstream. The inflammatory process is usually focal and irregular, primarily affecting the renal pelvis, calyces, and medulla. The infection causes medullary infiltration of white blood cells with renal inflammation, renal edema, and purulent urine. In severe infections, localized abscesses may form in the medulla and extend to the cortex. Primarily affected are the tubules; the glomeruli usually are spared. Necrosis of renal papillae can develop. After the acute phase, healing occurs with fibrosis and atrophy of affected tubules. The number of bacteria decreases until the urine again becomes sterile. Acute pyelonephritis rarely causes kidney failure.[44]

CLINICAL MANIFESTATIONS The onset of symptoms is usually acute, with fever, chills, and flank or groin pain. Symptoms characteristic of a

---

HEALTH PROMOTION

Urinary Tract Infection and Antibiotic Resistance

Uncomplicated urinary tract infection (UTI) is one of the most common bacterial infections. Of major concern is the worldwide emergence of bacterial strains resistant to specific antibiotics in both hospital- and community-acquired UTIs, causing increased cost, hospitalization, morbidity, and mortality. The resistance is caused in part by overuse of antibiotics. Risks for resistance are highest in regions with the highest rates of prescription and in those who have received trimethoprim-sulfamethoxazole (TMP-SMX [Bactrim]) treatment within the last 3 months, have a diagnosis of diabetes mellitus, have been recently hospitalized, and have community-specific antibiotic resistance rates of greater than 20%. The leading cause of UTI is *Escherichia coli*, followed by *Klebsiella pneumoniae*, and *Proteus mirabilis*, and antibiotics are the mainstay of treatment. These bacteria and other Gram-negative species produce β-lactamases and carbapenemases, causing resistance to penicillins, cephalosporins, and carbapenems (used for complicated UTI). TMP-SMX and fluoroquinolone (such as ciprofloxacin [Cipro] and levofloxacin [Levaquin]) have a high rate of resistance. Multidrug-resistant extended-spectrum β-lactamase (ESBL)–producing *E. coli* are occurring with no known risk factors. First-time uncomplicated UTI can be treated empirically with a 3-day regimen. Complicated infection requires individualized assessment of risk factors for medication resistance and medication tolerability and includes history, physical examination, urine culture and sensitivity, and possible radiological evaluation. Asymptomatic bacteriuria only requires treatment in exceptional cases. Awareness of medication resistance and knowledgeable prescribing are essential to prevent inappropriate use of antibiotics. New medications are being discovered that overcome bacterial resistance, and old medications in new combinations are being tested.

The North American Urinary Tract Infection Collaborative Alliance (NAUTICA) study indicates that antibiotic resistance rates for UTIs are higher in the United States than in Canada for four out of the five antibiotics tested. The study analyzed 813 isolates obtained from 586 patients in the United States and 227 patients in Canada. Overall, most of the bacteria found in the isolates were *E. coli* (54.4%), followed by *K. pneumoniae* (11.8%), Enterococcus species (7%), *P. mirabilis* (5.1%), *Pseudomonas aeruginosa* (2.9%), *Staphylococcus aureus* (2.3%), and *Enterobacter cloacae* (2.2%) (other bacteria accounted for the remaining 14.3% of the isolates). The antibiotic resistance rates were as follows: TMP-SMX, 20.8% among the US isolates and 16.7% among the Canadian isolates; nitrofurantoin (Macrobid), 13.7% among the US isolates and 11% among the Canadian isolates; levofloxacin, 8.9% among the US isolates and 5.3% among the Canadian isolates; and ciprofloxacin, 9.9% among the US isolates and 5.7% among the Canadian isolates. Only ampicillin had a higher antibiotic resistance rate among the Canadian isolates compared with the US isolates (44.9% versus 40.8%).

Data from Bush, K., Courvalin, P., Dantas, G., et al. (2011). *Nat Rev Microbiol, 9*(12), 894–896; Grigoryan, L., Trautner, B. W., & Gupta, K. (2014). *JAMA, 312*(16), 1677–1684; Gupta, K., & Bhadelia, N. (2014). *Infect Dis Clin North Am, 28*(1), 49–59; Ling, L. L., Schneider, T., Peoples, A. J., et al. (2015). *Nature, 517*(7535), 455–459; National Guideline Clearinghouse. (2008). *Guideline synthesis: Diagnosis and management of lower urinary tract infection.* Agency for Healthcare Research and Quality. https://www.guideline.gov; Splete, H. (2003). UTI patients show antibiotic resistance: lower resistance in Canada. *Internal Medicine News, 1*(39); Trautner, B. W., & Grigoryan, L. (2014). *Infect Dis Clin North Am, 28*(1), 15–31.

TABLE 30.3 Common Causes of Pyelonephritis

Predisposing Factor	Pathological Mechanisms
Kidney stones	Obstruction and stasis of urine contributing to bacteriuria and hydronephrosis; irritation of epithelial lining with entrapment of bacteria
Vesicoureteral reflux	Chronic reflux of urine up the ureter and into kidney during micturition, contributing to bacterial infection
Pregnancy	Dilation and relaxation of ureter with hydroureter and hydronephrosis; partly caused by obstruction from enlarged uterus and partly from ureteral relaxation caused by higher progesterone levels
Neurogenic bladder	Neurological impairment interfering with normal bladder contraction with residual urine and ascending infection
Instrumentation	Introduction of organisms into urethra and bladder by catheters and endoscopes introduced into urinary tract for diagnostic purposes
Female sexual trauma	Movement of organisms from urethra into bladder with infection and retrograde spread to kidney

UTI, including frequency, dysuria, and costovertebral tenderness, may precede systemic signs and symptoms. Older persons may have nonspecific symptoms, such as low-grade fever and malaise.

EVALUATION AND TREATMENT Differentiating symptoms of cystitis from those of pyelonephritis by clinical assessment alone is difficult. The specific diagnosis is established by urine culture, urinalysis, and clinical signs and symptoms. White blood cell casts indicate pyelonephritis, but they are not always present in the urine. Complicated pyelonephritis requires blood cultures and urinary tract imaging.[45] Uncomplicated acute pyelonephritis responds well to 2 to 3 weeks of microorganism-specific antibiotic therapy. Follow-up urine cultures are obtained at 1 and 4 weeks after treatment if symptoms recur. Antibiotic-resistant microorganisms or reinfection may occur in cases of urinary tract obstruction or reflux. Intravenous pyelography and voiding cystourethrography identify surgically correctable lesions.

Chronic Pyelonephritis

Chronic pyelonephritis is a persistent or recurrent infection of the kidney leading to scarring of one or both kidneys. The specific cause of chronic pyelonephritis is difficult to determine. Recurrent infections from acute pyelonephritis may be associated with chronic pyelonephritis. Generally, chronic pyelonephritis is more likely to occur in individuals who have renal infections associated with some type of obstructive pathological condition, such as renal stones and vesicoureteral reflux.

PATHOPHYSIOLOGY Chronic urinary tract obstruction prevents elimination of bacteria and starts a process of progressive inflammation, alterations of the renal pelvis and calyces, destruction of the tubules, atrophy or dilation and diffuse scarring, and, finally, impaired urine-concentrating ability, leading to CKD. The lesions of chronic pyelonephritis are sometimes termed *chronic interstitial nephritis* because the inflammation and fibrosis are located in the interstitial spaces between the tubules.

CLINICAL MANIFESTATIONS The early symptoms of chronic pyelonephritis are often minimal and may include hypertension, frequency, dysuria, and flank pain. Progression can lead to kidney failure, particularly in the presence of obstructive uropathy or diabetes mellitus.

EVALUATION AND TREATMENT Urinalysis, intravenous pyelography, and ultrasound are used diagnostically. Treatment is related to the underlying cause. Obstruction must be relieved. Antibiotics may be given, with prolonged antibiotic therapy for recurrent infection.

GLOMERULAR DISORDERS

 QUICK CHECK 30.3
1. What is glomerulonephritis? List two types.
2. What immune mechanisms are operative in glomerulonephritis?
3. Why is edema present in individuals with nephrotic syndrome?

Glomerulonephritis

Acute glomerulonephritis is an inflammation of the glomerulus caused by *primary glomerular injury*, including immunological responses, ischemia, free radicals, medications, toxins, vascular disorders, and infection. *Secondary glomerular injury* is a consequence of systemic diseases, including diabetes mellitus, hypertension, bacterial toxins, systemic lupus erythematosus, heart failure, and HIV-related kidney disease.

PATHOPHYSIOLOGY Immune mechanisms are a major cause of injury for primary and secondary causes of glomerulonephritis (Figure 30.6). The injury damages the glomerular capillary filtration membrane, including the endothelium, basement membrane, and epithelium (podocytes). The most common types of immune injury are (1) deposition of circulating antigen–antibody immune complexes into the glomerulus (type III hypersensitivity) and (2) reaction of antibodies in situ against planted antigens within the glomerulus (type II hypersensitivity, cytotoxic) (see Chapter 8). Nonimmune glomerular injury is related to ischemia, metabolic disorders (e.g., diabetes mellitus), toxin exposure, medications, vascular disorders (e.g., vasculitis), and infection with direct injury to glomerular cells. Different causes of injury may result in more than one type of glomerular lesion; thus, lesions are not necessarily disease specific (Table 30.4).

Immune injury is caused by activation of biochemical mediators of inflammation (i.e., complement and cytokines from leukocytes) and begins after the antigen–antibody complexes have deposited or formed in the glomerular capillary wall or mesangium. Complement is deposited with the antibodies, and activation can cause cell lysis or serve as a chemotactic stimulus for attraction of neutrophils, monocytes, and T cells. These phagocytes, along with activated platelets, further the inflammatory reaction by releasing mediators that injure the glomerular filtration membrane, including epithelial cells, glomerular basement membrane, and endothelial cells (podocytes and filtration slits).[46] The injury increases glomerular membrane permeability and reduces glomerular membrane surface area. The GFR decreases, resulting in increased serum creatinine levels. There also may be swelling and proliferation of mesangial cells and expansion of the extracellular matrix in the Bowman space, contributing to crescent formation (deposition of substances in the Bowman space, forming the shape of a crescent moon). The result is decreased glomerular blood flow, decreased driving hydrostatic pressure, decreased GFR, and hypoxic injury.[47]

Loss of negative electrical charge across the glomerular filtration membrane and increase in filtration pore size enhance movement of

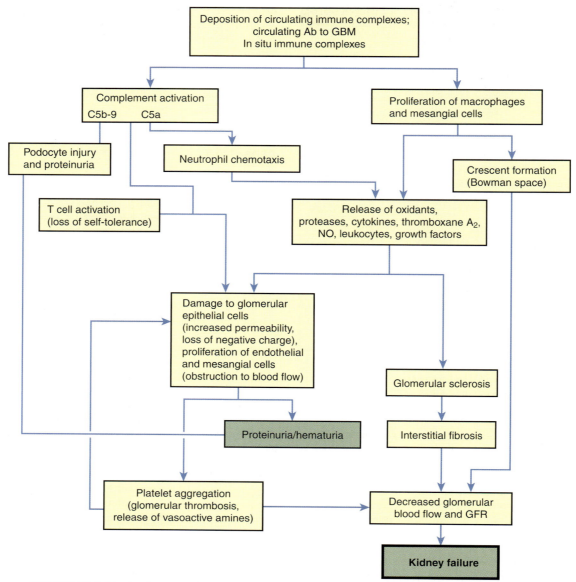

FIGURE 30.6 Mechanisms of Glomerular Injury. *Ab,* Antibody; *C5a,* small fragment produced from complement component C5; *C5b-9,* a complement complex; *GBM,* glomerular basement membrane; *GFR,* glomerular filtration rate; *NO,* nitric oxide.

proteins into the urine. Proteins are normally repelled because they also have a negative charge. Red blood cells also escape if pore size is large enough. Proteinuria or hematuria, or both, develops. The severity of glomerular damage and decline in glomerular function is related to the size, number, and location (focal or diffuse) of cells injured, duration of exposure, and type of antigen–antibody complexes.

CLINICAL MANIFESTATIONS The onset of glomerulonephritis may be sudden or insidious, and significant loss of nephron function can occur before symptoms develop. Acute glomerulonephritis may be silent, mild, moderate, or severe in symptom presentation. Severe or progressive glomerular disease causes oliguria (urine output of 30 mL/hour or less), hypertension, and kidney failure. Focal lesions tend to produce less severe clinical symptoms. Salt and water are reabsorbed, contributing to fluid volume expansion, edema, and hypertension.

Two major symptoms distinctive of more severe glomerulonephritis (i.e., associated with rapidly progressive glomerulonephritis) are (1) hematuria with red blood cell casts and (2) proteinuria exceeding 3 to 5 g/day with albumin (macroalbuminuria) as the major protein. Different types of acute glomerulonephritis may be associated with different patterns of urinary sediment and nephrotic or nephritic syndrome.

EVALUATION AND TREATMENT The diagnosis of glomerular disease is confirmed by the progressive development of clinical manifestations and laboratory findings of abnormal urinalysis with proteinuria, red blood cells, white blood cells, and casts. Microscopic evaluation from renal biopsy provides a specific determination of renal injury and type of pathological condition. Patterns of antigen–antibody complex deposition within the glomerular capillary filtration membrane have been established using light, electron, and immunofluorescent microscopy

TABLE 30.4 Types of Glomerular Lesions

Lesion	Characteristics
Glomerular Lesions	
Diffuse	Relatively uniform involvement of most or all glomeruli; most common form of glomerulonephritis
Focal	Changes in only some glomeruli, whereas others are normal
Segmental-local	Changes in one part of glomerulus with other parts unaffected
Lesion Characteristics	
Mesangial	Deposits of immunoglobulins in mesangial matrix, mesangial cell proliferation
Membranous	Thickening of glomerular capillary wall with immune deposits
Proliferative	Increase in number of glomerular cells
Sclerotic	Glomerular scarring from previous glomerular injury
Crescentic	Accumulation of proliferating cells within Bowman space, making crescent appearance
Interstitial fibrosis	Scarring between glomerulus and tubules

TABLE 30.5 Immunological Pathogenesis of Glomerulonephritis

Glomerular Injury	Mechanism
Soluble immune-complex glomerulonephritis (90%)	Formation of antibodies stimulated by presence of endogenous or exogenous antigens; results in circulating soluble antigen–antibody complexes deposited in glomerular capillaries or formation of complexes within the glomerular membrane; glomerular injury occurs with complement activation and release of immunological substances that lyse cells and increase membrane permeability; severity of glomerular injury related to number of complexes formed; type III hypersensitivity reaction
Anti–glomerular basement membrane glomerulonephritis (5%)	Antibodies are formed and act directly against glomerular basement membrane; immune response causes accumulation of inflammatory cells in Bowman space (in shape of a crescent moon) surrounding and compressing glomerular capillaries; generally associated with rapidly progressive kidney failure, such as Goodpasture's syndrome; type II hypersensitivity reaction
Alternative complement pathway	Relatively rare, mechanism associated with low levels of complement and membranoproliferative glomerulonephritis; type III hypersensitivity reaction
Cell-mediated immunity	Delayed hypersensitivity response that damages glomerulus; actual cellular mechanism not clearly understood; type IV hypersensitivity reaction

for different disease processes. The findings with light microscopy provide information about the distribution and extent of immune response injury (Table 30.5). Electron microscopy differentiates morphological changes within the glomerular capillary wall. Staining with fluorescein identifies different antibodies (i.e., immunoglobulin G [IgG] or immunoglobulin A [IgA]) and their configurations when viewed under ultraviolet (black) light with a microscope.

Reduced GFR during glomerulonephritis is evidenced by elevated plasma urea, cystatin C, and creatinine concentrations, or by reduced creatinine clearance (see Chapter 29). Edema, caused by excessive sodium and water retention, may require the use of diuretics or dialysis.

Management principles for treating glomerulonephritis are related to treating the primary disease, preventing or minimizing immune responses, and correcting accompanying problems, such as edema, hypertension, hypoalbuminemia, and dyslipidemia. Specific treatment regimens are necessary for particular types of glomerulonephritis. Antibiotic therapy is essential for the management of underlying infections that may be contributing to ongoing antigen–antibody responses. Corticosteroids decrease antibody synthesis and suppress inflammatory responses. Cytotoxic agents (e.g., cyclophosphamide) may be used to suppress the immune response in corticosteroid-resistant cases. Anticoagulants may be useful for controlling fibrin crescent formation in rapidly progressive glomerulonephritis.

Types of Glomerulonephritis

The classification of glomerulonephritis can be described according to cause, pathological lesions, disease progression (acute, rapidly progressive, chronic), or clinical presentation (nephrotic syndrome, nephritic syndrome, AKI, or CKD). In nearly all types of glomerulonephritis, the epithelial or podocyte layer of the glomerular capillary membrane is disturbed with loss of negative charges and changes in membrane permeability; the mesangial matrix may be expanded, or the basement membrane thickened. Features of the patterns of glomerular injury are summarized in Table 30.6. Many types of glomerular injury occur most often in children or young adults, including acute postinfectious glomerulonephritis and minimal change nephropathy (lipoid nephrosis). Details of these diseases are presented in Chapter 31.

Complications of diabetic nephropathy and systemic lupus erythematosus can affect the entire nephron and glomerular injury is significant. Different patterns of injury develop over the course of these diseases. Diabetic nephropathy develops from metabolic and vascular complications (see Chapter 19). Changes in the glomerulus are characterized by progressive thickening and fibrosis of the glomerular basement membrane, and nodular expansion of the mesangial matrix with albuminuria, podocyte loss, tubular epithelial cell atrophy, and progression to CKD (Figure 30.7). Diabetic nephropathy is the most common cause of CKD and end-stage kidney disease (ESKD; also called *end-stage renal failure*). Glomerular structure and function can return to normal after pancreatic transplantation and years of normoglycemia.[48] Lupus nephritis is caused by the formation of autoantibodies against double-stranded DNA with glomerular deposition of the immune complexes and alteration in B-cell and T-cell subsets. There is complement activation and a cascade of inflammatory events resulting in damage to the glomerular membrane with mesangial expansion.[49]

Chronic Glomerulonephritis

Chronic glomerulonephritis encompasses several glomerular diseases with a progressive course leading to CKD. There may be no history of kidney disease before the diagnosis. Hypercholesterolemia and proteinuria have been associated with progressive glomerular and tubular injury. The proposed mechanism is related to those observed in glomerulosclerosis and interstitial injury, such as hyperfiltration and inflammatory processes.[50] The primary cause may be difficult to establish because advanced pathological changes may obscure specific disease characteristics (see Figure 30.7). Diabetes mellitus and lupus erythematosus are examples of secondary causes of chronic glomerular injury.[51]

TABLE 30.6 Features of the Common Types of Glomerulonephritis

Type and Cause	Pathophysiology
Associated With Nephritic Syndrome	
Acute postinfectious/infection-related glomerulonephritis (group A β-hemolytic streptococcus or staphylococcus) • Occurs with untreated primary infection in throat or skin	Diffuse deposits of immune complexes (IgG and complement) in glomerular capillary wall; infiltration of leukocytes; endocapillary proliferation and mesangial proliferation Decreased capillary blood flow and GFR
Crescentic or rapidly progressive glomerulonephritis • In situ formation of anti–glomerular basement membrane antibodies or immune complex deposition • Nonspecific response to glomerular injury; can occur in any severe glomerular disease • Can be associated with Goodpasture's syndrome	Accumulation of immune deposits and inflammatory cells and debris that proliferate into Bowman space and form crescent-shaped lesions Decreased capillary blood flow and GFR Can result in kidney failure within 3 months Formation of Ab against both pulmonary capillary and GBM
Mesangial proliferative glomerulonephritis • IgA nephropathy	Deposits of immune complexes in mesangium with mesangial proliferation Decreased glomerular blood flow and GFR Abnormal glycosylated IgA-1 and complement bind to mesangial cells causing proliferation
Associated With Nephrotic Syndrome	
Minimal change disease (lipoid nephrosis) • Glomerular basement membrane appears normal • Usually idiopathic • No immune deposits	Uniform diffuse thinning of epithelial (podocyte) foot processes; loss of negative charge in basement membrane and increased permeability Severe proteinuria and nephrotic syndrome
Focal segmented glomerulosclerosis • Usually idiopathic	Similar to minimal change disease
Membranous nephropathy (autoimmune response to unknown renal antigen) • Usually idiopathic • Can be associated with systemic diseases (i.e., hepatitis B virus, systemic lupus erythematous, solid malignant tumours)	Thickening of glomerular capillary wall caused by antibody and complement deposition and release of inflammatory cytokines with focal segmental sclerosis and increased permeability, proteinuria, and nephrotic syndrome
Membranoproliferative glomerulonephritis • Usually idiopathic; associated with low complement levels	Mesangial cell proliferation; thickening of basement membrane; subendothelial deposits of immune complex occlude glomerular capillary blood flow Decreased GFR
IgA nephropathy (Berger's disease) Usually idiopathic; elevated IgA plasma levels	Mesangial deposits of IgA and proliferation of inflammatory cells into Bowman space, with sclerosis and fibrosis of glomerulus and crescent formation Decreased GFR and hematuria; usually focal, some diffuse lesions
Chronic glomerulonephritis • Can be a consequence of any type of glomerulonephritis; more common with crescentic or rapidly progressive glomerulonephritis	Glomerular fibrosis and scarring, interstitial and tubular fibrosis and vascular sclerosis; original glomerular lesions may not be definable; progression to end-stage kidney disease with uremia

Ab, Antibody; *GBM*, glomerular basement membrane; *GFR*, glomerular filtration rate; *IgA*, immunoglobulin A; *IgG*, immunoglobulin G.

Renal insufficiency usually begins to develop after 10 to 20 years, followed by nephrotic syndrome and an accelerated progression to ESKD. Symptom patterns vary depending on the underlying cause. The specific pathological condition is identified by renal biopsy and is best performed in early stages of CKD to identify specific treatment options.[52] Use of steroids and immunosuppressive agents can prolong remissions and preserve renal function. Dialysis or kidney transplantation ultimately may be needed.

Nephrotic and Nephritic Syndromes

Nephrotic syndrome is the excretion of 3.5 g or more of protein in the urine per day and is characteristic of glomerular injury. It occurs when filtration of proteins exceeds tubular reabsorption. *Primary causes of nephrotic syndrome* include minimal change nephropathy (lipoid nephrosis) (see Chapter 31), membranous glomerulonephritis, and focal segmented glomerulosclerosis.[53] *Secondary forms of nephrotic syndrome* occur in systemic diseases, including diabetes mellitus (see Chapter 19), amyloidosis, systemic lupus erythematosus, and Henoch-Schönlein purpura (see Chapter 31). Nephrotic syndrome also is associated with certain medications (e.g., nonsteroidal anti-inflammatory drugs [NSAIDs]), infections, malignancies, and vascular disorders. When present as a secondary complication with renal diseases, nephrotic syndrome often signifies a more serious prognosis.[53] Nephrotic syndrome is more common in children than adults (see Chapter 31).

Nephritic syndrome is characterized by hematuria and red blood cell casts in the urine. Proteinuria is usually less severe than in nephrotic syndrome. It occurs primarily with infection-related glomerulonephritis and rapidly progressive crescentic glomerulonephritis.

PATHOPHYSIOLOGY In nephrotic syndrome, disturbances in the glomerular basement membrane and podocyte injury lead to increased permeability to protein and loss of electrical negative charge. Loss of plasma proteins, particularly albumin and some immunoglobulins, occurs across the injured glomerular filtration membrane. Loss of plasma proteins decreases plasma oncotic

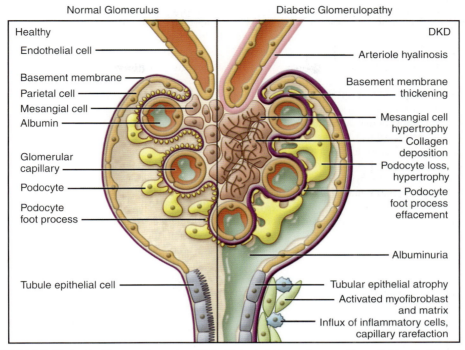

FIGURE 30.7 Diabetic Glomerulopathy. *DKD*, Diabetic kidney disease. (From Reidy, K., Kang, H. M., Hostetter, T., et al. [2014]. Molecular mechanisms of diabetic kidney disease. *Journal of Clinical Investigation, 124*[6], 2333–2340. Reproduced with permission.)

pressure, resulting in edema. The predominant cause of nephrotic syndrome is minimal change nephropathy, which is common in children (see Chapter 31). Hypoalbuminemia results from urinary loss of albumin combined with a diminished synthesis of replacement albumin by the liver. Albumin is lost in the greatest quantity because of its high plasma concentration and low molecular weight. Decreased dietary intake of protein from anorexia or malnutrition or accompanying liver disease may also contribute to lower levels of plasma albumin. Loss of albumin stimulates lipoprotein synthesis by the liver and dyslipidemia and can promote progression of glomerular disease. Loss of immunoglobulins may increase susceptibility to infections. Sodium retention is common.[53]

In nephritic syndrome, hematuria (usually microscopic) is present and red blood cell casts are present in the urine in addition to proteinuria, which is not severe. It is caused by increased permeability of the glomerular filtration membrane with pore sizes large enough to allow the passage of red blood cells and protein. Nephritic syndrome is associated with postinfectious glomerulonephritis, rapidly progressive (crescentic) glomerulonephritis, IgA nephropathy, lupus nephritis, and diabetic nephropathy. The pathophysiology is related to immune injury of the glomerulus as previously described. Hypertension and uremia occur in advanced stages of disease.

CLINICAL MANIFESTATIONS Many clinical manifestations of nephrotic and nephritic syndrome are related to loss of serum proteins and associated sodium retention (Table 30.7). They include edema, hypoproteinemia, proteinuria, dyslipidemia, lipiduria, vitamin D deficiency, and hypothyroidism.[54] Vitamin D deficiency is related to loss of serum transport proteins and decreased vitamin D activation by the kidney. Hypothyroidism can result from urinary loss of thyroid-binding protein and thyroxine. Alterations in coagulation factors can cause hypercoagulability and may lead to thromboembolic events.[55]

TABLE 30.7 Clinical Manifestations of Nephrotic Syndrome

Manifestation	Contributing Factors	Result
Significant proteinuria	Increased glomerular permeability, decreased proximal tubule reabsorption	Edema, increased susceptibility to infection from loss of immunoglobulins
Hypoalbuminemia	Increased urinary losses of protein	Edema
Edema	Hypoalbuminemia (decreased plasma oncotic pressure, sodium and water retention, increased aldosterone and antidiuretic hormone [ADH] secretion), unresponsiveness to atrial natriuretic peptides	Soft, pitting, generalized edema
Dyslipidemia	Decreased serum albumin level; increased hepatic synthesis of very low-density lipoproteins; increased levels of cholesterol, phospholipids, triglycerides	Increased atherogenesis
Lipiduria	Sloughing of tubular cells containing fat (oval fat bodies); free fat from dyslipidemia	Fat droplets that may float in urine

EVALUATION AND TREATMENT Nephrotic syndrome is diagnosed when the protein level in a 24-hour urine collection is greater than 3.5 g. Serum albumin level decreases (to less than 30 g/L), and concentrations of serum cholesterol, phospholipids, and triglycerides increase. Fat bodies may be present in the urine.

Nephrotic syndrome is commonly treated by consuming a moderate protein restriction (i.e., 0.8 g/kg body weight/day), low-fat, salt-restricted diet, as well as by prescribing diuretics. Diuretics are used to control hypertension and eliminate fluid. Care must be taken to observe for hypovolemia and hypokalemia or potassium toxicity in the presence of renal insufficiency. Spironolactone may be combined with loop diuretics to suppress aldosterone activity to conserve potassium. Heparinoids are used for prophylactic anticoagulation. Glucocorticoids are used to control immune-mediated disease or may be combined with immunosuppressive medications. Angiotensin-converting enzyme (ACE) inhibitors or angiotensin receptor blockers (ARBs) lower urine protein excretion.[56]

The evaluation and treatment of nephritic syndrome are similar to those described for nephrotic syndrome. The course of glomerulonephritis is usually more severe with nephritic syndrome. High-dose corticosteroids and cyclophosphamide represent the standard therapy for rapidly progressive crescentic glomerulonephritis. The addition of plasma exchange (plasmapheresis) also may be helpful.[57]

ACUTE KIDNEY INJURY

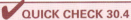
QUICK CHECK 30.4
1. What mechanisms cause prerenal acute kidney injury (AKI)?
2. How does intrarenal AKI differ from postrenal AKI?
3. Briefly describe the causes of anemia, cardiovascular disease, and bone and neurological changes associated with CKD.

Classification of Kidney Dysfunction

Kidney injury may be acute and rapidly progressive (within hours), and the process may be reversible. Acute kidney injury (AKI) commonly occurs as a result of ischemic damage to renal tubular epithelial cells (RTECs). The term acute tubular necrosis (ATN), which signifies a sudden deterioration in kidney function resulting from ischemic or toxin-related insult to the RTECs, was the common term in use. Recently, clinicians and researchers have debated the precision in using ATN because of the limited number of necrotic cells found on kidney biopsy. The term *acute tubular injury* has commonly been used instead of *acute tubular necrosis*, as it offers a broader and more inclusive definition that extends beyond the pathology of necrosis.[58] In this chapter we will continue to use ATN until a consensus on new terminology is reached.

Kidney failure also can be chronic, progressing to ESKD over a period of months or years. The terms *renal insufficiency, kidney failure, uremia,* and *azotemia* are associated with decreasing renal function but are not specific in relation to the cause of kidney disease. They are often used synonymously, although with some distinctions. Generally, renal insufficiency refers to a decline in renal function to about 25% of normal or a GFR of 25 to 30 mL/min. Levels of serum creatinine and urea are mildly elevated. The term *acute kidney injury* is preferred to the term *acute renal failure* because it captures the diverse nature of this syndrome, ranging from minimal or subtle changes in renal function to complete kidney failure requiring renal replacement therapy. Kidney failure refers to significant loss of renal function. When less than 10% of renal function remains, the term used is end-stage kidney disease (ESKD). Specific criteria for acute renal dysfunction are discussed in the next section. Uremia (uremic syndrome) is a syndrome of kidney failure and includes elevated blood urea and creatinine levels accompanied by fatigue, anorexia, nausea, vomiting, pruritus, and neurological changes. Uremia represents numerous consequences related to kidney failure, including retention of toxic wastes, deficiency states, electrolyte disorders, and immune activation promoting a proinflammatory state. Azotemia is characterized by increased blood urea nitrogen (BUN) levels (normal is 3.6 to 7.1 mmol/L) and frequently increased serum creatinine levels (normal is male 53 to 106 μmol/L, female 44 to 97 μmol/L). Renal insufficiency or kidney failure causes azotemia. Both azotemia and uremia indicate an accumulation of nitrogenous waste products in the blood, a common characteristic that explains the overlap in definitions of terms.

Classification of Acute Kidney Injury

AKI is a sudden decline in kidney function with a decrease in glomerular filtration and urine output with accumulation of nitrogenous waste products in the blood as demonstrated by an elevation in plasma creatinine and BUN levels. Classification criteria have been developed to guide the diagnosis of acute kidney dysfunction or failure and are described by the acronym RIFLE (R = risk, I = injury, F = failure, L = loss, and E = end-stage kidney disease [ESKD]), representing three levels of renal dysfunction of increasing severity (Table 30.8). A similar set of criteria has been published by the Acute Kidney Injury Network (AKIN) and Kidney Disease, Improving Global Outcomes (KDIGO).[59]

PATHOPHYSIOLOGY AKI results from ischemic injury related to extracellular volume depletion and decreased renal blood flow, toxic injury from chemicals, or sepsis-induced injury. The injury initiates an inflammatory response, vascular responses, and cell death. Alterations in renal function may be minimal or severe.[60] AKI can be categorized as prerenal (renal hypoperfusion), intrarenal (disorders involving renal parenchymal or interstitial tissue), or postrenal (urinary tract obstructive disorders) (Table 30.9 and Figure 30.8).

Prerenal acute kidney injury is the most common reason for AKI and is caused by inadequate kidney perfusion. Poor perfusion can result from hypotension, hypovolemia associated with hemorrhage or fluid loss (e.g., burns), sepsis, inadequate cardiac output (e.g., myocardial infarct [heart attack]), or renal vasoconstriction (e.g., caused by NSAIDs or radiocontrast agents) or renal artery stenosis. The GFR declines because of the decrease in filtration pressure. Failure to restore blood volume or blood pressure and oxygen delivery can cause ischemic cell

TABLE 30.8 RIFLE Criteria for Acute Kidney Dysfunction or Failure

Category	GFR Criteria	Urine Output (UO) Criteria
Risk	Increased creatinine × 1.5 or GFR decrease >25%	UO <0.5 mL/kg/hr × 6 hr
Injury	Increased creatinine × 2 or GFR decrease >50%	UO <0.5 mL/kg/hr × 12 hr
Failure	Increased creatinine × 3 or GFR decrease >75%	UO <0.3 mL/kg/hr × 24 hr or anuria × 12 hr
Loss	Persistent ARF = complete loss of kidney function >4 weeks	
ESKD	End-stage kidney disease (>3 months)	

ARF, Acute renal failure; *GFR*, glomerular filtration rate.
Adapted from Bellomo, R., Kellum, J. A., Mehta, R., et al. (2002). *Current Opinion in Critical Care, 8*(6), 505–508; Bellomo, R., Ronco, C., Kellum, J. A., et al. (2004). *Critical Care, 8*(4). R204–R212.

injury and ATN or acute interstitial necrosis, a more severe form of AKI. Reperfusion injury with cell death also can occur[61] (see Figure 4.11). AKI can occur during CKD if a sudden stress is imposed on already marginally functioning kidneys.

Intrarenal (intrinsic) acute kidney injury can result from ischemic ATN related to prerenal AKI, nephrotoxic ATN (e.g., exposure to radiocontrast media), acute glomerulonephritis, vascular disease (malignant hypertension, disseminated intravascular coagulation, and renal vasculitis), allograft rejection, or interstitial disease (medication allergy, infection, tumour growth). When ATN results from ischemia, it is often associated with necrosis of the tubular epithelium and the basement membrane. Moreover, because of normal discrepancies in regional blood flow and differences in energy and oxygen consumption in different areas of the nephron, tubular necrosis tends to be patchy. In the hospital setting, ATN is the most common cause of AKI, attributable to half of all cases.[58]

ATN caused by ischemia occurs most often after surgery (40 to 50% of cases) but also is associated with sepsis, obstetric complications, and severe hemorrhagic trauma or severe burns. Septic shock creates a hostile environment for the kidney because of changes in renal perfusion from systemic vasodilatation and intrarenal vasoconstriction. The decrease in renal perfusion is associated with a decrease in oxygen delivery and impairment of cellular waste removal. Moreover, sepsis can result in direct tubular damage from endotoxins and inflammatory cytokines. Hence sepsis-related tubular injury can occur in the absence of hypoperfusion and may be related to inflammation and changes in microcirculation and mitochondrial function.[58]

Abrupt cessation of blood supply to the kidney is rare but can result in kidney infarction. The culprits are usually atrial fibrillation, cardiac thrombus following myocardial infarction, paradoxical emboli from a patent foramen ovale, or thromboemboli from complex atherosclerotic plaques in the aorta.[58]

Hypotension associated with hypovolemia or shock produces ischemia and the inflammatory response, generating toxic oxygen free radicals that cause cellular swelling, injury, and necrosis. Under normal conditions, the kidney receives 20 to 25% of the total cardiac output. In response to shock and failure of peripheral circulation, the body will react by triggering the increased activity of the sympathetic nervous system and renin-angiotensin-aldosterone system. This reaction in turn causes severe vasoconstriction, particularly within the renal vasculature.[62]

TABLE 30.9 Categories of Acute Kidney Injury

Area of Dysfunction	Possible Causes
Prerenal	*Hypovolemia* Hemorrhagic blood loss (trauma, gastrointestinal bleeding, complications of childbirth) Loss of plasma volume (burns, peritonitis) Water and electrolyte losses (severe vomiting or diarrhea, intestinal obstruction, uncontrolled diabetes mellitus, inappropriate use of diuretics) *Hypotension or hypoperfusion* Septic shock Cardiac failure or shock Massive pulmonary embolism Stenosis or clamping of renal artery
Intrarenal	*Acute tubular necrosis (postischemic or nephrotoxic)* Glomerulopathies Acute interstitial necrosis (tumours or toxins) Vascular damage Malignant hypertension, vasculitis Coagulation defects Renal artery/vein occlusion Bilateral acute pyelonephritis
Postrenal	*Obstructive uropathies (usually bilateral)* Ureteral destruction (edema, tumours, stones, clots) Bladder neck obstruction (enlarged prostate) Neurogenic bladder

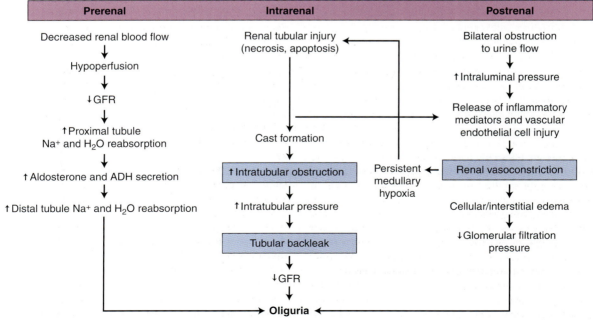

FIGURE 30.8 Acute Kidney Injury and Mechanisms of Oliguria. *ADH,* Antidiuretic hormone; *GFR,* glomerular filtration rate; H_2O, water; Na^+, sodium.

Nephrotoxic ATN can be produced by radiocontrast media and numerous antibiotics, particularly the aminoglycosides (neomycin [Neosporin], gentamicin [Garamycin], tobramycin [Nebcin]) because these medications accumulate in the renal cortex. Medications that interfere with the autoregulation of renal blood flow can also contribute to ATN. For instance, over-the-counter medications (i.e., NSAIDs) can decrease blood flow through the afferent arteriole and can impair medullary blood flow in patients who are prostaglandin-dependent. Other classes of medications that can potentially lead to ATN are ACE inhibitors and ARBs.[58]

Other substances, such as excessive myoglobin (oxygen-transporting substance from muscles released with crush injuries), can also contribute to ATN. Free circulating hemoglobin occurs in the setting of intravascular hemolysis. In small quantities, circulating hemoglobin will be completely bound by plasma haptoglobin to form a hemoglobin–haptoglobin compound that is then cleared by monocytes and macrophages. However, when significant quantities of hemoglobin are present in the plasma, the haptoglobin supply is quickly depleted. Filtered hemoglobin is taken up by proximal tubule cells, or it contributes to cast formation within the lumen. Numerous causes of hemolysis can lead to hemoglobinuria. Common aetiologies include transfusion reactions, autoimmune hemolytic anemia, mechanical shearing from prosthetic valves, and glucose-6 phosphate dehydrogenase deficiency. The term *rhabdomyolysis* specifically refers to the clinical syndrome associated with muscle necrosis and the release of intracellular contents into the extracellular space. The clinical spectrum can range from a relatively benign course to severe systemic illness with AKI due to heme pigment nephropathy.[58]

Other substances that can lead to ATN are carbon tetrachloride, heavy metals (mercury, arsenic), or methoxyflurane anaesthetic, and bacterial toxins may promote kidney failure. Dehydration, advanced age, concurrent renal insufficiency, and diabetes mellitus tend to enhance nephrotoxicity. Necrosis caused by nephrotoxins is usually uniform and limited to the proximal tubules.

Postrenal acute kidney injury is rare and usually occurs with urinary tract obstruction that affects the kidneys bilaterally (e.g., bladder outlet obstruction, prostatic hypertrophy, bilateral ureteral obstruction), tumours, or neurogenic bladder. A pattern of several hours of anuria with flank pain followed by polyuria is a characteristic finding. The obstruction causes an increase in intraluminal pressure upstream from the site of obstruction with a gradual decrease in GFR. This type of kidney failure can occur after diagnostic catheterization of the ureters, a procedure that may cause edema of the tubular lumen.

Oliguria (urine output of less than 400 mL/24 hours) can occur in AKI, and three mechanisms have been proposed to account for the decrease in urine output.[63] All three mechanisms probably contribute to oliguria in varying combinations and degrees throughout the course of the disease (see Figure 30.8). These mechanisms are:

1. *Alterations in renal blood flow.* Efferent arteriolar vasoconstriction may be produced by intrarenal release of angiotensin II or there may be redistribution of blood flow from the cortex to the medulla. Autoregulation of blood flow may be impaired, resulting in decreased GFR. Changes in glomerular permeability and decreased GFR also may result from ischemia.
2. *Tubular obstruction.* Necrosis of the tubules causes sloughing of cells, cast formation, or ischemic edema that results in tubular obstruction, which in turn causes a retrograde increase in pressure and reduces the GFR. Kidney failure can occur within 24 hours.
3. *Tubular backleak.* Glomerular filtration remains normal, but tubular reabsorption of filtrate is accelerated as a result of permeability caused by ischemia and increased tubular pressure from obstruction.

CLINICAL MANIFESTATIONS The clinical progression of AKI with recovery of renal function occurs in three overlapping phases: initiation phase, maintenance phase, and recovery phase. The *initiation phase* is the phase of reduced perfusion or toxicity in which kidney injury is evolving. Prevention of injury is possible during this phase. The *maintenance* or *oliguric phase* is the period of established kidney injury and dysfunction after the initiating event has been resolved and may last from weeks to months. Urine output is lowest during this phase and serum creatinine and BUN levels both increase. The *recovery* or *polyuric phase* is the interval when glomerular function returns but the regenerating tubules cannot concentrate the filtrate. Diuresis is common during this phase, with a decline in serum creatinine and urea concentrations and an increase in creatinine clearance.

Oliguria begins within 1 day after a hypotensive event and lasts 1 to 3 weeks, but it may regress in several hours or extend for several weeks, depending on the duration of ischemia or the severity of injury or obstruction. *Anuria* (urine output of less than 50 mL/day) is uncommon in ATN, involves both kidneys, and suggests bilateral renal artery occlusion, obstructive uropathy, or acute cortical necrosis. Kidney failure can present with *nonoliguric renal failure* and represents less severe injury, particularly with intrinsic kidney injury associated with nephrotoxins. The urine output may vary in volume, but the BUN and plasma creatinine concentrations increase (plasma creatinine concentration is inversely proportional to the GFR). Other manifestations include hyperkalemia, hyperphosphatemia, and metabolic acidosis from decreased urine excretion. Edema and heart failure can be associated with fluid retention.

As renal function improves, increase in urine volume (diuresis) is progressive. The tubules are still damaged early in the recovery phase but are recovering function. Polyuria can result in excessive loss of sodium, potassium, and water. Fluid and electrolyte balance must be carefully monitored, and excessive urinary losses replaced.

Serial measurements of plasma creatinine concentration provide an index of renal function during the *recovery phase*. Return to normal status may take from 3 to 12 months, and some individuals do not have full recovery of a normal GFR or tubular function.

EVALUATION AND TREATMENT The diagnosis of AKI is related to the cause of the disease. A history of surgery, trauma, or cardiovascular disorders is common, and exposure to nephrotoxins, obstructive uropathies (e.g., an enlarged prostate), or infection must be considered. The diagnostic challenge is to differentiate prerenal AKI from intrarenal AKI, and some evidence is available from urinalysis and measurement of plasma creatinine and BUN levels (Table 30.10). However, more than 50% of glomerular filtration must be lost before there is elevation of serum creatinine level. *Cystatin C*, a serum protein freely filtered at the glomerulus, can serve as a measure of GFR. Biomarkers are being developed to assess the extent of kidney injury before elevation of serum creatinine level.[64] Prevention of AKI is the most important therapeutic approach and involves avoidance of hypotension, hypovolemia, and nephrotoxicity.

The primary goal of therapy is to maintain the individual's life until renal function has recovered. Management principles directly related to physiological alterations generally include (1) correcting fluid and electrolyte disturbances, particularly hyperkalemia; (2) managing blood pressure; (3) preventing and treating infections; (4) maintaining nutrition; and (5) remembering that certain medications or their metabolites are not excreted and can be toxic. Renal replacement therapy (hemodialysis or peritoneal dialysis) may be indicated for uncontrollable hyperkalemia, acidosis, or severe fluid overload.[65,66]

TABLE 30.10 Differentiation of Acute Oliguric Kidney Failure

	Urine Volume	Urine Specific Gravity	Urine Osmolality	Urine Sodium (Na) Concentration	BUN/Plasma Creatinine Ratio	FE_{Na}
Prerenal failure	<400 mL	1.016–1.020	>500 mOsm	<10 mmol/L	>15:1	<1% (also seen in acute glomerulonephritis)
Intrarenal failure (i.e., acute tubular necrosis)	<400 mL	1.010–1.012	<400 mOsm	>30 mmol/L	<15:1	>1% (also seen in acute urinary tract obstruction and renal parenchymal disease)

NOTE: $FE_{Na} = \dfrac{UrineNa/plasmaNa}{Urine\ creatinine/plasma\ creatinine} = 100$.

BUN, Blood urea nitrogen.

COVID-19-Associated Acute Kidney Injury

Kidney involvement in patients with coronavirus disease 2019 (COVID-19) can range from proteinuria and hematuria to acute kidney injury that requires renal replacement therapy (RRT). COVID-19-associated AKI (COVID-19 AKI) increases mortality rates and is an independent risk factor for all-cause in-hospital death in patients with COVID-19.[67]

Pathophysiology and Effects of Treatment

Multiple causes of AKI exist in patients with COVID-19, including endothelial dysfunction, coagulopathy, and complement activation, which are general pathological mechanisms commonly found in critically ill patients. It is hypothesized that SARS-CoV-2 exhibit viral tropism to the kidney. The pathogenesis of COVID-19 AKI is multifactorial. Renal damage can be due to the direct effects of the SARS-CoV-2 virus on the kidney, or indirect, resulting from systemic consequences of viral infection. Indirect renal damage can also be secondary to the medical and pharmacological management strategies of COVID-19.

The receptor-binding domain of the SARS-CoV-2 spike protein gains entry to host cells by binding to membrane-bound ACE2—a protein also present on kidney tubular epithelial cells and podocytes—leads to viral activation of the complement system and thrombotic microangiopathy.[68] SARS-CoV-2 triggers activation of an inflammatory response that is termed a "cytokine storm", which further contributes to the pathogenesis of COVID-19-associated multi-organ dysfunction.

Renal dysfunction in patients with COVID-19 is directly linked to the systemic effects of SARS-CoV-2 infection and critical illness. For example, volume depletion, an important contributor to AKI, may result from insensible fluid losses caused by hyperpyrexia and the gastro-intestinal manifestations of COVID-19, such as diarrhea. Critically ill patients infected with COVID-19 might be exposed to nephrotoxins—specifically antibiotics—which can cause tubular injury or acute interstitial nephritis.[69] Individuals who develop secondary bacterial, fungal, or viral infections are also at increased risk of secondary sepsis-associated AKI.[70]

Mechanical ventilation for patients with severe COVID-19-associated pneumonia or ARDS increases the risk of AKI. Patients with COVID-19-associated ARDS are treated with positive end-expiratory pressure (PEEP). PEEP increases intrathoracic pressure, which ultimately results in increased renal venous pressure and reduced filtration. In addition, all forms of positive pressure ventilation can increase sympathetic tone, leading to secondary activation of the renin–angiotensin system.[71] Careful attention to volume status is needed in order to avoid hypovolemia or hypervolemia, because in the setting of ARDS after shock resolution, patients are often managed with a restrictive fluid strategy, whereas COVID-19 patients may initially present with relative volume depletion due to fever and gastro-intestinal losses.

Clinical Course and Prognosis

Patients with COVID-19 who develop AKI are more likely to be admitted to the critical care unit and require mechanical ventilation and vasopressors than patients who do not develop AKI. Approximately one-third of patients presented either with AKI or developed AKI within 24 hours of presentation;[72] other patients, however, may exhibit a median delay of 15 days from presentation,[73] which can differentiate COVID-19 AKI from AKI caused by other systemic infections.[67]

Prevention and Management of AKI

Apply standardized guidelines to manage AKI based on associated risks and stage. Prevention and management of AKI depends on the associated risk and stage of AKI. KDIGO-based strategies and other relevant guidelines are recommended for risk-based and stage-based prevention and management of COVID-19 AKI.[67] These include:

1. *Frequent assessment of kidney function.* Assessment of kidney function is necessary for accurate evaluation of risks and stage of AKI. The current gold standards for the evaluation of kidney function are serum creatinine and urine output.
2. *Optimize hemodynamic status.* Hypovolemia, hypotension, and vasoplegia may occur in patients with COVID-19. Fluid and vasopressor resuscitation using dynamic assessment of cardiovascular status may reduce the risk of renal injury and respiratory failure. Individualized fluid and hemodynamic management based on dynamic assessment of cardiovascular status is recommended.
3. *Fluid administration.* The composition of crystalloids for volume expansion is important. Clinical trials in non-COVID patients have shown reduced risk of AKI with use of balanced fluids for initial volume expansion, especially in sepsis. A balanced crystalloid solution is recommended as initial management for expansion of intravascular volume in patients at risk of or with COVID-19 AKI unless an indication for other fluids exists.
4. *Glucose monitoring and control.* Hyperglycemia due to insulin resistance and a hypercatabolic state are common in COVID-19. Monitoring for hyperglycemia and use of intensive glucose-lowering strategies are recommended for high-risk patients.
5. *Minimize or avoid nephrotoxic medications.* Nephrotoxic medications are frequently prescribed to patients with COVID-19. The risks and benefits of nephrotoxic medications and their alternatives need to be evaluated and followed closely. If contrast media is used, and to avoid nephrotoxicity, some clinicians may order sodium bicarbonate and N-acetylcysteine, even though evidence is not conclusive regarding their potential to prevent contrast-media-associated AKI. Optimization of intravascular volume status continues to be the only specific intervention that has proven to prevent contrast-media-associated AK.

6. *Nutritional management.* Patients with COVID-19 are at risk of malnutrition resulting from various factors, such as prolonged immobilization, catabolic changes, and reduced food intake. Current consensus recommendations for the nutritional management of critically ill patients should be followed. Early enteral feeding is preferred over parenteral nutrition, and the prone position is not a contraindication to enteral feeding.[59] KDIGO practice guidelines recommend that clinicians use anticoagulation for continuous renal replacement therapy, unless it is contraindicated. COVID-19 induces a hypercoagulable state potentially causing premature extracorporeal RRT circuit failure.

CHRONIC KIDNEY DISEASE

Chronic kidney disease (CKD) is the progressive loss of renal function associated with systemic diseases, such as diabetes mellitus (most significant risk factor), hypertension, or systemic lupus erythematosus, or with intrinsic kidney diseases, such as AKI, chronic glomerulonephritis, chronic pyelonephritis, obstructive uropathies, or vascular disorders. AKI can progress to CKD. The Canadian Medical Association and the US National Kidney Foundation define *kidney damage* as a GFR less than 60 mL/min/1.73 m² for 3 months or more, irrespective of cause. *Chronic kidney disease* is the preferred terminology to describe gradual loss of kidney function and declining GFR. Although the terms *renal insufficiency* and *chronic renal failure* are still often used to describe declining renal function, they do not have the specificity of the stages based on GFR recommended by the US National Kidney Foundation and the Kidney Foundation of Canada (Table 30.11). CKD decreases GFR and tubular functions with changes manifested throughout all organ systems (Table 30.12 and Figure 30.9).[82]

In 2017, around 39 000 Canadians were living with ESKD.[74] Indigenous peoples in Canada generally have higher rates and an earlier onset of ESKD compared to non-Indigenous Canadians.[75-77]

TABLE 30.11 Stages of Chronic Kidney Disease

Stage	Description	Signs/Symptoms
I	Normal kidney function Normal or high GFR (>90 mL/min)	Usually none Hypertension common
II	Mild kidney damage, mild reduction in GFR (60–89 mL/min)	Subtle Hypertension Increasing creatinine and urea levels
III	Moderate kidney damage GFR 30–59 mL/min	Mild As above
IV	Severe kidney damage GFR 15–29 mL/min	Moderate As above Erythropoietin deficiency anemia Hyperphosphatemia Increased triglycerides Metabolic acidosis Hyperkalemia Salt or water retention
V	End-stage kidney disease Established kidney failure GFR <15 mL/min	Severe As above

GFR, Glomerular filtration rate.

A retrospective cohort study[78] conducted in Ontario included adults with diabetes between 1994 and 2014, to identify kidney disease and quality indicators for care for early-stage disease. The study compared measures in Indigenous people in Ontario to those in non-Indigenous people in Ontario and included 21 968 Indigenous people with diabetes. The prevalence of chronic kidney disease was higher for Indigenous people in Ontario than for other Ontarians (20.7% vs. 18.4%), as was the prevalence of ESKD (2.9% vs. 1.0%). The incidence of end-stage kidney disease was higher among Indigenous people than among non-Indigenous people in Ontario (9.3 vs. 4.7 events per 10 000 person-years).[78] The two groups were similarly likely to receive recommended medications, but Indigenous people were less likely to receive laboratory tests for their kidney disease. Despite receiving similar quality of care for early-stage kidney disease, Indigenous people with diabetes in Ontario were 3 times more likely to have ESKD, with an earlier onset, than non-Indigenous people with diabetes in Ontario, despite receiving similar quality of care for early-stage kidney disease. They were also less likely to receive home dialysis therapy and were more likely to need to travel farther in order to receive in-centre dialysis treatment.[78]

Another retrospective analysis of a provincial electronic medical record clinical database from January 2012 to December 2013, included 2 478 individuals followed by the provincial chronic kidney care program (379 Indigenous and 2 099 non-Indigenous) who were older than 18 years of age and residents of Saskatchewan. This showed that Indigenous people have CKD at an earlier age and have more severe stages of CKD than non-Indigenous people in Saskatchewan. Chronic kidney disease secondary to type 2 diabetes is more prevalent in Indigenous people. Indigenous people are more likely to require dialysis, and travel further to receive kidney health services and dialysis.[75]

A retrospective cohort study of end-stage renal disease and death among youth with diabetes diagnosed before age 20 looked at incident cases of youth-onset diabetes diagnosed in 352 Indigenous and 2 288 non-Indigenous people. The study determined that Indigenous people with youth-onset diabetes experience higher long-term risks for ESKD and death than their non-Indigenous counterparts.[79]

The higher prevalence of ESKD among Indigenous peoples is associated with higher rates of obesity and diabetes. Compared to other Canadians with the condition, patients from the Indigenous community are more likely to be obese (40% vs. 27%) and to have diabetes (49% vs. 27%).[80] According to the Canadian Diabetes Association, Indigenous peoples living in Canada are among the highest-risk populations for diabetes and related complications.[81]

PATHOPHYSIOLOGY The kidneys have a remarkable ability to adapt to a loss of nephron mass. Symptomatic changes result from increased levels of creatinine, urea, and potassium. Alterations in salt and water balance usually do not become apparent until renal function declines to less than 25% of normal when adaptive renal reserves have been exhausted.

Different theories have been proposed to account for the adaptation to loss of renal function. The *intact nephron hypothesis* proposes that loss of nephron mass with progressive kidney damage causes the surviving nephrons to sustain normal kidney function. These nephrons are capable of a compensatory hypertrophy and expansion or hyperfunction in their rates of filtration, reabsorption, and secretion and can maintain a constant rate of excretion in the presence of overall declining GFR.[83] The intact nephron hypothesis explains adaptive changes in solute and water regulation that occur with advancing kidney failure. Although the urine of an individual with CKD may contain abnormal amounts of protein and red and white blood cells or casts, the major end products of excretion are similar to those of normally functioning

TABLE 30.12 Systemic Effects of Chronic Kidney Disease

System	Manifestations	Mechanisms	Treatment
Skeletal	Spontaneous fractures and bone pain Deformities of long bones	Osteitis fibrosa: bone inflammation with fibrous degeneration related to hyperparathyroidism Osteomalacia: bone resorption associated with vitamin D and calcium deficiency	Control of hyperphosphatemia to reduce hyperparathyroidism; administration of calcium and aluminum hydroxide antacids, which bind phosphate in the gut, together with a phosphate-restricted diet; vitamin D replacement; avoidance of magnesium antacids because of impaired magnesium excretion
Cardiopulmonary	Pulmonary edema, Kussmaul respirations	Fluid overload associated with pulmonary edema and metabolic acidosis leading to Kussmaul respirations	ACE inhibitors; combination of propranolol (Apo-Propranolol), hydralazine (Apo-Hydralazine), and minoxidil (Loniten) for those with high levels of renin; bilateral nephrectomy with dialysis or transplantation
Cardiovascular	Left ventricular hypertrophy, cardiomyopathy, and ischemic heart disease; hypertension, dysrhythmias, accelerated atherosclerosis; pericarditis with fever, chest pain, and pericardial friction rub	Extracellular volume expansion and hypersecretion of renin associated with hypertension; anemia increases cardiac workload; dyslipidemia promotes atherosclerosis; toxins precipitate into pericardium	Volume reduction with diuretics that are not potassium sparing (to avoid hyperkalemia); dialysis
Neurological	Encephalopathy (fatigue, reduced attention span, difficulty with problem solving); peripheral neuropathy (pain and burning in legs and feet, loss of vibration sense and deep tendon reflexes); loss of motor coordination, twitching, fasciculations, stupor, and coma with advanced uremia	Progressive accumulation of uremic toxins associated with end-stage kidney disease (ESKD) Stroke or intracerebral hemorrhage associated with chronic dialysis	Dialysis or successful kidney transplantation
Hematological	Anemia, usually normochromic–normocytic; platelet disorders with prolonged bleeding times	Reduced erythropoietin secretion and reduced red blood cell production; uremic toxins shorten red blood cell survival and alter platelet function	Dialysis; recombinant human erythropoietin and iron supplementation; conjugated estrogens; DDAVP (1-desamino-8-D-arginine vasopressin); transfusion
Gastro-intestinal	Anorexia, nausea, vomiting; mouth ulcers, stomatitis, urine odour of breath (uremic fetor), hiccups, peptic ulcers, gastro-intestinal bleeding, and pancreatitis associated with ESKD	Retention of metabolic acids and other metabolic waste products	Protein-restricted diet for relief of nausea and vomiting
Integumentary	Abnormal pigmentation and pruritus	Retention of urochromes, contributing to sallow yellow colour; high plasma calcium levels and neuropathy associated with pruritus	Dialysis with control of serum calcium levels
Immunological	Increased risk for infection that can cause death; increased risk for carcinoma	Suppression of cell-mediated immunity; reduction in number and function of lymphocytes, diminished phagocytosis	Routine dialysis
Reproductive	Sexual dysfunction: menorrhagia, amenorrhea, infertility, and decreased libido in women; decreased testosterone levels, infertility, and decreased libido in men	Dysfunction of ovaries and testes; presence of neuropathies	No specific treatment

With data from Almeras, C., & Argilés, A. (2009). *Seminars in Dialysis, 22*(4), 329–333; Keane, W. F. (2000). *Kidney International Supplements, 75,* S27–S31; Thomas, R., Kanso, A., & Sedor, J. R. (2008). *Primary Care, 35*(2), 329–344.

kidneys until the advanced stages of kidney failure, when there is a significant reduction of functioning nephrons.[84]

With severe or repeated injury, epithelial cells have an impaired proliferative response resulting in interstitial capillary loss and fibroblast proliferation. The progressive process of glomerulosclerosis and tubulointerstitial fibrosis contributes to CKD and ESKD.[85] The *particular location of kidney damage* also influences loss of kidney function. For example, tubular interstitial diseases primarily damage the tubular or medullary parts of the nephron, producing problems such as renal tubular acidosis, salt wasting, and difficulty diluting or concentrating the urine. When the damage is primarily vascular or glomerular, proteinuria, hematuria, and nephrotic syndrome are more prominent. A summary of factors involved in the progression of CKD is outlined in Table 30.13 and Figure 30.10.

Two factors that have consistently been recognized to advance renal disease are proteinuria and angiotensin II activity. Glomerular

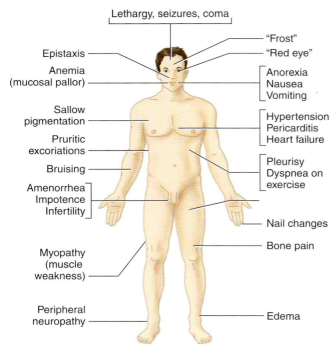

FIGURE 30.9 Common Signs and Symptoms of Kidney Failure. (From Goldman, L., & Schafer, A. I. [2012]. *Goldman's Cecil medicine* [24th ed.]. Saunders; redrawn from Forbes, C. D., & Jackson, W. F. [2003]. *Color atlas and text of clinical medicine* [3rd ed.]. Mosby.)

hyperfiltration and increased glomerular capillary permeability and loss of negative charge lead to proteinuria. *Proteinuria* contributes to tubulointerstitial injury by accumulating in the interstitial space of the nephron tubules and activating complement proteins and other mediators and cells, such as macrophages, that promote inflammation and progressive fibrosis.[86] Angiotensin II (from activation of the renin-angiotensin-aldosterone system) promotes glomerular hypertension and hyperfiltration caused by efferent arteriolar vasoconstriction and also promotes systemic hypertension. The chronically high intraglomerular pressure increases glomerular capillary permeability, contributing to proteinuria. Angiotensin II also may promote the activity of inflammatory cells and growth factors that participate in tubulointerstitial fibrosis and scarring.[87]

CLINICAL MANIFESTATIONS The clinical manifestations of CKD include uremia and azotemia with many systemic effects.[88] The many systemic manifestations associated with CKD are discussed in the following sections and summarized in Table 30.12 and Figure 30.9.

Creatinine and Urea Clearance

Creatinine is constantly released from muscle and excreted primarily by glomerular filtration. In CKD, as GFR declines, the plasma creatinine level increases by a reciprocal amount to maintain a constant rate of excretion. As GFR continues to decline, plasma creatinine concentration increases. The clearance of urea follows a similar pattern, but urea is both filtered and reabsorbed and its level varies with the state of hydration; therefore, urea concentration is not a good index of GFR. However, as the GFR decreases, plasma urea concentration also increases.

Fluid and Electrolyte Balance

Fluid and electrolyte and acid–base balance is significantly disturbed with CKD. When the GFR decreases to 25%, there is an adaptive loss of 20 to 40 mmol of sodium per day with osmotic loss of water. Dietary

TABLE 30.13 Factors Representing Progression of Chronic Kidney Disease

Factor	Characteristics
Proteinuria	Glomerular hyperfiltration of protein contributes to tubular interstitial injury by accumulating in interstitial space and promoting inflammation and progressive fibrosis.
Creatinine and urea clearance	In chronic kidney disease (CKD), the glomerular filtration rate (GFR) falls, and the plasma creatinine concentration increases by a reciprocal amount; because there is no regulatory adjustment for creatinine, plasma levels continue to rise and serve as an index of changing glomerular function.
	As GFR declines, urea clearance increases. (NOTE: Urea is both filtered and reabsorbed and varies with state of hydration.)
Sodium and water balance	In CKD, sodium load delivered to nephrons exceeds normal, so excretion must increase; thus, less is reabsorbed. Obligatory loss occurs, leading to sodium deficits and volume depletion. As GFR is reduced, ability to concentrate and dilute urine diminishes.
Phosphate and calcium balance	Changes in acid–base balance affect phosphate and calcium balance. Major disorders associated with CKD are reduced renal phosphate excretion, decreased renal synthesis of 1,25-dihydroxy-vitamin D_3, and hypocalcemia.
	Hypocalcemia leads to secondary hyperparathyroidism, GFR falls, and progressive hyperphosphatemia, hypocalcemia, and dissolution of bone result.
Hematocrit	Because of anemia that accompanies CKD, lethargy, dizziness, and low hematocrit are common.
Potassium balance	In CKD, tubular secretion of potassium increases until oliguria develops.
	Use of potassium-sparing diuretics also may precipitate elevated serum potassium levels.
	As disease progresses, total body potassium levels can rise to life-threatening levels and dialysis is required.
Acid–base balance	In early renal insufficiency, acid excretion and bicarbonate reabsorption are increased to maintain normal pH. Metabolic acidosis begins when GFR reaches 30–40%. Metabolic acidosis and hyperkalemia may be severe enough to require dialysis when end-stage kidney disease develops.
Dyslipidemia	Chronic dyslipidemia may induce glomerular and tubulointerstitial injury, contributing to progression of CKD.

intake must be maintained to prevent sodium deficits and volume depletion. As GFR continues to decline, there also is loss of tubular function to dilute and concentrate the urine and urine-specific gravity becomes fixed at about 1.010. Ultimately the kidney loses its ability to regulate sodium and water balance. Both sodium and water are retained, contributing to edema, proteinuria, and hypertension.

In early kidney failure, tubular secretion of potassium is maintained, and larger amounts of potassium are lost through the bowel. With the onset of oliguria, total body potassium concentration can increase to life-threatening levels and must be controlled by dialysis.

Metabolic acidosis develops when the GFR decreases to less than 20 to 25% of normal. The causes of acidosis are primarily related to decreased hydrogen ion elimination and decreased bicarbonate

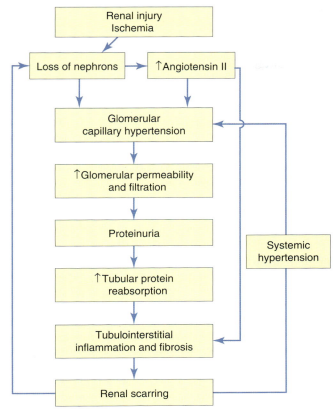

FIGURE 30.10 Mechanisms Related to the Progression of Chronic Kidney Disease.

reabsorption. With ESKD, metabolic acidosis may be severe enough to require alkali therapy and dialysis.[89]

Calcium, Phosphate, and Bone

Bone and skeletal changes develop with alterations in calcium and phosphate metabolism. These changes begin when the GFR decreases to 25% or less. Hypocalcemia is accelerated by impaired renal synthesis of 1,25-dihydroxy-vitamin D_3 (calcitriol) with decreased intestinal absorption of calcium. Renal phosphate excretion also decreases and the increased serum phosphate binds calcium, further contributing to hypocalcemia. Acidosis also contributes to a negative calcium balance. Decreased serum calcium level stimulates parathyroid hormone secretion with mobilization of calcium from bone. The combined effect of hyperparathyroidism related to elevated phosphate levels and vitamin D deficiency can result in renal osteodystrophies (i.e., osteoporosis, osteomalacia, and osteitis fibrosa) with increased risk for fractures.[90,91]

A recent Canadian study established that adequate vitamin D is an essential factor in the prevention of osteoporosis. To improve clinical outcomes such as fracture risk, an optimal serum level of 25-hydroxyvitamin D is probably above 75 nmol/L. In Canada, some vitamin D is obtained with safe exposure to the sun during the summer months, but exposure to sunlight and dietary intake are insufficient to maintain average serum 25-hydroxyvitamin D concentration above 75 nmol/L throughout the year.[92] For most Canadians, supplementation is needed to achieve this level. A daily intake of 25 μg of vitamin D_3 (1 000 international units [IU])—a safe, commonly available dose—will raise the average serum level of 25-hydroxyvitamin D by 15 to 25 nmol/L. The recommended vitamin D intake is 10 to 25 μg (400 to 1 000 units) daily for low-risk adults under 50 years of age and 20 to 50 μg (800 to 2 000 units) for high-risk adults and older persons, with the potential for consideration of higher doses. A dose of up to 50 μg (2 000 units) is safe and does not require monitoring, but if a higher dose is needed, closer monitoring is recommended.

The benefits of calcium supplementation are closely linked to adequate vitamin D intake.[93] Calcium is a mineral available in the food we consume and is instrumental for building and maintaining strong bones and teeth. Dietitians of Canada recommends that Canadian adults 19 to 50 years of age intake 1 000 mg of calcium per day (through two servings of milk or other calcium sources). It also recommends that adults aged 51 and older intake 1 200 mg of calcium per day (through three servings of milk or other calcium sources).[93] Supplementation with vitamin D and calcium increases bone density in postmenopausal women and in men over 50 years of age. Further, a daily dose of 20 μg (800 IU) of vitamin D_3 in combination with calcium (1 000 mg) reduces the risk for hip and nonvertebral fractures in older persons living in institutions. There is evidence that supplementation with 20 μg (800 units) of vitamin D_3 daily reduces the risk for falls.[91,92]

Osteoporosis Canada recommends that adults obtain their calcium through nutrition whenever possible, adding that excess calcium from diet is not harmful. If a person finds it difficult to obtain the recommended amounts of calcium through diet alone, a low-dose calcium supplement is recommended. The supplement label should state the amount of *elemental* calcium in each tablet (e.g., 400 mg of elemental calcium in a 1 000 mg tablet of calcium carbonate). It is the amount of elemental calcium that determines the true daily intake from a supplement.[94]

Protein, Carbohydrate, and Fat Metabolism

Protein, carbohydrate, and fat metabolism are altered in CKD. Proteinuria, metabolic acidosis, inflammation, and a catabolic state contribute to a negative nitrogen balance. Levels of serum proteins diminish, including albumin, complement, and transferrin, and there is loss of muscle mass. Insulin resistance and glucose intolerance are common and may be related to proinflammatory cytokines, and alterations in adipokines (high leptin and low adiponectin levels) that interfere with insulin action.[95]

Dyslipidemia is common among individuals with CKD. There is a high ratio of low-density lipoprotein (LDL) to high-density lipoprotein (HDL), a high level of triglycerides, and an accumulation of LDL particles with accelerated atherosclerosis and vascular calcification. Uremia causes a deficiency in lipoprotein lipase and a decreased level of hepatic triglyceride lipase. Decreased lipolytic activity results in a reduction in HDL level. The concentration of apolipoprotein B is also elevated, thereby accelerating atherogenesis.[80,96]

Cardiovascular System

Cardiovascular disease is a major cause of morbidity and mortality in CKD. Proinflammatory cytokines, oxidative stress, metabolic derangements, and uremic toxins are significant contributors. Hypertension is the result of excess sodium and fluid volume and arteriosclerosis. Endothelial cell dysfunction and calcium deposits lead to a loss of vessel elasticity and vascular calcification. Elevated renin concentration also stimulates the secretion of aldosterone, increasing sodium reabsorption. Dyslipidemia promotes atheromatous plaque formation. The resulting vascular disease increases the risk for ischemic heart disease, left ventricular hypertrophy, heart failure, stroke, and peripheral vascular disease in individuals with uremia. Declining erythropoietin production causes anemia, thereby increasing demands for cardiac output and adding to the cardiac workload. Pericarditis can develop from inflammation caused by the presence of uremic toxins. Accumulation of fluid in the pericardial space can compromise ventricular filling and cardiac output.[97] Fluid overload and hypertension can promote heart failure (cardiorenal syndrome).

Pulmonary System

Pulmonary complications are associated with fluid overload, heart failure, and dyspnea. Pulmonary edema develops and metabolic acidosis can cause Kussmaul respirations. Pulmonary hypertension can develop because of left ventricular dysfunction or uremic-associated vascular changes.[98]

Hematological System

Hematological alterations include normochromic–normocytic anemia, impaired platelet function, and hypercoagulability. Inadequate production of erythropoietin decreases red blood cell production, and uremia decreases red blood cell lifespan. Lethargy, dizziness, and low hematocrit values are common findings. Defective platelet aggregation, decreased platelet numbers, and altered vascular endothelium promote an increased bleeding tendency, increased risk for bruising, epistaxis, gastro-intestinal bleeding, or cerebrovascular hemorrhage. Alterations in thrombin and other clotting factors contribute to hypercoagulability; thus, control of coagulation is essential during dialysis.[99]

Immune System

Immune system dysregulation develops with the uremia of CKD. Chemotaxis, phagocytosis, antibody production, and cell-mediated immune responses are suppressed. Malnutrition, metabolic acidosis, and hyperglycemia may amplify immunosuppression. Release of inflammatory cytokines results in systemic inflammation. Failure of antioxidant systems also promotes inflammation. There are deficient responses to vaccination, increased risk for infection, and virus-associated cancers (e.g., human papillomavirus, hepatitis B and C viruses, Epstein-Barr virus).[88]

Neurological System

Neurological symptoms are common and progressive with CKD. Symptoms may include headache, pain, drowsiness, sleep disorders, impaired concentration, memory loss, and impaired judgement (known as *uremic encephalopathy*). In advanced stages of kidney failure, symptoms may progress to seizures and coma. Neuromuscular irritation can cause hiccups, muscle cramps, and muscle twitching. Peripheral neuropathies associated with uremic toxins also can develop with impaired sensations, particularly in the lower limbs. Symptoms improve with hemodialysis.[100]

Gastro-intestinal System

Gastro-intestinal complications are common in individuals with CKD. Uremic gastroenteritis can cause bleeding ulcers and significant blood loss. Nonspecific symptoms include anorexia, nausea, vomiting, constipation, or diarrhea. Uremic fetor is a form of bad breath caused by the breakdown of urea by salivary enzymes. Malnutrition is common.[101]

Endocrine and Reproductive Systems

Endocrine and reproductive alterations develop with progression of CKD. Both males and females have a decrease in levels of circulating sex steroids. Males often experience a reduction in testosterone levels and may have erectile dysfunction. Oligospermia and germinal cell dysplasia can result in infertility. Females have reduced estrogen levels, amenorrhea, and difficulty maintaining a pregnancy to term.[102] A decrease in libido and fertility can occur in both genders.[103]

Insulin resistance is common in uremia, and as CKD progresses the ability of the kidney to degrade insulin is reduced and the half-life of insulin is prolonged. Individuals with diabetes mellitus and CKD need to carefully manage their insulin dosages.[104]

CKD also causes alterations in thyroid hormone metabolism, particularly hypothyroidism, known as *nonthyroidal illness syndrome*. Uremia delays the response of thyroid-stimulating hormone receptors and triiodothyronine (T_3) levels are often low.[105]

Integumentary System

Skin changes are associated with other complications that develop with CKD. Anemia can cause pallor and bleeding into the skin and results in hematomas and ecchymosis. Retained urochromes manifest as a sallow skin colour. Hyperparathyroidism and uremic skin residues (known as *uremic frost*) are associated with inflammation, irritation, and pruritus with scratching, excoriation, and increased risk for infection. Half-and-half nails (half white and half red or brown) are common. Local bullous lesions and nephrogenic systemic fibrosis are less common.[106]

EVALUATION AND TREATMENT Early screening and evaluation of CKD is based on the risk factors, history, presenting signs and symptoms, and diagnostic testing. Elevated serum creatinine and serum urea nitrogen concentrations are consistent with CKD. Markers of kidney damage include measurement of urine protein level, particularly albumin, and examination of urine sediment. Ultrasound, CT scan, or plain X-ray films will show small kidney size. Renal biopsy confirms the diagnosis.

Management involves dietary restriction of protein, sodium, potassium, and phosphate; supplementation with vitamin D or vitamin D–receptor activators; maintenance of sodium and fluid balance; promotion of adequate caloric intake; management of dyslipidemias; and use of erythropoietin as needed. ACE inhibitors or ARBs are often used to control systemic hypertension, reduce proteinuria, provide renoprotection, and prevent progressive renal damage.[107,108]

ESKD related to diabetic nephropathy can be significantly reduced with glycemic control.[104] ESKD is treated with conservative care, continuous RRT, supportive therapy, and kidney transplantation.[109,110] Portable and wearable dialysis devices are in clinical trials.[111]

COMORBIDITIES

Comorbidities Relating to End-Stage Kidney Disease

Diabetes mellitus is a major cause of ESKD. Diabetic nephropathy (DN) accounts for 40% of all cases of ESKD. Chronic inflammation is common in patients with ESKD, demonstrated by a progressive increase in inflammatory markers as the renal function deteriorates.

ESKD is often associated with chronic diseases such as hypertension and diabetes. Serum markers of inflammation such has CRP and TNF-α levels are higher in diabetic and hypertensive patients when compared to ESKD patients who do not have these comorbidities. ESKD is classified as Stage 5 of chronic kidney disease (CKD), where the glomerular filtration rate (GFR) is less than 15 mL per minute per 1.73 m^2 body surface area, or where patients are on dialysis irrespective of their GFR. Old age (>60 years), obesity, family history of renal disease, and tobacco and drug usage are risk factors for ESKD. However, even when the risk factors are not underlying contributing factors to kidney disease, diabetes and hypertension are often found as comorbidities in ESKD patients and contribute to the worsening of kidney disease.

Complications of ESKD are secondary to inflammation and cardiovascular diseases, which trigger premature atherosclerosis, primarily resulting from endothelial dysfunction. Inflammation in ESKD patients is thought to be the result of decreased cytokine elimination, repeated infections, metabolic acidosis, and chronic hyperglycemia in diabetic patients. Prolonged inflammation and oxidative stress are established early in the process of failing kidney function, even among patients who have only moderate renal impairment, leading to an increase in inflammatory markers such as C-reactive protein (CRP) and cytokines.

Prolonged elevation of CRP is linked to endothelial injury and impaired vasodilation, both of which may lead to glomerular damage and progressive loss of kidney function. Elevated CRP and TNF-α levels have been found to be associated with mortality and cardiovascular complications in ESKD patients. At the same time, the proinflammatory cytokine interleukin-1-beta (IL-1β) plays a major role in fibrosis and inflammation and has been linked to kidney disease.

Data from Eloueyk, A. K., Alameddine, R. Y., Osta, B. A., et al. (2019). Correlations between serum inflammatory markers and comorbidities in patients with end-stage renal disease. *Journal of Taibah University Medical Sciences*, *14*(6), 547–552; Borthwick, L. A. (2016, July). The IL-1 cytokine family and its role in inflammation and fibrosis in the lung. *Seminars in Immunopathology*, *38*(4), 517–534; Rysz, J., Franczyk, B., Ławiński, J., et al. (2020). Oxidative stress in ESRD patients on dialysis and the risk of cardiovascular diseases. *Antioxidants*, *9*(11), 1079; Roumeliotis, S., Mallamaci, F., & Zoccali, C. (2020). Endothelial dysfunction in chronic kidney disease, from biology to clinical outcomes: a 2020 update. *Journal of Clinical Medicine*, *9*(8), 2359.

GERIATRIC CONSIDERATIONS

Aging and Chronic Kidney Disease

As life expectancy continues to increase, so does the prevalence of comorbidities and risk factors such as hypertension, diabetes, and atherosclerosis, predisposing to a high burden of CKD in older persons. Around half of older persons over 70 years of age have an estimated GFR <60 mL/min/1.73 m^2. There is a high prevalence of CKD in older persons, mainly as a result of increasing prevalence of traditional risk factors for CKD, such as diabetes, hypertension, and cardiovascular disease, in addition to the new definitions that have expanded the estimated glomerular filtration rate range for CKD. These new definitions for CKD are kidney damage evidenced by a reduction of the absolute estimated GFR to less than 60 mL/min/1.73 m^2 for at least 3 months. Recognizing that CKD is increasingly becoming a disease of older persons, there are concerns that this new standardization of estimated GFR has led to an increase in the number of older persons that fit the definition of CKD.

An important question that should be considered is whether older persons are classified as having CKD based on a single reduced estimated GFR value without other evidence of kidney damage. The difficulty in calculating the estimated GFR in older persons is made more complex by the number of equations available that can be used, and conflicting data about which equation is the best one to use.

Aging is a relatively accurate predictor of CKD, and 11% of individuals older than 65 years of age who do not have hypertension or diabetes have creatinine levels that fall into the stage 3 category or worse CKD. Nonetheless, due to the overall increased prevalence of CKD in older persons, KDIGO suggested in 2012[59] that CKD screening should be offered to patients with risk factors and those over 60 years of age.

Microvascular disease resulting from diabetes can cause CKD in about 40 to 50% of patients with diabetes, a process called diabetic nephropathy. Concomitant increase in both the aging and diabetic population has resulted in increased prevalence of older persons with diabetes who are at risk for CKD. Furthermore, there is high prevalence of CVD in dialysis patients, and mortality due to CVD in this population is 10 to 30 times higher than in the general population.

Older age is a risk factor for mortality in ESKD patients due to congestive heart failure, which is a common problem for patients who are on chronic dialysis. Preservation of the kidneys' hormonal function, electrolyte, and acid–base balance, as well as normal urinalysis in older persons with GFR <60 mL/min/1.73 m^2, is indicative of a kidney aging normally rather than a kidney with CKD.

As people get older, the common pathway for irreversible kidney damage is hypothesized to be increased intraglomerular hypertension resulting from the progressive loss of glomeruli, which eventually leads to hypertrophy and hyperfiltration of the remaining nephrons. The remaining nephrons continue to deteriorate and the loss of additional nephrons triggers hypertrophy and hyperfiltration of other nephrons, leading to continuous and progressive nephron loss until the kidney fails. Hormones such as angiotensin II and cytokines, released due to chronic diseases such as diabetes mellitus, cause vasoconstriction of the efferent arteriole, exacerbate intraglomerular hypertension, and result in glomerular fibrosis.

Data from McClure, M., Jorna, T., Wilkinson, L., et al. (2017). Elderly patients with chronic kidney disease: do they really need referral to the nephrology clinic? *Clinical Kidney Journal*, *10*(5), 698–702. https://doi.org/10.1093/ckj/sfx034; Kidney Disease, Improving Global Outcomes (KDIGO). (2013). KDIGO 2012 Clinical Practice Guideline for the Evaluation and Management of Chronic Kidney Disease. *Kidney International*, *3*(1). https://kdigo.org/wp-content/uploads/2017/02/KDIGO_2012_CKD_GL.pdf.

CASE STUDY

Part 1:

Helen is a 45-year-old female who is known to be diabetic and hypertensive for the past 5 years and has been taking Daonil 5 mg and Zestril 10 mg PO daily. She had a previous health history of urinary stones, for which she underwent extracorporeal shock wave lithotripsy last year.

Helen has been complaining of difficulty in passing urine and has been having severe flank pain, increased frequency of urinating, and fever (38°C) for a week. She went to the city clinic to seek medical guidance. The clinic nurse assessed Helen and noticed tenderness at the costovertebral angle. The physician ordered urinalysis and culture. The urine was sent to the laboratory to be tested for culture and sensitivity. Based on the assessment, the physician gave Helen a provisional diagnosis of urinary tract infection (UTI) and prescribed the following:

- Noroxin 400 mg PO bid for 7 days.
- Panadol 1 g q 6 hrs PRN for fever and pain.
- Increase fluid intake up to 3 L/day.

After starting the medical therapy, Helen notified the nurse that she developed rashes when she started taking the medications. After reporting to the physician, the nurse informed Helen that she had severe urinary tract infection and that the rashes indicated an allergic reaction to Noroxin, which then was discontinued. Instead, trimethoprim sulfamethoxazole (Bactrim forte) 1 tablet 100 mg PO q 12 hours for 10 days was prescribed. The nurse also gave Helen some instructions on how to prevent UTI recurrence and the importance of follow-up.

Critical Thinking and Clinical Judgement Questions—Part 1

1. Define the medical diagnosis of Helen.
2. a) Compare and contrast upper and lower urinary tract infections in terms of anatomical location and clinical manifestations. b) Which of these types did Helen develop? Justify your answer.
3. Briefly describe the pathophysiological changes that take place in urinary tract infection (UTI).
4. a) Identify the cause and risk factors that could lead to the development of UTI. b) Which of these factors are applicable to Helen?
5. Design nonantimicrobial recommendations for Helen related to the prevention of recurrent urinary tract infections, taking into consideration the possible complications that might develop.

Part 2:

Five years have passed, and Helen is now 50 years old. During the last two years, Helen suffered from recurring urinary stone formation and subsequent urinary tract infection. Nowadays, Helen is dyspneic and experiences an increase rate and depth of breathing, tiredness, and nausea. Her skin itches and she has frequent muscle twitching and cramps. Some parts of her body, especially the lower extremities, are swollen. Her husband made an appointment with the family doctor who referred her to Nephrology. The nephrologist explained to Helen and her family that her kidneys have been affected because of her recurrent renal problems. The results of the diagnostic tests, signs, and symptoms confirmed the diagnosis of renal failure.

Critical Thinking and Clinical Judgement Questions—Part 2

1. a) Briefly describe the difference between acute and chronic renal failure (CRF). b) Which type of renal failure did Helen develop? Justify your answer.
2. a) Identify the causes of acute and chronic renal failure. b) How do these relate to Helen?
3. Describe the stages of chronic renal failure.
4. Relate the clinical manifestations that Helen developed to the pathophysiological changes that take place in renal failure. What are the other manifestations that could be associated with CRF?
5. What is the relationship between UTI and CRF, and how does this relate to Helen?

DID YOU UNDERSTAND?

Urinary Tract Obstruction

1. Obstruction can occur anywhere in the urinary tract, and it may be anatomical or functional, including renal stones, an enlarged prostate gland, urethral strictures, or neurogenic bladder. Hypertrophy of the opposite kidney compensates for loss of function of the kidney with obstructive disease.
2. Relief of obstruction is usually followed by postobstructive diuresis and may cause fluid and electrolyte imbalance.
3. Persistent obstruction of the bladder outlet leads to residual urine volumes, low bladder wall compliance, and risk for vesicoureteral reflux and infection.
4. Kidney stones are caused by supersaturation of the urine with precipitation of stone-forming substances, changes in urine pH, or urinary tract infection (UTI).
5. The most common kidney stone is formed from calcium oxalate and most often causes obstruction by lodging in the ureter.
6. A neurogenic bladder is caused by a neural lesion that interrupts innervation of the bladder.
7. Upper motor neuron lesions result in overactive or hyper-reflexive bladder function.
8. Lower motor neuron lesions result in underactive, hypotonic, or atonic bladder function.
9. Partial obstruction of the bladder can result in OAB contractions with urgency. There is deposition of collagen in the bladder wall over time, resulting in decreased bladder wall compliance and ineffective detrusor muscle contraction.
10. Renal cell carcinoma is the most common renal neoplasm and usually presents with hematuria. The larger neoplasms tend to metastasize to the lung, liver, and bone.
11. Bladder tumours are commonly composed of transitional cells with a papillary appearance and a high rate of recurrence.

Urinary Tract Infection

1. UTIs are commonly caused by the retrograde movement of bacteria into the urethra and bladder. UTIs are uncomplicated when the urinary system is normal or complicated when there is an abnormality.
2. Cystitis is an inflammation of the bladder commonly caused by bacteria and may be acute or chronic.
3. Pyelonephritis is an infection of one or both upper urinary tracts (ureter, renal pelvis, and interstitium) often related to obstructive uropathies and may cause abscess formation and scarring with an alteration in renal function.

Glomerular Disorders

1. Glomerular disorders are a group of related diseases of the glomerulus that can be caused by immune responses, toxins or medications, vascular disorders, and other systemic diseases.
2. Acute glomerulonephritis commonly results from inflammatory damage to the glomerular filtration membrane as a consequence of immune reactions (e.g., after a streptococcal infection).
3. Immune mechanisms in glomerulonephritis include the deposition of circulating antigen–antibody complexes often with complement components or the in situ formation of antibodies, or both, specific for the glomerular basement membrane.
4. Diabetic nephropathy is the most common cause of glomerular injury progressing to chronic kidney disease (CKD) as well as end-stage kidney disease (ESKD).
5. Chronic glomerulonephritis is related to a variety of diseases that cause deterioration of the glomerulus and a progressive loss of renal function.
6. Nephrotic syndrome is the excretion of 3.5 grams or more of protein (primarily albumin) in the urine per day because of glomerular injury with increased capillary permeability and loss of membrane negative charge. Nephritic syndrome is characterized by hematuria and red blood cell casts with less severe proteinuria.

Acute Kidney Injury

1. Acute kidney injury (AKI) is a sudden decline in kidney function with a decrease in glomerular filtration rate (GFR) and urine output and with an elevation in plasma creatinine and blood urea nitrogen levels.
2. Prerenal AKI is caused by inadequate kidney perfusion with a decreased GFR, ischemia, and tubular necrosis.
3. Intrarenal AKI is associated with several systemic diseases but is commonly related to acute tubular necrosis.
4. Postrenal AKI is associated with diseases that obstruct the flow of urine from the kidneys.
5. Oliguria is urine output of less than 400 mL/24 hours.

Chronic Kidney Disease

1. CKD is the progressive loss of renal function. Plasma creatinine levels gradually become elevated as GFR declines.

31

Developmental Alterations of Renal and Urinary Tract Function

Mohamed Toufic El-Hussein, with originating chapter contributions by Patricia Ring and Sue E. Huether

Additional resources are available online at https://evolve.elsevier.com/Canada/Huether/pathophysiology.

CHAPTER OUTLINE

Structural Abnormalities, 757
   Hypospadias, 757
   Epispadias and Exstrophy of the Bladder, 757
   Bladder Outlet Obstruction, 758
   Ureteropelvic Junction Obstruction, 758
   Hypoplastic or Dysplastic Kidneys, 758
   Polycystic Kidney Disease, 758
   Renal Agenesis, 758
Glomerular Disorders, 758
   Glomerulonephritis, 758
   Immunoglobulin A Nephropathy, 759

Nephrotic Syndrome, 759
   Hemolytic Uremic Syndrome, 759
Nephroblastoma, 760
Bladder Disorders, 760
   Urinary Tract Infections, 760
   Vesicoureteral Reflux, 761
Urinary Incontinence, 761
   Types of Incontinence, 761

LEARNING OBJECTIVES

1. Describe the common congenital anomalies that occur within the renal and urological systems.
2. Describe the manifestations of nephrotic syndrome, glomerulonephritis, immunoglobulin A nephropathy, and hemolytic uremic syndrome in children.
3. Describe the risk factors, clinical manifestations, and pathophysiology of poststreptococcal glomerulonephritis.
4. Describe the pathophysiology and manifestations of hemolytic uremic syndrome.
5. Describe the clinical manifestations and treatments of urinary tract infections, cystitis, acute pyelonephritis, and chronic pyelonephritis.
6. Describe the structural alterations that result in vesicoureteral reflex.
7. Describe the pathogenesis of nephroblastoma.
8. Discuss the occurrence, patterns, and probable aetiologies of enuresis.

KEY TERMS

Acute poststreptococcal glomerulonephritis (APGN), 758
Acute pyelonephritis, 760
Ask-Upmark kidney, 758
Chordee (penile torsion), 757
Chronic pyelonephritis, 760
Congenital nephrotic syndrome (Finnish type), 759
Cystitis, 760
Daytime incontinence, 761
Enuresis, 761
Epispadias, 757
Exstrophy of the bladder, 757

Focal segmental glomerulosclerosis (FSGS), 759
Glomerulonephritis, 758
Hemolytic uremic syndrome (HUS), 759
Henoch-Schönlein purpura nephritis, 759
Horseshoe kidney, 757
Hypoplastic kidney, 758
Hypospadias, 757
Immunoglobulin A (IgA) nephropathy, 759
Minimal change nephropathy (MCN) (lipoid nephrosis), 759

Nephroblastoma (Wilms tumour), 760
Oligohydramnios, 758
Polycystic kidney disease (PKD), 758
Potter syndrome, 758
Primary incontinence, 761
Primary (idiopathic) nephrotic syndrome, 759
Renal agenesis, 758
Renal dysplasia, 758
Secondary incontinence, 761
Secondary nephrotic syndrome, 759

Secondary ureteropelvic junction (UPJ) obstruction, 758
Ureterocele, 758
Ureteropelvic junction (UPJ) obstruction, 758
Ureterovesical junction obstruction, 758
Urethral polyp, 758
Urethral valve, 758
Urinary incontinence, 761
Urinary tract infection (UTI), 760
Vesicoureteral reflux (VUR), 761

The incidence and type of renal and urinary tract disorders experienced by children vary with age and maturation. Newborn disorders may involve congenital malformations. During childhood, the kidney and genitourinary structures continue to develop, so renal dysfunction may be associated with mechanisms and manifestations that differ from those found in adults.

STRUCTURAL ABNORMALITIES

> ✓ **QUICK CHECK 31.1**
> 1. Describe hypospadias.
> 2. Why does bladder exstrophy occur?
> 3. Contrast dysplastic kidney and hypoplastic kidney.

Congenital abnormalities of the kidney and urinary tract range from minor, nonpathological, or easily correctable anomalies to those that are incompatible with life. For example, the kidneys may fail to ascend from the pelvis to the abdomen, causing ectopic kidneys—which usually function normally. The kidneys may fuse as they ascend, causing a single, U-shaped **horseshoe kidney**. Approximately one-third of individuals with horseshoe kidneys are asymptomatic, with the most common problems being hydronephrosis, infection, stone formation, and, rarely, renal malignancies.[1] Many are linked to gene defects.[2]

Hypospadias

Hypospadias is a congenital condition in which the urethral meatus is located on the ventral side or undersurface of the penis. The meatus can be located anywhere on the glans, on the penile shaft, at the base of the penis, at the penoscrotal junction, or on the perineum (Figure 31.1). The cause of this condition is multifactorial and includes genetic, endocrine, and environmental factors. Advanced maternal age and low birth weight also have been implicated.[3,4] **Chordee (penile torsion)** may accompany cases of hypospadias. In chordee, skin tethering and shortening of subcutaneous tissue cause the penis to bend or "bow ventrally" (Figure 31.2). Penile torsion is rotation of the penile shaft to either the right or the left. Partial absence of the foreskin and cryptorchidism (undescended testes; see Chapter 32) are associated with the anomaly.

Surgery is most effective, psychologically as well as physically, when performed between 6 and 12 months of age.[5,6]

Epispadias and Exstrophy of the Bladder

Epispadias and exstrophy of the bladder are the same congenital defect expressed to differing degrees. In male epispadias, the urethral opening is on the dorsal surface of the penis. In females, a cleft along the ventral urethra usually extends to the bladder neck.[7] Epispadias is seen predominantly in males.

In boys, the urethral opening may be small and situated behind the glans (anterior epispadias), or a fissure may extend the entire length of the penis and into the bladder neck (posterior epispadias).[8] Treatment is surgical reconstruction.

Exstrophy of the bladder is a rare, extensive congenital anomaly of herniation of the bladder through the abdominal wall. The bony part of the pelvis remains open (Figure 31.3), and the posterior portion of the bladder mucosa is exposed through the abdominal opening and appears bright red.[9]

Exstrophy of the bladder is caused by intrauterine failure of the abdominal wall and the mesoderm of the anterior bladder to fuse. The

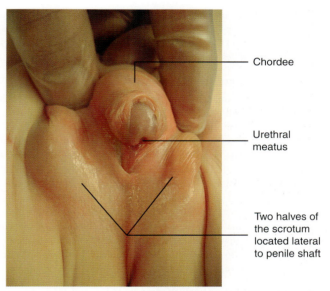

FIGURE 31.2 Hypospadias With Significant Chordee. (From Kliegman, R. M., Stanton, B. F., St. Geme, J. W., et al. [Eds.]. [2011]. *Nelson textbook of pediatrics* [19th ed.]. Saunders.)

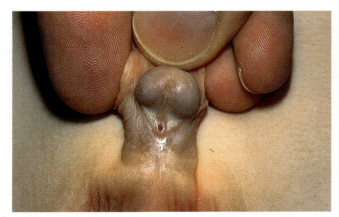

FIGURE 31.1 Hypospadias. (Courtesy H. Gil Rushton, MD, Children's National Medical Center, Washington, DC; from Hockenberry, M. J., & Wilson, D. [2015]. *Wong's nursing care of infants and children*. [10th ed.]. Mosby.)

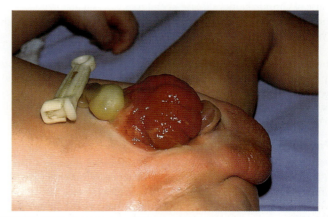

FIGURE 31.3 Exstrophy of Bladder. (Courtesy H. Gil Rushton, MD, Children's National Medical Center, Washington, DC; from Hockenberry, M. J., & Wilson, D. [2015]. *Wong's nursing care of infants and children*. [10th ed.]. Mosby.)

rectus muscles below the umbilicus are separated, and the pubic rami (bony projections of the pubic bone) are not joined. This causes a waddling gait when the child first learns to walk, but most children quickly learn to compensate. The clitoris in girls is divided into two parts with the urethra between each half. The penis in boys is epispadiac. Urine seeps onto the abdominal wall from the ureters, causing a constant odour of urine and excoriation of the surrounding skin. Because the exposed bladder mucosa becomes hyperemic and edematous, it bleeds easily and is painful.

The unrepaired exstrophic bladder is prone to cancerous changes as soon as 1 year after birth. Ideally, the bladder and pubic defect should be closed before the infant is 72 hours old. Surgical reconstruction is usually performed within the first year either as a complete primary repair or as staged procedures.[10] Diagnosis is often made by prenatal ultrasound.

Bladder Outlet Obstruction

Congenital causes of bladder outlet obstruction are rare and include urethral valves and polyps. A urethral valve is a thin membrane of tissue that blocks the urethral lumen and obstructs urinary outflow in males. Urethral polyps are rare.[11] The timing and presentation of these conditions depend on the degree of obstruction they cause.[12] Urethral valves or polyps are resected as soon as they are diagnosed.

Ureteropelvic Junction Obstruction

Ureteropelvic junction (UPJ) obstruction is a blockage of the tapered point where the renal pelvis transitions into the ureter. UPJ obstruction is the most common cause of hydronephrosis in neonates.[13] Secondary ureteropelvic junction (UPJ) obstruction is caused by kinking or secondary scarring in the presence of high-grade vesicoureteral reflux (VUR). There is an increased risk for VUR in children with UPJ obstruction in the obstructed or contralateral kidney, or both. Diagnosis of a UPJ obstruction can be made by ultrasound. Obstruction of the distal ureter (ureterovesical junction obstruction) causes dilation of the entire ureter, renal pelvis, and calyceal system. An ureterocele is a cystic dilation of the intravesical ureter. Open or endoscopic surgery to relieve an obstruction occurs if there is decline of renal drainage or function.[14]

Hypoplastic or Dysplastic Kidneys

A hypoplastic kidney is small with a decreased number of nephrons. These conditions may be unilateral or bilateral; the occurrence may be incidental or familial. Bilateral hypoplastic kidneys are a common cause of chronic kidney disease in children.[15] Segmental hypoplasia—the Ask-Upmark kidney—may be congenital or secondary to VUR. Systemic hypertension is a common presentation.[16]

Renal dysplasia usually results from abnormal differentiation of the renal tissues; for example, primitive glomeruli and tubules, cysts, and nonrenal tissue (such as cartilage) are found in the dysplastic kidney. Dysplasia may be secondary to antenatal obstruction of the urinary tract from ureteroceles, posterior urethral valves, or prune-belly syndrome (congenital absence of abdominal muscles).

Polycystic Kidney Disease

Polycystic kidney disease (PKD) is an autosomal dominant disease (*PDK1* or *PDK2* gene) or an autosomal recessive inherited disorder (*PKHD1* gene).[17] Affected kidneys have multiple cysts that interfere with renal function. Autosomal dominant polycystic kidney disease (ADPKD) usually presents in late childhood or adulthood with the development of cysts. Cysts in other organs, including the liver, pancreas, and ovaries, may occur. Hypertension, aortic and intracranial aneurysms, and heart valve defects may develop. Autosomal recessive polycystic kidney disease (ARPKD) is often first suspected on a prenatal ultrasound. Epithelial hyperplasia and fluid secretion result in collecting duct cysts.[18]

Renal Agenesis

Renal agenesis (the absence of one or both kidneys) may be unilateral or bilateral, and may occur randomly or be hereditary.

Males are more often affected, and it is usually the left kidney that is absent. The single remaining kidney is often completely normal so that the child can expect a normal, healthy life. By the time the child is several years old, the volume of this kidney may approach twice the normal size to compensate for the absence of a second kidney. In some instances, however, the single kidney is abnormally formed and associated with abnormalities of its collecting system. Because the child has a decreased number of nephrons, there is a risk for "hyperfiltration injury," increasing the chance of developing proteinuria, hypertension, and chronic kidney disease.[19]

Bilateral renal agenesis is a rare disorder that is incompatible with extrauterine life. Approximately 75% of affected children are males. Oligohydramnios (low amount of amniotic fluid) resulting from inadequate fetal urine production leads to underdeveloped lungs and Potter syndrome (wide-set eyes, parrot-beak nose, low-set ears, and receding chin).[20] Renal agenesis can be detected prenatally by ultrasound.

GLOMERULAR DISORDERS

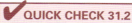

> ✓ **QUICK CHECK 31.2**
> 1. What is the cause of proteinuria?
> 2. What is Wilms tumour and what cellular components are involved?

Common glomerular disorders in children are glomerulonephritis, nephrotic syndrome, immunoglobulin A (IgA) nephropathy, and hemolytic uremic syndrome (HUS). Most glomerular diseases are acquired and immunologically mediated (see Chapter 30, Figure 30.6, and Table 30.5). The disease can be acute or chronic. The likelihood of developing kidney failure depends on the specific condition.

Glomerulonephritis

Glomerulonephritis includes a number of renal disorders in which proliferation and inflammation of the glomeruli are secondary to an immune mechanism (the pathophysiology is described in Chapter 30) and is the causative factor for 9% to 35% of end-stage kidney disease in children worldwide.[21]

Acute Poststreptococcal Glomerulonephritis

Acute poststreptococcal glomerulonephritis (APGN) is one of the most common immune complex–mediated renal diseases in children. It most commonly occurs after a throat or skin infection with a nephritogenic strain of group A beta-hemolytic streptococci, although other bacteria and viruses also may be responsible.[22] Occurrences have been observed after bacterial endocarditis, which may be associated with streptococcal or staphylococcal microorganisms, or after viral diseases, such as varicella-zoster virus and hepatitis B and C. Glomerulonephritis develops with the deposition of antigen–antibody complexes in the glomerulus. The antigen–antibody complex activates complement and the release of inflammatory mediators that damage endothelial and epithelial cells lying on the glomerular basement membrane. Damage to the glomerular basement membrane leads to hematuria and proteinuria.

Symptoms usually begin 1 to 2 weeks after an upper respiratory tract infection (more common during cold weather) and up to 6 weeks after skin infections such as impetigo (more common during warm weather).

The onset of symptoms is abrupt, varying with disease severity. The child typically has gross or microscopic hematuria, proteinuria, edema, and renal insufficiency. Oliguria may be present. Hypertension occurs because of increased vascular volume. Acute hypertension may cause headache, vomiting, somnolence, and other central nervous system manifestations. Cardiovascular symptoms are related to circulatory overload and are compounded by hypertension. These include dyspnea, tachypnea, and an enlarged, tender liver.

Prolonged proteinuria and abnormal glomerular filtration rate (GFR) indicate an unfavourable prognosis. More than 95% of affected children recover completely. Less than 1% of children develop end-stage kidney disease.[23]

Immunoglobulin A Nephropathy

Immunoglobulin A (IgA) nephropathy is the most common form of glomerulonephritis worldwide and occurs more often in males. It is characterized by deposition primarily of immunoglobulin A and complement proteins in the mesangium of the glomerulus. Children with the disease have recurrent gross hematuria concurrent with a respiratory tract infection. Most continue to have microscopic hematuria between the attacks of gross hematuria and have a mild proteinuria as well. Treatment is supportive. Some children recover completely, whereas 20% or more will eventually require dialysis and transplantation.[24] IgA nephropathy may recur following transplantation.[25]

Henoch-Schönlein purpura nephritis is a particular form of IgA nephropathy that involves a systemic vasculitis. In addition to palpable purpura, children may experience abdominal pain, arthralgia, hematuria, and/or proteinuria.[26]

Nephrotic Syndrome

Nephrotic syndrome is characterized by severe proteinuria, hypoalbuminemia, dyslipidemia, and edema. The syndrome is more common in children than in adults. When no identifiable cause is found, the condition is primary (idiopathic) nephrotic syndrome. If it results from a systemic disease or other causes (e.g., medications, toxins), it is called secondary nephrotic syndrome. Primary nephrotic syndrome is found predominantly in the preschool-age child, with a peak incidence of onset between 2 and 3 years of age. It is rare after 8 years of age. Boys are affected more often than girls.

PATHOPHYSIOLOGY The most common causes of primary nephrotic syndrome in children are minimal change nephropathy and focal segmental glomerulosclerosis. Minimal change nephropathy (MCN) (lipoid nephrosis) is characterized by fusion of the glomerular podocyte foot processes, which are seen by electron microscopy. The glomeruli appear normal by light microscopy. A systemic immune mechanism is a likely cause of the disease, but the true etiology is unknown.[27] Loss of the electrical negative charge and increased permeability within the glomerular capillary wall lead to albuminuria. Hypoalbuminemia (causing decreased plasma oncotic pressure) and sodium retention contribute to edema.[28] Dyslipidemia leads to hyperlipiduria and primarily results from increased hepatic lipid synthesis and decreased plasma lipid catabolism.

In idiopathic focal segmental glomerulosclerosis (FSGS), there is segmental loss of glomerular capillaries with proliferation of the mesangial matrix and adhesion of the capillaries to the Bowman capsule.

CLINICAL MANIFESTATIONS The onset of nephrotic syndrome can be insidious, with periorbital edema as the usual first sign. The edema is most noticeable in the morning and subsides during the day as fluid shifts to the abdomen, genitalia, and lower extremities. Parents may notice diminished, frothy, or foamy urine output; or when edema becomes pronounced with ascites, respiratory difficulty from pleural effusion or labial or scrotal swelling may occur. Edema of the intestinal mucosa may cause diarrhea, anorexia, and poor absorption. Edema often masks the malnutrition caused by malabsorption and protein loss. Pallor, with shiny skin and prominent veins, is also common. Blood pressure is usually normal. The child has an increased susceptibility to infection, especially pneumonia, peritonitis, cellulitis, and septicemia. Irritability, fatigue, and lethargy are common. Congenital nephrotic syndrome (Finnish type) is caused by an autosomal recessive mutation of the NPHS1 gene that encodes an immunoglobulin-like protein—nephrin—at the podocyte slit membrane.[29] Congenital nephrotic syndrome (Finnish type) presents with heavy proteinuria, hypoproteinemia, and edema in the first 3 months of life. These babies do not respond to steroid treatment and require albumin infusion and diuretics.[30]

EVALUATION AND TREATMENT Diagnostic testing, including kidney biopsy, may be required to determine whether the cause is an intrinsic kidney disease or a consequence of systemic disease. Basic management of nephrotic syndrome includes administering glucocorticosteroids (prednisone [Deltasone]); adhering to a low-sodium, well-balanced diet; performing good skin care; and, if edema becomes problematic, prescribing diuretics (furosemide [Lasix], metolazone [Zaroxolyn]). Immunosuppressive agents (i.e., cyclophosphamide [Procytox]) may be used with children who have frequent relapses or who are resistant to steroid therapy. Long-term outcomes depend on the underlying cause of the nephrotic syndrome. Children with minimal change disease tend to do very well, whereas those with other conditions may develop end-stage kidney disease.

Hemolytic Uremic Syndrome

Hemolytic uremic syndrome (HUS) is an acute disorder characterized by hemolytic anemia, thrombocytopenia, and acute kidney injury. HUS is the most common cause of acute kidney injury in children. The disease occurs most often in infants and children younger than 4 years of age but has been known to occur in adolescents and adults.

PATHOPHYSIOLOGY HUS has been associated with bacterial and viral agents, as well as endotoxins, especially that from Escherichia coli 0157:H7 and, more recently, E. coli 0104:H4 (Shiga toxins).[31] In HUS, the endothelial lining of the glomerular arterioles becomes swollen and occluded with platelets and fibrin clots. Narrowed vessels damage passing erythrocytes. These damaged red blood cells are removed by the spleen, causing acute hemolytic anemia. Fibrinolysis, the process of dissolution of a clot, acts on precipitated fibrin, causing the fibrin split products to appear in serum and urine. Platelet thrombi develop within damaged vessels, and platelet removal produces thrombocytopenia. Varying degrees of vascular occlusion cause altered renal perfusion and renal insufficiency or failure.[32]

CLINICAL MANIFESTATIONS A prodromal gastro-intestinal illness (fever, vomiting, diarrhea) or, less frequently, an upper respiratory tract infection often precedes the onset of HUS by 1 to 2 weeks. After a symptom-free 1- to 5-day period, the sudden onset of pallor, bruising or purpura, irritability, and oliguria heralds the commencement of the disease. Slight fever, anorexia, vomiting, diarrhea (with the stool characteristically watery and blood stained), abdominal pain, mild jaundice, and circulatory overload are accompanying symptoms. Seizures and lethargy indicate central nervous system involvement. Kidney failure is apparent within the first days of onset. The kidney failure causes metabolic acidosis, azotemia, hyperkalemia, and often hypertension.

EVALUATION AND TREATMENT Clinical evaluation includes history of pre-existing illness, presenting symptoms, and urine and blood analysis. Management is supportive. When kidney failure occurs, dialysis is indicated. Blood transfusions with packed red cells are needed to maintain reasonable hemoglobin levels. Seventy percent of children recover completely. Potential long-term sequelae include renal (hypertension, proteinuria, chronic kidney disease, and end-stage kidney disease) and nonrenal abnormalities (diabetes mellitus, neurological manifestations). In cases unresponsive to treatment, splenectomy may be indicated.[33]

NEPHROBLASTOMA

Nephroblastoma (Wilms tumour) is a rare embryonal tumour of the kidney arising from undifferentiated mesoderm. The peak incidence occurs between 2 and 3 years of age. Nephroblastoma is slightly more common in Black children than in White children. Maternal preconception toxin exposure (e.g., pesticides) may be associated with increased risk in offspring.[34]

PATHOGENESIS Nephroblastoma has both sporadic and inherited origins. The sporadic form occurs in children with no known genetic predisposition. Inherited cases, which are relatively rare, are transmitted in an autosomal dominant fashion. Syndromic and nonsyndromic causes of nephroblastoma have been linked to mutation of several tumour-suppressor genes (i.e., *WT1* and *WT2* mutations).[35]

Eighteen percent of children who have nephroblastoma also have other congenital anomalies. The anomalies associated with nephroblastoma include aniridia (lack of an iris in the eye), hemihyperplasia (an asymmetry of the body), and genito-urinary malformations (i.e., horseshoe kidneys, hypospadias, ureteral duplication, polycystic kidneys).[36] Children with both congenital anomalies and nephroblastoma are more likely to have the inherited bilateral form of the disease.

CLINICAL MANIFESTATIONS Most children with nephroblastoma present with an enlarging asymptomatic abdominal mass before the age of 5 years. Many tumours are actually discovered by the child's parent, who feels or notices an abdominal swelling, usually while dressing or bathing the child. The child appears healthy and thriving. Other presenting complaints include vague abdominal pain, hematuria, anemia, and fever. Hypertension may be present, often as a result of excessive renin secretion by the tumour.[37]

Nephroblastoma may occur in any part of the kidney and varies greatly in size at the time of diagnosis. The tumour generally appears as a solitary mass surrounded by a smooth, fibrous external capsule and also may contain cystic or hemorrhagic areas. A pseudocapsule generally separates the tumour from the renal parenchyma.

EVALUATION AND TREATMENT On physical examination, the tumour feels firm, nontender, and smooth, and is generally confined to one side of the abdomen. If the tumour is palpable past the midline of the abdomen, it may be large or may be arising from a horseshoe or ectopic kidney. Once an abdominal mass is detected, diagnostic imaging demonstrates a solid intrarenal mass.

Diagnosis is based on surgical biopsy. Imaging studies are used to evaluate the presence or absence of metastasis.[38] The most common sites of metastasis are regional lymph nodes and the lungs, and less common sites are the liver, brain, and bone.

Several staging systems for nephroblastoma have been developed and serve as guides to treatment. The most widely accepted system was developed by the National Wilms Tumor Study Group (Table 31.1). Primary treatment is usually surgical exploration and resection or

TABLE 31.1 Staging of Nephroblastoma Tumour[a]

Stage	Tumour Characteristics
I	Tumour limited to kidney; can be completely resected
II	Tumour ascending beyond kidney but is totally resected
III	Residual nonhematogenous tumour confined to abdomen
IV	Hematogenous metastases to organs such as lungs, liver, bone, or brain
V	Bilateral disease either at diagnosis or later, then staged for each kidney

[a]Staging system of the National Wilms Tumor Study Group.

chemotherapy and then surgical resection. Radiation therapy may be used for children with higher stages of disease and metastases. Survival is greater than 90% for localized disease and up to 80% for higher stages, although heart failure, kidney failure, and hypertension occur more frequently in long-term survivors than in the general population.[39]

BLADDER DISORDERS

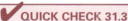

QUICK CHECK 31.3
1. How does the cause of urinary tract infections (UTIs) in newborns differ from that in older children?
2. How does vesicoureteral reflux occur?
3. What organic causes are operative in enuresis?

Urinary Tract Infections

Urinary tract infections (UTIs) are rare in newborns, and children with congenital renal abnormalities and noncircumcised males are at increased risk.[40] UTIs in children are most common in 7- to 11-year-old girls as a result of perineal bacteria, especially *E. coli*, ascending the urethra. Susceptibility, bacterial virulence, and, perhaps, genetics affect the severity of the disease.[41] An abnormal urinary tract (presence of reflux, obstruction, stasis, or stones) is particularly susceptible to infection. Sexually active female adolescents are at increased risk to have a UTI.

Cystitis, or infection of the bladder, results in mucosal inflammation and congestion. This causes detrusor muscle hyperactivity and thus a decrease in bladder capacity, resulting in urgency and frequency. It may also cause distortion of the ureterovesical junction, leading to transient reflux of infected urine up the ureters, causing acute or chronic pyelonephritis.

Differentiating whether an infection is in the bladder or in the kidneys is difficult based on symptoms alone. Infants may be asymptomatic or develop fever, lethargy, abdominal pain, vomiting, diarrhea, or asymptomatic jaundice. Children may present with fever of undetermined origin, frequency, urgency, dysuria, enuresis or incontinence in a previously dry child, flank or back pain, and sometimes hematuria. **Acute pyelonephritis** usually causes chills, high fever, and flank or abdominal pain, along with enlarged kidney(s) caused by inflammatory edema. **Chronic pyelonephritis** may be asymptomatic.

Diagnosis of UTIs is by urine culture. Dipstick analyses for nitrite, leukocyte esterase, and blood may be used as a screening tool. Any positive or strong suspicion of a UTI, including unexplained jaundice in infants,[42] requires urine culture. Diagnostic imaging may be necessary to rule out obstructions, renal scarring, or functional abnormalities. With treatment, UTI symptoms are usually relieved in 1 to 2 days, and the urine becomes sterile. A 2- to 4-day course of oral antibiotics is effective for uncomplicated UTI.[43] Longer treatment may be required if the child has a history of recurrent UTIs or has congenital abnormalities of the urinary tract. If there is no improvement in 2 days, the child should be re-evaluated.

Vesicoureteral Reflux

Vesicoureteral reflux (VUR) is the retrograde flow of urine from the bladder into the kidney or ureters, or both. This allows infected urine from the bladder to reach the kidneys. VUR occurs more often in girls by a ratio of 10:1 and is uncommon in Black individuals. Although reflux is considered abnormal at any age, the shortness of the submucosal tunnel of the ureter during infancy and childhood renders the antireflux mechanism relatively inefficient and delicate. Thus, reflux is seen commonly in association with infections during early childhood but rarely in older children and adults.

PATHOPHYSIOLOGY The normal distal ureter enters the bladder through the detrusor muscle and passes through a submucosal tunnel before opening into the bladder lumen via the ureteral orifice. As the bladder fills with urine, the ureter is compressed within the bladder wall, preventing reflux. Primary VUR results from a congenital abnormally short submucosal tunnel and ureter that permits reflux by the rising pressure of the filling bladder (Figure 31.4). Urine sweeps up into the ureter and then flows back into the empty bladder. The reflux perpetuates infection by preventing complete emptying of the bladder and providing a reservoir for infection. With bladder filling, the maximal intravesical pressure can be transmitted up the ureter to the renal pelvis and calyces. The combination of reflux and infection is an important cause of pyelonephritis. Renal parenchymal injury, scarring, hypertension, and chronic renal insufficiency can occur many years later, making early diagnosis and treatment important. Secondary reflux develops in association with acquired conditions (e.g., neurogenic bladder dysfunction, ureteral obstruction, voiding disorders, or surgery on the ureterovesical junction). Reflux may be unilateral or bilateral, and is graded using the International Reflux Grading System[44] (Figure 31.5):

- Grade I: reflux into a nondilated distal ureter
- Grade II: reflux into the upper collecting system without dilation
- Grade III: reflux into a dilated ureter or blunting of calyceal fornices
- Grade IV: reflux into a grossly dilated ureter and calyces
- Grade V: massive reflux with urethral dilation and tortuosity and effacement of the calyceal details

CLINICAL MANIFESTATIONS Children with reflux may be asymptomatic or have recurrent UTIs, unexplained fevers, poor growth and development, irritability, and feeding problems. The family history may reveal VUR or UTIs.

EVALUATION AND TREATMENT In addition to the history of recurrent UTIs and other symptoms, a voiding cystourethrogram is the primary diagnostic procedure. Most children with VUR respond to nonoperative management aimed at prevention and treatment of infection. Recurrent infection may require endoscopic, open, laparoscopic, and robotic procedures to stop the refluxing ureter.[45]

URINARY INCONTINENCE

Urinary incontinence refers to the involuntary passage of urine by a child who is beyond the age when voluntary bladder control should have been acquired. Bladder control is accomplished by most children before the age of 5 years, although it is largely influenced by cultural beliefs and parental toilet-training practices.

Types of Incontinence

Wetness that occurs during the day is called **daytime incontinence**. Nighttime wetting is called **enuresis**. **Primary incontinence** (enuresis) means the child has never been continent, whereas **secondary incontinence** (enuresis) means the child has been continent for at least 6 months before wetting recurs. A child may have daytime incontinence, enuresis, or a combination of both. (Types of incontinence and clinical manifestations are defined in Table 31.2.)

The incidence of incontinence (or enuresis) is difficult to determine because it is not a problem parents often discuss. Enuresis occurs in as many as 10% of 7-year-old males and resolves at a rate of 15% per year. Daytime incontinence occurs in up to 9% of early school-age children.[46]

PATHOGENESIS A combination of factors is likely responsible for incontinence or enuresis. Organic causes account for a minority of cases and include UTIs; neurological disturbances; congenital defects of the meatus, urethra, or bladder neck; and allergies. Disorders that increase the normal output of urine, such as diabetes mellitus and diabetes insipidus, or disorders that impair the concentrating ability of the kidney, such as chronic kidney disease or sickle cell disease, should be considered during evaluation. Other conditions that

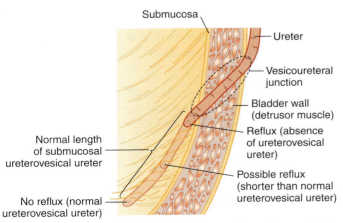

FIGURE 31.4 Normal and Abnormal Configurations of the Ureterovesical Ureter. A refluxing ureterovesical ureter has the same anatomical features as a nonrefluxing ureter, except for the shorter length of the intravesical ureter, which allows reflux of urine during filling of the bladder.

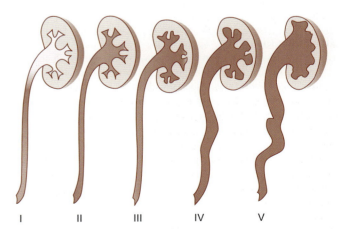

FIGURE 31.5 Grades of Vesicoureteral Reflux. (From Johnson, J. R., Feehally, J., & Floege, J. [2015]. *Comprehensive clinical nephrology* [5th ed.]. Saunders.)

TABLE 31.2 Classification of Incontinence

Type	Definition
Daytime voiding frequency	Decreased: 3 or fewer voids per day Increased: 8 or more voids per day
Dysfunctional voiding	Habitual contraction of urethral sphincter during voiding; observed by uroflow measurements
Enuresis	Incontinence of urine while sleeping
Incontinence, continuous	Continuous leakage, not in discrete portions
Incontinence, stress	Leakage with raised intra-abdominal pressure
Urgency	Sudden, unexpected, immediate need to void
Overactive bladder	Child with urgency; increased voiding frequency, incontinence, or both may or may not be present
Underactive bladder	Decreased voiding frequency with use of raised intra-abdominal pressure to void
Urge incontinence	Incontinence in children with urgency

From Nevéus, T., von Gontard, A., Hoebeke, P., et al. (2006). *Journal of Urology, 176*(1), 314–324.

may be associated with incontinence include perinatal anoxia, central nervous system trauma, seizures, attention-deficit/hyperactivity disorder,[47] developmental delay, imperforate anus, bladder trauma or surgery, obesity,[48] and occult spinal dysraphism. Altered sleep arousal or obstructive sleep apnea[49] may be associated with enuresis. Stressful psychological situations, such as a new sibling, may cause incontinence or enuresis to develop. Constipation is frequently present in children with urinary incontinence.[50] Incontinence or enuresis in which no structural or neurological abnormality is identified is common in children.

Genetic factors contribute to some types of incontinence. At least four gene loci associated with enuresis have been identified. Enuresis occurs with high frequency among parents, siblings, and other near relatives of symptomatic children. There is a high concordance rate in monozygotic twins with enuresis.[51]

EVALUATION AND TREATMENT Diagnostic evaluation of childhood incontinence includes a thorough history, voiding diary, physical examination, and urinalysis. Urodynamic flow studies or imaging may be required based on history and physical findings. Therapeutic management of incontinence or enuresis begins with education. If the child and family understand the probable etiology of the child's condition, they are better able to choose and participate in therapies that are most likely to succeed. Treatment of daytime incontinence includes behavioural therapy, including timed voiding; fluid management; treatment of constipation, UTIs, and other coexisting conditions if present; and medication (anticholinergic or alpha-blocker medications). Enuresis treatment also may include enuresis alarms or other medications (e.g., desmopressin acetate).[52]

DID YOU UNDERSTAND?

Structural Abnormalities
1. Hypospadias is a congenital condition in which the urethral meatus is located anywhere on the ventral surface of the glans, the penile shaft, the midline of the scrotum, or the perineum.
2. Exstrophy of the bladder is a congenital malformation in which the pubic bones are separated, the lower portion of the abdominal wall and anterior wall of the bladder are missing, and the posterior wall of the bladder is everted through the opening.
3. Ureteropelvic junction obstruction is blockage where the renal pelvis joins the ureter and is often caused by smooth muscle or urothelial malformation or by scarring that leads to hydronephrosis.
4. Polycystic kidney disease is a cystic genetic disorder resulting in multiple, bilateral renal cysts.
5. Renal agenesis is the failure of a kidney to grow or develop. The condition may be unilateral or bilateral and may occur as an isolated entity or in association with other disorders.

Glomerular Disorders
1. Glomerulonephritis is an inflammation of the glomeruli characterized by hematuria, edema, and hypertension. Glomerulonephritis may follow infections, especially those of the upper respiratory tract caused by strains of group A beta-hemolytic streptococcus. Increases in glomerular capillary permeability lead to hematuria and proteinuria.
2. Immunoglobulin A (IgA) nephropathy occurs with deposition of IgA in the glomerulus, causing glomerular injury with gross hematuria.
3. *Nephrotic syndrome* is a term used to describe a symptom complex characterized by proteinuria, hypoproteinemia, dyslipidemia, and edema.
4. Hemolytic uremic syndrome is an acute disorder characterized by hemolytic anemia, acute kidney injury, and thrombocytopenia.

Nephroblastoma
1. Nephroblastoma (Wilms tumour) is an embryonal tumour of the kidney that usually presents before the age of 5 years.
2. Bladder Disorders
3. Urinary tract infections (UTIs) can result from general sepsis in the newborn but are caused by bacteria ascending the urethra in older children. The bladder alone is infected in cystitis. The infection ascends to one or both kidneys in pyelonephritis.
4. Vesicoureteral reflux is the retrograde flow of bladder urine into the kidney or ureter, or both, increasing the risk for pyelonephritis. It can be unilateral or bilateral; primary or secondary.

Urinary Incontinence
1. Urinary incontinence is the involuntary passage of urine. It may occur during the day (incontinence) or at night (enuresis), or both. Maturational delay, UTIs, constipation, and many other factors may contribute.

32

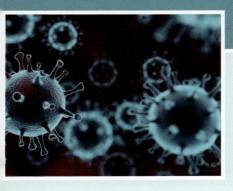

Structure and Function of the Reproductive Systems

Kelly Power-Kean, with originating chapter contributions by George W. Rodway and Sue E. Huether

Additional resources are available online at https://evolve.elsevier.com/Canada/Huether/pathophysiology.

CHAPTER OUTLINE

Development of the Reproductive Systems, 764
 Sexual Differentiation in Utero, 765
 Puberty and Reproductive Maturation, 767
The Female Reproductive System, 767
 External Genitalia, 767
 Internal Genitalia, 768
 Female Sex Hormones, 772
 Menstrual Cycle, 772
Structure and Function of the Breast, 775
 Female Breast, 775
 Male Breast, 777

The Male Reproductive System, 777
 External Genitalia, 777
 Internal Genitalia, 779
 Spermatogenesis, 780
 Male Sex and Reproductive Hormones, 780
Aging and Reproductive Function, 781
 Aging and the Female Reproductive System, 781
 Aging and the Male Reproductive System, 782

LEARNING OBJECTIVES

1. Describe the factors that promote sexual differentiation in utero.
2. Discuss the process of puberty, focusing on the three critical endocrine changes that occur and the role of the anterior pituitary gland.
3. Diagram normal female reproductive anatomy.
4. Describe the normal female reproductive cycle. Include changes in hormone levels and cellular events.
5. Diagram normal male reproductive anatomy.
6. Discuss the vascular and hormonal order of events needed for ejaculation of sperm.
7. Discuss the order of events that occurs during ovulation and menstruation.
8. Name the male and female hormones that regulate secondary sexual characteristics and reproductive functions.
9. Describe the functions of the female breast.
10. Discuss the cyclical, hormone-mediated changes in breast tissue that occur during the reproductive years and in pregnancy.
11. Discuss the normal age-related changes in the male and female reproductive systems.

KEY TERMS

Acinus (*pl.*, acini) of breast, 776
Activin, 775
Adrenarche, 767
Androgen, 767
Andropause, 782
Areola, 777
Breast, 775
Bulbourethral gland (Cowper gland), 780
Cervix, 769
Cornification, 775
Corpus (body of uterus), 769
Corpus cavernosum (*pl.*, corpora cavernosa), 779
Corpus luteum, 771
Corpus spongiosum, 779
Cul-de-sac, 768
Decornification, 775
Efferent tubule, 778
Ejaculatory duct, 780
Emission, 779
Endocervical canal, 769
Endometrium, 769
Epididymis (*pl.*, epididymides), 778
Erectile reflex, 779
Estradiol (E_2), 772
Estrogen, 772
Fallopian tube (uterine tube), 771
Fimbriae, 771
Follicle-stimulating hormone (FSH), 766
Follicular/proliferative phase, 774
Follistatin, 775
Fornix, 768
Fundus, 769
Glands of Montgomery, 777
Glans, 779
Gonad, 765
Gonadarche, 767
Gonadostat (gonadotropin-releasing hormone pulse generator), 767
Gonadotropin-releasing hormone (GnRH), 766
Granulosa cell, 772
Infundibulum, 771
Inguinal canal, 777
Inhibin, 775
Ischemic/menstrual phase, 774
Isthmus, 769
Leydig cell, 778
Libido, 781
Luteal/secretory phase, 774
Luteinizing hormone (LH), 766
Menarche, 772
Menopause, 772
Menstruation (menses), 774
Myometrium, 769
Nipple, 777
Ovarian cycle, 772
Ovarian follicle, 771
Ovary, 771
Ovulation, 774
Ovum (*pl.*, ova), 764
Oxytocin, 777
Penis, 779

Perimetrium (parietal peritoneum), 769
Prepuce (foreskin), 779
Primary spermatocyte, 780
Progesterone, 772
Prostate gland, 780
Puberty, 767
Rete testis, 778
Ruga (*pl.*, rugae), 768
Scrotum, 779
Secondary spermatocyte, 780
Semen, 779
Seminal vesicle, 779
Seminiferous tubule, 778
Sertoli cell (nondividing support cell), 780
Sex hormone, 764
Spermatid, 780
Spermatogenesis, 780
Spermatogonium (*pl.*, spermatogonia), 780
Spermatozoon (sperm cell), 764
Spinnbarkeit mucus, 770
Squamocolumnar junction, 770
Testis, 778
Testosterone, 766
Theca cell, 772
Thelarche, 767
Tubulus rectus, 778
Tunica albuginea, 778
Tunica dartos, 779
Tunica vaginalis, 778
Urethra, 779
Uterus, 769
Vagina, 768
Vas deferens, 779
Vasomotor flush, 782
Vulva, 767

The male and female reproductive systems have several anatomical and physiological features in common. Most obvious is their major function, reproduction. In this process a 23-chromosome female gamete, the ovum, and a 23-chromosome male gamete, the **spermatozoon (sperm cell)**, join to form a 46-chromosome zygote. The zygote can develop into a new individual. The male reproductive system produces sperm that can be transferred to the female reproductive tract. The female reproductive system produces the **ovum** (*pl.*, **ova**). If fertilization of the ovum occurs it is then called the *embryo* and *developing fetus*. These functions are determined by anatomical structures and complex hormonal and neurological factors.[1]

DEVELOPMENT OF THE REPRODUCTIVE SYSTEMS

  QUICK CHECK 32.1
1. When do sex hormones first influence sexual development?
2. Why are sex hormones needed for reproduction?

The structure and function of both male and female reproductive systems depend on steroid hormones called **sex hormones** and their precursors. Cholesterol is the precursor for steroid hormones, including the sex hormones. Other hormones support reproduction. Table 32.1

TABLE 32.1 Summary of Female and Male Sex and Reproductive Hormones

Hormone (Source)	Action in Females	Action in Males
Dehydroepiandrosterone (DHEA) (adrenal gland, ovary, other tissues)	Converted to androstenedione and then to estrogens, testosterone, or both	Converted to androstenedione and then to estrogens, testosterone, or both
Estrogens (estrone, estradiol, estriol) function through estrogen receptors alpha and beta (ovary and placenta, small amounts in other tissues)	Stimulates development of female sexual characteristics: maturation of breast, uterus, and vagina; promotes proliferative development of endometrium during menstrual cycle; during pregnancy promotes mammary gland development, fetal adrenal gland function, and uteroplacental blood flow (see Box 32.1)	Growth at puberty, growth plate fusion in bone, prevention of apoptosis of germ cells
Testosterone (adrenal glands from DHEA, ovaries)	Contributes to libido, learning, sleep, protein anabolism, growth of muscle and bone; growth of pubic and axillary hair; activation of sebaceous glands, accounting for some cases of acne during puberty	Stimulates spermatogenesis, stimulates development of primary and secondary sexual characteristics, promotes growth of muscle and bone (anabolic effect); growth of pubic and axillary hair; activates sebaceous glands, causing some cases of acne during puberty; supports libido
Gonadotropin-releasing hormone (GnRH) (hypothalamus-neuroendocrine cells)	Stimulates secretion of gonadotropins (FSH and LH) from anterior pituitary	Stimulates secretion of gonadotropins (FSH and LH) from anterior pituitary
Follicle-stimulating hormone (FSH) (anterior pituitary, gonadotroph cells)	Gonadotropin; promotes development of ovarian follicle; stimulates estrogen secretion	Gonadotropin; promotes development of testes and stimulates spermatogenesis by Sertoli cells
Luteinizing hormone (LH) (anterior pituitary, gonadotroph cells)	Gonadotropin; triggers ovulation; promotes development of corpus luteum	Gonadotropin; stimulates testosterone production by Leydig cells of testis
Inhibin (ovary and testes)	Inhibits FSH production in anterior pituitary (perhaps by limiting GnRH)	Inhibits FSH production in anterior pituitary
Human chorionic gonadotropin (hCG) (placenta)	Supports corpus luteum, which secretes estrogen and progesterone during first 7 weeks of pregnancy	
Activin (ovary)	Stimulates secretion of FSH and pituitary response to GnRH and FSH binding in dominant granulosa cells	
Progesterone (ovary and placenta)	Promotes secretory changes in endometrium during luteal phase of menstrual cycle; quiets uterine myometrium (muscle) activity and prevents lactogenesis during pregnancy	
Relaxin (corpus luteum, myometrium and placenta)	Inhibits uterine contractions during pregnancy and softens pelvic joints and cervix to ease childbirth	

summarizes the actions of sex and reproductive hormones. Sex hormones, like all hormones, act on target tissues by binding with cellular receptors (see Chapter 18). Hormonal effects on the reproductive systems begin during embryonic development. The effects of hormones continue in varying degrees throughout life.

Sexual Differentiation in Utero

Initially, in embryonic development, the reproductive structures of male and female embryos are homologous (the same) or undifferentiated. They consist of one pair of primary sex organs, or **gonads**, and two pairs of ducts—the mesonephric ducts (wolffian ducts) and the paramesonephric ducts (Müllerian ducts) (Figure 32.1). The Müllerian ducts are the precursor of the internal female sex organs (oviducts, uterus, cervix, and upper vagina). The initial formation of Müllerian ducts occurs regardless of genotypic sex. Formation of these ducts require no SRY signalling for development. SRY signalling is needed in males to cause regression of the Müllerian ducts. This process prevents the development of the female reproductive tract. The wolffian ducts are the precursor of male internal sex organs. These ducts secrete testosterone and promote development of the male sex organs.

The first sign of development of reproductive organs (male or female) occurs during the fifth week of gestation. Between 6 to 8 weeks of gestation, the male embryo will differentiate under the influence of testes-determining factor (TDF). TDF is a protein expressed by a gene in the sex-determining region on the Y chromosome (SRY). When expression of the SRY gene occurs, male gonadal development follows. TDF stimulates the male gonads to develop into the two testes. Between 8 to 9 weeks' gestation testosterone secretion begins. Müllerian inhibitory hormone (MIF), secreted by Sertoli cells in the testes, promotes degeneration of the Müllerian ducts. Without MIF, the Müllerian ducts would develop and the wolffian ducts would degenerate. The result would be a loss of male sex organ development. By 9 months' gestation, the male gonads (testes) have descended into the scrotum. The testes produce sperm after puberty.

Female gonadal development occurs in the absence of SRY expression and with the expression of other genes.[2] The presence of estrogen and the absence of testosterone and MIF cause a loss in the wolffian system. At 6 to 8 weeks' gestation the two female gonads develop into ovaries, which will produce ova. In females, the mesonephric ducts deteriorate. The upper ends of paramesonephric ducts become the fallopian tubules.

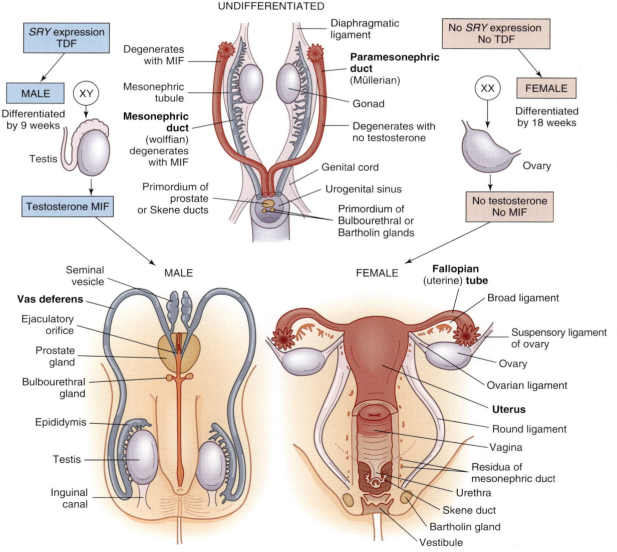

FIGURE 32.1 Internal Genitalia Development. Embryonic and fetal development of the internal genitalia. *MIF*, Müllerian inhibitory factor; *SRY*, sex-determining region on the Y chromosome (it produces TDF); *TDF*, testes-determining factor; see text for more details.

The lower ends of these ducts join to become the uterus, cervix, and upper two-thirds of the vagina (see Figure 32.1). The fallopian tubes will carry ova from the ovaries to the uterus during a woman's reproductive years. Lack of testosterone and the presence of estrogen promote the development of external genitalia (lower end of vagina, labia, and clitoris).

Like the internal reproductive structures, the external structures develop from homologous embryonic tissues. During the first 7 to 8 weeks' gestation, both male and female embryos develop an elevated structure called the *genital tubercle* (Figure 32.2). **Testosterone** is needed for the genital tubercle to differentiate into external male genitalia. Without testosterone the female genitalia develop. This development may occur even in the absence of ovaries possibly related to the presence of placental estrogens.

Anterior pituitary development begins between the fourth and fifth weeks of fetal life. The vascular connection between the hypothalamus and the pituitary occurs by the twelfth week. The production of **gonadotropin-releasing hormone (GnRH)** in the hypothalamus occurs by 10 weeks' gestation. GnRH controls the production of two gonadotropins, **luteinizing hormone (LH)** and **follicle-stimulating hormone (FSH)**, by the anterior pituitary gland. The excretion of high levels of FSH and LH occurs in the female fetus. FSH and LH stimulate the production of estrogen and progesterone by the ovary. The production of FSH and LH increases until about 28 weeks' gestation. At that time the production of estrogen and progesterone by the ovaries and placenta is high enough to result in the decline of gonadotropin production.[3] Production of primitive female gametes (ova) occurs only during fetal life. From puberty to

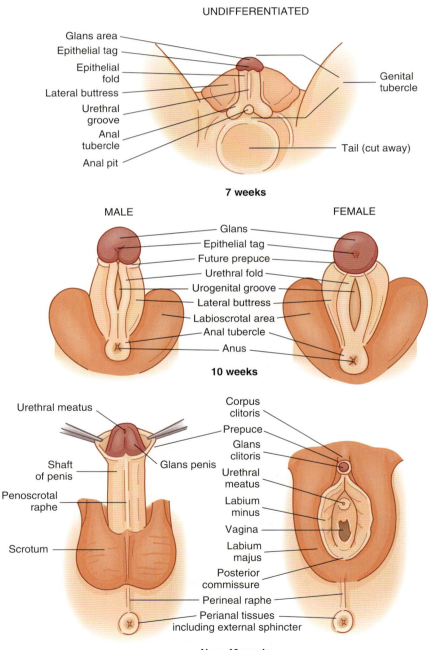

FIGURE 32.2 External Genitalia Development. Embryonic and fetal development of the external genitalia.

menopause, one female gamete matures per menstrual cycle. Production of the male gametes (sperm) begins at puberty. After puberty the production of millions of sperm occurs daily, usually for life.

By the end of pregnancy, a negative feedback system, which includes the gonadostat (also known as the **gonadotropin-releasing hormone pulse generator**), is active in the fetus. The gonadostat responds to high levels of placental estrogens by releasing low levels of GnRH. Soon after birth, steroid hormone levels drop. This decrease is due to the loss of maternal placental hormones. The secretion of hypothalamic pulsatile GnRH and the release of gonadotropins LH and FSH occurs. These hormone levels peak at 3 to 6 months for boys and at 12 to 18 months for girls and then fall steadily. The suppression of gonadotropins will occur until the onset of puberty.

Puberty and Reproductive Maturation

Puberty is the onset of sexual maturation and differs from adolescence. Adolescence is the stage of human development between childhood and adulthood. Adolescence includes social, psychological, and biological changes. In girls, puberty begins at about age 8 to 9 years with thelarche (breast development). In boys, puberty begins at about age 11 years but occurs earlier with increased weight and body mass index.[4] Genetics, environment, ethnicity, general health, and nutrition can influence the timing of puberty. There is an association between obesity and earlier puberty in girls. This early onset is perhaps from higher estrogen levels related to leptin, gonadotropin, and estrogen secretion.[5] Girls who have low body fat and reduced body weight and perform intense exercise may experience delayed maturation.[6]

Reproductive maturation involves the hypothalamic-pituitary-gonadal axis, the central nervous system, and the endocrine system (Figure 32.3). There is a sequential series of hormonal events that promote sexual maturation as puberty approaches. About 1 year before puberty in girls, nighttime pulses of gonadotropin secretion (i.e., LH and FSH) and an increased response in the pituitary to GnRH occur. This gonadotropin secretion and increased pituitary response stimulates gonadal maturation (gonadarche). Estradiol secretion occurs in girls and testosterone secretion in boys. Estradiol causes development of the breasts (thelarche), maturation of the reproductive organs (vagina, uterus, ovaries), and the deposit of fat in the female's hips. Estrogen and increased production of growth factors cause rapid skeletal growth in both genders. Testosterone causes growth of the testes, scrotum, and penis. The creation of a positive feedback loop occurs with gonadotropins stimulating the gonads to produce more sex hormones. The most important hormonal effects occur in the gonads. In males, the testes begin to produce mature sperm that can fertilize an ovum. Male puberty is complete with the first ejaculation that has mature sperm. In females, the ovaries begin to release mature ova. Female puberty is complete at the time of the first ovulatory menstrual period. Puberty can take up to 1 to 2 years to complete after menarche. Adrenarche is the increased production of adrenal androgens (dehydroepiandrosterone [DHEA] and androstenedione). The conversion of these hormones into testosterone and estrogen occurs before puberty in both sexes. Manifestations of this increase includes growth of axillary and pubic hair and activation of sweat and sebaceous glands. Puberty is complete when an individual is able to reproduce.

THE FEMALE REPRODUCTIVE SYSTEM

> **QUICK CHECK 32.2**
> 1. Where are the Bartholin glands found? What is their function?
> 2. Name three functions of the uterus.
> 3. What is the name of the cells where cervical cancer is most likely to grow?

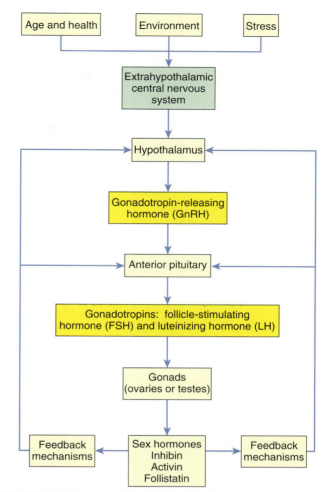

FIGURE 32.3 Hormonal Stimulation of the Gonads. The hypothalamic-pituitary-gonadal axis.

The function of the female reproductive system is to produce mature ova. If fertilization occurs, the female reproductive system supplies protection and nourishment of the fetus until it is expelled at birth. The most important internal reproductive organs in females are the ovaries, fallopian tubes, uterus, and vagina. The external genitalia protect body openings and play an important role in sexual functioning.

External Genitalia

Figure 32.4 shows the external female genitalia, known collectively as the vulva, or pudendum. The major structures are:

Mons pubis: Fatty layer of tissue over pubic symphysis (joint formed by union of the pubic bones). During puberty it becomes covered with pubic hair. The sebaceous and sweat glands also become more active. Estrogen causes fat deposition under the skin, gives the mons pubis a moundlike shape, and protects the pubic symphysis during sexual intercourse.

Labia majora (sing., labium majus): Two folds of skin starting at the mons pubis and extending back to the fourchette, forming a cleft. During puberty, the amount of fatty tissue increases, pubic hair grows on lateral surfaces, and sebaceous glands on hairless medial surfaces secrete lubricants. This structure is highly sensitive to temperature, touch, pressure, and pain. It is the equivalent to the male scrotum. It protects the inner structures of the vulva.

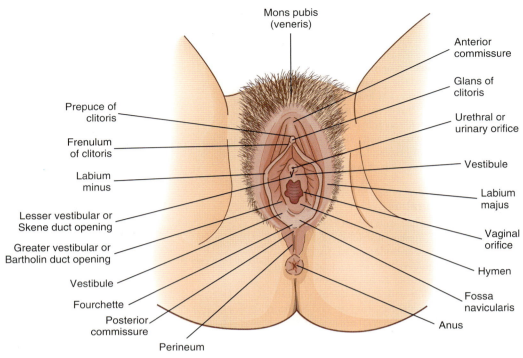

FIGURE 32.4 External Female Genitalia.

Labia minora (sing., labium minus): Two smaller, thinner, uneven folds of skin within the labia majora that form the clitoral hood (prepuce) and frenulum. It then splits to enclose the vestibule, and converges near the anus to form the fourchette. The labia minora are hairless, pink, and moist. They are supplied by nerves, blood vessels, and sebaceous glands that secrete bactericidal fluid. The fluid has a distinctive odour that lubricates and waterproofs vulvar skin. The labia swell with blood during sexual arousal.

Clitoris: Well innervated erectile organ between the labia minora. It is a small, cylindrical structure having a visible glans and a shaft that lies beneath the skin. The clitoris is equivalent to the penis. It secretes smegma. Smegma has a unique odour that may be sexually arousing to the male. Like the penis, the clitoris is a major site of sexual stimulation and orgasm. With sexual arousal, erectile tissue fills with blood. This filling process causes the clitoris to enlarge slightly.

Vestibule: An area protected by the labia minora. The vestibule holds the external opening of the vagina, called the *introitus* or vaginal orifice. A thin membrane, the *hymen*, may cover the introitus. The vestibule also has the opening of the urethra, or *urinary meatus* (orifice). Lubrication of these structures occurs by two pairs of glands: Skene glands and Bartholin glands. The ducts of the *Skene glands* (also called the *lesser vestibular* or *paraurethral glands*) open on both sides of the urinary meatus. The ducts of the *Bartholin glands* (*greater vestibular* or *vulvovaginal glands*) open on either side of the introitus. In response to sexual stimulation, Bartholin glands secrete mucus that lubricates the inner labial surfaces. This mucus also enhances the viability and motility of sperm. Skene glands help lubricate the urinary meatus and the vestibule. Secretions from both sets of glands help coitus. In response to sexual excitement, the vascular tissue beneath the vestibule also fills with blood and becomes engorged.

Perineum: An area with less hair, skin, and subcutaneous tissue. This structure lies between the vaginal orifice and anus. Unlike the rest of the vulva, this area has little subcutaneous fat. As a result, the skin is close to the underlying muscles. The perineum covers the muscular *perineal body*. This body is a fibrous structure that is made of elastic fibres and connective tissue. It serves as the common attachment for the bulbocavernosus, external anal sphincter, and levator ani muscles. The perineum varies in length from 2 to 5 cm or more and has elastic properties. The length of the perineum and the elasticity of the perineal body affect tissue resistance and injury during childbirth.

Internal Genitalia

Vagina

The **vagina** is an elastic, fibromuscular canal that is 9 to 10 cm long in a reproductive-age female. It extends up and back from the introitus to the lower part of the uterus. Figure 32.5 shows that the vagina lies between the urethra (and part of the bladder) and the rectum. Mucosal secretions from the upper genital organs, menstrual fluids, and products of conception leave the body through the vagina. The vagina also receives the penis during coitus. During sexual excitement, the vagina lengthens and widens and the anterior third becomes filled with blood.

The vaginal wall is composed of four layers:

1. Mucous membrane lining of squamous epithelial cells. This lining thickens and thins in response to hormones, particularly estrogen. The squamous epithelial membrane is continuous with the membrane that covers the lower part of the uterus. In women of reproductive age, the mucosal layer is composed of transverse wrinkles, or folds, called **rugae (sing., ruga)**. The rugae allow stretching during coitus and childbirth
2. Fibrous connective tissue having many blood and lymphatic vessels
3. Smooth muscle
4. Connective tissue and a rich network of blood vessels

The upper part of the vagina surrounds the cervix, the lower end of the uterus (see Figure 32.5). The **fornix** of the vagina is the recessed space around the cervix. The posterior fornix is "deeper" than the anterior fornix. This deepness is because of the angle at which the cervix meets the vaginal canal. In most women, this angle is about 90 degrees. A pouch called the **cul-de-sac** separates the posterior fornix and the rectum.

CHAPTER 32 Structure and Function of the Reproductive Systems

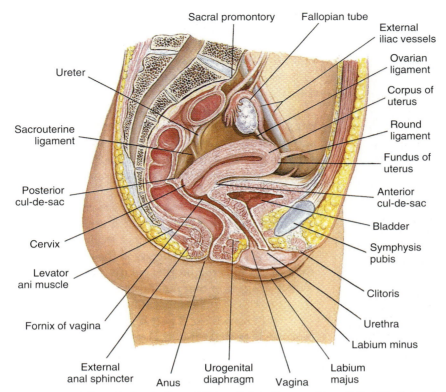

FIGURE 32.5 Internal Female Genitalia and Other Pelvic Organs. (From Ball, J. W., Dains, J. E., Flynn, J. A., et al. [2015]. *Seidel's guide to physical examination* [8th ed.]. Mosby.)

Its elasticity and relatively sparse nerve supply enhance the vagina's function as the birth canal. During sexual arousal, the vaginal wall becomes engorged with blood, like the labia minora and clitoris. Engorgement pushes some fluid to the surface of the mucosa, enhancing lubrication. The vaginal wall does not have mucus-secreting glands. Secretions drain into the vagina from the endocervical glands or from the Bartholin and Skene glands of the vestibule.

Two factors help to support the self-cleansing action of the vagina and to defend it from infection. They are (1) an acid–base balance that discourages the growth of most pathogenic bacteria and (2) the thickness of the vaginal epithelium. Before puberty, vaginal pH is about 7.0 (neutral) and the vaginal epithelium is thin. At puberty, the pH becomes more acidic (4.0 to 5.0), and the squamous epithelial lining thickens. These changes are supported until menopause (cessation of menstruation). At menopause the pH rises again to more alkaline levels and the epithelium thins. Therefore, protection from infection is greatest during the years when a woman is most likely to be sexually active. Both defence factors are greatest when estrogen levels are high and the vagina has a normal population of *Lactobacillus acidophilus*. This harmless resident bacterium helps to keep pH at acidic levels. Any condition that causes vaginal pH to rise lowers vaginal defences against infection. Douching or use of vaginal sprays or deodorants, the presence of low estrogen levels, or destruction of *L. acidophilus* by antibiotics can increase the vaginal pH.

Uterus

The **uterus** is a hollow, pear-shaped organ whose lower end opens into the vagina. It anchors and protects a fertilized ovum, supplies a best environment while the ovum develops, and pushes the fetus out at birth. In addition, the uterus plays an important role in sexual response and conception. During sexual excitement, the opening of the lower uterus (the cervix) dilates slightly. At the same time, the uterus increases in size and moves upward and backward, creating a tenting effect in the midvagina. This tenting effect results in the cervix "sitting" in a pool of semen. During orgasm, rhythmic contractions help movement of sperm through the cervical os while also enhancing physical pleasure.

At puberty, the uterus reaches its adult size and proportions. The uterus descends from the abdomen to the lower pelvis, between the bladder and the rectum (see Figure 32.5). The uterus of a mature, non-pregnant female is approximately 7 to 9 cm long and 6.5 cm wide. It has muscular 3.5 cm thick walls and enlarges about 1 cm in all dimensions after pregnancy.[7] Ligaments, peritoneal tissue folds, and the pressure of adjacent organs, especially the urinary bladder, sigmoid colon, and rectum hold the uterus in position. In most women, the uterus is tipped forward (anteverted) so that it rests on the urinary bladder. However, it may be tipped backward (retroverted). Various degrees of flexion are normal (Figure 32.6).

The uterus has two major parts: the body, or **corpus**, and the cervix (Figure 32.7). The **fundus** is the top of the corpus, above the insertion of the fallopian tubes. The diameter of the uterine cavity is widest at the fundus and narrowest at the **isthmus**, just above the **cervix** (see Figure 32.5). The cervix, or "neck of the uterus," extends from the isthmus to the vagina. The **endocervical canal** is the passageway between the upper opening (the internal os) and the lower opening (the external os) of the cervix (see Figure 32.7). The nerve supply of the entire uterus, like the upper vagina, is by motor and sensory fibres of the autonomic nervous system.

The uterine wall is composed of three layers (see Figure 32.7). The **perimetrium (parietal peritoneum)** is the outer serous membrane that covers the uterus. The **myometrium** is the thick, muscular middle layer. It is thickest at the fundus, apparently to help birth. The **endometrium**, or uterine lining, is made of a functional layer (superficial compact layer and spongy middle layer) and a basal layer. The functional layer of the endometrium responds to the sex hormones estrogen

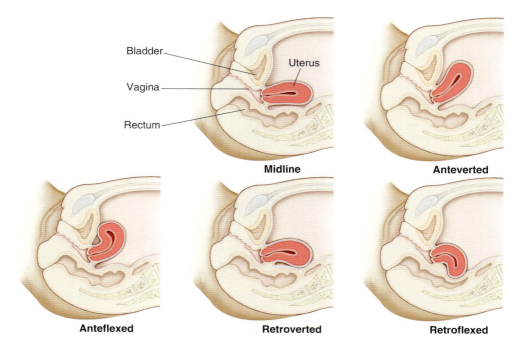

FIGURE 32.6 Variations in Uterine Positions.

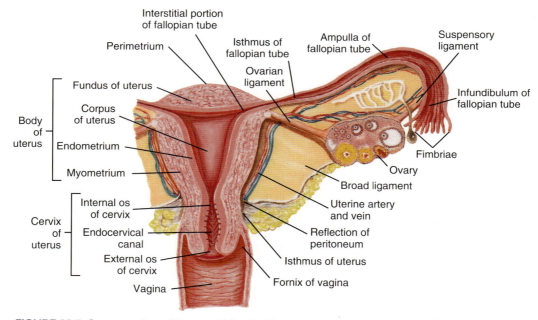

FIGURE 32.7 Cross-section of Uterus, Fallopian Tube, and Ovary. (From Ball, J. W., Dains, J. E., Flynn, J. A., et al. [2015]. *Seidel's guide to physical examination* [8th ed.]. Mosby.)

and progesterone. This layer proliferates and sheds monthly between puberty and menopause. Attached to the myometrium is the basal layer that renews the functional layer after shedding (menstruation).

The lining of the endocervical canal is made up of columnar epithelial cells. It is continuous with the lining of the outer cervix and vagina. Squamous epithelial cells line these two structures. The *transformation zone*, or **squamocolumnar junction** is the point where the two types of cells meet. The transformation zone is vulnerable to the human papillomavirus (HPV). HPV infection can lead to cervical dysplasia or carcinoma in situ (see Figure 33.16). The removal and examination of cells from the transformation zone occurs as a result of a Papanicolaou (Pap test) smear.[7]

The cervix acts as a mechanical barrier to infectious microorganisms from the vagina. The external cervical os is a very small opening that has thick, sticky mucus (the mucous "plug") during the luteal phase of the menstrual cycle and throughout pregnancy. During ovulation, the mucus changes under the influence of estrogen and forms watery strands, or **spinnbarkeit mucus**. This mucous helps the transport of sperm into the uterus. The downward flow of cervical secretions also moves microorganisms away from the cervix and uterus.

In women of reproductive age, the pH of these secretions is hostile to many bacteria. Further, mucosal secretions have enzymes and antibodies (mostly immunoglobulin A [IgA]) of the secretory immune system. Uterine pathophysiological disorders include infection, displacement of the uterus within the pelvis, benign growths (fibroids) of the uterine wall, hyperplasia of the endometrium, endometriosis, and cancer (see Chapter 33).

Fallopian Tubes

> **QUICK CHECK 32.3**
> 1. What hormones does the ovary produce?
> 2. Why is the ovary the most important female reproductive organ?

The two **fallopian tubes** (oviducts, **uterine tubes**) enter the uterus bilaterally just beneath the fundus (see Figure 32.7). They direct the ova from the spaces around the ovaries to the uterus. From the uterus, the fallopian tubes curve up and over the two ovaries. Each tube is 8 to 12 cm long and about 1 cm in diameter, except at its ovarian end where it is fringed or fimbriated (**infundibulum**). The **fimbriae** (fringes) move, creating a current that draws the ovum into the infundibulum. Once the ovum enters the fallopian tube, cilia (hairlike structures) and peristalsis (muscle contractions) keep it moving toward the uterus.

The ampulla, or distal third, of the fallopian tube is the usual site of fertilization (see Figure 32.7). Sperm released into the vagina travel upward through the endocervical canal and uterine cavity and enter the fallopian tubes. If an ovum is present in either tube, fertilization can occur. Whether or not the ovum encounters sperm, it continues to travel through the fallopian tube to the uterus. If fertilized, the ovum (then called a *blastocyst*) implants itself in the endometrial layer of the uterine wall. If not fertilized, the ovum fragments and leaves the uterus with menstrual fluids. Disorders that affect the fallopian tubes (e.g., congenital malformations, infection, and inflammation) block the path of both sperm and the ovum. The blockage may cause infertility or ectopic (tubal) pregnancy.

Ovaries

The **ovaries**, the female gonads, are the primary female reproductive organs (Figure 32.8). Their two main functions are secretion of female sex hormones and development and release of female gametes, or ova.

The almond-shaped ovaries are found on both sides of the uterus. The mesovarium portions of the broad ligament, ovarian ligaments, and suspensory ligaments support the uterus (see Figure 32.7). The ovaries are smaller than their male equivalent, the testes. In women of reproductive age, each ovary is about 3 to 5 cm long, 2.5 cm wide, and 2 cm thick and weighs 4 to 8 g. Size and weight vary slightly during each phase of the menstrual cycle.

At birth, the cortex of each ovary has approximately 1 to 2 million ova within primordial (immature) **ovarian follicles**. By puberty, the number ranges between 300 000 and 500 000. At puberty some of the follicles and the ova within them begin to mature. Between puberty and menopause, the ovarian cortex always has follicles and ova in various stages of development (primary and secondary follicles). Once every menstrual cycle (about every 28 days), one of the follicles reaches maturation and discharges its ovum through the ovary's outer covering, the germinal epithelium. During the reproductive years, 400 to 500 ovarian follicles mature completely and release an ovum (ovulation). The remaining follicles either do not develop or degenerate without maturing completely. They are known as atretic follicles[7] (see Figure 32.8).

After release of the mature ovum (ovulation), the follicle develops into the **corpus luteum** (see Figure 32.8). If fertilization occurs, the

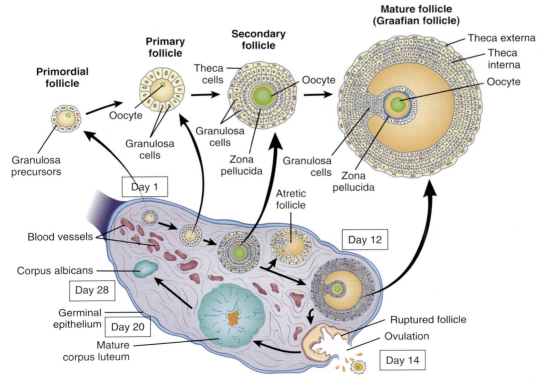

FIGURE 32.8 Cross-section of Ovary and Development of an Ovarian Follicle. Schematic representation (not to scale) of the structure of the ovary, showing the various stages in the development of the follicle and the corpus luteum. (Adapted from Berne, R. M., & Levy, M. N. [Eds.]. [2003]. *Physiology* [5th ed.]. Mosby.)

corpus luteum enlarges and begins to secrete hormones that support pregnancy. If fertilization does not occur, the corpus luteum secretes these hormones for about 14 days and then degenerates. This degeneration triggers the maturation of another follicle. The ovarian cycle is the process of follicular maturation, ovulation, corpus luteum development, and corpus luteum degeneration. This cycle continues from puberty to menopause, except during pregnancy or hormonal contraceptive use. At menopause, this process stops and the ovaries atrophy to the point that they cannot be felt during a pelvic examination.

The secretion of sex hormones occurs from cells present within the ovarian cortex. This includes two types of cells in the ovarian follicle, theca cells (produce androgens that migrate to granulosa cells) and granulosa cells (convert androgens to estradiol), and cells of the corpus luteum (secrete primarily progesterone, estrogen, and inhibin) (see Figure 32.8). These cells all have receptors for the gonadotropins (LH, FSH) or for the sex hormones.

Female Sex Hormones

The sex hormones are all steroid hormones. They are made from cholesterol (see Chapter 18). Both male and female sex hormones are present in all adults (see Table 32.1). The female body has low levels of testosterone and other androgens. The male body has low levels of estrogen. Individual effects of sex hormones depend on the amount and concentration in the blood.

Estrogens and Androgens

Estrogen is a generic term for any of three similar hormones derived from cholesterol: estradiol, estrone, and estriol. Estradiol (E2) is the most potent and plentiful of the three. It is mainly produced (95%) by the ovaries (ovarian follicle and corpus luteum). The cortices of the adrenal glands and the placenta secrete limited amounts during pregnancy. The conversion of androgens in ovarian and adipose tissue creates estrone. Estriol is the metabolite of estrone and estradiol.

Estrogen has several biological effects, many of which involve interactions with other hormones. Maturation of reproductive organs, development of secondary sex characteristics, growth, and maintenance of pregnancy require estrogen. There are many nonreproductive effects of estrogen. These effects include closure of long bones after the pubertal growth spurt (in both males and females), maintenance of bone and skin, and general organ function (see Table 32.1 and Box 32.1). After menopause, the ovaries dramatically reduce production of estradiol and secretion of estrone is greatly decreased (see "Aging and the Female Reproductive System"). Currently, most of the estradiol comes from intracellular synthesis in peripheral tissues. Estradiol acts locally to meet physiological needs according to cell type. The inactivation of estradiol occurs without systemic effects.[8]

Androgens are primarily male sex hormones produced in the testes. However, the adrenal cortex in both men and women, and the ovaries in women produce small amounts of androgens. Some androgens (DHEA and its metabolite androstenedione) are precursors of estrogens (estrone, estradiol) (see Table 32.1). At puberty, androgens contribute to the skeletal growth spurt and cause growth of pubic and axillary hair. Androgens also activate sebaceous glands, accounting for some cases of acne during puberty, and play a role in libido.

Progesterone

LH from the anterior pituitary stimulates the corpus luteum to secrete progesterone. Progesterone is the second major female sex hormone. With estrogen, progesterone controls the ovarian menstrual cycle. LH surge occurs when there is a peak level of estrogen, about 24 to 36 hours before ovulation. LH promotes luteinization of the granulosa in the dominant follicle. This action results in progesterone production and the development of blood vessels and connective tissue. During the follicular phase, the ovary and adrenal glands each contribute about 50% of the progesterone production. Conversely, a cyclical secretion of large amounts from the ovary occurs while the corpus luteum is active for about 9 to 13 days after ovulation. Table 32.2 lists the complementary and opposing effects of progesterone and estrogen. Progesterone secreted by the corpus luteum stimulates the thickened endometrium to become more complex. This thickening occurs in preparation for implantation of a blastocyte. If conception and implantation occurs, the corpus luteum persists and secretes progesterone (and estrogen) until the placenta is well established. This occurs at approximately 8 to 10 weeks' gestation when the placenta undertakes progesterone production.

Progesterone is also known as the *hormone of pregnancy*. Progesterone's effects in pregnancy include (1) maintaining the thickened endometrium; (2) relaxing smooth muscle in the myometrium, which prevents premature contractions and helps the uterus to expand; (3) thickening (hypertrophy) the myometrium, which prepares it for the muscular work of labour; (4) promoting growth of lobules and alveoli in the breast in preparation for lactation, but preventing lactation until the fetus is born and then promoting lactation in collaboration with prolactin after birth; (5) preventing additional maturation of ova by suppressing FSH and LH, thereby stopping the menstrual cycle; and (6) providing immune modulation, allowing tolerance against fetal antigens (the mother's immune system does not attack the fetus).[9]

Menstrual Cycle

>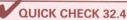
> **QUICK CHECK 32.4**
> 1. Why does menstruation occur?
> 2. What event is associated with the luteal/secretory phase of the menstrual cycle?

In addition to pregnancy, the obvious manifestation of female reproductive functioning is menstrual bleeding (the menses). Menses starts with menarche (first menstruation) and ends with menopause (cessation of menstrual flow for 1 year). The median age of first menarche varies based on ethnicity and country. Studies indicate a median

---

BOX 32.1 Summary of Nonreproductive Effects of Estrogen

Estrogens (including estrone, estradiol, estriol) function through estrogen receptors alpha and beta. Estrogen has different roles in different cells and tissues and have paracrine or intracrine function. Estrogen has the following nonreproductive effects:

- Maintains bone density
- Acts in liver to decrease cholesterol level, increase high-density lipoprotein (HDL) level, and decrease low-density lipoprotein (LDL) level (antiatherosclerotic); promotes fat deposition
- Maintains nervous system (neurotrophic and neuroprotective); helps memory and cognition
- Increases collagen content, dermal thickness, elasticity, water content, and healing ability of skin
- Protects against chronic kidney disease in individuals without diabetes
- Prevents vascular injury and early atheroma formation through endothelial mechanisms
- Inhibits platelet adhesiveness
- Can promote inflammation and has various effects on immunity

Estrogen associated with pregnancy or use in contraceptive pills promotes clotting. This clotting effect increases the risk of thromboembolism.

TABLE 32.2 Complementary and Opposing Effects of Estrogen and Progesterone

Structure	Effect of Estrogen	Effect of Progesterone
Vaginal mucosa	Growth of squamous epithelium; increase in glycogen content of cells; layering (cornification) of cells	Thinning of squamous epithelium; decornification
Cervical mucosa	Production of abundant fluid secretions that favour survival and enhance motility of sperm	Production of thick, sticky secretions that tend to plug cervical os
Fallopian tube	Increase of motility and ciliary action	Decrease of motility and ciliary action
Uterine muscle	Increase of blood flow; increase of contractile proteins; increase of uterine muscle and myometrial excitability to action potential; increase of sensitization to oxytocin	Relaxation of myometrium; decrease of sensitization to oxytocin
Endometrium	Stimulation of growth; increase in number of progesterone receptors	Activation of glands and blood vessels; decrease in number of estrogen receptors
Breasts	Growth of ducts; promotion of prolactin effects	Growth of lobules and alveoli; inhibition of prolactin effects

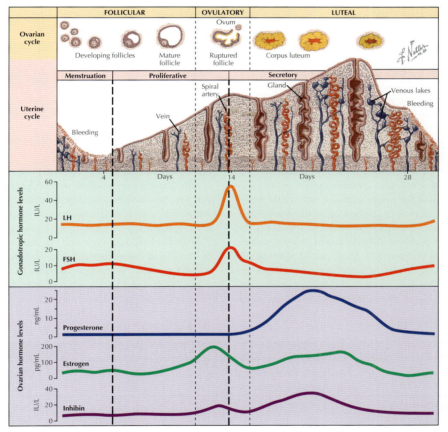

FIGURE 32.9 Female Reproductive Cycle. Correlation of events in follicular development, ovulation, hormonal interrelationships, and the menstrual cycle. Note: levels of estrogen (from ovarian follicle) and luteinizing hormone *(LH)* (from pituitary) are highest at the time of ovulation; progesterone from corpus luteum is highest during postovulation. *FSH*, Follicle-stimulating hormone. (From Mulroney, S. E., & Myers, A. K. [2009]. *Netter's essential physiology*. Saunders. Copyright © 2009 Elsevier Inc. All rights reserved. www.netterimages.com.)

age of 12.7 years in Canada; 12.3 years in the United States; in Europe, a range from 12.3 years in Greece to 13.3 years in Finland; 13.0 years in Australia; and 13.0 years in Russia.[10] Menarche appears to be related to body weight, especially percentage of body fat (ratio of fat-to-lean tissue). This increase may trigger a change in the metabolic rate and lead to hormonal changes associated with early menarche.[1] There is an increased sensitivity to leptin (a regulatory hormone of appetite and energy metabolism) during puberty. An increase in circulating leptin promotes the secretion of kisspeptin from the hypothalamus. This secretion leads to the release of GNRH which increases the release of FSH, LH, and estradiol. The increase in these hormones triggers ovulation and the start of puberty.[1]

Cycles are anovulatory at first and may vary in length from 10 to 60 days or more. As adolescence proceeds, regular patterns of menstruation and ovulation occur at intervals ranging from 21 to 45 days.[11] Menstruation continues to recur in a recognizable and characteristic pattern during adulthood. The length of the menstrual cycle varies considerably among women. The commonly accepted cycle average is 28 (25 to 30) days, with rhythmic intervals of 21 to 35 days considered normal (Figure 32.9). Approximately 2 to 8 years before menopause, cycles begin to lengthen again. Menstrual cyclicity and regular ovulation are dependent on variation of hormone levels.[12]

Phases of the Menstrual Cycle

The menstrual cycle (see Figure 32.9) consists of three phases. These phases are the ischemic/menstrual phase (menstruation), the follicular/proliferative phase (postmenstrual), and the luteal/secretory phase (premenstrual).

During **menstruation (menses)**, the functional layer of the endometrium disintegrates and is expelled through the vagina. The **follicular/proliferative phase** follows. This phase is named for two simultaneous processes: maturation of an ovarian follicle and proliferation of the endometrium (see Figure 32.9). During this phase, GnRH contributes to the increase of FSH level, which stimulates several follicles. The pulsatile secretion of FSH from the anterior pituitary gland rescues a dominant ovarian follicle from apoptosis. This occurs by days 5 to 7 of the cycle. Together, estrogen and FSH increase the number of FSH receptors in the granulosa cells of the primary follicle. The increase in receptors makes them more sensitive to FSH. FSH and estrogen combine to induce production of LH receptors on the granulosa cells. The production of LH receptors promotes LH stimulation to combine with FSH stimulation. This stimulation causes a more rapid secretion of follicular estrogen. As estrogen level increases FSH level drops. This drop in FSH concentration decreases the growth of less developed follicles (see Figure 32.8). Estrogen causes cells of the endometrium to proliferate and stimulates production of LH. A surge in the levels of both FSH and LH is needed for final follicular growth and ovulation.

Ovulation is the release of an ovum from a mature follicle. This release marks the beginning of the **luteal/secretory phase** of the menstrual cycle. The ovarian follicle begins its transformation into a corpus luteum (see Figure 32.8). This is the beginning of the *luteal phase*. Pulsatile secretion of LH from the anterior pituitary stimulates the corpus luteum to secrete progesterone. The secretion of progesterone starts the secretory phase of endometrial development. Glands and blood vessels in the endometrium branch and curl throughout the functional layer. The glands begin to secrete a thin, glycogen-containing fluid. This is the beginning of the *secretory phase*. If conception occurs, the nutrient-laden endometrium is ready for implantation. Three days after fertilization the secretion of human chorionic gonadotropin (hCG) occurs. hCG supports the corpus luteum once implantation occurs at about day 6 or 7. The detection of hCG in maternal blood and urine occurs 8 to 10 days after ovulation. The production of estrogen and progesterone will continue until the placenta can support hormonal production. If conception and implantation do not occur, the corpus luteum degenerates. The degeneration causes a decrease in its production of progesterone and estrogen. Without progesterone or estrogen to support it, the endometrium enters the ischemic ("blood-starved") phase and disintegrates. This is the beginning of the **ischemic/menstrual phase**. Then menstruation occurs, marking the beginning of another cycle.

Ovulatory cycles appear to have a minimum length of 24 to 26.5 days. The ovarian follicle requires 10 to 12.5 days to develop, and the luteal phase appears fixed at 14 days (±3 days). Menstrual blood flow usually lasts 3 to 7 days but is within normal ranges if it lasts up to 8 days or stops after 2 days. Bleeding is scant to heavy and varies from 30 to 80 mL. Most blood loss occurs during the first 3 days of menses. Menstrual discharge consists of blood, mucus, and desquamated endometrial tissue. This discharge does not clot under normal circumstances. It is usually dark and produces a characteristic musty odour. Environmental factors, such as severe emotional stress, illness, malnutrition, obesity, and seasonal variation, may affect the length of the menstrual cycle.[13]

Hormonal Controls

Hormonal control of the menstrual cycle depends on complex interactions among the hypothalamus, the anterior pituitary, and the ovaries (or hypothalamic-pituitary-ovarian [H-P-O] axis)[1] (Table 32.3). Hormonal control is dependent on negative and positive ovarian feedback mechanisms. GnRH controls the gonadotropin production of FSH and LH. The constant and pulsatile release of GnRH is critical to the timing of the menstrual cycle. The hypothalamus secretes GnRH, which travels to the anterior pituitary. This action stimulates the secretion of FSH and LH. The anterior pituitary releases FSH and LH in pulses that correspond to the secretion of GnRH.

TABLE 32.3 Hormonal Feedback Mechanism in the Menstrual Cycle

Phase of Cycle and Ovarian Hormone Levels	Feedback to Hypothalamus and Anterior Pituitary	Resultant GnRH, FSH, and LH Levels	Ovarian and Menstrual Events
Early follicular phase: estrogen levels low; minute amount of progesterone secreted	Negative and inhibitory	All low	Ovarian follicle develops; endometrium proliferates
Late follicular (preovulatory) phase: estrogen levels high; progesterone level increases with small surge before ovulation	Positive and stimulatory	All surge; LH dominates	Process of ovulation begins; endometrial proliferation complete
Ovulatory phase: estrogen levels dip; progesterone levels begin to rise	Negative and inhibitory	All fall sharply	Corpus luteum begins to develop; endometrium enters secretory phase
Early luteal phase: estrogen and progesterone levels high; progesterone dominates	Negative and inhibitory	All continue to decline, but gradually	Corpus luteum fully developed; endometrium ready for implantation
Late luteal phase: estrogen and progesterone levels fall sharply	Negative and inhibitory; feedback lessens slightly	All rise slightly	Corpus luteum regresses; endometrium disintegrates; menstruation begins
Menstrual phase: estrogen levels low; minute amount of progesterone secreted	Negative and inhibitory	All low	More ovarian follicles begin to develop; shedding of the functional layer of endometrium occurs

FSH, Follicle-stimulating hormone; *GnRH*, gonadotropin-releasing hormone; *LH*, luteinizing hormone.

During the early follicular phase, estrogen levels rise steadily. Through negative feedback the estrogen rise suppresses FSH production and positively increases the production of LH. During the late follicular phase, the preovulatory rise in progesterone level facilitates a positive feedback loop. Estrogen levels begin to increase, stimulating a surge of FSH and LH secretion from the anterior pituitary. The midcycle surge of LH and FSH induces ovulation.[14] Rising estrogen and progesterone levels during the luteal phase may inhibit the anterior pituitary. This inhibition will reduce LH and FSH secretion. Just before menstruation, FSH and LH levels begin to increase slightly. This increase is probably because of declining estrogen and progesterone levels (see Figure 32.9).

A variety of growth factors and autocrine/paracrine peptides influence hormonal control and follicular response. During the early follicular stage, FSH stimulates FSH receptors and LH receptors. FSH also stimulates the release of insulinlike growth factor 1 as well as the production of inhibin and activin in the ovary. **Activin** from granulosa cells stimulates the secretion of FSH, increases the pituitary response to GnRH, and increases FSH binding in the granulosa cells in the dominant follicle. FSH stimulates **inhibin** secretion from granulosa cells and it, in turn, suppresses FSH synthesis. In the follicular phase of the cycle, secretion of inhibin B mainly occurs and sharply spikes when ovulation occurs. In the luteal phase, secretion of inhibin A occurs and further suppresses FSH. Inhibin also restrains prolactin and growth hormone release, interferes with GnRH receptors, and promotes breakdown of intracellular gonadotropins. The balance between activin and inhibin regulates FSH secretion, and **follistatin** inhibits activin and boosts inhibin activity. Inhibin and activin also regulate LH stimulation of androgen synthesis in theca cells.[15] Research continues to advance understanding of the function and structural complexity of these polypeptides and their interaction with GnRH, gonadotropins, and sex hormones.

Ovarian Cycle

By stimulating follicles, gonadotropins start their growth and maturation. The most important hormonal event is a rise in FSH level. The decline in luteal-phase estrogen, progesterone, and inhibin secretion allows FSH levels to rise. At the same time there is a slight increase in LH levels (see Figure 32.9). FSH stimulates granulosa cell growth and initiates estrogen production in these cells. At this time, recruiting of a group of ovarian follicles occurs. These follicles begin to mature. The exact number depends on the remaining pool of inactive follicles. As the follicles mature, granulosa cells multiply, increasing estradiol secretion. Within a few days of the cycle, one follicle becomes dominant and the others atrophy. The mechanism for follicular recruitment or dominance is unknown. The dominant follicle begins to secrete progressively larger amounts of estrogen (estradiol). The estrogen exerts an increase in GnRH receptor concentration and an increase in pituitary sensitivity to GnRH. This process creates a positive feedback effect that causes a FSH and LH surge. Ovulation occurs 1 to 2 hours before the final progesterone surge, or about 12 to 36 hours after the onset of the FSH and LH surge. Progesterone, proteolytic enzymes, and prostaglandins trigger mechanisms controlling follicular rupture and release of the ovum.[14] The FSH and LH surge also changes the granulosa cells of the ovulatory follicle into the corpus luteum. The corpus luteum secretes both estrogen and progesterone in amounts that depend on adequate development of the follicle before ovulation. Progesterone acts both centrally and locally within the ovary to suppress new follicular growth during the early to midluteal phases. If pregnancy does not occur, the corpus luteum persists for 11 to 14 days and then regresses and eventually disappears. An increase in pulse frequency of GnRH from a low level reactivates hormonal control of the menstrual cycle.

Uterine Phases

The uterine phases of the menstrual cycle include the follicular/proliferative phase, the luteal/secretory phase, and menstruation. These phases involve the cyclic changes that occur in the endometrium controlled by estrogen and progesterone. The presence of receptors and many growth factors, peptides, and enzymes that act as intermediaries between the sex steroids and the endometrium influence the hormonal effects.[1] During the midfollicular/proliferative phase, increasing levels of estrogen contribute to endometrial repair and proliferation. This process increases endometrial thickness (luteal phase). Once ovulation occurs, serum progesterone levels increase. The endometrial tissue also develops secretory characteristics (secretory phase). If implantation of a fertilized ovum does not take place, endometrial tissue begins to break down. This breakdown occurs approximately 11 days after ovulation (ischemic phase of menstruation; see Figure 32.9). Shedding of tissue (menstrual bleeding) begins about 14 days after ovulation.

Cervical mucus also undergoes cyclic changes. During the proliferative phase, the cervical mucus is thin and watery. Peak estrogen levels occur just before ovulation and maximally stimulate the cervical glands to produce mucus. Cervical mucus becomes abundant and more elastic (spinnbarkeit). Increasing estrogen levels contribute to the development of tiny channels in cervical mucus, supplying access for sperm into the interior of the uterus. Changes in the consistency of cervical mucus can be used to identify fertile intervals.[1]

Vaginal Response

The vaginal endothelium also responds to the cyclic hormonal changes of the menstrual cycle. Under the influence of estrogen, cells of the vaginal epithelium grow maximally during the follicular/proliferative phase. After ovulation, layers of keratinized cells overgrow the basal epithelium. This process is known as **cornification**. Near the end of the luteal phase, leukocytes invade vaginal epithelium, removing the outer layers. This process is called **decornification**.

Body Temperature

Basal body temperature (BBT) undergoes characteristic biphasic changes during menstrual cycles in which ovulation occurs. During the follicular phase, the BBT fluctuates around 37°C (98°F). During the luteal phase, the average temperature increases by 0.5° to 2°C (0.4° to 1.0°F). At the end of the luteal phase, 1 to 3 days before the onset of menstruation, BBT declines to follicular-phase levels. The shift in temperature is related to ovulation, corpus luteum formation, and increased serum progesterone levels. Progesterone probably acts on the thermoregulatory centre of the hypothalamus to increase body temperature. Changes in BBT are used to document ovulatory cycles. When used alone BBT is not the best method to predict the exact timing of ovulation.[16]

STRUCTURE AND FUNCTION OF THE BREAST

>  **QUICK CHECK 32.5**
> 1. How does breast development differ between adult men and women?

The **breasts** are sebaceous glands that lie on the ventral surface of the thorax. They are found within the superficial fascia of the chest wall. They extend vertically from the second rib to the sixth or seventh intercostal space and laterally from the side of the sternum to the midaxillary line. Breast tissue also may extend into the axilla. This axilla tissue is known as the *tail of Spence*.

Female Breast

The female breast is composed of 15 to 20 pyramid-shaped lobes. Cooper ligaments separate and support the breasts (Figure 32.10).

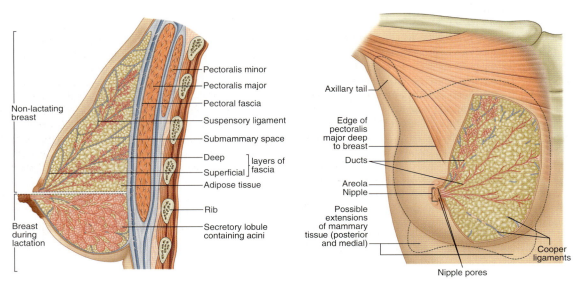

FIGURE 32.10 Schematic Diagram of the Breast. (From Standring, S. [2009]. *Gray's anatomy* [40th ed.]. Churchill Livingstone.)

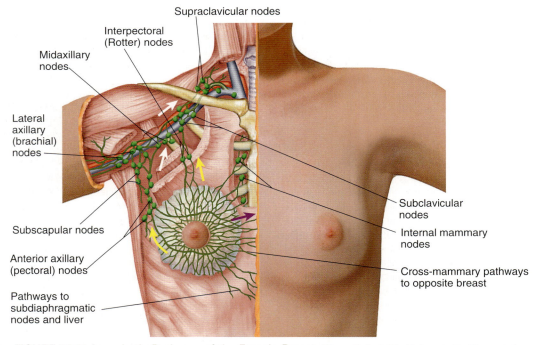

FIGURE 32.11 Lymphatic Drainage of the Female Breast. (From Ball, J. W., Dains, J. E., Flynn, J. A., et al. [2015]. *Seidel's guide to physical examination* [8th ed.]. Mosby.)

Each lobe has 20 to 40 lobules (alveoli), which subdivide further into many functional units called **acini** (*sing*., **acinus**). A layer of epithelial cells capable of secreting milk lines each acinus. A layer of subepithelial cells capable of contracting to squeeze milk from the acinus also is present. Biochemical signalling and density within the extracellular matrix are essential for differentiation and function of the acini glandular epithelium. The acini empty into a network of lobular collecting ducts. These collecting ducts empty into interlobular collecting and ejecting ducts. Collagen fibre alignment is needed for ductal elongation and organized branching.[17] The ducts reach the skin through openings (pores) in the nipple. Muscle strands and fatty connective tissue surround and separate the lobes and lobules. The amount of fatty connective tissue varies among individuals, depending on weight and genetic and endocrine factors, and contributes to the diversity of breast size and shape and the function of the mammary epithelium. Fat increases in the breast after menopause.[18]

The internal and lateral thoracic arteries and the intercostal arteries supply an extensive capillary network that surrounds the acini. Venous return follows arterial supply, with rapid emptying into the superior vena cava. The breasts receive sensory innervation from branches of the second through sixth intercostal nerves and the cervical plexus. As a result, breast pain may be referred to the chest, back, scapula, medial arm, and neck. Lymphatic drainage of the breast occurs largely through axillary nodes (Figure 32.11).

The **nipple** is a pigmented cylindrical structure usually found at the fourth or fifth intercostal space. On its surface lie multiple openings, one from each lobe. It measures 0.5 to 1.3 cm in diameter and is approximately 10 to 12 mm in height when erect. The **areola** is the pigmented circular area around the nipple. It may be 15 to 60 mm in diameter. Several sebaceous glands, the **glands of Montgomery**, are found within the areola. Secretions from these glands aid in lubrication of the nipple during lactation. The nipple and areola have smooth muscles, which receive motor innervation from the sympathetic nervous system. Sexual stimulation, breastfeeding, and exposure to cold cause the nipple to become erect.

The fetal and early postnatal development of breast tissue does not depend on hormones. However, fetal breast tissue does become progressively responsive to hormonal stimulation. During childhood, breast growth is latent, and growth of the nipple and areola keeps pace with body surface growth. At the onset of puberty in the female, estrogen secretion stimulates mammary growth. Breast development, or thelarche, is usually the first sign of puberty in the female. Several hormones mediate the full differentiation and development of breast tissue. These hormones include estrogen, progesterone, prolactin, growth hormone, thyroid and parathyroid hormones, insulin, and cortisol.

During the reproductive years, the breast undergoes cyclic changes in response to changes in the levels of estrogen and progesterone associated with the menstrual cycle. Estrogen promotes development of the lobular ducts. Progesterone stimulates development of cells lining the acini. Lactation (milk production) occurs after childbirth in response to increased levels of prolactin. Prolactin secretion increases by continued breastfeeding. **Oxytocin**, another hormone released after delivery, controls milk ejection (let down) from acini cells. During the follicular/proliferative phase of the menstrual cycle, high estradiol levels increase the vascularity of breast tissue and stimulate proliferation of ductal and acinar tissue. Sustainment of this effect occurs into the luteal/secretory phase of the cycle. During this phase, progesterone levels increase and contribute to the breast changes induced by estradiol. Specific effects of progesterone include dilation of the ducts and conversion of the acinar cells into secretory cells. Most women experience some degree of premenstrual breast fullness, tenderness, and increased breast nodularity. Breast volume may increase as much as 10 to 30 mL. Because the length of the menstrual cycle does not allow for complete regression of new cell growth, breast growth continues at a slow rate until approximately 35 years of age. Because of the cyclic changes that occur in breast tissue, the conduction of a breast examination should occur at the end of or a few days after the menstrual cycle. During this time hormonal effects are minimal, and breasts are at their smallest.

The function of the female breast is primarily to supply a source of nourishment for the newborn. Physiologically, breast milk is the best nourishment for newborns. Colostrum is produced in low quantities in the first few days postpartum. Colostrum is rich in immunological components, including secretory IgA, lactoferrin, leukocytes, and developmental factors, such as epidermal growth factor. The nutrient composition changes over time to meet the changing digestive capabilities and nutritional requirements of the infant. Secretory IgA and nonspecific antimicrobial factors, such as lysosomes and lactoferrin, protect the infant against infection.[19] During lactation, high prolactin levels interfere with hypothalamic-pituitary hormones that stimulate ovulation. This mechanism suppresses the menstrual cycle and can prevent ovulation.[20] In some parts of the world, breastfeeding is the major means of contraception (lactational amenorrhea method).[21] However, it is not absolute that ovulation will not occur, and this method will not ensure that pregnancy will not occur. Breasts are also a source of pleasurable sexual sensation and in Western cultures have become a sexual symbol.

Male Breast

Until puberty, development of the male breast is like that of the female breast. In the absence of sufficiently high levels of estrogen and progesterone, and with antagonistic effects of androgens, the male breast does not develop any further. The normal male breast consists mostly of fat with a small, underdeveloped nipple and a few ductlike structures in the subareolar area. The male breast may appear enlarged in obese men because of accumulation of fatty tissue. During puberty, some males experience benign gynecomastia (benign proliferation of male breast glandular tissue). This is a condition in which the breasts enlarge temporarily because of hormonal fluctuations. Differentiation of this condition from any underlying systemic disorders should occur.[22]

THE MALE REPRODUCTIVE SYSTEM

QUICK CHECK 32.6
1. Why do sperm take 12 days to travel the length of the epididymis?
2. What is the purpose of prostatic secretions?
3. Which cells produce testosterone?

The external genitalia in men perform the major functions of reproduction. The male gonads and the testes produce sperm. Delivery of sperm takes place via the penis. The internal male genitalia consist of conducting tubes and fluid-producing glands These structures aid in the transport of sperm from the testes to the urethral opening of the penis. The male reproductive and urinary structures are shown in Figure 32.12.

External Genitalia

Testes

The testes are the essential organs of male reproduction. Like the ovaries, the testes have two functions: (1) production of gametes (i.e., sperm) and (2) production of sex hormones (i.e., androgens and testosterone).

During embryonic and fetal life, the testes develop within the abdomen (see Figure 32.1). About 3 months before birth, the testes start to descend toward the developing scrotum. About 1 month before birth, they enter twin passageways called **inguinal canals**. The inguinal canals are vaginal processes created by outpouchings of the peritoneum

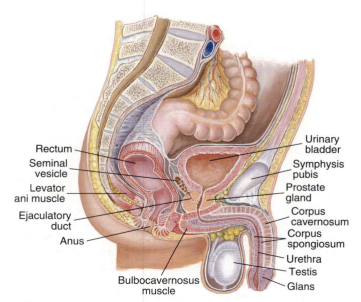

FIGURE 32.12 Structure of the Male Reproductive Organs. (From Ball, J. W., Dains, J. E., Flynn, J. A., et al. [2015]. *Seidel's guide to physical examination* [8th ed.]. Mosby.)

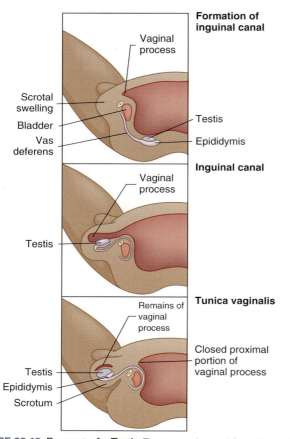

FIGURE 32.13 Descent of a Testis. The testes descend from the abdominal cavity to the scrotum during the last 3 months of fetal development.

(lining of the abdominal cavity). Figure 32.13 shows the descent of a testis. When descent is complete, the abdominal end of each vaginal process closes, and the inguinal canal disappears. Failure of the testes to descend through the inguinal canal is known as *cryptorchidism*. The scrotal end of each vaginal process becomes the outer covering of the testis, the **tunica vaginalis**.

Figure 32.14 shows a sagittal section of a mature testis. The adult **testis** is oval and varies considerably in length (3 to 6 cm), width (2 to 3.5 cm), depth (3 to 4 cm), and weight (10 to 40 g). The tunica vaginalis almost entirely surrounds the testis and separates the testis from the scrotal wall and the **tunica albuginea**. Inward extensions of the tunica albuginea separate the testis into about 250 compartments, or lobules. Each lobule has several tortuously coiled ducts called **seminiferous tubules**. Production of sperm takes place in these tubules. Tissue surrounding these ducts has **Leydig cells**. These cells occur in clusters and produce androgens, chiefly testosterone.

The two ends of each seminiferous tubule join and leave the lobule through the **tubulus rectus**. The tubulus rectus leads to the central portion of the testis, the **rete testis**. The sperm then move through the **efferent tubules**, or vasa efferentia, to the epididymis, where they mature.

Adrenergic fibres innervate the testes. The sole function of these fibres is to regulate blood flow to the Leydig cells. Arterial blood from the internal spermatic and differential arteries flows over the surface of the testes before entering the parenchyma (functional tissues). Surface flow cools the blood to temperatures that promote spermatogenesis, approximately 1° to 4°C (33.8° to 39.2°F) below rectal temperature.[23] Additionally, suspension of the testes outside the pelvic cavity occurs to help cooling.

Epididymis

The **epididymis** (*pl.*, **epididymides**) is a comma-shaped structure that curves over the posterior part of each testis (see Figure 32.14). It consists of a single, densely packed, and markedly coiled duct measuring

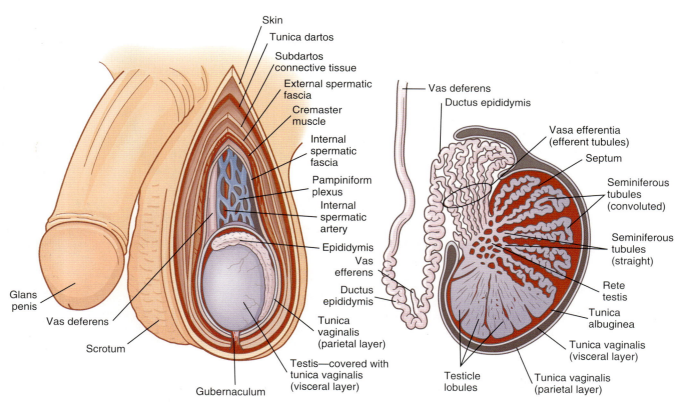

FIGURE 32.14 The Testes. External and sagittal views showing interior anatomy.

5 to 7 cm in length (but about 6 m in length when uncoiled). The epididymis has structural and physiological functions. Its structural function is to conduct sperm from the efferent tubules to the vas deferens. Physiological functions include sperm maturation, mobility, and fertility. When sperm enter the head of the epididymis, they are not fully mature or motile, nor can they fertilize an ovum. During the 12 days (or more) sperm take to travel the length of the epididymis, they receive nutrients and testosterone. This process enhances their ability for fertilization.[24] After travelling the length of the epididymis, sperm are stored in the epididymal tail and vas deferens. The **vas deferens** is a duct with muscular layers capable of powerful peristalsis. This structure transports sperm toward the urethra. The vas deferens enters the pelvic cavity through the spermatic cord (see Figure 32.14).

Scrotum

The **scrotum**, a skin-covered, fibromuscular sac, is equivalent to the female labia majora (see Figure 32.2). The scrotum encloses and protects the testes, epididymides, and spermatic cord. The skin of the scrotum is thin and has rugae (wrinkles or folds). The rugae enable the scrotum to enlarge or relax away from the body. At puberty, the scrotal skin darkens, develops active sebaceous glands, and becomes sparsely covered with hair. Just under the skin lies a layer of connective tissue (fascia) and smooth muscle, the **tunica dartos** (see Figure 32.14). The tunica dartos also forms a septum that separates the two testes. Exposure to cold temperatures causes the tunica dartos to contract, pulling the testes close to the warm body. In warm temperatures, the tunica dartos relaxes, suspending the testes away from body heat. These mechanisms promote best temperatures for spermatogenesis. In addition, scrotal sensitivity to touch, pressure, temperature, and pain protects the testes from potential harm. During sexual excitement, the scrotal skin and tunica thicken, the scrotum tightens and lifts, and the spermatic cords shorten, partially elevating the testes toward the body. As excitement plateaus, the engorged testes increase 50% in size, rotate anteriorly, and flatten against the body, signalling impending ejaculation.

Penis

The **penis** has two main functions: delivery of sperm to the female vagina and elimination of urine. (Chapter 29 reviews urine formation and excretion.) Embryonically, the penis is equivalent to the female clitoris (see Figure 32.2).

Figure 32.15 shows a sagittal section of the adult penis and its anatomical relation to other urogenital structures. Externally, the penis consists of a shaft with a tip (the **glans**) that has the opening of the urethra (see Figures 32.14 and 32.15). The skin of the glans folds over the tip of the penis, forming the **prepuce (foreskin)**. The skin of the penis is continuous with that of the groin, scrotum, and inner thighs. It is hairless, movable, and darker than surrounding skin.

Internally, the penis consists of the urethra and three compartments or sinusoids: two **corpora cavernosa** and the **corpus spongiosum** (see Figure 32.15) separated by Buck fascia. The fibrous tunica albuginea encloses these compartments. The **urethra** passes through the corpus spongiosum and ends at a sagittal slit in the glans.

The **erectile reflex** is a process in which erectile tissues within the corpora cavernosa and corpus spongiosum become engorged with blood. This process makes penetration of the female vagina possible. The erectile tissues consist of vascular spaces, or chambers, supplied with blood by arterioles (small arteries). Usually, constriction of the arterioles ensures that not much blood flows through the erectile tissues. Sexual stimulation, however, causes the arterioles to dilate and fill with blood. These actions expand the erectile tissues and cause an erection. Erection is supported by compression or constriction of veins that drain the corpora cavernosa and corpus spongiosum. When sexual stimulation ceases or orgasm and ejaculation occur, these veins open, blood flows out of the arterioles, and the penis becomes flaccid (soft and pendulous). Erection is under the control of the autonomic nervous system. However, stimulation or inhibition of erection can occur by central nervous system input.

Erections begin in utero and continue throughout life. Ejaculation does not occur until sperm production begins at puberty. Growth of the penis and scrotal contents continues well past puberty and may not be complete until the late teens or early twenties. Penis size, when flaccid, varies considerably. With an erection, difference in penis size diminishes. Sexual excitement causes the corpora cavernosa to increase in length and width and become rigid and the penis becomes erect. Stimulation of the glans, which has many sensitive nerve endings, supplies maximum erotic sensation. With sexual arousal, skin colour deepens, the glans doubles in size, and the urethral meatus dilates. Ejaculation occurs with frequent, strong contractions of the vas deferens, epididymis, seminal vesicles, prostate, urethra, and penis. Erection and ejaculation can occur independently of each other.[25]

Internal Genitalia

Figure 32.12 shows the anatomy of the internal genitalia and their relation to other pelvic organs. The internal genitalia consist of ducts and glands:

Ducts: consist of two vasa deferentia, ejaculatory duct, and urethra; conduct sperm and glandular secretions from the testes to the urethral opening of the penis

Glands: consist of prostate gland, two seminal vesicles, and two bulbourethral glands (Cowper glands); secrete fluids that serve as a vehicle for sperm transport and create nutritious alkaline medium that promotes sperm motility and survival

Together the sperm and the glandular fluids compose **semen**.

Sperm leave the epididymides and travel rapidly through the internal ducts (**emission**). Emission occurs just seconds before ejaculation when sexual arousal peaks. It always leads to ejaculation.

Emission occurs as smooth muscle in the walls of the epididymides and vasa deferentia begins to contract rhythmically. This action pushes sperm and epididymal secretions through the vasa deferentia. Each vas deferens is a firm, elastic, fibromuscular tube that begins at the tail of the epididymis, enters the pelvic cavity within the spermatic cord, loops up and over the bladder, and ends in the prostate gland (Figure 32.16). Movement of sperm occurs by peristaltic contractions of smooth muscle in the walls of the vas deferens.

As sperm leave the ampulla (wide part) of the vas deferens, the seminal vesicles secrete a nutritive, glucose-rich fluid into the ejaculate (semen). The **seminal vesicles** are glands about 4 to 6 cm long that lie behind the urinary bladder and in front of the rectum. The ducts of the seminal vesicles join the ampulla of the vas deferens to become

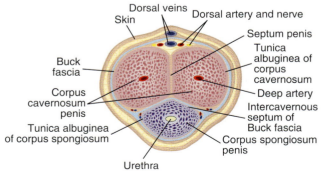

FIGURE 32.15 Cross-section of the Penis. (From Thompson, J. M., McFarland, G. K., Hirsch, J. E., et al. [Eds.]. [2002]. *Mosby's clinical nursing* [5th ed.]. Mosby.)

the ejaculatory duct. This duct contracts rhythmically during emission and ejaculation. As seen in Figures 32.13 and 32.16, the ejaculatory duct joins the urethra, where both pass through the prostate gland. During emission and ejaculation, a sphincter (muscle surrounding a duct) closes, preventing urine from entering the prostatic urethra.

The prostate gland is about the size of a walnut. It surrounds the urethra and is composed of glandular alveoli and ducts embedded in fibromuscular tissue. Nerves required for penile erection travel along the posterolateral surface of the prostate. While semen moves through the prostatic part of the urethra, the prostate gland contracts rhythmically and secretes prostatic fluid. This fluid is a thin, milky substance with an alkaline pH that helps sperm to survive in the acidic environment of the female reproductive tract. In addition, substances in seminal and prostatic fluids help to mobilize sperm after ejaculation.

Bulbourethral glands (Cowper glands) are the last pair of glands to add fluid to the ejaculate. Their ducts secrete mucus into the urethra near the base of the penis. Ejaculation occurs as semen reaches the base of the penis. During ejaculation, muscles rhythmically contract and expel semen. Normally a man ejaculates between 2 and 6 mL of semen, having 75 million to 400 million sperm. About 98% of the ejaculate consists of glandular fluids. Approximately 60% to 70% of the volume originates from the seminal vesicles and 20% from the prostate. Therefore, the ejaculate of a man who has undergone a vasectomy (a surgical procedure for permanent male birth control) is reduced by only about 2%.

Spermatogenesis

Spermatogenesis begins at puberty and continues for life. Spermatogenesis differs markedly from oogenesis (production of primordial ova), which occurs during fetal life only. Spermatogenesis takes place within the seminiferous tubules of the testes (see Figures 32.14 and 32.17). Diploid (46-chromosome) germ cells called spermatogonia (*sing.*, spermatogonium) line the basement membrane of each seminiferous tubule. These cells undergo continuous mitotic division (division into two identical cells; see Chapter 1). Some spermatogonia move away from the basement membrane and mature, becoming primary spermatocytes (Figure 32.17). These spermatogonia undergo meiosis, cell division that results in two haploid (23-chromosome) cells called secondary spermatocytes. (Chapter 2 describes and illustrates meiosis.) The secondary spermatocytes also undergo meiosis, resulting in four spermatids. The spermatids differentiate into spermatozoa, or sperm, each of which has 23 chromosomes (Figure 32.18).

The development of spermatids into sperm depends on the presence of Sertoli cells (nondividing support cells) within the seminiferous tubules. Spermatids attach themselves to the Sertoli cells (see Figure 32.17). It is from these cells they receive nutrients and hormonal signals necessary to develop into sperm.[26]

The process of spermatogenesis, from mitotic division of a spermatogonium to maturation of the spermatids, takes about 70 to 80 days. Mature sperm travel from the seminiferous tubules to the epididymides, where their ability for fertilization continues to develop. Although they are completely mature by the time they are ejaculated, the sperm do not become motile (capable of movement) until they are activated by biochemicals in semen and in the female reproductive tract (known as *sperm capacitation*).[1]

Male Sex and Reproductive Hormones

The male sex hormones are androgens. Leydig cells of the testes produce most of the testosterone, the primary male sex hormone, and other androgens. Production of these hormones also occurs in the adrenal glands (see Table 32.1 and discussion about adrenarche under "Puberty and Reproductive Maturation"). In men, sex hormone production is relatively constant and does not occur in a cyclic pattern, as it does in women.

The physiological actions of androgen are related to the growth and development of male tissues and organs.[1] Androgens are responsible for the fetal differentiation and development of the male urogenital system. They also have some effects on the fetal brain. After birth, the Leydig cells become quiescent until activated by the gonadotropins during puberty. Then androgens cause the sex organs to grow and secondary sex characteristics to develop.

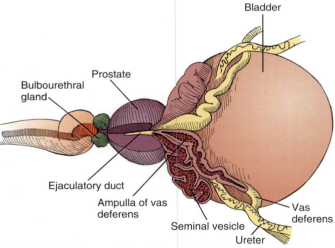

FIGURE 32.16 Prostate Gland, Seminal Vesicles, and Vas Deferens. (From Huguet, J. [2012]. *Hinman's atlas of urosurgical anatomy* [2nd ed., pp. 249–286]. Saunders.)

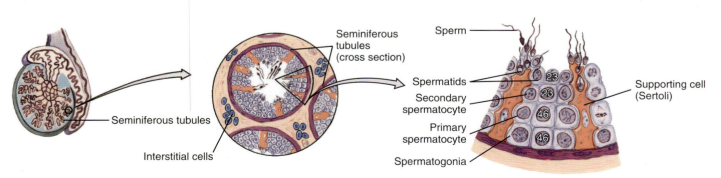

FIGURE 32.17 Seminiferous Tubule and Spermatogenesis. Cross section of a seminiferous tubule showing the different cell types. Interstitial cells that produce testosterone are between the seminiferous tubules. Spermatids in the lumen become sperm by a process called *spermiogenesis*. The numbers in white represent the number of chromosomes. (From Applegate, E. [2011]. *The anatomy and physiology learning system* [4th ed.]. Saunders.)

CHAPTER 32 Structure and Function of the Reproductive Systems

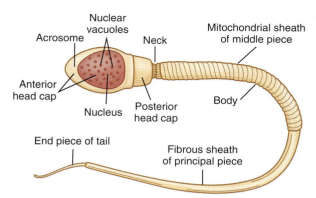

FIGURE 32.18 Mature Sperm Cell (Spermatozoon). Anatomy of mature sperm cell.

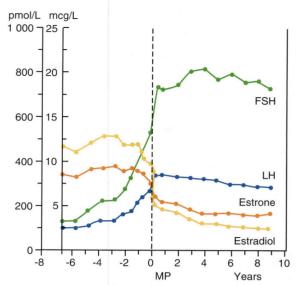

FIGURE 32.19 Perimenopausal Hormone Transition. Mean circulating hormone levels. *FSH*, Follicle-stimulating hormone; *LH*, luteinizing hormone; *MP*, menopause.

Testosterone affects nervous and skeletal tissues, bone marrow, skin and hair, and sex organs. It has an anabolic effect on skeletal muscle tissue. As a result, testosterone contributes to the difference in body weight and composition between men and women. Testosterone also stimulates growth of the musculature and cartilage of the larynx, causing a permanent deepening of the voice. Testosterone directly stimulates the bone marrow. Testosterone indirectly stimulates renal erythropoietin production to achieve increased hemoglobin and hematocrit levels. Because testosterone stimulates sebaceous gland activity, acne may develop. Hair becomes coarser in texture, and facial, axillary, and pubic hair grows in male patterns. Later in life, testosterone causes baldness in genetically susceptible individuals. Testosterone is needed for spermatogenesis and for secretion of fluid by the prostate gland, seminal vesicles, and Cowper glands. Testosterone is also associated with **libido** (sex drive). Other, less-understood effects of testosterone include alterations in fatty acid and cholesterol metabolism.

A complex feedback system involving the extrahypothalamic central nervous system, the hypothalamus, the anterior pituitary, the testes, and the androgen-sensitive end organs, regulates androgen production and spermatogenesis. These relationships are essentially the same in women (see Figure 32.3).

AGING AND REPRODUCTIVE FUNCTION

> **✓ QUICK CHECK 32.7**
> 1. What happens to estradiol levels in perimenopausal women?
> 2. What are the physical changes associated with menopausal decreases in estrogen level?
> 3. How does andropause affect muscle mass?

Aging and the Female Reproductive System

Menopause is a normal developmental and transitional event. It is universally experienced by the average age of about 51 years with a range of 40 to 60 years. Genetics are associated with timing of menopause. Menopause can occur 2 years sooner on average for smokers. Declining ovarian function and a resulting decrease in ovarian hormone secretion is the primary cause of these changes. The primary changes of menopause are:[1]

Perimenopause: This is the transitional period between reproductive and nonreproductive years and can last 1 to 8 years. About 5 to 10 years before menopause, approximately 90% of women note mild to extreme variability in frequency and quality of menstrual flow. Symptoms usually begin with a shortening of the menstrual cycle, which correlates with a shorter follicular phase. This phase is followed by unpredictable or irregular ovulation and a lengthening of the menstrual cycle. The perimenopause varies between women and from cycle to cycle in the same woman.

Menopause: The definition of menopause is the point that marks 12 consecutive months of amenorrhea. This means that it is decided retrospectively after a woman has not had a menstrual period for 1 year. Loss of ovarian function, low estrogen, and progesterone levels, and high FSH and LH levels occur (Figure 32.19).[1]

Ovarian changes: Around 37 to 38 years of age, women experience accelerated follicular loss. This process ends with the depletion in the supply of follicles at menopause. This accelerated loss is correlated with increased FSH stimulation, declining inhibin production, and slightly elevated estradiol levels (see Figure 32.19). The ovarian response to high FSH level recruits increasing numbers of follicles. These follicles only partially develop, with a net effect of irregular ovulation, lower progesterone levels, and depleted follicle reserve. The ovaries begin to decrease in size around age 30. This decrease accelerates after age 60.

Uterine changes: The increase in anovulatory cycles allows for proliferative growth of the endometrium. With this longer exposure to unopposed estrogen and greater thickness of the endometrium, 50% of perimenopausal women will experience dysfunctional uterine bleeding that is heavy and unpredictable. In the past, this has put women at high risk for hysterectomy. Newer treatment includes progesterone administration or endometrial ablation by laser or electrocautery. The development of new methods of decreasing the function of the endometrial tissue are being explored.

Breast tissue changes: Breast tissue becomes involuted, fat deposits and connective tissue increase, and a decrease in breast size and firmness occurs.

Urogenital tract changes: The ovaries shrink; the uterus atrophies; and the vagina shortens, narrows, and loses some elasticity. Lubrication of the vagina diminishes and vaginal pH increases. This pH change creates a higher incidence of vaginitis. The cervix atrophies; the cervical os shrinks; vaginal epithelium atrophies; labia major and minora become less prominent; loss of some pubic hair occurs; urethral tone declines along with muscle tone throughout the pelvic area; urinary frequency or urgency, urinary tract infections, and incontinence may occur. Regular sexual activity and orgasm may diminish some of these changes. Sexually active women have less vaginal atrophy.

Skeletal changes: Loss of bone mass occurs, leading to increased brittleness and porosity and possibly osteoporosis, particularly in the lumbar spine and femoral neck (see Chapter 39).

Cardiac changes: The risk for coronary heart disease increases significantly with an increase in total and LDL-cholesterol and a decrease in HDL-cholesterol (see Chapter 24).

Systemic changes: A rise in skin temperature, dilation of peripheral blood vessels, increased blood flow in the hands, increased skin conductance, and transient increase in heart rate followed by a temperature drop and profuse perspiration over the area of flush distribution are characteristics of **vasomotor flushes**. This usually occurs in the face and neck and may radiate into the chest and other parts of the body. Dizziness, nausea, headaches, and palpitations may go with the flush.[1] These flushes can vary in frequency, intensity, and duration and last for 1 to 15 years (mean 1 to 5 years) in up to 85% of perimenopausal to postmenopausal women. Rapid decreases in estrogen levels are thought to be the cause of flushes; estrogen replacement therapy can improve these symptoms. Rapid changes in estrogen levels also can increase emotional stress with unpredictable mood swings, depression and anxiety, weight gain, migraine headaches, and insomnia. Lower estrogen levels will decrease skin thickness and diminish skin elasticity. These changes cause increased skin dryness and wrinkling.

Menopause increases the risk for ovarian, breast, and uterine cancers. The risk is greater in women who began menstruating before age 12 or experience menopause after age 55. Women who menstruate longer than normal during a lifetime are exposed to more estrogen and have more ovulations. A longer exposure to estrogen increases a woman's risk for uterine and breast cancers. Having more ovulations than normal increases a woman's risk for ovarian cancer.[27]

The consideration of hormone therapy may be a choice for relief of severe menopausal symptoms. However, careful evaluation of risk and benefits of such therapy must occur. There is increased risk for serious disorders for some women including breast cancer, heart disease, and stroke. Risks vary depending on age, timing of menopause, health history, dosage, and route of delivery (oral versus patch). Nonhormonal therapy also may be a choice for symptom relief.

Aging and the Male Reproductive System

Men keep reproductive ability longer than women. No known discrete event, comparable to menopause, characterizes aging of the male reproductive system. Changes do occur, however, in testicular structure and function and sexual behaviour.[1] Emotional and physical changes associated with androgen deficiency in the aging male are known as **andropause**, but not all men experience it.[28] Contributing factors include decreased levels of testosterone, change in responsiveness of target tissues, decreased levels of sex hormone binding globulin, and changes in the hypothalamus and pituitary gland. Obesity also contributes to decreased testosterone production in aging men.[29]

Male sexual behaviour encompasses both sexual drive and erectile and ejaculatory ability. Libido, or sexual drive, is a complex phenomenon that requires a baseline hormonal milieu. Health status and environmental, social, and psychological factors significantly influence this phenomenon. However, in men older than 40 years of age, organic factors are involved in more than half of cases of male sexual dysfunction. Chronic disease and vascular, endocrine, and neurological disorders are common causes of organically based dysfunction of sexual capability. Primary changes[1] include:

Sexual drive (libido): influenced by changes in health status and testosterone levels

Erectile/ejaculatory capacity: longer stimulation needed to achieve full erection, slower and less forceful ejaculation, less pelvic muscle involvement; decreased vasocongestive response; longer refractory time, up to 24 hours

Testicular changes: decreased weight, atrophy, softening of testes; seminiferous tubules thicken in basement membrane area, have germ cell arrest, decrease in spermatogenic activity, and collapse; then sclerosis and fibrosis cause complete obstruction; semen volume, sperm concentration, total sperm count, sperm motility, and number of motile sperm decrease; morphological appearance of sperm changes; decreased fertility

Hormonal changes: hormone synthesis decreases, and target tissues decline in responsiveness; testosterone levels decline as number of Leydig cells decreases; gonadotropin levels increase

Associated change: functional deterioration of accessory sex organs occurs; loss of muscle mass, strength, and endurance and decrease in libido develop

DID YOU UNDERSTAND?

Development of the Reproductive Systems

1. Differentiation of female and male genitalia begins around 6 to 8 weeks of embryonic development. This occurs when the gonads of genetically male embryos begin to secrete male sex hormones, primarily testosterone, under the influence of *SRY* gene expression and testes-determining factor. Female gonadal development occurs in the absence of *SRY* gene expression. Until that time, the primitive reproductive organs of males and females are homologous (the same).
2. The structure and function of both male and female reproductive systems depend on interactions among the central nervous system (hypothalamus), the endocrine system (anterior pituitary), the gonads (ovaries, testes), and the hypothalamic-pituitary-gonadal axis. A set of complex neurological and hormonal interactions accelerate at puberty and lead to sexual maturation and reproductive capability.
3. Production of primitive female gametes (ova) occurs solely during fetal life. From puberty to menopause, one female gamete matures per menstrual cycle. Production of the male gametes (sperm) begins at puberty. The daily production of millions of sperm occurs after puberty, usually for life.
4. Puberty is the onset of sexual maturation. Adolescence is a stage of human development between childhood and adulthood.
5. At puberty, extrahypothalamic factors cause the hypothalamus to secrete gonadotropin-releasing hormone. This stimulates the anterior pituitary to secrete the gonadotropins follicle-stimulating hormone and luteinizing hormone that stimulate the gonads (ovaries and testes) to secrete female (estrogen and progesterone) or male sex hormones (testosterone). Puberty is complete in females with the first ovulatory menstrual period and is complete in males with the first ejaculation that has mature sperm.

The Female Reproductive System

1. The function of the female reproductive system is to produce mature ova. If fertilization occurs, the female reproductive system supplies protection and nourishment of the fetus until it is expelled at birth.

2. The external female genitalia are the mons pubis, labia majora, labia minora, clitoris, vestibule (urinary and vaginal openings), and perineum. They protect body openings and may play a role in sexual functioning.
3. The internal female genitalia are the vagina, uterus, fallopian tubes, and ovaries. The ovaries are the most essential because they produce the female gametes and female sex hormones.
4. The vagina is a fibromuscular canal that receives the penis during sexual intercourse and is the exit route for menstrual fluids and products of conception. The vagina leads from the introitus (its external opening) to the cervical part of the uterus.
5. The uterus is the hollow, muscular organ in which a fertilized ovum develops until birth. The uterine walls have three layers: the endometrium (lining), myometrium (muscular layer), and perimetrium (outer covering, which is continuous with the pelvic peritoneum). The endometrium proliferates (thickens) and sheds in response to cyclic changes in levels of female sex hormones. The cervix is the narrow, lower part of the uterus that opens into the vagina.
6. The two fallopian tubes extend from the uterus to the ovaries. Their function is to conduct ova from the spaces around the ovaries to the uterus. Fertilization normally occurs in the distal third of the fallopian tubes.
7. From puberty to menopause, the ovaries are the site of (a) ovum maturation and release and (b) production of female sex hormones (estrogen, progesterone) and androgens. The female sex hormones are involved in sexual differentiation and development, the menstrual cycle, pregnancy, and lactation. Androgens in women are precursors of female sex hormones and contribute to the prepubertal growth spurt, pubic and axillary hair growth, and activation of sebaceous glands.
8. Cells in the developing ovarian follicle (structure that encloses the ovum) produce estrogen (primarily estradiol). Cells of the corpus luteum, the structure that develops from the ruptured ovarian follicle after ovulation (ovum release) produce progesterone. The ovarian follicle, adrenal glands, and adipose tissue contribute to the production of androgens.
9. The average menstrual cycle lasts 25 to 30 days and consists of three phases. These phases correspond to ovarian and endometrial changes: the ischemic/menstrual phase (menstruation), the follicular/proliferative phase (postmenstrual), and the luteal/secretory phase (premenstrual).
10. Gonadotropins and follicular secretion of inhibin control the ovarian events of the menstrual cycle. High FSH levels stimulate follicle and ovum maturation (follicular phase); then a surge of LH causes ovulation. The development of the corpus luteum (luteal phase) follows.
11. Ovarian hormones cause the uterine (endometrial) phases of the menstrual cycle. During the follicular phase of the ovarian cycle, estrogen produced by the follicle causes the endometrium to proliferate (proliferative phase). During the luteal phase, estrogen supports the thickened endometrium, and progesterone causes it to develop blood vessels and secretory glands (secretory phase). During the ischemic/menstrual phase, the corpus luteum degenerates, production of both hormones drops sharply, and the "starved" endometrium degenerates and is shed, causing menstruation.
12. Cyclic changes in hormone levels also cause thinning and thickening of the vaginal epithelium, thinning, and thickening of cervical secretions, and changes in basal body temperature.

Structure and Function of the Breast

1. Until puberty, the female and male breasts are similar, consisting of a small, underdeveloped nipple, some fatty and fibrous tissue, and a few ductlike structures under the areola. At puberty a variety of hormones (estrogen, progesterone, prolactin, growth hormone, insulin, cortisol) cause the female breast to develop into a system of glands and ducts that can produce and eject milk.
2. The basic functional unit of the female breast is the lobe, a system of ducts that branches from the nipple to milk-producing units called *lobules*. Each breast has 15 to 20 lobes. Cooper ligaments separate and support the breasts. The lobules have *acini cells*, which are convoluted spaces lined with epithelial cells. Contraction of the subepithelial cells of each acinus moves milk into the system of ducts that leads to the nipple.
3. Milk production occurs in response to prolactin. Secretion of large amounts of this hormone occurs after childbirth. Milk ejection is under the control of oxytocin, another hormone of pregnancy and lactation.
4. During the reproductive years, breast tissue undergoes cyclic changes in response to hormonal changes of the menstrual cycle. At menopause, the tissue involutes, fat deposits and connective tissue increase, and the breasts reduce in size and firmness.
5. The male breast does not develop because of the absence of sufficiently high levels of estrogen and progesterone, and antagonistic effects of androgens.

The Male Reproductive System

1. The function of the male reproductive system is to produce male gametes (sperm) and deliver them to the female reproductive tract.
2. The external male genitalia are the testes, epididymides, scrotum, and penis.
3. The testes (male gonads) are paired glands suspended within the scrotum. The testes have two functions: spermatogenesis (sperm production) and production of male sex hormones (androgens, chiefly testosterone).
4. The epididymis is a long, coiled tube arranged in a comma-shaped compartment that curves over the top and rear of the testis. The epididymis receives sperm from the testis and stores them while they develop further. Sperm travel the length of the epididymis and then are ejaculated into the vas deferens, which transports sperm to the urethra.
5. The scrotum is a skin-covered, fibromuscular sac that encloses the testes and epididymides. The spermatic cord suspends these structures within the scrotum. The scrotum keeps these organs at best temperatures for sperm survival by contracting in cold environments and relaxing in warm environments.
6. The penis is a cylindrical organ consisting of three longitudinal compartments (two corpora cavernosa and one corpus spongiosum) and the urethra. The urethra runs through the corpus spongiosum. The corpora cavernosa and corpus spongiosum consist of erectile tissue. Externally the penis consists of a shaft and the *glans*.
7. The penis has two functions: delivery of sperm and elimination of urine.
8. The erectile reflex, in which tactile or psychogenic stimulation of the parasympathetic nerves causes arterioles in the corpora cavernosa and corpus spongiosum to dilate and fill with blood, causes the penis to enlarge and become firm, which makes sexual intercourse possible.
9. The internal genitalia are the vas deferens, ejaculatory duct, prostatic and membranous sections of the urethra, seminal vesicles, prostate gland, and bulbourethral glands.
10. Emission, which occurs at the peak of sexual arousal, is the movement of semen from the epididymides to the penis. Ejaculation, which is a continuation of emission, is the pulsatile ejection of semen from the penis.

11. Spermatogenesis is a continuous process because spermatogonia, the primitive male gametes, undergo continuous mitosis within the seminiferous tubules of the testes. Some spermatogonia develop into primary spermatocytes, which divide meiotically into secondary spermatocytes and then spermatids. The spermatids develop into sperm with the help of nutrients and hormonal signals from Sertoli cells.
12. Interactions among the hypothalamus, anterior pituitary, and gonads control the production of the male sex hormones (androgens). The male hormones are produced steadily rather than cyclically, however.

Aging and Reproductive Function

1. Perimenopause is the transitional period between reproductive and nonreproductive years in women.
2. Menopause, the point that marks 12 consecutive months of amenorrhea, includes atrophic changes in the ovaries, vagina, and breast; loss of bone mass; and increased risk for cardiovascular disease.
3. Andropause is androgen deficiency in the aging male and occurs in some men. There is a decrease in testosterone production with testicular atrophy, decreased fertility, and some loss of muscle mass and strength.

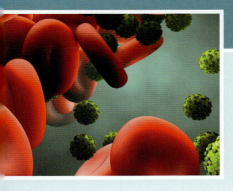

33

Alterations of the Female Reproductive System

Kelly Power-Kean, with originating chapter contributions by Kathryn L. McCance

Additional resources are available online at https://evolve.elsevier.com/Canada/Huether/pathophysiology.

CHAPTER OUTLINE

Abnormalities of the Female Reproductive Tract, 786
Alterations of Sexual Maturation, 786
    Delayed or Absent Puberty, 787
    Precocious Puberty, 787
Disorders of the Female Reproductive System, 787
    Hormonal and Menstrual Alterations, 788
    Infection and Inflammation, 793
    Pelvic Organ Prolapse, 797
    Benign Growths and Proliferative Conditions, 798
    Cancer, 802
    Sexual Dysfunction, 811
    Impaired Fertility, 811
Disorders of the Female Breast, 812
    Galactorrhea, 812
    Benign Breast Disease and Conditions, 813
    Breast Cancer, 814
CASE STUDY: Breast Cancer, 829

LEARNING OBJECTIVES

1. Describe delayed or precocious puberty.
2. Describe the primary causes, clinical indicators, and underlying pathological changes associated with dysmenorrhea, amenorrhea, and dysfunctional uterine bleeding.
3. Describe the mechanism and symptoms of polycystic ovary syndrome.
4. Name the manifestations of premenstrual syndrome. Describe the pathophysiological explanations for its occurrence.
5. Describe the various sites in which infection and inflammation can occur in the female reproductive system. Describe manifestations and treatments of each.
6. Describe the various disorders associated with pelvic relaxation. Include the clinical manifestations, risk factors, and treatments for each disorder.
7. Describe common benign cysts and growths of the female reproductive system. Include the causative factors and treatments for each.
8. Name the symptoms, risk factors, potential treatments, and diagnostic tests for cervical, vaginal, vulvar, endometrial, and ovarian cancer.
9. Name sources of female sexual dysfunction.
10. Identify the name, causative organism(s), and treatment for the major sexually transmitted infections.

KEY TERMS

Abnormal uterine bleeding (AUB), 790
Adenomyosis, 801
Amenorrhea, 789
Androgen insensitivity syndrome (AIS), 786
Anorgasmia (orgasmic dysfunction), 811
Atypia, 813
Atypical ductal hyperplasia (ADH), 814
Atypical hyperplasia (AH), 814
Atypical lobular hyperplasia (ALH), 814
Bartholinitis (Bartholin cyst), 797
Benign breast disease (BBD), 813
Carcinoma in situ, 824
Cervicitis, 796
Complete precocious puberty, 787
Corpus luteum cyst, 799
Cyst, 813
Cystocele, 797
Delayed puberty, 787
Dermoid cyst, 799
Diffuse papillomatosis, 813
Disorder of desire (hypoactive sexual desire, decreased libido), 811
Ductal carcinoma in situ (DCIS), 825
Dyspareunia (painful intercourse), 811
E-cadherin, 826
Endometrial polyp, 800
Endometriosis, 801
Enterocele, 798
Epithelial–mesenchymal transition (EMT), 824
Fibrocystic change (FCC), 813
Follicular cyst, 799
Functional cyst, 798
Galactorrhea (inappropriate lactation), 812
Genetic heterogeneity, 823
Hirsutism, 789
Infertility, 811
Intraductal papilloma, 813
Leiomyoma (myoma, uterine fibroid), 800
Lobular carcinoma in situ (LCIS), 826
Lobular involution, 818
Mammographic density (MD), 821
Menopausal hormone therapy (MHT), 819
Mild hyperplasia of the usual type, 813
Mucopurulent cervicitis (MPC), 796
Nonpuerperal hyperprolactinemia, 812
Ovarian torsion, 799
Papillary apocrine change, 813

Pelvic inflammatory disease (PID), 793	Premenstrual dysphoric disorder (PMDD), 792	Salpingitis, 794	Usual ductal hyperplasia (UDH), 813
Pelvic organ prolapse (POP), 797	Premenstrual syndrome (PMS), 792	Sclerosing adenosis, 813	Uterine prolapse, 797
Pessary, 797	Primary amenorrhea, 789	Secondary amenorrhea, 789	Vaginismus, 811
Polycystic ovary syndrome (PCOS), 791	Primary dysmenorrhea, 788	Secondary dysmenorrhea, 788	Vaginitis, 796
Precocious puberty, 787	Prolactin-inhibiting factor (PIF), 812	Sexual dysfunction, 811	Vaginosis, 796
Pregnancy-associated breast cancer (PABC), 814	Puberty, 786	Simple fibroadenoma, 814	Vascular mimicry, 825
	Radial scar (RS), 813	Terminal duct lobular unit (TDLU), 818	Vulvodynia, 796
	Rectocele, 798	Thelarche, 787	Xenoestrogen, 823
		Tumour dormancy, 824	

Alterations of the reproductive system span a wide range of concerns. These concerns include delayed sexual development, suboptimal sexual performance, and structural and functional abnormalities. Many common reproductive disorders have potentially serious physiological or psychological results. For example, sexual or reproductive dysfunction, such as impotence or infertility, can affect self-concept, relationships, and overall quality of life. Organic and psychosocial problems, such as alcoholism, depression, situational stressors, chronic illness, and medications, can affect ovulation, menstruation, sexual performance, and fertility. They may also be risk factors for the development of some types of reproductive tract cancers. Diagnosis and treatment of reproductive system disorders are often complicated by the stigma and symbolism associated with the reproductive organs and emotion-laden beliefs and behaviours related to reproductive health.[1] Embarrassment, guilt, fear, or denial may delay diagnosis and treatment.

ABNORMALITIES OF THE FEMALE REPRODUCTIVE TRACT

Normal development of the female reproductive tract requires absence of testosterone during embryonic and fetal life (see Chapter 32). The resulting fusion of the two paramesonephric (Müllerian) ducts produces the normal cervix and the uterus with an internal cavity. The distal portions of the paramesonephric ducts stay independent and form the two fallopian/uterine tubes. Alterations in the normal process include errors in cellular sensitivity to testosterone (androgen insensitivity) or failures of cell line migration. These alterations result in changes in the structure of the reproductive organs.

Androgen insensitivity occurs in 2 to 5 individuals per 100,000 male births.[2] **Androgen insensitivity syndrome (AIS)** is a disorder of hormone resistance. Characteristics of AIS include a female phenotype in an individual with an XY karyotype or male genotype, and with testes producing age-appropriate normal concentrations of androgens.[3] To date, more than 600 mutations have been reported with AIS.[2] Children with complete androgen insensitivity (CAIS) may have testes palpable within the labia majora.[3] Breast development may be normal but pubic and axillary hair is often sparse and the cervix, uterus, and ovaries are missing.[3] A short vagina that ends blindly also may be present. Milder forms of androgen insensitivity (also a common cause of male infertility)[4] are much more common and have less dramatic phenotypic manifestations. Many affected persons have normal male genitalia.

Other abnormalities of the uterus, cervix, and fallopian/uterine tubes have multifactorial origins. These factors are often the result of an interaction between genetic predisposition and environmental factors. Such interactions result in Müllerian duct abnormalities.[3] Some medications, chemicals, and toxins have been implicated as a cause of uterine abnormalities.

About 4% of the female population experiencing infertility has some sort of uterine abnormality.[5] Most uterine abnormalities stem from abnormal cell migration in the Müllerian ducts during fetal development (Figure 33.1). Uterine abnormalities are rarely diagnosed until the woman has trouble becoming pregnant or carrying a baby to term. In these women, the uterus is capable of menstruation but may have difficulty supporting a growing fetus.[6] Ultrasound during pregnancy or with magnetic resonance imaging (MRI) usually diagnoses uterine malformations. Their prognosis depends on the severity of the malformation and the location and size of the placenta and fetus. Some abnormalities can be surgically corrected to improve the outcome of later pregnancies.[6] Abnormalities of the lower genital tract also can result in women having two vaginas or a vaginal septum (a thin membrane dividing the vaginal vault). For most women, these structural abnormalities do not create functional problems. Surgical correction can take place if needed.

ALTERATIONS OF SEXUAL MATURATION

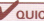

> **QUICK CHECK 33.1**
> 1. Why does puberty occur too late or too early in some individuals?
> 2. Define the normal age range for the onset of puberty.

The process of sexual maturation, or **puberty**, is started by the development of secondary sex characteristics, rapid growth, and the ability to reproduce. A variety of congenital and endocrine disorders can disrupt the timing of puberty. These disorders may cause puberty to occur too late (*delayed puberty*) or too early (*precocious puberty*). Both types involve an inappropriate onset of sex hormone production by the gonads.

The age of puberty is multifactorial, involving genetic and environmental components. The study of epigenetics and the regulation of puberty is only beginning.[7] A Canadian-based study revealed that variations related to menarche were statistically significant related to the province of residence, household income, and family type. The provinces of New Brunswick, Prince Edward Island, and Quebec had the highest proportions of early menarche. Ontario had the highest proportions of late menarche. Limited Canadian studies related to this topic exist. It is thought that these variations are associated with ethnic background diversity, lifestyle variations, and differences in socioeconomic classes.[7,8] Research has also shown that obesity decreases the age at onset of puberty by about 6 months. Although many factors are associated with obesity, much research is focusing on leptin-responsive pathways. These pathways affect the regulation of eating behaviours, onset of puberty, follicle-stimulating hormone (FSH), and luteinizing hormone (LH).[9] The normal range for the onset of puberty is now 8 to 13 years of age. Although there are conflicting and inconsistent reports, the age of pubertal onset appears to be decreasing for girls.[3] This earlier onset appears primarily in breast development, not age of menarche.

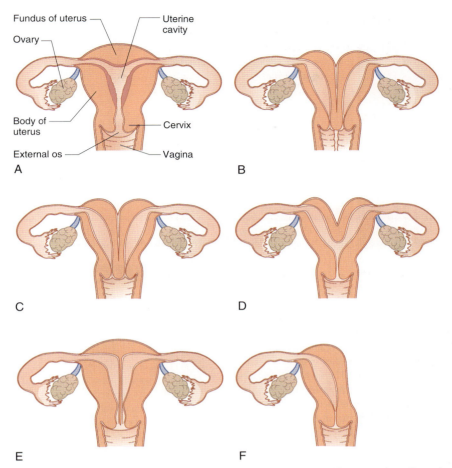

FIGURE 33.1 Uterine Malformations. Congenital uterine abnormalities. **A,** The normal configuration of the uterus and the ovaries. **B,** Double uterus with a double vagina and, **C,** a single vagina. **D,** Bicornuate uterus. **E,** A uterus with a midline septum. **F,** Unicornuate uterus. (From de Bruyn, R. [2010]. *Pediatric ultrasound* [2nd ed.]. Churchill Livingstone.)

Delayed or Absent Puberty

About 3% of children experience delayed development of secondary sex characteristics.[10] One of the first signs of puberty in girls is **thelarche**, or breast development. These signs should begin by 13 years of age. Normally, boys tend to mature later than girls, around 14 to 14.5 years of age. In boys, the first sign of maturity is enlargement of the testes and thinning of the scrotal skin. In **delayed puberty**, these secondary sex characteristics develop later.

In most cases, delayed puberty is a normal physiological event. Hormonal levels are normal, the hypothalamic–pituitary–gonadal (HPG) axis is intact, and maturation is slowly occurring. Unless the delayed puberty is causing psychosocial problems, treatment is usually not needed.[10]

Other cases are caused by the disruption of the HPG axis or by the outcomes of a systemic disease. Treatment depends on the cause (Table 33.1 and Box 33.1).

Precocious Puberty

Precocious puberty is a rare event. This condition affects about 1 in 10 000 girls and fewer than 1 in 50 000 boys. Precocious puberty is defined as sexual maturation occurring before the age of 6 years in Black girls or 7 years in White girls and before the age of 9 in boys. Precocious puberty for boys of all ethnic or racial groups is defined as sexual maturation occurring before age 9. Many conditions may cause precocious puberty (Box 33.2). These conditions include obesity, an increase in protein consumption, and endocrine disruptors in common household products, pesticides, plasticizers, and pharmaceuticals,[11] as well as lethal central nervous system (CNS) tumours. All cases of precocious puberty require thorough evaluation.

All forms of precocious puberty are treated by finding and removing the underlying cause or administering proper hormones (see Boxes 33.2 and 33.3). In many cases, the reversal of precocious puberty can occur. However, **complete precocious puberty**, the onset and progression of all pubertal features (i.e., thelarche, pubarche, and menarche), is a challenge to treat. This condition causes long bones to stop growing before the child has reached normal height.

DISORDERS OF THE FEMALE REPRODUCTIVE SYSTEM

> ### QUICK CHECK 33.2
> 1. Why does amenorrhea occur?
> 2. Why do anovulatory menstrual cycles lead to dysfunctional uterine bleeding?
> 3. Discuss insulin resistance, hyperinsulinemia, anovulation, and androgen production in polycystic ovary syndrome.
> 4. What are the current theories of pathophysiology for premenstrual syndrome/premenstrual dysphoric disorder?

TABLE 33.1 **Frequency and Common Causes of Delayed Puberty Other Than Constitutional Delay of Growth and Puberty**

Delayed Puberty	Hypergonadotropic Hypogonadism	Permanent Hypogonadotropic Hypogonadism	Functional Hypogonadotropic Hypogonadism
Frequency (%)			
Boys	5–10	10	20
Girls	25	20	20
Common causes	Turner's syndrome, gonadal dysgenesis, chemotherapy, or radiation therapy	Tumours or infiltrative diseases of the central nervous system, GnRH deficiency (isolated hypogonadotropic hypogonadism, Kallmann's syndrome), combined pituitary-hormone deficiency, chemotherapy, or radiation therapy	Systemic illness (inflammatory bowel disease, celiac disease, anorexia nervosa, or bulimia), hypothyroidism, excessive exercise

GnRH, Gonadotropin-releasing hormone.
Data from Palmert, M. R., & Dunkel, L. (2012). *New England Journal of Medicine*, 366(5), 443–453.

Hormonal and Menstrual Alterations

Dysmenorrhea

Primary dysmenorrhea is painful menstruation associated with the release of prostaglandins in ovulatory cycles, but not with pelvic disease. Approximately 50% of all women experience dysmenorrhea. About 10% experience 1 to 3 days of dysfunction because of pain severity. Primary dysmenorrhea begins with the onset of ovulatory cycles. Its prevalence is highest during adolescence.[12] The incidence steadily rises, peaks in women in the late teens and early twenties and decreases slowly thereafter. **Secondary dysmenorrhea** is related to pelvic pathological conditions. This condition manifests later in the reproductive years and may occur any time in the menstrual cycle.

PATHOPHYSIOLOGY Primary dysmenorrhea results mostly from excessive prostaglandin F_2 alpha ($PGF_2\alpha$). This is a potent myometrial stimulant and vasoconstrictor, found in secretory endometrium. Elevated levels of prostaglandins, especially $PGF_2\alpha$ and $PGE_2\alpha$, increase myometrial contractions, constrict endometrial blood vessels, and enhance nerve hypersensitivity. These symptoms result in pain.[12] These changes can lead to ischemia and endometrial shedding. Increased synthesis of prostaglandins may result from increased cyclo-oxygenase (COX) enzyme activity. Inflammatory mediators produced in leukocytes (leukotrienes) also contribute to increased levels of pain.[13] The first 48 hours of menstruation correlate with higher prostaglandin levels. Women who are anovulatory because they use oral contraceptives rarely have primary dysmenorrhea. Secondary dysmenorrhea may be caused by other disorders. These disorders include endometriosis (most common cause), endometritis (infection), pelvic inflammatory disease, adhesions, obstructive uterine or vaginal anomalies, inflammation, uterine fibroids, polyps, tumours, cysts, or intrauterine devices (IUDs).[14]

CLINICAL MANIFESTATIONS The chief symptom of dysmenorrhea is pelvic pain associated with the onset of menses. The severity is directly related to length and amount of menstrual flow. The pain often radiates into the groin. Added symptoms may include backache, anorexia, vomiting, diarrhea, syncope, and headache. The entry of prostaglandins and their metabolites into the systemic circulation are the cause of the latter symptoms. The discomfort commonly begins shortly before the onset of menstruation and rarely persists 1 to 3 days during menstrual flow.[14]

EVALUATION AND TREATMENT Differentiating primary dysmenorrhea from secondary dysmenorrhea occurs by obtaining a thorough medical history and performing a pelvic examination. Nonsteroidal

BOX 33.1 Causes of Delayed Puberty

Hypergonadotropic Hypogonadism (Increased Follicle-Stimulating Hormone [FSH] and Luteinizing Hormone [LH])
1. Gonadal dysgenesis, most commonly Turner's syndrome (45,X/46,XX; structural X or Y abnormalities; or mosaicism)
2. Klinefelter's syndrome (47,XXY)
3. Bilateral gonadal failure
   a. Traumatic or infectious
   b. Postsurgical, postirradiation, or postchemotherapy
   c. Autoimmune
   d. Idiopathic empty-scrotum or vanishing-testes syndrome (congenital anorchia) or resistant-ovary syndrome

Hypogonadotropic Hypogonadism (Decreased LH, Depressed FSH)
1. Reversible
   a. Physiological delay
   b. Weight loss or anorexia
   c. Strenuous exercise
   d. Severe obesity
   e. Illegal drug use, especially marijuana
   f. Primary hypothyroidism
   g. Congenital adrenal hyperplasia
   h. Cushing's syndrome
   i. Prolactinomas
2. Irreversible
   a. Gonadotropin-releasing hormone deficiency (Kallmann's syndrome) or idiopathic hypogonadotropic hypogonadism
   b. Hypopituitarism
   c. Congenital central nervous system defects
   d. Other pituitary adenomas
   e. Craniopharyngioma
   f. Malignant pituitary tumours

Eugonadism
These conditions are associated with amenorrhea but may have otherwise normal pubertal development:
1. Congenital anomalies
   a. Müllerian agenesis
   b. Vaginal septum or imperforate hymen
2. Androgen insensitivity syndrome
3. Inappropriate positive feedback

> **BOX 33.2 Primary Forms of Precocious Puberty**
>
> **Complete Precocious Puberty**
> Premature development of proper characteristics for the child's gender
> Hypothalamic–pituitary–ovarian axis functioning normally but prematurely
> In about 10% of cases, lethal central nervous system tumour may be the cause
>
> **Partial Precocious Puberty**
> Partial development of proper secondary sex characteristics
> Premature thelarche (breast budding) seen in girls between 6 months and 2 years of age
> Does not progress to complete puberty (ovulation and menstruation)
> Premature adrenarche (growth of axillary and pubic hair) tends to occur between 5 and 8 years of age
> Can progress to complete precocious puberty; estrogen-secreting neoplasms may be the cause or may be a variant of normal pubertal development
>
> **Mixed Precocious Puberty**
> Causes the child to develop some secondary sex characteristics of the opposite gender
> Common causes: adrenal hyperplasia or androgen-secreting tumours

Data from Burns, C. E., Dunn, A. M., Brady, M. A., et al. (Eds.). (2009). *Pediatric primary care* (4th ed.). Saunders; Jospe, N. (2005). Disorders of pubertal development. In Osborn, L. M., DeWitt, T. G., First, L. R., et al. (Eds.). (2005). *Pediatrics*. Mosby.

> **BOX 33.3 Causes of Mixed Precocious Puberty**
>
> | Female (Virilization) | Male (Feminization) |
> |---|---|
> | Congenital adrenal hyperplasia | Estrogen-producing tumours |
> | Androgen-secreting tumours | Adrenal |
> | Adrenal | Teratoma |
> | Ovarian | Hepatoma |
> | Teratoma | Testicular |
> | Exogenous androgens | Exogenous estrogens |
> | | Increased peripheral conversion of androgens to estrogens |

From Jospe, N. (2005). Disorders of pubertal development. In L. M. Osborn, T. G. DeWitt, L. R. First, et al. (Eds.), *Pediatrics*. Mosby.

anti-inflammatory drugs (NSAIDs, e.g., ibuprofen) are the treatment of choice because they reduce COX enzyme activity and thus prostaglandin production. NSAIDs are effective in most women with primary dysmenorrhea. Their use is most effective if started at the first sign of bleeding or cramping. In women who wish to use contraception, dysmenorrhea may be relieved with hormonal contraceptives. Hormonal contraception stops ovulation and creates an atrophic endometrium. As a result, prostaglandin synthesis and myometrial contractility is decreased. To help prevent or reduce symptoms, regular exercise and stress reduction are beneficial. Other helpful approaches with some effectiveness in pain relief include local application of heat; acupuncture; high-frequency transcutaneous electrical nerve stimulation (TENS); supplements, such as thiamine and vitamin E; and Chinese herbal treatment.[13]

Amenorrhea

Amenorrhea means lack of menstruation. The most common causes (aside from pregnancy) include hypothalamic dysfunction, polycystic ovarian syndrome, hyperprolactinemia, and ovarian failure. Primary amenorrhea is the failure of menarche and the absence of menstruation by age 13 years without the development of secondary sex characteristics or by age 15 years, regardless of the presence of secondary sex characteristics.[15] Secondary amenorrhea is the absence of menstruation for a time equivalent to three or more cycles in women who have previously menstruated.

PATHOPHYSIOLOGY One approach to understanding the pathophysiology of amenorrhea is to compartmentalize. *Compartment I disorders* are anatomical defects, including absence of the vagina and uterus. *Compartment II disorders* involve the ovary, primarily genetic disorders (such as Turner's syndrome) and AIS. The target organs (e.g., ovaries) in AIS are completely resistant to the action of androgens. This resistance results in a lack of estrogen. *Compartment III disorders* are of the anterior pituitary gland, including tumours. These disorders result in failure of signalling to the ovaries through FSH and LH secretion. *Compartment IV disorders* include CNS disorders and primarily involve hypothalamic defects that prevent secretion of gonadotropin-releasing hormone (GnRH). These defects result in no signalling to the pituitary to release FSH and LH.

CLINICAL MANIFESTATIONS The major clinical manifestation of primary amenorrhea is the absence of the first menstrual period. The cause of the amenorrhea decides whether secondary sex characteristics and height are affected.

EVALUATION AND TREATMENT Diagnosis of primary amenorrhea is based on the results of a history and physical examination and determination of the presence or absence of secondary sexual characteristics. Laboratory studies may be needed to document abnormal levels of gonadotropins or ovarian imaging. Structural abnormalities are documented using hormones or determined through the presence of genetic conditions.

Treatment involves correction of any underlying disorders and implementation of hormone replacement therapy (HRT) to induce the development of secondary sex characteristics. Although surgical alteration of the genitalia may occur to correct abnormalities, it should be postponed until the individual can make an informed decision.

Secondary Amenorrhea

Many disorders and physiological conditions are associated with secondary amenorrhea. Secondary amenorrhea is common (normal) during early adolescence, pregnancy, lactation, and the perimenopausal period. This condition is primarily because of anovulation. The most common causes (after pregnancy) are thyroid disorders (e.g., hypothyroidism); hyperprolactinemia; hypothalamic–pituitary–ovarian (HPO) interruption secondary to excessive exercise, stress, or weight loss; and polycystic ovary syndrome (PCOS).

PATHOPHYSIOLOGY The pathophysiology is dependent on the causes of secondary amenorrhea. Figure 33.2 summarizes these causes.

CLINICAL MANIFESTATIONS The major manifestation of secondary amenorrhea is the absence of menses after earlier menstrual periods. Depending on the underlying cause of the amenorrhea, infertility, vasomotor flushes, vaginal atrophy, acne, osteopenia, and hirsutism (abnormal hairiness) may be present.

EVALUATION AND TREATMENT Pregnancy is the most common cause of secondary amenorrhea and must be ruled out before any further evaluation. A thorough history and physical examination is important. The menstrual cycle may stop or become irregular in response to stress, extreme exercise, large dietary changes, eating

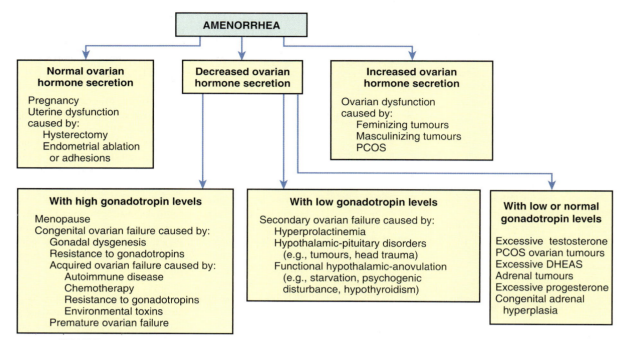

FIGURE 33.2 Causes of Secondary Amenorrhea. Hypothyroidism is a relatively common condition and should be ruled out as the cause of hyperprolactinemia before more extensive evaluation (i.e., computed tomography or magnetic resonance imaging) occurs. *DHEAS*, Dehydroepiandrosterone sulphate; *PCOS*, polycystic ovary syndrome.

disorders, or sleep abnormalities. Hypothyroidism also is a common cause and should be ruled out as well. Diagnosis of secondary amenorrhea involves finding underlying hormonal or anatomical alterations. Evaluation of thyroid-stimulating hormone (TSH) or prolactin levels may be needed. Depending on the cause of the amenorrhea, treatment may involve HRT or a corrective procedure, such as surgical removal of a pituitary tumour. The woman's child-bearing plans may influence the choice of treatment.

Abnormal Uterine Bleeding

Menstrual irregularity or abnormal bleeding patterns (Table 33.2) account for approximately 33% of all gynecological visits. The most common cause of cycle irregularity is failure to ovulate related to age, stress, or endocrinopathy. Table 33.3 presents common causes of abnormal bleeding based on age group and frequency.

Abnormal uterine bleeding (AUB) is bleeding that is abnormal in duration, volume, frequency, or regularity. It may be acute or chronic, and is classified by the cause of bleeding, using an internationally recognized PALM-COEIN system. PALM-COEIN stands for polyp, adenomyosis, leiomyoma, and malignancy and hyperplasia, and coagulopathy, ovulatory dysfunction, endometrial, iatrogenic, and not-yet classified. PALM consists of disorders of tissue or structure that are diagnosed by imaging or biopsy. COEIN consists of nonstructural causes of AUB. AUB is the leading cause for hysterectomies and for most endometrial ablation procedures.[16] Perimenopausal women are the most affected by AUB.

PATHOPHYSIOLOGY The majority of AUB is associated with lack of ovulation.[17] AUB may occur at any time during the reproductive years and many conditions are associated with irregular ovulation. More than 50% of cases occur in perimenopausal women ages 40 to 50 years when they are more likely to ovulate irregularly. Women who do not ovulate experience irregularities in their menstrual bleeding because of a lack of progesterone and, in some cases, an excess of estrogen. This results in excessive and irregular endometrial thickness and later excessive and irregular bleeding. PCOS, obesity, and thyroid disease also are common contributors. Abnormal bleeding can result from defects of the corpus luteum. These defects result in progesterone deficiencies or from abnormalities of the uterus or cervix. Some of these abnormalities include endometrial polyps, uterine fibroids, or uterine or cervical cancers.

Abnormal menstrual bleeding in ovulatory cycles is less common. Mechanisms underlying the bleeding are unclear. Some possible causes include defects of the corpus luteum and abnormalities of the uterus or cervix, such as polyps, fibroids, or cancer. Other causes may include excessive fibrinolytic activity, use of anticoagulants, diseases of coagulation, infection, and changes in prostaglandin production.

CLINICAL MANIFESTATIONS Unpredictable and variable bleeding in terms of amount and duration characterize AUB. Especially during perimenopause, abnormal bleeding also may involve flooding and the passing of large clots. These symptoms may lead to excessive blood loss. Excessive bleeding can lead to iron deficiency anemia and associated symptoms, including fatigue or shortness of breath.

EVALUATION AND TREATMENT Diagnosis of AUB occurs after other organic conditions that could cause abnormal bleeding are eliminated. If no cause is found, it is assumed that the bleeding is caused by lack of regular ovulation. NSAIDs are often first-line treatments for excessive menstrual bleeding. NSAIDS reduce prostaglandin synthesis within the endometrial tissues, leading to vasoconstriction and decreased bleeding. For the best effect they should be taken in the few days preceding the beginning of the menstrual period and be continued through the days of heaviest bleeding. NSAIDs are not as effective in controlling menstrual blood loss as hormonal therapies but they are readily available without a prescription.

Goals of therapy are to control bleeding, prevent hyperplasia, prevent or treat anemia, and treat endocrine problems if present. Common treatments include administration of oral contraceptive pills that have

TABLE 33.2 Abnormal Uterine Bleeding

Current Terminology	Outdated Terminology	Definition
Chronic AUB	Menometrorrhagia, Menorrhagia, Menorrhea, Polymenorrhea	Abnormal uterine bleeding for at least 4 out of 6 months; abnormal bleeding is characterized by increased amount, regularity, and/or timing
Acute AUB		Single episode of severe uterine bleeding that is sufficient to require immediate intervention to prevent further blood loss
Intermenstrual bleeding (AUB/IMB)	Metrorrhagia	Uterine bleeding that occurs between regular menstrual cycles; intermenstrual bleeding can be random or predictable
Heavy menstrual bleeding (HMB/AUB)	Hypermenorrhea	Increased menstrual volume that interferes with a woman's physical, emotional, and social quality of life

AUB, Abnormal uterine bleeding.
Data from Fraser, I. S., Critchley, H. O. D., Broder, M., et al. (2011). *Seminars in Reproductive Medicine, 29*(5), 383–390; Munro, M. G., Critchley, H. O. D., Broder, M. S., et al. (2011). *International Journal of Gynecology & Obstetrics, 113*(1), 3–13.

TABLE 33.3 Common Causes of Abnormal (Vaginal/Genital) Bleeding in Descending Order of Frequency

Age Group	Cause
Prepubescence	Sexual assault
	Trauma
	Foreign bodies
	Precocious puberty
Adolescence	Anovulation (immature hypothalamic–pituitary–ovarian axis)
	Trauma and sexual abuse
Reproductive years	Pregnancy
	Pelvic inflammatory disease
	Coagulation disorder
	Hormonal contraceptives
	Endometriosis
	Anovulation
	Intrauterine device
	Ovarian cysts
	Uterine polyps or tumours
	Polycystic ovary syndrome
	Bleeding disorders (e.g., von Willebrand's disease)
	Trauma/rape
Perimenopause	Anovulation
	Malignancy
	Pregnancy
	Endometriosis
	Benign neoplasms (myomas, adenomyosis)
Postmenopause	Malignancy
Other: non–age-specific	Chronic conditions
	Adrenal conditions
	Thyroid disorders
	Liver disease
	Diabetes mellitus
	Obesity
	Hypertension

estrogen and progesterone, prescription of long-term therapy with medroxyprogesterone (Provera), and placement of a levonorgestrel intrauterine device (LNG-IUD). The Health Canada black box warning about potential bone loss has greatly curtailed the use of Provera. The LNG-IUD has a dual use from Health Canada for birth control and suppression of abnormal menstrual bleeding. The device releases a steady amount of progesterone directly into the uterus to stabilize and suppress the uterine lining. The progesterone works to suppress the HPG axis and prevent ovulation.

Women who do not wish to have future pregnancies can opt for treatments that permanently suppress their uterine lining. These treatments include ablation. This treatment involves burning the uterine lining to prevent future proliferation of the endometrial cells, and complete removal of the uterus in hysterectomy. If a woman is menopausal and has not had a menstrual period for greater than 1 year investigation of vaginal bleeding should occur to rule out uterine and other cancers.

Polycystic Ovary Syndrome

Polycystic ovary syndrome (PCOS) is one of the most common endocrine disturbances affecting women (Figure 33.3). International criteria for the diagnosis of PCOS require at least two of the following conditions: few or anovulatory menstrual cycles, elevated levels of androgens, and polycystic ovaries. Thus, polycystic ovaries do not have to be present to diagnose PCOS. Their presence alone does not prove the diagnosis of PCOS. PCOS should not be confused with benign ovarian cysts. These cysts are common during the reproductive years and have a different etiology (see "Benign Ovarian Cysts"). PCOS is a leading cause of infertility in North America. PCOS has a large incidence of inheritability. Signs and symptoms of PCOS can vary over time, with metabolic syndrome becoming more common with age.[3]

PATHOPHYSIOLOGY The direct cause of PCOS is related to a genetic predisposition and an obesity-prone lifestyle. This lifestyle may lead to insulin resistance and an excess of insulin and androgens. A hyperandrogenic state is a key feature in the pathogenesis of PCOS. However, glucose intolerance or insulin resistance and hyperinsulinemia often occur at the same time. These symptoms significantly aggravate the hyperandrogenic state, thus contributing to the severity of signs and symptoms of PCOS.[18] PCOS predisposes to obesity, and pre-existing obesity predisposes to more severe PCOS.

Insulin resistance and resultant compensatory hyperinsulinemia overstimulates androgen secretion by the ovarian stroma. This process reduces hepatic secretion of serum sex hormone binding globulin (SHBG). The effect is an increase in free testosterone levels. Excessive androgens affect follicular growth. Insulin affects follicular decline by suppressing apoptosis and enabling the survival of follicles that would normally disintegrate (Figure 33.4). There also seems to be a genetic ovarian defect in PCOS that makes the ovary either more susceptible to or more sensitive to insulin's stimulation of ovarian androgen production.

Inappropriate gonadotropin secretion triggers the beginning of a vicious cycle that perpetuates anovulation. Typically, levels of FSH are low or below normal and the LH level is elevated. Persistent LH level elevation causes an increase in the concentration of androgens. These androgens include dehydroepiandrosterone sulphate [DHEAS] from

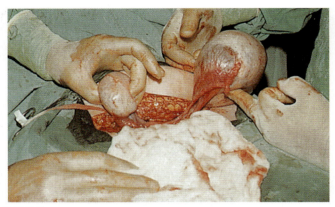

FIGURE 33.3 Polycystic Ovary. Surgical view of polycystic ovaries. (From Symonds, E. M., & Macpherson, M. B. A. [1997]. *Diagnosis in color: obstetrics and gynecology.* Mosby-Wolfe.)

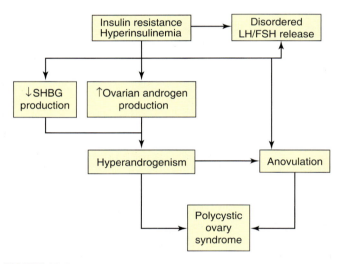

FIGURE 33.4 Insulin Resistance and Hyperinsulinemia in Polycystic Ovary Syndrome. See text for explanation. *FSH,* Follicle-stimulating hormone; *LH,* luteinizing hormone; *SHBG,* sex hormone–binding globulin.

BOX 33.4 Clinical Manifestations of Polycystic Ovary Syndrome

Presenting Signs and Symptoms (% of Women Affected)
Obesity (41%)
Menstrual disturbance (70% [e.g., abnormal uterine bleeding])
Oligomenorrhea (47%)
Amenorrhea (19%)
Regular menstruation (48%)
Hyperandrogenism (69–74%)
Infertility (73% of anovulatory infertility)
Asymptomatic (20% of those with polycystic ovary syndrome)

Hormonal Disturbances
Increased insulin (independent of obesity)
Decreased SHBG
Increased androgens (testosterone, androstenedione)
Increased DHEA (occurs in 50% of women)
Increased LH (genetic variant LH-β subunit)
Increased prolactin
Increased leptin, especially in obesity (independent of insulin)
Suggested decreased IGF-1 receptors on theca cells
Possible decreased estrogen receptors (intraovarian and along hypothalamic–pituitary axis)

Possible Late Sequelae
Dyslipidemia: increased low-density lipoproteins, decreased high-density lipoproteins, increased triglycerides
Diabetes mellitus (30% of women with or without obesity will develop type 2 diabetes mellitus by age 30)
Cardiovascular disease; hypertension
Endometrial hyperplasia and carcinoma (anovulatory women are hyperestrogenic)

Other
Women with PCOS are at increased risk for gestational diabetes mellitus, pregnancy-induced hypertension, preterm birth, and perinatal mortality

DHEA, Dehydroepiandrosterone; *IGF-1,* insulinlike growth factor 1; *LH,* luteinizing hormone; *PCOS,* polycystic ovary syndrome; *SHBG,* sex hormone–binding globulin. Adapted from Azziz, R., Carmina, E., Dewailly, D., et al. (2009). *Fertility and Sterility, 91*(2), 456–488; Boomsma, C. M., Fauser, B. C., & Macklon, N. S. (2008). *Seminars in Reproductive Medicine, 26*(1), 72–84; Diamanti-Kandarakis, E. (2008). *Expert Reviews in Molecular Medicine, 10*(2), e3; Spritzer, P. M., & Motta, A. B. (2015). *International Journal of Clinical Practice, 69*(11), 1236–1246.

the adrenal glands, and testosterone, androstenedione, and dehydroepiandrosterone [DHEA] from the ovary. Androgens are converted to estrogen in peripheral tissues. Increased testosterone levels cause an approximate 50% decrease in SHBG level. This decrease causes increased levels of free estradiol. Elevated estrogen levels trigger a positive feedback response in LH and a negative feedback response in FSH. Because FSH levels are not totally depressed, new follicular growth is continuously stimulated. However, the follicles do not reach full maturation and ovulation (see Figure 33.4).[3]

CLINICAL MANIFESTATIONS Clinical manifestations of PCOS usually appear within 2 years of puberty. These manifestations may, however, appear after a period of normal menstrual function and pregnancy. Symptoms are related to anovulation and hyperandrogenism. Symptoms include AUB or amenorrhea, hirsutism, acne, and infertility (Box 33.4). Hypertension and dyslipidemia also are often found in association with PCOS. PCOS is often accompanied by other endocrine disorders.[18]

EVALUATION AND TREATMENT Diagnosis of PCOS is based on evidence of androgen excess (hirsutism, male pattern hair distribution, acne), chronic anovulation (as shown by irregular menstrual patterns, amenorrhea, and infertility), insulin resistance (obesity may be a sign, as well as abnormal glucose tolerance testing), and inappropriate gonadotropin secretion (low serum FSH concentration, and elevated levels of LH and DHEA). Treatment of PCOS often includes use of combined oral contraceptives to control irregular menstrual cycles and to oppose estrogens and androgens. Insulin sensitizers, such as metformin (Glucophage), may be used to decrease insulin resistance, prevent diabetes and heart disease, and restore fertility. Insulin sensitizers combined with clomiphene citrate (Clomid) may be effective for ovulation induction for women who are trying to become pregnant. Reduction in weight can dramatically improve insulin sensitivity and return of ovulatory cycles.

Premenstrual Disorder Syndromes

Premenstrual syndrome (PMS) and **premenstrual dysphoric disorder (PMDD)** are the cyclic recurrence (in the luteal phase of the menstrual cycle) of distressing physical, psychological, or behavioural changes that impair interpersonal relationships or interfere with usual activities. The luteal phase of ovulatory cycles is linked with complex hormonal changes of the menstrual cycle. PMDD is a severe, sometimes disabling extension of PMS. The prevalence of PMS and PMDD is difficult to determine, possibly because of the wide-ranging nature of accepted symptoms. Symptoms for PMS and PMDD begin after ovulation during the luteal phase and persist up to 4 days into the menstrual cycle.[14] Estimates show that 91% of women experience some form of distress around their menstrual period. In addition, 30% experience enough distress to interrupt their daily routine, and approximately 3.1% meet the criteria for PMDD.

PATHOPHYSIOLOGY There are many theories to explain PMS/PMDD and their mechanisms. These theories include an increased vulnerability to *fluctuations* in ovarian-derived hormones, and hypothalamic–pituitary–adrenal (HPA) axis changes.[19] The neuroendocrine mechanisms of the hormonal environment of the menopausal transition that might trigger depression are poorly understood.[19] Irregular ovarian hormone fluctuation may be a mediator of risk for both vasomotor symptoms (hot flashes) and perimenopausal depression. Neurotransmitters, such as serotonin, gamma aminobutyric acid (GABA), and norepinephrine, have proven interactions with estrogen and progesterone, and proven mood and behaviour effects, including negative mood, irritability, aggression, and impulse control. Additionally, neurotransmitters may have mediating or moderating roles on symptom manifestation. Sex steroids also interact with the renin-angiotensin-aldosterone system (RAAS), which could explain some PMS/PMDD signs and symptoms (e.g., water retention, bloating, weight gain). Increased levels of inflammatory mediators may occur with menstrual symptom severity and PMS.[20]

A predisposition to PMS occurs in families, perhaps because of genetics or shared environment. A woman's menstrual experience is often like her mother's or her sister's experience. Evidence supports a relationship between severity and frequency of PMS/PMDD and reports of low well-being, major affective disorder, and personal characteristics, such as increased stress, poor nutrition, lack of exercise, low self-esteem, perfectionism, history of sexual abuse, and family conflict. In turn, when PMS/PMDD is distressing, negative quality of interpersonal relationships and self-image occur.

CLINICAL MANIFESTATIONS The pattern of symptom frequency and severity is more important than specific complaints. PMS/PMDD are associated with nearly 300 physical, emotional, and behavioural symptoms. Emotional symptoms, particularly depression, anger, irritability, and fatigue, have been reported as the most prominent and the most distressing. Physical symptoms seem to be the least prevalent and problematic. Premenstrual aggravation of underlying physical or psychological disease may occur and must be diagnosed and treated independently of PMS/PMDD.

EVALUATION AND TREATMENT Diagnosis of PMS/PMDD is based on health history and symptoms. Current treatment is symptomatic because the cause is complex and cannot be reduced to a single biological explanation. In addition, occurrence and severity are mediated by lifestyle, social, and psychological factors. Approaches may include stress reduction, exercise, family or individual counselling, biofeedback, diet (see *Health Promotion*: Nutrition and Premenstrual Syndrome), imagery, acupuncture, and rest. Two major forms of treatment include the use of hormonal cycle regulation and use of selective serotonin reuptake inhibitor (SSRI) antidepressants.[3] If a woman does not want immediate fertility, an estrogen and progesterone oral contraceptive pill has shown benefits in decreasing PMS/PMDD. In severe cases, the cessation of menses can occur using GnRH agonists.

HEALTH PROMOTION
Nutrition and Premenstrual Syndrome

Women who are affected by premenstrual syndrome (PMS) often look for ways to decrease or prevent their symptoms. Dietary interventions that can help are multiple: eating six small meals each day; increasing intake of complex carbohydrates, fibre, and water; and decreasing caffeine, alcohol, refined sugar, and animal fat consumption. A low-fat vegetarian diet has been associated with decreased symptoms. The reason for this is possibly because of an increase in serum sex hormone–binding globulin concentration that lowers serum estrogen levels. It also may be helpful to limit sodium intake. Some limited evidence suggests that moderate doses (50 mg/day) of vitamin B_6 may reduce emotional symptoms of depression, irritability, and fatigue.

High food intake of thiamine and riboflavin was seen to lower risk for PMS. Thiamine, riboflavin, niacin, vitamin B_6, folate, and vitamin B_{12} are needed to synthesize neurotransmitters. Limited data suggest that dietary minerals may be useful in preventing PMS. Prospective analyses suggest that higher plasma vitamin D levels may be inversely related to the development of specific menstrual symptoms. Vitamin D deficiency is associated with increased renin-angiotensin-aldosterone system activity, a system that regulates fluid balance and blood pressure. Vitamin D may lower the risk for unipolar depression.

Some researchers have suggested links between serotonin, endorphins, and high sugar intake and PMS risk. One interesting craving is chocolate. Some researchers suggest that a craving for chocolate is an unconscious desire for a compound called *phenylethylamine* in chocolate. This compound stimulates the release of the neurotransmitter dopamine, which regulates mood.

Data from Bernard, N. D., Scialli, A. R., Hurlock, D., et al. (2000). *Obstetrics & Gynecology, 95*(2), 245; Bertone-Johnson, E., Hankinson, S. E., Forger, N. G., et al. (2014). *BMC Womens Health, 14*, 56; Chocano-Bedoya, P. O., Manson, J. E., Hankinson, S. E., et al. (2011). *American Journal of Clinical Nutrition, 93*(5), 1080–1086; Chocano-Bedoya, P. O., Manson, J. E., Hankinson, S. E., et al. (2013). *American Journal of Epidemiology, 177*(10): 1118–1127; Eyles, D. W., Burne, T. H., & McGrath, J. J. (2012). *Frontiers in Neuroendocrinology, 34*, 47–64; Mahan, L. K., & Escott-Stump, S. (2000). *Krause's food, nutrition, and diet therapy* (10th ed.). Saunders; Murakami, K., Sasaki, S., Takahashi, Y., et al. (2008). *Nutrition, 24*(6), 554–561.

Infection and Inflammation

QUICK CHECK 33.3
1. Why is early treatment of pelvic inflammatory disease critical to reproductive health?
2. Why do benign ovarian cysts develop in women who ovulate?
3. What is the difference between a follicular cyst and a corpus luteum cyst?

Infections of the genital tract may result from exogenous or endogenous microorganisms. Exogenous pathogens are most often sexually transmitted. Endogenous causes of infection include microorganisms that are normally resident in the vagina, bowel, or vulva. Infection occurs if these microorganisms migrate to a new location or overgrow when the immune system and other defence mechanisms are impaired.

Skin disorders that can affect the vulva include reactive dermatitis, contact dermatitis, psoriasis, and impetigo. (For a discussion of skin disorders, see Chapter 41.) However, most infectious disorders that affect the vulva and vagina are sexually transmitted. Table 34.1 describes currently recognized sexually transmitted infections (STIs).

Pelvic Inflammatory Disease

Pelvic inflammatory disease (PID) is an acute inflammatory process caused by infection (Figure 33.5). PID may involve any organ, or combination of organs, of the upper genital tract. This includes

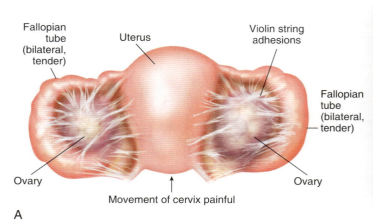
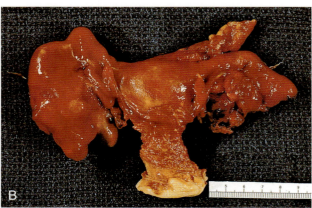

FIGURE 33.5 Pelvic Inflammatory Disease. **A,** Drawing depicting involvement of both ovaries and fallopian tubes. **B,** Total abdominal hysterectomy and bilateral salpingo-oophorectomy specimen showing unilateral pyosalpinx. ([A], from Ball, J. W., Dains, J. E., Flynn, J. A., et al. [2015]. *Seidel's guide to physical examination* [8th ed.]. Mosby; [B], from Morse, S. A., Holmes, K. K., & Ballard, R. C. [2010]. *Atlas of sexually transmitted diseases and AIDS* [4th ed.]. Mosby.)

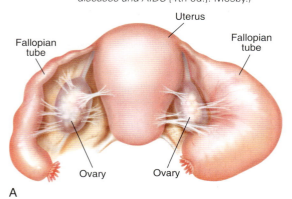
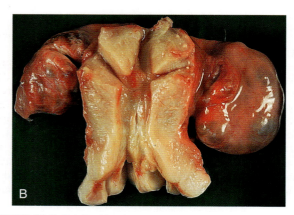

FIGURE 33.6 Salpingitis. **A,** Advanced pyosalpinx. Note the swollen fallopian tubes. **B,** Bilateral, retort-shaped, swollen, sealed tubes and adhesions of ovaries are typical of salpingitis. ([A], from Ball, J. W., Dains, J. E., Flynn, J. A., et al. [2015]. *Seidel's guide to physical examination* [8th ed.]. Mosby; [B], from Damjanov, I., & Linder, J. [Eds.]. [1996]. *Anderson's pathology* [10th ed.]. Mosby.)

the uterus, fallopian tubes, or ovaries and, in its most severe form, the entire peritoneal cavity. Many infectious disorders that affect the vulva and vagina are sexually transmitted. Examples of these infections include chlamydia and gonorrhea that migrate from the vagina to the uterus, fallopian tubes, and ovaries.[3] Microorganisms that make up the vaginal flora (e.g., anaerobes, *Gardnerella vaginalis*, *Haemophilus influenzae*, enteric Gram-negative rods, and *Streptococcus agalactiae*) also are implicated with PID. Additionally, cytomegalovirus (CMV), *Mycoplasma hominis*, *Ureaplasma urealyticum*, and *Mycoplasma genitalium* may be associated with PID. There are many risk factors for PID. These factors include infection by an earlier STI that was not treated (delaying treatment increases complications from PID); having multiple sex partners or a sex partner who has had multiple sex partners or a previous PID; being sexually active at age 25 or younger; using douches; and using an IUD for birth control.[21] Other causes of infection include spontaneous or induced abortions, normal or abnormal deliveries (called *puerperal infections*), or other surgical procedures.

PATHOPHYSIOLOGY Several defence mechanisms mediate the development of upper genital tract infections. These factors include the virulence of the microorganism, size of the inoculum, and immune defence status of the individual. PID develops when pathological microbes ascend from an infected cervix to infect the uterus and adnexae (uterine appendages). The first infection usually involves the endocervical mucosa, but it can start in the Bartholin gland and other glands. From these sites, the infection can move upward to involve the fallopian tubes and tubo-ovarian region (Figure 33.6). STIs from gonorrhea and chlamydia are the main infectious causes of PID; however, other infections that are not sexually transmitted (e.g., induced abortion, dilation and curettage of the uterus, and other surgical procedures) also can cause PID.[15] Many anaerobic bacteria have been implicated in increasing the risk for PID because they alter the pH of the vaginal environment and may decrease the integrity of the mucus blocking the cervical canal. Bacterial vaginosis (BV) is present in up to 66% of women with PID, and other anaerobes, such as *Bacteroides*, and *G. vaginalis*, *H. influenzae*, and genital tract mycoplasmas (*M. hominis*, *M. genitalium*, and *U. urealyticum*) are often isolated from women with PID. *Escherichia coli* may contribute to pelvic infections in older women. Therefore, although gonorrhea and chlamydia are the main pathogens in PID, the infection is polymicrobial in origin. Treatment of this infection is with broad spectrum of antibiotics to ensure that all the causative agents are eliminated.[22]

Salpingitis

Salpingitis is inflammation of the fallopian tubes (see Figure 33.6). The inflammatory process develops after the infection has been established.

> **BOX 33.5 Diagnostic Criteria for Pelvic Inflammatory Disease**
>
> **Minimum Criteria (One or More Needed for Diagnosis)**
> Cervical motion tenderness, *or*
> Uterine tenderness, *or*
> Adnexal tenderness
>
> **Additional Criteria That Increase Specificity of Diagnosis**
> Body temperature >38.3°C (>101°F)
> Mucopurulent cervical or vaginal discharge
> Numerous white blood cells on saline wet prep
> Elevated C-reactive protein
> Elevated erythrocyte sedimentation rate
> Documented infection with *Chlamydia trachomatis* or *Neisseria gonorrhoeae*
>
> **Definitive Criteria (Not Needed for Treatment)**
> Transvaginal ultrasound, magnetic resonance imaging, *or*
> Doppler studies showing thickened and fluid-filled tubes
> Laparoscopic visualization of PID-related abnormalities

PID, Pelvic inflammatory disease.
Data from Centers for Disease Control and Prevention. (2010). *MMWR: Morbidity & Mortality Weekly Report, 59*(RR-12); Yudin, M. H., & Ross, J. D. C. (2012). Pelvic inflammatory disease. In J. M. Zenilman, & M. Shahmanesh (Eds.), *Sexually transmitted diseases* (pp. 67–76). Jones & Bartlett Learning.

> **BOX 33.6 PHAC Outpatient Recommended Regimen for Pelvic Inflammatory Disease**
>
> 1. **Ceftriaxone** (Rocephin) 250 mg intramuscularly (IM) in a single dose
>   OR
>   **Cefoxitin** (Mefoxin Pws) 2 g IM in a single dose
>   PLUS
>   **Probenecid** (Benuryl) 1 g orally administered concurrently in a single dose
>   OR
>   **Other parenteral third-generation cephalosporin** (e.g., ceftizoxime [Cefizox] or cefotaxime [Cefotaxime Sodium])
>   PLUS
>   **Doxycycline** (Teva-Doxycycline) 100 mg orally twice a day for 14 days
>   *With or without*
>   **Metronidazole** (Flagyl) 500 mg orally twice a day for 14 days
>   Or
> 2. **Ofloxaxin** 400 mg orally twice a day for 14 days
>   OR
>   **Levofloxacin** 500 mg orally once a day for 14 days
>   *With or without*
>   **Metronidazole** 500 mg orally twice a day for 14 days

PHAC, Public Health Agency of Canada.
From Public Health Agency of Canada. (2013). *Canadian guidelines on sexually transmitted infections* (Section 4-4: Management and treatment of specific syndrome—pelvic inflammatory disease [PID], Table 5). https://www.canada.ca/en/public-health/services/infectious-diseases/sexual-health-sexually-transmitted-infections/canadian-guidelines/sexually-transmitted-infections/canadian-guidelines-sexually-transmitted-infections-22.html. Public Health Agency of Canada, Modified: 2017. Adapted and reproduced with permission from the Minister of Health, 2017.

The infection induces changes in the columnar epithelia that line the upper reproductive tract. The inflammation causes localized edema and sometimes necrosis of the area. Gonorrhea gonococci attach to the fallopian tubes and excrete a substance toxic to the tubal mucosa, causing further inflammation and damage. Chlamydia enters the tubal cells and replicates. The increased replication bursts the cell membrane, causing permanent scarring. Gonorrhea and chlamydia can spread to the abdominal cavity through the openings of the fallopian/uterine tubes. Other mechanisms that may contribute to PID include lymphatic drainage with parametrial spread of the infection. The acute complications of PID include peritonitis and bacteremia. These conditions can increase the risk for endocarditis, meningitis, and infectious arthritis. The chronic consequences of PID are many. These include infertility and tubal obstruction, ectopic pregnancy, pelvic pain of varying degrees, and intestinal obstruction from adhesions between the bowel and pelvic organs.[23]

CLINICAL MANIFESTATIONS The clinical manifestations of PID vary from sudden, severe abdominal pain with fever to no symptoms at all. An asymptomatic cervicitis may be present for some time before PID develops. The first sign of the ascending infection may be the onset of low bilateral abdominal pain. Pain is often characterized as dull and steady with a gradual onset. Symptoms are more likely to develop during or right after menstruation. The pain of PID may worsen with walking, jumping, or intercourse. Other manifestations of PID include dysuria (difficult or painful urination) and irregular bleeding.

EVALUATION AND TREATMENT PID often has limited or vague clinical symptoms, leading to undertreatment and long-term health effects.[24] Because PID is a substantial health risk to a woman, the Centers for Disease Control and Prevention (CDC) encourages clinicians to consider PID as a likely diagnosis when a sexually active woman has abdominal or pelvic tenderness and *one* of the following: cervical motion tenderness, uterine tenderness, or adnexal tenderness.[25] Box 33.5 lists the diagnostic criteria for PID. No laboratory results or studies are needed to begin treatment; however, more information can improve the specificity of diagnosis.[26]

The complications of PID can be significant; therefore, rapid treatment is recommended even before the causative pathogen can be named. Because treatment is empirical, it needs to be effective against a broad range of pathogens, especially chlamydia, gonorrhea, and anaerobic bacteria.[26] Treatment is usually done on an outpatient basis unless the woman has symptoms of advanced infection, cannot take oral medications, is pregnant, or shows other pathologies that cannot be excluded. Box 33.6 outlines the Public Health Agency of Canada's (PHAC's) recommended outpatient regimen.

Although alternative treatment regimens are available, the growing antibiotic resistance of gonorrhea limits antibiotic choices. The PHAC is closely watching gonorrhea's antibiotic sensitivity and updates treatment guidelines periodically to reflect new information.[26] To prevent recurrence, sexual partners of women with PID should also receive treatment, even if they are asymptomatic. Women receiving treatment should be re-evaluated by their care provider in 3 days to ensure antibiotic treatment is effective.[26] Because women with a history of PID are at increased risk for ectopic pregnancy, they should seek care as soon as they know they are pregnant because ectopic pregnancy is a major cause of maternal mortality.[27]

The diagnosis of PID is based on history, abdominal tenderness, the presence of uterine and cervical movement tenderness on bimanual pelvic examination, mucopurulent discharge at the cervical os, white blood cells on Gram stain or wet mount of cervical discharge, leukocytosis, and increased erythrocyte sedimentation rate. To support the diagnosis, tests for chlamydia and gonorrhea are done. When a woman has recurrent symptoms or symptoms unresponsive to outpatient treatment regimens, a temperature greater than 38°C (100.4°F), or an adnexal mass, the use of sonography, laparoscopy, and culdocentesis are indicated. However, other conditions that cause pelvic pain must be excluded. These include ectopic pregnancy, threatened abortion, ovarian torsion, ovarian cyst, or appendicitis. Recommendations for physical rest and avoidance of intercourse are often given as precautionary and comfort measures during initial recovery (i.e., 1 to 2 weeks).

Vaginitis

Vaginitis is irritation or inflammation of the vagina, typically caused by infection. Characteristics of vaginitis include an increase in white blood cells on saline wet prep examination. Vaginal irritation without white blood cells is known as **vaginosis**. The major causes of vaginitis are overgrowth of normal flora, STIs, and vaginal irritation related to low estrogen levels during menopause (a condition known as *atropic vaginitis*). The incidence of sexually transmitted vaginitis is highest in women 15 to 24 years of age.

The development of vaginitis is related to alterations in the vaginal environment. These changes include complications in local defence mechanisms, such as skin integrity, immune reaction, and particularly vaginal pH. The pH of the vagina (normally 4.0 to 4.5) depends on cervical secretions and the presence of normal flora that help support an acidic environment. Changes in the vaginal pH may predispose a woman to infection. Variables that affect the vaginal pH and thus the bactericidal nature of secretions and the predisposition to infection include douching, using soaps, spermicides, feminine hygiene sprays, and deodorant menstrual pads or tampons. In addition, having conditions associated with increased glycogen content of vaginal secretions, such as pregnancy and diabetes, may be involved.

Antibiotics often destroy normal vaginal flora, allowing overgrowth of *Candida albicans* and causing a yeast infection. Increased vaginal alkalinity also may enhance susceptibility to trichomoniasis and BV.

Diagnosis is based on history, physical examination, and microscopic examination of the discharge using a wet mount technique. A marked change in colour or if the discharge becomes copious, malodorous, or irritating suggests an infection.

Treatment involves developing and supporting an acidic environment, relieving symptoms (usually pruritus and irritation), and administering antimicrobial or antifungal medications to eradicate the infectious organism. If the infection can be sexually transmitted, the woman's partner also requires treatment. Research suggests that probiotics, especially *Lactobacillus crispatus*, can encourage proliferation of normal vaginal flora and decrease the incidence of vaginitis in women at risk for this disease.[28] A probiotic bacterial strain, *Lactobacillus plantarum* P17630, can attach to vaginal epithelium and reduce the adhesion of *C. albicans*, and may help reduce *Candida* recurrence.[29]

Cervicitis

Cervicitis is a nonspecific term used to describe inflammation of the cervix. The PHAC defines *cervicitis* as having two major diagnostic signs: a purulent or mucopurulent (mucus- and pus-containing) discharge from the cervical os or endocervical bleeding induced by gently introducing a cotton swab into the cervix.[30] Either sign or both may be present. Cervicitis can have infectious or noninfectious causes. Chemicals and substances introduced into the vagina can cause cervicitis as well as disruptions in the normal vaginal flora. However, there are conflicting definitions of *cervicitis* used clinically and in research. Age and risk factors are important in assessing a woman with cervicitis.

Younger women are at risk for STIs. As a result, they should be tested for chlamydia, gonorrhea, and trichomoniasis. Older women with cervicitis may have STIs but are at risk for irritation from abnormal vaginal flora related to low vaginal estrogen levels.

Mucopurulent cervicitis (MPC) is usually caused by one or more sexually transmitted pathogens, such as *Trichomonas*, *Neisseria*, *Chlamydia*, *Mycoplasma*, or *Ureaplasma*. Infection causes the cervix to become red and edematous. A mucopurulent exudate drains from the external cervical os, and the individual may report vague pelvic pain, bleeding, or dysuria. Bleeding can occur during sexual intercourse or with pelvic examinations. Because mucopurulent cervicitis is a symptom of PID, women at risk for STIs, especially those less than 26 years old, should receive treatment for PID while awaiting results of microbial testing.[30] If the woman is not at risk for STIs, a thorough evaluation often reveals another cause for the inflammation. Partners should be notified and examined if chlamydia, gonorrhea, or trichomoniasis was found or suspected in the affected woman. These partners should then be treated for the STIs. To avoid reinfection, women and their sex partners should abstain from sexual intercourse until therapy is completed (i.e., 7 days after a single-dose regimen or after completion of a 7-day regimen).[30] The infectious microorganisms are cultured or named by immunoassay. Definitive diagnosis indicates oral antibiotic therapy.

Vulvodynia

Vulvodynia (also referred to as *vulvitis*, *vestibulitis*, *vulvovestibulitis* or *vulvovestibulitisdynia*) is chronic vulvar pain and inflammation of the vulva or vaginal vestibule, or both.[3] The classification of vulvodynia is based on the location of the pain, whether it is localized or generalized, and whether the pain is provoked, unprovoked, or mixed.[31] *Localized* is characterized by pain from a cause that usually does not cause pain (allodynia) to the vulvar vestibule (entrance of vagina) area. *Generalized* is a diffuse pain pattern involving all the pudendal nerve distribution and beyond. *Provoked* means any touch or stimulation that elicits pain. *Unprovoked* is pain that occurs in the absence of touch or stimulation. *Mixed* is pain that varies with or without touch or stimulation. Individuals describe the pain as burning, stinging, irritation, or rawness. In many cases, it may represent several disorders without an identifiable cause. Vulvodynia affects 8 to 10% of all women.[32] It occurs across ethnicities, and the incidence seems to decrease with increasing age.

The cause of vulvodynia is unknown. Theories suggest that it is multifactorial in origin and include biological, psychological, and interpersonal factors.[33] Although the inflammation of vulvodynia may be caused by contact dermatitis (i.e., exposure to soaps, detergents, lotions, sprays, shaving, menstrual pads/tampons, perfumed toilet paper, tight-fitting clothes), the condition may be more complex and represent abnormalities in three interdependent systems: vestibular mucosa, pelvic floor musculature, and CNS pain regulatory pathways. The condition also may be an autoimmune reaction. The suggested pathophysiology of vulvodynia is a chronic disorder of the nerves that supply the vulva. An important trigger is chronic inflammation caused by contact irritants, recurrent infections, hormonal changes, and chronic skin conditions. Overall, with normal sensations there is a heightened sensitivity. Because of the poorly understood mechanisms of vulvodynia, it is often a difficult condition to evaluate and treat.

After ruling out and treating conditions that can contribute to or cause vulvar inflammation (e.g., *Candida*, STIs, seborrhea, psoriasis), there are few treatment options. Cotton swab testing is used to find painful areas. Studies on treatments are limited but suggest that women may receive help from topical lidocaine (Xylocaine), topical or systemic antidepressants, behavioural treatment, botulinum toxin type A (Botox) injections into the affected nerve, or vestibulectomy. Vestibulectomy is a procedure that is understandably unacceptable to

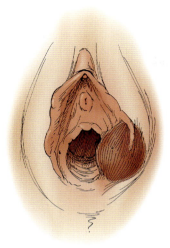

FIGURE 33.7 Inflammation of Bartholin Gland. (Modified from Fuller, J. K. [2013]. *Surgical technology* [6th ed.]. Saunders; Gershenson, D. M., DeCherney, A. H., Curry, S. L., et al. [2001]. *Operative gynecology* [2nd ed.]. Saunders.)

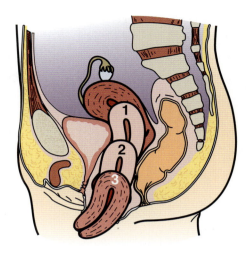

FIGURE 33.8 Degrees of Uterine Prolapse. Grade 1 is minimal and rarely requires correction. Grade 2 prolapse has moderate symptoms, and grade 3 prolapse is severe. The uterus is so low that the cervix protrudes from the vagina. (From Phillips, N. [2013]. *Berry & Kohn's operating room technique* [12th ed.]. Mosby.)

many women. Women also are recommended to avoid irritants, wear loose cotton clothing, and use proper antimicrobial or antifungal treatments for any recurrent vaginitis.

Bartholinitis

Bartholinitis, or Bartholin cyst, is an acute inflammation of one or both ducts that lead from the introitus (vaginal opening) to the Bartholin/greater vestibular glands (Figure 33.7). Most lesions of the Bartholin gland are cysts or abscesses. The usual causes are microorganisms that infect the lower female reproductive tract, such as streptococci, staphylococci, and sexually transmitted pathogens. Acute bartholinitis may be preceded by an infection, such as cervicitis, vaginitis, or urethritis.

Infection or trauma causes inflammatory changes that narrow the distal part of the duct. The narrowing may lead to obstruction and stasis of glandular secretions. The obstruction, or cyst, varies from 1 to 8 cm in diameter and is in the posterolateral part of the vulva. The affected area is usually red and painful, and pus may be visible at the opening of the duct. This exudate should be cultured. The individual may have fever and malaise. Diagnosis is based on the clinical manifestations and the identification of infectious microorganisms.

Characteristics of chronic bartholinitis include the presence of a small cyst that is slightly tender but otherwise is asymptomatic. Most Bartholin cysts require no treatment. Symptoms only occur if an exacerbation of infection causes an abscess to form in the gland itself.

Diagnosis is based on the clinical manifestations and the identification of infectious microorganisms. Treatment is controversial but involves broad-spectrum antibiotics. Some clinicians try to drain the cyst using hot soaks, needle aspiration, insertion of a catheter, or marsupialization (cutting a slit and suturing the edges) of the infected gland. No single treatment has proved superior for both relief and prevention of recurrence. Analgesics and warm sitz bath supply pain relief. If an abscess forms, it may be surgically drained.

Pelvic Organ Prolapse

The endopelvic fascia and perineal muscles support the bladder, urethra, and rectum. This muscular and fascial tissue loses tone and strength with aging and may fail to keep the pelvic organs in the proper position. Progressive descent of the pelvic support structures may cause pelvic floor disorders. These disorders include urinary and fecal incontinence, and pelvic organ prolapse. Pelvic organ prolapse (POP) is the descent of one or more of the following: the vaginal wall, the uterus, or the apex of the vagina (after a hysterectomy). Although more than 50% of women have some version of POP on physical examination, most women have no symptoms. Alteration in the function of the surrounding organs can occur when prolapse becomes severe. It is thought that POP is caused by direct trauma (such as childbirth); pelvic floor surgery; or damage to pelvic innervation, particularly the pudendal nerve. Risk factors in nulliparous women include occupational activities that require heavy lifting or chronic medical conditions, such as chronic lung disease or refractory constipation (chronically increased intra-abdominal pressure). The most often cited risk factors are aging, obesity, and hysterectomy. Other risk factors include a strong familial tendency and possibly a multifactorial genetic part.[34] Prolapse of the bladder, urethra, rectum, or uterus may occur many years after a first injury to the supporting structure.

Uterine prolapse is descent of the cervix or entire uterus into the vaginal canal. In severe cases the uterus falls completely through the vagina and protrudes from the introitus, creating ulceration and obvious discomfort. Figure 33.8 illustrates the different degrees (grades) of uterine prolapse, showing descent of the cervix or the entire uterus into the vaginal canal. Treatment of grade 1 prolapse does not occur unless it causes discomfort. Grades 2 and 3 prolapse usually cause feelings of fullness, heaviness, and collapse through the vagina. Symptoms of other pelvic floor disorders also may be present.

A common first-line treatment is a pessary. This is a removable mechanical device that holds the uterus in position. Strengthening of the pelvic fascia may occur through Kegel exercises (repetitive isometric tightening and relaxing of the pubococcygeal muscles) or by estrogen therapy in menopausal women. Maintaining a healthy body mass index (BMI), preventing constipation, and treating chronic cough may help prevent prolapse. Surgical repair, with or without hysterectomy, is the treatment of last resort.

Figure 33.9 shows POP associated with cystocele and rectocele. Cystocele is descent of a part of the posterior bladder wall and trigone into the vaginal canal. Its cause is usually childbirth-related injury. In severe cases, the bladder and anterior vaginal wall bulge outside the introitus. Symptoms are usually insignificant in mild to moderate cases. Vigorous activity, prolonged standing, sneezing, coughing, or

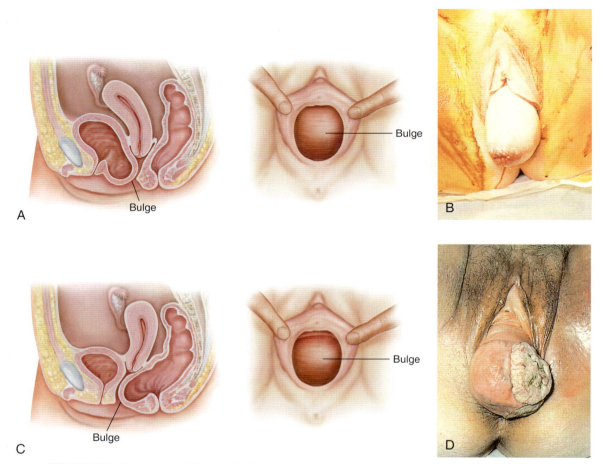

FIGURE 33.9 Cystocele and Rectocele. A, Grade 2: anterior vaginal wall prolapse (i.e., cystocele). **B,** Grade 4: prolapse. **C,** Grade 2: posterior wall prolapse (i.e., rectocele). **D,** Grade 4: associated with ulceration of vaginal wall. Grades 1 and 3 not shown. ([A] and [C], from Seidel, H. M., Ball, J. W., & Dains, J. E. [1999]. *Mosby's guide to physical examination* [4th ed.]. Mosby; [B] and [D], from Symonds, E. M., & Macpherson, M. B. A. [1994]. *Color atlas of obstetrics and gynecology*. Mosby-Wolfe.)

straining may aggravate increased bulging and descent of the anterior vaginal wall and urethra. Rest or assumption of a recumbent or prone position may supply relief. If the prolapse is large, women may describe symptoms of vaginal pressure. Medical management can include vaginal pessary, Kegel exercises, and estrogen therapy for postmenopausal women (see *Health Promotion:* Nonsurgical Management of Vaginal Prolapse). Severe injury unresponsive to medical treatment may require surgery.

A **rectocele** is the bulging of the rectum and posterior vaginal wall into the vaginal canal. Childbirth may increase damage, ultimately leading to a rectocele, but symptoms may not appear until after menopause. Genetic and familial predisposition and bowel habits contribute to rectocele development. Lifelong chronic constipation and straining may produce or aggravate a rectocele. A large rectocele may cause vaginal pressure, rectal fullness, and incomplete bowel evacuation. Defecation may be difficult and can be eased by applying manual pressure to the posterior vaginal wall. Medical treatment focuses on the management and prevention of constipation and, if needed, the use of a pessary. Rectocele alone (without associated enterocele, uterine prolapse, and cystocele) seldom requires surgery.

An **enterocele** is a herniation of the rectouterine pouch into the rectovaginal septum (between the rectum and the posterior vaginal wall). It can be congenital or acquired. Although congenital enterocele rarely causes symptoms or progresses in size, those acquired can result from muscular weakness caused by earlier surgery, especially those through the vagina, or from pelvic relaxation disorders, such as uterine prolapse, cystocele, and rectocele. Most large enteroceles are often found in grossly obese adults and older persons. Treatment is surgical. Box 33.7 summarizes the symptoms and treatment of POP.

Benign Growths and Proliferative Conditions
Benign Ovarian Cysts

Benign cysts of the ovary may occur at any time during the lifespan but are most common during the reproductive years and especially at the extremes of those years (Figure 33.10). An increase in benign ovarian cysts occurs when hormonal imbalances are more common, around puberty and menopause.[35] Benign ovarian cysts are quite common, responsible for one-third of gynecological hospital admissions. Two common causes of benign ovarian enlargement in ovulating women are follicular cysts and corpus luteum cysts. These cysts are called **functional cysts** because they are caused by variations of normal physiological events. Follicular and corpus luteum cysts are unilateral. They are typically 5 to 6 cm in diameter but can grow as large as 8 to 10 cm. Most women are asymptomatic.

The creation of benign cysts of the ovary occurs when a follicle or several follicles are stimulated but no dominant follicle develops and completes the maturation process. Every month about 120 follicles are stimulated, and generally, only one succeeds in ovulation of a mature

HEALTH PROMOTION
Nonsurgical Management of Vaginal Prolapse

Women with very mild symptoms of vaginal prolapse (mild pelvic discomfort and urinary symptoms) do not require treatment. However, relief may be achieved for women with moderate symptoms (increased pelvic discomfort, bowel and urinary symptoms, and sexual dysfunction), through weight loss, if necessary, refraining from heavy lifting, and smoking cessation.

Other strategies may be employed to improve symptoms, including performing regular Kegel exercises and the use of a pessary. Kegel exercises are a series of contractions that strengthen the pelvic floor. The woman is instructed to squeeze, at the same time, the two sets of pelvic floor muscles that are used to prevent the passage of gas and urine. This is done by completing 30 to 40 contractions spread over the duration of the day. The contractions are held for 3 seconds, gradually increasing to 10 seconds. Rest periods should occur in between contractions. A second way is the use of a pessary (a removable device that is inserted into the vagina to help in uterine support, like a diaphragm). These two less invasive treatments may diminish symptoms enough to delay the woman from seeking more aggressive surgical treatment.

Data from Harvard University. (2005). *What to do about pelvic organ prolapse*. https://www.health.harvard.edu/family-health-guide/what-to-do-about-pelvic-organ-prolapse.

BOX 33.7 Pelvic Organ Prolapse: Symptoms and Treatments

Symptoms	Treatment
Urinary	Depending on age of woman and cause and severity of condition:
Sensation of incomplete emptying of bladder	Isometric exercises to strengthen pubococcygeal muscles (Kegel exercises)
Urinary incontinence	
Urinary frequency/urgency	
Bladder "splinting" to accomplish voiding	Estrogen to improve tone and vascularity of fascial support (postmenopausal)
Bowel	
Constipation or feeling of rectal fullness or blockage	Pessary (a removable device) to hold pelvic organs in place
Difficult defecation	**Surgical**
Stool or flatus incontinence	Reconstructive: autologous grafts; synthetic mesh/sling
Urgency	
Manual "splinting" of posterior vaginal wall to carry out defecation	Obliterative (most extreme)
	Weight loss
Pain and Bulging	Avoidance of constipation
Vaginal, bladder, rectum	Treatment of cough/lung conditions
Pelvic pressure, bulging, pain	
Lower back pain	
Sexual	
Dyspareunia	
Decreased sensation, lubrication, arousal	

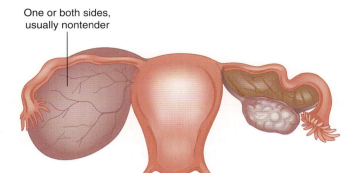

FIGURE 33.10 Depiction of Ovarian Cyst.

Follicular cysts (also called *ovarian cysts* or *functional cysts*) are filled with fluid and can be caused by a transient condition in which the dominant follicle does not rupture or one or more of the nondominant follicles does not regress. This disturbance is not well understood. It may be that the hypothalamus does not receive or send a message strong enough to increase FSH levels to the degree necessary to develop or mature a dominant follicle. The hypothalamus monitors blood levels of estradiol and progesterone. When FSH level is low, estradiol concentration does not increase enough to stimulate LH surge. Research shows that when progesterone is not being produced, the hypothalamus releases GnRH to increase the FSH level. FSH continues to stimulate follicles to mature, and the granulosa cells grow and, presumably, estradiol level increases. This abnormal cycle continues to stimulate follicular size and causes follicular cysts to develop. Although individuals may experience no symptoms, some have pelvic pain, a sensation of feeling bloated, tender breasts, and heavy or irregular menses. After several later cycles in which hormone levels once again follow a regular cycle and progesterone levels are restored, cysts usually will be absorbed or get smaller. Follicular cysts can be random or recurrent events.

A **corpus luteum cyst** may normally form by the granulosa cells left behind after ovulation. This cyst is highly vascularized but usually limited in size, and spontaneously regresses with the normal menstrual cycle. With an imbalance in hormones, low LH and progesterone levels may cause an abnormal or hemorrhagic cyst. In some cases, large cysts can rupture and cause hemorrhage.

Corpus luteum cysts are less common than follicular cysts. Luteal cysts typically cause more symptoms, particularly if they rupture. Manifestations include dull pelvic pain and amenorrhea or delayed menstruation, followed by irregular or heavier-than-normal bleeding. Rupture occasionally occurs and can cause massive bleeding with excruciating pain. Immediate surgery may be needed. Corpus luteum cysts usually regress spontaneously in nonpregnant women. The use of oral contraceptives may prevent future cysts from forming.

Dermoid cysts are ovarian teratomas that have elements of all three germ layers. They are common ovarian neoplasms. These growths may have mature tissue including skin, hair, sebaceous and sweat glands, muscle fibres, cartilage, and bone. Dermoid cysts are usually asymptomatic and found incidentally on pelvic examination. The removal of dermoid cysts should occur as they have malignant potential.

Torsion of the ovary is a rare complication of ovarian cysts or tumours or enlargement of the ovary. Torsion can occur in girls or women. If a cyst is sufficiently large, it can cause the ovary to twist on its ligaments. This action decreases blood supply to the ovary and causes extreme pain. **Ovarian torsion** is rare but is a gynecological emergency when present. It usually presents with acute, severe unilateral abdominal or pelvic pain. Recommendations for treatment include surgical intervention.

ovum. Normally, in the early follicular phase of the menstrual cycle, follicles of the ovary respond to hormonal signals from the brain. The pituitary gland produces FSH to mature follicles in the ovary. If the dominant follicle develops properly before ovulation, the corpus luteum becomes vascularized and secretes progesterone. Progesterone stops development of other follicles in both ovaries in that cycle. LH, proteolytic enzymes, and prostaglandins trigger follicular rupture and release of the ovum.

Endometrial Polyps

> ### QUICK CHECK 33.4
> 1. Why is cervical cancer considered a sexually transmitted infection?
> 2. What are the risk factors and pathogenesis for endometrial cancer?
> 3. What factors reduce the risk for ovarian cancer?
> 4. Discuss the new hypothesis for the pathogenesis of ovarian cancer.

An **endometrial polyp** is a benign mass of endometrial tissue and holds a variable number of glands, stroma, and blood vessels. Endometrial polyps are usually solitary and can occur anywhere within the uterus. Polyps are structurally diverse. They are classified as hyperplastic, atrophic (or inactive), or functional. Hyperplastic polyps are often pedunculated (have a stalk or appear mushroomlike) and may be mistaken for endometrial hyperplasia or, if large, adenosarcoma (Figure 33.11). Although polyps most often develop in women between ages 40 and 50 years, they can occur at all ages. Hyperestrogenic states, obesity, use of tamoxifen (Nolvadex; a medication that blocks the actions of estrogen), and hypertension are risk factors for developing polyps.

Most polyps are asymptomatic; however, they are a common cause of intermenstrual bleeding or even excessive menstrual bleeding. The use of hysteroscopy or ultrasonography confirms diagnosis. The removal of lesions can occur with the use of small, curved forceps but there is a high rate of spontaneous resolution. Coexistence of a separate endometrial atypical hyperplasia (AH) or adenocarcinoma is possible, but malignancy is extremely rare.

Leiomyomas

Leiomyomas, commonly called **myomas** or **uterine fibroids**, are benign tumours that develop from smooth muscle cells in the myometrium. Leiomyomas are the most common benign tumours of the uterus. They affect 70 to 80% of all women, and most remain small and asymptomatic. Prevalence increases in women ages 30 to 50 years but decreases with menopause. The incidence of leiomyomas in Black and Asian women is two to five times higher than that in White women.

The cause of uterine leiomyomas is unknown, although the size of the tumour appears to be related to hormonal fluctuations, including estrogen and progesterone, growth factors, and reduced apoptosis. Because leiomyomas are estrogen and progesterone sensitive, uterine leiomyomas do not occur before menarche, are common during the reproductive years, and generally shrink after menopause if present.

Tumours in pregnant women enlarge rapidly but often decrease in size after the end of the pregnancy. Risk factors include heredity, nulliparity, obesity, PCOS, diabetes, being of African descent, and hypertension.

PATHOPHYSIOLOGY Most leiomyomas occur in multiples in the fundus of the uterus, although they often occur singly and throughout the uterus. Leiomyomas are classified as subserous, submucous, or intramural, according to location within the various layers of the uterine wall (Figure 33.12). Most leiomyomas have normal karyotypes, but some have simple chromosomal abnormalities. Recently, mutations in the Mediator Subcomplex 12 *(MED12)* gene have been found in about 70% of uterine leiomyomas.[36] Uterine leiomyomas are usually firm and surrounded by a connective tissue layer. Degeneration and necrosis may occur when the leiomyoma outgrows its blood supply, which is more common in larger tumours and is often accompanied by pain.

CLINICAL MANIFESTATIONS The major clinical manifestations of leiomyomas are abnormal vaginal bleeding, pain, and symptoms

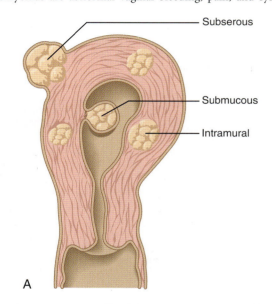

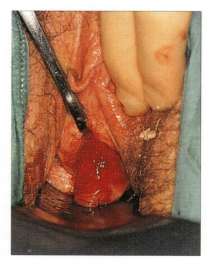

FIGURE 33.11 Endometrial Polyp. Polyp is protruding through the cervical os. (From Symonds, E. M., & Macpherson, M. B. A. [1994]. *Color atlas of obstetrics and gynecology*. Mosby.)

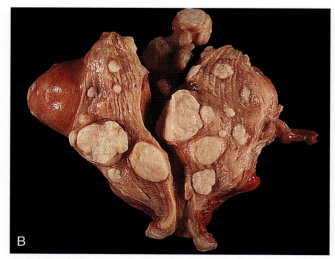

FIGURE 33.12 Leiomyomas. A, Uterine section showing whorl-like appearance and locations of leiomyomas, which are also called *uterine fibroids*. **B,** Multiple leiomyomas in sagittal section. Typical, well-circumscribed, solid, light grey nodules distort uterus. ([B], from Damjanov, I., & Linder, J. [2000]. *Pathology: a color atlas*. Mosby.)

related to pressure on nearby structures. Fibroids also may contribute to infertility and subfertility, as well as obstruction during birth if large enough. The leiomyoma can make the uterine cavity larger, thereby increasing the endometrial surface area. This enlargement may account for the increased menstrual bleeding associated with leiomyomas. Although pain is not an early symptom, it occurs with the devascularization of larger leiomyomas and is associated with blood vessel compression that limits blood supply to adjacent structures. Because the fibroid is relatively slow growing, enabling adjacent structures to adapt to pressure, symptoms of abdominal pressure develop slowly. Pressure on the bladder may contribute to urinary frequency, urgency, and dysuria. Pressure on the ureter may cause it to become distended "upstream" from the pressure point. Rectosigmoid pressure may lead to constipation. Larger fibroids may cause a sensation of abdominal or genital heaviness.

EVALUATION AND TREATMENT Uterine leiomyomas are suspected when bimanual examination shows irregular, nontender nodularity of the uterus. Pelvic sonography or MRI confirms the diagnosis. Treatment depends on symptoms, tumour size, age, reproductive status, and overall health of the individual. Most leiomyomas are asymptomatic. Management is by observation only. Shrinking the myoma or reducing the symptoms is the aim of treatment. Use of hormonal contraceptives may shrink or enhance growth and should be closely watched. Mifepristone (Mifegymiso; called *RU-486* in other countries), a progesterone receptor agonist, may be useful as a conservative treatment, while GnRH agonists may supply temporary management. Myomectomy or removal of the fibroid from the muscle of the uterus may be less invasive than a full hysterectomy. This treatment is the standard of cure for women wishing to preserve their fertility. Other treatments, such as uterine artery embolization (UAE), laser ablation, and levonorgestrel intrauterine device (LNG-IUD), all hold promise. A Cochrane review found UAE appears to have an overall satisfaction rate like hysterectomy and myomectomy.[37] UAE is associated with a higher rate of minor complications and a much higher risk of requiring future surgical intervention within 2 to 5 years of the first procedure.[37] Benefits and risks of all treatments should be considered, as well as a woman's desire for future pregnancy.

Adenomyosis

Adenomyosis is the presence of islands of endometrial glands surrounded by benign endometrial stroma within the uterine myometrium. It commonly develops during the late reproductive years. The highest incidence is among women in their 40s and in women taking tamoxifen. Parity also increases the risk for adenomyosis. Adenomyosis may be asymptomatic or may be associated with abnormal menstrual bleeding, anemia, dysmenorrhea, uterine enlargement, and uterine tenderness during menstruation. Secondary dysmenorrhea becomes increasingly severe as disease progresses. On examination, just before or after menstruation, the uterus is enlarged, globular, and tender. Diagnosis is confirmed with ultrasonography or MRI. Treatment is symptomatic, and like that for dysmenorrhea (i.e., NSAIDs, hormonal contraceptives, or LNG-IUD). Other options include surgical resection or, in severe cases, hysterectomy. UAE and LNG-IUDs have shown good first results but need further testing.

Endometriosis

Endometriosis is the presence of functioning endometrial tissue or implants outside the uterus. Like normal endometrial tissue, the ectopic (out-of-place) endometrium responds to the hormonal fluctuations of the menstrual cycle. The incidence of endometriosis is difficult to determine, especially in asymptomatic adolescent and fertile women.

The diagnosis of endometriosis is made in about 50% of women evaluated for pelvic pain, infertility, or pelvic mass. The frequency and severity of symptoms do not correlate with the extent or site of lesions. Many theories exist on the cause of endometriosis, including the implantation of endometrial cells during *retrograde menstruation*, in which menstrual fluids move through the fallopian tubes and into the pelvic cavity. It is now known, however, that retrograde menstruation occurs in almost all women, but not all women develop endometriosis. The main theories include coelomic metaplasia (peritoneal mesothelium, the Müllerian ducts, and the germinal epithelium of the ovary are all derived from coelomic wall epithelium), retrograde menstruation, embryonic cell rest (primitive "at rest" embryonic cells become activated), iatrogenic mechanical transplantation, and lymphatic and vascular dissemination.[38] There is a genetic predisposition to endometriosis. The identification of some genetic polymorphisms has occurred.

PATHOPHYSIOLOGY Endometriosis is a multifactorial estrogen-dependent condition that may affect 10 to 15% of women of child-bearing age (Figure 33.13).[39] Emerging evidence suggests that endometriosis can have heterogeneous characteristics. The pathogenesis is modulated by many factors, including genetic, epigenetic, environmental, and cellular factors.[39] The endometrium is highly dynamic tissue with regenerative tissue undergoing cyclic processes of growth, differentiation, shedding, and regeneration as part of the menstrual cycle. These processes depend on steroid hormones, growth factors, and leukocytes that affect the balance between proliferation and apoptosis. Although endometriosis is considered benign, approximately 1.0% of affected women have an increased risk for malignant transformation involving multiple pathways of development.[38] The defining feature of endometriosis is the presence and proliferation of endometrial-like tissue (implants), including stromal and glandular tissue, in locations outside of the uterine cavity. These locations are primarily in the ovaries, fallopian tubes, bladder, rectosigmoid colon, and uterine myometrium (adenomyosis), often causing infertility and pain (Figure 33.14).[38]

The pathophysiology of endometriosis is still poorly understood, but several characteristics are being investigated:

- High levels of estrogen production are seen in endometriosis. A key enzyme in estrogen production is aromatase, which has been correlated with the severity of endometriosis.
- There is evidence of switching of cell fates during development, where epithelial and mesenchymal markers highlight a contribution of the

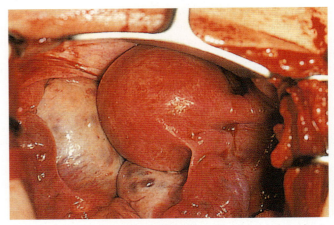

FIGURE 33.13 Endometriosis. The uterus is distended, and retrograde spill of menstrual loss has led to the development of endometriosis (*dark purple patches*). (From Symonds, E. M., & Macpherson, M. B. A. [1994]. *Color atlas of obstetrics and gynecology*. Mosby-Wolfe.)

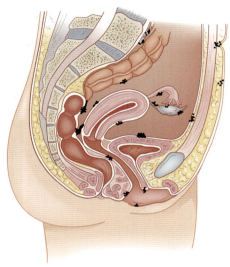

FIGURE 33.14 Pelvic Sites of Endometrial Implantation in Endometriosis. Endometrial cells may enter the pelvic cavity during retrograde menstruation.

mesenchymal–epithelial transition (MET) and of the epithelial–mesenchymal transition (EMT) in endometriosis (see Chapter 10).
- The roles of inflammation and of peritoneal leukocytes and their mediators may help the progression of endometriotic lesions.
- Some components of the innate immune system are involved in endometriosis (dendritic cells, macrophages, Toll-like receptors). Components of the adaptive immune system (T- and B-cell functions) can promote apoptosis, tissue damage, and multiorgan involvement.
- The development of lesions is dependent on new blood vessel development (angiogenesis).
- Genetic and epigenetic roles are present in endometriotic lesions and some ovarian cancers (clear cell carcinoma, endometrioid adenocarcinoma).
- Stem cells play a role in the development of endometriotic lesions. Changes in stem cell populations of endometriotic lesions are associated with genetic and epigenetic alterations.

Cyclic changes depend on the blood supply of the lesions (implants) and the presence of glandular and stromal cells. Given that the blood supply is sufficient, the ectopic endometrium proliferates, breaks down, and bleeds with the normal menstrual cycle. The bleeding is one cause of inflammation. The inflammation triggers a cascade of cellular inflammatory mediators, including cytokines, chemokines, growth factors, and protective factors such as secretory leukocyte protease inhibitor and superoxide dismutase.[40] The inflammation may lead to fibrosis, scarring, adhesions, and pain.

CLINICAL MANIFESTATIONS The clinical manifestations of endometriosis vary in frequency and severity and can mimic other pelvic disease (i.e., PID, ovarian cysts, irritable bowel syndrome). Symptoms include infertility, pelvic pain, dyschezia (pain on defecation), dyspareunia, (pain on intercourse), and, less commonly, constipation and abnormal vaginal bleeding. If implants are found within the pelvis, an asymptomatic pelvic mass having irregular, movable nodules and a fixed, retroverted uterus are found on examination. Most symptoms can be explained by the proliferation, breakdown, and bleeding of the ectopic endometrial tissue with later formation of adhesions. In most instances, however, the degree of endometriosis is not related to the frequency or severity of symptoms. Dysmenorrhea, for example, does not appear to be related to the degree of endometriosis. With involvement of the rectovaginal septum or the uterosacral ligaments, dyspareunia develops. Dyschezia, a hallmark symptom of endometriosis, occurs with bleeding of ectopic endometrium in the rectosigmoid musculature and later fibrosis.

Up to 25 to 40% of women with infertility have endometriosis. The relationship between endometriosis and infertility is strong. However, the *degree* of disease is not as closely associated. More simply, women with untreated minimal to mild disease may have high pregnancy rates or may experience infertility. The exact reason for infertility in women with endometriosis is unknown.

EVALUATION AND TREATMENT A presumptive diagnosis is based on the previously described symptoms, but pelvic laparoscopy is needed for a definitive diagnosis. A uniform classification system that includes both extent and severity exists. It includes stage I, minimal; stage II, mild; and stage III, moderate. The classification, however, still does not correlate well with a woman's symptoms. Treatment is based on preventing worsening of the disease, alleviating pain, and restoring fertility. Medical therapies include suppression of ovulation with various medications, such as noncyclic estrogen-progestin–combined oral contraceptive pills (COCs), depot medroxyprogesterone acetate (DMPA), danazol (Cyclomen), GnRH agonists, or mifepristone, and promotion of atrophy of the endometrium with progestins or an LNG-IUD. Conservative surgical treatment includes laparoscopic removal of endometrial implants with conventional or laser techniques and presacral neurectomy for severe dysmenorrhea. All treatments have risks or side effects, and recurrent symptoms will develop in most women within a few years, even with surgical treatments. Women should be fully informed of all options and understand the risk-to-benefit ratio of treatments, especially nonreversible treatments.

Cancer

Malignant tumours of the female reproductive system are common. Because the pelvis and abdomen are poorly innervated and designed to accommodate a growing fetus, cancers of the female reproductive tract can often grow large before causing pain. The early diagnosis of reproductive cancers more likely occurs if there are symptoms. For example, vaginal bleeding prompts women to seek treatment. Cervical cancer has minimal symptoms until late in the process but is easy to detect early with Pap smears. Globally, cervical cancer is ranked third in incidence. However, in Canada this cancer is ranked fourteenth in incidence.[41] Improved screening techniques, increased uptake of testing, and the universality of the Canadian health care system accounts for this significant difference. Investigators are researching new biomarkers for the screening, diagnosis, and surveillance for ovarian cancer. Obtaining an early diagnosis for ovarian cancer is very challenging.

Cervical Cancer

Cervical cancer is the fourth most common cancer in women worldwide and has the fourth highest death rate among cancers in women.[43] The Canadian Cancer Society estimated that 1 350 Canadian women were diagnosed with invasive cervical cancer in 2019. It also estimated that 410 Canadian women died of this disease in 2019.[41,42] In Canada, female populations found less likely to take part in regular cervical cancer screening include recent immigrants, Indigenous peoples, those of lower socioeconomic status, and those living in rural areas. The rates of invasive cervical cancer in Canada have steadily decreased since the 1960s, and death rates have declined significantly in Canada (and other developed countries). This decline is mainly attributable

HEALTH PROMOTION

Screening With the Papanicolaou Test and With the Human Papillomavirus DNA Test

Evidence shows that appropriate regular screening of women for cervical cancer with the Papanicolaou (Pap) test reduces mortality from cervical cancer. The benefits of screening women younger than 21 years are small because of the low prevalence of lesions that will progress to invasive cancer. Screening is not beneficial in women older than 65 years if they have had a history of recent negative tests.[*,†,‡] Regular Pap screening decreases cervical cancer incidence and mortality by at least 80%.[§]

When considering the harmful effects of Pap screening, evidence shows that regular screening leads to added diagnostic procedures (e.g., colposcopy) and treatment for low-grade squamous intraepithelial lesions (LSILs). These added procedures have long-term consequences for fertility and pregnancy. These harms are greatest for younger women, who have a higher prevalence of LSILs. LSIL lesions often regress without treatment. Increased harms exist in younger women because they have a higher rate of false-positive results.

Cervical screening may be undertaken with the human papillomavirus (HPV) DNA test (also called *HPV RNA* and *HPV test*). Evidence shows that screening with the HPV DNA test is most useful in screening for cervical cancer. However, HPV infections are common and often resolve on their own. As a result, HPV testing is not routinely used in provincial or territorial cervical cancer screening programs. Evidence shows that HPV testing is most useful in screening for cervical cancer in women 30 years of age or older.[**] This test is used only for women 30 years of age and older as a follow-up to abnormal Pap test results.[§]

Routine HPV testing may have harmful consequences. Evidence shows that HPV testing identifies many infections that will not lead to cervical dysplasia or cervical cancer. This point is especially true for women younger than 30 years, in whom rates of HPV infection may be higher. A positive test may expose these women to added unnecessary examinations and testing.

Regarding the joint use of the Pap test and the HPV DNA test, evidence shows that screening every 5 years with the Pap test and the HPV DNA test in women 30 years and older is more sensitive in detecting cervical abnormalities, compared with the Pap test alone. Screening with the Pap test and HPV DNA test reduces the incidence of cervical cancer.[‡]

There are also potential harmful consequences of joint testing. Evidence reveals that cotesting is associated with more false-positive results than the Pap test alone. Abnormal test results can lead to more frequent testing and invasive diagnostic procedures.[‡]

Regarding women who present for screening without a cervix, evidence shows that screening is not helpful in these women if the hysterectomy occurred for a benign condition.

*Sasieni, P., Castanon, A., & Cuzick, J. (2009). *British Medical Journal, 339*, b2968; †Sawaya, G. F., McConnell, K. J., Kulasingam, S. L., et al. (2003). *New England Journal of Medicine, 349*(16), 1501–1509; ‡Moyer, V. A. (2012). *Annals of Internal Medicine, 156*(12), 880–891, W312; §National Cancer Institute. (2015). *PDQ® cervical cancer screening*. Retrieved from https://www.cancer.gov/types/cervical/hp/cervical-screening-pdq#link/_115_toc; **Canadian Cancer Society. (2021). *Human papillomavirus (HPV) testing*. https://www.cancer.ca/en/cancer-information/diagnosis-and-treatment/tests-and-procedures/hpv-test/?region=on.

---

to the prevalence and frequency of screening with Pap tests.[42] (See *Health Promotion: Screening With the Papanicolaou Test and With the Human Papillomavirus DNA Test*.) The incidence rate of cervical cancer in Canada declined by 2.1% per year between 1984 and 2006, and 3.3% per year between 2010 and 2015.[42]

It is now known that HPV infection is a necessary condition in the development of almost all precancerous and cancerous cervical lesions. There are multiple subtypes of HPV. The "high-risk" (oncogenic) types of HPV (predominantly 16 and 18) have been most closely associated with high-grade dysplasia and cancer (also see Chapters 10 and 11). The precancerous lesion or dysplasia, also called *cervical intraepithelial neoplasia* (CIN) and *cervical carcinoma in situ* (CCIS), is a more advanced form of the cell changes. These changes can progress to become invasive cancer, but this process can be very slow. About 30 to 70% of those untreated for in situ carcinoma will develop invasive carcinoma over 10 to 12 years. However, in about 10% of women, progression from in situ to invasive cancer can occur in less than 1 year.[44] Other risk factors for cervical cancer include multiple sexual partners, a male partner with multiple previous or current sexual partners, young age at first sexual intercourse, high parity, persistent infection with HPV-16 or HPV-18, immunosuppression, use of oral contraceptives, certain human leukocyte antigen (HLA) subtypes, and use of nicotine.[45]

PATHOGENESIS As discussed earlier, HPV-16 and HPV-18 are the most important risk factors for cervical disease progression and cancer. HPV-16 accounts for about 60% of cervical cancer cases and HPV-18 for about another 10%. Other HPV types contribute to less than 5% of cases. Two types of epithelial cells line the cervix: squamous cells at the outer aspect and columnar glandular cells along the inner canal (Figure 33.15). Figure 33.16 illustrates the site of the cellular transformation zone that is called the *squamous–columnar junction*. HPVs infect immature basal cells of the squamous epithelium in the areas of epithelial breaks or injury, or immature metaplastic squamous cells present at the squamous–columnar junction. Establishing HPV infection in the mature squamous cells that cover the ectocervix, vagina, or vulva requires damage to the surface epithelium. The cervix, with its large areas of immature epithelium, is very vulnerable to HPV infection.[46] The ability of HPV to act as a carcinogen depends on the viral proteins E6 and E7. These proteins interfere with the activity of tumour-suppressor proteins that regulate cell growth and survival.[46] Replication of HPV occurs in the maturing squamous cells. Studies have shown that HPV activates the cell cycle by interfering with two tumour-suppressor genes, *Rb* and *p53*.[46] Although HPV is a causative factor for cervical cancer, it is not the *only* factor. Other important cocarcinogens must play a role. Despite the high percentage of young women infected with one or more HPV types during their reproductive years, only a few develop cancer. The other factors that appear to be associated include immune responses, hormonal responses, and other environmental factors that decide regression or persistence of the HPV infection.[46] Cervical cancer is a slowly progressive disease and moves from normal cervical epithelial cells to dysplasia to carcinoma in situ and, eventually, to invasive cancer (see Figure 33.16B). Table 33.4 summarizes the staging of cervical cancer. Testing for high-risk HPV is often positive for many years (10 years or more) before dysplasia progresses to high-grade squamous intraepithelial lesions (HSILs) that can develop into invasive cervical cancer (CIN III, Table 33.5).

CLINICAL MANIFESTATIONS Because cervical neoplasms are predominantly asymptomatic, about 90% of cervical cancers can be detected early using Pap and HPV testing. If symptoms exist, they may include a change in vaginal discharge or bleeding. Bleeding varies and may occur after intercourse or between menstrual periods. At times,

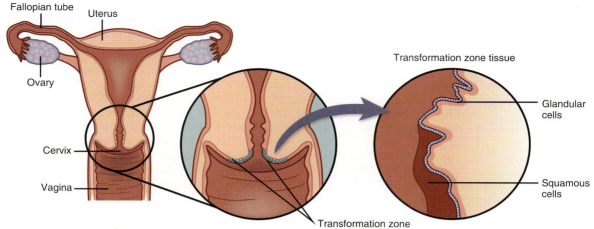

FIGURE 33.15 Cervix Is Lined by Two Types of Epithelial Cells: Squamous Cells and Columnar Glandular Cells.

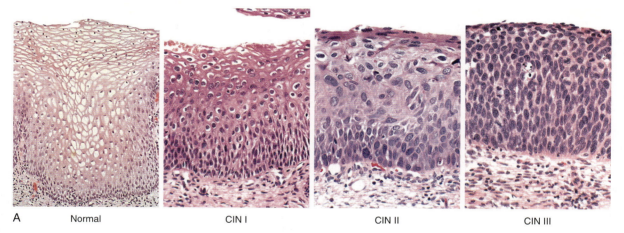

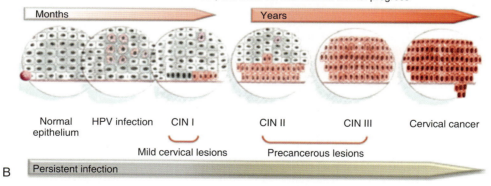

- CIN 2/3 lesions are more likely to progress to cervical cancer than CIN 1 lesions[1]

1. Oster A. *Int J of Gynecol Path*, 1993, 12:186-92. 2. Moscicki A et al, *Vaccine*, 2006, 2453:42-51. 3. Einstein M. *Cancer Immunol Immunother*, 2008, 57:443-51. 4. Winer R. et al. *J Int Dis*, 2005, 191:731-38. 5. Holowaty P. et al. *J Natl Cancer Inst*, 1999, 91:252-58. 6. Solomon D. et al. *JAMA*, 2002, 287:2114-19.

FIGURE 33.16 Cervical Intraepithelial Neoplasia (CIN). **A,** Normal multiparous cervix including the transformation zone where precancerous and cancerous changes occur. CIN stage I, note the white appearance of part of the anterior lip of the cervix associated with neoplastic changes; CIN stage II, lesions also are reflected in distant capillaries; CIN stage III, lesions are predominantly around the external os. **B,** Normal epithelium, HPV infection progressing to CIN stage I, and then with more time, persistent HPV infections progressing to precancerous lesions CIN II and CIN III, and eventually cervical cancer. Most cervical lesions do not progress to cervical cancer. *CIN,* Cervical intraepithelial neoplasia; *HPV,* human papillomavirus. ([A], from Kumar, V., Abbas, A. K., & Aster, J. C. [Eds.]. [2021]. *Robbins and Cotran pathologic basis of disease* [10th ed.]. Elsevier; [B], from Symonds, E. M., & Macpherson, M. B. A. [1994]. *Color atlas of obstetrics and gynecology.* Mosby.)

TABLE 33.4 Clinical Staging for Cancer of the Cervix

Stage		Characteristics
0		Cancer in situ, intraepithelial carcinoma; earliest stage of cancer; cancer confined to its original site
I		Carcinoma confined to cervix (extension to corpus disregarded)
	IA	Earliest form of stage I; there is very small amount of cancer, which is visible only under a microscope
	IA1	Area of invasion is <3 mm deep and <7 mm wide
	IA2	Area of invasion is between 3 and 5 mm deep, and <7 mm wide
	IB	Includes cancers that can be seen without a microscope; also includes cancers seen only with a microscope that have spread deeper than 5 mm into connective tissue of the cervix or are wider than 7 mm
	IB1	IB cancer that is no larger than 4 cm
	IB2	IB cancer that is >4 cm
II		Cancer has spread beyond the cervix to the upper part of the vagina; cancer does not involve the lower third of the vagina
	IIA	Cancer has spread beyond the cervix to the upper part of the vagina; cancer does not involve the lower third of the vagina
	IIB	Cancer has spread to the tissue next to the cervix, called the *parametrial tissue*
III		Cancer has spread to the lower part of the vagina or the pelvic wall; cancer may be blocking the ureters (tubes that carry urine from the kidneys to the bladder)
	IIIA	Cancer has spread to the lower third of the vagina but not to the pelvic wall
	IIIB	Cancer extends to the pelvic wall, blocks urine flow to the bladder, or both
IV		Most advanced stage of cervical cancer; cancer has spread to other parts of the body
	IVA	Cancer has spread to the bladder or rectum, which are organs close to the cervix
	IVB	Cancer has spread to distant organs beyond the pelvic area, such as the lungs

TABLE 33.5 Classification System for Squamous Cervical Precursor Lesions

Dysplasia/Carcinoma in Situ	Cervical Intraepithelial Neoplasia	Squamous Intraepithelial Lesion, Current Classification
Mild dysplasia	CIN I	Low-grade SIL (LSIL)
Moderate dysplasia	CIN II	High-grade SIL (HSIL)
Severe dysplasia	CIN III	High-grade SIL (HSIL)
Carcinoma in situ	CIN III	High-grade SIL (HSIL)

CIN, Cervical intraepithelial neoplasia; *SIL,* squamous intraepithelial lesion.
Data from Kumar, V., Abbas, A. K., & Aster, J. C. (Eds.). (2021). *Robbins and Cotran pathologic basis of disease* (10th ed.). Elsevier.

women will complain of abnormal menses or postmenopausal bleeding. A less common symptom may be a serosanguineous or yellowish vaginal discharge. A new or foul odour also may be present. Advanced disease may cause urinary or rectal symptoms and pelvic or back pain.

EVALUATION AND TREATMENT When dysplasia is detected, colposcopy is usually indicated to identify lesions and obtain needed biopsies.

HEALTH PROMOTION
Cervical Cancer Primary Prevention

Individuals not sexually active rarely develop genital HPV infections. HPV vaccination before sexual activity can reduce the risk for infection by HPV types targeted by the vaccine.

Health Canada has approved three vaccines to prevent HPV infection: Gardasil, Gardasil 9, and Cervarix. These vaccines supply strong protection against the HPV-targeted infections. These vaccines are not effective for treating established infections or disease caused by HPV. All three vaccines prevent infections with HPV-16 and HPV-18, the two high-risk HPVs that cause about 70% of cervical cancers. Gardasil also prevents infection with HPV-6 and HPV-11, which cause about 90% of genital warts. Gardasil 9 prevents infection with the same four high-risk HPV types plus five more high-risk types (31, 33, 45, 52, and 58). All three vaccines are administered as a series of three injections into muscle tissue over a 6-month period.

Importantly, consistent and correct condom use is associated with reduced HPV transmission. The virus can infect areas not covered by the condom.

From National Cancer Institute. (2019). *Human papillomavirus (HPV) vaccines.* https://www.cancer.gov/about-cancer/causes-prevention/risk/infectious-agents/hpv-vaccine-fact-sheet; Public Health Agency of Canada. (2017). *Human papillomavirus (HPV) prevention and HPV vaccines: questions and answers.* https://www.canada.ca/en/public-health/services/infectious-diseases/sexual-health-sexually-transmitted-infections/hpv-prevention-vaccines-questions-answers.html.

Lymphangiography, computed tomography (CT) scan, MRI, ultrasonography, or radioimmunodetection are methods used to further assess tissue involvement if invasive carcinoma is found.

Treatment depends on the degree of neoplastic change, the size and location of the lesion, and the extent of metastatic spread. Treatment for invasive carcinoma depends on the stage of the tumour. Treatment includes surgery, radiation therapy, chemotherapy, and targeted treatment. Prognosis is excellent with early detection and treatment. The prevention of HPV infection appears to be key for substantially reducing the risk for cervical cancer. The Health Canada–approved vaccines for two of the high-risk types of HPV show excellent promise (see *Health Promotion:* Cervical Cancer Primary Prevention).

Vaginal Cancer

Cancer of the vagina is the rarest (about 0.6 per 100 000 women yearly) of the female genital cancers. It can occur at any age but is found predominantly in women 50 years of age and older. More than 90% of women with vaginal cancer have squamous cell carcinoma. Most vaginal squamous cell carcinomas are associated with high-risk HPVs. Risk factors include being age 60 or older; diethylstilbestrol (DES) exposure in utero; HPV-16 (cause); human immunodeficiency virus (HIV); genital warts (associated most often with noncogenic types HPV-6 and HPV-11, which can infect female and male genital organs and the anal area); and earlier carcinoma of the cervix or vulva. The relationship between vaginal cancer and developing precancerous cell changes (called *vaginal intraepithelial neoplasia* [VAIN]) is controversial because these changes are associated with oncogenic HPV.[47,48] Approximately 30 to 50% of women with vaginal carcinomas have had a prior hysterectomy for benign, premalignant, or malignant disease.[48]

Vaginal cancer can be asymptomatic. Therefore, regular pelvic examinations, particularly for women with a history of intrauterine DES exposure, are extremely important. Clinical manifestations that occur include abnormal vaginal bleeding or discharge not related to menstrual periods, pain during intercourse, pain in the pelvic area, pain when urinating, and constipation.

Careful biopsy techniques confirm the tumour type and decide its size, location, and extent. Treatment depends on these findings and on the age of the individual. Treatments include surgery, chemotherapy, and radiation therapy.

Vulvar Cancer

Cancer of the vulva most often affects the labia majora and less often the labia minora, clitoris, or vaginal glands.[49] In Canada, 1 020 women were diagnosed with unspecified female genital organ cancers in 2016, which includes vulvar cancer.[50] Risk factors for vulvar cancer include HPV-16 (cause), HIV, HPV-18 (probable cause), increasing age, previous cancer (untreated high-grade vulvar intraepithelial neoplasia [VIN]), cervical cancer survivor, previous CIN, women with certain autoimmune conditions (increased risk for HPV-associated tumours), organ transplant recipients (perhaps because of immunosuppression to clear HPV), and tobacco use (may relate to inability to clear HPV infection).[51] The development of vulvar cancer is preceded by condyloma or squamous dysplasia.[52] Other possible risk factors include having many sexual partners, having first sexual intercourse at a young age, and having a history of abnormal Pap tests.[52] Risk factors for STIs are risk factors for vulvar cancer. Early detection is critical. Treatment includes surgery, radiation, chemotherapy, and biological therapy.

Endometrial Cancer

Carcinoma of the endometrium is the most common type of uterine cancer and the most prevalent gynecological malignancy (Figure 33.17). The Canadian Cancer Society estimated that 7 200 Canadian women were diagnosed with uterine cancer (which includes endometrial cancer) in 2019. It also estimated that 1 250 Canadian women died of this disease in 2019.[42] In Canada, the 5-year net survival for uterine cancer is 83%.[53] It is the sixth most common cancer worldwide, and the incidence is highest in high-income countries in North America and in Northern and Western Europe.[54,55]

The primary risk factor for endometrial cancer is unopposed estrogen exposure (without progesterone). Exposure to unopposed estrogen includes estrogen-only HRT, tamoxifen, early menarche, late menopause, never having children, and a failure to ovulate (i.e., PCOS and anovulatory cycles typical of the late reproductive years). Less is known about the association between endometrial cancer and other types of hormone therapy. Chronic hyperinsulinemia, hyperglycemia, body fatness and adult weight gain, chronic inflammation, and lack of physical activity represent an increased risk for endometrial cancer[56] (Figure 33.18).

Epidemiological studies suggest an association between type 2 diabetes mellitus and endometrial cancer, as well as other cancers. The presence of type 2 diabetes mellitus increases mortality.[57] Diabetes mellitus and cancer share several mechanisms, including insulin and insulinlike growth factor (IGF) signalling, dysregulation of ovarian steroid hormones, and chronic inflammation.[57,58]

Investigators recently found the use of long-cycle estrogen and progestin HRT was related to a tendency toward an elevated risk of developing endometrial cancer for exposure of less than 5 years.[59] For exposure of more than 10 years, the risk for endometrial cancer was elevated among users of long-cycle HRT and sequential HRT. The use of continuous HRT or estradiol plus an LNG-IUD system (Mirena) showed a decreased risk for endometrial cancer.[59] Other risk factors not directly related to estrogen include gallbladder disease and hypertension, although being overweight may be a mediating factor for these risks. A family history of colon, endometrial, or ovarian cancer could signal hereditary nonpolyposis colorectal cancer (HNPCC; also known as *Lynch syndrome*). Women with this family history may wish to explore genetic testing and more aggressive screening.[60]

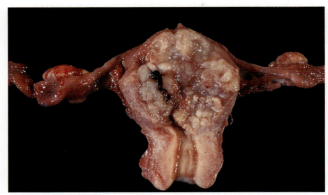

FIGURE 33.17 Endometrial Cancer. Tumour fills the endometrial cavity. Obvious myometrial invasion is shown. (From Damjanov, I., & Linder, J. [Eds.]. [1996]. *Anderson's pathology* [10th ed.]. Mosby.)

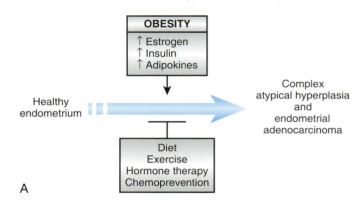

1 The panel interpreted BMI (including BMI at age 18–25 years), measures of abdominal girth, and adult weight gain as interrelated aspects of body fatness as well as fat distribution
2 Physical activity of all types; occupational, household, transport, and recreational
3 The effect is found in both caffeinated and decaffeinated coffee and cannot be attributed to caffeine

FIGURE 33.18 Food, Nutrition, Physical Activity, and Endometrial Cancer. A, Overview of the contribution of obesity to endometrial cancer progression and preventive strategies. The T-shaped bar shows factors that decrease the risk for endometrial cancer. See text for full discussion. **B,** Convincing and probable data for decreases and increases of endometrial cancer. *BMI,* Body mass index. ([A], Reprinted with permission from Schmandt, R. E., Iglesias, D. A., Co, N. N., et al. 2011. Understanding obesity and endometrial cancer risk: opportunities for prevention. *American Journal of Obstetrics & Gynecology, 205*(6), 518–525. [B], from World Cancer Research Fund/American Institute for Cancer Research. [2013]. *Continuous update project report: food, nutrition, physical activity, and the prevention of endometrial cancer.* https://www.dietandcancerreport.org.)

Ninety-five percent of endometrial cancers occur in postmenopausal women. There is a peak incidence occurring in the late 50s to early 60s. Although incidence rates are slightly higher in White women

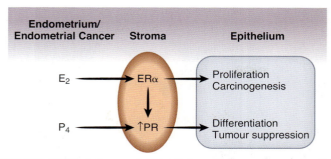

FIGURE 33.19 Actions of Estradiol and Progesterone in the Development of Endometrial Cancer. Estradiol (E_2) action through stromal estrogen receptor alpha (ERα) is critical for the development of endometrial cancer. Progesterone (P_4) acts through stromal progesterone receptor (PR) to oppose this carcinogenic effect of E_2. (From Kim, J. J., Kurita, T., & Bulun, S. E. [2013]. *Endocrine Reviews, 34*[1], 130–162.)

than in Black women, death rates in Black women are nearly twice as high as those for other ethnic or racial groups. Factors related to reductions in risk for endometrial cancer include delayed menarche; history of pregnancy or breastfeeding, or both; use of combined hormonal contraception; use of progestin-containing IUDs; and engagement in physical activity. So far, the lone dietary factor that may lower risk for endometrial cancer is drinking coffee regularly.[61] A recent meta-analysis suggests that protective effect of coffee consumption might be particularly beneficial for women with obesity.[61]

PATHOGENESIS Endometrial hyperplasia is associated with prolonged estrogenic stimulation of the endometrium. Endometrial hyperplasia and carcinoma share acquired genetic alterations in genes linked to carcinogenesis.[46] Frequent alterations in endometrial cancer include (1) altered estrogen receptor (ER) and progesterone receptor (PR) expression; (2) genetic mutation causing loss of function (inactivation) of the tumour-suppressor gene *PTEN*, which may enhance (3) the PI3K/AKT signalling pathway to become overactive, increasing the ability of the ER to "turn on" the expression of target genes; and (4) mutations to several genes, including fibroblast growth factor receptor (FGFR) and tumour protein 53 (TP53).[62] All of these events are predicted to affect PR actions in cancer pathogenesis. Progesterone inhibits estrogen-driven growth in the uterus.[62] The antagonistic effects of progesterone on the estrogen-induced proliferation and growth occur mostly during the luteal phase. These effects are dependent on the presence of functional PR expression.[62] Investigators are studying the importance of stromal PR and its role in progesterone inhibition of epithelial proliferation (Figure 33.19). The interactions between the epithelial and stromal cells of the endometrium may decide the eventual role in the actions of progesterone.[62] PR has two isoforms: PR-A and PR-B. These isoforms are both expressed in the epithelial and stromal cells of the endometrium. Their expression fluctuates during the menstrual cycle as well as during pregnancy. The delicate balance of the PR isoforms can tip the scales to foster endometrial hyperplasia and atypia. These isoforms also enhance expression of uterine growth factors.[62] Overall, depending on isoform expression, progesterone can be either an anti- or a pro-proliferative force on the endometrium. Misregulation of isoform expression can lead to abnormal function and precancerous changes.[62]

Two broad categories of endometrial carcinoma include type I and type II. About 80% of cases are type I. Table 33.6 summarizes type I and type II endometrial carcinoma.

CLINICAL MANIFESTATIONS, EVALUATION, AND TREATMENT Abnormal vaginal bleeding is the most common clinical manifestation of endometrial cancer. Postmenopausal women, obese women, and women with unopposed estrogenic conditions (i.e., anovulatory cycles) should be evaluated in the case of unscheduled or persistent irregular vaginal bleeding. Pain and weight loss are symptoms of more advanced disease. Transvaginal ultrasound (TVUS) is used to measure endometrial thickness. If the endometrium is abnormally thick (defined as greater than 5 mm), then further testing, such as an endometrial biopsy, is done. Treatment is based on the extent of the disease. Treatments include curettage for carcinoma in situ, total abdominal hysterectomy, chemotherapy, radiation, and (although controversial) progestins. The data supporting the use of metformin in the prevention and treatment of cancers are increasing, including those for endometrial cancer.[57]

Ovarian Cancer

Among gynecological malignancies, ovarian cancer is the leading cause of mortality in developed countries, with 295 414 new cases and 184 799 estimated deaths worldwide[55] (Figure 33.20). Globally, ovarian cancer is the eighth most common cancer and the eighth cause of death from cancer in women.[55] Incidence rates are highest in more developed regions and lowest in sub-Saharan Africa.[55] The Canadian Cancer Society estimated that 3 000 Canadian women were diagnosed with ovarian cancer in 2019. It also estimated that 1 900 Canadian women died of this disease in 2019.[51] An understanding of incidence patterns both within and between populations is essential to revealing potential causes of and risk factors for ovarian cancer (Figure 33.21). Worldwide, ovarian cancer accounts for more deaths than all other gynecological malignancies combined.[55] Risk factors for ovarian cancer are summarized in Table 33.7.

TABLE 33.6 Type I and Type II Endometrial Carcinoma

Characteristics	Type I	Type II
Age	55–65 years	65–75 years
Clinical setting	Unopposed estrogen Obesity Hypertension Diabetes	Atrophy Thin physique
Morphology	Endometrioid	Serous Clear cell Mixed Müllerian tumour
Precursor	Hyperplasia	Serous endometrial intraepithelial carcinoma
Mutated genes/ genetic abnormalities	PTEN ARID1A (regulator of chromatin) PIK3CA (PI3K) KRAS FGF2 (growth factor) MSI CTNNB1 (beta-catenin gene involved in Wnt signalling) TP53	TP53 Aneuploidy PIK3CA (PI3K) FBXW7 (regulator of MYC, cyclin E) CHD4 (regulator of chromatin) PPP2R1A (PP2A)
Behaviour	Indolent Spreads via lymphatics	Aggressive Intraperitoneal and lymphatic spread

MSI, Microsatellite instability, *MYC*, myelocytomatosis viral oncogene homologue; *PI3K*, phosphatidylinosityl-3-kinase; *PP2A*, protein phosphatase 2A.
Data from Kumar, V., Abbas, A. K., & Aster, J. C. (Eds.). (2021). *Robbins and Cotran pathologic basis of disease* (10th ed.). Elsevier.

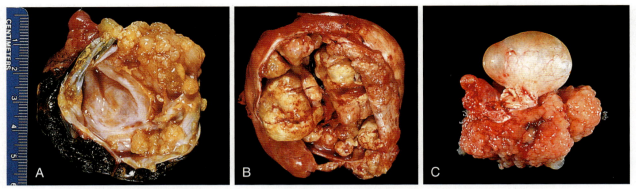

FIGURE 33.20 Ovarian Tumours. A serous borderline tumour displays a cyst cavity lined by papillary tumour growths, **A**. The cyst is opened **B**, to reveal a large bulky tumour mass called *cystadenocarcinoma* **C**, a tumour on the ovarian surface. Bilaterality of tumours is common, occurring in 20% of benign tumours, 30% of serous borderline tumours, and approximately 66% of serous carcinomas. A significant proportion of both borderline malignant and malignant tumours involve the surface of the ovary (C). (From Kumar, V., Abbas, A. K., & Aster, J. C. [Eds.]. [2021]. *Robbins and Cotran pathologic basis of disease* [10th ed.]. Elsevier.)

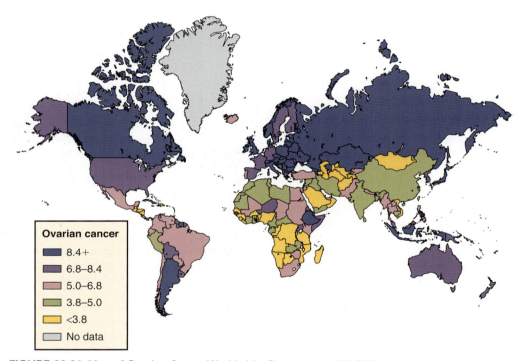

FIGURE 33.21 Map of Ovarian Cancer Worldwide. Rates are per 100 000 women and are age-standardized to the 1960 world standard population. Data were not included for white areas on the map. (Reproduced with permission from Ferlay, J., Soerjomataram, I., Ervik, M., et al. 2013. *GLOBOCAN 2012 v1.0, Cancer Incidence and Mortality Worldwide: IARC CancerBase No. 11* [Internet]. International Agency for Research on Cancer. https://globocan.iarc.fr, accessed on 28 September 2017.)

Despite study limitations, several factors related to ovulation have been consistently associated with increased or decreased risk of developing ovarian cancer. Risk is reduced by factors that suppress ovulation (pregnancy, breastfeeding, and combined hormonal contraceptive use). Ovarian cancer has been a very difficult disease to diagnose early and treat. The high mortality reflects a lack of early symptoms and a lack of effective screening tests.

PATHOGENESIS The biology of ovarian cancer is changing. Ovarian cancer is diverse in character, or *heterogeneous*. Many genetic and epigenetic changes are present in ovarian tumours. Previously, most ovarian cancers were thought to arise from epithelial cells that cover the ovarian surface or line subserosal cysts. Newer evidence suggests that tumours arise from three ovarian components: (1) from the fimbriae of fallopian tubes and from deposits of endometriosis; (2) from germ cells, which are pluripotent and migrate to the ovary from the yolk sac; and (3) from stromal cells, including the sex cords, which precede endocrine changes of the postnatal ovary.[46,63] Some ovarian tumours are still too difficult to classify. The normal ovary holds three major cell types: (1) germ cells that are derived from the endoderm and migrate to the gonadal ridge, where they proliferate and differentiate into oocytes; (2) the endocrine and interstitial hormone producing cells that produce estrogen and progesterone; and (3) epithelial cells derived from the Müllerian duct that cover the ovary and line inclusion cysts just beneath the ovarian surface. During normal ovulation, oocytes released from mature follicles enter the fallopian

TABLE 33.7 Risk Factors for Ovarian Cancer

Risk Factor	Description
Advancing age	Incidence of ovarian cancer increases with advancing age. Most cases occur in postmenopausal women.
Genetic factors	About 20% of all ovarian cancers are inherited. Of these, the majority are related to mutations in *BRCA1/BRCA2* genes, and others include mismatch repair genes (e.g., Lynch syndrome), *TP53* in the germ line (e.g., Li-Fraumeni syndrome), and Peutz-Jeghers syndrome. Fallopian tube cancer and peritoneal carcinomas also are part of the *BRCA*-associated disease spectrum.
Family history	A family history of ovarian cancer in a first-degree relative (e.g., mother, daughter, or sister) is the most important risk factor. The highest risk appears in women who have two or more first-degree relatives with ovarian cancer. Risk may be higher if the affected relative was diagnosed at a younger age, had breast cancer diagnosed before the age of 40, and had earlier breast cancer and a history of ovarian cancer. A cohort study showed ovarian cancer risk is higher in women whose sibling has or had liver, stomach, breast, prostate, connective tissue cancer, or melanoma; or whose parent has or had breast or liver cancer.
Overweight and obesity (BMI)	Meta-analysis found higher risk for ovarian cancer in premenopausal women with a body mass index (BMI) >30 and no effect in postmenopausal women. Another meta-analysis found a link between high BMI and ovarian cancer risk in women who had never used menopausal hormone therapy (MHT).
Height	Greater adult attained height (reflects factors that promote childhood growth) is classified by World Cancer Research Fund (WCRF) and the American Institute for Cancer Research (AICR) as a probable cause of ovarian cancer. A pooled analysis of Nordic data and meta-analyses showed ovarian cancer risk is 7–10% higher per 5-cm increment in height.
Reproductive/hormonal factors	Ovarian cancer risk is associated with factors affecting lifetime ovulations (and breaks between) or sex hormone levels (estrogens, progesterone, and androgens), or both. Structural changes to the ovary can occur with ovulation that may stimulate cancer development. These changes may be affected and enhanced by hormonal factors. Having more children, breastfeeding, or using oral contraceptives deceases the number of ovulations and therefore reduces the risk for ovarian cancer.
Menopausal hormone therapy	Current use of postmenopausal hormone replacement therapy (HRT, also known as *menopausal hormone therapy* [MHT]) is classified by the International Agency for Research on Cancer (IARC) as a cause of ovarian cancer (see Table 11.1). A meta-analysis found women using MHT for just a few years were more likely to develop ovarian cancer than women who had never used MHT. For every 1 000 women who take MHT for 5 years from about age 50, there will be 1 extra case of ovarian cancer. An estimated 1% of cases of ovarian cancer in the United Kingdom are linked to MHT use. In long-term (5+ years) users of estrogen-only MHT, compared with never-users, ovarian cancer risk is 53% higher. From a cohort study, ovarian cancer risk is 17% higher in long-term (5+ years) estrogen–progesterone MHT users when compared with never-users.
Endometriosis	Recent studies have shown that women with endometriosis have an increase in ovarian cancer risk.
Diabetes	Meta-analyses have shown ovarian cancer risk is 20–55% higher in women with diabetes compared with those without diabetes.
Previous cancer	Ovarian cancer risk is 24% higher in breast cancer survivors compared with the general population (possibly reflects *BRCA* mutations and Lynch syndrome or shared hormonal factors). It is higher in those diagnosed with breast cancer at a younger age versus those diagnosed older; the higher risk is limited to estrogen receptor (ER)–negative or ER-unknown breast cancer.
Smoking	An analysis showed an increased risk for mucinous ovarian tumours in current smokers. The risk decreased to normal after cessation of smoking. Recent results from the European Prospective Investigation into Cancer and Nutrition (EPIC) study showed smoking increases the risk for mucinous ovarian tumours.
Asbestos (occupational exposure)	Asbestos is classified by IARC as a cause of ovarian cancer (see Table 11.1).
Talc-based powder	Talc-based powder used peritoneally is classified by IARC as a probable cause of ovarian cancer (see Table 11.1). The risk for ovarian cancer with talc-based powders has been based on meta-analyses and pooled analyses of case-control studies. Not all body powders include talc.
Ionizing radiation	Use of X-radiation and gamma radiation is classified by IARC as a probable cause of ovarian cancer (see Table 11.1). A small number of individuals with ovarian cancer may be associated with radiotherapy for earlier cancer.
Factors that reduce risk for ovarian cancer	Taking contraceptives is classified by IARC as protective against ovarian cancer. Breastfeeding is classified by WCRF/AICR as possibly protective against ovarian cancer. Ovarian cancer risk is lower in women with the following factors supported by meta-analyses and pooled analyses: higher parity, hysterectomy, tubal ligation, and use of statins; there is controversial evidence linking systemic lupus erythematosus.

From Cancer Research UK. (n.d.). *Ovarian cancer risk factors.* https://www.cancerresearchuk.org/health-professional/cancer-statistics/statistics-by-cancer-type/ovarian-cancer/risk-factors; Cogliano, V. J., Baan, R., Straif, K., et al. (2011). *Journal of the National Cancer Institute, 103,* 1827–1839; Bray, F., Ferlay, J., Soerjomataram, I., et al. (2018). Global cancer statistics 2018: GLOBOCAN estimates of incidence and mortality worldwide for 36 cancers in 185 countries. *CA: A Cancer Journal for Clinicians, 68,* 394–424; International Agency for Research on Cancer. (2021). *List of classifications by cancer sites with sufficient or limited evidence in humans, Volumes 1 to 119.* https://monographs.iarc.fr/ENG/Classification/latest_classif.php; National Cancer Institute. (2021). *Ovarian epithelial, fallopian tube, and primary peritoneal cancer treatment (PDQ®)—Health professional version.* https://cancer.gov/cancertopics/pdq/treatment/ovarianepithelial/HealthProfessional; Parkin, D. M., Boyd, L., & Walker, L. C. (2011). *Cancer, 105*(Suppl. 2), S77–S81; World Cancer Research Fund/American Institute for Cancer Research. (2018). *Diet, Nutrition, Physical Activity and Cancer: a Global Perspective.* https://www.dietandcancerreport.org.

tube where fertilization usually occurs. The fimbriae of the fallopian tube cover the ruptured follicle and promote uptake of oocytes.[64] Both benign and malignant tumours come from each of the three ovarian cell types[65] (Figure 33.22). Epithelial ovarian cancers make up about 90% of malignant ovarian tumours and generally develop after age 40. Sex cord–stromal tumours arise from connective tissue, often secrete hormones, and can occur in women of all ages. These make up about 7% of ovarian tumours.[64] Tumours that arise from germ cells occur in the second and third decades and account for about 3 to 5% of ovarian tumours.[64] Borderline tumours of low malignant potential can contain

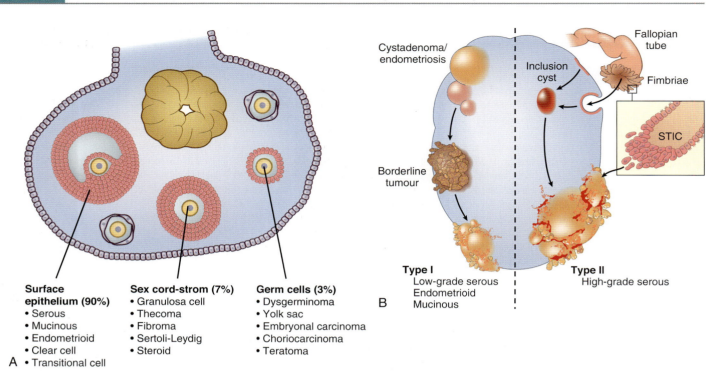

FIGURE 33.22 Heterogeneous Ovarian Tumours. **A**, Diverse ovarian tumours originate from different cell subtypes. **B**, Type I and type II ovarian tumours. Type I tumours progress from benign tumours through borderline tumours that give rise to low-grade carcinoma, and type II tumours arise from inclusion cysts/fallopian tube epithelium through intraepithelial precursors that often are unidentifiable. These tumours show high-grade features and are commonly of serous histology. *STIC*, Serous tubal intraepithelial carcinoma. ([B], from Kumar, V., Abbas, A. K., & Aster, J. C. [Eds.]. [2021]. *Robbins and Cotran pathologic basis of disease* [10th ed.]. Elsevier.)

structural and molecular evidence of transformed epithelial cells that do not invade the underlying stromal tissue. Approximately 10% of borderline tumours can recur after surgical resection and prove lethal.[64]

There are three major histological types of epithelial tumours: serous, mucinous, and endometrioid. These types all have a benign, borderline, and malignant category.[46] The most common histological subtype is high-grade serous cancers. These cancers may originate from a precursor lesion that arises from the fimbriae of the fallopian tubes. In women who underwent prophylactic salpingo-oophorectomies, studies showed that fallopian tubal lesions were present in almost 100% of women with early serous cancers associated with familial *BRCA* (breast cancer gene) mutations. Investigators recently proposed that the fallopian tube *is* the primary site of most serous carcinomas.[65] Although investigators historically proposed that the vast majority of serous carcinomas arose from cortical inclusion cysts, a newer hypothesis is that the cysts arise from implantation of detached fallopian tube epithelium at sites where ovulation has disrupted the surface of the ovary.[46] These findings have led to changes in management of women at high risk for ovarian cancer (*BRCA* mutation carriers and women with a strong family history of breast or ovarian cancer). These women are now recommended to have salpingo-oophorectomy and not just a simple oophorectomy.[46]

Histologically similar cancers diagnosed as primary peritoneal carcinomas share molecular findings (i.e., inactivation of p53 and BRCA1 and BRCA2 proteins). Therefore, tumours arising from fallopian tube and other locations from the peritoneal cavity, together with most ovarian epithelial cancers, are classified as "extrauterine adenocarcinomas of Müllerian epithelial origin." These cancers are included, staged, and treated similarly to ovarian cancer.[66]

The defining characteristics of malignant tumours are stromal invasion and increased epithelial atypia. Ovarian tumours are classified as type I (low-grade) and type II (high-grade) (see Figure 33.22B). Low-grade tumours arising in serous borderline tumours have several oncogene mutations. High-grade tumours have a high frequency of *TP53* mutations. Gene amplifications are found in many tumours, as well as deletions of tumour-suppressor genes. The majority of *BRCA* mutations are high-grade serous carcinomas with *TP53* mutations. *BRCA*-associated cancer risks are decided by the mutation location and variation of the *BRCA1/BRCA2* gene function.[63] Endometrioid ovarian carcinomas may arise in the setting of endometriosis and are sometimes associated with borderline tumour.[46]

CLINICAL MANIFESTATIONS Generally, individuals with ovarian cancer have no early symptoms. Because there are no effective screening techniques to detect it, the disease is usually advanced by the time treatment is explored. Some women may experience vague symptoms that include abdominal distension, loss of appetite, early satiety, and pelvic pain. These symptoms are important as *nonspecific* symptoms and can lead to delays in treatment. Symptoms of advanced disease include pain, abdominal swelling and distension, dyspepsia, vomiting, and alterations in bowel habits. Abnormal vaginal bleeding may occur if the postmenopausal endometrium is stimulated by a hormone-secreting tumour. The tumour also may cause ulcerations through the vaginal wall that result in bleeding. There also can be a feeling of pressure in the pelvis and leg pain. Given the location of the ovaries, assessing abnormalities on routine gynecological examination poses difficulty, especially in obese women. Ovarian cancer is considered a silent disease.

Tumour obstruction of vascular channels can cause venous and, occasionally, arterial thrombosis. Alterations in coagulation also occur, contributing to clot formation. Metastasis often causes pleural effusion (Figure 33.23).

CHAPTER 33 Alterations of the Female Reproductive System

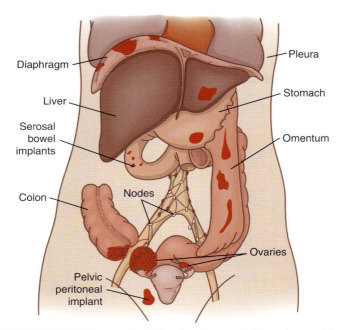

FIGURE 33.23 Metastasis of Ovarian Cancer. Pattern of spread for epithelial cancer of the ovary.

TABLE 33.8 FIGO[a] Staging of Carcinoma of the Ovary

Stage	Characteristics
I	Growth limited to ovaries
II	Growth involves one or both ovaries and involvement of other organs (i.e., uterus, bladder, colon)
III	Cancer involves one or both ovaries, and one or both of the following are present: (1) cancer has spread beyond pelvis to lining of abdomen, (2) cancer has spread to lymph nodes
IV	Growth involves one or both ovaries with distant metastases to lungs, liver, or other organs outside peritoneal cavity
Recurrent	Cancer recurs after completion of treatment

[a]The International Federation of Gynecology and Obstetrics.

EVALUATION AND TREATMENT There is no sensitive and specific test for ovarian cancer for screening low-risk women. Routine screening of women without risk factors has not been shown to be beneficial. Routine screening may cause harm because more women have unnecessary surgical procedures.[66] Solid evidence indicates that screening with a CA-125 blood test and TVUS does not result in a decrease in ovarian cancer mortality.[66] Pelvic examination may detect advanced disease.[66] Several biomarkers with potential application to screening are under investigation. The confirmation of a malignant tumour occurs by biopsy. The extent of disease is evaluated with imaging techniques. Table 33.8 describes the International Federation of Gynecology and Obstetrics (FIGO) staging system.

The first approach to treatment is surgery. Surgery is performed to decide the stage of disease and to remove as much of the tumour as possible. Treatment is most often provided by a multidisciplinary team from various disciplines including surgeons, pathologists, and oncologists.[67] Treatment is customized based on the stage of the cancer, the woman's desires, the cell type, and the sensitivity of the cancer cells. Radiation and chemotherapy are common treatments. New therapies under investigation include monoclonal antibodies, epidermal growth factor receptor, gene therapy, and small-molecular-weight inhibitors. Research into prevention and treatment of ovarian cancer is ongoing.

Sexual Dysfunction

Sexual dysfunction is the lack of satisfaction with sexual function resulting from pain or a deficiency in sexual desire, arousal, or orgasm/climax.[68] Sexual function and dysfunction result from a complex set of personal and biological factors that interact with culture. Implications of sexual dysfunction include both organic and psychosocial disorders. Studies have shown that 40 to 50% of adult women have some form of sexual dysfunction.[69] Chronic medical conditions can greatly affect both sexual desire and sexual function (Table 33.9).

Disorders of desire (hypoactive sexual desire, decreased libido) are the most common sexual dysfunction in women.[69] The prevalence of hypoactive sexual desire increases with age. The decreased desire may be a biological manifestation of depression, dissatisfaction with partner relationships, a history of sexual or physical abuse, alcohol or other substance abuse, prolactin-secreting pituitary tumours, or testosterone deficiency.[70] Medications, such as β-adrenergic blockers used for heart disease, may decrease sexual desire. Treatment may include counselling, psychotherapy, and antidepressants.

Anorgasmia (orgasmic dysfunction) is the inability of a woman to reach or achieve orgasm. This condition ranges from difficulty in arousal to lack of orgasm. Any chronic illness may affect arousal. Specific disorders that may block orgasm are diabetes, alcoholism, neurological disturbances, hormonal deficiencies, and pelvic disorders, such as infections, trauma, and surgical scarring. Other inhibitors include medications, such as narcotics, tranquilizers, antidepressants (especially SSRIs), and antihypertensive medications.

Dyspareunia (painful intercourse) is common. Women may experience pain at any time from the beginning of arousal to after intercourse. The pain may have a burning, sharp, searing, or cramping quality. Pain is described as external, vaginal, deep abdominal, or pelvic. A variety of psychosocial and organic causes have been found. Inadequate lubrication may make penetration or intercourse difficult or painful. Medications with a drying effect (such as antihistamines, certain tranquilizers, and marihuana) and disorders (such as diabetes, vaginal infections, and estrogen deficiency) can decrease lubrication. Other causes include skin problems around the introitus or affecting the vulva, and irritation or infection of the clitoris. Other contributors include disorders of the vaginal opening and disorders of the urethra or anus. Vaginal causes may include infections, thinning of the walls caused by aging or decreased estrogen level, or irritation caused by spermicides or douches. Pelvic-related causes include infection, tumours, and cervical or uterine abnormalities.

Vaginismus is an involuntary muscle spasm in response to attempted penetration. Common psychological causes include prior sexual trauma and fear of sex. Organic causes are like those that cause dyspareunia, including vulvovestibulitis. Even after the detection of underlying organic problem and successful treatment, vaginismus may persist.

Sexual dysfunction may develop as a coping mechanism. Women with a history of sexual trauma, including rape, incest, or molestation, often have problems with desire, arousal, or orgasm or experience pain with sexual activity. In extreme cases, total sexual aversion may develop. At other times, sexual dysfunction may be a symptom of marital or relationship problems. Because sexual dysfunction has many causes, assessment and treatment should be holistic and culturally sensitive.

Impaired Fertility

Infertility affects approximately 16% (or 1 in 6) of all couples in Canada. It is defined as the inability to conceive over 1 year of

TABLE 33.9 Possible Effects of Chronic Disease on Sexual Functioning in Women

Disease	Sexual Function
Cerebral palsy	Intact genital sensations, decreased lubrication; difficulty with sexual activity/positioning because of muscle spasticity, rigidity, or weakness; pain with positioning caused by contracture of knees and hips or because of increased spasms with arousal
Cerebrovascular accident	Difficulties in sexual positioning and sensitivity because of impaired motor strength, coordination, or paralysis; decreased libido with stroke on dominant side of brain
Diabetes	Diminished intensity of orgasm and gradual decline in ability to achieve orgasm; decreased lubrication or recurrent vaginal infections with resultant dyspareunia
Chronic kidney disease	Decreased arousal; increasingly rare and less intense orgasms; decreased lubrication
Rheumatoid arthritis	Painful sexual activity/positions because of swollen, painful joints, muscular atrophy, and joint contracture; decreased libido because of pain, fatigue, or medication; genital sensations are still intact
Systemic lupus erythematosus	Like rheumatoid arthritis; decreased lubrication and vaginal lesions result in painful penetration
Myocardial infarction	Most literature male-oriented; problems related to medications
Multiple sclerosis	Diminished genital sensitivity; decreased lubrication; declining orgasmic ability; difficulty with sexual activity because of muscle weakness, pain, or incontinence
Spinal cord injury	Reflex sexual response with injury above sacral area; disrupted response with lesion at or below sacrum; loss of sensation, decreased lubrication; spasticity, incontinence, or pain with arousal; continued orgasmic sensations or sensations diffused in general or to specific body parts, such as breast or lips

unprotected intercourse.[3] Factors in the man or woman, or in both partners may impair fertility. Female infertility results from dysfunction of the normal reproductive process: menses and ovulation, fallopian tube function (transport of the egg to the uterus and as a site of fertilization), and implantation of the fertilized egg into a receptive endometrium. Ovarian dysfunction includes defective ovulation because of hormonal effects (e.g., PCOS, depressed hypothalamic activity, secondary physical or emotional stress), diminished ovarian reserve (lack of immature eggs secondary to congenital, medical, or unexplained factors), or premature ovarian insufficiency (failure of ovarian function before the age of 40). Fallopian tube dysfunction may result from acute pelvic infections with chlamydia or gonorrhea. Adhesions from pelvic infection, abdominal surgery, or endometriosis may cause blockage of one or both fallopian tubes, preventing access of the sperm to the ovum. The fertilized ovum must implant on a receptive endometrium.[71] Greatly diminished receptivity may occur related to fibroids or inadequate molecular or cellular preparation of the implantation site.

Several diagnostic procedures are needed in the routine investigation of the infertile couple.[72] Initial workup includes analysis of semen, determination of ovulation, and hysterosalpingography of the fallopian tubes. Treatment of infertility is aimed toward correction of problems found during diagnostic workup. Treatment of anovulation includes hormonal medications that induce ovulation (e.g., clomiphene citrate, FSH, GnRH). Women with fallopian tube defects, who have failed other approaches or have no identifiable cause of their infertility, are often treated by assisted reproductive technology (ART).[72] The basic ART procedure is in vitro fertilization (IVF). IVF involves collecting eggs directly from the ovary, performing fertilization and early embryonic development in the laboratory, and then transferring the eggs into the uterus. Many variations of this procedure are available. Depending on the potential cause of infertility, proper modifications allow for the use of donor sperm, egg, or uterus (in the case of surrogacy). An essential treatment for infertility is prevention of STIs. STIs can result in scarring and adhesion formation in the reproductive tract of either the man or the woman.

DISORDERS OF THE FEMALE BREAST

> ### ✓ QUICK CHECK 33.5
> 1. What types of fibrocystic breast changes increase the risk for breast cancer?
> 2. What is the role of hormones and growth factors in the pathophysiology of breast cancer?
> 3. Why are reproductive factors, such as early menarche and late menopause, important for the pathogenesis of breast cancer?
> 4. Why is complete breast involution important for reducing risk for breast cancer?
> 5. Discuss the role of the microenvironment or stromal tissue on breast cancer development.

Galactorrhea

Galactorrhea (inappropriate lactation) is the constant and sometimes excessive secretion of a milky fluid from the breasts of a woman who is not pregnant or nursing an infant. Galactorrhea, which also can occur in men, may involve one or both breasts, and is not associated with breast cancer.

The incidence of galactorrhea is difficult to estimate because of differences among definitions of the condition, examination techniques, and the studied populations of women. Estimated prevalence is 0.1 to 32% of all women.

PATHOPHYSIOLOGY Galactorrhea is a manifestation of pathophysiological processes elsewhere in the body, rather than a primary breast disorder. These processes are chiefly hormone imbalances caused by hypothalamic–pituitary disturbances, pituitary tumours, or neurological damage. Exogenous causes include medications, estrogen, and manipulation of the nipples.

The most common cause of galactorrhea is **nonpuerperal hyperprolactinemia**, or excessive amounts of prolactin in the blood not related to pregnancy or childbirth. The cause of nonpuerperal hyperprolactinemia is any factor that (1) stimulates or overstimulates the prolactin-secreting units of the pituitary gland; (2) interferes with production of **prolactin-inhibiting factor (PIF)**, a neurotransmitter (probably dopamine) that inhibits prolactin secretion; or (3) interferes with pituitary receptors for PIF.

Certain medications can cause nonpuerperal hyperprolactinemia. They include the phenothiazines, reserpine (Serpasil), and methyldopa (Aldomet); exogenous estrogens, particularly in oral contraceptives; morphine; and the tricyclic antidepressants.

Hypothyroidism causes increased secretion of hypothalamic TSH, which stimulates prolactin release from the pituitary. Hypothyroidism also is associated with reduced metabolic clearance of prolactin, which prolongs its effects.

Many types of pituitary tumours cause hyperprolactinemia, particularly prolactinoma. Prolactinomas cause hyperprolactinemia by secreting prolactin, decreasing production of PIF, or applying pressure to the pituitary stalk. As a result, delivery of PIF to the anterior pituitary is prevented. Growth hormone–secreting pituitary tumours may cause galactorrhea through the intrinsic lactogenic effect that growth hormone appears to have on mammary tissue. Prolactin-secreting lung and kidney tumours also cause hyperprolactinemia.

Chronic stress may cause hyperprolactinemia by inhibiting PIF release. Head trauma, cervical spinal injuries, encephalitis, meningitis, herpes zoster, or thoracotomy scars may stimulate the suckling reflex. The suckling reflex increases prolactin secretion.

CLINICAL MANIFESTATIONS The manifestations of inappropriate lactation include the appearance of a milky breast secretion from one or both breasts of nonpregnant, nonlactating women. Most women with galactorrhea experience menstrual abnormality. If a pituitary process is involved, the woman usually experiences hirsutism and infertility. If a hypothalamic lesion is present, she may report CNS symptoms, such as intractable headache, visual field disturbances, sleep disturbances, and abnormal temperature, thirst, or appetite.

EVALUATION AND TREATMENT A thorough evaluation of galactorrhea in nulliparous women (women who have never been pregnant) or in parous women who have not breastfed for 12 months should occur. Evaluation includes a variety of diagnostic tests. At least two positive results of serum prolactin levels are needed to diagnose hyperprolactinemia. Prolactin levels higher than 25 to 30 µg/L are considered elevated. Those in the range of 75 to 100 µg/L are possibly caused by a pituitary tumour until proven otherwise. To rule out hypothyroidism, the measurement of serum thyroxine (T_4) and TSH levels takes place. LH and FSH levels are obtained if the individual is amenorrheic. MRI may aid in finding adenomas.

Treatment for galactorrhea consists of identification and treatment of the cause. Medical therapy is typical, and surgery or radiation therapy is rarely needed.

Benign Breast Disease and Conditions

Benign breast disease (BBD) is a spectrum of noncancerous changes in the breast. Numerous benign alterations in ducts and lobules occur in the breast. These alterations include lumps, cysts, sensitive nipples, and itching. The most common symptoms reported by women are pain, palpable mass, or nipple discharge. The majority of these prove to have a benign cause. Major determinants of the risk for breast cancer after a diagnosis of BBD include histological or biological features, or both; earlier biopsy; and degree of family history.[73] Benign epithelial lesions can be broadly classified as (1) nonproliferative breast lesions, (2) proliferative breast disease without atypia, and (3) atypical (atypia) hyperplasia (AH). The majority of nonproliferative benign lesions are not precursors of cancer and are not associated with an increased risk for breast cancer.[73] Some benign breast lesions (e.g., AH) present an increase in risk for development of breast cancer. These women should receive counselling about screening recommendations and risk reduction.[73]

Nonproliferative Breast Lesions

Nonproliferative epithelial breast lesions are usually not associated with an increased risk for breast cancer. The nonproliferative lesions include (1) simple breast cysts, (2) papillary apocrine change, and (3) mild hyperplasia of the usual type. Terms such as fibrocystic changes (FCCs; or physiological nodularity and cysts), fibrocystic disease, chronic cystic mastitis, and mammary dysplasia refer to nonproliferative lesions.[73] Simple cysts (fluid-filled sacs) are the most common nonproliferative breast lesion. These cysts are a specific type of lump that commonly occurs in women in their 30s, 40s, and early 50s. Cysts feel "squishy" when they occur close to the surface of the breast but when deeply embedded, they can feel hard. An estimated 50 to 80% of women normally experience some of these changes. The prevalence of fibrocystic lesions is probably related to hormonal changes. Genetic background, age, parity, history of lactation, and use of caffeine and exogenous hormones affects these lesions. Cystic changes can be induced in experimental animals by altering ratios of estrogens and progesterone. Breast cysts are thought to be the result of ovarian alterations, but the exact mechanism is unknown. Cysts also can be associated with unilateral nipple discharge. Cysts often rupture with release of secretory material into the adjacent tissue. The resulting chronic inflammation and scarring fibrosis contribute to the palpable firmness of the breast. Fibrous tissue increases progressively until menopause and regresses thereafter.

Papillary apocrine change is an increase in ductal epithelial cells that has apocrine changes or an eosinophilic cytoplasm. Mild hyperplasia of the usual type is an increase in the number of epithelial cells within a duct that is more than two cells, but not more than four cells, in depth.[73]

Proliferative Breast Lesions Without Atypia

Proliferative breast lesions without atypia are characterized by proliferation of ductal epithelium or stroma, or both, without cellular signs of abnormality (atypia or deviation from normal). A discussion of these structurally diverse lesions follows: (1) usual ductal hyperplasia, (2) intraductal papillomas, (3) sclerosing adenosis, (4) radial scar, and (5) simple fibroadenoma.

1. Usual ductal hyperplasia (UDH) is added or proliferating epithelial cells that fill and distend the ducts and lobules. They are usually found as an incidental finding from mammography. The cells can vary in size and shape, but they keep features of benign cells.[73] No treatment is needed.[73]
2. Intraductal papillomas can occur as solitary or multiple lesions. *Solitary papillomas* are a monotonous (sameness) array of papillary cells that grow from the wall of the cyst into the lumen of the duct. Growth occurs within a dilated duct often near or beside the nipple, causing benign nipple discharge. These papillomas *can* harbour areas of atypia requiring surgical excision. Diffuse papillomatosis (multiple papillomas) may present as breast masses, nodules on ultrasound, or the cause of nipple discharge. Diffuse papillomatosis is defined as a minimum of five papillomas within a localized segment of breast tissue.[74] Although the breast cancer risk is small, these lesions require surgical excision.
3. Sclerosing adenosis is a lobular lesion with increased fibrous tissue and scattered glandular cells.[75] It is a common but poorly understood benign breast lesion.[75] This lesion carries an approximate twofold increased chance of later breast cancer.[76] It is usually found as a suspicious lesion on mammography.
4. Radial scar (RS) refers to an irregular, radial proliferation of duct-like small tubules entrapped in a dense central fibrosis. The term

scar refers to the structural appearance only because these lesions are not associated with prior injury, biopsy, or surgery. *Radial scar* is also called *radial sclerosing lesions* and *sclerosing papillary proliferation*. The discovery of RSs usually occurs when a breast lesion or radiological abnormality is biopsied or removed. Controversy exists about the need for surgical excision.[3]

5. **Simple fibroadenomas** are benign solid tumours that hold glandular and fibrous lesions.[74] In about 20% of cases, multiple fibroadenomas can occur in the same breast or bilaterally.[74] The etiology for fibroadenomas is unknown. It appears to be hormonal because they can persist during the reproductive years and can increase in size during pregnancy or with estrogen therapy. They usually regress after menopause.[3] They are more common among women between 15 and 35 years of age. Fibroadenomas are considered proliferative lesions and the histological features influence the risk for breast cancer. There is no increased risk for breast cancer in most women with a simple fibroadenoma. It is not necessary to excise all biopsy-proven fibroadenomas.[3] Disadvantages of excisional surgery include scarring at the incision site, dimpling of the breast from the removal of the tumour, damage to the breast's duct system, and mammographic changes (e.g., architectural distortion, skin thickening, increased focal density).[46] If a biopsy-proven fibroadenoma is asymptomatic, it can then be left in place. Some women may wish to have the mass excised so that they will not worry further.[46]

Proliferative Breast Lesions With Atypia

Atypical hyperplasia (AH) is an increase in the number of cells (or proliferation) with the cells having some variation in structure—*atypia*. AH is a high-risk benign lesion found in about 10% of biopsies with benign findings.[46] These proliferative breast lesions with some atypia include atypical ductal hyperplasia and atypical lobular hyperplasia.[46] **Atypical ductal hyperplasia (ADH)** refers to abnormal proliferating cells in breast ducts. **Atypical lobular hyperplasia (ALH)** refers to proliferation of cells in the lumen of lobular units.

Studies show that women with AH have a 3- to 5-fold increased risk of breast cancer compared with women who have nonproliferative lesions.[77] Ongoing studies will further decide risk estimates with such factors, for example, as breast density[46] (Figure 33.24). About 58% of the subsequent breast cancers in women with AH occur in the ipsilateral breast (same side) as the biopsy.[77] Because some studies have shown a lack of agreement among pathologists in differentiating AH from carcinoma in situ,[78] it is important that pathologists follow standardized, published criteria. A diagnosis of either condition may be a factor for women to seek a second opinion. It appears that menopausal status at the time of benign breast biopsy influences the size of future breast cancer risk. For women who were premenopausal at the time of their breast biopsy, the risk for breast cancer was greater in those with ALH than among women with ADH.[79] Overall, the younger a woman is when she receives a diagnosis of AH, the higher the risk that breast cancer will develop.[80] Among women who were postmenopausal at the time of benign breast biopsy, the risk was similar with women with ALH and women with ADH.[79] Overall, ADH and ALH are viewed best as "markers" of a generalized bilateral increase in breast cancer risk.[81]

EVALUATION AND TREATMENT A multimodal approach that combines physical examination, mammography, ultrasonography, thermography, possibly MRI, and biopsy helps the diagnosis of breast problems. The dense breast tissue often seen in young women can make mammographic interpretation extremely difficult (see *Health Promotion*: Breast Cancer Screening Mammography).

Treatment consists largely of relieving symptoms. Decreased consumption of caffeinated beverages (e.g., cola, root beer) and chocolate, which can cause overstimulation for some women, may reduce pain and nodularity. Given time, the cysts may disappear without treatment.

Although still controversial, isoflavone exposure was associated with a decreased risk for proliferative benign fibrocystic changes, nonproliferative changes, and breast cancer.[82] Genistein, a soy isoflavone, has been reported to downregulate an enzyme important in cancer progression (i.e., telomerase) and contributes to inhibition in both breast benign and cancer cells.[83] Toxicologists have concluded that soy supplement intake will not induce proliferation of normal breast tissue and may even inhibit proliferation.[82] The North American Menopause Society found that soy foods generally appear to be breast protective and recommended moderate lifelong soy consumption.[84] Although quite controversial, another preventive factor may be iodine.[85]

Breast Cancer

In 2020, 2.2 million women were diagnosed with breast cancer. There were 7.8 million women alive who had been diagnosed with breast cancer in the previous 5 years (Figure 33.25).[86] Breast cancer is the most common cause of cancer death among women (684 996 deaths in 2020).[86] It is now responsible for one in four of all cancers in women.

Breast cancer is the most common cancer in Canadian women, excluding nonmelanoma skin cancers. It is the leading cause of death in women 40 to 44 years of age and the second leading cause of cancer death in women of all ages after lung cancer. The Canadian Cancer Society estimated that 26 900 Canadian women were diagnosed with breast cancer in 2019. It also estimated that 5 000 women died of this disease in 2019.[42] Breast cancer is more common in high-income, developed countries such as Canada, the United States, and some European countries. The risk of developing breast cancer increases with age. It occurs most often in women between the ages of 30 and 49.[42] Because the detection of DCIS most often occurs by mammography, the large increase in incidence of DCIS over the past 20 years can be attributed to screening.

Although breast cancer is a multifactorial disease involving a complex web of interacting factors, risk is related to timing, duration, and pattern of exposures. The broad classification of risk factors and possible causes of breast cancer are reproductive, hormonal, environmental, and familial (Table 33.10). However, two factors that appear as important are involution of the mammary gland and breast density (see the following discussion).

Reproductive Factors: Pregnancy

A clearer understanding of mammary gland structure (morphology) and function from fetal development to puberty, pregnancy, and aging will help explain fundamental changes to breast development and disease. A key element in that process is "branching morphogenesis". This is a process in which the mammary gland fulfills its function by producing and delivering copious amounts of milk by forming a root-like network of branched ducts from a rudimentary epithelial bud.[87] Branching morphogenesis begins in fetal development, pauses after birth, starts again in response to estrogens at puberty. It is changed by cyclic ovarian hormonal action. This systemic hormonal action causes local paracrine interactions between the developing epithelial ducts and their adjacent mesenchyme (embryonic) or postnatal stroma.[87] The local cellular crosstalk then directs the tissue remodelling, ultimately producing a mature ductal tree.[87]

A woman's age when her first child is born affects her risk of developing breast cancer. The younger she is, the lower the risk. Overall, lifetime risk for breast cancer is reduced in parous women compared with nulliparous women, but pregnancy must occur at a young age.[88] The influence of pregnancy on the risk for breast cancer also depends on family history, lactation postpartum, and overall parity.[89] Findings

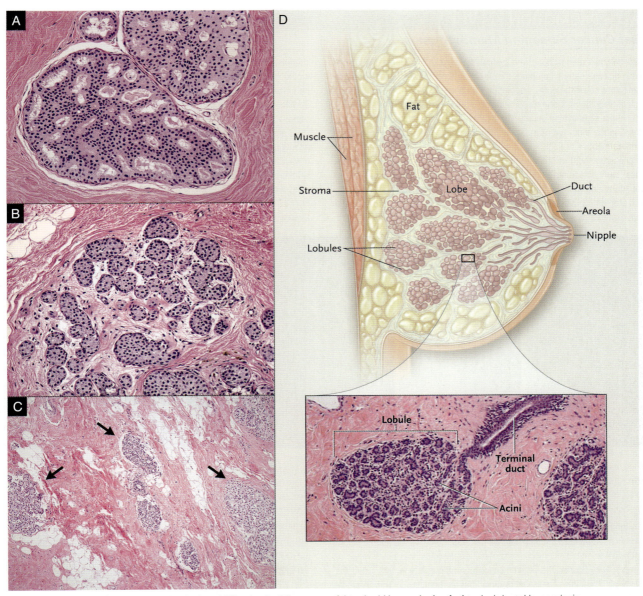

FIGURE 33.24 Anatomical and Histological Features of Atypical Hyperplasia. **A**, Atypical ductal hyperplasia with proliferation of monotonous cells in architecturally complex patterns, including secondary lumens and micropapillary formations. **B**, Atypical lobular hyperplasia (ALH), with expanded acini filled with monotonous polygonal cells and a loss of acinar lumen. **C**, Multifocal atypical hyperplasia (in this case ALH). ALH is present in more than one terminal duct lobular unit (TDLU), and units are clearly separated from one another by interlobular mammary stroma *(arrows)*. **D**, Illustration of the microanatomy of the breast, including a photomicrograph of a TDLU. (From Hartmann, L. C., Degnim, A. C., Santen, R. J., et al. [2015.] Atypical hyperplasia of the breast—risk assessment and management options. *New England Journal of Medicine, 372*[1], 1271–1272. Reprinted with permission.)

from a large prospective study found a *dual effect* from pregnancy. This includes a transient postpartum increase in breast cancer risk followed by a long-term reduction in risk (compared with nulliparous women).[90] **Pregnancy-associated breast cancer (PABC)** is defined as breast cancer that occurs during pregnancy. This risk may persist for at least 5 years postpartum and longer.[91,92] Delayed child-bearing, observed in Canada, the United States, and all developing countries, is expected to show a rise in diagnosed breast cancers.[89] A recent hypothesis for risk at any age is that gland *involution* after pregnancy and lactation uses some of the same tissue remodelling pathways activated during wound healing (i.e., proinflammatory pathways).[93] The proinflammatory environment, although physiologically normal, promotes tumour progression. The presence of macrophages in the involuting mammary gland may contribute to carcinogenesis. The normal involuting gland may be in an immunosuppressed state with T-cell suppression.[93,94] Discussion of involution is in the following section.

Although the proposal of many mechanisms exists for the *protective* effect of pregnancy, newer data on the genomic profile of parous women have shown pregnancy induces a long-lasting "genomic signature." This finding reveals chromatin remodelling derived from the early first pregnancy. The chromatin modifications are accompanied by higher expression of genes related to cell adhesion and differentiation.

HEALTH PROMOTION
Breast Cancer Screening Mammography

The idea behind screening healthy individuals for disease is the hope that we can diagnose disease early when more treatment options are available. Screening programs that cover the entire population of a country are a large undertaking and usually require extensive resources. Therefore, we need to make certain that the test has a high level of accuracy with reasonable costs and disadvantages, and the disease is not too rare. Those diagnosed because of screening respond well to treatment.

The encouragement of female breast cancer screening has existed for many decades. Early screening programs encouraged women to perform self-breast examinations and to have their clinician perform a breast examination in the office. Later data have shown that these screening techniques lead to false-positive examinations and are not associated with a reduction in mortality.

Another harm of screening mammography is overdiagnosis—a *diagnosis* that would never have harmed the woman during her lifetime. Such diagnoses can be either of a preinvasive lesion, such as ductal carcinoma in situ (DCIS), or of invasive breast cancer. With more women undergoing screening with mammography, we have seen a sharp increase in the number of women *diagnosed* with DCIS and early-stage breast cancer. DCIS is not an invasive carcinoma and not an immediate life-threatening cancer—it is confined to the duct. DCIS is almost always treated as if it is an invasive early-stage breast cancer. Women with DCIS are at increased risk for a later, invasive breast cancer diagnosis. However, most women with DCIS are never diagnosed with invasive cancer. Treatment of DCIS does not alter mortality. Women with DCIS have the same death rates as women without DCIS. Some discussion has centred on changing the name

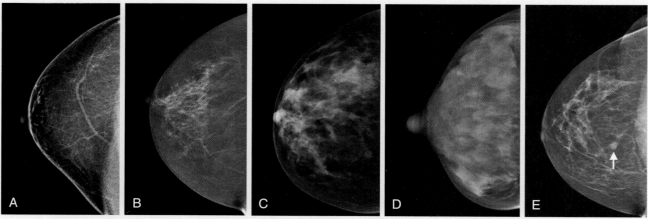

Mammograms. (A–D) Mammograms depicting varying breast densities from a craniocaudal view: **A**, almost entirely fat; **B**, scattered fibroglandular densities; **C**, heterogeneously dense; and **D**, extremely dense. **(E)** Mammogram showing invasive cancer. (Images provided by Christoph I. Lee, MD, MSHS. Reprinted from Fuller, M. S., Lee, C. I., Elmore, J. G. [2015]. Breast cancer screening: an evidence-based update. *Medical Clinics of North America, 99*[3], 451–468, with permission from Elsevier.)

Many groups continue to recommend mammography for breast cancer screening, although the benefits are less than we had hoped, and we are learning more about the harms. Mammography is an X-ray examination that takes views of each breast (see figure). The recommended age of first mammogram and the frequency of screening varies among guidelines and countries. The Canadian Task Force on Preventive Health periodically reviews the evidence, and issues guidelines to help aid discussions with women about screening.

The benefits, risks, and accuracy of mammography screening depend on many factors. These factors include women's age, breast density, and time interval between screening examinations. Possible risks of screening are important to consider because screening at a population level involves testing healthy individuals.

No medical test is perfect. The US National Cancer Institute reports that about 10% of screening mammograms are interpreted as "abnormal," requiring more testing. The great majority of women with these "abnormal" examinations do not have breast cancer. This is a false-positive result. The false-positive results lead to added diagnostic testing, which can result in anxiety and morbidity to women. Estimates show that at least 50% of women who are screened annually for a decade will have experienced at least one false-positive examination.

of DCIS lesions to better differentiate preinvasive DCIS from invasive cancer because the term *carcinoma* is like the term *cancer*. However, it is not likely that the name will be changed because of its current common usage.

Unfortunately, we are not able to name which women with a new diagnosis of DCIS or invasive breast cancer have the type of lesion that is so low risk that it will never harm them during their lifetime. Thus, most women undergo treatment with either lumpectomy and radiation therapy or mastectomy. This is overtreatment if the DCIS or invasive cancer was overdiagnosed. Estimates of the prevalence of overdiagnosis vary in the literature from less than 10 to 50%.

Women with abnormalities noted on screening mammography are often offered the choice of a breast biopsy versus watchful waiting with follow-up mammograms in 6 to 12 months. Some women think that a breast biopsy will give them an immediate and definitive diagnosis. However, this is not always the case. Disagreements by pathologists occur about the diagnoses of atypia and DCIS.

Balancing the benefits and harms of breast cancer screening is not an easy task for women or their clinicians. Encouragement should be provided to every woman to make an informed decision.

Joann G. Elmore, MD, MPH

From Elmore, J. G., Longton, G. M., Carney, P. A., et al. (2015). *JAMA, 313*(11), 1122–1132; Fuller, M. S., Lee, C. I., & Elmore, J. G. (2015). *Medical Clinics of North America, 99*(3), 451–468; Elmore, J., Wild, D., Nelson, H., et al. (2020). *Jekel's epidemiology, biostatistics, preventive medicine, and public health* (5th ed.). Elsevier; National Guideline C: *Breast cancer screening*. https://www.guideline.gov; National Care Institute. (2020). *Breast cancer screening: (PDQ®)–Health professional version*. https://www.cancer.gov/types/breast/hp/breast-screening-pdq; Pace, L. E., & Keating, N. L. (2015). *JAMA, 311*(13), 1327–1335; US Preventive Services Task Force. (2009). *Annals of Internal Medicine, 151*(10), 716–726.

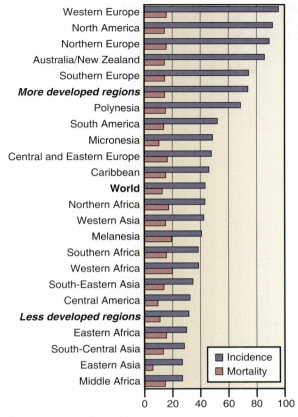

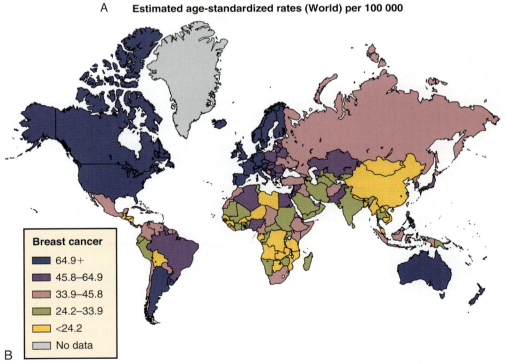

FIGURE 33.25 Breast Cancer Estimated Incidence and Mortality Worldwide in 2012. A, Estimated age-standardized rates (world) per 100 000 population. B, Incidence and mortality estimated age-standardized rates (world) per 100 000. These numbers show a sharp rise in breast cancer incidence since the 2008 estimates by more than 20%. It is the most common cancer in women both in more and in less developed regions, with slightly more cases in less developed (883 000 cases) than in more developed (794 000) regions. Incidence rates vary nearly fourfold across the world regions. (Reproduced with permission from Ferlay, J., Soerjomataram, I., Ervik, M., et al. 2020. *GLOBOCAN 2020 v1.0, Cancer Incidence and Mortality Worldwide: IARC CancerBase No. 11* [Internet]. International Agency for Research on Cancer. https://gco.iarc.fr/today/data/factsheets/cancers/20-Breast-fact-sheet.pdf.)

TABLE 33.10 Established Risk Factors for Breast Cancer

Relative Risk	Risk Factor
>4.0	Female
	Age
	Family history of breast cancer
	Personal history of breast cancer
	Inherited genetic mutations (*BRCA1/BRCA2* and others)
	High breast density
	Atypical hyperplasia
2.1–4.0	Family history (one first-degree relative)
	High-dose radiation to chest/breast
	Prior benign breast disease
1.1–2.0	No full-term pregnancies
	Late age at first full-term pregnancy (>30 years)
	Early menarche (<12 years)
	Late menopause (>55 years)
	Never breastfed children
	High alcohol consumption
	Smoking
	Recent oral contraceptive use
	Recent or current use of combined hormone replacement therapy
	Physical inactivity
	Obesity or adult weight gain (postmenopausal)

Data from American Cancer Society. (2010). *Cancer facts & figures 2010.*

Genes only activated during the first 5 years after pregnancy may contribute to increased risk, but the long-lasting genetic signature may explain pregnancy's preventive effect.[95]

Lobular Involution and Age and Postlactational Involution

Part of the uniqueness of the mammary gland is its profound physiological changes throughout the phases of a woman's life. These phases include puberty, pregnancy, lactation, postlactational involution, and aging. The human breast is organized into 15 to 20 major lobes, each with terminal lobules having milk-forming acini (see Figure 32.10). **Terminal duct lobular units (TDLUs)**, structures of the breast that are responsible for lactation, are the predominant source of breast cancers.[3] With aging, breast lobules regress or involute with a decrease in the number and size of acini per lobule. A replacement of the intralobular stroma with the denser collagen of connective tissue occurs.[96] With time, fatty tissue replaces the glandular elements and collagen. This process is called **lobular involution**. Over many years the parenchymal elements progressively atrophy and disappear. The first study of its kind found lobular involution was associated with reduced risk for breast cancer.[96] Breast cancer risk decreased with increasing *extent* of involution in both high- and low-risk subgroups. Risk was defined by family history of breast cancer, epithelial atypia, reproductive history, and age.[96] Based on pathological and epidemiological factors, these investigators propose that *delayed* involution (persistent glandular epithelium) is a major risk factor for breast cancer.[96] Tissue involution involves massive epithelial cell death, recruitment and activation of fibroblasts, stromal remodelling, and immune cell infiltration. The immune action includes macrophages with similarities to microenvironments present during wound healing and tumour progression.[97]

Investigators suggest that the effect of lobular involution on breast cancer risk is a reduction in tissue from the involuting process, or the issue may be aging. It is widely appreciated that as women age, their risk for breast cancer increases. However, the *rate* of increase of breast cancer *slows* at about 50 years of age. This decline has been attributed to a reduction in ovarian hormone production. However, involution may contribute to this slowing rate. Investigators found an inverse association between lobular involution and parity.[96] Other investigators have reported that the more children a woman has, the more likely she is to have persistent lobular tissue,[98] which Milanese and colleagues[96] found was associated with increased risk for breast cancer. However, research has shown that multiparity reduces the risk for breast cancer. This contradiction may be explained by studies documenting that full-term pregnancies after 35 years of age are correlated with an increased risk for breast cancer.[99] In the Milanese study, the age of the mother at each child's birth was unknown.

Henson and colleagues[100] proposed that late pregnancy with its concomitant increase in the proliferation of the ductal-alveolar epithelium is likely to interrupt the process of involution. Involution typically begins between 30 and 40 years of age. Failure to undergo TDLU involution among women with BBD has been associated with progression to breast cancer, independent of other breast cancer risk factors.[101] The activated stromal environment (with the influx of immune cells like that which occurs during wound healing) in involution is the "ideal niche" for carcinogenesis.

Major signalling pathways involved in mammary gland involution also are involved in breast cancer.[102] Certain proteases activated during involution change the extracellular matrix (ECM). In the ECM, proteases are implicated in loss of cell anchoring, which provides a microenvironment for tumour growth.[102] Further, the normal involuting gland may be in an immunosuppressed state with the transient presence of immune-regulating cells that promote T-cell suppression.[94] Overall, for breast cancer, the long-term protective effects of pregnancy from hormones released (with consequent genetic and epigenetic changes) during pregnancy affect remodelling of the stromal microenvironment by causing apoptosis and involution. However, a transient increase in breast cancer risk following pregnancy may be caused by the *process* of mammary gland involution. This process returns the tissue to its prepregnant state and is accompanied by the process of wound healing. This process results in a proinflammatory environment that, although physiologically normal, can promote carcinogenesis.[93] In postlactational involution, the mammary gland regresses, and remodels to its prepregnant state. During this process, fibroblasts secrete proteases that degrade the ECM proteins. As a result, the increased release of bioactive matrix fragments can promote tumour growth, motility, and invasion.[103] The ECM is very different between nulliparous, lactating, and involuting glands, as shown in Figure 33.26.

Oophorectomy, which is associated with a decrease in risk for breast cancer, leads to atrophy of breast parenchyma in young women, like older women.[100] Thus the risk reduction of oophorectomy may be caused by a quicker involution.[100]

Hormonal Factors

The link between breast cancer and hormones is based on six factors that affect risk: (1) the protective effect of an early (i.e., in the 20s) first pregnancy; (2) the protective effect of removal of the ovaries and pituitary gland; (3) the increased risk associated with early menarche, late menopause, and nulliparity; (4) the relationship between types of fat, free estrogen levels, and oxidative changes in estrogen metabolism; (5) the hormone-dependent development and differentiation of mammary gland structures; and (6) the efficacy of antihormone therapies for treatment and prevention of breast cancer. Throughout its existence, the mammary gland epithelium proceeds through critical "exposure periods" of rapid growth or cycles of proliferation This includes neonatal growth, pubertal development, pregnancy lactation, and involution (after pregnancy and postmenopause).[93] The lack of TDLU involution

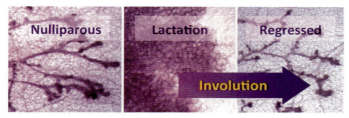

FIGURE 33.26 Extracellular Matrix is Different in Nulliparous, Lactating, and Involuting Glands. Several extracellular matrix (ECM) differences between nulliparous, lactational, and involuting mammary glands are related to collagen-fibre organization, cell motility and attachment, and cytokine regulation in a rodent model. Many protumourigenic ECM proteins are mediators of breast cancer progression specific to the involutional window, and systemic ibuprofen experimental treatment during involution decreases its tumour promotional changes. (Reprinted with permission from O'Brien, J. H., Vanderlinden, L. A., Schedin, P. J., et al. [2012]. Rat mammary extracellular matrix composition and response to ibuprofen treatment during postpartum involution by differential GeLC–MS/MS analysis. *Journal of Proteome Research, 11*, 4894–4905.)

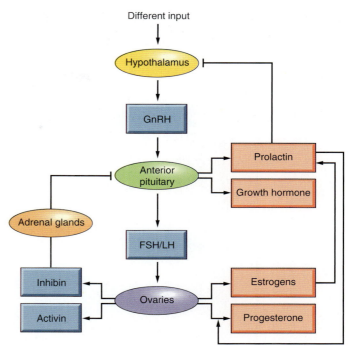

FIGURE 33.27 Female Endocrine System. The different mammary growth (mammotropic) hormone sites are shown in ovals, hormones are noted in blue boxes, and mammotropic hormones are noted in red boxes. *FSH*, Follicle-stimulating hormone; *GnRH*, gonadotropin-releasing hormone; *LH*, luteinizing hormone.

has been associated with increased breast cancer risk. The role of sex hormone levels and TDLU assessments is in its early stages of study. Investigators suggest that hormone levels may act, in part, to delay age-appropriate TDLU involution. This delay results in a higher quantity of at-risk epithelium.[101] These investigators found significant associations between higher TDLU counts, representing less involution, with higher levels of prolactin and lower levels of progesterone among premenopausal women. Higher levels of estradiol are seen among postmenopausal women.[101] Higher testosterone levels were suggestively associated with higher TDLU counts among postmenopausal women.

The understanding of the role of systemic hormones as powerful regulators of mammary gland development is shifting. Evidence points to the wide-ranging effects of systemic hormones. This is possibly not because of their *direct* hormone action but rather because of their *induced* actions from multiple secondary paracrine effectors—thus the term *hierarchical*. Unravelling is a complex model of hormone, paracrine, and adhesion molecule signalling pathways affecting both epithelial and stromal cell fate in both breast development and carcinogenesis (Figure 33.27). Key is *tissue remodelling*. This remodeling applies not only to pubertal growth but also immediately after pregnancy and during involution (see the earlier section).

The female reproductive hormones (estrogens, progesterone, and prolactin) have a major role and effect on mammary gland development and breast cancer. A vast majority of breast cancers are *initially* hormone dependent (estrogen positive [ER+], progesterone positive [PR+], or both), with estrogens playing a crucial role in their development.[104] Estrogens control processes critical for cellular functions by regulating activities and expression of key signalling molecules. These processes include regulation of receptor activity and receptor interaction with other intracellular proteins and DNA.[104] Estrogens thus play prominent roles in cellular proliferation, differentiation, and apoptosis.[104] Estrogens affect microtubules that are essential for establishing cell shape and cell polarity. These processes are necessary for epithelial gland organization.[104]

It is possible to consider four major hormonal hypotheses for breast cancer: (1) ovarian androgen excess (e.g., testosterone); (2) estrogen and progesterone levels (ovarian and hormone replacement); (3) elevated estrogen levels alone (ovarian and hormone replacement); and (4) local biosynthesis of estrogens in breast tissue. These hypotheses, however, may not be mutually exclusive. The following section discusses HRT or the newer term **menopausal hormone therapy (MHT)**.

The first hypothesis that breast cancer risk is increased among women who have an ovarian androgen excess also includes chronic anovulation and reduction of luteal phase (menstrual cycle) progesterone production. Therefore, it is also called the "ovarian hyperandrogenism/luteal inadequacy hypothesis." This hypothesis was based on the observation that women with breast cancer also show hyperplasia of the endometrium. This is a common symptom of ovarian androgen excess, chronic anovulation, and progesterone deficiency.[105] From the combination of prospective studies, case-control studies, and laboratory data, the association between circulating testosterone levels in postmenopausal women and later risk for breast cancer is now well established. Unclear is whether the association with testosterone levels is direct or indirect (i.e., enzyme conversion by aromatase of testosterone to estradiol) (Figure 33.28).

The androgen receptor has been implicated in prostate cancer and now in the development and progression of breast cancer.[106] Investigators used breast cancer cell lines and found that treatment of the breast cancer cells with 5α-dihydrotestosterone promotes cell proliferation and decreases apoptosis.[106] The reduction of testosterone levels in women with oophorectomy or hysterectomy also may be a protective factor.[107]

The second hypothesis is that breast cancer risk is increased among women with blood elevations of both estrogens and androgens. This has been called the "estrogen-plus-progesterone hypothesis." Evidence has revealed increased proliferation rates of breast epithelium during the luteal phase of the menstrual cycle when the ovaries produce both estradiol and progesterone. Substantial evidence supports a positive association of circulating estrogens, androgens, and prolactin with postmenopausal breast cancer risk.[107] New data show mammary stem cells (MaSCs) as critical targets for ovarian hormones. This especially occurs during the normal reproductive cycle when progesterone levels surge and during pregnancy when the proliferation of MaSCs is

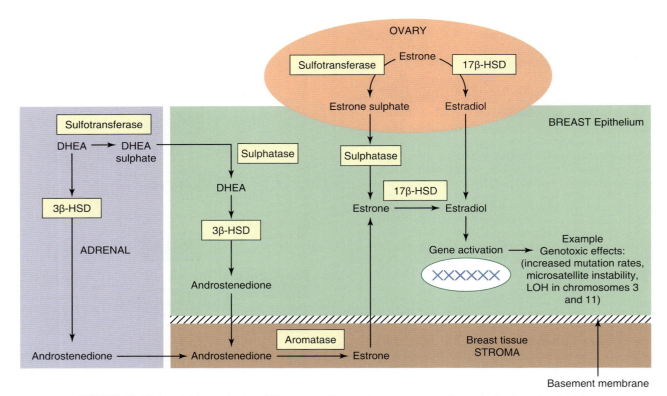

FIGURE 33.28 Local Biosynthesis of Estrogens. Four main enzyme complexes (yellow) are involved in estrogen formation in breast tissue: aromatase, sulphatase, 17β-estradiol hydroxysteroid dehydrogenase (17β-HSD), and 3β-hydroxysteroid dehydrogenase (3β-HSD). Data suggest that most abundant is sulphatase in both premenopausal and postmenopausal women with breast cancer. Numerous agents can block the aromatase action. Exploration of progesterone and various progestins to inhibit sulphatase and 17β-HSD or stimulate sulfotransferase (i.e., breast cancer cells cannot inactivate estrogens because they lack sulfotransferase) may supply new possibilities for treatment. *LOH*, Loss of heterozygosity (see Chapter 10). (Adapted from Russo, J., & Russo, I. [2004]. *Molecular basis of breast cancer: prevention and treatment.* Springer-Verlag.)

increased. Higher levels of progesterone among premenopausal women have been associated with lower TDLU counts.[101] Among postmenopausal women, higher levels of estradiol and testosterone have been associated with higher TDLU counts.[101] Select hormones may influence breast cancer risk through delaying TDLU involution.

The third hypothesis is called the "estrogen-alone hypothesis." Substantial prospective data have increased on the relationship between levels of circulating estrogens and breast cancer risk in postmenopausal women.[108,109] Overall, the positive association between levels of circulating estrogens in postmenopausal women and later risk for breast cancer is now well established.

The fourth hypothesis suggests that *local* (in situ; paracrine) formation of estrogens in breast tumours may be more significant than circulating estrogens in *plasma* for the growth and survival of estrogen-dependent breast cancer in postmenopausal women.[104] Investigators measured breast sex steroids in both benign and cancerous tissue.[110] Estrogen and androgen concentrations varied greatly in both tissue and blood levels in benign and cancerous tissue.[110] The estradiol-to-estrone ratio was lowest in premenopausal benign tissue. The ratio was much higher in premenopausal cancerous tissue and postmenopausal benign and cancerous tissue. Estradiol and estrone levels were substantially higher in tissue than in plasma in both premenopausal and postmenopausal women.[110] Hormone levels in breast adipose tissue revealed high levels of androstenedione and testosterone. There was also significant estrone and estradiol levels in breast adipocytes from postmenopausal breast cancer patients consistent with an obesity-inflammation-aromatase axis (obesity with inflammation, COX elevation, and increased aromatase, which converts androgens to estrogen) occurring locally in breast tissue.[110]

Overall, two main mechanisms of carcinogenicity of estrogens involve (1) a receptor-mediated hormonal activity shown to stimulate cellular proliferation, resulting in increased opportunities for accumulation of genetic damage; and (2) oxidative catabolism of estrogens mediated by various cytochrome complexes (cytochrome P-450 system) that eventually activate and generate reactive oxygen species that can cause oxidative stress and genomic damage directly. Oxidative metabolites of estrogens can develop ultimate carcinogens that react with DNA to cause mutations leading to carcinogenesis. Thus, imbalances in estrogen metabolites in breast tissue correlate with the development of tumours. This finding suggests possible biomarkers related to the risk of developing breast cancer.

Hormone Replacement Therapy and Breast Cancer Risk: Estrogen Plus Progesterone Therapy and Estrogen Only Therapy

The International Agency for Research on Cancer (IARC) lists estrogen-progestogen menopausal therapy and estrogen-progestogen contraceptives as carcinogenic agents with sufficient evidence in humans for breast cancer[111] (see Table 11.1). Evidence from the US Agency for Healthcare Research and Quality published a systematic review from 283 trials comparing effectiveness of treatments for menopausal symptoms.[112] In this report they state, "Over the long term, estrogen combined with progestogen has both beneficial effects (fewer osteoporotic fractures) and harmful effects (increased risk for breast cancer, gallbladder disease, venous thromboembolic events, and stroke). Estrogens given alone do not appear to increase breast cancer risk, although endometrial cancer risk is increased."[112] Evidence on the route of administration of MHT, oral versus transdermal (gel or patch), and the risk for breast cancer has limited research.

Insulin and Insulin like Growth Factors

IGFs regulate cellular functions involving cell proliferation, migration, differentiation, and apoptosis. Insulin like growth factor 1 (IGF-1) is a protein hormone with a structure like that of insulin. IGF-1 is a potent mitogen and after binding to the IGF-1R (receptor) triggers a signalling cascade leading to proliferation and antiapoptosis.[113]

Diabetes is associated with complex physiology of insulin resistance, increased insulin level, estrogen and growth hormone levels, inflammation, and signalling pathways leading to an increased risk for breast cancer.[114] Insulin therapy and sulphonylureas were found to be mildly associated with increased breast cancer risk.[114] A UK study showed that treating women with insulin glargine was not associated with breast cancer risk in the first 5 years. However, longer use may increase the risk.[115] Metformin appears to have a protective role. Much more investigation is needed to understand the role of insulin, IGFs, and diabetes mellitus and the risk for the development and reoccurrence of breast cancer.

Melatonin as a regulator of circadian rhythm is the main focus of shift work and light at night and breast cancer risk. However, tumour growth (in vivo) can be accelerated by light at night in part from continuous activation of IGF-1R signalling.[116] A recent case-control study of 1679 women showed that exposure to light at night during sleep is significantly associated with breast cancer risk.[116] Although inconclusive, shift work and its disruptive effects on circadian rhythms and sleep deprivation at night have been suggested as risk factors for breast cancer.[117]

Prolactin and Growth Hormone

Growth hormone induces the production of IGFs in the liver. IGF signalling is important for breast development and is implicated in breast carcinogenesis. Two studies, however, have reported a link between growth hormone level and breast cancer risk.[118,119] In the largest prospective analysis comparing circulating prolactin levels and breast cancer risk, those with the highest levels had the highest risk.[120] From a European Prospective Investigation into Cancer and Nutrition cohort, higher circulating prolactin level was associated with increased risk for in situ breast cancer.[121]

Oral Contraceptives

The IARC confirmed that combined estrogen-progestogen oral contraceptives increase the risk for breast, cervix, and liver cancers.[111,122] However, the efficacy of oral contraceptives in protecting against ovarian cancer and endometrial cancer is well established. The following "Pathogenesis" section discusses hormones in more detail.

Mammographic Density

Mammographic density (MD; also called *mammographic breast density*) is the radiological appearance of the breast, reflecting variations in breast composition (Figure 33.29). MD decreases with age and is associated with BMI, family history, and postmenopausal hormone use.[123] IGF-1R may play an important role in breast cancer in individuals with mammographic breast tissue density.[124] Investigators are studying whether MD is related to reduced lobular involution of breast tissue in dense breasts (reduced involution increases cancer risk). Having a

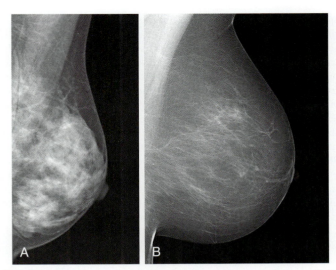

FIGURE 33.29 Breast Density Varies Among Women. The sensitivity of mammography for detecting malignancy is significantly reduced if the breast consists of a high proportion of fibroglandular (dense) breast tissue, **A**, compared with a breast that is fatty, **B**. (From O'Malley, F. P., Pinder, S. E., & Mulligan, A. M. [Eds.]. [2011]. *Breast pathology* [2nd ed.]. Saunders.)

combination of dense breasts and no lobular involution was found to be associated with higher breast cancer risk than having nondense or fatty breasts and complete involution.[125] Women with dense breasts whose percentage of MD is more than 60 to 75% of the breast have a fourfold to sixfold increased risk for breast cancer compared with those with little or no density.[126,127] Dense area percentage is a stronger breast cancer risk factor than absolute dense area.[128] Mammographic dense tissue has been thought to represent both epithelial and stromal components. One hypothesis is that the stromal-rich environment in MD may have an abundance of growth factors that could stimulate the epithelium in a noninvoluted breast This stimulation increases the risk for malignant transformation.[125] Finding tumours in women with MD is a challenge because they both appear white. As breast cancer surgeon Dr. Susan Love states, it is "… like trying to find a polar bear in a snow storm."

Environmental Factors

The environmental causes of breast cancer possibly affect the breast the most during critical phases or "windows" of development. These periods include early differential stages, that is, undifferentiated cells to alveolar buds and then lobules, puberty, pregnancy and lactation, involution, and menopause. During these early phases, mitotic activity and cell division are greater than later in life.

Radiation. Ionizing radiation is a known mutagen and established carcinogen for breast cancer. To date, only accidentally or medically induced radiation has been proven to exert a carcinogenic effect on the breast. According to the US Institute of Medicine (IOM), the two most strongly associated environmental factors are exposure to ionizing radiation and combined postmenopausal HRT.[129] There are many sources of ionizing radiation, including X-rays, CT scans, fluoroscopy, and other medical radiological procedures (see Chapter 11). The IOM conclusion of a causal relationship between radiation exposure in the same range as CT and cancer is consistent from a large varied literature.[130] The IOM makes it clear that *avoidance* of medical imaging is an important and concrete step that women (girls) can take to reduce their risk for breast cancer.[131] Scientists and clinicians also have expressed concern about the increasing number of CT scans performed, including those performed on children.[131] Radiological exposure of the upper spine, heart, ribs, lungs, shoulders, and esophagus also exposes breast tissue to radiation. Breast tissue may be exposed from abdominal CT scans; X-rays and fluoroscopy of infants may constitute whole-body irradiation. The duration of increased risk from radiation is unknown, but increased risk appears to have lasted at least 35 years in women treated for mastitis, those treated with fluoroscopy, and those who survived the atomic bombs during World War II. Breast cancer rates in atomic bomb survivors in Japan were highest among women younger than 20 years of age at time of exposure. Those who had early full-term pregnancies were at significantly lower risk than those who did not. Thus, interacting factors can modulate the risks from radiation.

An important topic currently is the effect of low-dose ionizing radiation. The debate is that low-energy X-rays may be more hazardous per unit dose than previously reported. Conventional X-ray mammography is one of the most valuable diagnostic tools for imaging of the breast. Currently, full-field digital mammography (FFDM) is often used. Continuous technical development has led to several new imaging techniques. These techniques include digital breast tomosynthesis (DBT), phase contrast X-ray imaging, and CT of the breast, as well as ultrasound and MRI. Despite technical innovations, except for ultrasound and MRI, these modalities require exposure of breast tissue to ionizing radiation. The breast is a very radiosensitive organ.[132] Therefore, it is critical to compare delivered radiation doses to the breast and measure X-ray–induced DNA damage. A new technique for the detection and quantification of in vivo DNA damage has been developed. DNA double-strand breaks (DSBs) are the most relevant lesion induced by ionizing irradiation.[132] After the induction of DSBs, phosphorylation of the histone variant H2AX (named γ-H2AX) occurs. Phosphorylated γ-H2AX forms visible foci, which are a reliable and sensitive tool for the determination of DNA damage. Recently, investigators found that mammography induces a slight but significant increase of γ-H2AX foci in systemic blood lymphocytes. A clear induction of DNA lesions was found both by FFDM and by DBT.[132] These data will be important in the comparison of different breast imaging techniques. Investigators are studying mammographic radiation–induced DNA damage in mammary epithelial cells from women with low or high family risk for breast cancer. This includes comparisons of the number of views performed during screening.[133] The presence of radiobiological effects occur in both low-risk and high-risk women, but they are greater in high-risk women.[133] Investigators are looking for markers that are activated by DNA damage. One new marker may be CAV1 (caveolin 1 protein; see Chapter 1). Caveolin protein acts as a sensor and early mediator in response to DNA damage and may be important as a biomarker for radiosensitivity.[134] Chapter 11 presents new biological understandings of low doses of radiation.

Women treated with chest radiation for a pediatric or young adult type of cancer have a substantially increased risk for breast cancer. Investigators from international studies have concluded that diagnostic chest irradiation or radiation therapy for benign or malignant diseases increases the risk for breast cancer for cumulative doses as low as 130 mGy. The breast cancer risk did not decrease when increasing the number of radiological treatment fractions for delivering the same total dose However, risk decreased greatly with increasing age of exposure to ionizing radiation.[135] International agencies are assessing the utility of screening MRI and mammography in these high-risk populations. The risk for secondary lung malignancy is an important concern for women treated with whole-breast radiation therapy after breast-conserving surgery for early-stage breast cancer.[136] Investigators studied secondary lung malignancy risk associated with several common methods of delivering whole-breast radiation therapy. Compared with supine whole-breast irradiation, prone breast irradiation is associated with a significantly lower predicted risk for secondary lung malignancy.[136]

The Canadian Task Force on Preventive Health Care has updated the recommendations for mammography because of overdiagnosis and overtreatment issues related to screening mammography (see *Health Promotion: Breast Cancer Screening Mammography*).

Diet. Prospective epidemiological studies on diet and breast cancer risk do not show an association that is consistent, strong, and statistically significant except for alcohol intake, being overweight, and weight gain after menopause (see the following section). Diet is thought to be an important breast cancer risk because of the international correlations of consumption of specific dietary factors (e.g., fats) and breast cancer incidence and mortality. Migrant studies also show greater incidence of breast cancer among descendants who moved to another country compared with those in the country of origin. International variations also can occur because of differences in reproductive history, physical activity, obesity, and other factors.

Dietary fat and breast cancer risk is the subject of much study, controversy, and debate.[3] Potential biological mechanisms between fat intake and breast cancer risk include: (1) fat may stimulate endogenous steroid hormone production (also affects weight gain, age of menarche), (2) fat interferes with immune or inflammatory function, and (3) fat influences gene expression. Although studies on fat and breast cancer risk have been inconsistent, the concern that any association with fat intake may be because of total energy intake exists. There is also limited evidence that modest reductions in fat intake (less than 20% of caloric intake) reduce breast cancer risk. Despite extensive investigation, there is no conclusive evidence overall that *adult* consumption of macronutrients including fat, carbohydrate, or fibre is strongly related to breast cancer incidence.

The association between individual foods and breast cancer is inconsistent. New data on *dietary patterns* are emerging. The Mediterranean diet includes high intake of vegetables, legumes, fruits, nuts, and minimally processed cereals; moderately high intake of fish; and high intake of monounsaturated lipids coupled with low intake of saturated fat, low to moderate intake of dairy products, low intake of meat products, and moderate intake of alcohol. The Mediterranean diet may favourably influence the risk for breast cancer.[137] The Western pattern includes higher intake of red and processed meats, refined grains, sweets and desserts, and high-fat dairy products.

Most studies have not supported a link between fibre intake and breast cancer. Carbohydrate quality, however, rather than absolute amount, may be important for breast cancer risk, especially for premenopausal women.

Evidence exists that alcohol consumption increases breast cancer risk. Beer, wine, and liquor all contributed to the positive association, and risks did not differ by menopausal status. In large prospective studies, high intake of folic acid appeared to decrease the enhanced risk for breast cancer caused by alcohol. The mechanisms by which alcohol intake increases the risk for breast cancer are unknown. Physiological studies have reported that alcohol intake leads to an estrogen level increase in women taking HRT as well as IGF-1 level increases. Alcohol may increase breast cancer risk through increasing MD, especially in women at high risk.[138] It is not known whether reducing or stopping alcohol consumption in midlife decreases the risk for breast cancer.

Research has occurred over the past three decades of the relationship between fruit and vegetable intake and reduction in breast cancer risk.

Soybeans are the main source of isoflavones. The isoflavone compounds, including daidzein and genistein, can bind ERs but are far less potent than estradiol. Soy may act like other antiestrogens (e.g., tamoxifen) by blocking the action of endogenous estrogens to reduce breast cancer risk. Thus, depending on the estradiol concentration, soy shows weak estrogenic or antiestrogenic activity. Many other mechanisms of action are proposed for isoflavones, including apoptosis and inhibition of angiogenesis. The North American Menopause Society states that soy foods generally appear to be breast protective and recommended moderate lifelong soy consumption.[84] A systematic review and meta-analysis suggested that intake of soy contributed to a significant reduction in breast cancer recurrence. However, soy was not significant in reduction of overall breast cancer mortality.[139] In addition, soy may optimize extrarenal 1,25-dihydroxycholecalciferol or vitamin D_3 (a prodifferentiating vitamin D metabolite), which could result in growth control and, conceivably, inhibition of tumour progression.

Iodine deficiency is hypothesized as contributing to the development of breast pathology and cancer.[85] Iodine plays a significant role in breast health.[85] Evidence reveals that iodine is an antioxidant and antiproliferative agent contributing to the integrity of normal mammary tissue.[85] Seaweed, which is iodine-rich, is an important dietary item in Asian communities and has been associated with the *low* evidence of BBD and breast cancer disease.[140] Molecular iodine (I_2) supplementation exerts an inhibitory effect on the development and size of benign and cancerous tissue.[141] Nutrition remains an important area of study.

Obesity. Excess body fatness is known to increase cancer risk from cellular pathways that involve hormonal regulation, cellular proliferation, and immunity.[142] Obesity, measured as BMI, has been associated with a *reduced* risk for *premenopausal* breast cancer. The Nurses' Health Study I and II reported, however, that weight gain or weight loss since age 18 did not significantly decrease the risk for premenopausal breast cancer.[143] Other data measuring adiposity using the waist–hip ratio has not shown a reduced risk but rather no association or an increased risk. Excess adiposity is positively associated with breast cancer recurrence and breast cancer–specific mortality among both premenopausal and postmenopausal women.[144]

Research has shown that excess body weight increased the risk of developing postmenopausal breast, colorectum, endometrium, kidney, and esophageal adenocarcinoma.[145]

Despite strong links with endogenous estrogen levels, body fat has been consistently but *weakly* related to increased postmenopausal risk.[146] This observation has been surprising because obese postmenopausal women have endogenous estrogen levels (estrone and estradiol) nearly double those of lean women.[146,147] This weak association is possibly related to two factors. First, the premenopausal reduction in breast cancer risk related to being overweight possibly persists, opposing the adverse effect of elevated levels of estrogens after menopause. Thus, *weight gain* should be more strongly related to postmenopausal breast cancer risk than reached weight.

Obesity is associated with poor survival among women with breast cancer. The association of obesity with mortality from breast cancer appears to be stronger than its association with incidence.[146] The increase in breast cancer risk with increasing BMI among postmenopausal women is most likely the result of increases in levels of estrogens by aromatase activity in adipose tissue.[142] However, studies of hormones secreted by adipose tissue, *leptin* and *adiponectin*, may underlie the association between obesity and breast cancer risk. Increasing BMI and central fat deposition are associated with increased risk for breast cancer in prospective studies. Research has shown leptin-stimulated breast carcinogenesis.[148] Leptin enhances breast cancer cell proliferation by inhibiting cell death (proapoptosis) signalling pathways and by increasing in vitro sensitivity to estrogens.[148] Leptin secreted by adipocytes and fibroblasts in the microenvironment act on breast cancer cells in a paracrine fashion.[148] Adiponectin has been shown to exert antiproliferative effects in vitro on human breast cancer cells.[149] Additionally, factors that may be related to recurrence of breast cancer in women with excess adiposity at the time of diagnosis include cytokines, IGF, and/or immune function.[148,149]

Environmental chemicals. Evidence linking chemicals to the cause of breast cancer is difficult to obtain. It is challenging because it is a life history of exposure that is important, not just a single chemical, but complex mixtures of chemicals, and their interaction with endogenous hormones. With industrial development, breast cancer rates increase. An estimated 23 000 chemical substances that were manufactured, imported, or used in Canada on a commercial scale since the mid-1980s have been named. Approximately 600 new chemical substances are added each year.[150] In 2006, Canada established the Chemicals Management Plan. This national science-based program aims to reduce the risks posed by chemicals to Canadians and their environment through various risk-management strategies.

Chemicals persist in the environment, accumulate in adipose tissue, interact with local adipose tissue physiology in an endocrine/paracrine manner, and remain in breast tissue for decades. Women who immigrate to North America from Asian countries experience an enormous percentage increase in risk for breast cancer within one generation. A generation later, the rate of their daughters' risk approaches that of women born in North America. This change in risk suggests that *in utero* exposures affect later disease risk. It is difficult to know whether these changes in risk come from nutritional content, pollutants, food additives, or other factors.

Xenoestrogens are synthetic chemicals that mimic the actions of estrogens. These substances are present in many pesticides, fuels, plastics, detergents, and medications. Many factors correlate with breast cancer (e.g., early menarche, delayed pregnancy and breastfeeding, late menopause) and are associated with lifetime exposure to estrogens. Investigators have reasoned that environmental chemicals affect estrogen metabolism and contribute to breast cancer. The most significant chemicals may be polychlorinated biphenyls (PCBs), such as dichlorodiphenyltrichloroethane (DDT), pesticides (dieldrin, aldrin, heptachlor, and others), bisphenol A (pervasive in polycarbonate plastics), tobacco smoke (active and passive), dioxins (vehicle exhaust, incineration, contaminated food supply), alkylphenols (detergents and cleaning products), metals, phthalates (makes plastics flexible, some cosmetics), parabens (antimicrobials), food additives (recombinant bovine somatotropin [rBST] and zeranol to enhance growth in cattle and sheep), MHT (i.e., HRT), and others.

Physical activity. Regular physical activity may reduce overall risk for breast cancer, especially in premenopausal or young postmenopausal women. Activity also may reduce the invasiveness of breast cancer.[151] A sedentary lifestyle may increase cancer risk. Mechanisms of these risks includes increased insulin resistance, increased inflammation, and decreased immune function.[151] Studies show that physical activity lowered the risk for breast cancer mortality in breast cancer survivors and improved their physiological and immune functions.[151]

Inherited Cancer Syndromes, Genes, Epigenetic Considerations

The causes of breast cancer have been difficult to define because each woman has a different genetic profile. Genetic heterogeneity is the term used to describe this phenomenon.[152] Genetic heterogeneity is common not only among individuals but also at the level of the tumour itself, involving both genetic and epigenetic processes. These genetic factors interact with environmental factors. These facts are sobering and make an understanding of the genetic driving force behind tumour initiation, progression, and metastasis very complicated. However, recently, an experiment using a mouse model of breast tumour heterogeneity allowed investigators to probe the molecular basis of stable differences in cell (clonal) populations. This research included information on how the molecular structure contributes to various aspects of the cancer process, including the ability to form circulating tumour cells (CTCs) and ultimately metastases[153] (see the following "Pathogenesis" section).

A history of breast cancer in first-degree relatives (mother or sister) increases a woman's risk about two to three times. Risk increases even more if two first-degree relatives are involved, especially if the disease occurred before menopause and was bilateral. A small total proportion of breast cancers (5 to 10%, although the prevalence is significant) are the result of highly penetrant dominant genes (i.e., hereditary breast cancers). The most important of the dominant genes are the breast cancer susceptibility genes (*BRCA1* [breast cancer 1], *BRCA2* [breast cancer 2]). *BRCA1*, found on chromosome 17, is a tumour-suppressor gene. Any mutation in the gene may inhibit or retard its suppressor function, leading to uncontrolled cell proliferation. *BRCA2* is found on chromosome 13. A family history of both breast cancer and ovarian cancer increases the risk that an individual with breast cancer carries a *BRCA1* mutation.[154] Carriers of the *BRCA1* gene also are at higher risk for ovarian cancer. The risks for breast or ovarian cancer, or both, however, are not equal in all mutation carriers and have been found to vary by several factors. These factors include type of cancer, age at onset, and mutation position.[154] This variation in penetrance has led to the hypothesis that other genetic factors, environmental factors, or both change cancer risk in mutation carriers. Men who develop breast cancer are more likely to have a *BRCA2* mutation than a *BRCA1* mutation (see Chapter 34). Options for those who have a positive test for *BRCA1* or *BRCA2* mutations include surveillance to find cancers early, prophylactic surgery (i.e., bilateral salpingo-oophorectomy), risk factor avoidance, promotion of breastfeeding, and chemoprevention. Several other genetic alterations can increase the risk for breast cancer.

PATHOGENESIS Most breast cancers are adenocarcinomas. This cancer first arises from the ductal/lobular epithelium as carcinoma in situ. Carcinoma in situ is a proliferation of epithelial cells confined to the ducts and lobules by the basement membrane. Tumours of the infiltrating (invasive) ductal type do not grow to a large size, but they metastasize early. This type accounts for 70% of breast cancers. Table 33.11 summarizes some types of breast cancer. Breast cancer is heterogeneous. It is a disease with diverse molecular, biological, phenotypic, and pathological changes.[155] Heterogeneity is an important concept because the biological attributes of a tumour are strongly influenced by its subpopulation of cells. They are also influenced by the tumour's surrounding neighbourhood or microenvironment.[156] Recent research suggests that breast cancer is heterogeneous from its first preinvasive stages[156] and within the same tumour.

The many genetic and epigenetic changes drive the sequential expansion of progressively more and more malignant cell populations.[158] Breast tissue stem cells are thought to be the cell of origin for all breast cancers. Gene expression profiling studies have found four major subtypes classified as luminal A, luminal B, HER2+, and basal-like.[157] Mounting evidence shows that there are "subtypes within subtypes". Emerging evidence suggests that the biology of specific subtypes reflects contributions from the microenvironment.[156] Many models of breast carcinogenesis have been suggested. Three interrelated themes related to breast cancer initiation also have emerged: (1) gene addiction, (2) phenotype plasticity, and (3) cancer stem cells.

Cancer gene addiction includes oncogene addiction. In this process these driver genes play key roles in breast cancer development and progression. In nononcogene addiction these genes may not start cancer but play roles in cancer development and progression.[159] Examples of key driver genes include *HER2* and *MYC*, and examples of tumour-suppressor genes are *TP53*, *BRCA1*, and *BRCA2*. Once a founding tumour clone is established, genomic instability may help through the establishment of other subclones and contribute to both tumour progression and therapy resistance.[46] Phenotypic plasticity is exemplified by a distinctive phenotype called epithelial–mesenchymal transition (EMT) (see Chapter 10). EMT is involved in the generation of tissues and organs during embryogenesis. This process is essential for driving tissue plasticity during development and is an unintentional process during cancer progression. The EMT-associated reprogramming is involved in many cancer cell characteristics. This includes suppression of cell death or apoptosis and senescence. It is reactivated during wound healing and is resistant to chemotherapy and radiation therapy.[160] Remodelling or reprogramming of the breast during postpregnancy involution is important because it involves inflammatory and "wound healing–like" tissue reactions known as *reactive stroma*. These tissue reactions increase the risk for tumour invasion and may help the transition of carcinoma in situ to invasive carcinoma. Activation of an EMT program during cancer development often requires signalling between cancer cells and neighbouring stromal cells.[160] In advanced primary carcinomas, cancer cells recruit a variety of cell types into the surrounding stroma. This includes fibroblasts, myofibroblasts, granulocytes, macrophages, mesenchymal stem cells, and lymphocytes (Figure 33.30). Overall, increasing evidence suggests that interactions of cancer cells with adjacent tumour-associated stromal cells induce malignant cell phenotypes (Figure 33.31).

Research is ongoing to define cancer stem cells in breast carcinogenesis. This includes cancer stem cell origin and renewability properties. Studies have begun to show the role of MaSCs and to describe how they drive development of the gland. Maintenance of allostasis, and the many cycles of proliferation and apoptosis needed to expand and maintain the breast during pregnancy, and return it to a quiet (quiescent) state after involution is also part of this role.[161] EMT generates multiple epithelial cell subsets with different states of stemness relative to more differentiated cells.[162] The ECM and the basement membrane, in particular, are no longer just considered the "bricks and mortar" of a tissue. They are now a place where stem cells exist and correct tissue architecture. This process occurs together with the reservoir of growth factors, cytokines, and proteinases, and is critical for mammary tissue to develop and function properly.[161] Many of the biological traits of high-grade malignancy including motility, invasiveness, and self-renewal, have been traced to subpopulations of stem cells within carcinomas.[162] Hormones may act as accelerators as well as initiators, delay involution, and influence the susceptibility of the breast epithelium to environmental carcinogens because hormones control the differentiation of the mammary gland epithelium and, thereby, regulate the rate of stem cell division.

Two new important concepts under investigation related to metastases are tumour dormancy and vascular mimicry. Tumour dormancy has been noted in the care of people with cancer. With this occurrence, microscopic and occult cancerous lesions enter a latent or dormant phase in various stages of tumour progression. In fact, these microscopic and occult cancerous lesions are often found in healthy people.[163] Ironically, in healthy people these are the slow-growing tumours (some called "pseudodisease") detected by present screening methods that would not advance to routine clinical presentation over the individual's lifetime.[163] Current debates surround the concern that individuals often undergo unnecessary treatment for a disease they were never destined to experience.[163] Evidence exists that organ-specific molecular signalling can decide whether a metastatic lesion will expand or remain dormant. Significant to different signalling profiles that may decide this outcome are stress-activated kinases, transcription factors (such as p53), and cell cycle inhibitors. Thus, an increase in cell stress–activated signalling may occur, for example, with certain treatment modalities such as surgery. Evidence has been accumulating that removal of a malignant tumour from a host is curative for many but in some

TABLE 33.11 Types of Breast Carcinomas and Major Distinguishing Features

Histological Type	Distinguishing Features
Carcinoma of Mammary Ducts	
Papillary	Well-delineated cystic masses in multiple areas; hemorrhage often present; majority appear in 40- to 60-year age group; often involves skin
Intraductal (comedo)	Often accompanied by evidence of inflammation; well-circumscribed tumours within duct; well-differentiated tumour cells; rarely ulcerates skin
Infiltrating Carcinoma	
Ductal (no specific type)	Fibrous, firm, glistening, grey-tan mass with chalky streaks, mixture of patterns; may cause discharge from nipple; represents about 70–80% of all breast cancers
Mucinous	Usually large (>3 cm in diameter), circumscribed, and encapsulated, glistening appearance, varies in colour; two types: pure and mixed; mucin surrounds this pure tumour; infrequent; found in lateral half of breast; tends to occur in women after age 70 years
Medullary	Encapsulated and grows very large (7–8 cm in diameter); commonly surrounded by lymphocytic inflammatory infiltrate; occurs after age 50 years
Tubular	Well-differentiated with orderly tubules in centre (stroma) of mass; can be associated with noninfiltrating ductal carcinoma; occurs in women about 50 years of age; nodal metastasis infrequent; occurrence rare
Adenoid cystic	Very rare; well-circumscribed, painless mass arising from nipple and areola
Metaplastic	Involves cartilage or bone, mixed tumours, or osteogenic sarcomas
Squamous cell	Frequent in Blacks; originates in ductal epithelium
Carcinoma of Mammary Lobules	
Lobular carcinoma in situ	Found in individuals with fibrocystic disease; localized to upper breast quadrants; 15–35% risk of becoming invasive; occurs often in mid-40s; infiltrating variety occurs in early 50s
Infiltrating lobular	Infiltrates from duct; firm mass with chalky streaks
Paget's disease	Eczema of nipple that extends to areola; cancer usually found underneath nipple; poorly circumscribed; large Paget cells arise from duct and directly invade nipple; history of scaly, red rash spreading from nipple; lesion palpable beneath nipple, often bilateral; occurs in middle age
Inflammatory carcinoma	Not a histological type; diffuse within breast tissue, diffuse edema of overlying skin; extremely undifferentiated, very rare; most metastasize to axilla
Sarcoma of the Breast	
Cystosarcoma phyllodes	Usually large (>17 cm in diameter); mostly localized but can rupture through skin; rarely metastasizes to lymph nodes; history of painless nodule present for years before it forms a large mass; ulceration and bleeding of skin often present; occurs in wide age range (13–77 years)
Fibrosarcoma	Well-circumscribed, firm, and usually does not involve skin or nipple; well-differentiated to extremely undifferentiated; arises from connective tissue; extremely rare (e.g., liposarcoma, angiosarcoma)

circumstances is insufficient to prevent the cancer from recurring. As a result, this can lead to rapid cancer recurrence.[164] Recognition of immune cells in the ECM or stroma and the overall immune response for their role in regulating tumour growth and are being investigated for their role in tumour dormancy.

Cancer metastases require that primary tumour cells evolve the ability to intravasate into the lymphatic system or vasculature, and extravasate into and colonize secondary sites.[3] Investigators developed a mouse model of breast tumour heterogeneity and isolated a distinct clone of specialized cells that efficiently enter the vasculature and express two proteins, Serpine2 and SLPI. These proteins were necessary and sufficient to program these cells for vascular mimicry. **Vascular mimicry** is a blood supply pathway in tumours that is formed by tumour cells. This blood supply is independent of endothelial cell–lined blood vessels, therefore it *mimics* real blood vessels (Figure 33.32). This blood supply pathway helps perfusion of the primary tumours and correlates with poor clinical outcome. The increase in these blood supply pathways was associated with an increase in CTCs and a later increase in lung metastases. Additionally, treatment with the anticoagulant warfarin (Coumadin) increased the number of CTCs and lung metastases. These results suggested that the anticoagulant function of Serpine2 and secretory leukocyte protease inhibitor (SLPI) both support blood flow through the extravascular network and promote intravasation. These remarkable findings show Serpine2- and SLPI-driven vascular mimicry as a critical mechanism or driver of metastatic progression in cancer.[153]

Ductal and Lobular Carcinoma in Situ

Ductal carcinoma in situ (DCIS) is a heterogeneous group of proliferations limited to breast ducts and lobules without invasion of the basement membrane. About 84% of all in situ disease is DCIS. The remaining are mostly lobular carcinoma in situ (LCIS). DCIS occurs predominantly in females but can occur in males. Since 1980, the widespread adoption of screening mammography has led to an epidemic of diagnoses of DCIS.[165] DCIS presents as microcalcifications (low grade) (Figure 33.33B) or rod-shaped branching (high grade) on a mammogram (Figure 33.33A).

Still controversial, DCIS does not appear to progress from sequential steps of low grade or risk types to higher grade or risk types during its route to cancer or cancer recurrence.[166] This property, therefore, suggests a stable population.[166] Because of these findings, some argue that the term is misleading and should be replaced by *ductal intraepithelial neoplasia*, similar to the term used in prostate cancer. DCIS is a very common type of noninvasive cancer, with one in five breast cancers diagnosed as DCIS.[167] Because of the large numbers of cases diagnosed yearly in Canada, the debate is whether mammography is causing the overdiagnosis of potential pseudodisease. For example, the Canadian National Breast Screening Study-2 of women aged 50 to 59 years found a fourfold increase in DCIS cases in those screened by clinical breast examination (CBE). Mammography compared with those screened by CBE alone, with no difference in breast cancer mortality.[167]

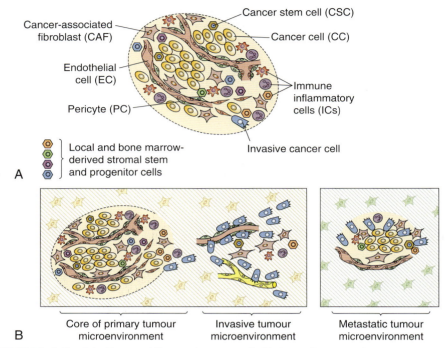

FIGURE 33.30 Cells of the Tumour Microenvironment. A, Distinct cell types make up most solid tumours including breast tumours. Both the main cellular tissue, called *parenchyma*, and the surrounding tissue, or stroma, of tumours have cell types that enable tumour growth and progression. For example, the immune-inflammatory cells present in tumours can include both tumour-promoting and tumour-killing subclasses of cells. **B,** The microenvironment of tumours. Multiple stromal cell types create a succession of tumour microenvironments that change as tumours invade normal tissue, eventually seeding and colonizing distant tissues. The organization, numbers, and phenotypic characteristics of the stromal cell types and the extracellular matrix *(hatched background)* evolve during progression and enable primary, invasive, and metastatic growth. (Not shown are the premalignant stages.) (Data from Hanahan, D., & Weinberg, R. [2011]. *Cell, 144,* 646–674.)

The difficulty for this clinical dilemma is that the natural history of DCIS is poorly understood because nearly all cases are treated. More directed research is needed on DCIS. Areas of research include genetic expression profiling, best treatment to achieve disease regression, and studies of tumour characteristics and risk profiling. A newer mission of the DCIS Discovery Enterprise at MD Anderson Cancer Center in Houston, Texas, is to prevent invasive disease while also reducing unnecessary surgery or radiation.

Key to understanding the progression of breast cancer after treatment of DCIS are the characteristics of the lesion and the delivered treatment. According to the US National Cancer Institute, the best evidence indicates that most lesions of DCIS will not evolve to invasive cancer. It is also known that those that become invasive can be managed successfully, even after that transition.[168] The detection and treatment of nonpalpable DCIS often represents overdiagnosis and overtreatment.[168] Surprisingly, the overall death rate for women with DCIS is lower than that for women in the population as a whole.[46,168] This favourable outcome may reflect the benign nature of the condition or the benefits of treatment. It may also be a marker for socioeconomic factors associated with longevity.[46,168] Attempts to define low-risk DCIS cases that can be managed with fewer therapies are critical.[168]

Lobular carcinoma in situ (LCIS) originates from the TDLU. Unlike DCIS, LCIS has a uniform appearance. The cells expand but do not distort involved spaces. This preserves the lobular structure. The cells grow in a noncohesive (discohesive) fashion usually because of a loss of the tumour-suppressive adhesion protein **E-cadherin**.[46] The discovery of LCIS as an incidental lesion from a biopsy and not from mammography occurs because it is not associated with calcifications or stromal reactions that produce mammographic densities. LCIS has an incidence of about 1 to 6% of all carcinomas and did not increase with mammographic screening.[46] With biopsies in both breasts, LCIS is bilateral in 20 to 40% of cases, compared with 10 to 20% of cases of DCIS.[46] The cells of AH, LCIS, and invasive lobular carcinoma are structurally identical.[46] Loss of cellular adhesion because of dysfunction of E-cadherin results in a rounded shape without attachment to adjacent cells, increasing the risk for invasion. E-cadherin functions as a tumour-suppressor protein. Loss of this function in neoplastic proliferations from various mechanisms occurs, including mutation.

LCIS is a risk factor for invasive carcinoma. LCIS develops in 25 to 35% of women over a period of 20 to 30 years. Unlike DCIS, the risk is almost as high in the contralateral breast as in the ipsilateral breast. Treatments include close clinical follow-up and mammographic screening, tamoxifen, and bilateral prophylactic mastectomy.

CLINICAL MANIFESTATIONS Most carcinomas of the breast occur in the upper outer quadrant, where most of the glandular tissue of the breast is found. Obstruction of the normal lymphatic pathways or destruction of lymphatic vessels by surgery or radiotherapy causes the lymphatic spread of cancer to the opposite breast, to lymph nodes in the base of the neck, and to the abdominal cavity (see Figure 32.11). The less common inner quadrant tumours may spread to mediastinal nodes or Rotter nodes, which are found between the pectoral muscles

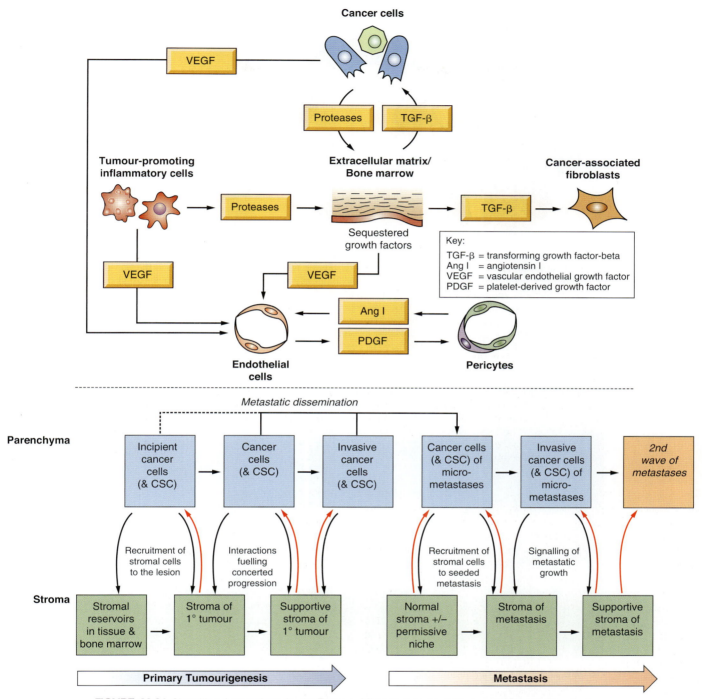

FIGURE 33.31 **Signalling Interactions in the Tumour Microenvironment During Malignant Progression.** *Upper panel:* Numerous cell types form the tumour microenvironment and are orchestrated and supported by reciprocal interactions. *Lower panel:* The reciprocal interactions between the breast main tissue or parenchyma and the surrounding stroma are important for cancer progression and growth. Certain organ sites of "fertile soil" or "metastasis niches" help metastatic seeding and colonization. Cancer stem cells are involved in some or all stages of tumour development and progression. *CSC,* Cancer stem cell. (Adapted from Hanahan, D., & Weinberg, R. [2011]. *Cell, 144,* 646–674.)

(see Figure 32.11). Internal mammary chain nodes also are common sites of metastasis. Metastases from the vertebral veins can involve the vertebrae, pelvic bones, ribs, and skull. The lungs, kidneys, liver, adrenal glands, ovaries, and pituitary gland are also sites of metastasis.

The first sign of breast cancer is usually a painless lump. Lumps caused by breast tumours do not have any classic characteristics. Other presenting signs include palpable nodes in the axilla, retraction of tissue (dimpling) (Figure 33.34), or bone pain caused by metastasis to the vertebrae.

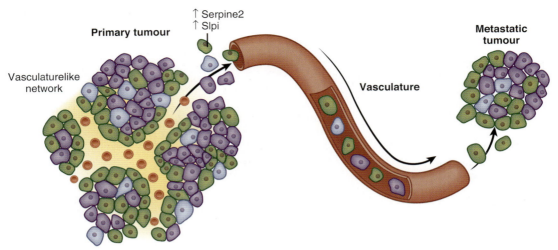

FIGURE 33.32 Vascular Mimicry Drives Metastasis. The steps to carry out metastasis include *intravasation*, in which tumour cells escape from the primary tumour into the vasculature and move through the bloodstream; or *extravasation*, in which tumour cells escape from the vasculature to colonize in distant tissue. Vascular mimicry promotes metastasis. Tumour cells adopt characteristics like those of the endothelial cells that line blood vessels, and mimic vascularlike networks within tumours and between tumours and blood vessels. Wagenblast and colleagues found that two proteins, Serpine2 and SLPI, promoted metastasis by stimulating vascular mimicry. Tumour cells expressing these proteins *(green)* form the vascularlike network that allows other tumour cells *(purple, blue)* to move to secondary sites. (Adapted from Hendrix, M. J. C. [2015]. *Nature, 520*, 300–302; Wagenblast, E., Soto, M., Gutiérrez-Ángel, C. A., et al. [2015]. *Nature, 520*, 358–362.)

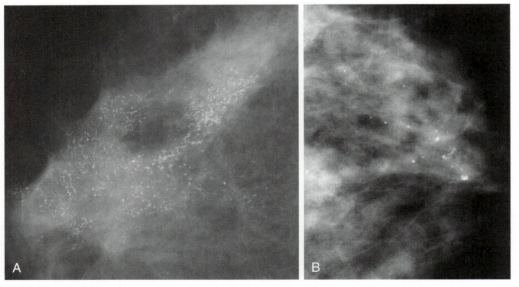

FIGURE 33.33 Ductal Carcinoma In Situ. A, Malignant microcalcifications. Extensive area of pleomorphic microcalcifications; granular, rod-shaped, and branching microcalcifications can be found. The appearances are typical of high-grade ductal carcinoma in situ (DCIS). **B,** Craniocaudal mammography reveals fine and coarse granular calcifications. Histopathological analysis revealed low-grade DCIS. ([A], from O'Malley, F. P., Pinder, S. E., & Mulligan, A. M. [Eds.]. [2011]. *Breast pathology* [2nd ed.]. Saunders; [B], from Donegan, W. L., & Spratt, J. S. [2002]. *Cancer of the breast* [5th ed.]. Saunders.)

Table 33.12 summarizes the clinical manifestations of breast cancer. Manifestations vary according to the type of tumour and stage of disease.

EVALUATION AND TREATMENT
Means of evaluating breast alterations and cancer include CBE, mammography, ultrasound, thermography, MRI, biopsy, hormone receptor assays, and gene expression profiling.

Treatment is based on the extent or stage of the cancer. The extent of the tumour at the primary site, the presence and extent of lymph node metastases, and the presence of distant metastases are all evaluated to decide the stage of disease. Treatment includes surgery, radiation, chemotherapy, hormone therapy, and biological therapy.

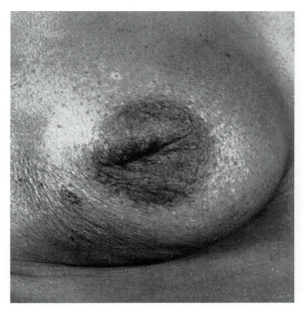

FIGURE 33.34 Retraction of Nipple Caused by Carcinoma. (From Ackerman, L. V., del Regato, J. A., Spjut, H. J., et al. [1985]. *Cancer: diagnosis, treatment, and prognosis* [6th ed.]. Mosby.)

TABLE 33.12 Clinical Manifestations of Breast Cancer

Clinical Manifestation	Pathophysiology
Local pain	Local obstruction caused by tumour
Dimpling of skin	Can occur with invasion of dermal lymphatics because of retraction of Cooper ligament or involvement of pectoralis fascia
Nipple retraction	Shortening of mammary ducts
Skin retraction	Involvement of suspensory ligament
Edema	Local inflammation or lymphatic obstruction
Nipple/areolar eczema	Paget's disease
Pitting of skin (like surface of an orange [peau d'orange])	Obstruction of subcutaneous lymphatics, resulting in accumulation of fluid
Reddened skin, local tenderness, and warmth	Inflammation
Dilated blood vessels	Obstruction of venous return by a fast-growing tumour; obstruction dilates superficial veins
Nipple discharge in a nonlactating woman	Spontaneous and intermittent discharge caused by tumour obstruction
Ulceration	Tumour necrosis
Hemorrhage	Erosion of blood vessels
Edema of arm	Obstruction of lymphatic drainage in axilla
Chest pain	Metastasis to lung

CASE STUDY

Joanne Talbot is a 43-year-old White premenopausal woman who visited her primary care provider for her annual physical and scheduled Pap test. The patient states that she is feeling well but did discover a small painless lump in the upper outer quadrant of her right breast 2 months ago. She initially thought the lump could be associated with her premenstrual symptoms but has noted that the lump has remained unchanged over the 4-week period.

History of Present Illness: Joanne states she is feeling "pretty good". She is not experiencing any breast tenderness, pain, nipple discharge, or changes in the breast appearance. She experiences regular menses every 28 days. Her last menstrual period was finished 7 days ago. She has never had a mammogram and assesses her breasts occasionally while she is in the shower. Her last Pap test was 3 years ago, and the results were normal.

OBS GYN Hx: G3P3A0, children are ages 6, 8, and 10 years and all were healthy full-term deliveries. She breastfed all three of her children for 6 months each. Her first pregnancy was at age 33. She experienced menarche at age 11. She has been taking an oral contraceptive since the birth of her last child 6 years ago.

Past Medical Hx: Hypothyroidism × 3 years.

Family Hx: Maternal grandmother was diagnosed with breast cancer premenopausal at age 44. Her mother was diagnosed with breast cancer premenopausal at age 46 and died from breast cancer 10 years ago at the age of 72. Her father is alive at age 82 and has DM2, hypertension, and dyslipidemia. She has no siblings.

Medications: Synthroid 150 µg once daily, tri-cyclen 28 (oral contraceptive), occasional OTC ibuprofen, no vitamin or herbal supplements

Social history: Married 22 years with 3 children; husband is an engineer; nonsmoker, nondrinker, no recreational drugs, works full time as a primary school teacher, exercises four times per week by walking 45 minutes, drinks three coffees per day and three carbonated caffeine-based soft drinks per day, eats a well-balanced diet, experiences no increased daily stressors.

Review of Systems: Unremarkable with exception of breast lump as stated above, no heat/cold intolerance; no goitre; hypothyroid well controlled.

Physical Exam: Appears stated age, well-groomed and in no acute distress, HEENT unremarkable; ROM neck full, no cervical, supraclavicular or infraclavicular adenopathy; one 2-cm mobile, firm, nontender right anterior axillary lymph node; no thyroidomegaly; respiratory, cardiovascular, musculoskeletal, neurological, and gastrointestinal exams unremarkable; breast symmetric, no dimpling or skin lesions, no nipple retraction or discharge, no edema, no swelling, no discoloration. Breast tissue dense, one 2.5-cm mass palpated in the upper lateral quadrant of the right breast, firm, fixed, nontender.

Vital signs: BP 128/74 LA sitting; pulse 70 regular; RR 14 unlaboured; temperature 36.8°C oral; BMI 26.

Critical Thinking and Clinical Judgement Questions

1. The primary care provider suspects a diagnosis of breast cancer. Based on the information provided, identify five possible risk factors that predispose this patient to that diagnosis.
2. Based on the information provided, identify five possible protective factors that have been identified in this patient's history and physical examination.
3. What clinical signs and symptoms does this patient present with that are consistent with the diagnosis of breast cancer?
4. Name the diagnostic tests the primary care provider could order to confirm the diagnosis of breast cancer. Indicate what each test is assessing and provide the expected results to confirm the diagnosis of breast cancer.

DID YOU UNDERSTAND?

Abnormalities of the Female Reproductive Tract
1. Normal development of the female reproductive tract requires absence of testosterone during embryonic and fetal life.
2. Alterations in the normal process include errors in cellular sensitivity to testosterone (androgen insensitivity) or failures of cell line migration. This results in changes in the structure of the reproductive organs.
3. Androgen insensitivity syndrome is a disorder of hormone resistance. It is characterized by a female phenotype in an individual with an XY karyotype or male genotype.
4. Other abnormalities of the uterus, cervix, and fallopian/uterine tubes have multifactorial origins and are often the result of an interaction between genetic predisposition and environmental factors.

Alterations of Sexual Maturation
1. Sexual maturation, or puberty, is marked by the development of secondary sex characteristics, rapid growth, and, ultimately, the ability to reproduce. The normal range for the onset of puberty is now 8 to 13 years of age but can vary geographically.
2. Delayed puberty is the onset of sexual maturation after these ages. Precocious puberty is the onset before these ages. Treatment for delayed and precocious puberty depends on the cause.

Disorders of the Female Reproductive System
1. Hormonal imbalances, infectious microorganisms, inflammation, structural abnormalities, and benign or malignant proliferative conditions can alter the female reproductive system.
2. Primary dysmenorrhea is painful menstruation not associated with pelvic disease. It results from excessive synthesis of prostaglandin $F_2\alpha$. Secondary dysmenorrhea results from endometriosis, pelvic adhesions, inflammatory disease, uterine fibroids, or adenomyosis.
3. Primary amenorrhea is the continued absence of menarche and menstrual function by 13 years of age without the development of secondary sex characteristics or by 15 years of age if these changes have occurred.
4. Secondary amenorrhea is the absence of menstruation for a time equivalent to three or more cycles in women who have previously menstruated. Secondary amenorrhea is associated with many disorders and physiological conditions.
5. Abnormal uterine bleeding is heavy or irregular bleeding in the absence of organic disease.
6. Polycystic ovary syndrome is a condition in which excessive androgen production. Inappropriate secretion of gonadotropins may trigger this disorder. This hormonal imbalance prevents ovulation and causes enlargement and cyst formation in the ovaries, excessive endometrial proliferation, and often hirsutism. Insulin resistance and hyperinsulinemia play a key role in androgen excess.
7. Premenstrual syndrome is the cyclic recurrence of physical, psychological, or behavioural changes distressing enough to disrupt normal activities or interpersonal relationships. The most distressing symptoms include emotional symptoms, particularly depression, anger, irritability, and fatigue. Physical symptoms tend to be less problematic. Treatment is symptomatic and includes stress reduction, exercise, biofeedback, lifestyle changes, counselling, and medication.
8. Infection and inflammation of the female genitalia can result from microorganisms that are present in the environment and often sexually transmitted or from overproliferation of microorganisms that normally populate the genital tract.
9. Pelvic inflammatory disease (PID) is an acute inflammatory process caused by infection. Many infections are sexually transmitted and microorganisms that make up the vaginal flora are implicated. PID is a substantial health risk to women, and untreated PID can lead to infertility.
10. Vaginitis is irritation or inflammation of the vagina, typically caused by infection. Sexually transmitted pathogens or *Candida albicans*, which causes candidiasis, is the usual cause.
11. Cervicitis, which is infection of the cervix, can be acute (mucopurulent cervicitis) or chronic. Its most common cause is a sexually transmitted pathogen.
12. Vulvodynia is chronic vulvar pain lasting 3 months or longer without visible dermatosis. The cause is unknown with many theories implicated.
13. Bartholinitis, also called *Bartholin cyst*, is an infection of the ducts that lead from the Bartholin glands to the surface of the vulva. Infection blocks the glands, preventing the outflow of glandular secretions.
14. The relaxation of muscles and fascial supports usually cause the pelvic relaxation disorders. These disorders include uterine displacement, uterine prolapse, cystocele, rectocele, and urethrocele. This relaxation is usually a result of advancing age or following childbirth or other trauma. They are more likely to occur in women with a familial or genetic predisposition.
15. Benign ovarian cysts develop from mature ovarian follicles that do not release their ova (follicular cysts) or from a corpus luteum that persists abnormally instead of degenerating (corpus luteum cyst). Cysts usually regress spontaneously.
16. Endometrial polyps consist of benign overgrowths of endometrial tissue. Polyps often cause abnormal bleeding in the premenopausal woman.
17. Leiomyomas, also called *myomas* or *uterine fibroids*, are benign tumours arising from the smooth muscle layer of the uterus, the myometrium.
18. Adenomyosis is the presence of endometrial glands and stroma within the uterine myometrium.
19. Endometriosis is the presence of functional endometrial tissue (i.e., tissue that responds to hormonal stimulation) at sites outside the uterus. Endometriosis causes an inflammatory reaction at the site of implantation and is a cause of infertility.
20. Cancers of the female genitalia involve the uterus (particularly the endometrium), the cervix, and the ovaries. Cancer of the vagina is rare.
21. Cervical cancer arises from the cervical epithelium. HPV is the usual trigger. The cellular transformational zone is known as the *squamous–columnar junction*. The progressively serious neoplastic alterations are cervical intraepithelial neoplasia (CIN) (cervical dysplasia), cervical carcinoma in situ, and invasive cervical carcinoma. Cocarcinogens include immune responses, hormonal responses, and other environmental factors that decide regression or persistence of the HPV infection.
22. Primary cancer of the vagina is rare. Risk factors include being 60 or older, diethylstilbestrol exposure in utero, HPV-16, human immunodeficiency virus (HIV), genital warts, and earlier carcinoma of the cervix or vulva. The relationship between cancer of the vagina and developing precancerous cell changes called *vaginal intraepithelial neoplasia* is controversial.
23. Risk factors for vulvar cancer include HPV-16 (cause), HIV, HPV-18 (probable cause), increasing age, earlier cancer, cervical cancer survivor, earlier CIN, certain autoimmune conditions, organ transplant recipient, and tobacco use.

24. Carcinoma of the endometrium is the most common type of uterine cancer. It is the most prevalent gynecological malignancy. Primary risk factors for endometrial cancer include exposure to unopposed estrogen (e.g., estrogen-only hormone replacement therapy [HRT], tamoxifen, early menarche, late menopause, nulliparity, failure to ovulate), chronic hyperinsulinemia, hyperglycemia, body fatness and adult weight gain, chronic inflammation, and lack of physical exercise.
25. Risk factors for ovarian cancer include advancing age, genetic factors, family history, overweight and obesity, height, reproductive or hormonal factors, HRT, endometriosis, diabetes, earlier cancer, smoking, asbestos, talc-based powder, and ionizing radiation. Ovarian cancer causes more deaths than any other genital cancer in women.
26. The biology of ovarian cancer is changing, and ovarian cancer is heterogeneous.
27. Sexual dysfunction is the lack of satisfaction with sexual function resulting from pain or a deficiency in sexual desire, arousal, or orgasm/climax.
28. Sexual function and dysfunction result from a complex set of personal and biological factors that interact with culture.
29. Infertility, or the inability to conceive after 1 year of unprotected intercourse, affects approximately 16% of all couples. Impairment of fertility can occur related to factors in the male, female, or both partners.
30. Female infertility results from dysfunction of the normal reproductive process: menses and ovulation, fallopian tube function, ovarian dysfunction, and implantation of the fertilized egg into a receptive endometrium.

Disorders of the Female Breast

1. Most disorders of the female breast are disorders of the mammary gland.
2. Galactorrhea, or *inappropriate lactation*, is the persistent secretion of a milky substance by the breasts of a woman who is not in the postpartum state or nursing an infant. Its most common cause is nonpuerperal hyperprolactinemia related to a rise in serum prolactin levels.
3. Benign breast conditions are many and involve both ducts and lobules. Benign epithelial lesions are classified according to their future risk of developing breast cancer as (a) nonproliferative breast lesions, (b) proliferative breast disease, and (c) atypical (atypia) hyperplasia.
4. Nonproliferative breast lesions include simple breast cysts, papillary apocrine change, and mild hyperplasia of the usual type.
5. Proliferative breast lesions without atypia are diverse and include usual ductal hyperplasia, intraductal papillomas, sclerosing adenosis, radial scar, and simple fibroadenoma.
6. Proliferative breast lesions with atypia include atypical ductal hyperplasia and atypical lobular hyperplasia.
7. Ductal carcinoma in situ (DCIS) refers to a heterogeneous group of proliferations limited to breast ducts and lobules without invasion of the basement membrane. Lobular carcinoma in situ (LCIS) originates from the duct lobular unit.
8. Breast cancer is the most common form of cancer in women and second to lung cancer as the most common cause of cancer death. However, the inclusion of DCIS with invasive breast cancer statistics is controversial. Breast cancer is a heterogeneous disease with diverse molecular, phenotypic, and pathological changes.
9. The major risk factors for breast cancer are reproductive factors. These risk factors include nulliparity; hormonal factors and growth factors, such as excessive estradiol and insulinlike growth factor 1; familial factors, such as a family history of breast cancer; and environmental factors, such as ionizing radiation. Two factors appearing as important are delayed involution of the mammary gland and breast density. Physical activity and lack of postmenopausal weight gain may be risk-reducing factors.
10. A dominating movement in the field of cancer research is that epithelial function depends on the *entire* tissue including the stroma or microenvironment. Breast cancer is now known as a tissue-based disease with a possible abnormal, aberrant wound healing and inflammatory stromal (reactive stroma) part.
11. Models of breast carcinogenesis include three interrelated themes: gene addiction, phenotype plasticity, and cancer stem cells. The exact molecular events leading to breast cancer invasion are complex and not completely understood. These events involve genetic and epigenetic alterations and cancer cell and stromal interactions. New concepts for breast cancer metastases include tumour dormancy and vascular mimicry.
12. Most breast cancers arise from the ductal epithelium. They may then metastasize to the lymphatics, opposite breast, abdominal cavity, lungs, bones, kidneys, liver, adrenal glands, ovaries, and pituitary glands.
13. The first clinical manifestation of breast cancer is usually a small, painless lump in the breast. Other manifestations include palpable lymph nodes in the axilla, dimpling of the skin, nipple and skin retraction, nipple discharge, ulcerations, reddened skin, and bone pain associated with bony metastases.

34

Alterations of the Male Reproductive System

Kelly Power-Kean, with originating chapter contributions by George W. Rodway

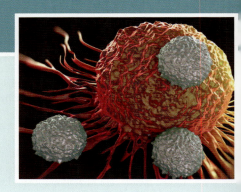

Additional resources are available online at https://evolve.elsevier.com/Canada/Huether/pathophysiology.

CHAPTER OUTLINE

Alterations of Sexual Maturation, 833
  Delayed or Absent Puberty, 833
  Precocious Puberty, 833
Disorders of the Male Reproductive System, 833
  Disorders of the Urethra, 833
  Disorders of the Penis, 833
  Disorders of the Scrotum, Testis, and Epididymis, 836

Disorders of the Prostate Gland, 840
  Sexual Dysfunction, 852
Disorders of the Male Breast, 855
  Gynecomastia, 855
  Carcinoma, 855
Sexually Transmitted Infections, 856
CASE STUDY: Benign Prostatic Hyperplasia, 859

LEARNING OBJECTIVES

1. Describe delayed or precocious puberty.
2. Describe the various sites in which infection and inflammation can occur in the male reproductive system. Describe manifestations and treatments of each.
3. Describe risk factors for penile cancer.
4. Explain the differences between a varicocele, hydrocele, and spermatocele.
5. Describe symptoms, risk factors, diagnoses, and pathological changes that occur in disorders of the testes. Include cryptorchidism, torsion, orchitis, and testicular cancer.
6. Compare the pathology and symptoms of benign prostatic hyperplasia with prostate cancer.
7. Describe the various types of prostatitis.
8. Name sources of male sexual dysfunction.
9. Describe the incidence, symptoms, and changes that occur in male gynecomastia and male breast cancer.
10. Identify the name, causative organism(s), and treatment for the major sexually transmitted infections.

KEY TERMS

Acute bacterial prostatitis (ABP, category I), 843
Androgen receptor (AR) signalling, 848
Balanitis, 836
Benign prostatic hyperplasia (BPH, benign prostatic hypertrophy), 841
Bladder outflow obstruction, 842
Chemical epididymitis, 840
Chronic bacterial prostatitis (CBP, category II), 843
Chronic prostatitis/chronic pelvic pain syndrome (CP/CPPS, category III), 843
Complete precocious puberty, 833
Condyloma acuminatum, 836
Cryptorchidism, 838
Delayed puberty, 833
Ectopic testis, 838
Epididymitis, 840
Fibroblast, 850
Gynecomastia, 855
Hydrocele, 837
Intraprostatic conversion, 844
Nonbacterial prostatitis, 843
Orchitis, 839
Paraphimosis, 834
Penile intraepithelial neoplasia (PeIN), 836
Peyronie disease ("bent nail syndrome"), 834
Phimosis, 834
Precocious puberty, 833
Priapism, 834
Prostatic intraepithelial neoplasia (PIN), 850
Prostatitis, 842
Sexual dysfunction, 852
Sexually transmitted infections (STIs), 856
Spermatocele (epididymal cyst), 838
Stroma, 850
Testicular appendage, 838
Torsion of the testis, 838
Urethral stricture, 834
Urethritis, 834
Varicocele, 836

Alterations of the reproductive system span a wide range of concerns, including delayed sexual development, suboptimal sexual performance, and structural and functional abnormalities. Many common male reproductive disorders carry potentially serious physiological or psychological consequences. For example, sexual or reproductive dysfunction, such as erectile dysfunction or infertility, can dramatically affect self-concept, relationships, and overall quality of life. Organic and psychosocial problems, such as alcoholism, depression, situational stressors, chronic illness, and medications, can affect sexual performance and may be risk factors for the development of some types of reproductive tract cancers. Aside from skin cancer, prostate cancer is the second leading cause of cancer deaths and is the most often diagnosed cancer in men. Incidence rates for prostate cancer changed substantially between the mid-1980s and mid-1990s. These rates fluctuate widely from year to year, reflecting changes in prostate cancer screening with the prostate-specific antigen (PSA) blood test.[1] Diagnosis and treatment of male reproductive system disorders is often complicated by the stigma and symbolism associated with the reproductive organs. This includes emotion-laden beliefs and behaviours related to reproductive health. Embarrassment, guilt, fear, or denial may delay treatment or diagnosis.

ALTERATIONS OF SEXUAL MATURATION

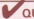
QUICK CHECK 34.1
1. Why does puberty occur too late or too early in some individuals?
2. Why do all forms of precocious puberty require evaluation?

The development of secondary sex characteristics, rapid growth, and the ability to reproduce mark the process of sexual maturation, or puberty. A variety of congenital and endocrine disorders can disrupt the timing of puberty. The inappropriate onset of sex hormone production causes puberty that occurs too late (delayed puberty) or too early (precocious puberty). While the mean age of pubertal onset appears to be decreasing for girls, the age of pubertal onset has remained unchanged for boys.

Delayed or Absent Puberty

About 2% of children experience delayed development of secondary sex characteristics.[2] Boys tend to mature later than girls, around 14 to 14.5 years of age. In boys, the first sign of maturity is the enlargement of testes and thinning of the scrotal skin. In **delayed puberty**, these secondary sex characteristics develop later.

In about 95% of cases, delayed puberty is a normal physiological event. Hormonal levels are normal, the hypothalamic–pituitary–gonadal axis is intact, and maturation is slowly occurring. Unless the delayed puberty is causing psychosocial problems treatment is not needed.[3]

The disruption of the hypothalamic–pituitary–gonadal axis or the outcomes of a systemic disease cause the other 5% of cases. Treatment depends on the cause (see Box 33.1). Referral to a pediatric endocrinologist is necessary.[3]

Precocious Puberty

Precocious puberty is a rare event, affecting fewer than 1 in 50 000 boys. Precocious puberty for boys of all ethnic groups is defined as sexual maturation occurring before age 9.[4] A recent study reports that the mean ages of beginning male genital and pubic hair growth and early testicular volumes are leaning toward younger ages than earlier studies have suggested and may be dependent on genetic factors.[5] Precocious puberty may be caused by many conditions (see Box 33.2), including deadly central nervous system tumours. All cases of precocious puberty require thorough evaluation.

All forms of precocious puberty are treated by finding and removing the underlying cause or administering proper hormones. In many cases, the reversal of precocious puberty can occur. However, **complete precocious puberty** (development consistent with the gender of the individual) is difficult to treat. This condition can cause long bones to stop growing before the child has reached normal height.

DISORDERS OF THE MALE REPRODUCTIVE SYSTEM

QUICK CHECK 34.2
1. Why are priapism and severe paraphimosis considered urological emergencies?
2. What are the risk factors for cancer of the penis?

Disorders of the Urethra

Urethritis and urethral strictures are common disorders of the male urethra. Urethral carcinoma, an extremely rare form of cancer, can occur in men older than 60 years.

Urethritis

Urethritis is an inflammatory process that is usually caused by a sexually transmitted microorganism. Infectious urethritis caused by *Neisseria gonorrhoeae* is often called *gonococcal urethritis*. Urethritis caused by other microorganisms is called *nongonococcal urethritis*. Nonsexual origins of urethritis include inflammation or infection because of urological procedures, insertion of foreign bodies into the urethra, anatomical abnormalities, or trauma.

Noninfectious urethritis is rare and is associated with the ingestion of wood or ethyl alcohol or turpentine. It may also occur with Reiter syndrome, a form of reactive arthritis.[1]

Symptoms of urethritis include urethral tingling, itching or a burning sensation, and urinary frequency and urgency. The individual may note a purulent or clear mucous like discharge from the urethra. Urine nucleic acid detection amplification tests allow early detection of *N. gonorrhoeae* and *Chlamydia trachomatis*.[6] Treatment consists of proper antibiotic therapy for infectious urethritis and avoidance of future exposure or mechanical irritation.

Urethral Strictures

A **urethral stricture** is a narrowing of the urethra caused by scarring. The scars may be congenital but can be present at any age. Strictures have a wide range of etiological factors, including untreated urethral infection, trauma, and urological instrumentation. Infections also can occur from long-term use of indwelling catheters. Prostatitis and infection secondary to urinary stasis are common complications. Severe and prolonged obstruction can result in hydronephrosis and kidney failure.

The clinical manifestations of urethral stricture are caused by bladder outlet obstruction. Urethral stricture often manifests itself as lower urinary tract symptoms (LUTS) or urinary tract infections with significant impairment in the quality of life. The primary symptom is diminished force and calibre of the urinary system. Other symptoms include urinary frequency and hesitancy, mild dysuria, double urinary stream, or spraying, and dribbling after voiding. The diagnosis of urethral stricture is based on history, physical examination, flow rates, and cystoscopy. Treatment is usually surgical and may involve urethral dilation, urethrotomy, or a variety of open surgical techniques. The choice of surgical intervention depends on the age of the individual and the severity of the problem.

Disorders of the Penis
Phimosis and Paraphimosis

Phimosis and paraphimosis are both disorders in which the foreskin (prepuce) is "too tight" to move easily over the glans penis.

Phimosis is a condition in which the foreskin cannot be retracted back over the glans. **Paraphimosis** is a condition in which the foreskin is retracted and cannot be moved forward (reduced) to cover the glans (Figure 34.1). Both conditions can cause penile pathological conditions.

The inability to retract the foreskin is normal in infancy. Congenital adhesions are usually the cause. During the first 3 years of life, congenital adhesions (between the foreskin and glans) separate naturally with penile erections. In this situation circumcision is not indicated. Phimosis can occur at any age and is usually caused by poor hygiene and chronic infection.[1] It rarely occurs with normal foreskin.

Reasons for seeking treatment include edema, erythema, and tenderness of the prepuce and purulent discharge. The inability to retract the foreskin is a less common complaint. After the infection has been eradicated circumcision can take place if needed. Complications of phimosis include inflammation of the glans (balanitis) or prepuce (posthitis) and paraphimosis. There is a higher incidence of penile carcinoma in uncircumcised males. Chronic infection and poor hygiene are usually the underlying factors in such cases. Approximately 50% of penile carcinomas are attributable to human papillomavirus (HPV).[7]

Paraphimosis can constrict the penis, causing edema of the glans. If manual reduction of the foreskin cannot occur, surgery must be performed to prevent necrosis of the glans caused by constricted blood vessels. Severe paraphimosis is a surgical emergency.

Peyronie Disease

Peyronie disease ("bent nail syndrome") is a fibrotic condition that causes lateral curvature of the penis during erection (Figure 34.2). Peyronie disease develops slowly. Characteristics of this condition include tough, fibrous thickening of the fascia in the erectile tissue of the corpora cavernosa. A dense, fibrous plaque is usually palpable on the dorsum of the penile shaft. The problem usually affects middle-aged men. This condition is associated with painful erection, painful intercourse (for both partners), and poor erection distal to the involved area.[1] In some cases, erectile dysfunction or unsatisfactory penetration occurs. When the penis is flaccid, there is no pain.

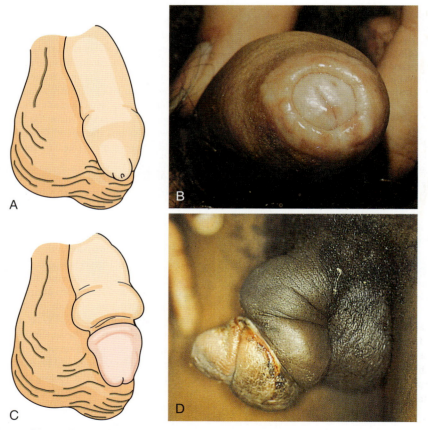

FIGURE 34.1 Phimosis and Paraphimosis. A, Phimosis: the foreskin has a narrow opening that is not large enough to allow retraction over the glans. **B,** Lesions on the prepuce secondary to infection cause swelling, and retraction of foreskin may be impossible. Circumcision is usually needed. **C,** Paraphimosis: the foreskin is retracted over the glans but cannot be reduced to its normal position. Here it has formed a constricting band around the penis. **D,** Ulcer on the retracted prepuce with edema. ([A and C], from Monahan, F. D., Sands, J., Neighbors, M., et al. [2007]. *Phipps' medical-surgical nursing: health and illness perspectives* [8th ed.]. Mosby; [B], from Taylor, P. K. [1995]. *Diagnostic picture tests in sexually transmitted diseases.* Mosby; [D], from Morse, S. A., Holmes, K. K., & Ballard, R. C. [2011]. *Atlas of sexually transmitted diseases and AIDS* [4th ed.]. Saunders.)

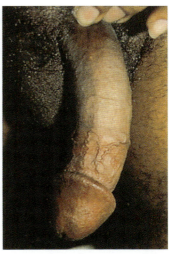

FIGURE 34.2 Peyronie Disease. This person complained of pain and deviation of his penis to one side on erection. (From Taylor, P. K. [1995]. *Diagnostic picture tests in sexually transmitted diseases*. Mosby.)

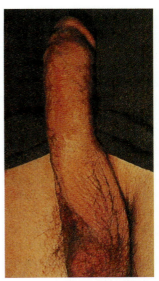

FIGURE 34.3 Priapism. (From Lloyd-Davies, R. W., Parkhouse, H., Crow, J., et al. [1994]. *Color atlas of urology* [2nd ed.]. Wolfe Medical.)

A local vasculitis-like inflammatory reaction occurs, and decreased tissue oxygenation results in fibrosis and calcification. The exact cause is unknown. Peyronie disease is associated with Dupuytren's contracture (a flexion deformity of the fingers or toes caused by shortening or fibrosis of the palmar or plantar fascia), diabetes, tendency to develop keloids, and, in rare cases, use of beta-blocker medications.[1]

There is no definitive treatment for Peyronie disease. Treatment can include pharmacological agents and surgery. Spontaneous remissions occur in as many as 50% of individuals. However, men suffering with Peyronie disease and who have significant penile deformity precluding successful coitus should have an assessment for surgical correction.[1]

Priapism

Priapism is an uncommon condition of prolonged penile erection. It is usually painful and is not associated with sexual arousal (Figure 34.3).

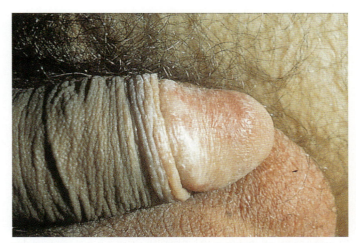

FIGURE 34.4 Balanitis. (From Taylor, P. K. [1995]. *Diagnostic picture tests in sexually transmitted diseases*. Mosby.)

Priapism is idiopathic in 60% of cases. The remaining 40% of cases can be associated with spinal cord trauma, sickle cell disease, leukemia, pelvic tumours, infections, or penile trauma.

Priapism is a urological emergency. Treatment within hours is effective and prevents erectile dysfunction. Conservative approaches include iced saline enemas, ketamine administration, and spinal anaesthesia. Needle aspiration of blood from the corpus through the dorsal glans is often effective. This process is followed by catheterization and pressure dressings to support decompression. More aggressive surgical treatments include the creation of vascular shunts to support blood flow. Erectile dysfunction results in up to 50% of prolonged cases.

Balanitis

Balanitis is an inflammation of the glans penis (Figure 34.4). This condition usually occurs in conjunction with posthitis, an inflammation of the prepuce. Inflammation of the glans and the prepuce is called *balanoposthitis*. It is associated with poor hygiene and phimosis. The accumulation under the foreskin of glandular secretions (smegma), sloughed epithelial cells, and *Mycobacterium smegmatis* can irritate the glans directly or lead to infection. Skin disorders (e.g., psoriasis, lichen planus, eczema) and candidiasis must be differentiated from inflammation resulting from poor hygienic practices. Balanitis is most often seen in men with poorly controlled diabetes mellitus and candidiasis. Antimicrobials are used to treat the infection. After the inflammation has subsided, circumcision can be considered to prevent recurrences.

Tumours of the Penis

Tumours of the penis are not common. The most frequent are the benign epithelial tumour condyloma acuminatum and penile carcinomas.

Condyloma acuminatum is a benign tumour caused by HPV, a sexually transmitted infection (STI). HPV type 6 and, less often, type 11 are the most frequent types and can cause a common wart and moist surface of the external genitalia. Giant condylomata (Buschke-Löwenstein tumour) affect older men and may grow up to 20 cm in size.[8] Atypia may be seen in longstanding, giant condylomata. Assessment of other HPV subtypes may be indicated to distinguish from a noninvasive warty carcinoma.[8]

Penile Cancer

Carcinoma of the penis is rare in Canada. The Canadian Cancer Society estimated that 160 Canadian men were diagnosed with penile cancer in 2016. It also estimated that 60 Canadian men died of this disease in 2017.[9] It does account for about 10% of cancers in African and South American men. It can affect men 40 to 70 years of age, with two-thirds of men diagnosed at 65 years of age and older.[1] Although the exact cause is unknown, risk factors include HPV infection, smoking, low socioeconomic status, poor personal hygiene, and psoriasis (possibly autoimmune diseases linked to the lack of clearance of HPV). Circumcision at birth decreases the risk for penile cancer. Penile cancer is more common in men with phimosis and those with acquired immune deficiency syndrome (AIDS).[1]

Squamous cell carcinoma accounts for 95% of invasive penile cancers. Other premalignant lesions, or in situ forms of epidermal carcinoma, which occur on the penis include leukoplakia (white plaque), Paget's disease (red, inflamed areas), erythroplasia of Queyrat (raised red areas), and Buschke-Löwenstein patches (large venous areas). Recently, penile intraepithelial neoplasia (PeIN; atypical cells) has been redesignated into two subcategories. These subcategories are differentiated PeIN and undifferentiated PeIN, including warty basaloid and mixed warty-basaloid subtypes.[10] HPV-6 and HPV-11 associated with genital warts (condylomata acuminata) have low cancer risks.[11] At times, the penis might be the site of metastatic spread of solid tumours from the bladder, prostate, rectum, or kidney. Early squamous cell carcinoma and premalignant epidermal lesions are easily treated. Delays in seeking treatment are attributed to denial, embarrassment, failure to detect lesions under a phimotic foreskin, fear, guilt, and ignorance.

Squamous cell carcinoma usually begins as a small, flat, ulcerative, or papillary lesion on the glans or foreskin that grows to involve the entire penile shaft. Extensive lesions are associated with metastases and a poor prognosis.[1] The regional femoral and iliac lymph nodes are common metastatic sites. The urethra and bladder are rarely involved. Weight loss, fatigue, and malaise occur in chronic suppurative lesions.

The specific diagnosis is made by biopsy after examination to document the location, size, and fixation of the lesion. After a positive biopsy, the extent of cancer spread is decided by imaging studies. Distant metastases are uncommon. Box 34.1 presents the stages of carcinoma of the penis.

Penile carcinoma is managed primarily with surgery. Newer, innovative surgical techniques can preserve as much penile tissue as possible without compromising cancer control. Treatment with neoadjuvant systemic chemotherapy, as well as other treatments, continue to be explored to improve poor long-term survival rates.[12,13] When the disease is inoperable and bulky inguinal metastases have occurred, palliative treatment with radiation or chemotherapy may be used. Options for individuals with carcinoma in situ include local excision, radiation, laser surgery, cryosurgery, chemosurgery, or chemotherapy with topical (5%) 5-fluorouracil (Efudex).[1]

Disorders of the Scrotum, Testis, and Epididymis

> ✓ **QUICK CHECK 34.3**
> 1. Why is a genetic link suggested for testicular cancer?
> 2. Why is testicular torsion considered a urological emergency?
> 3. Why is epididymitis rare in prepubescent males?

Disorders of the Scrotum

Men may seek treatment for painful or painless scrotal masses. Masses may be serious (cancer or torsion) or benign (hydrocele or cyst). Masses may require immediate surgical intervention or allow for careful observation. Varicocele, hydrocele, and spermatocele are common intrascrotal disorders. A **varicocele** is an abnormal dilation of the testicular veins and the pampiniform plexus within the scrotum. This finding is often described as a "bag of worms" (Figure 34.5). Varicoceles are one of the most identified scrotal abnormalities and abnormal findings among infertile men. Advancements in diagnostic techniques show that the incidence of varicoceles is significantly greater than previously reported.[14] Most (90%) occur on the left side because of discrepancies in venous drainage and may be painful or tender. Varicocele occurs in 10 to 15% of males. This condition usually occurs after puberty.[1] Because most develop in adolescence, physiological changes in testosterone level may contribute to increasing blood flow to the testicle,

---

BOX 34.1 Staging for Penile Cancer

Stage 0: Tis or Ta, N0, M0
The cancer has not grown into tissue below the top layers of skin and has not spread to lymph nodes or distant sites.

Stage I: T1a, N0, M0
The cancer has grown into tissue just below the superficial layer of skin but has not grown into blood or lymph vessels. It is a grade 1 or 2. It has not spread to lymph nodes or distant sites.

Stage II: Any of the Following:
T1b, N0, M0
The cancer has grown into tissue just below the superficial layer of skin and is high grade or has grown into blood or lymph vessels. It has not spread to lymph nodes or distant sites.
Or

T2, N0, M0
The cancer has grown into one of the internal chambers of the penis (the corpus spongiosum or corpora cavernosa). The cancer has not spread to lymph nodes or distant sites.
Or

T3, N0, M0
The cancer has grown into the urethra. It has not spread to lymph nodes or distant sites.

Stage IIIA: T1 to T3, N1, M0
The cancer has grown into tissue below the superficial layer of skin (T1). It also may have grown into the corpus spongiosum, the corpora cavernosa, or the urethra (T2 or T3). The cancer has spread to a single groin lymph node (N1). It has not spread to distant sites.

Stage IIIB: T1 to T3, N2, M0
The cancer has grown into the tissues of the penis and may have grown into the corpus spongiosum, the corpora cavernosa, or the urethra (T1 to T3). It has spread to two or more groin lymph nodes. It has not spread to distant sites.

Stage IV: Any of the Following:
T4, any N, M0
The cancer has grown into the prostate or other nearby structures. It may or may not have spread to groin lymph nodes. It has not spread to distant sites.
Or

Any T, N3, M0
The cancer has spread to lymph nodes in the pelvis or spread in the groin lymph nodes and grown through the lymph nodes' outer covering and into surrounding tissue. The cancer has not spread to distant sites.
Or

Any T, any N, M1
The cancer has spread to distant sites.

T, Primary tumour size; *N*, regional lymph nodes; *M*, distant metastasis.

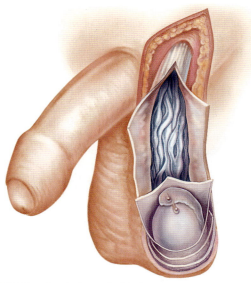

FIGURE 34.5 Depiction of a Varicocele. Dilation of veins within the spermatic cord. (From Ball, J. W., Dains, J. E., Flynn, J. A., et al. [2015]. *Seidel's guide to physical examination* [8th ed.]. Mosby.)

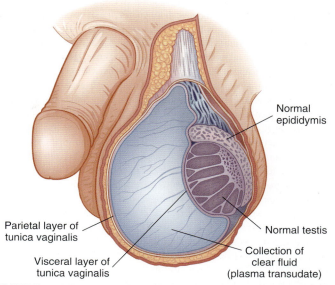

FIGURE 34.6 Depiction of a Hydrocele. Accumulation of clear fluid between the visceral (inner) and parietal (outer) layers of the tunica vaginalis.

causing venous dilation.[15] Unilateral right-sided varicoceles are rare and result from compression or obstruction of the inferior vena cava by a tumour or thrombus.[1]

The cause of varicocele is poorly understood. Blood pools in the veins rather than flowing into the venous system. Varicocele decreases blood flow through the testis, interfering with spermatogenesis and causing infertility. Varicoceles can alter testosterone and follicle-stimulating hormone (FSH) levels, cause oxidative stress, decrease sperm count, and affect sperm quality.[15,16] Varicocele surgical repair occurs when the male has a grade II or III varicocele and an abnormal semen analysis and the female has no known cause of infertility. If varicocele is mild and fertility is not an issue, a scrotal support is usually sufficient to relieve symptoms of scrotal heaviness or "dragging." To confirm diagnosis colour Doppler ultrasonography is used.[17]

A *hydrocele* is a collection of fluid between the layers of the tunica vaginalis (Figure 34.6). It is the most common cause of scrotal swelling. Hydroceles occur in 6% of male newborns. They are congenital malformations that often resolve spontaneously in the first year of life.[1] In North America, common infectious causes include epididymitis and viruses. Worldwide, however, filariasis is a major cause, especially with recent travel to tropical countries.[18] Other causes include trauma, torsion of the testicle or testicular appendage, and recent scrotal surgery.

Hydroceles vary in size, and most are asymptomatic. The most important feature on physical examination is a tense, smooth, scrotal mass that easily transilluminates. Transillumination, or holding a light behind the scrotum, can help distinguish a hydrocele from a hernia or a solid mass. Treatment includes watchful waiting in infants and for those older than 1 year. Most hydroceles resolve spontaneously by the end of the first year of life.[19] Symptomatic or communicating hydroceles need definitive treatment. Treatment includes surgical resection, aspiration, and sclerotherapy (injection of a sclerosing agent into the scrotal sac [cystic dilation]) to excise the tunica vaginalis.[20]

Spermatoceles (epididymal cysts) are benign cystic collections of fluid of the epididymis. They are found between the head of the epididymis and the testis. Spermatoceles are filled with a milky fluid having sperm and are usually painless (Figure 34.7). Removal of spermatoceles that cause significant pain or discomfort can occur. Both

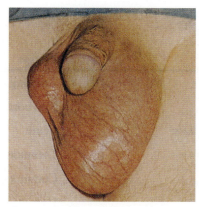

FIGURE 34.7 Spermatocele. Retention cyst of the head of the epididymis or of an aberrant tubule or tubules of the rete testis. The spermatocele lies outside the tunica vaginalis; therefore, on palpation it can be readily distinguished and separated from the testis. (From Lloyd-Davies, R. W., Parkhouse, H., Crow, J., et al. [1994]. *Color atlas of urology* [2nd ed.]. Wolfe Medical.)

spermatoceles and epididymal cysts present clinically as discrete, firm, freely mobile masses distinct from the testis that may be transilluminated. Spermatoceles are usually asymptomatic or produce mild discomfort that is relieved by scrotal support. Neither hydroceles nor spermatoceles are associated with infertility.

Cryptorchidism and Ectopy

Cryptorchidism is a group of abnormalities in which the testis does not descend completely. An **ectopic testis** is one that has strayed from the normal pathway of descent. An abnormal connection at the distal end of the gubernaculum testis that leads the gonad to an abnormal position may cause ectopy. This usually occurs at the superficial inguinal site. In cryptorchidism, the descent of one or both testes is stopped. Unilateral stoppage occurs more often than bilateral arrest. The testes may remain in the abdomen, or testicular descent may stop in the inguinal canal or the puboscrotal junction. Cryptorchidism is a common congenital anomaly, with an incidence of approximately 3% in full-term infants and 30% of premature infants.[21] The incidence of cryptorchidism in adults is 0.7 to 0.8%.[22] Cryptorchidism is commonly associated with vasal or epididymal abnormalities. These congenital anomalies affect about 33 to 66% of newborns with cryptorchidism. Other structural anomalies include posterior urethral valves (less than 5%), upper genital tract abnormalities (less than 5%), and hypospadias. The presence of both hypospadias and cryptorchidism raises the suspicion of mixed gonadal dysgenesis (intersex infant). It is thought that cryptorchidism may result from an absence or abnormality of the gubernaculum. This is a cordlike structure that extends from the lower pole of the testis to the scrotum. A congenital gonadal or dysgenetic defect that makes the testis insensitive to gonadotropins (a likely explanation for unilateral cryptorchidism) or lack of maternal gonadotropins (a likely explanation for bilateral cryptorchidism of prematurity) are the usual causes.[22]

Mechanical possibilities include a short spermatic cord, fibrous bands, or adhesions in the normal path of the testes, or a narrowed inguinal canal. Chromosomal studies do not support a genetic cause. Physiological cryptorchidism, also called *retractile testis* or *migratory testis*, is an involuntary retraction of the testes out of the scrotum. This condition occurs with excitement, physical activity, or exposure to cold. It is caused by the small mass of prepubertal testis and the strength of the cremaster muscle. This phenomenon is common and self-limiting (descent occurs at puberty).

Physical examination shows the absence of one or both testes in the scrotum and an atrophic scrotum on the affected side. If the undescended testis is in a vulnerable position, over the pubic bone for example, an individual may complain of severe pain secondary to trauma. The adult male with bilateral cryptorchidism may be infertile.

Testicular cancer also is a well-established complication of cryptorchidism. In men with a history of unilateral cryptorchidism, neoplasms also develop more commonly in the contralateral testis. This finding suggests that cryptorchidism affects the testes and is a process more significant than simply the position of the testis in childhood. The risk for testicular cancer is 35 to 50 times greater for men with cryptorchidism or a history of cryptorchidism than for the general male population. Because definite histological change occurs in the cryptorchid testis by 1 year of age, surgical correction is recommended before that age.[23] Treatment often begins with administration of gonadotropin-releasing hormone (GnRH) or human chorionic gonadotropin (hCG). These hormones may start descent and make surgery unnecessary. GnRH is available as a nasal spray in Europe only and may enhance germ cell counts even when the testis does not descend.[24] If hormonal therapy is not successful (success rates range from 6 to 75%), the testis is located and moved surgically (orchiopexy) in young children or removed (orchiectomy) in adults and children more than 10 years of age.[22] The testis that is properly placed in the scrotum provides adequate hormonal function and gives the scrotum a normal appearance. A successful operation does not ensure fertility if the testis is congenitally defective. Approximately 20% of males with unilateral undescended testis remain infertile even though orchiopexy occurs by age 1 year. Most individuals with treated or untreated bilateral testicular maldescent have poor fertility.

Torsion of the Testis and Testicular Appendages

In **torsion of the testis**, the testis rotates on its vascular pedicle, interrupting its blood supply (Figure 34.8). Torsion of the testis is one of several conditions that cause an acute scrotum, which is testicular pain and swelling. **Testicular appendages** include the appendix testis (a remnant of the Müllerian duct) and the appendix epididymis (a remnant of the wolffian duct). Torsion of the appendages can also cause acute scrotum and be confused with testicular torsion, a urological emergency.

Torsion of the testis can occur at any age but is most common among neonates and adolescents, particularly at puberty.[25] Onset may be spontaneous or follow physical exertion or trauma. Torsion twists the arteries and veins in the spermatic cord, reducing or stopping circulation to the testis. Vascular engorgement and ischemia develop, causing scrotal swelling and pain not relieved by rest or scrotal support. Diagnostic testing includes urinalysis (to assess for infection) and colour Doppler ultrasonography.[22,25] Torsion of the testis is a surgical emergency. In order to preserve testicular function, surgery must be performed within 6 hours after the onset of symptoms if it cannot be reduced manually (scrotal elevation).

Orchitis

Orchitis is an acute inflammation of the testes (Figure 34.9). This condition is uncommon except as a complication of systemic infection or as an extension of an associated epididymitis.[26] Infectious organisms may reach the testes through the blood or the lymphatics or, most commonly, by ascent through the urethra, vas deferens, and epididymis. Most cases of orchitis are cases of epididymo-orchitis (inflammation of both the epididymis and testis). Occasionally in middle-aged men, a nonspecific, apparently noninfectious inflammatory process (called *granulomatous orchitis*) can occur, presumably a granulomatous response to spermatozoa.

Mumps is the most common infectious cause of orchitis. This condition usually affects post pubertal males. The onset is sudden, occurring 3 to 4 days after the onset of parotitis. Signs and symptoms include high fever, reaching 40°C (104°F), marked prostration, bilateral or unilateral erythema, edema and tenderness of the scrotum, and leukocytosis. An acute hydrocele may develop. Urinary signs and symptoms, which occur in epididymitis, are absent. Atrophy with irreversible damage to spermatogenesis may result in 30% of affected testes. Bilateral orchitis does not affect hormonal function but may cause permanent sterility.

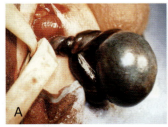
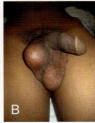
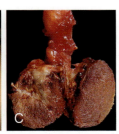

FIGURE 34.8 Torsion of the Testis. ([A and B], from Kliegman, R. M., Stanton, B. F., St. Geme, J. W., et al. [Eds.]. [2011]. *Nelson textbook of pediatrics* [19th ed.]. Saunders; [C], from Damjanov, I., & Linder, J. [Eds]. [1996]. *Anderson's pathology* [10th ed.]. Mosby.)

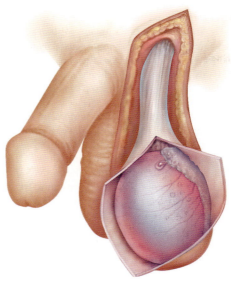

FIGURE 34.9 Depiction of Orchitis. (From Ball, J. W., Dains, J. E., Flynn, J. A., et al. [2015]. *Seidel's guide to physical examination* [8th ed.]. Mosby.)

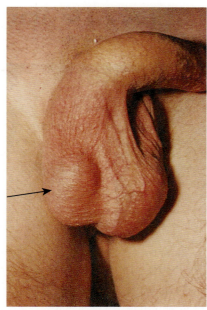

FIGURE 34.10 Testicular Tumour (*arrow*). (From Wolfe, J. [1984]. *400 self-assessment picture tests in clinical medicine*. Wolfe Medical.)

Treatment is supportive and includes bed rest, scrotal support, elevation of the scrotum, hot or cold compresses, and analgesic agents for relief of pain. Aspiration occurs if an acute hydrocele develops. Testicular abscess usually requires orchiectomy (removal of the testis). Appropriate antimicrobial medications should be used for bacterial orchitis. Corticosteroids are used in proven cases of nonspecific granulomatous orchitis.

Cancer of the Testis

Testicular cancer is a highly treatable, usually curable cancer that most often develops in young and middle-aged men. For men with seminoma (all stages combined), the cure rate exceeds 90%. For men with low-stage seminoma or nonseminoma, the cure rate approaches 100%.[27] Testicular cancers are uncommon, accounting for approximately 1% of all male cancers; yet they are the most common solid tumour of young adult men.[27] Cancer of the testis occurs most commonly in men between the ages of 15 and 35 years. The Canadian Cancer Society estimated that 1 150 Canadian men will be diagnosed with testicular cancer in 2020. It also estimated that 35 Canadian men died of this disease in 2020.[28] Testicular cancer is more common in White men than in men of African or Asian ancestry. It occurs more often in men with a higher socioeconomic status.[27] Testicular tumours are slightly more common on the right side than on the left and they are bilateral in 1 to 3% of cases (Figure 34.10).

PATHOPHYSIOLOGY Ninety percent of testicular cancers are germ cell tumours, arising from the male gametes. Germ cell tumours include seminomas (most common), embryonal carcinomas, teratomas, and choriosarcomas. Testicular tumours also can arise from specialized cells of the gonadal stroma (Leydig, Sertoli, granulosa, theca cells).

The cause of testicular neoplasms is unknown (see *Risk Factors: Cancer of the Testis*). The fact that the incidence is higher among brothers, identical twins, and other close male relatives suggests a genetic predisposition. The disease is relatively rare among Africans, Blacks, Asians, and native New Zealanders. Risk factors include history of cryptorchidism, abnormal testicular development, human immunodeficiency virus (HIV) and AIDS, Klinefelter's syndrome, and history of testicular cancer.[27]

> **RISK FACTORS**
> *Cancer of the Testis*
>
> - HIV and AIDS
> - History of cryptorchidism
> - Abnormal testicular development
> - Klinefelter's syndrome
> - History of testicular cancer

CLINICAL MANIFESTATIONS Painless testicular enlargement commonly is the first sign of testicular cancer. Occurring gradually, a sensation of testicular heaviness or a dull ache in the lower abdomen may be present. Occasionally acute pain occurs because of rapid growth, resulting in hemorrhage and necrosis. Ten percent of affected men have epididymitis, 10% have hydroceles, and 5% have breast enlargement (gynecomastia). The testicular mass is usually discovered by the individual or by his sexual partner. At the time of first diagnosis, approximately 10% of individuals already have symptoms related to metastases. Lumbar pain also may be present. The cause of this pain is retroperitoneal node metastasis. Signs of metastasis to the lungs include cough, dyspnea, and bloody sputum (hemoptysis). Supraclavicular node involvement may cause difficulty swallowing (dysphagia) and neck swelling. Alterations in vision or mental status, papilledema, and seizures may be experienced when metastasis to the central nervous system occurs.

EVALUATION AND TREATMENT An incorrect diagnosis at the first examination occurs in as many as 25% of men with testicular cancer. Epididymitis and epididymo-orchitis are the most common misdiagnoses; others include hydrocele and spermatocele. Evaluation begins with careful physical examination, including palpation of the scrotal contents with the individual in the erect and supine positions. Signs of testicular cancer include abnormal consistency, induration, nodularity, or irregularity of the testis. The abdomen and lymph nodes are palpated to seek evidence of metastasis. Tumour type is identified after orchiectomy. The Canadian Cancer Society recommends that all men should know how their testicles normally look and feel and should talk to their primary health care provider if they notice any changes in their testicles.[29] Testicular biopsy is not recommended because it may cause dissemination of the tumour and increase the risk for local recurrence. Primary testicular cancer can be assessed rapidly and accurately by scrotal ultrasonography. Tumour markers are higher than normal in the presence of a tumour and may help detect a tumour that is too small to be felt during physical examination or to be seen on imaging. Radiological imaging and measurement of serum markers are used in clinical staging of the disease. Besides surgery, treatment involves radiation and chemotherapy singly or in combination. Factors influencing the prognosis include histological studies of the tumour stage of the disease and selection of proper treatment. Most individuals treated for cancer of the testis can expect a normal lifespan. Some men have persistent paresthesias, Raynaud phenomenon, or infertility. Approximately 10% of men treated for testicular cancer will experience a relapse. If the relapse is discovered early and treated, 99% can be cured. Orchiectomy does not affect sexual function.

Epididymitis

Epididymitis, or inflammation of the epididymis, generally occurs in sexually active young males (younger than 35 years) and is rare before puberty (Figure 34.11). In young men, the usual cause is a sexually transmitted microorganism, such as *N. gonorrhoeae* or *C. trachomatis*. A Gram-negative organism is isolated in most samples from older men living in the community who have urinary tract infections.[30] Men who practise unprotected anal intercourse may get sexually transmitted epididymitis that results from infection with *Escherichia coli*, *Haemophilus influenzae*, tuberculosis, or *Cryptococcus* or *Brucella* species. In men older than 35 years, Enterobacteriaceae (intestinal bacteria) and *Pseudomonas aeruginosa* associated with urinary tract infections and prostatitis also may cause epididymitis. Epididymitis also may result from a chemical inflammation caused by the reflux of sterile urine into the ejaculatory ducts. This inflammation is then called **chemical epididymitis**.[31] It is associated with urethral strictures, congenital posterior valves, and excessive physical straining in which increased abdominal pressure is transmitted to the bladder. Chemical epididymitis is usually self-limiting and does not require evaluation or intervention unless it persists.

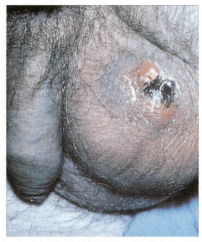

FIGURE 34.11 Epididymitis Secondary to Gonorrhea or Nongonococcal Urethritis. This infection spread to the testes and rupture through the scrotal wall is threatened. (From Taylor, P. K. [1995]. *Diagnostic picture tests in sexually transmitted disease*. Mosby.)

PATHOPHYSIOLOGY The pathogenic microorganism usually reaches the epididymis by ascending the vasa deferentia from an already infected urethra or bladder. The resulting inflammatory response causes symptoms of bacterial epididymitis. Epididymitis caused by heavy lifting or straining results from reflux of urine from the bladder into the vas deferens and epididymis. Urine is extremely irritating to the epididymis and starts the inflammatory response called *chemical epididymitis*.

CLINICAL MANIFESTATIONS The main symptom of epididymitis is scrotal or inguinal pain caused by inflammation of the epididymis and surrounding tissues. The pain is usually acute and severe. Flank pain may occur if, as the urethra passes over the spermatic cord, edematous swelling of the cord obstructs the urethra. The individual may have pyuria, bacteriuria, and a history of urinary symptoms, including urethral discharge. The scrotum on the involved side is red and edematous. The tail of the epididymis near the lower pole of the testis usually swells first; then swelling ascends to the head of the epididymis. The spermatic cord also may be swollen and tender.

Complications include abscess formation, infarction of the testis, recurrent infection, and infertility. The probable cause of infarction is thrombosis (obstruction by blood clots) of the prostatic vessels secondary to severe inflammation. Recurrent epididymitis may result from inadequate first treatment or failure to identify or treat predisposing factors. Chronic epididymitis can cause scarring of the epididymal endothelium and infertility. Once scarring has occurred, treatment with antibiotics is ineffective because adequate antibiotic levels cannot be achieved within the epididymis.

EVALUATION AND TREATMENT A history of recent urinary tract infections or urethral discharge suggests the diagnosis of epididymitis. Common physical findings include a swollen epididymis or testis associated with acute and severe pain.[1] The relief of pain when the inflamed testis and epididymis are elevated (Prehn sign) is also diagnostic. Definitive diagnosis is based on culture or Gram stain of a urethral swab. Epididymal aspiration may be necessary to obtain a specimen, especially if the individual has been taking antibiotics and has sterile urine.

Treatment includes antibiotic therapy for the infection itself. Analgesics, ice, and scrotal elevation can supply symptomatic relief. If the individual does not steadily improve, he should be re-evaluated for possible complications, such as abscess formation, sepsis, or continued infection. Complete resolution of swelling and pain may take several weeks to months. Antibiotic treatment of the individual's sexual partner should occur if the causative microorganism is a sexually transmitted pathogen.

Disorders of the Prostate Gland

> ✓ **QUICK CHECK 34.4**
> 1. Why is the worldwide variation of prostate cancer incidence important?
> 2. What is the current understanding of hormones in the pathophysiology of prostate cancer?
> 3. Describe what is meant by prostate cancer cell and stromal interactions for carcinogenesis.
> 4. What causes impaired spermatogenesis?

Benign Prostatic Hyperplasia

Benign prostatic hyperplasia (BPH), also called **benign prostatic hypertrophy**, is the enlargement of the prostate gland (Figure 34.12). Because the major prostatic changes are caused by hyperplasia, not hypertrophy, *benign prostatic hyperplasia* is the preferred term. This condition becomes problematic when prostatic tissue compresses the urethra, where it passes through the prostate, resulting in frequency of LUTS. Like prostate cancer, BPH occurs more often in Westernized

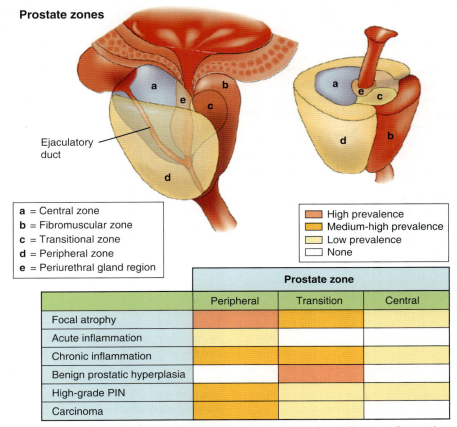

FIGURE 34.12 Prostate Zones, Benign Prostatic Hyperplasia (BPH), and Prostate Cancer Locations. Benign prostatic hyperplasia (BPH) occurs in the peripheral zone of the prostate gland that can enlarge (not shown). BPH nodules and atrophy are associated with inflammation in the transition zone. Most cancer lesions occur in the peripheral zone. Carcinoma can involve the central zone but rarely occurs in isolation, suggesting that prostatic intraepithelial neoplasia (PIN) lesions do not easily progress to carcinoma in this region. (Adapted from De Marzo, A. M., Platz, E. A., Sutcliffe, S., et al. [2007]. Inflammation in prostate carcinogenesis. *Nature Reviews: Cancer, 7,* 256–269.)

countries (e.g., Canada, the United States, and the United Kingdom). BPH appears to be more common in Black men than White men, and family history may increase the risk. Being overweight or obese with central fat distribution (i.e., around the abdomen) increases the risk of developing BPH. The worldwide prevalence of BPH is over 210 million men. Approximately 50% for men over 50, and 80% for men over 80 experience LUTS from BPH.[32] BPH is common and involves a complex pathophysiology with several endocrine and local factors and remodelled microenvironment. Its relationship to aging is well documented. At birth, the prostate is pea sized, and growth of the gland is gradual until puberty. At that time, there is a period of rapid development that continues until the third decade of life when the prostate reaches adult size (see Chapter 32). Around 40 to 45 years of age, benign hyperplasia begins and continues slowly until death. Although androgens, such as dihydrotestosterone (DHT), are necessary for normal prostatic development, their role in BPH is still unclear. Among all the androgen-metabolizing enzymes within the prostate, 5α-reductase is the most powerful. This reductase corresponds to an age dependent DHT level. Therefore, although levels of 5α-reductase and DHT in the epithelium decrease with age, they stay constant in the stroma (microenvironment) of the prostate gland.

PATHOGENESIS Current causative theories of BPH focus on aging and levels and ratios of endocrine factors. These factors include androgens and estrogens (androgen/estrogen ratio), the role of chronic inflammation, and the effects of autocrine/paracrine growth-stimulating and growth-inhibiting factors. These factors include insulinlike growth factors (IGFs), epidermal growth factors, fibroblast factors, and transforming growth factor-beta (TGF-β), and several others. Recent data show that human prostate stromal cells can actively contribute to the inflammatory process from the induction of inflammatory cytokines and chemokines[33] (see "Cancer of the Prostate").

With aging, circulating androgens are associated with BPH and enlargement. Other effects related to estrogens include apoptosis, aromatase expression, and paracrine regulation that may be important for stimulating inflammation.[34] BPH is a multifactorial disease and not all men respond well to currently available treatments. This finding suggests factors other than androgens are involved. Testosterone, the primary circulating androgen in men, also can be metabolized through aromatase cytochrome P450 (CYP19) into the potent estrogen estradiol-17β. The prostate is an estrogen target tissue, and estrogens directly and indirectly affect growth and differentiation of the prostate. The precise role of endogenous and exogenous estrogens in directly affecting prostate growth and differentiation in the context of BPH is understudied. Estrogens and selective estrogen receptor modulators have been shown to promote or inhibit prostate proliferation, signifying potential roles in BPH.[35,36] Taken together, these interactions lead to an increase in prostate volume. The remodelled stroma promotes local inflammation with altered cytokine, reactive oxygen, or nitrogen species, and chemoattractants.[37] The resultant increased oxygen demands of proliferating cells cause a local hypoxia that induces angiogenesis and changes to fibroblasts.

BPH begins in the periurethral glands, which are the inner glands or layers of the prostate. The prostate enlarges as nodules form and grow (nodular hyperplasia), and glandular cells enlarge (hypertrophy). The development of BPH occurs over a prolonged period, and changes within the urinary tract are slow and insidious.

CLINICAL MANIFESTATIONS As nodular hyperplasia and cellular hypertrophy progress, tissues that surround the prostatic urethra compress it. This usually causes bladder outflow obstruction. These symptoms are sometimes called the spectrum of LUTS. Symptoms include the urge to urinate often, some delay in starting urination, and decreased force of the urinary stream. As the obstruction progresses, often over several years, the bladder cannot empty all the urine. The increasing volume leads to long-term urine retention. The volume of urine retained may be great enough to produce uncontrolled "overflow incontinence" with any increase in intra-abdominal pressure. At this stage, the force of the urinary stream is significantly reduced, and much more time is needed to start and complete voiding.[1] Hematuria, bladder or kidney infection, bladder calculi, acute urinary retention hydroureter, hydronephrosis, and renal insufficiency are common complications.[38]

Progressive bladder distension causes diverticular outpouchings of the bladder wall. The ureters may be obstructed where they pass through the hypertrophied detrusor muscle, potentially causing hydroureter, hydronephrosis, and bladder or kidney infection.

EVALUATION AND TREATMENT A medical history, physical examination, and laboratory tests, including urinalysis confirm the diagnosis. Careful review of symptoms is necessary. Digital rectal examination (DRE) and measurement of PSA level are conducted to determine hyperplasia. PSA level alone cannot confirm symptoms attributable to BPH because PSA level is elevated in both BPH and prostate cancer. Annual DREs are used to screen men older than 50 years for BPH, sooner in high-risk men.[39] If marked enlargement, moderate to severe symptoms, or complications are present, transrectal ultrasound (TRUS) is used to determine bladder and prostate volume and residual urine. Urinalysis, serum creatinine and blood urea nitrogen levels, uroflowmetry, postvoid residual (PVR) urine, pressure-flow study, and cystometry are used to determine kidney and bladder function.[39] BPH has been treated successfully with medications. α_1-Adrenergic blockers (prazosin [Minipress] and tamsulosin [Flomax CR]) are used to relax the smooth muscle of the bladder and prostate. Antiandrogen agents, such as finasteride (Proscar), selectively block androgens at the prostate cellular level and cause the prostate gland to shrink.[39] These medications have been shown to improve BPH-related symptoms and reduce the risk for future urinary retention and BPH-related surgery by shrinking the prostate. α_1-Adrenergic blockers do not affect PSA and have no effect on prostate cancer risk. However, antiandrogen agents lower PSA by 50% after 6 months of therapy.[40,41] Newer, minimally invasive treatments include interstitial laser treatment, transurethral radiofrequency procedures (such as transurethral needle ablation [TUNA]), and Cooled ThermoTherapy.

Prostatitis

Prostatitis is an inflammation of the prostate. The incidence and prevalence of prostatitis is not known. Inflammation is usually limited to a few of the gland's excretory ducts.

BOX 34.2 NIH Classification of Prostatitis Syndrome

This system, developed for clinical research purposes, can be simplified for use in primary care practice (see text).

Category I, or acute bacterial prostatitis (ABP), is an acute infection of the prostate and is manifested by systemic signs of infection and positive urine culture.

Category II, or chronic bacterial prostatitis (CBP), is a chronic bacterial infection in which bacteria are received in significant numbers from a purulent prostatic fluid. These bacteria are thought to be the most common cause of recurrent urinary tract infection in men.

Category III, or chronic pelvic pain syndrome (CPPS), is diagnosed when no pathological bacteria can be localized to the prostate (culture of expressed prostatic fluid or postprostatic massage urine specimen) and is further divided into IIIa and IIIb. Category IIIa refers to inflammatory CPPS, where a significant number of white blood cells (WBCs) are localized to the prostate, while category IIIb is noninflammatory.

Category IV refers to asymptomatic inflammatory prostatitis in which bacteria or WBCs are localized to the prostate, but individuals are asymptomatic.

Prostatitis syndromes have been classified by the US National Institutes of Health as (1) acute bacterial prostatitis (ABP), (2) chronic bacterial prostatitis (CBP), (3) chronic pelvic pain syndrome (CPPS), and (4) asymptomatic inflammatory prostatitis (Box 34.2). ABP and CBP are mostly caused by Gram-negative Enterobacteriaceae and *Enterococci* species that originate in the gastro-intestinal flora. The most common organism is *E. coli*, which is found in most infections.[42] *Klebsiella* species, *P. aeruginosa*, and *Serratia* species are common Gram-negative cultured microorganisms. Nonbacterial prostatitis (chronic prostatitis/chronic pelvic pain syndrome [CP/CPPS]) syndromes are caused by a cascade of inflammatory, immunological, neuroendocrine, and neuropathic mechanisms whereby the initiating cause is unknown.

Bacterial prostatitis. Acute bacterial prostatitis (ABP, category I) is an ascending infection of the urinary tract that tends to occur in men between the ages of 30 and 50 years. It is also associated with BPH in older men. Infection stimulates an inflammatory response in which the prostate becomes enlarged, tender, firm, or boggy. The onset of prostatitis may be acute and unrelated to earlier illnesses, or it may follow catheterization or cystoscopy.

Clinical manifestations of ABP are those of urinary tract infection or pyelonephritis. Sudden onset of malaise, low back and perineal pain, high fever (up to 40°C [104°F]), chills, dysuria, inability to empty the bladder, nocturia, and urinary retention are common symptoms. The individual also may have symptoms of lower urinary tract obstruction, such as slow, small, "narrowed" urinary stream, which may be a medical emergency. Acute inflammatory prostatic edema can compress the urethra, causing urinary obstruction. Systemic signs of infection include sudden onset of a high fever, fatigue, arthralgia, and myalgia. Prostatic pain may occur, especially when the individual is in an upright position. This occurs because the pelvic floor muscles tighten with standing, and compression of the prostate gland occurs. Some individuals experience low back pain, painful ejaculation, and rectal or perineal pain. Palpation shows an enlarged, extremely tender, and swollen prostate that is firm, indurated, and warm to the touch.

Because ABP is usually associated with a bladder infection caused by the same microorganism, urine cultures show its identity. Prostatic massage may express enough secretions from the urethra for direct bacterial examination. Massage may be painful and increases the risk that the infection will ascend to adjacent structures or enter the bloodstream and cause septicemia.

To resolve the infection and control its spread, individuals may need antibiotics. In severe cases, hospitalization and treatment with intravenous antibiotics, followed by oral antibiotics may be needed. Analgesics, antipyretics, bed rest, and adequate hydration are also therapeutic. Complications include urinary retention that resolves with antibiotic therapy; prostatic abscess that may rupture into the urethra, rectum, or perineum; epididymitis; bacteremia; and septic shock. Urinary retention requiring drainage is best managed with a suprapubic catheter. Foley catheterization is contraindicated during acute infection.

Chronic bacterial prostatitis (CBP, category II) is characterized by recurrent urinary tract symptoms and persistence of pathogenic bacteria (usually gram negative) in urine or prostatic fluid. This form of prostatitis is the most common recurrent urinary tract infection in men. Symptoms may be like those of an acute bladder infection: frequency, urgency, dysuria, perineal discomfort, low back pain, myalgia, arthralgia, and sexual dysfunction. The prostate may be only slightly enlarged or boggy, but it may be fibrotic because repeated infections can cause it to be firm and irregular in shape.

When the first urine sample is bacteria-free, prostatic massage is used to express secretions. Subsequently, the first 10 mL of voided urine is collected and examined microscopically. Prostatic secretions showing more than 10 white blood cells (WBCs) per high-power field (hpf) and macrophages holding fat are indicative of bacterial infection. Diagnosis is confirmed by culture. A pelvic X-ray or transurethral ultrasound may show prostatic calculi.

Because CBP is often caused by prostatic calculi, treatment is difficult. Calculi are silent and are found in up to 50% of men with prostatitis. Infected calculi can serve as a source of bacterial persistence and relapsing urinary tract infection. Calculi harbour pathogens within the stone and pathogens cannot be eradicated from the urinary tract. Surgical intervention can provide a permanent cure.[1]

Chronic prostatitis/chronic pelvic pain syndrome. Chronic prostatitis/chronic pelvic pain syndrome (CP/CPPS, category III) is diagnosed when no pathogenic bacteria can be localized to the prostate. This syndrome is further subdivided into categories IIIa and IIIb (see Box 34.2). Category IIIa refers to inflammatory CPPS in which WBC count is elevated and localized to the prostate. Compared with category III, symptoms tend to be milder but are persistent and annoying. Presumably, noninfectious prostatitis or pain is caused by reflux of sterile urine into the ejaculatory ducts because of high-pressure voiding.[43] Spasms of the external or internal sphincters can trigger reflux. Category IIIb is noninflammatory. Category IV exists when individuals are asymptomatic but have an increase in bacteria and WBCs localized to the prostate. Microorganisms suspected of causing CP/CPPS include *E. coli, Enterobacter, P. aeruginosa,* and, a new suspect, *Helicobacter pylori*.[44]

Men with **nonbacterial prostatitis** may complain of pain or a dull ache that is continuous or spasmodic in the suprapubic, infrapubic, scrotal, penile, or inguinal area. Other symptoms are pain on ejaculation and urinary symptoms, such as frequency of urination. The prostate gland generally feels normal on palpation.

Nonbacterial prostatitis is a diagnosis of exclusion. The use of digital examination of the prostate, bacterial cultures of the urogenital tract, microscopic examination of expressed prostatic fluid, urethroscopy, and urodynamic studies verify the diagnosis of nonbacterial prostatitis.

There is no generally accepted treatment for nonbacterial prostatitis. Hot sitz baths, bed rest, and pharmacological therapies, including anti-inflammatory medications, can relieve symptoms.

Cancer of the Prostate

Prostate cancer is the most diagnosed, nonskin cancer in men in Canada. It was estimated that in 2020, 23 300 men would be diagnosed with prostate cancer.[45] The incidence varies greatly worldwide (Figure 34.13). It is still considered to be the second most

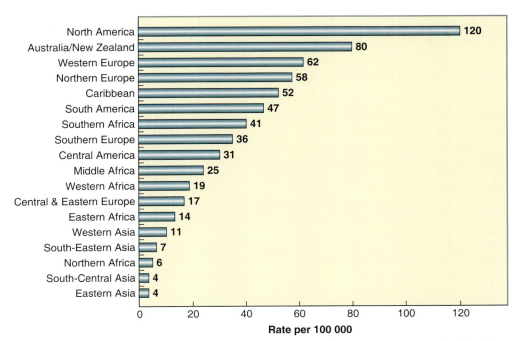

FIGURE 34.13 Selected World Population Age-Standardized (to the World Population) Incidence Rates of Prostate Cancer. (From Jemal, A., Center, M. M., DeSantis, C., et al. [2010]. Global patterns of cancer incidence and mortality rates and trends. *Cancer Epidemiology, Biomarkers & Prevention, 19*[8], 1893–1907.)

frequently diagnosed cancer in men and the fifth leading cause of death worldwide.[46] An estimated 1.2 million cases of prostate cancer were diagnosed worldwide in 2018, accounting for 13.5% of the cancers diagnosed in men.[45] Incidence rates vary by more than 25-fold worldwide. The highest rates are recorded mostly in developed countries in regions such as Oceania, Europe, and North America, largely because of wide use or overuse of PSA testing. Screening with PSA can amplify the incidence of prostate cancer by allowing detection of prostate lesions that, although meeting the pathological criteria for malignancy, may have low potential (e.g., latent, indolent, preclinical) for growth and metastasis. In countries with higher use of PSA testing, such as Canada, the United States, Australia, and the Nordic countries, trends in incidence rates follow similar patterns.[45]

Different from Western countries, incidence and death rates are rising in several Asian and Central and Eastern European countries. Death rates have been decreasing in several countries, including Australia, Canada, the United Kingdom, the United States, Italy, and Norway, in part because of improved treatment. Males of African descent in the Caribbean region have the highest mortality from prostate cancer in the world.[45] Most cases of prostate cancer have a good prognosis even without treatment, but some cases are aggressive. The lifetime risk of dying of prostate cancer is 3.4%. Prostate cancer is rare before age 50 years, and very few men die from this cancer before 60 years of age. The highest incidence of prostate cancer is in men older than 65.[47] With aging, most of the androgen-metabolizing enzymes undergo significant alteration and older age, race (Black), and family history remain the well-established risk factors.

Dietary factors. Although evidence exists for a dietary role in prostate cancer, the epidemiological evidence is inconsistent.[1] The problem has been complicated by the lack of biomarkers for certain nutrients, difficulties in measuring and quantifying diet, and a limitation of clinical trials to study diet over time. The effects of diet on signalling pathways, hormones, oxidative stress, and reactive oxygen species (ROS) are important. Obesity seems to be negatively associated with more indolent prostate cancer and positively associated with more aggressive disease and a worse outcome.[48] The nutrients in the epidemiology of prostate cancer that have received the most attention include carotenoids, fat, vitamin E, vitamin D, calcium, and selenium (Box 34.3).

Hormones. Prostate cancer develops in an androgen-dependent epithelium and is usually androgen sensitive. Androgens are made not only in the testis, accounting for 50 to 60% of the total testosterone in the prostate, but also in the prostate gland itself. In a process called **intraprostatic conversion**, the hormone dehydroepiandrosterone (DHEA) produced by the adrenal glands[49] is converted to testosterone and then into DHT in the prostate (Figure 34.14). Additionally, prostate cancer cells have been reported to make androgens from cholesterol (i.e., de novo).[50] However, these overall relative contributions from intratumoural sources are still to be decided. Population studies have not supplied clear and convincing patterns involving associations between circulating hormone concentrations (i.e., not concentrations in tissue) and prostate cancer risk.[51] There is universal agreement that androgens are important for prostatic growth, development, and maintenance of tissue balance. However, their role in cancer is controversial. Evidence in support of the involvement of androgens in prostate cancer development comes from clinical trials with 5α-reductase inhibitors. However, the involvement of 5α-reductase, which is critical in androgen activity in the prostate, is contradictory and inconsistent[51,52] (see Figure 34.14). A prevention study has provided some of the strongest hormonal data with the medication finasteride (Apo-Finasteride), which inhibits 5α-reductase. The 7-year intervention study reduced prostate cancer risk in healthy men by about 25%.[53] It is important to note that more high-grade tumours were found in those men who developed prostate cancer while on the medication. In men younger than 50 years of age, circulating levels of androgens and estrogens appear to be higher in men of African descent than in men of European descent.

Despite the well-documented importance of androgens, their pathophysiological process in prostate diseases is incomplete.[54] Androgens also are metabolized to estrogens (Figure 34.14B) through the action of the enzyme aromatase, and a growing body of evidence implicates estrogens in the etiology of prostate disease (see the following "Pathogenesis" section).

Vasectomy. In a meta-analysis of prospective studies, vasectomy has been identified as a possible risk factor for prostate cancer.[55] Three mechanisms by which vasectomy could increase risk are (1) elevation of circulating androgens; (2) activation of immunological mechanisms involving antisperm antibodies; and (3) reduction of seminal fluid levels of 5α-DHT, the active metabolite of testosterone in the prostate, in vasectomized men. These results suggest an elevation of circulating free testosterone level following vasectomy. However, with these combined mechanisms, it is unlikely that vasectomy plays a causal role.[56]

Chronic inflammation. A 5-year longitudinal study of the influence of chronic inflammation and prostate cancer was undertaken with 144 men, 33 of whom presented with chronic inflammation in their first biopsy.[57] Biopsies revealed prostatic hyperplasia and proliferative inflammatory atrophy (PIA) in those with chronic inflammation. Upon repeat biopsy, 29 new cancers were diagnosed, representing a new cancer incidence of 20%.[57] In contrast, of the 33 men initially showing no inflammation, 2 (6%) were found to have adenocarcinoma. Certain metabolic comorbidities, including obesity, diabetes, sleep apnea, and erectile dysfunction, may be linked to both BPH and inflammation.[58] The causes of chronic inflammation are emerging. (Figure 34.15 shows possible causes). Thus, chronic inflammation may be an important risk factor for prostatic adenocarcinoma.[1] Chronic inflammation involves autocrine/paracrine growth-stimulating and growth-inhibiting factors. These factors include IGFs, epidermal growth factors, fibroblast factors, and TGF-β, as well as several others. Recent data show that human prostate stromal cells can actively contribute to the inflammatory process from the induction of inflammatory cytokines and chemokines.[59] Importantly, a continuous input from TGF-β and IGF in the tumour microenvironment or stroma will result in cancer progression. Understanding of these events can help prevention, diagnosis, and therapy of prostate cancer[1] (Figure 34.16).

Genetic and epigenetic factors. Other possible causes are those of genetic predisposition (familial and hereditary forms). Genetic studies suggest that strong familial predisposition may be responsible for 5 to 10% of prostate cancers.[1] Compared with men with no family history, those with one first-degree relative with prostate cancer have twice the risk. Those with two first-degree relatives have five times the risk.[60] Germline mutations in the breast cancer predisposition gene 2 (*BRCA2*) are the genetic events known to date that confer the highest risk for prostate cancer (8.6-fold in men 65 years of age and younger). Although the role of *BRCA2* and *BRCA1* in prostate tumourigenesis is still unrevealed, harmful mutations in both genes have been associated with more aggressive disease and poor clinical outcomes.[61] Men with *BRCA2* (tumour suppressor) germline mutations have a two-to-five-times relative risk for prostate cancer. *BRCA1* mutations are associated with a

BOX 34.3 Summary of Diet for Prostate Cancer

- Lower rates of prostate cancer are found in countries whose residents consume a low-fat and high-vegetable diet. When men from a low-risk country move to North America and eat a Western diet, their rates of prostate cancer increase significantly. It is inconclusive what the exact culprits that increase this risk are, but fat and sugar intake seem to be related.
- Obesity is linked to advanced and aggressive prostate cancer.
- High body mass index (BMI) is associated with more aggressive disease and a worse outcome.
- Calorie-dense or excessive carbohydrate intake and obesity, independent of dietary fat intake, may increase the risk of developing prostate cancer.
- Dietary fat may increase levels of androgens, increase oxidative stress, and increase reactive oxygen species (ROS).
- Monounsaturated fats may decrease the risk for prostate cancer.
- High levels of linoleic acid (found in corn oil) act as a proinflammatory eicosanoid. This substance is implicated in promotion of cell proliferation and angiogenesis as well as inhibition of apoptosis.
- The Western diet has increased omega-6 to omega-3 ratios and therefore is proinflammatory. Carcinogenic nitrosamines are formed after consumption of processed meat that has nitrites and from heme iron present in large quantities of red meat.
- Even given the preceding knowledge, it is important to realize that studies showing an association between meat intake and prostate cancers have been largely inconclusive. Some studies reveal red meat is positively associated with increased prostate cancer risk with an association with more aggressive disease states. However, despite some studies showing a 43% elevation in prostate cancer risk with high consumption of red meat, others show no association with prostate cancer risk.
- Although the role of red meat in prostate and breast cancer is still inconclusive, one explanation for the possible associations reported is the accumulation of carcinogens during the cooking process. Cooking meat at high temperatures produces heterocyclic amines and aromatic hydrocarbons that are carcinogenic.
- Vitamin E has long been considered a candidate for prostate cancer prevention based on in vitro and in vivo animal studies. Vitamin E belongs to the family of tocopherols and tocotrienols that exist as α, β, γ, and δ isoforms. Among these, δ-tocopherol is the major dietary isoform, and supplements contain α-tocopherol. Vitamin E is a fat-soluble vitamin obtained from vegetable oils, nuts, and egg yolk. It is a potent intracellular antioxidant known to inhibit peroxidation and DNA damage. The Alpha-Tocopherol, Beta-Carotene Cancer Prevention Study showed that supplementation with vitamin E could reduce the incidence of prostate cancer among men who smoked. In vitro studies show that α-tocopherol succinate induces cell cycle arrest in human prostate cancer cells (i.e., induces apoptosis) and inhibits the androgen receptor (AR). Mouse studies show vitamin E can inhibit the growth-promoting effects of a high-fat diet. Vitamin E in combination with selenium does not reduce the incidence of prostate cancer in LADY mice models. A prospective large clinical trial, the Selenium and Vitamin E Cancer Prevention Trial (SELECT), showed no reduction in prostate cancer period prevalence but an increased risk for prostate cancer with vitamin E alone.
- Selenium is a trace mineral and exists in food as selenomethionine and selenocysteine. It is essential for the functioning of many antioxidant enzymes and proteins in the body. Humans receive selenium in their diet through plant (dependent on soil concentrations) and animal products. SELECT showed that neither selenium nor vitamin E, taken alone or together, helped to prevent prostate cancer.
- Vitamin D may play an important role in prostate cancer prevention.
- Soy anticancer properties include inhibition of cell proliferation and angiogenesis and reduction in prostate-specific antigen (PSA) and AR levels. Countries whose residents have a high intake of soy have much lower rates of prostate cancer.
- Tomatoes or tomato products ingested daily seem to reduce prostate cancer risk. In vitro studies show lycopene found in tomatoes inhibits DNA strand breaks. It is unresolved whether lycopene itself or a metabolic product causes its biological effect. In clinical studies, tomato paste, which is high in lycopene, reduced plasma PSA levels in those men with benign prostatic hyperplasia. Lycopene administration is associated with cell cycle arrest (apoptosis) and growth factor signalling. In 2007, the US Food and Drug Administration evaluated 13 available studies and found the relationship between lycopene and reduced risk for prostate cancer inadequate.
- Vegetables including broccoli, cabbage, cauliflower, Brussels sprouts, Chinese cabbage, and turnips (all crucifers) may be protective (several epidemiological studies) against prostate cancer. A diet high in broccoli reduced cancer risk. By contrast, four studies revealed no cancer-preventive effects. Cruciferous vegetables have anticancer properties mediated by the phytochemicals phenethyl isothiocyanate, sulforaphane, and indole-3-carbinol. Sulforaphane is a naturally occurring isothiocyanate that was first isolated in broccoli. It protects against carcinogen-induced cancer in many rodents. Mice given 240 mg of broccoli sprouts per day showed a significant reduction in growth of prostate cancer cells. Sulforaphane treatment lowered AR protein and gene expression.
- Green tea has polyphenols, including epigallocatechin gallate (EGCG). Green tea consumption has been associated with a reduced incidence of several cancers, including prostate cancer. Green tea consumed within a balanced controlled diet in humans improved overall antioxidant potential. The potential anticancer effect of green tea from in vitro and experimental studies shows these compounds bind directly to carcinogens and induce phase II enzymes that inhibit heterocyclic amines. EGCG administration decreased NF-$\kappa\beta$ activity. Green tea was shown to inhibit insulinlike growth factor 1 (IGF-1) and increase IGF-binding protein 3 (IGFBP3), leading to inhibition of prostate cancer development and progression. In two small, randomized studies in individuals with high-grade prostatic neoplasia, it showed no effects. However, treatment with a mixture of bioactive compounds that share molecular anticarcinogenic targets may enhance the effect on these targets at low concentrations of individual compounds.
- Epidemiological studies have consistently shown that regular consumption of fruits and vegetables is strongly associated with reduced risk of developing chronic diseases, such as cancer. It is now accepted that the actions of any specific phytonutrient alone do not explain the observed health benefits of diets rich in fruits and vegetables. Clinical trials showed that consumption of phytonutrients did not show consistent preventive effects. Synergistic inhibition of prostate cancer cell growth has been evident when using combinations of low concentrations of various carotenoids or carotenoids with retinoic acid and the active metabolite of vitamin D. Combinations of several carotenoids (e.g., lycopene, phytoene, and phytofluene) or carotenoids and polyphenols (e.g., carnosic acid and curcumin) and/or other compounds (e.g., vitamin E) synergistically inhibit the androgen receptor activity and activate the electrophile/antioxidant response element (EpRE/ARE) transcription system. The activation of EpRE/ARE is up to fourfold higher than the sum of activities of single ingredients.
- Examples of important potential processes that can be targeted in the regulation of tumourigenesis include cholesterol synthesis and metabolites, ROS and hypoxia, macrophage activation and conversion, indoleamine 2,3-dioxygenase regulation of dendritic cells, vascular endothelial growth factor regulation of angiogenesis, fibrosis inhibition, and endoglin and Janus kinase signalling.
- Curcumin has anticarcinogenic potential with well-characterized anti-inflammatory, antiangiogenic, and antioxidant properties. Recent studies report curcumin modulates the Wingless signalling pathway (Wnt) that supports its antiproliferative potential. Curcumin is characteristic of regulating multiple

Continued

BOX 34.3 Summary of Diet for Prostate Cancer—cont'd

targets, a desirable feature in current medication design and medication development. Together with its potential in treating castration-resistant prostate cancer and its safety profile, this feature enables curcumin to serve as an ideal compound for the design and syntheses of agents with improved potential for enhancing clinical therapies used to treat prostate cancer.
- Overall, multiple signalling pathways are involved in prostate cancer development and progression, many of which are affected by dietary and lifestyle factors.

References

Alexander, D. D., Mink, P. J., Cushing, C. A., et al. (2010). A review and meta-analysis of prospective studies of red and processed meat intake and prostate cancer. *Nutrition Journal, 9*, 50. doi:10.1186/1475-2891-9-50.

Astorg, P. (2004). Dietary N-6 and N-3 polyunsaturated fatty acids and prostate cancer risk: a review of epidemiological and experimental evidence. *Cancer Causes and Control, 15*(4), 367–386. doi:10.1023/B:CACO.0000027498.94238.a3.

Beier, R., Bürgin, A., Kiermaier, A., et al. (2000). Induction of cyclin E-cdk2 kinase activity, E2F-dependent transcription and cell growth by Myc are genetically separable events. *EMBO Journal, 19*(21), 5813–5823. doi:10.1093/emboj/19.21.5813.

Casey, S. C., Amedei, A., Aquilano, K., et al. (2015). Cancer prevention and therapy through the modulation of the tumor microenvironment. *Seminars in Cancer Biology, 35*(Suppl.), S199–S223. doi:10.1016/j.semcancer.2015.02.007.

Chen, Q. H. (2015). Curcumin-based anti-prostate cancer agents. *Anti-cancer Agents in Medicinal Chemistry, 15*(2), 138–156.

Dagnelie, P. C., Schuurman, A. G., Goldbohm, R. A., et al. (2004). Diet, anthropometric measures and prostate cancer risk: a review of prospective cohort and intervention studies. *BJU International, 93*(8), 1139–1150. doi:10.1111/j.1464-410X.2004.04795.x.

Demark-Wahnefried, W., & Moyad, M. A. (2007). Dietary intervention in the management of prostate cancer. *Current Opinion in Urology, 17*(3), 168–174. doi:10.1097/MOU.0b013e3280eb10fc.

Freedland, S. J., & Aronson, W. J. (2005). Obesity and prostate cancer. *Urology, 65*(3), 433–439. doi:10.1016/j.urology.2004.08.035.

Giovannucci, E., Liu, Y., Platz, E. A., et al. (2007). Risk factors for prostate cancer incidence and progression in the health professionals follow-up study. *International Journal of Cancer, 121*(7), 1571–1578. doi:10.1002/ijc.22788.

Greenwald, P. (2004). Clinical trials in cancer prevention: current results and perspectives for the future. *Journal of Nutrition, 134*(12, Suppl.), 3507S–3512S.

Hill, P., Wynder, E. L., Barbaczewski, L., et al. (1979). Diet and urinary steroids in Black and White North American men and Black South African men. *Cancer Research, 39*(12), 5101–5105.

Kim, D. J., Gallagher, R. P., Hislop, T. G., et al. (2000). Premorbid diet in relation to survival from prostate cancer (Canada). *Cancer Causes and Control, 11*(1), 65–77.

Kobayashi, N., Barnard, R. J., Henning, S. M., et al. (2006). Effect of altering dietary omega-6/omega-3 fatty acid ratios on prostate cancer membrane composition, cyclooxygenase-2, and prostaglandin E2. *Clinical Cancer Research, 12*(15), 4660–4670. doi:10.1158/1078-0432.CCR-06-0459.

Kolonel, L. N. (2001). Fat, meat, and prostate cancer. *Epidemiologic Reviews, 23*(1), 72–81.

Kristal, A. R., Arnold, K. B., Schenk, J. M., et al. (2008). Dietary patterns, supplement use, and the risk of symptomatic benign prostatic hyperplasia: results from the prostate cancer prevention trial. *American Journal of Epidemiology, 167*(8), 925–934. doi:10.1093/aje/kwm389.

Linnewiel-Hermoni, K., Khanin, M., Danilenko, M., et al. (2015). The anti-cancer effects of carotenoids and other phytonutrients resides in their combined activity. *Archives of Biochemistry and Biophysics, 572*, 28–35. doi:10.1016/j.abb.2015.02.018.

Lloyd, J. C., Antonelli, J. A., Phillips, T. E., et al. (2010). Effect of isocaloric low fat diet on prostate cancer xenograft progression in a hormone deprivation model. *Journal of Urology, 183*(4), 1619–1624. doi:10.1016/j.juro.2009.12.003.

Matsumara, K., Tanaka, T., Kawashima, H., et al. (2008). Involvement of the estrogen receptor beta in genistein-induced expression of p21 (waf1/cip1) in PC-3 prostate cancer cells. *Anticancer Research, 28*(2A), 709–714.

Ngo, T. H., Barnard, R. J., Cohen, P., et al. (2003). Effect of isocaloric low-fat diet on human LAPC-4 prostate cancer xenografts in severe combined immunodeficient mice and the insulin-like growth factor axis. *Clinical Cancer Research, 9*(7), 2734–2743.

Ngo, T. H., Barnard, R. J., Tymchuk, C. N., et al. (2002). Effect of diet and exercise on serum insulin, IGF-1, and IGFBP-1 levels and growth of LNCaP cells in vitro (United States). *Cancer Causes and Control, 13*(10), 929–935.

Ni, J., & Yeh, S. (2007). The roles of alpha-vitamin E and its analogues in prostate cancer. *Vitamins and Hormones, 76*, 493–518. doi:10.1016/S0083-6729(07)76019-3.

Punnen, S., Hardin, J., Cheng, I., et al. (2011). Impact of meat consumption, preparation, and mutagens on aggressive prostate cancer. *PLoS ONE, 6*(11), e27711. doi:10.1371/journal.pone.0027711.

Rodriguez, C., Freedland, S. J., Deka, A., et al. (2007). Body mass index, weight change, and risk of prostate cancer in the Cancer Prevention Study II Nutrition Cohort. *Cancer Epidemiology, Biomarkers and Prevention, 16*(1), 63–69. doi:10.1158/1055-9965.EPI-06-0754.

Salem, S., Salahi, M., Mohseni, M., et al. (2011). Major dietary factors and prostate cancer risk: a prospective multicenter case-control study. *Nutrition and Cancer, 63*(1), 21–27. doi:10.1080/01635581.2010.516875.

Sinha, R., Park, Y., Graubard, B. I., et al. (2009). Meat and meat-related compounds and risk of prostate cancer in a large prospective cohort study in the United States. *American Journal of Epidemiology, 170*(9), 1165–1177. doi:10.1093/aje/kwp280.

Teiten, M., Gaascht, F., Cronauer, M., et al. (2011). Anti-proliferative potential of curcumin in androgen dependent prostate cancer cells occurs through modulation of the Wingless signaling pathway. *International Journal of Oncology, 38*(3), 603–611. doi:10.3892/ijo.2011.905.

Wang, P., Wang, B., Chung, S., et al. (2014). Increased chemopreventive effect by combining arctigenin, green tea polyphenol and curcumin in prostate and breast cancer cells. *RSC Advance, 4*(66), 35242–35250. doi:10.1039/C4RA06616B.

Wright, J. L., Neuhouser, M. L., Lin, D. W., et al. (2011). AMACR polymorphisms, dietary intake of red meat and dairy and prostate cancer risk. *Prostate, 71*(5), 498–506. doi:10.1002/pros.21267.

Zhou, D. Y., Ding, N., Du, Z. Y., et al. (2014). Curcumin analogues with high activity for inhibiting human prostate cancer cell growth and androgen receptor activation. *Molecular Medicine Reports, 10*(3), 1315–1322. doi:10.3892/mmr.2014.2380.

---

moderate prostate cancer risk at younger ages, with a relative risk range of two to four for ages less than 65 years.[61] A common type of somatic mutation that develops into chromosomal rearrangements is the *ETS* gene. The most common epigenetic alteration in prostate cancer is hypermethylation of the glutathione-S-transferase (*GSTP1*) gene found on chromosome 11. Repeated independent, peer-reviewed studies have reported a consistently high sensitivity and specificity of *GSTP1* hypermethylation in prostatectomy or biopsy tissue.[62] There is no clear evidence of a causal link between BPH and prostate cancer, even though they may often occur together. Variations in several other genes related to inflammatory pathways might affect the probability of developing prostate cancer.

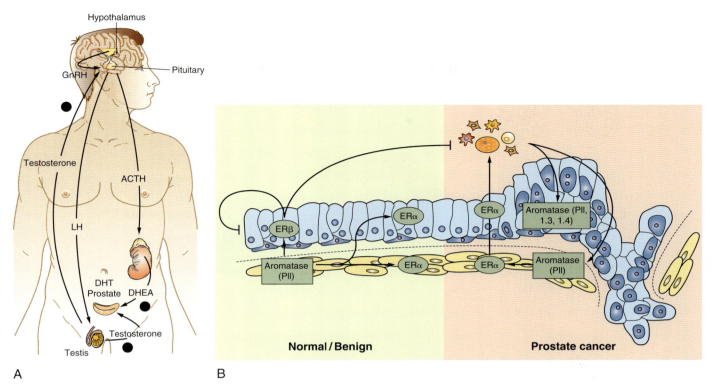

FIGURE 34.14 Sources of Androgens and Aromatase and Estrogen Signalling in the Prostate.
A, Body sources of androgens in the prostate gland. Hypothalamic GnRH causes the release of LH from the anterior pituitary gland. LH stimulates the testes to produce testosterone, which then accumulates in the blood. Pituitary ACTH release stimulates the adrenal glands, which secrete the androgen precursor DHEA into the blood. DHEA is converted into testosterone and then into DHT in the prostate. **B,** Aromatase and estrogen signalling in the prostate. In normal and benign tissue, aromatase is expressed within the stroma and regulated by promoter PII. Estrogen then exerts its effects in an autocrine fashion through the stromal ERα receptor and in a paracrine fashion through both ERα and ERβ receptors. With prostate cancer, aromatase is now expressed within the tumour cells and in stromal cells, and regulated by aromatase promoters 1.3, 1.4, and PII. Thus, estrogen exerts its effects in an autocrine way through stromal and epithelial ERα and ERβ. Consequently, the increased levels of estrogen and abnormal ERα signalling promote inflammation, which increases aromatase expression and the development of a positive feedback cycle. Inflammation drives aromatase expression, thus increasing estrogen, which in turn promotes further inflammation. *ACTH*, Adrenocorticotropic hormone; *DHEA*, dehydroepiandrosterone; *DHT*, dihydrotestosterone; *ERα*, estrogen receptor alpha; *ERβ*, estrogen receptor beta; *GnRH*, gonadotropin-releasing hormone; *LH*, luteinizing hormone. ([A], adapted from Labrie, F. [2011]. *Nature Reviews: Urology, 8*, 73–80; [B], from Ellem, S. J., & Risbridger, G. P. [2010]. *Journal of Steroid Biochemistry and Molecular Biology, 118*[4–5], 246–251.)

PATHOGENESIS More than 95% of prostatic neoplasms are adenocarcinomas.[63] Most of these tumours occur in the periphery of the prostate (see Figures 34.12 and 34.17). Prostatic adenocarcinoma is a heterogeneous group of tumours with a diverse spectrum of molecular and pathological characteristics and diverse clinical behaviours and challenges.[64] The biological aggressiveness of the neoplasm appears to be related to the degree of differentiation rather than the size of the tumour (Box 34.4). Several genetic alterations have been found for prostate carcinoma. These alterations include acquired genomic structural changes, somatic mutations, and epigenetic alterations.[64]

Hormonal factors. Just as the testicles are the male equivalent of the female ovaries, the prostate is the male equivalent of the female uterus. In both situations, they originate from the same embryonic cells. This correspondence may be important in understanding the role of the associated hormones testosterone, DHT, and estrogens in prostate cancer development. Testicular testosterone synthesis and serum testosterone levels fall as men age, but the levels of estradiol remain unchanged or increase with age.[65] The relationship between hormones and the pathophysiology of prostate carcinogenesis is incomplete and controversial.[66,77] The main issues and controversies include (1) sources of androgen production outside of the testes, or extratesticular sources (e.g., from adrenal DHEA and from prostate tissue cholesterol [de novo] itself); (2) the role of prostatic androgen receptor (AR); (3) the role of estrogens, aromatase enzyme, and the estrogen receptors (ERα and ERβ); and (4) the role of the surrounding microenvironment or stroma.

Prostate cancer is a hormone-dependent disease. Cell growth and survival of early-stage prostate cancer can respond to androgens, which is the background evidence for androgen-deprivation therapy (ADT). However, evidence to associate *plasma* androgens with prostate cancer progression is lacking thus far. Prostatic tissue can produce its own steroids, including androgens and estrogens.[67] Therefore, the local tissue levels of sex steroids have become a major focus of intraprostatic hormonal profiles. Prostate tissue has many metabolizing enzymes for the local production of active androgens and estrogens. Carcinogenesis can alter these intraprostatic enzymes and alter the normal balance.

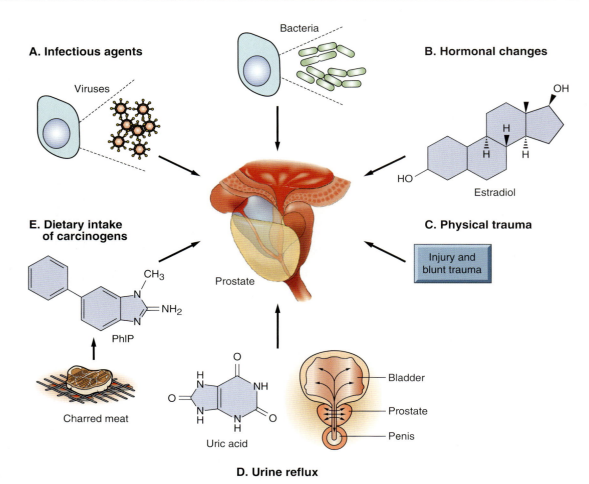

FIGURE 34.15 Possible Causes of Prostate Inflammation. A, Infection, including viruses, bacteria, fungi, and parasites. **B,** Hormones, for example, estrogen at key times during development. **C,** Physical trauma, any type of blunt physical injury. **D,** Urine reflex. **E,** Certain dietary factors (see text).

The androgenic hormone responses in the normal prostate and prostate cancer are mediated by **androgen receptor (AR) signalling**.[52] Exactly how AR drives the growth of prostate cancer cells is not fully known. Several mechanisms have been suggested.[52] Specific pathways of signalling are important because they can supply novel therapeutic targets. A recent study using animal models found that loss of AR function prevented prostatic carcinogenesis, malignant transformation, and metastasis. Tissue-specific evaluation of androgen hormone action showed that epithelial AR was not necessary for prostate cancer progression. However, stromal AR was essential for prostate cancer progression, malignant transformation, and metastasis.[54]

Testicular testosterone provides the main source of androgens in the prostate (see Figure 34.14) and is the major *circulating* androgen. DHT predominates in prostate tissue and binds to the AR with greater affinity than does testosterone.[68] The adrenal cortex contributes the far less potent DHEA, which promotes synthesis of androgens in the prostate. In the target tissues and, to a lesser extent, in the testes themselves, testosterone is converted to DHT by the enzyme 5α-reductase (Figure 34.18). Thus, DHT is the most potent intraprostatic androgen.

Normally, a small amount of estrogen is produced daily—estrone and estradiol—by the aromatization of androstenedione and testosterone, respectively. This reaction is catalyzed by the enzyme aromatase. The testes release a small quantity of estradiol (see Figure 34.18). The rest of the estrogens in males are produced by adipose tissue, liver, skin, brain, and other nonendocrine tissue. Thus, testosterone is a precursor of two hormones—DHT and estradiol.

Studies show that aromatase is expressed in stromal tissue in the benign human prostate gland.[1,52] It appears that both normal prostate and benign prostate have the ability to locally metabolize androgens to estrogens through aromatase. This finding leads to the following question: How does aromatase gene expression contribute to the etiology and progression of prostate cancer? Investigators have shown altered aromatase expression in prostate cancer[69,70] (Figure 34.14B).

Accumulating evidence shows that estrogens take part in the pathogenesis and development of BPH and prostate cancer by activating estrogen receptor alpha (ERα). In contrast, estrogen receptor beta (ERβ) is involved in the differentiation and maturation of prostatic epithelial cells, and thus possesses antitumour effects in prostate cancer.[70] The effect of estrogen is determined by the two receptors ERα and ERβ. ERα leads to abnormal proliferation, inflammation, and the development of premalignant lesions.[70] In contrast, ERβ leads to antiproliferative, anti-inflammatory, and potentially anticarcinogenic effects that act in concert or balance the actions of ERα and androgens.[70] Increased expression of ERα has been found to be associated with prostate cancer progression, metastasis, and the so-called castration-resistant (medical treatment that suppresses androgens) phenotype.[71] A specific oncogene is regulated by ERs, and those hormones that stimulate the ERα

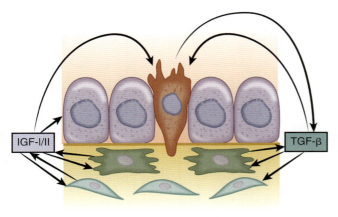
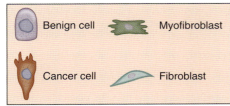

FIGURE 34.16 **Working Model Stromal–Epithelial Interaction in Prostate Cancer Development and Progression.** Normally, signalling events between transforming growth factor-beta *(TGF-β)* and insulinlike growth factor *(IGF)* are tightly controlled, keeping the epithelial cells under allostatic balance. TGF-β binds to receptors on the cell surface known as receptor type I (TBR-I) and type II (TBR-II). A reduction in TBRs in the stromal cells will result in an increase in IGF production. The increase in IGF has a proliferative effect on the prostate epithelial cells (which have already undergone a cancer initiation process because of the hormones testosterone and estradiol). TGF-β and IGF in the stromal cells next to prostate epithelial cells will perpetuate a vicious cycle to promote cancer progression. (Adapted from Lee, C., Jia, Z., Rahmatpanah, F., et al. [2014]. *Biomedical Research International, 2014*, 502093.)

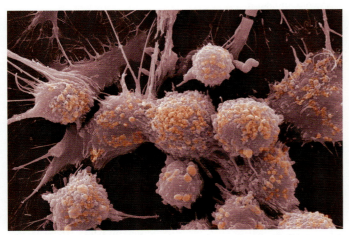

FIGURE 34.17 **Photomicrograph of Prostate Cancer Cells.** Pink ruffled cells are prostate cancer cells. (Dr. Gopal Murti/Science Source.)

receptorlike (i.e., agonists) endogenous estrogens can stimulate oncogene expression.[72,73]

Most of the androgen-metabolizing enzymes undergo a significant age-dependent alteration. In epithelium, both the blood levels of 5α-reductase activity and the DHT level decrease with age. In stroma (prostate), not only the 5α-reductase activity but also the stromal DHT level is rather constant over the lifetime. In contrast to

> BOX 34.4 **Determining the Grade of Prostate Cancer With the Gleason Score**
>
> *Grade 1.* The cancer cells closely resemble normal cells. They are small, uniform in shape, evenly spaced, and well differentiated (i.e., they remain separate from one another).
> *Grade 2.* The cancer cells are still well differentiated, but they are arranged more loosely and are irregular in shape and size. Some of the cancer cells have invaded the neighbouring prostate tissue.
> *Grade 3.* This grade is the most common. The cells are less well differentiated (some have fused into clumps) and are more variable in shape.
> *Grade 4.* The cells are poorly differentiated and highly irregular in shape. Invasion of the neighbouring prostate tissue has progressed further.
> *Grade 5.* The cells are undifferentiated. They have merged into large masses that no longer resemble normal prostate cells. Invasion of the surrounding tissue is extensive.

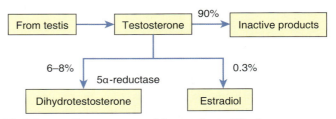

FIGURE 34.18 Testosterone and Conversion to Dihydrotestosterone.

the relatively unaltered DHT level over time, the estrogen concentration follows an age-dependent increase. Thus, the age-dependent decrease of the DHT accumulation in epithelium and the concomitant increase of the estrogen accumulation in stroma lead to a tremendous increase with age of the estrogen/androgen ratio in the human prostate. In animal studies, chronic exposure to testosterone plus estradiol is strongly carcinogenic, whereas testosterone alone is weakly carcinogenic.[52] In mice studies, elevated testosterone level in the absence of estrogen leads to the development of hypertrophy and hyperplasia but not malignancy.[1,74] High estrogen and low testosterone levels have been shown to lead to inflammation with aging and the emergence of precancerous lesions.[74] The mechanism is not clearly understood and may involve estrogen-generated oxidative stress and DNA toxicity. The mechanism requires androgen-mediated and estrogen receptor–mediated processes, such as changes in sex steroid metabolism and receptor status. In addition, there are changes in the balance between autocrine/paracrine growth-stimulatory and growth-inhibitory factors, such as the IGFs.[52]

Investigators have summarized the following key findings on hormones and prostate cancer: (1) androgens are clearly involved in the progression of prostate cancer; (2) it is only with the addition of estrogen to testosterone in rats that cancer can be reliably induced; (3) in vivo and in vitro studies have found multiple mechanisms connecting hormonal involvement with genotoxicity, epigenetic toxicity, hyperprolactinemia, chronic inflammation, and estrogen receptor–mediated changes.[75]

Prostate epithelial neoplasia. A precursor lesion, **prostatic intraepithelial neoplasia (PIN)**, has been described. PIN may be more concentrated in prostates having cancer and is noted in proximity to cancer.[76] However, the final fate of PIN is unknown, including the possibilities of latency, invasion, and even regression. The current working model of prostate carcinogenesis suggests that repeated cycles of injury and cell death occur to the prostate epithelium because of damage

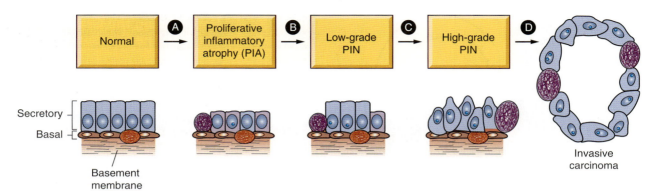

FIGURE 34.19 Cellular and Molecular Model of Early Prostate Neoplasia Progression. **A**, This stage includes infiltration of lymphocytes, macrophages, and neutrophils caused by repeated infections, dietary factors, urine reflux, injury, onset of autoimmunity (which triggers inflammation), and wound healing. **B**, Epigenetic alterations mediate telomere shortening. **C**, Genetic instability and accumulation of genetic alterations. **D**, Continued proliferation of genetically unstable cells leading to cancer progression. *PIN*, Prostatic intraepithelial neoplasia.

(i.e., from oxidative stress) from inflammatory responses.[77] The direct injury is hypothesized as a response to infections; autoimmune disease; circulating carcinogens or toxins, or both, from the diet; or urine that has refluxed into the prostate (see Figure 34.15). The resultant manifestation of this injury is focal atrophy or PIA. Biological responses cause an increase in proliferation and a massive increase in epithelial cells that have a phenotype between basal cells and mature luminal cells[77] (Figure 34.19). In a small subset of cells, some may have "stem cell" or tumour-initiating properties and telomere shortening (see Chapter 10). A subset of PIN cells may activate telomerase enzyme, causing the cells to become immortal.[78] Molecular genetic and epigenetic changes can increase genetic instability that might progress to high-grade PIN and early prostate cancer formation. This model of prostate carcinogenesis needs much more research.

Stromal environment. The prostate gland is composed of secretory luminal epithelium, basal epithelium, neuroendocrine cells, and various cell types that form supportive tissue or stroma. **Stroma**, or tissue microenvironment, produces autocrine/paracrine factors as well as structural supporting molecules that help regulate normal cell behaviour and organ allostasis.[64] Stromal components in the tumour microenvironment are important contributors to tumour progression and metastasis.[64] Reciprocal interactions between tumour cells and stromal components influence the metastatic, dormancy-related, and stem cell–like potential of tumour cells.[79] The stromal compartment of the tumour is complex and includes inflammatory/immune cells, vascular endothelial cells, pericytes, fibroblasts, adipocytes, and components of the extracellular matrix.[64,79] Tumour-infiltrating inflammatory cells release a host of growth factors, chemokines, cytokines, and proinvasive matrix-degrading enzymes that promote tumour growth and progression.[79] Angiogenesis occurs in response to factors secreted from tumour cells, resulting in continued growth and progression. Adipocytes in the tumour microenvironment produce adipokines, which are important for tumour growth.[80] **Fibroblasts** in the tumour microenvironment supply the structural framework of the stroma. They are still quiet or dormant, but proliferate during wound healing, inflammation, and cancer.[81] Tumour cells release paracrine factors that activate fibroblasts to become cancer-associated fibroblasts (CAFs). CAFs secrete factors that modulate tumour growth and change the stroma to enhance metastasis and dampen responses to anticancer therapies.[81] These findings suggest that alteration occurs in the prostate microenvironment with therapeutic agents and approaches. In particular, natural products such as berberine, resveratrol, onionin A, epigallocatechin gallate, genistein, curcumin, naringenin, desoxyrhapontigenin, piperine, and zerumbone require further investigation into their abilities to target the tumour microenvironment for the treatment and prevention of cancer.[82]

Epithelial–mesenchymal transition (EMT) was first described in embryonic development, and it is seen in several solid tumours[83] (see Chapter 10). Cells that undergo EMT become more migratory and invasive and gain access to vascular vessels.[84] Numerous studies have shown that these transition states (EMT and mesenchymal–epithelial transition [MET]) are a consequence of tumour–stromal interactions.[85] Investigators studying prostate cancer cells in vitro correlated EMT with increased growth, migration, and invasion.[86] These investigators demonstrated that the microenvironment is a critical site for the transition of human prostate cancer cells from epithelial to mesenchymal structure, resulting in increased metastatic potential for bone and adrenal gland.[86]

Prostate cancer is known to be diverse and composed of multiple genetically distinct cancer cell clones. Recent studies, however, show that most metastatic cancers arise from a single precursor cancer cell.[87]

From all of these observations, the following multifactorial general hypothesis of prostate carcinogenesis emerges: (1) androgens act as strong tumour promoters through AR-mediated mechanisms to enhance the carcinogenic activity of strong endogenous DNA toxic carcinogens, including reactive estrogen metabolites and estrogen, and prostate-generated ROS; (2) reciprocal interactions between tumour cells and the stromal microenvironment promote prostate cancer pathogenesis; and (3) possibly unknown environmental–lifestyle carcinogens may contribute to prostate cancer. All these factors are modulated by diet and genetic determinants. These factors include hereditary susceptibility genes and polymorphic genes, which encode receptors and enzymes involved in the metabolism and action of steroid hormones.[52]

The most common sites of distant metastasis are the lymph nodes, bones, lungs, liver, and adrenals. The pelvis, lumbar spine, femur, thoracic spine, and ribs are the most common sites of bone metastasis. Local extension is usually posterior, although late in the disease the tumour may invade the rectum or encroach on the prostatic urethra and cause bladder outlet obstruction (Figure 34.20). Figure 34.21 illustrates the spread of cancer through blood vessels.

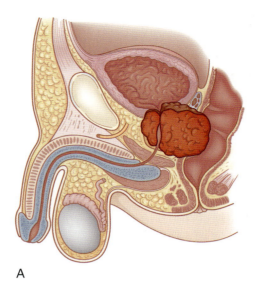

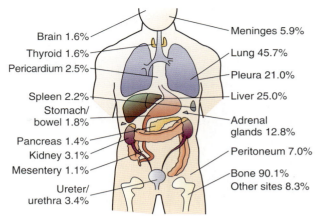

FIGURE 34.21 **Distribution of Hematogenous Metastases in Prostate Cancer.** Based on an autopsy study of 1589 patients with metastatic prostate cancer. (Adapted from Budendorf, L., Schöpfer, A., Wagner, U., et al. [2000]. Metastatic patterns of prostate cancer: an autopsy study of 1,589 patients. *Human Pathology, 31*[5], 578–583.)

EVALUATION AND TREATMENT Screening for prostatic cancer includes DRE and PSA blood tests. There is lack of evidence, however, whether screening with PSA or DRE reduces mortality from prostate cancer.[1] It is unclear whether detection of prostate cancer at an early stage leads to any change in the natural history or outcome.[1] Observational studies in some countries show a trend toward lower mortality. The relationship between the intensity and trends of screening is not clear and the associations with screening are inconsistent.[1] The observed trends may be a result of screening or improved treatment. Two randomized trials show no effect on mortality through 7 years and are inconsistent beyond 7 to 10 years.[88,89] Strong evidence shows implementation of PSA or DRE detects some prostate cancers that would never have caused significant clinical problems.[89] These screening tests lead to some degree of overtreatment. The screening tests can harm patients. These tests may lead to radical prostatectomy and radiation therapy that result in irreversible side effects in many men.[89] The most common side effects are erectile dysfunction and urinary incontinence. The screening process can cause considerable anxiety, especially in men who have a prostate biopsy but no identified prostate cancer. Screening can lead to biopsies, which are associated with complications. Complications include fever, pain, hematuria, hematospermia, positive urine cultures for bacteria, and, rarely, sepsis. About 20 to 70% of men who had no problems before radical prostatectomy or external-beam radiation therapy will have reduced sexual function or urinary problems, or both.

Prostate cancer usually grows very slowly and is predominantly a tumour of older men, with the median age of diagnosis at 72 years.[89] Until recently, many primary care providers and organizations encouraged yearly PSA screening for men beginning at age 50. However, with more understanding about the benefits and detriments, several organizations have cautioned men against routine population screening (Figure 34.22). Some organizations continue to recommend PSA screening. Some tumours found through PSA screening do not cause symptoms, grow slowly, and are unlikely to threaten a man's life. The PSA screening test often suggests that prostate cancer may be present when there is no cancer. This is called a "false positive" result. False-positive results lead to unnecessary follow-up tests. Detecting these benign tumours is called overdiagnosis.

Across age ranges, Black men, and men with a family history of prostate cancer have an increased risk of developing and dying

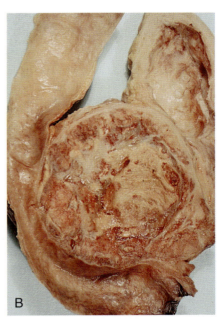

FIGURE 34.20 **Carcinoma of Prostate. A,** Schematic of carcinoma of the prostate. **B,** Carcinoma of the prostate extending into the rectum and urinary bladder. ([B] from Damjanov, I., & Linder, J. [Eds]. [2000]. *Pathology: a color atlas.* Mosby.)

CLINICAL MANIFESTATIONS Prostatic cancer often causes no symptoms until it is far advanced. The first manifestations of disease are those of bladder outlet obstruction. These symptoms include slow urinary stream, hesitancy, incomplete emptying, frequency, nocturia, and dysuria. Unlike the symptoms of obstruction caused by BPH, the symptoms of obstruction caused by prostatic cancer are progressive and do not remit. Local extension of prostatic cancer can obstruct the upper urinary tract ureters as well. Rectal obstruction also may occur, causing the individual to experience large bowel obstruction or difficulty in defecation. Symptoms of late disease include bone pain at sites of bone metastasis, edema of the lower extremities, enlargement of lymph nodes, liver enlargement, pathological bone fractures, and mental confusion associated with brain metastases. Prostatic cancer and its treatment can affect sexual functioning.

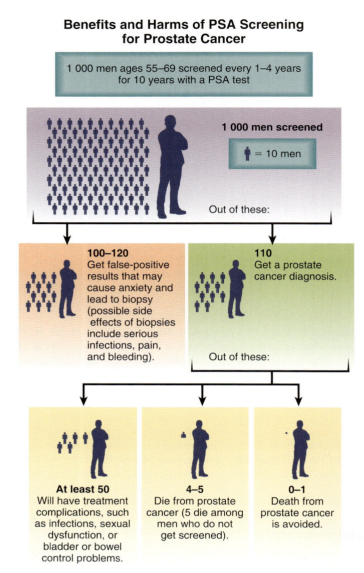

FIGURE 34.22 Benefits and Harms of PSA Screening for Prostate Cancer. The US Preventive Services Task Force (PSTF) recommends against PSA-based screenings for prostate cancer (grade D recommendation). *PSA*, Prostate-specific antigen. (Adapted from Moyer, V. A., & U.S. Preventive Services Task Force. [2012]. Screening for prostate cancer: U.S. Preventive Services Task Force recommendation statement. Annals of Internal Medicine, 157[2]:120–134. doi:10.7326/0003-4819-157-2-201207170-00459.)

of prostate cancer. Black men are approximately twice as likely to die of prostate cancer compared with men of other races in North America. The reason for this disparity is unknown. Black men are a very small minority of participants in randomized clinical trials of screening, and thus no firm conclusions can be made about the balance of benefits and harms of PSA-based screening in this population. As such, it is questionable practice to selectively recommend PSA-based screening for Black men in the absence of data that support a more favourable balance of risks and benefits.[90] Because of this "overtreatment" phenomenon, active surveillance with delayed intervention is gaining traction as a practical management approach in contemporary practice.

Treatment of prostatic cancer depends on the stage of the neoplasm, the expected effects of treatment, and the age, general health, and life expectancy of the individual. Options include no treatment; surgical treatments, such as total prostatectomy, transurethral resection of the prostate, or cryotherapy; nonsurgical treatments, such as radiation therapy, hormone therapy, corticosteroids, high intensity focused ultrasound or chemotherapy; watchful waiting; and any combination of these treatment modalities.[90,91] In addition, new approaches are using immunotherapy. Palliative treatment is aimed at relieving urinary, bladder outlet, or colon obstruction; spinal cord compression; and pain. Box 34.5 shows staging for prostate cancer. Survival varies with each stage or the grade of prostate cancer. Prognosis and survival rates have improved steadily over the past 50 years. Over the past 25 years, the 5-year relative survival rate for all stages combined has increased from 68% to almost 100%. In Canada, the 5-year net survival for prostate cancer is 93%.[92]

Stress incontinence can occur after surgery and mild urge incontinence can occur after radiation therapy. Prostate cancer and its treatment can affect sexual functioning. Sensation of orgasm is not usually affected, but smaller amounts of ejaculate will be produced, or men may experience a "dry" ejaculate because of retrograde ejaculation.

Sexual Dysfunction

In males, the normal sexual response involves erection, emission, and ejaculation. **Sexual dysfunction** is the impairment of any or all these processes and can be caused by various physiological, psychological, and emotional factors.

Until the late 1970s, most cases of male sexual dysfunction were considered psychogenic. Now there is evidence that 89 to 90% of cases involve organic factors and include (1) vascular, endocrine, and neurological disorders; (2) chronic disease, including kidney failure and diabetes mellitus; (3) penile diseases and penile trauma; and (4) iatrogenic factors, such as surgery and pharmacological therapies. Most of these disorders cause erectile dysfunction.[1]

PATHOPHYSIOLOGY Sexual dysfunction can have a specific physiological cause, can be associated with many chronic diseases and their treatment, or may be related to low energy levels, stress, or depression. For example, vascular disease may cause erectile dysfunction, and endocrine disorders or conditions that cause decreased testosterone levels or testicular atrophy can diminish sexual functioning or libido. In addition, neurological disorders and spinal cord injuries can interfere with sympathetic, parasympathetic, and central nervous system mechanisms needed for erection, emission, and ejaculation.

Medication-induced sexual dysfunction consists of decreased desire, decreased erectile ability, or decreased ejaculatory ability. Alcohol and other central nervous system depressants, antihypertensives, antidepressants, antihistamines, and hormonal preparations are commonly used medications that affect sexual functioning. Other pharmacological agents may diminish the quality or quantity of sperm or cause priapism.

CLINICAL MANIFESTATIONS AND TREATMENT Evaluation of sexual dysfunction includes a thorough history and physical examination. Particular attention is given to medication history and examination of the genitalia, prostate, and nervous system. Basic laboratory tests are used to show the presence of endocrinopathies or other underlying disorders that can cause dysfunction. Psychological evaluation is indicated for younger men with a sudden onset of sexual dysfunction or for men of any age who can achieve but not keep an erection. If

BOX 34.5 Staging for Prostate Cancer

Stage I

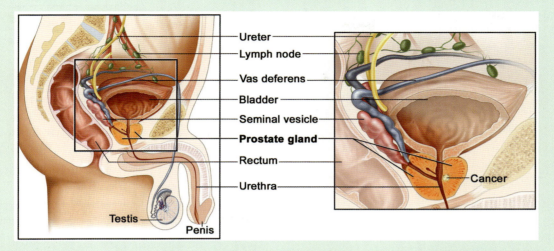

In stage I, cancer is found in the prostate only. In this stage, cancer:
- Is found by performing a needle biopsy (done for a high prostate-specific antigen [PSA] level) or by examining a small amount of tissue during surgery for other reasons (such as benign prostatic hyperplasia). The PSA level is lower than 10, and the Gleason score is 6 or lower; *or*
- Is found on half or less of one lobe of the prostate. The PSA level is lower than 10, and the Gleason score is 6 or lower; *or*
- Cannot be felt during a digital rectal examination and cannot be seen in imaging tests. Cancer is found in half or less of one lobe of the prostate. The PSA level and the Gleason score are not known.

Stage II
In stage II, cancer is more advanced than in stage I, but has not spread outside the prostate. Stage II is divided into stages IIA and IIB.

Stage IIA
In stage IIA, cancer:
- Is found by performing a needle biopsy (done for a high PSA level) or by examining a small amount of tissue during surgery for other reasons (such as benign prostatic hyperplasia). The PSA level is lower than 20, and the Gleason score is 7; *or*
- Is found by performing a needle biopsy (done for a high PSA level) or by examining a small amount of tissue during surgery for other reasons (such as benign prostatic hyperplasia). The PSA level is at least 10 but lower than 20, and the Gleason score is 6 or lower; *or*
- Is found in half or less of one lobe of the prostate. The PSA level is at least 10 but lower than 20, and the Gleason score is 6 or lower; *or*
- Is found in half or less of one lobe of the prostate. The PSA level is lower than 20, and the Gleason score is 7; *or*
- Is found in more than half of one lobe of the prostate.

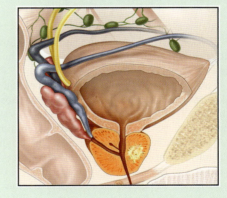

Stage IIB
In stage IIB, cancer:
- Is found on opposite sides of the prostate. The PSA can be any level, and the Gleason score can range from 2 to 10; *or*
- Cannot be felt during a digital rectal examination (DRE) and cannot be seen in imaging tests. The PSA level is 20 or higher, and the Gleason score can range from 2 to 10; *or*
- Cannot be felt during a DRE and cannot be seen in imaging tests. The PSA can be any level, and the Gleason score is 8 or higher.

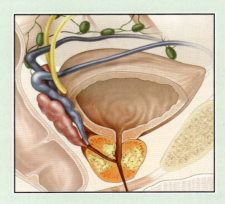

Continued

> **BOX 34.5 Staging for Prostate Cancer—cont'd**
>
> **Stage III**
> In stage III, cancer has spread beyond the outer layer of the prostate and may have spread to the seminal vesicles. The PSA can be any level, and the Gleason score can range from 2 to 10.
>
>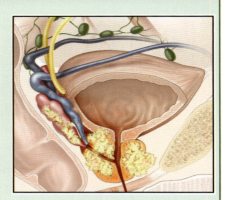
>
> **Stage IV**
> In stage IV, the PSA can be any level, and the Gleason score can range from 2 to 10. Also, in this stage, cancer:
> - Has spread beyond the seminal vesicles to nearby tissue or organs, such as the rectum, bladder, or pelvic wall; *or*
> - May have spread to the seminal vesicles or to nearby tissue or organs, such as the rectum, bladder, or pelvic wall. Cancer has spread to nearby lymph nodes; *or*
> - Has spread to distant parts of the body, which may include lymph nodes or bones. Prostate cancer often spreads to the bones.
>
>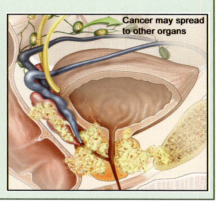

Data from National Cancer Institute. (2020). *Prostate cancer treatment (PDQ®)—Patient version*. https://www.cancer.gov/types/prostate/patient/prostate-treatment-pdq. Figures © 2010 by Terese Winslow; U.S. Government has certain rights.

no physiological cause is found and the condition does not improve with psychotherapy, the man is referred for further investigation of organic causes.

Treatments for organic sexual dysfunction include both medical and surgical approaches. The advent of phosphodiesterase type 5 inhibitors (PDE5i) has revolutionized the erectile dysfunction treatment landscape and supplied effective, minimally invasive therapies to restore male sexual function. The original PDE5i, sildenafil (Viagra), has created much enthusiasm over its ability to help a man keep an erection. For approximately 1% of men, however, this improvement in sexual function is accompanied by heart attacks and death. Whether these effects are the result of sexual performance or sildenafil has been controversial. Research has shown that sildenafil increases blood concentrations of the enzyme cyclic guanosine monophosphate (cGMP)–dependent protein kinase G (PKG), which increases blood flow to the penis. PKG, however, plays a dual role: first, it increases platelet aggregation; and then, minutes later, it decreases clot size. The first clot could cause some men with heart disease to experience cardiac arrest.

Currently available PDE5i medications in Canada include sildenafil, vardenafil (Levitra), tadalafil (Cialis), and avanafil (Stendra), each of which has unique side effect profiles. For instance, sildenafil is associated with cardiac issues and an increased rate of visual changes, vardenafil with QT prolongation, and tadalafil with lower back pain.[93] Nonsurgical approaches include correction of underlying disorders, particularly medication-induced dysfunction and endocrinopathy-related (e.g., reduced testosterone level associated with chronic kidney disease) dysfunction. Use of vasodilators and cessation of smoking can help individuals with vasculogenic erectile dysfunction. Surgical approaches include penile implants, penile revascularization, and correction of other anatomical defects contributing to sexual dysfunction.

Impairment of Sperm Production and Quality

Spermatogenesis requires adequate secretion of FSH and luteinizing hormone (LH) by the pituitary and sufficient secretion of testosterone by the testes. Inadequate secretion of gonadotropins may be caused by many alterations (e.g., hypothyroidism, hyperadrenocorticolism, hyperprolactinemia, or hypogonadotropic hypogonadism). In the absence of adequate gonadotropin levels, the Leydig cells are not stimulated to secrete testosterone, and sperm maturation is not promoted in the Sertoli cells. Spermatogenesis also depends on a proper response by the testes. Defects in testicular response to the gonadotropins result in decreased secretion of testosterone and inhibin B. These responses occur because of normal feedback mechanisms and high levels of circulating gonadotropins. In the absence of adequate testosterone levels, spermatogenesis is impaired. Newer studies show the importance of inhibin B as a valuable marker of the competence of Sertoli cells and spermatogenesis.[1] Impaired spermatogenesis also can be caused by testicular trauma, infection, atrophy of the testes, systemic illness involving high fever, ingestion of various medications, exposure to environmental toxins, and cryptorchidism.

Fertility is adversely affected if spermatogenesis is normal, but the sperm are chromosomally or morphologically abnormal or are produced in insufficient quantities. Chromosomal abnormalities are caused by genetic factors and by external variables, such as exposure to radiation or toxic substances. Because the Y chromosome plays a key role in testis determination and control of spermatogenesis, understanding how the genes interact can elucidate exact causes of infertility. The most common mutations are microdeletion of the Y chromosome.[94] Research related to mapping the critical genes and gene pathways is the current focus of male infertility. Common mechanisms may be involved in infertility and testicular cancer. In utero environmental exposure to endocrine disruptors modulates the genetic makeup of the gonad and may result in both infertility and testicular cancer.[22]

Sperm motility also may affect fertility. Motility appears to be affected by the characteristics of the semen. Dysfunction of the prostate, excessive viscosity of the semen, presence of medications or toxins in the semen, and presence of antisperm antibodies are associated with impaired sperm motility. However, new data show that motile density may not be a good indicator of infertility.[95] Approximately 17% of infertile males have antisperm antibodies in their semen. These antibodies may be (1) cytotoxic antibodies, which attack sperm and reduce their number in the semen, or (2) sperm-immobilizing antibodies, which impair sperm motility and reduce their ability to traverse the endocervical canal.

Treatment for impaired spermatogenesis involves correcting any underlying disorders, avoiding radiation and possibly electromagnetic radiation (hypothesis from cellphones) and toxins, and using hormones to enhance spermatogenesis. In addition, semen can be changed to improve sperm motility; modifications are followed by artificial insemination.

DISORDERS OF THE MALE BREAST

> ✓ **QUICK CHECK 34.5**
> 1. What is the cause of male gynecomastia?
> 2. What are the risk factors for male breast cancer?
> 3. What factors increase the incidence of sexually transmitted infections (STIs)?
> 4. What are the long-term health consequences of getting syphilis for men who have sex with men?

Gynecomastia

Gynecomastia is the overdevelopment of breast tissue in a male. Gynecomastia accounts for approximately 85% of all masses that develop in the male breast and affects 32 to 40% of the male population. If only one breast is involved, it is typically the left. Incidence is greatest among adolescents and men older than 50 years.

Gynecomastia results from hormonal alterations, which may be idiopathic or caused by systemic disorders, medications, or neoplasms. Gynecomastia usually involves an imbalance of the estrogen/testosterone ratio. The normal estrogen/testosterone ratio can be altered in one of two ways. First, estrogen levels may be excessively high, although testosterone levels are normal. This is the case in medication-induced and tumour-induced hyperestrogenism. Second, testosterone levels may be extremely low, although estrogen levels are normal, as is the case in hypergonadism. Gynecomastia also can be caused by alterations in breast tissue responsiveness to hormonal stimulation. Breast tissue may have increased responsiveness to estrogen or decreased responsiveness to androgen. Alterations of responsiveness may cause many cases of idiopathic gynecomastia.

Besides puberty and aging, estrogen/testosterone imbalances are associated with hypogonadism, Klinefelter's syndrome, and testicular neoplasms. Hormone-induced gynecomastia is usually bilateral. Pubertal gynecomastia is a self-limiting phenomenon that usually disappears within 4 to 6 months. Senescent gynecomastia usually regresses spontaneously within 6 to 12 months.

Systemic disorders associated with gynecomastia include cirrhosis of the liver, infectious hepatitis, chronic kidney disease, chronic obstructive lung disease, hyperthyroidism, tuberculosis, and chronic malnutrition. It may be that these disorders ultimately alter the estrogen/testosterone ratio, starting the gynecomastia.

Gynecomastia is often seen in males receiving estrogen therapy, either in preparation for a gender-change operation or in the treatment of prostatic carcinoma. Other medications that can cause gynecomastia include digitalis (Digoxin), cimetidine (Tagamet), spironolactone (Aldactone), reserpine (Serpasil), thiazide (Hydrochlorothiazide), isoniazid (Rifater), ergotamine (Bellergal Spacetabs), tricyclic antidepressants, amphetamines, vincristine (Oncovin), and busulfan (Busulfex). Gynecomastia is usually unilateral in these instances.

Malignancies of the testes, adrenals, or liver can cause gynecomastia if they alter the estrogen/testosterone ratio. Pituitary adenomas and lung cancer also are associated with gynecomastia.

PATHOPHYSIOLOGY The enlargement of the breast consists of hyperplastic stroma and ductal tissue. Hyperplasia results in a firm, palpable mass that is at least 2 cm in diameter and found beneath the areola.

EVALUATION AND TREATMENT The diagnosis of gynecomastia is based on physical examination. Identification and treatment of the cause are likely to be followed by resolution of the gynecomastia. The man should be taught to perform breast self-examination and is re-examined at 6- and 12-month intervals if the gynecomastia persists.

Carcinoma

Breast cancer in males accounts for less than 1% of all breast cancers.[96] The Canadian Cancer Society estimated that 240 men were diagnosed with breast cancer in 2020. It also estimated that 55 men died of this disease in 2020.[96] About 20% of men with breast cancer have a first-degree relative with breast cancer.[97] Male breast cancer (MBC) is seen most commonly after the age of 60 years, with the peak incidence between 60 and 69 years (men tend to be diagnosed at an older age than women). Klinefelter's syndrome is the strongest risk factor for developing MBC. Other risk factors include germline mutation in *BRCA1* or *BRCA2*, but familial cases usually have *BRCA2* mutations.[98] Obesity increases the risk for MBC. Testicular disorders, including cryptorchidism, mumps, orchitis, and orchiectomy, are related to risk.[99] The relationship between these factors and the risk for disease is not clearly defined.

Recent data on the most frequent molecular subtypes of MBC appear to be different than those for female breast cancers. Luminal A and luminal B are most common; and basal-like, unclassifiable triple-negative, and *HER2*-driven MBCs are rare.[100,101] Male breast tumours often resemble carcinoma of the breast in women. The majority of MBCs express estrogen and progesterone receptors. The malignant male breast lesion is usually a unilateral solid mass found near the nipple. Because the nipple is commonly involved, crusting and nipple discharge are typical clinical manifestations. Other findings include skin retraction, ulceration of the skin over the tumour, and axillary node involvement. Patterns of metastasis are like those in females.

The diagnosis of cancer is confirmed by biopsy. Because of delays in seeking treatment, MBC tends to be advanced at the time of diagnosis and therefore is likely to have a poor prognosis. Treatment protocols are like those for female breast cancer, but endocrine therapy is used more often for males because a higher percentage of male tumours are hormone dependent. The mainstay of treatment is modified mastectomy with axillary node dissection to assess stage and prognosis. Because 90% of tumours are hormonal-receptor positive, tamoxifen (Nolvadex) is standard adjuvant therapy. Orchiectomy is performed to treat metastatic disease. For metastatic disease, hormonal therapy is the main treatment, but chemotherapy also can supply palliation.[98]

SEXUALLY TRANSMITTED INFECTIONS

Sexually transmitted infections (STIs) are a variety of clinical syndromes and infections caused by pathogens that can be acquired and transmitted through sexual activity. Trends in all reportable STIs in Canada have revealed a dramatic increase in the last decade. Similar increases in reportable STI rates have been seen in Australia, the United Kingdom, and the United States.[102] From 2008 to 2017, rates of gonorrhea and infectious syphilis were higher among males compared to females, with males comprising most infectious syphilis cases in all years. Young Canadians have the highest reported rates of STIs; however, increased rates have been reported among middle-aged and older adults[102] (Table 34.1). STIs can lead to severe reproductive health problems, for example, infertility and ectopic pregnancy.[102] Untreated or undertreated chlamydial infections are the primary cause of preventable infertility and ectopic pregnancy. In addition to ectopic pregnancy and infertility, other complications of STIs include pelvic inflammatory disease (PID), chronic pelvic pain, neonatal morbidity and mortality, genital cancer, and epidemiological synergy with HIV transmission (Table 34.2). Long-term sequelae of untreated or undertreated STIs may be disastrous and can affect a person's physical, emotional, and financial well-being. Treatment guidelines for STIs can be found on the Centers for Disease Control and Prevention website (https://www.cdc.gov/std/treatment-guidelines/toc.htm).

Anyone can become infected with an STI, but young people and gay and bisexual men are at greatest risk.[102] Young people between the ages of 20 and 24 years have the highest reported rates of chlamydia, and females between the ages of 20 and 24 years and males between the ages of 20 and 29 years account for the highest rates of gonorrhea. Both young men and women are negatively affected by STIs, but young women have the most serious long-term health consequences. Undiagnosed STIs may cause PID, which may lead to chronic abdominal pain, infertility, and ectopic pregnancy.[102] In Canada, it has been suggested that recent increases in the incidence of syphilis are largely related to transmission among men who have sex with men (MSM) who engage in high-risk sexual practices. The majority of all reported cases of infectious syphilis was among men aged 30 years and older. Primary and secondary syphilis are the most infectious stages of the disease and, if not treated adequately, can lead to visual impairment and stroke.[102] Syphilis infection raises the risk of getting and transmitting HIV infection and is a common and concerning occurrence.[102]

Individual risk behaviours, such as higher numbers of lifetime sex partners and environmental, social, and cultural factors, contribute to health disparities of MSM, for example, difficulty accessing health care. Homophobia and stigma also can make it difficult for gay and bisexual men to find culturally sensitive and appropriate care and treatment.[102] STI screening is critical. It is recommended that women who are sexually active and younger than 25 years of age or have multiple sex partners be tested annually for chlamydia and gonorrhea. A woman should request syphilis, HIV, chlamydia, and hepatitis B testing early in her pregnancy. These tests also should be requested if a woman has a new partner or multiple sex partners.[102] Recommended tests include syphilis, chlamydia, gonorrhea, and HIV once a year for gay, bisexual, or other MSM. More frequent testing is recommended for men at high risk.

TABLE 34.1 Currently Recognized Sexually Transmitted Infections

Causal Microorganism	Infection	Causal Microorganism	Infection
Bacteria		Herpes simplex virus (HSV)	Genital herpes
Campylobacter	Campylobacter enteritis	Human immunodeficiency virus (HIV)	Acquired immune deficiency syndrome (AIDS)
Klebsiella granulomatis	Granuloma inguinale		
Chlamydia trachomatis	Urogenital infections; lymphogranuloma venereum	Human papillomavirus (HPV)	Condylomata acuminata, cervical dysplasia, and cervical cancer
Polymicrobial		Molluscum contagiosum virus	Molluscum contagiosum
Gardnerella vaginalis interaction with anaerobes (*Bacteroides* and *Mobiluncus* spp.) and genital mycoplasmas	Bacterial vaginosis	**Protozoa**	
		Entamoeba histolytica	Amebiasis; amebic dysentery
		Giardia lamblia	Giardiasis
Haemophilus ducreyi	Chancroid	*Trichomonas vaginalis*	Trichomoniasis
Mycoplasma	Mycoplasmosis	**Ectoparasites**	
Neisseria gonorrhoeae	Gonorrhea		
Shigella	Shigellosis	*Pthirus pubis*	Pediculosis pubis (crab louse)
Treponema pallidum	Syphilis	*Sarcoptes scabiei*	Scabies
Viruses		**Fungus**	
Cytomegalovirus	Cytomegalic inclusion disease	*Candida albicans*	Candidiasis
Hepatitis B virus (HBV)	Hepatitis		
Hepatitis C virus (HCV)	Hepatitis		

CHAPTER 34 Alterations of the Male Reproductive System

TABLE 34.2 Photographs of Sexually Transmitted Infections and Precursors to Sexually Transmitted Infections

Bacterial Sources
Gonococcal Infections

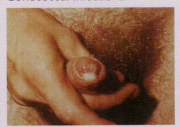

Symptomatic Gonococcal Urethritis.[a]

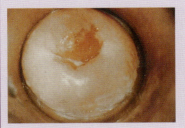

Endocervical Gonorrhea.[a]

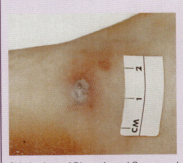

Skin Lesions of Disseminated Gonococcal Infection.[a]

Bacterial Vaginosis

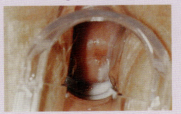

Vaginal Examination Showing Mild Bacterial Vaginosis.[a]

Syphilis

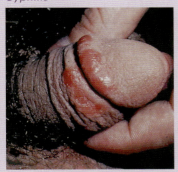

Erythematous Penile Plaques of Secondary Syphilis.[b]

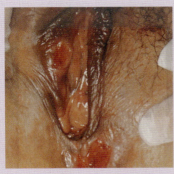

Multiple Primary Syphilitic Chancres of Labia and Perineum. (Courtesy Barbara Romanowski, MD.)[a]

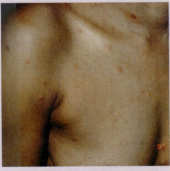

Papular Secondary Syphilis.[a]

Lymphogranuloma

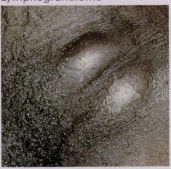

"Groove Sign" in Man With Lymphogranuloma Venereum (LV).[b]

Chlamydial Infections

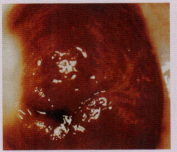

Beefy Red Mucosa in Chlamydial Infection.[a]

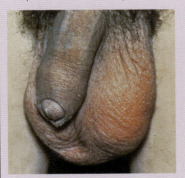

Chlamydial Epididymitis. (Courtesy Richard E. Berger.)[a]

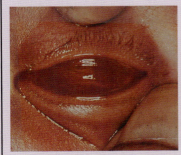

Chlamydial Ophthalmia: Erythematous Conjunctiva in Infant.[a]

Continued

TABLE 34.2 Photographs of Sexually Transmitted Infections and Precursors to Sexually Transmitted Infections—cont'd

Viral Sources
Genital Herpes

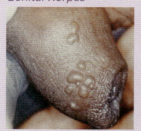
Early Lesions of Primary Genital Herpes.[a]

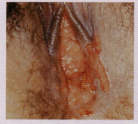
Primary Vulvar Herpes. (Courtesy Barbara Romanowski, MD.)[a]

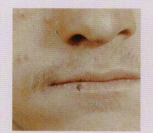
Generalized Herpes Simplex in Patient With Atopic Dermatitis. (Courtesy David Mandeville and Peter Lane, MD.)[a]

Human Papillomavirus

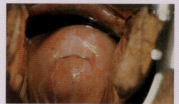
Human Papillomavirus (HPV) Infection of the Cervix.[b]

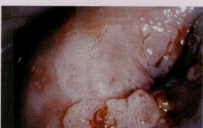
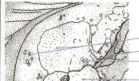
Exophytic (Outward-Growing) Condyloma, Subclinical Human Papillomavirus (HPV) Infection, and High-Grade Cervical Intraepithelial Neoplasia (CIN).[b]

- Subclinical HPV infection
- Cervical os
- Cervical intraepithelial neoplasia
- Exophytic condyloma

Condylomata Acuminata

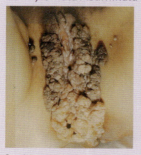
Condylomata Acuminata: Vulva and Perineum.[a]

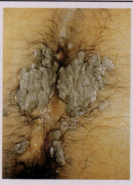
Condylomata Acuminata: Penile.[a]

Condylomata Acuminata: Perianal.[a]

Parasite Sources
Trichomoniasis

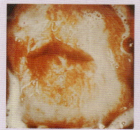
"Strawberry Cervix" Seen With Trichomoniasis.[a]

Scabies

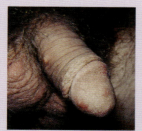
Nodular Lesions of Scabies on Male Genitalia.[b]

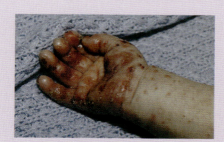
Scabies of Palm With Secondary Pyoderma in Infant.[a]

TABLE 34.2 Photographs of Sexually Transmitted Infections and Precursors to Sexually Transmitted Infections—cont'd

Pediculosis Pubis (*Pthirus pubis* [Crablouse])

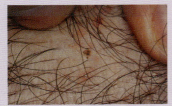

Pthirus pubis Feeding on Its Host.[a]

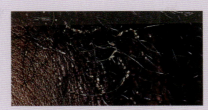

Pubic Hair With Multiple Nits.[a]

[a]From Morse, S. A., Holmes, K. K., & Ballard, R. C. (2010). *Atlas of sexually transmitted diseases and AIDS* (4th ed.). Elsevier.
[b]From Morse, S. A., Moreland, A. A., & Holmes, K. K. (1996). *Atlas of sexually transmitted diseases and AIDS* (2nd ed.). Elsevier.

CASE STUDY

Elias D'Youville is a 75-year-old male who states that he is not getting enough sleep at night because he must urinate at least four times each night after he has gone to bed. He also states that each time he goes to the bathroom, only a little bit of urine comes out. He is also experiencing urgency and has had trouble making it to the bathroom on time. He is wondering what is going on with his urinary system and wants the primary care provider to figure it out.

History of Present Illness: Elias has also experienced four urinary tract infections over the past year and had one episode of pyelonephritis where he had to be hospitalized for a week. He currently is complaining of a 2-month history of urinary frequency, urgency, occasional incontinence and nocturia. He is afebrile and reports no dysuria, nausea, vomiting, hematuria, or penile discharge. His last urinary tract infection was 1 month ago and was treated with antibiotics.

Past Medical Hx: COPD for 6 years, dyslipidemia × 10 years and osteoarthritis × 15 years. No surgical history.

Family Hx: His father had type 2 diabetes mellitus and died at age 68 of a myocardial infarction. His mother had hypertension and breast cancer. She lived until the age of 78. He has one sister who is in good health. He has one older brother, age 82, who has been diagnosed with benign prostatic hyperplasia (BPH). He has two daughters who are in good health.

Medications: Ibuprofen PRN for osteoarthritis pain, rosuvastatin for dyslipidemia and ipratropium bromide MDI for COPD, no vitamin, or herbal supplements

Social History: A retired mechanic, widower for 5 years, consumes alcohol socially during holidays and on special occasions, 1 pack per day cigarette smoker × 45 years but quit 20 years ago, no recreational drugs, drinks four to five cups of coffee or tea daily, no exercise, not sexually active since his wife's death, eats a well-balanced diet.

Review of Systems: Unremarkable with the exception of urinary symptoms. Occasionally finds it difficult to start urination and has been having post-void dribble for about 8 months.

Physical Exam: Appears stated age; well-groomed overweight Black male in no distress. Integumentary, HEENT, neck/lymph nodes, respiratory, cardiovascular, neurological, and gastro-intestinal examination unremarkable except for a slightly distended bladder. Bilateral decreased ROM and discomfort of knees, peripheral pulses 2+ bilaterally. Normal male genitalia, no discharge, erythema, or lesions. No inguinal lymphadenopathy, no herniation. Digital rectal examination for a large smooth prostate with no nodules or tenderness. Rectal exam negative for hemorrhoids, normal anal sphincter tone, Stool for OB negative.

Vital signs: BP 132/84 LA sitting; pulse 79 regular; RR 18 unlaboured; temperature 36.8°C oral; BMI 30.

Critical Thinking and Clinical Judgement Questions

1. The primary care provider suspects a diagnosis of benign prostatic hyperplasia. Identify four possible contributing factors for this diagnosis.
2. Based on the information provided, identify five clinical signs and symptoms in this patient that are consistent with a diagnosis of a benign prostatic hyperplasia.
3. Name the diagnostic tests that the primary care provider could order to confirm the diagnosis of benign prostatic hyperplasia, and indicate what each test is assessing.
4. Discuss how the primary care provider would distinguish between BPH, prostate cancer, and prostatitis.

DID YOU UNDERSTAND?

Alterations of Sexual Maturation

1. Sexual maturation, or puberty, begins in boys between the ages of 9 and 14.5 years.
2. Delayed puberty is the onset of sexual maturation after 14.5 years. Precocious puberty is sexual maturation occurring before age 9. Treatment for delayed, precocious, or absent puberty depends on the cause.

Disorders of the Male Reproductive System

1. Disorders of the urethra include urethritis and urethral strictures.
2. Most cases of urethritis result from sexually transmitted pathogens. Urological instrumentation, foreign body insertion, trauma, or an anatomical abnormality can cause urethral inflammation with or without infection.
3. Urethritis causes urinary symptoms, dysuria, frequency, urgency, urethral tingling, or itching, and clear or purulent discharge.
4. The scarring that causes urethral stricture can be attributed to trauma or severe untreated urethritis.
5. Manifestations of urethral stricture include those of bladder outlet obstruction: urinary frequency and hesitancy, diminished force, and calibre of the urinary stream, dribbling after voiding, and nocturia.
6. Phimosis and paraphimosis are penile disorders involving the foreskin (prepuce). In phimosis, the foreskin cannot be retracted over

the glans. In paraphimosis, the foreskin is retracted and cannot be reduced. Phimosis is caused by poor hygiene and chronic infection and can lead to paraphimosis. Paraphimosis can constrict the penile blood vessels, preventing circulation to the glans.
7. Peyronie disease consists of fibrosis affecting the corpora cavernosa, which causes penile curvature during erection. Fibrosis prevents engorgement on the affected side, causing a lateral curvature that can prevent intercourse.
8. Priapism is a prolonged, painful erection that is not stimulated by sexual arousal. The corpora cavernosa (but not the corpus spongiosum) fill with blood that will not drain from the area, probably because of venous obstruction. Priapism is associated with spinal cord trauma, sickle cell disease, leukemia, and pelvic tumours. It can also be idiopathic.
9. Balanitis is an inflammation of the glans penis. It is associated with phimosis, inadequate cleansing under the foreskin, skin disorders, and pathogens (e.g., *Candida albicans*).
10. Carcinoma of the penis is rare in Canada. Penile carcinoma in situ tends to involve the glans; invasive carcinoma of the penis involves the shaft as well.
11. A varicocele is an abnormal dilation of the testicular veins within the spermatic cord caused either by congenital absence of valves in the internal spermatic vein or by acquired valvular incompetence.
12. A hydrocele is a collection of fluid between the testicular and scrotal layers of the tunica vaginalis. Hydroceles can be idiopathic or caused by trauma or infection of the testes.
13. A spermatocele is a cyst found between the testis and epididymis that is filled with fluid and sperm.
14. Cryptorchidism is a congenital condition in which one or both testes do not descend into the scrotum. Uncorrected cryptorchidism is associated with infertility and significantly increased risk for testicular cancer.
15. Testicular torsion is the rotation of a testis, which twists blood vessels in the spermatic cord. This rotation interrupts the blood supply to the testis, resulting in edema and, if not corrected within 6 hours, necrosis, and atrophy of testicular tissues.
16. Orchitis is an acute inflammation of the testes. Complications of orchitis include hydrocele and abscess formation.
17. Testicular cancer is the most common malignancy in males 15 to 35 years of age. Although its cause is unknown, high androgen levels, genetic predisposition, and history of cryptorchidism, trauma, or infection may contribute to tumourigenesis.
18. Epididymitis, an inflammation of the epididymis, is usually caused by a sexually transmitted pathogen that ascends through the vasa deferentia from an already infected urethra or bladder.
19. Benign prostatic hyperplasia (BPH) is the enlargement of the prostate gland. This condition becomes symptomatic as the enlarging prostate compresses the urethra, causing symptoms of bladder outlet obstruction and urine retention.
20. Prostatitis is an inflammation of the prostate. Prostatitis syndromes have been classified by the US National Institutes of Health as (a) acute bacterial prostatitis (ABP), (b) chronic bacterial prostatitis (CBP), (c) chronic pelvic pain syndrome (CPPS), and (d) asymptomatic inflammatory prostatitis.
21. Prostate cancer is the most-often diagnosed nonskin cancer in men in Canada. Its incidence varies greatly worldwide. Possible causes include genetic predisposition, environmental and dietary factors, inflammation, and alterations in levels of hormones (testosterone, dihydrotestosterone, and estradiol) and growth factors. Incidence is greatest in men in developed countries, men older than 65 years, and Black men.
22. Most cancers of the prostate are adenocarcinomas that develop at the periphery of the gland.
23. Sexual dysfunction in males can be caused by any physical or psychological factor that impairs erection, emission, or ejaculation.
24. Spermatogenesis can be impaired by disruptions of the hypothalamic–pituitary–testicular axis that reduce testosterone secretion and by testicular trauma, infection, or atrophy from any cause. Sperm production is also impaired by neoplastic disease, cryptorchidism, or any factor that causes testicular temperature to rise (e.g., circulatory impairment, wearing tight clothing).

Disorders of the Male Breast

1. Gynecomastia is the overdevelopment (hyperplasia) of breast tissue in a male. It is first seen as a firm, palpable mass at least 2 cm in diameter and is in the subareolar area.
2. Gynecomastia affects 32 to 40% of the male population. The incidence is greatest among adolescents and men older than 50 years of age.
3. Gynecomastia is caused by hormonal or breast tissue alterations that cause estrogen to dominate. These alterations can result from systemic disorders, medications, neoplasms, or idiopathic causes.
4. Breast cancer is relatively uncommon in males, but it has a poor prognosis because men tend to delay seeking treatment until the disease is advanced. The incidence is greatest in men in their 60s.
5. Most breast cancers in men are estrogen-receptor positive.

Sexually Transmitted Infections

1. Sexually transmitted infections (STIs) are contracted through intimate as well as sexual contact and include systemic infections, such as tuberculosis and hepatitis, which can spread to a sexual partner.
2. The etiology of an STI may be bacterial, viral, protozoan, parasitic, or fungal.

35

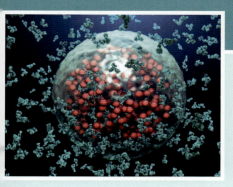

Structure and Function of the Digestive System

Mohamed Toufic El-Hussein, with originating chapter contributions by Sue E. Huether

Additional resources are available online at https://evolve.elsevier.com/Canada/Huether/pathophysiology.

CHAPTER OUTLINE

The Gastro-intestinal Tract, 862
 Mouth and Esophagus, 862
 Stomach, 864
 Large Intestine, 871
 Intestinal Microbiome, 873
 Splanchnic Blood Flow, 873

Accessory Organs of Digestion, 873
 Liver, 874
 Gallbladder, 877
 Exocrine Pancreas, 877
GERIATRIC CONSIDERATIONS: Aging and the Gastro-Intestinal System, 880

LEARNING OBJECTIVES

1. Describe the process leading to the breakdown of food, nutrient uptake by the body's cells, and elimination of waste products.
2. Describe the normal structure and function of the gastro-intestinal tract.
3. List the enzymes responsible for the digestion and absorption of carbohydrates, fats, and proteins.
4. Identify the specific locations of absorption for the major nutrients.
5. List the functional divided segments of the small and large intestines.
6. Describe haustral segmentation and peristalsis.
7. Describe the three major neural reflexes of the small intestine and explain their effects on motility, digestion, and absorption.
8. Describe the movement of chyme and feces through the large intestine, ending in defecation.
9. Describe the characteristic actions of normal intestinal flora.
10. Briefly describe splanchnic blood flow.
11. List the accessory organs of digestion and briefly explain their functions related to digestion.
12. Identify the major functions of the liver.
13. Discuss the formation and secretion of bile.
14. Discuss how bilirubin is metabolized.
15. Discuss the process of metabolism of fats, proteins, and carbohydrates.
16. Describe the function of the gallbladder.
17. Discuss the exocrine functions of the pancreas.

KEY TERMS

Ampulla of Vater, 877
Antrum, 864
Ascending colon, 871
Bile, 875
Bile acid pool, 875
Bile acid–dependent fraction, 875
Bile acid–independent fraction, 875
Bile canaliculi, 874
Bile salt, 875
Bilirubin, 876
Body of the stomach, 864
Brush border, 869
Cardiac orifice, 864
Cecum, 871
Chief cell, 867
Cholecystokinin, 865
Choleresis, 876
Choleretic agent, 876
Chyme, 864
Colon, 871
Common bile duct, 874
Conjugated bilirubin, 876
Crypts of Lieberkühn, 869
Cystic duct, 877
Deamination, 876
Defecation reflex (rectosphincteric reflex), 873
Descending colon, 871
Disse space, 875
Duodenum, 868
Enteric (intramural) plexus, 862
Enterocytes, 869
Enterohepatic circulation, 875
Enterokinase, 878
Esophageal phase of swallowing, 864
Esophagus, 864
Exocrine pancreas, 877
External anal sphincter, 871
Fecal mass, 872
Fundus, 864
Gallbladder, 877
Gastric emptying, 866
Gastric gland, 867
Gastrin, 865
Gastrocolic reflex, 872
Gastroileal reflex, 870
Gastro-intestinal (GI) tract, 862
Glisson capsule, 874
Haustral segmentation, 869
Haustrum (*pl.*, haustra), 872
Hepatic artery, 874
Hepatic portal vein, 874
Hepatic vein, 874
Hepatocyte, 874
Ileocecal valve (sphincter), 868
Ileogastric reflex, 870
Ileum, 868
Internal anal sphincter, 871
Intestinointestinal reflex, 870
Intrinsic factor, 867
Jejunum, 868
Kupffer cell (tissue macrophage), 875
Lacteal, 869
Lamina propria, 869
Large intestine, 871
Liver, 874
Liver lobule, 874

Lower esophageal sphincter (cardiac sphincter), 864
Major duodenal papilla, 873
Mesentery, 868
Metabolic detoxification (biotransformation), 877
Microvillus (*pl.*, microvilli), 869
Motilin, 865
Mouth, 862
Mucosal barrier, 867
Myenteric plexus (Auerbach plexus), 865
Natural killer cells (pit cells), 874
Oropharyngeal (voluntary) phase of swallowing, 864
Pancreas, 877
Pancreatic duct (Wirsung duct), 877
Paneth cell, 873
Parietal cell, 867
Pepsin, 867
Peristalsis, 862
Peritoneal cavity, 868
Peritoneum, 868
Peyer patch, 873
Primary bile acid, 875
Primary peristalsis, 864
Pyloric sphincter, 864
Pylorus (gastroduodenal junction), 864
Rectosigmoid (O'Beirne) sphincter, 871
Rectum, 873
Reticuloendothelial system, 876
Retropulsion, 866
S cell, 878
Saliva, 862
Salivary α-amylase (ptyalin), 862
Salivary gland, 862
Secondary bile acid, 875
Secondary peristalsis, 864
Secretin, 865
Sigmoid colon, 871
Sinusoid, 874
Small intestine, 868
Sphincter of Oddi, 868
Splanchnic blood flow, 873
Stellate cells, 874
Stomach, 864
Submucosal plexus (Meissner plexus), 865
Swallowing, 864
Teniae coli, 872
Transverse colon, 871
Trypsin inhibitor, 878
Unconjugated bilirubin, 876
Upper esophageal sphincter, 864
Urobilinogen, 876
Valsalva manoeuvre, 873
Vermiform appendix, 871
Villus (*pl.*, villi), 869

The digestive system includes the gastro-intestinal (GI) tract and accessory organs of digestion: the salivary glands, liver, gallbladder, and exocrine pancreas (Figure 35.1). The digestive system breaks down ingested food, prepares it for uptake by the body's cells, absorbs fluid, and eliminates wastes. Food breakdown begins in the mouth with chewing and continues in the stomach, where food is churned and mixed with acid, mucus, enzymes, and other secretions. From the stomach, the fluid and partially digested food pass into the small intestine, where biochemical agents and enzymes secreted by the intestinal cells, liver, gallbladder, and exocrine pancreas break it down into absorbable components of proteins, carbohydrates, and fats. These nutrients pass through the walls of the small intestine into blood vessels and lymphatics that carry them to the liver for storage or further processing.

Ingested substances and secretions that are not absorbed in the small intestine pass into the large intestine, where fluid continues to be absorbed. Fluid wastes travel to the kidneys and are eliminated in the urine. Solid wastes pass into the rectum and are eliminated from the body through the anus. Except for chewing, swallowing, and defecation of solid wastes, the movements of the digestive system (**peristalsis**) are all controlled by hormones and the autonomic nervous system. The autonomic innervation, both sympathetic and parasympathetic, is controlled by centres in the brain and by local stimuli that are mediated at plexuses (networks of nerve fibres) within the GI walls. The GI tract and gut microbiome provide important immune and protective functions. Aging can alter the structure and function of the GI tract (see *Geriatric Considerations:* Aging and the Gastro-intestinal System).

THE GASTRO-INTESTINAL TRACT

QUICK CHECK 35.1
1. What are the functions of saliva?
2. What are the phases of swallowing and how are they controlled?

The **gastro-intestinal (GI) tract** (alimentary canal) consists of the mouth, esophagus, stomach, small intestine, large intestine, rectum, and anus (see Figure 35.1). It carries out the following digestive processes:
- Ingests food
- Propels food and wastes from the mouth to the anus
- Secretes mucus, water, and enzymes
- Mechanically digests food particles
- Chemically digests food particles
- Absorbs digested food
- Eliminates waste products by defecation
- Provides immune and microbial protection against infection

Histologically, the GI tract consists of four layers. From the inside out they are the mucosa, submucosa, muscularis, and serosa (or adventitia). These concentric layers vary in thickness, and each layer has sublayers (Figure 35.2). A network of intrinsic nerves that controls mobility, secretion, sensation, and blood flow is located solely within the GI tract and controlled by local and autonomic nervous system stimuli through the **enteric (intramural) plexus** located in different layers of the GI walls (see Figure 35.2).

Mouth and Esophagus

The **mouth** is a reservoir for the chewing and mixing of food with saliva. There are 32 permanent teeth in the adult mouth, and they are important for speech and mastication. As food particles become smaller and move around in the mouth, the taste buds and olfactory nerves are continuously stimulated, adding to the satisfaction of eating. The tongue's surface contains thousands of chemoreceptors, or taste buds, which can distinguish salty, sour, bitter, sweet, and savoury (umami) tastes. Tastes and food odours help to initiate salivation and the secretion of gastric juice in the stomach.

Salivation

The three pairs of **salivary glands**—the submandibular, sublingual, and parotid glands (Figure 35.3)—secrete about 1 L of saliva per day. **Saliva** consists mostly of water with mucus, sodium, bicarbonate, chloride, potassium, and **salivary α-amylase (ptyalin)**, an enzyme that initiates carbohydrate digestion in the mouth and stomach.

Both sympathetic and parasympathetic divisions of the autonomic nervous system control salivation. Cholinergic parasympathetic fibres stimulate the salivary glands, and atropine (an anticholinergic agent) inhibits salivation and makes the mouth dry. β-Adrenergic stimulation from sympathetic fibres also increases salivary secretion. The salivary gland secretion is not regulated by hormones.

The composition of saliva depends on the rate of secretion (Figure 35.4). Aldosterone can increase epithelial exchange of sodium for potassium, increasing sodium conservation and potassium excretion. The bicarbonate concentration of saliva sustains a pH of about 7.4, which neutralizes bacterial acids and prevents tooth decay. Saliva also

CHAPTER 35 Structure and Function of the Digestive System

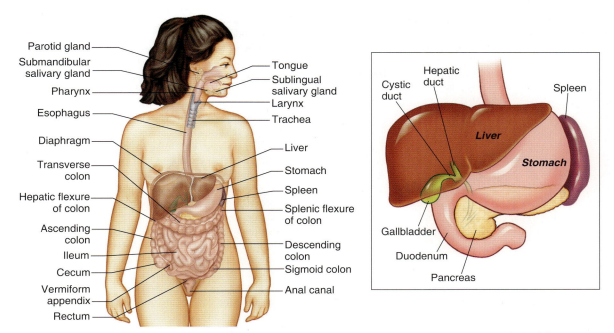

FIGURE 35.1 Structures of the Digestive System. (From Patton, K. T. [2019]. *Anatomy and physiology* [10th ed.]. Elsevier.)

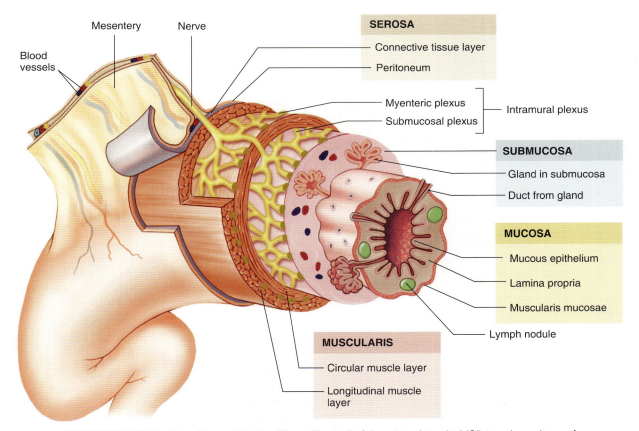

FIGURE 35.2 Wall of the Gastro-intestinal Tract. The wall of the gastro-intestinal (GI) tract is made up of four layers with a network of nerves between the layers. This generalized diagram shows a segment of the GI tract. Note that the serosa is continuous with a fold of serous membrane called the *mesentery*. Note also that digestive glands may empty their products into the lumen of the GI tract by way of ducts. (From Patton, K. T. [2019]. *Anatomy & physiology* [10th ed.]. Elsevier.)

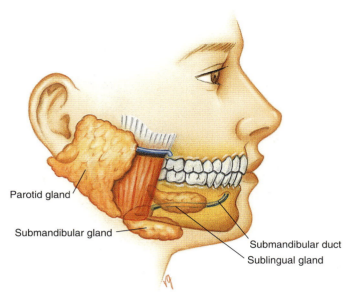

FIGURE 35.3 Salivary Glands. (From Gerdin, J. [2012]. *Health careers today* [5th ed.]. Mosby.)

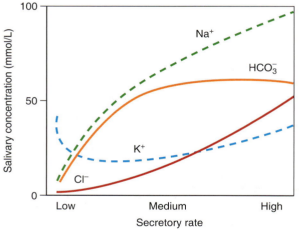

FIGURE 35.4 Salivary Electrolyte Concentrations and Flow Rate. Changes in concentrations of sodium (Na^+), potassium (K^+), chloride (Cl^-), and bicarbonate (HCO_3^-) increase flow rate of saliva. *Green line*, sodium; *orange line*, bicarbonate; *red line*, chloride; *blue line*, potassium. At low rates of salivary flow (i.e., between meals), sodium, chloride, and bicarbonate are reabsorbed in the collecting ducts of the salivary glands, and the saliva contains fewer of these electrolytes (i.e., is more hypotonic). At higher flow rates (i.e., stimulated by food), reabsorption decreases and saliva is hypertonic. By this mechanism, sodium, chloride, and bicarbonate are recycled until they are released to help with digestion and absorption.

contains mucin, immunoglobulin A (IgA), and other antimicrobial substances, which help prevent infection. Mucin provides lubrication. Exogenous fluoride (e.g., fluoride in drinking water) is also secreted in the saliva, providing additional protection against tooth decay.

Swallowing

The **esophagus** is a hollow, muscular tube approximately 25 cm long that guides substances from the oropharynx to the stomach (see Figure 35.1). Swallowed food is moved to the stomach by peristalsis, the coordinated sequential contraction and relaxation of outer longitudinal and inner circular layers of muscles. The pharynx and upper third of the esophagus contain striated muscle (voluntary) that is directly innervated by skeletal motor neurons that control swallowing. The lower two-thirds contain smooth muscle (involuntary) that is innervated by preganglionic cholinergic fibres from the vagus nerve. The fibres are activated in a downward sequence and coordinated by the swallowing centre in the medulla. Peristalsis is stimulated when afferent fibres distributed along the length of the esophagus sense changes in wall tension caused by stretching as food passes. The greater the tension, the greater the intensity of esophageal contraction. Occasionally, intense contractions cause pain similar to "heartburn" or angina.

Each end of the esophagus is opened and closed by a sphincter. The **upper esophageal sphincter** keeps air from entering the esophagus during respiration. The **lower esophageal sphincter (cardiac sphincter)** prevents regurgitation from the stomach and caustic injury to the esophagus.

Swallowing is coordinated primarily by the swallowing centre in the medulla. During the **oropharyngeal (voluntary) phase of swallowing**, the following steps occur:
1. Food is broken up and formed into a bolus by the tongue and forced posteriorly toward the pharynx.
2. The superior constrictor muscle of the pharynx contracts so the food cannot move into the nasopharynx.
3. Respiration is inhibited, and the epiglottis slides down to prevent the food from entering the larynx and trachea.

This entire sequence takes place in less than 1 second.

The **esophageal phase of swallowing** proceeds as follows:
1. The bolus of food enters the esophagus.
2. Waves of relaxation travel the esophagus, preparing for the movement of the bolus.
3. **Peristalsis**, the sequential waves of muscular contractions that travel down the esophagus, transports the food to the lower esophageal sphincter, which is relaxed at that point.
4. The bolus enters the stomach, and the sphincter muscles return to their resting tone.

This phase takes 5 to 10 seconds, with the bolus moving 2 to 6 cm/sec. Peristalsis that immediately follows the oropharyngeal phase of swallowing is called **primary peristalsis**. If a bolus of food becomes stuck in the esophageal lumen, **secondary peristalsis**—a wave of contraction and relaxation independent of voluntary swallowing—occurs. This secondary peristalsis occurs in response to stretch receptors (stimulated by increased wall tension) that activate impulses from the swallowing centre of the brain.

The lower esophageal sphincter is normally constricted and serves as a barrier between the stomach and esophagus. The muscle tone of the lower sphincter changes with neural and hormonal stimulation and relaxes with swallowing. Cholinergic vagal input and the digestive hormone gastrin increase sphincter tone. Nonadrenergic, noncholinergic vagal impulses relax the lower esophageal sphincter, as do the hormones progesterone, secretin, and glucagon.[1]

Stomach

> ✓ **QUICK CHECK 35.2**
> 1. Why are there three layers of stomach muscle and how do they function?
> 2. What hormones stimulate gastric motility?
> 3. What are the phases of gastric secretion?

The **stomach** is a hollow, muscular organ just below the diaphragm that stores food during eating, secretes digestive juices, mixes food with these juices, and propels partially digested food, called **chyme**, into the duodenum of the small intestine. The anatomy of the stomach is presented in Figure 35.5. The stomach's major anatomical boundaries

CHAPTER 35 Structure and Function of the Digestive System

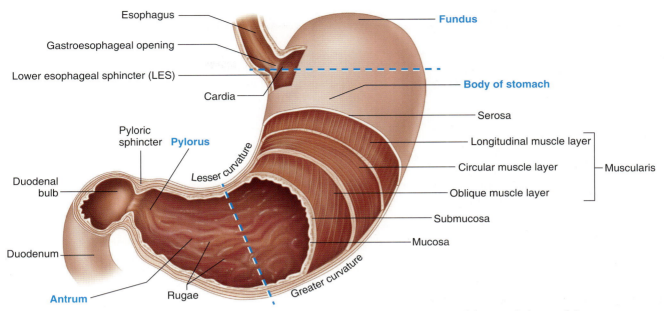

FIGURE 35.5 **Stomach.** A portion of the anterior wall has been excised to reveal the muscle layers of the stomach wall. Note that the mucosa lining the stomach forms folds called *rugae*. The dashed lines distinguish the fundus, body, and antrum of the stomach. (Modified from Patton, K. T., & Thibodeau, G. A. [2018]. *The human body in health & disease* [7th ed.]. Elsevier.)

are the lower esophageal sphincter, where food passes through the **cardiac orifice** at the gastroduodenal junction into the stomach, and the **pyloric sphincter**, which relaxes as food is propelled through the **pylorus (gastroduodenal junction)** into the duodenum. Functional areas are the **fundus** (upper portion), **body of the stomach** (middle portion), and **antrum** (lower portion).

The stomach has three layers of smooth muscle: an outer, longitudinal layer; a middle, circular layer; and an inner, oblique layer (the most prominent) (see Figure 35.5). These layers become progressively thicker in the body and antrum where food is mixed and pushed into the duodenum. The glandular epithelium is discussed under "Gastric Secretion".

The stomach's blood supply comes from a branch of the celiac artery (Figure 35.6) and is so abundant that nearly all arterial vessels must be blocked before ischemic changes occur in the stomach wall. A series of small veins drain blood from the stomach toward the hepatic portal vein.

Sympathetic and parasympathetic divisions of the autonomic nervous system innervate the stomach. Some of the autonomic fibres are extrinsic—that is, they originate outside of the stomach and are controlled by nerve centres in the brain. The vagus nerve provides parasympathetic innervation, and branches of the celiac plexus innervate the stomach sympathetically. The **myenteric plexus (Auerbach plexus)** and the **submucosal plexus (Meissner plexus)** are intrinsic and part of the enteric (intramural) nervous system. They originate within the stomach and respond to local stimuli.

Gastric Motility

In its resting state, the stomach is small and contains about 50 mL of fluid. There is no wall tension, and the muscle layers in the fundus contract very little. Swallowing causes the fundus to relax (receptive relaxation) to receive a bolus of food from the esophagus (see "Swallowing"). Relaxation is coordinated by efferent, nonadrenergic, noncholinergic vagal fibres and is helped by **gastrin** and **cholecystokinin**—two polypeptide hormones secreted by the GI mucosa. (The actions of digestive

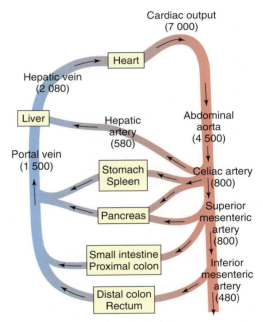

FIGURE 35.6 **Major Blood Vessels and Organs Supplied With Blood in the Splanchnic Circulation.** Numbers in parentheses reflect approximate blood flow values (mL/min) for each major vessel in an 80-kg normal, resting, adult human subject. Arrows indicate the direction of blood flow. (Modified from Johnson, L. R. [2001]. *Gastrointestinal pathophysiology*. Mosby.)

hormones are summarized in Table 35.1.) Food is stored in vertical or oblique layers as it arrives in the fundus, whereas fluids flow relatively quickly down to the antrum.

Gastric (stomach) motility increases with the initiation of peristaltic waves, which sweep over the body of the stomach toward the antrum. The rate of peristaltic contractions is approximately three per minute

TABLE 35.1 Selected Hormones[a] and Neurotransmitters of the Digestive System

Source	Hormone/Neurotransmitter	Stimulus for Secretion	Action
Mucosa of stomach	Gastrin	Presence of partially digested proteins in stomach	Stimulates gastric glands to secrete hydrochloric acid, pepsinogen, and histamine; growth of gastric mucosa
	Histamine	Gastrin	Stimulates acid secretion
	Somatostatin	Acid in stomach	Inhibits acid, pepsinogen, and histamine secretion and release of gastrin
	Acetylcholine	Vagus and local nerves in stomach	Stimulates release of pepsinogen and acid secretion
	Gastrin-releasing peptide (bombesin)	Vagus and local nerves in stomach	Stimulates gastrin and release of pepsinogen and acid secretion
	Ghrelin	High during fasting	Stimulates growth hormone secretion and hypothalamus to increase appetite
Mucosa of small intestine	Motilin	Presence of acid and fat in duodenum	Increases gastro-intestinal (GI) motility
	Secretin	Presence of chyme (acid, partially digested proteins, fats) in duodenum	Stimulates pancreas to secrete alkaline pancreatic juice and liver to secrete bile; decreases GI motility; inhibits gastrin and gastric acid secretion
	Serotonin (5-hydroxytryptamine)	Intestinal distension; vagal stimulation; presence of acids, amino acids, or hypertonic fluids; released from enterochromaffin cells throughout intestine	Stimulates intestinal secretion, motility, and sensation (i.e., pain and nausea), vasodilation; activates gut immune responses
	Cholecystokinin	Presence of chyme (acid, partially digested proteins, fats) in duodenum	Stimulates gallbladder to eject bile and pancreas to secrete alkaline fluid; decreases gastric motility; constricts pyloric sphincter; inhibits gastrin
	Enteroglucagon	Intraluminal fats and carbohydrates	Weakly inhibits gastric and pancreatic secretion and enhances insulin release, lipolysis, ketogenesis, and glycogenolysis
	Gastric inhibitory peptide (GIP)	Fat and glucose in small intestine	Inhibits gastric secretion and emptying; stimulates insulin release
	Peptide YY	Intraluminal fat and bile acids	Inhibits postprandial gastric acid and pancreatic secretion and delays gastric and small bowel emptying
	Pancreatic polypeptide	Protein, fat, and glucose in small intestine	Decreases pancreatic and enzyme secretion
	Vasoactive intestinal peptide	Intestinal mucosa and muscle	Relaxes intestinal smooth muscle

[a]The digestive hormones are not secreted into the gastro-intestinal (GI) lumen but instead into the bloodstream, where they travel to target tissues. There are more than 30 peptide hormone genes expressed in the GI tract and more than 100 hormonally active peptides.
Modified from Johnson, L. R. (2014). *Gastrointestinal physiology* (8th ed.). Mosby. Data from Feldman, M., Friedman, L. S., & Brandt, L. J. (2015). *Sleisenger and Fordtran's gastrointestinal and liver disease* (10th ed.). Saunders.

and is influenced by neural and hormonal activity. Gastrin, **motilin** (an intestinal hormone), and the vagus nerve increase the rate of contraction by lowering the threshold potential of muscle fibres. (The neural and biochemical mechanisms of muscle contraction are described in Chapter 38.) Sympathetic activity and **secretin** (another intestinal hormone) are inhibitory and raise the threshold potential. The rate of peristalsis is communicated by pacemaker cells that initiate a wave of depolarization (basic electrical rhythm), which moves from the upper part of the stomach to the pylorus.

Gastric mixing and emptying of gastric contents (chyme) from the stomach take several hours. Mixing occurs as food is propelled toward the antrum. As food approaches the pylorus, the speed of the peristaltic wave increases, forcing the contents back toward the body of the stomach. This **retropulsion** effectively mixes food with digestive juices, and the oscillating motion breaks down large food particles. With each peristaltic wave, a small portion of the gastric contents (chyme) passes through the pylorus and into the duodenum. The pyloric sphincter is about 1.5 cm long and is always open about 2.0 mm. It opens wider during antral contraction. Normally there is no regurgitation from the duodenum into the antrum.

The rate of **gastric emptying** (movement of gastric contents into the duodenum) depends on the volume, osmotic pressure, and chemical composition of the gastric contents. Larger volumes of food increase gastric pressure, peristalsis, and rate of emptying. Solids, fats, and non-isotonic solutions (i.e., hypertonic or hypotonic gastric tube feedings) delay gastric emptying. (Osmotic pressure and tonicity are described in Chapters 1 and 5.) Products of fat digestion, which are formed in the duodenum by the action of bile from the liver and enzymes from the pancreas, stimulate the secretion of cholecystokinin. This hormone inhibits food intake, reduces gastric motility, and decreases gastric emptying so that fats are not emptied into the duodenum at a rate that exceeds the rate of bile and enzyme secretion. Osmoreceptors in the wall of the duodenum are sensitive to the osmotic pressure of duodenal contents. The arrival of hypertonic or hypotonic gastric contents activates the osmoreceptors, which delay gastric emptying to help the formation of an isosmotic duodenal environment. The rate at which acid enters the duodenum also influences gastric emptying. Secretions from the pancreas, liver, and duodenal mucosa neutralize gastric hydrochloric acid in the duodenum. The rate of emptying is adjusted to the duodenum's ability to neutralize the incoming acidity.[2]

Gastric Secretion

The secretion of gastric juice is influenced by numerous stimuli that together ease the process of digestion. The phases of gastric secretion are the *cephalic phase* (stimulated by the thought, smell, and taste of food), the *gastric phase* (stimulated by distension of the stomach), and the *intestinal phase* (stimulated by histamine and digested protein). All phases promote the secretion of acid by the stomach.

Gastric secretion is stimulated by the process of eating (gastric distension), by the actions of the hormone gastrin and paracrine pathways (e.g., histamine, ghrelin, somatostatin), and by the effects of the neurotransmitter acetylcholine (ACh) and other chemicals (e.g., ethanol, coffee, protein). The stomach secretes large volumes of gastric juices or gastric secretions, including mucus, acid, enzymes, hormones, intrinsic factor, and gastroferrin. **Intrinsic factor** is necessary for the intestinal absorption of vitamin B_{12}, and gastroferrin assists the small intestine to absorb iron. The hormones are secreted into the blood and travel to target tissues. The other gastric secretions are released directly into the stomach lumen.[3]

In the fundus and body of the stomach, the **gastric glands** of the mucosa are the primary secretory units (Figure 35.7). The composition of gastric juice depends on volume and flow rate (Figure 35.8). Potassium level remains relatively constant, but its concentration is greater in gastric juice than in plasma. The rate of secretion varies with the time of day. Generally, the rate and volume of secretion are lowest in the morning and highest in the afternoon and evening. Loss of gastric juices through vomiting, drainage, or suction may decrease body stores of sodium and potassium and result in fluid, electrolyte (e.g., hyponatremia, hypokalemia, dehydration), and acid–base imbalances (e.g., metabolic alkalosis) (see Chapters 5 and 36).[4]

Gastric secretion is inhibited by somatostatin, by unpleasant odours and tastes, and by rage, fear, or pain. A discharge of sympathetic impulses inhibits parasympathetic impulses. Increased secretions are associated with aggression or hostility and may contribute to some forms of gastric pathology.

Gastric acid. The major functions of gastric hydrochloric acid are to dissolve food fibres, act as a bactericide against swallowed microorganisms, and convert pepsinogen to pepsin. The production of acid by the **parietal cells** requires the transport of hydrogen and chloride from the parietal cells to the stomach lumen. Acid is formed in the parietal cells, primarily through the hydrolysis of water (Figure 35.9). At a high rate of gastric secretion, bicarbonate moves into the plasma, producing an "alkaline tide" in the venous blood, which also may result in a more alkaline urine.[4]

Acid secretion is stimulated by the vagus nerve, which releases ACh and stimulates the secretion of gastrin; then gastrin stimulates the release of histamine from enterochromaffin cells (mast cells; see Chapter 6) in the gastric mucosa. Histamine stimulates acid secretion by activating histamine receptors (H2 receptors) on acid-secreting parietal cells. Caffeine stimulates acid secretion, as does calcium. Acid secretion is inhibited by somatostatin, secretin, and other intestinal hormones.[3]

Pepsin. ACh, gastrin, and secretin stimulate the **chief cells** to release pepsinogen during eating. Pepsinogen is quickly converted to **pepsin** in the acidic gastric environment (optimum pH for pepsin activation = 2.0). Pepsin is a proteolytic enzyme—that is, it breaks down protein and forms polypeptides in the stomach. Once chyme has entered the duodenum, the alkaline environment of the duodenum inactivates pepsin.

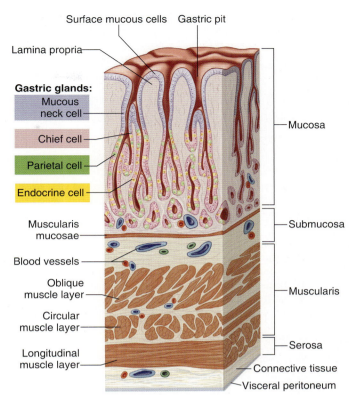

FIGURE 35.7 Gastric Pits and Gastric Glands. Gastric pits are depressions in the epithelial lining of the stomach. At the bottom of each pit are one or more tubular *gastric glands*. Chief cells produce pepsinogen, which is converted to pepsin (a proteolytic enzyme); parietal cells secrete hydrochloric acid and intrinsic factor; G cells produce gastrin; endocrine cells (enterochromaffin-like cells and D cells) secrete histamine and somatostatin. (From Patton, K. T., Thibodeau, G. A., & Douglas, M. M. [2012]. *Essentials of anatomy & physiology*. Mosby.)

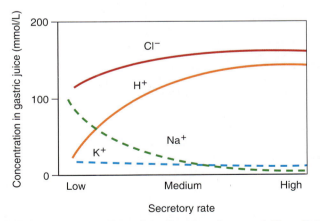

FIGURE 35.8 Gastric Electrolyte Concentrations and Flow Rate. Sodium (Na^+) concentration is lower in the gastric juice than in the plasma, whereas hydrogen (H^+), potassium (K^+), and chloride (Cl^-) concentrations are higher. *Red line,* Chloride; *orange line,* hydrogen; *green line,* sodium; *blue line,* potassium.

Mucus. The gastric mucosa is protected from the digestive actions of acid and pepsin by intercellular tight junctions, a coating of mucus called the **mucosal barrier**, and gastric mucosal blood flow. Prostaglandins protect the mucosal barrier by stimulating the secretion of mucus and bicarbonate and by inhibiting the secretion of acid. A

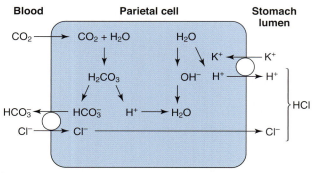

FIGURE 35.9 Hydrochloric Acid Secretion by Parietal Cell. Cl^-, Chloride; CO_2, carbon dioxide; H^+, hydrogen; H_2CO_3, carbonic acid; H_2O, water; HCl, hydrochloric acid; HCO_3^-, bicarbonate; K^+, potassium; OH^-, hydroxyl ion.

break in the protective barrier may occur from ischemia or by exposure to *Helicobacter pylori*, Aspirin, nonsteroidal anti-inflammatory medications (which inhibit prostaglandin synthesis), ethanol, or regurgitated bile. Breaks cause inflammation and ulceration.

Few substances are absorbed in the stomach. The stomach mucosa is impermeable to water, but the stomach can absorb alcohol and Aspirin.

Small Intestine

> **✓ QUICK CHECK 35.3**
> 1. What cells arise from the crypts of Lieberkühn?
> 2. How are fats absorbed from the small intestine?
> 3. Which reflexes inhibit intestinal motility? Which promote it?

The **small intestine** is coiled within the peritoneal cavity and is about 5 to 6 m long. Functionally, it is divided into three segments: the **duodenum**, **jejunum**, and **ileum** (Figure 35.10). The duodenum begins at the pylorus and ends where it joins the jejunum at a suspensory ligament called the *Treitz ligament*. The end of the jejunum and beginning of the ileum are not distinguished by an anatomical marker. These structures are not grossly different, but the jejunum has a slightly larger lumen than the ileum. The **ileocecal valve**, or **sphincter**, controls the flow of digested material from the ileum into the large intestine and prevents reflux into the small intestine.

The duodenum lies behind the peritoneum, or retroperitoneally, and is attached to the posterior abdominal wall. The ileum and jejunum are suspended in loose folds from the posterior abdominal wall by a peritoneal membrane called the **mesentery**. The mesentery eases intestinal motility and supports blood vessels, nerves, and lymphatics.

The **peritoneum** is the serous membrane surrounding the organs of the abdomen and pelvic cavity. It is comparable to the pericardium around the heart and the pleura around the lungs. The visceral peritoneum lies on the surface of the organs, and the parietal peritoneum lines the wall of the body cavity. The space between these two layers is called the **peritoneal cavity** and normally contains just enough fluid to lubricate the two layers and prevent friction during organ movement.

The arterial supply to the duodenum arises primarily from the gastroduodenal artery, a branch of the celiac artery. The jejunum and ileum are supplied by branches of the superior mesenteric artery. The superior mesenteric vein drains blood from the entire small intestine and empties into the hepatic portal circulation. The regional lymph nodes and lymphatics drain into the thoracic duct.

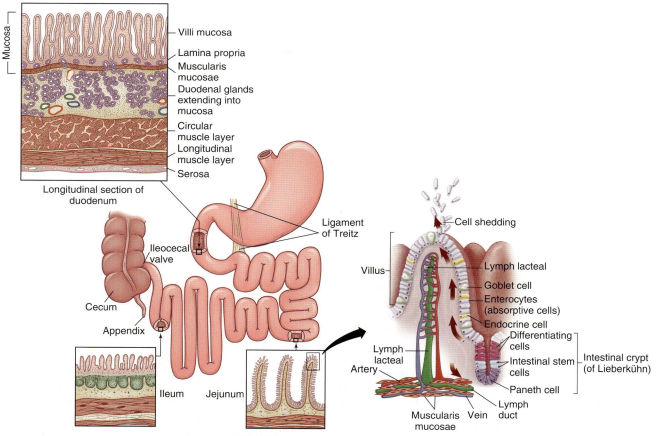

FIGURE 35.10 The Small Intestine.

Enteric nerves from both divisions of the autonomic nervous system innervate the small intestine. Secretion, motility, pain sensation, and intestinal reflexes (e.g., relaxation of the lower esophageal sphincter) are mediated parasympathetically by the vagus nerve. Sympathetic activity inhibits motility and produces vasoconstriction. Intrinsic reflexive activity is mediated by the myenteric plexus (Auerbach plexus) and the submucosal plexus (Meissner plexus) of the enteric nervous system.

The smooth muscles of the small intestine are arranged in two layers: a longitudinal outer layer and a thicker inner circular layer (see Figures 35.2 and 35.10). Circular folds of the small intestine slow the passage of food, thereby providing more time for digestion and absorption. The folds are most numerous and prominent in the jejunum and proximal ileum (see Figure 35.10).

Absorption occurs through **villi** (*sing.*, **villus**), which cover the circular folds and are the functional units of the intestine. A villus is composed of absorptive columnar cells (**enterocytes**) and mucus-secreting goblet cells of the mucosal epithelium. Each villus (see Figure 35.10) secretes some of the enzymes necessary for digestion and absorbs nutrients. Near the surface, columnar cells closely adhere to each other at sites called *tight junctions*. Water and electrolytes are absorbed through these intercellular spaces. The surface of each columnar epithelial cell on the villus contains tiny projections called **microvilli** (*sing.*, **microvillus**) (see Figure 35.10). Together the microvilli create a mucosal surface known as the **brush border**. The villi and microvilli greatly increase the surface area available for absorption. Coating the brush border is an "unstirred" layer of water that is important for the absorption of water-soluble substances, including emulsified micelles of fat. The **lamina propria** (a connective tissue layer of the mucous membrane) lies beneath the epithelial cells of the villi and contains lymphocytes and plasma cells, which produce immunoglobulins (see "The Gastro-intestinal Tract and Immunity").

Central arterioles ascend within each villus and branch into a capillary array that extends around the base of the columnar cells and cascades down to the venules that lead to the hepatic portal circulation (see Figure 35.10). A central **lacteal**, or lymphatic capillary, also is contained within each villus and is important for the absorption and transport of fat molecules. Contents of the lacteals flow to regional nodes and channels that eventually drain into the thoracic duct.[5]

Between the bases of the villi are the **crypts of Lieberkühn**, which extend to the submucosal layer. Undifferentiated cells arise from stem cells at the base of the crypt and move toward the tip of the villus, maturing to become columnar epithelial secretory cells (water, electrolytes, and enzymes) and goblet cells (mucus). After completing their migration to the tip of the villus, they function for a few days and then are shed into the intestinal lumen and digested. Discarded epithelial cells are an important source of endogenous protein. The entire epithelial population is replaced about every 4 to 7 days. Many factors can influence this process of cellular proliferation. Starvation, vitamin B_{12} deficiency, and cytotoxic medications or irradiation suppress cell division and shorten the villi. Decreased absorption across the epithelial membrane can cause diarrhea and malnutrition. Nutrient intake and intestinal resection stimulate cell production.

Intestinal Digestion and Absorption

The process of digestion is initiated in the stomach by the actions of gastric hydrochloric acid and pepsin. The chyme that passes into the duodenum is a liquid with small particles of undigested food. Digestion continues in the proximal portion of the small intestine by the action of pancreatic enzymes, intestinal enzymes, and bile salts. In the proximal small intestine, carbohydrates are broken down to monosaccharides and disaccharides; proteins are degraded further to amino acids and

---

BOX 35.1 Dietary Fat

Saturated Fatty Acids (e.g., Palmitic Acid [$C_{16}H_{32}O_2$])
Each carbon atom in the chain is linked by single bonds to adjacent carbon and hydrogen atoms.
1. They are solid at room temperature; they include animal fat and tropical oils (coconut and palm oils).
2. They increase low-density lipoprotein (LDL) cholesterol ("bad" cholesterol) blood levels.
3. They increase the risk of coronary artery disease.

Unsaturated Fatty Acids
1. They are soft or liquid at room temperature.
2. Omega-6 fatty acids are found in plants and vegetables (olive, canola, and peanut oils).
3. Omega-3 fatty acids are found in fish and shellfish.

Monounsaturated Fatty Acids (e.g., Oleic Acid [$C_{18}H_{34}O_2$])
They contain one double bond in the carbon chain.
1. They are found in both plants and animals.
2. They may be beneficial in reducing blood cholesterol level, glucose level, and systolic blood pressure.
3. They do not lower high-density lipoprotein (HDL) cholesterol ("good" cholesterol) blood levels.
4. Low HDL levels have been associated with coronary heart disease.

Polyunsaturated Fatty Acids (e.g., Linoleic Acid [$C_{18}H_{32}O_2$])
They contain two or more double bonds in the carbon chain.
1. They are found in plants and fish oils.
2. Omega-6 fatty acids lower total and LDL cholesterol blood levels.
3. High levels of polyunsaturated fatty acids may lower LDL levels.
4. Omega-3 fatty acids lower blood triglyceride levels and reduce platelet aggregation and, therefore, blood coagulation.
5. They are necessary for growth and development and may prevent coronary artery disease, hypertension, and inflammatory and immune disorders.

---

peptides; and fats are emulsified and reduced to fatty acids (Box 35.1) and monoglycerides (Figure 35.11). These nutrients, along with water, vitamins, and electrolytes, are absorbed across the intestinal mucosa by active transport, diffusion, or facilitated diffusion. Products of carbohydrate and protein breakdown move into villus capillaries and then to the liver through the hepatic portal vein. Digested fats move into the lacteals and eventually reach the liver through the systemic circulation. Intestinal motility exposes nutrients to a large mucosal surface area by mixing chyme and moving it through the lumen. Different segments of the GI tract absorb different nutrients. Digestion and absorption of all major nutrients and many medications occur in the small intestine. Sites of absorption are shown in Figure 35.12. Box 35.2 outlines the major nutrients involved in this process.

Intestinal Motility

The movements of the small intestine help digestion and absorption. Chyme leaving the stomach and entering the duodenum stimulates intestinal movements that help blend secretions from the liver, gallbladder, pancreas, and intestinal glands. A churning motion brings the luminal contents into contact with the absorbing cells of the villi. Propulsive movements then move the chyme toward the large intestine.

Intestinal motility is affected by the following two movements:
1. **Haustral segmentation**. Localized rhythmic contractions of circular smooth muscles divide and mix the chyme, enabling the chyme to have contact with digestive enzymes and the absorbent mucosal surface, and then propel it toward the large intestine.

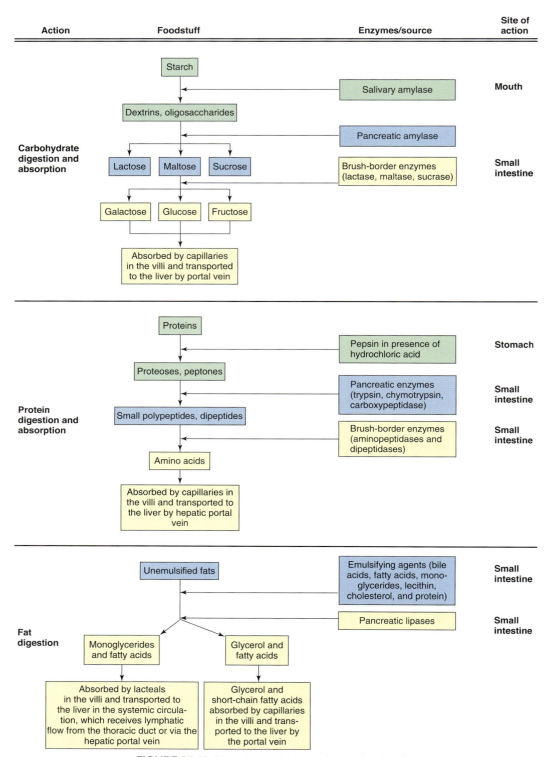

FIGURE 35.11 Digestion and Absorption of Foodstuffs.

2. **Peristalsis**. Waves of contraction along short segments of longitudinal smooth muscle allow time for digestion and absorption. The intestinal villi move with contractions of the muscularis mucosae, a thin layer of muscle separating the mucosa and submucosa, with absorption promoted by the swaying of the villi in the luminal contents.

Neural reflexes along the length of the small intestine help with motility, digestion, and absorption. The **ileogastric reflex** inhibits gastric motility when the ileum becomes distended. This reflex prevents the continued movement of chyme into an already distended intestine. The **intestinointestinal reflex** inhibits intestinal motility when one part of the intestine is overdistended. Both of these reflexes require

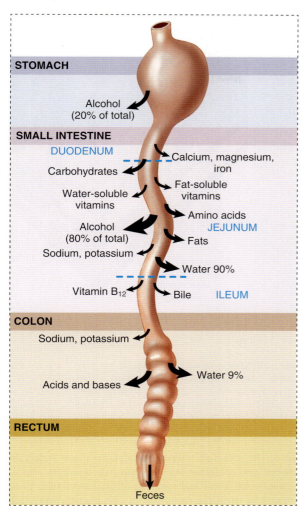

FIGURE 35.12 Sites of Absorption of Major Nutrients.

> **BOX 35.2 Major Nutrients Absorbed in the Small Intestine**
>
> **Water and Electrolytes**
> - Approximately 85 to 90% of the water that enters the gastro-intestinal tract is absorbed in the small intestine.
> - Sodium passes through tight junctions and is actively transported across cell membranes; it is exchanged for bicarbonate to maintain electroneutrality in the ileum; sodium absorption is enhanced by cotransport with glucose.
> - Potassium moves passively across tight junctions with changes in the electrochemical gradient.
>
> **Carbohydrates**
> - Only monosaccharides are absorbed by intestinal mucosa; therefore, complex carbohydrates must be hydrolyzed to simplest form.
> - Salivary and pancreatic amylases break down starches to oligosaccharides (sucrose, maltose, lactose) in stomach and duodenum; brush-border enzymes hydrolyze them in intestine so they can pass through the unstirred water layer by diffusion.
> - Fructose diffuses into the bloodstream; glucose and galactose diffuse or are actively transported.
> - Cellulose remains undigested and stimulates large intestine motility.
>
> **Proteins**
> - From 90 to 95% of protein is absorbed; major hydrolysis is accomplished in the small intestine by the pancreatic enzymes trypsin, chymotrypsin, and carboxypeptidase.
> - Brush-border enzymes break down proteins into smaller peptides that can cross cell membranes. In the cytosol, they are metabolized into amino acids, specifically neutral amino acids, basic amino acids, and proline and hydroxyproline.
>
> **Fats**
> Digestion and absorption occur in four phases:
> 1. *Emulsification and lipolysis:* agents cover small fat particles and prevent them from reforming into fat droplets; then lipolysis divides them into diglycerides, monoglycerides, free fatty acids, and glycerol.
> 2. *Micelle formation:* products are made water soluble.
> 3. *Fat absorption:* fat products move from micelle to absorbing surface of intestinal epithelium and diffuse through resynthesis.
> 4. *Triglycerides and phospholipids:* they then become chylomicrons that eventually enter the systemic circulation.
>
> **Minerals**
> - *Calcium:* it is absorbed by passive diffusion and transported actively across cell membranes bound to a carrier protein; absorption primarily in ileum.
> - *Magnesium:* 50% is absorbed by active transport or passive diffusion in jejunum and ileum.
> - *Phosphate:* it is absorbed by passive diffusion and active transport in small intestine.
> - *Iron:* it is absorbed by epithelial cells of duodenum and jejunum; vitamin C assists iron absorption.
>
> **Vitamins**
> - They are absorbed mainly by sodium-dependent active transport, with vitamin B_{12} bound to intrinsic factor and absorbed in terminal ileum.

extrinsic innervation. The **gastroileal reflex**, which is activated by an increase in gastric motility and secretion, stimulates an increase in ileal motility and relaxation of the ileocecal valve (sphincter). It empties the ileum and prepares it to receive more chyme. The gastroileal reflex is probably regulated by the hormones gastrin and cholecystokinin.

During prolonged fasting or between meals, particularly overnight, slow waves sweep along the entire length of the intestinal tract from the stomach to the terminal ileum. This interdigestive myoelectric complex appears to propel residual gastric and intestinal contents into the colon.

The ileocecal valve (sphincter) marks the junction between the terminal ileum and the large intestine. This valve is intrinsically regulated and is normally closed. The arrival of peristaltic waves from the last few centimetres of the ileum causes the ileocecal valve to open, allowing a small amount of chyme to pass. Distension of the upper large intestine causes the sphincter to constrict, preventing further distension or retrograde flow of intestinal contents.

Large Intestine

> ✓ **QUICK CHECK 35.4**
> 1. What is the major arterial blood supply to the large intestine?
> 2. What is the function of haustra?
> 3. What is the Valsalva manoeuvre?

The **large intestine** is approximately 1.5 m long and consists of the cecum, appendix, colon (ascending, transverse, descending, and sigmoid), rectum, and anal canal (Figure 35.13). The **cecum** is a pouch that receives chyme from the ileum. Attached to it is the **vermiform**

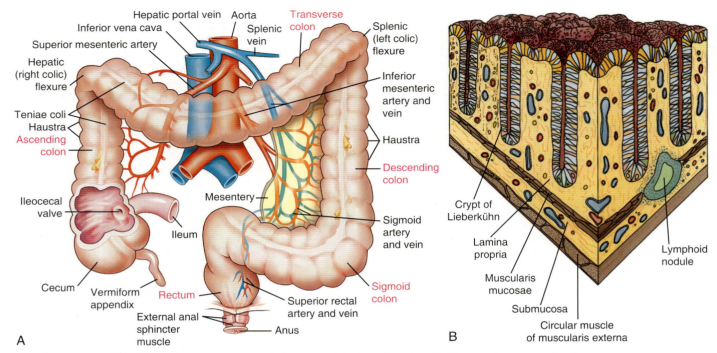

FIGURE 35.13 Large Intestine. A, Structure of the large intestine. B, Microscopic cross-section illustrating cellular structures of the large intestine. The wall of the large intestine is lined with columnar epithelium in contrast to the villi characteristics of the small intestine. The longitudinal layer of muscularis is reduced to become the teniae coli. ([A], modified from Patton, K. T., & Thibodeau, G. A. [2018]. *The human body in health & disease* [7th ed.]. Elsevier; [B], from Gartner, L. P., & Hiatt, J. L. [2007]. *Color textbook of histology* [3rd ed.]. Saunders.)

appendix, an appendage having little or no physiological function. From the cecum, chyme enters the **colon**, which loops upward, traverses the abdominal cavity, and descends to the anal canal. The four parts of the colon are the **ascending colon**, **transverse colon**, **descending colon**, and **sigmoid colon**. Two sphincters control the flow of intestinal contents through the cecum and colon: the ileocecal valve, which admits chyme from the ileum to the cecum, and the **rectosigmoid (O'Beirne) sphincter**, which controls the movement of wastes from the sigmoid colon into the rectum. A thick (2.5 to 3 cm) portion of smooth muscle surrounds the anal canal, forming the **internal anal sphincter**. Overlapping it distally is the striated skeletal muscle of the **external anal sphincter** (anus).

In the cecum and colon, the longitudinal muscle layer consists of three longitudinal bands called **teniae coli** (see Figure 35.13). They are shorter than the colon and give it a gathered appearance. The circular muscles of the colon separate the gathers into outpouchings called **haustra** (*sing.*, **haustrum**). The haustra become more or less prominent with the contractions and relaxations of the circular muscles. The mucosal surface of the colon has rugae (folds), particularly between the haustra, and Lieberkühn crypts but no villi. Columnar epithelial cells and mucus-secreting goblet cells form the mucosa throughout the large intestine. The columnar epithelium absorbs fluid and electrolytes, and the mucus-secreting cells lubricate the mucosa.

The enteric nervous system controls motor and secretory activity independently of the extrinsic nervous system. Extrinsic parasympathetic innervation occurs through the vagus nerve and extends from the cecum up to the first part of the transverse colon. Vagal stimulation increases rhythmic contraction of the proximal colon. Extrinsic parasympathetic fibres reach the distal colon through the sacral parasympathetic splanchnic nerves. The internal anal sphincter is usually contracted, and its reflex response is to relax when the rectum is distended. The myenteric plexus provides the major innervation of the internal anal sphincter, but responds to sympathetic stimulation to maintain contraction and parasympathetic stimulation that helps with relaxation when the rectum is full. Sympathetic innervation of this sphincter arises from the celiac and superior mesenteric ganglia and the sphincter nerve. The external anal sphincter is innervated by the pudendal nerve arising from sacral levels of the spinal cord. Sympathetic activity in the entire large intestine modulates intestinal reflexes, conveys somatic sensations of fullness and pain, participates in the defecation reflex, and constricts blood vessels. The blood supply of the large intestine and rectum is derived primarily from branches of the superior and inferior mesenteric arteries[6] (see Figure 35.6), and venous blood drains through the inferior mesenteric vein.

The primary type of colonic movement is segmental. The circular muscles contract and relax at different sites, shuttling the intestinal contents back and forth between the haustra, most commonly during fasting. The movements massage the intestinal contents, called the **fecal mass** at that point, and ease the absorption of water. Propulsive movement occurs with the proximal-to-distal contraction of several haustral units. Peristaltic movements also occur and promote the emptying of the colon. The **gastrocolic reflex** initiates propulsion in the entire colon, usually during or immediately after eating, when chyme enters from the ileum. The gastrocolic reflex causes the fecal mass to pass rapidly into the sigmoid colon and rectum, which stimulates defecation. Gastrin may participate in stimulating this reflex. Epinephrine inhibits contractile activity.

Approximately 500 to 700 mL of chyme flows from the ileum to the cecum per day. Most of the water is absorbed in the colon by diffusion and active transport. Aldosterone increases membrane permeability to sodium, thereby increasing both the diffusion of sodium into the cell and the active transport of sodium to the interstitial fluid. (See

Chapters 5 and 18 for a discussion of aldosterone secretion.) The colon does not absorb monosaccharides and amino acids, but some short-chain free fatty acids, which are produced by fermentation, are absorbed.

Absorption and epithelial transport occur in the cecum, ascending colon, transverse colon, and descending colon. By the time the fecal mass enters the sigmoid colon, the mass consists entirely of wastes and is called the *feces*, composed of food residue, unabsorbed GI secretions, shed epithelial cells, and bacteria.

The movement of feces into the sigmoid colon and rectum stimulates the defecation reflex (rectosphincteric reflex). The rectal wall stretches, and the tonically constricted internal anal sphincter (smooth muscle with autonomic nervous system control) relaxes, creating the urge to defecate. The defecation reflex can be overridden voluntarily by contraction of the external anal sphincter and muscles of the pelvic floor. The rectal wall gradually relaxes, reducing tension, and the urge to defecate passes. Retrograde contraction of the rectum may displace the feces out of the rectal vault until a more convenient time for evacuation. Pain or fear of pain associated with defecation (e.g., rectal fissures or hemorrhoids) can inhibit the defecation reflex.

Squatting and sitting help with defecation because these positions straighten the angle between the rectum and anal canal and increase the efficiency of straining (increasing intra-abdominal pressure). Intra-abdominal pressure is increased by initiating the Valsalva manoeuvre —that is, inhaling and forcing the diaphragm and chest muscles against the closed glottis to increase both intrathoracic and intra-abdominal pressure, which is transmitted to the rectum.

The Gastro-intestinal Tract and Immunity

The GI tract plays a major role in immune defences by killing many microorganisms.[7] The mucosa of the intestine cover a large surface area, and mucosal secretions produce antibodies, particularly IgA, and enzymes that provide defences against microorganisms. Small intestinal Paneth cells, located near the base of the crypts of Lieberkühn, produce defensins and other antimicrobial peptides and lysozymes important to mucosal immunity. Small intestinal Peyer patches (lymph nodules containing collections of lymphocytes, plasma cells, and macrophages) are most numerous in the ileum and produce antimicrobial peptides and IgA as a component of the gut-associated lymph tissue in the small intestine (see Figures 35.2 and 7.3). Peyer patches are important for antigen processing and immune defence (see Chapter 7).

Intestinal Microbiome

The type and number of bacterial flora vary greatly throughout the normal GI tract and among individuals. There are an increasing number of bacteria from the proximal to the distal GI tract, with the highest number in the colon. Genetics, diet, environmental pollution, personal hygiene, vaccination, and antibiotics and other medications affect the normal composition of bacterial flora. The intestinal bacteria do not have major digestive or absorptive functions but do play a role in metabolism of bile salts, estrogens, androgens, lipids, carbohydrates, various nitrogenous substances, and medications. They produce antimicrobial peptides, hormones, neurotransmitters, anti-inflammatory metabolites, and vitamins; destroy toxins; prevent pathogen colonization; and alert the immune system to protect against infection. They are important to overall health and when they are altered (dysbiosis) or translocated, they cause disease.[8]

The intestinal tract is sterile at birth but becomes colonized within a few hours. Within 3 to 4 weeks after birth, the normal flora is established. The number and diversity of bacteria decrease with aging, increasing the risk for infection. The normal flora does not have the virulence factors associated with pathogenic microorganisms, thus permitting immune tolerances.[9]

Bacteria in the stomach are relatively sparse because of the secretion of acid that kills ingested pathogens or inhibits bacterial growth (with the exception of *H. pylori*). Bile acid secretion, intestinal motility, and antibody production suppress bacterial growth in the duodenum. In the duodenum and jejunum, there is a low concentration of aerobes (10^{-1} to 10^{-4}/mL), primarily streptococci, lactobacilli, staphylococci, and other enteric bacteria. Anaerobes are found distal to the ileocecal valve but not proximal to the ileum. They constitute about 95% of the fecal flora in the colon and contribute one-third of the solid bulk of feces. *Bacteroides* and *Firmicutes* are the most common intestinal bacteria.

Splanchnic Blood Flow

The splanchnic blood flow provides blood to the esophagus, stomach, small and large intestines, liver, gallbladder, pancreas, and spleen (see Figure 35.6). Blood flow is regulated by cardiac output and blood volume, the autonomic nervous system, hormones, and local autoregulatory blood flow mechanisms. The splanchnic circulation serves as an important reservoir of blood volume to maintain circulation to the heart and lungs when needed. The superior and inferior mesenteric arteries provide the blood supply to the large intestine (see Figures 35.6 and 35.13).

ACCESSORY ORGANS OF DIGESTION

> ✓ **QUICK CHECK 35.5**
> 1. Where does blood in the hepatic portal vein originate?
> 2. What is the function of hepatocytes?
> 3. What is the function of Kupffer cells?

The liver, gallbladder, and exocrine pancreas all secrete substances necessary for the digestion of chyme. These secretions are delivered to the duodenum through the sphincter of Oddi at the major duodenal papilla (of Vater) (Figure 35.14). The liver produces bile, which contains salts necessary for fat digestion and absorption. Between meals,

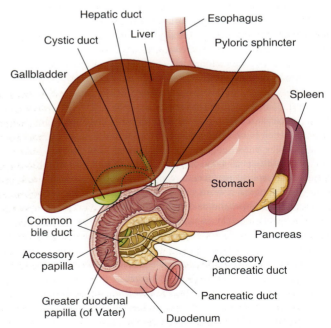

FIGURE 35.14 Location of the Liver, Gallbladder, and Exocrine Pancreas, Which Are the Accessory Organs of Digestion.

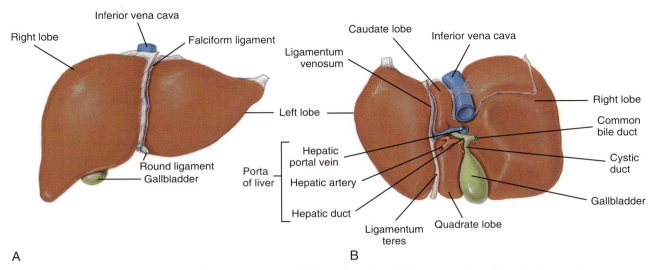

FIGURE 35.15 Gross Structure of the Liver. A, Anterior surface. B, Visceral surface. (From Applegate, E. [2011]. *The anatomy and physiology learning system* [4th ed.]. Saunders.)

bile is stored in the gallbladder. The exocrine pancreas produces (1) enzymes needed for the complete digestion of carbohydrates, proteins, and fats and (2) an alkaline fluid that neutralizes chyme, creating a duodenal pH that supports enzymatic action.

The liver also receives nutrients absorbed by the small intestine and metabolizes or synthesizes them into forms that can be absorbed by the body's cells. It then releases the nutrients into the bloodstream or stores them for later use.

Liver

The **liver** weighs 1200 to 1600 g. It is located under the right diaphragm and is divided into right and left lobes. The larger right lobe is divided further into the caudate and quadrate lobes (Figure 35.15). The *falciform ligament* separates the right and left lobes and attaches the liver to the anterior abdominal wall. The *round ligament (ligamentum teres)* extends along the free edge of the falciform ligament, extending from the umbilicus to the inferior surface of the liver. The *coronary ligament* branches from the falciform ligament and extends over the superior surface of the right and left lobes, binding the liver to the inferior surface of the diaphragm. The liver is covered by the **Glisson capsule**, which contains blood vessels, lymphatics, and nerves. When the liver is diseased or swollen, distension of the capsule causes pain because it is innervated by sensory neurons.

The metabolic functions of the liver require a large amount of blood. The liver receives blood from both arterial and venous sources. The **hepatic artery** branches from the celiac artery and provides oxygenated blood at the rate of 400 to 500 mL/min (about 25% of the cardiac output). The **hepatic portal vein** receives deoxygenated blood from the inferior and superior mesenteric veins, the splenic vein, and the gastric and esophageal veins, and delivers about 1000 to 1500 mL/min to the liver. The hepatic portal vein, which carries 70% of the blood supply to the liver, is rich in nutrients that have been absorbed from the intestinal tract (Figure 35.16).

Within the liver lobes are multiple, smaller anatomical units called **liver lobules** (Figure 35.17). They are formed of cords or plates of **hepatocytes**, which are the functional cells of the liver. These cells can regenerate; therefore, damaged or resected liver tissue can regrow. Small capillaries (**sinusoids**) are located between the plates of hepatocytes. They receive a mixture of venous and arterial blood from branches of the hepatic artery and portal vein. Blood from the sinusoids drains to a central vein in the

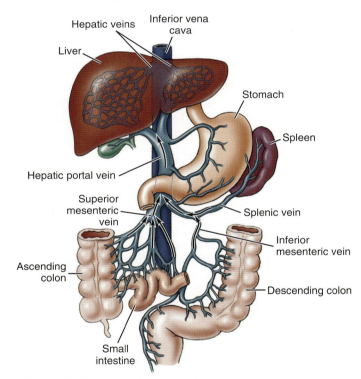

FIGURE 35.16 Hepatic Portal Circulation. In this unusual circulatory route, a vein is located between two capillary beds. The hepatic portal vein collects blood from capillaries in visceral structures located in the abdomen and empties into the liver. Hepatic veins return blood to the inferior vena cava. (From Herlihy, B. [2018]. *The human body in health and illness* [6th ed.]. Elsevier.)

middle of each liver lobule. Venous blood from all the lobules then flows into the **hepatic vein**, which empties into the inferior vena cava. Small channels (**bile canaliculi**) conduct bile, which is produced by the hepatocytes, outward to bile ducts and eventually drain into the **common bile duct** (see Figure 35.17). This duct empties bile into the ampulla of Vater, and then into the duodenum through an opening called the *major duodenal papilla* (which is surrounded by the sphincter of Oddi).

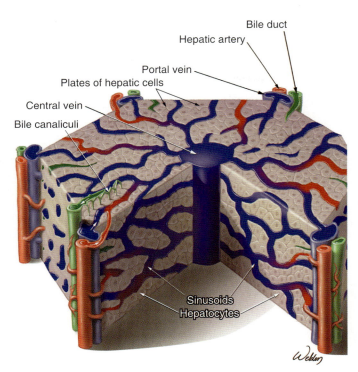

FIGURE 35.17 Schematic View of the Liver Lobule. The central vein is shown in the centre of the lobule, separated by cords of hepatocytes forming sinusoids from six portal areas at the periphery. The portal areas contain a portal vein, hepatic artery, and bile duct. Blood flows toward the centre of the lobule, while bile flows toward the portal triads at the margins. Note the hepatic artery providing oxygenated blood to the hepatic sinusoids as well as the peribiliary plexus. (From Polin, R. A., Fox, W. W., & Abman, S. H. [2011]. *Fetal and neonatal physiology* [4th ed.]. Saunders.)

The sinusoids of the liver lobules are lined with highly permeable endothelium. This permeability enhances the transport of nutrients from the sinusoids into the hepatocytes, where they are metabolized. Various cells carry out immune functions of the liver. The sinusoids are lined with phagocytic **Kupffer cells (tissue macrophages)** and are part of the mononuclear phagocyte system. Kupffer cells are important for healing of liver injury, are bactericidal, and are important for bilirubin production and lipid metabolism.[10] **Stellate cells** contain retinoids (vitamin A), are contractile in liver injury, regulate sinusoidal blood flow, may proliferate into myofibroblasts, participate in liver fibrosis, produce erythropoietin, can act as antigen-presenting cells, remove foreign substances from the blood, and trap bacteria.[11] **Natural killer cells (pit cells)** also are found in the sinusoidal lumen; they produce interferon gamma and are important in tumour defence.[12] Between the endothelial lining of the sinusoid and the hepatocyte is the **Disse space**, which drains interstitial fluid into the hepatic lymph system.

Secretion of Bile

> **QUICK CHECK 35.6**
> 1. Trace the route of bile salts and acids from formation to recycling.
> 2. What are the sources of the two types of bilirubin?
> 3. What is the function of the gallbladder?
> 4. How do pancreatic beta cells differ from acinar cells?

The liver assists intestinal digestion by secreting 700 to 1 200 mL of bile per day. **Bile** is an alkaline, bitter-tasting, yellowish green fluid that contains bile salts (conjugated bile acids), cholesterol, bilirubin

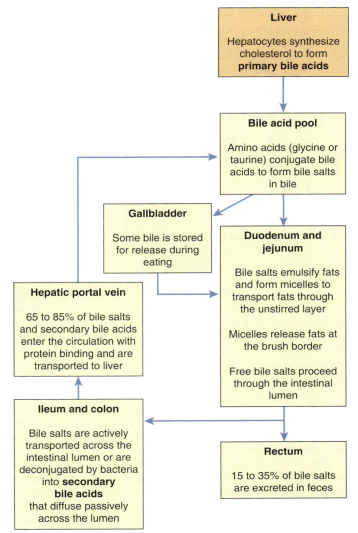

FIGURE 35.18 Enterohepatic Circulation of Bile Salts.

(a pigment), electrolytes, and water. It is formed by hepatocytes and secreted into the canaliculi. **Bile salts**, which are conjugated bile acids, are required for the intestinal emulsification and absorption of fats. Having eased fat emulsification and absorption, most bile salts are actively absorbed in the terminal ileum and returned to the liver through the portal circulation for resecretion. The pathway for recycling of bile salts is called the **enterohepatic circulation** (Figure 35.18).

Bile has two fractional components: the acid-dependent fraction and the acid-independent fraction. Hepatocytes secrete the **bile acid–dependent fraction**, which consists of bile acids, cholesterol, lecithin (a phospholipid), and bilirubin (a bile pigment). The **bile acid–independent fraction**, which is secreted by the hepatocytes and epithelial cells of the bile canaliculi, is a bicarbonate-rich aqueous fluid that gives bile its alkaline pH.

Bile salts are conjugated in the liver from primary and secondary bile acids. The **primary bile acids** are cholic acid and chenodeoxycholic (chenic) acid. These acids are synthesized from cholesterol by the hepatocytes. The **secondary bile acids** are deoxycholic and lithocholic acid. These acids are formed in the small intestine by intestinal bacteria, after which they are absorbed and flow to the liver (see Figure 35.18). Both forms of bile acids are conjugated with amino acids (glycine or taurine) in the liver to form bile salts. Conjugation makes the bile acids more water soluble, thus restricting their diffusion from the duodenum and ileum. The primary and secondary bile acids together form the **bile acid pool**.

Some bile salts are deconjugated by intestinal bacteria to secondary bile acids. These acids diffuse passively into the portal blood from both the small and large intestines. An increase in the plasma concentration of bile acids accelerates the uptake and resecretion of bile acids and salts by the hepatocytes. The cycle of hepatic secretion, intestinal absorption, and hepatic resecretion of bile acids completes the enterohepatic circulation.

Bile secretion is called **choleresis**. A **choleretic agent** stimulates the liver to secrete bile. One strong stimulus is a high concentration of bile salts. Other choleretics include cholecystokinin, vagal stimulation, and secretin, which increases the rate of bile flow by promoting the secretion of bicarbonate from canaliculi and other intrahepatic bile ducts.

Metabolism of Bilirubin

Bilirubin is a byproduct of the destruction of aged red blood cells. It gives bile a greenish black colour and produces the yellow tinge of jaundice. Aged red blood cells are absorbed and destroyed by macrophages (Kupffer cells) of the mononuclear phagocyte system (also called the **reticuloendothelial system**), primarily in the spleen and liver. Within these cells, hemoglobin is separated into its component parts: heme and globin (Figure 35.19). The globin component is further degraded into its constituent amino acids, which are recycled to form new protein. The heme moiety is converted to biliverdin by the enzymatic (heme oxygenase) cleavage of iron. The iron attaches to transferrin in the plasma and can be stored in the liver or used by the bone marrow to make new red blood cells. The biliverdin is enzymatically converted to bilirubin in the Kupffer cell and then is released into the plasma, where it binds to albumin and is known as **unconjugated bilirubin**, or free bilirubin, which is lipid soluble. Bilirubin also may have a role as an antioxidant and provide cytoprotection.[13]

In the liver, unconjugated bilirubin moves from plasma in the sinusoids into the hepatocyte. Within hepatocytes, unconjugated bilirubin joins with glucuronic acid to form **conjugated bilirubin**, which is water soluble and is secreted in the bile. When conjugated bilirubin reaches the distal ileum and colon, it is deconjugated by bacteria and converted to **urobilinogen**. Urobilinogen is then reabsorbed in the intestines and excreted in the urine as urobilin. A small amount is eliminated in feces, as stercobilin, which contributes to the stool's brown pigmentation.

Vascular and Hematological Functions

Because of its extensive vascular network, the liver can store a large volume of blood. The amount stored at any one time depends on pressure relationships in the arteries and veins. The liver also can release blood to maintain systemic circulatory volume in the event of hemorrhage.

The liver also has hemostatic functions. It synthesizes most clotting factors (see Chapter 20). Vitamin K, a fat-soluble vitamin, is essential for the synthesis of the clotting factors. Because bile salts are needed for reabsorption of fats, vitamin K absorption depends on adequate bile production in the liver.

Metabolism of Nutrients

Fats. Ingested fat absorbed by lacteals in the intestinal villi enters the liver through the lymphatics, primarily as triglycerides. In the liver the triglycerides can be hydrolyzed to glycerol and free fatty acids and used to produce metabolic energy (adenosine triphosphate), or they can be released into the bloodstream bound to proteins (lipoproteins). Blood carries the lipoproteins to adipose cells for storage. The liver also synthesizes phospholipids and cholesterol, which are needed for the hepatic production of bile salts, steroid hormones, components of plasma membranes, and other special molecules.

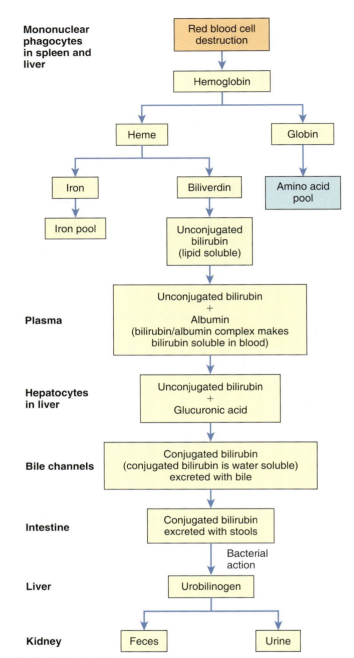

FIGURE 35.19 Bilirubin Metabolism. See text for explanation.

Proteins. Protein synthesis requires the presence of all the essential amino acids (obtained only from food), as well as nonessential amino acids. Proteins perform many important functions in the body; these functions are summarized in Table 35.2.

Within hepatocytes, amino acids are converted to carbohydrates (keto acids) by the removal of ammonia (NH_3), a process known as **deamination**. The ammonia is converted to urea by the liver and passes into the blood to be excreted by the kidneys. Depending on the nutritional status of the body, the keto acids either are converted to fatty acids for fat synthesis and storage or are oxidized by the Krebs cycle (also called the *tricarboxylic acid cycle*; see Chapter 1) to provide energy for the liver cells.

The plasma proteins, including albumins and globulins (with the exception of gamma globulin, which is formed in lymph nodes and

TABLE 35.2 Importance of Proteins in the Body

Function	Example
Contraction	Actin and myosin enable muscle contraction and cellular movement.
Energy	Proteins can be metabolized for energy.
Fluid balance	Albumin is a major source of plasma oncotic pressure.
Protection	Antibodies and complement protect against infection and foreign substances.
Regulation	Enzymes control chemical reactions; hormones regulate many physiological processes.
Structure	Collagen fibres provide structural support to many parts of body.
	Keratin strengthens skin, hair, and nails.
Transport	Hemoglobin transports oxygen and carbon dioxide in blood.
	Plasma proteins, particularly albumin, serve as transport molecules (i.e., for hormones, cations, bilirubin, and medications).
	Proteins in cell membranes control movement of materials into and out of cells.
Coagulation	Hemostasis is regulated by clotting factors and proteins that balance coagulation and anticoagulation.

lymphoid tissue), are synthesized by the liver. They play an important role in preserving blood volume and pressure by maintaining plasma oncotic pressure. The liver also synthesizes several nonessential amino acids and serum enzymes, including aspartate aminotransferase (AST; previously *serum glutamic oxaloacetic transaminase [SGOT]*), alanine aminotransferase (ALT; previously *serum glutamic pyruvic transaminase [SGPT]*), lactate dehydrogenase (LDH), and alkaline phosphatase (ALP).

Carbohydrates. The liver contributes to the stability of blood glucose levels by releasing glucose during hypoglycemia (low blood glucose level) and absorbing glucose during hyperglycemia (high blood glucose level) and storing it as glycogen (glycogenesis) or converting it to fat. When all glycogen stores have been used, the liver can convert amino acids and glycerol to glucose (gluconeogenesis).

Insulin is a hormone synthesized in the pancreas by the beta cells of the islets of Langerhans and plays a vital role in glycogenesis. The primary stimulus for the secretion of insulin from the beta cells is glucose. The presence of insulin stimulates the diffusion of glucose into adipose and muscle tissue and inhibits the production of glucagon. Declining glucose levels, on the other hand, stimulate the alpha cells of the pancreatic islets to secrete insulin antagonist, glucagon. Glucagon is a hyperglycemic hormone because it raises blood glucose levels. Glucagon works on the liver and fat tissue. Liver cells respond by accelerating glycogenolysis and gluconeogenesis, whereas fats cells mobilize their fatty stores (lipolysis) and release fatty acid and glycerol to the blood. Glucagon-stimulated glycogenolysis and gluconeogenesis are responsible for up to 75% of glucose production in the fasting state.

Metabolic Detoxification

The liver alters exogenous and endogenous chemicals (e.g., medications), foreign molecules, and hormones to make them less toxic or less biologically active. This process, called **metabolic detoxification** or **biotransformation**, diminishes intestinal or renal tubular reabsorption of potentially toxic substances, and helps with their intestinal and renal excretion. In this way alcohol, barbiturates, amphetamines, steroids, and hormones (including estrogens, aldosterone, antidiuretic hormone, and testosterone) are metabolized or detoxified, preventing excessive accumulation and side effects. Although metabolic detoxification is usually protective, the end products of metabolic detoxification sometimes become toxins or active metabolites. Toxins of alcohol metabolism, for example, are acetaldehyde and hydrogen, which can damage the liver's ability to function (see Chapter 4 and Figure 4.19).

Storage of Minerals and Vitamins

The liver stores certain vitamins and minerals, including iron and copper, in times of excessive intake and releases them in times of need. The liver can store vitamins B_{12} and D for several months and vitamin A for several years. The liver also stores vitamins E and K. Iron is stored in the liver as ferritin, an iron–protein complex, and is released as needed for red blood cell production. Common tests of liver function are listed in Table 35.3.

Gallbladder

The **gallbladder** is a saclike organ on the inferior surface of the liver (Figure 35.20). Its primary function is to store and concentrate bile between meals. During the interdigestive period, bile flows from the liver through the right or left hepatic duct into the common hepatic duct and meets resistance at the closed sphincter of Oddi, which controls flow into the duodenum and prevents backflow of duodenal contents into the pancreatobiliary system. Bile then flows through the **cystic duct** into the gallbladder, where it is concentrated and stored. The mucosa of the gallbladder wall readily absorbs water and electrolytes, leaving a high concentration of bile salts, bile pigments, and cholesterol. The gallbladder holds about 90 mL of bile.

Within 30 minutes after eating, the gallbladder begins to contract, forcing stored bile through the cystic duct and into the common bile duct. The sphincter of Oddi relaxes, and bile flows into the duodenum through the major duodenal papilla. During the cephalic and gastric phases of digestion, gallbladder contraction is mediated by cholinergic branches of the vagus nerve. Hormonal regulation of gallbladder contraction is derived primarily from the release of *cholecystokinin* secreted by the duodenal and jejunal mucosa in the presence of fat. Vasoactive intestinal peptide, pancreatic polypeptide, and sympathetic nerve stimulation relax the gallbladder.

Exocrine Pancreas

The **pancreas** is approximately 20 cm long, with its head tucked into the curve of the duodenum and its tail touching the spleen. The body of the pancreas lies deep in the abdomen, behind the stomach (see Figure 35.20). The pancreas is unique in that it has both endocrine and exocrine functions. The endocrine pancreas secretes hormones: insulin, glucagon, somatostatin, and pancreatic polypeptide (see Chapter 18).

The **exocrine pancreas** is composed of acinar cells that secrete enzymes and networks of ducts that secrete alkaline fluids. Both have important digestive functions. The acinar cells are organized into spherical lobules around small secretory ducts (see Figure 35.20). Secretions drain into a system of ducts that leads to the **pancreatic duct (Wirsung duct)**, which empties into the common bile duct at the **ampulla of Vater**, and then into the duodenum. In some individuals, an accessory duct (the duct of Santorini) branches off the pancreatic duct and drains directly into the duodenum at the minor duodenal papilla.

Arterial blood is supplied to the pancreas by branches of the celiac and superior mesenteric arteries. Venous blood leaves the head of the pancreas through tributaries to the portal vein, with the body and tail being drained through the splenic vein. All hormonal pancreatic secretions also pass through the hepatic portal vein into the liver.

Pancreatic innervation arises from parasympathetic neurons of the vagus nerve. These fibres activate postganglionic fibres, which stimulate enzymatic and hormonal secretion. Sympathetic postganglionic fibres from the celiac and superior mesenteric plexuses innervate the blood vessels, cause vasoconstriction, and inhibit pancreatic secretion.

TABLE 35.3 Common Tests of Liver Function

Test	Normal Value	Interpretation
Serum Enzymes		
Alkaline phosphatase (ALP)	35–120 units/L	It increases with biliary obstruction and cholestatic hepatitis.
Gamma-glutamyltranspeptidase (GGT)	Males: 8–38 units/L Females: 5–31 units/L	It increases with biliary obstruction and cholestatic hepatitis.
Aspartate aminotransferase (AST)	0–35 units/L	It increases with hepatocellular injury (and injury in other tissues, such as skeletal and cardiac muscle).
Alanine aminotransferase (ALT)	4–36 units/L	It increases with hepatocellular injury and necrosis.
Lactate dehydrogenase (LDH)	100–190 units/L	Isoenzyme LD_5 is elevated with hypoxic and primary liver injury.
5′-Nucleotidase	2–16 units/L	It increases with an increase in ALP and in cholestatic disorders.
Bilirubin Metabolism		
Serum bilirubin		
Unconjugated (indirect)	3.4–120 µmol/L	It increases with hemolysis (lysis of red blood cells).
Conjugated (direct)	1.7–5.1 µmol/L	It increases with hepatocellular injury or obstruction.
TOTAL	5.1–17 µmol/L	It increases with biliary obstruction.
Urine bilirubin	0	It increases with biliary obstruction.
Urine urobilinogen	0–34 µmol/L	It increases with hemolysis or shunting of portal blood flow.
Serum Proteins		
Albumin	35–50 g/L	It decreases with hepatocellular injury.
Globulin	23–34 g/L	It increases with hepatitis.
TOTAL	64–83 g/L	
Albumin/globulin (A/G) ratio	1.5:1 to 2.5:1	The ratio reverses with chronic hepatitis or other chronic liver disease.
Transferrin	Males: 2–5 g/L Females: 1.9–4.4 g/L	Liver damage occurs with decreased values; iron deficiency with increased values.
Alpha fetoprotein (AFP)	0–40 µg/L	Elevated values occur in primary hepatocellular carcinoma.
Blood-Clotting Functions		
Prothrombin time (PT)	11–12.5 sec or 85–100% of control	It increases with chronic liver disease (cirrhosis) or vitamin K deficiency.
Activated partial thromboplastin time (aPTT)	30–40 sec	It increases with severe liver disease or heparin therapy.
Bromosulfophthalein (BSP) excretion	<6% retention in 45 min	Increased retention occurs with hepatocellular injury.

The aqueous secretions of the exocrine pancreas are isotonic and contain potassium, sodium, bicarbonate, and chloride. The highly alkaline pancreatic juice neutralizes the acidic chyme that enters the duodenum from the stomach and provides the alkaline medium needed for the actions of digestive enzymes and intestinal absorption of fat.

In the pancreas, transport of water and electrolytes through the ductal epithelium involves both active and passive mechanisms. The ductal cells actively transport hydrogen into the blood and bicarbonate into the duct lumen. Potassium and chloride are secreted by diffusion according to changes in electrochemical potential gradients. As the secretion flows down the duct, water is osmotically transported into the juice until it becomes isosmotic. At low flow rates bicarbonate is exchanged passively for chloride, but at higher flow rates there is less time for this exchange and bicarbonate concentration increases. Because eating stimulates the flow of pancreatic juice, the juice is most alkaline when it needs to be: during digestion.

The pancreatic enzymes can hydrolyze proteins (proteases), carbohydrates (amylases), and fats (lipases) (see Figure 35.11). The proteolytic (protein-digesting) enzymes include trypsin, chymotrypsin, carboxypeptidase, and elastase. These enzymes are secreted in their inactive forms—that is, as trypsinogen, chymotrypsinogen, procarboxypeptidase, and proelastase, respectively—to protect the pancreas from the digestive effects of its own enzymes. For further protection, the pancreas produces **trypsin inhibitor**, which prevents the activation of proteolytic enzymes while they are in the pancreas. Once in the duodenum, the inactive forms (proenzymes) are activated by **enterokinase**, an enzyme secreted by the duodenal mucosa. Trypsinogen is the first proenzyme to be activated. Its conversion to trypsin stimulates the conversion of chymotrypsinogen to chymotrypsin and procarboxypeptidase to carboxypeptidase. Each of these enzymes splits specific peptide bonds to reduce polypeptides to smaller peptides.

Secretion of the aqueous and enzymatic components of pancreatic juice is controlled by hormonal and vagal stimuli. Secretin stimulates the acinar and duct cells to secrete the bicarbonate-rich fluid that neutralizes chyme and prepares it for enzymatic digestion. As chyme enters the duodenum, its acidity (pH of 4.5 or less) stimulates the **S cells** (secretin-producing cells) of the duodenum to release secretin, which is absorbed by the intestine and delivered to the pancreas in the bloodstream. In the pancreas, secretin causes ductal and acinar cells to release alkaline fluid. Secretin also inhibits the actions of gastrin, thereby decreasing gastric hydrochloric acid secretion and motility. The overall effect is to neutralize the contents of the duodenum.

Enzymatic secretion follows, stimulated by cholecystokinin, which activates ACh from the vagus nerve and release of ACh from pancreatic stellate cells. Cholecystokinin is released in the duodenum in response to the essential amino acids and fatty acids already present in chyme. Once in the small intestine, activated pancreatic enzymes inhibit the release of more cholecystokinin and ACh. This feedback mechanism inhibits the secretion of more pancreatic enzymes. Pancreatic polypeptide is released after eating and inhibits postprandial pancreatic exocrine secretion. (See Table 35.1 for a summary of hormonal stimulation of pancreatic secretions.) Selected tests of pancreatic function are listed in Table 35.4.

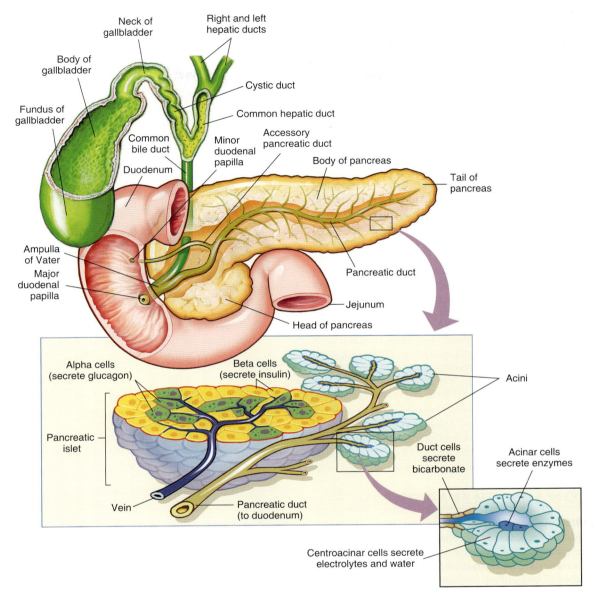

FIGURE 35.20 Associated Structures of the Gallbladder, Pancreas, and Pancreatic Acinar Cells and Duct. (Modified from Patton, K. T. [2018]. *Anatomy & physiology* [10th ed.]. Elsevier.)

TABLE 35.4 Common Laboratory Tests of Exocrine Pancreatic Function

Test	Normal Value	Clinical Significance
Serum amylase	31–107 units/L	Elevated levels occur with pancreatic inflammation.
Serum lipase	0–160 units/L	Elevated levels occur with pancreatic inflammation (may be elevated with other conditions. Differentiates pancreatitis from other conditions by measuring amylase isoenzyme study).
Urine amylase	2–19 units/hr 24–408 units/24 hr	Elevated levels occur with pancreatic inflammation.
Secretin test	Volume 1.8 mL/kg/hr Bicarbonate concentration: >80 mmol/L	Decreased volume occurs with pancreatic disease because a secretin stimulates pancreatic secretion. Decreased concentration or secretion can occur with pancreatic injury related to pancreatitis. Lack of buffering of gastric acid can lead to intestinal ulcers and decrease activation of digestive enzymes and medications that require a higher pH.
	Bicarbonate output: >10 mmol/L/30 sec	See above.
Stool fat	2–5 g/24 hr	This test measures fatty acids. Decreased pancreatic lipase increases stool fat.

GERIATRIC CONSIDERATIONS
Aging and the Gastro-intestinal System

Age-related changes in gastro-intestinal (GI) function vary among individuals and within organ systems. Changes can include:

Oral Cavity and Esophagus
1. Tooth enamel and dentin deteriorate, so cavities are more likely.
2. Teeth are lost as a result of periodontal disease and brittle roots that break easily.
3. Taste buds decline in number.
4. Sense of smell diminishes.
5. Salivary secretion decreases.
6. Dysphagia is much more common.
7. Eating is less pleasurable, appetite is reduced, and food is not sufficiently chewed or lubricated; therefore, swallowing is difficult.

Stomach
1. Gastric motility, blood flow, and volume and acid content of gastric juice may be reduced, particularly with gastric atrophy, and gastric emptying may be delayed.
2. Protective mucosal barrier decreases.

Intestines
1. There is a change in the composition of the intestinal microbiota and, as a result, increased susceptibility to disease.
2. Size of Peyer patches and degree of mucosal immunity decline, which increases the risk for infection and inflammation.
3. The brain–gut axis (bidirectional neuroendocrine communication) may be disrupted, and enteric neurons may degenerate with changes in GI motility, secretion, and absorption as well as the older person's appetite and overall nutritional status.
4. Intestinal villi may become shorter and more convoluted, with diminished ability to repair themselves.
5. Intestinal absorption, motility, and blood flow may decrease, prolonging transit time and altering nutrient absorption.
6. Rectal muscle mass decreases and the anal sphincter weakens.
7. Constipation, fecal impaction, and fecal incontinence may develop and are related to immobility, low-fibre diet, and changes in enteric nervous system structure and functions.

Liver
1. There is decreased hepatic regeneration; size and weight of liver decrease.
2. The ability to detoxify medications decreases.
3. Blood flow decreases, influencing the efficiency of medication metabolism.

Pancreas and Gallbladder
1. Fibrosis, fatty acid deposits, and pancreatic atrophy occur.
2. Secretion of digestive enzymes, particularly proteolytic enzymes, decreases.
3. No changes in gallbladder and bile ducts occur, but there is an increased prevalence of gallstones and cholecystitis.

Data from Britton, E., & McLaughlin, J. T. (2013). *Proceedings of the Nutrition Society, 72*(1), 173–177; Lakshminarayanan, B., Stanton, C., O'Toole, P. W., et al. (2014). *Journal of Nutrition, Health and Aging, 18*(9), 773–786; Rayner, C. K., & Horowitz, M. (2013). *Current Opinion in Clinical Nutrition & Metabolic Care, 16*(1), 33–38; Saffrey, M. J. (2013). *Developmental Biology, 382*(1), 344–355; Saffrey, M. J. (2014). *Age (Dordr), 36*(3), 9603.

DID YOU UNDERSTAND?

The Gastro-intestinal Tract

1. The gastro-intestinal (GI) tract is a hollow tube that extends from the mouth to the anus.
2. The major functions of the GI tract are the mechanical and chemical breakdown of food and the absorption of digested nutrients.
3. The wall of the GI tract is made up of four layers: mucosa, muscularis, submucosa, and serosa.
4. The peritoneum is a double layer of membranous tissue. The visceral layer covers the abdominal organs, and the parietal layer extends along the abdominal wall. The peritoneal cavity is the space between the two layers.
5. Digestion begins in the mouth, with chewing and salivation. The digestive component of saliva is α-amylase, which initiates carbohydrate digestion.
6. The esophagus is a hollow, muscular tube that transports food from the mouth to the stomach. Peristalsis—waves of sequential relaxations and contractions of the tunica muscularis—propels food through the esophagus.
7. The lower esophageal sphincter opens to allow swallowed food into the stomach and then closes to prevent regurgitation of food back into the esophagus.
8. The stomach is a hollow, baglike structure that secretes digestive juices, mixes and stores food, and propels partially digested food (chyme) through the pylorus into the duodenum.
9. The hormones gastrin and motilin stimulate gastric emptying; the hormones secretin and cholecystokinin delay gastric emptying.
10. The vagus nerve stimulates gastric (stomach) secretion and motility.
11. Gastric glands in the fundus and body of the stomach secrete intrinsic factor, which is needed for vitamin B_{12} absorption, and hydrochloric acid, which dissolves food fibres, kills microorganisms, and activates the enzyme pepsin.
12. Acid secretion is stimulated by the vagus nerve, gastrin, and histamine and is inhibited by sympathetic stimulation and cholecystokinin.
13. Chief cells in the stomach secrete pepsinogen, which is converted to pepsin in the acidic environment created by hydrochloric acid.
14. Mucus is secreted throughout the stomach and protects the stomach wall from acid and digestive enzymes.
15. The small intestine is 5 to 6 m long and has three segments: the duodenum, jejunum, and ileum.
16. The ileocecal valve connects the small and large intestines and prevents reflux into the small intestine.
17. Villi are small fingerlike projections that extend from the small intestinal mucosa and increase its absorptive surface area.
18. The duodenum receives chyme from the stomach through the pyloric valve. The presence of chyme stimulates the liver and gallbladder to deliver bile and the pancreas to deliver digestive enzymes. Digested substances are absorbed across the intestinal wall and then transported to the liver, where they are metabolized further.
19. Carbohydrates, amino acids, and fats are absorbed primarily by the duodenum and jejunum; bile salts and vitamin B_{12} are absorbed by

the ileum. Vitamin B$_{12}$ absorption requires the presence of intrinsic factor.
20. Minerals and water-soluble vitamins are absorbed by both active and passive transport throughout the small intestine.
21. Peristaltic movements created by longitudinal muscles move the chyme along the intestinal tract, and contractions of the circular muscles (haustral segmentation) mix the chyme.
22. The ileogastric reflex inhibits gastric motility when the ileum is distended.
23. The intestinointestinal reflex inhibits intestinal motility when one intestinal segment is overdistended.
24. The gastroileal reflex increases intestinal motility when gastric motility increases.
25. The large intestine consists of the cecum, appendix, colon (ascending, transverse, descending, and sigmoid), rectum, and anal canal.
26. The mucosa of the large intestine contains mucus-secreting cells and mucosal folds, but no villi.
27. The large intestine massages the fecal mass and absorbs water and electrolytes.
28. Distension of the ileum with chyme causes the gastrocolic reflex, or the mass propulsion of feces to the rectum.
29. Defecation is stimulated when the rectum is distended with feces. The tonically contracted internal anal sphincter relaxes, and if the voluntarily regulated external sphincter relaxes, defecation occurs.
30. The intestinal tract is sterile at birth and becomes totally colonized within 3 to 4 weeks.
31. The splanchnic blood flow provides blood to the esophagus, stomach, small and large intestines, gallbladder, pancreas, and spleen.

Accessory Organs of Digestion

1. The liver is the second largest organ in the body. It has digestive, metabolic, hematological, vascular, and immunological functions.
2. The liver is divided into the right and left lobes and smaller units called *liver lobules*. Liver lobules consist of plates of hepatocytes, which are the functional cells of the liver.
3. Bile is produced by the liver and is necessary for fat digestion and absorption. Bile's alkalinity helps to neutralize chyme, thereby creating a pH that enables the pancreatic enzymes to digest proteins, carbohydrates, and fats.
4. The hepatocytes synthesize 700 to 1 200 mL of bile per day and secrete it into the bile canaliculi, which are small channels between the hepatocytes. The bile canaliculi drain bile into the common bile duct and then into the duodenum through an opening called the *major duodenal papilla* (which is surrounded by the sphincter of Oddi).
5. Sinusoids are capillaries located between the plates of hepatocytes. Blood from the portal vein and hepatic artery flows through the sinusoids to a central vein in each lobule and then to the hepatic vein and inferior vena cava.
6. Kupffer cells, which are part of the mononuclear phagocyte system, line the sinusoids and destroy microorganisms in sinusoidal blood; they are important in bilirubin production and lipid metabolism.
7. The primary bile acids are synthesized from cholesterol by the hepatocytes. The primary acids are then conjugated to form bile salts. The secondary bile acids are the product of bile salt deconjugation by bacteria in the intestinal lumen.
8. Most bile salts and acids are recycled. The absorption of bile salts and acids from the terminal ileum and their return to the liver are known as the *enterohepatic circulation of bile*.
9. Bilirubin is a pigment liberated by the lysis of aged red blood cells in the liver and spleen. Unconjugated bilirubin is fat soluble and can cross cell membranes. Unconjugated bilirubin is converted to water-soluble, conjugated bilirubin by hepatocytes and is secreted with bile.
10. The liver produces clotting factors and can store a large volume of blood.
11. The liver metabolically transforms or detoxifies hormones, toxic substances, and medications to less active substances.
12. The gallbladder is a saclike organ located on the inferior surface of the liver. The gallbladder stores bile between meals and ejects it when chyme enters the duodenum.
13. Stimulated by cholecystokinin, the gallbladder contracts and forces bile through the cystic duct and into the common bile duct. The pancreas is a gland located behind the stomach. The endocrine pancreas produces hormones (glucagon, insulin) that help with the formation and cellular uptake of glucose. The exocrine pancreas secretes an alkaline solution and the enzymes (trypsin, chymotrypsin, carboxypeptidase, α-amylase, lipase) that digest proteins, carbohydrates, and fats.
14. Secretin stimulates pancreatic secretion of alkaline fluid, and cholecystokinin and acetylcholine stimulate secretion of enzymes. Pancreatic secretions originate in acini and ducts of the pancreas and empty into the duodenum through the common bile duct or an accessory duct that opens directly into the duodenum.

36

Alterations of Digestive Function

Mohamed Toufic El-Hussein, with originating chapter contributions by Sue E. Huether

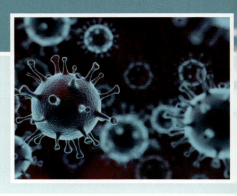

Additional resources are available online at https://evolve.elsevier.com/Canada/Huether/pathophysiology.

CHAPTER OUTLINE

Disorders of the Gastro-intestinal Tract, 883
  Clinical Manifestations of Gastro-intestinal Dysfunction, 883
  Disorders of Motility, 887
  Gastritis, 892
  Peptic Ulcer Disease, 893
  Malabsorption Syndromes, 897
  Inflammatory Bowel Disease, 898
  Diverticular Disease of the Colon, 900
  Appendicitis, 901
  Mesenteric Vascular Insufficiency, 901
  Disorders of Nutrition, 902
Disorders of the Accessory Organs of Digestion, 905
  Common Complications of Liver Disorders, 906

Disorders of the Liver, 910
Disorders of the Gallbladder, 914
Disorders of the Pancreas, 915
Digestive Symptoms and Intestinal Inflammation in COVID-19 Patients, 917
Cancer of the Digestive System, 917
  Cancer of the Gastro-intestinal Tract, 917
  Cancer of the Accessory Organs of Digestion, 921
  COMORBIDITIES: Comorbidities Related to Digestive Function, 923
  GERIATRIC CONSIDERATIONS: Age-Related Gastric Changes, 924
CASE STUDY, 924

LEARNING OBJECTIVES

1. Describe the pathophysiological alterations that lead to diarrhea, constipation, and abdominal pain.
2. Differentiate between parietal pain, visceral pain, and referred pain of the abdomen.
3. Discuss the signs and symptoms and physiological response to acute gastro-intestinal bleeding.
4. List and briefly explain the various disorders of motility of the gastro-intestinal tract.
5. Identify the consequences of obstruction at various sites in the gastro-intestinal tract.
6. Describe the causes, manifestations, treatments, outcomes, and complications of gastritis.
7. Compare the three main types of peptic ulcers: duodenal, gastric, and stress.
8. Discuss the postgastrectomy syndromes as they relate to long-term complications of partial or complete gastrectomy.
9. Discuss the clinical effects of pancreatic insufficiency, lactase deficiency, and bile salt deficiency.
10. Compare and contrast ulcerative colitis and Crohn's disease.
11. Discuss the pathophysiology, clinical manifestations, and treatment of diverticulitis, appendicitis, irritable bowel syndrome, and vascular insufficiency.
12. Discuss the pathophysiology, clinical manifestations, and treatment of obesity.
13. Compare and contrast short-term and long-term starvation.
14. Discuss the five major complications of liver dysfunction: portal hypertension, ascites, hepatic encephalopathy, jaundice, and hepatorenal syndrome.
15. Discuss the pathophysiology of viral hepatitis and fulminant hepatitis.
16. Discuss the causation, treatment options, and prognosis for alcoholic and biliary cirrhosis.
17. Discuss the pathophysiology of cholelithiasis and cholecystitis.
18. Compare and contrast acute and chronic pancreatitis.
19. Discuss the risk factors, incidence, manifestations, treatment, morbidity, and mortality of the various cancers of the digestive system.

KEY TERMS

Achalasia, 887
Acute colonic pseudo-obstruction, 891
Acute gastritis, 892
Acute liver failure (fulminant liver failure), 910
Acute pancreatitis, 915
Adiponectin, 904
Afferent loop obstruction, 896
Alcoholic cirrhosis, 911
Alcoholic fatty liver (steatosis), 910
Alcoholic steatohepatitis (alcoholic hepatitis), 911
Alkaline reflux gastritis, 896
Anemia, 897
Anorexia, 883
Appendicitis, 901
Ascites, 906
Barrett esophagus, 918
Biliary cirrhosis, 912
Bone and mineral disorder, 897
Cachexia, 905

Cholangiocellular carcinoma (cholangiocarcinoma), 922
Cholecystitis, 914
Cholelithiasis, 914
Chronic active hepatitis, 913
Chronic gastritis, 892
Chronic pancreatitis, 916
Cirrhosis, 910
Colorectal polyp, 920
Constipation, 884
Crohn's disease (CD), 899
Curling ulcer, 895
Cushing's ulcer, 895
Diarrhea, 896
Diverticula, 900
Diverticulitis, 900
Diverticulosis, 900
Dumping syndrome, 896
Duodenal ulcer, 894
Dysphagia, 887
Eosinophilic esophagitis, 889
Esophageal varices, 906
Familial adenomatous polyposis (FAP), 920
Gallstone, 914
Gastric ulcer, 895
Gastritis, 892
Gastroesophageal reflux disease (GERD), 888
Gastroparesis, 889
Ghrelin, 904
Gluconeogenesis, 905
Glycogenolysis, 905
Hematochezia, 886
Hemolytic jaundice, 908
Hepatic encephalopathy, 908
Hepatocellular carcinoma (HCC), 921
Hepatopulmonary syndrome, 906
Hepatorenal syndrome, 908
Hereditary nonpolyposis colorectal cancer (HNPCC), 920
Hiatal hernia, 889
Hyperbilirubinemia, 908
Icteric phase of hepatitis, 913
Incubation phase, 913
Intestinal obstruction, 890
Irritable bowel syndrome (IBS), 899
Ischemic ulcer, 895
Jaundice (icterus), 908
Lactase deficiency, 897
Lactase non-persistence, 897
Large bowel obstruction, 891
Leptin, 904
Leptin resistance, 904
Long-term starvation, 905
Lower gastro-intestinal bleeding, 886
Lynch syndrome, 920
Malabsorption, 897
Maldigestion, 897
Malnutrition, 905
Melena, 886
Microscopic colitis, 899
Mixed hiatal hernia (type 3), 889
Motility diarrhea, 885
Nausea, 883
Neoplastic polyp, 920
Nonalcoholic fatty liver disease (NAFLD), 912
Nonalcoholic steatohepatitis (NASH), 912
Obesity, 902
Obstructive jaundice, 908
Occult bleeding, 886
Osmotic diarrhea, 885
Pancreatic cancer, 922
Pancreatic insufficiency, 897
Pancreatitis, 915
Paraesophageal hiatal hernia (type 2), 889
Paralytic ileus, 890
Parietal pain, 886
Peptic ulcer, 893
Peptide YY, 904
Portal hypertension, 906
Portopulmonary hypertension, 906
Primary biliary cirrhosis, 912
Prodromal (preicteric) phase of hepatitis, 913
Projectile vomiting, 884
Pyloric obstruction (gastric outlet obstruction), 889
Recovery phase of hepatitis, 913
Rectal carcinoma, 921
Refeeding syndrome, 905
Referred pain, 886
Retching, 883
Secondary biliary cirrhosis, 912
Secretory diarrhea, 885
Short-term starvation, 905
Sliding hiatal hernia (type 1), 889
Small bowel obstruction (SBO), 890
Small intestinal carcinoma, 920
Splenomegaly, 906
Starvation, 905
Steatorrhea, 885
Stress-related mucosal disease (stress ulcer), 895
Ulcerative colitis (UC), 899
Upper gastro-intestinal bleeding, 886
Varices, 906
Viral hepatitis, 912
Visceral pain, 886
Vomiting (emesis), 883
Weight loss, 897
Zollinger-Ellison syndrome, 893

The gastro-intestinal (GI) tract is a continuous, hollow organ that extends from the mouth to the anus. It includes the esophagus, stomach, small intestine, large intestine, and rectum. The accessory organs of digestion include the salivary glands, liver, gallbladder, and pancreas.

Disorders of the GI tract disrupt one or more of its functions. Structural and neural abnormalities can slow, obstruct, or accelerate the movement of intestinal contents at any level of the GI tract. Inflammatory and ulcerative conditions of the GI wall disrupt secretion, motility, and absorption. Inflammation or obstruction of the liver, pancreas, or gallbladder can alter metabolism and result in local and systemic symptoms. Many clinical manifestations of GI tract disorders are nonspecific and can be caused by a variety of impairments.

DISORDERS OF THE GASTRO-INTESTINAL TRACT

QUICK CHECK 36.1
1. How does osmotic diarrhea differ from secretory diarrhea?
2. How is visceral pain "referred"?
3. What are the best clinical indicators of acute GI bleeding blood loss?

Clinical Manifestations of Gastro-intestinal Dysfunction
Anorexia
Anorexia is lack of a desire to eat despite physiological stimuli that would normally produce hunger. This nonspecific symptom is often associated with nausea, abdominal pain, diarrhea, and psychological stress. Side effects of medications and disorders of other organ systems, including cancer, heart disease, and kidney disease, are often accompanied by anorexia.

Vomiting
Vomiting (emesis) is the forceful emptying of stomach and intestinal contents (chyme) through the mouth.[1] The vomiting centre lies in the medulla oblongata. Stimuli initiating the vomiting reflex include severe pain; distension of the stomach or duodenum; the presence of ipecac or copper salts in the duodenum; stimulation of the vestibular system through cranial nerve VIII (motion sickness); side effects of many medications; torsion or trauma affecting the ovaries, testes, uterus, bladder, or kidney; motion; and activation of the chemoreceptor trigger zone (CTZ) (area postrema) in the medulla (e.g., morphine). Nausea and retching (dry heaves) are distinct events that usually precede vomiting. Nausea is a subjective experience associated with various conditions, including abnormal pain and labyrinthine stimulation (i.e., spinning movement). Specific neural pathways have not been identified, but hypersalivation and tachycardia are common associated symptoms. Retching is the muscular event of vomiting without the expulsion of vomitus.

Vomiting begins with deep inspiration. The glottis closes, the intrathoracic pressure falls, and the esophagus becomes distended. Simultaneously, the abdominal muscles contract, creating a pressure gradient from abdomen to thorax. The lower esophageal sphincter (LES) and body of the stomach relax, but the duodenum and antrum of the stomach spasm. The reverse peristalsis and pressure gradient force chyme from the stomach and duodenum up into the esophagus. Because the upper esophageal sphincter is closed, chyme does not enter the mouth. As the abdominal muscles relax, the contents of the esophagus drop back into the stomach. This process may be repeated several times before vomiting occurs. A diffuse sympathetic discharge causes the tachycardia, tachypnea, and diaphoresis that accompany retching and vomiting. The parasympathetic system mediates copious salivation, increased gastric motility, and relaxation of the upper and lower esophageal sphincters.

With vomiting, the duodenum and antrum of the stomach produce reverse peristalsis, while the body of the stomach and the esophagus relax. When the stomach is full of gastric contents, the diaphragm is forced high into the thoracic cavity by strong contractions of the abdominal muscles. The higher intrathoracic pressure forces the upper esophageal sphincter to open, and chyme is expelled from the mouth. Then the stomach relaxes and the upper part of the esophagus contracts, forcing the remaining chyme back into the stomach. The LES then closes. The cycle is repeated if there is a volume of chyme remaining in the stomach.

Spontaneous vomiting not preceded by nausea or retching is called *projectile vomiting*. It is caused by direct stimulation of the vomiting centre by neurological lesions (e.g., increased intracranial pressure, tumours, or aneurysms) involving the brainstem or can be a symptom of GI obstruction (pyloric stenosis). The metabolic consequences of vomiting are fluid, electrolyte, and acid–base disturbances, including hyponatremia, hypokalemia, hypochloremia, and metabolic alkalosis (see Chapter 5).

Constipation

Constipation is difficult or infrequent defecation. It is a common problem, particularly among older persons, and usually means a decrease in the number of bowel movements per week, hard stools, and difficult evacuation. The definition of *constipation* must be individually determined since normal bowel habits range from one to three evacuations per day to one per week. Constipation is not significant until it causes health risks or impairs quality of life.

PATHOPHYSIOLOGY Constipation can occur as a primary or secondary condition.[2] Primary constipation is generally classified into three categories. *Normal transit (functional) constipation* involves a normal rate of stool passage, but there is difficulty with stool evacuation. *Functional constipation* is associated with a sedentary lifestyle, low-residue diet (the habitual consumption of highly refined foods), or low fluid intake. *Slow-transit constipation* involves impaired colonic motor activity with infrequent bowel movements, straining to defecate, mild abdominal distension, and palpable stool in the sigmoid colon. *Pelvic floor dysfunction* or *outlet dysfunction* refers to an inability or difficulty expelling stool because of dysfunction of the pelvic floor muscles or anal sphincter. Examples include pelvic floor dyssynergia, rectal fissures, strictures, or hemorrhoids.

Secondary constipation can be caused by diet, medications, or neurogenic disorders (e.g., stroke, Parkinson's disease, spinal cord lesions, multiple sclerosis, Hirschsprung's disease) in which neural pathways or neurotransmitters are altered and colon transit time delayed. Opiates (particularly codeine), antacids containing calcium carbonate or aluminum hydroxide, anticholinergics, iron, and bismuth tend to inhibit bowel motility. Endocrine or metabolic disorders associated with constipation include hypothyroidism, diabetes mellitus, hypokalemia, and hypercalcemia. Pelvic hiatal hernia (herniation of the bowel through the floor of the pelvis), diverticuli, irritable bowel syndrome (constipation predominant), and pregnancy are associated with constipation. Aging may result in decreased mobility, changes in neuromuscular function, use of medications, and comorbid medical conditions causing constipation.[2] Constipation as a notable change in bowel habits can be an indication of colorectal cancer.

CLINICAL MANIFESTATIONS Indicators of constipation include two of the following for at least 3 months: (1) straining with defecation at least 25% of the time; (2) lumpy or hard stools at least 25% of the time; (3) sensation of incomplete emptying at least 25% of the time; (4) manual manoeuvres to facilitate stool evacuation for at least 25% of defecations; and (5) fewer than three bowel movements per week.[3] Changes in bowel evacuation patterns, such as less frequent defecation, smaller stool volume, hard stools, difficulty passing stools (straining), or a feeling of bowel fullness and discomfort, require investigation. Fecal impaction (hard, dry stool retained in the rectum) is associated with rectal bleeding, abdominal or cramping pain, nausea and vomiting, weight loss, and episodes of diarrhea. Straining to evacuate stool may cause engorgement of the hemorrhoidal veins and hemorrhoidal disease or thrombosis with rectal pain, bleeding, and itching. Passage of hard stools can cause painful anal fissures.

EVALUATION AND TREATMENT The history, current use of medications, physical examination, and stool diaries provide precise clues regarding the nature of constipation. The individual's description of frequency, stool consistency, associated pain, and presence of blood or whether evacuation was stimulated by enemas or cathartics (laxatives) is important. Palpation may disclose colonic distension, masses, and tenderness. Digital examination of the rectum and anorectal manometry are performed to assess sphincter tone and detect anal lesions. Colonic transit time and imaging techniques can assist in identifying the cause of constipation. Colonoscopy is used to visualize the lumen directly.

The treatment for constipation is to manage the underlying cause or disease for each individual. Management of constipation usually consists of bowel retraining, in which the individual establishes a satisfactory bowel evacuation routine without becoming preoccupied with bowel movements. The individual also may need to engage in moderate exercise, drink more fluids, and increase fibre intake. Fibre supplements, stool softeners, and laxative agents are useful for some individuals. Enemas can be used to establish bowel routine, but they should not be used habitually. Biofeedback may be beneficial in some instances for forming new bowel evacuation habits. When there is failure to respond to dietary or medical therapies, surgery (colectomy) is considered as a last resort.[4]

Diarrhea

Diarrhea is the presence of loose, watery stools. Acute diarrhea is more than three loose stools developing within 24 hours and lasting less than 14 days. Persistent diarrhea lasts longer than 14 to 30 days, and chronic diarrhea lasts longer than 4 weeks.[5,6] Diarrhea can have high rates of morbidity and mortality in children younger than 5 years of age, particularly in developing countries (see Chapter 37) and in older persons. Many factors determine stool volume, including water content of the colon, diet, the presence of nonabsorbed food, nonabsorbable material, and intestinal secretions. Stool volume in the normal adult averages less than 200 g per day. Stool volume in children depends on age and size. An infant may pass up to 100 g per day. The adult intestine processes approximately 9 L of luminal contents per day: 2 L are ingested and the remaining 7 L consist of intestinal secretions. Of this volume, 99% of the fluid is absorbed: 90% (7 to 8 L) in the small intestine and 9% (1 to 2 L) in the colon. Normally, approximately 150 mL of water is excreted daily in the stool.

PATHOPHYSIOLOGY Diarrhea in which the volume of feces is increased is called *large-volume diarrhea*. It generally is caused by excessive amounts of water or secretions or both in the intestines. *Small-volume diarrhea*, in which the volume of feces is not increased, usually results from excessive intestinal motility.

The three major mechanisms of diarrhea are osmotic, secretory, and motile.

1. **Osmotic diarrhea.** A nonabsorbable substance in the intestine draws excess water into the intestine and increases stool weight and volume, producing large-volume diarrhea. Causes include lactase and pancreatic enzyme deficiency; excessive ingestion of synthetic, nonabsorbable sugars; full-strength tube-feeding formulas; or dumping syndrome associated with gastric resection.
2. **Secretory diarrhea.** Excessive mucosal secretion of fluid and electrolytes produces large-volume diarrhea. Infectious causes include viruses (e.g., rotavirus), bacterial enterotoxins (e.g., *Escherichia coli* and *Vibrio cholerae*), exotoxins from overgrowth of *Clostridium difficile* following antibiotic therapy (see *Health Promotion: Clostridium difficile and Diarrhea*), and small bowel bacterial overgrowth.[7] Small-volume diarrhea is usually caused by an inflammatory disorder of the intestine, such as ulcerative colitis (UC), Crohn's disease (CD), or microscopic colitis, but also can result from colon cancer or fecal impaction.
3. **Motility diarrhea** is caused by resection of the small intestine (short bowel syndrome), surgical bypass of an area of the intestine or fistula formation between loops of intestine, irritable bowel syndrome–diarrhea predominant, diabetic neuropathy, hyperthyroidism, and laxative abuse. Excessive motility decreases transit time and opportunity for fluid absorption, resulting in diarrhea.

CLINICAL MANIFESTATIONS Diarrhea can be acute or chronic, depending on its cause. Systemic effects of prolonged diarrhea are dehydration, electrolyte imbalance (hyponatremia, hypokalemia), and weight loss. Manifestations of acute bacterial or viral infection include fever, with or without vomiting or cramping pain. Most infectious diarrhea usually lasts less than 2 weeks. The exceptions are *C. difficile*, *Aeromonas*, or *Yersinia enterocolitica*.[8] Fever, cramping pain, and bloody stools accompany chronic diarrhea caused by inflammatory bowel disease (IBD) or dysentery. **Steatorrhea** (fat in the stools), bloating, and diarrhea are common signs of malabsorption syndromes. (Steatorrhea can also indicate alterations in liver and pancreatic functions.) Anal and perineal skin irritation can occur.

EVALUATION AND TREATMENT A thorough history is taken to document the onset, frequency, and duration of diarrhea, the volume of stools, and the presence of blood in the stools. Malabsorption syndromes

HEALTH PROMOTION
Clostridium difficile and Diarrhea

Clostridium difficile is a Gram-positive, spore-forming, anaerobic bacillus that causes infectious diarrhea by producing toxins. *C. difficile* is the most frequent cause of health care–associated infectious diarrhea in Canada and other developed countries.

The reported incidence of health care–associated *C. difficile* infection in Canada has risen over the last decade. *C. difficile* infection manifestations range from uncomplicated diarrhea to life-threatening pseudomembranous colitis, bowel perforation, and sepsis. In Canadian hospitals, the mortality rate associated with *C. difficile* infection increased almost fourfold from 1997 to 2005 (1.5% of cases to 5.7% of cases, respectively, $p < 0.001$).

The main mode of transmission for *C. difficile* in health care settings is person-to-person spread through the fecal–oral route. Momentary contamination of the hands of health care personnel with *C. difficile* spores and environmental contamination play an important role in the transmission of *C. difficile* in health care settings. *C. difficile*, unlike other bacterial pathogens, persists longer in the environment and resists routine disinfection processes. For this reason, environmental contamination is a significant factor in cross-transmission between patients and health care providers.

Often a *C. difficile* infection is associated with previous antibiotic use. Judicious administration of antibiotics is believed to have a role in preventing and terminating the incidence of *C. difficile* infection.

Measures to Prevent C. difficile Infections in Health Care Facilities
- Facility design should include single rooms for the routine care of inpatients that includes private toilets inside the room, designated patient sinks, alcohol-based hand rub dispensers, and designated handwashing sinks for staff.
- Special disposal systems should be used to manage the disposal of fecal matter when bedpans or commodes are required to avoid environmental contamination with *C. difficile* spores.
- For patients with acute diarrhea due (suspected or confirmed) to *C. difficile* infection, contact precautions must be implemented immediately until the diarrhea is resolved or its cause is determined not to be infectious.
- Patients with uncontrolled diarrhea or fecal incontinence should be given preference for single private rooms where possible.
- Signage should be placed at the entrance to the infected patient's room, cubicle, and designated bed space to indicate the need to apply contact precautions.
- Frequent hand hygiene should be performed using effective techniques:
  - following patient care or contact with patient's environment
  - after removing gloves at point of care and just prior to leaving the patient's room
  - following contact with fecal matter, bedpans, and commodes
- Handwashing with soap and water should be performed at the point of care and at an assigned staff handwashing sink. If an assigned staff handwashing sink is not available at the point of care, alcohol-based hand rub (with an alcohol concentration between 60 and 90%) must be used, and hand hygiene with soap and water must be performed as soon as a staff handwashing sink is available.
- Hand wipes (impregnated with plain soap, antimicrobials, or alcohol) may be used as an alternative to soap and water when an assigned staff handwashing sink is not readily available, or when the handwashing sink is not appropriate (e.g., contaminated, no running water, no soap), when hands are not visibly soiled. When hands are visibly soiled, alcohol-based hand rub should be used after the use of hand wipes, and hands should be washed with soap and water once a suitable staff handwashing sink is available.
- Unless medically indicated (e.g., for essential diagnostic and therapeutic tests or treatment) the transfer of patients suspected or confirmed to have *C. difficile* infection within and between facilities should be avoided.
- The number of visitors for a patient on contact precautions must be restricted to essential visitors (e.g., immediate family member or parent, guardian, or primary caretaker) only.

From Public Health Agency of Canada. (2013). *Clostridium difficile infection: infection prevention and control guidance for management in acute care settings*. https://www.phac-aspc.gc.ca/nois-sinp/guide/c-dif-acs-esa/index-eng.php.

usually manifest as steatorrhea. Exposure to contaminated food or water is indicated if the individual has travelled in foreign countries or areas where drinking water might be contaminated. Iatrogenic diarrhea is suggested if the individual has undergone abdominal radiation therapy, intestinal resection, or treatment with selected medications (e.g., antibiotics, diuretics, antihypertensives, laxatives, anticoagulants, or chemotherapy). Physical examination helps identify underlying systemic disease. Stool studies, abdominal imaging, endoscopy, and intestinal biopsies provide more specific data, particularly for persistent diarrhea.

Treatment for diarrhea includes restoration of fluid and electrolyte balance, administration of antimotility (e.g., loperamide [Imodium]) medication, water absorbent medication (e.g., attapulgite [Kaopectate] and polycarbophil [Equalactin]), or both, and treatment of causal factors. Nutritional deficiencies need to be corrected in cases of chronic diarrhea or malabsorption.[9]

Abdominal Pain

Abdominal pain is the presenting symptom of a number of GI diseases and can be acute or chronic.[10] The causal mechanisms of abdominal pain are *mechanical*, *inflammatory*, or *ischemic*. Generally, the abdominal organs are not sensitive to mechanical stimuli, such as cutting, tearing, or crushing. These organs are, however, sensitive to stretching and distension, which activate nerve endings in both hollow and solid structures. Pain accompanies rapid distension rather than gradual distension. Traction on the peritoneum caused by adhesions, distension of the common bile duct, or forceful peristalsis resulting from intestinal obstruction causes pain because of increased tension. Capsules that surround solid organs, such as the liver and gallbladder, contain pain fibres that are stimulated by stretching if these organs swell. Abdominal pain may be generalized to the abdomen or localized to a particular abdominal quadrant. The nature of the pain is often described as sharp, dull, or colicky.

Abdominal pain is usually associated with tissue injury and inflammation. Biochemical mediators of the inflammatory response, such as histamine, bradykinin, and serotonin, stimulate organic nerve endings and produce abdominal pain. The edema and vascular congestion that accompany chemical, bacterial, or viral inflammation also cause painful stretching. Hindrance of blood flow from the distension of bowel obstruction or mesenteric vessel thrombosis produces the pain of ischemia, and increased concentrations of tissue metabolites stimulate pain receptors.

Abdominal pain can be parietal (somatic), visceral, or referred. **Parietal pain**, from the parietal peritoneum, is more localized and intense than visceral pain, which arises from the organs themselves. Parietal pain lateralizes because, at any particular point, the parietal peritoneum is innervated from only one side of the nervous system. **Visceral pain** arises from a stimulus (distension, inflammation, ischemia) acting on an abdominal organ. Inflammatory mediators associated with chronic low-grade inflammation can cause pain hypersensitivity.[11] The pain is usually poorly localized, diffuse, or vague with a radiating pattern, because nerve endings in abdominal organs are sparse and multisegmented. Pain arising from the stomach, for example, is experienced as a sensation of fullness, cramping, or gnawing in the midepigastric area. **Referred pain** is visceral pain felt at some distance from a diseased or affected organ. It is usually well localized and is felt in the skin dermatomes or deeper tissues that share a central afferent pathway with the affected organ. For example, acute cholecystitis (gallbladder inflammation) may have pain referred to the right shoulder or scapula.

Gastro-intestinal Bleeding

Upper gastro-intestinal bleeding is bleeding in the esophagus, stomach, or duodenum, and is characterized by frank, bright-red bleeding or dark, grainy digested blood ("coffee grounds") that has been affected by stomach acids (Table 36.1). Upper GI bleeding is commonly caused by bleeding varices (varicose veins) in the esophagus, peptic ulcers, arteriovenous malformations, or a Mallory-Weiss tear at the esophageal-gastric junction caused by severe retching.[12] **Lower gastro-intestinal bleeding**, or bleeding from the jejunum, ileum, colon, or rectum, can be caused by polyps, diverticulitis, inflammatory disease, cancer, or hemorrhoids. **Occult bleeding** is usually caused by slow, chronic blood loss that is not obvious and results in iron deficiency anemia as iron stores in the bone marrow are slowly depleted.[13] Acute, severe GI bleeding is life-threatening depending on the volume and rate of blood loss, associated disease and age of the affected individual, and effectiveness of treatment.

Physiological response to GI bleeding depends on the amount and rate of the loss (Figure 36.1). Changes in blood pressure and heart rate are the best indicators of massive blood loss in the GI tract. During the early stages of blood volume depletion, the peripheral arteries and arterioles constrict to shunt blood to vital organs, including the brain. Signs of large-volume blood loss are postural hypotension (a drop in blood pressure that occurs with a change from the recumbent position to a sitting or upright position), lightheadedness, and loss of vision. Tachycardia develops as a compensatory response to maintain cardiac output and tissue perfusion. If blood loss continues, hypovolemic shock develops (see Chapter 24). Diminished blood flow to the kidneys causes decreased urine output and may lead to oliguria (low urine output), tubular necrosis, and kidney failure. Ultimately, insufficient cerebral and coronary blood flow causes irreversible anoxia and death.

The presentations of GI bleeding are summarized in Table 36.1. The accumulation of blood in the GI tract is irritating and increases peristalsis, causing vomiting or diarrhea, or both. If bleeding is from the lower GI tract, the diarrhea is frankly bloody. Bleeding from the upper GI tract also can be rapid enough to produce **hematochezia** (bright-red stools), but generally some digestion of the blood components will have occurred, producing **melena**—black or tarry stools that are sticky and have a characteristic foul odour. The digestion of blood proteins originating from massive upper GI bleeding is reflected by an increase in blood urea nitrogen (BUN) levels (see Figure 36.1).

The hematocrit and hemoglobin values are not the best indicators of acute GI bleeding because plasma volume and red cell volume are lost proportionately. As the plasma volume is replaced, the hematocrit and hemoglobin values begin to reflect the extent of blood loss. The interpretation of these values is modified to account for exogenous replacement of fluids and the hydration status of the tissues.

TABLE 36.1 Presentations of Gastro-intestinal Bleeding

Presentations	Definition
Acute Bleeding	
Hematemesis	Bloody vomitus; either fresh, bright-red blood or dark, grainy digested blood with "coffee grounds" appearance
Melena	Black, sticky, tarry, foul-smelling stools caused by digestion of blood in gastro-intestinal tract; should be distinguished from black stools caused by dietary iron supplements, blackberries, or bismuth (e.g., Pepto-Bismol)
Hematochezia	Fresh, bright-red blood passed from rectum
Occult Bleeding	Trace amounts of blood in normal-appearing stools or gastric secretions; detectable only with positive fecal occult blood test (guaiac test)

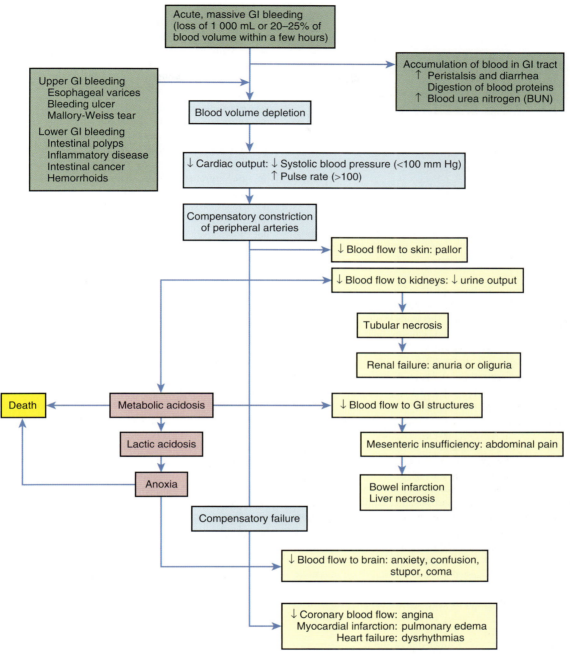

FIGURE 36.1 Pathophysiology of Gastro-Intestinal Bleeding. *GI*, Gastro-intestinal.

Disorders of Motility

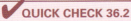 **QUICK CHECK 36.2**
1. Why is heartburn associated with gastroesophageal reflux?
2. What causes postoperative paralytic ileus?
3. How does peritonitis develop with bowel obstruction?

Dysphagia

PATHOPHYSIOLOGY Dysphagia is difficulty swallowing. It can result from *mechanical obstruction* of the esophagus or a functional disorder that impairs esophageal motility. Intrinsic obstructions originate in the wall of the esophageal lumen (esophageal dysphagia) and include tumours, strictures, and diverticular herniations (outpouchings). Extrinsic mechanical obstructions originate outside the esophageal lumen and narrow the esophagus by pressing inward on the esophageal wall. The most common cause of extrinsic mechanical obstruction is tumour.

Functional dysphagia is caused by neural or muscular disorders that interfere with voluntary swallowing or peristalsis. Disorders that affect the striated muscles of the hypopharyngeal area and upper esophagus interfere with the oropharyngeal (voluntary) phase of swallowing (oropharyngeal dysphagia). Typical causes are dermatomyositis (a muscle disease) and neurological impairments caused by cerebrovascular accidents, Parkinson's disease, multiple sclerosis, muscular dystrophy, or achalasia.[14]

Achalasia is a rare form of dysphagia related to loss of inhibitory neurons in the myenteric plexus with smooth muscle atrophy in the

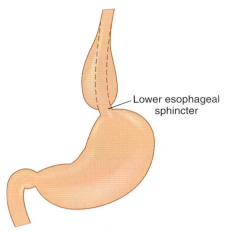

FIGURE 36.2 Achalasia. Increased lower esophageal sphincter muscle tone and loss of peristaltic function prevent food from entering the stomach, causing esophageal distension.

middle and lower portions of the esophagus. The myenteric neurons are attacked by a cell-mediated and antibody-mediated immune response against an unknown antigen. This leads to altered esophageal peristalsis and failure of the LES to relax, causing functional obstruction of the lower esophagus with varying severity.[15] Food accumulates above the obstruction, distends the esophagus, and causes dysphagia (Figure 36.2). Cough and aspiration can occur. As hydrostatic pressure increases, food is slowly forced past the obstruction into the stomach. Chronic esophageal distension requires dilation or surgical myotomy of the LES.

CLINICAL MANIFESTATIONS Distension and spasm of the esophageal muscles during eating or drinking may cause a mild or severe stabbing pain at the level of obstruction. Discomfort occurring 2 to 4 seconds after swallowing is associated with upper esophageal obstruction. Discomfort occurring 10 to 15 seconds after swallowing is more common in obstructions of the lower esophagus. If obstruction results from a growing tumour, dysphagia begins with difficulty swallowing solids and advances to difficulty swallowing semisolids and liquids. If motor function is impaired, both solids and liquids are difficult to swallow. Regurgitation of undigested food, unpleasant taste sensation, vomiting, aspiration, and weight loss are common manifestations of all types of dysphagia. Aspiration of esophageal contents can lead to cough and pneumonia.

EVALUATION AND TREATMENT Knowledge of the person's history and clinical manifestations contributes significantly to a diagnosis of dysphagia. Further evaluation of swallowing should be performed by a speech language pathologist to determine what the person can eat/drink, and whether the swallowing reflex is intact, to prevent potential aspiration. Recommendations are then made based on the outcome of this assessment. (Note that this evaluation is *not* performed by the nurse.)

Imaging is used to visualize the contours of the esophagus and identify structural defects. High-resolution manometry and intraluminal impedance monitoring document the duration and amplitude of abnormal pressure changes associated with obstruction or loss of neural regulation. Esophageal endoscopy is performed to examine the esophageal mucosa and obtain biopsy specimens.

The individual is taught to manage symptoms by eating small meals slowly, taking fluid with meals, and sleeping with the head elevated to prevent regurgitation and aspiration. Food and medications may need to be formulated so they can be swallowed. Anticholinergic medications (e.g., botulinum toxin type A [Botox]) may relieve symptoms of dysphagia. Mechanical dilation of the esophageal sphincter and surgical separation of the lower esophageal muscles with a longitudinal incision (myotomy) are the most effective treatments for achalasia.[16]

Gastroesophageal Reflux Disease (GERD)

Gastroesophageal reflux disease (GERD) is the reflux of acid and pepsin or bile salts from the stomach into the esophagus that causes esophagitis. The prevalence of GERD is estimated at 18 to 27% in North America.[17] Risk factors for GERD include older age, obesity, hiatal hernia, and medications or chemicals that relax the LES (anticholinergics, nitrates, calcium channel blockers, nicotine).[18] GERD may be a trigger for asthma or chronic cough. Gastroesophageal reflux that does not cause symptoms is known as *physiological reflux*. In *nonerosive reflux disease*, individuals have symptoms of reflux disease but no visible esophageal mucosal injury (functional heartburn).[19]

PATHOPHYSIOLOGY Abnormalities in LES function, esophageal motility, and gastric motility or emptying can cause GERD. The resting tone of the LES tends to be lower than normal from either transient relaxation or weakness of the sphincter. Vomiting, coughing, lifting, bending, obesity, or pregnancy increases abdominal pressure, contributing to the development of reflux esophagitis. Hiatal hernia can weaken the LES. Delayed gastric emptying can contribute to reflux esophagitis by (1) lengthening the period during which reflux is possible and (2) increasing gastric acid content. Disorders that delay emptying include gastroparesis, gastric or duodenal ulcers, which can cause pyloric edema, and strictures that narrow the pylorus.

The severity of the esophagitis depends on the composition of the gastric contents and the esophageal mucosa exposure time. An acid pocket is an area of postprandial unbuffered gastric acid immediately distal to the gastroesophageal junction. It is enlarged in hiatal hernia and can contribute to GERD. If the gastric content is highly acidic or contains bile salts and pancreatic or intestinal enzymes, reflux esophagitis can be severe. In individuals with weak esophageal peristalsis, refluxed chyme remains in the esophagus longer than usual. The prolonged presence of refluxed chime in the esophagus increases the amount of time the esophageal mucosa is exposed to acids, enzymes, and bile. The refluxate causes mucosal injury and inflammation with hyperemia, increased capillary permeability, edema, tissue fragility, and erosion. Fibrosis and thickening may develop. Precancerous lesions (Barrett esophagus) can be a long-term consequence. Precancerous lesions can progress to adenocarcinoma.[20]

CLINICAL MANIFESTATIONS The clinical manifestations of erosive reflux esophagitis are heartburn (pyrosis), acid regurgitation, dysphagia, chronic cough, asthma attacks (see Chapter 27), laryngitis, and upper abdominal pain within 1 hour of eating. The symptoms worsen if the individual lies down or if intra-abdominal pressure increases (e.g., as a result of coughing, vomiting, or straining at stool). Edema, strictures, esophageal spasm, or decreased esophageal motility may result in dysphagia with weight loss. Alcohol or acid-containing foods, such as citrus fruits, can cause discomfort during swallowing.

EVALUATION AND TREATMENT Diagnosis of GERD is based on history and clinical manifestations. Esophageal endoscopy shows hyperemia, edema, erosion, and strictures. Dysplastic changes (Barrett esophagus) can be identified by tissue biopsy. Impedance or pH monitoring measures the movement of stomach contents upward into the esophagus and the acidity of the refluxate. Because heartburn also may be experienced as chest pain, cardiac ischemia must be ruled out.

Proton pump inhibitors are the agents of choice for controlling symptoms and healing esophagitis. Other therapies include H2 receptor antagonists or prokinetics and antacids. Weight reduction, smoking cessation, elevation of the head of the bed 15 cm, and avoiding tight clothing also help to alleviate symptoms. Laparoscopic fundoplication is the most common surgical intervention when medical treatment fails.[21]

Eosinophilic esophagitis is an idiopathic inflammatory disease of the esophagus characterized by infiltration of eosinophils associated with atopic disease, including asthma and food allergies. It occurs in adults and children. Dysphagia, food impaction, vomiting, and weight loss are common symptoms. Endoscopy with biopsy identifies the eosinophilic infiltration and differentiation from GERD. Treatment is symptomatic, including elimination diets and steroids.

Hiatal Hernia

PATHOPHYSIOLOGY Hiatal hernia is a type of diaphragmatic hernia with protrusion (herniation) of the upper part of the stomach through the diaphragm and into the thorax (Figure 36.3).[22] Sliding hiatal hernia (type 1) is the most common. With this type of hernia, the proximal portion of the stomach moves into the thoracic cavity through the esophageal hiatus, an opening in the diaphragm for the esophagus and vagus nerves. A congenitally short esophagus, fibrosis or excessive vagal nerve stimulation, or weakening of the diaphragmatic muscles at the gastroesophageal junction contributes to the hernia. GERD is associated with this type of herniation. Coughing, bending, tight clothing, ascites, obesity, and pregnancy accentuate the hernia.

Paraesophageal hiatal hernia (type 2) is the herniation of the greater curvature of the stomach through a secondary opening in the diaphragm alongside the esophagus. The position of a portion of the stomach above the diaphragm causes congestion of mucosal blood flow, leading to gastritis and ulcer formation. Strangulation of the hernia is a major complication. It can present with vomiting and epigastric and retrosternal epigastric pain and is a surgical emergency.[23]

Mixed hiatal hernia (type 3) is less common and is a combination of sliding and paraesophageal hiatal hernias. It tends to occur in conjunction with several other diseases, including reflux esophagitis, peptic ulcer, cholecystitis (gallbladder inflammation), cholelithiasis (gallstones), chronic pancreatitis, and diverticulosis.

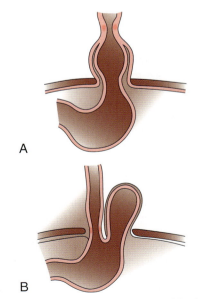

FIGURE 36.3 Types of Hiatal Hernia. **A**, Sliding hiatal hernia (type 1). **B**, Paraesophageal hiatal hernia (type 2). Not shown is mixed hiatal hernia (type 3).

CLINICAL MANIFESTATIONS Hiatal hernias are often asymptomatic. Generally, a wide variety of symptoms develop later in life and are associated with other GI disorders, including GERD. Symptoms include heartburn, regurgitation, dysphagia, and epigastric pain. Ischemia from hernia strangulation causes acute, severe chest or epigastric pain, nausea, vomiting, and GI bleeding.

EVALUATION AND TREATMENT Diagnostic procedures include radiology with barium swallow, endoscopy, and high-resolution manometry. A chest X-ray film often will show the protrusion of the stomach into the thorax, indicating paraesophageal hiatal hernia.

Treatment for sliding hiatal hernia is usually conservative. The individual can diminish reflux by eating small, frequent meals and avoiding the recumbent position after eating. Abdominal supports and tight clothing should be avoided, and weight control is recommended for obese individuals. Antacids alleviate reflux esophagitis. Individuals who are uncomfortable at night benefit from sleeping with the head of the bed elevated 15 cm. Surgery (fundoplication) is performed if medical management fails to control symptoms.

Gastroparesis is delayed gastric emptying in the absence of mechanical gastric outlet obstruction. It is most commonly associated with diabetes mellitus, surgical vagotomy, or fundoplication. It can be idiopathic. The pathophysiology is not well understood but involves abnormalities of the autonomic nervous system, smooth muscle cells, enteric neurons, and GI hormones. Diabetic gastroparesis represents a form of neuropathy involving the vagus nerve. Symptoms include nausea, vomiting, abdominal pain, and postprandial fullness or bloating. Treatment options include dietary management; prokinetic medications; and, in some cases, gastric electrical stimulation or surgical venting gastrostomy.[24]

Pyloric Obstruction

PATHOPHYSIOLOGY Pyloric obstruction (gastric outlet obstruction) is the narrowing or blocking of the opening between the stomach and the duodenum. This condition can be congenital (e.g., infantile hypertrophic pyloric stenosis; see Chapter 37) or acquired. Acquired obstruction is caused by peptic ulcer disease or carcinoma near the pylorus. Duodenal ulcers are more likely than gastric ulcers to obstruct the pylorus. Ulceration causes obstruction resulting from inflammation, edema, spasm, fibrosis, or scarring. Tumours cause obstruction by growing into the pylorus.

CLINICAL MANIFESTATIONS Early in the course of pyloric obstruction, the individual experiences vague epigastric fullness, which becomes more distressing after eating and at the end of the day. Nausea and epigastric pain may occur as the muscles of the stomach contract in attempts to force chyme past the obstruction. These symptoms disappear when the chyme finally moves into the duodenum. As obstruction progresses, anorexia develops, sometimes accompanied by weight loss. Severe obstruction causes gastric distension and atony (lack of muscle tone and gastric motility). Gastric distension stimulates gastric secretion, which increases the feeling of fullness. Rolling or jarring of the abdomen produces a sloshing sound called the *succussion splash*. At this stage, vomiting is a cardinal sign of obstruction. It is usually copious and occurs several hours after eating. The vomitus contains undigested food but no bile. Prolonged vomiting leads to dehydration, which is accompanied by a hypokalemic and hypochloremic metabolic alkalosis caused by loss of gastric potassium and acid, respectively. Because food does not enter the intestine, stools are infrequent and small. Prolonged pyloric obstruction causes severe malnutrition, dehydration, and extreme debilitation.

EVALUATION AND TREATMENT Diagnosis is based on clinical manifestations, a history of ulcer disease, and examination of residual gastric contents. Endoscopy is performed if gastric carcinoma is the suggested cause of pyloric obstruction.

Obstructions resulting from ulceration often resolve with conservative management. A large-bore nasogastric tube is used to aspirate stomach contents and relieve distension. Then nasogastric suction is maintained for 2 to 3 days to decompress the stomach and restore normal motility. Gastric secretions that contribute to inflammation and edema can be suppressed with proton pump inhibitors or H2 receptor antagonists. Fluids and electrolytes (saline and potassium) are given intravenously to promote rehydration and correct hypokalemia and alkalosis (see Chapter 5). Severely malnourished individuals may require parenteral hyperalimentation (intravenous nutrition). Surgery or the placement of pyloric stents may be required to treat gastric carcinoma or persistent obstruction caused by fibrosis and scarring.[25,26]

Intestinal Obstruction and Paralytic Ileus

Intestinal obstruction can be caused by any condition that prevents the normal flow of chyme through the intestinal lumen (Table 36.2).[27]

TABLE 36.2 Common Causes of Intestinal Obstruction

Cause	Pathophysiology
Hernia	Protrusion of intestine through weakness in abdominal muscles or through inguinal ring
Intussusception	Telescoping of one part of intestine into another; this usually causes strangulation of blood supply; more common in infants 10–15 months of age than in adults (see Figure 36.4D)
Torsion (volvulus)	Twisting of intestine on its mesenteric pedicle, with occlusion of blood supply; often associated with fibrous adhesions; occurs most often in middle-aged and older men
Diverticulosis	Inflamed saccular herniations (diverticuli) of mucosa and submucosa through tunica muscularis of colon; diverticuli are interspersed between thick, circular, fibrous bands; most common in obese individuals older than 60 years (see Figure 36.9)
Tumour	Tumour growth into intestinal lumen; adenocarcinoma of colon and rectum is most common tumoral obstruction; most common in individuals older than 60 years
Paralytic (adynamic) ileus	Loss of peristaltic motor activity in intestine; associated with abdominal surgery, peritonitis, hypokalemia, ischemic bowel, spinal trauma, or pneumonia
Fibrous adhesions	Peritoneal irritation from surgery, trauma, or Crohn's disease leads to formation of fibrin and adhesions that attach to intestine, omentum, or peritoneum and can cause obstruction; most common in small intestine
Fecal mass (impaction)	Hardened stool impacted in the rectum or distal sigmoid colon, with subsequent obstruction; associated with lack of mobility due to aging or spinal cord injury; fecal impaction is related to reduction of colonic mass movements and an inability to use abdominal muscles to assist in defecation

TABLE 36.3 Large and Small Bowel Obstruction

Type of Obstruction	Cause
Small bowel obstruction	Adhesions: secondary to previous abdominal surgeries—75%
	Hernia: inguinal, ventral, or femoral—10%
	Tumours: may be associated with intussusception—10%
	Mesenteric ischemia—3–5%
	Crohn's disease—<1%
Large bowel obstruction	Colon/rectal cancer—90%
	Volvulus—4–5%
	Diverticular disease—3–5%
	Other causes (inflammatory bowel disease, adhesions, hernia)

Data from Mizell, J. S., & Turnage, R. H. (2016). Intestinal obstruction. In M. Feldman, L. S. Friedman, & L. J. Brandt (Eds.), *Sleisenger & Fordtran's gastrointestinal and liver disease: pathophysiology, diagnosis, management* (10th ed., pp. 2154–2170). Saunders.

Obstructions can occur in either the small or the large intestine (Table 36.3). The small intestine is more commonly obstructed because of its narrower lumen. Classifications of intestinal obstruction are summarized in Table 36.4. Intestinal obstruction is classified by cause as simple or functional. *Simple obstruction* is mechanical blockage of the lumen by a lesion, and it is the most common type of intestinal obstruction. Paralytic ileus, or *functional obstruction*, is a failure of intestinal motility often occurring after intestinal or abdominal surgery, acute pancreatitis, or hypokalemia. Acute obstructions usually have mechanical causes, such as adhesions or hernias (Figure 36.4). Chronic or partial obstructions are more often associated with tumours or inflammatory disorders, particularly of the large intestine.

PATHOPHYSIOLOGY The major pathophysiological alterations are presented in Figure 36.5. Postoperative paralytic ileus results from inhibitory neural reflexes associated with inflammatory mediators and the influence of exogenous (i.e., meperidine [Demerol] or morphine) and endogenous opioids (endorphins) that affect the entire GI tract. Small bowel obstruction (SBO) is caused by postoperative adhesions, tumours, CD, and hernias. SBO leads to distension caused by impaired absorption and increased secretion with accumulation of fluid and gas inside the lumen proximal to the obstruction.[28] Distension decreases the intestine's ability to absorb water and electrolytes and increases the net secretion of these substances into the lumen. Copious vomiting or sequestration of fluids in the intestinal lumen prevents their reabsorption and produces severe fluid and electrolyte disturbances. Extracellular fluid volume and plasma volume decrease, causing dehydration, increased hematocrit level, hypotension, and tachycardia. Severe dehydration leads to hypovolemic shock. Metabolic alkalosis initially develops as a result of excessive loss of hydrogen ions that would normally be reabsorbed from the gastric juice and vomiting. With prolonged obstruction or obstruction lower in the intestine, metabolic acidosis is more likely to occur because bicarbonate from pancreatic secretions and bile cannot be reabsorbed. Hypokalemia from vomiting and decreased potassium absorption can be extreme, promoting acidosis and atony of the intestinal wall. Metabolic acidosis also may be accentuated by ketosis, the result of declining carbohydrate stores caused by starvation. Lack of circulation permits the buildup of significant amounts of

TABLE 36.4 Classifications of Intestinal Obstruction

Criteria for Classification	Definition
Onset	
Acute	Sudden onset; often caused by torsion, intussusception, or herniation
Chronic	Protracted onset; more commonly from tumour growth or progressive formation of strictures
Extent of Obstruction	
Partial	Incomplete obstruction of intestinal lumen
Complete	Complete obstruction of intestinal lumen
Location of Obstructing Lesion	
Intrinsic	Obstruction develops within intestinal lumen; examples: gut wall edema or hemorrhage, foreign bodies (gallstones), tumours, or gut wall fibrosis
Extrinsic	Obstruction originates outside intestine; examples: tumours, torsion, fibrosis, hernia, intussusception
Effects on Intestinal Wall	
Simple	Luminal obstruction without impairment of blood supply
Strangulated	Luminal obstruction with occlusion of blood supply
Closed loop	Obstruction at each end of a segment of intestine
Casual Factors	
Mechanical	Blockage of intestinal lumen by intrinsic or extrinsic lesions; usually treated surgically
Functional (paralytic ileus)	Paralysis of intestinal musculature caused by trauma, peritonitis, electrolyte imbalances, or spasmolytic agents; usually treated by decompression with suction or surgery if death of tissue occurs

lactic acid, which worsen the metabolic acidosis. If pressure from the distension is severe enough, it occludes the arterial circulation and causes ischemia, necrosis, perforation, and peritonitis. Fever and leukocytosis are often associated with overgrowth of bacteria, ischemia, and bowel necrosis. Bacterial proliferation and translocation across the mucosa to the systemic circulation cause peritonitis or sepsis. The release of inflammatory mediators into the circulation causes remote organ failure.

Large bowel obstruction is less common and often related to cancer. Diverticulitis, IBD, and other causes of obstruction are less common. *Acute colonic pseudo-obstruction* (Ogilvie syndrome) is a rare massive dilation of the large bowel that is related to excessive sympathetic motor input or decreased parasympathetic motor input with absence of mechanical obstruction. It occurs primarily in people who are critically ill and immobilized older persons.

CLINICAL MANIFESTATIONS
Signs and symptoms of *small intestine obstruction* include colicky pains caused by intestinal distension followed by nausea and vomiting. Pain intensifies for seconds or minutes as a peristaltic wave of muscle contraction meets the obstruction. Pain may be continuous with severe distension and then diminish in intensity. If ischemia occurs, the pain loses its colicky character and becomes more constant and severe. Sweating and tachycardia occur as a sympathetic nervous system response to hypotension. Fever, severe leukocytosis, abdominal distension, and rebound tenderness develop as ischemia progresses to necrosis, perforation, and peritonitis.

Obstruction at the pylorus causes early, profuse vomiting. Obstruction in the proximal small intestine causes mild distension and vomiting of bile-stained fluid. Lower obstruction in the small intestine causes more pronounced distension because a greater length of intestine is proximal to the obstruction. In this case, vomiting may not occur early but may occur later and contain fecal material. Partial obstruction can cause diarrhea or constipation, but complete obstruction usually causes constipation only. Complete obstruction increases the number of bowel sounds, which may be tinkly and accompanied by peristaltic rushes and crampy abdominal pain. Signs of hypovolemia and metabolic acidosis may be observed as early as 24 hours after the occurrence of complete obstruction. Distension may be severe enough to push against the diaphragm and decrease lung volume. It can also lead to atelectasis and pneumonia, particularly in debilitated individuals.

Large intestine obstruction usually presents with hypogastric pain and abdominal distension. Pain can vary from vague to excruciating, depending on the degree of ischemia and the development of peritonitis. Vomiting occurs late in the obstructive process. Small and large intestinal perforation presents the same with acute, persistent abdominal pain, nausea, vomiting, and fever.[29] *Acute colonic pseudo-obstruction* is characterized by abdominal distension, abdominal pain, and nausea and vomiting. Bowel sounds are usually present.

EVALUATION AND TREATMENT
Evaluation is based on clinical manifestations and imaging studies. Successful management requires early identification of the site and type of obstruction. Replacement of fluid and electrolytes and decompression of the lumen with gastric or intestinal suction are essential forms of therapy. Laparoscopic procedures can release adhesions. Immediate surgical intervention is required for strangulation, complete obstruction, or perforation. Colonic stents may be placed for malignant obstruction. Neostigmine (Prostigmin), a parasympathomimetic, is used for colonic pseudo-obstruction and colonoscopic decompression may be required.[30]

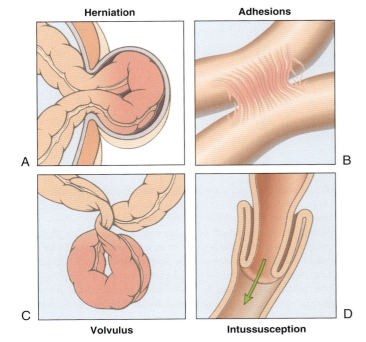

FIGURE 36.4 Intestinal Obstructions. **A**, Hernia. **B**, Constrictions from adhesions. **C**, Volvulus. **D**, Intussusception. From Kumar, V., Abbas, A., & Aster, J. [2021]. *Robbins basic pathology* [10th ed.]. Saunders.

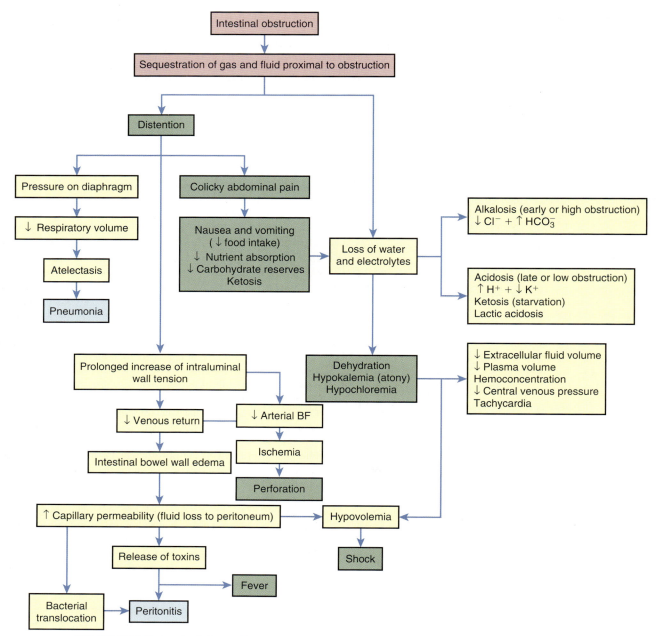

FIGURE 36.5 Pathophysiology of Intestinal Obstruction. *BF,* Blood flow; *Cl⁻,* Chloride; *H⁺,* hydrogen; *HCO₃⁻,* bicarbonate; *K⁺,* potassium.

Gastritis

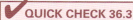

QUICK CHECK 36.3
1. What is the most common cause of chronic gastritis?
2. Compare the three types of peptic ulcers.
3. What causes a stress ulcer?

Gastritis is an inflammatory disorder of the gastric mucosa. It can be acute or chronic and affect the superficial mucosa of the fundus or antrum, or both.

Acute gastritis is caused by injury of the protective mucosal barrier caused by medications, chemicals, or *Helicobacter pylori* infection. Nonsteroidal anti-inflammatory drugs (NSAIDs; e.g., ibuprofen [Advil], naproxen [Apo-Naproxen], indomethacin [Indocin], and Aspirin) inhibit the action of cyclooxygenase-1 (COX-1) and cause gastritis because they inhibit prostaglandin synthesis, which normally stimulates the secretion of mucus. Alcohol, histamine, digitalis, and metabolic disorders, such as uremia, are contributing factors. *H. pylori*–associated acute gastritis causes inflammation, increased gastric secretion in antral gastritis, decreased gastric section in fundal gastritis, pain, nausea, and vomiting. The clinical manifestations of acute gastritis can include vague abdominal discomfort, epigastric tenderness, and bleeding. Healing usually occurs spontaneously within a few days. Discontinuing injurious medications, using antacids, or decreasing acid secretion with H2 receptor antagonists facilitates healing.

Chronic gastritis tends to occur in older persons and causes chronic inflammation, mucosal atrophy, and epithelial metaplasia.

Chronic gastritis is classified as type A, immune (fundal), or type B, nonimmune (antral), depending on the pathogenesis and location of the lesions. When both types of chronic gastritis occur, it is known as type AB, or pangastritis, and the antrum is more severely involved. Type C gastritis is associated with reflux of bile and pancreatic secretions into the stomach, causing chemical injury.

Chronic immune (fundal) gastritis is the rarest form of gastritis and is associated with loss of T lymphocyte (T cell) tolerance and development of autoantibodies to gastric H^+–K^+ ATPase. The gastric mucosa degenerates extensively in the body and fundus of the stomach, leading to gastric atrophy. Loss of parietal cells diminishes acid and intrinsic factor secretion. Pernicious anemia can develop from decreased vitamin B_{12} absorption (see Chapter 21). The feedback mechanism that normally inhibits gastrin secretion is impaired, causing elevated plasma levels of gastrin. Chronic fundal gastritis occurs in association with other autoimmune diseases (e.g., rheumatoid arthritis, autoimmune thyroid disease, or type 1 diabetes mellitus) and is a risk factor for gastric carcinoma, particularly in individuals who develop pernicious anemia.

Chronic nonimmune (antral gastritis) generally involves the antrum only and is more common than fundal gastritis. It is caused by *H. pylori* bacteria, and it also is associated with use of alcohol, tobacco, and NSAIDs.[31] There are high levels of hydrochloric acid secretion with an increased risk for duodenal ulcers. *H. pylori* also can progress to autoimmune atrophic gastritis and involves the fundus, thus becoming pangastritis. There is greater risk for the development of gastric cancer in these cases.[32]

Signs and symptoms of chronic gastritis often include vague symptoms: anorexia, fullness, nausea, vomiting, and epigastric pain. Gastric bleeding may be the only clinical manifestation of gastritis. Gastroscopic examination and biopsy may show a longstanding inflammatory process and gastric atrophy in an individual with no history of abdominal distress. Failure to stimulate acid secretion confirms achlorhydria (diminished secretion of hydrochloric acid). The gastric secretions also can be evaluated for the presence of intrinsic factor. Symptoms can usually be managed by eating smaller meals in conjunction with a soft, bland diet and by avoiding alcohol and Aspirin. *H. pylori* infection is treated with antibiotics, and vitamin B_{12} is administered to correct pernicious anemia.

Peptic Ulcer Disease

A **peptic ulcer** is a break or ulceration in the protective mucosal lining of the lower esophagus, stomach, or duodenum. Ulcers develop when mucosal protective factors are overcome by erosive factors commonly caused by NSAIDs and *H. pylori* infection. Risk factors for peptic ulcer disease are summarized in *Risk Factors*: Peptic Ulcer. Psychological stress may be a risk factor for peptic ulcer disease, but the exact mechanism of causation is not known.[33]

In Canada, it is estimated that 8 to 10 million people are infected with *H. pylori*. In Indigenous communities, approximately 75% of people are infected with *H. pylori*. *H. pylori* eradication therapy costs around $90 per person in Canada and is 80 to 90% effective. A second round of therapy in instances of resistance costs around $275.[34]

The *H. pylori* infection rate increases with age in Canada. The infection rate for 30-year-olds is 1 in 5 people, or 1 million people. The infection rate for people 80 years or older is 1 in 2 people, or 0.5 million people.[34]

H. pylori infection is one of the causes of functional dyspepsia. The Canadian population groups considered to be at a high risk for *H. pylori* infection number over 4.1 million; these groups have been identified based on origin of birth, area of residence, or both. Testing and eradication costs for these groups are estimated to be $350 million.[34]

H. pylori infection is considered to be a carcinogen by World Health Organization because it is associated with the development of stomach cancer. In communities with a high prevalence of *H. pylori* infection, treated individuals have a 1 in 10 chance of reinfection after one year.[34]

Peptic ulcers can be single or multiple, acute or chronic, and superficial or deep. Superficial ulcerations are called *erosions* because they erode the mucosa but do not penetrate the muscularis mucosae (Figure 36.6). True ulcers extend through the muscularis mucosae and damage blood vessels, causing hemorrhage, or perforate the GI wall.

Zollinger-Ellison syndrome is a rare syndrome that also is associated with peptic ulcers caused by a gastrin-secreting neuroendocrine tumour or multiple tumours (gastrinoma) of the pancreas or duodenum. Increased secretion of gastrin causes excess secretion of gastric acid, resulting in gastric and duodenal ulcers, gastroesophageal reflux with abdominal pain, and diarrhea.[35]

RISK FACTORS
Peptic Ulcer

- Infection of the gastric and duodenal mucosa with *Helicobacter pylori*
- Chronic use of nonsteroidal anti-inflammatory drugs
- Alcohol
- Smoking
- Advanced age
- Chronic diseases, such as emphysema, rheumatoid arthritis, cirrhosis, obesity, and diabetes
- Type O blood
- Psychological stress

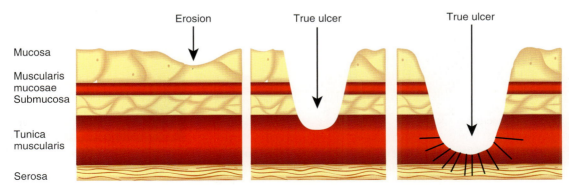

FIGURE 36.6 Lesions Caused by Peptic Ulcer Disease.

Duodenal Ulcers

Duodenal ulcers occur with greater frequency than other types of peptic ulcers and are commonly caused by *H. pylori* infection and NSAID use.[36] Idiopathic duodenal ulcers are rare and can be associated with altered mucosal defences, rapid gastric emptying, elevated serum gastrin levels, or acid production stimulated by smoking.[36]

PATHOPHYSIOLOGY Causative factors, singly or in combination, cause acid and pepsin concentrations in the duodenum to penetrate the mucosal barrier and cause ulceration (Figure 36.7). The host response to *H. pylori* infection is activation of T and B lymphocytes (T and B cells) with infiltration of neutrophils. Release of inflammatory cytokines damages the gastric epithelium. An *H. pylori* virulence factor (cytotoxin-associated gene A [*CagA*]) produces vacuolating cytotoxin A (VacA), causing apoptosis of gastric epithelial cells and promoting inflammation. *H. pylori* mucosal infection underlies gastric and duodenal ulcer and gastric cancer.[37]

CLINICAL MANIFESTATIONS The characteristic manifestation of a duodenal ulcer is chronic intermittent pain in the epigastric area. The pain begins 2 or 3 hours after eating, when the stomach is empty. It is not unusual for pain to occur in the middle of the night and disappear by morning. Pain is relieved rapidly by ingestion of food or antacids, creating a typical pain-food-relief pattern. Some individuals with duodenal ulcer may have no symptoms; the first manifestation may be hemorrhage or perforation, particularly with a history of NSAID or anticoagulant use.

Complications of duodenal ulcer include bleeding, perforation, and obstruction of the duodenum or outlet of the stomach. Bleeding is the most common cause of mortality, particularly among older persons. Perforation occurs with destruction of all layers of the duodenal wall and causes sudden, severe epigastric pain.[38] Obstruction may be the result of edema from inflammation or scarring from chronic injury. It is not clear why individuals infected with *H. pylori* duodenal ulcers are negatively associated with gastric cancer.[39]

Duodenal ulcers often heal spontaneously but recur within months without treatment. Exacerbations tend to develop in the spring and fall. Relief of pain accompanies healing. Constant, unremitting pain may be caused by complications, such as intestinal obstruction or perforation. Bleeding from duodenal ulcers causes hematemesis or melena.[40]

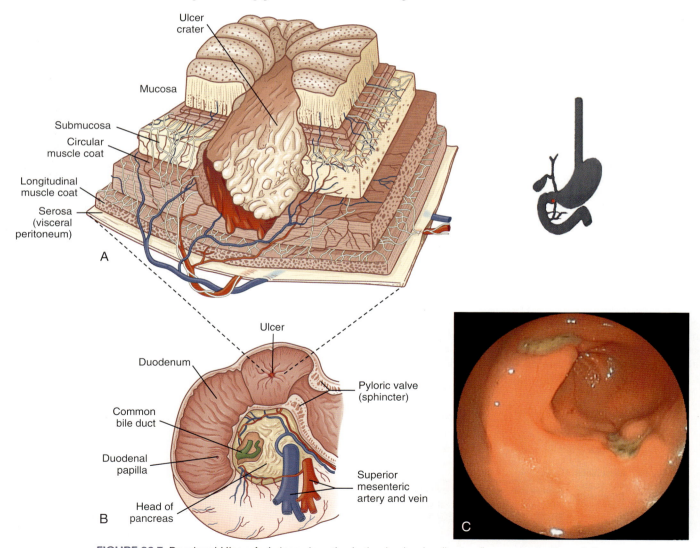

FIGURE 36.7 Duodenal Ulcer. **A,** A deep ulceration in the duodenal wall extending as a crater through the entire mucosa and into the muscle layers. **B,** Sequence of ulcerations from normal mucosa to duodenal ulcer. **C,** Bilateral (kissing) duodenal ulcers in a person using nonsteroidal anti-inflammatory drugs. ([C], Med_Chaos. https://commons.wikimedia.org/wiki/File:Gastric_Ulcer_Antrum.jpg.)

EVALUATION AND TREATMENT Several diagnostic approaches are used to differentiate duodenal ulcers from gastric ulcers or gastric carcinoma. Endoscopic evaluation allows visualization of lesions and biopsy. Radioimmune assays of gastrin levels are evaluated to identify ulcers associated with gastric carcinomas. *H. pylori* is detected using the urea breath test, *H. pylori*–specific serum immunoglobulin G (IgG) and immunoglobulin A (IgA) antibodies, and measurement of *H. pylori* stool antigen levels. Findings from gastric biopsy detect *H. pylori* infection and confirm eradication after treatment.[41]

Management of duodenal ulcers is aimed at relieving the causes and effects of hyperacidity and preventing complications. Antacids neutralize gastric contents and relieve pain. Acid secretion can be suppressed with medications that block H2 receptors and inhibit the secretion of acid. Proton pump inhibitors inhibit acid production. *H. pylori* is treated with a combination of antibiotics and proton pump inhibitors, but antibiotic resistance is an increasing problem.[42] Surgical resection may be required for bleeding or perforating ulcers, obstruction, or peritonitis.

Gastric Ulcers

Gastric ulcers are ulcers of the stomach and occur about equally in males and females, usually between the ages of 55 and 65 years. They are about one-fourth as common as duodenal ulcers (Table 36.5).

PATHOPHYSIOLOGY Generally, gastric ulcers develop in the antral region, adjacent to the acid-secreting mucosa of the body. The primary defect is an abnormality that increases the mucosal barrier's permeability to hydrogen ions. Gastric secretion may be normal or less than normal, and there may be a decreased mass of parietal cells. Chronic gastritis is often associated with development of gastric ulcers and may precipitate ulcer formation by limiting the mucosa's ability to secrete a protective layer of mucus (Figure 36.8). Other factors include:
- decreased mucosal synthesis of prostaglandins
- duodenal reflux of bile and pancreatic enzymes damage the mucosal membrane
- use of NSAIDs (decreases prostaglandin synthesis)
- *H. pylori* infection.

A break in the mucosal barrier permits hydrogen ions to diffuse into the mucosa, where they disrupt permeability and cellular structure. A vicious cycle can be established as the damaged mucosa liberates histamine, which stimulates the increase of acid and pepsinogen production, blood flow, and capillary permeability. The disrupted mucosa becomes edematous and loses plasma proteins. Destruction of small vessels causes bleeding.

CLINICAL MANIFESTATIONS The clinical manifestations of gastric ulcers are similar to those of duodenal ulcers (see Table 36.5). The pattern of pain is common, but the pain of gastric ulcers also occurs immediately after eating. Gastric ulcers also tend to be chronic rather than alternating between periods of remission and exacerbation and cause more anorexia, vomiting, and weight loss than duodenal ulcers. The evaluation and treatment of gastric ulcers are similar to the evaluation and treatment of duodenal ulcers.

Stress-Related Mucosal Disease

A stress-related mucosal disease (stress ulcer) is an acute form of peptic ulcer that tends to accompany the physiological stress of severe illness or major trauma. Usually, multiple sites of ulceration are distributed within the stomach or duodenum. Stress ulcers may be classified as ischemic ulcers or Cushing's ulcers.

Ischemic ulcers develop within hours of an event such as hemorrhage, multisystem trauma, severe burns, heart failure, or sepsis. Shock, anoxia, inflammation, and sympathetic responses cause ischemia of the stomach and duodenal mucosa, disrupting the mucosal barrier. Stress ulcers that develop as a result of burn injury are often called Curling ulcers. Cushing's ulcer is a stress ulcer associated with severe brain trauma or brain surgery. Decreased mucosal blood flow and hypersecretion of acid caused by overstimulation of the vagal nuclei damage the mucosal barrier, causing erosions and ulceration.

The primary clinical manifestation of stress-related mucosal disease is bleeding, which is uncommon, but occurs more readily with the presence of coagulopathy and more than 48 hours of mechanical ventilation. Prophylactic treatment regimens are used to prevent this disease.[43] Stress ulcers seldom become chronic.

Surgical Treatment of Ulcer

Advances in the medical treatment of peptic ulcer disease with acid suppression and eradication of *H. pylori* have reduced the number of cases requiring surgery. The most common indications for ulcer surgery are recurrent or uncontrolled bleeding and perforation of the stomach or duodenum. The primary objectives of surgical treatment are to reduce stimuli for acid secretion, decrease the number of acid-secreting cells in the stomach, and correct complications of ulcer disease.

TABLE 36.5 Characteristics of Gastric and Duodenal Ulcers

Characteristics	Gastric Ulcer	Duodenal Ulcer
Incidence		
Age at onset	50–70 years	20–50 years
Family history	Usually negative	Positive
Gender (prevalence)	Equal in women and men	Greater in men
Stress factors	Increased	Average
Ulcerogenic medications	Normal use	Increased use
Cancer risk	Increased	Not increased
Pathophysiology		
Abnormal mucus	May be present	May be present
Parietal cell mass	Normal or decreased	Increased
Acid production	Normal or decreased	Increased
Serum gastrin	Increased	Normal
Serum pepsinogen	Normal	Increased
Associated gastritis	More common	Usually not present
Helicobacter pylori	May be present (60–80%) Stimulates reduced acid secretion, gastric atrophy, and risk for gastric cancer	Often present (95–100%) Stimulates acid hypersecretion
Clinical Manifestations		
Pain	Located in upper abdomen; Intermittent; Pain-antacid-relief pattern; Food–pain pattern (when food in stomach)	Located in upper abdomen; Intermittent; Pain-antacid/food-relief pattern; Pain when stomach empty; Nocturnal pain common
Clinical course	Chronic ulcer without pattern of remission and exacerbation; Heals more slowly	Pattern of remissions and exacerbation for years; Heals more quickly

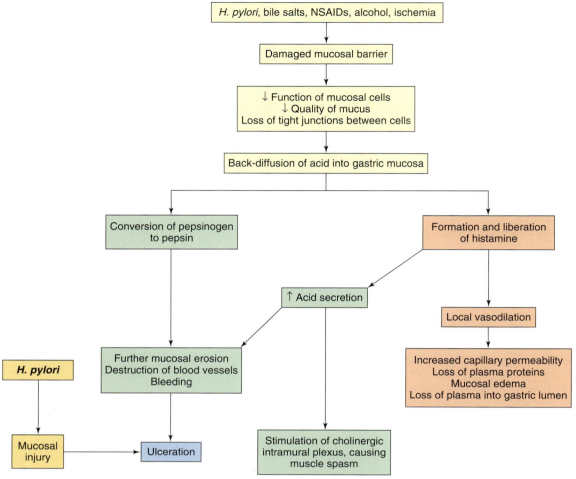

FIGURE 36.8 Pathophysiology of Gastric Ulcer Formation. *H. pylori, Helicobacter pylori; NSAIDs,* nonsteroidal anti-inflammatory drugs.

Acute complications of gastrectomy or anastomosis are relatively uncommon except in debilitated persons. Chronic complications, however, are likely to develop if a large portion of the stomach has been removed. These complications and their pathophysiological mechanisms are described in the next section.

Postgastrectomy Syndromes

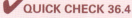 **QUICK CHECK 36.4**
1. Why are Crohn's disease and ulcerative colitis called *inflammatory bowel diseases*?
2. How is leptin resistance associated with obesity?
3. When does proteolysis begin in long-term starvation?

Postgastrectomy syndromes are a group of signs and symptoms that occur after gastric resection for the treatment of peptic ulcer, gastric carcinoma, or bariatric surgery for extreme obesity. They are caused by anatomical and functional changes in the stomach and upper small intestine[44] and include the following:

- **Dumping syndrome**. Rapid emptying of hypertonic chyme from the surgically residual stomach (the stomach component remaining after surgical resection following gastric or bariatric surgery) into the small intestine 10 to 20 minutes after eating; promoted by loss of gastric capacity, loss of emptying control when pylorus is removed, and loss of feedback control by duodenum when it is removed; responds to dietary management. Symptoms include cramping pain, nausea, vomiting, osmotic diarrhea, weakness, pallor, and hypotension.
- **Alkaline reflux gastritis**. Stomach inflammation caused by reflux of bile and alkaline pancreatic secretions containing proteolytic enzymes that disrupt the mucosal barrier in the remnant stomach. Symptoms include nausea, bilious vomiting, and sustained epigastric pain that worsens after eating and is not relieved by antacids; responds somewhat to avoidance of Aspirin and alcohol,[45] but surgical correction may be required.
- **Afferent loop obstruction**. Intermittent severe pain and epigastric fullness after eating as a result of volvulus, hernia, adhesion, or stenosis of the duodenal stump on the proximal side of the gastrojejunostomy; vomiting relieves symptoms; management includes low-fat diet, but decompression or surgery revision is required for complete obstruction.[46]
- **Diarrhea**. Either frequent, persistent elimination of loose stools or intermittent, precipitous, and unpredictable elimination of a large volume of stool; related to rapid gastric emptying and osmotic attraction of water into the gut, especially after large intake of high-carbohydrate liquids; small, dry meals and anticholinergic medications are effective control measures.

- **Weight loss.** Commonly caused by inadequate caloric intake because individual cannot tolerate carbohydrates or a normal-sized meal; stomach is also less able to mix, churn, and break down food. In the case of bariatric surgery for extreme obesity, weight loss is the intended outcome, but nutrient deficiencies, including vitamins and minerals, must be supplemented.[47]
- **Anemia.** Iron malabsorption may result from decreased acid secretion or lack of duodenum after Billroth II procedure (gastrojejunostomy); deficiencies of iron and vitamin B_{12} or folate may result.
- **Bone and mineral disorders.** Related to altered calcium absorption and metabolism, with increased risk for fractures and deformity and malabsorption of vitamins and nutrients, such as vitamin D.

Malabsorption Syndromes

Malabsorption syndromes interfere with nutrient absorption in the small intestine. Historically they have been classified as maldigestion or malabsorption. **Maldigestion** is failure of the chemical processes of digestion that take place in the intestinal lumen or at the brush border of the intestinal mucosa. **Malabsorption** is failure of the intestinal mucosa to absorb (transport) the digested nutrients. Often these two syndromes are interrelated, or occur together, making classification difficult. Generally, however, maldigestion is caused by deficiencies of the enzymes needed for digestion or inadequate secretion of bile salts and inadequate reabsorption of bile in the ileum. Malabsorption is the result of mucosal disruption caused by gastric or intestinal resection, vascular disorders, or intestinal disease.

Pancreatic Exocrine Insufficiency

The pancreatic enzymes (lipase, amylase, trypsin, chymotrypsin) are required for the digestion of proteins, carbohydrates, and fats. **Pancreatic insufficiency** is the deficient production of these enzymes, particularly lipase, by the pancreas. Causes include chronic pancreatitis, pancreatic carcinoma, pancreatic resection, and cystic fibrosis. Significant damage to or loss of pancreatic tissue must occur before enzyme levels decrease sufficiently to cause maldigestion. Although pancreatic insufficiency causes poor digestion of all nutrients, fat maldigestion is the chief problem. Absence of pancreatic bicarbonate in the duodenum and jejunum causes an acidic pH that worsens maldigestion by precipitating bile salts and preventing activation of the pancreatic enzymes that are present. A large amount of fat in the stool (steatorrhea) is the most common sign of pancreatic insufficiency. There is also a deficit of fat-soluble vitamins (A, D, E, and K) and weight loss.[48]

Lactase Deficiency (Lactose Intolerance)

Deficiency of disaccharidase at the brush border of the small intestine is caused by a genetic defect in which a single enzyme, usually lactase, is lacking. **Lactase deficiency** inhibits the breakdown of lactose (milk sugar) into monosaccharides and therefore prevents lactose digestion and absorption across the intestinal wall. Secondary (acquired) lactase deficiency can be caused by several diseases of the intestine, including gluten-sensitive enteropathy, enteritis, and bacterial overgrowth.

The undigested lactose remains in the intestine, where bacterial fermentation causes formation of gases. Undigested lactose also increases the osmotic gradient in the intestine, causing irritation and osmotic diarrhea. Clinical manifestations of lactose consumption with lactase deficiency are bloating, crampy pain, diarrhea, and flatulence. The disorder is diagnosed by a lactose-tolerance test. Avoiding milk products (more than 250 mL of milk) and adhering to a lactose-free diet relieve symptoms.[48]

According to a 2013 study, no data exist on the prevalence, correlates, and potential impact of perceived lactose intolerance among Canadians. To address this lack of data, the study's author undertook an online survey of 2251 Canadians aged 19 years and older on whether they perceive themselves to be lactose intolerant. In all, 16% of respondents self-reported as lactose intolerant. Lactose intolerance was more common in women and in non-Whites and less common in those older than 50 years of age.[49]

Lactase non-persistence, also known as adult hypolactasia, affects 70% of the world adult population.[50] **Lactase non-persistence (LNP)** is an autosomal recessive inheritance of low lactase levels. Lactase activity is often high in fully mature human babies. Genetic polymorphism can act in cis to the lactase gene to determine either high or low messenger RNA expression, which is reflected in lactase persistence activity or lactase non-persistence. Evidence of the recessive inheritance of lactase non-persistence was first observed in 1974 from studies conducted in Finland.

In patients with lactase non-persistence, a 50-g-lactose load yields a net secretion into the stomach, duodenum, and jejunum. (In one study, the lactose test solution was diluted fivefold in the mid ileum; 12 g and 24 g were the net fluid accumulation in the jejunum and ileum, whereas 6 g were the net secretion in the jejunum.) In the colon, fermentation of the unabsorbed lactose into short chain fatty acids results in interference with net absorption. Carbon dioxide and hydrogen produced by this fermentation leads to the bloating, frothy diarrhea, and flatulence. The absence of symptoms in a person with lactase non-persistence may not reflect that the lactose was digested, and that the subject received the nutrient contents of the milk. Lactase non-persistence and potential lactose intolerance are factors in global milk-drinking habits. Countries with a high prevalence of LNP in their populations tend to consume lower quantities of dairy foods in their diets.

Bile Salt Deficiency

Conjugated bile acids (bile salts) are necessary for the digestion and absorption of fats. Bile salts are conjugated in the bile that is secreted from the liver. When bile enters the duodenum, the bile salts aggregate with fatty acids and monoglycerides to form micelles. Micelle formation makes fat molecules more soluble and allows them to pass through the unstirred layer at the brush border of the small intestinal villi (see Chapter 35). A minimum concentration of bile salts, termed the *critical micelle concentration*, is required to allow formation of micelles. Therefore, conditions that decrease the production or secretion of bile result in decreased micelle formation and fat malabsorption. These conditions include advanced liver disease, which decreases the production of bile salts; obstruction of the common bile duct, which decreases flow of bile into the duodenum (cholestasis); intestinal stasis (lack of motility), which permits overgrowth of intestinal bacteria that deconjugate bile salts; and diseases of the ileum, which prevent the reabsorption and recycling of bile salts (enterohepatic circulation).[51]

Clinical manifestations of bile salt deficiency are related to poor intestinal absorption of fat and fat-soluble vitamins (A, D, E, and K). The absence of bile secretion can cause the feces to turn grey or pale. Increased fat in the stools (steatorrhea) leads to diarrhea and decreased levels of plasma proteins. The losses of fat-soluble vitamins and their effects include the following:
- Vitamin A deficiency results in night blindness.
- Vitamin D deficiency results in decreased calcium absorption with bone demineralization (osteoporosis), bone pain, and fractures.
- Vitamin K deficiency prolongs prothrombin time, leading to spontaneous development of purpura (bruising) and petechiae.
- Vitamin E deficiency has uncertain effects but may cause testicular atrophy and neurological defects in children.

The most effective treatment for fat-soluble vitamin deficiency is to increase consumption of medium-chain triglycerides in the diet, for

TABLE 36.6 Features of Ulcerative Colitis and Crohn's Disease

Feature	Ulcerative Colitis	Crohn's Disease
Incidence		
Age at onset	Any age; 10–40 years most common	Any age; 10–30 years most common
Family history	Less common	More common
Gender	Prevalence equal in women and men	Prevalence about equal in women and men
Cancer risk	Increased	Increased
Nicotine use	Later and less severe disease; nicotine withdrawal may cause exacerbation	Increases disease risk and greater disease severity
Pathophysiology		
Location of lesions	Large intestine, continuous lesions; Left side more common	Mouth to anus, "skip" lesions common; Right side more common
Inflammation	Mucosal layer involved	Entire intestinal wall involved
Granulomata	Rare	Transmural granulomata common; cobblestone appearance
Ulceration	Friable mucosa, superficial ulcers, crypt abscesses common	Deep fissuring ulcers and fistulae common
Anal and perianal fistulae	Rare	Common; abscesses
Narrowed lumen and possible obstruction	Rare	Common; obstruction
Clinical Manifestations		
Abdominal pain	Mild to severe	Moderate to severe
Diarrhea	Common; 4 times/day	May or may not be present
Bloody stools	Common	Less common
Weight loss	Less common	Common
Abdominal mass	Rare	Common
Small intestine malabsorption	None	Common
Clinical course	Remissions and exacerbations	Remissions and exacerbations
Comorbidities	Extraintestinal manifestations	Extraintestinal manifestations

example, by using coconut oil for cooking. Vitamins A, D, and K are given parenterally. Oral bile salts are an effective therapy.

Inflammatory Bowel Disease

UC and CD are chronic relapsing IBDs. The disease is more prevalent among White populations and Ashkenazi Jews.[52] In addition to the disease processes that impact the bowels, patients with IBD suffer from financial and nonfinancial costs due to their illness. Risk factors and theories of causation include susceptibility genes, environmental factors, alterations in epithelial cell barrier functions, and an altered immune response to intestinal microflora[53,54] (Table 36.6). Environmental factors or infections are thought to alter the barrier function of the mucosal epithelium, leading to loss of immune tolerance to normal intestinal antigens. There is possible loss of discrimination of potentially harmful pathogens from commensal microorganisms in the intestinal mucosa. The loss of tolerance activates dendritic cells, triggering their transport to mesenteric lymph nodes, where they promote differentiation of naive T cells to T-helper 1 (Th1), Th2, and Th17 cells, or T-regulatory cells. Production of pro-inflammatory cytokines and chemokines, including tumour necrosis factor (TNF), interleukins, toxic oxygen free radicals, and interferon gamma (IFN-γ), damages the intestinal epithelium.[55] The risk for colon cancer increases significantly after 30 to 35 years of IBD, particularly in untreated disease.[56] Future research is directed at an integration of these factors to refine our understanding of disease cause and trajectory, particularly interactions between genetics, the microflora, mucosa, and immune responses.[57,58]

Canada has the highest incidence rates of IBD in the world; approximately 270 000 Canadians were living with IBD in 2018 of which 135 000 patients had Crohn's disease, and 120 000 individuals had ulcerative colitis. The direct annual cost of providing the needs management for Canadians with IBD is approximately $1.28 billion.[59] The direct cost of treating IBD is linked to other indirect costs of illness. In 2018, the indirect health-related costs related to IBD were approximately $1.29 billion. Indirect costs are incurred by productivity losses, particularly premature retirement, and out-of-pocket expenses ($629 million in permanent lost wages accrued annually). Absenteeism ($88 million annually), premature death ($34 million annually), and out-of-pocket expenses ($541 million annually) are other factors that indirectly impact the cost of management for patients with IBD.[59]

It is estimated that by 2030, 1% (400 000) of the Canadian population will develop IBD. Older persons aged 65 and over with Crohn's or colitis are the fastest-growing group of Canadians with IBD. The Canadian health care system is not yet prepared to meet this growing challenge. Older persons with Crohn's or colitis are likely to have age-related medical conditions such as diabetes and cardiovascular disease, and as such may experience complications of longer disease duration.[59]

Canadians with Crohn's or colitis in rural areas are more likely to develop long-term complications due to lack of adequate gastroenterologist care. Crohn's and colitis impact Canadians of all ethnicities and religions, but the rate of new diagnoses is higher among Ashkenazi Jewish and South Asian people.[59]

According to the *2018 Impact of Inflammatory Bowel Disease in Canada* report, more than 7 000 Canadian children under the age of 18 have been diagnosed with Crohn's or colitis. In the last 10 years, the prevalence of Crohn's and colitis in Canadian children has increased by more than 50%. Different disease-related complications are developed by children who have Crohn's or colitis, and affected children often respond differently to treatments. Children are also at a greater risk of side effects of medication than adults.[59]

IBD has a significant impact on quality of life because of the associated personal, emotional, and social burdens. The impact of IBD on quality of life cannot readily be quantified as a cost, but must be discussed with patients with IBD to help in determining resources.

Ulcerative Colitis

Ulcerative colitis (UC) is a chronic inflammatory disease that causes ulceration of the colonic mucosa, most commonly in the rectum and sigmoid colon. The lesions appear in susceptible individuals between 20 and 40 years of age. UC is less common in people who smoke.[60]

PATHOPHYSIOLOGY The primary lesion of UC begins with inflammation at the base of the crypt of Lieberkühn in the large intestine. The disease begins in the rectum (proctitis) and may extend proximally to the entire colon (pancolitis). The mucosa is hyperemic and may appear dark red and velvety and is involved in a continuous fashion. Small erosions form and coalesce into ulcers. Abscess formation, necrosis, and ragged ulceration of the mucosa ensue. Edema and thickening of the muscularis mucosae may narrow the lumen of the involved colon. Mucosal destruction and inflammation cause bleeding, cramping pain, and an urge to defecate. Frequent diarrhea, with passage of small amounts of blood and purulent mucus, is common. Loss of the absorptive mucosal surface and rapid colonic transit time cause large volumes of watery diarrhea.

CLINICAL MANIFESTATIONS The course of UC consists of intermittent periods of remission and exacerbation. Mild UC involves less mucosa, so that the frequency of bowel movements, bleeding, and pain is minimal. Severe forms may involve the entire colon and are characterized by abdominal pain, fever, elevated pulse rate, frequent diarrhea (10 to 20 stools/day), urgency, obviously bloody stools, and continuous, crampy pain. Dehydration, weight loss, anemia, and fever result from fluid loss, bleeding, and inflammation. Complications include anal fissures, hemorrhoids, and perirectal abscess. Severe hemorrhage is rare. Edema, strictures, or fibrosis can obstruct the colon. Perforation is an unusual but possible complication. Extraintestinal manifestations include cutaneous lesions (erythema nodosum), polyarthritis, episcleritis, uveitis, disorders of the liver, and alterations in coagulation.[61]

EVALUATION AND TREATMENT Diagnosis of UC is based on the medical history, clinical manifestations, and laboratory, serological, radiological, endoscopic, and biopsy findings. Infectious causes are ruled out by stool culture. The symptoms of UC may be similar to those of CD, making differential diagnosis challenging.[62] Treatment is individualized and depends on the severity of symptoms and the extent of mucosal involvement. A goal is to promote mucosal healing and avoid surgery. Mild to moderate disease is treated with 5-aminosalicylate therapy followed by steroids. Thioprine and immunomodulatory agents (cyclosporine [Sandimmune] and TNF-blocking agents [i.e., tacrolimus (Advagraf, Prograf)]) or vedolizumab (Entyvio) are used for serious disease.[63] New immunotherapies are emerging.[64] Severe, unremitting disease can require hospital admission for administration of intravenous fluids and steroids. Extreme malnutrition may require total parenteral nutrition (TPN). Surgical resection of the colon may be performed if other forms of therapy are unsuccessful or if there are acute serious complications (sepsis, hemorrhage, perforation, or obstruction). Surgical approaches for severe UC include total proctocolectomy, with end ileostomy or ileorectal anastomosis, or ileal pouch anal anastomosis (IPAA).[65] *Pouchitis* is a complication of restorative proctocolectomy with ileal pouch–anal anastomosis performed as surgical treatment for both UC and CD. Antibiotic treatment is usually successful.[66]

Crohn's Disease

Crohn's disease (CD) (granulomatous colitis, ileocolitis, or regional enteritis) is an idiopathic inflammatory disorder that affects any part of the GI tract from the mouth to the anus. In a small percentage of cases, CD is difficult to differentiate from UC (see Table 36.6). The distal small intestine and proximal large colon are most commonly involved.[53]

PATHOPHYSIOLOGY Inflammation begins in the intestinal submucosa and spreads with discontinuous transmural involvement ("skip lesions"). The ascending colon and the transverse colon are the most common sites of the disease, but both the large and small intestines may be involved, particularly the ileum. One side of the intestinal wall may be affected and not the other. The ulcerations of CD can produce fissures that extend inflammation into lymphoid tissue. The typical lesion is a granuloma (granulomas are described in Chapter 6) with a cobblestone appearance from projections of inflamed tissue surrounded by ulceration. Fistulae may form in the perianal area between loops of intestine or extend into the bladder, rectum, or vagina. Strictures may develop, promoting obstruction. Smoking increases the risk of developing severe disease and may cause a poorer response to treatment.[67]

CLINICAL MANIFESTATIONS Individuals with CD may have no specific symptoms for several years. Symptoms vary according to the location of the disease but are similar to those for UC. Diarrhea is one of the most common symptoms and, occasionally, rectal bleeding if the colon is involved. Weight loss and abdominal pain accompany CD. If the ileum is involved, the individual may be anemic as a result of malabsorption of vitamin B_{12}. There also may be deficiencies in folic acid and vitamin D absorption. In addition, proteins may be lost, leading to hypoalbuminemia. Extraintestinal complications are similar to those occurring in UC.

EVALUATION AND TREATMENT The diagnosis and treatment of CD are similar to the diagnosis and treatment of UC; however, imaging of the small intestine is used in the diagnosis of CD, including either a small bowel series or a capsule endoscopy (camera pill). There are no specific biomarkers or definitive treatments. Smoking cessation is a component of therapy. Immunomodulators (i.e., anti-TNF) are effective for initial therapy or for resistance to other medications.[68] Surgery may be performed to manage complications such as fistula, abscess, or obstruction. Routine colonoscopy for cancer screening should be performed for longstanding colonic disease.

Microscopic Colitis

Microscopic colitis is a relatively common cause of diarrhea primarily in females and older persons. Although the mucosa appears normal, there are two histological forms: lymphocytic and collagenous. Lymphocytic colitis shows an increase in the number of intraepithelial lymphocytes. Collagenous colitis is characterized by a thickened subepithelial collagen layer, alteration of the vascular mucosal pattern, and mucosal nodularity. The cause is unknown. Risk factors include age (50 years or older), female gender, weight loss, absence of abdominal pain, and use of proton pump inhibitors or NSAIDs.[69]

The symptoms of frequent, chronic daily watery diarrhea are the same for both types and can be accompanied by abdominal pain and weight loss. Antidiarrheal agents and budesonide (an anti-inflammatory steroid) are the best documented treatments. The disease is negatively associated with colorectal cancer.[70]

Irritable Bowel Syndrome

Irritable bowel syndrome (IBS) currently is a symptom-based disease characterized by recurrent abdominal pain with altered bowel habits.

There is increasing evidence of organic causes of disease. In North America the prevalence is about 12% and is probably underestimated.[71] It is more common in women (1.5 to 3 times greater than in men) with a higher prevalence during youth and middle age. Individuals with symptoms of IBS also are more likely to have anxiety, depression, and reduced quality of life.[72]

The pathophysiology of IBS is unknown and there are no specific biomarkers for the disease. There is increasing evidence to explain the varying symptom presentations, particularly in relation to altered gut microflora, gut immune responses, gut neuroendocrine cell function, the brain–gut axis, genetic susceptibility, and epigenetic factors.[73,74] The presentations are summarized as follows:

- *Visceral hypersensitivity or hyperalgesia*, particularly with distension of the rectum but also other areas of the gut, may originate in either the peripheral or the central nervous system. The mechanism may be related to dysregulation of the bidirectional "brain–gut axis" (alterations in gut or central nervous system processing of gut nociceptive information).[75] Factors include genetic-related changes in the function of serotonin-secreting cells of gut–brain pain modulation, alterations in gut microbiota metabolite production with activation of the gut immune system, increased visceral sensitivity and permeability, and altered motility.[76]
- *Abnormal GI permeability, motility, and secretion* are associated with IBS. Individuals with diarrhea-type IBS have more rapid colonic transit times and increased intestinal permeability. Those with bloating and constipation have delayed transit times and decreased intestinal permeability. The mechanism may be related to dysregulation of the brain–gut axis, alterations in the function of gut neuroendocrine cells or dorsal root ganglion neurons, or changes in the activity of mast cells.[77]
- *Postinflammatory (infectious or noninfectious) IBS* is diagnosed if two or more of the following occur: fever, vomiting, diarrhea, and a positive stool culture. Intestinal infection (bacterial enteritis) and low-grade inflammation have been associated with symptoms of IBS and appear to be related to alteration of gut microbiota, immune activation in gut tissues, and changes in intestinal permeability.[78,79]
- *Alteration in gut microbiota (dysbiosis)* influences the sensory, motor, and immune systems of the gut and interacts with higher brain centres and may contribute to symptoms of IBS.[80] Small intestine overgrowth of normal gut bacteria may be associated with IBS symptoms in some cases.[75] Nonabsorbable antibiotics and prebiotics and probiotics may be helpful in some individuals.
- *Food allergy or food intolerance* is associated with IBS in some cases. Food antigens may activate the mucosal immune system, alter intestinal flora, or mediate hypersensitivity reactions and IBS symptoms. Food elimination approaches are helpful in some cases.[81]
- *Psychosocial factors (epigenetic factors)*—including early life trauma or abuse or emotional stress interacting with neuroendocrine, neuroimmune, autonomic nervous system, and pain modulatory responses—contribute to the symptoms of IBS.[74,82]

CLINICAL MANIFESTATIONS IBS is characterized by lower abdominal pain or discomfort and bloating. Women report more abdominal pain and constipation, and men report more diarrhea.[83] IBS can be grouped as diarrhea-predominant, constipation-predominant, or alternating diarrhea and constipation. Symptoms including gas, bloating, and nausea are usually relieved with defecation and do not interfere with sleep.

EVALUATION AND TREATMENT The diagnosis of IBS is based on signs, symptoms, and personal history and includes the exclusion of structural or biochemical causes of disease. Diagnostic procedures to rule out other causes of symptoms may include endoscopic evaluations, computed tomography (CT) scans or abdominal ultrasound, blood tests, and tests for lactose intolerance, celiac disease (see Chapter 37), or other disorders. The person may be evaluated for food allergies, parasites, or bacterial growth. The Rome III criteria for diagnosing IBS guide evaluation (Box 36.1).

There is no cure for IBS and treatment is individualized. Treatment of symptoms may include laxatives and fibre, antidiarrheals, antispasmodics, prosecretory medications, low-dose antidepressants, visceral analgesics, and serotonin agonists or antagonists. Alternative therapies include prebiotics and probiotics to manipulate the microflora, hypnosis, acupuncture, yoga, cognitive-behavioural therapy, and dietary interventions. Research continues to advance the management and understanding of the pathophysiology of this complex syndrome.[84,85]

Diverticular Disease of the Colon

Diverticula are herniations or saclike outpouchings of the mucosa and submucosa through the muscle layers, usually in the wall of the sigmoid colon (Figure 36.9). They rarely occur in the small intestine.[86] **Diverticulosis** is asymptomatic diverticular disease. **Diverticulitis** represents inflammation. The cause of diverticular disease is unknown. It is associated with increased intracolonic pressure, abnormal neuromuscular function, and alterations in intestinal motility. Approximately 300 000 hospital admissions per year are related to diverticular disease.[87] Predisposing factors include older age, genetic predisposition, obesity, smoking, diet, lack of physical activity, and medication use, such as Aspirin and NSAIDs.[88] Lack of dietary fibre may or may not contribute to diverticular disease.[89]

> **BOX 36.1 Rome III—Diagnostic Criteria for Irritable Bowel Syndrome**
>
> Recurrent abdominal pain or discomfort* at least 3 days/month in the last 3 months associated with two or more of the following:
> - Improvement with defecation
> - Onset associated with a change in frequency of stool
> - Onset associated with a change in form (appearance) of stool†
> - Onset of symptoms more than 6 months before diagnosis
>
> *"Discomfort" means an uncomfortable sensation not described as pain.
> †Diagnostic criterion.
> Saps, M., Velasco-Benitez, C. A., Langshaw, A. H., & Ramírez-Hernández, C. R. (2018). Prevalence of functional gastrointestinal disorders in children and adolescents: comparison between Rome III and Rome IV criteria. *The Journal of pediatrics*, 199, 212–216.

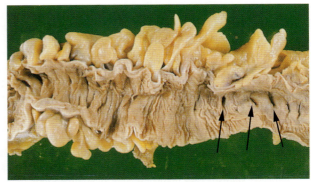

FIGURE 36.9 Diverticular Disease. In diverticular disease, the outpouches *(arrows)* of mucosa seen in the sigmoid colon appear as slit-like openings from the mucosal surface of the opened bowel. (From Stevens, A., Lowe, J., & Scott, I. [2009]. *Core pathology* [3rd ed.]. Mosby.)

PATHOPHYSIOLOGY Diverticula can occur anywhere in the GI tract, particularly at weak points in the colon wall, usually where arteries penetrate the tunica muscularis. The most common sites are the left sigmoid colon (prevalent in Western countries) and the right colon (prevalent in Asian countries). A common associated finding is thickening of the circular muscles and shortening of the longitudinal (teniae coli) muscles surrounding the diverticula. Increased collagen and elastin deposition, not muscle hypertrophy, is associated with muscle thickening, which contributes to increased intraluminal pressure and herniation. According to Laplace's law (see Chapter 23), wall pressure increases as the diameter of a cylindrical structure decreases. Therefore, pressure within the narrow lumen can increase enough to rupture the diverticula, causing inflammation and diverticulitis. Bacteria and local ischemia also may be contributing factors. Complicated diverticulitis includes abscess, fistula, obstruction, bleeding, or perforation.

CLINICAL MANIFESTATIONS Symptoms of uncomplicated diverticular disease may be vague or absent. Cramping pain of the lower abdomen can accompany constriction of the thickened colonic muscles. Diarrhea, constipation, distension, or flatulence may occur. If the diverticula become inflamed or abscesses form, the individual develops fever, leukocytosis (increased white blood cell count), and tenderness of the lower-left quadrant.

EVALUATION AND TREATMENT Diverticula are often discovered during diagnostic procedures performed for other problems. Ultrasound, sigmoidoscopy, or colonoscopy permits direct observation of the lesions. Abdominal CT is used for diagnosis of complicated cases.

An increase of dietary fibre intake often relieves symptoms, and probiotics and mesalazine (Pentasa) are being evaluated. Uncomplicated diverticulitis is usually treated with bowel rest and analgesia. Antibiotics are not required.[90] Laparoscopic resection and other minimally invasive approaches are implemented for more severe complications.[91]

Appendicitis

Appendicitis is an inflammation of the vermiform appendix, which is a projection from the apex of the cecum. It is the most common surgical emergency of the abdomen, usually occurs between 10 and 19 years of age (although it may develop at any age), and has an incidence in the United States of 7 to 10 per 10 000 persons.[92]

PATHOPHYSIOLOGY The exact mechanism of the cause of appendicitis is controversial. Obstruction of the lumen with stool, tumours, or foreign bodies with consequent bacterial infection is the most common theory. The obstructed lumen does not allow drainage of the appendix, and as mucosal secretion continues, intraluminal pressure increases. The increased pressure decreases mucosal blood flow, and the appendix becomes hypoxic. The mucosa ulcerates, promoting bacterial or other microbial invasion with further inflammation and edema. Inflammation may involve the distal or entire appendix. Gangrene develops from thrombosis of the luminal blood vessels, followed by perforation.[93]

CLINICAL MANIFESTATIONS Gastric or periumbilical pain is the typical symptom of an inflamed appendix. The pain may be vague at first and in the periumbilical area, increasing in intensity over 3 to 4 hours. It may subside and then migrate to the right lower quadrant, indicating extension of the inflammation to the surrounding tissues. Nausea, vomiting, and anorexia follow the onset of pain, and a low-grade fever is common. Diarrhea occurs in some individuals, particularly children; others have a sensation of constipation. Perforation, peritonitis, and abscess formation are the most serious complications of appendicitis.

EVALUATION AND TREATMENT In addition to clinical manifestations, there is pain with abdominal palpation and rebound tenderness, usually referred to the lower-right quadrant. The white blood cell count is greater than 10 000 cells/mm^3 with increased neutrophils and C-reactive protein. Abdominal ultrasound, CT scans, and magnetic resonance imaging (MRI) (particularly for pregnant women and children) assist with diagnostic accuracy and help rule out nonappendiceal disease.[94] Antibiotics and appendectomy are the treatment for simple or perforated appendicitis. There is controversy regarding antibiotics first, then surgery.[95] Laparoscopic surgery provides quick recovery for simple appendicitis. Recovery is more complicated in cases of perforation, abscess formation, peritonitis, or older age.

Mesenteric Vascular Insufficiency

Mesenteric vascular insufficiency is rare, with an incidence of about 2 to 3 cases per 100 000 persons.[96] Three branches of the abdominal aorta supply the stomach and intestines: the celiac artery and the superior and inferior mesenteric arteries (see Figure 35.6). The inferior mesenteric vein drains into the splenic vein, and the splenic vein and superior mesenteric vein join the portal vein. *Mesenteric venous thrombosis* is the least common of the causes of mesenteric vascular insufficiency. Malignancies, right ventricular failure, and deep vein thrombosis are risk factors. Mesenteric venous thrombosis presents with abdominal pain and is treated with anticoagulants.[97]

Acute mesenteric arterial insufficiency results in a significant reduction in mucosal blood flow to the large and small intestines and can be acute or chronic.[98,99] Pre-existing morbidities include dissecting aortic aneurysms, arterial thrombi, or emboli. Embolic obstruction is associated with atrial fibrillation, mitral valve disease, heart valve prostheses, and myocardial infarction. The superior mesenteric artery has a more direct line of flow from the aorta; therefore, emboli enter it more readily than the inferior branch, causing ischemia and necrosis of the small intestine. Ischemia and necrosis (intestinal infarction) alter membrane permeability. Initially, there is increased motility, nausea and vomiting, urgent bowel evacuation, and severe abdominal pain. Ischemia leads to decreased motility and distension. The damaged intestinal mucosa cannot produce enough mucus to protect itself from digestive enzymes. Mucosal alteration causes fluid to move from the blood vessels into the bowel wall and peritoneum. Fluid loss causes hypovolemia, and further decreases intestinal blood flow. As intestinal infarction progresses, shock, fever, bloody diarrhea, and leukocytosis develop. Bacteria invade the necrotic intestinal wall, causing gangrene and peritonitis.

Chronic mesenteric ischemia is rare but can develop with atherosclerotic stenosis or occlusion[96] or secondary to heart failure, acute myocardial infarction, hemorrhage, thrombus formation, or any condition that decreases arterial blood flow. Chronic occlusion is often accompanied by formation of collateral circulation. The collateral vessels may be able to nourish the resting intestine, but after eating, when the intestine requires more blood, the arterial supply may be insufficient. Ischemia develops, causing cramping abdominal pain (abdominal angina), a cardinal symptom. Some individuals suffer significant weight loss because they stop eating to control the pain. Progressive vascular obstruction eventually causes continuous abdominal pain and necrosis of the intestinal tissue.

Diagnosis of acute and chronic mesenteric ischemia is based on clinical manifestations, laboratory findings, and imaging studies. A bruit can often be heard over a partially occluded artery. Treatment includes aggressive rehydration and the use of antibiotics, anticoagulants, vasodilators, and inhibitors of reperfusion injury. Surgery, including endovascular techniques, is required to remove necrotic tissue, repair sclerosed vessels, and revascularize affected tissue. Acute occlusion is a surgical emergency and mortality is high (50 to 90%). Early diagnosis and aggressive treatment result in the best survival rates.[100]

Disorders of Nutrition

Obesity

Obesity is a complex chronic disease related to abnormal or excess body fat (adiposity) that ultimately increases the risk of long-term medical complications and reduces the life span. **Obesity** is defined based on the body mass index (BMI; weight/height as a BMI exceeding 30 kg/m and is subclassified into class 1 (30–34.9), class 2 (35–39.9) and class 3 (≥40). Obesity is known to occur in families and genotypes, and gene–environment interactions are important predisposing factors.[101] Environmental factors include culture, socioeconomic status, food intake habits, and level of physical activity. Metabolic abnormalities associated with obesity include Cushing's syndrome, Cushing's disease, polycystic ovarian syndrome, hypothyroidism, and hypothalamic injury.

In 2015, 61.9% of Canadian adults were overweight or obese. In 2018, 7.3 million adults (26.8%) in Canada who reported height and weight were classified as obese, whereas 9.9 million adults (36.3%) were classified as overweight. As such, the total population with increased health risks due to excess weight was calculated to be about 63.1% in 2018. The percentage of Canadian adults who were overweight or obese was higher in men (69.4%) than in women (56.7%).[102] Obesity rates among children and youth in Canada have nearly tripled in the last 30 years. Children and youth who are obese are at higher risk of developing a range of health problems, and weight issues in childhood are likely to persist into adulthood.[103] Therefore, parents should encourage children to develop healthy eating habits and be physically active (see *Health Promotion*: Promotion of Physical Activity in Canadian Schools).

HEALTH PROMOTION

Promotion of Physical Activity in Canadian Schools

Many Canadian children and youth have a risk of developing cardiovascular disease, obesity, and diabetes because they do not get enough physical activity. Moreover, several studies have concluded that children who do not get enough physical activity are more likely to struggle with cognitive and academic challenges. The *Canadian 24-Hour Movement Guidelines for Children and Youth (Ages 5–17 Years)* emphasized the use of a new movement paradigm where the integration of all movement behaviours happen throughout a whole day, thereby shifting the focus from the person to the whole. The core of the new guidelines is to encourage children and youth to "Sweat, Step, Sleep and Sit" the right amounts during each 24-hour period:

- **SWEAT** by engaging in moderate to vigorous physical activity to accumulate at least 60 minutes per day of moderate to vigorous physical activity including aerobic activities. For at least 3 days per week children and youth (aged 5 to 17 years) should engage in vigorous physical activities involving muscle and bone strengthening activities.
- **STEP:** Try to involve children and youth (aged 5 to 17 years) with light physical activity and several hours of a variety of structured and unstructured light physical activities.
- **SLEEP:** Facilitate uninterrupted sleep for 9 to 11 hours per night for children aged 5 to 13 years and 8 to 10 hours per night for children aged 14 to 17 years, with consistent bed and wake-up times.
- **SIT:** Avoid sedentary behaviour. For example, do not allow more than 2 hours per day of recreational screen time, and limit sitting for prolonged periods (e.g., reduce the time your children sit in cars or on school buses and limit the time they spend sitting or indoors for extended periods). Encourage children to swap inactive time (e.g., using a computer or sitting on a bus) with activities such as dancing, or walking to school. Start by encouraging them to be active 10 minutes a day; then increase the amount of time each week until daily activity becomes part of their healthy lifestyle. Try increasing active periods by 10 minutes and reducing screen time by 10 minutes every few days to make being active a part of their daily routine.

Schools can provide ample opportunities for students to improve both health and academic outcomes by promoting physical activity, healthy behaviours, and healthy eating as part of a Comprehensive School Health (CSH) approach. CSH is an internationally recognized approach that was created to improve students' educational outcomes without neglecting students' health. The CSH framework is designed in an integrated and holistic way, taking into consideration four categories: (1) teaching and learning; (2) social and physical environments; (3) healthy school policy; and (4) partnerships and services. Schools can apply several interventions to help children improve their levels of physical activity within these categories. Factors such as geography and socioeconomic status should also be considered to address the needs of individual school communities.

The Heart and Stroke Foundation of Canada also recommends that children and youth accumulate at least 60 minutes of daily physical activity through a variety of activities and programs (both structured and unstructured). It recommends that schools integrate knowledge into physical activities to develop positive attitudes toward physical activity; for example, it suggests incorporating physical activity into lesson plans for subjects other than physical education (e.g., math, science, languages, etc.). As well, it recommends that schools encourage students to engage in physical activity and active play during recess and lunch breaks and provide students with incentives such as free healthy drinks and fruits. By promoting active transportation (e.g., walking and cycling), schools can also increase students' level of physical activity.

Schools should be located in areas that are accessible to large numbers of students. Municipalities must take into consideration ways to help students use active transportation by developing active and safe routes to school and by providing amenities like bike racks and crossing guards. The benefits of these measures extend beyond children and youth to families and the entire community.

School facilities should be available during nonschool hours to provide additional programs (e.g., childcare, cooking classes) for the whole community, giving parents the opportunity to engage in supporting the healthy development of their children.

Given that health, well-being, and learning are intimately connected, schools have the ability to make a dramatic difference in the lives of Canadian children and youth. However, to accomplish this goal, schools need funding and policies for the delivery of programs that foster physical activity.

The *Canadian 24-Hour Movement Guidelines for Adults (Ages 18–64 Years)* recommend that a healthy 24 hours should include performing physical activities of various intensities, including moderate-to-vigorous aerobic physical activities to accumulate of at least 150 minutes per week in addition to activities that use major muscle groups at least twice a week for muscle strengthening. Light physical activities and breaking up long periods of sitting as often as possible were also recommended. Standing instead of sitting, and limiting sedentary time to 8 hours or less, is also encouraged. Recreational screen time for more than 3 hours is discouraged. Getting 7 to 9 hours of good-quality sleep daily with consistent bed and wake-up times is important. Finally, the core recommendation to keep in mind is to *move more*—including moderate-to-vigorous physical activity, but light activity and standing matter too.

Data from Canadian Society for Exercise Physiology (CSEP). (2021). *Canadian 24-hour movement guidelines for children and youth (ages 5–17): an integration of physical activity, sedentary behaviour, and sleep.* https://csepguidelines.ca/children-and-youth-5-17/; Canadian Society for Exercise Physiology (CSEP). (2021). *Canadian 24-hour movement guidelines for adults (ages 18–64): an integration of physical activity, sedentary behaviour, and sleep.* https://csepguidelines.ca/adults-18-64/; Heart & Stroke Canada. (2020). Heart healthy activity. https://www.heartandstroke.ca/healthy-living/healthy-kids/heart-healthy-activity; Heart and Stroke Foundation of Canada. (2011). *Position statment: Physical activity, heart disease and stroke.* https://www.heartandstroke.ca/-/media/pdf-files/canada/2017-position-statements/physicalactivity-ps-eng.ashx.

While BMI is commonly used to classify obesity, it falls short of identifying adiposity-related complications. Waist circumference, on the other hand, is associated with an increase in cardiovascular risk, but not a good predictor of visceral adipose tissue. Assessing both the BMI and waist circumference helps with identifying the higher-risk phenotype of obesity more accurately than BMI or waist circumference alone, especially in individuals with lower BMI.

A comprehensive history of patients' unique conditions that lead to obesity should be explored. BMI and waist circumference measurements, thorough physical examination, and laboratory investigations can aid in recognizing individuals who will benefit from treatment.

The Edmonton Obesity Staging System is a guide used in clinical decision making that helps with obesity assessment of each BMI category. The Edmonton Obesity Staging System is a 5-stage system of obesity classification that considers metabolic, physical, and psychological parameters to determine the optimal obesity treatment, and has been shown to be a better predictor of all-cause mortality when compared with BMI or waist circumference measurements alone.[104,105]

Obesity management should concentrate on improved health and well-being, and not just weight loss. The existing literature focuses on weight-loss outcomes, and most of the current recommendations are weight-loss centred. However, more research is needed to shift the focus of obesity management toward improving patient-centred health outcomes, rather than weight loss alone. Canadian nurses are impacted by the biased beliefs about obesity, which in turn impact the quality of care delivered to obese patients. The negative cultural narrative regarding obesity seems to have a lot of false assumptions by directing the blame to people living with obesity. This has created an obesity stigma that negatively influences the level and quality of care for people living with obesity.

The clinical practice guideline for obesity in adults[106] stipulates 5 steps to guide nurses in the care of individuals with obesity, as follows:
1. Nurses should recognize obesity as a chronic disease. As such, nurses should ask the patient for their permission before offering advice so as to approach obese individuals in an unbiased manner.
2. Nurses should assess an individual living with obesity by utilizing appropriate measurements to identify the causes, complications, and potential barriers to obesity treatment.
3. Nurses should discuss with the individual the treatment options such as nutrition therapy, physical activity, and adjunctive therapies that may be required, including psychological, pharmacological, and surgical interventions.
4. Nurses should establish an agreement with the person living with obesity regarding goals of therapy, focusing mainly on the value that the person derives from health-based interventions.
5. Nurses should engage with the person with obesity in continued follow-up and reassessments, and encouragement of advocacy to improve care for this chronic disease.

Obesity is a major risk factor for morbidity, death, and high health care costs.[107] Three leading causes of death associated with obesity are coronary artery disease, type 2 diabetes mellitus, and cancer (colorectal, breast in postmenopausal women, endometrial, prostate, renal, and esophageal). Obesity also is a risk factor for hypertension, stroke, dyslipidemia, gallstones, nonalcoholic steatohepatitis (NASH), gastroesophageal reflux, osteoarthritis, infectious disease, and sleep apnea.[108] Rapidly advancing research regarding risk factors, causal mechanisms, complications, and treatment is in progress.

PATHOPHYSIOLOGY The pathophysiology of obesity involves the interaction of peripheral and central pathways and numerous cytokines, hormones, and neurotransmitters. In the periphery, white adipocytes (fat cells) store triglycerides and increase in size and number.

Adipocytes also secrete hormones and cytokines, known as *adipocytokines*.[109] These adipocytokines and other hormones (Box 36.2) participate in regulation of food intake, lipid storage, insulin sensitivity, vascular homeostasis, blood pressure regulation, angiogenesis, coagulation, bone metabolism, inflammatory and immune responses, female reproduction, and regulation of energy metabolism. Visceral white fat accumulation causes dysfunction in the regulation and interaction of these cytokines and hormones and contributes to the complications and consequences of obesity.

Neuroendocrine regulation of appetite, eating behaviour, energy metabolism, and body fat mass are controlled by a dynamic circuit of signalling mediators from the periphery acting centrally on the hypothalamus and brainstem to regulate hunger and satiety.[110] Peripheral sources of mediators include insulin from the beta cells of the pancreas; ghrelin from the stomach; peptide YY from the intestines; glucagonlike peptide-1 from intestinal endocrine cells; and the adipokines leptin, adiponectin, and resistin. Obesity is associated with increased circulating plasma levels of leptin, insulin, resistin, and ghrelin. There are decreased levels of adiponectin and peptide YY (see Box 36.2).

Within the hypothalamus are the orexigenic neurons (increase food intake and decrease metabolism) and the anorexigenic neurons (decrease food intake and increase metabolism). They interact with peripheral mediators to control food intake and energy expenditure. The hypothalamus also communicates with higher brain centres related to reward, pleasure, and addictive behaviour. These centres can

---

BOX 36.2 Examples of Adipocytokines and Other Hormones Related to Complications of Obesity

Cytokines From Adipose Cells
Adipocytokines

Leptin: Suppresses appetite at hypothalamus; promotes insulin sensitivity
Adiponectin: Insulin sensitizing for regulation of blood glucose level; promotes anti-inflammatory and antihypertensive vascular effects; reduces atherosclerosis and oncogenesis; increases metabolic rate
Resistin: Promotes insulin resistance and increases blood glucose levels
Visfatin: Mimics insulin and binds to insulin receptors

Proinflammatory Cytokines

Tumour necrosis factor-alpha: A proinflammatory hormone; suppresses appetite; induces insulin resistance
Interleukin-6, -8, and -10: Proinflammatory mediators; suppress appetite; induce insulin resistance
Monocyte chemotactic protein-1: Involved in macrophage recruitment
Plasminogen activator inhibitor-1: Promotes clot formation by inhibiting plasminogen and urokinase (also released by endothelial cells)
Retinol binding protein 4: Promotes insulin resistance

Other Hormones

Insulin: Secreted from pancreatic beta cells; suppresses appetite at hypothalamus; promotes glucose utilization in muscle and fat
Amylin: Secreted from pancreatic beta cells; suppresses appetite and postprandial glucagon secretion
Ghrelin: Secreted from stomach; stimulates appetite and controls gastric motility and acid secretion
Peptide YY: Secreted from intestine; reduces appetite and inhibits gastric motility
Incretin: Stimulates insulin release; inhibits glucagon release; slows gastric emptying to reduce postprandial hyperglycemia
Glucagonlike peptide 1: Gastric inhibitory peptide (glucose-dependent insulinotropic peptide)

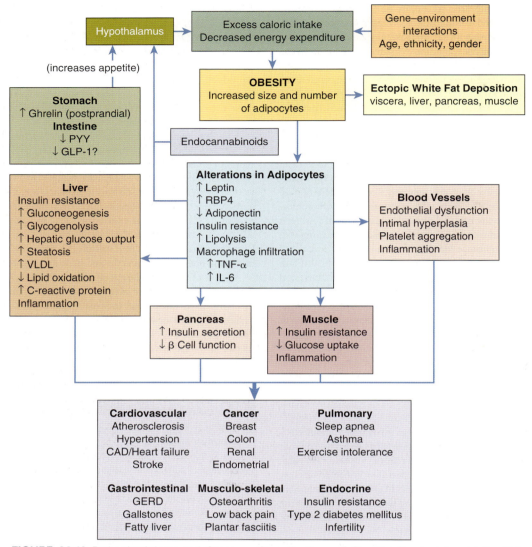

FIGURE 36.10 Pathophysiology and Common Complications of Obesity. See text for details. *CAD,* Coronary artery disease; *GERD,* gastroesophageal reflux disease; *GLP-1,* glucagonlike peptide-1; *IL-6,* interleukin-6; *PYY,* intestinal peptide YY; *RBP4,* retinol-binding protein 4; *TNF-α,* tumour necrosis factor-alpha; *VLDL,* very-low-density lipoprotein.

override hypothalamic control of food intake and satiety, increasing consumption of highly palatable foods and resulting in increased fat stores.[111,112] Interaction of altered levels of hormones and adipocytokines with hypothalamic neurons is an important determinant of excessive fat mass and the complications of obesity.

Leptin, a product of the obesity gene (*Ob* gene), acts on the hypothalamus to suppress appetite and functions to regulate body weight within a fairly narrow range. Leptin levels increase as the number of adipocytes increases; however, for unknown reasons, high leptin levels are ineffective at decreasing appetite and energy expenditure, a condition known as **leptin resistance**.[113] Leptin resistance fails to inhibit orexigenic hypothalamic satiety signalling and promotes overeating and excessive weight gain. Leptin resistance is also associated with insulin resistance (hyperinsulinemia or glucose intolerance) and the cardiovascular complications of obesity. Simultaneously there is an increase in **ghrelin**, which stimulates orexigenic neurons and increases appetite. Decreased levels of **adiponectin** and **peptide YY** decrease stimulation of anorexigenic neurons. Adiponectin also is insulin sensitizing, promotes glucose uptake, and has anti-inflammatory actions. A decrease in adiponectin is associated with insulin resistance, coronary artery disease, and hypertension, contributing to the complications of obesity.

Enlarged adipocytes increase lipolysis (with release of fatty acids) and secrete proinflammatory adipokines from T cells and activated macrophages. The result is a low-grade systemic inflammation. The inflammatory state and accelerated lipolysis contribute to the development of insulin resistance and metabolic syndrome (hypertriglyceridemia, reduced high-density lipoproteins, increased low-density lipoproteins, hypertension, and insulin resistance).[114,115] Figure 36.10 summarizes the pathophysiology and major consequences of obesity.

CLINICAL MANIFESTATIONS Obesity usually presents with two different forms of adipose tissue distribution, visceral and peripheral.[116] Visceral obesity (also known as *intra-abdominal, central,* or *masculine obesity*) occurs when the distribution of body fat is localized around the abdomen and upper body, resulting in an apple shape.[117] Visceral obesity has an increased risk for systemic inflammation, metabolic syndrome, obstructive sleep apnea syndrome, cardiovascular complications, nonalcoholic steatohepatitis cancer, osteoarthritis, and type 2 diabetes mellitus.[118,119] (Diabetes mellitus is discussed in Chapter 19).

Peripheral obesity (also known as *gluteal-femoral*, *feminine*, or *subcutaneous obesity*) occurs when the distribution of body fat is extraperitoneal and distributed around the thighs and buttocks and through the muscle, resulting in a pear shape, and is more common in women. Peripheral and subcutaneous fat is less metabolically active, is less lipolytic, and releases fewer adipocytokines (particularly adiponectin) than visceral fat. Risk factors are still present for the complications of obesity, but they are less severe than those for visceral obesity.

Normal weight obesity (NWO) describes individuals with normal body weight and BMI with percentage of body fat greater than 30%. These individuals are at risk for metabolic dysregulation, increases in inflammatory cytokines, insulin resistance, increased risk for cardiovascular disease, and higher mortality.[120] NWO is estimated to occur in 2 to 28% of women and 3% of men.[121]

Metabolically healthy obesity (MHO) describes about 10 to 30% of individuals who are obese but have no metabolic-obesity–associated complications and decreased risk for morbidity and mortality. MHO is more prevalent among women and declines with age with adverse long-term outcomes.[122] Research is in progress to better understand the genetics, body fat distribution patterns, metabolic pathways, lifestyle practices, and therapeutic options for these individuals.

EVALUATION AND TREATMENT There are several methods for measuring or estimating body fat mass, including CT and MRI techniques; bioimpedance analysis; underwater weighing; and anthropometric measurements, such as skinfold thickness, circumferences, and various body diameters (i.e., waist-to-hip ratios and waist circumference; BMI tables).[123] The BMI and waist-to-hip ratios are most commonly used because they are the easiest to measure and are most cost effective. *Overweight* is defined as a BMI greater than 25 kg/m^2, and *obesity* is defined as a BMI greater than 30 kg/m^2. BMI charts are available for children ages 2 to 20 years; they can be used for comparison during adulthood because obese children generally become obese adults.[124] No specific diagnostic criteria for obesity have been established. The complications of obesity affect nearly every body system (see Figure 36.10).

Obesity is a chronic disease for which various approaches to treatment have been used; these include correction of metabolic abnormalities, individually tailored weight reduction diets and exercise programs, psychotherapy, behavioural modification, and antiobesity medications.[125,126] Weight loss (bariatric) surgery is the most effective treatment for decreasing obesity-related morbidity.[127,128] Unravelling the causes of obesity will lead to more specific prevention and pharmacotherapeutic strategies.

Obesity contributes to changes in the intestinal flora and is a comorbidity that increases the severity of COVID-19.[129] Studies have demonstrated that at least 25% of patients who die from COVID-19 are obese, similar to the rates of death in patients with cardiovascular disease who get infected with COVID-19.[130] Adipose tissue acts as a reservoir for SARS-CoV-2 and has higher levels of angiotensin-converting enzyme II (ACE2). Obese individuals experience dysregulation of myeloid and lymphoid responses within adipose tissue, which dysregulate the release of cytokines. Obese individuals also have increased levels of proinflammatory adipokines, leukotrienes, and chemerin which exacerbates their risk for cytokine storm syndrome and death.[131]

Malnutrition and Starvation

Malnutrition is lack of nourishment from inadequate amounts of calories, protein, vitamins, or minerals and is caused by improper diet, alterations in digestion or absorption, chronic disease, or a combination of these factors. **Starvation** is a reduction in energy intake leading to weight loss. Short-term starvation and long-term starvation have different effects. Therapeutic short-term starvation is part of many weight-reduction programs because it causes an initial rapid weight loss that reinforces the individual's motivation to diet. Therapeutic long-term starvation is used in medically controlled environments to facilitate rapid weight loss in morbidly obese individuals. Pathological long-term starvation can be caused by poverty (particularly in developing countries); chronic diseases of the cardiovascular, pulmonary, hepatic, renal, and digestive systems; malabsorption syndromes; and cancer.

Short-term starvation, or extended fasting, consists of several days of total dietary abstinence or deprivation. Once all available energy has been absorbed from the intestine, glycogen in the liver is converted to glucose through **glycogenolysis**, the metabolism of glycogen into glucose. This process peaks within 4 to 8 hours, and gluconeogenesis begins. **Gluconeogenesis** is the formation of glucose from noncarbohydrate molecules: lactate, pyruvate, amino acids, and the glycerol portion of fats. Like glycogenolysis, gluconeogenesis takes place within the liver. Both of these processes deplete stored nutrients and thus cannot meet the body's energy needs indefinitely. Proteins continue to be catabolized to a minimal degree, providing carbon for the synthesis of glucose needed by brain and blood cells.

Long-term starvation begins after several days of dietary abstinence and eventually causes death. The major characteristics of long-term starvation are decreased energy expenditure, a decreased dependence on gluconeogenesis, and an increased use of ketone bodies (products of lipid and pyruvate metabolism) as a cellular energy source. Depressed insulin and glucagon levels promote lipolysis in adipose tissue. Lipolysis liberates fatty acids, which supply energy to cardiac and skeletal muscle cells, as well as ketone bodies, which sustain brain tissue. Fatty acid or ketone body oxidation meets most energy needs of the cells (Some glucose is still needed as fuel for brain tissue). Once the supply of adipose tissue is depleted, proteolysis begins. The breakdown of muscle protein is the last process to supply energy for life. Death results from severe alterations in electrolyte balance and loss of renal, pulmonary, and cardiac function.[132]

Adequate ingestion of appropriate nutrients is the obvious treatment for starvation. In medically induced starvation, the body is maintained in a ketotic state until the desired amount of adipose tissue has been lysed. Starvation imposed by chronic disease, long-term illness, or malabsorption is treated with enteral or parenteral nutrition. Care must be taken to prevent **refeeding syndrome** during the treatment of long-term starvation.[133] With refeeding, insulin release, hypophosphatemia, hypomagnesemia, and hypokalemia can cause life-threatening complications.

Cachexia (also known as *cytokine-induced malnutrition*) is physical wasting with loss of weight and muscle atrophy, fatigue, and weakness. Inflammatory cytokines induce skeletal muscle wasting and a blunted response to ghrelin. Adiponectin suppresses appetite. Cancer, acquired immune deficiency syndrome (AIDS), tuberculosis, and other major chronic progressive diseases contribute to cachexia (see Chapter 10).[134]

DISORDERS OF THE ACCESSORY ORGANS OF DIGESTION

> ✓ **QUICK CHECK 36.5**
> 1. How does portal hypertension cause varices and promote formation of ascites?
> 2. What are two factors that cause hepatic encephalopathy?
> 3. Why is the concentration of unconjugated bilirubin elevated in hemolytic jaundice?
> 4. Describe how failure of liver function causes kidney failure (hepatorenal syndrome).

The accessory organs of digestion (liver, gallbladder, pancreas) secrete substances necessary for digestion and, in the case of the liver, carry out metabolic functions needed to maintain life. Disorders of these organs include inflammatory disease, obstruction of ducts, and tumours. (Cancer of the digestive system is described at the end of this chapter.)

Common Complications of Liver Disorders

Of all the accessory organ disorders, acute or chronic liver disease leads to the most significant systemic, life-threatening complications. These complications are common to all liver disorders and include portal hypertension, ascites, hepatic encephalopathy, jaundice, and hepatorenal syndrome.

Portal Hypertension

Portal hypertension is abnormally high blood pressure in the portal venous system caused by resistance to blood flow. Pressure in this system is normally 3 mm Hg; portal hypertension is an increase to at least 10 mm Hg.

PATHOPHYSIOLOGY Portal hypertension is caused by disorders that obstruct or impede blood flow through any component of the portal venous system or vena cava. *Intrahepatic causes* result from vascular remodelling with shunts, thrombosis, inflammation, or fibrosis of the sinusoids, as occurs in cirrhosis of the liver, biliary cirrhosis, viral hepatitis, or schistosomiasis (a parasitic infection). *Posthepatic causes* occur from hepatic vein thrombosis or cardiac disorders that impair the pumping ability of the right side of the heart. The impaired ability of the right side of the heart causes blood to collect and increases pressure in the veins of the portal system. The most common cause of portal hypertension is fibrosis and obstruction caused by cirrhosis of the liver. Long-term portal hypertension causes several pathophysiological problems that are difficult to treat and can be fatal. These problems include varices, splenomegaly, ascites, hepatic encephalopathy, and hepatopulmonary syndrome.[135]

Varices are distended, tortuous collateral veins. Prolonged elevation of pressure in the portal vein cause collateral veins to open between the portal vein and systemic veins and their transformation into varices, particularly in the lower esophagus and stomach, but also over the abdominal wall (known as the *caput medusae* [Medusa head]) and rectum (hemorrhoidal varices) (Figure 36.11). Rupture of varices can cause life-threatening hemorrhage.[136]

Splenomegaly is enlargement of the spleen caused by increased pressure in the splenic vein, which branches from the portal vein. Thrombocytopenia is the most common symptom of congestive splenomegaly. The enlarged spleen can be palpated. Hepatopulmonary syndrome (vasodilation, intrapulmonary shunting, and hypoxia) and portopulmonary hypertension (pulmonary vasoconstriction and vascular remodelling) are complications of liver disease and portal hypertension. The pathophysiology is complex and involves different effects of vasoactive substances. There may be no clinical manifestations, although dyspnea, cyanosis, and clubbing may occur.[137]

CLINICAL MANIFESTATIONS Vomiting of blood (hematemesis) from bleeding esophageal varices is the most common clinical manifestation of portal hypertension. Bleeding is usually from varices that have developed slowly over a period of years. Slow, chronic bleeding from varices causes anemia or melena (dark, tarry stools). Rupture of esophageal varices causes hemorrhage and voluminous vomiting of dark-coloured blood. The ruptured varices are usually painless. Rupture is caused by a combination of erosion by gastric acid and elevated venous pressure. Mortality from ruptured esophageal varices ranges from 30 to 60%. Recurrent bleeding of esophageal varices indicates a poor

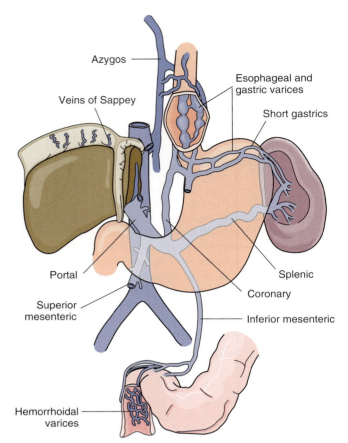

FIGURE 36.11 Varices Related to Portal Hypertension. Portal vein, its major tributaries, and the most important shunts (collateral veins) between the portal and caval systems. The shunted blood returns to the systemic venous system, bypassing the liver. (From Monahan, F. D., Sands, J. K., Neighbors, M., et al. [2007]. *Phipps' medical-surgical nursing: concepts and clinical practice* [8th ed.]. Mosby.)

prognosis. Hemorrhoidal varices present as hematochezia and copious rectal bleeding. Most individuals die within 1 year.

EVALUATION AND TREATMENT Portal hypertension is often diagnosed at the time of variceal bleeding and confirmed by upper GI endoscopy and evaluation of portal venous pressure. The individual usually has a history of jaundice, hepatitis, alcoholism, or cirrhosis. Pressure in the portal venous system can be reduced with nonselective beta-blocking medications to assist in preventing variceal bleeding.[138]

Emergency management of bleeding varices includes use of vasopressors and compression of the varices with an inflatable tube or balloon, sclerotherapy, variceal ligation, or portacaval shunt. Surgical construction of transjugular intrahepatic portosystemic shunts (TIPS procedure: anastomosis of the portal vein to the inferior vena cava) may decompress the varices. This treatment can precipitate encephalopathy. Liver transplant is the most successful option for liver failure.[139]

Ascites

Ascites is the accumulation of fluid in the peritoneal cavity. Ascites traps body fluid in the peritoneal space, from which it cannot escape. The effect is to reduce the amount of fluid available for normal physiological functions. Cirrhosis is the most common cause of ascites, but other causes include heart failure, constrictive pericarditis, abdominal malignancies, nephrotic syndrome, and malnutrition.[135] Of individuals who develop ascites caused by cirrhosis, 25% die within 1 year.

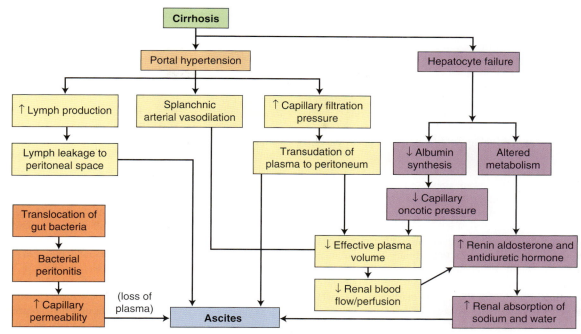

FIGURE 36.12 Mechanisms of Ascites Caused by Cirrhosis.

Continued heavy drinking of alcohol is associated with this mortality and is related to cirrhosis.

PATHOPHYSIOLOGY Several factors contribute to the development of ascites, including portal hypertension, decreased synthesis of albumin by the liver, splanchnic arterial vasodilation, and renal sodium and water retention. Portal hypertension and reduced serum albumin levels cause capillary hydrostatic pressure to exceed capillary osmotic pressure (see Chapter 5), pushing water into the peritoneal cavity. Portal hypertension also increases the production of hepatic lymph, which "weeps" into the peritoneal cavity. Splanchnic arterial vasodilation, associated with increased nitric oxide produced by the diseased liver, can decrease effective circulating blood volume, activating aldosterone and antidiuretic hormone, which promote renal sodium and water retention. The sodium and water retention expands plasma volume, thereby accelerating portal hypertension and ascites formation. Translocation of bacteria and release of endotoxins cause peritonitis with an inflammatory response that increases mesenteric capillary permeability and fluid movement into the peritoneal cavity, promoting ascites. Figure 36.12 summarizes the mechanisms by which cirrhosis of the liver cause ascites.

CLINICAL MANIFESTATIONS The accumulation of ascitic fluid causes abdominal distension, increased abdominal girth, and weight gain (Figure 36.13). Large volumes of fluid (10 to 20 L) displace the diaphragm and cause dyspnea by decreasing lung capacity. Respiratory rate increases, and the individual assumes a semi-Fowler position to relieve the dyspnea. Some peripheral edema is usually present. Approximately 10% of individuals with ascites develop bacterial peritonitis, which causes fever, chills, abdominal pain, decreased bowel sounds, and cloudy ascitic fluid.

EVALUATION AND TREATMENT Diagnosis is usually based on clinical manifestations and identification of liver disease. Dietary salt restriction and use of potassium-sparing diuretics can reduce ascites. Stronger diuretics, such as furosemide (Lasix) or ethacrynic acid (Edecrin), may be used, and vasopressin receptor 2 antagonists are effective for dilutional hyponatremia. Albumin may be given. Paracentesis is used to aspirate ascitic fluid for bacterial culture, biochemical analysis, and microscopic examination. The goal of treatment is to relieve discomfort. If the restoration of liver function is possible, the ascites diminishes spontaneously. Levels of serum electrolytes are monitored carefully because the individual is at risk for hyponatremia and hypokalemia.

Palliative measures include paracentesis to remove 1 or 2 L of ascitic fluid and relieve respiratory distress. However, the removal of too much fluid relieves pressure on blood vessels and carries the risk for hypotension, shock, or death. Despite repeated paracentesis, ascitic fluid reaccumulates because of the persistent portal hypertension and reduced plasma albumin levels associated with irreversible disease. Peritonitis is treated with antibiotics. Other procedures include peritoneovenous shunt (peritoneal fluid into veins) and TIPS (bypass of blood flow from

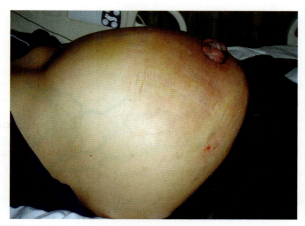

FIGURE 36.13 Massive Ascites in an Individual With Cirrhosis. Distended abdomen, dilated upper abdominal veins, and inverted umbilicus are classic manifestations. (From Goldman, L., & Schafer, A. I. [2012]. *Goldman's Cecil medicine* [24th ed.]. Saunders.)

the portal venous branch to the hepatic venous branch).[140] Individuals with ascites and portal hypertension have a poor prognosis, and liver transplant is the best treatment option.[141]

Hepatic Encephalopathy

Hepatic encephalopathy (portal-systemic encephalopathy) is a complex neurological syndrome characterized by impaired behavioural, cognitive, and motor function. The syndrome may develop rapidly during acute fulminant hepatitis or slowly during the course of cirrhosis and the development of portal hypertension or after portosystemic bypass or shunting.

PATHOPHYSIOLOGY Hepatic encephalopathy results from a combination of biochemical alterations that affect neurotransmission and brain function. Liver dysfunction and the development of collateral vessels that shunt blood around the liver to the systemic circulation permit toxins absorbed from the GI tract and normally removed by the liver to accumulate and circulate freely to the brain. The accumulated toxins alter cerebral energy metabolism, interfere with neurotransmission, and cause edema. The most hazardous substances are end products of intestinal protein digestion, particularly ammonia, which cannot be converted to urea by the diseased liver. Other substances include inflammatory cytokines, short-chain fatty acids, serotonin, tryptophan, and manganese. These substances cause astrocyte swelling and alter the blood–brain barrier, promoting cerebral edema. Infection, hemorrhage, electrolyte imbalance (including zinc deficiency), constipation, and use of sedatives and analgesics can precipitate hepatic encephalopathy in the presence of liver disease.[141]

CLINICAL MANIFESTATIONS Subtle changes in personality, memory loss, irritability, disinhibition, lethargy, and sleep disturbances are common initial manifestations of hepatic encephalopathy. Symptoms then can progress to confusion, disorientation to time and space, flapping tremor of the hands (asterixis), slow speech, bradykinesia, stupor, convulsions, and coma. Coma is usually a sign of liver failure and ultimately results in death. Variceal bleeding and ascites may develop concurrently. Symptoms may be episodic, recurrent, or persistent.[142] Hepatic encephalopathy is often associated with bleeding varices and ascites.

EVALUATION AND TREATMENT Diagnosis of hepatic encephalopathy is based on a history of liver disease, clinical manifestations, psychometric tests, and exclusion of other causes of brain dysfunction. Electroencephalography and blood chemistry tests provide supportive data. Tracking levels of serum ammonia assesses treatment effectiveness and liver function.

Correction of fluid and electrolyte imbalances and withdrawal of depressant medications metabolized by the liver are the first steps in the treatment of hepatic encephalopathy. Dietary protein is maintained to prevent malnutrition, but at levels that reduce blood ammonia levels.[143] Lactulose (Apo-Lactulose) prevents ammonia absorption in the colon. Neomycin (Neosporin) eliminates ammonia-producing intestinal bacteria but can be nephrotoxic. Glutamase inhibitors reduce gut ammonia. Rifaximin (Xifaxan) decreases intestinal production of ammonia and is used for lactulose nonresponders. Extracorporeal liver support systems remove toxins from the blood and are an option for managing overt hepatic encephalopathy.[144]

Jaundice

Jaundice, or icterus, is a yellow or greenish pigmentation of the skin caused by hyperbilirubinemia (plasma bilirubin concentrations greater than 42.5 to 51 μmol/L). Hyperbilirubinemia and jaundice can result from (1) extrahepatic (posthepatic) obstruction to bile flow, (2) intrahepatic obstruction, or (3) prehepatic excessive production of unconjugated bilirubin (i.e., excessive hemolysis of red blood cells)[145] (Figure 36.14). Jaundice in newborns is caused by impaired bilirubin uptake and conjugation (see Chapter 37).

PATHOPHYSIOLOGY Obstructive jaundice can result from extrahepatic or intrahepatic obstruction.[146] *Extrahepatic obstructive jaundice* develops if the common bile duct is occluded (e.g., by a gallstone, tumour, or inflammation). Bilirubin conjugated by the hepatocytes cannot flow through the obstructed common bile duct into the duodenum. Therefore, it accumulates in the liver and enters the bloodstream, causing hyperbilirubinemia and jaundice. *Intrahepatic obstructive jaundice* involves disturbances in hepatocyte function and obstruction of bile canaliculi. The uptake, conjugation, or excretion of bilirubin can be affected, with elevated levels of both conjugated and unconjugated bilirubin. Obstruction of bile canaliculi diminishes flow of conjugated bilirubin into the common bile duct. In mild cases, some of the bile canaliculi open. Consequently, the amount of bilirubin in the intestinal tract may be only slightly decreased.

Excessive hemolysis (destruction) of red blood cells can cause hemolytic jaundice (*prehepatic* or *nonobstructive jaundice*). Increased unconjugated bilirubin is formed through metabolism of the heme component of destroyed red blood cells and exceeds the conjugation ability of the liver, causing blood levels of unconjugated bilirubin to rise. Decreased bilirubin uptake or conjugation also causes unconjugated hyperbilirubinemia, as occurs with reaction to some medications (e.g., rifampin [Rifadin]) and in genetic disorders such as Gilbert's syndrome. Because unconjugated bilirubin is not water soluble, it is not excreted in the urine. The causes of jaundice are summarized in Table 36.7.

CLINICAL MANIFESTATIONS Conjugated bilirubin is water soluble and appears in the urine. The urine may darken several days before the onset of jaundice. The complete obstruction of bile flow from the liver to the duodenum causes grey or light-coloured stools. With partial obstruction, the stools are normal in colour and bilirubin is present in the urine.

Fever, chills, and pain often accompany jaundice resulting from viral or bacterial inflammation of the liver (e.g., viral hepatitis). Yellow discoloration may first occur in the sclera of the eye and then progress to the skin as bilirubin attaches to elastic fibres. Pruritus (itching) often accompanies jaundice because bilirubin accumulates in the skin.

EVALUATION AND TREATMENT Laboratory evaluation of serum establishes whether elevated plasma bilirubin is conjugated, unconjugated, or both. The history and physical examination identify underlying disorders, such as cirrhosis, exposure to hepatitis virus, and gallbladder or pancreatic disease. The treatment for jaundice consists of correcting the cause.

Hepatorenal Syndrome

Hepatorenal syndrome is functional kidney failure that develops as a complication of advanced liver disease. The kidney failure is not caused by primary kidney disease or other extrinsic factors but rather by portal hypertension, cardiac impairment, and other circulatory alterations associated with advanced liver disease, such as cirrhosis or fulminant hepatitis with portal hypertension. Manifestations include oliguria, sodium and water retention (usually with ascites and peripheral edema), hypotension, and peripheral vasodilation.[147] The kidney usually has a normal structure.

PATHOPHYSIOLOGY Type 1 hepatorenal syndrome accompanies a sudden decrease in blood volume secondary to massive GI or variceal

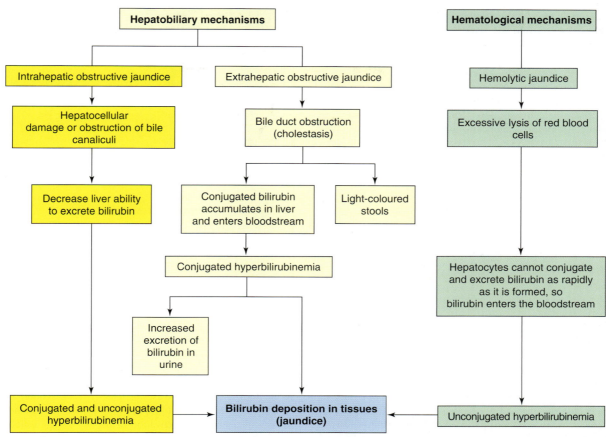

FIGURE 36.14 Mechanisms of Jaundice.

TABLE 36.7	Common Types of Jaundice	
Type	**Mechanism**	**Causes**
Hemolytic (prehepatic) jaundice (predominantly unconjugated bilirubin)	Destruction of erythrocytes (increased bilirubin production)	Hemolytic anemias (e.g., sickle cell) Severe infection Toxic substances in circulation (e.g., snake venom) Transfusion of incompatible blood
Disorders of bilirubin metabolism (unconjugated bilirubin)	Decreased bilirubin uptake Decreased bilirubin conjugation	Medication induced (e.g., rifampin [Rifadin] and cyclosporine [Sandimmune]) Hereditary disorder (e.g., Gilbert's syndrome)
Obstructive (posthepatic) jaundice (predominantly conjugated bilirubin)	Obstruction of passage of conjugated bilirubin from liver to intestine	Obstruction of bile duct by gallstones or tumour (extrahepatic obstructive jaundice) Obstruction of bile flow through liver (intrahepatic obstructive jaundice) Medications
Hepatocellular (intrahepatic) jaundice (both conjugated and unconjugated bilirubin)	Failure of liver cells (hepatocytes) to conjugate bilirubin and of bilirubin to pass from liver to intestine	Genetic defect of hepatocytes (decreased enzymes), such as occurs in premature infants (see Chapter 37) Severe infections (e.g., hepatitis) Alcoholic liver disease or biliary cirrhosis

bleeding and hypotension caused by bleeding and peripheral vasodilation associated with failing liver function. Hypotension also can be caused by the excessive use of diuretics to treat ascites or decreased cardiac output. The decrease in blood volume and hypotension result in decreased renal perfusion, decreased glomerular filtration, and oliguria (see Chapter 30). *Type 2 hepatorenal syndrome* develops slowly and is related to ascites. Ineffective circulating blood volume causes decreased glomerular filtration and oliguria. Intrarenal vasoconstriction may result from the selective effects of vasoactive substances that accumulate in the blood because of liver failure or a compensatory response to portal hypertension and the pooling of blood in the splanchnic circulation.[148]

CLINICAL MANIFESTATIONS The onset of hepatorenal manifestations may be acute or gradual. Oliguria and complications of advanced liver disease, including jaundice, ascites, peripheral edema, hypotension, and GI bleeding, are usually present. Systolic blood pressure is usually below 100 mm Hg. Nonspecific symptoms of hepatorenal syndrome include anorexia, weakness, and fatigue.[148]

EVALUATION AND TREATMENT Despite oliguria, serum potassium levels do not become dangerously elevated until the end stages of the hepatorenal syndrome. Blood urea level increases, followed by an increase in creatinine concentration. Urine osmolality increases, but urine sodium concentrations are below normal. Urine specific gravity is greater than 1.015.

The prognosis is usually poor and is related to a failing liver requiring liver transplant. Bridge treatments include albumin administration and a vasopressin analogue (Pressyn).[147]

Disorders of the Liver

> **QUICK CHECK 36.6**
> 1. How does alcohol damage the liver?
> 2. What kind of liver changes are common to alcoholic cirrhosis and nonalcoholic fatty liver disease?
> 3. What are the major pathological differences between alcoholic and primary biliary cirrhosis?

Liver disease is the fourth leading cause of death in Canada. The most common cause of liver failure is a condition known as fatty liver disease, but hepatitis B and C are also major causes of chronic liver disease. The causes of liver disease are different in children as compared with adults. In children, the leading causes of acute liver failure include acetaminophen toxicity, metabolic disorders, and autoimmune disease. It is estimated that more than 2 million Canadians—regardless of age, sex, ethnic origin, or lifestyle—will be affected by a liver or biliary tract disease in their lifetime.[149]

Acute Liver Failure

Acute liver failure (fulminant liver failure) is a rare clinical syndrome resulting in severe impairment or necrosis of liver cells without pre-existing liver disease or cirrhosis. Acute liver failure also can occur with concurrent liver disease (acute or chronic liver failure),[150] including complication of viral hepatitis, particularly hepatitis B virus (HBV) infection; compounded by infection with the hepatitis delta virus; as well as metabolic liver disorders. Edematous hepatocytes and patchy areas of necrosis and inflammatory cell infiltrates disrupt the parenchyma. The death of hepatocytes may be caused by viral or toxic injury or immunological and inflammatory damage with necrosis or apoptosis.

Acute liver failure usually develops 6 to 8 weeks after the initial symptoms of viral hepatitis or a metabolic liver disorder, or within 5 days to 8 weeks of acetaminophen (Tylenol) overdose. Anorexia, vomiting, abdominal pain, and progressive jaundice are initial signs followed by ascites and GI bleeding. Hepatic encephalopathy is manifested as lethargy and altered motor functions. Coma is related to cerebral edema, ischemia, and brainstem herniation. Liver function tests show elevations in the levels of both direct and indirect serum bilirubin, serum transaminases, and blood ammonia. Prothrombin time is prolonged. Kidney failure and pulmonary distress can occur.[151] Treatment of acute liver failure requires rapid evaluation and critical care. The hepatic necrosis is irreversible, and 60 to 90% of affected children die. Liver transplantation may be lifesaving;[152] in Canada, over 400 liver transplant operations are performed every year.[149] Artificial liver support devices are being evaluated. Survivors usually do not develop cirrhosis or chronic liver disease.

> **BOX 36.3 Causes of Cirrhosis**
>
> Hepatitis virus: B and C (common)
> Excessive alcohol intake (common)
> Idiopathic (common)
> Nonalcoholic fatty liver disease, also known as *nonalcoholic steatohepatitis*
> Autoimmune disorders
>   Autoimmune hepatitis
>   Primary biliary cirrhosis
>   Primary sclerosing cholangitis
> Hereditary metabolic disorder
> α_1-Antitrypsin deficiency
>   Hemochromatosis
>   Wilson's disease
>   Glycogen or lipid storage diseases
> Prolonged exposure to chemicals or toxins (e.g., carbon tetrachloride, cleaning and industrial solvents, copper salts)
> Hepatic venous outflow obstruction
>   Budd-Chiari syndrome
>   Right ventricular failure

Cirrhosis

Cirrhosis is an irreversible inflammatory and fibrotic liver disease. Many disorders can cause cirrhosis and are listed in Box 36.3. The process of cellular injury depends on the cause of cirrhosis, and the pathological mechanisms are not all clearly understood. Structural changes result from injury (e.g., viruses or toxicity from alcohol) and fibrosis, which is a consequence of infiltration of leukocytes, release of inflammatory mediators, and activation of hepatic stellate cells and myofibroblasts.[153,154] Chaotic fibrosis alters or obstructs biliary channels and blood flow, producing jaundice and portal hypertension. New vascular channels form shunts, and blood from the portal vein bypasses the liver, contributing to portal hypertension, metabolic alterations, and toxin accumulation. The process of regeneration is disrupted by hypoxia, necrosis, atrophy, and (ultimately) liver failure. The formation of fibrous bands and regenerating nodules distorts the architecture of the liver parenchyma and gives the liver a cobbly appearance. The liver may be larger or smaller than normal and is usually firm or hard when palpated.

There are no data on the prevalence of cirrhosis in Canada. However, from 2000 to 2007, noncancer liver–related deaths increased from 2 673 to 3 227 per year, an increase of 20.7%. Over the same period, all deaths from chronic liver disease increased from 3 964 to 5 049 per year, an increase of 27.9%. This significant increase in mortality occurred over only 8 years.[153]

Cirrhosis develops slowly over a period of years. Its severity and rate of progression depend on the cause. If toxins, such as alcohol metabolites, are involved, the rate of cell death and the severity of inflammation depend on the amount of toxin present. Removal of the toxin slows the progression of liver damage and enhances the process of regeneration.[154]

Alcoholic liver disease. Alcoholic liver disease is related to the toxic effects of alcohol (see Chapter 4) and coexisting liver disease. The incidence of alcoholic cirrhosis is greatest in middle-aged men; however, women develop more severe liver injury than men.[155] Although alcoholic cirrhosis is the most prevalent of the various types of cirrhosis, the occurrence of cirrhosis among persons with alcoholism is relatively low (approximately 25%). The spectrum of alcoholic liver disease includes alcoholic fatty liver, alcoholic steatohepatitis, and alcoholic cirrhosis.

PATHOPHYSIOLOGY **Alcoholic fatty liver (steatosis)** is the mildest form of alcoholic liver disease. It can be caused by relatively small

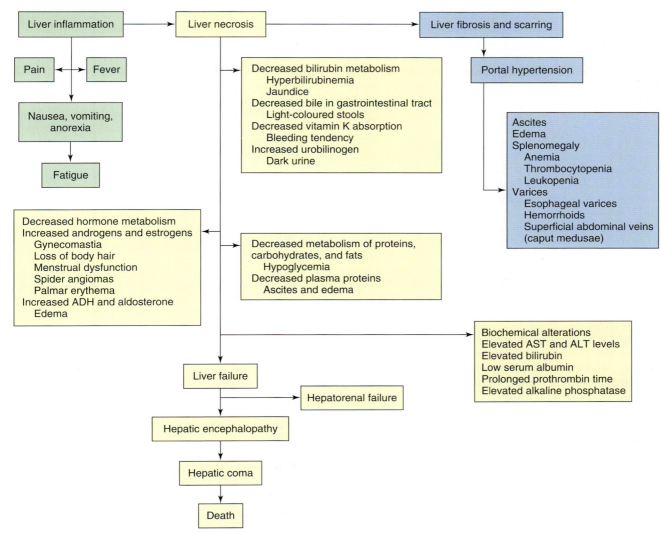

FIGURE 36.15 Clinical Manifestations of Cirrhosis. *ADH*, Antidiuretic hormone; *ALT*, alanine transaminase; *AST*, aspartate transaminase.

amounts of alcohol, may be asymptomatic, and is reversible with cessation of drinking.[156] Fat deposition (deposition of triglycerides) within the liver is caused primarily by increased lipogenesis, cholesterol synthesis, and decreased fatty acid oxidation by hepatocytes. Lipids mobilized from adipose tissue or dietary fat intake may contribute to fat accumulation.

Alcoholic steatohepatitis (alcoholic hepatitis) is a precursor of cirrhosis characterized by increased hepatic fat storage, inflammation, and degeneration and necrosis of hepatocytes with infiltration of neutrophils and lymphocytes. The injured hepatocytes contain Mallory bodies (hyaline endoplasmic reticulum), indicating the onset of fibrosis. The inflammation and necrosis caused by alcoholic steatohepatitis stimulate the irreversible fibrosis characteristic of the cirrhotic stage of disease.[157]

Alcoholic cirrhosis is caused by the toxic effects of alcohol metabolism on the liver, immunological alterations, inflammatory cytokines, oxidative stress from lipid peroxidation, and malnutrition. Alcohol is transformed to acetaldehyde, and excessive amounts significantly alter hepatocyte function and activate hepatic stellate cells, a primary cell involved in liver fibrosis. Mitochondrial function is impaired, decreasing oxidation of fatty acids. Enzyme and protein synthesis may be depressed or altered, and hormone and ammonia degradation is diminished. Acetaldehyde inhibits export of proteins from the liver, alters metabolism of vitamins and minerals, and induces malnutrition.[155,158] Kupffer cell (macrophage) activation attracts neutrophils, promoting inflammation; endotoxins accumulate from translocation of gut bacteria; and cell-mediated immunity is suppressed. Cellular damage initiates an inflammatory response that, along with necrosis, results in activation of hepatic stellate cells and excessive collagen formation. Fibrosis and scarring alter the structure of the liver and obstruct biliary and vascular channels.

CLINICAL MANIFESTATIONS Fatty infiltration causes no specific symptoms or abnormal liver function test results. The liver is usually enlarged, however, and the individual has a history of continuous alcohol intake during the previous weeks or months. Anorexia, nausea, jaundice, and edema develop with advanced fatty infiltration or the onset of alcoholic steatohepatitis (Figure 36.15).

The clinical manifestations of alcoholic steatohepatitis can be mild or severe. Nonspecific symptoms include fatigue, weight loss, and anorexia. Manifestations of acute illness include nausea, anorexia, fever, abdominal pain, and jaundice. Cirrhosis is a multiple-system disease and causes hepatomegaly, splenomegaly, ascites, portal hypertension, GI hemorrhage, hepatic encephalopathy, and esophageal varices. Anemia results from blood loss, malnutrition, and hypersplenism. Kidney failure is often a late complication of hepatorenal syndrome. Toxic effects of alcohol also can cause testicular atrophy, reduced libido, azoospermia, and decreased testosterone levels in men. The presence of numerous and severe manifestations increases the risk for death. Cirrhosis increases the risk for hepatocellular carcinoma.

EVALUATION AND TREATMENT The diagnosis of alcoholic steatohepatitis or cirrhosis is based on the individual's history and clinical manifestations. The results of liver function tests are abnormal, and serological studies show elevated levels of serum enzymes and bilirubin, decreased levels of serum albumin, and prolonged prothrombin time that is not easily corrected with vitamin K therapy. Liver biopsy can confirm the diagnosis of cirrhosis, but biopsy is not necessary if clinical manifestations of cirrhosis are evident.

There is no specific treatment for alcoholic steatohepatitis or cirrhosis. Rest, vitamin supplements, a nutritious diet, corticosteroids, antioxidants, medications that slow fibrosis, and management of complications (such as ascites, GI bleeding, and encephalopathy) slow disease progression. Cessation of alcohol consumption slows the progression of liver damage, improves clinical symptoms, and prolongs life. Although the liver damage is irreversible, measures that halt the inflammation and destruction of liver cells prolong life. Liver transplantation is the treatment of end-stage liver disease. Artificial liver support systems continue to be evaluated and hepatocyte transplantation is being explored.[159,160]

Nonalcoholic fatty liver disease and nonalcoholic steatohepatitis. Nonalcoholic fatty liver disease (NAFLD) is infiltration of hepatocytes with fat, primarily in the form of triglycerides, but it occurs in the absence of alcohol intake. It is associated with obesity (including obese children), high levels of cholesterol and triglycerides, metabolic syndrome, and type 2 diabetes mellitus. Some individuals with NAFLD will develop nonalcoholic steatohepatitis (NASH) with hepatocellular injury, inflammation, and fibrosis. NASH is difficult to distinguish from alcohol-induced liver fibrosis. NAFLD is usually asymptomatic and may remain undetected for years. The most severe forms of NASH progress to cirrhosis and end-stage liver disease. Treatment is individualized and includes the use of behavioural modification, dietary counselling, and regular exercise.[161,162]

Biliary cirrhosis. Biliary cirrhosis differs from alcoholic cirrhosis in that the damage and inflammation leading to cirrhosis begin in bile canaliculi and bile ducts, rather than in the hepatocytes. The two types of biliary cirrhosis are *primary* and *secondary*. Although both involve bile duct pathological changes, they differ with respect to cause, risk factors, and mechanisms of obstruction and inflammation.

Primary biliary cirrhosis is a chronic, autoimmune, cholestatic liver disease. It is caused by autoimmune T-cell and highly specific antimitochondrial antibody destruction of the small intrahepatic bile ducts and primarily affects middle-aged women. Primary biliary cirrhosis often accompanies other autoimmune diseases. Pathogenesis includes inflammation, destruction, fibrosis, and obstruction of the intrahepatic bile ducts. Primary biliary cirrhosis can be detected by biochemical evidence of cholestatic liver disease. Test findings include the presence of antinuclear antibodies, anticentromere antibodies, and the GP210 antinuclear antibody as well as elevated alkaline phosphatase levels for at least 6 months' duration. Ultrasound imaging of the liver, or liver biopsy, assists with diagnosis. Manifestations progress insidiously from pruritus, hyperbilirubinemia, jaundice, and light or clay-coloured stools to cirrhosis, portal hypertension, and encephalopathy. Life expectancy is 5 to 10 years after onset of symptoms if not treated.

Treatment with ursodeoxycholic acid (Ursodiol) slows disease progression, and pruritus may be relieved by cholestyramine (Olestyr), which binds bile salts in the intestine. Liver transplant is highly effective.[163]

Secondary biliary cirrhosis is caused by prolonged partial or complete obstruction of the common bile duct or branches by gallstones, tumours, fibrotic strictures, or chronic pancreatitis; biliary atresia and cystic fibrosis are causative in children. Necrotic areas develop and lead to proliferation and inflammation of portal ducts, producing edema, fibrosis, and cirrhosis if not treated. Surgery or endoscopy relieves obstruction, prolongs survival, and diminishes or resolves symptoms.

Viral Hepatitis

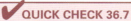

> **QUICK CHECK 36.7**
> 1. How does hepatitis A virus differ from hepatitis B virus?
> 2. What vaccines are available to prevent viral hepatitis?
> 3. What are the three phases of hepatitis viral infection?
> 4. What complications are associated with chronic active hepatitis?

Viral hepatitis is a relatively common systemic disease that primarily affects the liver. Different strains of viruses cause different types of hepatitis. Characteristics of the different types of viruses that cause hepatitis are presented in Table 36.8. Viral hepatitis in children is presented in Chapter 37.

Hepatitis B infection is a reportable disease. All public health jurisdictions record all positive hepatitis B blood tests (HBsAg-positive is the marker for active infection) and report data on acute and "indeterminate" cases to the Canadian Notifiable Disease Surveillance System (CNDSS).[153]

Canada draws a large proportion of its immigrants from areas of the world where hepatitis B is highly prevalent, including China, the Philippines, and other areas of South East Asia, as well as the Middle East and Africa. Based on the size and origin of the immigrant population in the 2006 census, the estimated number of people infected with hepatitis B in Canada ranges from 242 749 to 444 500, which corresponds to between 0.81 to 1.44% of the Canadian population.[153]

As the province with the highest proportion of hepatitis B carriers in Canada (50%), Ontario is the only province that has attempted to determine the effect of hepatitis B on population morbidity and mortality. Hepatitis B infection is the fifth leading cause of morbidity and mortality among all infectious diseases in Ontario. And yet, Ontario has the most restrictive reimbursement criteria for hepatitis B medications.[153]

PATHOPHYSIOLOGY All five types of viral hepatitis (A, B, C, D, and E) can cause acute, icteric illness. The pathological lesions of hepatitis include hepatic cell necrosis, scarring (with chronic disease), and Kupffer cell hyperplasia, and infiltration by mononuclear phagocytes occurs with varying severity. Cellular injury is promoted by cell-mediated immune mechanisms (i.e., T-cytotoxic cells, T-regulatory cells, and natural killer cells). Regeneration of hepatic cells begins within 48 hours of injury. The inflammatory process can damage and obstruct bile canaliculi, leading to cholestasis and obstructive jaundice. In milder cases, the liver parenchyma is not damaged. Damage tends to be most severe in cases of hepatitis B and C. Acute fulminating hepatitis can cause acute liver failure and severe hepatic encephalopathy, which manifests as confusion, stupor, coma, and coagulopathy. Hepatitis B and C are the most common causes, with hepatitis E occurring more commonly in pregnant women.[164]

Co-infection of hepatitis B virus (HBV), hepatitis C virus (HCV), hepatitis D virus (HDV), and human immunodeficiency virus (HIV)

TABLE 36.8 Characteristics of Viral Hepatitis

Characteristic	Hepatitis A	Hepatitis B	Hepatitis D	Hepatitis C	Hepatitis E
Virus	27-nm RNA virus	42-nm DNA virus	36-nm RNA virus	30- to 60-nm RNA virus	32-nm RNA virus
Antigens or antibodies	Anti-HAV	HBsAg, HBcAg, HBeAg	Anti-HDV	Anti-HCV	Anti-HEV
Incubation period	30 days	60–180 days	30–180 days	35–60 days	15–60 days
Route of transmission	Fecal–oral (most common), parenteral, sexual	Parenteral, sexual, across placenta	HBV co-infection Parenteral (?), fecal–oral, sexual	Parenteral, sexual, across placenta	Fecal–oral
Onset	Nonspecific Acute with fever	Insidious	Insidious	Insidious	Acute
Carrier state	Negative	Positive	Positive	Positive	Negative
Severity	Mild	Severe; may be prolonged or chronic	Severe	Unknown	Severe in pregnant women
Chronic hepatitis	No	Yes Increased risk for HCC	Yes	Yes Increased risk for HCC	No
Age group affected	Children and young adults	Any	Any	Any	Children and young adults
Prophylaxis	Hygiene, immune serum globulin, HAV vaccine	Hygiene, HBV vaccine, blood screening	Hygiene, HBV vaccine	Hygiene, blood screening, interferon-alpha	Hygiene, safe water
Pathophysiology	Hepatocyte injury caused by cellular immune responses (T cells, NK cells, and cytokines)	Viral replication, co-infection with viral mutation, inflammation, and cellular necrosis	Co-infection with HBV, severe cell injury, inflammation progressing to cirrhosis	Hepatocyte injury caused by immune response, inflammation, and fibrosis leading to cirrhosis	Viral replication, liver is cytotoxic, immune response causes inflammation and cholestasis
Treatment	Immune globulin within 2 weeks of exposure Symptomatic support	Interferon-alpha, peginterferon-alpha, antivirals (lamivudine [3TC], adefovir [Hepsera], entecavir [Baraclude], telbivudine [Sebivo], tenofovir [Viread])	Interferon-alpha	Interferon-alpha, peginterferon-alpha, antivirals (ribavirin [Virazole], boceprevir [Victrelis], telaprevir [Incivek], simeprevir [Olysio], daclatasvir [Daklinza], sofosbuvir [Sovaldi]), combinations of antivirals, sofosbuvir/ledipasvir for 12 weeks in genotypes 1, 4, 5 and 6.	Symptomatic support similar to HAV

HAAg, Hepatitis A antigen; *HAV*, hepatitis A virus; *HBcAg*, hepatitis B core antigen; *HBeAg*, hepatitis B e antigen; *HBsAg*, hepatitis B surface antigen; *HBV*, hepatitis B virus; *HCC*, hepatocellular carcinoma; *HCV*, hepatitis C virus; *HDV*, hepatitis D virus; *HEV*, hepatitis E virus; *NK cells*, natural killer cells.

occurs because these viruses share the same route of transmission (contact between infected body fluids and broken skin or mucous membranes, or intravenously). Progression of liver disease is more rapid in these cases.[165]

CLINICAL MANIFESTATIONS The clinical manifestations of the various types of hepatitis are very similar. The spectrum of manifestations ranges from absence of symptoms to fulminating hepatitis, with rapid onset of liver failure and coma. Acute viral hepatitis causes abnormal liver function test results. The serum aminotransferase values, aspartate transaminase (AST) and alanine transaminase (ALT), are elevated but not consistent with the extent of cellular damage. The clinical course of hepatitis usually consists of three phases. The **incubation phase** and manifestations vary depending on the virus (see Table 36.8):

1. **Prodromal (preicteric) phase.** Begins about 2 weeks after exposure and ends with the appearance of jaundice; marked by fatigue, anorexia, malaise, nausea, vomiting, headache, hyperalgia, cough, and low-grade fever; infection is highly transmissible during this phase.

2. **Icteric phase.** Begins 1 to 2 weeks after the prodromal phase and lasts 2 to 6 weeks; jaundice, dark urine, and clay-coloured stools are common; the liver is enlarged, smooth, and tender, and percussion or palpation of the liver causes pain; GI and respiratory symptoms subside, but fatigue and abdominal pain may persist or become more severe. This is the actual phase of illness. Individuals who develop chronic HBV, HDV, or HCV infection do not become jaundiced and may not be diagnosed.

3. **Recovery phase.** Begins with resolution of jaundice, about 6 to 8 weeks after exposure; symptoms diminish, but the liver remains enlarged and tender; liver function returns to normal 2 to 12 weeks after the onset of jaundice.

Chronic active hepatitis is the persistence of clinical manifestations and liver inflammation after acute stages of HBV, HBV/HDV co-infection, and HCV infection. Liver function tests remain abnormal for longer than 6 months, and hepatitis B surface antigen (HBsAg) persists. Chronic active HBV or HCV is a predisposition to cirrhosis and primary hepatocellular carcinoma.[166,167] Chronic active hepatitis constitutes a carrier state, and HBV and HCV can be transmitted from mothers to infants.

EVALUATION AND TREATMENT Diagnosis of hepatitis A virus (HAV) and HCV is based on the presence of anti-HAV and anti-HCV antibodies. The most specific diagnostic test for HBV is serological analysis for specific hepatitis virus antigens (i.e., HBsAg, which is the marker for HBV). Other markers for HBV include antibody to hepatitis B surface antigen (anti-HBs), hepatitis B e antigen (HBeAg), antibody to hepatitis B e antigen (anti-HBe), antibody to hepatitis B core antigen (anti-HBc), immunoglobulin M (IgM), and immunoglobulin G (IgG).[168] The assay for HDV is the measurement of total antibody to hepatitis D antigen (anti-HDV) and serum HDV RNA.[169]

According to the *Management of Chronic Hepatitis C: 2018 Guideline* update from the Canadian Association for the Study of the Liver, anti-HCV antibody testing is the diagnostic test of choice for initial screening. If positive and to confirm chronic infection, a confirmatory HCV RNA polymerase chain reaction test is needed. In patients with spontaneous or treatment-induced clearance and patients with suspected acute infection, HCV RNA is the screening test of choice because anti-HCV antibody tests will continue to test positive for life, even after spontaneous or treatment-induced clearance of HCV. A small percentage of patients will spontaneously clear infection shortly after contracting the virus, with no long-term complications. These individuals will test positive for anti-HCV antibodies, but negative for HCV RNA, and are not protected from reinfection. After 6 months, the infection becomes chronic and spontaneous clearance of HCV is extremely uncommon.[140]

All patients with chronic HCV infection should be considered candidates for antiviral therapy. Direct-acting antiviral agents can induce sustained virological response, effectively and safely; thus, there is no medical justification to restrict therapy, except in patients with severe comorbidities and short life span that are not secondary to HCV infection. As such, all individuals with chronic HCV infection should be considered candidates for antiviral therapy. Initiation of treatment should be started promptly in patients with advanced liver fibrosis. Patients with mild fibrosis should also be considered for antiviral therapy because viral eradication in these patients improves their quality of life and prevents the risk of infecting others.[140]

The treatment of HCV with interferon-free direct-acting antiviral agent–based therapy has shown to be cost-effective at all stages of fibrosis. While some provinces in Canada limit access to treatment to those patients who have hepatic fibrosis, there is no medical or epidemiological evidence to support these restrictions based on fibrosis stage. The decrease in price has led to more patients having access to these medications. Laboratory testing to confirm and characterize the infection and determine the HCV RNA viral load, and HCV genotype and subtype (i.e., 1a versus 1b), is helpful in the management of patients with chronic HCV infection. In addition, liver function tests and abdominal ultrasound to assess the stage of fibrosis should be done.[140]

Documentation of detectable HCV RNA is needed to confirm HCV infection. Treatment regimens vary, depending on the level of HCV RNA. However, the HCV RNA levels must not impact the therapeutic decision-making. Current medical therapy is effective against all HCV genotypes; therefore, genotyping is not always needed before therapy if a pan-genotypic regimen is used, in patients who do not have cirrhosis. However, many medications are genotype- and/or subtype-specific, and even with pan-genotypic regimens, efficacy varies by genotype, therefore, genotyping before starting therapy is still recommended.

Considering the efficacy, safety, and tolerability of interferon-free direct-acting antiviral agent regimens, therapy containing pegylated interferon-α are no longer recommended for patients with HCV infection. As such interferon-free regimens are recommended as first-line therapy for all indications. According to WHO,[170] treatment with pan-genotypic DAA agent is recommended to all individuals diagnosed with HCV infection who are 12 years of age or older, and to persons with chronic HCV infection aged 18 years and above. Adolescents aged 12 to 17 years and those weighing at least 36 kg with chronic HCV infection should also receive pan-genotypic DAA agent, (WHO) sofosbuvir/ledipasvir for 12 weeks in genotypes 1, 4, 5 and 6. WHO recommends sofosbuvir/ribavirin for 12 weeks in genotype 2 and sofosbuvir/ribavirin for 24 weeks in genotype 3. In children aged less than 12 years with chronic HCV infection, the WHO recommends deferring treatment until 12 years of age. Treatment with interferon-based regimens should no longer be used. Hepatitis E virus (HEV) is diagnosed from the presence of serum anti-HEV IgG and HEV RNA. HEV is usually a self-limiting disease except in undeveloped countries, where it causes chronic hepatitis, with increased risk in pregnant women. Liver enzyme levels and function tests also can indicate other viral liver diseases, medication toxicity, or alcoholic hepatitis.[171]

Treatments for different types of viral hepatitis are summarized in Table 36.8. Physical activity may be restricted, and a low-fat, high-carbohydrate diet is beneficial if bile flow is obstructed. For chronic hepatitis, treatment is directed at suppressing viral replication before irreversible liver cell damage or hepatic carcinoma occurs. Cyclic and combination therapy may prevent medication resistance, and new agents are being developed.[172,173]

After ingestion and GI uptake, HAV replicates in the liver and is secreted into the bile, feces, and sera. To prevent transmission of hepatitis A, proper hand hygiene and the use of gloves for disposing of bedpans and fecal matter are imperative. HAV may be shed in the feces for up to 3 months after onset of symptoms. Molecular procedures are available for direct surveillance of HAV in food.[174] Direct contact with blood or body fluids of individuals with HBV or HBV/HDV co-infection or HCV should be avoided. The administration of immunoglobulin before exposure or early in the incubation period can prevent hepatitis A and hepatitis B. A combined vaccine is available to protect against HAV and HBV infection. There is no vaccine for HCV.[175] A vaccine for HEV exists and is widely used in China, but it is not currently licensed in Canada or other industrialized countries.[176] Pre-exposure vaccination is recommended for health care workers, liver transplant recipients, and others who are at risk for contact with infected body fluids, particularly children.

Disorders of the Gallbladder

> ✓ **QUICK CHECK 36.8**
> 1. How do gallstones form?
> 2. Compare acute and chronic pancreatitis.
> 3. What factors are associated with cancer of the esophagus?
> 4. What dietary factors are associated with gastric cancer?

Obstruction and inflammation are the most common disorders of the gallbladder. Obstruction is caused by **gallstones**, which are aggregates of substances in the bile. The gallstones may remain in the gallbladder or be ejected, with bile, into the cystic duct. Gallstones that become lodged in the cystic duct obstruct the flow of bile into and out of the gallbladder and cause inflammation. Gallstone formation is termed **cholelithiasis**. Inflammation of the gallbladder or cystic duct is known as **cholecystitis**.

Cholelithiasis (Gallstones)

Cholelithiasis (gallstones) is a prevalent disorder in developed countries. Up to 20% of Canadian women and 10% of men have had cholelithiasis by the age of 60. Moreover, 70 to 80% of the Indigenous population is affected by this disorder. Risk factors include obesity, middle age, female gender, use of oral contraceptives, rapid weight loss,

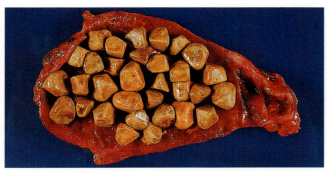

FIGURE 36.16 Resected Gallbladder Containing Mixed Gallstones. (From Kissane, J. M. [Ed.]. [1990]. *Anderson's pathology* [9th ed.]. Mosby).

Indigenous ancestry, genetic predisposition, and gallbladder, pancreatic, or ileal disease.[177,178]

PATHOPHYSIOLOGY Gallstones are formed from impaired metabolism of cholesterol, bilirubin, and bile acids. All gallstones contain cholesterol, unconjugated bilirubin, bilirubin calcium salts, fatty acids, calcium carbonates and phosphates, and mucin glycoproteins. Gallstones are of three types, depending on chemical composition: *cholesterol* (70% cholesterol and the most common [70 to 80%]); *pigmented* (black [hard] and brown [soft] with less than 30% cholesterol); and *mixed*.[179] *Cholesterol gallstones* form in bile that is supersaturated with cholesterol produced by the liver. Supersaturation sets the stage for cholesterol crystal formation, or the formation of "microstones." More crystals then aggregate on the microstones, which grow to form "macrostones." This process usually occurs in the gallbladder, which may have decreased motility. The stones may lie dormant or become lodged in the cystic or common duct, causing pain when the gallbladder contracts and cholecystitis. The stones can accumulate and fill the entire gallbladder (Figure 36.16). *Pigmented brown gallstones* form from calcium bilirubinate and fatty acid soaps that bind with calcium. They are associated with biliary stasis, bacterial infections, and biliary parasites. They are more common in East Asia. *Pigmented black gallstones* are rare. They are associated with chronic liver disease and hemolytic disease and are composed of calcium bilirubinate with mucin glycoproteins.[180]

CLINICAL MANIFESTATIONS Cholelithiasis is often asymptomatic. Epigastric and right hypochondrium pain and intolerance to fatty foods are the cardinal manifestations of cholelithiasis. Vague symptoms include heartburn, flatulence, epigastric discomfort, and food intolerances, particularly to fats and cabbage. The pain (biliary colic) occurs 30 minutes to several hours after eating a fatty meal. It is caused by the lodging of one or more gallstones in the cystic or common duct during contraction of the gallbladder. It can be intermittent or steady and usually occurs in the right upper quadrant, radiating to the mid-upper area of the back. Jaundice indicates that the stone is located in the common bile duct.

EVALUATION AND TREATMENT Diagnosis is based on medical history, physical examination, and imaging evaluation. An oral cholecystogram usually outlines the stones. Intravenous cholangiography is used to differentiate cholelithiasis from other causes of extrahepatic biliary obstruction if the cholecystogram is negative. Endoscopic or percutaneous cholangiography and endoscopic or transabdominal ultrasonography are diagnostic options. Oral bile acids (ursodeoxycholic acid or chenodeoxycholic acid) may prevent or dissolve cholesterol stones, but the stones may recur when the medication is discontinued. Dietary factors may prevent the development of gallstones, including reducing the intake of polyunsaturated fat, monounsaturated fat, and caffeine, and increasing the consumption of fibre.[181] Endoscopic removal of gallstones by sphincterotomy or endoscopic papillary balloon dilation is the preferred treatment for uncomplicated gallstones causing obstruction of the bile ducts. Large stones may be managed by lithotripsy.[182]

Cholecystitis

Cholecystitis can be acute or chronic, but both forms are almost always caused by a gallstone lodged in the cystic duct.[183] Obstruction causes the gallbladder to become distended and inflamed. The pain is similar to that caused by gallstones. Pressure against the distended wall of the gallbladder decreases blood flow and may result in ischemia, necrosis, and perforation. Fever, leukocytosis, rebound tenderness, and abdominal muscle guarding are common findings. Serum bilirubin and alkaline phosphatase levels may be elevated. Cholescintigraphy is the most sensitive imaging for cholecystitis. The acute abdominal pain of cholecystitis must be differentiated from that caused by pancreatitis, myocardial infarction, and acute pyelonephritis of the right kidney. Narcotics may be required to control pain, and antibiotics often are prescribed to manage bacterial infection in severe cases. Acute attacks usually require laparoscopic gallbladder resection (cholecystectomy). Obstruction also may lead to reflux of bile into the pancreatic duct, causing acute pancreatitis.[184]

Disorders of the Pancreas

Pancreatitis, or inflammation of the pancreas, is a relatively rare and potentially serious disorder. The incidence is about equal in men and women, is more common between 50 and 60 years of age, and is more likely to occur in Black people. Risk factors include obstructive biliary tract disease (particularly cholelithiasis), alcoholism, obesity, peptic ulcers, trauma, dyslipidemia, hypercalcemia, smoking, certain medications, and genetic factors (hereditary pancreatitis, cystic fibrosis). The cause is unknown in 15 to 25% of cases. Pancreatitis can be acute or chronic.

According to the Canadian Digestive Health Foundation, acute care inpatient costs for pancreas diseases are ranked as the fifth most expensive digestive disease in Canada; it costs $120 million per year for 13 000 patients. In Canada, pancreatitis affects 1 million people. Acute pancreatitis affects more than 600 000 people, while chronic pancreatitis affects more than 300 000 people. In Canada, similar to other Western countries, obesity is the main risk factor for developing acute pancreatitis.[185]

Acute Pancreatitis

Acute pancreatitis is usually a mild disease and resolves spontaneously, but about 20% of those with the disease develop a severe, acute pancreatitis requiring hospitalization. Pancreatitis develops because of obstruction to the outflow of pancreatic digestive enzymes caused by bile and pancreatic duct obstruction (e.g., gallstones). Acute pancreatitis also results from direct cellular injury from alcohol, medications, or viral infection.[186]

PATHOPHYSIOLOGY In obstructive disease, there is backup of pancreatic secretions and activation and release of enzymes (activated trypsin activates chymotrypsin, lipase, and elastase) within the pancreatic acinar cells. The activated enzymes cause autodigestion of pancreatic cells and tissues, resulting in inflammation. The autodigestion causes vascular damage, coagulation necrosis, fat necrosis (see Chapter 4), and formation of pseudocysts (walled-off collections of pancreatic

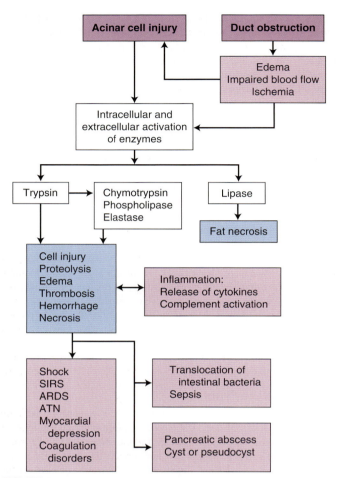

FIGURE 36.17 Pathophysiology of Acute Pancreatitis. *ARDS*, Acute respiratory distress syndrome; *ATN*, acute tubular necrosis; *SIRS*, systemic inflammatory response syndrome.

CLINICAL MANIFESTATIONS The cardinal manifestation of acute pancreatitis is epigastric or midabdominal constant pain ranging from mild abdominal discomfort to severe, incapacitating pain. The pain may radiate to the back. Pain is caused by (1) edema, which distends the pancreatic ducts and capsule; (2) chemical irritation and inflammation of the peritoneum; (3) irritation or obstruction of the biliary tract; and (4) inflammation of nerves. Fever and leukocytosis accompany the inflammatory response. Nausea and vomiting are caused by paralytic ileus secondary to the pancreatitis or peritonitis. Jaundice can occur from obstruction of the bile duct (e.g., a gallstone) or from pancreatic edema pressing on the duct. Abdominal distension accompanies bowel hypomotility and the accumulation of fluids in the peritoneal cavity. Hypovolemia, hypotension, tachycardia, myocardial insufficiency, and shock occur because plasma volume is lost as inflammatory mediators released into the circulation increase vascular permeability and dilate vessels. Tachypnea and hypoxemia develop secondary to ascites, pulmonary edema, atelectasis, or pleural effusions. Hypovolemia can decrease renal blood flow sufficiently to impair renal function and can cause kidney failure. Tetany may develop as a result of hypocalcemia when calcium is deposited in areas of fat necrosis or as a decreased response to parathormone. Transient hyperglycemia also can occur if glucagon is released from damaged alpha cells in the pancreatic islets. In severe acute pancreatitis, some individuals develop flank or periumbilical ecchymosis, a sign of poor prognosis. Multiple organ failure or SIRS accounts for most deaths of those with severe acute pancreatitis.

EVALUATION AND TREATMENT Diagnosis is based on clinical findings, identification of associated disorders, laboratory studies, and imaging results. Elevated serum amylase concentration is characteristic but is not diagnostic of severity or specificity of disease. Elevated serum lipase level is the primary diagnostic marker for acute pancreatitis.

The goal of treatment for acute pancreatitis is to stop the process of autodigestion and prevent systemic complications. Narcotic medications may be needed to relieve pain. To decrease pancreatic secretions and "rest the gland," oral food and fluids may be withheld initially, and continuous gastric suction instituted. Nasogastric suction may not be necessary with mild pancreatitis, but it helps to relieve pain and prevent paralytic ileus in individuals who are nauseated and vomiting. Feeding is usually initiated within 24 to 48 hours if ileus is not present. Parenteral fluids are essential to restore blood volume and prevent hypotension and shock. In severe pancreatitis, enteral nutrition with use of jejunal tube feeding usually is well tolerated, may decrease pancreatic enzyme secretion, prevents gut bacterial overgrowth, and maintains gut barrier function. Medications that decrease gastric acid production (e.g., H2 receptor antagonists) can decrease stimulation of the pancreas by secretin. Antibiotics are used if there is infection. The risk for mortality increases significantly with the development of infection or pulmonary, cardiac, and renal complications.[188]

Chronic Pancreatitis

Chronic pancreatitis is a process of progressive fibrotic destruction of the pancreas. Chronic alcohol abuse is the most common cause. Obstruction from gallstones, smoking, and genetic factors increase the risk for chronic pancreatitis.[189] Toxic metabolites and chronic release of inflammatory cytokines contribute to the destruction of acinar cells and islets of Langerhans. The pancreatic parenchyma is destroyed and replaced by fibrous tissues, strictures, calcification, ductal obstruction, and pancreatic cysts. The cysts are walled-off areas or pockets of pancreatic juice, necrotic debris, or blood within or adjacent to the pancreas. New imaging techniques have advanced evaluation of disease severity.[190]

secretions). Edema within the pancreatic capsule leads to ischemia and can contribute to necrosis. There also may be independent activation of inflammation within acinar cells contributing to the local and systemic responses occurring in acute pancreatitis[187] (Figure 36.17). In cases of alcohol abuse, the pancreatic acinar cell metabolizes ethanol with the generation of toxic metabolites that injure pancreatic acinar cells, causing release of activated enzymes. Chronic alcohol use may also cause formation of protein plugs in pancreatic ducts and spasm of the sphincter of Oddi, resulting in obstruction. The obstruction leads to intrapancreatic release of activated enzymes, autodigestion, inflammation, and pancreatitis.

Systemic effects of acute pancreatitis are related to release of proinflammatory cytokines (e.g., interleukin-6, tumour necrosis factor-alpha, and platelet-activating factor) into the bloodstream. There is activation of leukocytes, injury to vessel walls, and coagulation abnormalities with development of vasodilation, hypotension, and shock. Complications can include acute respiratory distress syndrome (ARDS), heart failure, kidney failure, coagulopathies, intra-abdominal hypertension, and systemic inflammatory response syndrome (SIRS) (see Chapter 24). Paralytic ileus and GI bleeding can occur. Translocation of intestinal bacteria to the bloodstream may cause peritonitis or sepsis. Recurrent inflammation activates pancreatic stellate cells, causing pancreatic fibrosis, strictures, and duct obstruction that lead to chronic pancreatitis.[51]

Continuous or intermittent abdominal pain and weight loss are common. The pain is difficult to manage and is associated with increased intraductal pressure, ischemia, neuritis, intra-abdominal hypertension (compartment syndrome), ongoing injury, and both peripheral and central pain sensitization.[191] Manifestations of pancreatic enzyme deficiency, such as steatorrhea or a malabsorption syndrome, are present in late stages of chronic pancreatitis. To correct enzyme deficiencies and prevent malabsorption, oral enzyme replacements are taken before and during meals. Loss of islet cells can cause insulin-dependent diabetes and requires treatment. Cessation of alcohol intake is essential for the management of both acute and chronic pancreatitis. Endoscopic or surgical drainage of cysts or partial resection of the pancreas may be required to relieve pain and to prevent cystic rupture.[192] Chronic pancreatitis is a risk factor for pancreatic cancer.

Digestive Symptoms and Intestinal Inflammation in COVID-19 Patients

COVID-19 is a viral infection that causes respiratory manifestations. Diarrhea and other gastro-intestinal symptoms are also observed in patients with COVID-19. The link between intestinal problems and COVID-19 was observed in patients in Wuhan, China.[193]

There is no evidence regarding the efficacy of antidiarrheal medications in COVID-19 patients. Diarrhea should raise a red flag of a possible SARS-CoV-2 infection and should be further investigated to rule out COVID-19. Patients with diarrhea of unknown cause should be suspected of being infected with COVID-19 instead of waiting for respiratory symptoms to appear. Patients with COVID-19 and digestive symptoms may delay their admission to the hospital, leading to a poorer clinical outcome, in comparison with patients who did not suffer from GI symptoms. One study determined that patients with digestive symptoms had an average time of 9 days from the onset of symptoms until hospital admission, whereas patients with respiratory symptoms had an admission time of 7.3 days.[194] Therefore, patients with GI symptoms are likely to wait longer to be diagnosed with SARS-CoV-2 in the absence of respiratory symptoms. In addition to diarrhea, COVID-19 patients may also develop anorexia, vomiting, or abdominal pain. As the severity of COVID increases, gastro-intestinal symptoms become more pronounced. In patients with diarrhea, the fecal test may remain positive for SARS-CoV-2 twelve days after the disease onset, and the stool test may continue to be positive despite negative respiratory tests.[195]

Gastro-intestinal symptoms of COVID 19 are associated with inflammation and intestinal damage leading to loss of intestinal barrier integrity, and stimulation of intestinal signalling pathways that regulate inflammation through dendritic cells. Gut microbes activate innate and adaptive immune cells to release proinflammatory cytokines into the circulatory system, leading to systemic inflammation.

The presence of SARS-CoV-2 in the feces of asymptomatic patients implies that COVID-19 could be transmitted through the fecal route. SARS-CoV-2 shedding in stool samples is detectable over a longer period than in nasopharyngeal swabs.[193] Patients who have experienced SARS-CoV-2 should undergo a thorough evaluation to prevent the potential risk of transmission if they are selected to be donors for fecal microbiota transplant. Candidates for fecal microbiota transplantation and healthy donors must be screened for the COVID-19 virus.[193] Fecal calprotectin in COVID-19 patients supports the growing evidence that SARS-CoV-2 infection causes an inflammatory response in the intestine. Studies demonstrated that calprotectin and serum IL-6 concentrations were significantly higher in COVID-19 patients who initially developed diarrhea. To diagnose and follow-up COVID-19-related diarrhea, calprotectin measurement can play a role in monitoring the disease. The incidence of diarrhea may be secondary to virus-induced inflammation, which results from the entry of inflammatory cells, including neutrophils and lymphocytes, into the intestinal mucosa, thus causing disruption of the gut microbiota.[193]

SARS-CoV-2 enters cells by binding its protein S to ACE2 receptors on the epithelial cells in the lungs, small intestine and colon, tubular cells of the kidney, neuronal and glial cells in the brain, enterocytes, vascular endothelial cells, smooth muscle cells, and cardiomyocytes. SARS-CoV-2 also uses the receptors for transmembrane protease serine 2 (TMPRSS2), an enzyme expressed in the small intestinal epithelial cells, to enter to those cells. The SARS-CoV-2 activity causes ACE2 modifications in the gut that increase susceptibility to intestinal inflammation and diarrhea. A high expression of ACE2 and TMPRSS2 is detected in enterocytes, and the esophagus and lungs.[193]

Primary inflammatory stimuli trigger the release of microbial products and cytokines, which can cause microbial dysbiosis that can induce an inflammatory environment, releasing intestinal cytokines into the circulatory system, and increasing the systemic inflammation of COVID-19. Taken together, a combined inflammation can potentially initiate an immune reaction that can cause even more harm than the virus itself. It is essential to understand the host cytokine pathways and microbiota interactions with cytokine responses in SARS-CoV-2 infection to develop novel treatment approaches, and to investigate how intestinal bacteria interact in response to SARS-CoV-2 infection.[193]

SARS-CoV-2 infects individuals regardless of their age, but older persons with comorbidities are more vulnerable to becoming seriously ill.[196] Loss of microbial diversity associated with aging increases susceptibility to inflammation.[197] Comorbidities determine the risk of severe complications and death after COVID-19 infection, and these comorbidities (e.g., asthma, hypertension, smoking, male gender, or Alzheimer's disease or dementia) increase the risk of COVID-19 complications and severity.[198] Changes in gut microbiota associated with aging are also linked to these comorbidities. The dysregulation of the gut microbiota results in changes in the immune system and increases the risk of developing more severe consequences of COVID-19. This causes a higher mortality rate in this portion of the population. The gut microbiota in humans is often stable throughout adult life but starts to change in older persons; gut microbiota diversity decreases and dysbiosis increases, increasing the risk of cognitive deficits, depression, and inflammatory markers.

CANCER OF THE DIGESTIVE SYSTEM

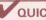

QUICK CHECK 36.9
1. What are the primary risk factors for colorectal carcinoma?
2. Compare tumours of the right colon with those of the left colon.
3. What is the most common cause of liver cancer?

Cancer of the Gastro-intestinal Tract

Table 36.9 contains information on the various GI cancers by organ, percentage of death compared with all cancer deaths, risk factors, type of cell, and common manifestations. The biology of cancer is presented in Chapter 10.

Cancer of the Esophagus

Carcinoma of the esophagus is a rare type of cancer with an estimated incidence of 1.7% in males and 0.5% in females. The Canadian Cancer Society estimated that over 2 300 Canadians (1 800 men and 530 women) were diagnosed with esophageal cancer in 2017. It also estimated that 2 200 Canadians (1 650 men and 480 women) died of

TABLE 36.9 Cancer of the Gut, Liver, and Pancreas

Organ	Projected Deaths Out of All Cancer Deaths in Canada, 2020 (%)	Risks	Cell Type	Common Manifestations
Esophagus	Males: 1.6% Females: 0.5%	Malnutrition Alcohol Tobacco Chronic reflux	Squamous cell Adenocarcinoma	Chest pain Dysphagia
Stomach	Males: 2.3% Females: 1.4%	Salty food Fried red meat Nitrates–nitrosamines	Adenocarcinoma Squamous cell	Anorexia Malaise Weight loss Upper abdominal pain Vomiting Occult blood
Colorectal	Males: 12.9% Females: 10.9%	Polyps Long-term inflammatory bowel disease Diverticulitis Highly refined carbohydrates; low-fibre, high-fat diets	Adenocarcinoma (left colon grows as ring; right colon grows as mass)	Pain Mass Anemia Bloody stool Obstruction Distension
Liver	Males: 1.9%[a] Females: 0.7%[a]	HBV, HCV, HDV Cirrhosis Intestinal parasite Aflatoxin from mouldy peanuts and corn	Hepatomas Cholangiomas	Pain Anorexia Bloating Weight loss Portal hypertension Ascites Jaundice
Pancreas	Males: 2.7% Females: 2.6%	Chronic pancreatitis Cigarette smoking Alcohol (?) Diabetic women	Adenocarcinoma (exocrine part of gland, ductal epithelium)	Weight loss Weakness Nausea Vomiting Abdominal pain Depression ± jaundice May have insulin-secreting tumours with symptoms of hypoglycemia

[a]Liver deaths are underestimated.
From American Cancer Society. (2015). *Cancer facts & figures 2015*. https://www.cancer.org/research/cancer-facts-statistics/all-cancer-facts-figures/cancer-facts-figures-2015.html; Canadian Cancer Society, & Government of Canada. (2019). *Canadian cancer statistics 2019*. https://www.cancer.ca/en/cancer-information/cancer-101/canadian-cancer-statistics/past-editions-canadian-cancer-statistics/?region=on.

this disease in 2017.[199] Risk factors are summarized in *Risk Factors: Esophageal Cancer*.

RISK FACTORS
Esophageal Cancer

- Age greater than 60 years
- Male
- Tobacco use
- Alcoholism
- Dietary factors: deficiencies of trace elements and vitamins
- Malnutrition associated with poor economic conditions or special dietary habits (e.g., very hot drinks, fish preserved in lye, diet deficient in fruits and vegetables)
- Reflux esophagitis with dysplasia
- Sliding hiatal hernia
- Obesity

PATHOPHYSIOLOGY Carcinoma of the esophagus includes squamous cell carcinoma and adenocarcinoma. The main risk factors for squamous cell carcinoma include chronic alcohol use combined with smoking or chewing tobacco, hot and irritant (alcohol) drinks, food containing nitrosamines, and achalasia.[200] Squamous cell carcinomas are more common in the thoracic and cervical areas of the esophagus.

Adenocarcinomas are more prevalent in males and are associated with cigarette smoking, obesity, and GERD. Adenocarcinoma development is often secondary to infiltration by a gastric carcinoma or to the presence of Barrett dysplasia, also known as **Barrett esophagus** (columnar rather than squamous epithelium in the lower esophagus) and can progress to metaplasia.[201] Adenocarcinoma is more common at the gastroesophageal junction. The CagA-positive strain of *H. pylori* may be a protection against esophageal carcinoma.[202]

CLINICAL MANIFESTATIONS The two frequent symptoms of esophageal carcinoma are chest pain and dysphagia. The most common type of pain is heartburn. It is initiated by eating spicy or highly seasoned foods and by assuming the recumbent position. Odynophagia (pain on swallowing) may be initiated by the swallowing of cold liquids. Spontaneous chest pain is more difficult to diagnose positively. Some individuals with esophageal cancer complain of a constant retrosternal pain that radiates to the back. Dysphagia (difficulty swallowing) usually gives the feeling of pressure and may radiate posteriorly between the scapulae. Dysphagia usually progresses rapidly. Esophageal carcinoma is asymptomatic during the early stages and presents at an advanced stage. Esophageal cancer metastasizes rapidly and, therefore, has a poor prognosis.

EVALUATION AND TREATMENT Individuals with dysphagia undergo endoscopy so that specimens can be obtained and examined for neoplastic change. Endoscopic ultrasound and CT studies of the thorax are used for diagnosis and staging. Prevention of gastroesophageal reflux and removal of high-grade dysplasia are essential to the management of Barrett esophagus.[203] It is impossible to remove all lymph nodes with the tumour, but removal of the primary lesion and the local lymph nodes can benefit the individual with esophageal cancer. If the malignancy has not spread beyond these sites, cure is likely. If metastasis has occurred, however, an incomplete resection is of little survival benefit. Treatment is combined radiation and chemotherapy.[204,205]

Cancer of the Stomach

The Canadian Cancer Society estimated that 4 200 Canadians (2 700 men and 1 450 women) were diagnosed with stomach cancer (also called *gastric cancer*) in 2020. It also estimated that 1 950 Canadians (12 000 men and 760 women) died of this disease in 2019.[206]

In Canada, the incidence rates of stomach cancer continue to decline in both males (2.2% per year) and females (1.3% per year); current rates are about half of what they were in 1985. This decline may be due to long-term improvements in diets and decreases in smoking and heavy alcohol use. The declining incidence rates of stomach cancer may also be related to the more recent recognition and treatment of infection caused by the bacterium *H. pylori*, an important risk factor for stomach cancer.[207]

The case fatality rate for stomach cancer is 75%.[208] Stomach cancer is more prevalent in Asia, particularly China.[209] Loss of tumour-suppressor genes and other genetic alterations may be important in stomach cancer.[210]

PATHOPHYSIOLOGY Gastric adenocarcinomas are associated with atrophic gastritis and *H. pylori* that carry the *CagA* gene product VacA. It also causes gastric B-cell mucosa–associated lymphoid tissue lymphoma. Hereditary diffuse adenocarcinoma is rare and occurs at a younger age.[211] Most adenocarcinomas are sporadic and associated with consumption of heavily salted and preserved foods (e.g., nitrates in pickled foods or in salted foods such as bacon), low intake of fruits and vegetables, and use of tobacco and alcohol. Dietary salt enhances the conversion of nitrates to carcinogenic nitrosamines in the stomach. Salt and nitrates converted to nitrites are caustic to the stomach, delay gastric emptying, and can cause chronic atrophic gastritis. Insufficient acid secretion by the atrophic mucosa creates a relatively alkaline environment that permits bacteria to multiply and act on nitrates. The resulting increase in nitrosamines damages the DNA of mucosal cells, further promoting metaplasia and neoplasia.

Gastric adenocarcinoma usually begins in the glands of the distal stomach mucosa. Duodenal reflux also may contribute to an intestinal-like metaplasia. The reflux contains caustic bile salts that destroy the mucosal barrier that normally protects the stomach.

CLINICAL MANIFESTATIONS The early stages of stomach cancer are generally asymptomatic or produce vague symptoms such as loss of appetite (especially for meat), malaise, and indigestion. Later manifestations of stomach cancer include unexplained weight loss, upper abdominal pain, vomiting, change in bowel habits, and anemia caused by persistent occult bleeding. The prognosis is poor because symptoms do not occur until the tumour has spread and caused distant metastases, particularly to the liver and peritoneal structures. Generally, the first manifestations of carcinoma are caused by distant metastases, and the disease is already in an advanced stage.

EVALUATION AND TREATMENT There are no specific biomarkers for stomach cancer. Micro RNAs are being evaluated as a specific diagnostic and prognostic marker.[212] Most symptoms suggest a problem in the upper GI tract, and a barium X-ray film shows the lesion. Direct endoscopic visualization, lavage, and cellular examination or biopsy establish the diagnosis. Screening and treatment for *H. pylori* infection are the best preventive approaches to stomach cancer. Surgery is the usual treatment for early stages of disease. Staging is determined by pathological findings after resection. Early diagnosis and chemotherapy combined with radiation improves postsurgical outcomes.[213]

Cancer of the Colon and Rectum

In Canada, from the mid-1980s to the mid-1990s, overall incidence rates for colorectal cancer declined for both sexes (this decline was more prominent for females). Incidence rates then rose through 2000, only to decline slightly thereafter. This change is most likely due to the increased use of colorectal cancer screening, which can identify and remove precancerous polyps and in turn reduce incidence. The decline in colorectal cancer incidence rates appears mostly in older persons, as rates are increasing among adults under the age of 50 years.[207]

As of 2014, nine provinces had organized colorectal cancer screening programs, and the remaining province has announced the intention to implement one. Participation rates vary within and between the existing organized programs and do not meet the target of 60%. Colorectal cancer is linked to several modifiable risk factors, including obesity, physical inactivity, consumption of red and processed meat, and smoking.[214] Diabetes may also increase risk for colorectal cancer. (See *Risk Factors:* Cancer of the Colon and Rectum.)

The Canadian Cancer Society estimated that 26 900 Canadians (14 900 men and 12 000 women) were diagnosed with colorectal cancer in 2020. This number represents 12% of all predicted new cancer cases in 2020. The Canadian Cancer Society also estimated that 9 700 Canadians (5 300 men and 4 400 women) died of this disease in 2020. This total represents 12% of all cancer deaths in 2020.[214] Colorectal cancer incidence rates for both males and females are highest in Newfoundland and Labrador. For females, high rates are also seen in Nova Scotia, Prince Edward Island, and Manitoba. The lowest rates for

---

RISK FACTORS

Cancer of the Colon and Rectum

- Advanced age
- High-fat (especially egg consumption) diet, red and processed meat, low-fibre diet
- High consumption of alcohol
- Cigarette smoking
- Obesity
- Familial polyposis or family history of colorectal cancer
- Low levels of physical activity
- Inflammatory bowel disease
- Type 2 diabetes mellitus

both sexes are in British Columbia.[207] In males, colorectal cancer is now the second most common cancer, and it accounts for approximately 14% of all new male cases. In females, colorectal cancer is the third most common cancer, and it accounts for approximately 12% of all new female cases.[207] Colorectal cancer typically occurs in women 10 years later than in men. Worldwide, the prevalence and death rate of colorectal cancer are highest in Black populations, possibly because of lack of access to screening and treatment.[215]

PATHOPHYSIOLOGY   Most colorectal cancers are sporadic (acquired) or associated with a family history of colorectal cancer. They are caused by multiple gene alterations and environmental interactions (see Chapter 3 for epigenetics and Chapter 10 for mechanisms of oncogenesis). Familial adenomatous polyposis (FAP) is a mutation of the *APC* gene (adenomatous polyposis coli, a tumour-suppressor gene) and is the most common hereditary cause of colorectal cancer. Hereditary nonpolyposis colorectal cancer (HNPCC), or Lynch syndrome, is associated with several DNA mismatch repair (MMR) gene mutations. Both FAP and HNPCC have a rare, family-linked autosomal dominant inheritance trait that accounts for about 3 to 5% of colorectal cancers.[216,217] Sporadic tumours are also thought to involve the loss of function or mutation of tumour-suppressor genes (i.e., *APC*, *kRAS*, *p53* genes). Colorectal cancer begins with the formation of an adenoma and is termed "tumour initiation." The progression to carcinoma is termed *tumour progression* and is a multistep process of genetic mutations that may take 8 to 10 years.

Colorectal polyps are closely associated with the development of cancer. A polyp, or papilloma, is a projection arising from the mucosal epithelium. The most common types of polyps are hyperplastic (a non-neoplastic, or benign, polyp). Adenomatous polyps are neoplastic. They can be pedunculated (have a stalk) or sessile (flat with no stalk). Neoplastic polyps are premalignant lesions and are further classified as tubular (the most prevalent), villous (usually sessile), or tubulovillous adenomas (Figure 36.18). Serrated sessile polyps have a sawtooth appearance and can be difficult to detect. Serrated sessile polyps are associated with oncogene mutations and should be removed.[218] The larger the polyp, the greater the risk for colorectal cancer. Although lesions larger than 1.5 cm occur less often, they are more likely to be malignant than those smaller than 1.0 cm. Thus, screening colonoscopy with polypectomy is performed when polyps are found.

Adenocarcinomas of the colon and rectum usually arise from adenomatous polyps and undergo a multistep cascade of genetic events that leads to carcinoma and metastasis[219] (see Figure 10.7). Most colorectal cancers are moderately differentiated adenocarcinomas. These tumours have a long preinvasive phase and when they invade, they tend to grow slowly. Colorectal carcinoma begins from epithelial stem cells located in the glands at the base of the intestinal crypts. Because the lymphatic channels are located under the muscularis mucosae, the lesions must traverse this layer before the multistep process of metastasis can occur. Once the malignant cells of an adenoma traverse the muscularis mucosae, tumour cells enter the bloodstream and lymphatics and become invasive, spreading to other organs. Adenomas can be detected early, however, because the submucosa may not be penetrated for several years.

Small intestinal carcinoma is very rare and is usually located in the duodenum.[220]

CLINICAL MANIFESTATIONS   Symptoms of colorectal cancer depend on the location, size, and shape of the lesion and are silent in the early stages (Figure 36.19). Tumours of the right (ascending) colon and left (descending) colon evolve into two distinct tumour types.[221] On the right side (proximal colon), the lesions are polypoid and extend along one wall of the cecum and ascending colon. These tumours may be

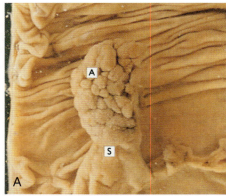
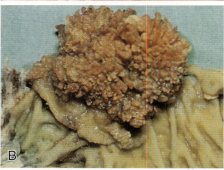

FIGURE 36.18 Neoplastic Polyps. **A,** Tubular adenomata *(A)* are rounded lesions 0.5 to 2 cm in size that are generally red and sit on a stalk *(S)* of normal mucosa that has been dragged up by traction of the polyp in the bowel lumen. **B,** Villous adenomata are velvety lesions about 0.6 cm thick that occupy a broad area of mucosa generally 1 to 5 cm in diameter. (From Stevens, A., Lowe, J., & Scott, I. [2009]. *Core pathology* [3rd ed.]. Mosby.)

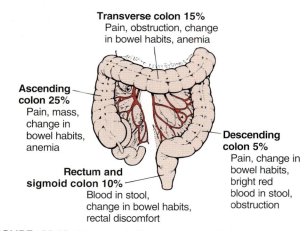

FIGURE 36.19 Signs and Symptoms of Colorectal cancer by Location of Primary Lesion. Clinical manifestations are listed in order of frequency for each region (lymphatics of colon also shown).

silent, evolving to pain, palpable mass in the lower-right quadrant, anemia, fatigue, and dark red or mahogany-coloured blood mixed with the stool. These tumours can become large and bulky with necrosis and ulceration, contributing to persistent blood loss and anemia. Obstruction is unusual because the growth does not readily encircle the colon. These tumours are more common in women.

Tumours of the left, or descending, colon (distal colon) start as small, elevated, buttonlike masses. This type grows circumferentially, encircling the entire bowel wall, and eventually ulcerating in the middle as the tumour penetrates the blood supply. Obstruction is common but occurs slowly, and stools become narrow and pencil shaped. Manifestations include progressive abdominal distension, pain, vomiting, constipation, need for laxatives, cramps, and bright red blood on the surface of the stool. These tumours are more common in men.

Systematic lymphatic distribution occurs along the aorta to the mesenteric and pancreatic lymph nodes. Liver metastasis is common and follows invasion of the mesenteric veins (left colon) or superior veins (right colon), which drain into the portal circulation.

Rectal carcinomas (about 30% of colorectal carcinomas) are defined as tumours occurring up to 15 cm from the anal opening. Tumours of the rectum can spread through the rectal wall to nearby structures: the prostate in men and the vagina in women. Penetration occurs more readily in the lower third of the rectum because it has no serosal covering. Systemic and pulmonary metastases occur through the hemorrhoidal plexus, which drains into the vena cava.

EVALUATION AND TREATMENT   Individuals with hereditary polyposis should begin screening at an early age (10 to 12 years) using colonoscopy, with removal of polyps when they are found. Specific, sensitive, and affordable molecular markers are being evaluated to assist with early diagnosis and evaluation of therapy. Carcinoembryonic antigen (CEA) is evaluated during and after cancer treatment. Screening procedures for detection of nonhereditary colorectal cancer are summarized in Box 36.4. Aspirin and celecoxib (Celebrex) may reduce the incidence of colorectal cancer in the general population, but risk for GI bleeding must be considered. Vitamin D, calcium, fibre, folate, dietary modification, weight control, exercise, and other nondietary lifestyle changes can decrease the risk for colorectal cancer.[222]

The staging of colorectal cancer involves imaging and operative exploration.[223] Physical examination of the abdomen detects liver enlargement and ascites; appropriate lymph nodes are palpated. Imaging is useful for pretreatment staging.[223] Operative staging consists of careful exploration during surgery and biopsy of possible metastases. The World Health Organization's TNM classification is widely used for staging of colorectal cancer[224] (see https://www.cancer.ca/en/cancer-information/cancer-type/colorectal/staging/?region=on; see also Figure 10.23).

Treatment for all stages of cancer of the colon is surgical. Chemotherapy and radiation therapy may be given before surgery in the hope that they will shrink the tumour or alter the malignant cells, or both, so that these cells will not survive after surgery. Resection and anastomosis can be performed for cancer of the ascending, transverse, descending, or sigmoid colon and upper rectum. These surgeries are performed through abdominal incisions and assisted with radiofrequency ablation. Natural defecation is preserved. Growths in the lower portion of the rectum require removal of the entire rectum with the formation of a permanent colostomy. Chemotherapy, including immunotherapy, is used to treat metastatic disease and cases with a high risk for recurrence. New chemotherapeutic agents are improving personalized, first-line therapy. Immunotherapy, vaccines, and viral vectors for the treatment of colon cancer are under continuing investigation.[225,226] Resection of liver metastases or hepatic intra-arterial chemotherapy may prolong survival.[227,228]

Cancer of the Accessory Organs of Digestion
Cancer of the Liver

Cancer of the liver is a leading cause of cancer death worldwide and is highest in East and Southeast Asia.[229] Liver cancer is one of the fastest rising cancers in Canada. While it is still considered a rare cancer, accounting for an estimated 1% of all new cancer diagnoses and deaths in 2013, the incidence rate of liver cancer has tripled in Canadian men and doubled in women since 1970.[230] Primary liver cancer is rare before the age of 40 years and is most common after 60 years. Cancer in the liver is usually caused by metastatic spread from a primary site elsewhere in the body.[231] Risk factors for primary liver cancer are summarized in *Risk Factors: Primary Liver Cancer*. Risks associated with HBV and HCV are decreasing with antiviral therapy.[232]

The Canadian Cancer Society estimated that approximately 3 100 Canadians (2 300 men and 810 women) were diagnosed with liver cancer in 2020. It also estimated that 1 450 Canadians (1 150 men and 279 women) died of this disease in 2020.[233] As these numbers indicate, men are more affected by liver cancer than women. From 1992 to 2012, the incidence rate of liver cancer rose for males (2.8% per year) and females (1.7% per year). These increases may be at least partially explained by rising immigration from regions of the world where risk factors for liver cancer, such as hepatitis B and C infection and exposure to aflatoxin, are more common.[207]

In Canada, between 2001 and 2010, the mortality rate of liver cancer increased significantly for both males (3.1% per year) and females (2.2% per year). The upward trend in mortality rates is associated with the increase in liver cancer incidence rates.[207]

PATHOPHYSIOLOGY   Primary carcinomas of the liver are hepatocellular or cholangiocellular. Hepatocellular carcinoma (HCC) develops

---

> **BOX 36.4   Screening for Colorectal Cancer**
>
> Beginning at age 50, both men and women should follow one of these testing schedules:
>
> **Tests That Find Polyps and Cancer**
> - Flexible sigmoidoscopy every 5 years, *or*
> - Colonoscopy every 10 years, *or*
> - Double-contrast barium enema every 5 years,[†] *or*
> - CT colonography (virtual colonoscopy) every 5 years[*]
>
> **Tests That Primarily Find Cancer**
> - Every 2 years fecal occult blood test,[†] *or*
> - Yearly fecal immunochemical test,[†] *or*
> - Stool DNA or RNA tests (sDNA, sRNA), interval uncertain[†]

[*] All positive tests should be followed up with colonoscopy.
[†] The multiple stool take-home test should be used.
From American Cancer Society. (2015). *Cancer facts & figures 2015*. https://www.cancer.org/research/cancer-facts-statistics/all-cancer-facts-figures/cancer-facts-figures-2015.html; Canadian Cancer Society. (2020). *Screening for colorectal cancer*. https://www.cancer.ca/en/cancer-information/cancer-type/colorectal/screening/?region=on; Koga, Y., Yamazaki, N., & Matsumura, Y. (2014). *Expert Review of Molecular Diagnostics*, 14(1), 107–120.

> **RISK FACTORS**
> **Primary Liver Cancer**
>
> - Exposure to mycotoxins (aflatoxins), particularly those produced by *Aspergillus flavus*, a mould found on spoiled corn, peanuts, and grain
> - Alcohol abuse
> - Obesity
> - Chronic liver disease, especially cirrhosis
> - Infection with hepatitis B virus, hepatitis C virus, and hepatitis D virus, particularly in conjunction with cirrhosis; these infections act either as carcinogens or as cocarcinogens in chronically infected hepatocytes

in the hepatocytes and can be nodular (consisting of multiple, discrete nodules), massive (consisting of a large tumour mass having satellite nodules), or diffuse (consisting of small nodules distributed throughout most of the liver). It is closely associated with chronic hepatitis and cirrhosis. Because carcinoma of the liver invades the hepatic and portal veins, it often spreads to the heart and lungs. Other sites of metastases are the brain, kidney, and spleen.

Cholangiocellular carcinoma (cholangiocarcinoma) is rare (less than 1% of liver cancers), develops in the bile ducts, and occurs less often than HCC.[234] It is associated with primary sclerosing cholangitis (a rare autoimmune disease often associated with UC) and is geographically associated with areas where liver fluke infestation is prevalent, such as Southeast Asia. Cholangiocellular carcinoma can occur anywhere along the bile duct and extend directly into the liver, usually as a solitary lesion. A combined form of HCC is known as combined (mixed) hepatocellular–cholangiocellular carcinoma. It is difficult to distinguish an invasion of cholangiocellular carcinoma from a metastatic adenocarcinoma except by neoplastic changes found in nearby ducts.

CLINICAL MANIFESTATIONS HCC is usually asymptomatic. Manifestations can develop slowly or abruptly and include vague abdominal symptoms such as nausea and vomiting, fullness, pressure, and dull ache in the right hypochondrium. In individuals with cirrhosis, deepening jaundice or abrupt lack of appetite is a sign of hepatocellular carcinoma. Obstruction by the tumour can cause sudden worsening of portal hypertension and development of ascites. As the tumour enlarges, it causes pain. Cholangiocellular carcinoma more commonly presents insidiously as pain, loss of appetite, weight loss, and gradual onset of jaundice. Some carcinomas of the liver rupture spontaneously, causing hemorrhage. Others are discovered accidentally during laboratory evaluation, imaging, or surgery for other diseases or trauma.

EVALUATION AND TREATMENT There is no specific test for the diagnosis of liver cancer. Biopsy is not recommended because of the risk for tumour seeding. For high-risk individuals, alpha fetoprotein associated with HBV and abdominal ultrasound are common screening tools. Diagnosis is based on clinical manifestations, laboratory findings, imaging, and exploratory laparotomy. In individuals without cirrhosis, liver scans can document filling defects. CT or ultrasonography is used to detect solid tumours, but neither can distinguish benign from malignant tumours. Primary prevention may be achieved by vaccinating against HBV, preventing and treating HBV and HCV, screening all donated blood for the presence of HBV, and reducing contamination of food with aflatoxins.[235]

Surgical resection is possible only if the tumour is localized to a removable lobe of the liver. Surgery is hazardous and usually not undertaken if the individual has cirrhosis. Radiofrequency (thermal) ablation has emerged as the most effective method for local tumour destruction. Most individuals develop metastases after surgical resection, but long-term survival is possible. Chemotherapeutic agents, immunotherapy, and radiotherapy are treatment options.[236] Liver transplant offers a cure if the waiting time is short. The prognosis for those with symptomatic liver cancer is poor.[237]

Cancer of the Gallbladder

Risk factors for gallbladder cancer include gallstones, advancing age, female gender (2:1), anomalous pancreaticobiliary ductal junction, and obesity. Gallbladder cancer occurs rarely before the age of 40 years and is most common between the ages of 50 and 60 years. Primary carcinoma of the gallbladder is rare and associated with larger gallstones. Most gallbladder cancer is caused by metastasis.

The Canadian Cancer Society estimated that 365 Canadians (130 men and 235 women) were diagnosed with gallbladder cancer in 2016. It also estimated that 273 Canadians (100 men and 173 women) died of this disease in 2016.[238]

PATHOPHYSIOLOGY Most primary carcinomas of the gallbladder are adenocarcinomas, and more rarely squamous cell carcinomas. The pathogenesis is not clear. Chronic inflammation may trigger dysplasia and progression to metaplasia. The molecular mechanisms involve mutation of several genes, including tumour-suppressor genes and oncogenes, and alterations in the extracellular matrix.[239] Invasion of the liver and lymph nodes occurs early. Direct invasion of the stomach and the duodenum can cause pyloric obstruction. Infection often accompanies cancer of the gallbladder. Generalized peritonitis, gangrene, perforation, and liver abscesses are potential complications of infection.

CLINICAL MANIFESTATIONS Early stages of gallbladder cancer are asymptomatic, and the disease usually presents at an advanced stage. When symptoms develop, there is usually steady pain in the upper-right quadrant for about 2 months. Other manifestations include diarrhea, belching, weakness, loss of appetite, weight loss, and vomiting. Obstructive jaundice can occur if an enlarging tumour presses on the extrahepatic ducts.

EVALUATION AND TREATMENT Early diagnosis of gallbladder cancer is rare and is often found incidentally. Therefore, older persons with gallstones, particularly women, are evaluated for disease. Inflammatory disorders, such as cholangitis (bile duct inflammation) and peritonitis, often obscure an underlying malignancy. Diagnostic procedures include ultrasonography and further imaging with suspicious findings.[240] Complete surgical resection of the gallbladder is the only effective treatment for early stages of disease, and recurrence is common. Complete removal of tumour tissue and lymph nodes with chemoradiation therapy is performed for more advanced stages. Because advanced malignancies cannot be resected, gallbladders containing stones are removed as a preventive measure. The prognosis of unresectable gallbladder cancer is extremely poor. Molecular therapies are under development.[241]

Cancer of the Pancreas

The Canadian Cancer Society estimated that 6 000 Canadians (3 100 men and 2 900 women) were diagnosed with pancreatic cancer in 2020. It also estimated that 5 300 Canadians (2 700 men and 2 600 women) died of this disease in 2020.[242]

The incidence of pancreatic cancer rises steadily with age. Males are affected slightly more often than females, and Black individuals more often than White individuals. Mortality is nearly 100% at 5 years. The cause of pancreatic cancer is not known, but there are modest risks associated with tobacco smoking, certain dietary factors (e.g., high-fat foods and processed meat), obesity, diabetes mellitus, chronic pancreatitis, family history of pancreatic cancer, HNPCC (Lynch syndrome), and *BRCA1* and *BRCA2* mutations.[243]

PATHOPHYSIOLOGY Pancreatic cancer can arise from exocrine or endocrine cells. Most pancreatic tumours arise from metaplastic exocrine cells in the ducts and are called *ductal adenocarcinomas*. Chronic pancreatitis and inflammatory cytokines support tumour growth.[243] There is significant expansion of the extracellular matrix (stroma) from activation of pancreatic stellate cells, a type of fibroblast in the pancreas, that contributes to therapeutic resistance.[244] Tumours arising in small ducts invade nearby glandular tissue, penetrate the covering of the pancreas, and extend into surrounding tissues.[245] Tumours of the head of the pancreas quickly spread to obstruct the common bile duct and portal vein. These tumours can then infiltrate the superior mesenteric artery, the vena cava, and the aorta and form emboli. Tumours of the body and tail of the pancreas infiltrate the posterior abdominal wall. Lymphatic invasion occurs early and rapidly. Venous invasion causes metastases to the liver. Tumour implants on the peritoneal surface can obstruct veins and promote development of ascites.

CLINICAL MANIFESTATIONS Early stages of pancreatic cancer are asymptomatic. When symptoms occur there usually has been a malignant transformation. Typically, vague upper abdominal pain that radiates to the back develops. Jaundice arises in most cases, usually caused by obstruction of the bile duct. Because obstruction impairs enzyme secretion and flow to the duodenum, pancreatic cancer causes fat and protein malabsorption, resulting in weight loss. Distant metastases are found in the cervical lymph nodes, the lungs, and the brain. Most individuals die of hepatic failure, malnutrition, or systemic diseases.

EVALUATION AND TREATMENT There is no specific biomarker for pancreatic cancer and the diagnosis is usually made after the tumour has spread. Several molecular markers are under investigation.[246] Endoscopic ultrasound and CT are used initially for diagnosis.[246] Laparotomy is often used to establish a definitive diagnosis, evaluate the extent of disease, and determine whether palliative bypass surgery (i.e., cholecystojejunostomy and gastrojejunostomy) is needed. Many surgeons recommend a total pancreatectomy because cancer of the pancreas seldom consists of a single lesion. Adjuvant chemotherapy, immunotherapy, radiochemotherapy, and combination therapy may produce favourable controls in locally advanced cancer.[247] Pain management includes opioids and celiac plexus nerve block. Supportive therapy involves an interdisciplinary team.[248] Five-year survival is about 20% with resectable disease (a small subset) and less than 6% for metastatic disease. There is a need for new approaches for earlier diagnosis and more effective treatment.

COMORBIDITIES

Comorbidities Related to Digestive Function
Liver Disease
Nonalcoholic fatty liver disease (NAFLD) is the most common chronic liver disease in the developed world and is associated with multiple comorbidities. Patients with NAFLD are at increased risk of cirrhosis and HCC. Patients with NAFLD are also at increased risk of metabolic syndrome, cardiovascular disease, and malignancy.

The management of NAFLD can reverse or limit the worsening of some of these comorbidities. It is worth noting that the primary cause of death in patients with NAFLD, especially in patients without advanced fibrosis or cirrhosis, is due to cardiovascular disease and extrahepatic malignancy, and not from liver disease itself.[a]

NAFLD is considered the hepatic manifestation of metabolic syndrome and is strongly associated with type 2 diabetes mellitus, cardiovascular disease, chronic kidney disease, and obstructive sleep apnea. Patients with ultrasound-based evidence of NAFLD are 2 to 5 times more likely to develop type 2 diabetes mellitus. NAFLD results in increased insulin requirements and is associated with a twofold increase in all-cause mortality in patients with diabetes mellitus. Improving hepatic steatosis can improve blood glucose control and decrease insulin requirements.[a]

Inflammatory Bowel Disease
Inflammatory bowel disease (IBD) is another GI ailment that is associated with many chronic comorbidities. IBD shares pathogenic immune-mediated inflammatory pathways with other inflammatory diseases. For example, chronic systemic inflammation plays a role in the pathogenesis of atherosclerosis, acute arterial events, and rheumatological diseases. In IBD, gut-related microvascular alterations diminish its vasodilatory capacity, causing tissue hypoperfusion. It can also lower rates of mucosal healing and increase incidence of refractory inflammatory ulcerations.

In a large French cohort study,[b] researchers established an increased risk of acute arterial events in patients with Crohn's disease and ulcerative colitis, including ischemic heart disease, cerebrovascular disease, and peripheral artery disease. Patients are much more likely to be hospitalized because of cardiovascular complications than because of IBD-related complications.

There is an increased risk of ischemic heart disease during the first year after initial IBD diagnosis. An association between early implementation of IBD treatment after the diagnosis and a lower risk of ischemic heart disease has also been established. Therefore, early implementation of IBD treatment can reduce risks of ischemic heart disease.[c]

IBD leads to iron deficiency mainly because of inadequate dietary intake, malabsorption, and chronic blood loss. Iron deficiency anemia is the most common nutritional deficiency in patients with IBD. IBD patients are at risk for osteoporosis because of the marked side-effects of prolonged steroid use and inflammation-induced bone loss. Chronic inflammation of the colonic mucosa was shown to be associated with malnutrition and colorectal cancer. IBD is also associated with an increased likelihood of mental disorders such as generalized anxiety, depression, and further mood disorders compared with the general population.[d]

Comorbidities in inflammatory bowel disease include:

- **Classic:** Psoriasis and psoriatic arthritis, psychological and psychiatric disorders, osteoporosis
- **Emerging:** Metabolic syndrome and its components, cardiovascular diseases, atherosclerosis, fatigue, chronic obstructive pulmonary disease, sexual dysfunction, Parkinson's disease
- **Related to lifestyle**: Smoking, alcohol consumption, anxiety and stress, substance misuse
- **Related to treatment**: Skin cancer, lymphoma, dyslipidemia.[e]

---

[a] Glass, L. M., Hunt, C. M., Fuchs, M., et al. (2019). Comorbidities and nonalcoholic fatty liver disease: the chicken, the egg, or both? *Federal Practitioner, 36*(2), 64–71. https://www.ncbi.nlm.nih.gov/pmc/articles/PMC6411365/.

[b] Nguyen, N. H., Ohno-Machado, L., & Sandborn, W. J. (2018). Infections and cardiovascular complications are common causes for hospitalization in older patients with inflammatory bowel diseases. *Inflammatory Bowel Disease, 24*(4), 916–923. https://doi.org/10.1093/ibd/izx089.

[c] Kirchgesner, J., Beaugerie, L., Carrat, F., et al. (2017). Increased risk of acute arterial events in young patients and severely active IBD: a nationwide French cohort study. *Gut, 67*(7), 1261–1268. https://doi.org/10.1136/gutjnl-2017-314015.

[d] Bähler, C., Schoepfer, A. M., Vavricka, S. R., et al. (2017). Chronic comorbidities associated with inflammatory bowel disease: prevalence and impact on healthcare costs in Switzerland. *European Journal of Gastroenterology & Hepatology, 29*(8), 916–925. doi:10.1097/MEG.0000000000000891.

[e] Argollo, M., Gilardi, D., Peyrin-Biroulet, C., et al. (2019). Comorbidities in inflammatory bowel disease: a call for action. *Lancet: Gastroenterology & Hepatology, 4*(8), 643–654. https://doi.org/10.1136/gutjnl-2017-314015.

GERIATRIC CONSIDERATIONS
Age-Related Gastric Changes

Altered gastric microbiota, reduced mucosal protective mechanisms, decreased gastric blood flow, and compromised repair mechanisms are all features of age-related gastric changes. As such, older persons are more susceptible to the development of gastric ulcer, atrophic gastritis, and peptic ulcer disease.

Older persons have a higher risk of medication-related gastro-intestinal side effects, which often results in decreased medication adherence and an increase in rates of morbidity and mortality. Parkinson's disease and diabetes mellitus in older persons have the greatest impact on gastric emptying.

Previously, advanced age was thought to be related to chronic atrophic gastritis; however, current literature supports the theory that atrophic changes of the gastric mucosa are associated with *H. pylori* infection, rather than age itself. Chronic atrophic gastritis in the elderly is associated with *H. pylori* infection. The disease results in the partial loss of glands in the gastric mucosa, leading to hypochlorhydria (a low level of stomach acid) or achlorhydria (absence of hydrochloric acid in the gastric secretions). Decrease in acid secretion in the elderly because of chronic atrophic gastritis leads to small intestinal bacterial overgrowth (SIBO) and malabsorption. SIBO implies presence of bacteria, above 10^5 to 10^6 organisms/mL in small bowel aspirate. This condition is common in older persons and is associated with chronic diarrhea, malabsorption, weight loss, and secondary nutritional deficiencies.

The main contributing factors are a higher prevalence of *H. pylori* infection among older persons, increased NSAID/aspirin use, and polypharmacy, including medications associated with increased risk of peptic ulcer disease (e.g., anti-coagulants, selective serotonin reuptake inhibitors [SSRIs], and oral steroids).

Physiological changes associated with old age that may also contribute to SIBO are reduced blood flow through the GI system and decreased secretion of key components of gastro-intestinal protective mechanisms, such as bicarbonates, mucin, and prostaglandins. Motility of the small intestine is not affected by age itself, but is associated with medications, polypharmacy, and presence of concomitant diseases such as autonomic neuropathy from longstanding diabetes.

The prevalence of constipation in the general population is anywhere from 2 to 28%. Among older persons, this number goes up to 40%, and up to 50% among elderly nursing home residents.

An increased prevalence of constipation in older persons is not related to decrease in colon transition time as much as it is to decreased mobility, cognitive impairment, comorbid medical problems, polypharmacy (especially opioid and anticholinergic medication use), and dietary changes. Older persons usually associate constipation with straining rather than with decreased frequency of bowel movements.

CASE STUDY

Part 1

Mr. Kent is a 45-year-old man who works as a taxi driver and shares a one-bedroom flat with his partner. Mr. Kent is a heavy smoker who abuses alcohol and sometimes uses drugs.

Two months ago, Mr. Kent started complaining of edema of the lower extremities, abdominal pain, difficulty sleeping, shortness of breath, dyspnea, orthopnea, and insomnia. Because Mr. Kent's condition persisted, he decided to seek medical help.

At the clinic, Mr. Kent's vital signs are as follows: BP: 150/80 mm Hg, P: 104/min, RR: 26/min, and T: 37.3°C.

CT scan and liver biopsy results showed that Mr. Kent has a cirrhotic liver with scar tissue.

Critical Thinking and Clinical Judgement Questions—Part 1

1. Define liver cirrhosis. How would you classify Mr. Kent's liver cirrhosis?
2. a) What factors could have led to cirrhosis in Mr. Kent? b) Are there other factors that can lead to liver cirrhosis?
3. Relate the clinical manifestations exhibited by Mr. Kent to the pathophysiology of liver disease.
4. What other clinical manifestations may be present in a patient with liver cirrhosis? Explain the rationale for each.
5. Explain the significance behind each of the diagnostic tests carried out for Mr. Kent.

Part 2

Physical exam revealed that Mr. Kent had a grossly distended abdomen, bilateral ankle edema, slow activity and response, an unbalanced gait, jaundiced sclera, and pruritus. Mr. Kent asked the nurse about his condition, and she replied that she could not tell him anything before some investigations were done.

Mr. Kent was admitted to hospital with the following orders: bed rest, head of the bed elevated 30 degrees; to be weighed upon admission (80 kg) and daily thereafter.

The nurse noticed that Mr. Kent's weight kept increasing by half a kilogram daily for one week. His belly was getting larger day by day. He was placed on a high-caloric, low-sodium (500 mg) diet. Fluids were restricted to 1 000 mL each day. He was started on accurate intake and output measurement, as well.

Critical Thinking and Clinical Judgement Questions—Part 2

1. Discuss the rationale behind each of the additional management measures that were implemented for Mr. Kent.
2. a) Why do you think Mr. Kent's weight was increasing in the first week of admission? b) What are the other complications of liver cirrhosis? Briefly explain the scientific basis behind each complication.

DID YOU UNDERSTAND?

Disorders of the Gastro-intestinal Tract

1. Anorexia is lack of a desire to eat despite physiological stimuli that would normally produce hunger.
2. Vomiting is the forceful emptying of the stomach effected by gastro-intestinal (GI) contraction and reverse peristalsis of the esophagus. It is usually preceded by nausea and retching, except for projectile vomiting, which is associated with direct stimulation of the vomiting centre in the brain.
3. Constipation is difficult or infrequent defecation often caused by unhealthy dietary and bowel habits combined with lack of exercise. Constipation can result from a disorder that impairs intestinal motility or obstructs the intestinal lumen.
4. Diarrhea is the presence of frequent loose, watery stools and can be caused by excessive fluid drawn into the intestinal lumen by osmosis (osmotic diarrhea), excessive secretion of fluids by the intestinal mucosa (secretory or infectious diarrhea), or excessive GI motility (motility diarrhea).
5. Abdominal pain is caused by stretching, inflammation, or ischemia (insufficient blood supply). Abdominal pain originates in the organs themselves (visceral pain) or in the peritoneum (parietal

pain) and can be acute or chronic. Obvious manifestations of GI bleeding are hematemesis (vomiting of blood), melena (dark, tarry stools), and hematochezia (frank bleeding from the rectum).
6. Dysphagia is difficulty swallowing. It can be caused by a mechanical or functional obstruction of the esophagus. Achalasia is a form of functional dysphagia caused by loss of esophageal innervation.
7. Gastroesophageal reflux disease is the regurgitation of chyme from the stomach into the esophagus, resulting in an inflammatory response (reflux esophagitis) when the esophageal mucosa is repeatedly exposed to acids and enzymes in the regurgitated chyme.
8. Hiatal hernia is the protrusion of the upper part of the stomach through the hiatus (esophageal opening in the diaphragm) at the gastroesophageal junction. Hiatal hernia can be sliding or paraesophageal or a combination of both.
9. Gastroparesis is delayed gastric emptying in the absence of mechanical gastric outlet obstruction.
10. Pyloric obstruction is the narrowing or blockage of the pylorus, which is the opening between the stomach and the duodenum. Intestinal obstruction prevents the normal movement of chyme through the intestinal tract. It can be mechanical (i.e., caused by torsion, herniation, or tumour) or functional as a result of paralytic ileus.
11. The most severe consequences of intestinal obstruction are fluid and electrolyte losses, hypovolemia, shock, intestinal necrosis, and perforation of the intestinal wall.
12. Gastritis is an acute or chronic inflammation of the gastric mucosa.
13. Regurgitation of bile, use of anti-inflammatory drugs or alcohol, *Helicobacter pylori* infection, and some systemic diseases are associated with gastritis.
14. A peptic ulcer is a circumscribed area of mucosal inflammation and ulceration caused by excessive secretion of gastric acid, disruption of the protective mucosal barrier, or infection with *H. pylori*.
15. Zollinger-Ellison syndrome is a rare syndrome associated with peptic ulcers caused by a gastrin-secreting neuroendocrine tumour or multiple tumours (gastrinoma) of the pancreas or duodenum.
16. There are three types of peptic ulcers: duodenal, gastric, and stress ulcers.
17. Duodenal ulcers, the most common peptic ulcers, are associated with *H. pylori* infection, chronic use of nonsteroidal anti-inflammatory drugs, increased numbers of parietal (acid-secreting) cells in the stomach, elevated gastrin levels, and rapid gastric emptying. Gastric ulcers develop near parietal cells, generally in the antrum, and tend to become chronic.
18. Stress ulcers develop suddenly after severe illness, systemic trauma, or neural injury. Ulceration follows mucosal damage caused by ischemia (decreased blood flow to the gastric mucosa).
19. Cushing's ulcer is a stress ulcer caused by head trauma. Ulceration follows hypersecretion of hydrochloric acid caused by overstimulation of the vagal nuclei.
20. Curling ulcer is associated with burn trauma.
21. Dumping syndrome is the rapid emptying of chyme into the small intestine. It causes an osmotic shift of fluid from the vascular compartment to the intestinal lumen, which decreases plasma volume.
22. Alkaline reflux gastritis is stomach inflammation caused by the reflux of bile and pancreatic secretions from the duodenum into the stomach. These substances disrupt the mucosal barrier and cause inflammation.
23. Malabsorption syndromes result in impaired digestion or absorption of nutrients and usually cause diarrhea.
24. Pancreatic exocrine insufficiency causes malabsorption associated with impaired digestion. The pancreas does not produce sufficient amounts of the enzymes that digest protein, carbohydrates, and fats into components that can be absorbed by the intestine.
25. Deficient lactase production in the brush border of the small intestine inhibits the breakdown of lactose. It prevents lactose absorption and causes osmotic diarrhea.
26. Bile salt deficiency causes fat malabsorption and steatorrhea (fatty stools). Bile salt deficiency can result from inadequate secretion of bile, excessive bacterial deconjugation of bile, or impaired reabsorption of bile salts caused by ileal disease.
27. Ulcerative colitis (UC) is a chronic inflammatory bowel disease that causes ulceration, abscess formation, and necrosis of the colonic and rectal mucosa. Cramping pain, bleeding, frequent diarrhea, dehydration, and weight loss accompany severe forms of the disease. A course of frequent remissions and exacerbations is common.
28. Crohn's disease (CD) is similar to UC, but it affects the GI tract from the mouth to the anus and tends to involve all the layers of the intestinal lumen. Irritable bowel syndrome (IBS) is described as a functional disorder with recurring abdominal pain and bloating. IBS can be diarrhea prevalent or constipation prevalent or may alternate between diarrhea and constipation. Diverticula are outpouchings of colonic mucosa through the muscle layers of the colon wall. Diverticulosis is the presence of these outpouchings; diverticulitis is inflammation of the diverticula.
29. Appendicitis is the most common surgical emergency of the abdomen. Obstruction of the lumen leads to increased pressure, ischemia, and inflammation of the appendix. Mesenteric vascular insufficiency in the intestine is most often associated with occlusion or obstruction of the mesenteric vessels or insufficient intestinal arterial blood flow. The resulting ischemia and necrosis produce abdominal pain, fever, bloody diarrhea, hypovolemia, and shock.
30. Obesity is a metabolic disorder with an increase in body fat mass and a BMI greater than 30.
31. Visceral obesity and normal weight obesity increase the risk of developing systemic inflammation, dyslipidemia, and insulin resistance with predisposition to atherosclerosis, hypertension, cardiovascular disease, cancer, and type 2 diabetes mellitus. Malnutrition is lack of nourishment from inadequate amounts of calories, protein, vitamins, or minerals. Starvation is an extreme state of malnutrition. Cachexia is physical wasting associated with chronic disease.
32. Short-term starvation, or lack of dietary intake for 3 or 4 days, stimulates mobilization of stored glucose by two metabolic processes: glycogenolysis (splitting of glycogen into glucose) and gluconeogenesis (formation of glucose from noncarbohydrate molecules).
33. Long-term starvation triggers the breakdown of ketone bodies and fatty acids. Eventually proteolysis (protein breakdown) begins, and death ensues if nutrition is not restored.

Disorders of the Accessory Organs of Digestion

1. Portal hypertension, ascites, hepatic encephalopathy, jaundice, and hepatorenal syndrome are complications of many liver disorders.
2. Portal hypertension is an elevation of portal venous pressure to at least 10 mm Hg. It is caused by increased resistance to venous flow in the portal vein and its tributaries, including the sinusoids and hepatic vein.
3. Portal hypertension is the most serious complication of liver disease because it can cause potentially fatal complications, such as bleeding varices, ascites, and hepatic encephalopathy.
4. Varices (esophageal, gastric, hemorrhoidal) are distended, tortuous, collateral veins resulting from prolonged elevation of pressure in the portal vein.
5. Splenomegaly is enlargement of the spleen caused by increased pressure in the splenic vein, which branches from the portal vein.

6. Ascites is the accumulation and sequestration of fluid in the peritoneal cavity, often as a result of portal hypertension and decreased concentrations of plasma proteins.
7. Hepatic encephalopathy (portal-systemic encephalopathy) is impaired cerebral function caused by bloodborne toxins (particularly ammonia) not metabolized by the liver. Manifestations of hepatic encephalopathy range from confusion and asterixis (flapping tremor of the hands) to loss of consciousness, coma, and death.
8. Jaundice (icterus) is a yellow or greenish pigmentation of the skin or sclera of the eyes caused by increases in plasma bilirubin concentration (hyperbilirubinemia).
9. Obstructive jaundice is caused by obstructed bile canaliculi (intrahepatic obstructive jaundice) or obstructed bile ducts outside the liver (extrahepatic obstructive jaundice). Bilirubin accumulates proximal to the sites of obstruction, enters the bloodstream, and is carried to the skin and deposited.
10. Hemolytic jaundice is caused by destruction of red blood cells at a rate that exceeds the liver's ability to metabolize unconjugated bilirubin.
11. Hepatorenal syndrome is functional kidney failure caused by advanced liver disease, particularly cirrhosis with portal hypertension. Kidney failure is caused by a sudden decrease in blood flow to the kidneys usually caused by massive GI hemorrhage, liver failure, or inadequate circulating blood volume associated with ascites. The chief clinical manifestation is oliguria.
12. Acute liver failure is severe impairment or necrosis of liver cells with or without pre-existing liver disease or cirrhosis. It is commonly associated with acetaminophen overdose or as a complication of viral hepatitis.
13. Cirrhosis is an inflammatory disease of the liver that causes disorganization of lobular structure, fibrosis, and nodular regeneration. Cirrhosis can result from hepatitis or exposure to toxins, such as acetaldehyde (a product of alcohol metabolism). The disease causes progressive irreversible liver damage, usually over a period of years.
14. Alcoholic liver disease includes fatty liver and alcoholic steatohepatitis from accumulations of fat in the liver and is a precursor to alcoholic cirrhosis.
15. Alcoholic cirrhosis impairs the hepatocytes' ability to oxidize fatty acids, synthesize enzymes and proteins, degrade hormones, and clear portal blood of ammonia and toxins. The inflammatory response includes excessive collagen formation, fibrosis, and scarring, which obstruct bile canaliculi and sinusoids. Bile obstruction causes jaundice. Vascular obstruction causes portal hypertension, shunting, and varices.
16. Nonalcoholic fatty liver disease and nonalcoholic steatohepatitis involve accumulation of fat in the liver not associated with alcohol intake and are commonly associated with obesity.
17. Secondary biliary cirrhosis develops from prolonged obstruction of bile flow with increased pressure in the hepatic bile ducts that causes pooling of bile and necrosis of tissue. Relief of obstruction allays symptoms of jaundice and pruritus. Viral hepatitis is an infection of the liver caused by a strain of the hepatitis virus (i.e., hepatitis A virus, hepatitis B virus, hepatitis C virus, and hepatitis E virus). Although they differ with respect to modes of transmission and severity of acute illness, all can cause hepatic cell necrosis, Kupffer cell hyperplasia, and infiltration of liver tissue by mononuclear phagocytes. These changes obstruct bile flow and impair hepatocyte function.
18. The clinical manifestations of viral hepatitis depend on the stage of infection. Cholelithiasis (the formation of gallstones) is a common disorder of the gallbladder. Gallstones form in the bile as a result of the aggregation of cholesterol crystals (cholesterol stones) or precipitates of unconjugated bilirubin (pigmented stones). Gallstones that fill the gallbladder or obstruct the cystic or common bile duct cause abdominal pain and jaundice.
19. Cholecystitis is an acute or chronic inflammation of the gallbladder usually associated with obstruction of the cystic duct by gallstones.
20. Acute pancreatitis (pancreatic inflammation) is a serious but relatively rare disorder. Pancreatic duct obstruction and injury permits leakage of digestive enzymes into pancreatic tissue, where they become activated and begin the process of autodigestion, inflammation, and destruction of tissues. Chronic pancreatitis results from structural or functional impairment of the pancreas. It causes recurrent abdominal pain and digestive disorders.

Cancer of the Digestive System
1. Cancer of the esophagus is rare and tends to occur in people older than 60 years of age. Alcohol and tobacco use, reflux esophagitis, and nutritional deficiencies are associated with esophageal carcinoma.
2. Dysphagia and chest pain are the primary manifestations of esophageal cancer. Early treatment of tumours that have not spread into the mediastinum or lymph nodes results in a good prognosis.
3. Gastric adenocarcinomas are associated with *H. pylori* that carries the *CagA* gene product cytotoxin-associated vacuolating antigen A, a diet high in salt and food preservatives (nitrates, nitrites), and atrophic gastritis.
4. Approximately 50% of all stomach cancers are located in the prepyloric antrum. Clinical manifestations (weight loss, upper abdominal pain, vomiting, hematemesis, anemia) develop only after the tumour has penetrated the wall of the stomach.
5. Rectal carcinomas occur up to 15 cm from the opening of the anus. The tumour spreads transmurally to the vagina in women or the prostate in men.
6. Metastatic invasion of the liver is more common than primary cancer of the liver.
7. Primary liver cancers are associated with chronic liver disease (cirrhosis, hepatitis B). Hepatocellular carcinomas arise from the hepatocytes, whereas cholangiocellular carcinomas arise from the bile ducts. Primary liver cancer spreads to the heart, lungs, brain, kidney, and spleen through the circulation.
8. Cancer of the pancreas is the fourth leading cause of cancer deaths in Canada. Most tumours are adenocarcinomas that arise in the exocrine cells of ducts in the head, body, or tail of the pancreas. Symptoms may not be evident until the tumour has spread to surrounding tissues.

Geriatric Considerations: Age-Related Gastric Changes
1. Aging is associated with decreased secretion of hydrochloric acid and pepsin and an associated small rise in gastric pH.
2. Aging leads to a decline in the absorption of some substances.
3. Older persons are at high risk of pill-induced esophagitis due to polypharmacy, and other age-related physiological changes such as decreased saliva production and impaired esophageal motility.
4. The incidence of gastric ulcer is increasing in older persons due the increased prevalence of aspirin/nonsteroidal anti-inflammatory medication use and *Helicobacter pylori* infection in this population. Bleeding complications and mortality are more than 100 times higher in older persons compared to those who are younger.

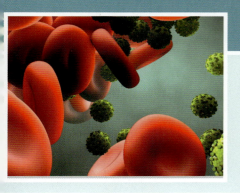

37

Developmental Alterations of Digestive Function

Mohamed Toufic El-Hussein, with originating chapter contributions by Sharon Sables-Baus and Sara J. Fidanza

Additional resources are available online at https://evolve.elsevier.com/Canada/Huether/pathophysiology.

CHAPTER OUTLINE

Key Terms, 927
Disorders of the Gastro-intestinal Tract, 928
    Congenital Impairment of Motility, 928
    Acquired Impairment of Motility, 931
    Impairment of Digestion, Absorption, and Nutrition, 932
    Diarrhea, 936
Disorders of the Liver, 937
    Disorders of Biliary Metabolism and Transport, 937

    Inflammatory Disorders, 938
    Portal Hypertension, 939
    Metabolic Disorders, 939
Gastro-intestinal Malignancies in Children, 939
    Hepatoblastoma, 940
    Pancreatic Tumours, 940

LEARNING OBJECTIVES

1. Describe the common congenital malformations of the intestinal tract: cleft lip and palate, esophageal atresia, pyloric stenosis, meconium ileus, small and large bowel obstructions, congenital aganglionic megacolon, and malformations of the anus and rectum.
2. Describe the pathophysiology and treatment for intussusception.
3. Discuss the reasons for an infant's increased susceptibility to gastroesophageal reflux.
4. Discuss the pathophysiology of cystic fibrosis and explain how the treatment attempts to compensate for the pathophysiological findings.
5. Discuss the pathophysiology, clinical manifestations, evaluation, and treatment of gluten-sensitive enteropathy and protein energy malnutrition.
6. Discuss the multiple factors implicated in failure to thrive.
7. Discuss the pathophysiology of necrotizing enterocolitis.
8. Identify the causes and consequences of diarrhea in infants and children.
9. Compare and contrast physiological and pathological jaundice.
10. Define biliary atresia and describe the resulting damage sustained by the liver and the significance of that damage.
11. Discuss the etiology of hepatitis A, B, and C.
12. Briefly explain what is meant by cirrhosis of the liver.
13. Discuss the different types of portal hypertension and list their clinical manifestations.
14. Discuss the three common metabolic disorders in children that produce liver damage: galactosemia, fructosemia, and Wilson's disease.

KEY TERMS

Anorectal malformation (ARM), 931
Biliary atresia (BA), 937
Celiac crisis, 934
Celiac disease (CD), 934
Cirrhosis, 938
Cleft lip (CL), 928
Cleft palate (CP), 928
Cystic fibrosis (CF), 933
Diarrhea, 937
Distal intestinal obstruction syndrome (DIOS), 930
Esophageal atresia (EA), 928
Esophageal atresia/tracheoesophageal fistula (EA/TEF), 928

Extrahepatic portal hypertension, 939
Failure to thrive (FTT), 935
Fructosemia, 939
Galactosemia, 939
Gastroesophageal reflux (GER), 931
Gastroesophageal reflux disease (GERD), 931
Glycogen storage disease (GSD), 939
Growth faltering (GF), 935
Hepatitis A virus (HAV), 938
Hepatitis B virus (HBV), 938
Hepatitis C virus (HCV), 938
Hepatitis D virus (HDV), 938
Hepatoblastoma, 940

Hirschsprung's disease, 930
Idiopathic intestinal pseudo-obstruction, 930
Infantile hypertrophic pyloric stenosis (IHPS), 929
Intrahepatic portal hypertension, 939
Intussusception, 932
Jaundice (icterus), 937
Kernicterus, 937
Kwashiorkor, 935
Lactose intolerance, 935
Marasmus, 935
Meckel diverticulum, 930
Meconium, 930
Meconium disease (MD), 930
Meconium ileus (MI), 930

Meconium plug syndrome (MPS), 930
Necrotizing enterocolitis (NEC), 936
Nonceliac gluten sensitivity (NCGS), 934
Nonsyndromic (isolated) CP, 928
Physiological jaundice (hyperbilirubinemia) of the newborn, 937
Protein-energy malnutrition (PEM), 935
Rotavirus, 937
Syndromic CLP, 928
Wilson's disease, 939

Disorders of the gastro-intestinal (GI) tract, liver, and pancreas in children include congenital anomalies with structural and functional alterations, enzyme deficiencies, infections, and malignancies. These disorders lead to impairment of motility, digestion, absorption, nutrition, and normal growth and development.

DISORDERS OF THE GASTRO-INTESTINAL TRACT

> **QUICK CHECK 37.1**
> 1. What structures are affected in cleft palate and cleft lip?
> 2. What is esophageal atresia?
> 3. What produces pyloric stenosis?

Congenital Impairment of Motility
Cleft Lip and Cleft Palate

There are numerous types of congenital orofacial anomalies, the most common of which is cleft lip (CL) or cleft palate (CP), or both (CLP). A cleft is a congenital anomaly that features a defect of the lip, alveolus, and/or palate and could be unilateral or bilateral. In Canada specifically, 1 in 700 children are born with a cleft of the lip, palate, or both.[1,2] CL and CP can occur in isolation or as part of a broad range of chromosomal, mendelian, or teratogenic syndromes. When CL occurs as part of a chromosomal, mendelian, or teratogenic syndrome, the defect may be referred to as syndromic CLP. If CP occurs alone, the defect may be referred to as nonsyndromic or isolated CP. Both anomalies can be unilateral or bilateral, partial or complete.[3]

PATHOPHYSIOLOGY. Cleft lip (CL) and cleft palate (CP) are embryonic developmental anomalies and vary in severity (Figure. 37.1). There may be genetic and environmental triggers for syndromic and nonsyndromic CLP. Epigenetic influences include maternal smoking, alcohol, steroid, or statin use, and folate deficiency or disordered metabolism. CL and CP also may be associated with other malformations (i.e., cardiac, skeletal, or central nervous system). This phenomenon, called *multifactorial inheritance*, is discussed in Chapter 2.

CL is caused by the incomplete fusion of the nasomedial or intermaxillary process beginning in the fourth week of embryonic development, a period of rapid development. The cleft causes structures of the face and mouth to develop without the normal restraints of encircling lip muscles. The cleft is usually just beneath the centre of one nostril. The defect may occur bilaterally and may be symmetrical or asymmetrical.

CP is often associated with CL but may occur without it. The fissure may affect only the uvula and soft palate or may extend forward to the nostril and involve the hard palate and the maxillary alveolar ridge. It may be unilateral or bilateral, with the cleft occupying the midline posteriorly and as far forward as the alveolar process, where it deviates to the involved side. Clefts involving the palate only are usually, but not necessarily, in the midline. When these facial bones are involved, the nasal cavity may freely communicate with the oral cavity. Teeth in the CP area may be missing or deformed. There is increased risk for middle ear infections.

CLINICAL MANIFESTATIONS. Clefts of the lip or palate, or both, are immediately recognizable disruptions of normal facial structure. Feeding difficulty is the most significant clinical manifestation because of the oronasal communication and inability to generate negative pressure that infants need for normal sucking.[4] They may also experience swallowing difficulty.

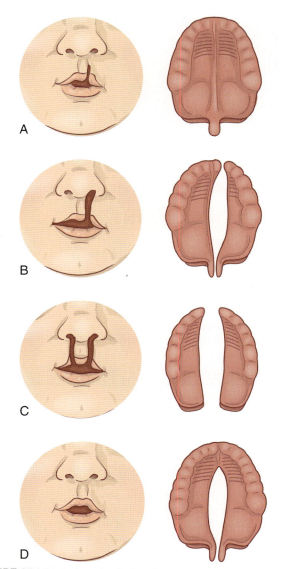

FIGURE 37.1 Variations in Clefts of the Lip and Palate. **A,** Notch in vermilion border. **B,** Unilateral cleft lip and palate. **C,** Bilateral cleft lip and cleft palate. **D,** Cleft palate.

EVALUATION AND TREATMENT. Prenatal diagnosis is made by ultrasound, and postnatal imaging confirms the extent of bone deformity. The nature and extent of the cleft, the infant's condition, and the method of surgical correction proposed determine the course of treatment.

A baby with a complete CP requires consultation with a feeding and swallowing specialist to ensure adequate and safe nutritional intake. Bottles with nipples that are specialized for feeding an infant with a CP are required. Breastfeeding may be possible for some infants.[5] An orthodontic prosthesis for the roof of the mouth may facilitate sucking for some infants.

Esophageal Atresia

Esophageal atresia (EA) is the most common congenital atresia of the esophagus. The esophagus ends in a blind pouch. EA is usually accompanied by a fistula between the esophagus and the trachea (esophageal atresia/tracheoesophageal fistula [EA/TEF]).[6,7] Either defect can occur alone (Figure. 37.2). Environmental risk factors include maternal exposure to methimazole (Tapazole), exogenous sex hormones,

CHAPTER 37 Developmental Alterations of Digestive Function

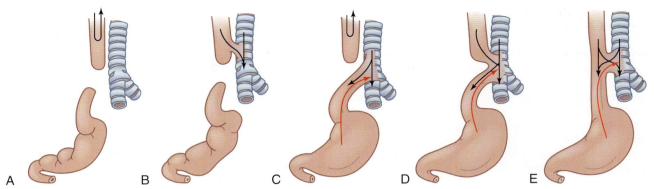

FIGURE 37.2 Five Types of Esophageal Atresia and Tracheoesophageal Fistulae. **A**, Simple esophageal atresia. Proximal esophagus and distal esophagus end in blind pouches, and there is no tracheal communication. Nothing enters the stomach; regurgitated food and fluid may enter the lungs. **B**, Proximal and distal esophageal segments end in blind pouches, and a fistula connects the proximal esophagus to the trachea. Nothing enters the stomach; food and fluid enter the lungs from the mouth. **C**, Proximal esophagus ends in a blind pouch, and a fistula connects the trachea to the distal esophagus. Air enters the stomach; regurgitated gastric secretions enter the lungs through the fistula. **D**, Fistula connects both proximal and distal esophageal segments to the trachea. Air, food, and fluid enter the stomach and the lungs from the mouth; regurgitated gastric secretions enter the lungs through the fistula. **E**, Simple tracheoesophageal fistula between otherwise normal esophagus and trachea. Air, food, and fluid enter the stomach and the lungs from the mouth through the fistula; and regurgitated gastric secretions enter the lungs through the fistula. Between 85 and 90% of esophageal anomalies are type **C**; 6 to 8% are type **A**; 3 to 5% are type **E**; and fewer than 1% are type **B** or **D**.

infectious diseases, alcohol, or smoking; maternal diabetes; advanced maternal age; and maternal employment in agriculture.[8]

PATHOPHYSIOLOGY. The pathogenesis of esophageal abnormalities is unknown. Defective growth of endodermal cells and impaired embryonic foregut development of the trachea and esophagus lead to atresia.[9]

CLINICAL MANIFESTATIONS. Antenatal diagnosis of EA/TEF increases with the findings of polyhydramnios (excessive amniotic fluid).[7,8] Swallowed amniotic fluid is usually absorbed into the placental circulation; therefore, if the fetus cannot swallow, amniotic fluid accumulates in the uterus. EA will be diagnosed at birth on the basis of drooling, inability to swallow secretions or choking with feeding, and respiratory distress. Confirmation is established by inability to pass a gastric tube into the stomach. If a fistula connects the trachea with the distal esophagus, the abdomen fills with air and becomes distended, possibly interfering with breathing (Figure. 37.2C–E).

Pulmonary complications are compounded by reflux of air and gastric secretions into the tracheobronchial tree through the fistula, causing severe chemical irritation. Infants with EA but no fistulae have scaphoid (boat-shaped), gasless abdomens. In infants with fistulae but without atresia (see Figure. 37.2E), the usual symptoms are recurrent aspiration, pneumonia, and atelectasis (lung collapse) that remains unexpressed for days or even months.

EVALUATION AND TREATMENT. Infants that present with EA are evaluated with ultrasound, echocardiogram, and vertebral and limb radiographs. Following diagnosis, a tube should be placed into the upper pouch and continuous suction applied to decrease risk for aspiration. The head of the bed should be elevated slightly to assist drainage of the upper pouch. The infant should not be fed orally. Surgical repair is completed in most cases.[9] The overall survival rate for infants with esophageal defects is 95%.[10]

Infantile Hypertrophic Pyloric Stenosis

Infantile hypertrophic pyloric stenosis (IHPS) is an acquired narrowing and distal obstruction of the pylorus and a common cause of postprandial vomiting. The etiology is unclear but probably multifactorial, involving genetic and environmental factors.[11]

PATHOPHYSIOLOGY. Individual muscle fibres thicken, so the entire pyloric sphincter becomes enlarged and inflexible. The mucosal lining of the pyloric opening is folded and narrowed by the encroaching muscle. Because of the extra peristaltic effort necessary to force the gastric contents through the narrow pylorus, the muscle layers of the stomach may become hypertrophied as well.

CLINICAL MANIFESTATIONS. Between 2 and 8 weeks after birth, an infant who has fed well and gained weight begins forceful, nonbilious vomiting immediately after feeding.[12,13] The infant then demands to be refed. Constipation occurs because little food reaches the intestine. Infants with pyloric stenosis are irritable because of hunger, and they may have esophageal discomfort caused by repeated vomiting and esophagitis.

EVALUATION AND TREATMENT. The force and timing of the vomiting can help distinguish IHPS from gastroesophageal reflux (GER), for which episodes of vomiting are not forceful and occur 10 minutes or more after a feeding. The hypertrophied pylorus is palpable as a firm, small, movable mass, approximately the size of an olive, and is felt in the right upper quadrant in 70 to 90% of infants with pyloric stenosis. The standard treatment for hypertrophic pyloric stenosis is a laparoscopic pyloromyotomy, which involves the separation and splitting of the muscles of the pylorus.[14]

Obstructions of the Duodenum, Jejunum, and Ileum

High intestinal obstruction should be considered whenever persistent vomiting occurs. With duodenal obstruction, there will be upper abdominal distension, visible peristaltic waves, a decrease in the size and frequency of meconium stools, progressive weight loss, persistent vomiting, and dehydration. The obstruction may be partial or complete and is usually located at or near the major duodenal papilla. The classic "double bubble" sign is seen on imaging of the abdomen and represents duodenal obstruction. The larger, proximal "bubble" is air in a dilated stomach. The more distal, smaller "bubble" is air in a dilated proximal duodenum.

Meckel Diverticulum

Diverticula are small outpouches, or sacs, that have formed and pushed outward through weak spots of the intestinal wall. Meckel diverticulum is a remnant of the embryonic yolk sac and the most prevalent congenital abnormality of the small bowel (usually in the ileum). It is a true diverticulum in that it contains all layers of the intestinal wall. Ectopic gastric mucosal cells are contained in the diverticuli and may cause peptic ulcer and painless bleeding or mimic colonic diverticulitis. Although most Meckel diverticuli are asymptomatic, the most common symptom is painless rectal bleeding. Intestinal obstruction, intussusception, and volvulus can occur, more commonly in adults. Diagnosis is made by symptom presentation and radionucleotide scintigraphy. The scan shows the gastric mucosal cells in the diverticuli. Treatment in those with symptoms is surgical resection.[15–18]

Meconium Syndromes

> **QUICK CHECK 37.2**
> 1. Describe the pathological defect in meconium ileus.
> 2. Why is there poor bowel motility with Hirschsprung's disease?
> 3. Describe the defect in intussusception.

Meconium is a substance that fills the entire intestine before birth. It is a dark greenish mass of desquamated cells, mucus, and bile that accumulates in the bowel of a fetus and is typically discharged during the first 12 to 48 hours after birth.

Meconium ileus (MI) is an intestinal obstruction in the neonatal period caused by meconium formed in utero that is abnormally thick and sticky, which leads to a partial or complete obstruction at the level of the terminal ileum. There are two forms of MI: simple and complex. Complex MI is a surgical emergency and there is usually an associated GI pathology, such as bowel atresia, necrosis, or perforation. MI occurs in 10 to 15% of infants with cystic fibrosis (CF) and is thought to result from abnormal mucous production in the intestine or impaired pancreatic enzymes, or both[19,20] (see Chapter 28).

Meconium plug syndrome (MPS), also called *functional immaturity of the colon*, is a transient disorder of the newborn colon characterized by delayed passage (greater than 24 to 48 hours) of meconium and intestinal dilatation. Meconium disease (MD) is often associated with severe prematurity and low birth weight. It results from a combination of extremely sticky meconium in the colon or terminal ileum and poor intestinal motility, resulting in mechanical bowel obstruction.

Distal intestinal obstruction syndrome (DIOS), formerly called *meconium ileus equivalent*, is seen in about 7.4% of children and adults with CF.[21] It is characterized by complete or incomplete intestinal obstruction of viscid fecal accumulation in the terminal ileum and proximal colon.[22]

PATHOPHYSIOLOGY. The terminal ileum is plugged with thick, viscous meconium resulting from the formation of an insoluble, calcium–glycoprotein compound in abnormal mucus. The segment of the ileum proximal to the obstruction is distended with liquid contents, and its walls may be hypertrophied. The segment distal to the obstruction is collapsed and filled with small pellets of pale-coloured stool. Peristalsis fails to propel this viscous material through the ileum, and it becomes impacted. Volvulus, atresia, or perforation of the bowel sometimes accompanies MI.

CLINICAL MANIFESTATIONS. Abdominal distension usually develops during the first few hours after birth. As air is swallowed, the distension increases, and the infant begins to vomit bile-stained material. Infants with CF may have signs of pulmonary involvement, such as tachypnea, intercostal retractions, and grunting respirations. The distended abdomen shows patterns of dilated intestinal loops that feel doughlike when palpated. Some of the loops contain scattered, firm, movable masses.

EVALUATION AND TREATMENT. Radiological examination confirms the presence of meconium in the ileum or ileocecum. The sweat test measures the amount of chloride in the sweat, is performed to detect or rule out CF, and is accurate in 90% of infants. Defective chloride channels in CF cause increased chloride concentration in sweat. In most cases, the obstruction is relieved by intestinal lavage and administration of oral laxatives.[22,23] If this is not possible, the meconium is removed surgically.[24]

Idiopathic Intestinal Pseudo-Obstruction

Idiopathic intestinal pseudo-obstruction is a disorder of impaired intestinal motility. The pseudo-obstruction is caused by nerve or peristaltic muscle dysfunction that affects the movement of food, fluid, or air through the intestine. Children present with abdominal swelling or bloating, crampy abdominal pain, nausea, vomiting, constipation, or diarrhea. Idiopathic intestinal pseudo-obstruction is difficult to diagnose, and treatment includes intestinal decompression, nutritional support, and symptom management.[25–27]

Hirschsprung's Disease

Hirschsprung's disease, or *aganglionic megacolon*, is a functional obstruction of the colon. It is the most common cause of colon obstruction, accounting for about one-third of all GI obstructions in infants. The incidence is approximately 1 in 5 000 live births and varies among ethnic groups. There is a predominance in males.[28,29]

PATHOPHYSIOLOGY. Hirschsprung's disease is characterized by the absence of parasympathetic intrinsic ganglion cells in the submucosal and myenteric plexuses along with the absence of peristaltic movement in the bowels (see Figure 35.13 for normal colon structure). In 80% of cases, the aganglionic segment is limited to the rectal end of the sigmoid colon. The abnormally innervated colon impairs fecal movements, causing the proximal colon to become distended—hence the term *megacolon* (Figure. 37.3).

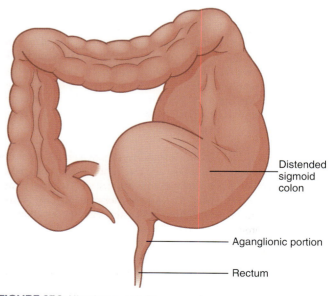

FIGURE 37.3 Hirschsprung's Disease.

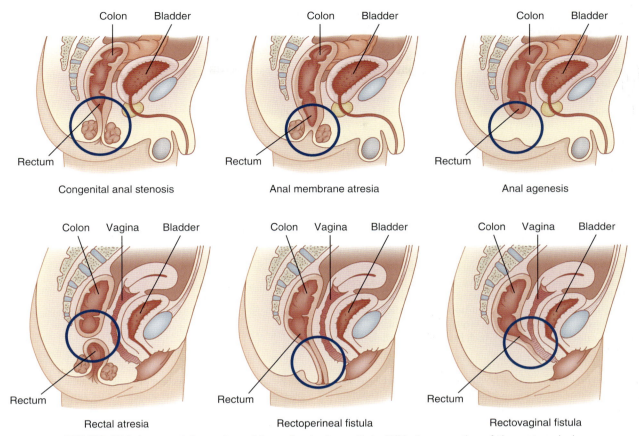

FIGURE 37.4 Anorectal Stenosis and Imperforate Anus. Note: With the exception of the rectovaginal fistula, all of the malformations shown occur in both males and females.

CLINICAL MANIFESTATIONS. The infant typically becomes symptomatic during the first 24 to 72 hours after birth with delayed passage of meconium. Mild to severe constipation is the usual manifestation of Hirschsprung's disease, with poor feeding, poor weight gain, and progressive abdominal distension. However, diarrhea may be the first sign because only water can travel around the impacted feces.

The most serious complication in the neonatal period is enterocolitis related to fecal impaction. Bowel dilation stretches and partly occludes the encircling blood and lymphatic vessels, causing edema, ischemia, infarction of the mucosa, and significant outflow of fluid into the bowel lumen. Copious liquid stools result. Infarction and destruction of the mucosa enable enteric microorganisms to penetrate the bowel wall. Frequently, Gram-negative sepsis occurs, accompanied by fever and vomiting. Severe and rapid fluid and electrolyte changes may take place, causing hypovolemic or septic shock or death.

EVALUATION AND TREATMENT. Radiocontrast enema and anorectal manometry are screening tools for the diagnosis of Hirschsprung's disease. The definitive diagnosis is made by rectal biopsy showing an absence of ganglion cells in the submucosa of the colon.[30] Surgery is the definitive treatment in all cases of Hirschsprung's disease, and bowel training may be prolonged.[28,31-34]

Anorectal Malformations

Anorectal malformations (ARMs) represent a spectrum of anomalies of the anus and rectum (Figure. 37.4). ARMs include anorectal stenosis, imperforate anus, anorectal atresia, and rectal atresia. Persistent cloaca is the most severe type of ARM and occurs exclusively in girls. The rectum, urethra, and vagina fail to develop separately; instead, they drain through a single, common channel onto the perineum.[35-38]

Types of imperforate anus include an anal opening that is narrow or misplaced, a membrane (covering) may be present over the anal opening, the rectum may not connect to the anus, the rectum may connect to part of the urinary tract or to the reproductive system through an opening called a fistula, or the anal opening is not present. Treatment recommendations depend on the type of imperforate anus, the presence and type of associated abnormalities, and the child's overall health status. Anal stenosis can be treated by dilations. Infants with an imperforate anus and other anorectal malformations require surgical correction.[37,39]

Acquired Impairment of Motility
Gastroesophageal Reflux

Gastroesophageal reflux (GER) is the passage of gastric contents into the esophagus independent of swallowing. GER is normal and nonpathological in healthy infants and may be asymptomatic or exhibited by regurgitation and vomiting.[40] The frequency of GER is highest in premature infants and occurs in about 70% of healthy infants; however, GER resolves without treatment in 95% of infants by 12 to 14 months of age.[41] Gastroesophageal reflux disease (GERD) is different from GER and occurs when it is the cause of troublesome symptoms or complications, or both, described as esophageal or extraesophageal in nature.[42] Children at greatest risk for complicated GERD are those with prematurity, neurological impairment, EA, obesity, hiatal hernia, achalasia, chronic lung diseases, and certain genetic disorders, including CF.

PATHOPHYSIOLOGY. GERD is influenced by genetic, environmental, anatomical, hormonal, and neurogenic factors. Although transient lower esophageal sphincter relaxations are the most common pathophysiological cause of GER, inadequate adaptation of sphincter tone to changes in abdominal pressure also may be implicated. Factors that maintain lower esophageal sphincter integrity in children include the location of the gastroesophageal junction in a high-pressure zone within the abdomen, mucosal gathering within the sphincter, and the angle at which the esophagus is inserted into the stomach. Reflux persists if any one of these pressure-maintaining factors is altered. Reflux of acidic gastric contents results in inflammation of the esophageal epithelium (esophagitis) and stimulation of the vomiting reflex.

CLINICAL MANIFESTATIONS. The clinical manifestations of GERD include excessive regurgitation or vomiting; food refusal/anorexia; unexplained crying, choking, or gagging; sleep disturbance; dysphagia; and abdominal or epigastric pain, or both.[42] Esophageal complications of GER can be significant, such as esophagitis, hemorrhage, stricture, Barrett's esophagus (metaplasia) (see Chapter 36), and, rarely, adenocarcinoma. Extraesophageal symptoms include cough and wheezing, laryngitis, pharyngitis, dental erosions, sinusitis, recurrent otitis media, and Sandifer syndrome (a neurological disorder).[43] This constellation of symptoms is often indistinguishable from those of cow's milk protein allergy, which may coexist with or overlap GERD.

EVALUATION AND TREATMENT. The clinical manifestations are often adequate to confirm a diagnosis of GERD. Esophageal pH monitoring with a probe for 24 hours and endoscopy are routinely used for diagnosis.

Normal physiological GER resolves without treatment. In breastfed babies, maternal elimination of cow's milk protein is recommended, whereas formula-fed infants may require feeding volume and frequency adjustments using extensively hydrolyzed protein or amino acid–based formulas. Using thickened feedings has shown to improve symptoms of GER. Prone positioning is only recommended for infants older than 1 year of age because of the risk for sudden unexpected infant death. Medications are used to buffer or decrease gastric acid secretion, increase motility, or increase lower esophageal sphincter pressure to treat GER.[44,45]

Intussusception

Intussusception is the telescoping of a proximal segment of intestine into a distal segment, causing an obstruction. It is the most common cause of small bowel obstruction in children. Most cases occur between 5 and 7 months of age. Intussusception is more common in males and can occur in children with polyps or tumours (lead points), CF, Meckel diverticulum, intestinal adhesions, or immediately after abdominal surgery.[46] There is a small risk for intussusception associated with rotavirus vaccination, but the vaccine is generally safe.[47]

In Canada, as a precaution, infants with a history of intussusception should not be given rotavirus vaccine. About 4% of infants with intussusception will have another episode in the following year; there is no evidence that children who have a history of intussusception are at an increased risk for another intussusception after receiving rotavirus vaccine.[48]

PATHOPHYSIOLOGY. In intussusception, the ileum commonly telescopes into the cecum and part of the ascending colon by collapsing through the ileocecal valve, although intussusception can occur anywhere from the duodenum to the rectum. The proximal portion of the intestine (the intussusceptum) collapses into the distal portion (the

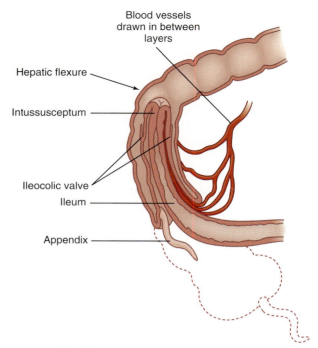

FIGURE 37.5 Ileocolic Intussusception.

intussuscipiens) in the direction of peristaltic flow (Figure. 37.5). The intussusceptum then drags its mesentery into the enveloping lumen, causing an intussusception. Initially, the mesentery is constricted, obstructing venous return. Compression of the mesenteric vessels between the two layers of intestinal wall and at the U-shaped angle at either end of the intussusceptum leads within hours to venous stasis, engorgement, edema, exudation, and further vascular compression. Edema and compression obstruct the flow of chyme through the intestine. Unless the intussusception is treated, ischemia and necrosis follow.

CLINICAL MANIFESTATIONS. The classic symptoms of intussusception include colicky abdominal pain, irritability, knees drawn to the chest, abdominal mass, vomiting, and bloody (currant-jelly) stools.

EVALUATION AND TREATMENT. Diagnosis is based on clinical manifestations, onset of symptoms, and ultrasonographic or radiological imaging studies. An enema reduction is usually effective for large bowel intussusception and prevents the progression to ischemia and perforation. Laparotomy remains the treatment of choice for small bowel intussusception.[49] Untreated intussusception in infants is nearly always fatal. Most infants recover if the intussusception is reduced within 24 hours.[50]

Appendicitis

Appendicitis is common in children between the ages of 10 and 11 years.[51] The mechanisms of disease, symptoms, and treatment are similar to those for adults and can be reviewed in Chapter 36.

Impairment of Digestion, Absorption, and Nutrition

> **QUICK CHECK 37.3**
> 1. Why do individuals with cystic fibrosis have pancreatic insufficiency?
> 2. Why does loss of villi occur with gluten-sensitive enteropathy?
> 3. Compare kwashiorkor and marasmus.

TABLE 37.1 Pathophysiology, Clinical Manifestations, and Complications of Cystic Fibrosis

Organ Involved	Secretory Dysfunction	Clinical Manifestations	Complications
Sweat glands	Elevated concentration of sodium and chloride in sweat	Hyponatremia; hypochloremia	Heat prostration; shock
Intestine			
Newborn	Viscid meconium	Meconium ileus with intestinal obstruction	Meconium peritonitis; growth failure
Older child and adult	Inspissated (dried out) mucofecal masses (intestinal sludging)	Partial intestinal obstruction with severe cramping pains	Volvulus (obstruction), intussusception (prolapse) Distal intestinal obstruction syndrome Growth failure
Pancreas (enzyme deficiency)	Inspissation and precipitation of pancreatic secretions, causing obstruction of pancreatic ducts Insulin deficiency	Absence of pancreatic enzymes, causing malabsorption of food and fatty, bulky stools Decreased vitamin A, D, E, and K absorption Glucose intolerance	Hypoproteinemia; iron deficiency anemia; malnutrition Vitamins A, D, E, and K deficiency and rectal prolapse Diabetes mellitus (see Chapter 19)
Liver	Inspissation and precipitation of bile and biliary system	Focal biliary cirrhosis; shrunken, "hobnail" liver; fatty liver	Portal hypertension with esophageal varices and hematemesis
Salivary glands	Inspissation and precipitation of secretions in small ducts of submaxillary and sublingual salivary glands	Mild patchy fibrosis of salivary glands	None
Respiratory Tract			
Paranasal structures	Viscid mucus	Retention of mucus; clouding seen on sinus roentgenograms	Mucopyoceles (pus accumulations) with nasal deformity or orbital cavity extension
Nose	Nasal polyps	Obstruction of nasal air flow	Sinusitis
Lungs	Viscid mucus in bronchioles and bronchi	Obstruction of bronchioles causing bronchiolectasis, bronchiectasis, and chronic lung infection	Atelectasis, hemoptysis; pneumothorax; cor pulmonale; respiratory failure
Reproductive Tract			
Male	Viscid genital tract secretions during embryological development, causing failure of formation of normal vas deferens; aspermia	Sterility	None
Female	Distension of endocervical epithelial cells with cytoplasmic mucin	Decreased fertility	Polypoid cervicitis (cervical inflammation) while taking oral contraceptives

Data from Marcdante, K. J., & Kliegman, R. M. (2015). *Nelson essentials of pediatrics* (7th ed.). Saunders.

Cystic Fibrosis

Cystic fibrosis (CF) is an autosomal recessive disease that involves multiple organ systems and leads to death at an earlier age, although new treatments are extending life expectancy. This section focuses on GI complications of CF; Chapter 28 discusses CF's epidemiology and pulmonary involvement.

PATHOPHYSIOLOGY. The GI presentation of CF is caused by a dysfunction of the cystic fibrosis transmembrane regulator (CFTR) protein, which is located on epithelial membranes and regulates chloride and sodium ion channels. It is found throughout the airways, sweat glands, digestive tract, pancreas, hepatobiliary system, and reproductive system (also called *mucoviscidosis* or *fibrocystic disease of the pancreas*). The hallmark pathophysiological triad of CF includes obstruction, infection, and inflammation that are evident throughout the GI tract and within the airways. The full spectrum of involvement is summarized in Table 37.1.

Dysfunction of the CFTR protein results in altered sodium, chloride, and potassium resorption, all of which remain external to the surface of the epithelial membrane, with reduced clearance from tubular structures lined by affected epithelia.[52] Maldigestion of proteins, carbohydrates, fats, and fat-soluble vitamins occurs because mucous obstruction of the pancreatic ducts blocks the flow of pancreatic enzymes, causing intestinal malabsorption and degenerative and fibrotic changes in the pancreas and GI tract. Diabetes mellitus commonly develops from damage to insulin-producing beta cells and insulin resistance.[53]

CLINICAL MANIFESTATIONS. Clinical manifestations are summarized in Table 37.1. GI symptoms often precede pulmonary manifestations. Approximately 85% of those with CF present early in life with pancreatic insufficiency (PI). PI is the cause of nutrient malabsorption and failure to thrive in children with CF. Steatorrhea and abdominal distension are common symptoms with potential sequelae that include DIOS, fibrotic colonopathy, or focal biliary cirrhosis. Children who are pancreatic sufficient are at greater risk of developing pancreatitis.[54] Those with CF are at greater risk for many GI complications, including GI cancers and hepatobiliary abnormalities, which may lead to pancreatic transplant or death.

EVALUATION AND TREATMENT. Genetic screening and the sweat test are required for diagnosis. Evaluation of pancreatic sufficiency also is

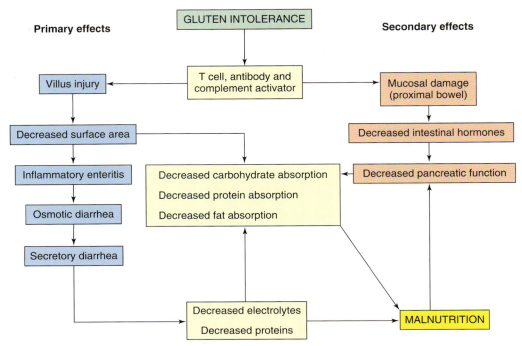

FIGURE 37.6 Pathophysiology of Celiac Disease.

essential. The extent of pancreatic function is determined by 72-hour fecal fat measurements, which are not easily obtained. Therefore, the most common measurement of fat malabsorption is fecal elastase. A serum test for trypsinogen also can be used to detect pancreatic insufficiency in children older than 8 years of age.

The goal of treatment for PI is to reduce malabsorption of nutrients and improve growth. Most children with CF take pancreatic enzyme replacement therapy (PERT) for the rest of their lives. PERT is administered before or with every meal, snack, or enteral feeding supplementation. High doses of PERT are associated with DIOS; therefore, minimal effective doses are indicated. High-caloric, high-protein diets with frequent snacks and vitamin supplements are used to treat malnutrition. Nutritional status and growth should be carefully monitored, and growth hormone may be included with nutritional supplements.[55]

Celiac Disease

Celiac disease (CD), formerly called *celiac sprue*, is an autoimmune disease that damages small intestinal villous epithelium when there is ingestion of gluten (gliadin), the protein component of cereal grains. CD is a common multiorgan disease with a strong genetic predisposition associated with human leukocyte antigen DQ2 (HLA-DQ2) and HLA-DQ8.[56] Nonceliac gluten sensitivity (NCGS), or wheat allergy, should not be confused with CD; although it presents similarly after the ingestion of gluten, the individual does not have positive autoantibodies or classic intestinal villous atrophy, but instead has variable HLA status with similar symptoms as CD.[57]

The pathogenesis of CD is complex and involves genetic and immunological factors. Environmental factors include early infections, gut microbiota in infants, feeding patterns, and timing and amount of gluten. CD presents with greater frequency in children with type 1 diabetes mellitus, autoimmune thyroid or liver disease, Down syndrome, Turner's syndrome, Williams syndrome, selective immunoglobulin A (IgA) deficiency, Addison's disease, and first-degree relatives with CD.[58]

PATHOPHYSIOLOGY. The major pathophysiological characteristic of CD is T-cell–mediated autoimmune injury to the small intestinal epithelial cells of genetically susceptible individuals. There is atrophy and flattening of villi, crypt hyperplasia in the upper small intestine, and malabsorption of most nutrients in the presence of cereal gluten, particularly wheat, rye, and barley (Figure. 37.6).[59]

Destruction of mucosal cells causes inflammation, and water and electrolytes are secreted, leading to watery diarrhea. Potassium loss leads to muscle weakness. Unabsorbed fatty acids combine with calcium, and secondary hyperparathyroidism increases phosphorus excretion, resulting in bone resorption. Calcium is no longer able to bind oxalate in the intestine and is absorbed, which causes hyperoxaluria

Fat malabsorption in the jejunum is the major cause of steatorrhea (fatty stools). Deficiencies of fat-soluble vitamins are common in children with CD. Vitamin K malabsorption leads to hypoprothrombinemia.

CLINICAL MANIFESTATIONS. The onset of clinical manifestations of CD depends on the age of the infant when gluten-containing substances are added to the diet. Severity of symptoms can vary tremendously, and many children older than 3 years of age present with non–gastro-intestinal symptoms.[58] GI and extraintestinal symptoms of CD are listed in Box 37.1.

An unusual complication of CD in infancy is celiac crisis. Celiac crisis is characterized by severe diarrhea, dehydration, and hypoproteinemia as a result of malabsorption and protein loss.

EVALUATION AND TREATMENT. Diagnosis includes confirmation with serological autoantibody measurement against tissue transglutaminase IgA (tTG IgA) (most sensitive and specific), antiendomysial antibody (anti-EMA) IgA, or deaminated gliadin peptides (DGPs), which are more sensitive in children younger than 2 years of age. A negative genetic screening for HLA haplotypes would rule out CD.[60] Currently, there is controversy regarding treatment for those children who are HLA-positive but asymptomatic. If an autoantibody or genetic screen is positive, a small intestinal biopsy is obtained to detect the classic mucosal changes caused by gluten-induced enteropathy. A wide variety of screening tests for malabsorption also may be useful. Even

BOX 37.1 Symptoms of Celiac Disease

Gastro-intestinal Symptoms	Extraintestinal Symptoms
Diarrhea	Fatigue
Abdominal pain and distension	Weight loss, growth failure
Vomiting	Delayed puberty
	Dermatitis herpetiformis
Anorexia	Dental enamel hypoplasia, aphthous stomatitis
Constipation	Arthritis
	Osteoporosis
	Fractures
	Neurological manifestations: ataxia, neuropathy, seizures

Data from Ferraz, E. G., de Jesus Campos, E., Sarmento, V. A., et al. (2012). *Pediatric Dentistry, 34*(7), 485–488; Guandalini, S., & Assiri, A. (2014). *JAMA Pediatrics, 168*(3), 274; Hadjivassiliou, M., Duker, A. P., & Sanders, D. S. (2014). *Handbook of Clinical Neurology, 120,* 607–619.

though there are very useful screening tools to diagnose CD, many children remain undiagnosed.

Treatment consists of lifelong adherence to a gluten-free diet, which includes elimination of wheat, rye, barley, and malt. **Lactose intolerance** also may be present from damage to villi; therefore, lactose (milk sugar) also may be excluded from the diet but should be resumed after treatment. Infants are routinely given vitamin D, iron, and folic acid supplements to treat deficiencies. Bone mineral density screening is required. For most children, the long-term prognosis is excellent. There is an increased incidence of malignant disease, particularly lymphoma, in individuals who fail to respond or are nonadherent to a gluten-free diet.[61]

Malnutrition

Pediatric malnutrition is an imbalance between nutrient requirements and intake that results in energy, protein, and micronutrient deficits that negatively impact growth and development. Malnutrition also involves impaired absorption and altered nutrient utilization. **Kwashiorkor** (deficiency of dietary protein) and **marasmus** (all forms of inadequate nutrient intake) are the two most common types of malnutrition in children. Collectively, they are known as **protein-energy malnutrition (PEM)**. PEM describes the effects of malnutrition but not the etiology or interactions that contribute to nutrient depletion.

Both kwashiorkor and marasmus are states of long-term starvation and are the result of widespread nutritional deficiencies among children in developing countries and economically destitute populations, particularly when associated with human immunodeficiency virus (HIV) infection.[62] Kwashiorkor usually occurs in infants or children from 1 to 4 years of age who have been weaned from breast milk to a high-starch, protein-deficient diet. The death rate of kwashiorkor is higher than that for marasmus.

Marasmus can occur at any age, but it is common in children younger than 1 year. In marasmus, starvation is attributable to lack of protein and carbohydrates, and in neglected children it can have a psychogenic basis. In developing countries and impoverished populations, early weaning of breastfed infants to overdiluted commercial formulas is a risk factor for marasmus.

Although PEM is common in developing countries, it is underestimated in hospitalized children. A new paradigm used to define pediatric malnutrition includes etiology (illness or environmental), identification of pathogenesis and chronicity, associations with inflammation, and resulting impact on functional outcomes.[63] PEM is a known complication of chronic diseases, such as chronic fever; infectious diseases like tuberculosis; malignancy; digestive and malabsorptive disorders; cardiac, pulmonary, kidney, and neurological diseases; burns or hypermetabolic states; anorexia and bulimia; and psychogenic illness.

PATHOPHYSIOLOGY. The pathogenesis of kwashiorkor is uncertain but includes inadequate dietary protein, leaky gut syndrome (compromised gut barrier), and intestinal inflammation.

The lack of sufficient plasma proteins results in generalized edema with a substantial loss of potassium. The liver swells with stored fat because no hepatic proteins are synthesized to form and release lipoproteins. Pancreatic atrophy and fibrosis may be present. Kwashiorkor also causes malabsorption, reduced bone density, and impaired renal function. If the condition is not reversed, the prognosis is very poor.

The metabolic response in marasmus is different, allowing sustained protein and lipid supply during periods of decreased dietary intake. Metabolic processes, including liver function, are preserved, but growth is severely developmentally delayed. Caloric intake is too low to support protein synthesis for growth or the storage of fat. Muscle and fat wasting occur, and anemia is common and can be severe.[64]

CLINICAL MANIFESTATIONS. Children with kwashiorkor have appropriate stores of protein and fat but these are mobilized inadequately. They have marked generalized edema, dermatoses, hypopigmented hair, distended abdomen, hepatomegaly, and almost normal weight for age (because of edema). Children with marasmus demonstrate greater wasting of protein and fat stores yet have improved survival. Marasmus is characterized by muscle wasting, fatty liver and hepatomegaly, diarrhea, dermatosis, low hemoglobin level, and infection. There is loss of subcutaneous fat and an absence of edema. Both conditions lead to delays in physical, behavioural, and cognitive development and academic performance

EVALUATION AND TREATMENT. Evaluation of PEM is based on nutritional history and clinical manifestations, including anthropometric measurements. Laboratory monitoring is used to assess for macronutrient and micronutrient deficiencies, aminotransaminase alterations, and response to refeeding. The provision of deficient nutrients will resolve clinical symptoms in 4 to 6 weeks. Use of antibiotics has been shown to improve recovery of PEM and decrease mortality.[65] Developmental sequelae of PEM may be irreversible; therefore, early intervention is recommended. Nutritional rehabilitation with appropriate environmental stimulation for infants and young children has been shown to resolve or improve cerebral shrinkage, physical growth, and psychomotor development.

Failure to Thrive or Growth Faltering

Failure to thrive (FTT) or **growth faltering (GF)** is a physical sign demonstrating that a child is not receiving adequate nutrition for optimal growth and development. It is manifested as a deceleration in weight gain, a low weight/height or body-mass-index ratio, or a low weight/height/head circumference ratio. FTT is a common problem and can present at any time in childhood.[66] Approximately 80% of children with FTT present before 18 months of age.[66]

PATHOPHYSIOLOGY. Currently, there is a move away from describing FTT as organic versus nonorganic; instead, it is considered a multifactorial condition that includes biological, psychosocial, and environmental contributions that are illness related or nonillness related (Box 37.2). An underlying medical condition is never found in more than 80% of

> **BOX 37.2 Factors Associated With Failure to Thrive or Growth Faltering**
>
> Mechanical feeding difficulties (oromotor dysfunction, congenital anomalies, central nervous system disorders)
> Inadequate caloric intake or caloric absorption: infant feeding problems, underlying chronic disease or malabsorption syndromes
> Incorrect preparation of formula (too diluted, too concentrated)
> Unsuitable feeding habits (food fads, excessive juice)
> Behaviour problems that affect eating
> Disturbed parent–child relationship; parental stress, parental lack of knowledge; child neglect

Data from Kyle, U. G., Shekerdemian, L. S., & Coss-Bu, J. A. (2015). *Nutrition in Clinical Practice, 30*(2), 227–238; Mehta, N. M., Corkins, M. R., Lyman, B., et al. (2013). *Journal of Parenteral and Enteral Nutrition, 37*(4), 460–481.

cases of FTT. Categories of FTT include inadequate caloric intake, inadequate caloric absorption, and excessive caloric expenditure. Infants and children are at risk for FTT if their parents or primary caregivers are unable to provide nurturance.

CLINICAL MANIFESTATIONS. Clinical manifestations of FTT are delayed growth accompanied by manifestations of malnutrition or an underlying disease, or both. Infants who present with FTT frequently have feeding problems. Symptoms include delayed growth; pallid or dry, cracked skin; sparse hair; poorly developed musculature; decreased subcutaneous fat; and swollen abdomen with malabsorption, diarrhea, anorexia, and signs of vitamin deficiencies such as rickets. Social or emotional manifestations include reduced energy level, reduced responsiveness and interaction with the environment, social isolation, spasticity and rigidity when held or touched, inability to make eye contact or smile, refusal to eat, and rejection of foods. There may be long-term side effects on cognitive, behavioural, and academic performance.[67]

EVALUATION AND TREATMENT. FTT is suggested if a child falls below the third percentile for weight, or shows stagnation in length or weight.[68] Underlying medical conditions are evaluated. If illness is ruled out, a thorough review of psychosocial, emotional, and environmental components of care is necessary. Screening tools are available to assist with evaluation of nutrition status and to guide therapy, particularly in hospitalized children.[69]

Treatment of FTT includes treating an underlying illness (if one is found), increasing volume or caloric density of formula, increasing frequency of breastfeeding (if found to be insufficient), structuring meals and snacks, and adding high-calorie foods and additives. Eliminating fruit juice, soda, or excessive milk also will improve appetite and absorption of nutrients Nutrient deficiencies are supplemented. If the child is unable to gain weight, an oral enteral supplement may be added to the diet, or a nasogastric or gastrostomy tube can be used to supplement oral intake.

If the cause is not medical, management then involves the immediate total care of the child and measures to address (1) the psychosocial and emotional problems of the caregivers and (2) parent–child interactions. Counselling, parental modelling, and long-term family support are sometimes needed.[70]

Necrotizing Enterocolitis

Necrotizing enterocolitis (NEC) is an ischemic inflammatory condition that causes bowel necrosis and perforation. NEC is not a specific diagnosis but a constellation of signs and symptoms with several proposed etiologies. It is the most common severe neonatal GI emergency that predominantly affects the smallest and most premature infants.[71,72] Approximately 12% of infants born weighing less than 1500 g will develop NEC; of those, about 30% will not survive.[73]

PATHOPHYSIOLOGY. The exact etiology of NEC is unclear. Factors contributing to the development of NEC include infections, abnormal bacterial colonization, intestinal ischemia, immature immune responses, exaggerated inflammatory responses, immature intestinal motility and barrier function, perinatal stress, effects of medications and feeding practices, and genetic predisposition. The immature mucosal barrier delays digestion and motility is slower, allowing for the accumulation of noxious substances that damage the intestine, increase permeability, and increase the risk for infection. Translocation of intestinal bacteria and other substances contributes to injury, inflammation, and development of systemic inflammatory disease. Immature intestinal innate immunity and an unfavourable balance between normal and pathogenic bacteria promote intestinal inflammation and release of proinflammatory cytokines. Accumulation of gas in the intestine can cause pressure that decreases blood flow, and an imbalance between vasodilator and vasoconstrictor inputs in the immature gut may lead to vasoconstriction, promoting ischemia, injury, and necrosis.[74]

CLINICAL MANIFESTATIONS. Manifestations of NEC usually appear suddenly and within weeks of premature birth, and sooner for term neonates. Signs and symptoms of "classic" NEC include feeding intolerance, abdominal distension and bloody stools after 8 to 10 days of age, septicemia with elevated white blood cell count, and falling platelet levels. Unstable temperature, bradycardia, and apnea are nonspecific signs. In late preterm or term infants, NEC is more likely to be associated with other predisposing factors, such as low Apgar scores, chorioamnionitis, exchange transfusions, prolonged rupture of membranes, congenital heart disease, or neural tube defects.

EVALUATION AND TREATMENT. Abdominal radiographs show pneumatosis intestinalis or portal venous gas, or both. Symptoms usually progress rapidly, often within hours, from subtle signs to abdominal discoloration, intestinal perforation, and peritonitis or even death. Systemic hypotension requires intensive medical support or bowel resection, or both. Preventive strategies include encouragement of breast milk feeding, judicious fluid management to prevent vascular fluid overload, confirmation of patent ductus arteriosus (see Chapter 25), administration of arginine and glutamine supplements to support intestinal epithelial cell growth, and utilization of enteral probiotics to support normal gut bacteria.[71,75]

Treatments include cessation of feeding, implementation of gastric suction to decompress the intestines, maintenance of fluid and electrolyte balance, and administration of antibiotics to control sepsis. Surgical resection is the treatment of choice for perforation, and peritoneal drainage may be used as an adjunct to laparotomy.[76] Overall mortality is high, particularly for infants who have surgery.[72]

Diarrhea

> ✓ **QUICK CHECK 37.4**
> 1. Why is diarrhea such a serious disorder in infants and children?
> 2. What is biliary atresia?
> 3. What are the three most common metabolic disorders that cause liver damage in children?

Diarrhea is an increase in the water content, volume, or frequency of stools and can be acute or chronic. Diarrhea is usually defined as three or more watery or loose stools in 24 hours.[77] Children with acute gastroenteritis often remain mildly symptomatic for up to 4 weeks; therefore, diarrhea that persists longer than 4 weeks is considered chronic. Diarrhea is a common GI problem during infancy and early childhood and is the leading cause of death in young children, particularly among preterm infants and children in developing countries, with 760 000 deaths per year.[78,79] Severe, acute infectious diarrhea occurs one to three times during the first 3 years of life. Most episodes are self-limiting and resolve within 72 hours.

The pathophysiological mechanisms of diarrhea in children are similar to those described for adults—osmotic, secretory, motility, or inflammatory diarrhea (see Chapter 36). Prolonged diarrhea is more dangerous in infants and children, however, because they have much smaller fluid reserves and more rapid peristalsis and metabolism than adults. Therefore, dehydration can develop rapidly if any disturbance increases fluid secretion into the GI lumen (secretory diarrhea), draws fluid into the lumen by osmosis (osmotic diarrhea), reduces intestinal transit time with luminal fluid retention (motility diarrhea), or causes inflammation that results in malabsorption and increased luminal osmotic load from nutrients, fluid, and blood, which may increase gut motility (inflammatory diarrhea).[80]

Diarrhea in Infants and Children

There are numerous causes of diarrhea in infants and young children, including bacterial and systemic infections, malabsorption syndromes, autoimmune disorders, congenital malformations, and genetic disorders.[80] Acute infection is a common cause of childhood diarrhea worldwide.

Acute infectious diarrhea in infants and young children is usually associated with viral or bacterial gastroenteritis. Viruses include rotaviruses, noroviruses, and adenoviruses. Rotavirus is the most common cause in young children and is associated with a higher death rate in low-income countries. Rotavirus vaccine is an effective preventive strategy.[81] *Clostridium difficile* is often associated with previous antibiotic therapy.

Infectious diarrhea has a rapid onset, with watery stools sometimes mixed with blood, abdominal cramping, fever, vomiting, and weight loss. Severe dehydration, acidosis, and shock can occur quickly from diarrhea and vomiting.[82] Hemolytic uremic syndrome and kidney failure can develop when diarrhea is associated with *Shigella* toxin and *Escherichia coli* infection (see Chapter 31). Other causes of acute diarrhea in children include antibiotic therapy, appendicitis, chemotherapy, inflammatory bowel disease, parasitic infestation, parenteral infections, and ingestion of toxic substances.

Treatment of diarrhea requires evaluation of cause through history, stool testing for common pathogens, and laboratory analysis. Treatment of underlying illness is warranted when identified. Other treatments include fluid and electrolyte replacement, and antibiotics if a pathogen is found. Antispasmodics may relieve abdominal cramping, and probiotics can reduce duration and improve morbidity and mortality.[83] Intravenous solutions are used only when oral solutions are not tolerated.[82] Prevention includes clean water, environmental sanitation, and good hygiene.

DISORDERS OF THE LIVER

Disorders of Biliary Metabolism and Transport

Neonatal Jaundice

Jaundice (icterus) is a yellow pigmentation of the skin caused by an increased level of bilirubin in the bloodstream (total serum bilirubin) that exceeds the 95th percentile for the infant's age in hours.

Physiological jaundice (hyperbilirubinemia) of the newborn, or *neonatal bilirubinemia*, is a frequently encountered problem in otherwise healthy newborns caused by lack of maturity of bilirubin uptake and conjugation. Poor caloric intake or dehydration, or both, associated with inadequate breastfeeding also may contribute to the high levels of bilirubin. Although up to 60% of term newborns have clinical jaundice in the first week of life, with a higher percentage in the preterm population, few have significant underlying disease. High bilirubin levels in the newborn period can be associated with hemolytic disease of the newborn, metabolic and endocrine disorders, anatomical abnormalities of the liver, and infections. For older infants and children, the most common causes of unconjugated hyperbilirubinemia are hemolytic processes resulting in bilirubin overproduction. *Pathological jaundice* is a bilirubin concentration greater than 342 μmol/L in the newborn period associated with a severe illness, or a total serum bilirubin level that rises by more than 85.5 μmol/L during the newborn period.

Risk factors for development of pathological jaundice include fetal–maternal blood type incompatibility (ABO and Rh incompatibility, hemolytic disease of the newborn), premature birth, exclusive breastfeeding in some infants, maternal age greater than or equal to 25 years, male gender, delayed meconium passage, glucose-6-phosphate dehydrogenase deficiency, and excessive birth trauma such as bruising or cephalohematomas.[84,85]

PATHOPHYSIOLOGY. Pathological jaundice results from the complex interaction of factors that cause (1) increased bilirubin production (e.g., hemolysis), (2) impaired hepatic uptake or excretion of unconjugated bilirubin, or (3) delayed maturation of liver bilirubin conjugating mechanisms.[85] The most common cause is hemolytic disease of the newborn (ABO blood incompatibility) (see Chapters 8 and 22), and all pregnant women should be tested for ABO and Rh incompatibility. Unconjugated bilirubin (indirect bilirubin) is lipid soluble and bound to albumin in the blood, and in the free form it readily crosses the blood–brain barrier in infants. Chronic bilirubin encephalopathy (kernicterus) is caused by the deposition of toxic, unconjugated bilirubin in brain cells and usually does not occur in healthy, full-term infants. The mechanism of injury is not clearly known. Elevated conjugated bilirubin level is a sign of underlying disease.

CLINICAL MANIFESTATIONS. Physiological jaundice develops during the second or third day after birth and usually subsides in 1 to 2 weeks in full-term infants and in 2 to 4 weeks in premature infants. After this period, increasing bilirubin values and persistent jaundice indicate pathological hyperbilirubinemia. Manifestations include yellowing of skin, dark urine, light-coloured stools, and weight loss. Premature infants with respiratory distress, acidosis, or sepsis are at greater risk for kernicterus (brain damage related to unconjugated hyperbilirubinemia) and the development of athetoid cerebral palsy and speech and hearing impairment.[85]

EVALUATION AND TREATMENT. Jaundice is detected by clinical assessment. Both total and direct (conjugated) bilirubin levels are monitored as described previously. Other causes of jaundice must be eliminated to confirm physiological jaundice. Treatment depends on the degree of hyperbilirubinemia. Physiological jaundice is commonly treated by phototherapy and several techniques are available.[86] Pathological jaundice requires an exchange transfusion and treatment of the underlying disorder.

Biliary Atresia

Biliary atresia (BA) is a rare congenital malformation (from 1 in 8 000 to 1 in 18 000 live births) characterized by the absence or obstruction of intrahepatic or extrahepatic bile ducts; the most common cause of BA is neonatal cholestasis.[87] The etiology of duct injury is not clear but is thought to be related to an embryonic, congenital, or genetic abnormality or an acquired, perinatal, viral-induced progressive inflammation with innate autoimmune destruction. The disease expression is a continuum in which the principal process is one of bile duct destruction.[88] The atresia or obstruction of the bile ducts leads to plugging, inflammation, fibrosis of the bile canaliculi, and cholestasis. Progressive obstruction leads to secondary biliary cirrhosis (see Chapter 36), portal hypertension, or liver failure.

Jaundice is the primary clinical manifestation of BA, along with hepatomegaly and acholic (clay-coloured) stools. Fat absorption is impaired because of the lack of bile salts. Abdominal distension caused by hepatomegaly and ascites may cause anorexia and FTT. Fat-soluble vitamin (A, D, E, K) deficiencies require supplementation. Manifestations of cirrhosis and liver failure include ascites, hypoalbuminemia, hypercoagulation, pruritus, esophageal varices, and GI bleeding that may lead to death.

Early diagnosis of BA is essential, with the best outcome occurring when it is diagnosed and treated in the first 30 to 45 days of life. Late diagnosis of BA does not respond well to current surgical treatment. Diagnosis of BA is based on clinical manifestations, abnormal liver function tests, liver biopsy results, and intraoperative cholangiogram. Serum aminotransaminase and alkaline phosphatase levels are elevated and conjugated (direct) serum bilirubin levels rise progressively. BA can be relieved by hepatoportoenterostomy (also called the *Kasai procedure*). Even with initial restoration of bile flow, however, obliteration of intrahepatic bile ducts can continue and cirrhosis results. Liver transplantation is a successful long-term therapy for BA.[89] Eighty percent of children with BA die before the age of 3 years if not treated.

Inflammatory Disorders
Hepatitis
Viral hepatitis is discussed in Chapter 36, and the characteristics of the types of viruses that cause hepatitis are presented in Table 36.8.

Hepatitis A virus. Approximately 30 to 50% of reported cases of hepatitis A virus (HAV) occur in children,[90] particularly children of nursery school age.

Outbreaks tend to occur in day care centres with large numbers of children who are not toilet trained and staff members who practice poor handwashing techniques.[91] Vertical transmission from mother to newborn or from a transfusion is rare. HAV in children is usually mild and asymptomatic, but it may involve nausea, vomiting, and diarrhea. Jaundice appears in more than 70% of older children. Almost all children recover from hepatitis A without residual liver damage.

Hepatitis B virus. Risk factors for hepatitis B virus (HBV) include infants of mothers who are chronic hepatitis B surface antigen (HBsAg) carriers; children who immigrated with their families or through adoption from endemic areas; children who live with HBsAg-positive household members; and children who abuse parenteral medications or engage in unprotected sex. Ninety percent of newborns are infected by their mothers (vertical transmission); 25 to 50% of children between the ages of 1 and 5 years of age who are acutely infected will develop chronic infection.[92] Chronic hepatitis may develop because the infant's immune system is immature. Infected infants are at risk for cirrhosis and hepatocellular carcinoma.[93] Hepatitis D virus (HDV) infection depends on active infection with HBV. Exacerbation of HBV is more common in children with superinfected HDV. There is evidence that the risk for fulminant hepatitis is higher in individuals with combined infection of HBV and HDV than in those with HBV infection alone.[94] There also is a higher risk for hepatocellular carcinoma and increased mortality in this group. Aggressive HBV vaccination programs have reduced the incidence of HBV; HDV reduction has mirrored this response.[95] To prevent perinatal transmission of HBV, immunoprophylaxis and HBV vaccination within the first 12 hours of birth are recommended with close follow-up visits.[96] Treatment is conservative and antivirals are used for chronic disease. Children aged 2 to 17 years who are HBsAg seropositive for more than 6 months with elevated serum alanine transaminase and HBV DNA levels for more than 3 months may be eligible for treatment with antivirals. Maternal antiviral therapy may be given during the third trimester when there is impending liver decompensation.[97]

Hepatitis C virus. Hepatitis C virus (HCV) in children is most commonly transmitted vertically and is enhanced with maternal co-infection with HIV. Risk factors for vertical transmission include internal fetal monitoring, prolonged rupture of membranes, and fetal anoxia.[98] HCV transmission also can occur through exposure to infected blood or contaminated materials (as in injection medication use or tattooing and body piercing) and, less commonly, following sexual encounters with HCV-infected partners. Transmission from blood transfusions has become a negligible risk with universal HCV screening of blood. Because of adverse drug events, only children with persistently elevated serum aminotransferases or those with progressive liver disease are treated with antiviral medications.

Chronic hepatitis. HBV and HCV are the main causes of chronic hepatitis in children. Manifestations of chronic hepatitis include malaise, anorexia, fever, GI bleeding, hepatomegaly, edema, and transient joint pain. Often there are no symptoms. Serum alanine aminotransferase and bilirubin levels are elevated. There may be evidence of impairment of synthetic functions of the liver: prolonged prothrombin time, thrombocytopenia, and hypoalbuminemia. Diagnosis is based on the clinical manifestations and liver biopsy results. There is no curative therapy for chronic HBV. Children are treated with antiviral medications and should continue to be monitored.[99] Liver transplant may ultimately be required for chronic hepatitis.

There also are autoimmune forms of chronic hepatitis, *autoimmune hepatitis* or *primary sclerosing cholangitis*, with unknown etiologies. The pathogenic mechanism is thought to be immunological, environmental, or genetic in nature. These diseases present with elevations in the levels of aminotransferases, autoantibodies, and immunoglobulin G (IgG). Autoimmune hepatitis is more common in female children, and both are treated with immunosuppressive therapy; about 50 to 80% will achieve remission and long-term survival.

Treatment and self-care, including reducing alcohol intake, can prevent progressive liver disease and improve quality of life. Treatment of HCV is shifting from older, poorly tolerated interferon-based therapies, which cure approximately 55% of those treated, to new well-tolerated short-course (8 to 12 weeks) interferon-free direct-acting antiviral drugs with cure rates approaching more than 95%. However, treatment can only occur if undiagnosed people get tested and if diagnosed people are engaged in care.[100]

Cirrhosis
Cirrhosis is fibrotic scarring of the liver in response to inflammation and tissue damage resulting in obstruction to the flow of blood and bile. Most forms of chronic liver diseases in children can progress to cirrhosis, but they seldom do so. The complications of cirrhosis in children are the same as those in adults: portal hypertension, the opening of collateral vessels between the portal and systemic veins, and varices. In addition, children with cirrhosis experience growth failure caused by nutritional deficits, as well as developmental delay, particularly in gross motor function because of ascites and weakness. The cause of cirrhosis may influence its severity and course. Some types of cirrhosis can be stabilized if the cause is identified and treated early.[98] The

risk for cirrhosis is increasing in obese children who have nonalcoholic fatty liver disease (NAFLD).

Portal Hypertension

Portal hypertension is increased pressure in the portal venous system (see Chapter 36) and a major cause of morbidity and mortality in children with liver disease. There are two basic causes of portal hypertension in children: (1) increased resistance to blood flow within the portal system and (2) increased volume of portal blood flow. The second cause is rare in children and is not discussed here. Increased resistance to flow can occur anywhere in the portal circulatory system. Portal hypertension can accompany cirrhosis, intra-abdominal infections, portal vein thrombosis, congenital anomalies of the portal vein, and congenital hepatic fibrosis.

Types of Portal Hypertension

Extrahepatic portal hypertension. Extrahepatic (prehepatic) portal venous obstruction causes 50 to 70% of the cases of extrahepatic portal hypertension in children. In approximately two-thirds of these children, no specific cause can be found.[101] Obstruction is almost always in the portal vein and is usually caused by thrombosis as a complication of abdominal trauma, pancreatitis, abdominal infections, and some systemic disorders; however, these causes are rare. Life-threatening bleeding and coagulation disorders can occur. Mesoportal bypass (anastomosis of portal vein to mesenteric vein) restores normal physiological portal flow to the liver and corrects portal hypertension.[102]

Intrahepatic portal hypertension. Liver fibrosis is the primary cause of intrahepatic portal hypertension. The fibrosis can lead to cirrhosis with increased resistance to portal blood flow by constricting and reducing the compliance of hepatic sinusoids. Chronic hepatitis, BA, NAFLD, and congenital hepatic fibrosis are causes of liver fibrosis in children.[103–106]

The clinical manifestations of portal hypertension are (1) splenomegaly, (2) upper GI tract bleeding, (3) ascites, (4) hepatopulmonary syndrome, (5) hepatorenal syndrome, and (6) hepatic encephalopathy (see Chapter 36).

The objectives of the clinical investigation are to (1) locate the site of the venous block and (2) identify the disease responsible for the portal hypertension. The following may be included in the diagnostic evaluation: thorough physical examination; laboratory evaluation of liver function, white blood cell count, and platelet count; ultrasonographic imaging; endoscopic evaluation; and biopsy. Treatment in children is the same as that in adults (see Chapter 36). The outcome of portal hypertension depends almost entirely on its cause. Children with extrahepatic disease are expected to recover with little morbidity. For children with intrahepatic disease, the prognosis varies.

Metabolic Disorders

More than 5000 genetically determined metabolic pathways have been identified in liver tissue. The earliest possible identification of metabolic disorders is essential because (1) early treatment may prevent permanent damage to vital organs, such as the liver or brain; (2) precise genetic counselling may be possible with prenatal diagnosis; and (3) complications can be minimized, even if cure is not possible. Galactosemia, fructosemia, glycogen storage disease (GSD), and Wilson's disease are the most common metabolic disorders. They are treatable and have hepatic clinical manifestations. The mechanisms of disease, clinical manifestations, and evaluation and treatment of these disorders are presented in Table 37.2.

GASTRO-INTESTINAL MALIGNANCIES IN CHILDREN

Globally, cancers in children (0 to 14 years of age) differ from those occurring in adults in terms of their origin and their malignant

TABLE 37.2 Galactosemia, Fructosemia, and Wilson's Disease

	Galactosemia	Fructosemia	Wilson's Disease
Mechanism of disease	Deficiency of galactose-1-phosphate uridylyltransferase Autosomal recessive trait Inability to convert galactose to glucose Toxic accumulation of galactose in body tissues, liver, and brain	Deficiency of fructose-1-phosphate aldolase Autosomal recessive trait Inability to metabolize fructose, sucrose, or honey; occurs when breast milk is replaced with cow's milk Toxic accumulation of fructose in body tissues	Autosomal recessive: defect on chromosome 13 (ATP 7B) Defect in copper excretion by liver Impaired transport of copper into bile/blood caused by diminished transport protein (ceruloplasmin) Toxic accumulations of copper in liver, brain, kidney, corneas
Clinical manifestation	High levels of blood galactose Vomiting Hypoglycemia May have failure to thrive Symptoms of cirrhosis at 2–6 months jaundice Intellectual disabilities if not treated Cataracts if not treated	High levels of blood fructose Vomiting Hypoglycemia May have failure to thrive Hepatomegaly Jaundice Seizures	Intention tremors Indistinct speech Dystonia Greenish yellow rings in cornea Hepatomegaly Jaundice Anorexia Renal tubular defects
Evaluation	Newborn screening Presence of reducing substances in urine when infant is receiving lactose	Detailed dietary history Liver or intestinal mucosa biopsy	Low plasma ceruloplasmin level
Treatment	Galactose-free diet	Fructose, sucrose, honey-free diet Vitamin C supplementation	Chelation therapy to remove copper from body Decreased dietary intake of copper Liver transplant

behaviour. Tumours in children generally have shorter latency periods and are more aggressive and invasive than tumours in adults.

Hepatoblastoma

Hepatoblastoma is the most common pediatric liver cancer, representing more than 90% of malignant liver tumours diagnosed in children under 5 years of age.[107,108] It usually affects young children within the first 3 years of life, and boys are more affected than girls. Children with hepatoblastoma typically present with an abdominal mass that causes pain and discomfort. Parents often report that their child has lost their appetite and is losing weight. Patients also develop weakness and fatigue in addition abdominal swelling and hepatomegaly on physical examination.

Hepatoblastomas are heterogeneous tumours that usually display combinations of epithelial, mesenchymal, undifferentiated, and/or other components. The most common epithelial component is the embryonal pattern, which is characterized by histological patterns recapitulating liver development, and is sometimes associated with genetic disorders.[108]

Hepatoblastoma is often associated with aberrant activation of developmental pathways similar to other embryonal tumours in children. Hepatoblastoma therapy generally includes a combination of surgical resection and chemotherapy. If surgical removal presents a high risk for mortality owing to the size and location of this tumour inside the liver, cure is still possible with liver transplantation. Unfortunately, the prognosis is still poor for children with unresectable or disseminated hepatoblastoma.[109]

Pancreatic Tumours

Malignant pancreatic tumours are a heterogeneous assortment of benign or malignant neoplasms, arising from exocrine cells or endocrine cells that are extremely rare in pediatric age. While pancreatic cancer is one of the most frequent fatal malignancies in adults, only very small series and a few case reports have been published in the pediatric oncology literature.[110] The main clinical symptom is abdominal pain associated with a palpable mass on examination. Patients also often report a lack of appetite and vomiting.

DID YOU UNDERSTAND?

Overview
1. Alterations of digestive function in children include congenital obstructions of the intestinal tract; disorders of digestion, absorption, or nutrition; or liver disease.

Disorders of the Gastro-intestinal Tract
1. Cleft lip and cleft palate (failure of the bony palate to fuse in the midline) may occur separately or together. The fissure may affect the uvula, soft palate, hard palate, nostril, and maxillary alveolar ridge, with difficulty sucking and swallowing.
2. Esophageal atresia, a condition in which the esophagus ends in a blind pouch, may occur with or without tracheoesophageal fistula. As the infant swallows oral secretions or ingests milk, the pouch fills, causing either drooling or aspiration into the lungs.
3. Infantile hypertrophic pyloric stenosis is an obstruction of the pyloric outlet caused by hypertrophy of circular muscles in the pyloric sphincter.
4. Meckel diverticulum is a congenital malformation of the GI tract involving all layers of the small intestinal wall; it usually occurs in the ileum.
5. Meconium ileus is a newborn condition in which intestinal secretions and amniotic waste products produce a thick, tarry plug that obstructs the intestine; it occurs in 10 to 15% of newborns with cystic fibrosis (CF).
6. Idiopathic intestinal pseudo-obstruction is a disorder of impaired intestinal motility.
7. Hirschsprung's disease (aganglionic megacolon) is caused by a malformation of the parasympathetic nervous system in a segment of the colon needed for peristalsis, resulting in colon obstruction.
8. Malformations of the anus and rectum range from mild congenital stenosis of the anus to complex deformities, all of which are classified as imperforate anus.
9. Gastroesophageal reflux disease is the presence of symptoms related to the return of stomach contents into the esophagus caused by relaxation or incompetence of the lower esophageal sphincter that results from immaturity of the gastroesophageal sphincter.
10. Intussusception is the telescoping of a proximal segment of intestine into a distal segment, causing an obstruction.
11. CF is an inherited fibrocystic disease that involves mucosal chloride and sodium ion channels in many organs, including the GI tract and pancreas; CF causes pancreatic enzyme deficiency with maldigestion.
12. Celiac disease is caused by hypersensitivity to gluten protein, with autoimmune injury and loss of the villous epithelium. It results in malabsorption and growth failure.
13. Pediatric malnutrition is an imbalance between nutrient requirements and intake that results in energy, protein, and micronutrient deficits, which negatively impact growth and development.
14. Kwashiorkor is a severe protein deficiency. Marasmus is a deficiency of all dietary nutrients, including carbohydrates.
15. Failure to thrive or growth faltering is a multifactorial condition that includes biological, psychosocial, and environmental contributions; it may or may not be illness related; and it results in inadequate physical growth and development of a child.
16. Necrotizing enterocolitis is an ischemic inflammatory disorder in neonates, particularly premature infants, thought to result from immaturity, infection, stress, and anoxia of the bowel wall.
17. Acute diarrhea in infants and children is three or more watery or loose stools in 24 hours; it is commonly caused by viral or bacterial enterocolitis.
18. Chronic diarrhea (diarrhea persisting longer than 4 weeks) can be caused by a wide variety of underlying conditions and often leads to growth failure and slow development.
19. Primary lactose intolerance is the inability to digest milk sugar because of a lack of the enzyme lactase, resulting in osmotic diarrhea.

Disorders of the Liver
1. Physiological jaundice of the newborn is caused by mild hyperbilirubinemia that subsides in 1 or 2 weeks. Pathological jaundice is caused by severe hyperbilirubinemia and can cause brain damage (kernicterus).
2. Biliary atresia is a congenital malformation of the bile ducts that obstructs bile flow and causes jaundice, cirrhosis, and liver failure.
3. Acute hepatitis is usually caused by a virus, and hepatitis A is the most common form of childhood hepatitis. Chronic hepatitis B or C usually occurs by maternal transmission.

4. Cirrhosis results from fibrotic scarring of the liver and is rare in children, but it can develop from most forms of chronic liver disease.
5. Portal hypertension in children usually is caused by extrahepatic obstruction, and the cause is often unknown. Intrahepatic obstruction is related to diseases that cause liver fibrosis.
6. The four most common metabolic disorders that cause liver damage in children are galactosemia, fructosemia, glycogen storage disease, and Wilson's disease. All are inherited as genetic traits and allow toxins to accumulate in the liver.

38

Structure and Function of the Musculoskeletal System

Stephanie Zettel, with originating chapter contributions by Geri C. Reeves

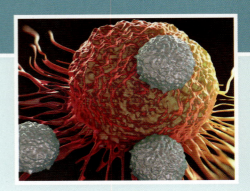

Additional resources are available online at https://evolve.elsevier.com/Canada/Huether/pathophysiology.

CHAPTER OUTLINE

Structure and Function of Bones, 943
  Elements of Bone Tissue, 943
  Types of Bone Tissue, 947
  Characteristics of Bone, 948
  Maintenance of Bone Integrity, 949
Structure and Function of Joints, 950
  Fibrous Joints, 950
  Cartilaginous Joints, 950
  Synovial Joints, 953

Structure and Function of Skeletal Muscles, 953
  Whole Muscle, 953
  Components of Muscle Function, 958
  Tendons and Ligaments, 961
Aging and the Musculoskeletal System, 961
  Aging of Bones, 961
  Aging of Joints, 962
  Aging of Muscles, 962

LEARNING OBJECTIVES

1. Identify the different cells of bone tissue and their corresponding functions.
2. Discuss the methods by which bones are grouped and classified.
3. Briefly discuss the process of bone remodelling and bone repair.
4. Discuss the methods by which joints are classified.
5. Describe the structure and function of articular cartilage in synovial joints.
6. List and describe the different types of skeletal muscles.
7. Describe the motor unit of a muscle.
8. Describe the structure of the myofibril and sarcomere.
9. Describe the cellular and molecular mechanisms of muscle contraction.
10. Discuss the factors that affect muscle contraction.
11. Describe the process of muscle metabolism.
12. Identify types of muscle contraction.
13. Describe the function of ligaments and tendons.
14. Discuss the effects of aging on bone, joints, and muscle.

KEY TERMS

Agonist, 961
α-Glycoprotein, 947
Amphiarthrosis (slightly movable joint), 950
Antagonist, 961
Appendicular skeleton, 948
Articular cartilage, 951
Axial skeleton, 948
Basement membrane, 956
Basic multicellular unit, 949
Bone albumin, 947
Bone fluid, 947
Bone matrix, 943
Calcification, 943
Canaliculus (*pl.*, canaliculi), 947
Chondrocyte, 951
Collagen fibre, 945
Compact bone (cortical bone), 947
Concentric (shortening) contraction, 961
Contraction, 958
Coupling, 958
Cross-bridge theory, 958
Diaphysis, 948
Diarthrosis (freely movable joint), 950
Dynamic (isotonic) contraction, 961
Eccentric (lengthening) contraction, 961
Endomysium, 953
Endosteum, 948
Enthesis, 961
Epimysium, 953
Epiphysis, 948
Excitation, 958
Fascia, 953
Fascicle, 953
Fibril, 945
Fibrous joint, 950
Flat bone, 949
Fusiform muscle, 953
Glycoprotein, 947
Golgi tendon organ, 955
Gomphosis, 950
Ground substance, 943
Growth plate (epiphyseal plate), 948
Haversian canal, 947
Haversian system, 947
Hydroxyapatite (HAP), 947
Integrin, 945
Irregular bone, 949
Isometric (static) contraction, 961
Joint (articular) capsule, 950
Joint (articulation), 950
Joint (synovial) cavity, 950
Lacuna, 945
Lamella (*pl.*, lamellae), 947
Ligament, 961
Long bone, 948
Metaphysis, 948
Mineralization, 947
Motor unit, 954
Muscle fibre action potential, 955
Muscle fibre (muscle cell), 955
Muscle membrane, 956
Myoblast, 955

Myofibril, 955
Myoglobin, 956
Osteoblast, 943
Osteocalcin, 947
Osteoclast, 945
Osteocyte, 945
Osteoid, 943
Osteoprotegerin (OPG), 945
Oxygen debt, 960
Pennate muscle, 953
Perimysium, 953
Periosteum, 947
Physiological tetanus, 960
Podosome, 945
Proteoglycan, 945
Receptor activator of nuclear factor kappa-B ligand (RANKL), 945
Relaxation, 960
Remodelling, 949
Repetitive discharge, 960
Resorb, 943
Ruffled border, 945
Sarcolemma, 956
Sarcomere, 956
Sarcopenia, 962
Sarcoplasm, 956
Sarcoplasmic reticulum, 956
Sarcotubular system, 956
Sarcotubule, 956
Satellite cell, 955
Short bone, 949
Sialoprotein, 947
Skeletal muscle (voluntary, striated, or extrafusal muscle), 954
Spindle, 955
Spongy bone (cancellous bone), 947
Static (holding) contraction, 961
Suture, 950
Symphysis, 950
Synarthrosis (immovable joint), 950
Synchondrosis, 950
Syndesmosis, 950
Synovial fluid, 951
Synovial joint, 953
Synovial membrane, 950
Tendon, 961
Tidemark, 952
Trabecula (*pl.*, trabeculae), 947
Transverse tubule, 956
Type I fibre (red slow-twitch fibre), 955
Type II fibre (white fast-twitch fibre), 955
Voluntary muscle, 954

Regular function and movement, as well as normal activities of daily living, depend on the integrity of the musculoskeletal system. The musculoskeletal system is actually two systems: (1) the skeleton, composed of bones and joints, and (2) soft tissues (skeletal muscles, tendons, and ligaments). Each system contributes to mobility. The skeleton supports the body and provides leverage to the skeletal muscles in order to make movement of various parts of the body possible. Contraction of the skeletal muscles and bending or rotation at the joints facilitate movements of the various body parts.

STRUCTURE AND FUNCTION OF BONES

✓ **QUICK CHECK 38.1**
1. Name the different types of bone cells.
2. What are the major cells involved in bone resorption?
3. Briefly describe the process of remodelling.
4. What are the stages of bone healing?

Bones give form to the body, support tissues, and allow movement by providing points of attachment for muscles. Many bones meet in movable joints that determine the type and extent of movement possible. Bones also protect many of the body's vital organs. For example, the bones of the skull, thorax, and pelvis are hard exterior shields that protect the brain, heart and lungs, and reproductive and urinary organs, respectively.

The marrow cavities within certain bones serve as sites of blood cell formation. In adults, blood cells originate exclusively in the marrow cavities of the skull, vertebrae, ribs, sternum, shoulders, and pelvis. The development of blood cells is discussed in Chapter 20. Bones also have a crucial role in mineral homeostasis (storing minerals [i.e., calcium, phosphate, carbonate, magnesium] that are essential for the proper performance of many delicate cellular mechanisms), play a role in hormone homeostasis, and assist in maintaining normal immunological function.

Elements of Bone Tissue

Mature bone is a rigid connective tissue consisting of cells, fibres, a gelatinous material termed 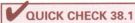 ground substance, and large amounts of crystallized minerals, mainly calcium, that give bone its rigidity. Ground substance consists of proteoglycans and hyaluronic acid secreted by chondroblasts. The structural elements of bone are summarized in Table 38.1.

Bone cells enable bone to grow, repair itself, change shape, and continuously synthesize new bone tissue and **resorb** (dissolve or digest) old tissue. The fibres in bone are made of collagen, which gives bone its tensile strength (the ability to hold itself together). Ground substance acts as a medium for the diffusion of nutrients, oxygen, metabolic wastes, biochemicals, and minerals between bone tissue and blood vessels.

Bone formation begins during fetal life with the growth of cartilage—the precursor of bone tissue. In mature bone, the formation of new tissue begins with the production of an organic matrix by the bone cells. This **bone matrix** consists of ground substance, collagen, and other proteins (see Table 38.1) that take part in bone formation and maintenance.

The next step in bone formation is **calcification**, in which minerals are deposited and then crystallize. Minerals bind tightly to collagen fibres, producing tensile and compressional strength in bone that allow it to withstand pressure and weight-bearing.

Bone Cells

Bone contains three types of cells: osteoblasts, osteocytes, and osteoclasts (Figure. 38.1). Both osteoblasts and osteocytes originate from osteoprogenitor cells found in the mesenchymal stem cell (MSC) lineage. Unlike osteoblasts and osteocytes, osteoclasts originate from hematopoietic stem cells. Osteoblasts are the bone-forming cells. Once this function is complete, osteoblasts become osteocytes. Osteocytes, the most numerous cells within bone, are osteoblasts that have become imprisoned within the mineralized bone matrix. They have multiple important duties in maintaining bone homeostasis, including synthesizing new bone matrix molecules and initiating osteoclast function. Osteoclasts primarily resorb (remove) bone during processes of growth and repair.

Osteoblasts. Originating from MSCs, **osteoblasts** are the primary bone-producing cells, and are involved in many functions related to the skeletal system (see Table 38.1). Osteoblasts are responsive to parathyroid hormone (PTH) and produce *osteocalcin* (a small protein hormone present in bone and dentin that has numerous metabolic functions in the body) when stimulated by 1,25-dihydroxy-vitamin D_3.[1] Osteoblasts are active on the outer surfaces of bones, where they form a single layer of cells. Osteoblasts initiate new bone formation by their synthesis of **osteoid** (nonmineralized bone matrix). Osteoblasts also mineralize newly formed bone matrix. Stimulation of new bone formation and orderly mineralization of bone matrix occur by concentrating some of the plasma proteins (growth factors) found in the bone matrix and by facilitating the deposit and exchange

TABLE 38.1 Structural Elements of Bone

Structural Elements	Function
Bone Cells	
Osteoblasts	Synthesize collagen and proteoglycans, mineralize osteoid matrix; produce receptor activator of nuclear factor kappa-B ligand (RANKL), which in turn stimulates osteoclast resorption of bone; also produce osteoprotegerin, which inhibits osteoclast formation by binding to RANKL
Osteoclasts	Resorb bone; major role in bone homeostasis
Osteocytes	Transform osteoblasts trapped in osteoid; signal both osteoblasts and osteoclasts; maintain bone matrix; mechanosensory receptors to reduce or augment bone mass; produce sclerostin, which inhibits bone growth
Bone Matrix	
Bone morphogenic proteins (BMPs)	Induce and regulate bone and cartilage formation; affect all other organ systems; a subfamily of transforming growth factor-beta cytokine growth factors
BMP-1	Plays a key role in extracellular matrix formation; is unrelated to other BMPs (is a metalloprotease)
BMP-2	Promotes chondrogenesis, bone formation; clinically used to enhance bone formation in spine surgery
BMP-3 (osteogenin)	Inhibits bone formation
BMP-4	Is involved in osteoblast differentiation; involved in cartilage repair, endochondral bone formation; enhances chondrogenesis
BMP-6	Found in human plasma; promotes osteoblast differentiation from mesenchymal stem cells (MSCs)
BMP-7	Is involved in osteogenic cell formation from MSCs; enhances bone formation in spine surgery; induces formation of brown fat
BMP-9	Promotes osteoblast formation from MSCs
BMP-13	Inhibits bone formation by reducing calcium mineralization
Collagen fibres	Lend support and tensile strength
Proteoglycans	Control transport of ionized materials through matrix
Glycoproteins	
Albumin	Transports essential elements to matrix; maintains osmotic pressure of bone fluid
α-Glycoproteins	Promote calcification
Laminin	Stabilizes basement membranes in bones
Osteocalcin	Inhibits calcium phosphate precipitation (attracts calcium ions to incorporate into hydroxyapatite crystals); serum osteocalcin is a sensitive marker of bone formation; is a vitamin K–dependent protein present in bone
Osteonectin	Binds calcium in bone; necessary for normal bone formation
Sialoprotein	Promotes calcification, osteoblast formation
Minerals	
Calcium	Crystallizes, providing bone rigidity and compressive strength
Phosphate	Regulates vitamin D, promoting mineralization; a balance of organic and inorganic phosphate required for proper bone mineralization
Alkaline phosphatase	Promotes mineralization
Vitamins	
Vitamin D	Assists with differentiation, mineralization of osteoblasts
Vitamin K	Increases bone calcification; reduces serum osteocalcin

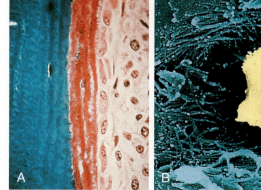
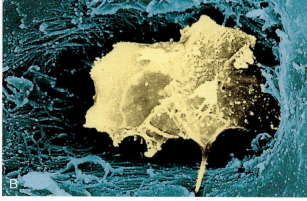
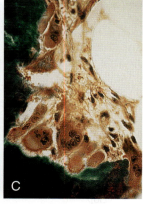

FIGURE 38.1 Bone Cells. **A,** Osteoblasts are responsible for the production of collagenous and noncollagenous proteins that compose osteoid. Active osteoblasts are aligned on the osteoid. Note the eccentrically located nuclei. **B,** Electron photomicrograph of an osteocyte. Osteocytes reside within the lacunae of compact bone. **C,** Osteoclasts actively resorb mineralized tissue. The scalloped surface in which the multinucleated osteoclasts rest is termed *Howship lacuna*. ([A and C], from Damjanov, I., & Linder, J. [Eds.]. [1996]. *Anderson's pathology* [10th ed.]. Mosby; [B], from Wikimedia Commons, courtesy Robert M. Hunt.)

of calcium and other ions at the site. Enzymes, signalling proteins, and growth factors, including bone morphogenic proteins (BMPs) and other members of the transforming growth factor-beta (TGF-β) superfamily, are critical components of bone formation, maintenance, and remodelling (Table 38.2).

Osteoblasts use intercellular calcium signalling to include osteoclastic activity. One of the most important discoveries linking osteoblast and osteoclast function is the cytokine **receptor activator nuclear factor kappa-B ligand**, or RANKL (see "OPG/RANKL/RANK System"). RANKL is expressed by osteoblasts and osteocytes and is necessary for forming osteoclasts[2-4] (see "Osteoclasts"). Thus, the cells of the osteoblastic lineage (osteoblasts, osteocytes) form a network of cells in bone that sense the shape and structure of bone and determine where it is appropriate that bone be formed or resorbed, according to Wolff's law (e.g., bone is shaped according to its function).

Osteoblasts synthesize and secrete osteoid when active, and in the resting state they are termed *satellite cells*. If appropriately stimulated, however, the resting osteoblasts are capable of resuming activity.

Osteocytes. **Osteocytes**, the most abundant cells in bone, are transformed osteoblasts trapped or surrounded in osteoid as it hardens because of minerals that enter during calcification (Figure 38.1B). The osteocyte is within a space in the hardened bone matrix called a **lacuna**. Each osteocyte contains long, thin cytoplasmic extensions, called *processes*, which run through the canaliculi, providing communication with osteoblasts lying on the bone surface. Osteocytes also use gap junctions that connect the cytoplasm of adjacent cells as another form of extracellular communication.

Osteocytes have numerous functions, which include (1) acting as mechanoreceptors and synthesizing certain matrix molecules, (2) playing a major role in controlling osteoblast differentiation and production of growth factors, and (3) maintaining bone homeostasis.[5] As the major source of sclerostin, RANKL, and osteoprotegerin (OPG), osteocytes are thought to be key regulators of both bone formation and bone resorption.[6-8] They also help concentrate nutrients in the matrix. Osteocytes obtain nutrients from capillaries in the canaliculi, which contain nutrient-rich fluids. Exchanges among these cells, hormone catalysts, and minerals maintain optimal levels of calcium, phosphorus, and other minerals in blood plasma.

As a mechanoreceptor, the osteocyte responds to changes in weight-bearing or other stressors ("loading") on bone. The primary cilia on the osteocyte act as the primary mechanoreceptors in bone.[9,10] These cilia detect changes in bone, such as mechanical stress, hormonal imbalance, loading, or unloading, and produce multiple molecular signals, thus beginning the process of bone remodelling.[4,11]

Osteoclasts. **Osteoclasts** are large (typically 20 to 100 μm in diameter), multinucleated cells that develop from the hematopoietic monocyte/macrophage lineage. Osteoclasts are the major resorptive cells of bone. They migrate over bone surfaces to resorption areas where enzymes have broken down the osteoid. Osteoblasts, in the presence of PTH, secrete enzymes such as collagenases, which are necessary for the resorptive process. Osteoclasts travel over the prepared bone surfaces, creating irregular, scalloped cavities known as *Howship lacunae* or *resorption bays*, as they resorb bone areas and then acidify hydroxyapatite (HAP) to dissolve it.

A specific area of the cell membrane forms adjacent to the bone surface and develops multiple infoldings to permit intimate contact with the resorption bay. These infoldings, known as the **ruffled border**, greatly increase the surface areas of cells under their scalloped or ruffled borders. Osteoclasts resorb bone by secretion of hydrochloric acid, acid proteases (such as cathepsin K), and matrix metalloproteinases (MMPs) that help digest collagen, along with the action of cytokines (see Table 38.2). Osteoclasts also resorb bone through the action of lysosomes (digestive vacuoles) filled with hydrolytic enzymes in their mitochondria.

Osteoclasts bind to the bone surfaces through attachments called **podosomes**, which are footlike structures that cluster together along a sealing membrane that forms a "belt" containing multiple proteins, enzymes, and **integrin** receptors.[12,13] Once resorption is complete, the osteoclasts retract and loosen from the bone surface under the ruffled border through the action of calcitonin. Calcitonin binds to receptor areas of the osteoclasts' cell membranes to effectively loosen the osteoclasts from the bone surfaces. Osteoclasts then disappear by the process of degeneration, either by reverting to the form of their parent cells or by undergoing cell movements away from the site, in which the osteoclast becomes an inactive, or "resting," osteoclast.

In addition to resorption of bone, osteoclasts assist the endocrine and renal systems in maintaining appropriate serum calcium and phosphorus levels. Osteoclasts also appear to have a role in the body's immune response.[12]

OPG/RANKL/RANK System

Osteoprotegerin (OPG) is a glycoprotein belonging to the tumour necrosis factor (TNF) superfamily and inhibits bone remodelling/resorption, inhibiting osteoclast formation. Numerous cells, including osteoblasts and osteocytes, produce it. OPG is key in the interaction between osteoblasts and osteoclasts.[14] Osteoblasts and osteoclasts cooperate (a process called *coupling*) to maintain normal bone homeostasis. RANKL is an essential cytokine needed for the formation and activation of osteoclasts. RANKL, like an automobile's accelerator, increases bone loss. OPG, similar to an automobile's brakes, decreases bone loss because upon activation, it promotes bone formation. The binding of RANKL to its receptor, RANK, on osteoclast precursor cells, triggers their proliferation and increases bone resorption. When OPG is secreted by osteoblasts and B lymphocytes,[15] it serves as a decoy by binding to RANK, preventing RANKL binding to RANK, and thus preventing bone resorption. Therefore, the overall balance between RANKL and OPG determines the amount of bone loss. In turn, cytokines and hormones regulate the balance between RANKL and OPG.[16] Alterations of the OPG/RANKL/RANK system can lead to dysregulation and pathological conditions, including primary osteoporosis, immune-mediated bone diseases, malignant bone disorders, and inherited skeletal diseases (see Figure 38.5).

Bone Matrix

Bone matrix is made of the extracellular elements of bone tissue, specifically collagen fibres, structural proteins (such as proteoglycans and certain glycoproteins), carbohydrate–protein complexes, ground substance, and minerals.

Collagen fibres. **Collagen fibres** make up the bulk of bone matrix. They are formed as follows:

1. Osteoblasts synthesize and secrete type I collagen and osteocalcin.
2. Collagen molecules assemble into three thin chains (alpha chains) to form **fibrils**.
3. Fibrils organize into the staggered pattern, with each fibril overlapping its nearest neighbour by about one-fourth of its length. This process creates gaps into which mineral crystals are deposited.
4. After mineral deposition, fibrils interlink and twist to form ropelike fibres.
5. The fibres join to form the framework that gives bone its tensile and supportive strength.

Proteoglycans. **Proteoglycans** are large complexes of numerous polysaccharides attached to a common protein core. They strengthen bone by forming compression-resistant networks between the collagen fibres. Proteoglycans also control the transport and distribution

TABLE 38.2 Selected Factors Affecting Bone Formation, Maintenance, and Remodelling

Factor	Function
Transforming growth factor-beta (TGF-β)	Regulates bone formation, many other cellular processes through signalling; a superfamily of polypeptides
Platelet-derived growth factor (PDGF)	Increases number of osteoblasts
Fibroblast growth factor-2 (FGF-2)	FGF-2 increases osteoblast population, but not function; inhibits alkaline phosphatase activity, osteocalcin, type I collagen, and osteopontin
Insulinlike Growth Factor (IGF)	
IGF-1	Increases peak bone mass during adolescence; decreases osteoblast apoptosis; maintains bone matrix
IGF-2	Increases BMP-9–induced endochondral ossification
Smad proteins	Mediate signalling cascade of TGF-β, especially in embryonic bone development; play role in crosstalk between BMP/TGF-β and Wnt signalling pathways
Bone morphogenic proteins (BMPs)	Have many functions outside skeletal system; stimulate endochondral bone and cartilage formation and function, promote osteoblast maturation; augment bone remodelling by affecting both osteoblasts and osteoclasts; members of TGF-β superfamily of polypeptides
Tumour necrosis factors (TNFs)	Play major role in regulating bone metabolism, especially osteoclast function; superfamily of cytokines
Osteoprotegerin (OPG)	Inhibits bone remodelling/resorption; produced by several cells, including osteoblasts; is a decoy receptor for RANKL (binds to RANKL, inhibiting RANK/RANKL interactions, suppressing osteoclast formation and bone resorption); also may directly interfere with ability of osteoclasts' podosomes to attach to bone matrix
Receptor activator of nuclear factor kappa-B (RANK)	Stimulates differentiation of osteoclast precursors; activates mature osteoclasts
Receptor activator of nuclear factor kappa-B ligand (RANKL)	Promotes osteoclast differentiation/activation; inhibits osteoclast apoptosis
Bone morphogenic protein antagonists	Prevent BMP signalling
Noggin	Binds BMP-2 and -4, reducing osteoblast function
Gremlin	Has multiple effects in and out of skeletal system, but also binds BMP-2, -4, and -7, thus reducing BMP signalling; may play role in development of osteoporosis
Twisted gastrulation	Acts as either a BMP agonist or a BMP antagonist
Activin (a BMP-related protein)	Affects both osteoblasts and osteoclasts; may promote bone formation and fracture healing; expressed by both osteoblasts and chondrocytes; helps regulate bone mass
Annexins	Help mineralize matrix vesicles; may influence bone formation; a class of calcium-binding proteins
Inhibin	Is dominant over activin and BMPs; helps regulate bone mass and strength by affecting formation of osteoblasts and osteoclasts
Leptin	Plays a role in bone formation and resorption
Wnt Antagonists	
Dickkopf (Dkk) family	Disrupt Wnt signalling, leading to reduced bone mass
Sclerostin	Is a protein secreted by osteocytes, osteoblasts, and osteoclasts; binds to BMP-6 and -7; interferes with Wnt signalling pathway, inhibiting bone formation by osteoblasts
Transcription Factors	
β-Catenin pathway	Is a protein with multiple functions; one of most important is activation of genetic transcription factors; balance between Wnt/β-catenin signalling promotes normal bone formation/resorption
Wnt (complex signalling pathway)	Is important in differentiating osteoblasts, bone formation; has overlapping effects with BMPs, helps regulate bone formation and remodelling; crosstalks with other signalling pathways
Nuclear factor of activated B cells (NF-κB)	Affects embryonic osteoclastogenesis; plays role in certain osteoclast, osteoblast, and chondroblast functions
Matrix Metalloproteinases (MMPs)	
Family of endopeptidases (enzymes) that includes collagenases, gelatinases, stromelysins, matrilysins	Help maintain equilibrium of extracellular matrix (ECM); break down almost all components of ECM
A disintegrin and metalloproteinase (ADAM)	Are proteolytic enzymes; also have cell-signalling functions, usually linked to cell membrane
A disintegrin and metalloproteinase with thrombospondin motifs (ADAMTs)	Are similar to ADAMs but are secreted into circulation, are found around cells; various subgroups affect multiple tissues
Cysteine protease	Expressed by osteoclasts as cathepsin K; assists in bone remodelling by cleaving proteins, such as collagen type I, collagen type II, and osteonectin
MMP Inhibitors	
Tetracyclines (especially doxycycline [Teva-Doxycycline]), bisphosphonates	Block enzymatic function of MMPs
Tissue inhibitors of metalloproteinases (TIMPs)	Balance effect of MMPs in maintaining ECM equilibrium

From Boyce, B. F., Yao, Z., & Xing, L. (2010). *Annals of the New York Academy of Science, 1192*, 367–375; Genetos, D. C., Wong, A., Weber, T. J., et al. (2014). *PLoS ONE, 9*(9), e107482; Kim, Y-S., Paik, I. Y., Rhie, Y. J., et al. (2010). *Journal of Korean Medical Science, 25*, 985–991; Norrie, J. L., Lewandowski, J. P., Bouldin, C. M., et al. (2014). *Developmental Biology, 393*(2), 270–281; Stewart, A., Guan, H., & Yang, K. (2010). *Journal of Cellular Physiology, 223*(3), 658–666; Wang, R. N., Green, J., Wang, Z., et al. (2014). *Genes and Diseases, 1*(1), 87–105; Zhao, H., Liu, X., Zou, H., et al. (2014). *Cytokine, 71*(2), 199–206.

of electrically charged particles (ions), particularly calcium, through the bone matrix, thereby playing a role in bone calcium deposition and calcification. Proteoglycans are important constituents of ground substance.

Glycoproteins. Glycoproteins are carbohydrate–protein complexes that control the collagen interactions that lead to fibril formation. They also may function in calcification. Four glycoproteins are present in bone: **sialoprotein**, which binds easily with calcium; **osteocalcin**, which binds preferentially to crystallized calcium; **bone albumin**, which is identical to serum albumin and possibly transports essential nutrients to and from bone cells and maintains the osmotic pressure of **bone fluid**; and **α-glycoprotein**, which probably plays a significant role in calcification and also may facilitate bone resorption by activating osteoclasts (see Table 38.1).

Bone Minerals

After collagen synthesis and fibre formation, **mineralization**, the final step, occurs in areas known as matrix vesicles that "bud" from the surfaces of osteoblasts, chondrocytes (cartilage cells), and odontoblasts (cells that form dentin in teeth).[17] Mineralization has two distinct phases: (1) formation of the initial mineral deposit (initiation) and (2) proliferation or accretion of additional mineral crystals on the initial mineral deposits (growth). The majority of the minerals in the body are an analogue of the naturally occurring mineral **hydroxyapatite (HAP)**. The HAP crystals then penetrate the matrix vesicle membrane and enter into the extracellular space.[17]

Table 38.3 lists the conversion sequence (in stages) in which calcium and phosphate form amorphous (fluid) calcium phosphate compounds to solid hexagonal crystals of HAP. As the calcium and phosphorus concentrations increase in the bone matrix, dicalcium phosphate dihydrate (DCPD) is the first precipitate to form. Once DCPD precipitation begins, the remaining phases of bone crystal formation proceed with the production of insoluble HAP. The collagen fibres contain approximately 80 to 90% of this HAP. Furthermore, amorphous calcium phosphate is distributed throughout the bone matrix.

Types of Bone Tissue

Bone consists of two types of bony (osseous) tissue: **compact bone (cortical bone)** and **spongy bone (cancellous bone)** (Figure 38.2). Cortical bone is about 85% of the skeleton; cancellous bone makes up the remaining 15%. Both types of bone tissue contain the same structural elements, with a few exceptions (see below). In addition, both compact tissue and spongy tissue are present in every bone. The major difference between the two types of tissue is the organization of the elements.

Compact bone is highly organized, solid, and extremely strong. The basic structural unit in compact bone is the **haversian system** (Figure. 38.3). Each haversian system consists of the following:
1. A central canal called the **haversian canal**
2. Concentric layers of bone matrix called **lamellae** (*sing.*, **lamella**)
3. Tiny spaces (lacunae) between the lamellae
4. Bone cells (osteocytes) within the lacunae
5. Small channels or canals called **canaliculi** (*sing.*, **canaliculus**)

Spongy bone is less complex and lacks haversian systems. In spongy bone, the lamellae are not arranged in concentric layers but in plates or bars termed **trabeculae** (*sing.*, **trabecula**) that branch and unite with one another to form an irregular meshwork. The direction of stress on the particular bone determines the pattern of the meshwork. The spaces between the trabeculae consist of red bone marrow. The osteocyte-containing lacunae are distributed between the trabeculae and interconnected by canaliculi. Capillaries pass through the marrow to nourish the osteocytes.

TABLE 38.3 Sequence of Calcium and Phosphate Compound Formation and Crystallization[a]

Formula	Name	Abbreviation
Ca(HPO$_4$)•2H$_2$O	Dicalcium phosphate dihydrate	DCPD
Ca$_4$H(PO$_4$)$_3$	Octacalcium phosphate	OCP
Ca$_9$(PO$_4$)$_6$ (var.)	Amorphous calcium phosphate	ACP
Ca$_3$(PO$_4$)$_2$	Tricalcium phosphate	TCP
Ca$_5$(PO$_4$)$_3$OH	Hydroxyapatite	HAP

[a]Compounds are listed in the order in which precipitation and crystal formation occur.

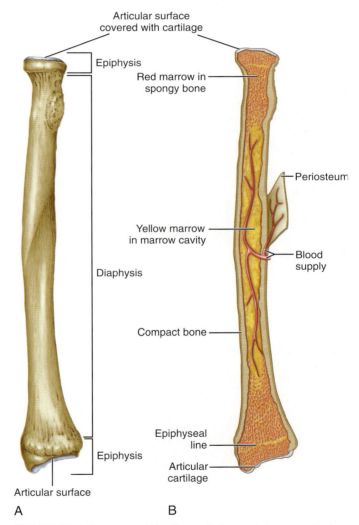

FIGURE 38.2 Anatomy of the Bone. **A**, External anatomy of a long bone. **B**, Internal structure of a long bone showing spongy (cancellous) and compact bone. (From Solomon, E. [2016]. *Introduction to human anatomy and physiology* [4th ed.]. Saunders.)

All bones are covered with a double-layered connective tissue called the **periosteum**. The outer layer of the periosteum contains blood vessels and nerves, some of which penetrate to the inner structures of the bone through channels called *Volkmann canals* (see Figure 38.3). Collagenous fibres (Sharpey fibres) that penetrate the bone anchor the periosteum to the bone. Sharpey fibres also help hold or attach tendons and ligaments to the periosteum of bones.

Characteristics of Bone

The 206 bones of the human skeleton are distributed between the axial skeleton and the appendicular skeleton. The **axial skeleton**—the skull, vertebral column, and thorax—consists of 80 bones. The other 126 bones of the **appendicular skeleton** comprise the upper and lower extremities, the shoulder girdle (pectoral girdle), and the pelvic girdle (os coxae) (Figure 38.4). The skeleton contributes approximately 14% of an adult's body weight.

Bones are long, flat, short (cuboidal), or irregular. **Long bones** are longer than they are wide and consist of a narrow tubular midportion (**diaphysis**) that merges into a broader neck (**metaphysis**) and a broad end (**epiphysis**) (see Figure 38.2).

The diaphysis consists of a shaft of thick, rigid compact bone that is able to tolerate bending forces. Contained within the diaphysis is the elongated marrow (medullary) cavity. The marrow cavity of the diaphysis contains primarily fatty tissue, or *yellow marrow*. The yellow marrow assists red bone marrow in hematopoiesis only during times of stress. The yellow marrow cavity of the diaphysis is continuous with marrow cavities in the spongy bone of the metaphysis and diaphysis. The marrow contained within the epiphysis is red because it contains primarily blood-forming tissue (see Chapter 20). A layer of connective tissue, the **endosteum**, lines the outer surfaces of both types of marrow cavity.

The broadness of the epiphysis allows weight-bearing to be distributed over a wide area. The epiphysis is made up of spongy bone covered by a thin layer of compact bone. In a child, the epiphysis is separated from the metaphysis by a cartilaginous **growth plate (epiphyseal plate)**. After puberty, the epiphyseal plate calcifies and the epiphysis

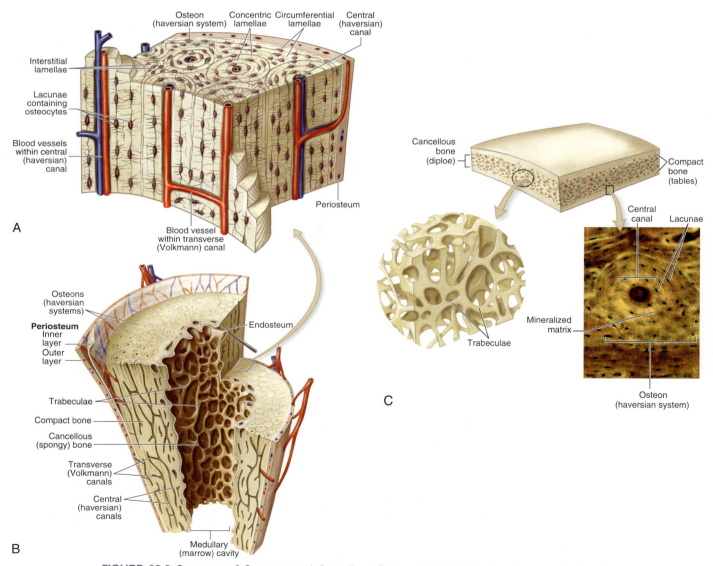

FIGURE 38.3 Structure of Compact and Cancellous Bone. **A**, Magnified view of compact bone. **B**, Longitudinal section of a long bone showing both cancellous and compact bone. **C**, Section of a flat bone. Outer layers of compact bone surround cancellous bone. Fine structure of compact and cancellous bone is shown in the electron photomicrograph. (From Patton, K. T., & Thibodeau, G. A. [2019]. *Anatomy & physiology* [10th ed.]. Mosby. Photo by Steve Gschmeissner/Science Source.)

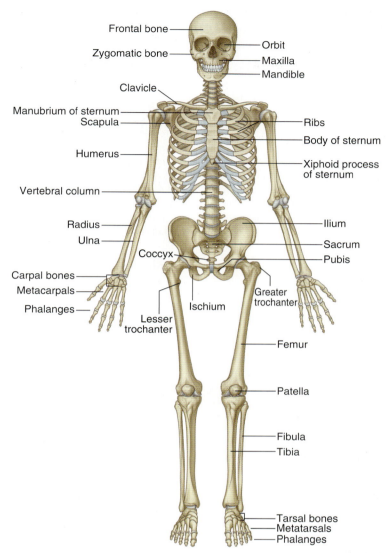

FIGURE 38.4 Anterior View of the Skeleton. (From Drake, R., Vogl, A. W., Mitchell, A. W. M., et al. [2015]. *Gray's atlas of anatomy* [2nd ed.]. Churchill Livingstone.)

and metaphysis merge. By adulthood, the line of demarcation between the epiphysis and metaphysis is undetectable.

In **flat bones**, such as the ribs and scapulae, two plates of compact bone are nearly parallel to each other. Between the compact bone plates is a layer of spongy bone. **Short bones**, such as the bones of the wrist or ankle, are often cuboidal. They consist of spongy bone covered by a thin layer of compact bone.

Irregular bones, such as the vertebrae, mandibles, or other facial bones, have various shapes that include thin and thick segments. The thin part of an irregular bone consists of two plates of compact bone surrounding spongy bone. The thick part consists of spongy bone surrounded by a layer of compact bone.

Maintenance of Bone Integrity
Remodelling

The internal structure of bone is maintained by **remodelling**, a three-phase process in which existing bone is resorbed and new bone is laid down to replace it. Clusters of bone cells, termed **basic multicellular units**, carry out remodelling. The basic multicellular units are made up of bone precursor cells that differentiate into osteoclasts and osteoblasts. Precursor cells are located on the free surfaces of bones and along the vascular channels (especially the marrow cavities).

In phase 1 (activation) of the remodelling cycle, a stimulus (e.g., hormone, medication, vitamin, physical stressor) activates the cytokine system, particularly the TNF superfamily, to form osteoclasts.[14] Osteoclasts attach to the bone matrix by actin microfilaments and multiple other proteins that form footlike structures called *podosomes*. Once attached, the osteoclasts' integrin receptors anchor its microfilaments to the extracellular matrix, thus providing receptor pathways between the osteocyte and bone matrix. Lysosomal enzymes produced by osteoclasts "digest" bone; the osteoclasts then release the degraded bone products into the vascular system.[12] After bone is resorbed, the osteoclast leaves behind an elongated cavity termed a *resorption cavity*. The resorption cavity in compact bone follows the longitudinal axis of the haversian system, whereas the resorption cavity in spongy bone parallels the surface of the trabeculae.

New bone formation begins as osteoblasts lining the walls of the resorption cavity express osteoid and alkaline phosphatase, forming sites for calcium and phosphorus deposition. As the osteoid mineralizes, new bone is formed. Successive layers (lamellae) in compact bone are laid down until the resorption cavity is reduced to a narrow haversian canal around a blood vessel. In this way, old haversian systems are destroyed and new haversian systems are formed. New trabeculae form in spongy bone. The entire process of remodelling takes about 3 to 6 months.

Repair

The remodelling process can repair microscopic bone injuries, but gross injuries, such as fractures and surgical wounds (osteotomies), heal by the same stages as soft tissue injuries, except that new bone, instead of scar tissue, is the final result (see Chapter 6). The stages of bone healing are listed here and shown in Figure 38.5:

1. Inflammation or hematoma formation
2. Procallus formation
3. Callus formation
4. Replacement, by basic multicellular units, of the callus with lamellar or trabecular bone
5. Remodelling of the periosteal and endosteal surfaces of the bone to the size and shape of the bone before injury

The speed with which bone heals depends on many factors: (1) the severity of the bone disruption; (2) the type and amount of bone tissue that need to be replaced (spongy bone heals faster); (3) the blood and oxygen supply available at the site; (4) the presence of growth and thyroid hormones, insulin, vitamins, and other nutrients; (5) the existence of systemic disease; (6) the effects of aging (see "Osteoporosis" in Chapter 39); and (7) the availability of effective treatment, including immobilization and the prevention of complications such as infection. In general, however, hematoma formation occurs within hours of fracture or surgery, formation of procallus by osteoblasts within days, callus formation within weeks, and replacement and contour modelling within years—up to 4 years in some cases.

STRUCTURE AND FUNCTION OF JOINTS

QUICK CHECK 38.2
1. How do the following joints differ from each other: synarthrosis, amphiarthrosis, and diarthrosis?
2. Name at least two characteristics of each of the joints in the previous question that either facilitate or hinder movement.
3. Name three functions of articular cartilage.

The site where two or more bones are attached is a **joint**, or **articulation** (Figure. 38.6). Joints provide stability and mobility to the skeleton, and its function depends on both its location and its structure. Generally, joints that stabilize the skeleton have a simpler structure than those that enable the skeleton to move. Most joints provide some degree of both stability and mobility.

Joints are classified based on the degree of movement they permit or on the connecting tissues that hold them together. A joint that cannot move is a **synarthrosis** (immovable joint), whereas an **amphiarthrosis** is a slightly movable joint, and a **diarthrosis** is a freely movable joint. Similarly, based on connective structures, joints can be fibrous, cartilaginous, or synovial. The classification of each joint also depends on the shape and contour of the articulating surfaces (ends) of the bones and the type of motion the joint permits.

Fibrous Joints

A joint in which bone is united directly to bone by fibrous connective tissue is called a **fibrous joint**. These joints have no joint cavity and allow little, if any, movement. Fibrous joints are further subdivided into three types: sutures, syndesmoses, and gomphoses. A **suture** has a thin layer of dense fibrous tissue that binds together interlocking flat bones in the skulls of young children. Sutures form an extremely tight union that permits no motion. By adulthood, the fibrous tissue has been replaced by bone. A **syndesmosis** is a joint in which the two bony surfaces are united by a ligament or membrane. The fibres of ligaments are flexible and stretch, permitting a limited amount of movement. The paired bones of the lower arm (radius and ulna) and the lower leg (tibia and fibula) and their ligaments are syndesmotic joints. A **gomphosis** is a special type of fibrous joint in which a conical projection fits into a complementary socket and is held in place by a ligament. The teeth held in the maxilla or mandible are gomphosis joints.

Cartilaginous Joints

There are two types of cartilaginous joints: symphyses and synchondroses. A **symphysis** is a cartilaginous joint in which bones are united by a pad or disc of fibrocartilage. A thin layer of hyaline cartilage usually covers the articulating surfaces of these two bones, and the thick pad of fibrocartilage acts as a shock absorber and stabilizer. Examples of symphyses are the symphysis pubis, which joins the two pubic bones, and the intervertebral discs, which join the bodies of the vertebrae. A **synchondrosis** is a joint in which hyaline cartilage, rather than fibrocartilage, connects the two bones. The joints between the ribs and the sternum are synchondroses. The hyaline cartilage of these joints is called *costal cartilage*. Slight movement at the synchondroses between the ribs and the sternum allows the chest to move outward and upward during breathing.

Joint (Articular) Capsule

The **joint (articular) capsule** is fibrous connective tissue that covers the ends of bones where they meet in a joint; Sharpey fibres firmly attach the proximal and distal capsule to the periosteum, and ligaments and tendons also may reinforce the capsule. It is composed of parallel, interlacing bundles of dense, white fibrous tissue richly supplied with nerves, blood vessels, and lymphatic vessels. Nerves in and around the joint capsule are sensitive to rate and direction of motion, compression, tension, vibration, and pain.

Synovial Membrane

The **synovial membrane** is a smooth, delicate inner lining of joint capsule found in the nonarticular portion of the synovial joint and any ligaments or tendons that traverse this cavity. It is composed of two layers: the vascular subintima and the thin cellular intima. The vascular subintima merges with the fibrous joint capsule and is made up of loose fibrous connective tissue, elastin fibres, fat cells, fibroblasts, macrophages, and mast cells; the cellular intima consists of rows of synovial cells embedded in fibre-free intercellular matrix and contains two types of cells—A and B. A cells (macrophages) ingest and remove (phagocytose) bacteria and particles of debris in the joint cavity; B cells (fibroblasts) are the most numerous and secrete hyaluronate, which gives synovial fluid its viscous quality. The synovial membrane is richly supplied with blood and lymphatic vessels and is capable of rapid repair and regeneration.

Joint (Synovial) Cavity

The **joint (synovial) cavity** is an enclosed, fluid-filled space between articulating surfaces of two bones, also called *joint space*. It enables two bones to move "against" one another and is surrounded by synovial membrane and filled with synovial fluid.

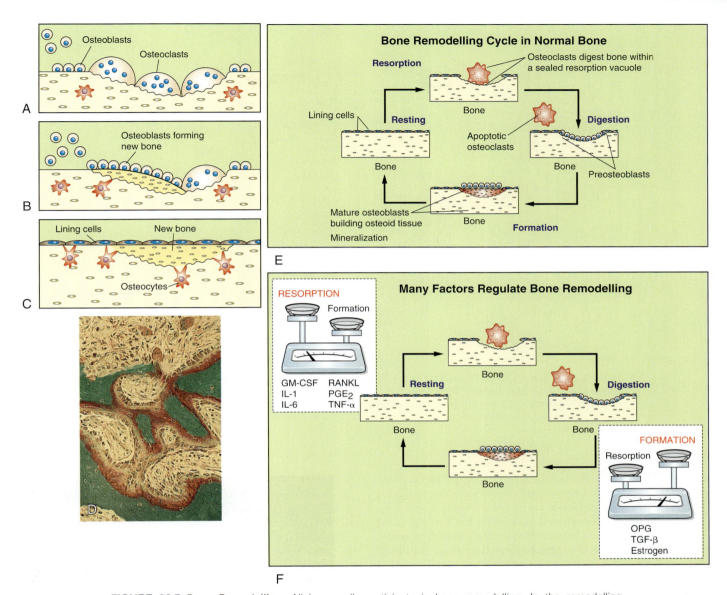

FIGURE 38.5 **Bone Remodelling.** All bone cells participate in bone remodelling. In the remodelling sequence bone sections are removed by bone-resorbing cells (osteoclasts) and replaced with a new section laid down by bone-forming cells (osteoblasts). Bone remodelling is necessary because it allows the skeleton to respond to mechanical loading, maintains quality control (repair and prevent microdamage), and allows the skeleton to release growth factors and minerals (calcium and phosphate) stored in bone matrix to the circulation. The cells work in response to signals generated in the environment (see [F]). Only the osteoclastic cells mediate the first phase of remodelling. They are activated, scoop out bone. **A,** and resorb it; then the work of the osteoblasts begins. **B,** They form new bone that replaces bone removed by the resorption process. **C,** The sequence takes 4 to 6 months. **D,** Micrograph of active bone remodelling seen in the settings of primary or secondary hyperparathyroidism. Note the active osteoblasts surmounted on red-stained osteoid. Marrow fibrosis is present. **E,** Bone remodelling cycle in normal bone with **F.** Numerous signalling factors are necessary for remodelling. Factors most important for resorption include granulocyte-macrophage colony-stimulating factor *(GM-CSF)*, interleukin-1 *(IL-1)* and IL-6, receptor activator of nuclear factor kappa-B ligand *(RANKL)*, prostaglandin E_2 *(PGE$_2$)*, and tumour necrosis factor-alpha *(TNF-α)*. Important factors for bone formation include osteoprotegerin *(OPG)*, transforming growth factor-beta *(TGF-β)*, and estrogen. (Adapted from Nucleus Medical Art. [D], from Damjanov, I., & Linder, J. [Eds.]. *Anderson's pathology* [10th ed.]. Mosby.)

Synovial Fluid

Synovial fluid is superfiltrated plasma from blood vessels that lubricates the joint surfaces, nourishes the pad of the articular cartilage, and covers the ends of the bones. Hyaluronic acid in the synovial fluid gives it important biomechanical properties. It also contains free-floating synovial cells and various leukocytes that phagocytose joint debris and microorganisms.

Articular Cartilage

Articular cartilage is a layer of hyaline cartilage that covers the end of each bone; it may be thick or thin, depending on the size of the joint,

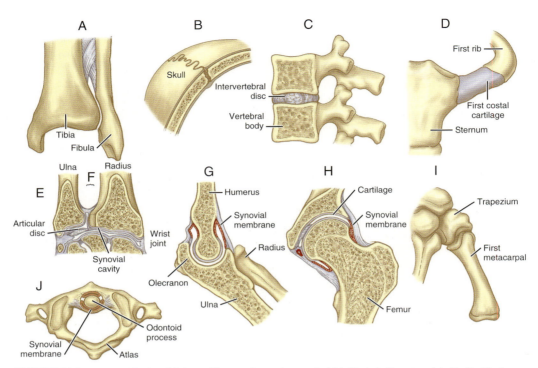

FIGURE 38.6 Various Kinds of Joints. *Fibrous:* **A,** syndesmosis (tibiofibular); **B,** suture (skull). *Cartilaginous:* **C,** symphysis (vertebral bodies); **D,** synchondrosis (first rib and sternum). *Synovial:* **E,** condyloid (wrist); **F,** gliding (radioulnar); **G,** hinge or ginglymus (elbow); **H,** ball and socket (hip); **I,** saddle (carpometacarpal of thumb); **J,** pivot (atlantoaxial). (From Dorland. [2012]. *Dorland's medical illustrated dictionary* [32nd ed.]. Saunders.)

the fit of the two bone ends, and the amount of weight and shearing force the joint normally withstands. The function of articular cartilage is to reduce friction in the joint and to distribute the forces of weight-bearing. Articular cartilage is composed of **chondrocytes** (cartilage cells) (about 2% of the tissue) and an intercellular matrix consisting of type II collagen (about 10 to 30% of weight), proteoglycans (about 5 to 10% of weight), and water. The water content ranges from 60 to almost 80% of the net weight of the cartilage, and individual molecules rapidly enter or exit the articular cartilage to contribute to the resiliency of the tissue.

At the surface of articular cartilage, the collagen fibres run parallel to the joint surface and are closely compacted into a dense, protective mat. (Loss of this dense, compacted configuration at the surface subjects the underlying fibres to splitting and thinning, in which case the cartilage is unable to tolerate weight-bearing.) In the middle layer (the proliferative zone) of the cartilage, the fibres are arranged tangential to the surface, which allows them to deform and absorb some of the weight-bearing (Figure. 38.7). In the bottom layer (the hypertrophic zone) of the cartilage, the fibres are perpendicular to the joint surface, allowing them to resist shear forces, and are embedded in a calcified layer of cartilage called the *tidemark*.[18] The **tidemark** anchors the collagen fibres to the underlying (subchondral) bone. Collagen fibres are important components of the cartilage matrix because they account for approximately 60% of the dry weight and because they (1) anchor the cartilage securely to underlying bone, (2) provide a taut framework for the cartilage, (3) control the loss of fluid from the cartilage, and (4) prevent the escape of protein polysaccharides (proteoglycans) from the cartilage. The proteoglycans give articular cartilage its stiff quality and regulate the movement of synovial fluid through the cartilage. The proteoglycans are macromolecules consisting of proteins, carbohydrates (glycosaminoglycans), and hyaluronic acid.

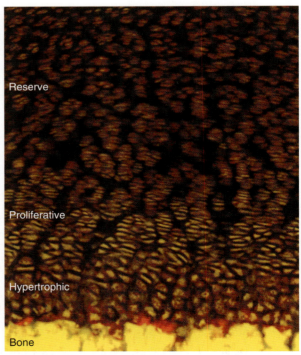

FIGURE 38.7 Collagen Zones. The three collagen zones (reserve, proliferative, and hypertrophic) are distinctly shown in a growth plate. (Reprinted with permission from Elsevier from Hjorten, R., Hansen, U., Underwood, R. A., et al. [2007]. Type XXVII collagen at the transition of cartilage to bone during skeletogenesis. *Bone, 41*[4], 535–542.)

CHAPTER 38 Structure and Function of the Musculoskeletal System

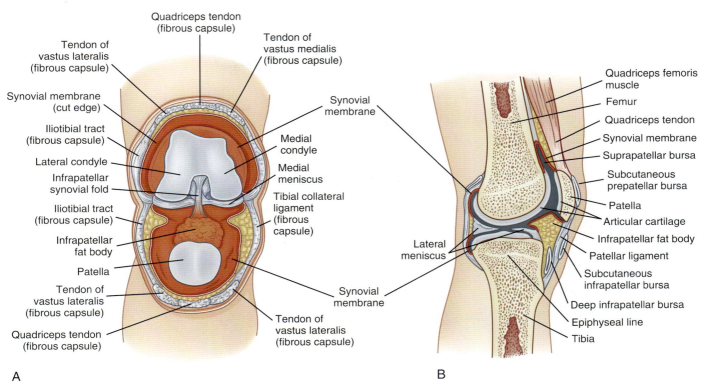

FIGURE 38.8 Knee Joint (Synovial Joint). A, Frontal view. B, Lateral view.

Synovial Joints

Structure of Synovial Joints

Synovial joints (diarthroses) are the most movable and the most complex joints in the body (Figure 38.8).

Movement of Synovial Joints

Synovial joints are described as uniaxial, biaxial, or multiaxial according to the shapes of the bone ends and the type of movement occurring at the joint (Figure 38.9). Usually, one of the bones is stable and serves as an axis for the motion of the other bone. The body movements made possible by various synovial joints are either circular or angular (Figure 38.10).

STRUCTURE AND FUNCTION OF SKELETAL MUSCLES

 QUICK CHECK 38.3
1. Name three differences between slow-twitch and fast-twitch muscle fibres.
2. Why is adenosine triphosphate used for muscle contraction?
3. Define the differences between tendons and ligaments.
4. Describe significant changes in the musculoskeletal system with aging.

Skeletal muscles arise from mesodermal precursor cells that then form myoblasts. The millions of individual fibres of skeletal muscle contract and relax to perform the work necessary to move the body (Figure 38.11). Muscle constitutes 40% of an adult's body weight and 50% of a child's weight. Muscle is 75% water, 20% protein, and 5% organic and inorganic compounds. Thirty-two percent of all protein stores for energy and metabolism are contained in muscle. Between the ages of 30 and 60, muscle mass decreases by about 225 g of muscle each year. For each 225 grams of muscle lost, about 450 g of fat is typically gained.

Whole Muscle

There are more than 600 skeletal muscles in the body. The body's muscles vary dramatically in size and shape. They range from 2 to 60 cm in length and are shaped according to function. **Fusiform muscles** are elongated muscles shaped like straps and can run from one joint to another. The biceps brachii and psoas major are examples of fusiform muscles. **Pennate muscles** are broad, flat, and slightly fan shaped, with fibres running obliquely to the muscle's long axis. The multipennate deltoid muscle, which flexes and extends the arm, is a good example of a muscle shaped according to its function.

Each skeletal muscle is a separate organ, encased in a three-part connective tissue framework called **fascia**. The layers of connective tissue protect the muscle fibres, attach the muscle to bony prominences, and provide a structure for a network of nerve fibres, blood vessels, and lymphatic channels. The layers are:

1. The outermost layer, the **epimysium**, is located on the surface of the muscle and tapers at each end to form the tendon (Figure 38.12). Tendons allow short muscles to exert power on a distant joint, whereas a thick muscle would interfere with the joint's mobility.
2. The **perimysium** further subdivides the muscle fibres into bundles of connective tissue, or **fascicles**.
3. The smallest unit of muscle visible without a microscope is the **endomysium**, which surrounds the muscle.

The ligaments, tendons, and fascia are made up of connective tissue that also buffers the limbs from the effects of sudden strains or changes

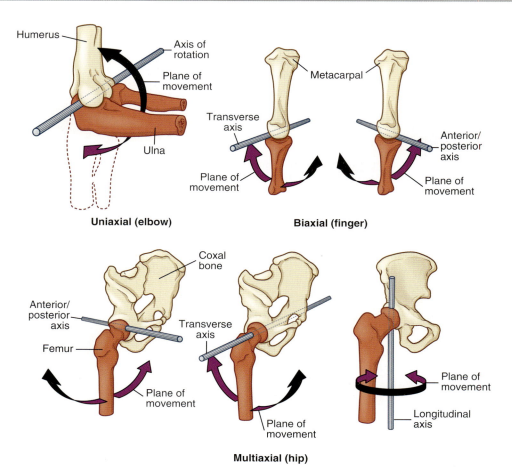

FIGURE 38.9 Movements of Synovial (Diarthrodial) Joints.

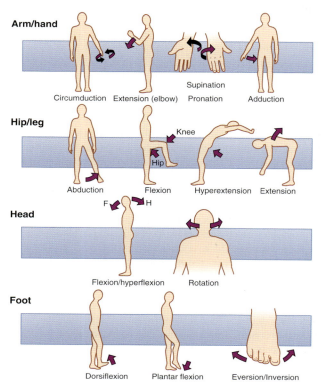

FIGURE 38.10 Body Movements Made Possible by Synovial (Diarthrodial) Joints.

in speed. The rapid recovery necessary for strenuous exercise is supported by the elastic property of muscle and its connective tissue.

Skeletal muscle has been designated as **voluntary** (controlled directly by the nervous system), **striated** (has a striped pattern when viewed under a light microscope), or **extrafusal** (to distinguish from other contractile fibres in the sensory organ of the muscle). Components that are visible on gross inspection of the whole muscle include the motor and sensory nerve fibres. These function together with the muscle, innervating portions of it and providing the electrical impulses needed for motor function.

Motor Unit

From the anterior horn cell of the spinal cord, the axons of motor nerves branch to innervate a specific group of muscle fibres. Each anterior horn cell, its axon (part of the lower motor neuron; see Chapter 13), and the muscle fibres innervated by it are called a **motor unit** (Figure 38.13). The motor units are composed of lower motor neurons, which extend to skeletal muscles. Often termed the *functional unit* of the neuromuscular system, the motor unit behaves as a single entity and contracts as a whole when it receives an electrical impulse.

The whole muscle may be controlled by several motor nerve axons. These branch to innervate many motor units within the muscle. The whole muscle then may be made up of many motor units. The number of motor units per individual muscle varies greatly. In the calf, for example, 1 motor axon innervates approximately 2 000 muscle fibres, out of a total of 1 200 000 muscle fibres. This is a high innervation ratio of muscle fibres to axons and contrasts markedly with the low innervation

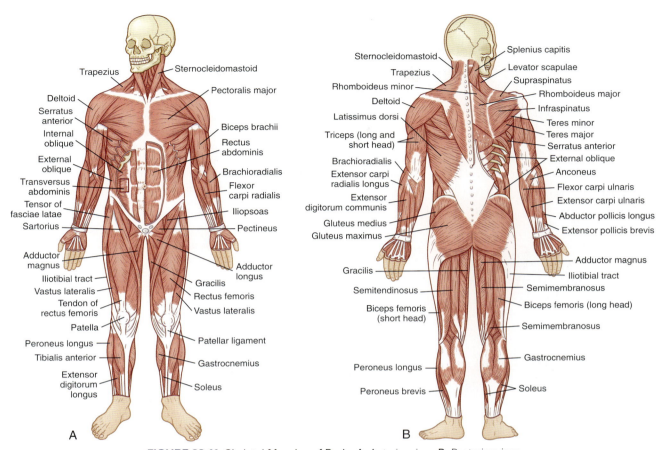

FIGURE 38.11 Skeletal Muscles of Body. A, Anterior view. B, Posterior view.

ratio found in laryngeal muscles, where two to three muscle fibres constitute each motor unit, and the innervation ratio can be of great functional significance. The greater innervation ratio of a particular organ improves its endurance. In other words, higher innervation ratios prevent fatigue, whereas lower innervation ratios allow for precision of movement.

Sensory receptors. Although muscles function as effector organs, they also contain sensory receptors and are involved in sending different signals to the central nervous system. Among these are the muscle spindles and Golgi tendon organs. **Spindles** are mechanoreceptors that lie parallel to muscle fibres and respond to muscle stretching. **Golgi tendon organs** are dendrites that terminate and branch to tendons near the neuromuscular junction. The muscle spindles, Golgi tendon organs, and free nerve endings provide a means of reporting changes in length, tension, velocity, and tone in the muscle. This system of afferent signals is responsible for the muscle stretch response and maintenance of normal muscle tone.

Muscle fibres. Each **muscle fibre** is a single **muscle cell** that is cylindrical in structure and surrounded by a membrane capable of excitation and impulse propagation. The muscle fibre contains bundles of **myofibrils**, the fibre's functional subunits, in a parallel arrangement along the longitudinal axis of the muscle (Figure 38.14). At birth, the muscle fibres have completed development from precursor cells called **myoblasts**. All **voluntary muscles** are derived from the mesodermal layer of the embryo. Genetic transcription factors, most notably myoblast determination protein (MyoD), induce skeletal muscle differentiation. Myoblasts are the main cells responsible for muscle growth and regeneration. Myoblasts are *satellite cells* when in a dormant state. **Satellite cells** are crucial in muscle growth, maintenance, repair, and regeneration. Once muscle is injured, satellite cells become activated and increase the number of transcriptional factors necessary to form myoblasts and assist in repair.[19]

The type of peripheral nerve influences the muscle fibre and motor unit considerably. Whether motor nerves are fast or slow determines the type of muscle fibres in the motor unit. White muscle (**type II fibres [white fast-twitch fibres]**) is innervated by relatively large type II alpha motor neurons with fast conduction velocities. These fibres rely on a short-term anaerobic glycolytic system for rapid energy transfer. Red muscle (**type I fibres [red slow-twitch fibres]**) depends on aerobic oxidative metabolism. Table 38.4 describes the specific characteristics of type I and type II fibres.

The overlap of muscle fibres that appears with staining gives a checkerboard appearance to muscle biopsy specimens. This overlap provides an equal distribution of fibre types throughout the muscle and helps to compensate for muscle fibre loss and fatigue of individual motor units during activity. Despite this overlap, some muscles contain proportionally more of one fibre type than another. Postural muscles have more type I fibres, allowing them the high resistance to fatigue that is necessary to maintain the same position for extended periods. The ocular muscles have more type II muscle fibres, allowing them to respond rapidly to visual changes.

The number of muscle fibres varies according to location. Large muscles, such as the gastrocnemius, have more fibres (1 200 000) than smaller muscles, such as the lumbrical muscles in the hand (10 000). The diameter of muscle fibres also varies. The closely packed polygons are small (10 to 20 µm) until puberty, when they attain the normal adult diameter of 40 to 80 µm. Women usually have smaller-diameter fibres than men. Small muscles, such as the ocular muscles, are 15 µm in diameter; larger, more proximal muscles are 40 µm in diameter.

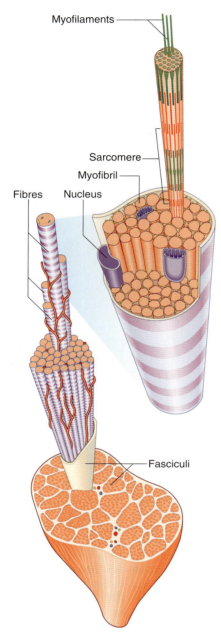

FIGURE 38.12 Levels of Organization Within a Skeletal Muscle Showing Muscle Fibres and Their Coverings. (From Standring, S. [2008]. *Gray's anatomy* [40th ed.]. Churchill Livingstone.)

Fibre size can have functional significance. Studies have shown that larger fibre diameter is associated with generation of greater forces. Fibre diameter can be increased by exercise or occupational overuse, activities that cause hypertrophied muscle.

The major components of the muscle fibre include the muscle membrane, myofibrils, sarcotubular system, sarcoplasm, and mitochondria (see Figure 38.14). The **muscle membrane** is a two-part membrane. It includes the **sarcolemma**, which contains the plasma membrane of the muscle cell, and the cell's **basement membrane**. The sarcolemma is 7.5 μm thick and is capable of propagating electrical impulses to initiate contraction. At the motor nerve end plate, where the nerve impulse is transmitted, the sarcolemma forms the highly convoluted synaptic cleft. The sarcolemma is made up of lipid molecules and protein systems. The protein systems perform special functions, such as transport of nutrients and protein synthesis. They also provide the sodium–potassium pump and include the cell's cholinergic receptor. The basement membrane is 50 μm thick and is composed primarily of proteins and polysaccharides. It also serves as the cell's microskeleton and maintains the shape of the muscle cell. The basement membrane also may function in some way to restrict further diffusion of electrolytes once they have crossed the sarcolemma.

The **sarcoplasm** is the cytoplasm of the muscle cell and contains myoglobin plus the intracellular components that are common to all cells (see Chapter 1). **Myoglobin** is a protein found primarily in skeletal and heart muscle. Related to hemoglobin in the blood, myoglobin stores oxygen and iron in the muscle. The sarcoplasm is an aqueous substance that provides a matrix that surrounds the myofibrils. It contains numerous enzymes and proteins that are responsible for the cell's energy production, protein synthesis, and oxygen storage. The mitochondria house enzyme systems for energy production, particularly those that regulate processes such as the citric acid cycle and adenosine triphosphate (ATP) formation. Many other structures are present in the sarcoplasm. The ribosomes contain primarily RNA and participate in the process of protein synthesis. The cell nucleus, satellite cells, glycogen granules, and lipid droplets are suspended in the sarcoplasmic matrix. Blood vessels, nerve endings, muscle spindles, and Golgi tendon organs are also directly located within this structure.

Unique to the muscle is the **sarcotubular system**, a network that includes the transverse tubules and the sarcoplasmic reticulum, which crosses the interior of the cell. The **sarcoplasmic reticulum** is constructed like the endoplasmic reticulum in other cells. The sarcoplasmic reticulum is composed of tubules that run parallel to the myofibrils. The longitudinal tubules are termed **sarcotubules**. In muscle cells, the sarcoplasmic reticulum contains a network of intracellular receptors known as *ryanodine receptors* (RyRs). In response to a nerve impulse, RyR1 (found in skeletal muscle cells) releases intracellular calcium and initiates muscle contraction at the

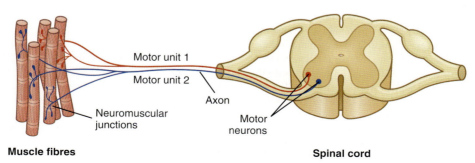

FIGURE 38.13 Motor Units of a Muscle. Each motor unit consists of a motor neuron and all the muscle fibres (cells) supplied by the neuron and its axon branches.

TABLE 38.4 Characteristics of Human Skeletal Muscle Fibres

Characteristics	Type I (Red) (Oxidative Fibres [OFs])	Type II (White) Type II-1A (Fast Oxidative Glycolic Fibres [FOGs])
Anatomical location	Deep axial portion of muscle	Surface portion of muscle
Fibre diameter	Small	Large
Motor neuron size	Small	Large
Contraction speed	Slow	Fast
Motor neuron type	Type I, α	Type II-A, II-B, II-X, and II-D
		II-A: fatigue resistant; II-B: fast fatigable; II-X and II-D: intermediate fatigability
Glycogen content (at rest)	Low	High
Oxidative capacity	High	High (for short periods)
Myosin-ATPase activity	Low	High
Metabolism	Oxidative (also most effective in removing glucose from bloodstream)	Some oxidative pathways, mostly glycolysis
Used for	Maintaining body posture, skeletal support, aerobic activity	Short, intense activity (e.g., sprinting)
Aerobic metabolic capacity	High	Low
Fatigue resistance	High	Intermediate to low
Myoglobin content	High	Low
Capillary supply	Profuse	Intermediate to low
Mitochondria	Many	Few
Intensity of contraction	Low	High
Example (most muscles are mixed)	Soleus muscle	Laryngeal
Satellite cell content	High	Low

ATPase, Adenosinetriphosphatase.
From Schiaffino, S., & Reggiani, C. (2011). *Physiological Reviews, 91*, 1447–1531; Verdijk, L. B., Snijders, T., Drost, M., et al. (2014). *Age, 36*(2), 545–547.

sarcomere, a portion of the myofibril. The **transverse tubules**, which also contain calcium release channels and are closely associated with the sarcotubules, run across the sarcoplasm and communicate with the extracellular space. Together, the tubules of this membrane system allow for uptake and regulation of intracellular calcium, release of calcium during muscle contraction, and storage of calcium during muscle relaxation.[20-22]

Myofibrils. The myofibrils are the functional units of muscle contraction. Each myofibril contains sarcomeres, which appear at intervals (see Figure 38.14). The speed with which sarcomeres lengthen and shorten during movement directly influences the strength and function of skeletal muscles. Sprinters tend to have more fast-twitch fibres than slow-twitch fibres in their leg muscles, and endurance runners have more slow-twitch fibres in their leg muscles. Sarcomeres are composed of several proteins. The two most abundant are actin and myosin, but three other giant, muscle-specific proteins (titin, nebulin, and obscurin) play important roles in myofibril formation and function (Table 38.5).

The myofibrils are the most abundant subcellular muscle component and comprise 85 to 90% of the total volume. On cross-section, they are irregular polygons with a mean diameter of less than 1 μm. Each myofibril contains serially repeating sarcomeres, separated by Z bands (also called *Z discs*), which give the muscle its striped, cross-striated appearance. Each sarcomere has a dark A band and is flanked by two light I bands (Figure. 38.15). The A band is 1.5 to 1.6 μm long and contains the thick myosin filaments. The A band has a lighter zone called the *H band*, and the *M line*, or *M band*, is in the centre of the H band. The I band, which contains actin, is divided at the midpoint of each sarcomere by the Z band. Its length varies with the start of muscle contraction. The Z band marks the boundaries of the sarcomere.[23]

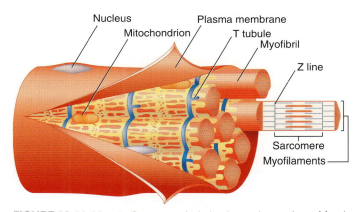

FIGURE 38.14 Muscle Structure. A skeletal muscle consists of fascicles (bundles) of muscle fibres. Each fibre is a cell containing myofibrils that consist of actin and myosin filaments. The filaments are organized into repeating units called sarcomeres. (From Solomon, E. [2016]. *Introduction to human anatomy and physiology* [4th ed.]. Saunders.)

Myofibrils are composed of myofilaments. Each myofilament is structured in a closely packed hexagonal arrangement, with two thin filaments for every thick filament. The thick filament, along with C protein and M line protein, is made up of myosin. Myosin has two subunits—heavy and light meromyosin, which resemble twisted golf club shafts. The thin filaments are twisted double strands consisting of actin, troponin, and tropomyosin (see Chapter 23 and Figure 23.13).

Muscle proteins. Table 38.5 summarizes the location and function of some of the important muscle proteins, and many more are yet to be discovered.

TABLE 38.5 Contractile Proteins of Skeletal Muscle Sarcomere

Protein	Location	Function
Actinin	Z disc	Attaches actin to Z discs; helps coordinate sarcomere contraction; cross-links thin filaments in adjacent sarcomeres
Actin	I band (thin filaments)	Is involved in contraction; activates myosin-ATPase; interacts with myosin
α-Actin	Z disc	Is main ligand of titin; links and controls filament length
β-Actin	Z disc	Has regulatory and structural functions; links filaments, controls filament length
Myosin	A band (thick filament)	Is involved in contraction force; two distinct types: myosin heavy chain (MyHC) and myosin light chain (MyLC); hydrolyzes ATP and develops tension
Titin[a] (largest and third most abundant muscle protein)	Half of sarcomere (from Z disc to M band)	Coordinates assembly of proteins that comprise sarcomere; regulates resting length of sarcomere; important for myofibril assembly, stabilization, and maintenance
Nebulin[a]	I band (with α-actin)	Interacts with myosin to produce contraction; binding site for actin, desmin, titin, other proteins; stabilizes and regulates length of actin filaments; plays role in assembly, structure, and maintenance of Z discs
Obscurin[a]	Surrounds sarcomere (mainly at Z disc and M band)	May mediate interaction of sarcoplasmic reticulum and myofibrils; plays role in muscle response to injury; has role in formation and stabilization of M bands and A band

[a]Also may function as molecular scaffolds for myofibril formation.
ATP, Adenosine triphosphate; *ATPase*, adenosinetriphosphatase.
Data from Herzog, J. A., Leonard, T. R., Jinha, A., et al. (2014). *Molecular & Cellular Biomechanics, 11*(1), 1–17; Luther, P. K. (2009). *Journal of Muscle Research and Cell Motility, 30*, 171–185; Pappas, C. T., Krieg, P. A., & Gregorio, C. C. (2010). *Journal of Cell Biology, 189*(5), 859–870; Schiaffino, S., & Reggiani, C. (2011). *Physiological Reviews, 91*, 1447–1531.

Nonprotein constituents of muscle. Substances such as nitrogen, creatine, creatinine, phosphocreatine, purines, uric acid, and amino acids all serve in the complex process of muscle metabolism. Energy is provided by glycogen and its derivatives.

Creatine metabolism and creatinine metabolism have been used to measure muscle mass. Plasma creatine is taken up by muscle and converted into the high-energy phosphate compound phosphocreatine by the enzyme creatine kinase. Creatinine is formed in muscle from creatine at a constant rate of 2% per day. (Measurement of plasma creatinine concentration is discussed in Chapter 29.) Creatine excretion is increased in muscle wasting. This change reflects the reduction in total body creatine stores and the loss of muscle mass.

Inorganic compounds, anions (phosphate, chloride), and cations (calcium, magnesium, sodium, potassium) are important in the regulation of protein synthesis, muscle contraction, and enzyme systems as well as in the stabilization of cell membranes. Total body potassium level in adults, measured by the K40 method, has been used to estimate muscle mass, also called *lean body mass*. Total body potassium levels reflect changes in muscle mass seen during growth, malnutrition, and muscle wasting.

Components of Muscle Function

The ultimate function of muscle is to accomplish work. Although variously expressed in such measures as foot-pounds or kilogram-metres, work usually refers to the amount of energy liberated or force exerted over a distance (work = force × distance). Muscles usually contract or tense while doing work. Muscle contraction occurs on the molecular level and leads to the observable phenomenon of muscle movement.

Muscle Contraction at the Molecular Level

The four steps of muscle contraction are (1) excitation, (2) coupling, (3) contraction, and (4) relaxation. The process involves the electrical properties of all cells and the movement of ions across the plasma membrane (see Chapter 1). The muscle fibre is an excitable tissue. At rest, an electrical charge of −90 mV is continually maintained across the sarcolemma. This resting potential, generated by the separation of positive and negative charges on either side of the membrane, creates an electrochemical equilibrium caused by the selective permeability of the sarcolemma to electrolytes in the intracellular and extracellular fluids, particularly potassium and sodium.

Excitation, the first step of muscle contraction, begins with the spread of an action potential from the nerve terminal to the neuromuscular junction. The rapid depolarization of the membrane initiates an electrical impulse in the muscle fibre membrane called the **muscle fibre action potential**. As the action potential advances along the sarcolemmal membrane, it spreads to the transverse tubules. (The velocity of conduction is much slower in muscle fibres than in myelinated nerve fibres—only 3 to 5 m/sec compared with 54 to 90 m/sec in nerve fibres.) A receptor on the transverse tubule opens, allowing calcium to enter the cell.[24]

The second stage, **coupling**, follows the depolarization of the transverse tubules. This triggers the release of calcium ions from the sarcoplasmic reticulum through RyR1 channels into the sarcoplasm. The calcium then binds to a protein on the actin filament. (Calcium affects troponin and tropomyosin, muscle proteins that bind with actin when the muscle is at rest.) In the presence of calcium, however, both these proteins are attracted to calcium ions, leaving the actin free to bind with myosin. The release of intracellular calcium ions is the critical link between a nerve impulse (electrical excitation) and muscle contraction.[25]

Contraction begins as the calcium ions combine with troponin, a reaction that overcomes the inhibitory function of the troponin–tropomyosin system. Myosin binds to actin, forming cross-bridges. The myosin heads attach to the exposed actin-binding sites, pulling actin (the thin filament) inward. The thin filament, actin, then slides toward the thick filament, myosin. The two ends of the myofibril shorten after contraction when the myosin heads attach to the actin molecules, forming a cross-bridge that constitutes an actin–myosin complex. ATP, located on the actin–myosin complex, is released when the cross-bridges

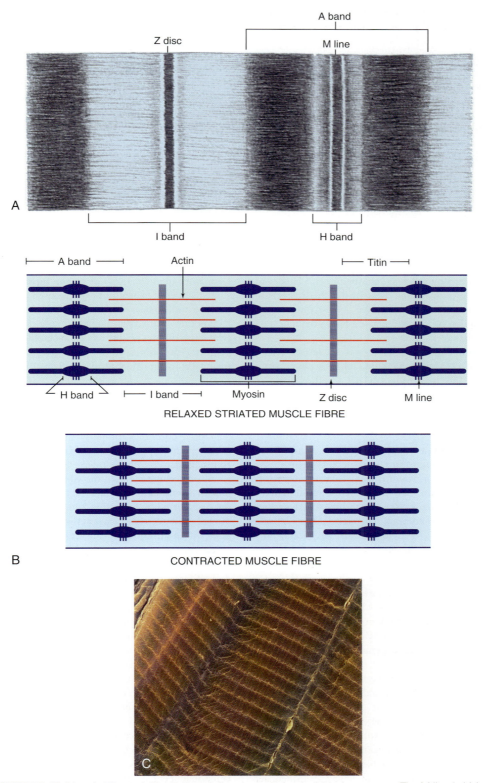

FIGURE 38.15 Muscle Fibres. A, The Z discs define the end of an individual sarcomere. The M line (which lies within the H band) is made of cross-connecting elements of the cytoskeleton. B, Actin is the primary protein of the I band (thin filament). Nebulin also extends along the I band and contains binding sites for actin and myosin. Myosin (thick filament) extends through the A band. Titin extends from the Z disc to the M band, binding with myosin; strong titin anchoring within the I band is necessary for proper muscle function. During contraction, the I bands and H bands shorten, moving the Z discs closer together. C, Electron photomicrograph of human muscle tissue corresponding to schematics in (A) and (B). ([A], modified from Thompson, J. M., McFarland, G. K., Hirsch, J. E., et al. [2002]. *Mosby's clinical nursing* [5th ed.]. Mosby; [C], SPL/Science Source.)

TABLE 38.6 Energy Sources for Muscular Activity

Sources	Reactions
Short-term (anaerobic) sources	$ATP \rightarrow ADP + P_i + Energy$
	$Phosphocreatine + ADP \rightleftharpoons Creatine + ATP$
	$Glycogen/glucose + P_i + ADP \rightarrow Lactate + ATP$
Long-term (aerobic) sources	$Glycogen/glucose + ADP + P_i + O_2 \rightarrow H_2O + CO_2 + ATP$
	$Free\ fatty\ acids + ADP + P_i + O_2 \rightarrow H_2O + CO_2 + ATP$
	Creatine kinase catalyzes reversible reaction of ATP to ADP: $Creatine\ phosphate + ATP \xrightleftharpoons[]{Creatine\ Kinase} Creatine + ATP$

ADP, Adenosine diphosphate; *ATP*, adenosine triphosphate; CO_2, carbon dioxide; H_2O, water; O_2, oxygen; P_i, inorganic phosphate. Data from Barclay, C. J. (2017). Energy demand and supply in human skeletal muscle. *Journal of Muscle Research and Cell Motility, 38*(2), 143–155. https://doi.org/10.1007/s10974-017-9467-7.

attach. The process of contraction was first described by A.F. Huxley in the 1950s and is commonly known as the **cross-bridge theory** because the actin and myosin proteins form cross-bridges as they contract. The useful distance of contraction of a skeletal muscle is approximately 25 to 35% of the muscle's length.

The last step, **relaxation**, begins as calcium ions are actively transported back into the sarcoplasmic reticulum, removing ions from interaction with troponin. The cross-bridges detach, and the sarcomere lengthens. (The cross-bridge theory of muscle contraction is discussed in Chapter 23.)

Muscle Metabolism

Skeletal muscle requires a constant supply of ATP and phosphocreatine. These substances are necessary to fuel the complex processes of muscle contraction, driving the cross-bridges of actin and myosin together and transporting calcium from the sarcoplasmic reticulum to the myofibril. Other internal processes of the muscular system that require ATP include protein synthesis, which replenishes muscle constituents and accommodates growth and repair. The rate of protein synthesis is related to hormone levels (particularly insulin), the presence of amino acid substrates, and overall nutritional status. At rest, the rate of ATP formation by oxidation of glucose or acetoacetate is sufficient to maintain internal processes, given normal nutritional status. During activity, the need for ATP increases 100-fold. The metabolic pathways for muscle activity in Table 38.6 show reactions to the immediate need for increased ATP caused by contraction. Activity lasting longer than 5 seconds expends the available stored ATP and phosphocreatine.

Stored glycogen and blood glucose are converted anaerobically to sustain brief activity without increasing the demand for oxygen. Anaerobic glycolysis is much less efficient than aerobic glycolysis, using six to eight times more glycogen to produce the same amount of ATP. With increased activity, such as intense exercise, or with ischemia, an increase in the amount of lactic acid occurs because of the breakdown of glycogen, thus causing a shift in muscle pH (see Table 38.6). This short-term mechanism buys time by allowing ATP formation in spite of inadequate energy stores or oxygen supply. When the anaerobic threshold is reached and more oxygen is required, physiological changes occur, including an increase in lactic acid level and increases in oxygen consumption, heart rate, respiratory rate, and muscle blood flow.

Strenuous exercise requires oxygen, which activates the aerobic glycogen pathway for ATP formation. During maximal exercise, free fatty acid mobilization and the aerobic glycogen pathways provide ATP over an extended time. These pathways require oxygen both to maintain maximal activity and to return the muscle to the resting state. Maximal exercise increases oxygen uptake by 15 to 20 times over the resting state. When this system becomes exhausted or inadequate to respond to the need for ATP, fatigue and weakness finally force the muscle to reduce activity with a resultant buildup of lactic acid in muscle fibres. Creatine supplementation may provide some protective effects on muscle in older athletes as well as after strenuous physical activity.[26]

Sustaining maximal muscular activity accumulates an **oxygen debt**, which is the amount of oxygen needed to oxidize the residual lactic acid, convert it back to glycogen, and replenish ATP and phosphocreatine stores. For example, after running at maximal speed for 10 seconds, the average person has consumed 1 L of oxygen. At rest, oxygen consumption for the same period is approximately 40 mL. As the person recovers, the measured oxygen debt is 4 L greater than the amount used during activity.

Oxygen consumption is measured to calculate the metabolic cost of activity in normal and diseased muscle. It is an indirect measure of energy expenditure, along with timed tests of activity, heart rate, and respiratory quotient (ratio of carbon dioxide to expired oxygen consumed). Energy expenditure is measured directly by heat production because heat is released whenever work is accomplished.

Another factor that changes energy requirements is muscle fibre type. Type II fibres readily rely on anaerobic glycolytic metabolism and fatigue. Type I fibres can resist fatigue for longer periods because of their capacity for oxidative metabolism.

Muscle Mechanics

Muscle contraction cannot be viewed in isolation. Several factors determine how force is transmitted from the cross-bridges on individual muscle fibres to accomplish whole-muscle contraction. First, when a motor unit responds to a single nerve stimulus, it develops a phasic contraction, also called a *twitch*. Because the motor unit contracts in an all-or-nothing manner, the contraction that is generated will be a maximal contraction. The central nervous system smoothly grades the force generated by recruiting additional motor units and varying the discharge frequency of each active motor unit. This adding of motor units within the muscle is called **repetitive discharge**.

Recruitment and repetitive discharge of motor units allow the muscle to activate the number of motor units needed to generate the desired force. The total force developed is the sum of the force generated by each motor unit. If the motor units are stimulated again, and the muscle unit has not been able to relax between stimulation and the next contraction, the second contraction will fuse with the first, causing **physiological tetanus** (not to be confused with the disease tetanus).

Other variables, such as fibre type, innervation ratio, muscle temperature, and muscle shape, influence the efficiency of muscular contraction. The two muscle fibre types differ in their responses to electrical activity. Tetanus and duration of phasic contractions, which take microseconds to accomplish, are achieved more rapidly in type II (white fast-twitch) than in type I (red slow-twitch) muscle fibres. Low innervation ratios promote control and coordination, whereas high ratios promote strength and endurance. Muscles work best at normal body temperature, 37°C (98.6°F). Finally, muscles with a large cross-sectional area, such as the fan-shaped pennate muscles, develop greater contractile forces than smaller-diameter muscles. The initial length of a muscle and the range of shortening that occurs when the muscle contracts also determine the force it can generate. The long fusiform muscles have a greater range of shortening and can contract up to 57% of their resting length. A certain amount of elongation is necessary to generate sufficient tension and muscular force. The elongation that occurs during the swing of a golf club or tennis racket is an example of how stretch improves contractile force.

Types of Muscle Contraction

During **isometric** (or **static**) **contraction**, the muscle maintains constant length as tension is increased (Figure 38.16). Isometric contraction occurs, for example, when the arm or leg is pushed against an immovable object. The muscle contracts, but the limb does not move. Isometric contraction is also called **static (holding) contraction**.

During **dynamic** (formerly **isotonic**) **contraction**, the muscle maintains a constant tension as it moves. Dynamic contractions can be **eccentric (lengthening)** or **concentric (shortening)**. Positive work is accomplished during concentric contraction, and energy is released to exert force or lift a weight. In contrast, during an eccentric contraction the muscle lengthens and absorbs energy (such as extending the elbow while lowering a weight). Eccentric contraction requires less energy to accomplish and has been said to result in the development of pain and stiffness after unaccustomed exercise.

Movement of Muscle Groups

Muscles do not act alone but in groups, often under automatic control. When a muscle contracts and acts as a prime mover, or **agonist**, its reciprocal muscle, or **antagonist**, relaxes. To illustrate this, hold the right arm in the horizontal position in front of the body and bend the elbow; use the other hand to feel the biceps on the top and the triceps on the bottom of the arm. When the elbow is bent, the biceps are firm, and the triceps are soft. As the arm is extended, the muscles change. When the elbow is completely extended, the biceps are soft and the triceps firm. Completing this movement causes the agonist and antagonist to change automatically; only the movement is commanded, not the alternate contraction and relaxation of the specific muscle groups.

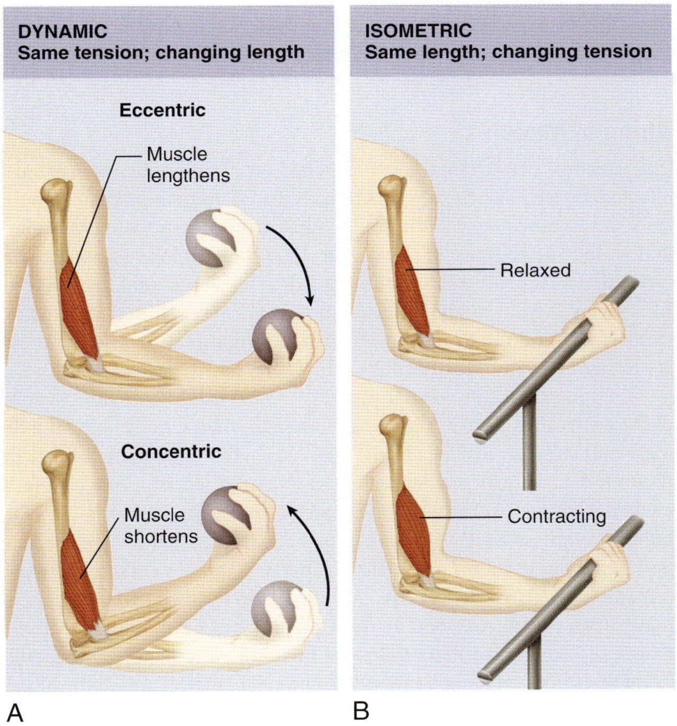

Other associated actions may be seen during walking; as the foot leaves the ground, the paravertebral and gluteal muscles on the opposite sides of the body contract to maintain balance. One notices the loss of the associated muscle's action when paralysis offsets this process and decreases balance. If a person is paralyzed, difficulty in maintaining balance is noticeable.

Tendons and Ligaments

Tendons are important musculoskeletal structures that attach muscle to bone at a site called an **enthesis**. **Ligaments** attach bone to bone, helping to form joints as well as stabilizing them against excessive movement. Both tendons and ligaments are primarily composed of types III, IV, V, and VI collagen and fibroblasts (termed *tenocytes* in tendons).[27] The fibroblasts in a tendon are arranged in parallel rows; fibroblasts appear less organized in ligaments. Collagen fibres and fibroblasts form fascicles, with multiple fascicles then forming a whole tendon or ligament. In the proteoglycan matrix of tendons, collagen oligomeric matrix protein assists in providing gliding and viscoelastic properties. Compared with tendons, ligament fibres typically contain a greater proportion of elastin.

Two main functions of tendons are (1) transferring forces from muscle to bone and (2) acting as a type of biological spring for muscles to allow additional stability during movement. Ligaments stabilize joints by restricting movement. Although both tendons and ligaments can withstand significant distraction (stretching) force, they tend to buckle when compressive force is applied.

Both tendons and ligaments have complex structures at the attachment site of two dissimilar tissues. Figure 38.17 illustrates the transition of tissue between tendon/ligament and bone. These complex structures and differences in mechanical and structural characteristics (either tendon and bone or ligament and bone) make healing and repair of damaged tissue complicated (see *Health Promotion:* Tendon and Ligament Repair).

> ### HEALTH PROMOTION
> #### Tendon and Ligament Repair
>
> Injury of tendons and ligaments constitutes one of the greatest challenges in musculoskeletal rehabilitation. When these types of structures are damaged, attempts to engineer suitable tissue replacements have proved disappointing. The structures and intricate protein composition of tendons and ligaments are the basis for their complex biomechanical properties. One reason for poor clinical outcome in synthetic tendon structures has been the inability to replicate any material that can bear the high mechanical stresses that occur at the interface between two dissimilar materials (i.e., either tendon and bone or ligament and bone). One promising area of investigation is finding or engineering a biodegradable material, or "scaffold," implanted with specific cells that would regenerate into normal tendon or ligament. The scaffold must be strong enough to withstand the forces at the tissue–bone interface and then gradually break down as it is completely replaced by new cells. Currently, investigators are using synthetic polymers, silk, and collagen as scaffolds, with tendon or ligament fibroblasts and mesenchymal stem cells as the implanted cells. Once these biochemical hurdles are overcome, the repair of damaged tendons and ligaments will be revolutionized.

Data from Jahr, H., Matta, C., & Mobasheri, A. (2015). Physicochemical and biomechanical stimuli in cell-based articular cartilage repair. *Current Rheumatology Reports, 17*(3), 22.

AGING AND THE MUSCULOSKELETAL SYSTEM

Aging of Bones

Aging is accompanied by the loss of bone tissue. Bones become less dense, less strong, and more brittle with aging. The bone remodelling

FIGURE 38.16 Dynamic and Isometric Contraction. **A,** In dynamic contraction, the muscle shortens, producing movement. **B,** In isometric contraction, the muscle pulls forcefully against a load but does not shorten. (From Patton, K. T., & Thibodeau, G. A. [2019]. *Anatomy & physiology* [10th ed.]. Mosby.)

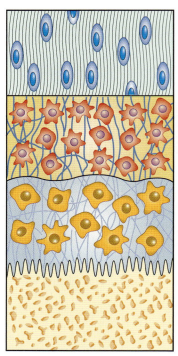

FIGURE 38.17 Cartilage–Bone, Tendon/Ligament–Bone, Meniscus–Bone, and Muscle–Tendon Interfaces. This diagram depicts the cartilage–bone, tendon/ligament–bone, meniscus–bone, and muscle–tendon interfaces and their compositions. Gradients of matrix composition, interdigitation of tissue zones, and interconnecting collagen fibres all enable load transfer between disparate tissues. From Yang, P. J., & Temenoff, J. S. [2009]. Tissue engineering, part B: reviews, 15[2], 128.

cycle takes longer to complete, and the rate of mineralization also slows. With aging, women experience loss of bone density, accelerated with the rapid bone loss that occurs during early menopause from increased osteoclastic bone resorption, fewer osteocytes, and decreased numbers of osteoblasts.[28] By age 70, susceptible women have, on average, lost 50% of their peripheral cortical bone mass (see Chapter 39). Bone mass losses to such an extent can lead to deformity, pain, stiffness, and high risk for fractures. Men also experience bone loss but at later ages and at a much slower rate than seen in women. Also, initial bone mass in men is approximately 30% higher than in women; therefore, bone loss in men causes less risk for disability than it does for women. Men's peak bone mass is related to their race, heredity, hormonal factors, physical activity, and calcium intake during childhood. Bone loss in both genders is related to smoking, calcium deficiency, alcohol intake, and physical inactivity. Bone mass can be gained in healthy young women up to the third decade through participation in physical activity, intake of dietary calcium and other minerals, and use of oral contraceptives. Height is also lost with aging because of intervertebral disc degeneration and, sometimes, osteoporotic spinal fractures.

Stem cells in the bone marrow perform less efficiently with aging, predisposing older persons to acute and chronic illnesses. Such illnesses cause weakness and confusion in older persons and may increase the risk for injury or falling.

Aging of Joints

With aging, cartilage becomes more rigid, fragile, and susceptible to fraying because of increased cross-linking of collagen and elastin, decreased water content in the cartilage ground substance, and reduced concentrations of glycosaminoglycans. Decreased range of motion of the joint is related to the changes in ligaments and muscles. Bones in joints develop evidence of osteoporosis with fewer trabeculae and thinner, less dense bones, making them prone to fractures. Intervertebral disc spaces decrease in height. The rate of loss of height accelerates at age 70 and beyond. Tendons shrink and harden.

Aging of Muscles

The function of skeletal muscle depends on many influences that are affected by cellular factors, such as reduced mitochondrial volume associated with aging.[29] Other influences include the nervous, vascular, and endocrine systems. In the young child, the development of muscle tissue depends greatly on continuing neurodevelopmental maturation. Muscle loss begins at about age 50; however, muscle function remains trainable even into advanced age. Maintaining musculoskeletal fitness at any age can improve overall health.[30,31]

Age-related loss in skeletal muscle, or sarcopenia, is a direct cause of the age-related decrease in muscle strength. As the body ages, muscle mass and strength decline slowly; thus, strength is maintained through the fifth decade, with a slow decline in dynamic and isometric strength evident after age 70. The amount of type II fibres also decreases. There is reduced synthesis of RNA, loss of mitochondrial function,[29,32] and reduction in the size of motor units. The regenerative function of muscle tissue remains normal in older persons. As much as 30 to 40% of skeletal muscle mass and strength may be lost from the third to ninth decade. Muscle fatigue also may contribute to loss of function with aging.[32] Sarcopenia occurs secondary to progressive neuromuscular changes and diminishing levels of anabolic hormones. There is an age-related decline in the synthesis of mixed proteins, myosin heavy chains, and mitochondrial protein.[33] Changes in these muscle proteins are related to reduced levels of insulin-like growth factor 1, testosterone, and dehydroepiandrosterone sulphate.

Maximal oxygen intake declines with age. Basal metabolic rate is reduced and lean body mass decreases in older persons.

DID YOU UNDERSTAND?

Structure and Function of Bones
1. Bones provide support and protection for the body's tissues and organs and are important sources of minerals and blood cells.
2. Bone formation begins with the production of an inorganic matrix by bone cells. Bone minerals crystallize in and around collagen fibres in the matrix, giving bone its characteristic hardness and strength.
3. Bone tissue is continuously being resorbed and synthesized by basic multicellular units of osteoclasts and osteoblasts, respectively.
4. Osteoblasts are multifunctional mononuclear cells derived from osteogenic mesenchymal stromal cells; they are the primary bone-producing cells and are involved in many functions related to the skeletal system.
5. Osteocytes are the most numerous cells in bone and represent the final stage of an osteoblast's life. Though imbedded in the bone matrix, osteocytes have important functions in directing bone remodelling.
6. Osteoclasts are large (typically 20 to 100 μm in diameter), multinucleated cells that develop from the hematopoietic monocyte/macrophage lineage. Osteoclasts are the major resorptive cells of bone.
7. Bones in the body are made up of compact bone tissue and spongy bone tissue. Compact bone is highly organized into haversian systems that consist of concentric layers of crystallized matrix surrounding a central canal that contains blood vessels and nerves. Dispersed throughout the concentric layers of crystallized matrix are small spaces containing osteocytes. Smaller canals, called *canaliculi*, interconnect the osteocyte-containing spaces. The crystallized matrix in spongy bone is arranged in bars or plates. Spaces containing *osteocytes* are dispersed between the bars or plates and interconnected by canaliculi.
8. There are 206 bones in the body divided into the axial skeleton and the appendicular skeleton. Bones are classified by shape as long, short, flat, or irregular. Long bones have a broad end (epiphysis), broad neck (metaphysis), and narrow midportion (diaphysis) that contains the medullary cavity.
9. Bone injuries are repaired in stages. Hematoma formation provides the fibrin framework for formation and organization of granulation tissue. The granulation tissue provides a cartilage model for the formation and crystallization of bone matrix. Remodelling restores the original shape and size to the injured bone.

Structure and Function of Joints
1. A joint is the site where two or more bones attach. Joints provide stability and mobility to the skeleton.
2. Joints are classified as synarthroses, amphiarthroses, or diarthroses, depending on the degree of movement they allow. Joints are also classified by the type of connecting tissue holding them together. Fibrous joints are connected by dense fibrous tissue, ligaments, or membranes. Cartilaginous joints are connected by fibrocartilage or hyaline cartilage. Synovial joints are connected by a fibrous joint capsule. Within the capsule is a small fluid-filled space. The fluid in the space nourishes the articular cartilage that covers the ends of the bones meeting in the synovial joint.
3. Articular cartilage is a highly organized system of collagen fibres and proteoglycans. The fibres firmly anchor the cartilage to the bone, and the proteoglycans control the loss of fluid from the cartilage.
4. Joints help move bones and muscle.

Structure and Function of Skeletal Muscles
1. Skeletal muscle is made up of millions of individual fibres.
2. Between the ages of 30 and 60, muscle mass decreases by about 225 g of muscle each year. For each 225 g of muscle lost, about 450 g of fat is typically gained.
3. Whole muscles vary in size (2 to 60 cm) and shape (fusiform, pennate). They are encased in a three-part connective tissue framework. The fundamental unit of muscle contraction is the motor unit, defined as those muscle fibres innervated by a single motor nerve, its axon, and an anterior horn cell.
4. Satellite cells are dormant myoblasts; however, when activated, they can regenerate muscle.
5. Muscle fibres contain bundles of myofibrils arranged in parallel along the longitudinal axis and include the muscle membrane, myofibrils, sarcotubular system, sarcoplasm, and mitochondria. There are two types of muscle fibres, type I and type II, determined by motor nerve innervation.
6. Myofibrils and myofilaments contain the major muscle proteins actin and myosin, which interact to form cross-bridges during muscle contraction. The nonprotein muscle constituents provide an energy source for contraction and regulate protein synthesis and enzyme systems as well as stabilize cell membranes.
7. Muscle contraction includes excitation, coupling, contraction, and relaxation.
8. Muscle strength is graded by the all-or-nothing phenomenon and recruitment. Speed of contraction is affected by several factors: muscle fibre type, temperature, stretch, and weight of the load.
9. Skeletal muscle requires a constant supply of adenosine triphosphate (ATP) and phosphocreatine to fuel muscle contraction and for growth and repair. ATP and phosphocreatine can be generated aerobically or anaerobically.
10. There are two types of muscle contraction: isometric (static) and dynamic (formerly *isotonic*). Muscle shortening occurs during contraction but can also be seen during pathological and physiological contracture.
11. The site at which tendons attach muscle to bone is called an *enthesis*.
12. Ligaments attach bone to bone, helping to form joints as well as stabilizing them against excessive movement. Both tendons and ligaments are mostly composed of types III, IV, V, and VI collagen and fibroblasts (termed *tenocytes* in tendons).

Aging and the Musculoskeletal System
1. Sarcopenia, or age-related loss in skeletal muscle, is a direct cause of decrease in muscle strength. A slow decline in dynamic and isometric strength is evident after age 70.
2. The regenerative function of muscle tissue remains normal in older persons.
3. Reduced basal metabolic rate and decreased lean body mass are also noted in older persons.

39

Alterations of Musculoskeletal Function

Stephanie Zettel, with originating chapter contributions by Benjamin A. Smallheer

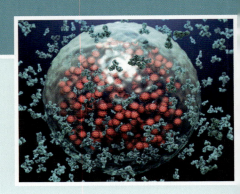

Additional resources are available online at https://evolve.elsevier.com/Canada/Huether/pathophysiology.

CHAPTER OUTLINE

Musculoskeletal Injuries, 965
- Skeletal Trauma, 965
- Support Structures, 968

Disorders of Bones, 973
- Metabolic Bone Diseases, 974
- Infectious Bone Disease: Osteomyelitis, 981

Disorders of Joints, 982
- Osteoarthritis, 982
- Classic Inflammatory Joint Disease, 985

Disorders of Skeletal Muscle, 994

Secondary Muscular Dysfunction, 994
- Fibromyalgia, 994
- Chronic Fatigue Syndrome, 996
- Muscle Membrane Abnormalities, 996
- Metabolic Muscle Diseases, 996
- Inflammatory Muscle Diseases: Myositis, 997
- Toxic Myopathies, 999

Musculoskeletal Tumours, 1000
- Bone Tumours, 1000
- Muscle Tumours, 1004

LEARNING OBJECTIVES

1. Compare and contrast the different types of fractures.
2. Describe the process of bone healing following a fracture.
3. Define dislocation and subluxation.
4. Differentiate between a strain, a sprain, and an avulsion.
5. Differentiate between the types of joint inflammation.
6. Describe the pathophysiology, physical manifestations, evaluation, and treatment of rhabdomyolysis.
7. Describe the pathophysiology and manifestations of malignant hyperthermia and compartment syndrome.
8. Differentiate between osteoporosis and osteomalacia.
9. Describe the pathophysiology and clinical manifestations of ankylosing spondylitis and Paget's disease.
10. Describe the pathophysiology of osteomyelitis and differentiate between exogenous and endogenous osteomyelitis.
11. Differentiate between inflammatory and noninflammatory joint disease and discuss a specific example of each.
12. Describe the pathophysiology of osteoarthritis and rheumatoid arthritis.
13. Describe the pathophysiology of gout.
14. Identify the causes of contractures.
15. Discuss techniques for limiting or decreasing muscle atrophy caused by inactivity.
16. Describe the most common precipitating factors and pathophysiology of fibromyalgia.
17. Describe myotonia and periodic muscle paralysis.
18. Identify the metabolic diseases associated with the musculoskeletal system.
19. Discuss and define the term *myositis*.
20. Identify the various types of musculoskeletal tumours.

KEY TERMS

Acid maltase deficiency, 997
Acute gouty arthritis, 993
Age-related bone loss, 977
Ankylosing spondylitis (AS), 989
Asymptomatic hyperuricemia, 993
Avulsion, 969
Biofeedback, 994
Bone tumour, 1000
Bowing fracture, 965
Bursa (*pl.*, bursae), 969
Caplan's syndrome, 988
Central sensitization, 994
Chondrogenic (cartilage-forming) tumour, 1003
Chondrosarcoma, 1003
Chronic fatigue syndrome (CFS), 996
Closed (incomplete) fracture, 965
Collagenic (collagen-forming) tumour, 1003
Comminuted fracture, 965
Compartment syndrome, 972
Complete fracture, 965
Contiguous osteomyelitis, 981
Contracture, 994
Delayed union, 968
Direct (primary) healing, 967
Dislocation, 968
Disuse atrophy, 994
Dual X-ray absorptiometry (DXA), 978
Endochondral bone formation, 967
Enthesis, 968
Epicondyle, 969
Epicondylopathy, 969
Ewing sarcoma, 1003
External fixation, 968
Fatigue fracture, 966
Fibromyalgia (FM), 994
Fibrosarcoma, 1003
Fracture, 965
Giant cell tumour (GCT), 1003
Glucocorticoid-induced osteoporosis, 977
Glycogen storage disease (GSD), 997
Gout, 991
Gouty arthritis, 991

CHAPTER 39 Alterations of Musculoskeletal Function

Greenstick fracture, 965
Hematogenous osteomyelitis, 981
Heterotopic ossification (HO), 970
Hyperbaric oxygen therapy, 982
Idiopathic inflammatory myopathy (IIM), 998
Immobilization (of a fracture), 968
Incomplete fracture, 965
Indirect (secondary) healing, 967
Inflammatory joint disease (arthritis), 985
Internal fixation, 968
Involucrum, 981
Joint effusion, 984
Joint stiffness, 984
Kyphosis, 977
Lateral epicondylopathy (tennis elbow), 969
Leiomyosarcoma, 1003
Ligament, 968
Linear fracture, 965
Malignant hyperthermia (MH), 973
Malunion, 968
McArdle's disease, 997
Medial epicondylopathy (golfer's elbow), 969
Muscle strain, 970
Myalgic encephalomyelitis (ME), 996
Myelogenic tumour, 1003
Myoadenylate deaminase deficiency (MDD), 997
Myoglobinuria, 970
Myositis ossificans, 970
Myositis, 997
Myotonia, 996
Nonunion, 968
Oblique fracture, 965
Open (compound) fracture, 965
Osteoarthritis (OA), 982
Osteogenic (bone-forming) tumour, 1002
Osteomalacia, 979
Osteomyelitis, 981
Osteophyte, 982
Osteoporosis (porous bone), 974
Osteoprotegerin (OPG), 976
Osteosarcoma, 1002
Paget's disease of bone (PDB, osteitis deformans, or Paget's disease), 980
Pannus, 986
Pathological (insufficiency or fragility) fracture, 966
Peak bone mass, 975
Periodic paralysis, 996
Pleomorphic liposarcoma, 1003
Pompe's disease (PD), 997
Postmenopausal osteoporosis, 976
Progressive relaxation training, 994
Receptor activator of nuclear factor kappa-B (RANK), 976
Receptor activator of nuclear factor kappa-B ligand (RANKL), 976
Reduction (of a fracture), 965
Regional osteoporosis, 976
Rhabdomyolysis, 970
Rhabdomyoma, 1004
Rhabdomyosarcoma, 1003
Rheumatoid arthritis (RA), 985
Rheumatoid factor (RF), 985
Rheumatoid nodule, 988
Secondary osteoporosis, 976
Sequestrum, 981
Spiral fracture, 965
Sprain, 969
Strain, 969
Stress fracture, 966
Subluxation, 968
Syndesmophyte, 990
Synovial sarcoma, 1003
Systemic exertional intolerance disease (SEID), 996
Tendinopathy, 969
Tendon, 968
Tophaceous gout, 993
Tophus (*pl.*, tophi), 991
Torus fracture, 965
Toxic myopathy, 999
Transchondral fracture, 967
Transverse fracture, 965
Volkmann ischemic contracture, 973

Musculoskeletal injuries include fractures, dislocations, sprains, and strains. Metabolic disorders, infections, inflammatory or noninflammatory diseases, or tumours may cause alterations in bones, joints, and muscles. The most common disease affecting bone is osteoporosis; much attention and debate has been focused on its risk factors and pathophysiology. Soft tissue disorders—including muscle, tendon, and ligament injuries; tumours; and metabolic derangements—also affect the musculoskeletal system.

MUSCULOSKELETAL INJURIES

> **QUICK CHECK 39.1**
> 1. How are fractures classified?
> 2. What is the primary pathology of epicondylopathy?
> 3. What are some causes of compartment syndrome?
> 4. Why is myoglobinuria a dangerous complication of rhabdomyolysis?

Musculoskeletal injuries have a major impact on the affected individuals, families, and the larger society because of the physical and psychological effects of limitation on mobility and daily activities, pain, and decreased quality of life. In addition, there are direct costs of diagnosis and treatments, and indirect economic costs related to loss of employment and decreased productivity.

Skeletal Trauma
Fractures

A **fracture** is a break in the continuity of a bone. A break occurs when force is applied that exceeds the tensile or compressive strength of the bone. The incidence of fractures varies for individual bones according to age and gender, with the highest incidence of fractures in young males (between the ages of 15 and 24 years) and older persons (65 years of age and older). Fractures of healthy bones, particularly the tibia, clavicle, and lower humerus, tend to occur in young persons as the result of trauma. Fractures of the hands and feet are often caused by accidents in the workplace. The incidence of fractures of the upper femur, upper humerus, vertebrae, and pelvis is highest in older persons and is often associated with osteoporosis. Hip fractures, the most serious outcome of osteoporosis, are prevalent worldwide amongst a range of populations.[1]

Classification of fractures. There are numerous classification systems for various types of fractures, but the simplest systems describe the basic features of the broken bone. Fractures are complete or incomplete, and they are open or closed (Figure 39.1). The bone is broken entirely in a **complete fracture**, whereas in an **incomplete fracture**, the bone is damaged but still in one piece. Complete and incomplete fractures are also **open** (formerly referred to as **compound**) **fractures** if the skin is open and **closed** (formerly called *simple* or *incomplete*) **fractures** if it is not. A **comminuted fracture** is a fracture in which a bone breaks into more than two fragments. The direction of the fracture line is another useful way to classify fractures. A **linear fracture** runs parallel to the long axis of the bone. An **oblique fracture** occurs at a slanted angle to the shaft of the bone. A **spiral fracture** encircles the bone, and a **transverse fracture** occurs straight across the bone.

Incomplete fractures tend to occur in the more flexible, growing bones of children. The three main types of incomplete fractures are greenstick, torus, and bowing fractures. A **greenstick fracture** perforates one cortex and splinters the spongy bone. The name is derived from the damage sustained by a young tree branch (a green stick) when it is bent sharply. The outer surface is disrupted, but the inner surface remains intact. Greenstick fractures typically occur in the metaphysis or diaphysis of the tibia, radius, and ulna. In a **torus fracture**, the cortex buckles but does not break. **Bowing fractures** usually occur when

CHAPTER 39 Alterations of Musculoskeletal Function

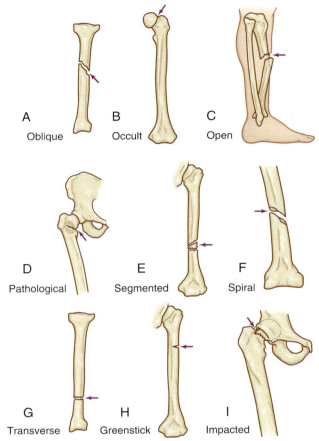

FIGURE 39.1 Examples of Types of Bone Fractures. A, Oblique: fracture at oblique angle across both cortices. *Cause:* Direct or indirect energy, with angulation and some compression. **B,** Occult: fracture that is hidden or not readily discernible. *Cause:* Minor force or energy. **C,** Open: skin broken over fracture; possible soft tissue trauma. *Cause:* Moderate to severe energy that is continuous and exceeds tissue tolerance. **D,** Pathological: transverse, oblique, or spiral fracture of bone weakened by tumour pressure or presence. *Cause:* Minor energy or force, which may be direct or indirect. **E,** Segmented: fracture with two or more pieces or segments. *Cause:* Direct or indirect moderate to severe force. **F,** Spiral: fracture that curves around cortices and may become displaced by twist. *Cause:* Direct or indirect twisting energy or force, with distal part held or unable to move. **G,** Transverse: horizontal break through bone. *Cause:* Direct or indirect energy toward bone. **H,** Greenstick: break in only one cortex of bone. *Cause:* Minor direct or indirect energy. **I,** Impacted: fracture with one end wedged into opposite end of inside fractured fragment. *Cause:* Compressive axial energy or force directly to distal fragment. (Redrawn from Mourad, L. [2002]. Musculoskeletal system. In J. M. Thompson, G. K. McFarland, J. E. Hirsch, et al. [Eds.], *Mosby's clinical nursing* [7th ed.]. Mosby.)

TABLE 39.1 Types of Fractures

Type of Fracture	Definition
Typical Complete Fractures	
Closed	Noncommunicating wound between bone and skin
Open	Communicating wound between bone and skin
Comminuted	Multiple bone fragments
Linear	Fracture line parallel to long axis of bone
Oblique	Fracture line at an angle to long axis of bone
Spiral	Fracture line encircling bone (as a spiral staircase)
Transverse	Fracture line perpendicular to long axis of bone
Impacted	Fracture fragments pushed into each other
Pathological	Fracture at a point where bone has been weakened by disease, for example, by tumours or osteoporosis
Avulsion	Fragment of bone connected to a ligament or tendon detaches from main bone
Compression	Fracture wedged or squeezed together on one side of bone
Displaced	Fracture with one, both, or all fragments out of normal alignment
Extracapsular	Fragment close to joint but remains outside joint capsule
Intracapsular	Fragment within joint capsule
Typical Incomplete Fractures	
Greenstick	Break in one cortex of bone with splintering of inner bone surface; commonly occurs in children and older persons
Torus	Buckling of cortex
Bowing	Bending of bone
Stress	Microfracture
Transchondral	Separation of cartilaginous joint surface (articular cartilage) from main shaft of bone

longitudinal force is applied to bone. This type of fracture is common in children and usually involves the paired radius–ulna or the fibula–tibia. A complete diaphyseal fracture occurs in one of the bones of the pair, which disperses the stress sufficiently to prevent a complete fracture of the second bone, which bows rather than breaks. A bowing fracture resists correction **(reduction)** because the force necessary to reduce it must be equal to the force that bowed it. Treatment of bowing fractures is also difficult because the bowed bone interferes with reduction of the fractured bone. Table 39.1 summarizes the types of fractures.

Fractures are also pathological, stress, or transchondral fractures. A **pathological** (also known as **insufficiency** or **fragility**) **fracture** is a break at the site of a pre-existing abnormality, resulting from force that would not fracture a normal bone. In any bone that lacks normal ability to deform and recover, these fractures can occur with normal weight-bearing or activity. Rheumatoid arthritis (RA), osteoporosis, Paget's disease, osteomalacia, rickets, hyperparathyroidism, and radiation therapy all cause bone to lose its normal ability to deform and recover. Pathological fractures are generally a result of bone weakness caused by another disease such as cancer, metabolic bone disorders, or infection. Although usually considered insufficiency fractures, breaks in the bone attributable to osteoporosis are also pathological fractures. Any disease process that weakens a bone (especially the cortex) predisposes the bone to pathological fracture.

During activities that subject a bone to repeated strain, such as certain athletics, a **stress fracture** can occur in normal or abnormal bone. The forces placed on the bone are cumulative, eventually causing a fracture. A **fatigue fracture** is caused by repetitive, sometimes abnormal stress or torque applied to a bone with normal ability to deform and recover. Fatigue fractures usually occur in individuals who engage in a new or different activity that is both strenuous and repetitive (e.g., joggers, skaters, dancers, military recruits). Because gains in muscle strength occur more rapidly than gains in bone strength, the newly developed muscles place exaggerated stress on the bones that are not yet ready for the additional stress. The imbalance between muscle and bone development causes microfractures to develop in the cortex. If the activity is controlled and increased gradually, new bone formation catches up to the increased demands and microfractures do not occur.

A **transchondral fracture** consists of fragmentation and separation of a portion of the articular cartilage. (Joint structures are defined in Chapter 38.) Single or multiple sites may be fractured, and the fragments may consist of cartilage alone or cartilage and bone. Typical sites of transchondral fracture are the distal femur, the ankle, the patella, the elbow, and the wrist. Transchondral fractures are most prevalent in adolescents.

PATHOPHYSIOLOGY Fracture healing is a complex process that occurs primarily in one of two ways: direct or indirect healing.[2] Both types of healing require integration of cells, signalling pathways, and various molecules. In **direct** (or **primary**) **healing**, intramembranous bone formation occurs when adjacent bone cortices are in contact with one another. Direct bone healing most often occurs when surgical fixation is used to repair a broken bone. No callus formation occurs with this process. **Indirect** (or **secondary**) **healing** involves both intramembranous and endochondral bone formation, development of callus, and eventual remodelling of solid bone.[3] Bone formation that begins with an underlying cartilage scaffold is **endochondral bone formation**.

Callus is a hallmark of indirect fracture healing. Indirect fracture healing most often occurs when the treatment for a fracture involves a cast or other nonsurgical method. There is a disruption of the periosteum and blood vessels in the cortex, marrow and surrounding soft tissues when a bone is broken. Bleeding occurs from the damaged ends of the bone and from the neighbouring soft tissue. A clot (hematoma) forms within the medullary canal, between the fractured ends of the bone, and beneath the periosteum (Figure 39.2). Bone tissue immediately adjacent to the fracture dies. This dead tissue (along with any debris in the fracture area) stimulates an intense inflammatory response characterized by vasodilation, exudation of plasma and leukocytes, and infiltration by inflammatory leukocytes, growth factors, and mast cells that simultaneously decalcify the fractured bone ends. Within 48 hours after injury, vascular tissue from surrounding soft tissue and the marrow cavity invades the fracture area, and blood flow to the entire bone increases. The next step is activation of bone-forming cells in the periosteum, endosteum, and marrow to produce subperiosteal procallus along the outer surface of the shaft and over the broken ends of the bone (see Figure 39.2). Osteoblasts within the procallus synthesize collagen and matrix, which becomes mineralized to form callus. As the repair process continues, remodelling occurs, during which unnecessary callus is resorbed and trabeculae are formed along lines of stress as the repair tissues align with the tissue cells of the host (Figure 39.3). Except for the liver, bone is unique among all body tissues in that it will form new bone, not scar tissue, when it heals after a fracture.

CLINICAL MANIFESTATIONS The signs and symptoms of a fracture include (1) unnatural alignment (deformity), (2) swelling, (3) muscle spasm, (4) tenderness, (5) pain and impaired sensation, and (6) decreased mobility. The pull of attached muscles, gravity, and the direction and magnitude of the force that caused the fracture determine the position of the broken bone segments.

There is often numbness at the fracture site immediately after a bone is fractured because of trauma to the nerve or nerves at the injury site. The numbness may last several minutes, during which time the injured person can continue to use the fractured bone. However, once the numbness dissipates, the subsequent pain is quite severe and may be incapacitating until relieved with medication and treatment of the fracture. Pain can be the result of muscle spasms at the fracture site, overriding of the fracture segments, or damage to adjacent soft tissues.

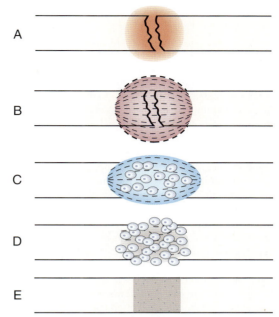

FIGURE 39.2 Bone Healing (Schematic Representation). **A**, Bleeding at broken ends of the bone with subsequent hematoma formation. **B**, Organization of hematoma into fibrous network. **C**, Invasion of osteoblasts, lengthening of collagen strands, and deposition of calcium. **D**, Callus formation; new bone is built while osteoclasts destroy dead bone. **E**, Remodelling is accomplished while excess callus is reabsorbed and trabecular bone is deposited. (From Monahan, F. D., Sands, J., Neighbors, M., et al. [2007]. *Phipps' medical-surgical nursing: health and illness perspectives* [8th ed.]. Mosby.)

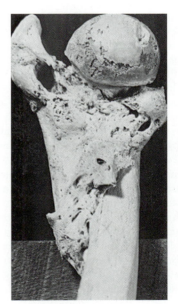

FIGURE 39.3 Exuberant Callus Formation Following Fracture. (From Rosai, J. [1996]. *Ackerman's surgical pathology* [8th ed.]. Mosby.)

Pathological fractures can cause angular deformity, painless swelling, or generalized bone pain. Stress fractures are painful because of accelerated remodelling; initially, pain occurs during activity and is usually relieved by rest. Stress fractures also cause local tenderness and soft tissue swelling. Transchondral fractures may be entirely asymptomatic or may be painful during movement. Range of motion in the joint is limited, and movement may evoke audible clicking sounds (crepitus).

EVALUATION AND TREATMENT Adequate immobilization with a splint or cast is often all that is required for healing of fractures that are *not* misaligned. Treatment of a displaced fracture involves realigning the bone fragments (reduction) close to their normal or anatomical position and holding the fragments in place (immobilization) so that bone union can occur. Several methods are available to reduce a fracture: *closed manipulation*, *traction*, and *open reduction*. Many displaced fractures can be reduced by closed manipulation and reduction: manipulation or movement of the bone occurs without opening the skin. Closed reduction is used when the contour of the bone is in fair anatomical alignment and can be manually placed into normal alignment, and then maintained with immobilization. Splints and casts are used to immobilize and hold a closed reduction in place.

Traction can also accomplish or maintain reduction. Weights apply firm, steady traction (pull) and countertraction to the long axis of the bone when there is displacement of bone fragments from their normal anatomical position. Traction stretches and fatigues muscles that have pulled the bone fragments out of place, more readily allowing the distal fragment to align with the proximal fragment. Traction can be applied to the skin (skin traction) or directly to the involved bone (skeletal traction). Skin traction involves only a few kilograms of pulling force to realign the fragments or when the traction will be used only for a brief time, such as before surgery or, for children with femoral fractures, for 3 to 7 days before applying a cast. Skeletal traction involves a pin or wire drilled through the bone distal to the fracture site, and a traction bow, rope, and weights that are attached to the pin or wire to apply tension and to provide the pulling force required to overcome the muscle spasm and help realign the fracture fragments. Surgical repair (open reduction and internal fixation) or external fixation devices are more commonly used to realign displaced fractures.

Open reduction is a surgical procedure that exposes the fracture site; the fragments are then manipulated into alignment under direct visualization. Some form of hardware, such as a screw, plate, nail, or wire, maintains the reduction (internal fixation). External fixation, a procedure in which pins or rods are surgically placed into uninjured bone near the fracture site and then stabilized with an external frame of bars, treats fractures that would not be adequately stabilized with a cast. Bone grafts—using donor bone from the individual (autograft), a cadaver (allograft), or bone substitutes (ceramic composites, bioactive cement)—can fill voids in the bone.

Improper reduction or immobilization of a fractured bone may result in nonunion, delayed union, or malunion. Nonunion is failure of the bone ends to grow together. The gap between the broken ends of the bone fills with dense fibrous and fibrocartilaginous tissue instead of new bone. Occasionally, the fibrous tissue contains a fluid-filled space that resembles a joint and is termed a *false joint*, or *pseudoarthrosis*. Delayed union is union that does not occur until approximately 8 to 9 months after a fracture. Malunion is the healing of a bone in an incorrect anatomical position.

Dislocation and Subluxation

Dislocation and subluxation are usually caused by trauma. Dislocation is the displacement of one or more bones in a joint in which the opposing joint surfaces entirely lose contact with one another. If contact between the opposing joint surfaces is only partially lost, the injury is called a subluxation.

Dislocation and subluxation are most common in persons younger than 20 years of age and are generally associated with fractures. However, they may be the result of congenital or acquired disorders that cause (1) muscular imbalance, as occurs with congenital dislocation of the hip or neurological disorders; (2) incongruities in the articulating surfaces of the bones, as occur with rheumatoid arthritis; or (3) joint instability.

Shoulder, elbow, wrist, finger, hip, and knee joints are most commonly dislocated and subluxated. The glenohumeral joint is the shoulder joint that is most often injured. Finger dislocations are common injuries in contact sports such as basketball, football, and rugby.

Traumatic dislocation of the elbow joint is common in the immature skeleton. In adults, an elbow dislocation commonly occurs with a fracture of the ulna or head of the radius. Traumatic dislocation of the wrist usually involves the distal ulna and carpal bones. Any one of the eight carpal bones can be dislocated after an injury. Dislocation in the hand usually involves the metacarpophalangeal (MCP) and interphalangeal joints.

Considerable trauma is needed to dislocate the hip. Anterior hip dislocation is rare in healthy persons; it is caused by forced abduction—for example, when an individual lands on his or her feet after falling from an elevated height. Posterior dislocation of the hip can occur as a result of an automobile accident in which the flexed knee strikes the dashboard, causing the head of the femur to be pushed posteriorly from the hip joint.

The knee is an unstable weight-bearing joint that depends heavily on the soft tissue structures around it for support. It is exposed to many different types of motion (flexion, extension, rotation) and is one of the most commonly injured joints. A knee dislocation can be anterior, posterior, lateral, medial, or rotary. It is often the result of an injury that occurs during contact sports activities, such as soccer, lacrosse, or football.

PATHOPHYSIOLOGY Dislocations and subluxations are often accompanied by fracture because stress is placed on areas of bone not usually subjected to stress. In addition, as the joint loses its normal congruity, there may be bruising or tearing of adjacent nerves, blood vessels, ligaments, supporting structures, and soft tissue. Dislocations of the shoulder may damage the shoulder capsule and the axillary nerve. Damage to axillary nerves can cause anaesthesia or dysesthesia in the sensory distribution of the nerve and paralysis of the deltoid muscle. Dislocations may also disrupt circulation, leading to ischemia and possibly even permanent disability of the affected extremity tissues.

CLINICAL MANIFESTATIONS Signs and symptoms of dislocations or subluxations include (1) pain, (2) swelling, (3) limitation of motion, and (4) joint deformity. Pain may be caused by effusion of inflammatory exudate into the joint or by associated tendon and ligament injury. Joint deformity is typically caused by muscle contractions that exert pull on the dislocated or subluxated joint. Limitation of motion results from effusion into the joint or the displacement of bones.

EVALUATION AND TREATMENT Evaluation of dislocations and subluxations is based on clinical manifestations and radiographic evaluation. Treatment consists of reduction and immobilization for 2 to 6 weeks to allow healing of damaged structures, followed by exercises to restore normal range of motion in the joint. Depending on the joint and severity of injury, complete healing can take months to sometimes years.

Support Structures

Sprains and Strains of Tendons and Ligaments

Tendon and ligament injuries often accompany fractures and dislocations. A tendon is fibrous connective tissue (composed primarily of type I collagen) that attaches skeletal muscle to a bone or other structure; the area of attachment on a bone is an **enthesis**. The enthesis serves to evenly distribute tension differences between the bone and tendon. The zone where muscle transitions into tendon is the *myotendinous junction*. Functionally, muscles and tendons work together as a single, integrated unit allowing motion.[4,5] A **ligament** is a band of fibrous connective tissue that connects bones where they meet in a joint. Ligaments are structurally similar to tendons, although ligaments have a higher proportion of small-diameter collagen fibrils. The primary difference between tendons and ligaments is their anatomical location.[6] Tendons and ligaments support the bones and joints and either facilitate or limit motion, respectively. Either structure can be completely separated from bone at their points of attachment, torn, lacerated, or ruptured.

Tearing or stretching of a muscle or tendon is a **strain**. Major trauma can tear or rupture a tendon at any site in the body. The tendons of the hands and feet, the knee (patellar), the upper arm (biceps and triceps), the thigh (hamstring), the ankle, and the heel (Achilles) are most commonly injured.

Ligament tears are **sprains**. Ligament tears and ruptures can occur at any joint but are most common in the wrist, ankle, elbow, and knee joints. A complete separation of a tendon or ligament from its bony attachment site is an **avulsion** and is commonly seen in young athletes, especially sprinters, hurdlers, and distance runners.

Strains and sprains are classified as first degree (mild), second degree (moderate), and third degree (severe). In first-degree injuries, the fibres are stretched but the muscle (strain) or joint (sprain) remains stable. In second-degree strains or sprains, there is more tearing of the tendon or ligament fibres, with muscle weakness (strain) or some joint instability (sprain) but incomplete tearing of fibres. Third-degree strains and sprains result in an inability to contract the muscle normally (strain) and cause significant joint instability (sprain).

PATHOPHYSIOLOGY When a tendon or ligament is torn, an inflammatory exudate develops between the torn ends. Multiple growth factors that direct the repair process are released. Later, granulation tissue containing macrophages, fibroblasts, and capillary buds grows inward from the surrounding soft tissue and cartilage to begin the repair process. Within 4 to 5 days after the injury, collagen formation begins. At first, collagen formation is random and disorganized. As the collagen fibres interweave and connect with pre-existing tendon fibres, they become organized, parallel to the lines of the musculotendinous unit. Eventually, vascular fibrous tissue fuses the new and surrounding tissues into a single mass. Collagen fibres reconnect the tendon and bone, forming a type of enthesis.[6] Usually, a healing tendon or ligament lacks sufficient strength to withstand some stress for 4 to 5 weeks after the injury; mechanical stability of a joint may take more than 3 months to achieve.[7] If powerful muscle pull does occur during healing, the tendon or ligament ends may separate again, which causes the tendon or ligament to heal in a lengthened shape or with an excessive amount of scar tissue, resulting in poor tendon or ligament function.

CLINICAL MANIFESTATIONS Tendon and ligament injuries are painful and are usually accompanied by soft tissue swelling, changes in tendon or ligament contour, and dislocation or subluxation of bones. Pain is generally sharp and localized, and tenderness persists over the distribution of the tendon or ligament. Movement or weight-bearing increases pain. Even with prompt treatment, depending on the tendon or ligament involved, significant injuries may result in decreased mobility, instability, and weakness of the affected joints.

EVALUATION AND TREATMENT Evaluation is based on mechanism of injury, clinical manifestations, stress radiography, arthroscopy, or arthrography. Initial treatment consists of PRICE (*p*rotection, *r*est, *i*ce, *c*ompression, and *e*levation) for the first 48 to 72 hours. Once swelling and acute pain subside, in most cases, support of the affected tendon or ligament with a compression dressing or brace will provide appropriate reinforcement while the tissues heal. Rehabilitation is crucial to regaining good functional outcome.[8] In severe (third-degree) injuries, treatment may include suturing the tendon or ligament ends in close approximation. If this is not feasible because of the extent of damage, tendon or ligament grafting may be necessary. Prolonged, functional rehabilitation programs help ensure return of near-normal functions, but recovery may be complicated by post-traumatic arthritis.

Tendinopathy, Epicondylopathy, and Bursitis

Trauma can also cause painful inflammation of tendons (tendinopathy [tendonitis]) and bursae (bursitis). Other causes of damage to tendons (or *tendinopathy*) include reduced tissue perfusion, mechanical irritation, crystal deposits, postural misalignment, and hypermobility of a joint. Vascular ingrowth in tendinopathy (neovascularization) occurs in conjunction with nerve ingrowth, facilitating pain transmission most notably in Achilles and patellar tendinopathy.[9]

Lateral epicondylopathy ("tennis elbow") or medial epicondylopathy ("golfer's elbow"), involves a common degenerative process[10,11] (Figure 39.4). The bony prominence at the end of a bone where tendons or ligaments attach is an **epicondyle**. When force is sufficient to cause microscopic tears (microtears) in tissue, the result is **tendinopathy** or **epicondylopathy**. Microtears in the tendon, the presence of disorganized collagen fibres, and neovascularization indicate an incomplete tissue repair. Initial inflammatory changes cause thickening of the tendon sheath, limiting movements and causing pain.[12] Microtears cause bleeding, edema, and pain (because of the presence of substance P) in the involved tendon or tendons. At times, after repeated microtears, calcium may be deposited in the tendon origin area.

Lateral epicondylopathy (tennis elbow) is the result of irritation and overstretching of the extensor carpi radialis brevis tendon and forearm extensor muscles and leads to tissue degradation, loss of grip strength, and pain.[13] **Medial epicondylopathy (golfer's elbow)** results from similar forces affecting the forearm muscles responsible for forearm flexion and pronation (see Figure 39.4). Repetitive load-bearing activities or acute injuries that involve flexion, extension, pronation, or supination of the elbow and forearm can lead to either lateral or medial elbow symptoms.

Clinical manifestations of epicondylopathy are usually localized to one side of the joint. In general, there is local tenderness and more pain with active motion than with passive motion. With tendinopathy (or tendonitis), the pain is localized over the involved tendon. Stressing the tendon with simple activities, such as lifting even a few kilograms of weight, can increase pain. Pain and sometimes weakness limit joint movement.

Bursae are small sacs lined with synovial membrane and filled with synovial fluid that are located between bony prominences and soft tissues such as tendons, muscles, and ligaments (Figure 39.5). Bursae can be either "constant" (those formed during embryological development) or "adventitious" (bursae that develop as a result of chronic friction and degeneration of fibrous tissue between adjacent structures). The primary function of a bursa is to separate, lubricate, and cushion these structures. When irritated or injured, these sacs become inflamed and swell. Because most bursae lie outside joints, joint movement is rarely compromised with bursitis. Acute bursitis occurs primarily in middle age and is caused by trauma. Chronic bursitis can result from repeated trauma. Septic bursitis is the result of wound infection or bacterial infection of the skin overlying the bursae. Bursitis commonly occurs in the shoulder, hip, knee, and elbow but also can affect the spine, wrist, foot, and ankle.

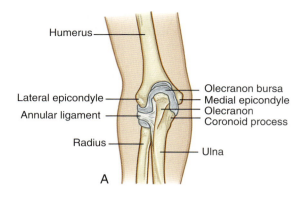

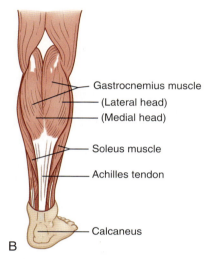

FIGURE 39.4 Epicondylopathy and Tendinopathy. A, Lateral and medial epicondyles of the distal humerus, sites of tennis elbow (lateral) and golfer's elbow (medial). B, Achilles tendon, common site of tendinopathy.

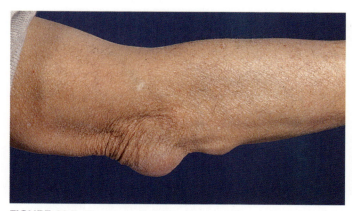

FIGURE 39.5 Olecranon Bursitis. Note swelling at the point of the elbow (olecranon). A smaller, rheumatoid nodule also is present. (From Hochberg, M. C., Silman, A. J., Smolen, J. S., et al. [2015]. *Rheumatology* [6th ed.]. Elsevier.)

PATHOPHYSIOLOGY Bursitis is usually an inflammation that is reactive to overuse or excessive pressure, but can also be caused by infection, autoimmune diseases, crystal deposition, or acute trauma. The inflamed bursal sac becomes engorged, and the inflammation can spread to adjacent tissues. The inflammation may decrease with rest, ice, and aspiration of the fluid. (Inflammation is discussed in Chapter 6.)

CLINICAL MANIFESTATIONS Joint motion is rarely limited in bursitis, except by pain. Shoulder pain may impair arm abduction. Bursitis in the knee produces pain when climbing stairs, and crossing the legs is painful in bursitis of the hip. Lying on the side of the inflamed trochanteric bursa is also very painful. Signs of infectious bursitis may include the presence of pain, a puncture site, warmth and erythema, prior corticosteroid injection, severe inflammation, or an adjacent source of infection, such as from total joint replacement surgery.

EVALUATION AND TREATMENT The diagnosis of tendinopathy, epicondylopathy, and bursitis is primarily based on clinical history and physical examination. Other imaging techniques, such as ultrasound or magnetic resonance imaging (MRI), may be used to evaluate the severity of the problem. Treatment may include temporary immobilization of the joint with a sling, splint, or cast; administration of systemic analgesics; application of ice or heat; or local injection of an anaesthetic, a corticosteroid, platelet-rich plasma (PRP), or a combination of local anaesthetic/corticosteroid. Physical therapy to prevent loss of function begins after acute inflammation subsides (see *Health Promotion*: Managing Tendinopathy).

Muscle Strains

Muscle strain is a general term for local muscle damage. Mild injury such as muscle strain is usually seen after traumatic or sports injuries. It is often the result of sudden, forced motion causing the muscle to become stretched beyond normal capacity. Strains often involve the tendon as well. Penetrating injuries, such as knife and gunshot wounds, can cause traumatic rupture (see Chapter 4). Muscles are ruptured more often than tendons in young people; the opposite is true in the older population. Muscle strain may be chronic when the muscle is repeatedly stretched beyond its usual capacity. There is evidence of tissue disruption with subsequent signs of muscle regeneration and connective tissue repair when a biopsy is performed. Hemorrhage into the surrounding tissue and signs of inflammation also may be present.

Muscle healing occurs in three phases:

1. *Destruction*, in which the myofibres of the damaged muscle contract and necrose, beginning an inflammatory reaction. The gap between torn fibres is filled by a hematoma.
2. *Repair*, which begins with monocytes phagocytizing the dead tissue and activating satellite cells, which become myoblasts. The myoblasts infiltrate the scar tissue, and new capillary formation begins at the site of injury. The first two phases occur within a week of injury.
3. *Remodelling* occurs as the myofibres mature, form contractile tissue, and attach to the ends of scar tissue.[14] Regeneration may take up to 6 weeks, and the affected muscle should be protected during that time.

Table 39.2 summarizes the degrees of acute muscle strain, together with their manifestations and treatment.

A late complication of some muscle injuries is myositis ossificans, also known as heterotopic ossification (HO). Its exact pathophysiology remains unknown, but the basic problem seems to be the inability of mesenchymal cells to differentiate into osteoblastic stem cells and inappropriate differentiation of fibroblasts into bone-forming cells. Though uncommon, HO is associated with burns, joint surgery, and trauma to the musculoskeletal system or central nervous system (CNS). HO may involve the muscle or tendons, ligaments, or bones near the muscle, causing stiffness or deformity of an extremity. Soft tissue calcifications may be seen on plain radiographs.

Rhabdomyolysis

Once used interchangeably with the term *myoglobinuria*, rhabdomyolysis is the rapid breakdown of muscle that causes the release of intracellular contents, including the protein pigment myoglobin,

HEALTH PROMOTION
Managing Tendinopathy

Tennis and golfer's elbow, Achilles tendinopathy, and other tendon problems account for a large percentage of sports-related overuse injuries. Successful treatment of these conditions is challenging because of the mechanisms of tendon healing as well as inconsistent results, with many interventions still not completely understood. Persistent pain is common and may be the result of an ingrowth of nerves that accompanies ingrowth of new blood vessels during the healing process. Recent studies suggest that the traditional approach of corticosteroid injections is helpful only for the short term. Other therapies that show promise include:

Prolotherapy: An irritant such as glucose or lidocaine (2% Lidocaine Hydrochloride Injection USP) is injected into the affected tendon, inducing an inflammatory response, thereby stimulating growth of new tendon fibres.

Eccentric exercises: The tendon is "prestretched," increasing its resting length and resulting in less strain during movement. The load on the tendon is gradually increased, causing the tendon itself to strengthen.

Extracorporeal shockwave therapy: External acoustic or sonic waves are focused on the affected area. The shockwaves stimulate soft tissue healing and inhibit pain receptors.

Needling: This treatment involves multiple insertions of a sterile needle into affected tissue. The pain sensation is reduced by stimulating A-nerve fibres, or "dry needling," since no fluid is introduced.

Platelet-rich plasma (PRP): This autologous source of concentrated platelets comes from the centrifugation of plasma. The resulting solution contains high concentrations of cytokines and growth factors, such as platelet-derived growth factor (PDGF) and transforming growth factor-beta (TGF-β), which promote the growth of new, healthy tissue.

Autologous tenocyte injections: Autologous injection of tenocytes at the site of tendinopathy is thought to provide necessary mediators of tissue healing.

From Andarawis-Puri, N., Flatow, E. L., & Soslowsky, L. J. (2015). *Journal of Orthopaedic Research, 33*(6), 780–784; Krey, D., Borchers, J., & McCamey, K. (2015). *The Physician and Sportsmedicine, 43*(1), 80–86; Langer, P. R. (2015). *Clinics in Podiatric Medicine and Surgery, 32*(2), 183–193; Mautner, K., & Kneer, L. (2014). *Physical Medicine and Rehabilitation Clinics of North America, 25*(4), 865–880; Wang, A., Mackie, K., Breidahl, W., et al. (2015). *American Journal of Sports Medicine, 43*(7), 1775–1783.

TABLE 39.2 Muscle Strain

Type	Manifestations	Treatment
First degree (example: bench press in untrained athlete)	Muscle overstretched, pain but no muscle deformity	Ice should be applied 5 or 6 times in first 24–48 hours; gradual resumption of full weight-bearing after initial rest for up to 2 weeks
		Exercises individualized to specific injury
Second degree (example: any muscle strain with bruising and pain)	Muscle intact with some tearing of fibres, swelling, pain	Treatment similar to that for first-degree strains
Third degree (example: traumatic injury)	Caused by tearing of fascia, marked weakness, deformity	Surgery to approximate ruptured edges; immobilization and non-weight-bearing status for 6 weeks

into the extracellular space and bloodstream. Physical interruptions in the sarcolemma membrane, called delta lesions, are the route by which muscle constituents are released. (The sarcolemma membrane, the plasma membrane of the muscle cell, is described in Chapter 38.) **Myoglobinuria**, first described in victims of crush injuries in London during World War II, refers to the presence of the muscle protein myoglobin in the urine.

PATHOPHYSIOLOGY Rhabdomyolysis is sometimes incorrectly used interchangeably with *crush injury* (a description of injuries resulting from crushing of a body part), *compartment syndrome* (the consequences of increased intracompartmental pressures of a muscle), or *crush syndrome* (the systemic pathophysiological events caused by rhabdomyolysis, primarily involving the kidneys and coagulation syndrome).[15,16] Although relatively rare, rhabdomyolysis has many causes (Box 39.1) and can result in serious complications, including hyperkalemia (because of the release of intracellular potassium into the circulation) and cardiac dysrhythmias. The most clinically significant complication is acute kidney failure (myoglobin precipitates in the tubules, obstructing flow through the nephron and producing injury).[17] Other complications include metabolic acidosis (from liberation of intracellular phosphorus and sulphate) and even disseminated intravascular coagulation (likely caused by activation of the clotting cascade by sarcolemma damage and release of intracellular components from the damaged muscles).

CLINICAL MANIFESTATIONS A *classic triad* of muscle pain, weakness, and dark urine is considered typical of rhabdomyolysis, but those affected may have no complaint of pain or muscle weakness.[15] Abnormally dark urine caused by myoglobinuria may be the first and only symptom; however, the presence of myoglobin in urine is not a reliable test for rhabdomyolysis.[18] The renal threshold for myoglobin is low (approximately 285 nmol/L of urine); therefore, only 200 g of muscle needs to be damaged to cause visible changes in the urine. Myoglobin is rapidly cleared, and levels may return to normal within 24 hours of injury. Along with the release of myoglobin, creatine kinase (CK) and other serum enzymes are released in massive quantities (normal CK levels are 5 to 25 units/L for women and 5 to 35 units/L for men). The efflux of intracellular proteins and enzymes includes loss of potassium, phosphate, nucleotides, creatinine, and creatine. Serum hypocalcemia occurs early in the course of myoglobinuria and is followed by late hypercalcemia. The risk for kidney failure increases proportionately to the increase in the levels of serum CK, potassium, and phosphorus.

EVALUATION AND TREATMENT The most important and clinically useful measurement in rhabdomyolysis is serum CK level. A level 5 to 10 times the upper limit of normal (about 1 000 units/L) identifies rhabdomyolysis.[17] Once CK levels exceed 15 000 units/L, acute kidney injury is likely. Other laboratory tests may include electrolytes (elevated serum potassium level [hyperkalemia] can cause

BOX 39.1 Selected Causes of Rhabdomyolysis

Direct Trauma
Blunt trauma or crush injury (motor vehicle crashes, collapsed buildings)
Burns (thermal)
Electrical injury
Excessive compression (from immobility attributable to stroke or alcohol or medication intoxication)

Medications, Drugs, and Substances
Alcohol
Amphetamines
Anaesthetic and paralytic agents (halothane [Fluothane], propofol [Diprivan], succinylcholine [Anectine]—malignant hyperthermia syndrome)
Antihistamines (diphenhydramine [Benadryl], doxylamine [Unisom])
Antihyperlipidemic agents (statins, clofibrate [Atromid S], bezafibrate [Bezalip SR])
Antipsychotics and antidepressants (amitriptyline [Elavil], doxepin [Apo-Doxepin], fluoxetine [Apo-Fluoxetine], haloperidol [Apo-Haloperidol], lithium [PMS-Lithium Carbonate], protriptyline [Triptil], perphenazine [Perphenazine], promethazine [Histantil], chlorpromazine [Chlorprom], trifluoperazine [Novo-flurazine], venlafaxine [Effexor])
Caffeine
Cocaine
Corticosteroids
Fibrinates (antilipid agents: bezafibrate, ciprofibrate [Modalim], clofibrate, ezetimibe [Ach-exetimibe], gemfibrozil [Dom-gemfibrozil])
Heroin
HIV integrase inhibitor (raltegravir [Isentress])
Hypnotics and sedatives (benzodiazepines, barbiturates)
LSD (lysergic acid diethylamide)
Methadone
Methamphetamine
Methylenedioxymethamphetamine (MDMA; "ecstasy")
Miscellaneous medications (amphotericin B [Abelcet], arsenic, azathioprine [Imuran], ε-aminocaproic acid [Amicar], halothane, quinidine [Quin-G], penicillamine [Cuprimine], propofol, salicylates, succinylcholine, theophylline [Slo-bid], terbutaline [Bricanyl], thiazides, vasopressin [Pressyn])
Phencyclidine
Protease inhibitors
Statins (atorvastatin [Lipitor], fluvastatin [Lescol], lovastatin [Mevacor], pravastatin [Pravachol], rosuvastatin [Crestor], simvastatin [Zocor])

Excessive Muscular Contraction
Status epilepticus
Delirium tremens
Acute psychosis
Severe dystonia
Sporadic strenuous exercise (e.g., marathons, squats)
Tetanus

Infectious Agents
Bacteria (group B streptococci, *Streptococcus pneumoniae, Staphylococcus epidermidis, Borrelia burgdorferi, Escherichia coli, Clostridium perfringens, Clostridium tetani, Streptococcus viridans; Bacillus, Brucella, Legionella, Listeria, Leptospira, Mycoplasma, Plasmodium, Rickettsia, Salmonella,* and *Vibrio* species)
Fungal organisms (Aspergillus, Candida species)
Viruses (influenza types A and B, coxsackievirus, dengue, Epstein-Barr, HIV, cytomegalovirus, parainfluenza, varicella-zoster, West Nile)

Toxins
Carbon monoxide
Envenomation (black widow spider, Africanized honey bees, vipers)
Hemlock
Methanol
Toluene

Hereditary Enzyme Disorders (Rare)
McArdle's disease (myophosphorylase deficiency)
Tarui's disease (type VII glycogen storage disease)
Phosphoglycerate mutase deficiency (glycogen storage disease type X)
Carnitine palmitoyltransferase deficiency (CPT1 deficiency)

Miscellaneous Causes
Diabetic ketoacidosis
Endocrinopathy
Heatstroke
Hypothermia
Nonketotic hyperosmolar coma
Polymyositis
Severe electrolyte disorders (near-drowning or water intoxication; severe vomiting or diarrhea)

Data from Cervellin, G., Comelli, I., & Lippi, G. (2010). *Clinical Chemistry and Laboratory Medicine, 48*(6), 749–756; Croce, F., Vitello, P., Dalla Pria, A., et al. (2010). *International Journal of STD & AIDS, 21*(11), 783–785; Halpern, P., Moskovich, J., Avrahami, B., et al. (2011). *Human & Experimental Toxicology, 30*(4), 259–266; Keltz, E., Khan, F. Y., & Mann, G. (2014). *Muscle, Ligaments and Tendons Journal, 3*(4), 303–312; Torres, P. A., Helmstetter, J. A., Kaye, A. M., et al. (2015). *Ochsner Journal, 15*(1), 58–69; Zutt, R., van der Kooi, A. J., Linthorst, G. E., et al. (2014). *Neuromuscular Disorders, 24*(8), 651–659.

life-threatening cardiac abnormalities) and blood urea nitrogen (BUN)/creatinine ratio (decreased ratio because of creatine released from damaged muscle being converted to creatinine). Additional laboratory tests—such as measurement of hemoglobin, hematocrit, and platelet levels and determination of activated partial thromboplastin time—may be indicated in the presence of other trauma or suspected bleeding.

The goals of treatment are maintaining adequate urinary flow and prevention of kidney injury/failure. Rapid intravenous hydration maintains adequate kidney flow. Other issues, such as hyperkalemia, may require temporary hemodialysis. Common treatments for rhabdomyolysis such as mannitol (Osmitrol) to cause an osmotic diuresis or bicarbonate to alkalinize the urine are not consistent with improved outcomes.[15,16]

Compartment Syndrome

Compartment syndrome is the result of increased pressure within a muscle compartment. Several layers of fibrous fascia (that do not expand) surround skeletal muscles. Increased pressure on the muscle tissue causes diminished capillary blood flow, resulting in local tissue hypoxia and necrosis. Causes of compartment syndrome include conditions that increase the contents of the compartment (such as bleeding after a fracture), decrease the compartment volume (such as a tight bandage or cast), or a combination of both conditions that result in disturbing the muscle's microvasculature (Box 39.2).[19–21] Any condition that disrupts the vascular supply to an extremity (such as severe burns, bleeding disorders, crush injury, snake or insect bites, extremely tight bandages, or casts) can cause increased pressure within the muscle compartments.

BOX 39.2 Factors Affecting Development of Compartment Syndrome

Increased Intracompartmental Pressure
Fracture (open or closed)
Traction
Crush syndrome
Vigorous exercise or nonroutine activity/overuse in nonathletes
High-energy soft tissue injury (blast injuries, blunt force trauma)
Fluid infusion
Arterial puncture
Ruptured abdominal aortic aneurysm
Ruptured ganglion/other cyst
Envenomation (venomous snakes, black widow spiders)
Nephrotic syndrome
Viral myositis
Acute hematogenous osteomyelitis
Orthopedic procedures (e.g., osteotomy, joint replacement)
Seizures
Tetany

Reduced Compartment Volume
Burns
Repair of muscle herniation
Circumferential dressings
Casts that are too tight

Conditions That Disturb Microcirculation
Diabetes
Hypothyroidism
Bleeding disorders (hemophilia, von Willebrand's disease, leukemia, vitamin K deficiency, viral hemorrhagic fevers [dengue])
Excessive anticoagulation
Malignancies

Data from Raza, H., & Mahapatra, A. (2015). Acute compartment syndrome in orthopedics: causes, diagnosis, and management. *Advances in Orthopedics, 2015*, 543412; Shadgan, B., Menon, M., Sanders, D., et al. (2010). Current thinking about acute compartment syndrome of the lower extremity. *Canadian Journal of Surgery, 53*(5), 329–334.

PATHOPHYSIOLOGY The weight of a limb extremity can generate enough pressure to produce muscle ischemia (Figures 39.6 and 39.7). Muscle ischemia causes edema, rising compartment pressure, and tamponade, leading to muscle infarction and neural injury and eventually resulting in cell loss.

CLINICAL MANIFESTATIONS The anterior and deep posterior tibial compartments in the leg, the forearm, the gluteal compartments in the buttocks, and the abdominal wall are the compartments that are most often affected by compartment syndrome. Clinical examination of the "6 Ps" of compartment syndrome: Pain (out of proportion to the injury), Pressure (swelling, tenseness of the affected area), Pallor, Paresthesia, Paresis (of the involved extremity), and Pulselessness, help in its diagnosis. None of these signs is truly dependable, although pain with passive extension of the fingers or toes in the affected extremity and paresthesia tend to be most suggestive of compartment syndrome.[19,22]

Volkmann ischemic contracture can develop when compartment syndrome is unrecognized or is not adequately treated. This condition involves irreversible neurovascular damage, and contracture deformities of the fingers, hand, and wrist can lead to partial or complete disability of the affected limb.

EVALUATION AND TREATMENT Direct measurement of intracompartmental pressure, using a manometer or an electronic transducer, is essential to confirm the diagnosis.[23,24] Laboratory tests, ultrasonography, and imaging studies may help exclude other conditions but generally are not helpful in diagnosing compartment syndrome. Once intracompartmental pressures reach 30 mm Hg, surgical intervention is warranted to relieve pressure within the compartment.

Surgical intervention consists of performing a fasciotomy of the affected area to decompress the compartment and allow return of normal blood supply. Skin grafts are often required to close the resultant opening, but vacuum-assisted wound closure devices also have been used successfully in accelerating wound closure.

Malignant Hyperthermia

Malignant hyperthermia (MH) is an autosomal dominant inherited muscle disorder characterized by a hypermetabolic reaction to certain volatile anaesthetics or certain depolarizing muscle relaxants (such as succinylcholine [Anectine]) that activate a prolonged release of intracellular calcium from the sarcoplasmic reticulum. Advances in molecular genetics indicate that a mutation in the ryanodine receptor of skeletal muscle (RyR1) is responsible for the majority of cases, though other genetic mutations also may be involved.[25,26] There is a disruption of the normal excitation-coupling process of muscle contraction in MH. Mutations of RyR1 receptors release uncontrolled amounts of calcium from the sarcoplasmic reticulum into the cytoplasm, causing continuous muscle contraction.[27] This process also causes hypermetabolism with extremely high body temperature, muscle rigidity, rhabdomyolysis, and death if not quickly treated with dantrolene (Dantrium) infusion.[28]

Though reported in all countries, ages, and both genders, young males tend to be more susceptible to MH. Common signs and symptoms are respiratory acidosis (with elevated end tidal carbon dioxide), tachycardia, masseter and skeletal muscle spasm, and elevated body temperature.[27,29]

EVALUATION AND TREATMENT Careful and thorough preoperative assessment should alert the anaesthesiologist to the possibility of an individual being susceptible to MH. A family history of anaesthetic problems and previous untoward anaesthetic experiences (muscle cramping, unexplained fevers, dark urine) are criteria that require further clarification before administration of a volatile anaesthetic, such as halothane (Fluothane), or of the muscle relaxant succinylcholine. Currently, the muscle contracture test is considered the best predictor of developing MH. A muscle biopsy is obtained from the individual, and the tissue is then separately exposed to standardized amounts of halothane and caffeine. If the muscle bundles exhibit a contracture at specified limits, the individual is considered susceptible to MH.[29] Molecular and DNA testing are promising future means of identifying at-risk individuals.

Priorities in treatment of MH include identifying and treating the underlying disorder and preventing life-threatening kidney failure. MH and myoglobinuria can be treated by infusing dantrolene sodium (Dantrium). Secondary problems include electrolyte imbalance, volume depletion, acidosis, hyperuricemia, hyperkalemia, and calcium imbalance; these need specific treatment. Short-term dialysis also may be necessary.

DISORDERS OF BONES

> ✓ **QUICK CHECK 39.2**
> 1. What are the causes associated with osteoporosis in women and men?
> 2. How does osteoporosis differ from osteomalacia? Name three differences.
> 3. What are the risk factors for osteomyelitis?

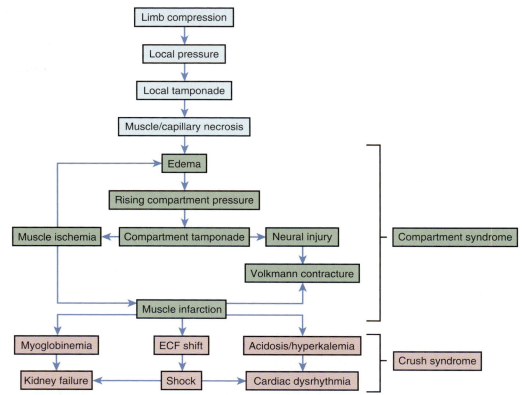

FIGURE 39.6 Pathogenesis of Compartment Syndrome and Crush Syndrome Caused by Prolonged Muscle Compression. *ECF,* Extracellular fluid.

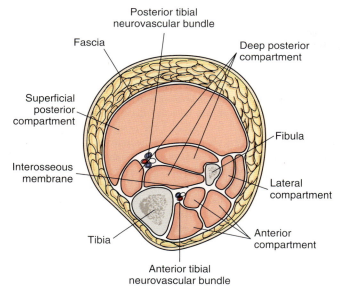

FIGURE 39.7 Muscle Compartments of the Lower Leg. (From Monahan, F. D., Sands, J., Neighbors, M., et al. [2007]. *Phipps' medical-surgical nursing: health and illness perspectives* [8th ed.]. Mosby.)

Metabolic Bone Diseases

Metabolic bone disease is characterized by abnormal bone structure that is caused by altered or inadequate biochemical reactions, which may be attributable to genetics, diet, or hormones.

Osteoporosis

Osteoporosis, or **porous bone**, is generally described as decreased bone mineral density (BMD) and an increased risk for fractures because of alterations in bone microarchitecture. Osteoporosis is a complex, multifactorial, chronic disease that often progresses silently for decades until fractures occur. It is the most common disease that affects bone but is not necessarily a consequence of the aging process because some older adults retain strong, relatively dense bones. In osteoporosis, old bone is resorbed faster than new bone is made, causing the bones to lose density, becoming thinner and more porous. A progressive loss of bone mass may continue until the skeleton is no longer strong enough to support itself. Eventually, bones can fracture spontaneously. As bone becomes more fragile, falls or bumps that would not have caused a fracture previously now cause bone to break (a fragility fracture). The most common sites for osteoporosis-related fractures are the spine, femoral neck, and wrist.[30]

Bone tissue can be normally mineralized in osteoporosis, but the mass (density) of bone is decreased and the structural integrity of trabecular bone is impaired. Cortical bone becomes more porous and thinner, making bone weaker and prone to fractures (Figures 39.8 and 39.9). The World Health Organization (WHO) has defined *osteoporosis* as "a systematic skeletal disease characterized by low bone density and microarchitectural deterioration of bone tissue with a consequent increase in bone fragility."[31]

Bone density is based on the number of standard deviations that an adult's bone density differs from the mean BMD of a young-adult reference population (a T-score). Table 39.3 lists these categories. Bone density between 1.5 and 2.5 standard deviations below normal is considered osteopenia. A T-score of 2.5 or more standard deviations below normal bone density is considered osteoporotic. Severe or established

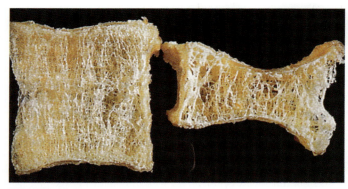

FIGURE 39.8 Vertebral Body. Osteoporotic vertebral body *(right)* shortened by compression fractures compared with a normal vertebral body. Note that the osteoporotic vertebra has a characteristic loss of horizontal trabeculae and thickened vertical trabeculae. (From Kumar, V., Abbas, A. K., & Aster, J. C. [Eds.]. [2021]. *Robbins and Cotran pathologic basis of disease* [10th ed.]. Saunders.)

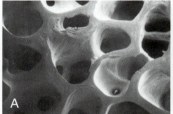 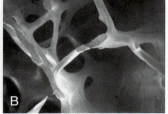

FIGURE 39.9 Electron Microscopic Comparison of Normal and Osteoporotic Bone. A, Normal trabecular structure. B, Osteoporotic bone; note the loss of supporting trabeculae. (Reprinted with permission from Golob, A. L., & Laya, M. B. [2015]. Osteoporosis: screening, prevention, and management. *Medical Clinics of North America, 99*[3], 587–606.)

TABLE 39.3 T-Score and World Health Organization Diagnosis of Bone Density

T-Score	Diagnosis
0 to −0.99 SD	Normal BMD
−1.0 to −2.49 SD	Low bone density (osteopenia)
≤2.5 SD	Osteoporosis
≤2.5 SD with any fracture	Severe osteoporosis

BMD, Bone mineral density; *SD,* standard deviation.

osteoporosis is identified when there has been a fragility fracture associated with low bone density. The disease can be (1) generalized, involving major portions of the axial skeleton, or (2) regional, involving one segment of the appendicular skeleton.

Skeletal allostasis depends on a narrow range of plasma calcium and phosphate concentrations, which are maintained by the endocrine system. Therefore, endocrine dysfunction ultimately can cause metabolic bone disease. In addition to declining levels of sex steroids, the hormones most commonly associated with osteoporosis are parathyroid hormone (PTH), cortisol, thyroid hormone, and growth hormone. (Endocrine function is discussed in Chapters 18 and 19.)

Other factors that can adversely affect normal bone homeostasis include multiple medications (such as glucocorticoids, proton pump inhibitors, thiazolidinediones, antiseizure medications, aromatase inhibitors, selective serotonin reuptake inhibitors [SSRIs], and anticoagulants), vitamin D deficiency, underlying diseases (rheumatoid disease, Paget's disease, cancer, diabetes), low physical activity, and abnormal body mass index.[32–36]

Throughout a lifetime, old bone is removed (resorption) and new bone is added (formation) to the skeleton. During childhood and teenage years, new bone is added faster than old bone is removed. Consequently, bones become larger, heavier, and denser. Bone formation continues at a pace faster than resorption until **peak bone mass** or maximum bone density and strength is reached, around age 30. Up to 90% of peak bone mass is obtained by age 20. After age 30, bone resorption slowly exceeds bone formation. In women, bone loss is most rapid in the first years after menopause but persists throughout the postmenopausal years. The *2010 Clinical Practice Guidelines for the Diagnosis and Management of Osteoporosis in Canada* included a new recommendation that all men and women aged 65 and older be routinely screened for osteoporosis.[37] Fractures are the major complication of osteoporosis, and it has been estimated that the fracture risk for osteoporosis is a worldwide problem with significant economic and health implications.[38–40] Hip fractures in particular can have devastating effects on an individual's life. In addition to direct medical costs, studies have shown decreased quality of life as well as excess loss of life-years for those experiencing hip or osteoporotic fractures.[41–43] The major complications for persons with osteoporosis are fractures. Bone structure in men allows for improved torque strength, and although men lose bone density with aging, it is at a slower, steadier rate than that of women.[44] Nevertheless, men are more likely to die after a hip fracture than are women.[45,46]

Vertebral fractures tend to occur in the later years of life; however, they are more difficult to diagnose because people may be unaware of the fracture. There is still no clear standardization for measuring the degree of compression necessary to define a vertebral fracture. The true prevalence of such fractures is unknown, but fractures do increase in frequency by the sixth and seventh decades. Approximately one in six women and one in twelve men will sustain a vertebral fracture.[47]

Age-related loss of bone density and osteoporosis is most common in White women but affects all races. Asian and Black women have only about half the fracture rate of White women, but that percentage is expected to increase with improved life expectancy.[48] In spite of lower incidence, mortality in Black women after a hip fracture is higher than among White women. Other factors may include lower calcium intake, a high percentage of lactose intolerance, and increased prevalence of diseases such as sickle cell disease and lupus that increase the risk of developing osteoporosis.[49] Both Black women and Black men have generally been undertreated for osteoporosis.

Fracture prevention is a primary goal of osteoporosis treatment. Measuring BMD by using dual X-ray absorptiometry (DXA) to calculate an individual's T-score continues to be the most common method of evaluating bone health and predicting fracture risk. Unfortunately, the technology to perform DXA scans is not available in all areas of the world. As a result, several tools that do not require BMD testing have been developed and validated to predict future fracture risk. These tools are summarized in Table 39.4. Interestingly, when BMD measurement is not available, there is little difference in fracture prediction between the Internet-based FRAX and the other tools, including the simplest screening tool—the Osteoporosis Self-assessment Tool, or OST.[50]

Bone quality is not defined by bone mass alone (as measured by BMD) but also by the microarchitecture of the bone. Thus, other variables include crystal size and shape, brittleness, vitality of bone cells, structure of the bone proteins, integrity of the trabecular network, and the ability to repair tiny cracks. Because bone density relates to *quantity* of bone, *quality* of bone is not accurately identified by bone density testing alone. As a result, bone density testing may not accurately identify those who will eventually be susceptible to fractures.

TABLE 39.4	Comparison of Fracture Risk Assessment Tools Not Utilizing Bone Mineral Density				
Risk Factor	FRAX	SCORE	OSIRIS	ORAI	OST
Age	X	X	X	X	X
Weight	X	X	X	X	X
Previous low-energy fracture	X	X	X		
Estrogen therapy		X	X	X	
Rheumatoid arthritis	X	X			
Height	X				
Parental hip fracture	X				
Smoking	X				
Alcohol	X				
Glucocorticoid therapy	X				
Secondary osteoporosis	X				
Sex	X				
Ethnicity		X			

FRAX, World Health Organization's "Fracture Risk Assessment Tool"; ORAI, osteoporosis risk assessment instrument; OSIRIS, osteoporosis index of risk; OST, osteoporosis self-assessment tool; SCORE, simple calculated osteoporosis risk estimation.
Chart from Rubin, K. H., Abrahamsen, B., Friis-Holmberg, T., et al. (2013). Comparison of different screening tools (FRAX, OST, ORAI, OSIRIS, SCORE and age alone) to identify women with increased risk of fracture. A population-based prospective study. Bone, 56(1), 18.

Postmenopausal osteoporosis is bone loss that occurs in middle-aged and older women. It can occur because of estrogen deficiency as well as from estrogen-independent age-related mechanisms (e.g., secondary causes such as hyperparathyroidism and decreased mechanical stimulation) (see Health Promotion: Management of Postmenopausal Osteoporosis). Estrogen deficiency can also increase with stress, excessive exercise, and low body weight. Postmenopausal changes include alterations in the OPG/RANKL/RANK system, resulting in a substantial increase in bone turnover—that is, a remodelling imbalance between the activity of osteoclasts (bone destroyers) and osteoblasts (bone formers). Increased production and activity of osteoclasts causes removal or resorption of bone and results in a cascade of proinflammatory cytokines. Increased cytokine activation, especially tumour necrosis factor (TNF), can occur with declining estrogen levels.[51] In addition, estrogen helps osteoclast apoptosis (programmed cell death), so a decrease in estrogen levels is associated with *survival* of the bone-removing osteoclasts. Biologically, these processes involve the receptor activator of nuclear factor kappa-B ligand (RANKL), osteoprotegerin (OPG) signalling pathways, and insulinlike growth factor (IGF) (see Chapter 38 and Figures 38.5 and 39.10). Other causes may include a combination of inadequate dietary calcium intake and lack of vitamin D (and possibly decreased magnesium), lack of exercise, low body mass, and family history. IGF is known to help in fracture healing and collagen synthesis and improves conditions for bone mineralization. IGF levels significantly decline by age 60. Excessive phosphorus intake, chiefly through the intake of highly processed foods, hampers the calcium–phosphorus balance by interfering with PTH and fibroblast growth factor-23 (FGF-23).[52,53]

Sex hormones, particularly estradiol (estrogen), are major determinants of bone density in both females and males.[54,55] Androgens (i.e., testosterone and dihydrotestosterone) have long been recognized as stimulants of bone formation. Increasing age in both men and women is associated with declining levels of estradiol and androgen, leading to losses in BMD. Other factors, such as inadequate dietary calcium intake, decreases in weight-bearing exercise, and sarcopenia, also are associated with osteoporosis. Other risk factors are identified in *Risk Factors: Osteoporosis*.

Insufficient intake or malabsorption of dietary minerals is a factor in the development of osteoporosis. Calcium absorption from the intestine decreases with age, and studies of individuals with osteoporosis show that their calcium intake is lower than that of age-matched controls. Other mineral deficiencies, including magnesium, also may be important. Vitamin deficiencies, particularly vitamin D, as well as either deficiencies or excesses of protein also contribute to bone loss. Decreased serum levels of trace elements (zinc, copper, iron, magnesium, and manganese) have been associated not only with lower peak bone mass in developing bone but also with later development of osteoporosis.[56-58] Excessive intake of caffeine, phosphorus, alcohol, and nicotine along with low body fat (weight less than 57 kg) has been shown to lower BMD.[59-61] **Secondary osteoporosis** is osteoporosis caused by other conditions, including hormonal imbalances (endocrine disease, diabetes, hyperparathyroidism, hyperthyroidism), medications (e.g., heparin, corticosteroids, phenytoin, barbiturates, lithium), and other substances (e.g., tobacco, ethanol). Other conditions, including rheumatoid disease, human immunodeficiency virus (HIV), malignancies, malabsorption syndrome, and liver or kidney disease, also increase the risk of developing osteoporosis (see *Risk Factors: Osteoporosis*).

Secondary osteoporosis sometimes develops temporarily in individuals receiving large doses of heparin by decreasing osteoblast formation and increasing bone resorption by reducing OPG and, thus, increasing osteoclast formation.[62] Osteoporosis caused by heparin therapy usually resolves when therapy ceases. Other medications increasing risk for osteoporosis include glucocorticoids, proton pump inhibitors, aromatase inhibitors, lithium, methotrexate, anticonvulsants, cyclophosphamide (Procytox), thiazolidinediones, and cyclosporine.

Regional osteoporosis—osteoporosis confined to a segment of the appendicular skeleton—often has no known cause. Classic regional osteoporosis is associated with disuse or immobilization of a limb because of fractures or bone or joint inflammation. A negative calcium balance develops early and continues throughout the period of immobilization. After 8 weeks of immobilization, significant osteoporosis is present. One result of weightlessness has been a uniform distribution of osteoporosis observed in astronauts and in individuals treated with air suspension therapy.

Transient regional osteoporosis has no known aetiology and is characterized by bone marrow edema and, sometimes, severe pain. Transient regional osteoporosis is usually self-limiting, and tends to occur in middle-aged men and in women during their late second or third trimester of pregnancy.[63,64] Bone marrow edema can be seen on MRI, and areas of localized bone demineralization are evident in plain radiographs.[65] The lower extremity is most often affected but other areas can also be involved. Treatment is primarily symptomatic and the condition usually resolves spontaneously over 3 to 6 months, with no long-term side effects.

PATHOPHYSIOLOGY Osteoporosis develops when there is a disruption in the remodelling cycle (coupling)—bone resorption and bone formation—leading to an imbalance in the coupling process. Osteoclasts are differentiated cells that function to resorb bone. The

RISK FACTORS
Osteoporosis

Genetic
Family history of osteoporosis
White race
Increased age
Female gender

Anthropometric
Small stature
Fair or pale-skinned
Thin build
Low bone mineral density

Hormonal and Metabolic
Early menopause (natural or surgical)
Late menarche
Nulliparity
Obesity
Hypogonadism
Gaucher's disease
Cushing's syndrome
Weight below healthy range
Acidosis

Dietary
Low dietary calcium and vitamin D
Low endogenous magnesium
Excessive protein*
Excessive sodium intake
Anorexia
Malabsorption

Lifestyle
Sedentary

Smoker
Alcohol consumption (excessive)
Low-impact fractures as an adult
Inability to rise from a chair without using one's arms

Concurrent
Hyperparathyroidism

Illness and Trauma
Renal insufficiency, hypocalciuria
Rheumatoid arthritis
Spinal cord injury
Systemic lupus erythematosus

Liver Disease
Marrow disease (myeloma, mastocytosis, thalassemia)

Medications
Corticosteroids
Phenytoin (Dilantin)
Gonadotropin-releasing hormone agonists
Loop diuretics
Methotrexate (Apo-Methotrexate)
Thyroid medications
Heparin
Cyclosporine (Sandimmune)
Medroxyprogesterone acetate (Depo-Provera)
Retinoids

*Low levels of protein intake also have been reported.

HEALTH PROMOTION
The Management of Postmenopausal Osteoporosis

Osteoporosis is the most common bone disease of adults and the foremost cause of fractures in postmenopausal women. Following are some treatment guidelines:
- Post-menopausal women at high risk of fractures should be treated with pharmacological therapies to maintain bone density.
- Bisphosphonates (alendronate, risedronate) are the first-line drugs for initial treatment of osteoporosis to reduce fracture risk and maintain bone density.
- Fracture risk should be re-evaluated every 3–5 years.
- Denosumab, a monoclonal antibody against the RANKL receptor that works to prevent the development of osteoclasts, is an alternative therapy for prevention of bone density loss in postmenopausal osteoporosis.
- Parathyroid hormone and parathyroid hormone analogues (teriparatide and abaloparatide, respectively) are useful therapies for those postmenopausal women who are at very high risk of fractures.
- Selective estrogen receptor modulators (raloxifene) can reduce the risk of vertebral fractures.
- Menopausal hormonal therapy can reduce the risk of vertebral fractures in those who are at risk for fractures.
- Calcitonin nasal spray should be used in those who are at risk and cannot tolerate the above medications.
- Calcium and vitamin D should be used as adjunct therapy in women with low bone density and high risk for fractures.

Data from Eastell, R., Rosen, C. J., Black, D. M., et al. (2019). Pharmacological management of osteoporosis in postmenopausal women: an Endocrine Society Clinical Practice Guideline. *Journal of Clinical Endocrinology & Metabolism, 104*(5), 1595–1622. https://doi.org/10.1210/jc.2019-00221.

---

osteoclast differentiation pathway is dependent on various processes, including proliferation, maturation, fusion, and activation. These processes, in turn, are dependent on the availability of stem cells to allow differentiation to occur and are controlled by hormones, cytokines, and paracrine stromal cell interactions. Thus, proper intracellular communication within bone among its molecular regulators is necessary for normal bone homeostasis. Numerous interleukins, TNF, transforming growth factor-beta (TGF-β), prostaglandin E_2, and hormones interact to control osteoclasts (Figure 39.10). The cytokine **receptor activator of nuclear factor kappa-B ligand (RANKL)**; its **receptor activator of nuclear factor kappa-B (RANK)**; and its decoy receptor **osteoprotegerin (OPG)**, a glycoprotein (see Chapter 36 and Figure 36.5) have also contributed to further understanding of osteoclast biology.

Glucocorticoid-induced osteoporosis (e.g., prednisone, cortisone) is the most common type of secondary osteoporosis. Glucocorticoids have a direct impact on bone quality by improving osteoclast survival, inhibiting osteoblast formation and function, and increasing osteocyte apoptosis.[66–68] Glucocorticoids increase RANKL expression and inhibit OPG production by osteoblasts. Overall, these alterations result in decreased thickness of the bone cortex and fewer, thinner, and more widely spaced trabeculae in the marrow.[69]

Age-related bone loss begins in the third to fourth decade.[70] The cause remains unclear, but decreased serum growth hormone and insulinlike growth factor 1 (IGF-1) levels, along with increased binding of RANKL and decreased OPG production, affect osteoblast and osteoclast function.[71] Loss of trabecular bone in men proceeds in a linear fashion with thinning of trabecular bone rather than complete loss, as is noted in women (Figure 39.11).[72] Men have approximately 30% greater bone mass than women, which may be a factor in their later involvement with osteoporosis (Figure 39.12). In addition, men have a more gradual decrease in the levels of testosterone and estradiol (and possibly progesterone), thereby maintaining their bone mass longer than women. Reduced physical activity in older persons is also a likely factor.

CLINICAL MANIFESTATIONS The specific clinical manifestations of osteoporosis depend on the bones involved. The most common manifestations, however, are pain and bone deformity because of fracture. Unfortunately, these manifestations occur only in an advanced disease state. Fractures are likely to occur because the trabeculae of spongy bone become thin and sparse, and compact bone becomes porous. As the bones lose volume, they become brittle and weak and may collapse or become misshapen. Vertebral collapse causes **kyphosis** (hunchback) and diminishes height (Figure 39.13). Fractures of the long bones (particularly the femur),[73] distal radius, ribs, and vertebrae are most common. Fracture of the neck of the femur—the so-called broken hip—tends to occur in older women with osteoporosis. Fatal complications of fractures include fat or pulmonary embolism, pneumonia, hemorrhage, and shock. Approximately 20% of persons may die as a result of surgical complications. Osteoporosis in men, as in women, also may be related to hypogonadism, with estradiol levels being more

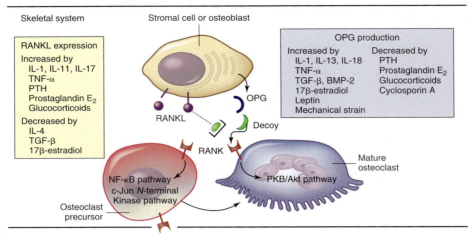

FIGURE 39.10 OPG/RANKL/RANK System. Expression of RANKL, a cytokine and part of the TNF family, and OPG, a glycoprotein receptor antagonist, is modulated by various cytokines, hormones, medications, and mechanical strains (see inserts). In bone, RANKL is expressed by both stromal cells and osteoblasts. RANKL stimulates the receptor RANK on osteoclast precursor cells and mature osteoclasts and activates intracellular signalling pathways to promote osteoclast differentiation and activation as well as cytoskeletal reorganization and survival (PKB/Akt pathway), which increase resorption and bone loss. OPG, secreted by stromal cells and osteoblasts, acts as a "decoy" receptor and blocks RANKL binding to and activation of RANK. *BMP*, Bone morphogenetic protein; *IL*, interleukin; *OPG*, osteoprotegerin; *PKB/Akt pathway*, protein kinase B pathway; *PTH*, parathyroid hormone; *RANK*, receptor activator of nuclear factor kappa-B; *RANKL*, receptor activator of nuclear factor kappa-B ligand; *TGFβ*, transforming growth factor-beta; *TNF-α*, tumour necrosis factor-alpha. (Adapted from Hofbauer, L. C., & Schoppet, M. [2004]. Clinical implications of the osteoprotegerin/RANKL/RANK system for bone and vascular diseases. *JAMA, 292*[4], 490–495.)

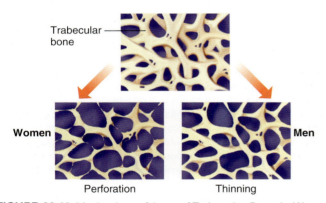

FIGURE 39.11 Mechanism of Loss of Trabecular Bone in Women and Trabecular Thinning in Men. Bone thinning predominates in men because of reduced bone formation. Loss of connectivity and complete trabeculae predominates in women.

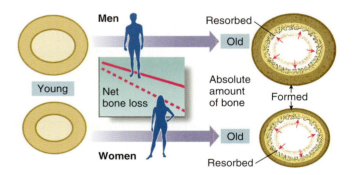

FIGURE 39.12 Bone Loss in Men and Women. Absolute amount of bone resorbed on the inner bone surface and formed on the outer bone surface is more in men than women during aging.

clinically important than testosterone levels in both genders. Adequate dietary intake of calcium, vitamin D, magnesium, and other trace minerals (see *Health Promotion:* Calcium, Vitamin D, and Bone Health); adherence to a regular regimen of weight-bearing exercise; and avoidance of alcoholism, tobacco, and glucocorticoids seem to help prevent primary osteoporosis.

EVALUATION AND TREATMENT In general, osteoporosis is detected radiographically as increased radiolucency of bone. By the time abnormalities are detected by radiological examination, up to 25 to 30% of bone tissue may have been lost.

Dual X-ray absorptiometry (DXA) is the current gold standard for detecting and monitoring osteoporosis; however, bone density is not necessarily indicative of bone quality. The utility of DXA in predicting fracture risk has recently been enhanced by development of a trabecular bone score (TBS). TBS evaluates pixel variations in the grey-level areas of lumbar spine images from DXA scans and has been shown to correlate with high-resolution peripheral quantitative computed tomography (HRpQCT) and be a reliable predictor of fractures.[74–77] High-resolution imaging techniques, such as quantitative computed tomography (QCT) scans and HRpQCT imaging, show changes of trabecular and cortical microarchitecture in osteopenic women.[78] Newer MRI techniques also show promise for providing more detailed information about cortical and trabecular bone and have the added safety of no radiation exposure.[78,79] Other evaluation procedures include measurement of serum and urinary biochemical markers to monitor bone turnover (Box 39.3).

The goals of osteoporosis treatment are risk reduction and the prevention of fractures. Bisphosphonates are first-line medications for treating osteoporosis; they primarily work by inhibiting hydroxyapatite breakdown, reducing bone resorption. New medications formulated to prevent or treat osteoporosis are currently being prescribed

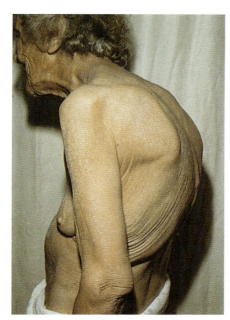

FIGURE 39.13 Kyphosis. This older adult woman's condition was caused by a combination of spinal osteoporotic vertebral collapse and chronic degenerative changes in the vertebral column. (From Kamal, A., & Brocklehurst, J. C. [1992]. *Color atlas of geriatric medicine* [2nd ed.]. Mosby.)

HEALTH PROMOTION
Calcium, Vitamin D, and Bone Health

Vitamin D helps to increase the absorption of calcium, which helps to build stronger bones. Among Canadians 40 years of age and older, less than half report taking calcium and vitamin D supplements; however, experts recommend that all Canadian adults take a vitamin D supplement year-round.

Osteoporosis Canada recommends the following related to intake of calcium and vitamin D:
- Healthy adults between 19 to 50 years of age, including pregnant or breastfeeding women, require 400 to 1000 IU daily.
- Those over 50 or younger adults at high risk (with osteoporosis, multiple fractures, or conditions affecting vitamin D absorption) should receive 800 to 2000 IU daily.
- Specific recommendations for each age group are:

Age	Calcium	Vitamin D
4–8 years	1000 mg	600 IU
9–18 years	1300 mg	600 IU
19–50 years	1000 mg	400–1000 IU
50+ years	1200 mg	800–2000 IU

Data from Osteoporosis Canada. (2021). *Vitamin D and effects on fractures, falls and bone mineral density.* https://osteoporosis.ca/vitamin-d-and-effects-on-fractures-falls-and-bone-mineral-density/.

BOX 39.3 Biochemical Markers of Bone Turnover

Biochemical markers of bone turnover are useful in monitoring osteoporosis treatment. Markers of resorption include urinary N-telopeptide, C-telopeptide, and deoxypyridinoline. Markers of bone formation include bone-specific alkaline phosphatase and osteocalcin. However, these tests have diurnal variability within the same individual, so there must be significant changes in levels to indicate a difference in bone turnover.

---

and evaluated. There are new treatments that help rebuild the skeleton. Selective steroid agents—for example, raloxifene (Evista)—also may be prescribed (see Chapter 33). Regular, moderate weight-bearing exercise can slow the rate of bone loss and, in some cases, reverse demineralization because the mechanical stress of exercise stimulates bone formation. An exercise program to enhance strength and balance has the added benefits of reducing the risk for falls and promoting bone quality.

The anabolic or bone-building medication PTH has been widely studied and is a major regulator of calcium homeostasis. PTH acts directly on osteocytes, stimulates bone formation, and promotes migration of progenitor bone cells from the marrow into the bloodstream, increasing the production of osteoblasts when intermittently administered.[80,81]

Osteomalacia

Osteomalacia is a metabolic disease characterized by inadequate and delayed mineralization of osteoid in mature compact and spongy bone. In osteomalacia, the remodelling cycle proceeds normally through osteoid formation, but mineral calcification and deposition do not occur. Bone volume remains unchanged, but the replaced bone consists of soft osteoid instead of rigid bone. Rickets is similar to osteomalacia in pathogenesis, but it occurs in the growing bones of children, whereas osteomalacia occurs in adult bone. (Chapter 40 describes rickets.)

Both osteomalacia and rickets are relatively rare in Canada (rates of incidence are higher in the north—Yukon, Northwest Territories, and Nunavut), but are significant health problems in other parts of the world, such as Great Britain, Ethiopia, Pakistan, Iran, and India. Concomitant diseases, such as HIV, chronic kidney or liver disease, certain cancers, and impaired nutrient absorption from bariatric surgery, can result in vitamin D deficiency and secondary osteomalacia. In Canada, other causes include prematurity with very low birth weight and adhering to a rigid macrobiotic vegetarian diet. Breastfed infants with darker skin who do not receive vitamin D supplementation have been shown to be at risk for developing nutritional rickets.[82]

Many factors contribute to the development of osteomalacia, but the most important is a deficiency of vitamin D. The major risk factors in vitamin D deficiency are diets deficient in vitamin D, decreased endogenous production of vitamin D, intestinal malabsorption of vitamin D, renal tubular diseases, certain types of tumours (particularly of mesenchymal origin), and anticonvulsant therapy. Classic vitamin D deficiency is rare in Canada because of the addition of synthetic vitamin D to dairy products and bread.

Disorders of the small bowel, hepatobiliary system, and pancreas are causes of vitamin D deficiency in Canada. In malabsorptive disease of the small bowel, both vitamin D and calcium absorption are decreased, so vitamin D is lost in feces. Liver disease interferes with the metabolism of vitamin D to its more active form, and diseases of the pancreas and biliary system cause a deficiency of bile salts, which are necessary for normal intestinal absorption of vitamin D.

The mechanism by which anticonvulsant medication therapy results in vitamin D deficiency is not completely understood, but researchers think that the anticonvulsants phenobarbital (PMS-Phenobarbital) and phenytoin interfere with calcium absorption and increase degradation of vitamin D metabolism in the liver. Renal osteodystrophy is another cause of osteomalacia.

PATHOPHYSIOLOGY Crystallization of minerals in osteoid requires adequate concentrations of calcium and phosphate. When the concentrations are too low, crystallization (and hence ossification) does not proceed normally.

Vitamin D deficiency disrupts mineralization because vitamin D normally regulates and enhances the absorption of calcium ions from the intestine. A lack of vitamin D causes the plasma calcium concentrations to fall. Low plasma calcium levels stimulate increased synthesis and secretion of PTH. The increase in circulating PTH level raises not only the plasma calcium concentration, but it also stimulates increased renal clearance of phosphate. When the concentration of phosphate in the bone decreases below a critical level, mineralization cannot proceed normally. A complex interplay of matrix proteins, hormones, metallopeptidases, and certain proteins is also involved in the development of osteomalacia.

Abnormalities occur in both spongy and compact bone. Trabeculae in spongy bone become thinner and fewer, whereas haversian systems in compact bone develop large channels and become irregular. Because osteoid continues to be produced but not mineralized, abnormal quantities of osteoid accumulate, coating the trabeculae and the linings of the haversian canals. Excessive osteoid also can accumulate in areas beneath the periosteum. The excess of osteoid leads to gross deformities of the long bones, spine, pelvis, and skull.

CLINICAL MANIFESTATIONS Osteomalacia causes varying degrees of diffuse muscular and skeletal pain and tenderness. Pain is noted particularly in the hips, and the individual may be hesitant to walk.[83] Muscular weakness is common and may contribute to a waddling gait. Facial deformities and bowed legs or "knock-knees" may be present. Bone fractures and vertebral collapse occur with minimal trauma. Low back pain may be an early complaint, but pain may also involve ribs, feet, other areas of the vertebral column, and other sites. Fragility fractures may occur. Uremia may be present in renal osteodystrophy.

EVALUATION AND TREATMENT Laboratory data may include elevated BUN and creatinine levels, normal or low serum calcium levels, and a serum inorganic phosphate level that is usually more than 5.5 mg. Alkaline phosphatase and PTH levels are usually elevated. Radiographic findings may show symmetric bowing deformities and fractures with callus formation, particularly in the lower extremities. These types of fractures, known as pseudofractures, along with radiolucent bands perpendicular to the surface of involved bones can help differentiate osteomalacia from fragility fractures that are seen in osteoporosis. A bone biopsy is used to obtain information on bone structure and remodelling and evaluate the presence of subclinical renal osteodystrophy to determine bone architecture, turnover, and even aluminum deposits.[84,85]

Treatment of osteomalacia may vary, depending on its aetiology, but the following general principles are included:

1. Adjustment of serum calcium and phosphorus levels to normal.
2. Suppression of secondary hyperthyroidism.
3. Chelation of bone aluminum if needed.
4. Administration of calcium carbonate to decrease hyperphosphatemia.
5. Administration of vitamin D supplements (oral or infusion).
6. Administration of bisphosphonate.
7. Implementation of renal dialysis, if indicated.

Paget's Disease

Paget's disease of bone (PDB, osteitis deformans, or Paget's disease), the second most common bone disease after osteoporosis, is a state of increased metabolic activity in bone characterized by localized abnormal and excessive bone remodelling. Chronic accelerated remodelling eventually enlarges and softens the affected bones, causing bowing deformity, fracture, or neurological problems.

Paget's disease can occur in any bone but most often affects the vertebrae, skull, sacrum, sternum, pelvis, and femur. The disease process may occur in one or more bones without causing significant clinical manifestations.

Paget's disease occurs with equal frequency in men more than 55 years of age and women older than 40 years of age. It is often symptomless and diagnosis is often suspected when an elevated serum alkaline phosphatase level or abnormal X-ray is noted.[86] Radioisotope bone scan, X-rays, and computed tomography (CT) confirm the diagnosis.[87] Serum plasma procollagen-1 N-peptide (PINP) is another serum marker that may provide a more accurate diagnosis.[88]

The cause of Paget's disease is due to both genetic and environmental factors. Environmental factors include viruses, particularly from the paramyxovirus family (i.e., mumps, parainfluenza, and measles viruses), but no definitive microorganism has yet been identified.[89,90] Ten to 30% of the individuals diagnosed with Paget's disease have mutations of a specific gene, *sequestosome-1 (SQSTM1)*.[91,92] Interaction between genetic and environmental factors appears to increase osteoclast activity in Paget's disease.

PATHOPHYSIOLOGY Certain chromosomes on *SQSTM1* affect osteoclast differentiation and function, although the exact locus of the genetic abnormality is still under investigation.[90,93] Paget's disease begins with excessive resorption of spongy bone and deposition of disorganized bone. The trabeculae diminish, and bone marrow is replaced by extremely vascular fibrous tissue.

The resorption phase of Paget's disease is followed by the formation of abnormal new bone at an accelerated rate. The collagen fibres are disorganized, and glycoprotein levels in the matrix decrease. Mineralization may extend into the bone marrow. Bone formation is excessive around partially resorbed trabeculae, causing them to thicken and enlarge. The net result of this accelerated remodelling process is increased bone fragility and an increased risk for bone tumours.[94]

CLINICAL MANIFESTATIONS In the skull, abnormal remodelling is first evident in the frontal or occipital regions; then it encroaches on the outer and inner surfaces of the entire skull. The skull thickens and assumes an asymmetric shape. Thickened segments of the skull may compress areas of the brain, producing altered mentality and dementia. Impingement of new bone on cranial nerves causes sensory abnormalities, impaired motor function, deafness (because of involvement of the middle ear ossicles or compression of the auditory nerve), atrophy of the optic nerve, and obstruction of the lacrimal duct. Headache is commonly noted.

Extensive alterations of the facial bones are rare except in the jaw, where sclerosis and thickening of the maxilla and mandible displace teeth and produce malocclusion. In long bones, resorption begins in the subchondral regions of the epiphysis and extends into the metaphysis and diaphysis. Occasionally, Paget's disease affects both ends of a tubular bone. In the femur, Paget's disease produces an exaggerated lateral curvature. In the tibia, anterior curvature is also exaggerated. Stress fractures are common in the lower extremities.

Clinical manifestations of Paget's disease in the vertebral column depend on the level of involvement and are caused by compression of adjacent structures. In the cervical spine, cord compression can lead to spastic quadriplegia. Approximately 1% of persons with Paget's disease develop osteogenic sarcoma.

EVALUATION AND TREATMENT Evaluation of Paget's disease is made based on radiographic findings of irregular bone trabeculae with a thickened and disorganized pattern. Early disease is detected by bone scanning that shows increased uptake of bone radionuclides. Plasma alkaline phosphatase and urinary hydroxyproline levels are elevated.

Many individuals require no treatment if the disease is localized and does not cause symptoms. Treatment during active disease is for relief of pain and prevention of deformity or fracture. Bisphosphonates

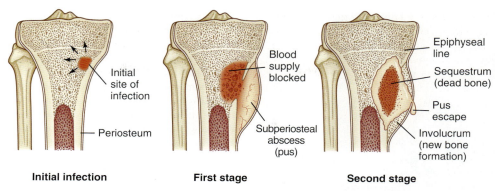

FIGURE 39.14 Osteomyelitis Showing Sequestration and Involucrum.

are the treatment of choice; a one-time infusion of zoledronic acid can provide long-term reduction of biochemical markers and even remission.[95–98] Newer agents, including monoclonal antibodies (denosumab), interleukin-6 (IL-6) receptor inhibitors (tocilizumab [Actemra]), cathepsin K inhibitors, and Dickkopf-1 inhibitors, are under study for treatment of Paget's disease.[87,94]

Infectious Bone Disease: Osteomyelitis

Osteomyelitis is a bone infection most often caused by bacteria; however, fungi, parasites, and viruses also can cause bone infection (Figure 39.14). Multiple classification systems can describe osteomyelitis; the simplest refers to the mode of infection. A bone infection caused by pathogens carried through the bloodstream is hematogenous osteomyelitis. Acute hematogenous osteomyelitis occurs more often in children and is characterized by fever, pain, and voluntary immobility of the affected limb. (Osteomyelitis in children is discussed in Chapter 40.) Contiguous osteomyelitis occurs when infection spreads to an adjacent bone and is often caused by open fractures, penetrating wounds, or surgical procedures. Other causes of osteomyelitis include metabolic and vascular diseases (diabetes, peripheral vascular disease), lifestyle risks (smoking, alcohol, or drug abuse), and advanced age.[99] In infants, incidence rates among males and females are approximately equal. In children and older persons, however, males are most commonly affected. A new category of autoimmune, noninfectious osteomyelitis, known as chronic nonbacterial osteomyelitis, has recently been identified as a cause of chronic bone pain in children.[100]

Staphylococcus aureus remains the primary microorganism responsible for osteomyelitis.[101–103] Other microorganisms include group B streptococcus, *Haemophilus influenzae*, *Salmonella*, and Gram-negative bacteria. Group B streptococcus and *H. influenzae* tend to infect young children; *Salmonella* infection is associated with sickle cell anemia; and Gram-negative infections are most common in older persons and immunocompromised individuals with impaired immunity. Mycobacterial, viral, and fungal infections occur in immunocompromised individuals.

Cutaneous, sinus, ear, and dental infections are the primary sources of bacteria in hematogenous bone infections. Soft tissue infections, disorders of the gastro-intestinal tract, infections of the genitourinary system, and respiratory tract infections are also sources of bacterial contamination. In addition, infections that occur after total joint replacement procedures are sometimes the cause. The vulnerability of specific bone depends on the anatomy of its vascular supply.

In adults, hematogenous osteomyelitis is more common in the spine, pelvis, and small bones. Microorganisms reach the vertebrae through arteries, veins, or lymphatic vessels. The spread of infection from pelvic organs to the vertebrae is well documented. Vaginal, uterine, ovarian, bladder, and intestinal infections can lead to iliac or sacral osteomyelitis.

Superficial animal or human bites inoculate local soft tissue with bacteria that later spread to underlying bone. Deep bites can introduce microorganisms directly onto bone. The most common infecting organism in human bites is *S. aureus*. In animal bites, the most common infecting organism is *Pasteurella multocida*, which is part of the normal mouth flora of cats and dogs.

Direct contamination of bones with bacteria can also occur in open fractures or dislocations with an overlying skin wound. Intervertebral disc surgery and operative procedures involving implantation of large foreign objects, such as metallic plates or artificial joints, are associated with contiguous osteomyelitis. Osteomyelitis of the arm and hand bones tends to occur in persons who abuse medications. In general, persons who are chronically ill, have diabetes or alcoholism, or are receiving large doses of steroids or immunosuppressive medications are particularly susceptible to chronic osteomyelitis or recurring episodes of this disease.

PATHOPHYSIOLOGY Regardless of the source of the pathogen, the pathological features of bone infection are similar to those in any other body tissue (see Chapter 6). First, the invading pathogen provokes an intense inflammatory response. *S. aureus*, in addition to producing toxins that destroy neutrophils, also forms colonies of microorganisms, called *biofilms*, that adhere to surfaces (such as implants) and increase antibiotic resistance. Biofilms can also reduce the duration of osteoblast activity while enhancing osteoclast activity and promoting inflammation[104–106] (see Chapter 8). The biofilm and inflammation primarily alter the normal balance between osteoblast and osteoclast activity through activation of the cytokine pathway.[103,107] Vascular engorgement, edema, leukocyte activity, and abscess formation all characterize inflammation in bone. Once inflammation begins, the small terminal vessels thrombose and exudate seals the bone's canaliculi. Inflammatory exudate extends into the metaphysis and the marrow cavity and through small metaphyseal openings into the cortex. In children, exudate that reaches the outer surface of the cortex forms abscesses that lift the periosteum of underlying bone. Lifting of the periosteum disrupts blood vessels that enter bone through the periosteum, which deprives underlying bone of its blood supply. This leads to necrosis and death of the area of bone infected, producing sequestrum, an area of devitalized bone. Lifting of the periosteum also stimulates an intense osteoblastic response. Osteoblasts lay down new bone that can partially or completely surround the infected bone. This layer of new bone surrounding the infected bone is called an involucrum (Figure 39.15). Openings in the involucrum allow the exudate to escape into surrounding soft tissue and ultimately through the skin by way of sinus tracts.

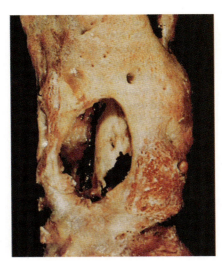

FIGURE 39.15 Resected Femur in a Person With Draining Osteomyelitis. The drainage tract in the subperiosteal shell of viable new bone (involucrum) reveals the inner native necrotic cortex (sequestrum). (From Kumar, V., Abbas, A. K., & Aster, J. C. [Eds.]. [2021]. *Robbins and Cotran pathologic basis of disease* [10th ed.]. Saunders.)

In adults, this complication is rare because the periosteum is firmly attached to the cortex and resists displacement. Instead, infection disrupts and weakens the cortex, which predisposes the bone to pathological fracture.

CLINICAL MANIFESTATIONS Clinical manifestations of osteomyelitis vary with the age of the individual, the site of involvement, the initiating event, the infecting organism, and the type of infection—acute, subacute, or chronic. Osteomyelitis is acute if diagnosed within 2 weeks after symptom onset and is associated with abrupt onset of inflammation (see Figure 39.15). Subacute osteomyelitis is disease that has been present for 1 to several months, and chronic disease is that which has been present for many months to even years.[99,108]

If an acute infection is not completely eliminated, the disease may become subacute or chronic. In subacute osteomyelitis, signs and symptoms are usually vague. In the chronic stage, infection is indolent or silent between exacerbations. The microorganisms persist in small abscesses or fragments of necrotic bone and produce occasional exacerbations of acute osteomyelitis. The progression from acute to subacute osteomyelitis may be the result of inadequate or inappropriate therapy, or the development of medication-resistant microorganisms.

In the adult, hematogenous osteomyelitis has an insidious onset. The symptoms are usually vague and include fever, malaise, anorexia, weight loss, and pain in and around the infected areas. Edema may or may not be evident. Recent infection (urinary, respiratory, cutaneous) or instrumentation (catheterization, cystoscopy, myelography, discography) usually precedes onset of symptoms.

Single or multiple abscesses (Brodie abscesses) characterize subacute or chronic osteomyelitis. Brodie abscesses are circumscribed lesions 1 to 4 cm in diameter that are usually found in the ends of long bones and surrounded by dense ossified bone matrix. The abscesses develop when the infectious microorganism has become less virulent, or the individual's immune system is resisting the infection.

In contiguous osteomyelitis, signs and symptoms of soft tissue infection predominate. Inflammatory exudate in the soft tissues disrupts muscles and supporting structures and forms abscesses. Low-grade fever, lymphadenopathy, local pain, and swelling usually occur within days of contamination by a puncture wound.

EVALUATION AND TREATMENT Laboratory data show an elevated white cell count and an elevated level of noncardiac C-reactive protein (CRP). Radiographic studies include radionuclide bone scanning, CT, functional imaging using a combination of radionuclide scanning (using fluorodeoxyglucose [FDG]) and single-photon emission computed tomography (SPECT), positron emission tomography (PET), and MRI. MRI scanning with gadolinium contrast shows both bone and soft tissue, providing more accurate assessment of infection. MRI also shows early changes of bone marrow edema. FDG-SPECT imaging is highly sensitive for evaluating osteomyelitis of the extremities.[109]

Treatment of osteomyelitis includes bone biopsy to identify the causative organism, use of antimicrobial agents, and debridement of infected bone.[102,110] Biodegradable antibiotic-impregnated bioabsorbable beads have also benefited many individuals; newer therapies include the promise of injectable scaffolds impregnated with antibiotics and other antimicrobial substances.[111] Chronic conditions may require surgical removal of the inflammatory exudate followed by continuous wound irrigation with antibiotic solutions in addition to systemic treatment with antibiotics. Hyperbaric oxygen therapy with 100% oxygen may stimulate healing by suppressing proinflammatory cytokines and prostaglandins. Implants for total joint replacements may be removed to treat the infected joint more thoroughly.

DISORDERS OF JOINTS

> ✓ **QUICK CHECK 39.3**
> 1. How does noninflammatory joint disease differ from inflammatory joint disease? Describe two principal features of each.
> 2. How does rheumatoid arthritis affect the skin, heart, lungs, and kidneys?
> 3. How do monosodium urate crystals cause gout to develop?

The Canadian Rheumatology Association (https://rheum.ca) recognizes several groups of joint disease (arthropathies). Most of these disorders can be placed into two major categories: noninflammatory joint disease and inflammatory joint disease. With the improvement in detection methods, however, inflammatory pathways are now being identified in conditions previously classified as noninflammatory, such as osteoarthritis.

Osteoarthritis

Osteoarthritis (OA) is the most common age-related disorder of synovial joints. Local areas of loss and damage of articular cartilage, inflammation, new bone formation of joint margins (osteophytosis), subchondral bone changes, variable degrees of mild synovitis, and thickening of the joint capsule (Figure 39.16) are all clinical manifestations of OA and affect the entire joint. The pathology depends on load-bearing areas. Advancing disease shows narrowing of the joint space attributable to cartilage loss, bone spurs (osteophytes), and sometimes changes in the subchondral bone. OA can arise in any synovial joint but is commonly found in the knees, hips, hands, and spine. It is less common in people younger than 40 years of age, and its prevalence increases with age. Although the exact causes of OA are unclear, obesity and trauma are well-known risk factors.[112] Specific microRNAs that affect gene expression in chondrocytes may play a role in developing OA.[113,114] OA involves a complex interaction of transcription factors, cytokines, growth factors, matrix molecules, the immune system, mechanical stresses on joints, and enzymes[115–117] (see the following "Pathophysiology" section). Emerging understanding of synovitis and inflammation in OA has led to the recognition of the role played by the body's immune system in OA.[118]

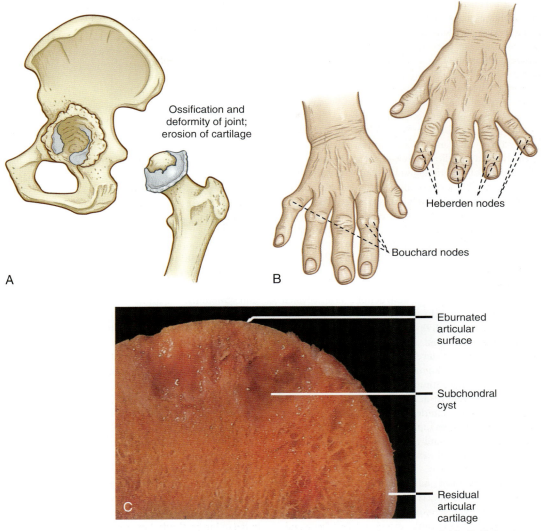

FIGURE 39.16 Osteoarthritis. **A,** Cartilage and degeneration of the hip joint from osteoarthritis. **B,** Heberden nodes and Bouchard nodes. **C,** Severe osteoarthritis with small islands of residual articular cartilage next to exposed subchondral bone. ([C] from Kumar, V., Abbas, A. K., & Aster, J. C. [2021]. *Robbins and Cotran pathologic basis of disease* [10th ed.]. Saunders.)

Although incidence rates are quite similar in men and women, after age 50, women typically are more severely affected. OA usually occurs in those persons who put exceptional stress (or joint loading) on joints (e.g., obese persons, gymnasts, long-distance runners or marathoners); persons participating in such sports as basketball, soccer, or football have been shown to develop OA at earlier ages than usual. Obesity is an independent risk factor for developing OA of the knee.[119–122] Chondrocyte death because of mitochondrial release of reactive oxygen species is caused by increased stress on joints.[116] A previously torn anterior cruciate ligament or meniscectomy increases the risk for accelerated OA of the knee.[123,124]

Types of Osteoarthritis

PATHOPHYSIOLOGY The primary defect in OA is loss of articular cartilage.[125] Early in the disease, the articular cartilage loses its glistening appearance, becoming yellow-grey or brownish grey. As the disease progresses, surface areas of the articular cartilage flake off, and deeper layers develop longitudinal fissures (fibrillation). The cartilage becomes thin and may be absent over some areas, leaving the underlying bone (subchondral bone) unprotected. Consequently, the unprotected subchondral bone becomes sclerotic (dense and hard). Cysts sometimes develop within the subchondral bone and communicate with the longitudinal fissures in the cartilage. Pressure builds in the cysts until the cystic contents are forced into the synovial cavity, breaking through the articular cartilage on the way. As the articular cartilage erodes, cartilage-coated osteophytes may grow outward from the underlying bone and alter the bone contours and joint anatomy. These spurlike bony projections enlarge until small pieces, called *joint mice*, break off into the synovial cavity. If osteophyte fragments irritate the synovial membrane, synovitis and joint effusion result. Interestingly, joint pain may be more related to inflammation of the synovium than subsequent cartilage damage or the radiographic extent of arthritis.[126,127] The joint capsule also becomes thickened and at times, adheres to the deformed underlying bone, which may contribute to the limited range of motion of the joint (see Figure 39.16).

The loss of articular cartilage occurs through a cascade of signalling, cytokine, and anabolic growth factor pathways.[128,129] Enzymatic processes (including matrix metalloproteinases [MMPs]) assist in breaking the macromolecules of proteoglycans, glycosaminoglycans, and collagen into large, diffusible fragments. Then the fragments are taken up by the cartilage cells (chondrocytes) and digested by the cell's own lysosomal enzymes. (Processes of cellular uptake and lysosomal digestion are described in Chapter 1.) The loss of proteoglycans from articular cartilage is a hallmark of the osteoarthritic process.

Enzymatic destruction of articular cartilage begins in the matrix with destruction of proteoglycans and collagen fibres. Enzymes, particularly stromelysin and acid metalloproteinases, affect proteoglycans by interfering with assembly of the proteoglycan subunit or the proteoglycan aggregate (see Chapter 38); levels of these enzymes are markedly elevated in OA. Changes in the conformation of proteoglycans disrupt the pumping action that regulates movement of water and synovial fluid into and out of the cartilage. Without the regulatory action of the proteoglycan pump, cartilage takes on too much fluid and becomes less able to withstand the stresses of weight-bearing. With aging, the proteoglycan content decreases, and water content in cartilage can increase by as much as 8%, affecting the strength of the cartilage. People with OA, even those with fairly extensive cartilage destruction, have elevated levels of proteoglycans or fragments in their synovial fluid, perhaps indicative of the degree of disease activity. MicroRNAs, small nucleic acids that do not code for proteins (but appear to regulate the RNAs that do), may have a direct effect on developing OA by targeting specific genes involved in cartilage development and homeostasis.[114,130,131] Disruptions in cellular signalling pathways, particularly the TGF-β superfamily, play a significant role in developing OA.[129] Other studies indicate that cytokines, such as interleukin-1 (IL-1) and TNF (see Chapter 7 for discussion of cytokines), play a major role in cartilage degradation[128] as a result of release and activation of proteolytic and collagenolytic enzymes associated with an imbalance of cell responses to growth factor activity.[132,133]

Cell-signalling proteins, particularly adipokines such as adiponectin and collagenases (enzymes that degrade collagen), contribute to collagen breakdown in cartilage.[134] Collagen breakdown destroys the fibrils that give articular cartilage its tensile strength and exposes the chondrocytes to mechanical stress and enzyme attack. The osteochondral junction formed by cartilage and its underlying subchondral bone allows alterations in one tissue to affect the adjacent one (biomechanical coupling). When articular cartilage is damaged, abnormal subchondral bone remodelling occurs.[135,136] Thus, a cycle of destruction begins that involves all the components of a joint: cartilage, bone, and the synovium.

CLINICAL MANIFESTATIONS Clinical manifestations of OA typically appear during the fifth or sixth decade of life; although often asymptomatic, articular surface changes are common after the age of 40. Pain in one or more joints—usually with weight-bearing, use of the joint, or load bearing—is the first and most predominant symptom of the disease. Resting the joint often relieves pain. Paresthesias (numbness, tingling, or prickling sensations) might also be present. Sometimes pain is referred to another part of the body. For example, OA of the lumbosacral spine may mimic sciatica, causing severe pain in the back of the thigh along the course of the sciatic nerve. OA in the lower cervical spine may cause brachial neuralgia (pain in the arm) and is aggravated by movement of the neck. Osteoarthritic conditions in the hip cause pain that may be referred to the lower thigh and knee area. Sleep deprivation adds to the stress of the persistent pain of OA. Physical examination of the person with OA usually shows general involvement of both peripheral and central joints. Peripheral joints most often involved are in the hands, wrists, knees, and feet. Central joints most often afflicted are in the lower cervical spine, lumbosacral spine, shoulders, and hips.

Joint structures are capable of generating a limited number of signs and symptoms. The primary signs and symptoms of osteoarthritic joint disease are pain, stiffness, enlargement or swelling, tenderness, limited range of motion, muscle wasting, partial dislocation, and deformity (see Risk Factors: Osteoarthritis).

Joint stiffness is generally defined as difficulty initiating joint movement, immobility, or a loss of range of motion. The stiffness usually occurs as joint movement begins, and it dissipates rapidly after a few minutes. Stiffness lasting longer than 30 minutes is uncommon in OA. Enlargement and bulging of bone contour, commonly described as swelling, may be caused by bone enlargement or the proliferation of osteophytes around the margins of the joint. In the hands, these areas are called Heberden and Bouchard nodes, where they are typical features of OA (see Figure 39.16). The release of cartilage extracellular matrix into the joint initiates inflammation of the joint lining, known as synovitis, which then activates the body's complement system.[137] Swelling also occurs if inflammatory exudate or blood enters the joint cavity, thereby increasing the volume of synovial fluid. This condition, or **joint effusion**, has numerous causes: (1) the presence of osteophyte fragments in the synovial cavity, (2) drainage of cysts from diseased subchondral bone, or (3) acute trauma to joint structures, resulting in hemorrhage and inflammatory exudation into the synovial cavity (Figure 39.16C).

There is some limit to the joint's range of motion, depending on the extent of cartilage degeneration. Frequently, sounds of crepitus, creaking, or grating accompany joint movement. Hypermobility and subluxation of joints occur in OA secondary to a neurological disorder. Abnormal knee alignment (either varus or valgus) is a risk factor and can increase progression of the disease.[138,139]

As OA of the lower extremity progresses, the person may begin to limp (Figure 39.17). Having a limp is distressing because it affects the person's independence and ability to perform the usual activities of daily living. The affected joint is also more symptomatic after use, such as at the end of a period of strenuous activity.

EVALUATION AND TREATMENT Evaluation consists primarily of clinical assessment and radiological studies. More expensive studies, including CT scan, arthroscopy, and MRI, are rarely needed. Newer imaging technologies, such as compositional MRI, show promise in identifying structural changes in cartilage; improvements in technology may also allow better monitoring of OA treatment.

Treatment is either conservative or surgical. Conservative treatment includes both pharmacological and nonpharmacological therapies;

RISK FACTORS
Osteoarthritis

- Trauma, sprains, strains, joint dislocations, and fractures
- Long-term mechanical stress—athletics, ballet dancing, repetitive physical tasks, and obesity
- Inflammation in joint structures
- Joint instability from damage to supporting structures
- Neurological disorders (e.g., diabetic neuropathy, Charcot neuropathic joint) in which pain and proprioceptive reflexes are diminished or lost
- Congenital or acquired skeletal deformities
- Hematological or endocrine disorders, such as hemophilia, which causes chronic bleeding into the joints, or hyperparathyroidism, which causes bone to lose calcium
- Medications (e.g., colchicine, indomethacin [Indocin], steroids) that stimulate the collagen-digesting enzymes in the synovial membrane

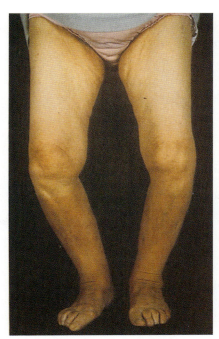

FIGURE 39.17 Typical Varus Deformity of Knee Osteoarthritis. (From Doherty, M. [1994]. *Color atlas and text of osteoarthritis*. Wolfe.)

surgery is a last resort. Both exercise and weight loss are two of the most important nonpharmacological treatments in improving knee OA symptoms. Exercise can reduce pain and improve physical function in people with knee OA.[140-144] Exercises to improve muscle tone, range of motion, and balance, as well as those that stretch the joint capsule and decrease fear of falling have potential for reducing OA symptoms.[145,146] Braces and foot orthoses may help correct biomechanical abnormalities, thereby reducing pain and improving mobility.[147] Dietary and nutritional supplements can sometimes also improve symptoms. Nutraceuticals, such as chondroitin and glucosamine, have shown success in relieving OA pain in some individuals.[148] Other nonsurgical therapies include analgesic and anti-inflammatory medication therapy to reduce swelling and pain. Acetaminophen (Tylenol) was once considered first-line treatment, but it is now less effective than nonsteroidal anti-inflammatory drugs (NSAIDs), such as ibuprofen (Advil). However, prolonged use of such medications significantly increases the risk for some common and serious associated side effects.[149] Intra-articular injection of corticosteroids and high-molecular-weight viscose supplements, such as hyaluronic acid, also decreases knee pain with OA.[150,151] Recently, because of its high concentration of growth factors, PRP also has been injected into osteoarthritic knee joints with some success in reducing pain and markers of inflammation.[152] Current evidence does not support low-level laser therapy for knee OA.[153] Newer agents, including inhibitors of cytokines, MMPs, and leptin, are under investigation and may prove more effective in treating OA. Surgery is used to improve joint movement, correct deformity or malalignment, or create a new joint with artificial implants. Estimates suggest one in four individuals has a lifetime risk of developing symptomatic OA of the hip.[154] More than 62 000 hip replacements and over 75 000 knee replacements were performed in Canada in 2018–2019.[155] This represents an increase of 20.1% and 22.5%, respectively, over the last 5 years.

Classic Inflammatory Joint Disease

Inflammatory joint disease is commonly called **arthritis**. Inflammatory damage or destruction in the synovial membrane or articular cartilage and systemic signs of inflammation (fever, leukocytosis, malaise, anorexia, hyperfibrinogenemia) are all typical of inflammatory joint disease.

Inflammatory joint disease can be infectious or noninfectious. The cause of infectious inflammatory joint disease is invasion of the joint by bacteria, mycoplasmas, viruses, fungi, or protozoa. These agents can invade the joint through a traumatic wound, surgical incision, or contaminated needle, or they can be delivered by the bloodstream from sites of infection elsewhere in the body—typically bones, heart valves, or blood vessels. Immune reactions or the deposition of crystals of monosodium urate (MSU) in and around the joint are cause of the most common form of noninfectious inflammatory joint disease. RA, psoriatic arthritis, and ankylosing spondylitis (AS) are noninfectious inflammatory diseases caused by immune reactions and hypersensitivity reactions; gouty arthritis is a noninfectious inflammatory disease caused by crystal deposition.

Rheumatoid Arthritis

Rheumatoid arthritis (RA) is a chronic, systemic, inflammatory autoimmune disease distinguished by joint swelling and tenderness and destruction of synovial joints, leading to disability and premature death.[156] (Autoimmune disease is described in Chapter 8.) The first joint tissue to be affected is the synovial membrane, which lines the joint cavity (see Chapter 36, Figure 36.9). The two primary types of synovial cells (synovial fibroblasts, SFs) are fibroblastlike synovial cells and macrophagelike synovial cells. Though the initiating mechanism of RA is still unknown, its pathology is fairly well understood. Some factor activates the SFs that line the joint cavity.[157-159] The SFs undergo significant changes and develop an exaggerated immune response. Once activated, both types of SF abnormally proliferate and produce proinflammatory cytokines, enzymes, and prostaglandins that perpetuate the inflammatory process,[160] including increasing their lining depth from the normal 1 to 2 cells deep up to 10 to 20 cells thick. This thickened synovial tissue, called "pannus," invades the bone and acts like a localized tumour, where other factors (including increased osteoclast activity) cause bone destruction.[161] Some of the most significant synovial changes involve altered signalling pathways for immune reactions, where SFs attach to articular cartilage and attack it, causing more inflammation; the release of enzymes, such as MMPs, inflammatory chemokines, and cytokines (interleukins and TNF); and ingrowth of blood vessels. Increased blood vessel formation improves the opportunity for activated SFs to enter the bloodstream and affect other joints.[162-164] Eventually, inflammation spreads to the fibrous joint capsule and surrounding ligaments and tendons, causing pain, joint deformity, and loss of function (Figure 39.18). The joints most commonly affected are in the fingers, feet, wrists, elbows, ankles, and knees, but the shoulders, hips, and cervical spine also may be involved, as well as the tissues of the lungs, heart, kidneys, and skin.

The incidence and prevalence of RA have decreased over the past five decades; RA now affects about 1% of the adult population in developed countries.[165] The frequency of RA increases with age. Besides inflammation and destruction of the joints, RA can cause fever, malaise, rash, lymph node or spleen enlargement, and Raynaud's phenomenon (transient lack of circulation to the fingertips and toes).

Despite intensive research, the exact cause of RA remains obscure. It is likely a combination of genetic factors interacting with inflammatory mediators. There is a strong genetic predisposition to developing RA. The chronic inflammation characteristics of RA result from an intricate interplay of chemokines that are powerful mediators of inflammation. Ligand/receptor chemokines attract T lymphocytes (T cells) and produce inflammatory changes.[162] A key genetic element has been localized to the human leukocyte antigen (HLA) areas of the major histocompatibility complex in all ethnic groups. Recent research

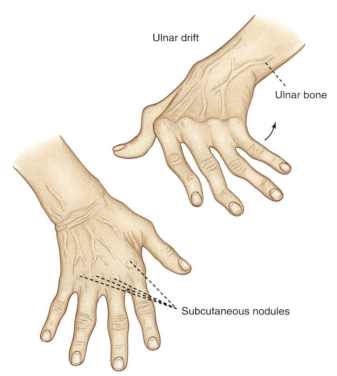

FIGURE 39.18 Rheumatoid Arthritis of the Hand. Note swelling from chronic synovitis of metacarpophalangeal joints, marked ulnar drift, subcutaneous nodules, and subluxation of metacarpophalangeal joints with extension of proximal interphalangeal joints and flexion of distal joints. Note also deformed position of thumb. Hand has wasted appearance. (From Mourad, L. A. [1991]. *Orthopedic disorders.* Mosby.)

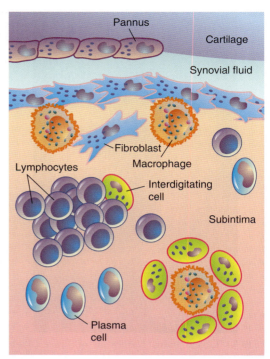

FIGURE 39.19 Synovitis. Inflamed synovium showing typical arrangements of macrophages and fibroblastic cells.

reveals the possibility of specific amino acid malpositions in the HLA molecule as a major factor in developing rheumatic diseases.[166] A surprising new discovery is the presence of T-cell abnormalities in individuals with RA, indicating a defect in telomere repair that may result in faster aging of telomeres and consequent less efficient immune function. With long-term or intensive exposure to the antigen, normal antibodies (immunoglobulins [Igs]) become autoantibodies—antibodies that attack host tissues (self-antigens). Because they are usually present in individuals with RA, the altered antibodies are termed **rheumatoid factors (RFs).** The RFs usually consist of two classes of immunoglobulin antibodies (antibodies for IgM and IgG) but occasionally involve antibodies for IgA. Their main antigenic targets are portions of the Ig molecules. RFs bind with their target self-antigens in blood and synovial membrane, forming immune complexes (antigen–antibody complexes). (See Chapter 7 for a discussion about antigen–antibody binding in the immune response.)

Environmental factors, including geographical area of birth, diet, socioeconomic status, and especially smoking, have been identified as risk factors for developing and having higher disease activity of RA.[167,168] RA and other autoimmune diseases are more prevalent among women. Additionally, because disease symptoms lessen during pregnancy and are increased again in the postpartal period, researchers are including hormonal involvement in their studies.

PATHOPHYSIOLOGY Although no specific events (such as trauma, illness, or environmental conditions) have been identified that would cause immune abnormalities to develop into localized tissue and joint inflammation, the pathology of RA is fairly well understood. During inflammation, arginine (an α-amino acid) can be enzymatically modified into another α-amino acid, citrulline. This process (citrullination) changes the structure and function of the protein. Other proteins, such as fibrin and vimentin, become citrullinated during cell death and tissue inflammation.[169] In turn, the citrullinated proteins can be seen as antigens by the body's immune system.[170] Thus, both T cells and B cells (B lymphocytes) play a role in the autoimmune response. T cells express RANKL, which promotes osteoclast formation and causes bony erosion.

Basically, cartilage damage in RA is the result of at least three processes: (1) neutrophils and other cells in the synovial fluid become activated, degrading the surface layer of articular cartilage; (2) inflammatory cytokines, particularly tumour necrosis factor-alpha (TNF-α), interleukin-1beta (IL-1β), IL-6, IL-7, and IL-21 induce enzymatic (metalloproteinase) breakdown of cartilage and bone; and (3) T cells also interact with SFs through TNF-α, converting synovium into a thick, abnormal layer of granulation tissue known as **pannus** (see Chapter 7). Macrophages, components of pannus (Figure 39.19), stimulate the release of IL-1, PDGF, and fibronectin. The B cells are stimulated to produce more RFs. The newly targeted self-antigens (Igs) are in relatively constant supply and can thus perpetuate inflammation and the formation of immune complexes indefinitely (Figure 39.20).

Inflammatory and immune processes have several damaging effects on the synovial membrane. Along with the swelling caused by leukocyte infiltration, the synovial membrane undergoes hyperplastic thickening as its cells proliferate and abnormally enlarge. As synovial inflammation progresses to involve its blood vessels, small venules become occluded by hypertrophied endothelial cells, fibrin, platelets, and inflammatory cells, which decrease vascular flow to the synovial tissue. Compromised circulation, coupled with increased metabolic needs as a result of hypertrophy and hyperplasia, causes hypoxia and metabolic acidosis. Acidosis stimulates the release of hydrolytic enzymes from synovial cells into the surrounding tissue, initiating erosion of the articular cartilage and inflammation in the supporting ligaments and tendons. Pannus formation does not lead to synovial or

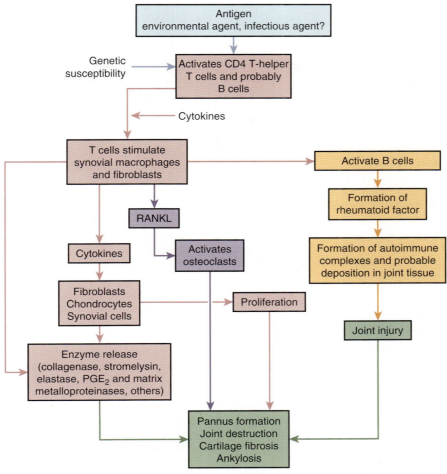

FIGURE 39.20 Emerging Model of Pathogenesis of Rheumatoid Arthritis. Rheumatoid arthritis is an autoimmune disease of a genetically susceptible host triggered by an unknown antigenic agent. Chronic autoimmune reaction with activation of CD4+ T-helper cells and possibly other lymphocytes and the local release of inflammatory cytokines and mediators eventually destroy the joint. T cells stimulate cells in the joint to produce cytokines that are key mediators of synovial damage. Apparently, immune complex deposition also plays a role. Tumour necrosis factor and interleukin-1, as well as some other cytokines, stimulate synovial cells to proliferate and produce other mediators of inflammation, such as prostaglandin E_2 *(PGE$_2$)*, matrix metalloproteinases, and enzymes that all contribute to destruction of cartilage. Activated T cells and synovial fibroblasts also produce receptor activator of nuclear factor kappa-B ligand *(RANKL)*, which activates the osteoclasts and promotes bone destruction. Pannus is a mass of synovium and synovial stroma with inflammatory cells, granulation tissue, and fibroblasts that grows over the articular surface and causes its destruction.

articular regeneration but rather to formation of scar tissue that immobilizes the joint.

CLINICAL MANIFESTATIONS The onset of RA is usually insidious, although only 10% of cases have an acute onset.[171] RA begins with general systemic manifestations of inflammation, including fever, fatigue, weakness, anorexia, weight loss, and generalized aching and stiffness. Local manifestations also appear gradually over a period of weeks or months. Typically, the joints become painful, tender, and stiff. Pain early in the disease is caused by pressure from swelling. Later in the disease, pain is caused by sclerosis of subchondral bone and new bone formation. Pain and inability to perform normal functions are the main reasons people seek medical help.[172] Stiffness usually lasts for about 1 hour after rising in the morning and is thought to be related to synovitis. Initially the joints most commonly involved are the MCP joints, proximal interphalangeal joints, and wrists, with later involvement of larger weight-bearing joints.

Widespread, symmetric joint swelling is caused by increasing amounts of inflammatory exudate (leukocytes, plasma, plasma proteins) in the synovial membrane, hyperplasia of inflamed tissues, and formation of new bone. On palpation, the swollen joint feels warm, and the synovial membrane feels boggy. The skin over the joint may have a ruddy, cyanotic hue and may look thin and shiny.

An inflamed joint may lose some of its mobility. Even mild synovitis can lead to reduced range of motion, which becomes evident after inflammation subsides. Extension becomes limited and is eventually lost if flexion contractures develop. Limited range of motion can progress to permanent deformities of the fingers, toes, and limbs, including ulnar deviation of the hands, boutonnière and swan neck deformities of the finger joints, plantar subluxation of the metatarsal heads of the foot, and hallux valgus (angulation of the great toe toward the other toes). Flexion contractures of the knees and hips are also common.

Joint deformities cause the physical limitations experienced by persons with RA (see Figure 39.18). Loss of joint motion is quickly followed by secondary atrophy of the surrounding muscles. With secondary muscle atrophy, the joint becomes unstable, which further aggravates joint pathology.

Two complications of chronic RA are caused by too much inflammatory exudate in the synovial cavity. One complication is the formation of cysts in the articular cartilage or subchondral bone. Occasionally, these cysts communicate with the skin surface (such as in the sole of the foot) and can drain through passages called *fistulae*. The second complication is rupture of a cyst or of the synovial joint itself, usually caused by strenuous physical activity that places excessive pressure on the joint. Rupture releases inflammatory exudate into adjacent tissues, thereby spreading inflammation.

Extrasynovial rheumatoid nodules, seen in up to 30% of individuals with RA, are the most common extra-articular manifestations. Each nodule is a collection of inflammatory cells surrounding a central core of fibrinoid and cellular debris. T cells are the predominant leukocytes in the nodule. B cells, plasma cells, and phagocytes are found around the periphery. Nodules are most often found in subcutaneous tissue over the extensor surfaces of elbows and fingers. Less common sites are the scalp, back, feet, hands, buttocks, and knees.

Rheumatoid nodules also may invade the skin, cardiac valves, pericardium, pleura, lung parenchyma, and spleen. These nodules are identical to those encountered in some individuals with rheumatic fever and are characterized by central tissue necrosis surrounded by proliferating connective tissue. Also noted are large numbers of lymphocytes and occasional plasma cells. Acute glaucoma may result with nodules forming on the sclera. Pulmonary involvement may result in diffuse pleuritis or multiple intraparenchymal nodules. Together, the occurrence of pulmonary nodules and pneumoconiosis (chronic inflammation of the lungs from inhalation of dust) creates the syndrome called Caplan's syndrome. Diffuse pulmonary fibrosis may occur because of immunologically mediated immune complex deposition.

Rheumatoid nodules within the heart may cause valvular deformities, particularly of the aortic valve leaflets, and pericarditis. Lymphadenopathy of the nodes close to the affected joints may develop. Rheumatoid nodules within the spleen result in splenomegaly. Involvement of blood vessels results in an acute necrotizing vasculitis, characteristic of that noted in other immunological/inflammatory states. Thromboses of such involved vessels may lead to myocardial infarctions, cerebrovascular occlusions, mesenteric infarction, kidney damage, and vascular insufficiency in the hands and fingers (Raynaud's phenomenon). Fortunately, the development of vascular changes (particularly systemic vasculitis) is decreasing in frequency as more effective RA treatments are becoming available.[173] Changes in skeletal muscle are often noted in the form of nonspecific atrophy secondary to joint dysfunction.

EVALUATION AND TREATMENT The diagnosis of RA relies on clinical evaluation of joint swelling; however, limitation of movement and control of pain often prevent identification of individuals who would benefit from treatment in early stages of the disease. Early treatment can be effective in preventing the systemic and joint abnormalities of chronic disease. The autoantibodies, RF and anticitrullinated protein antibody (ACPA), can be present for years to decades before synovial or radiographic involvement becomes apparent.[174,175] Compared with RF, ACPA is a much more specific serum marker for RA. The American College of Rheumatology and the European League Against Rheumatism revised their RA classification criteria in 2010 to better identify the early stage of RA, and these continue to serve as the current criteria.[156] Table 39.5 illustrates these criteria. Similarly, the Canadian Rheumatology Association revised its clinical guidelines on the management of RA in 2012 to reflect recent research on effective methods in achieving remission from the condition.[176] Clinical examination and history are the mainstays of RA diagnosis, but new imaging techniques show promise for earlier diagnosis, leading to earlier treatment with a better chance for avoiding disability and joint destruction (see *Health Promotion*: Musculoskeletal Molecular Imaging).

Early treatment of RA begins with disease-modifying antirheumatic drugs (DMARDs), such as methotrexate, azathioprine (Imuran), sulfasalazine (Salazopyrin), hydroxychloroquine (Plaquenil), leflunomide (Arava), and cyclosporine (Sandimmune). These agents slow the progression of RA and may prevent complications such as joint deformities and extra-articular complications. Methotrexate remains the first line of treatment. More recent targeted treatment for RA involves the use of agents aimed at interrupting the pathogenesis of the disease. Known as biological DMARDs (bDMARDs), these medications affect specific processes in the development of RA and include TNF inhibitors, such as etanercept (Enbrel), adalimumab (Humira), and infliximab (Remicade). These medications also include newer monoclonal antibodies such as golimumab (Simponi) and certolizumab (Cimzia). Other agents interfere with cytokine function (anakinra [Kineret] inhibits IL-1 function, and tocilizumab targets IL-6), inhibit T-cell activation (abatacept [Orencia]), or deplete B cells (rituximab [Rituxan]).

Education for individuals with RA is fundamental to treatment. Other treatments and therapies include NSAIDs, glucocorticoids, intra-articular steroid injections, physical and occupational therapy with therapeutic exercise, and use of assistive devices. Surgery is used to treat deformities or mechanical deficiencies of joints and can include synovectomy or joint replacement surgery.

> **HEALTH PROMOTION**
> ***Musculoskeletal Molecular Imaging***
>
> With improved understanding of the molecular and cellular mechanisms responsible for the effects of rheumatoid arthritis (RA), new imaging techniques promise benefits in earlier and more accurate diagnosis and monitoring of cartilage and bone involvement. Although anatomical imaging remains the mainstay of musculoskeletal radiology, significant progress has been made in functional and molecular imaging, as well as in hybrid imaging, with an expanding armament of technologies becoming available or already in development. Imaging on that same molecular level can provide a "biological readout" of disease progression and response to treatment. Nuclear medicine imaging, PET, and MRI all incorporate some element of molecular imaging.
>
> New modalities of molecular imaging use various probes and contrast agents that have an affinity for specific targets, such as cells, hormones, antigens, and enzymes. Certain monoclonal antibodies have already been successfully labelled with various nuclides and could be used to identify disease progression. Bioluminescent and fluorescent imaging techniques have the advantage of being radiation-free tests and are being used to view in vivo activity, osteoblast activity, osteocalcin expression in bone damage, and osteoclast activity and gene expression during inflammation. A significant area of promise for molecular imaging in RA is recognition of the initial molecular events that occur before cartilage and joint damage becomes apparent. Better monitoring of response to medications also may allow more accurate dosing with the potential for fewer side effects. Because certain bioluminescent and fluorescent agents have specific affinities for particular cells, more efficient bone regeneration may be possible by targeted delivery of appropriate growth factors or stem cells to damaged bone and cartilage.

Data from Farrell, T. P., Niamh, C. A., Walsh, J. P., et al. (2018). Musculoskeletal imaging: current practice and future directions. *Seminars in Musculoskeletal Radiology, 22*(5), 564–581.

TABLE 39.5 The 2010 American College of Rheumatology/European League Against Rheumatism Classification Criteria for Rheumatoid Arthritis

Target population to be tested:
1. Persons who have at least one joint with definite clinical synovitis (swelling)[a]
2. Persons who have synovitis not better explained by another disease[b]

Classification criteria for RA (score-based algorithm: add scores of categories A to D; a score of ≥6/10 is needed for positive RA diagnosis)[c]

Clinical Finding	Score
A. Joint involvement[d]	
1 large joint[e]	0
2–10 large joints	1
1–3 small joints (with or without involvement of large joints)[f]	2
4–10 small joints (with or without involvement of large joints)	3
>10 joints (at least 1 small joint)[g]	5
B. Serology (at least 1 test result is needed for classification)[h]	
Negative RF *and* negative ACPA	0
Low-positive RF *or* low-positive ACPA	2
High-positive RF *or* high-positive ACPA	3
C. Acute-phase reactants (at least 1 test result is needed for classification)[i]	
Normal CRP *and* normal ESR	0
Abnormal CRP *or* abnormal ESR	1
D. Duration of symptoms[j]	
<6 weeks	0
≥6 weeks	1

[a]The criteria are aimed at classification of newly presenting persons. In addition, persons with erosive disease typical of RA with a history compatible with prior fulfillment of the 2010 criteria should be classified as having RA. Persons with longstanding disease—including those whose disease is inactive (with or without treatment) and who, based on retrospectively available data, have previously fulfilled the 2010 criteria—should be classified as having RA.
[b]Differential diagnoses vary among persons with different presentations, but may include conditions such as systemic lupus erythematosus, psoriatic arthritis, and gout. If it is unclear about the relevant differential diagnoses to consider, an expert rheumatologist should be consulted.
[c]Although persons with a score <6/10 are not classifiable as having RA, their status can be reassessed, and the criteria might be fulfilled cumulatively over time.
[d]Joint involvement refers to any *swollen* or *tender* joint on examination, which may be confirmed by imaging evidence of synovitis. Distal interphalangeal joints, first metacarpophalangeal joints, and first metatarsophalangeal joints are *excluded from assessment*. Categories of joint distribution are classified according to the location and number of involved joints, with placement into the highest category possible based on the pattern of joint involvement.
[e]"Large joints" refer to shoulders, elbows, hips, knees, and ankles.
[f]"Small joints" refer to the metacarpophalangeal joints, proximal interphalangeal joints, second through fifth metatarsophalangeal joints, thumb interphalangeal joints, and wrists.
[g]In this category, at least one of the involved joints must be a small joint; the others can include any combination of large and additional small joints, as well as other joints not specifically listed elsewhere (e.g., temporomandibular, acromioclavicular, sternoclavicular).
[h]Negative refers to unit values that are less than or equal to the upper limit of normal (ULN) for the laboratory and assay; low-positive refers to values that are higher than the ULN but ≤3 times the ULN for the laboratory and assay; high-positive refers to unit values that are >3 times the ULN for the laboratory and assay. Where rheumatoid factor (RF) information is only available as positive or negative, a positive result should be scored as low-positive for RF.
[i]Normal/abnormal is determined by local laboratory standards.
[j]Duration of symptoms refers to individual's self-report of the duration of signs and symptoms of synovitis (e.g., pain, swelling, tenderness) of joints that are clinically involved at the time of assessment, regardless of treatment status.

ACPA, Anti-citrullinated protein antibody; CRP, C-reactive protein; ESR, erythrocyte sedimentation rate; RA, rheumatoid arthritis.
Data from Aletaha, D., Neogi, T., Silman, A. J., et al. (2010). 2010 rheumatoid arthritis classification criteria: an American College of Rheumatology/European League Against Rheumatism collaborative initiative. *Arthritis & Rheumatology*, 62(9), 2574.

Ankylosing Spondylitis

Ankylosing spondylitis (AS) is the most common of a group of inflammatory arthropathies known as *spondyloarthropathies* (SpAs). The Assessment of SpondyloArthritis International Society (ASAS) recommends classifying SpAs to include individuals who do not have visible radiographic changes of the skeleton, as well as those who do. Consequently, there are two subgroups: (1) mainly axial disease, including AS, and (2) peripheral SpA.[177] AS is a chronic inflammatory joint disease characterized by stiffening and fusion (ankylosis) of the spine and sacroiliac joints. Like RA, ankylosing spondylitis is a systemic, autoimmune inflammatory disease. Although inflammation is the primary pathological process in both RA and AS, the two diseases differ in the primary site of inflammation and the end result. In RA, the primary site of inflammation is the synovial membrane, resulting in the destruction and instability of synovial joints. In AS, excessive bone formation occurs. The primary pathological site is the enthesis (the point at which ligaments, tendons, and the joint capsule are inserted into bone), and the end result is fibrosis, ossification, and fusion of the joint, primarily the sacroiliac joints and the vertebral column (axial skeleton).

AS occurs worldwide, with the lowest prevalence in South Asian countries and the highest prevalence in North America and Europe; it affects men more often than women.[178] In women, AS may affect the peripheral joints of the appendicular skeleton rather than the axial skeleton, progress less rapidly, and cause less dramatic spinal changes. Primary AS usually develops in late adolescence and young adulthood, with peak incidence at about 20 years of age. Secondary AS affects older age groups and is often associated with other inflammatory diseases (e.g., psoriatic arthropathy, inflammatory bowel disease, Reiter syndrome).

The exact cause of AS is unknown, but it has a high association with histocompatibility antigen human leukocyte antigen (HLA-B27). Misfolding of HLA-B27 in the endoplasmic reticulum may play a key role in developing AS. As misfolded proteins accumulate, they may cause an unfolded protein response that disrupts normal cellular functions and causes a stress response of the endoplasmic reticulum (also see Chapter 4). That stress response increases production of interleukin-17 and -23 (IL-17, IL-23), potent cytokines that also may act on T-helper 17 (Th17) cells, promoting their survival.[179,180] Th17 cells are important mediators in human immune diseases. Additional studies have revealed that HLA-B27 itself has many forms; to date, more than 100 subtypes have been identified.[181] Certain variations in the endoplasmic reticulum aminopeptidase 1 protein appear to increase the likelihood of developing AS in people who are HLA-B27 positive.

PATHOPHYSIOLOGY AS begins with inflammation of fibrocartilage in cartilaginous joints. In men, the sacroiliac joint is often affected first, usually before any damage can be radiographically detected.[179] Knee pain may be the initial symptom in women.[182] Inflammatory cells infiltrate the fibrous tissue of the joint capsule, the cartilage that surrounds intervertebral discs, the entheses, and the periosteum. As inflammatory cells (chiefly macrophages) and lymphocytes infiltrate and erode bone and fibrocartilage in joint structures, repair begins. Repair of cartilaginous structures begins with the proliferation of fibroblasts. Fibroblasts synthesize and secrete collagen. The collagen becomes organized into fibrous scar tissue that eventually undergoes calcification and ossification. With time, all the cartilaginous structures of the joint are replaced by ossified scar tissue, causing the joint to fuse, or lose flexibility.

Repair of eroded bone begins with osteoblast activation and proliferation. Osteoblasts lay down new bone (callus), which is remodelled and replaced by compact, lamellar bone. Bone repair changes the contour of the bone's surface because the new bone grows outward (outside the normal border of unaffected bone) to form a new enthesis with the end of the eroded ligament. The new enthesis, which forms on top of the old one, is called a **syndesmophyte**. As calcification of the spinal ligaments progresses, the vertebral bodies lose their concave anterior contour and appear square. The spine assumes the classic bamboo spine appearance of AS.

CLINICAL MANIFESTATIONS The most common signs and symptoms of early AS are low back pain and stiffness. Typically, the individual with primary disease develops low back pain during their early 20s. The pain is at first insidious but progressively becomes persistent. Pain is often worse after prolonged rest and is alleviated by physical activity. Early morning stiffness usually accompanies the low back pain, and the individual typically has difficulty sitting up or twisting the spine.

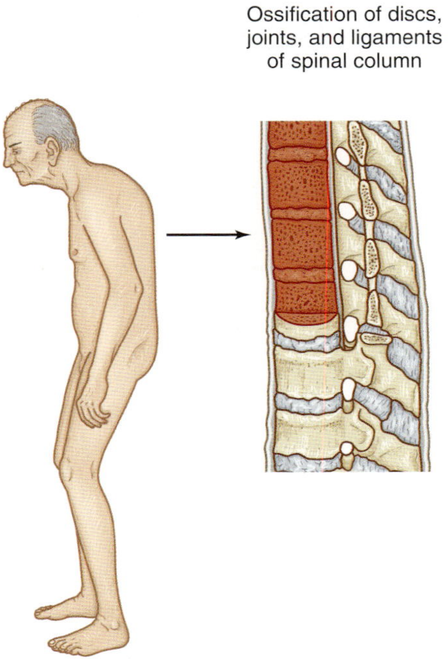

FIGURE 39.21 Ankylosing Spondylitis. Characteristic posture and primary pathological sites of inflammation and resulting damage. (Redrawn from Mourad, L. A. [1991]. *Orthopedic disorders*. Mosby.)

Forward flexion, rotation, and lateral flexion of the spine are restricted and painful. The underlying inflammation and reflex muscle spasm, rather than soft tissue or bony fusion, cause the early pain and resultant loss of motion.

As the disease progresses, the normal convex curve of the lower spine (lumbar lordosis) diminishes and concavity of the upper spine (kyphosis) increases. The individual becomes increasingly stooped. The thoracic spine becomes rounded, the head and neck are held forward on the shoulders, and the hips are flexed (Figure 39.21).

Inflammation in the tendon insertions of the many costosternal and costovertebral muscles can cause pleuritic chest pain and restricted chest movement. The pain is usually worse on inspiration. Movement of the diaphragm is normal and full. Pressure on the anterior chest wall over the sternum, ribs, and costal cartilages may cause tenderness. Tenderness over the pelvic brim may cause discomfort at night and interfere with sleep because turning onto the iliac crests causes pain. Tenderness over the ischial tuberosities may make sitting on hard seats unbearable. Tenderness in the heels may contribute to a limp or cautious placement of the feet during walking.

Along with low back pain and sacroiliac pain, inflammation of the bowels, anterior uveitis, aortic regurgitation, fibrosis of the upper lobes of the lung, Achilles tendonitis, and immune-related (IgA) kidney disease frequently accompany AS.[183] Elevated erythrocyte sedimentation rate (ESR) and elevated level of CRP also are common.

EVALUATION AND TREATMENT There are specific criteria for the diagnosis of AS. The requirement for radiographic (X-ray) evidence of sacroiliitis has posed problems with diagnosing AS; MRI can discover sacroiliitis an average of 7.7 years before there is evidence on X-rays.[184] Both MRI and plain radiographic findings are important in detecting early disease and for evaluating individuals younger than 45 years of age with back pain of at least 3 months' duration.[185]

In addition to sacroiliitis on imaging, one or more of the following features allow a diagnosis of spondyloarthritis: (1) inflammatory back pain, (2) arthritis, (3) anterior uveitis, (4) heel pain, (5) dactylitis, (6) psoriasis, (7) Crohn's disease or ulcerative colitis, (8) good response to NSAIDs, (9) family history of spondyloarthritis, (10) positive HLA-B27, or (11) elevated CRP. If the individual has a positive HLA-B27, at least two of the previously mentioned items must be present along with sacroiliitis on MRI or radiographic imaging to make a diagnosis.[186]

Treatment of individuals with AS consists of education about the disease, as well as physical therapy to maintain skeletal mobility and prevent the natural progression of contractures. Prevention of deformity and maintenance of mobility require a continuous program of physical therapy. Supervised group exercises reduce pain, as well as maintain and improve chest expansion and respiratory function, spine mobility, and complete range of motion in the proximal joints.[187]

NSAIDs will often provide temporary symptom relief within 48 hours. Analgesic medications suppress some of the pain and stiffness and facilitate exercise. The medications do not prevent disease progression, but they do provide relief from symptoms. Biological response modifying agents, such as TNF inhibitors (certolizumab, golimumab) or B-cell depleting agents (rituximab), are increasingly being used to treat AS. Newer agents that target cytokines of Th17 and small nanoparticles that alter certain inflammatory pathways are showing promise in treating AS.[188,189] Surgical procedures, such as osteotomy, total hip replacement, and cervical spinal fusion, and radiation therapy are sometimes used to provide relief for individuals with end-stage disease or intolerable deformity. Individuals should stop smoking to lessen pulmonary problems.

Gout

Gout, a condition traditionally known as the "disease of kings", is a syndrome caused by either overproduction or underexcretion of uric acid and has characteristics of inflammation and pain of the joints. It is also the most common type of inflammatory arthritis.[195] Incomplete purine metabolism results in excess serum uric acid levels (hyperuricemia). Underexcretion of uric acid is responsible for about 90% of the cases of an elevated uric acid level and appears to have a strong genetic basis.[190,191]

When uric acid reaches a certain concentration in fluids, it crystallizes, forming insoluble precipitates that deposit themselves in connective tissues throughout the body. Crystallization in synovial fluid triggers the TNF-α inflammatory pathway, causing the release of various chemokines and interleukins, and resulting in painful inflammation of the joint, a condition known as **gouty arthritis**. Urate crystal deposits cause oxidative stress reactions in other tissues as well. With time, crystal deposition in subcutaneous tissues causes the formation of small, white nodules, or **tophi**, that are visible through the skin. Tophi indicate joint damage and result in an increased death rate, primarily because of cardiovascular events.[192] Hyperuricemia positively correlates with hypertension, heart disease, type 2 diabetes, kidney disease, and metabolic syndrome.[193]

In classic gouty arthritis, MSU crystals form and deposit themselves in joints and their surrounding tissues, initiating a powerful inflammatory response.[194] Pseudogout results from the formation of calcium pyrophosphate-dihydrate crystals. The effect of either crystal is the same—the onset of an acute inflammatory response (see Chapter 6).

Gout is rare in children and premenopausal women and is uncommon in males younger than 30 years. Male gender, increasing age, and high intake of alcohol, red meat, and fructose are all risk factors for gout.[196] The peak age of onset in males is between 40 and 50 years of age. For females, the risk of getting gout increases with age due to decreased concentrations of estrogen in the blood (estrogen protects against gout and causes uric acid to be flushed out of the urine), increased use of

TABLE 39.6 Mean Urate Concentrations by Age and Gender

Characteristic	Mean Urate Levels (μmol/L)
Prepuberty	208.18
Males (at puberty)	Steep rise to 309.3
Females (puberty to after premenopause)	Slow rise to ≈237.9
Females (after menopause)	279.6
Hyperuricemia	
Males	416.4
Females	356.8

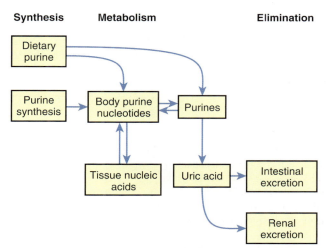

FIGURE 39.22 Uric Acid Synthesis and Elimination. Uric acid is derived from purines ingested or synthesized from ingested foods, as well as being recycled after cell breakdown. Uric acid is then eliminated through the kidneys and gastro-intestinal tract. (Redrawn from Klippel, J. H., & Dieppe, P. A. [Eds.]. [1998]. *Rheumatology* [2nd ed.]. Mosby.)

diuretics, more co-existing diseases (hypertension, renal insufficiency), more frequent involvement of other joints, and fewer recurrent episodes.[195] Plasma urate concentration is the single most important determinant of the risk of developing gout (Table 39.6).

Uric acid is a weak acid that is ionized at normal body pH and thus occurs in the blood or tissues in the form of urate ion. When ionized, uric acid can form salts with various cations, but 98% of extracellular uric acid is in the form of MSU (uric acid salt). At any time, the proportion of uric acid or urate is pH dependent, and the ratio of these two forms varies considerably in urine.

The solubility of urate and uric acid is critical to the development of crystals. Urate is more soluble in plasma, synovial fluid, and urine than in aqueous solutions. The solubility of uric acid in urine rises dramatically as the pH increases. There is little change, however, in the solubility of urate within the normal pH range that exists in the plasma, synovial fluid, and other tissues. The pH can be 5.0 in the collecting tubules of the kidney, thus favouring formation of uric acid. Decreasing temperatures cause both urate and uric acid solubility to fall. Figure 39.22 illustrates the pathways of uric acid production.

PATHOPHYSIOLOGY The pathophysiology of gout is closely linked to purine metabolism (or cellular metabolism of purines) and kidney function. Most mammals, except humans, have the enzyme uricase, which catalyzes the conversion of uric acid to allantoin, thus preventing

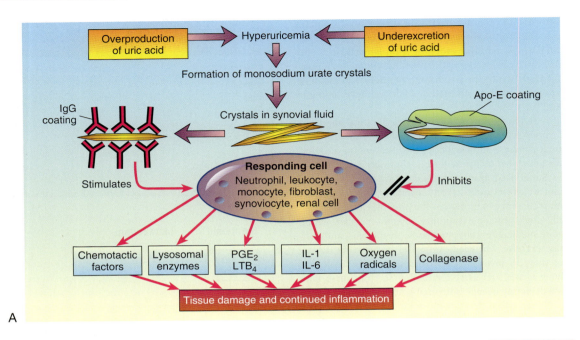
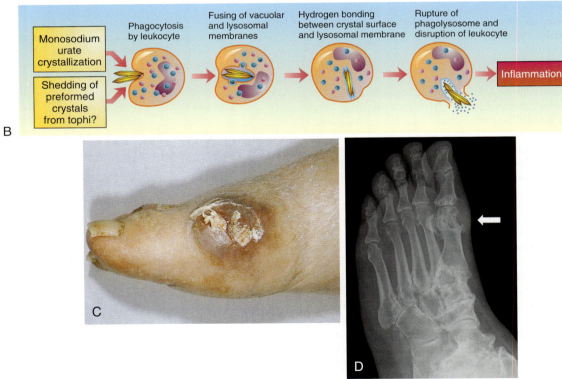

FIGURE 39.23 Pathogenesis of Acute Gouty Arthritis. **A,** Depending on the urate crystal coating, a variety of cells may be stimulated to produce a wide range of inflammatory mediators. **B,** Sequence of events in the production of the inflammatory response to urate crystals. **C,** Gouty tophus on right foot. **D,** Bone destruction of first metatarsal because of gout. *Apo-E,* Apolipoprotein E; *IgG,* immunoglobulin G; *IL,* interleukin; LTB_4, leukotriene B_4; PGE_2, prostaglandin E_2. ([C] from Dieppe, P. A., Kirwan, J., Cooper, C., et al. [1991]. *Arthritis and rheumatism in practice.* London: Gower; [D] Reprinted with permission from Chhana, A., & Dalbeth, N. [2014]. Structural joint damage in gout. *Rheumatic Disease Clinics of North America, 40*[2], 291–309.)

overproduction of uric acid. Environmental and genetic factors also play a role in an individual's urate concentration. At the cellular level, purines are synthesized to purine nucleotides, which are used in the synthesis of nucleic acids, adenosine triphosphate (ATP), cyclic adenosine monophosphate, and cyclic guanosine monophosphate. Uric acid is a breakdown product of purine nucleotides (urate synthesis and elimination are illustrated in Figure 39.23).

The kidneys eliminate most uric from the body. The glomerulus filters the urate, and the renal tubules both reabsorb and excrete it. In primary gout, urate excretion by the kidneys is sluggish. The sluggish excretion may be the result of a decrease in glomerular filtration of urate or acceleration in urate reabsorption. In addition, MSU crystals are deposited in renal interstitial tissues, causing impaired urine flow. (Kidney function is described in Chapter 29.)

There are several proposed mechanisms by which the joints accumulate MSU crystals and induce gouty arthritis, including:

1. MSU precipitates at the periphery of the body, where lower body temperatures may reduce the solubility of MSU.
2. Albumin or glycosaminoglycan levels decrease, which causes decreased urate solubility.
3. Changes in ion concentration and decreases of pH enhance urate deposition.
4. Trauma promotes urate crystal precipitation.

The MSU crystals may form in the synovial fluid or in the synovial membrane, cartilage, or other connective tissues in joints and elsewhere, such as in the heart, earlobes, and kidneys. An acute attack of gout is actually the result of the *formation* of crystals rather than the release of crystals from connective tissues into the synovial fluid.

MSU crystals can stimulate and perpetuate the inflammatory response (see Figure 39.23A,B). The presence of the crystals triggers the acute inflammatory response, releasing proinflammatory cytokines and TNFs, during which neutrophils migrate out of the circulation and begin to phagocytose (ingest) the crystals.

Importantly, deposits of MSU in joints and other tissues are often present years before an acute gout attack occurs. Early identification and intervention in treating gout can reduce morbidity and mortality associated with the disease. Traditionally, plain radiographs (X-rays) have been used to assess joints affected by gout, but only damaged joints can be seen. Newer technologies, including high-resolution ultrasound, dual-energy computed tomography, and MRI, can assess the presence of MSU crystals before joint, tendon, or ligament damage occurs.[197] Imaging modalities can also be used when joints cannot be aspirated to look for MSU crystals microscopically. Earlier identification allows timely as well as ongoing evaluation of treatment.[198]

CLINICAL MANIFESTATIONS The clinical manifestations of gout are (1) an increase in serum urate concentration (hyperuricemia); (2) recurrent attacks of monoarticular arthritis (inflammation of a single joint); (3) deposits of MSU monohydrate (tophi) in and around the joints; (4) kidney disease involving glomerular, tubular, and interstitial tissues and blood vessels; and (5) the formation of kidney stones. These manifestations appear in three clinical stages:

1. **Asymptomatic hyperuricemia.** The serum urate level is elevated but arthritic symptoms, tophi, and kidney stones are not present; this stage may persist throughout life.
2. **Acute gouty arthritis.** Attacks develop with increased serum urate concentrations; tends to occur with sudden or sustained increases of hyperuricemia but also can be triggered by trauma, medications, and alcohol.
3. **Tophaceous gout.** This third and chronic stage of the disease can begin as early as 3 years or as late as 40 years after the initial attack of gouty arthritis. Progressive inability to excrete uric acid expands the urate pool until MSU crystal deposits (tophi) appear in cartilage, synovial membranes, tendons, and soft tissue.

Trauma is the most common aggravating factor of an acute gouty exacerbation. Attacks of gouty arthritis occur abruptly, usually in a peripheral joint (Figure 39.23C). The primary symptom is severe pain. Approximately 50% of the initial attacks occur in the metatarsophalangeal joint of the great toe (a condition known as *podagra*). The other 50% can occur in almost any joint, but most often involve the heel, ankle, instep of the foot, knee, wrist, or elbow. The pain usually occurs at night. Within a few hours, the affected joint becomes hot, red, and extremely tender and may be slightly swollen. Lymphangitis and systemic signs of inflammation (leukocytosis, fever, ESR) are occasionally present. Untreated, mild attacks usually subside in several hours but may persist for 1 or 2 days. Severe attacks may persist for several days or weeks. When the individual recovers, the symptoms resolve completely.

Tophaceous deposits produce irregular swellings of the fingers, hands, knees, and feet. The helix of the ear is the most common site of tophi, which are the characteristic diagnostic lesions of chronic gout. Tophi also may develop along the ulnar surface of the forearm, the tibial surface of the leg, the Achilles tendon, olecranon bursa, or other areas. Tophi may produce marked limitation of joint movement and can eventually cause grotesque deformities of the hands and feet (see Figure 39.23C). Although the tophi themselves are painless, they often cause progressive stiffness and persistent aching of the affected joint. Tophi in the extremities can cause nerve compression—carpal tunnel syndrome in the wrists, tarsal tunnel syndrome in the ankles. Tophi also may erode and drain through the skin.

Kidney stones are 1000 times more prevalent in individuals with primary gout than in the general population. The stones can be the size of a grain of sand or a piece of gravel, or they can accumulate in massive deposits called *staghorn calculi*. They range in colour from pale yellow to brown to reddish black, depending on their composition. Some stones consist of pure MSU; others consist of calcium oxalate or calcium phosphate. Kidney stones can form in the collecting tubules, pelvis, or ureters, causing obstruction, dilation, and atrophy of the more proximal tubules and leading eventually to acute kidney failure. Stones deposited directly in renal interstitial tissue initiate an inflammatory reaction that leads to chronic kidney disease and progressive kidney failure.

EVALUATION AND TREATMENT Evaluation of gout may include history and physical examination, blood tests, joint fluid test, ultrasound, and other imaging. The goals of treatment are to terminate the acute gouty attack as promptly as possible, decrease serum uric acid levels (to dissolve MSU crystals), prevent acute attacks of gout by removing tophi, and, finally, cure gout.[199] Acute gouty arthritis should be treated with anti-inflammatory medications within 24 hours after the attack. The medications of choice are NSAIDs, corticosteroids, and colchicine.[200] Newer medications include interleukin inhibitors.[201] In people who are unable to tolerate NSAIDs, colchicine is useful but can be poorly tolerated because of a number of side effects. Once infection has been ruled out, steroids may be injected into the joint to relieve pain. Local application of ice reduces pain during an acute attack.[202] Weight-bearing on the involved joint is avoided until the acute attack subsides. A diet that includes mostly vegetables and fruit with little meat, avoidance of alcohol, and weight loss can help lower serum uric acid concentration.[203] Current recommendations include decreasing serum urate levels to less than 356.9 μmol/L (or less than 297.4 μmol/L if the individual has marked MSU crystal deposits on clinical examination or imaging studies).[197] High fluid intake, particularly water, can increase urinary output. Long-term use of antihyperuricemic medications, including newer agents such as pegloticase (Krystexxa), helps reduce serum urate concentrations. Allopurinol (Zyloprim) and febuxostat (Adenuric) both lower serum urate levels by inhibiting the activity of xanthine oxidase.

DISORDERS OF SKELETAL MUSCLE

> **QUICK CHECK 39.4**
> 1. What is the main objective clinical finding in fibromyalgia?
> 2. How do metabolic muscle diseases develop? What causes them?
> 3. Name one toxic myopathy and explain why it develops.

Muscle weakness and muscle fatigue are common symptoms of many muscle diseases (or myopathies). In many cases, neural, traumatic, and psychogenic causes provide an adequate explanation for the failure to generate force (weakness) or sustain force (fatigue) seen in myopathies, but the causes of many myopathies remain unknown. The complex interaction between muscles and nerves affects muscular function as well. The following discussion focuses only on inherited and acquired disorders of skeletal muscles.

Secondary Muscular Dysfunction

Muscular symptoms arise from a variety of causes unrelated to the muscle itself. For example, secondary muscular phenomena (contracture, stress-related muscle tension, immobility) are common disorders that influence muscular function.

Contractures

Contractures result from the loss of full passive range of motion secondary to joint, muscle, or other soft tissue limitations[204] and can be pathological or physiological. A physiological muscle contracture occurs in the absence of a muscle action potential in the sarcolemma. Muscle shortening happens because of failure of the calcium pump in the presence of plentiful ATP. A physiological contracture is present in McArdle's disease (muscle myophosphorylase deficiency) and MH. The contracture is usually temporary if the underlying pathology is reversed.

A pathological contracture is a permanent muscle shortening caused by muscle spasm or weakness. Heel cord (Achilles tendon) contractures are examples of pathological contractures. Contractures occur with plentiful ATP and despite a normal action potential. Contractures are most common in stroke, neuromuscular diseases (such as muscular dystrophy), Charcot-Marie-Tooth disease, amyotrophic lateral sclerosis, and CNS injury. Lower-extremity contractures are more common than those in the upper extremity. Prolonged splinting in a single position or an imbalance between agonist–antagonist muscles also can cause joint stiffness and contractures. Contractures may also develop secondary to scar tissue contraction in the flexor tissues of a joint, as in scarring of burned tissues in the antecubital area of the forearm, leading to a flexion contracture.

Stress-Induced Muscle Tension

Abnormally increased muscle tension has been associated with chronic anxiety as well as a variety of stress-related muscular symptoms, including neck stiffness, back pain, and headache.[205] Abnormalities in the CNS, reticular activating system, and autonomic nervous system (ANS) also play a role. For example, as an individual progressively relaxes, the amplitude of the knee jerk reflex diminishes. Conversely, individuals with absent reflexes increase tension by such manoeuvres as clenching the teeth or strengthening the handgrip. The underlying pathophysiology may be related to the fact that as a muscle contracts, the muscle spindle is activated. This gamma-feedback system produces a series of impulses that are transmitted to the brain by the sensitive 1 A afferent fibres. Unconscious tension increases the activity of the reticular activating system, which stimulates firing of the efferent loop of the gamma fibres, producing further muscle contraction, and increasing muscle tension. ANS function that regulates increased blood flow to the muscle during sympathetic activity may be related to increased muscle contraction tension.

Various forms of treatment can reduce the muscle tension associated with stress. Progressive relaxation training, yoga, meditation, and biofeedback are examples of stress reduction therapies. Biofeedback uses integrated electromyography (EMG) to make recordings from the skin surface. The goal is to teach the individual to control maladaptive tension. Biofeedback is particularly useful in individuals who have a connection between skeletal muscle tension and pain. Progressive relaxation training emphasizes the individual's ability to perceive the difference between tension and relaxation. This technique involves sequential tensing and a relaxing environment. The individual practises this routine daily, often with the use of audio instructions. By teaching the individual to recognize excessive contraction of skeletal muscle, one hopes to enhance the person's ability to relax specific muscle groups to relieve tension and thus reduce CNS arousal as well as ANS arousal.

Disuse Atrophy

The term disuse atrophy describes the pathological reduction in normal size of muscle fibres after prolonged inactivity from bed rest, trauma (casting), or local nerve damage as can be seen with spinal cord trauma or poliomyelitis. Decreased muscle activity reduces muscle mass through both decreased muscle protein synthesis and increased muscle protein breakdown.[206] Reduced protein synthesis is primarily responsible for muscle atrophy. The effects of muscular deconditioning associated with lack of physical activity may be apparent in a matter of days. A normal individual on bed rest loses muscle strength from baseline levels at a rate of 3% per day. Bed rest is also associated with cardiovascular, skeletal, and other organ system changes. Likewise, as people age, their muscles atrophy and become weaker (sarcopenia).

Measures to prevent atrophy include frequent forceful isometric muscle contractions and passive lengthening exercises. Artificial gravity (through the use of a "human centrifuge") has potential in maintaining muscle strength. One of the simplest ways to improve disuse atrophy is to restore a load to the muscle, such as returning to walking, starting active motion to a limb, and adding resistance to movements.[207] If reuse is not restored within 1 year, regeneration of muscle fibres becomes impaired.

Fibromyalgia

Fibromyalgia (FM) is a chronic musculoskeletal syndrome characterized by diffuse pain, fatigue, increased sensitivity to touch (i.e., tender points), the absence of systemic or localized inflammation, and the presence of fatigue and nonrestorative sleep; anxiety and depression also are frequently present. FM has often been misdiagnosed or completely dismissed by clinicians because there are few objective clinical findings on examination. A common misdiagnosis has been chronic fatigue syndrome (CFS). Of affected individuals, 80 to 90% are women, and the peak age of onset is 30 to 50 years of age. New research supports the possible role of inflammation in FM.[208-210] FM and its symptoms are viewed as the result of CNS dysfunction, where there is an amplification of pain transmission and interpretation, or central sensitization. Although the incidence is unknown, the prevalence is 2 to 8% and increases with age.[211] Certain autoimmune diseases, especially systemic lupus erythematosus and irritable bowel syndrome, coincide with FM and may coexist if not initially present with FM.

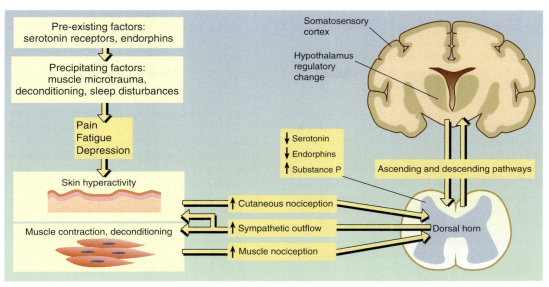

FIGURE 39.24 Theoretical Pathophysiological Model of Fibromyalgia.

PATHOPHYSIOLOGY Genetic factors have a role in the development of FM. Relatives of individuals with FM have an increased risk of developing FM. Studies of genetic factors include alterations in genes affecting serotonin, catecholamines, and dopamine—all of these substances are involved in the stress response and sensory processing.[212–214] In spite of these studies, there is much more to discover about the role of genetic factors in FM. External stressors, such as infection, psychosocial stress, and physical or emotional trauma, are also proposed mechanisms precipitating FM.[215]

Functional magnetic resonance imaging and PET scans of the brains of individuals with FM indicate activity in different areas of the brain than normally seen in healthy individuals exposed to painful stimuli.[216] Figure 39.24 illustrates these functional abnormalities within the CNS. Other pathophysiological evidence includes hypothalamic–pituitary axis alterations that show abnormal response to stress.[217]

CLINICAL MANIFESTATIONS The prominent symptom of FM is diffuse, persistent pain. Persistent pain is pain that is present for more than 3 months. Traditionally, to be classified as FM, there is an additional requirement of tenderness in 11 of 18 specific points along with widespread pain. The 2012 classification of FM was simplified and expanded to include other important nonpain symptoms.[218] The pain often begins in one location, especially the neck and shoulders, but then becomes more generalized. People describe the pain as "burning" or "gnawing." Fatigue is profound. The effect on everyday life is considerable. Fatigue is most notable when arising from sleep and in midafternoon. Headaches and memory loss are common complaints. There is a strong association between FM, Raynaud's phenomenon, and irritable bowel syndrome. Individuals with FM are light sleepers and awake frequently, which may explain why individuals feel nonrefreshed upon waking.

Almost 25% of individuals seek psychological support for depression. Anxiety, particularly with regard to their diagnosis and future, is almost universal.

EVALUATION AND TREATMENT Because the manifestations of chronic, generalized pain and fatigue are present in many musculoskeletal (e.g., rheumatic) disorders, these disorders should be considered in the differential diagnosis of FM. In an effort to simplify and more accurately diagnose FM, a panel of experts from across Canada developed the Canadian Guidelines for the Diagnosis and Management of Fibromyalgia Syndrome.[219] According to these guidelines, the symptom complex for FM includes:

- Pain that has been present at a similar level for at least 3 months, with insidious onset, usually localized to a particular area (often in muscles and joints); pain might also be neuropathic in nature (i.e., burning); there is no other underlying pathology to explain the pain
- Other associated symptoms: fatigue, nonrestorative sleep, cognitive dysfunction, changes in mood.

FM treatment should be highly individualized and can include mind–body interventions (such as biofeedback), movement therapies, and relaxation techniques as well as medication.[220] FM requires multiple medication regimens for improved outcomes. Exercise regimens are beneficial in reducing symptoms. Recommended exercises for individuals with FM include aerobic activities (including kickboxing and weightlifting), stretching, and gentle strengthening programs. Medications such as NSAIDs, opioids, cannabinoids, antidepressants, and anticonvulsants with pain-modulating effects, as well as medications that alter the level of neurotransmitters in the brain are also helpful. Two of the most important aspects of treatment are physical activity and patient education (Box 39.4).[221–223]

> **BOX 39.4 Educating and Providing Reassurance for Individuals With Fibromyalgia**
>
> Stress that the illness is real, not imagined.
> Explain that fibromyalgia is presumably not caused by infection.
> Explain that fibromyalgia is not a deforming or deteriorating condition.
> Explain that fibromyalgia is neither life-threatening nor markedly debilitating, although it is an irritating presence.
> Discuss the role of sleep disturbances and the relationship of neurohormones to pain, fatigue, abnormal sleep, and mood.
> Reassure that although the cause is unknown, some information is known about the physiological changes responsible for the symptoms.
> Use muscle "spasms" and, perhaps, "low muscle blood flow" to lay the groundwork for exercise recommendations.
> Assist the individual to use aerobic exercise to reduce stress and increase rapid eye movement sleep.

Chronic Fatigue Syndrome

Chronic fatigue syndrome (CFS) is a chronic debilitating disease that is likely best described as neuroimmunoendocrine disease that has clinical manifestations of cognitive impairment, severe postexertional fatigue (including physical, emotional, or cognitive activity), unrefreshing sleep, and decreased physical activity that affects daily functioning.[223,224] Other frequent symptoms include sore throat, tender lymph nodes, pain, and psychiatric complaints. CFS has often been a diagnosis of exclusion because it cannot be objectively identified by any laboratory or specific clinical tests.[225] Because of the difficulty finding objective data to diagnose CFS, the disease is also known as myalgic encephalomyelitis (ME) and has been considered a psychiatric disorder. CFS/ME has remained a controversial diagnosis until recently.

Though there seems to be some psychological involvement in CFS/ME, there is emerging evidence for a physiological basis. There are a number of physiological abnormalities associated with CFS/ME. Some of these processes include skeletal muscle abnormalities, mitochondrial dysfunction, diminished activity of several types of immune cells, abnormal cytokine regulation, and dysfunction of the hypothalamic–pituitary–adrenal (HPA) axis.[226–229] Because of the continued controversy surrounding CFS/ME and the difficulties diagnosing and treating it, the Institute of Medicine recommended a new term for the condition in 2015: systemic exertional intolerance disease (SEID).[230] Treatment for SEID remains challenging and must be individualized because there are both physical and psychological components to the disease. Learning how to adapt to stressors and improving physical activity may assist in improving symptoms.[231,232]

Muscle Membrane Abnormalities

Two defects of the muscle membrane (plasma membrane of the muscle fibre) have been linked to clinical syndromes: the hyperexcitable membrane seen in myotonic disorders and the intermittently unresponsive membrane seen in periodic paralyses. Although these are rare disorders, research into their pathological processes has led to an improved understanding of cell membrane channelopathies (ion channels are described in Chapter 13).

Myotonia

Myotonias are genetically inherited diseases caused by alterations in skeletal muscle sodium and calcium ion channels that result in delayed relaxation after voluntary muscle contraction, such as handgrip, eye closure, or muscle percussion.[233,234] Definitive diagnosis is possible by genetic testing. Needle EMG is useful in determining the likelihood of disease; the distinctive "dive bomber" noise, audible on needle EMG, is caused by the prolonged depolarization of the muscle membrane.

Myotonia comprises various disorders: myotonia congenita, paramyotonia congenita, myotonic muscular dystrophy, and some forms of periodic paralysis. With the exception of myotonic muscular dystrophy, most are mild in symptomatology. Treatment includes sodium channel blocking agents, such as mexiletine (Mexitil Cap). In Canada, little information is available on the use of pharmacological agents for treating myotonia. In a small randomized control trial, methylphenidate was found to decrease excessive somnolence seen in this disorder. There are some promising disease-modifying therapies entering clinical trials.[235] Other treatment modalities include genetic counselling as well as lifestyle and dietary modifications.[236]

Periodic Paralysis

Periodic paralysis encompasses a rare group of muscle diseases characterized by episodes of flaccid weakness. Most are hereditary (autosomal dominant) and caused by calcium or sodium channel abnormalities (pore gating anomalies) because of specific genetic mutations. In normal skeletal muscle, the cellular inflow and outflow of potassium are balanced to maintain the cell's resting membrane potential. Sodium channels, in response to nerve stimulation, create the action potentials that initiate muscle contraction. Calcium channels interact with ryanodine receptors to initiate fast muscle contraction.[237] In susceptible individuals, some instigating factor (such as hyperthyroidism, strenuous exercise, or intake of a high-carbohydrate meal) allows increased muscle uptake of potassium from the plasma. This results in slightly decreased plasma potassium levels, but it triggers depolarization of the sarcolemma and allows more potassium to enter the cell, causing hypokalemia.[238] Exposure to cold or rest after strenuous exercise can trigger hypokalemic periodic paralysis. During an attack of hypokalemic periodic paralysis, the resting muscle membrane potential is both unresponsive to neural stimuli and reduced from −90 to −45 mV. This condition can last hours to days.

Thyrotoxic periodic paralysis (TPP) results from a potassium channelopathy that causes increased flow of potassium into the cell; it does not indicate a potassium deficiency.[239,240] Most common in Asian males, TPP is increasing in all ethnic groups.[240] The main consequence of increased concentration of intracellular potassium is depolarization of the muscle and resulting weakness. Prevention is aimed at correcting the hyperthyroidism. β-Adrenergic blockers, such as propranolol (Apo-Propranolol), are sometimes given until thyroid function is normal. Oral and intravenous administration of potassium can relieve acute hypokalemic attacks.

Hyperkalemic periodic paralysis is another genetic disorder with episodes of flaccid paralysis. Several factors can activate it, including pregnancy, alcohol, illness, certain medications, eating potassium-rich foods, exposure to cold, and rest after exercising.[241] Although the most striking feature of the condition is flaccid paralysis, many individuals have myotonia present on examination.[241] The sodium channel fails to completely inactivate, causing more sodium to enter the cell and forcing potassium into the extracellular space, thus blocking sodium channels from depolarizing. Though hyperkalemic periodic paralysis episodes are typically shorter in duration than those of hypokalemic periodic paralysis, there is often a lifelong trend to have increasing frequency of attacks. In addition, hyperkalemic periodic paralysis can cause permanent muscle weakness. Respiratory insufficiency can be a life-threatening situation.

Preventive measures include avoiding alcohol and diet soda, potassium-rich foods, or activities that provoke symptoms. Maintaining adequate water intake, eating carbohydrate-rich foods, and keeping warm seem to help some individuals.[242] In acute hyperkalemic periodic paralysis, inhaled albuterol (Ventolin) or glucose/insulin therapy can reduce symptoms. Preventive medications include potassium-lowering agents, such as hydrochlorothiazide (Urozide) or mexiletine.

Metabolic Muscle Diseases

Disorders in muscle metabolism can be caused by endocrine abnormalities or diseases of energy metabolism, such as glycogen storage disease, enzyme deficiencies, and abnormalities in lipid metabolism and mitochondrial function. The term *metabolic myopathies* refers to a group of hereditary muscle disorders caused by defective genes.

Endocrine Disorders

The systemic effects of hormonal imbalance often overshadow the individual's muscular symptoms. For example, individuals with thyrotoxicosis may have signs of proximal weakness, paresis of the extraocular muscles (exophthalmic ophthalmoplegia), and, rarely, hypokalemic periodic paralysis. Hypothyroidism is often associated with a decrease in muscle mass and strength, with weak, flabby skeletal muscles and sluggish movements.

Thyroid hormone regulates muscle protein synthesis and electrolyte balance. Alterations in muscle protein synthesis and electrolyte balance may therefore explain the changes in muscle mass and contractility of endocrine disorders. The muscular symptoms subside with appropriate treatment of the primary hormonal disorder.

Diseases of Energy Metabolism

Muscles rely on carbohydrates (such as glycogen) and lipids (free fatty acids) for energy. When stored glycogen or lipids cannot be metabolized because of lack of enzymes necessary to generate ATP for muscle contraction, the individual experiences cramps, fatigue, and exercise intolerance. Disorders of muscle metabolism can be self-limiting, such as McArdle's disease and some lipid disorders, or they can cause widespread irreparable muscle destruction, as in acid maltase deficiency.

McArdle's disease. **McArdle's disease**, or *myophosphorylase deficiency*, is also known as *glycogen storage disease type V*. It was the first myopathy in which a single enzyme defect was identified. It is now one of nine diseases identified to date that have an underlying defect in glycogen synthesis, glycogenolysis, or glycolysis in common. These diseases are often referred to as **glycogen storage diseases (GSDs)** because each defect results in the abnormal deposition and accumulation of glycogen in skeletal muscle. Individuals with McArdle's disease lack muscle phosphorylase, an enzyme responsible for the breakdown of glycogen in muscle. Normally, after the body uses the short-term ATP and phosphocreatine stores, intramuscular lactic acid accumulated as glycogen is used (see Chapter 18). The individual with McArdle's disease is not able to metabolize glycogen or produce lactic acid.

The altered energy production manifests itself in exercise intolerance, fatigue, and painful muscle cramps. When exercise is carried to an extreme, painful muscle contracture and myoglobinuria can develop. Some individuals describe a "second wind" phenomenon, in which exercise tolerance increases if they slow their pace once the initial sensation of fatigue commences.[243] The muscles of people with McArdle's disease are able to readily utilize glucose and lactate from the bloodstream. Lactate, after it is converted to pyruvate, is an energy substrate that undergoes oxidization more quickly than either fructose or glucose.[244,245] Higher levels of lactate found in skeletal muscles of those with McArdle's disease may account for this "second wind." As the disease progresses, some individuals have pronounced muscle weakness and wasting. Other organs are not involved, because the absence of phosphorylase is limited to muscle. In general, individuals with McArdle's disease learn to adapt their daily routine to avoid muscle symptoms.

Acid maltase deficiency. **Acid maltase deficiency** (*glycogen storage disease type II*, or *Pompe's disease*) is an autosomal recessive neuromuscular disease caused by mutations of the acid α-glucosidase gene. This deficiency results in an accumulation of glycogen in the lysosomes of muscle cells and other tissues because of the lack of the enzyme acid maltase (also known as acid α-glucosidase [GAA]).[246,247] The exact mechanism of disease progression is still unknown, but mitochondrial dysfunction and abnormal autophagy of cells appear to play a major role in the disease's clinical manifestations.

The infantile form, which is more severe, is called **Pompe's disease (PD)** and is recognized shortly after birth by hypotonia, dysreflexia, and an enlarged heart, tongue, and liver. Hypertrophy of these tissues is the result of glycogen deposition. Muscle biopsy is an important diagnostic tool in identifying PD.[248] In the past, children died of cardiac or respiratory failure within 1 year of diagnosis, but new treatments have improved survival. Late-onset Pompe's disease occurs from childhood into adulthood. Muscular symptoms of late-onset Pompe's disease are highly variable and can range from muscle cramping and weakness to varying degrees of respiratory insufficiency.[249] The mainstay of treatment is enzyme replacement therapy with recombinant GAA, but dietary modifications also may improve the course of the disease.[250]

Myoadenylate deaminase deficiency. An enzyme deficiency that produces changes in skeletal muscle and is associated with exercise intolerance is **myoadenylate deaminase deficiency (MDD)**. More often referred to as *adenosine monophosphate deaminase deficiency* (AMDD), this autosomal recessive condition has a wide variation in symptoms.[251] Because individuals with MDD lack myoadenylate deaminase, they have a poor capacity for sustained energy production, yet some with the condition have been able to perform as high-level athletes. The most common symptoms appear to be postexercise muscle cramping or pain, or both, and easy fatigability. Myoadenylate deaminase is the catalytic enzyme that forms phosphocreatine and ATP during exercise through a metabolic pathway that binds the purine and phosphate molecules that constitute ATP. Individuals with MDD differ from those with McArdle's disease in that, during the ischemic exercise test, lactate production is normal in MDD when ATP and phosphocreatine are synthesized. The enzyme defect is quite common, but in practice it may be rarely recognized as a cause of exercise intolerance.

Lipid deficiencies. Disorders of lipid metabolism are uncommon but account for severe changes in muscle metabolism. These disorders are caused by abnormalities in the transport and processing of fatty acids for energy. The lipid content of muscle cells consists of free fatty acids, which are oxidized in the mitochondria. These acids require carnitine and the enzyme carnitine palmitoyltransferase (CPT) to transport long-chain fatty acids to the mitochondria. There are two types of CPT: CPT1 is found in liver, muscle, and brain tissue; only deficiencies of the liver type have been found in humans. Children younger than 18 months are most often affected. CPT2 deficiency, most often seen in adolescents or young adults, is an autosomal recessive disorder that invariably causes attacks of severe myalgia and may cause myoglobinuria.[252] Carnitine deficiency causes abnormal lipid deposition in skeletal muscles.

Measuring the CPT and carnitine content in muscle is essential to diagnosis. Cells in the muscle biopsy show vacuoles and lipid deposits. Treatments with riboflavin, medium-chain triglycerides, oral carnitine, prednisone (Deltasone), and propranolol have been beneficial to some individuals. Bezafibrate (Bezalip SR), a medication used to lower lipid levels, also has shown promise in treating CPT2 deficiency.[252]

Inflammatory Muscle Diseases: Myositis
Viral, Bacterial, and Parasitic Myositis

Viral, bacterial, and parasitic infections of varying severity are known to produce inflammatory changes in skeletal muscle, a group of conditions collectively described by the term **myositis**. In tuberculosis and sarcoidosis, chronic inflammatory changes and granulomata are found in muscle as well as in other affected tissues. In the parasitic infection trichinellosis, *Trichinella* larvae reside in infected meat (primarily pork, but wildlife and even horses can carry the microorganism), migrate to the intestinal mucosa after ingestion, and then travel through the circulatory system to various tissues. The larvae that penetrate into skeletal muscle are able to survive and grow, causing symptoms such as severe pain, rash, and muscle stiffness. Treatment includes the administration of corticosteroids, immunotherapeutic agents, and the antiparasitic agent thiabendazole (Mertect). Toxoplasmosis, a common parasitic infection, is also associated with a generalized polymyositis that responds rapidly to therapy.

In the tropics, more prevalent disorders include bacterial infections with *S. aureus* and parasites such as cysticercus, the larva of the tapeworm *Taenia solium*. Viral infections can be associated with an acute myositis. Muscle pain, tenderness, signs of inflammation, and CK elevation are common manifestations of viral myositis. The self-limiting

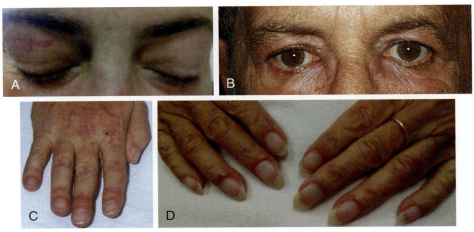

FIGURE 39.25 Clinical Manifestations of Dermatomyositis. **A** and **B**, Heliotrope (violaceous) discoloration around the eyes and periorbital edema. **C**, Gottron lesions. **D**, Increased erythema around nail beds. ([A, C, D] from Dimachkie, M. M., Barohn, R. J., & Amato, A. A. [2014]. *Neurol Clin, 32*[3], 595–628; (B) from Habif, T. P. [1996]. *Clinical dermatology* [3rd ed.]. Mosby.)

symptoms of muscle aches and pains during a bout of influenza may actually be a subacute form of viral myopathy.

Polymyositis, Dermatomyositis, and Inclusion Body Myositis

Idiopathic inflammatory myopathies (IIMs) are a group of autoimmune diseases that target skeletal muscle in both children and adults. There are generally four diseases included in this group: (1) dermatomyositis (DM), (2) polymyositis (PM), (3) necrotizing myopathy (NM), and (4) sporadic inclusion body myositis (IBM). The most common form, DM, has been further subclassified into additional subgroups, including the juvenile form—juvenile dermatomyositis. The exact cause of IIMs is unknown, but recent investigations suggest strong links between genetic, environmental, and immunological factors.[253,254] Though still relatively rare, IIMs seem to have a geographical distribution, with greater incidence in northern latitudes, further supporting the hypotheses of genetic and environmental influences in their development.[255,256] The pathophysiology of IIMs remains fully unknown, but it involves interplay between specific autoantibodies, cytokine-mediated inflammation of muscle, and genetic factors.[257,258]

Several characteristics differentiate IBM from the other IIMs in that IBM affects men more often than women and can cause asymmetric weakness. Compared with DM and PM, IBM does not respond as well to anti-inflammatory and immunosuppressive medications.

CLINICAL MANIFESTATIONS IIMs are characterized by progressive, symmetric proximal (shoulder girdle and quadriceps) muscle weakness and myalgia that develops over weeks to months. Because of their progressive nature, these illnesses can be initially confused with other myopathies. A thorough evaluation is required to exclude other disorders. Clinical features common in both PM and DM are joint pain, dysphagia, reduced esophageal motility, vasculitis, Raynaud's phenomenon, cardiomyopathy, and interstitial pulmonary fibrosis. Reduced mobility with frequent falls is a common symptom in IBM because both proximal and distal muscles are affected. Some individuals have other coexisting collagen vascular disorders, such as RA, systemic lupus erythematosus, and progressive systemic sclerosis (formerly called *scleroderma*).

Although PM and DM have similar histories of onset, DM includes cutaneous manifestations. The presence of skin involvement is significant in that it can precede muscle involvement by months or even years.[259] The two most classic signs of skin involvement are (1) rashes—a typical heliotrope (reddish purple) rash that generally covers the eyelids and periorbital tissue (Figure 39.25), and (2) erythematous, scaly lesions that cover joints such as the knees and elbows, known as *Gottron lesions*. Other differences between PM and DM include their suspected pathology. PM may be caused by T-cell invasion of the muscle fibres.[260] DM, PM, and NM are associated with an increased risk for malignancy.[261] Both PM and DM seem to respond to prednisone, with or without the addition of immunosuppressives as well as intravenous Ig administration.[262]

IBM is the most common acquired muscle disease affecting individuals older than age 50. IBM differs from both PM and DM in several important ways. Muscle biopsy and histopathological studies of IBM show degenerative changes of muscle, accumulation of multiple proteins within muscle fibres, and evidence of endoplasmic reticular stress with misfolding of proteins.[263,264] Clinical presentation may show earlier onset of asymmetric atrophy and weakness of the quadriceps as well as the wrists and finger flexors. Additionally, IBM generally does not improve with standard immunosuppressants or immune-modifying medications.[265]

EVALUATION AND TREATMENT Muscle biopsy results are striking in DM, with most individuals showing inflammatory cells grouped around blood vessels and atrophy of cells in muscle fascicles. This change, perifascicular atrophy, is absent in PM. CK level is often extremely elevated in both disorders and is a helpful indicator of disease activity. Levels of other muscle enzymes, including aldolase, aspartate aminotransferase (AST), alanine aminotransferase (ALT), and lactate dehydrogenase (LDH), are also found to be elevated in most individuals. The presence of serum antinuclear antibodies (ANAs) also may be helpful in diagnosis. Muscle biopsy is indispensable for a diagnosis of PM or DM as opposed to other myotonic disease.[261] MRI reveals inflammation and edema of the muscles, as well as changes in muscles that may not show clinical evidence of disease. Contrast-enhanced ultrasound can differentiate between IBM and myositis.[266,267] EMG is useful in guiding the site for muscle biopsy.

Treatment primarily includes immunosuppressive medications, although they are not always successful, particularly in the case of IBM. Most clinicians choose corticosteroids initially, usually prednisone on a daily or alternating day schedule, tapering the dosage as the symptoms subside. Successful treatment with azathioprine, methotrexate, creatine

BOX 39.5 Agents That Can Cause Toxic Myopathy

Medications, Drugs, and Substances
- Alcohol
- Amiodarone (Cordarone; and other medications that inhibit CYP3A4 when combined with a statin)
- Amphotericin B
- Azathioprine
- Chloroquine (Teva-Chloroquine)
- Clofibrate
- Colchicine
- Diuretics
- Ethanol
- Finasteride (CO Finasteride)
- Illicit drugs and drugs of abuse (heroin, cocaine, amphetamine, meperidine, pentazocine)
- Ipecac (withdrawn from Canadian and US markets)
- Isotretinoin (Accutane)
- Labetalol (Trandate)
- 3,4-Methylenedioxymethamphetamine (MDMA, "ecstasy")
- Omeprazole (Losec)
- Pentachlorophenol (PCP)
- Propofol
- Retrovirals (AZT [zidovudine])
- Statins
- Steroids (especially with prolonged high doses; doses >25 mg/day; fluorinated steroids)
- Vincristine (Oncovin)

Endocrine Disorders
- Adrenal disorders (Addison's disease, Cushing's disease)
- Hyperparathyroidism
- Hyperthyroidism (creatine kinase may be normal)
- Hypothyroidism (creatine kinase may be mildly elevated)

Infectious Agents
- Coxsackie A and B viruses
- Human immunodeficiency virus (HIV)
- Influenza
- Lyme disease
- *Staphylococcus aureus* muscle infection (frequent cause of pyomyositis)
- Toxoplasmosis
- Trichinosis

Miscellaneous
- Licorice
- Certain edible wild mushrooms
- Lead poisoning
- Malignant hyperthermia
- Organophosphates
- Red yeast rice
- Snake venom
- European migratory quail (quail eat toxic hemlock, hellebore seeds)
- Any medication that alters serum concentrations of sodium, potassium, calcium, phosphorus, or magnesium

Data from Pasnoor, M., Barohn, R. J., & Dimachkie, M. M. (2014). Toxic myopathies. *Neurologic Clinics, 32*, 647–670; Valiyil, V. R., & Christopher-Stine, O. (2010). Drug-related myopathies of which the clinician should be aware. *Current Rheumatology Reports, 12*(3), 213–220.

(Creatine Systemic), and cyclosporine also has been reported.[261,268] High-dose intravenous IgG administration is sometimes used during active disease. Individuals with muscle weakness require careful physiotherapy to design a regular exercise program that prevents contractures and maximizes functional ability.

Toxic Myopathies

Muscle damage caused by medications or toxins is also called **toxic myopathy**. Alcohol, lipid-lowering agents (fibrates and statins), antimalarial medications, steroids, thiol derivatives, and narcotics (particularly heroin) can all cause symptoms. Many medications, diseases, and infectious and environmental agents can cause myopathy. The combination of certain medications can also cause muscle injury.[269] Box 39.5 lists some of the causes of toxic myopathy.

Alcohol remains the most common cause of toxic myopathy. Two clinical syndromes are prevalent: (1) an acute attack of muscle weakness, pain, and swelling after a drinking binge or (2) a more chronic, progressive proximal weakness in a long-term drinker.[270] The incidence of acute alcoholic myopathy has been estimated as being up to 20% of individuals admitted with acute alcoholic withdrawal.

The pathological abnormalities include necrosis of individual muscle fibres; whole segments can be found in the same stage of degeneration. The mechanism by which alcohol affects the muscle fibre is unclear, but there is evidence to support both a direct toxic effect and nutritional deficiency.

Acute alcoholic myopathy can range from benign cramps and pain resolving in a matter of hours to severe weakness and markedly increased CK level associated with myoglobinuria and kidney failure. Individuals are prone to repeated attacks following recovery. The only treatment is abstinence from alcohol and improved nutrition. The individual with chronic alcoholic myopathy often has coexisting peripheral neuropathy that complicates the diagnosis.

The most severe complication of toxic myopathy is rhabdomyolysis (acute muscle fibre necrosis with leakage of muscle protein into the bloodstream) that leads to myoglobinuria and acute kidney failure. Most individuals with toxic myopathy present with acute muscle weakness. Pain is an unreliable indicator because many toxic myopathies are painless but necrotizing toxic myopathies can cause severe pain. Dark-coloured urine may indicate rhabdomyolysis, a serious complication that can lead to death. Other serious complications can include involvement of respiratory and cardiac muscles.

Measurement of serum creatine levels is helpful in determining muscle damage. Other tests such as EMG may show characteristic changes in function. MRI can demonstrate muscle edema, and features of myopathy can be seen on muscle biopsy.

Repeated intramuscular injections are also associated with changes in muscle fibres. Local necrosis of muscle fibres and elevated CK level have been reported after intramuscular injections of cephalothin (Averon-1), lidocaine, diazepam (Apo-Diazepam), and digoxin (Toloxin); injections of saline did not produce these effects. Injection of medication over long periods causes the development of a chronic focal myopathy. There is a proliferation of connective tissue in both the muscle fibre and the overlying skin and subcutaneous tissue. Over time, segments of the muscles, particularly the deltoid and quadriceps, become fibrotic bands. Pathophysiological mechanisms for these changes include repeated needle trauma and infection, along with the nonphysiological acidity or alkalinity of the injected material. Treatment primarily consists of removing or stopping the offending agent and providing supportive care. Supportive care may include hemodialysis and respiratory or cardiovascular support, depending on severity of symptoms.

MUSCULOSKELETAL TUMOURS

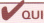

QUICK CHECK 39.5
1. From what cells do bone tumours originate?
2. Compare five major characteristics of benign bone tumours with those of malignant bone tumours.
3. How does the presence of metastatic tumours affect treatment options and prognosis of persons with osteosarcoma?

Bone Tumours

Many different types of tumours involve the skeleton. Although the skeleton is the major site for metastatic spread of multiple myeloma and breast, lung, and prostate cancers, primary bone tumours are relatively rare. **Bone tumours** may originate from bone cells, cartilage, fibrous tissue, marrow, or vascular tissue. Based on the tissue of origin, bone tumours are osteogenic, chondrogenic, collagenic, or myelogenic. Box 39.6 contains the classification of major primary bone tumours. Each type arises from one of the four stem cells that are ultimately derived from the primitive mesoderm (Figure 39.26). In addition, bone tumours may be of histiocytic, notochordal, lipogenic, or neurogenic origin.

The mesoderm contributes the primitive fibroblast and reticulum cells. The fibroblast is the progenitor of the osteoblast and chondroblast cells. Each cell synthesizes a specific type of intercellular ground substance, and the type of ground substance produced by the cell generally characterizes the tumour derived from that cell. For example, osteogenic tumours usually contain cells that have the appearance of osteoblasts and produce an intercellular substance that can be recognized as osteoid. Chondrogenic tumours contain chondroblasts and produce an intercellular substance similar to chondroid (cartilage). Collagenic tumours contain fibrous tissue cells and produce an intercellular substance similar to the type of collagen found in fibrous connective tissue.

Tumours are also classified as benign or malignant, based on characteristics of the tumour cells (see Chapter 10). The criteria used to identify tumour cells as malignant are (1) an increased nuclear/cytoplasmic ratio, (2) an irregular nuclear border, (3) an excess of chromatin, (4) a prominent nucleolus, and (5) an increase in the number of cells undergoing mitosis. However, many young, rapidly growing normal cells and cells subjected to inflammation and change in their blood supply also exhibit many of these same characteristics. (Chapter 10 describes general characteristics of tumours.)

BOX 39.6 Classification of Major Primary Tumours Involving Bone

Category and Fraction (%)	Behaviour	Tumour Type	Common Locations	Age (Years)	Morphology
Hematopoietic (20)	Malignant	Myeloma Lymphoma	Vertebrae, pelvis	50–60	Malignant plasma cells or lymphocytes replacing marrow space
Cartilage forming (30)	Benign	Osteochondroma	Metaphysis of long bones	10–30	Bony excrescence with cartilage cap
		Chondroma	Small bones of hands and feet	30–50	Circumscribed hyaline cartilage nodule in medulla
		Chondroblastoma	Epiphysis of long bones	10–20	Circumscribed, pericellular calcification
		Chondromyxoid fibroma	Tibia, pelvis	20–30	Collagenous to myxoid matrix, stellate cells
	Malignant	Chondrosarcoma (conventional)	Pelvis, shoulder	40–60	Extends from medulla through cortex into soft tissue, chondrocytes with increased cellularity and atypia
Bone forming (26)	Benign	Osteoid osteoma	Metaphysis of long bones	10–20	Cortical, interlacing microtrabeculae of woven bone
		Osteoblastoma	Vertebral column	10–20	Posterior elements of vertebrae, histology similar to osteoid osteoma
	Malignant	Osteosarcoma	Metaphysis of distal femur, proximal tibia	10–20	Extends from medulla to lift periosteum, malignant cells produce woven bone
Unknown origin (15)	Benign	Giant cell tumour	Epiphysis of long bones	20–40	Destroys medulla and cortex, sheets of osteoclasts
		Aneurysmal bone cyst	Proximal tibia, distal femur, vertebrae	10–20	Vertebral body, hemorrhagic spaces separated by cellular, fibrous septae
	Malignant	Ewing sarcoma	Diaphysis of long bones	10–20	Sheets of primitive small round cells
		Adamantinoma	Tibia	30–40	Cortical, fibrous, bone matrix with epithelial islands
Notochordal (4)	Malignant	Chordoma	Clivus, sacrum	30–60	Destroys medulla and cortex, foamy cells in myxoid matrix

From Kumar, V., Abbas, A. K., & Aster, J. C. (Eds.). (2021). *Robbins and Cotran pathologic basis of disease* (10th ed.). Elsevier. Adapted from Unni, K. K., & Inwards, C. Y. (2010). *Dahlin's bone tumors* (6th ed.). Lippincott Williams & Wilkins; by permission of Mayo Foundation.

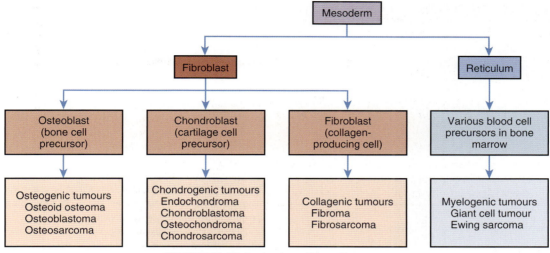

FIGURE 39.26 Derivation of Bone Tumours.

Epidemiology

The incidence rate of bone tumours varies with age. In children younger than 15 years, the rate of bone tumours is relatively low, constituting approximately 5% of all malignancies. Adolescents have the highest incidence of bone tumours, and adults between the ages of 30 and 35 have the lowest incidence. After age 35, the incidence rate slowly increases until at age 60 it nearly equals the incidence rate in adolescents, primarily related to secondary metastatic tumours.

The most recent incidence statistics for bone cancer in Canada are from 2016 (https://www.cancer.ca/en/cancer-information/cancer-type/bone/statistics/?region=on). The Canadian Cancer Society estimated that 240 Canadians (145 men and 100 women) were diagnosed with bone cancer in 2016. It also estimated that 183 Canadians (108 men and 75 women) died of this disease in 2016.[271]

Patterns of Bone Destruction

The general pathological features of bone tumours include bone destruction, erosion or expansion of the cortex, and periosteal response to changes in underlying bone. The least amount of pathological damage occurs with benign bone tumours, which push against neighbouring tissue. Because they usually have a symmetric, controlled growth pattern, benign bone tumours tend to compress and displace neighbouring normal bone tissue, which weakens the bone's structure until it is incapable of withstanding the stress of ordinary use, leading to pathological fracture. Other tumours invade and destroy adjacent normal bone tissue by producing substances that promote resorption by increasing osteoclast activity or by interfering with a bone's blood supply. Three patterns of bone destruction by bone tumours exist: (1) the geographical pattern, (2) the moth-eaten pattern, and (3) the permeative pattern (Table 39.7).

Tumours that erode the cortex of the bone usually stimulate a periosteal response—that is, new bone formation at the interface between the surface of the bone and the periosteum. Slow erosion of the cortex usually stimulates a uniform periosteal response. Additional layers of bone are added to the exterior surface of the bone to buttress the cortex. Eventually, the additional layers expand the bone's contour. Aggressive penetration of the cortex, often seen with malignant tumours, usually elevates the periosteum and stimulates erratic patterns of new bone formation. Examples of erratic patterns include concentric layers of new bone; a sunburst pattern, in which delicate rays of new bone radiate toward the periosteum from a single focus on the underlying surface; and rays of new bone that grow perpendicularly, creating a brush or bristle pattern.

EVALUATION A malignant bone tumour must be identified early to allow survival of the individual and preservation of the affected limb. However, individuals often have only vague symptoms that may be attributed to minor trauma, degenerative changes, or inflammatory conditions. In addition, other conditions may obscure the diagnosis.

Thorough diagnostic studies are needed to determine the exact type and extent of bone tumour present, which also helps determine the optimal treatment regimen. Serum alkaline phosphatase levels are elevated in bone lytic tumours and significantly elevated in osteosarcoma. Radiological studies, including plain radiographic films,

TABLE 39.7 Patterns of Bone Destruction Caused by Bone Tumours

Type	Features
Geographical pattern	Least aggressive type
	Generally indicative of slow-growing or benign tumour
	Well-defined margins on tumour, easily separated from surrounding normal bone
	Uniform and well-defined lytic area in bone
	Margin smooth or irregular, demarcated by short zone of transition between normal and abnormal bone tissue
Moth-eaten pattern	Characteristic of rapidly growing, malignant bone tumours
	More aggressive pattern
	Tumour margin less defined or demarcated; cannot easily be separated from normal bone
	Areas of partially destroyed bone adjacent to completely lytic areas
Permeative pattern	Caused by aggressive malignant tumour with rapid growth potential
	Margins of tumour poorly demarcated
	Abnormal bone merges imperceptibly with normal bone

TABLE 39.8 Surgical Staging System for Bone Tumours of Mesenchymal Origin

Stage	Grade	Site (T)	Metastasis (M)
IA	Low (G_1)	Intracompartmental (T_1)	None (M_0)
IB	Low (G_1)	Extracompartmental (T_2)	None (M_0)
IIA	High (G_2)	Intracompartmental (T_1)	None (M_0)
IIB	High (G_2)	Extracompartmental (T_2)	None (M_0)
IIIA	Low (G_1)	Intracompartmental or extracompartmental (T_1 or T_2)	Regional or distant (M_1)
IIIB	High (G_2)	Intracompartmental or extracompartmental (T_1 or T_2)	Regional or distant (M_1)

Data from Jawad, M. U., & Scully, S. P. (2010). In brief: classifications in brief: Mirels' classification: Metastatic disease in long bones and impending pathologic fracture. *Clinical Orthopaedics and Related Research, 468*(7), 2000–2002; Simon, S. R. (Ed.). (1994). *Orthopaedic basic science.* American Academy of Orthopaedic Surgeons.

radionucleotide bone scans, CT scan, MRI, and PET combined with CT (PET/CT), are used to evaluate bone lesions. MRI and PET/CT have become the examination of choice for the local staging of bone tumours, especially the staging of peripheral osteosarcomas (Table 39.8). MRI and PET/CT are used to monitor the response of osteosarcomas to radiation or chemotherapy and to detect recurrent disease. A PET/CT, particularly when augmented by injection of the radioisotope FDG, provides earlier, more detailed information on tumour location, differentiation, metastases, and response to therapy than other imaging modalities.[272] (Chapter 10 discusses tumour staging.)

Additional diagnostic studies for specific bone tumours include a complete blood count and ESR (to rule out infection or myeloma) and measurement of serum levels of calcium and phosphorus to detect hypercalcemia. Serum glucose levels may be elevated in chondrosarcoma. Bone-specific alkaline phosphatase is elevated when there is bone metastasis.[273] Acid phosphatase level may be moderately elevated in bone metastases, multiple myeloma, and advanced Paget's disease. Serum protein electrophoresis and immunoelectrophoresis exclude other diseases. To determine the exact tumour type, core needle biopsy is usually done at the time of surgery.[274]

Types

A large number of lesions are classified as bone tumours. Bone tumours are typically classified according to their origin—osteogenic, chondrogenic, collagenic, and myelogenic tumours. They are described in the following sections (Figure 39.27).

Osteogenic tumours: osteosarcoma. The formation of bone or osteoid tissue with a sarcomatous tissue characterize **osteogenic (bone-forming) tumours**. The tissue can have the appearance of callus or compact or spongy bone. The most common malignant bone-forming tumour is the **osteosarcoma**.

The incidence of osteosarcomas peaks around the second decade, with a slight preference for males.[275,276] Sixty percent of osteosarcomas occur in persons younger than 20 years. A secondary peak incidence for osteosarcoma occurs in the 50- to 60-year age group, primarily in individuals with a history of radiation therapy several years previously for pelvic or other malignancies or for Paget's disease of bone.[277,278] Though considered a bone-forming tumour because of formation of immature osteoid that shows a "lacelike" pattern of bone growth, the radiological appearance of sarcoma is quite variable and often shows a moth-eaten (lytic) pattern of destruction with the tumour extending into the adjacent soft tissue.[279] Occasionally, the tumour may spread to nonadjacent bone or across a joint with normal-appearing areas of bone between tumours (i.e., "skip lesions"). Radionuclide bone scans are used to find skip lesions. MRI and PET/CT are useful in determining bony changes associated with the tumour.

The borders of the tumour are indistinct and merge into adjacent normal bone. Osteosarcomas contain osteoid produced by anaplastic stromal cells, which are atypical, abnormal cells not seen in normal developing bone; they are neither normal nor embryonal. Many

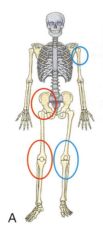
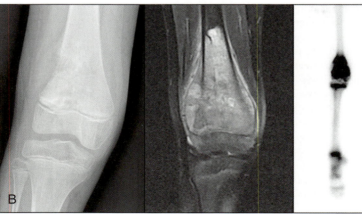
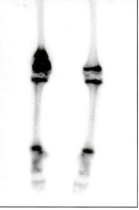

FIGURE 39.27 Osteosarcoma. **A,** Common locations of Ewing sarcoma and osteosarcoma. *Blue,* osteosarcoma; *red,* Ewing sarcoma. **B,** Comparison of plain radiograph, MRI, and nuclear bone scan appearances of osteosarcoma of the distal femur. Note destruction of the bone cortex and soft tissue component. ([A] adapted from Bontrager, K. L., & Lampugnano, J. P. [Eds.]. [2013]. *Textbook of radiographic positioning and related anatomy.* Elsevier. [B] Reprinted with permission from HaDuong, J.H., Martin, A.A., Skapek, S.X., & Mascarenhas, L. [2015]. Sarcomas. *Pediatric Clinics of North America, 62,* 179–200.)

tumours are heterogeneous; for example, the osteosarcoma also may contain chondroid (cartilage) and fibrinoid tissue that may form the bulk of the tumour. The osteoid is deposited as thick masses or "streamers," which infiltrate the normal compact bone, destroy it, and replace it with masses of osteoid. Bone tissue produced by osteosarcomas never matures to compact bone.

Ninety percent of osteosarcomas are located in the metaphyses of long bones, especially the distal femoral metaphysis, with 50% around the knee area. The tumour typically impregnates the cortex, lifts the periosteum, and forms a soft tissue mass that is not covered by a smooth shell of new bone. Lifting of the periosteum stimulates bizarre patterns of new bone formation called a *periosteal reaction*. Distinct osteosarcomas occur on the surface of long bones, called parosteal, periosteal, and high-grade surface osteosarcomas; dedifferentiated parosteal and central osteosarcomas also occur.

The most common initial symptoms are pain and an enlarging mass.[280] Initially, the pain is slight and intermittent, but within a short time the pain increases in severity and duration. Pain is usually worse at night and gradually requires medication. Systemic symptoms are uncommon. Often, a coincidental history of trauma is noted. Occasionally, the individual may present with a pathological fracture.

Bone biopsy is critical to diagnosis. Because the most frequent site of metastasis is the lung, a chest CT or MRI of the thorax also should be performed. There are no specific laboratory tests that aid in diagnosing sarcoma, but laboratory studies are helpful in assessing overall health before beginning treatment. Once osteosarcoma has been diagnosed, measuring serum alkaline phosphatase and LDH levels can be useful in following response to treatment. The best clinical outcomes occur in those who receive both preoperative and postoperative chemotherapy in addition to surgery.[281,282] Surgery is directed at salvaging the affected limb.[276,280]

Surgery is the major treatment of choice, with the tumour's location and size, the extent of malignancy, and evidence of metastasis dictating the type and extent of surgery (see Table 39.8). Preoperative chemotherapy has greatly increased the number of individuals qualifying for limb salvage surgery. Limb-salvaging procedures have been made possible by advances in reconstructive techniques and endoprosthetics. If an amputation is done, individuals are monitored closely with chest radiographs and CT. Pulmonary metastases are surgically resected, and chemotherapy is now a common therapy given both before and after surgery, using combinations of chemotherapeutic agents. Despite advances in chemotherapy and surgical techniques, overall long-term survival in osteosarcoma with metastases has not significantly improved in the past 30 to 40 years. Osteosarcomas are very difficult to treat with current chemotherapeutic agents.[283,284]

Other sarcomas include **Ewing sarcoma** (consisting of malignant small round blue cells that originate in the bone, surround soft tissue, and affect mainly children and adolescents) and **synovial sarcoma** (originating in the joints), each of which demonstrates specific genetic alterations.[285,286] Others include **rhabdomyosarcoma** (a soft tissue sarcoma that likely originates in the skeleton but with features more like skeletal muscle) and sarcomas that have no definite morphological pattern, such as **leiomyosarcoma** (a soft tissue sarcoma) and **pleomorphic liposarcoma** (a rare and aggressive cancer that affects mainly fat cells in many different sizes and shapes within the same tumour).

Chondrogenic tumours: chondrosarcoma. **Chondrogenic (cartilage-forming) tumours** produce cartilage or chondroid, a primitive cartilage or cartilagelike substance. The most common chondrogenic tumour is chondrosarcoma.

Chondrosarcoma is the second most common primary malignant bone tumour[287] and is a tumour of middle-aged and older adults. Chondrosarcomas that develop from a pre-existing benign bone lesion (such as an enchondroma) are known as secondary chondrosarcomas. Individuals with certain conditions, such as multiple osteochondromas, may be at greater risk of developing secondary chondrosarcoma. Secondary chondrosarcomas are rare, occurring most often in young adults between 20 and 30 years of age. The tumour is more common in men than in women.

A chondrosarcoma is a large, cartilage-producing, ill-defined malignant tumour that infiltrates trabeculae in spongy bone. It occurs most often in the metaphysis or diaphysis of long bones, especially the femur or proximal humerus, and in the bones of the pelvis.[288] If located near the end of the bone, the tumour will infiltrate into the joint space. The tumour expands and enlarges the contour of the bone, causes extensive erosion of the cortex, and grows into the soft tissues.

Symptoms associated with a chondrosarcoma have an insidious onset. Local swelling and pain are the usual presenting symptoms. At first the pain is dull and intermittent, then gradually intensifies and becomes constant; it may awaken the person at night.

Diagnostic studies include radiographs, which must be reviewed carefully for an accurate diagnosis. MRI is useful in determining the extent of soft tissue involvement.[289,290] Biopsy is done at the time of surgery. (If biopsy is conducted before scheduled surgical incision, seeding of tumour cells could occur.) Sufficient tumour material must be obtained to facilitate an accurate diagnosis.

Surgical excision is generally regarded as the treatment of choice because chemotherapy is generally ineffective.[287] Tumours more centrally located (in the appendicular skeleton) are more likely to metastasize. Consequently, individuals with tumours located in the limbs may have a better prognosis than those with pelvic lesions. Recent advances in understanding the pathophysiology of bone sarcomas have led to development of targeted therapies that show promise for improving outcomes.[291,292]

Collagenic tumours: fibrosarcoma. **Collagenic (collagen-forming) tumours** originate from mesenchymal cells and produce fibrous connective tissue. Fibrosarcoma is the most common collagenic tumour and can affect bone or soft tissue.

Fibrosarcomas represent 4% of the primary malignant bone tumours, with a broad age distribution. They may occur at any age but are most common in adults between 30 and 50 years of age. The incidence is slightly greater in females. Fibrosarcoma also may be a secondary complication of radiation therapy, Paget's disease, and long-standing osteomyelitis.

Fibrosarcoma is a rare, malignant, solitary tumour that most often affects the metaphyseal region of the femur or tibia. The tumour is composed of a firm, fibrous mass of tissue that contains collagen, malignant fibroblasts, and occasional osteoclastlike giant cells. Secondary fibrosarcoma, which tends to have a worse prognosis, can occur after prior radiation to an area. The tumour begins in the marrow cavity of the bone and infiltrates the trabeculae. It demonstrates a permeative growth pattern, destroys the cortex, and extends into the soft tissue. Metastasis to the lung is common.

Symptoms associated with the tumour have an insidious onset, which delays diagnosis. Pain and swelling are the usual presenting symptoms and usually indicate that the tumour has infiltrated the cortex. Local tenderness, a palpable mass, and limitation of motion also may be present. A pathological fracture in the affected bone is often the reason for seeking medical help. Diagnostic studies include radiographs and MRI.

Radical surgery and amputation are the treatments of choice for fibrosarcoma. There is a high probability of metastases. Radiation therapy is generally considered ineffective treatment for this tumour. Promising investigations of MMP inhibitors and even injectable compounds may alter future treatment of fibrosarcoma.[293,294]

Giant cell tumour (myelogenic tumours). **Giant cell tumour (GCT)**, along with myeloma (see Chapter 21), are **myelogenic tumours**, ones that originate from various bone marrow cells. GCT is the sixth most common of the primary bone tumours, accounting for 4 to 5% of bone tumours. It is generally benign but can become malignant after radiation treatment. GCTs have a wide age distribution; however, they are rare in persons younger than 10 years of age or older than 70 years of age. Most GCTs are found in persons between 20 and 40 years of age. Unlike most other bone tumours, GCTs affect females more often than males.

The GCT is a solitary, circumscribed tumour that causes extensive bone resorption because of its osteoclastic origin and RANKL overexpression.[295] GCTs are typically located in the epiphyseal regions of the femur, tibia, radius, or humerus.[296] The tumour has a slow, relentless growth rate and is usually contained within the original contour of the affected bone. It may, however, extend into the articular cartilage. When the tumour extends, it is usually covered by periosteum or periosteal bone growth; it may extend into surrounding soft tissue. GCTs have a low rate of metastasis to other organs or tissues, although they have a high rate of recurrence.

The most common symptoms associated with GCT are pain, local swelling, and limitation of movement. Diagnostic studies include radiographs, CT, and MRI. Cryosurgery and resection of the tumour with the use of adjuvant polymethylmethacrylate for bone grafts decrease recurrence and are more successful treatments than curettage and radiation.[295] The monoclonal antibody denosumab has been approved for treating GCTs in cases of recurrence or where surgery is not feasible.[297,298] Depending on the extent of the tumour and its recurrence, amputation may be necessary.

Muscle Tumours

Rhabdomyoma

Rhabdomyoma is an extremely rare benign tumour of muscle that generally occurs in the tongue, neck muscles, larynx, uvula, nasal cavity, axilla, vulva, and heart. These tumours are usually treated by surgical excision and typically do not recur.

Rhabdomyosarcoma

About 3 to 5% of childhood cancers are malignant tumours of striated muscle called *rhabdomyosarcoma*. Infants, children, and teenagers account for more than 85% of cases; there is a slight preference for males. This tumour is highly malignant with rapid metastasis. Rhabdomyosarcomas are located in the muscle tissue of the head, neck, and genito-urinary tract in 75% of cases, with the remainder found in the trunk and extremities. Recent animal studies have established a link between chemical, biological, and physical triggers of rhabdomyosarcoma.[299] Recent advances in treatment have improved the 5-year survival for children to greater than 80% in cases of localized tumours.[300] Unfortunately, survival in adults remains poor.

Three specific types of rhabdomyosarcoma can be determined on pathological section: anaplastic (formerly known as *pleomorphic*), embryonal, and alveolar. Each type differs from the other molecularly; they are all aggressive tumours and are typically more resistant to therapy. Although rare, the anaplastic, or spindle cell, type is considered to be one of the most highly malignant tumours of the extremities seen in adulthood. Microscopically, embryonal tumours resemble a tadpole or tennis racquet and are most often seen in infancy and childhood. Alveolar-type tumours appear latticelike, similar to lung tissue alveoli, and are more often found in adolescents and adults.

The diagnosis of rhabdomyosarcoma is made by careful incisional biopsy or core needle aspiration and examination of the specimen by a pathologist. CT scan also helps define the tissue borders. PET/CT is useful in identifying involvement of bones, lymph nodes, and bone marrow. Staging is based on the tumour's size, location, presence of metastases, and lymph node involvement. Pathological grading of the tumour is helpful in determining prognosis and treatment. Treatment consists of a combination of surgical excision, systemic chemotherapy, and radiation therapy. Cure is unlikely when distant metastases are present.

Other Tumours

Metastatic tumours in muscles are rare despite the extensive vascular supply of skeletal muscles. It is suggested that local pH or metabolic changes within muscles prevent metastatic involvement from other tumours. When adjacent carcinomas do cause muscle damage, it is usually related to the compression of tissue and resultant muscle atrophy.

CASE STUDY

Fractures from a Fall

Mrs. Johnson, an 82-year-old woman with osteoarthritis and osteoporosis, is admitted to the hospital for a recent fall at home while she was going down stairs, during which she sustained an open fracture to the greater trochanter of her right hip and her right humerus. She complained of persistent right ankle pain which confirmed an additional tibia and fibula fracture on X-ray. She has a previous history of falls (she has OA and osteoporosis), having injured the same hip 2 years ago. Her medical history also includes a diagnosis of hypertension with heart failure and type 2 diabetes. Her BMI is 30. She is on a diuretic and an ACE inhibitor for her hypertension and heart failure, and her diabetes is managed well with metformin 500 mg twice a day. Her recent BMD is very low.

Critical Thinking and Clinical Judgement Questions

1. What risk factors contributed to Mrs. Johnson's fractured hip and why?
2. Mrs. Johnson is worried about what she should be taking to treat her arthritis. a) How is her arthritis different from inflammatory arthritis varieties such as gout and RA? b) What should the nurse tell her?

3. a) What are the differences between her fractures? b) How might each of them heal differently?
4. What are some complications that Mrs. Johnson might experience as a result of her injuries and how might they present?
5. Mrs. Johnson would benefit from more screening and follow-up post-discharge. What sort of follow-up and screening would be of most benefit for Mrs. Johnson?

DID YOU UNDERSTAND?

Musculoskeletal Injuries

1. The most serious musculoskeletal injury is a fracture. A bone can be completely or incompletely fractured. A closed fracture leaves the skin intact. An open fracture has an overlying skin wound. The direction of the fracture line can be linear, oblique, spiral, or transverse. Greenstick, torus, and bowing fractures are examples of incomplete fractures that occur in children. Stress fractures occur in normal or abnormal bone that is subjected to repeated stress. Fatigue fractures occur in normal bone subjected to abnormal stress. Normal weight-bearing can cause an insufficiency (or fragility) fracture in abnormal bone.
2. Dislocation is complete loss of contact between the articular surfaces of two bones. Subluxation is partial loss of joint contact between two bones. As a bone separates from a joint, it may damage adjacent nerves, blood vessels, ligaments, tendons, and muscle.
3. Tendon tears are called *strains*, and ligament tears are called *sprains*. A complete separation of a tendon or ligament from its attachment is called an *avulsion*.
4. Rhabdomyolysis, often manifested by the presence of myoglobinuria, can be a life-threatening complication of severe muscle trauma, genetic predisposition, or toxic effects of certain medications.

Disorders of Bones

1. Metabolic bone diseases are characterized by abnormal bone structure. In osteoporosis, the density or mass of bone is reduced because the bone remodelling cycle is disrupted. Osteomalacia is a metabolic bone disease characterized by inadequate bone mineralization. Excessive and abnormal bone remodelling occurs in Paget's disease.
2. Osteomyelitis is a bone infection *most often* caused by bacteria. Bacteria can enter bone from outside the body (exogenous osteomyelitis) or from infection sites within the body (hematogenous osteomyelitis).

Disorders of Joints

1. Because of improved imaging technology, inflammation has been identified as an important feature of osteoarthritis (OA).
2. OA is a common age-related disorder of synovial joints. The primary defect in OA is loss of articular cartilage.
3. Rheumatoid arthritis (RA) is an inflammatory joint disease characterized by inflammatory destruction of the synovial membrane, articular cartilage, joint capsule, and surrounding ligaments and tendons. Rheumatoid nodules also may invade the skin, lung, and spleen and involve small and large arteries. RA is a systemic disease that affects the heart, lungs, kidneys, and skin, as well as the joints.
4. Ankylosing spondylitis is a chronic, systemic autoimmune disease characterized by stiffening and fusion of the sacroiliac and spine joints.
5. Gout is a syndrome caused by defects in uric acid metabolism with high levels of uric acid in the blood and body fluids. Uric acid crystallizes in the connective tissue of a joint, where it initiates inflammatory destruction of the joint.

Disorders of Skeletal Muscle

1. A pathological contracture is permanent muscle shortening caused by muscle spasticity, as seen in central nervous system injury or severe muscle weakness.
2. Stress-induced muscle tension is presumably caused by increased activity in the reticular activating system and gamma loop in the muscle fibre. The use of progressive relaxation training and biofeedback has been advocated to reduce muscle tension.
3. Fibromyalgia (FM) is a chronic musculoskeletal syndrome characterized by diffuse pain and tender points. Theories have proposed that the muscle is the end organ responsible for the pain and fatigue, although they have not been confirmed. Most cases of FM involve women, and the peak age of onset is 30 to 50 years of age. Genetic factors are being increasingly recognized as agents in developing FM.
4. Atrophy of muscle fibres and overall diminished size of the muscle are seen after prolonged inactivity. Isometric contractions and passive lengthening exercises decrease atrophy to some degree in immobilized persons.
5. Because of ion channel disorders, hyperexcitable membranes cause the physical and electrical phenomenon of myotonia. The disorder is treated with medications that reduce muscle fibre excitability. The biochemical defect is related to changes in the muscle membrane and sarcoplasmic reticulum.
6. Metabolic muscle diseases are caused by endocrine disorders, glycogen storage diseases, enzyme deficiencies, and abnormal lipid function. The muscle depends on a complex system of carbohydrates and fats converted by enzymes to produce energy for the muscle cell. Abnormalities in these pathways can inhibit function or cause damage to the muscle fibre. These illnesses are rare, yet they account for significant functional abnormalities.
7. Viral, bacterial, and parasitic infections of muscles produce the characteristic clinical and pathological changes associated with inflammation. These infections are usually treatable and self-limiting.
8. Polymyositis (generalized muscle inflammation) and dermatomyositis (polymyositis accompanied by skin rash) are characterized by inflammation of connective tissue and muscle fibres and muscle fibre necrosis. Cell-mediated and humoral immune factors have been implicated. Treatment with immunosuppressive agents is effective in many cases.
9. The most common cause of toxic myopathy is alcohol abuse. It has been suggested that alcohol use affects muscle fibres both directly (by causing necrosis) and indirectly (by the concomitant nutritional deficiencies typically associated with excessive use of alcohol). Medication administration can also lead to toxic myopathy; a needle used during an injection, secondary infection, and alterations in the acidity and alkalinity of muscle fibres can mechanically damage muscle fibres.

Musculoskeletal Tumours

1. Bone tumours originate from bone cells, cartilage cells, fibrous tissue cells, or vascular marrow cells. Each cell produces a specific type

of ground substance that is used to classify the tumour as osteogenic (bone cell), chondrogenic (cartilage cell), collagenic (fibrous tissue cell), or myelogenic (vascular marrow cell). Malignant bone tumours are usually large, aggressively destroy surrounding bone, invade surrounding tissue, and initiate independent growth outside the site of origin. Benign bone tumours are generally less destructive, limit their growth to the anatomical confines of the bone, and have a well-demarcated border. Certain benign tumours can become malignant.

2. Sarcomas of muscle tissue are rare. Rhabdomyosarcoma has a uniformly poor prognosis, particularly in adults, because of an aggressive invasion and early, widespread dissemination. The usual treatment includes surgical excision, radiation therapy, and systemic chemotherapy.

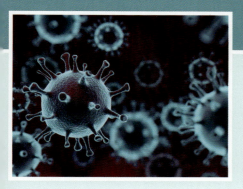

40

Developmental Alterations of Musculoskeletal Function

Stephanie Zettel, with originating chapter contributions by Kathryn L. McCance

Additional resources are available online at https://evolve.elsevier.com/Canada/Huether/pathophysiology.

CHAPTER OUTLINE

Congenital Defects, 1008
　Clubfoot, 1008
　Developmental Dysplasia of the Hip, 1008
　Osteogenesis Imperfecta, 1009
Bone Infection, 1010
　Osteomyelitis, 1010
　Septic Arthritis, 1010
Juvenile Idiopathic Arthritis, 1012
Osteochondroses, 1012
　Legg-Calvé-Perthes Disease, 1013
　Osgood-Schlatter Disease, 1014

Scoliosis, 1014
Muscular Dystrophy, 1015
　Duchenne Muscular Dystrophy, 1015
　Becker Muscular Dystrophy, 1016
　Facioscapulohumeral Muscular Dystrophy, 1017
　Myotonic Muscular Dystrophy, 1017
Musculoskeletal Tumours, 1017
　Benign Bone Tumours, 1017
　Malignant Bone Tumours, 1018
Nonaccidental Trauma, 1019
　Fractures in Nonaccidental Trauma, 1019

LEARNING OBJECTIVES

1. Describe the following congenital defects of the skeletal system: clubfoot, developmental dysplasia of the hip, and osteogenesis imperfecta.
2. Describe the pathogenesis of infection in osteomyelitis and septic arthritis.
3. Discuss the diagnostic features of juvenile rheumatoid arthritis.
4. Describe the two forms of osteochondrosis.
5. Describe the pathophysiology of Legg-Calvé-Perthes disease and Osgood-Schlatter disease.
6. List the three types of scoliosis and discuss the treatment of idiopathic scoliosis.
7. Identify the types of muscular dystrophy and their occurrence.
8. Describe the pathophysiology and manifestations of the muscular dystrophies.
9. Discuss the clinical manifestations and treatment of osteochondromas and nonossifying fibromas.
10. Describe the most common malignant bone tumours of childhood: osteosarcoma and Ewing sarcoma.
11. Describe the incidence and characteristic features of nonaccidental trauma in children.

KEY TERMS

Acetabular dysplasia, 1008
Acute hematogenous osteomyelitis, 1010
Becker muscular dystrophy (BMD), 1016
Clubfoot, 1008
Congenital equinovarus, 1008
Developmental dysplasia of the hip (DDH), 1008
Dislocated hip, 1008
Duchenne muscular dystrophy (DMD), 1015

Dystrophin, 1015
Ewing sarcoma, 1018
Facioscapulohumeral muscular dystrophy (FSHD), 1017
Hereditary multiple exostoses (HME), 1017
Involucrum, 1010
Juvenile idiopathic arthritis (JIA), 1012
Legg-Calvé-Perthes (LCP) disease, 1013

Malignant bone tumour, 1018
Muscular dystrophy, 1015
Myotonic muscular dystrophy (MMD), 1017
Nonossifying fibroma, 1018
Nonstructural scoliosis, 1014
Oligoarthritis, 1012
Osgood-Schlatter disease, 1014
Osteochondroma, 1017
Osteochondrosis, 1012

Osteogenesis imperfecta (OI; brittle bone disease), 1009
Osteomyelitis, 1010
Osteosarcoma, 1018
Polyarthritis, 1012
Scoliosis, 1014
Septic arthritis, 1010
Still disease, 1012
Structural scoliosis, 1014
Subluxated hip, 1008

Musculoskeletal problems in children are either congenital or acquired. Both pathology and treatment can cause long-term problems because of the growing nature of the immature skeleton. In addition, the emotional trauma of an injured or malformed child is substantial and dramatically affects the emotional health of both the child and their family.

CONGENITAL DEFECTS

> **QUICK CHECK 40.1**
> 1. Why is an early diagnosis of developmental dysplasia of the hip imperative?
> 2. How does osteomyelitis develop?
> 3. How has methicillin-resistant *Staphylococcus aureus* changed musculoskeletal infections in children?
> 4. How does juvenile idiopathic arthritis differ from the adult form?

Clubfoot

Clubfoot describes a range of foot deformities in which the foot turns inward and downward. It can affect one or both feet. Technically called **congenital equinovarus** (Table 40.1), the heel is positioned varus (inwardly deviated) and equinus (plantar flexed) (Figures 40.1 and 40.2). The clubfoot deformity can be positional (which can be easily corrected with passive movement), idiopathic, or teratological (i.e., as a result of another syndrome, such as spina bifida). The idiopathic clubfoot occurs in 1 per 1000 live births, with males twice as likely as females to be affected.

The clubfoot deformity can be corrected by an above-knee casting regimen popularized by Ponseti.[1] In almost 90% of idiopathic and up to 70% of teratological clubfeet, the Ponseti method of serial casting infants' feet is effective (Figure 40.1B). The hindfoot equinus portion of the deformity often requires lengthening of the Achilles tendon, which can be performed in a clinic with the use of a local anaesthetic. Achilles tenotomy (complete transection of the tendon) can be safely performed with local anaesthetic until 8 or 9 months after birth. After this age, a formal lengthening and repair procedure using a general anaesthetic is required. Bracing is required until age 3. Idiopathic feet resistant to these procedures require repeat casting or, in very rare cases, a surgical posteromedial release (PMR). The PMR includes lengthening of the Achilles, posterior tibialis, and flexor tendons, and surgical release of the capsules of the ankle, subtalar, and midfoot joints. Teratological clubfeet require surgical intervention more often than idiopathic clubfeet (see Figure 40.1B) and more prolonged bracing, often through childhood. The Ponseti technique has revolutionized clubfoot treatment around the world. The ability to correct such a crippling deformity without the need for surgery has helped countless children.[2]

Developmental Dysplasia of the Hip

Developmental dysplasia of the hip (DDH) describes imperfect development of the hip joint and can affect the femur, the acetabulum, or both (Figure 40.3). Dysplasia may develop later in the newborn or infant period, although it is most often present congenitally. Like clubfoot, DDH is either idiopathic or teratological. Teratological hips (i.e., those attributable to another disorder such as cerebral palsy, spina bifida, or arthrogryposis) are more difficult to treat and often need operative intervention. In idiopathic DDH, 70% of cases involve the left side only and 10 to 15% are bilateral. Girls are four times as likely as boys to be affected. Positive family history, breech presentation, and oligohydramnios (low levels of intrauterine fluid) all predispose children to DDH. Children in these groups are considered high risk and must be carefully evaluated with physical examination and ultrasound.[3,4] Variants of idiopathic DDH are **dislocated hip** (no contact between the femoral head and acetabulum), **subluxated hip** (partial contact only), and **acetabular dysplasia** (the femoral head is located properly but the acetabulum is shallow). Idiopathic instability of the hip ranges from 3 to 7 per 1000 live births, but a true dislocation is present in only 1 of 1000 live births.

Clinical examination is the mainstay of diagnosis and is best performed on an infant who is relaxed, for accuracy. Absolute indications for treatment include a positive Barlow sign (hip reduced, but dislocatable) (Figure 40.4A) or positive Ortolani sign (hip dislocated, but reducible) (Figure 40.4B). Other indicators for further evaluation are limitation of abduction[5] or apparent shortening of the femur (Galeazzi sign). Asymmetric skin folds at the groin also can be a clinical sign of hip pathology.

In children younger than 4 months, bracing with a Pavlik harness is successful in 90% of DDH cases. A Barlow-positive hip (hip reduced, but dislocatable) is easier to treat with a Pavlik harness, and success rates approach 95 to 98% (Figure 40.5). An Ortolani-positive hip (hip dislocated, but reducible) must be followed closely with ultrasound and examination; the success rate with Pavlik harness is 70%. If a stable reduction does not occur within 2 to 3 weeks of treatment, casting or surgery is the only option. A partially reduced hip applies pressure on the rim of the acetabulum by the femoral head and can worsen dysplasia, making treatment more difficult. Older children (6 to 12 months) or those who failed bracing with a Pavlik harness require closed reduction of the hip and spica (body) casting with a general anaesthetic. Children wear the spica cast for 3 months. Children older than 12 months require surgery on the joint, the femur, or the acetabulum, or

TABLE 40.1 Terms Used to Describe Foot Abnormalities

Term	Definition
Position[a]	
Abduction	Lateral deviation away from the midline of the body
Adduction	Lateral deviation toward the midline of the body
Eversion	Twisting of the foot outward along its long axis
Inversion	Twisting of the foot inward on its long axis
Dorsiflexion	Bending of the foot upward and backward
Plantar flexion	Bending of the foot downward and forward
Abnormality	
Talipes	Congenital abnormality of the foot (clubfoot)
Pes	Acquired deformity of the foot
Varus	Inversion and adduction of the heel and forefoot
Valgus	Eversion and abduction of the heel and forefoot
Equinus	Plantar flexion of the foot in which the heel is lower than the toes
Calcaneus	Dorsiflexion of the foot in which the heel is lower than the toes
Planus	Flattening of the medial longitudinal arch of the foot (flatfoot)
Cavus	Elevation of the medial longitudinal arch of the foot (high arch)
Equinovarus	Coexistent equinus and varus deformities
Calcaneovarus	Coexistent calcaneus and varus deformities
Equinovalgus	Coexistent equinus and valgus deformities
Calcaneovalgus	Coexistent calcaneus and valgus deformities

[a]The positions listed can all be achieved by voluntary movement of the normal foot; an abnormality exists if the foot is fixed in one or more of the positions while at rest.

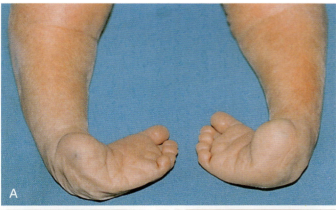
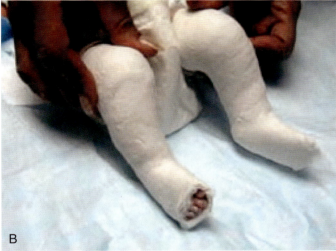

FIGURE 40.1 A, Infant with bilateral congenital talipes equinovarus. B, Ponseti casting. ([A], courtesy Dr. A. E. Chudley, Section of Genetics and Metabolism, Department of Pediatrics and Child Health, Children's Hospital and University of Manitoba, Winnipeg, Manitoba. In K. L. Moore, T. V. N. Persaud, & M. G. Torchia [Eds.]. [2016]. *The developing human* [10th ed.]. Saunders. [B], Reprinted with permission from Scher, D. M. (2005). The Ponseti method for clubfoot correction. *Operative Techniques in Orthopaedics, 15*(4), 345–349.)

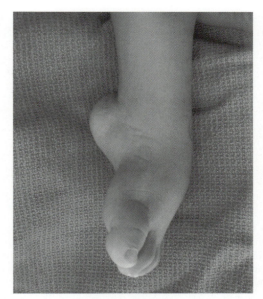

FIGURE 40.2 Idiopathic Clubfoot. Idiopathic clubfoot displaying forefoot adduction (toward midline of body) and supination (upturning) and hindfoot equinus (pointed downward). Note skin creases along arch and back of heel.

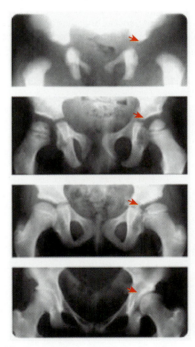

FIGURE 40.3 Hip Dysplasia in Children. Developmental dysplasia of the hip with residual acetabular dysplasia. Radiographs at birth and 3, 10, and 19 years of age (top to bottom) show persisting dysplasia.

all three (see Figure 40.3). The incidence of good or excellent outcome falls to only 20% by age 4, underscoring the need for early diagnosis and treatment.[6]

Osteogenesis Imperfecta

Osteogenesis imperfecta (OI; brittle bone disease) is a spectrum of disease caused by genetic mutation in the gene that encodes for type I collagen, the main component of bone and blood vessels. The Sillence classification defines six types:
- Types I and IV are milder forms and are inherited in an autosomal dominant pattern.
- Types II and III are more severe and are inherited in a recessive pattern.
- Types V and VI are very rare and are autosomal recessive.

Children with type II often die during infancy because of extreme bone fragility.

The classic clinical manifestations of OI are osteopenia (decreased bone mass) and an increased rate of fractures. Children can also have fatigue, pain, hearing loss, and abnormal dentition. With recurrent fractures, bone deformity (bowing) often occurs. In type III OI, the most severe form compatible with life, children have short stature and triangular faces, possibly blue sclerae, and poor dentition. Because type I collagen also is the main component of blood vessels, vascular deformity, such as aortic aneurysm, can occur. Type IV OI can be subtle, with the child presenting with more normal stature and with fractures often not occurring until the child is older; it can be misdiagnosed as child abuse. Analysis of skin fibroblasts is diagnostic in 85% of children with OI.

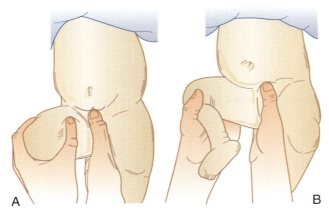

FIGURE 40.4 Congenital Dislocation of the Hip. **A**, Barlow manoeuvre *(left side)*. With one hand pressing the symphysis in front and the sacral spine in back, lateral pressure is applied to the thigh with the thumb of the other hand while pressure is applied with the palm to the knee on the side being examined. The hip that has been flexed to 90 degrees is then adducted. A positive sign is a sensation of abnormal movement, indicating dislocation of the femoral head from the acetabulum. The hands are reversed for examining the other hip. This sign and the Ortolani sign may be found only in the first weeks of life. **B**, Ortolani manoeuvre *(right side)*. Sign of jerking into correct position. After Barlow manoeuvre (A), the hip should be abducted to about 80 degrees while the femur is lifted anteriorly with the fingers along the thigh. A positive sign is a sensation of a jerk or snap with reduction into the joint socket. (Adapted from Specht, E. E. [1974]. Congenital dislocation of the hip. *American Family Physician, 9*, 88–96.)

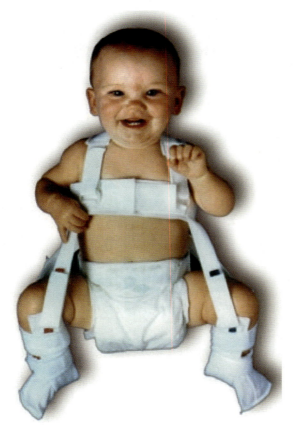

FIGURE 40.5 Pavlik Harness for Bilateral Hip Dislocation. (Wheaton Pavlik Harness. Courtesy Wheaton Brace Co., Carol Stream, IL.)

Treatment is a combination of medical and surgical approaches (Figure 40.6). For fractures and deformity, intramedullary rodding of the long bones improves position and also splints new fractures. Telescoping rods, which grow with the child, are improving in efficacy. Unfortunately, these children may have to undergo multiple surgeries and re-roddings with growth. The medical treatment, classically involving calcium and vitamin D supplementation, is under intense study. Pamidronate (Aredia) and other bisphosphates, such as alendronate (Fosamax), which decrease bone resorption by inhibiting osteoclasts, are now frequently used.

BONE INFECTION

Osteomyelitis

Osteomyelitis, or bone infection, is caused by either bacterial or granulomatous (e.g., tuberculosis) infective processes (Box 40.1, Figures 40.7 and 40.8). Antibiotic medications and often surgical interventions are used to treat these infections. Morbidity and mortality resulting from osteomyelitis declined drastically until the 1980s. Unfortunately, with the escalation of methicillin-resistant *Staphylococcus aureus* (MRSA) infections, serious increases in morbidity and mortality have developed.

Acute hematogenous osteomyelitis is the most common form in children. The infection usually begins as an abscess in the metaphysis of a long bone where blood flow is sluggish and bacteria can collect. With increasing pressure, the infection will rupture out of the periosteum and spread along the diaphysis of the bone. A new shell of bone can develop under the elevated periosteum. The portion of bone that is separated from adequate blood supply by the infection can die, thereby leading to an involucrum. All three of these changes are apparent on radiograph and signify the need for surgical debridement as well as antibiotic treatment.

These radiographic bone changes take 2 to 3 weeks to develop. Initially, osteomyelitis presents as pain, swelling, and warmth. Common signs and symptoms include fever, decreased appetite, fatigue, elevated white blood cell (WBC) count (50 to 70%), elevated C-reactive protein (CRP) (98%) level, and elevated erythrocyte sedimentation rate (ESR) (90%). Blood culture is positive in only 40 to 60% of cases. Without changes on plain radiograph, magnetic resonance imaging (MRI) can help define the location and extent of the infectious process. In infants, where osteomyelitis can be multifocal in up to 40% of cases, a bone scan identifies other locations of infection that may need surgical intervention.

Treatment of osteomyelitis consists of appropriate antibiotic management for 6 weeks. If blood cultures are negative, bone aspirate must be analyzed to determine the bacterial source of the infection. With MRSA or bone changes on MRI, surgical debridement is required. MRSA often leads to more systemic illness, such as endocarditis (infection of the heart valves), organ failure, and infected thrombotic events.[7]

Septic Arthritis

Septic arthritis is a bacterial or granulomatous infection of the joint space. This is always a surgical emergency. The bacteria, and the lysosomes created by WBCs fighting the bacteria, can quickly destroy the articular cartilage of the joint and affect the blood supply to the epiphyseal bone nearby. Both complications have poor outcomes and can lead to a lifetime of disability.

Septic arthritis can occur primary or secondary to osteomyelitis that spreads from the metaphysis of the bone into the joint space. The

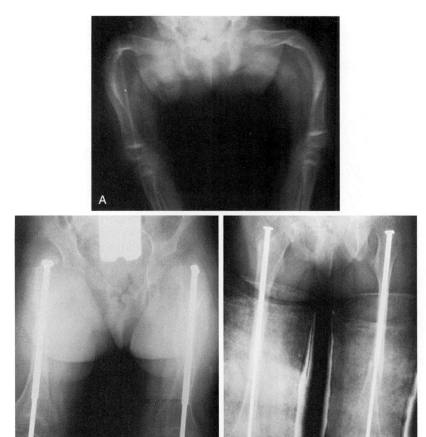

FIGURE 40.6 Osteogenesis imperfecta treated with osteotomies and *telescoping medullary rods*. **A**, Severe deformity of both femurs. **B**, Same individual after multiple osteotomies with telescoping medullary rod fixation. **C**, Same individual 4 years later demonstrating growth of femurs, no recurrence of deformity, and elongation of rods. (Plaster casts are in place for immobilization of tibial osteotomies.) (From Crenshaw, A. H. [Ed.]. [1992]. *Campbell's operative orthopaedics* [8th ed., vol. 3]. Mosby.)

BOX 40.1 Causative Microorganisms of Osteomyelitis According to Age

Newborns
Staphylococcus aureus (both methicillin-sensitive [MSSA] and methicillin-resistant [MRSA])
Group B streptococcus
Gram-negative enteric rods

Infants
S. aureus (MSSA and MRSA)
Haemophilus influenzae (decreasingly less common secondary to immunization)

Older Children
S. aureus (MSSA and MRSA)
Pseudomonas
Salmonella
Neisseria gonorrhoeae

Adolescents and Adults
Pseudomonas
Mycobacterium tuberculosis

---

metaphyses of the pediatric hip, shoulder, proximal radius, and distal lateral tibia are all located within the joint capsule, and therefore osteomyelitis in these regions must be carefully monitored for secondary septic arthritis. The most common sites for septic arthritis are knees, hips, ankles, and elbows.

Children with septic arthritis present with severe joint pain, "pseudoparalysis" or marked guarding to motion of the joint, inability to bear weight, and malaise, often with anorexia. Children appear quite ill with this diagnosis. Nonpyogenic arthritis, such as juvenile idiopathic arthritis (JIA), can be difficult to distinguish clinically from septic arthritis because both can lead to malaise and elevated ESR. The Kocher criteria are often used to distinguish septic joints from joint pain of another cause. There is a greater than 90% chance of a septic joint if three of the five following criteria are met:[8,9]

1. WBC greater than 12 000 cells/μL.
2. Inability to bear weight on the joint.
3. Fever greater than 38.5°C (101.3°F).
4. ESR greater than 40 mm/hr.
5. CRP greater than 0.190 μmol/L.

Fever and CRP level greater than 0.190 μmol/L appear to have the most influence in the differential diagnosis.

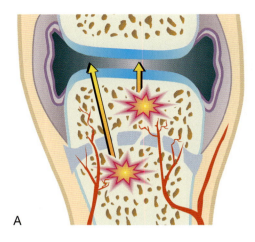

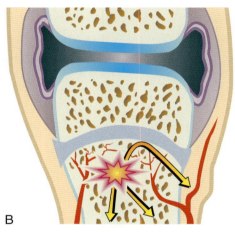

FIGURE 40.7 Pathogenesis of Acute Osteomyelitis Differs With Age. **A,** In infants younger than 1 year the epiphysis is nourished by arteries penetrating through the physis, allowing development of the condition within the epiphysis. **B,** In children up to 15 years of age, the infection is restricted to below the physis because of interruption of the vessels.

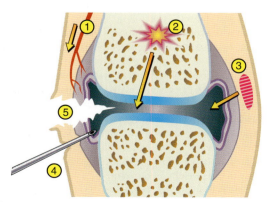

FIGURE 40.8 Routes of Infection to the Joint. (1) Hematogenous route. (2) Dissemination from osteomyelitis. (3) Spread from an adjacent soft tissue infection. (4) Diagnostic or therapeutic measures. (5) Penetrating damage by puncture or cutting.

Blood cultures are positive in 30 to 40% of cases. Joint aspirate that is positive for a WBC count of greater than 7000 per high-power field defines the diagnosis, and culture of this fluid often determines bacterial etiology. As in osteomyelitis, S. aureus is the most common bacteria; however, MRSA is now present in up to 30% of affected children.[7,10]

After surgical debridement of the joint, antibiotics are required for 2 to 3 weeks. Long-term follow-up to assess articular or physeal damage is required.

JUVENILE IDIOPATHIC ARTHRITIS

Juvenile idiopathic arthritis (JIA) is the childhood form of rheumatoid arthritis (see Chapter 39) and accounts for 5% of all cases of rheumatoid arthritis. JIA has three distinct modes of onset: oligoarthritis (fewer than three joints), polyarthritis (more than three joints), and Still disease (severe systemic onset) (Table 40.2). JIA differs from rheumatoid arthritis in several ways:

- Large joints are most commonly affected.
- Chronic uveitis (inflammation of the anterior chamber of the eye) is common if the blood test for antinuclear antibody (ANA) is positive; slit lamp examination by a trained ophthalmologist is required every 6 months to avoid vision loss.
- Serum tests may be negative for rheumatoid factor (RF); RF-positive children have a worse prognosis.
- Subluxation and ankylosis may occur in the cervical spine if disease progresses.
- Rheumatoid arthritis that continues through adolescence can have severe effects on growth and adult morbidity.

Many children with oligoarthritis who are "seronegative" (blood tests negative for RF or ANA) will resolve their symptoms over time. Systemic onset, or "seropositivity," of the disease is more likely consistent with lifelong arthritis. Therefore, treatment is supportive, not curative. Nonsteroidal anti-inflammatory drugs are a mainstay of treatment, and methotrexate (Apo-Methotrexate) is also being used with success. The goals are to minimize inflammation and deformity.

OSTEOCHONDROSES

> ✓ **QUICK CHECK 40.2**
> 1. What is the pathophysiology of osteochondrosis?
> 2. What is the cause of Duchenne muscular dystrophy (DMD)?
> 3. Discuss the clinical manifestations of DMD.
> 4. Which dystrophy is really a systemic disease?
> 5. What is the difference between Becker and Duchenne muscular dystrophies?

The osteochondroses are a series of childhood diseases involving areas of significant tensile or compressive stress (e.g., tibial tubercle, Achilles insertion, hip epiphysis). The pathophysiology is partial loss of blood supply, death of bone (osseous necrosis), progressive bony weakness, and then microfracture. The cause of the decreased blood supply is controversial; trauma, a change in clotting sensitivity, vascular injury, genetic predisposition, or a combination of these factors is presently considered most likely. Additionally, during the years of rapid bone growth, blood supply to the growing ends of bones (epiphyses) may become insufficient, resulting in necrotic bone, usually near joints. Because bone is normally undergoing a continuous rebuilding process, the necrotic areas can self-repair over a period of weeks or months.

Use of anti-inflammatory medications, modification of activities, immobilization, and rest are recommended during active stages of the

TABLE 40.2 Characteristics of Juvenile Idiopathic Arthritis Related to Mode of Onset

	Systemic Onset	Pauciarticular (Two or Three Subtypes)	Polyarticular (Two Subtypes)
Percentage of patients	30	45	25
Age at onset	Bimodal distribution 1–3 years of age 8–10 years of age	Type I: younger than 10 years Type II: older than 10 years	Throughout childhood and adolescence
Gender ratio (female/male)	1.5 : 1	Type I: almost all female Type II: 1 : 9	Mostly female
Joints involved	Any Only 20% have joint involvement at time of diagnosis	Usually confined to lower extremities—knee, ankle, and eventually sacroiliac; sometimes elbow	Any joint; usually symmetric involvement of small joints Hip involvement in 50% Spine involvement in 50%
Extra-articular manifestations	Fever, malaise, myalgia, rash, pleuritis or pericarditis, adenomegaly, splenomegaly, hepatomegaly Systemic signs minimal	Type I: chronic iridocyclitis; mucocutaneous lesions Type II: acute iridocyclitis; sacroiliitis common; eventual ankylosing spondylitis in many	Possible low-grade fever, malaise, weight loss, rheumatoid nodules, or vasculitis
Laboratory test results	Elevated ESR, CRP levels; RF negative; ANA rarely positive; anemia; leukocytosis	Elevated ESR, CRP levels; ANA positive Type I: HLA-DRW5 positive Type II: HLA-B27 positive Type III: HLA-TMo positive	Elevated ESR, CRP levels Type I: RF positive Type II: RF negative
Long-term prognosis	Mortality: 1–2% of all JIA patients Joint destruction in 40%	Continuous disease; eventual remission in 60% Type I: ocular damage; functional blindness in 10% Type II: ankylosing spondylitis Type III: best outlook for recovery	Longer duration; more crippling; remission in 25% Type I: high incidence of crippling arthritis Type II: outlook good

ANA, Antinuclear antibody; *CRP*, C-reactive protein; *ESR*, erythrocyte sedimentation rate; *HLA*, human leukocyte antigen; *JIA*, juvenile idiopathic arthritis; *RF*, rheumatoid factor.
From Hockenberry, M. J., & Wilson, D. (2015). *Wong's nursing care of infants and children* (11th ed.). Mosby.

disease. Reparative correction by revascularization is the rule, although years may be required for full healing, and deformity from compression during the period of osseous necrosis can persist.

Legg-Calvé-Perthes Disease

Legg-Calvé-Perthes (LCP) disease is a common osteochondrosis usually occurring in children between the ages of 3 and 10 years, with a peak incidence at 6 years. The disorder is bilateral in 10 to 20% of children, and boys are affected five times more often than girls. Boys have a more poorly developed blood supply to the femoral head than do girls of the same age, and this is thought to be the reason for male predilection. The role of genetics is unclear, but LCP disease is more common in northern European and Japanese children and rare in Black children; family history is positive in 20% of cases. This self-limited disease of the hip, which runs its natural course in 2 to 5 years, is presumably created by recurrent interruption of the blood supply to the femoral head. The ossification centre first becomes necrotic (osteonecrosis) and then is gradually replaced by live bone.

PATHOPHYSIOLOGY There are several causative theories, including a generalized disorder of epiphyseal cartilage growth, thyroid hormone deficiency, trauma, infection, and blood clotting disorders. Boys with a hypercoagulable state are three times more likely to acquire LCP disease than girls with the same disorder.[11] Another study suggests the risk for LCP disease is greater in children who are obese, have a history of metabolic diseases, and who are hypothyroid.[12] Increased risk positively correlates with smoke from indoor use of a wood stove.[13]

In the first stage of LCP disease, the soft tissues of the hip (synovial membrane and joint capsule) are swollen, edematous, and hyperemic, often with fluid present in the joint (Figure 40.9). In the second necrotic stage, the anterior 50% or more of the epiphysis of the femoral head dies because of a lack of blood supply, and the metaphyseal bone at the junction of the femoral neck and capital epiphyseal plate is softened because of increased blood supply and decalcification. Granulation tissue (procallus) and blood vessels then invade the dead bone. The third, or regenerative healing, stage ordinarily lasts 2 to 4 years. The dead bone in the femoral head is replaced by procallus, and new bone is established (see Figure 40.9). In the fourth, or residual, stage, remodelling takes place, and the newly formed bone is organized into a live spongy bone.

CLINICAL MANIFESTATIONS Injury or trauma precedes the onset of LCP disease in approximately 30 to 50% of children with LCP disease. For several months, the child complains of a limp and pain that can be referred to the knee, inner thigh, and groin, following the path of the obturator nerve. The pain is usually aggravated by activity and relieved by rest and administration of anti-inflammatory medications.

The typical physical findings include spasm on rotation of the hip, limitation of internal rotation and abduction, and hip flexion–adduction deformity. A child may have an early abnormal "Trendelenburg gait", where they have defective hip abductor function, and the weakness of the gluteus medius muscle causes a drooping of the pelvis to the contralateral side while walking. If the hip pain or limp has been present for a prolonged period, muscles of the hip and thigh atrophy.

EVALUATION AND TREATMENT The goals of treatment are to preserve normal congruity of the femoral head and acetabulum and maintain spasm-free and pain-free range of motion in the hip joint. Currently, most children can be managed with anti-inflammatory medications and activity modification during periods of synovitis. Serial radiographs monitor the progress of the disease and ensure that the femoral head remains congruent in the acetabulum. Surgery

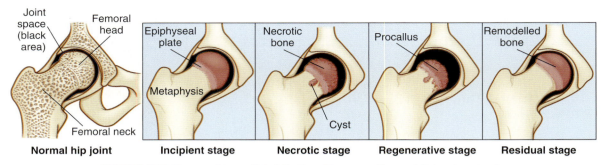

FIGURE 40.9 Stages of Legg-Calvé-Perthes Disease, a Form of Osteochondrosis.

may be necessary if the femoral head becomes subluxated or incongruent with the acetabulum (Figure 40.10).[14–16] Children older than age 6 (by bone age) have a worse prognosis attributable to poorer remodelling potential. Older children require surgery more often to avoid poor congruence of the hip. Poor congruence predisposes to early osteoarthritis, with nearly 50% requiring hip replacement surgery by age 40.

Osgood-Schlatter Disease

Osgood-Schlatter disease consists of osteochondrosis of the tibia tubercle and associated patellar tendonitis. Osgood-Schlatter disease occurs most often in preadolescents and adolescents who participate in sports and is more prevalent in boys than in girls. Osgood-Schlatter disease is one of the most common ailments reported in the 30 million children who are involved in sports.[17]

The severity of the lesion varies from mild tendonitis to a complete separation of the anterior tibial apophysis, a part of the tibial tubercle. The mildest form of Osgood-Schlatter disease causes ischemic (avascular) necrosis in the region of the bony tibial tubercle, with hypertrophic cartilage formation during the stages of repair. In more severe cases, the abnormality involves a true apophyseal separation of the tibial tubercle with avascular necrosis.

The child complains of pain and swelling in the region around the patellar tendon and tibial tubercle, which becomes prominent and is tender to direct pressure. The pain is most severe after physical activity that involves vigorous quadriceps contraction (jumping or running) or direct local trauma to the tibial tubercle area.

The goal of treatment for Osgood-Schlatter disease is to decrease the stress at the tubercle. Often a period of 4 to 8 weeks of restriction from strenuous physical activity, administration of anti-inflammatory medications, and stretching of the quadriceps muscle are sufficient. Bracing with a tubercle band can be very helpful. If the pain is not relieved, a cast or knee immobilizer is required, a situation that is particularly difficult if the condition is bilateral.

Gradual resumption of activity is permitted after 8 weeks but return to unrestricted athletic participation requires an additional 8 weeks to allow for revascularization, healing, and ossification of the tibial tubercle.[14,18] With skeletal maturity and closure of the apophysis, Osgood-Schlatter disease resolves.

Sever Disease

Sever disease is the "Osgood-Schlatter" of the calcaneus (heel bone). The insertion of the Achilles pulls on the cartilaginous apophysis of the calcaneus, causing pain. It is more common in athletic children and children who have underlying Achilles tendon tightness, for example, soccer players between the ages of 8 and 12. It is relieved by a heel lift in the shoe, rest, stretching, and anti-inflammatory medications.

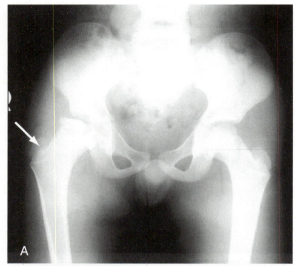
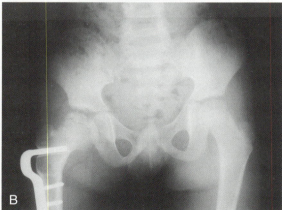

FIGURE 40.10 Pelvis of a 7-Year-Old Boy With Legg-Calvé-Perthes Disease. **A,** The femoral head is flat and extruded from the edge of the joint. This hip is at risk for early arthritis if left to revascularize and heal in this position. **B,** Surgical replacement of the femoral head. As the Perthes heals, the ball has assumed a round shape that matches the socket well.

SCOLIOSIS

Scoliosis is a rotational curvature of the spine most obvious in the anteroposterior plane (Figure 40.11). It is either nonstructural or structural. Nonstructural scoliosis results from a cause other than the spine itself, such as posture, leg length discrepancy, or splinting from pain. Structural scoliosis is a curvature of the spine associated with

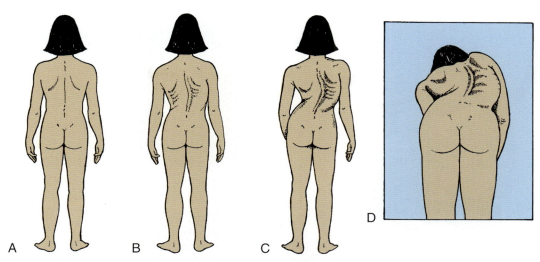

FIGURE 40.11 Scoliosis in Children. Normal spine alignment and abnormal spinal curvatures associated with scoliosis. **A**, Normal. **B**, Mild. **C**, Severe. **D**, Rotation and curvature of scoliosis.

TABLE 40.3 Major Muscular Dystrophy Syndromes

Disease	Mode of Inheritance	Age at Clinical Onset	Distribution of Weakness
Duchenne muscular dystrophy/Becker muscular dystrophy (DMD/BMD)	X-linked, sporadic	2–3 years/5–7 years	Proximal with pseudohypertrophy
Facioscapulohumeral muscular dystrophy (FSHD)	Autosomal dominant	Early adolescence	Face, arms, legs
Myotonic muscular dystrophy (MMD)	Autosomal dominant	Variable—birth to adulthood	Distal muscles, face

From Moxley, R. T., 3rd., Ashwal, S., Pandya, S., et al. (2005). *Neurology, 64*(1), 13–20.

vertebral rotation. Nonstructural scoliosis can become structural if the underlying cause is not found and treated.

There are three main types of structural scoliosis: (1) idiopathic; (2) congenital (attributable to bony deformity such as hemivertebrae); and (3) teratological (caused by another systemic syndrome such as cerebral palsy). Eighty percent of all scoliosis is idiopathic, which may have a genetic component. Although girls and boys are equally affected, once the curve becomes more than 20 degrees, girls are five times more likely to be affected. Ninety-eight percent of curves are apex right thoracic. If a left thoracic curve appears in the adolescent with idiopathic scoliosis, MRI rules out a neurological cause. MRI should be performed in scoliotic children with loss of abdominal reflexes and those who have exertional headaches or a congenital curve.[18,19]

Idiopathic curves progress while a child is growing, and progression can be very rapid during growth spurts. When idiopathic curves progress to 25 degrees or greater, and the child is skeletally immature, bracing is required. The total number of hours a brace is worn correlates to efficacy of treatment; 82% of children who wore the brace as prescribed had minimal progression.[20] In braced curves, 72% required no surgery compared with only 48% of those who wore no brace.[21]

Curves of more than 50 degrees will progress after skeletal maturity, so spinal fusion is required to stop progression. Bracing is the only non-operative measure known to slow scoliotic progression. Chiropractic manipulation, physical therapy, exercise, and diet regimens have not been shown to alter natural history. Bracing is less successful in teratological or congenital curves; therefore, these conditions may require surgical intervention more often.

MUSCULAR DYSTROPHY

The muscular dystrophies are a group of inherited disorders that cause progressive muscle fibre loss leading to weakness, mostly of the voluntary muscles. Some dystrophies cause disease in infancy, others in childhood, and others not until adulthood. Muscular dystrophies have different inheritance patterns and different biochemical alterations that cause each specific type. Three are discussed in detail in this chapter. Individuals with Duchenne muscular dystrophy (DMD) have a mutation in a specific gene that leads to alterations in the muscle protein dystrophin. Individuals with myotonic muscular dystrophy (MMD) have a genetic alteration that leads to systemic disease. Although there is no cure for any of the muscular dystrophies, aggressive preventive management has increased the life expectancy and quality of life of children with these disorders. Common forms of muscular dystrophy are described in Table 40.3.

Duchenne Muscular Dystrophy

PATHOPHYSIOLOGY Duchenne muscular dystrophy (DMD) is X-linked, generally occurring in boys, and is present in about 1 in 3 500 male births. It is the most common childhood dystrophy. DMD is caused by mutations in the dystrophin gene, which lead to alterations or deletions of the muscle protein dystrophin.

The protein dystrophin mediates anchorage of the actin cytoskeleton of skeletal muscle fibres to the basement membrane through a membrane–glycoprotein complex. With lack of dystrophin, the poorly anchored fibres tear themselves apart under the repeated stress of contraction. Free calcium then enters the muscle cells, causing cell death and fibre necrosis (Figure 40.12).

CLINICAL MANIFESTATIONS Boys with DMD will present in the preschool years with muscle weakness, difficulty walking, and large calves (pseudohypertrophy) caused by normal muscle fibre replacement with fat and connective tissue (Figure 40.12B–C). Although the calves are large, the muscle is actually weak. Clinical weakness starts in the pelvic girdle, initially causing difficulty rising from the floor (Gower sign) and

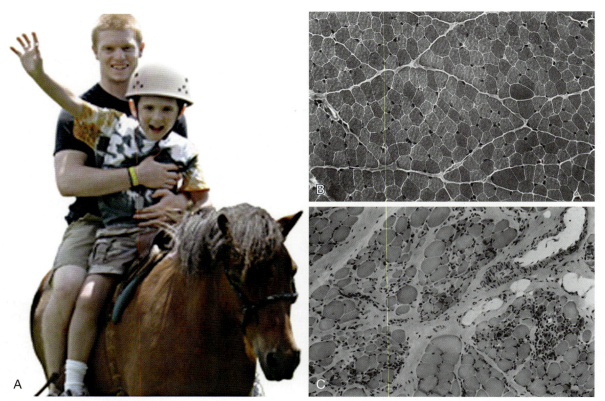

FIGURE 40.12 Duchenne Muscular Dystrophy. **A**, Young boy with Duchenne muscular dystrophy (DMD) on horseback. **B**, Transverse section of gastrocnemius muscle from a healthy boy. **C**, Transverse section of gastrocnemius muscle from a boy with DMD. Normal muscle fibre is replaced with fat and connective tissue. (From Jorde, L. B., Carey, J. C., & Bamshad, M. J. [2010]. *Medical genetics* [4th ed.]. Mosby.)

climbing stairs, and a waddling gait because of weakness in the lumbar and gluteal muscles. Boys with DMD often toe-walk because of weakness of the anterior tibial and peroneal muscles, causing the feet to assume a talipes equinovarus position. The weakness worsens over the subsequent few years, resulting in the loss of ability to ambulate by 8 to 13 years of age. Muscle weakness also leads to contractures of the knees, hips, and other joints, and scoliosis develops in most boys with DMD. Once scoliosis begins, it is relentlessly progressive. Curves of more than 20 degrees are treated surgically to maintain pulmonary function. Muscle weakness and inactivity, particularly once a person is in a wheelchair full time, lead to osteoporosis and pathological fractures. If fracture occurs, bisphosphonates may be used to strengthen bone, although long-term studies on safety have not been performed in this population.

As children age, muscle weakness progresses and respiratory weakness leads to breathing difficulty, particularly when sleeping. Susceptibility to respiratory tract infections and progressive deterioration of pulmonary function generally lead to premature death, usually in the 20s. Cardiomyopathy also may occur and, despite treatment, is generally progressive. Bowel and bladder functions are often mildly affected, with constipation and urinary urgency as frequent symptoms. Mild to moderate cognitive problems are common but not universal.

EVALUATION AND TREATMENT Diagnosis involves measuring the blood creatine kinase (CK) level, which can be 100 times the normal level, with confirmation by genetic testing for mutations in the dystrophin gene (however, a high CK level does not confirm the diagnosis, because many other alterations can also increase CK).

Management involves maintaining function for as long as possible. Treatment with steroids can prolong the ability to walk by several years and improves life expectancy.[22] Deflazacort (Alnacort) is a corticosteroid that is not easily accessible in Canada and has been approved for use in treating DMD in the United States.[23,24] It is a steroid that may have fewer side effects than prednisone (Deltasone). There is also promising new research into the use of gene therapy and delivering the *Wnt7a* gene to a susceptible individual with the goal of increasing growth of the muscles.[25] Treatment also involves range-of-motion exercises, bracing, and surgical release of contracture deformities and scoliosis when necessary. Children with DMD require a multidisciplinary approach to care, including attention to heart and breathing problems, weight loss/gain, constipation, rehabilitative/developmental problems, psychosocial needs, and neurological and orthopedic problems (Figure 40.13).

The care for individuals with DMD across Canada is multidisciplinary and includes corticosteroid treatment (which tends to prolong ambulation and preserve both cardiac and respiratory function) as well as routine calcium and vitamin D supplementation, and the use of night splints to prevent foot drop.[24] If appropriate, families should receive genetic counselling for recurrence risk and prenatal screening. Family support is necessary throughout the lifespan of the child because needs vary depending on the stage of the disease.

Becker Muscular Dystrophy

Although **Becker muscular dystrophy (BMD)** has been designated historically as a separate muscular dystrophy, it is actually caused by alterations of the same dystrophin gene (i.e., dystrophinopathies) and protein as seen in DMD. Children with BMD present later and have a longer life expectancy than those with DMD; however, they are part of the same clinical spectrum.

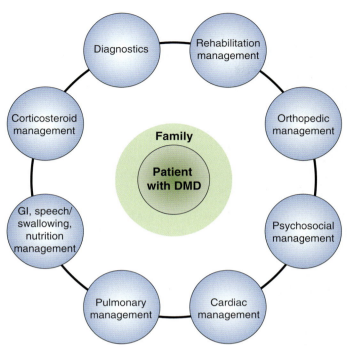

FIGURE 40.13 Multisystem Approach for Evaluation and Treatment of Duchenne Muscular Dystrophy. *GI*, Gastro-intestinal. (Adapted from Bushby, K., Finkel, R., Birnkrant, D. J., et al. [2010]. Diagnosis and management of Duchenne muscular dystrophy part 1: diagnosis and pharmacological and psychosocial management. *Lancet, 9*(1), 77–93; Bushby, K., Finkel, R., Birnkrant, D. J., et al. [2010]. Diagnosis and management of Duchenne muscular dystrophy part 2: implementation of multidisciplinary care. *Lancet, 9*(2), 177–189.)

Facioscapulohumeral Muscular Dystrophy

Facioscapulohumeral muscular dystrophy (FSHD), one of the most common muscular dystrophies, is inherited in an autosomal dominant fashion. It is more variable in presentation than DMD. FSHD is usually observed in *late* childhood. Progression is usually slow, and lifespan is normal or near normal. FSHD occurs because of a deletion on chromosome 4 that is not associated with any particular gene and causes disease by still unknown mechanisms.

Muscle weakness, which is often asymmetric, usually begins in the face and is then observed in the shoulders and legs. Individuals with FSHD often have weak eye closure, are not able to whistle or inflate a balloon, and have scapular winging.

Diagnosis is by genetic testing, although sometimes biopsies or electrodiagnostic testing may also be performed as part of the diagnostic evaluation. FSHD also may be associated with mild hearing loss, retinal abnormalities, and mild cardiac problems. Unlike DMD or BMD, children with FSHD often have muscle pain, particularly in their arms and shoulders.

Treatment involves administration of nonsteroidal anti-inflammatory drugs to decrease pain and inflammation. Massage and heat treatments also may be helpful. Bracing may be performed for function; for example, dorsiflexion of the feet with ankle-foot orthotics to prevent tripping or to provide support and comfort.

Myotonic Muscular Dystrophy

PATHOPHYSIOLOGY Myotonic muscular dystrophy (MMD) is a multisystem disease that can occur because of mutations in either of two genes resulting in type 1 (*DMPK* gene) and type 2 (*CNBP* gene) MMD. MMD1 may demonstrate a genetic mechanism called *anticipation*, in which children born to a mother with MMD usually have a more severe form of the disease.

CLINICAL MANIFESTATIONS MMD affects the brain, skeletal and smooth muscles, the eyes, the heart, and the endocrine system, manifesting as distal muscle weakness, learning problems or intellectual disability, or both. Additionally, children can have dysphagia, constipation, cardiac dysrhythmias that if untreated may be life-threatening, diabetes, and cataracts. Boys with MMD also may manifest testicular atrophy and early male-pattern baldness. A hallmark of the disease is myotonia—individuals have difficulty relaxing muscles; for example, they may have difficulty relaxing their hand grip after a handshake or opening their eyes after closing them tightly.

Children with mild disease do not develop symptoms until adolescence or older and may display mild muscle weakness (usually more pronounced in the distal muscles), cataracts, and myotonia, but have normal lifespans. Children with a more classic form of the disease also have onset of symptoms in the teenage years but have progressive muscle weakness, cataracts, and cardiac conduction abnormalities; they may have a shortened lifespan and require a wheelchair for mobility. The congenital form, the most severe, may be present at birth or become obvious over the first few years of life.

EVALUATION AND TREATMENT Diagnosis is via genetic testing for the two genes known to cause MMD. In each case, an abnormal segment of DNA, caused by an abnormally large trinucleotide (repeat expansion of a cytosine–thymine–guanine (CTG) triplet in an untranslated region of a gene) causes abnormal functioning of muscle and other cells. Type 1 is more common and can present in infancy (the congenital form). Infants with MMD may have life-threatening breathing and swallowing problems and developmental delay or intellectual disability, although MMD is not observed until childhood or even adolescence.

Steroids are not useful for the treatment of MMD; however, maintaining muscle function is important, including range-of-motion exercises, bracing, and surgical release of contractures when necessary. Children need to be followed closely by neurologists and primary care providers with treatment for the various aspects of the disease, such as dysphagia, heart dysrhythmias, and constipation, as well as other problems.

MUSCULOSKELETAL TUMOURS

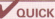 **QUICK CHECK 40.3**
1. What are the most common benign bone tumours of children?
2. What are the two malignant bone tumours found in children?
3. What is the most lethal bone tumour in children?

Benign Bone Tumours

The two most common forms of benign bone tumours in children are osteochondroma and nonossifying fibroma.

Osteochondroma

Osteochondroma (or exostosis) can occur as a solitary lesion or as an inherited syndrome of hereditary multiple exostoses (HME). HME is an autosomal dominant condition with exostoses occurring throughout the skeleton. Osteochondromas appear as bony protuberances because of *EXT1* and *EXT2* genetic anomalies near active growth plates of the proximal humerus, distal femur, or proximal tibia. The most common presentation is a palpable mass that is painful when traumatized. Rarely, the lesion can cause neurological or vascular problems, or tendon rupture from local compression. The lesions can lead to growth disturbance and mildly short stature. Knee valgus (knock-knee), ankle valgus, and hip problems are common. Upper extremity lesions can lead to a pronounced deformity in the forearm with a very short ulna bone. These lesions grow until skeletal maturity; growth or pain after skeletal maturity is a sign of possible malignant transformation, especially in the pelvis or scapular region. Transformation to chondrosarcoma is very rare, occurring in less than 1% of children.

Nonossifying Fibroma

Of all benign bone tumours, 50% are nonossifying fibromas or fibrous cortical defects. Nonossifying fibromas are sharply demarcated, cortically based lesions of fibrocytes that have replaced normal bone. The lesion can occur in any bone, at any age. Nearly 30% of all children have at least one.

Microscopically, these benign nonmetastasizing lesions appear as whorled bundles of fibroblasts and osteoclastlike giant cells. As the tumour grows, lipids make the fibroblasts foamy in appearance, and they are known as *foam cells*.

Treatment is observational only. If these lesions grow too large, however, they will compromise the biomechanical strength of the bone and lead to pathological fractures. Curettage and bone grafting is suggested after pathological fracture or if impending fracture (nonossifying fibroma greater than 50% of the diameter of the bone or greater than 3 or 4 cm) is noted radiographically.

Malignant Bone Tumours

Malignant bone tumours are uncommon tumours in childhood, accounting for fewer than 5% of childhood malignancies and occurring mostly during adolescence. The two main tumours are osteosarcoma and Ewing sarcoma (see Chapter 39).

Osteosarcoma

Osteosarcoma is the most common malignant bone tumour found during childhood and originates in bone-producing mesenchymal cells. Tumours can be broadly classified as those arising within the bone and those arising on the surface of bone. Approximately 75% of these tumours occur in persons between the ages of 10 and 25 years, with most being diagnosed between 15 and 19 years of age during the adolescent growth spurt. Incidence is the same for males and females.

Osteosarcoma may develop as a result of rapid local growth, which increases the likelihood of mutation. It can be induced by ionizing radiation, even with relatively low doses, and can be a tragic consequence of therapeutic radiation for other forms of cancer. The latent period after radiation exposure is 5 to 40 years. There also has been a link to individuals with retinoblastoma (a hereditary eye tumour). Osteosarcoma has not been linked to chemical carcinogens or viruses. No DNA or RNA virus has been isolated.

Molecular analysis has demonstrated deletion of genetic material on the long arm of chromosome 13, which led to the identification of a tumour-suppressor gene as being part of the mechanism for tumour development. The oncogene *src* also has been associated with osteosarcoma.

PATHOPHYSIOLOGY Osteosarcoma occurs mainly in the metaphyses of long bones near sites of active physeal growth. The tumour most commonly occurs at the distal femur, proximal tibia, or proximal humerus. As a tumour of mesenchymal cells, osteosarcoma demonstrates production of osteoid cells.

Osteosarcoma is a bulky tumour that extends beyond the bone into a soft tissue mass. It may encircle the bone and destroy the trabeculae of the diseased area. Osteosarcoma disseminates through the bloodstream, usually to the lung. As many as 25% of children diagnosed with osteosarcoma exhibit lung metastases at diagnosis. Other sites of metastatic spread include other bones and visceral organs.

CLINICAL MANIFESTATIONS The most common presenting complaint is pain. Night pain, awakening a child from sleep, is a particularly foreboding sign. There may be swelling, warmth, and redness caused by the vascularity of the tumour. Symptoms also may include cough, dyspnea, and chest pain if lung metastasis is present. If a lower extremity is involved, a child may limp or suffer a pathological fracture. Although osteosarcoma is not the result of trauma, trauma may call attention to a pre-existing tumour.

EVALUATION AND TREATMENT The five histological types of osteosarcoma are determined by the predominant cell type. The tumour is graded according to degree of malignancy; the higher the grade, the worse the prognosis.

Surgery and chemotherapy are the primary treatments for osteosarcoma. The tumour is resistant to radiation. Traditionally, surgery includes amputation at the joint above the involved bone; however, more recent limb salvage procedures have gained acceptance, and amputation may be avoided in many children.

Chemotherapy is an important component of treatment. Children routinely receive chemotherapy preoperatively; then the disease is restaged with MRI and surgical biopsy to determine rate of "tumour kill." If more than 90% of tumour cells are killed by chemotherapy, the prognosis is markedly improved. Chemotherapy is then used after surgery for any additional cell spill during surgery. The use of chemotherapy with surgery has increased the 5-year survival rate to 60% or more.[26]

A number of approaches have been used to treat pulmonary metastases. Because pulmonary metastases are generally solitary, thoracotomy with wedge resection has proved to be the most effective treatment.

Ewing Sarcoma

Ewing sarcoma is the second most common and the most lethal malignant bone tumour that occurs during childhood. This tumour is named after James Ewing, who first identified it as a separate clinical diagnosis in 1921. The most common period of diagnosis is between 5 and 15 years of age; it is rare after age 30. Ewing sarcoma is slightly more common in males than females. Cytogenic studies have shown a translocation of chromosomes 11 and 22 resulting in a fusion protein (EWS-FLI 1) forming at the chromosomal junction.

PATHOPHYSIOLOGY Ewing sarcoma is most commonly located in the midshaft of long bones or in flat bones. The most common sites include the femur, pelvis, and humerus (Figure 40.14).

Ewing sarcoma arises from the bone marrow and can penetrate the cortex of the bone to form a soft tissue mass. Unlike osteosarcoma, Ewing sarcoma does not make bone and radiographically appears as a permeative, destructive lesion (Figure 40.15). Ewing sarcoma metastasizes to nearly every organ. Metastasis occurs early and is usually apparent at diagnosis or within 1 year. The most common sites are the lung, other bones, lymph nodes, bone marrow, liver, spleen, and central nervous system.

CLINICAL MANIFESTATIONS As with osteosarcoma, the most common complaint is pain that increases in severity. A soft tissue mass is often present. Additional symptoms may include fever, malaise, and anorexia. The radiographic appearance is similar to that of osteomyelitis, and diagnosis is only confirmed with biopsy.

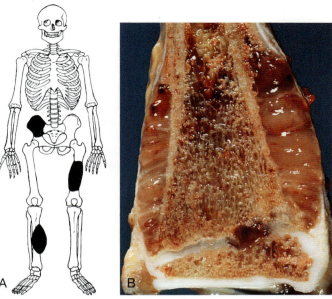

FIGURE 40.14 Ewing Sarcoma. A, Most common anatomical sites. **B,** Close-up view of Ewing sarcoma of the distal end of the tibia. Tumour extends into the soft tissue. (From Damjanov, I., & Linder, J. [Eds.]. [1996]. *Anderson's pathology* [10th ed.]. Mosby.)

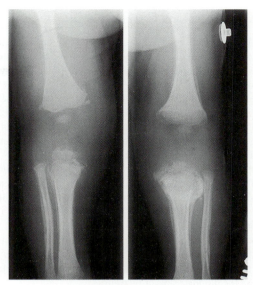

FIGURE 40.16 Corner Fracture. Bilateral knee radiograph showing healing corner fractures of bilateral proximal tibias and distal femurs. Note the varying amount of callus formation signifying fractures at different stages of healing.

NONACCIDENTAL TRAUMA

✓ **QUICK CHECK 40.4**
1. What is the most common orthopedic injury in nonaccidental trauma?

Fractures in Nonaccidental Trauma

Children who are not yet ambulatory and present with a long bone fracture have more than a 75% chance of that fracture being caused by nonaccidental trauma (NAT).[27] "Corner" metaphyseal fractures are nearly always from abuse but occur only 25% of the time (Figure 40.16). Fractures at multiple stages of healing also suggest abuse; however, OI or other causes of systemic osteomalacia must be ruled out. The most common presentation is a transverse tibia fracture. After walking age, only 2% of long bone fractures are the result of NAT.[28]

EVALUATION NAT necessitates early consultation with child protective services. The child should undergo skeletal survey (especially if less than 2 years of age) and have a complete physical examination to evaluate for pattern bruising, burns, or multiple soft tissue injuries. A thorough history must be obtained for all identified injuries. It is important to remember that social isolation can lead to an increased likelihood of abuse, but no social status is immune. One study reported that racial differences may exist in the evaluation and reporting of NAT. Skeletal trauma is present in a significant number of abused children.[29–31]

When the cause of injury is unclear, bone scan can be helpful in diagnosing subtle injuries, especially rib fractures. Posterior rib fractures are especially likely to be the result of abuse. An MRI and a computed tomography scan of the brain to check for subdural hematoma and retinal examination to look for hemorrhages are essential.

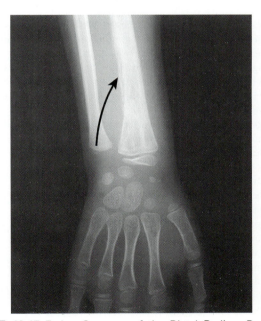

FIGURE 40.15 Ewing Sarcoma of the Distal Radius. Radiograph of an 8-year-old boy showing a permeative lesion of the distal radius. Note the loss of bone cortex on the ulnar border *(arrow),* suggesting an aggressive process. Bone biopsy revealed Ewing sarcoma.

EVALUATION AND TREATMENT Evaluation is determined from genetic testing, elevated sedimentation rate, and lactate dehydrogenase levels. Biopsy is used to conclusively establish the diagnosis of a small round cell tumour.

Treatment includes radiation, chemotherapy, and, if possible, surgical debridement. Chemotherapy is continued for 12 to 18 months after resection. Present 5-year survival with this tritherapeutic approach is 60%; however, tumours of the pelvis have a markedly worse prognosis. Metastasis at diagnosis is another poor prognostic indicator, with 5-year survival rate dropping to less than 40%.

TREATMENT The treating health care provider must have a nonjudgemental attitude. The child and family involved in NAT are emotionally delicate and require not only physical but also emotional care. Social workers need to be involved early to ensure that the child receives appropriate medical care. Fortunately, fractures tend to heal quickly for those in this age group. Neurological injury and social disease, however, are much more difficult to cure.

DID YOU UNDERSTAND?

Congenital Defects
1. Clubfoot is a common deformity in which the foot is twisted out of its normal shape or position. Clubfoot can be positional, idiopathic, or teratological.
2. Developmental dysplasia of the hip (DDH) is an abnormality in the development of the femoral head, acetabulum, or both. Like clubfoot, DDH can be idiopathic or teratological. It is a serious and disabling condition in children if not diagnosed and treated early; best outcomes occur when treated before walking age.
3. Osteogenesis imperfecta (brittle bone disease) is an inherited disorder of collagen that affects primarily bones (it also may cause vascular deformity) and results in serious fractures of many bones.

Bone Infection
1. Osteomyelitis is a local or generalized bacterial or granulomatous (e.g., tuberculosis) infection of bone and bone marrow. Bacteria are usually introduced by direct extension from a nearby infection, through the bloodstream, or by trauma.
2. Septic arthritis can occur de novo or secondary to osteomyelitis in very young children in which the metaphysis is still located within the joint capsule of certain joints.

Juvenile Idiopathic Arthritis
1. Juvenile idiopathic arthritis is an inflammatory joint disorder characterized by pain and swelling. Large joints are most commonly affected.

Osteochondroses
1. Avascular diseases of the bone are collectively referred to as osteochondroses and are caused by an insufficient blood supply to growing bones.
2. Legg-Calvé-Perthes disease is one of the most common osteochondroses. This disorder is characterized by epiphyseal necrosis or degeneration of the head of the femur followed by regeneration or recalcification. Children older than 7 years of age at onset have a worse prognosis.
3. Osgood-Schlatter disease is characterized by tendonitis of the anterior patellar tendon and inflammation or partial separation of the tibial tubercle caused by chronic irritation, usually as a result of overuse of the quadriceps muscles. The condition is seen primarily in muscular, athletic adolescent males.

Scoliosis
1. Scoliosis is a rotational curvature of the spine most obvious in the anteroposterior plane and can be classified as nonstructural or structural. Nonstructural scoliosis results from a cause other than the spine itself, such as posture, leg length discrepancy, or splinting from pain. Structural scoliosis is a curvature of the spine associated with vertebral rotation.

Muscular Dystrophy
1. The muscular dystrophies are a group of genetically transmitted diseases characterized by progressive atrophy of skeletal muscles. There is an insidious loss of strength in all forms of the disorder with increasing disability and deformity. The most common type in childhood is Duchenne muscular dystrophy.

Musculoskeletal Tumours
1. The two most common forms of benign bone tumours are osteochondroma and nonossifying fibroma.
2. The two main types of malignant childhood bone tumours are osteosarcoma and Ewing sarcoma.
3. Osteosarcoma, the most common malignant childhood bone tumour, originates in bone-producing mesenchymal cells and is most often located near active growth plates, such as the distal femur, proximal tibia, or proximal humerus.
4. Most children with osteosarcoma are diagnosed between 15 and 19 years of age, and osteosarcoma occurs equally in males and females.
5. Ewing sarcoma originates from cells within the bone marrow space and is most often located in the midshaft of long bones or in flat bones. The most common sites include the femur, pelvis, and humerus.
6. Ewing sarcoma is more common in males and is diagnosed most often between the ages of 5 and 15 years.
7. Pain is the usual presenting symptom for either osteosarcoma or Ewing sarcoma.
8. The primary treatments for osteosarcoma are surgery and chemotherapy. The primary treatment for Ewing sarcoma is a combination of chemotherapy, radiation, and surgery.

Nonaccidental Trauma
1. Nonaccidental trauma (NAT) must be considered with any long bone injury in the preambulatory child.
2. The presence of soft tissue injury, corner fractures, and multiple fractures at different stages of healing is extremely helpful for making a diagnosis of NAT.
3. When NAT is suspected, a child must be evaluated radiographically for other fractures, heat trauma, and retinal hemorrhage.
4. All social strata are at risk.
5. The health care provider is legally responsible to report suspected NAT.

41

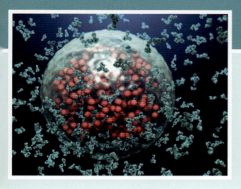

Structure, Function, and Disorders of the Integument

Stephanie Zettel, with originating chapter contributions by Sue Ann McCann and Sue E. Huether

Additional resources are available online at https://evolve.elsevier.com/Canada/Huether/pathophysiology.

CHAPTER OUTLINE

Structure and Function of the Skin, 1022
    Layers of the Skin, 1022
    Clinical Manifestations of Skin Dysfunction, 1024
Disorders of the Skin, 1029
    Inflammatory Disorders, 1029
    Papulosquamous Disorders, 1030
    Vesiculobullous Diseases, 1033
    Infections, 1034
    Vascular Disorders, 1038
    Benign Tumours, 1039
    Skin Cancer, 1039

Burns, 1042
Cold Injury, 1046
Disorders of the Hair, 1047
    Alopecia, 1047
    Hirsutism, 1049
Disorders of the Nail, 1049
    Paronychia, 1049
    Onychomycosis, 1049
GERIATRIC CONSIDERATIONS: Aging and Changes in Skin Integrity, 1049

LEARNING OBJECTIVES

1. Describe the structural layers and primary function of the skin.
2. Describe the pathophysiology of pressure ulcers, including the risk factors associated with their development.
3. Describe a keloid and how it differs from a normal scar.
4. Discuss risk factors and treatments for pruritus.
5. Compare and contrast the various forms of dermatitis.
6. Describe the various papulosquamous disorders.
7. Compare and contrast acne vulgaris and acne rosacea.
8. Discuss the clinical manifestations and treatment of discoid lupus erythematosus (DLE).
9. Compare and contrast the various types of pemphigus.
10. Discuss the pathophysiology and treatment of Stevens-Johnson syndrome and toxic epidermal necrolysis (TEN).
11. Describe the skin lesions produced by the following infectious agents: streptococcus, staphylococcus, herpesvirus, papillomavirus, tinea, and candidiasis.
12. Discuss the pathophysiology of cutaneous vasculitis, urticaria, and scleroderma.
13. Compare and contrast seborrheic keratosis, keratoacanthoma, and actinic keratosis.
14. Describe the incidence, risk factors, manifestations, treatments, and prognosis of cancers of the skin.
15. Describe the depth and extent of injury for first-, second-, and third-degree burns.
16. Discuss the consequences of body fluid shifts, cardiovascular compromise, and immunological alterations related to severe burn injuries.
17. Describe the mechanism of injury for frostbite.
18. Differentiate between male- and female-pattern alopecia.
19. Identify the causative organisms of nail infections.

KEY TERMS

Acne rosacea, 1033
Acne vulgaris, 1032
Actinic keratosis, 1039
Allergic contact dermatitis, 1029
Alopecia, 1047
Alopecia areata, 1049
Androgenic alopecia, 1048
Apocrine sweat gland, 1022
Atopic dermatitis (allergic dermatitis), 1030
Basal cell carcinoma (BCC), 1040
Bullous erythema multiforme, 1034
Burn shock, 1044
Candidiasis, 1037
Capillary seal, 1045
Carbuncle, 1035
Cellulitis, 1035
Chronic urticarial, 1038
Clawlike prolongation, 1029
Condylomata acuminata (venereal warts), 1036
Cutaneous melanoma, 1041
Cutaneous vasculitis, 1038
Deep partial-thickness burn, 1043
Dermal appendage, 1022
Dermatitis, 1029
Dermis, 1022
Discoid (cutaneous) lupus erythematosus (DLE), 1033
Eccrine sweat gland, 1022
Eczema, 1029
Epidermis, 1022
Erysipelas, 1035
Erythema multiforme, 1034
Erythrodermic (exfoliative) psoriasis, 1031
Escharotomy, 1044
First-degree burn, 1043
Fluid resuscitation, 1045
Folliculitis, 1035
Fourth-degree burn, 1044
Furuncle, 1035
Guttate psoriasis, 1031
Herald patch, 1032
Herpes simplex virus (HSV), 1035
Herpes zoster (shingles), 1036

Hirsutism, 1049
Human papillomavirus (HPV), 1036
Hypertrophic scar, 1029
Immunoglobulin A pemphigus, 1034
Impetigo, 1035
Inverse psoriasis, 1031
Irritant contact dermatitis, 1030
Kaposi sarcoma (KS), 1042
Keloid, 1029
Keratoacanthoma, 1039
Lichen planus (LP), 1032
Lip cancer, 1041
Localized scleroderma (morphea), 1038
Lupus erythematosus, 1033
Lyme disease, 1035
Mycosis fungoides, 1042
Nails, 1022
Necrotizing fasciitis, 1035
Nevus (*pl.*, nevi), 1039
Onychomycosis (tinea unguium), 1049
Papillary capillary, 1022
Papulosquamous disorder, 1030
Paraneoplastic pemphigus, 1034
Paronychia, 1049
Pemphigus, 1033
Pemphigus erythematosus, 1034
Pemphigus foliaceus, 1034
Pemphigus herpetiformis, 1034
Pemphigus vegetans, 1034
Pemphigus vulgaris, 1034
Pityriasis rosea, 1032
Plaque psoriasis, 1031
Pressure ulcer, 1024
Primary cutaneous lymphoma, 1042
Psoriasis, 1031
Psoriatic arthritis, 1031
Psoriatic nail disease, 1031
Pustular psoriasis, 1031
Sebaceous gland, 1022
Seborrheic dermatitis, 1030
Seborrheic keratosis, 1039
Second-degree burn, 1043
Squamous cell carcinoma (SCC), 1040
Stasis dermatitis, 1030
Stevens-Johnson syndrome, 1034
Subcutaneous layer (hypodermis), 1022
Systemic scleroderma, 1038
Third-degree burn (full-thickness burn), 1044
Tinea infection, 1037
Total body surface area (TBSA), 1044
Toxic epidermal necrolysis (TEN), 1034
Urticaria (hives), 1038
Urticarial lesion, 1038
Varicella (chickenpox), 1036
Wart, 1036

The skin covers the entire body and is the largest organ of the body, accounting for about 20% of body weight. Combined with the accessory structures of hair, nails, and glands, skin forms the integumentary system. The skin's primary function is protection from the environment by serving as a barrier against microorganisms, ultraviolet radiation (UVR), loss of body fluids, and the stress of mechanical forces. The skin regulates body temperature and is involved in immune surveillance and the activation of vitamin D. Touch and pressure receptors provide important protective functions and pleasurable sensations. The commensal (normal) microorganisms of the skin also protect against pathological bacteria.

STRUCTURE AND FUNCTION OF THE SKIN

> **QUICK CHECK 41.1**
> 1. Describe the two layers of the skin.
> 2. How do the skin blood vessels and sweat glands regulate body temperature?
> 3. What are some changes that occur in skin with aging?

Layers of the Skin

The skin is formed of two major layers: (1) a superficial or outer layer of **epidermis** and (2) a deeper layer of **dermis** (the true skin) (Figure 41.1). The **subcutaneous layer (hypodermis)**, the lowest-lying layer of connective tissue, contains macrophages, fibroblasts, fat cells, nerves, fine muscles, blood vessels, lymphatics, and hair follicle roots. Each skin layer contains cells that represent progressive stages of skin cell differentiation and function as the skin grows. These are summarized in Table 41.1.

Dermal Appendages

The **dermal appendages** include the nails, hair, sebaceous glands, and the eccrine and apocrine sweat glands. The **nails** are protective keratinized plates that appear at the ends of fingers and toes. They have the following structures: (1) the proximal nail fold, (2) the eponychium (cuticle), (3) the matrix from which the nail grows and its nail root, (4) the hyponychium (nail bed), (5) the nail plate, and (6) the paronychium (lateral nail fold) (Figure 41.2). Nail growth continues throughout life at 1 mm or less per day.

Hair colour, density, grain, and pattern of distribution vary considerably among people and depend on age, sex, and ethnicity. Hair follicles arise from the matrix (or bulb) located deep in the dermis. They extend from the dermis at an angle and have an erector pili muscle attached near the mid-dermis that straightens the follicle when contracted, causing the hair to stand up. Hair growth begins in the bulb, with cellular differentiation occurring as the hair progresses up the follicle. Hair is fully hardened, or cornified, by the time it emerges at the skin surface. Hair colour is determined by melanin-secreting follicular melanocytes. Hair growth is cyclic, with periods of growth and rest that vary over different body surfaces.

The **sebaceous glands** open onto the surface of the skin through a canal. They are found in the greatest numbers on the face, chest, and back, with modified glands on the eyelids, lips, nipples, glans penis, and prepuce. Sebaceous glands secrete sebum, composed primarily of lipids, which oils the skin and hair and prevents drying. Androgens stimulate the growth of sebaceous glands, and their enlargement is an early sign of puberty.

The **eccrine sweat glands** are distributed over the body, with the greatest numbers in the palms of the hands, soles of the feet, and forehead. They open onto the surface of the skin and are important in thermoregulation and cooling of the body through evaporation. There are fewer **apocrine sweat glands**, but these glands produce significantly more sweat than the eccrine glands. They are located near the bulb of hair follicles in the axillae, scalp, face, abdomen, and genital area. Their ducts open into the hair follicle. The interaction of sweat with commensal (normal) flora bacteria contributes to the odour of perspiration.

Blood Supply and Innervation

The blood supply to the skin is from the **papillary capillaries**, or plexus, of the dermis. These capillary loops are supplied by a deeper arterial plexus. Branches from the deep plexus also supply hair follicles and sweat glands. A subpapillary network of veins drains the capillary loops. Arteriovenous anastomoses in the dermis facilitate the regulation of body temperature. Heat loss is regulated by (1) variations in skin blood flow through the opening and closing of arteriovenous anastomoses and (2) the evaporative heat loss of sweat. The sympathetic nervous system regulates both vasoconstriction and vasodilation through α-adrenergic receptors in the skin. The lymphatic vessels of the skin arise in the papillary dermis and drain into larger subcutaneous trunks, removing cells, proteins, and immunological mediators.

The structure and function of the skin change with advancing age. A summary of aging changes is included in the box titled *Geriatric Considerations: Aging and Changes in Skin Integrity.*

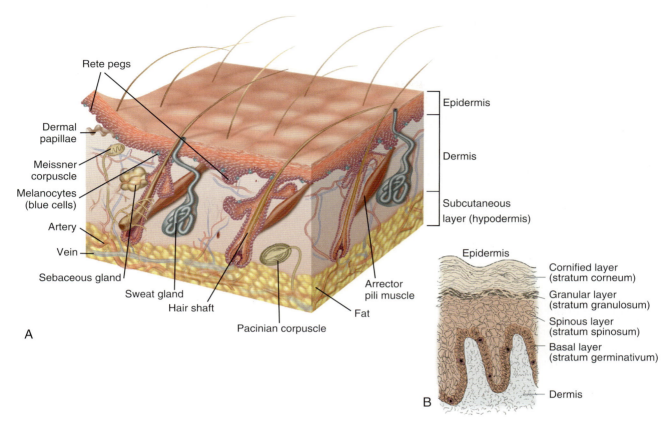

FIGURE 41.1 Structure of the Skin. **A,** Cross-section showing major skin structures. **B,** Layers of the epidermis. ([A], from Kumar, V., Abbas, A. K., & Aster, J. C. [Eds.]. [2021]. *Robbins and Cotran pathologic basis of disease* [10th ed.]. Saunders; [B], from Baker, S. R. [2007]. *Local flaps in facial reconstruction* [3rd ed.]. Saunders.)

TABLE 41.1 Layers of the Skin

Structure	Cell Types	Characteristics
Epidermis	Keratinocytes	Most important layer of skin; normally very thin (0.12 mm) but can thicken and form corns or calluses with constant pressure or friction; includes rete pegs that extend into papillary layer of dermis
	Langerhans cells	Cells with dendrite process and immune functions
Stratum corneum	Keratinocytes	Tough superficial layer covering body
Stratum lucidum	Keratinocytes	Clear layers of cells containing eleidin, which becomes keratin as cells move up to corneum layer
Stratum granulosum	Keratinocytes	Keratohyalin gives granular appearance to this layer
	Melanocytes	
Stratum spinosum	New keratinocytes	Polygonal shaped with spinous processes projecting between adjacent keratinocytes
Stratum basale (germinativum)	Keratinocytes	Basal layer where keratinocytes divide and move upward to replace cells shed from surface
	Melanocytes	Melanocytes synthesize pigment melanin
	Merkel cells	Function of Merkel cells is not clearly known; they are associated with sensory nerve endings
Dermis	Macrophages	Irregular connective tissue layer with rich blood, lymphatic, and nerve supply; contains sensory receptors and sweat glands (apocrine, eccrine, sebaceous), macrophages (phagocytic and important for wound healing), and mast cells (release histamine and have immune functions) (see Chapter 6)
Papillary layer (thin)	Mast cells	
Reticular layer (thick)	Histiocytes	Histiocytes are wandering macrophages that collect pigments and inflammatory debris
Subcutaneous Layer (Hypodermis)		Subcutaneous tissue or superficial fascia of varying thickness that connects overlying dermis to underlying muscle; contains macrophages, fibroblasts, fat cells, nerves, blood vessels, lymphatics, and hair follicle roots

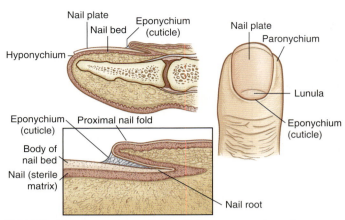

FIGURE 41.2 Structures of the Nail. (Redrawn from Thompson, J. M., McFarland, G. K., Hirsch, J. E., et al. [2002]. *Mosby's clinical nursing* [5th ed.]. Mosby.)

Clinical Manifestations of Skin Dysfunction

> **QUICK CHECK 41.2**
> 1. What areas are at greatest risk for pressure ulcers?
> 2. How does a keloid differ from a normal scar?
> 3. What stimulates pruritus?

Lesions

Identification of the morphological structure of the skin, including differentiation between primary and secondary lesions, and assessment of the appearance of the skin in combination with obtaining a health history are essential to identify underlying pathophysiology. Tables 41.2 and 41.3 describe and illustrate the basic lesions of the skin. Table 41.4 describes clinical manifestations of select skin lesions.

Pressure ulcers. **Pressure ulcers** (sometimes called *pressure sores*) are ischemic ulcers resulting from unrelieved pressure, shearing forces, friction, and moisture. The term *decubitus ulcer* refers to ulcers that develop when unrelieved pressure interrupts normal blood flow to the skin and its underlying tissues. The risks for pressure ulcers are summarized in *Risk Factors:* Pressure Ulcer.[1]

Pressure ulcers usually develop over bony prominences, such as the sacrum, heels, ischia, and greater trochanters. Continuous pressure on tissue between the bony prominence and a resistant outside surface distorts capillaries and occludes the blood supply. Pressure ulcers can also occur in soft tissues from unrelieved pressure, for example, from nasal cannulas or endotracheal tubes. If the pressure is relieved within a few hours, a brief period of reactive hyperemia (redness) occurs and there may be no lasting tissue damage. If the pressure continues unrelieved, platelet aggregation occurs with damage to the endothelial cells lining the capillaries, and microthrombi block blood flow and cause anoxic necrosis of surrounding tissues (Figure 41.3). Shearing and friction are mechanical forces moving parallel to the skin (dragging) and can extend to the bony skeleton, causing detachment and injury of tissues. Pressure injuries are staged or graded, and one classification scheme is:[2]

Stage 1—Nonblanchable erythema of intact skin, usually over a bony prominence; darkly pigmented skin may not have visible blanching. Presence of blanchable erythema or changes in sensation, temperature, or firmness may precede visual changes. Colour changes do not include purple or maroon discolouration; these may indicate deep tissue pressure injury.

RISK FACTORS
Pressure Ulcer

External Factors
- Prolonged pressure
- Immobilization
- Lying in bed or sitting in chair or wheelchair without changing position or relieving pressure over an extended period
- Lying for hours on hard X-ray, emergency department, and operating room tables
- Prolonged moisture exposure
- Neurological disorders (coma, spinal cord injuries, cognitive impairment, or cerebrovascular disease)
- Fractures or contractures
- Debilitation: older persons in hospitals and nursing homes
- Pain
- Sedation
- Friction and shearing forces
- Coarse bed sheets used for turning by dragging, which produces friction and a shearing force
- Inadequate caretaking staff
- Lack of communication and education regarding pressure ulcer care

Disease and Tissue Factors
- Impaired perfusion; ischemia
- Fecal or urinary incontinence; prolonged exposure to moisture
- Malnutrition, dehydration
- Chronic diseases accompanied by anemia, edema, kidney failure, malnutrition, peripheral vascular disease, or sepsis
- Previous history of pressure ulcers
- Thin skin associated with aging or prolonged use of steroids

Data from Bogie, K., Powell, H. L., & Ho, C. (2012). *Handbook of Clinical Neurology, 109,* 235–246; Coleman, S., Gorecki, C., Nelson, E. A., et al. (2013). *International Journal of Nursing Studies, 50*(7), 974–1003; García-Fernández, F. P., Agreda, J. J., Verdú, J., et al. (2014). *Journal of Nursing Scholarship, 46*(1), 28–38; Michel, J. M., Willebois, S., Ribinik, P., et al. (2012). *Annals of Physical and Rehabilitation Medicine, 55*(7), 454–465.

Stage 2—Partial-thickness skin loss with exposed dermis. The wound is still vascular and pink or red and can also have an intact or ruptured serum-filled blister. There is no fat, granulation, or eschar (dead tissue that sheds from healthy skin) tissue.

Stage 3—Full-thickness skin loss where fat and granulation tissue are visible in the ulcer. Eschar and tunnelling may be visible. Fascia, muscle, tendons, bones, and ligaments are not exposed.

Stage 4—Full-thickness skin and tissue loss with exposure of muscle, bone, or supporting structures (tendons or joint capsules); can include undermining and tunnelling.

Unstageable—Obscured full-thickness skin and tissue loss with base of ulcer covered by slough or eschar, or both, in the wound bed.

Deep tissue pressure injury—Intact or nonintact skin with localized area of persistent nonblanchable deep red, maroon, purple discolouration, or epidermal separation revealing a dark wound bed or blood-filled blister. Pain and temperature change often precede skin colour changes. Discolouration may appear differently in darkly pigmented skin. This injury results from intense or prolonged pressure and shear forces at the bone–muscle interface. The wound may evolve rapidly to reveal the actual extent of tissue injury or may resolve without tissue loss. If necrotic tissue, subcutaneous tissue, granulation tissue, fascia, muscle, or other underlying structures are visible, this indicates a full thickness pressure injury.

TABLE 41.2 Primary Skin Lesions

Macule
A flat, circumscribed area that is a change in colour of skin; less than 1 cm in diameter
Examples: Freckles, flat moles (nevi), petechiae, measles, scarlet fever

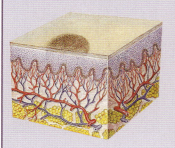 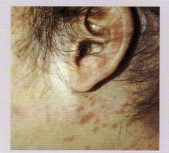

Macules[a]

Papule
An elevated, firm, circumscribed area less than 1 cm in diameter
Examples: Wart (verruca), elevated moles, lichen planus, fibroma, insect bite

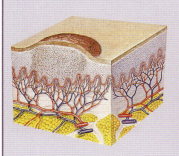 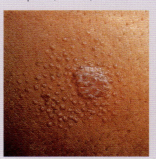

Lichen planus[b]

Patch
A flat, nonpalpable, irregular-shaped macule more than 1 cm in diameter
Examples: Vitiligo, port-wine stains, Mongolian spots, café-au-lait spots

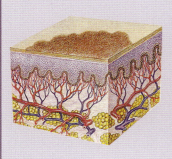 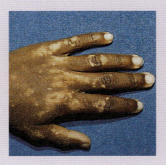

Vitiligo[c]

Plaque
Elevated, firm, and rough lesion with flat top surface greater than 1 cm in diameter
Examples: Psoriasis, seborrheic and actinic keratoses

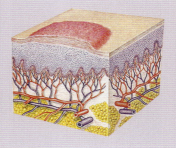 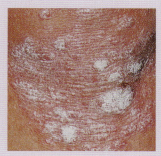

Plaque[d]

Wheal
Elevated, irregular-shaped area of cutaneous edema; solid, transient; variable diameter
Examples: Insect bites, urticaria, allergic reaction

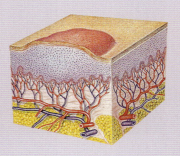 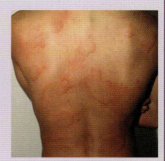

Wheal[e]

Nodule
Elevated, firm, circumscribed lesion; deeper in dermis than a papule; 1–2 cm in diameter
Examples: Erythema nodosum, lipomas

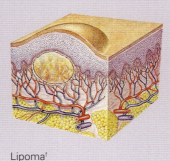 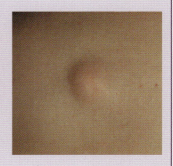

Lipoma[f]

Continued

TABLE 41.2 Primary Skin Lesions—cont'd

Tumour
Elevated, solid lesion; may be clearly demarcated; deeper in dermis; more than 2 cm in diameter
Examples: Neoplasms, benign tumour, lipoma, neurofibroma, hemangioma

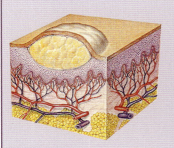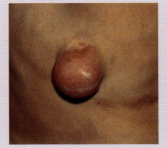

Neurofibroma[f]

Vesicle
Elevated, circumscribed, superficial; does not extend into dermis; filled with serous fluid; less than 1 cm in diameter
Examples: Varicella (chickenpox), herpes zoster (shingles), herpes simplex

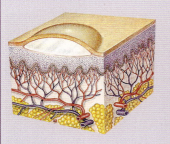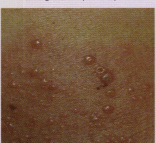

Vesicles[g]

Bulla
Vesicle more than 1 cm in diameter
Examples: Blister, pemphigus vulgaris

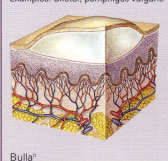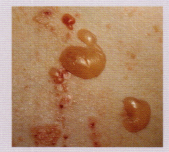

Bulla[h]

Pustule
Elevated, superficial lesion; similar to a vesicle but filled with purulent fluid
Examples: Impetigo, acne

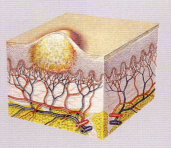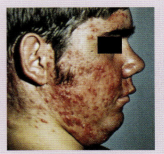

Acne[c]

Cyst
Elevated, circumscribed, encapsulated lesion; in dermis or subcutaneous layer; filled with liquid or semisolid material
Examples: Sebaceous cyst, cystic acne

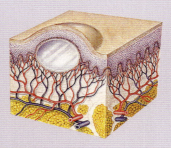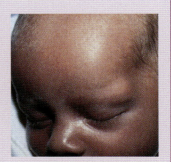

Sebaceous cyst[c]

Telangiectasia
Fine (0.5–1.0 mm), irregular red lines produced by capillary dilation; can be associated with acne rosacea (face), venous hypertension (spider veins in legs), systemic sclerosis, or developmental abnormalities (port-wine birthmarks)
Example: Telangiectasia in rosacea

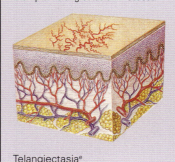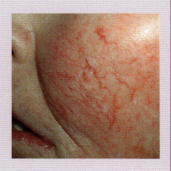

Telangiectasia[e]

[a]Farrar, W. E., Wood, M. J., Innes, J. A., et al. (1992). *Infectious diseases* (2nd ed.). Gower.
[b]James, W. D., Berger, T. G., & Elston, D. M. (2011). *Andrews' diseases of the skin* (11th ed.). Saunders.
[c]Weston, W. L., & Lane, A. T. (2002). *Color textbook of pediatric dermatology* (3rd ed.). Mosby.
[d]Habif, T. P. (2010). *Clinical dermatology: a color guide to diagnosis and therapy* (5th ed.). Mosby.
[e]Bolognia, J. L., Jorizzo, J., & Schaffer, J. (2012). *Dermatology* (3rd ed.). Saunders.
[f]Weston, W. L., Lane, A. T., & Morelli, J. G. (2007). *Color textbook of pediatric dermatology* (4th ed.). Mosby.
[g]Black, M. M., Ambros-Rudolph, C., Edwards, L., et al. (2008). *Obstetric and gynecologic dermatology* (3rd ed.). Mosby.
[h]Marks, J. G., & Miller, J. J. (2006). *Lookingbill & Marks' principles of dermatology* (4th ed.). Saunders.

TABLE 41.3 Secondary Skin Lesions

Scale
Heaped-up, keratinized cells; flaky skin; irregular shape; thick or thin; dry or oily; variation in size
Examples: Flaking of skin with seborrheic dermatitis following scarlet fever, or flaking of skin following a medication reaction; dry skin

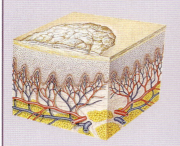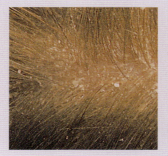

Fine scaling[a]

Lichenification
Rough, thickened epidermis secondary to persistent rubbing, itching, or skin irritation; often involves flexor surface of extremity
Example: Chronic dermatitis

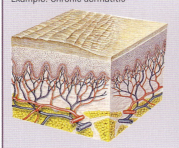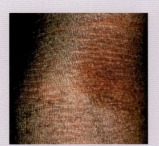

Atopic dermatitis of arm[b]

Keloid
Irregular-shaped, elevated, progressively enlarging scar; grows beyond boundaries of wound; caused by excessive collagen formation during healing
Examples: Keloid formation following surgery

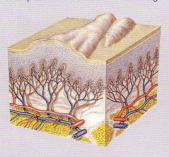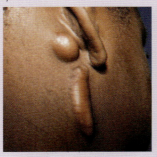

Keloid[c]

Scar
Thin to thick fibrous tissue that replaces normal skin following injury or laceration to the dermis
Examples: Healed wound or surgical incision

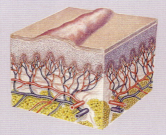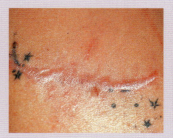

Hypertrophic scar[d]

Excoriation
Loss of epidermis; linear, hollowed-out, crusted area
Examples: Abrasion or scratch, scabies

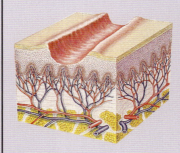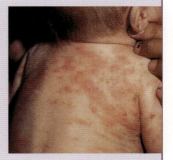

Scabies[c]

Fissure
Linear crack or break from the epidermis to the dermis; may be moist or dry
Examples: Athlete's foot, cracks at the corner of mouth, anal fissure, dermatitis

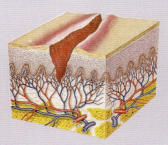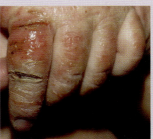

Fissures from infected dermatitis[c]

Continued

TABLE 41.3 Secondary Skin Lesions—cont'd

Erosion
Loss of part of the epidermis; depressed, moist, glistening; follows rupture of a vesicle or bulla or chemical injury
Example: Chemical injury

Erosion on leg[e]

Ulcer
Loss of epidermis and dermis; concave; varies in size
Examples: Pressure ulcer, stasis ulcers

Pressure ulcer on heel[f]

Atrophy
Thinning of skin surface and loss of skin markings; skin appears translucent and paperlike
Examples: Aged skin, striae

Aged skin[g]

[a]Baran, R., Dawber, R. P. R., & Levene, G. M. (1991). *Color atlas of the hair, scalp, and nails*. Mosby.
[b]James, W. D., Berger, T. G., & Elston, D. M. (2011). *Andrews' diseases of the skin* (11th ed.). Saunders.
[c]Weston, W. L., Lane, A. T., & Morelli, J. (2007). *Color textbook of pediatric dermatology* (4th ed.). Mosby.
[d]Nouri, K., & Leal-Khouri, S. (2003). *Techniques in dermatologic surgery*. Mosby.
[e]Bolognia, J. L., Jorizzo, J., & Schaffer, J. (2012). *Dermatology* (3rd ed.). Saunders.
[f]Robinson, J. K., Hanke, C. W., Siegel, D. M., et al. (2015). *Surgery of the skin* (3rd ed.). Saunders.
[g]Ball, J. W., Dains, J. E., Flynn, J. A., et al. (2015). *Seidel's guide to physical examination* (8th ed.). Mosby.

TABLE 41.4 Clinical Manifestations of Select Skin Lesions

Type	Clinical Manifestation
Comedone	Plug of sebaceous and keratin material lodged in opening of hair follicle; open comedone has dilated orifice (blackhead) and closed comedone has narrow opening (whitehead)
Burrow	Narrow, raised, irregular channel caused by parasite
Petechiae	Circumscribed area of blood less than 0.5 cm in diameter
Purpura	Circumscribed area of blood greater than 0.5 cm in diameter
Telangiectasia	Dilated, superficial blood vessels

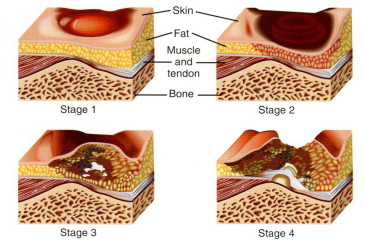

FIGURE 41.3 Progression of Pressure Ulcer. Sustained pressure over a bony prominence compresses the tissue and reduces blood flow, resulting in progressive ischemia and necrosis of tissue.

Superficial damage results in a layer of dead tissue that forms as an abrasion, blister, erosion, or nonblanchable red or darkened skin or as a reddish blue discolouration when there is deeper tissue damage. Superficial ulcers are more common on the sacrum as a result of shearing or friction forces (forces parallel to the skin). Deep ulcers develop closer to the bone as a result of tissue distortion and vascular occlusion from pressure perpendicular to the tissue (over the heels, trochanter, and ischia). Bacteria colonize the dead tissue, and infection is usually localized and self-limiting. Proteolytic enzymes from bacteria and macrophages dissolve necrotic tissues and cause a foul-smelling discharge that resembles, but is not, pus. The necrotic tissue initiates an inflammatory response with potential pain, fever, and leukocytosis. If the ulceration is large, toxicity and pain lead to a host of possible complications, including loss of appetite, debility, local or systemic infections, and renal insufficiency.

The primary goal for those at risk for pressure ulcers is prevention and early detection. Preventive techniques include frequent assessment of the skin with repositioning and turning of the individual; promotion of movement; implementation of pressure reduction (type of positioning and use of specialty beds), pressure removal (positioning interval), and pressure distribution devices (positioning aids); and elimination of excessive moisture and drainage. Adequate nutrition, oxygenation, and fluid balance must be maintained.[3,4]

Superficial ulcers should be covered with flat, moisture-retaining dressings (e.g., hydrogel dressings) that cannot wrinkle and cause increased pressure or friction. Successful healing requires continued adequate relief of pressure, debridement of necrotic tissue, opening of deep pockets for drainage, and repair of damaged tissue by construction of skin flaps for large, deep ulcers. Infection requires treatment with antibiotics, and pain should be controlled.[5,6]

Keloids and Hypertrophic Scars

Keloids are rounded, firm, elevated scars with irregular clawlike margins that extend beyond the original site of injury. They are most common in darkly pigmented skin types and generally appear weeks to months after a stable scar has formed. **Hypertrophic scars** are elevated erythematous fibrous lesions that do not extend beyond the border of injury. Hypertrophic scars appear within 3 to 4 months and usually regress within 1 year. Both lesions are caused by abnormal wound healing with excessive fibroblast activity and collagen formation, and loss of control of normal tissue repair and regeneration.[7] Genetic susceptibility is likely.[8]

Excessive or poorly aligned tension on a wound, introduction of foreign material into the skin, infection, and certain types of trauma (e.g., burns) are all provocative factors. Those parts of the body at risk include shoulders, back, chin, ears, and lower legs. Individuals 10 to 30 years of age develop lesions much more commonly than do prepubescent children or older persons.

Keloids start as pink or red, firm, well-defined, rubbery plaques that persist for several months after trauma. Later, uncontrolled overgrowth causes extension beyond the site of the original wound, and the overgrowth becomes smoother, irregularly shaped, hyperpigmented, harder, and more symptomatic. The fibrous tissue that accumulates in keloids has increased cellularity, and there is metabolic activity of fibroblasts. The tendency to form **clawlike prolongations** is typical (Figure 41.4). Various treatments are available for the management of keloids and hypertrophic scars; however, there also is a need for research to improve treatment outcomes.[7]

Pruritus

Pruritus, or itching, is a symptom associated with many primary skin disorders, such as eczema, psoriasis, or insect infestations, or it can be

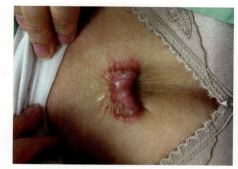

FIGURE 41.4 Keloid. (Courtesy Dr. M. G. Jeschke.)

a manifestation of systemic disease (e.g., chronic kidney disease, cholestatic liver disease, thyroid disorders, iron deficiency, neuropathies, or malignancy) or the use of opiate drugs. It may be acute or chronic (neuropathic itch), localized or generalized, and migratory (moves from one location to another).[9] Multiple stimuli can produce itching, and there is interaction between itch and pain sensations. There are many itch mediators, including histamine, serotonin, prostaglandins, bradykinins, neuropeptides, acetylcholine, and interleukin-2 (IL-2) and IL-31. Small unmyelinated type C nerve fibres transmit itch sensations, and specific spinal pathways may carry itch sensations to the brain.[10] Management of pruritus is challenging and depends on the cause; therefore, the primary condition must be treated. Both topical and systemic therapies are used.[11]

DISORDERS OF THE SKIN

> **QUICK CHECK 41.3**
> 1. Why does inflammation occur with contact dermatitis?
> 2. What factors are associated with atopic dermatitis?
> 3. What lesions are associated with papulosquamous disorders?
> 4. Give three examples of papulosquamous disorders.

Disorders of the skin may be precipitated by trauma, abnormal cellular function, infection, immune responses and inflammation, and systemic diseases.

Inflammatory Disorders

The most common inflammatory disorders of the skin are eczema and dermatitis. **Eczema** and **dermatitis** are general terms that describe a particular type of inflammatory response in the skin and can be used interchangeably. Eczematous disorders are generally characterized by pruritus, lesions with indistinct borders, and epidermal changes. These lesions can appear as erythema, papules, or scales; they can present in an acute, subacute, or chronic phase. Edema, serous discharge, and crusting occur with continued irritation and scratching. In chronic eczema, the skin becomes thickened, leathery, and hyperpigmented from recurrent irritation and scratching. The location of eczema is related to the underlying cause. Eczematous inflammations need to be differentiated from other rashes and dermatoses, particularly psoriasis.

Allergic Contact Dermatitis

Allergic contact dermatitis is a common form of T-cell–mediated or delayed hypersensitivity. (See Chapter 8 for different types of allergic responses.) The response is an interaction of skin barrier function, reaction to irritants, and neuronal responses, such as pruritus. Genetic susceptibility involves several genes, including loss-of-function mutations in the gene encoding the epidermal protein filaggrin. Various

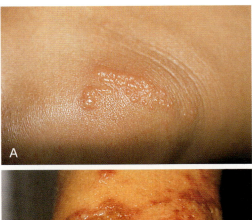
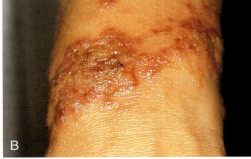

FIGURE 41.5 Poison Ivy. A, Poison ivy on knee. **B,** Poison ivy dermatitis. (Courtesy Department of Dermatology, School of Medicine, University of Utah, Salt Lake City, UT.)

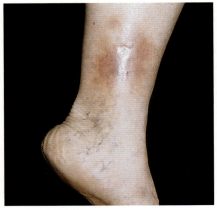

FIGURE 41.6 Stasis Ulcer. (Courtesy Department of Dermatology, School of Medicine, University of Utah, Salt Lake City, UT.)

allergens (e.g., microorganisms, chemicals, foreign proteins, latex, medications, metals) can form the sensitizing antigen. Contact with poison ivy is a common example (Figure 41.5). As the allergen contacts the skin, the allergen is bound to a carrier protein, forming a sensitizing antigen. The Langerhans cells (antigen-presenting dendritic cells) process the antigen and present it to T lymphocytes (T cells). T cells then become sensitized to the antigen, inducing the release of inflammatory cytokines and the symptoms of dermatitis.[12] In latex allergy, there is either a type IV hypersensitivity reaction to chemicals used in latex rubber processing or a type I immediate hypersensitivity reaction with immunoglobulin E (IgE) antibodies formed in response to latex rubber protein.[13]

In delayed hypersensitivity (type IV), several hours pass before an immunological response is apparent. The T cells play an important role because they differentiate and secrete lymphokines that affect macrophage (Langerhans cells) movement and aggregation, coagulation, and other inflammatory responses (see Chapter 8). Sensitization usually develops with first exposure to the antigen, and symptoms of dermatitis occur with re-exposure.

The manifestations of allergic contact dermatitis include erythema and swelling with pruritic (itching) vesicular lesions in the areas of allergen contact. The pattern of distribution provides clues to the source of the antigen (e.g., hands exposed to chemical solutions or boundaries from rings and bracelets). The antigen must be removed for the inflammatory response to resolve and tissue repair to begin. Treatment may require topical or systemic steroids.

Irritant Contact Dermatitis

Irritant contact dermatitis is a nonspecific inflammatory dermatitis caused by activation of the innate immune system by proinflammatory properties of chemicals. The severity of the inflammation is related to the concentration of the irritant, length of exposure, and disruption of the skin barrier.[14] Chemical irritation from acids and prolonged exposure to soaps, detergents, and various agents used in industry can cause inflammatory lesions. The skin lesions resemble allergic contact dermatitis. Removing the source of irritation and using topical agents provide effective treatment.

Atopic Dermatitis

Atopic dermatitis (allergic dermatitis) is common in individuals with a history of hay fever or asthma and is associated with IgE antibodies. It is more common in infancy and childhood; however, some individuals are affected throughout life. Chapter 42 presents specific details about this disorder.

Stasis Dermatitis

Stasis dermatitis usually occurs on the lower legs as a result of chronic venous stasis and edema and is associated with varicosities, phlebitis, and vascular trauma (see Chapter 24). Pooling of venous blood traps neutrophils that may release oxidants and proteolytic enzymes. Increased venous pressure widens interendothelial pores with deposition of red blood cells, fibrin, and other macromolecules, making them unavailable for repair while promoting inflammation.[15] First, erythema and pruritus develop, followed by scaling, petechiae, and hyperpigmentation. Progressive lesions become ulcerated, particularly around the ankles and pretibial surface (Figure 41.6).

Treatment includes elevating the legs as often as possible, not wearing tight clothes around the legs, and not standing for long periods. Defined infections are treated with antibiotics. Treatment for chronic lesions with ulceration includes moist dressings, external compression or dressings, and vein ablation surgery.[16]

Seborrheic Dermatitis

Seborrheic dermatitis is a common chronic inflammation of the skin involving the scalp, eyebrows, eyelids, ear canals, nasolabial folds, axillae, chest, and back (Figure 41.7). In infants it is known as *cradle cap*. The cause is unknown. Proposed theories include genetic predisposition, phospholipases from *Malassezia* yeasts, immunosuppression, and epidermal hyperproliferation.[17]

The lesions develop from infancy to old age with periods of remission and exacerbation. The lesions appear as scaly, white or yellowish inflammatory plaques with mild pruritus. Topical therapy includes antifungal shampoos, calcineurin inhibitors, and low-dose steroids for acute flares. Corticosteroids should not be used for maintenance therapy.

Papulosquamous Disorders

Psoriasis, pityriasis rosea, lichen planus, acne vulgaris, acne rosacea, and lupus erythematosus exhibit papules, scales, plaques, and erythema. Collectively they are described as papulosquamous disorders.

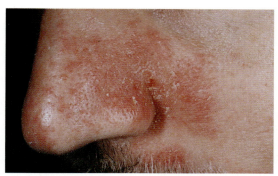

FIGURE 41.7 Seborrheic Dermatitis. (Courtesy Department of Dermatology, School of Medicine, University of Utah, Salt Lake City, UT.)

Psoriasis

Psoriasis is a chronic, relapsing, proliferative, inflammatory disorder that involves the skin, scalp, and nails and can occur at any age. Psoriasis affects about 1 to 4% of the population in countries north of the equator. The onset is generally established by 40 years of age. A family history of psoriasis is common, and the genetic mechanisms are complex. The onset of psoriasis later in life is less familial and more secondary to comorbidities, such as obesity, smoking, hypertension, and diabetes.[18,19]

The inflammatory cascade of psoriasis involves the complex interactions between macrophages, fibroblasts, dendritic cells, natural killer cells, T helper cells, and T regulatory cells. These immune cells lead to the secretion of numerous inflammatory mediators, such as interferon (IFN), tumour necrosis factor-alpha (TNF-α), and various other cytokines, including IL-12, IL-23, and IL-17. These inflammatory markers are the target for several therapeutic medications known as biologics (biotherapy).[20]

Both the dermis and the epidermis thicken because of cellular hyperproliferation, altered kerotinocyte differentiation, and expanded dermal vasculature. The turnover time for shedding the epidermis decreases to 3 to 4 days from the normal of 14 to 20 days, with many more germinative cells and increased transit time through the dermis. There is no cell maturation and keratinization, and the epidermis thickens and plaques form. The loosely cohesive keratin gives the lesion a silvery appearance. Capillary dilation and increased vascularization accommodate the increased cell metabolism but also cause erythema. The disease can be mild, moderate, or severe, depending on the size, distribution, and inflammation of the lesions. Psoriasis characteristically has both remissions and exacerbations.

The types of psoriasis include plaque (psoriasis vulgaris), inverse, guttate, pustular, and erythrodermic. **Plaque psoriasis** is the most common and affects 80 to 90% of individuals with psoriasis. The typical plaque psoriatic lesion is a well-demarcated, thick, silvery, scaly, erythematous plaque surrounded by normal skin (Figure 41.8). Small erythematous papules enlarge and coalesce into larger inflammatory lesions on the face, scalp, elbows, and knees and at sites of trauma (Koebner phenomenon). **Inverse psoriasis** is rare and involves lesions that develop in skin folds (i.e., axilla or groin). In **guttate psoriasis**, small papules appear suddenly on the trunk and extremities (Figure 41.9) a few weeks after a streptococcal respiratory tract infection. Guttate psoriasis may resolve spontaneously in weeks or months. **Pustular psoriasis** appears as blisters of noninfectious pus (collections of neutrophils), and **erythrodermic (exfoliative) psoriasis** exists with pruritus or pain with widespread red, scaling lesions that cover a large area of the body. **Psoriatic arthritis** of hands, feet, knees, and ankle joints develops in 5 to 30% of cases. **Psoriatic nail disease** is possible in all psoriasis subtypes with pitting, onycholysis, subungal hyperkeratosis, and nail plate dystrophy. A number of comorbidities correlate with the inflammatory mechanisms of psoriasis (see *Health Promotion*: Psoriasis and Comorbidities).

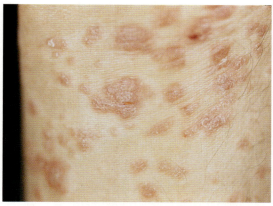

FIGURE 41.8 Psoriasis. Typical oval plaque with well-defined borders and silvery scale. (Courtesy Department of Dermatology, School of Medicine, University of Utah, Salt Lake City, UT.)

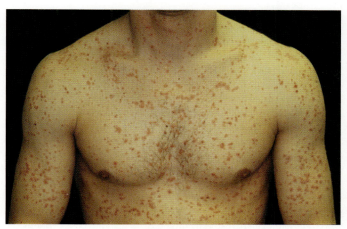

FIGURE 41.9 Guttate Psoriasis Following Streptococcal Infection. Numerous uniformly small lesions may abruptly occur following streptococcal pharyngitis. (Courtesy Department of Dermatology, School of Medicine, University of Utah, Salt Lake City, UT.)

HEALTH PROMOTION
Psoriasis and Comorbidities

In addition to skin and joint manifestations, including rheumatoid arthritis, severe psoriasis occurs with inflammatory bowel disease and metabolic syndrome, which includes hypertension, insulin resistance, dyslipidemias, abdominal obesity, nonalcoholic fatty liver disease, and increased risk for atherosclerosis and myocardial infarction that is independent of traditional risk factors for these diseases. The underlying mechanisms are related to increased levels of systemic proinflammatory mediators, such as tumour necrosis factor-alpha (TNF-α) and chemokines, which play a major role in the chronic inflammation, oxidative stress, and angiogenesis of psoriasis. The increased prevalence of cancer, particularly lymphoma, may be related to the pathogenesis of psoriasis or could be a consequence of immune modulation therapies. Crohn's disease is also associated with psoriasis, and there may be a genetic overlap between these two diseases. Treatment considerations need to include screening, monitoring, and managing these comorbidities.

Data from Baeta, I. G. R., Bittencourt, F. V., Gontijo, B., et al. (2014). *Anais Brasileiros de Dermatologia, 89*(5), 735–744; Boehncke, W. H., & Schön, M. P. (2015). *Lancet, 6736*(14), 61909–61917; Gisondi, P., Galvan, A., Idolazzi, L., et al. (2015). *Frontiers in Medicine (Lausanne), 2*, 1; Ni, C., & Chiu, M. W. (2014). *Clinical, Cosmetic and Investigational Dermatology, 7*, 119–132.

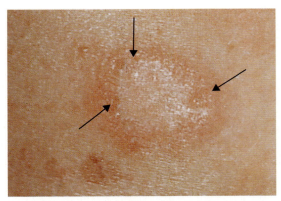

FIGURE 41.10 Pityriasis Rosea Herald Patch. A collarette pattern has formed around the margins *(arrows)*. (Courtesy Department of Dermatology, School of Medicine, University of Utah, Salt Lake City, UT.)

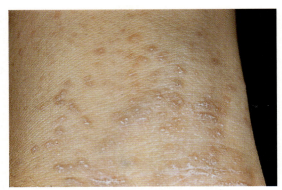

FIGURE 41.11 Hypertrophic Lichen Planus on Arms. (Courtesy Department of Dermatology, School of Medicine, University of Utah, Salt Lake City, UT.)

Treatment is individualized and related to maintaining skin moisture, reducing epidermal cell turnover and pruritus, and promoting immunomodulation. Treatment for mild psoriasis includes skin-directed therapy, such as medium- to high-strength topical corticosteroids, vitamin D analogues, emollients, and keratolytic agents (such as salicylic acid), and narrow-band ultraviolet (UV) light therapy. Systemic therapy is indicated for moderate to severe disease or in the presence of psoriatic arthritis. Current medications used in Canada to treat this condition include methotrexate (Apo-Methotrexate), oral retinoids, acitretin (Soriatane), and cyclosporine (Sandimmune) (short term). Newer biologics enable more specific treatment that targets inflammation itself. These biologics include the anti-TNF medications infliximab (Remicade), adalimumab (Humira), and etanercept (Enbrel). Ustekinumab (Stelara) is the most recent injectable biological treatment targeting IL-12 and IL-23. The IL-17 inhibitors are currently under investigation for their safety and efficacy.[21,22] A potential complication of biotherapy is the development of antimedication antibodies.[23]

Pityriasis Rosea

Pityriasis rosea is a self-limiting inflammatory disorder that occurs more often in young adults. A herpeslike virus (e.g., human herpesvirus 6 [HHV6] and HHV7) is most likely the cause.[24] Pityriasis rosea begins as a single circular, demarcated and salmon-pink lesion (**herald patch**), approximately 3 to 10 cm in diameter, and usually located on the trunk. Early lesions are macular and papular. Secondary lesions develop within 14 to 21 days and extend over the trunk and upper part of the extremities (Figure 41.10), but rarely on the face. The small erythematous rose-coloured papules expand into characteristic bilateral and symmetrically distributed oval lesions. The pattern of distribution on the back follows the skin lines around the trunk and resembles a drooping pine tree. Sloughing of the scales begins from the margin of the lesions, forming a collarette pattern. Itching is the most common symptom. Occasionally, headache, fatigue, or sore throat precedes the development of the lesions.

The diagnosis of pityriasis rosea follows the clinical appearance of the lesion. Secondary syphilis, psoriasis, medication eruption, nummular eczema, and seborrheic dermatitis are among the differential diagnosis considerations. The disorder is usually self-limiting and resolves in a few months with symptomatic treatment for pruritus or cosmetic concerns. UV light (with some risk for hyperpigmentation) or systemic corticosteroids may be used to control pruritus. Acyclovir (Zovirax) and erythromycin (Erythrocin) also may be used for treatment.[25]

Lichen Planus

Lichen planus (LP) is a benign autoimmune inflammatory disorder of the skin and mucous membranes.[26] The age of onset is usually between 30 and 70 years. The cause is unknown, but T cells, adhesion molecules, inflammatory cytokines, perforin, and antigen-presenting cells are involved. LP is also linked to numerous medications and hepatitis C virus.[27] The disorder begins with nonscaling, purple-coloured, flat-topped, polygonal pruritic papules 2 to 4 mm in size, usually located symmetrically on the wrists, ankles, lower legs, and genitalia (Figure 41.11). New lesions are pale pink and evolve into a dark violet colour. Persistent lesions may be thickened and red, forming hypertrophic LP. Oral lesions (oral LP) appear as lacy white rings that must be differentiated from leukoplakia or oral candidiasis.[28] Usually, oral lesions do not ulcerate, but localized or extensive painful ulcerations can occur, and there may be increased risk for oral cancer.[28] Chronic ulcerated lesions become malignant in 1% of individuals with the disease. Thinning and splitting of nails are common, and part or the entire nail may be shed.

Pruritus is the most distressing symptom. The lesions are self-limiting and may last for months or years, with an average duration of 6 to 18 months. Postinflammatory hyperpigmentation is a common consequence of the lesion. Approximately 20% of individuals have a recurrence. Diagnosis is based on the clinical appearance and histopathology of the lesion. Treatment is individualized and includes topical, intralesional, or systemic corticosteroids (second line for resistant LP), and systemic acitretin with or without adjuvant light therapy. Antihistamines are effective for itching, and short-term use of topical or systemic corticosteroids may be used to control inflammation. Mucous membrane lesions respond well to topical steroids, topical retinoids or immunomodulators (or both), and systemic glucocorticoids.[29]

Acne Vulgaris

> **✓ QUICK CHECK 41.4**
> 1. Describe the inflammatory lesion associated with lupus erythematosus.
> 2. Compare the three forms of pemphigus.
> 3. What is the characteristic lesion of erythema multiforme?

Acne vulgaris is an inflammatory disorder of the pilosebaceous follicle (the sebaceous gland contiguous with a hair follicle) that usually occurs during adolescence. It is discussed in Chapter 42.

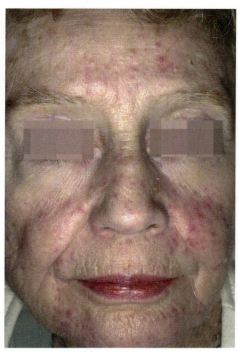

FIGURE 41.12 Granulomatous Rosacea. Pustules and erythema occur on the forehead, cheeks, and nose. (From Habif, T. P. [2016]. *Clinical dermatology* [6th ed.]. Saunders.)

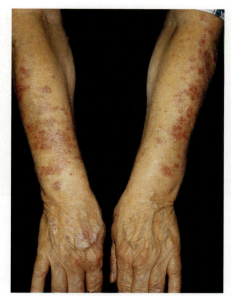

FIGURE 41.13 Subacute Cutaneous Lupus (Discoid Lupus Erythematosus). (Courtesy Department of Dermatology, School of Medicine, University of Utah, Salt Lake City, UT.)

Acne Rosacea

Acne rosacea is a chronic inflammation of the skin that develops in middle-aged adults. There are four subtypes of lesions: erythematotelangiectatic, papulopustular, phymatous, and ocular (eyelids and ocular surface). The exact cause is unknown, although evidence suggests the involvement of factors that trigger an altered innate immune response (i.e., sun exposure and damage, drinking alcohol or hot beverages, hormonal fluctuations, and *Demodex folliculorum* [mites]).[30] The most common lesions are erythema, papules, pustules, and telangiectasia. They occur in the middle third of the face, including the forehead, nose, cheeks, and chin (Figure 41.12). The lesions are associated with chronic, inappropriate vasodilation resulting in flushing and sun sensitivity. Sebaceous hypertrophy, fibrosis, and telangiectasia may be severe enough to produce an irreversible bulbous appearance of the nose (rhinophyma). Disorders of the eye often accompany rosacea, particularly conjunctivitis and keratitis, which can result in visual impairment. Facial application of fluorinated topical steroids may increase the severity of telangiectasias.

Photoprotection, using sunscreens, is essential along with avoidance of other triggers. Both topical (metronidazole [Flagyl], azelaic acid [Finacea]) and oral medications (tetracyclines and doxycycline [Teva-Doxycycline]) may be effective. Surgical excision of excessive tissue may be required for rhinophyma.[31]

Lupus Erythematosus

Lupus erythematosus is a systemic, inflammatory autoimmune disease with cutaneous manifestations (see Chapter 8). Discoid (or cutaneous) lupus erythematosus (DLE) is limited to the skin and can progress to systemic lupus erythematosus.[32]

Discoid (cutaneous) lupus erythematosus. Discoid (cutaneous) lupus erythematosus (DLE) usually occurs in genetically susceptible adults, particularly women in their late 30s or early 40s, but people of any age can be affected. The disease can be acute, subacute, intermittent, or chronic. Differentiation of subtypes is by physical examination, laboratory studies, histological analysis, and antibody serology direct immunofluorescence.[33] The lesions may be single or multiple and vary in size. Often the lesions are located on light-exposed areas of the skin, and photosensitivity is common. The face is the most common site of lesion involvement, with a butterfly pattern of distribution found over the nose and cheeks.

The cause is unknown but is related to genetic and environmental factors and an altered immune response to an unknown antigen or to ultraviolet B (UVB) wavelengths. There is development of self-reactive T cells and B cells (B lymphocytes), decreased number of regulatory T cells, and increased levels of proinflammatory cytokines. Autoantibodies and immune complexes cause tissue damage and inflammation[34] (Figure 41.13). On skin biopsy with immunofluorescent observation, there are lumpy deposits of Igs, especially IgM (lupus band test).[35]

The early lesion is asymmetric, with a 1- to 2-cm raised red plaque with a brownish scale. The scale penetrates the hair follicle and leaves a visible follicle opening (carpet-tack appearance) when removed. The lesions persist for months and then resolve spontaneously or atrophy. Healing progresses outward from the centre of the lesion, with residual telangiectasia and hypopigmented scarring. Atrophy of the dermis and epidermis can cause a depressed scar. Treatment options include protection from the sun and use of topical steroids, calcineurin inhibitors, antimalarial medications (e.g., hydroxychloroquine sulphate [Plaquenil sulphate]), and immunosuppressors. These medications must be used with caution to prevent serious side effects.[35]

Vesiculobullous Diseases

Vesiculobullous skin diseases share a common characteristic of vesicle, or blister, formation. Two such diseases are pemphigus and erythema multiforme.

Pemphigus

Pemphigus (meaning "to blister or bubble") is a group of rare autoimmune blistering diseases of the skin and oral mucous membranes caused by circulating autoantibodies directed against the cell surface

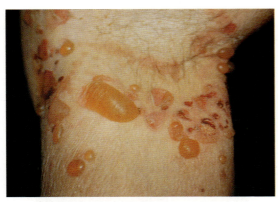

FIGURE 41.14 Bullous Pemphigoid. Generalized eruption with blisters arising from an edematous, erythematous annular base. (Courtesy Department of Dermatology, School of Medicine, University of Utah, Salt Lake City, UT.)

adhesion molecule desmoglein at the desmosomal cell junction in the suprabasal layer of the epidermis. IgG autoantibodies and complement component C3 bind to the desmoglein adhesion molecules, resulting in the destruction of cell-to-cell adhesion (acantholysis) in the basal layer of the epidermis (see Table 41.1) with fluid accumulation and the resulting symptom of blister formation (Figure 41.14). Pemphigus can occur in all age groups but is more prevalent in persons between 40 and 50 years of age. There is a genetic predisposition as well as environmental (viral infections, medication-induced, dietary intake, or physical effects such as radiation or surgery) and endogenous (emotional or hormonal stressors) influences. Pemphigus presents in varying forms, often with painful, superficial erosions prone to infection:[36,37]

- **Pemphigus vulgaris** is the most common form. Oral lesions precede the onset of skin blistering, which is more prominent on the face, scalp, and axilla. The blisters rupture easily because of the thin, fragile overlying portion of the epidermis.
- **Pemphigus vegetans** is a variant of pemphigus vulgaris in which large blisters develop in tissue folds of the axilla and groin.
- **Pemphigus foliaceus** is a milder form of the disease and involves acantholysis at the more superficial, subcorneal level of the epidermis (see Table 41.1), with blistering, erosions, scaling, crusting, and erythema usually of the face and chest. Oral mucous membranes are rarely involved.
- **Pemphigus erythematosus** is a subset of pemphigus foliaceus often associated with systemic lupus erythematosus with positive antinuclear antibodies. The lesions are generally less widely distributed.
- **Paraneoplastic pemphigus** is the most severe form of pemphigus and is associated with lymphoproliferative neoplasms.
- **Immunoglobulin A pemphigus** is the most benign form of pemphigus characterized by tissue-bound and circulating IgA antibodies targeting desmosomal or nondesmosomal cell surface components in the basement membrane of the epidermis.
- **Pemphigus herpetiformis** is a very rare form of pemphigus that resembles dermatitis herpetiformis (blistering lesions that have the appearance of herpes lesions) but with immunological and histological findings consistent with pemphigus.

The diagnosis of pemphigus is made from the clinical and histological findings of the skin. Immunofluorescence demonstrates the presence of antibodies at the site of blister formation. The clinical course of the disease may range from rapidly fatal to relatively benign. The primary treatment for pemphigus is systemic corticosteroids in combination with adjuvant immunosuppressants. Newer methods of treatment and a clearer understanding of the pathogenesis have improved the prognosis and decreased mortality.[38]

Erythema Multiforme

Erythema multiforme is a syndrome characterized by inflammation of the skin and mucous membranes, often associated with a T-cell–mediated immunological reaction to a medication or microorganisms (e.g., herpes simplex virus [HSV]) that targets small blood vessels in the skin or mucosa.[39] **Bullous erythema multiforme** involves the mucous membranes. It is relatively rare and occurs more often during the second to fourth decade of life; however, it can occur at any age. Immune complex formation and deposition of C3, IgM, and fibrinogen around the superficial dermal blood vessels, basement membrane, and keratinocytes are common histological findings. Edema develops in the superficial dermis, so vesicles and bullae form. The lesions vary in clinical presentation and may involve the skin or mucous membranes, or both. The characteristic "bull's-eye," or "target," lesions occur on the skin surface with a central erythematous region surrounded by concentric rings of alternating edema and inflammation. The lesions usually occur suddenly in groups over a period of 2 to 3 weeks. Urticarial plaques, 1 to 2 cm in diameter, can develop without the target lesion. A vesiculobullous form is characterized by mucous membrane lesions and erythematous plaques on the extensor surfaces of the extremities. Single or multiple vesicles or bullae may arise on a part of the plaque accompanied by pruritus and burning. The lesions heal within 3 to 4 weeks.

The most common forms of erythema multiforme are usually associated with severe medication reactions and include **Stevens-Johnson syndrome** (severe mucocutaneous bullous form involving 10% of body surface area) and **toxic epidermal necrolysis (TEN)** (severe mucocutaneous bullous form involving 30% of body surface area). T-cytotoxic cells in a human leukocyte antigen–restricted fashion mediate the immune mechanism related to medication reactions[40,41] (see Chapter 42 for pediatric considerations).

Prodromal symptoms of erythema multiforme, including fever, headache, malaise, sore throat, and cough, develop in approximately one-third of the cases. The bullous lesions form erosions and crusts when they rupture. There is necrosis of the epidermis in TEN. The mouth, air passages, esophagus, urethra, and conjunctiva may be involved when mucous membranes are affected. Blindness can result from corneal ulcerations. Difficulty eating, breathing, and urinating may develop with severe consequences. The disease can involve the kidneys and extend from the upper respiratory passages into the lungs. Severe forms of the disease can be fatal.

Recognizing the person's medication history that preceded the target lesion and performing a skin biopsy establish the diagnosis. Mild acute forms of the disease last 10 to 14 days and require no treatment. Any ongoing medication therapy should be withdrawn and re-evaluated and underlying infections treated. Monitoring of fluid and electrolyte balance is important in severe forms of the disease, and mucous membranes should be carefully managed with a bland diet, warm saline eyewashes, topical anaesthetics, or corticosteroids to maintain comfort and prevent infection. Cutaneous blisters can be treated with wet compresses of Burrow's solution. Ophthalmic, kidney, and lung involvement require special care. Resolution occurs in 8 to 10 days, usually without scarring. Mucosal lesions may take 6 weeks to heal.

Infections

> ✓ **QUICK CHECK 41.5**
> 1. Name two bacterial skin infections and describe the typical lesions.
> 2. Compare herpes zoster and varicella.
> 3. What features distinguish urticarial lesions?

Cutaneous infections are common forms of skin disease. They generally remain localized, although serious complications can develop with systemic involvement that can be life-threatening. The types of skin infection include bacterial, viral, and fungal. The commensal (normal) flora of the skin consists of aerobes, yeast, and anaerobes and often provides protection against pathogens that cause skin infections, including *Staphylococcus* and *Streptococcus*.

Bacterial Infections

Most bacterial infections of the skin are caused by local invasion of pathogens. Coagulase-positive *Staphylococcus aureus* and, less often, beta-hemolytic streptococci are the common causative microorganisms. Community-acquired methicillin-resistant *Staphylococcus aureus* (CA-MRSA [see Chapter 8]) also is a cause of serious skin infection, particularly skin abscesses.[42]

Folliculitis. Folliculitis is an infection of the hair follicle and can be caused by bacteria, viruses, or fungi, although *S. aureus* is the common culprit. The infection develops from proliferation of the microorganism around the opening and inside the follicle. Inflammation is a result of the release of chemotactic factors and enzymes from the bacteria. The lesions appear as pustules with a surrounding area of erythema. They are most prominent on the scalp and extremities and rarely cause systemic symptoms. Prolonged skin moisture, skin trauma (e.g., shaving facial hair), occlusive clothing, topical agents, and poor hygiene are associated contributing factors. Cleaning with soap and water and topical application of antibiotics are effective treatments.

Furuncles and carbuncles. Furuncles, or "boils," are inflammations of hair follicles (Figure 41.15). They may develop after folliculitis that spreads through the follicular wall into the surrounding dermis. The invading microorganism is usually *S. aureus*, including CA-MRSA (see Chapter 8). The infecting strain may spread to the skin from the anterior nares. Any skin area with hair can be infected, and one or several lesions may be present. The initial lesion is a deep, firm, red, painful nodule 1 to 5 cm in diameter. Within a few days, the erythematous nodules change to a large, fluctuant, and tender cystic nodule accompanied by cellulitis. No systemic symptoms are present, and the lesion may drain large amounts of pus and necrotic tissue.

Carbuncles are a collection of infected hair follicles and usually occur on the back of the neck, the upper back, and the lateral thighs. The lesion begins in the subcutaneous tissue and lower dermis as a firm mass that evolves into an erythematous, painful, swollen mass that drains through many openings. Abscesses may develop. Chills, fever, and malaise can occur during the early stages of lesion development.

Furuncles and carbuncles are treated with warm compresses to provide comfort and promote localization and spontaneous drainage. Abscess formation, recurrent infections, extensive lesions, or lesions associated with cellulitis or systemic symptoms require incision and drainage and are treated with systemic antibiotics.

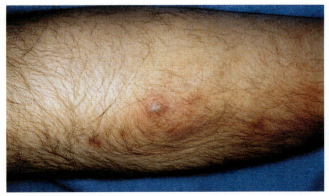

FIGURE 41.15 Furuncle of the Forearm. (Courtesy Department of Dermatology, School of Medicine, University of Utah, Salt Lake City, UT.)

Cellulitis. Cellulitis is an infection of the dermis and subcutaneous tissue usually caused by *S. aureus*, CA-MRSA, or group B streptococci.[43] Cellulitis can occur as an extension of a skin wound, as an ulcer, or from furuncles or carbuncles. The infected area is warm, erythematous, swollen, and painful. The infection is usually in the lower extremities and responds to systemic antibiotics, as well as therapy to relieve pain. Cellulitis also can be associated with other diseases, including chronic venous insufficiency and stasis dermatitis.

Cellulitis must be differentiated from necrotizing fasciitis. Necrotizing fasciitis is a rare, rapidly spreading infection. It is commonly caused by *Streptococcus pyogenes* starting in the fascia, muscles, and subcutaneous fat with subsequent necrosis of the overlying skin. Treatment requires antibiotics and, often, surgical debridement.[44]

Erysipelas. Erysipelas is an acute superficial infection of the upper dermis most often caused by *S. pyogenes*, beta-hemolytic streptococci, and *S. aureus*. The face, ears, and lower legs are involved. Chills, fever, and malaise precede the onset of lesions by 4 hours to 20 days. The initial lesions appear as firm, red spots that enlarge and coalesce to form a clearly circumscribed, advancing, bright red, hot lesion with a raised border. Vesicles may appear over the lesion and at the border. Pruritus, burning, and tenderness are present. Cold compresses provide symptomatic relief, and systemic antibiotics are required to arrest the infection.[45]

Impetigo. Impetigo is a superficial lesion of the skin that is caused by coagulase-positive *Staphylococcus* or beta-hemolytic streptococci. The disease occurs in adults but is more common in children (see Chapter 42).

Lyme disease. Lyme disease is a multisystem inflammatory disease caused by the spirochete *Borrelia burgdorferi* transmitted by *Ixodes* tick bites and is the most frequently reported vectorborne illness. The highest incidence of Lyme disease is among children. The microorganism is difficult to culture, escapes immunodefences, and hides in tissue. It spreads to other tissues by entering capillary beds.[46]

Symptoms of the disease occur in three stages, although 50% of infected individuals are symptom free.[47] *Localized infection* occurs soon after the bite (within 3 to 32 days) with erythema migrans (bull's-eye rash), a T-cell–mediated response usually with fever. Within days to weeks after the onset of the illness, there is *disseminated infection* with secondary erythema migrans, usually with myalgias, arthralgias, and more rarely meningitis, neuritis, or carditis. *Late persistent infection* (more common in Europe) can continue for years with arthritis, encephalopathy, polyneuropathy, or heart failure. The diagnosis of Lyme disease is based on the clinical presentation and history of the tick bite, if known. Serological tests confirm the diagnosis, although there is a delayed antibody response and the test may be negative during the first 3 weeks after infection.[48] Antibiotics (e.g., doxycycline [Teva-Doxycycline], which is not used in children younger than 8 years of age or in pregnant or breastfeeding women, or amoxicillin [Amoxil]) are common treatment.[49] Re-infection can occur. There is currently no vaccine for Lyme disease.[50]

Viral Infections

Herpes simplex virus. Skin infections with herpes simplex virus (HSV) are commonly caused by two types of HSV: HSV-1 and HSV-2. Either type can occur in different parts of the body, including oral and genital locations. Their differences are distinguished by laboratory tests. HSV-1, transmitted by contact with infected saliva, is generally associated with oral infections (cold sore or fever blister) or infection of the cornea (herpes keratitis), mouth (gingivostomatitis), and orolabia (lips/labialis), but it can also cause genital herpes. With initial (primary) infection, the virus embeds itself in sensory nerve endings, and it moves by retrograde axonal transport to the posterior root ganglion,

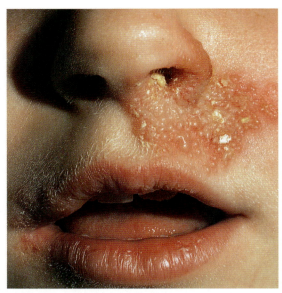

FIGURE 41.16 Herpes Simplex of the Lips (Labialis). Typical presentation with tense vesicles appearing on the lips and extending onto the skin. (From Habif, T. P. [2004]. *Clinical dermatology: a color guide to diagnosis and therapy* [4th ed.]. Mosby.)

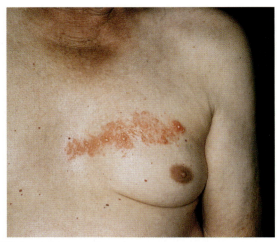

FIGURE 41.17 Herpes Zoster. Diffuse involvement of a dermatome. (Courtesy Department of Dermatology, School of Medicine, University of Utah, Salt Lake City, UT.)

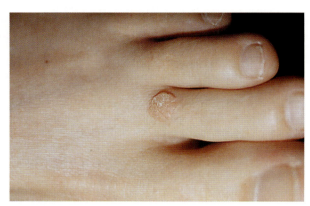

FIGURE 41.18 Verruca Vulgaris (Near Toes). (Courtesy Department of Dermatology, School of Medicine, University of Utah, Salt Lake City, UT.)

where the virus develops lifelong latency. During the secondary phase, the lesions occur at the same site from reactivation of the virus. The virus travels down the peripheral nerve to the site of the original infection, where it is shed. Exposure to UV light, skin irritation, fever, fatigue, or stress may cause reactivation.[51]

The lesions for HSV-1 appear as a rash or clusters of inflamed and painful vesicles (e.g., within the mouth, over the tongue, on the lips, around the nose) (Figure 41.16). Increased sensitivity, paresthesias, pruritus, and mild burning may occur before onset of the lesions. The vesicles rupture, forming a crust. Lesions may last from 2 to 6 weeks but usually resolve within 2 weeks. Treatment is symptomatic and includes topical or oral antiviral agents.[52]

Genital infections are more commonly caused by HSV-2. The virus is spread by skin-to-skin mucous membrane contact during viral shedding. Risk for infection is high in immunosuppressed persons or in persons who have sexual contact with infected individuals. Vertical transmission from mother to neonate accounts for significant neonatal neurological morbidity and mortality.[53] The initial infection is asymptomatic. With recurrent exposure, the lesions begin as small vesicles that progress to ulceration within 3 to 4 days with pain, itching, and weeping. Treatment is symptomatic and includes topical or oral antiviral agents. A vaccine has been effective in controlling recurrent infection, and progress is being made with prophylactic vaccines.[54]

Herpes zoster and varicella. Herpes zoster (shingles) and varicella (chickenpox; see Chapter 42) are caused by the same herpesvirus—varicella-zoster virus (VZV). VZV occurs as a primary infection followed years later by activation of the virus to cause herpes zoster (shingles). During this time, the virus remains latent in trigeminal and posterior root ganglia.

Herpes zoster has initial symptoms of pain and paresthesia localized to the affected dermatome (the cutaneous area innervated by a single spinal nerve; see Chapter 13), followed by vesicular eruptions that follow a facial, cervical, or thoracic lumbar dermatome (Figure 41.17). Compresses, calamine lotion, or baking soda alleviate local symptoms. Approximately 15 to 20% of individuals experience postherpetic neuralgia (pain) with reactivation of the virus.[55] Antiviral medications, tricyclic antidepressants, and analgesics are helpful treatments. The varicella vaccine is safe and effective in both children and adults, particularly those older than age 60. In children, the vaccine prevents chickenpox; and in adults, particularly the older person, the vaccine prevents herpes zoster (shingles).[56]

Warts. Warts (verrucae) are benign lesions of the skin caused by the many different types of human papillomavirus (HPV) that infect the stratified epithelium of skin and mucous membranes. The lesions can occur anywhere and are flat, round, or fusiform and elevated with a rough, greyish surface. Warts are transmitted by touch. Common warts (verruca vulgaris) occur most often in children and are usually on the fingers (Figure 41.18). Plantar warts are usually located at pressure points on the bottom of the feet. Treatment for warts includes cryotherapy or topical salicylic acid; new agents are now also available.[57,58]

Condylomata acuminata (venereal warts) are highly contagious and sexually transmitted. The cauliflowerlike lesions occur in moist areas, along the glans of the penis, vulva, and anus. Oncogenic types of HPV are a primary cause of cervical and other types of cancer[59] (see Chapter 33).

Fungal Infections

The fungi causing superficial skin infections are called *dermatophytes*, and they thrive on keratin (stratum corneum, hair, nails). Fungal disorders are *mycoses*; when caused by dermatophytes, the mycoses are called *tinea* (dermatophytosis or ringworm).

Tinea infections. Classification of tinea infections is according to their location on the body (Figure 41.19). Table 41.5 summarizes the most common sites.

Culture, microscopic examination of skin scrapings prepared with potassium hydroxide (KOH) wet mount, or observation of the skin with a UV light (Wood's lamp) are all involved with the diagnosis of tinea. Cultures establish the particular type of fungus; identification is necessary for diagnosis of hair and nail infections. Fungi have characteristic spores and filaments known as *hyphae* that are more prominent when prepared in KOH. The spores fluoresce blue-green when exposed to UV light. Treatment is related to the type of fungi and includes both topical and systemic antifungal medication.[60]

Candidiasis. Candidiasis is caused by the yeastlike fungus *Candida albicans* and normally can be found on mucous membranes, on the skin, in the gastro-intestinal tract, and in the vagina. *C. albicans* can, under certain circumstances, change from a commensal (normal) microorganism to a pathogen, particularly in the critically ill and those who are immunosuppressed.[61]

Factors that predispose to infection include (1) local environment of moisture, warmth, maceration, or occlusion; (2) systemic administration of antibiotics; (3) pregnancy; (4) diabetes mellitus; (5) Cushing's disease; (6) debilitated states; (7) infants younger than 6 months of age, as a result of decreased immune reactivity; (8) immunosuppressed persons; and (9) certain neoplastic diseases of the blood and monocyte/macrophage system. The commensal (normal) bacteria on the skin, mainly cocci, inhibit proliferation of *C. albicans*. *C. albicans* can activate the complement system by the alternative pathway and produce small abscesses. Candidiasis affects only the outer layers of mucous membranes and skin and occurs in the mouth, vagina, uncircumcised penis, nail folds, interdigital areas, and large skin folds. Table 41.6 lists the points of differentiation of various sites of candidiasis habitation.

The initial lesion is a thin-walled pustule that extends under the stratum corneum with an inflammatory base that may burn or itch. The accumulation of inflammatory cells and scale produces a whitish yellow curdlike substance over the infected area. The lesion ceases to spread when it reaches dry skin.[62] Topical antifungal agents are a common treatment.

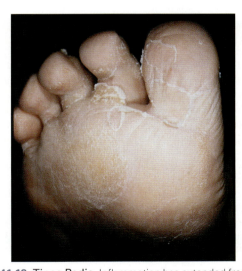

FIGURE 41.19 Tinea Pedis. Inflammation has extended from the web area onto the dorsum of the foot. (Courtesy Department of Dermatology, School of Medicine, University of Utah, Salt Lake City, UT.)

TABLE 41.5 Common Sites of Tinea Infections

Site	Clinical Manifestations
Tinea capitis (scalp)	Scaly, pruritic scalp with bald areas; hair breaks easily
Tinea corporis (skin areas, excluding scalp, face, hands, feet, groin)	Circular, clearly circumscribed, mildly erythematous scaly patches with slightly elevated ringlike border; some forms are dry and macular, and other forms are moist and vesicular
Tinea cruris (groin, also known as "jock itch")	Small, erythematous, and scaling vesicular patches with well-defined borders that spread over inner and upper surfaces of thighs; occurs with heat and high humidity
Tinea pedis (foot; also known as "athlete's foot")	Lesions between toes, which may spread to soles of feet, nails, and skin or toes; slight scaling; macerated, painful skin, occasionally with fissures and vesiculation
Tinea manus (hand)	Dry, scaly, erythematous lesions, or moist, vesicular lesions that begin with clusters of intensely pruritic, clear vesicles; often associated with fungal infection of feet
Tinea unguium or onychomycosis (nails)	Superficial or deep inflammation of nail that develops yellow-brown accumulations of brittle keratin over all or portions of nail

TABLE 41.6 Sites of Candidiasis Infection

Site	Risk Factors	Clinical Manifestations	Treatment
Vagina (vulvovaginitis)	Heat, moisture, occlusive clothing Pregnancy Systemic antibiotic therapy Diabetes mellitus Sexual intercourse with infected male	Vaginal itching; white, watery, or creamy discharge Red, swollen vaginal and labial membranes with erosions Lesions, which may spread to anus and groin	Miconazole (Monistat) cream Clotrimazole (Canesten) tablets or cream Nystatin (Nyaderm) tablets Ketoconazole (Nizoral) cream Loose cotton clothing
Penis (balanitis)	Uncircumcised Sexual intercourse with infected female	Pinpoint, red, tender papules and pustules on glans and shaft of penis	Any of the creams listed above Topical steroids for severe inflammation
Mouth	Diabetes mellitus Immunosuppressive therapy Inhaled steroid therapy	Red, swollen, painful tongue and oral mucous membranes Localized erosions and plaques appear with chronic infection	Nystatin (Nyaderm) oral suspension Clotrimazole troches Ketoconazole

Vascular Disorders

Vascular abnormalities commonly occur with skin diseases; they may be congenital or may involve vascular responses to local or systemic vasoactive substances. Blood vessels may increase in number, dilate, constrict, or become obliterated by disease processes.

Cutaneous Vasculitis

Vasculitis (angiitis) is an inflammation of the blood vessel wall that can result in bleeding aneurysm formation, or occlusion with ischemia or infection of surrounding tissue. The extensive vascular bed in the skin results in vasculitic syndromes that may be localized and self-limiting or generalized with multiorgan involvement. The initiating site may be the blood, the vessel wall, or the adjacent tissue. Small vessels are usually affected.

Cutaneous vasculitis develops from the deposit of immune complexes in small blood vessels as a toxic response to medications (phenothiazines, barbiturates, sulfonamides), allergens, or streptococcal or viral infection, or as a component of systemic vasculitic syndromes. The deposits activate complement, which is chemotactic for polymorphonuclear leukocytes, and proinflammatory cytokines.

The disorder is *cutaneous leukocytoclastic angiitis* (from the presence of leukocytes [i.e., neutrophils] in and around vessel walls). A systemic form (cutaneous systemic vasculitis) can involve other organs, including the kidneys, lungs, and gastro-intestinal tract. The pattern of skin involvement includes palpable purpura in the lower legs and feet (from the leakage of blood from damaged vessels) that may progress to hemorrhagic bullae with necrosis and ulceration from occlusion of the vessel. Lesions appear in clusters and persist for 1 to 4 weeks. The disease may be self-limiting and occur as a single episode. Biopsy confirms the diagnosis.

Identifying and removing the antigen (chemical, medication, or source of infection) is the first step of treatment. Corticosteroids and immunosuppressants may be used when symptoms are severe.[63]

Urticaria

Urticaria (hives) is a circumscribed area of raised erythema and edema of the superficial dermis. Urticarial lesions are most commonly associated with type I hypersensitivity reactions to medications (penicillin, Aspirin), certain foods (strawberries, shellfish, food dyes), environmental exposure (pollen, animal dander, insect bites), systemic diseases (intestinal parasites, lupus erythematosus), or physical agents (heat or cold) (see Chapter 8). The lesions are mediated by histamine release from sensitized mast cells or basophils, or both, which causes the endothelial cells of skin blood vessels to contract. The leakage of fluid from the vessel appears as wheals, welts, or hives, and there may be few or many that may be distributed over the entire body. Most lesions resolve spontaneously within 24 hours, but new lesions may appear. All possible causes of the reaction should be removed. Antihistamines usually reduce hives and provide relief of itching. Corticosteroids and β-adrenergic agonists may be required for severe attacks. Chronic urticaria (recurrent wheals for more than 6 weeks) is either idiopathic or autoimmune in origin and involves inappropriate activation of mast cells.[64] Angioedema (welts or swelling deeper within the skin or mucous membranes) can be both idiopathic or autoimmune in origin and more commonly affects the eyes and mouth.

Scleroderma

Localized scleroderma (morphea) means sclerosis of the skin and underlying tissue. The disease is rare and more common in females, and the cause is unknown. Genetic predisposition, autoimmunity, and an immune reaction to a toxic substance are possible initiating mechanisms of the disease. Autoantibodies are often recovered from the skin and serum of individuals with scleroderma. Impaired regulation of collagen gene expression by fibroblasts most likely underlies the persistent fibrosis. There are subtypes of localized scleroderma, but all involve thickening of the skin. The systemic form of scleroderma, as compared to the localized variety, has the following characteristic features: (1) sclerodactyly, (2) Raynaud's phenomenon, (3) abnormalities of the nail bed capillaries, or (4) internal organ involvement.[65]

Systemic scleroderma involves the connective tissues of the skin and many organs, including the kidneys, gastro-intestinal tract, and lungs. There are massive deposits of type I collagen with progressive fibrosis accompanied by inflammatory reactions as well as vascular changes in the capillary network with a decrease in the number of capillary loops, dilation of the remaining capillaries, formation of perivascular infiltrates, and development of occlusion and ischemia.[66]

The clinical features of systemic scleroderma can be summarized using the CREST acronym as a guide:

*C*alcinosis—calcium deposits in the subcutaneous tissue that cause pain

*R*aynaud's phenomenon—episodes of arteriolar vasoconstriction or spasm in response to cold or stress

*E*sophageal changes—swallowing difficulty related to acid reflux and increased esophageal fibrosis

*S*clerodactyly—tightening of skin over the fingers and toes leading to tapering of the digits with scarring and tissue atrophy

*T*elangiectasias—dilation of capillaries causing small (0.5 cm), weblike red marks on skin surface

The cutaneous lesions are most often on the face and hands, the neck, and the upper chest, although the entire skin can be involved. The skin is hard, hypopigmented, taut, shiny, and tightly connected to the underlying tissue. The tightness of the facial skin projects an immobile masklike appearance, and the mouth may not open completely. The nose may assume a beaklike appearance. The hands are shiny and sometimes red and edematous (Figure 41.20). Progression to body organs may occur, and death is caused by subsequent respiratory failure, kidney failure, cardiac dysrhythmias, or esophageal or intestinal obstruction or perforation.[67]

Suitable clothing and a warm environment are essential for protecting the hands. Trauma and smoking should be avoided. Treatment is individualized and based on severity and progression of the disease. Immunosuppression, UV treatment, and other therapies are common.[68]

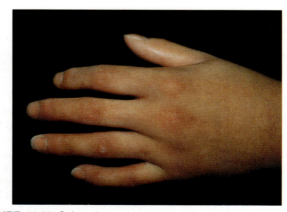

FIGURE 41.20 Scleroderma. Note the inflammation and shiny skin resulting from a combination of Raynaud's phenomena and scleroderma affecting the fingers (acrosclerosis). (Courtesy Department of Dermatology, School of Medicine, University of Utah, Salt Lake City, UT.)

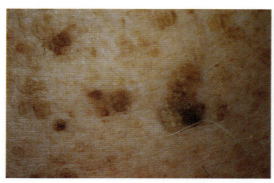

FIGURE 41.21 Seborrheic Keratosis. Typical lesion that is broad, flat, and comparatively smooth surfaced. (Courtesy Department of Dermatology, School of Medicine, University of Utah, Salt Lake City, UT.)

TABLE 41.7	Classification of Nevi
Type	**Common Characteristics**
Junctional nevus	Flat, well-circumscribed; vary in size up to 2 cm; dark-coloured hairs may be present; originate in basal layer of epidermis and can eventually reach cutaneous surface; most likely to develop into melanoma
Compound nevus	Most common in adolescents; majority of pigmented lesions in children; rarely does this lesion develop into melanoma; usually 1 cm in size; hairs may be present; surface is elevated and smooth
Intradermal nevus	Small, less than 1 cm, with regular edges and bristlelike hairs; colour ranges from fair skin tone to light brown; has slight likelihood of developing into melanoma

Benign Tumours

> **QUICK CHECK 41.6**
> 1. List two diseases caused by arthropod bites.
> 2. Compare keratoacanthoma and actinic keratosis.

Most benign tumours of the skin are associated with aging. Benign tumours include seborrheic keratosis, keratoacanthoma, actinic keratosis, and moles.

Seborrheic Keratosis

Seborrheic keratosis is a benign proliferation of cutaneous basal cells that produces flat or slightly elevated lesions that may be smooth or warty in appearance. The pathogenesis is unknown. These benign tumours are usually in older persons and occur as multiple lesions on the chest, back, and face. The colour varies from tan to waxy yellow, flesh coloured, or dark brown-black. Lesion size varies from a few millimetres to several centimetres, and they are often oval and greasy appearing with a hyperkeratotic scale (Figure 41.21). Cryotherapy with liquid nitrogen and laser therapy are effective treatments.

Keratoacanthoma

A **keratoacanthoma** is a benign, self-limiting tumour of squamous cell differentiation arising from hair follicles. It usually occurs on sun-damaged skin of older persons. Incidence is highest among smokers and males. The most commonly affected sites are the face, back of the hands, forearms, neck, and legs. The lesion develops in stages (proliferative, mature, and involution) over a period of 1 to 2 months with a histological pattern resembling squamous cell carcinoma (SCC).

Although the lesions resolve in 3 to 4 months, they can be removed by curettage or excision to improve cosmetic appearance and reduce the risk for evolution to SCC. A biopsy is performed to rule out SCC.

Actinic Keratosis

Actinic keratosis is a premalignant lesion composed of aberrant proliferations of epidermal keratinocytes caused by prolonged exposure to UVR. The prevalence is highest in individuals with unprotected, fair skin and is rare in those with darkly pigmented skin. The lesions appear as rough, poorly defined papules, which may be felt more than seen. Surrounding areas may have telangiectasias. Treatment options include cryoablation, photodynamic therapy, laser surgery, and topical therapies, such as 5-fluorouracil (Adrucil), diclofenac (Voltaren), imiquimod cream (Aldara), and ingenol mebutate (Picato).[69]

Excisions also may be performed, providing tissue for cellular analysis. The lesions should continue to be evaluated for progression to SCC. Protection from the sun with clothing or a sun-blocking agent to prevent lesions from developing elsewhere is advised.

Nevi (Moles)

Nevi (*sing.*, **nevus**) (also known as *moles* or *birthmarks*) are benign pigmented or nonpigmented lesions. Melanocytic nevi, formed from melanocytes, may be congenital or acquired and small (less than 1 cm) or large (greater than 20 cm). Congenital melanocytic nevi may be removed to reduce risk for cutaneous malignant melanoma.[70] During the early stages of development, the cells accumulate at the junction of the dermis and epidermis and are macular lesions. Over time, the cells move deeper into the dermis and the nevi become nodular and symmetric without irregular borders. Nevi may appear on any part of the skin, vary in size, occur singly or in groups, and may undergo transition to malignant melanoma. Classification of nevi is summarized in Table 41.7. Nevi irritated by clothing or trauma, or large lesions may be excised. Multiple and changing moles require regular evaluation.[71]

Skin Cancer

> **QUICK CHECK 41.7**
> 1. What is the most common skin cancer?
> 2. What malignancy can arise from melanocytes?
> 3. How is Kaposi sarcoma related to AIDS?

Basal cell carcinoma (BCC) and SCC (collectively known as *nonmelanoma skin cancers*) are the most prevalent forms of cancer. Malignant melanoma is the most serious and most common cause of death from skin cancer. Important trends related to skin cancer are described in Box 41.1.

Chronic exposure to UVR causes most skin cancers. Lesions are most common on the face, neck, hands, and other areas with intense sunlight exposure. Protection from the sun and avoidance of tanning beds, particularly during childhood, significantly reduce the risk for skin cancer in later years. Genetic mutations in oncogenes and tumour-suppressor genes (see Chapter 10) are associated with skin cancers. These mutations lead to loss of keratinocyte repair functions and apoptosis resistance of DNA-damaged cells.[72] People with darkly pigmented skin and those who avoid sunlight are significantly less likely to develop these malignant tumours. In people with darkly pigmented skin, basal cells contain more of the pigment melanin, a protective factor against sun exposure. Vitamin D may be an important tumour suppressor for the skin, but more research is needed.[73]

BOX 41.1 Important Trends for Skin Cancer

Incidence

In 2020, an estimated:
- 8 000 Canadians will be diagnosed with melanoma skin cancer.
- 1 300 Canadians will die from melanoma skin cancer.
- 4 400 men will be diagnosed with melanoma skin cancer and 870 will die from it.
- 3 600 women will be diagnosed with melanoma skin cancer and 450 will die from it.

Mortality
- Total estimated deaths from skin cancer in 2015 were 13 340:9 940 from malignant melanoma and 3 400 from other nonepithelial skin cancers.

Survival
- Basal and squamous cell carcinoma can be cured when detected early.
- Five-year survival for melanoma: it can be cured if diagnosed and removed early.

Risk Factors
- Excessive exposure to ultraviolet radiation from the sun or tanning salons
- Fair complexion
- Darkly pigmented skin: in people with darkly pigmented skin, skin cancer is less common, is diagnosed at a more advanced stage, and has a higher morbidity and mortality than in people with fair skin; it is often found on the palms of hands and soles of feet
- Occupational exposure to coal tar, pitch, creosote, arsenic compounds, and radium
- Immunosuppression

Warning Signs
- Any unusual skin condition, especially a change in the size, borders, or colour of a mole or other darkly pigmented growth or spot

Prevention and Early Detection
- Avoid the sun when ultraviolet light is strongest (e.g., 10 a.m. to 3 p.m.), avoid sun tanning beds, seek shade, use sunscreen preparations, especially those containing ingredients such as PABA (*para*-aminobenzoic acid), and wear protective clothing.
- Basal and squamous cell skin cancers often form a pale, waxlike pearly nodule, or a red, scaly, sharply outlined patch.
- Melanomas usually have dark brown or black pigmentation; they start as small molelike growths that increase in size, change colour, become ulcerated, and bleed easily from slight injury.

Treatment
- Options for treatment include surgery, electrodesiccation (tissue destruction by heat), radiation therapy, cryosurgery (tissue destruction by freezing).
- Malignant melanomas require wide and often deep excisions and removal of nearby lymph nodes; selective lymphadenectomy or immunotherapy can be used; vaccines and gene therapy are in development.

Survival
- For basal cell and squamous cell cancers, cure is virtually ensured with early detection and treatment; malignant melanoma, however, metastasizes quickly and accounts for a lower 5-year survival rate.

Data from Canadian Cancer Society. (2020). *Melanoma skin cancer statistics*. https://www.cancer.ca/en/cancer-information/cancer-type/skin-melanoma/statistics/?region=on.

Basal Cell Carcinoma

Basal cell carcinoma (BCC) of the skin is the most common cancer in the world, making it the most common skin cancer by default. BCC is most likely caused by UVR exposure and is also associated with arsenic in food or water.

BCCs have numerous subtypes, including superficial, nodular, pigmented, morpheaform, and combinations of each; thus, they can have very different clinical presentations—from superficial erythematous papules; to thick, pigmented nodules resembling melanomas; to erosive, necrotic, and ulcerating lesions (Figure 41.22). As the tumour grows, it usually has a depressed centre, a rolled border, and small blood vessels on the surface (telangiectasias) (see Figure 41.22). Early tumours are so small, they are not clinically apparent. The lesion grows slowly, often ulcerates, develops crusts, and is firm to the touch. If left untreated, basal cell lesions invade surrounding tissues and, over months or years, can destroy a nose, eyelid, or ear (for treatment, see Box 41.1). Metastasis is rare because these tumours do not invade blood or lymph vessels.

Squamous Cell Carcinoma

Squamous cell carcinoma (SCC) of the skin is a tumour of the epidermis and is the second most common human cancer. There are two types: (1) in situ (including Bowen's disease) and (2) invasive. UVR exposure causes SCC, and actinic keratosis is a precursor lesion. Other risk factors include arsenic at a higher level in drinking water, exposure to X-rays and gamma rays, immunosuppression, and fair skin. P53 gene mutations are common in SCC and produce tumour cells resistant to apoptosis.[72]

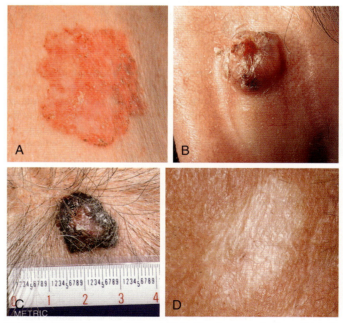

FIGURE 41.22 Types of Basal Cell Carcinoma. **A**, Superficial. **B**, Nodular. **C**, Pigmented. **D**, Morpheaform—recurrent tumour. ([A and D], from Bolognia, J. L., Jorizzo, J., & Schaffer, J. [2012]. *Dermatology* [3rd ed.]. Saunders; [B and C], from James, W. D., Berger, T. G., & Elston, D. M. [2009]. *Andrews' diseases of the skin: clinical dermatology* [11th ed.]. Saunders.)

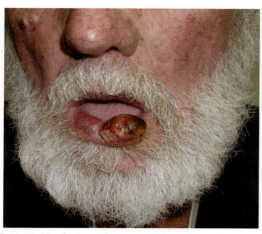

FIGURE 41.23 Lip Cancer. Biopsy confirmed squamous cell carcinoma. Lip vermilion shows diffuse actinic keratosis. (From Bagheri, S. C., Bell, B., & Khan, H. A. [2012]. *Current therapy in oral and maxillofacial surgery*. Saunders.)

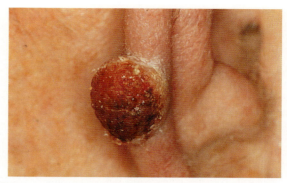

FIGURE 41.24 Squamous Cell Carcinoma. The sun-exposed ear is a common site for squamous cell carcinoma. (Courtesy Department of Dermatology, School of Medicine, University of Utah, Salt Lake City, UT.)

Premalignant lesions include actinic keratosis, leukoplakia (whitish discoloured areas), scars, radiation-induced keratosis, tar and oil keratosis, and chronic ulcers. In situ SCC is usually only in the epidermis (intraepidermal) but may extend into the dermis. Bowen's disease is a dysplastic epidermal lesion often found on unexposed areas of the body, such as the penis, and has flat, reddish, scaly patches. These lesions rarely invade surrounding tissue and, although they rarely metastasize, they do so more often than BCCs. Other components of the skin (e.g., sweat glands, hair follicles) can develop into skin cancer, but this outcome is relatively uncommon.

SCC is the most common cause of lip cancer, prevalent in older White men, with about 3 000 new cases per year.[74] The lower lip is the most common site. Long-term environmental exposure results in dryness, chapping, hyperkeratosis, and predisposition to malignancy. Immunosuppression, pipe smoking, and chronic alcoholism increase the risk for lip cancer. The most common lesion is termed *exophytic* and usually develops in the outer part of the lip along the vermilion border. The lip becomes thickened and evolves to an ulcerated centre with a raised border (Figure 41.23). These lesions have an irregular surface, follow cracks in the lip, and tend to extend toward the inner surface.

Invasive SCC can arise from premalignant lesions of the skin; it rarely develops from normal-appearing skin and is usually only in the epidermis (intraepidermal) but may extend into the reticular layer of the dermis (see Table 41.1). Invasive SCCs grow more rapidly than BCCs and can spread to regional lymph nodes. These tumours are firm and increase in both elevation and diameter. The surface may be granular and bleed easily (Figure 41.24). Treatment includes surgical excision and radiotherapy with consideration of adjuvant chemotherapy or epithelial growth factor receptor inhibitors for advanced disease.[75]

Cutaneous Melanoma

Cutaneous melanoma is a malignant tumour of the skin originating from melanocytes, cells that synthesize the pigment melanin, and arise from the neural crest. Malignant melanoma is the most serious skin cancer (see Box 41.1).[76]

Melanoma can also develop in the uvea of the eye and on mucous membranes.[77] There is an increased incidence worldwide. Risk factors include (1) a personal or family history (or both), (2) UVR exposure (including sunbed use before age 30), (3) immunosuppression, (4) fair hair, (5) fair skin with repeated sunburns, (6) freckles, (7) being a younger female, (8) being an older male, (9) geographical location, (10) past pesticide exposure, and (11) three or more clinically atypical (dysplastic) nevi[78] (see *Health Promotion: Melanoma in People With Darkly Pigmented Skin*). Melanoma is the most common cancer in White women 25 to 29 years old.[79]

HEALTH PROMOTION

Melanoma in People with Darkly Pigmented Skin

The risk for melanoma is lower in people with darkly pigmented skin. However, they have more advanced disease when diagnosed and a higher death rate. Associated factors include location of the lesion on palms, soles, and subungual sites (e.g., acral lentiginous melanoma) and lower socioeconomic status and education level. These melanomas may represent molecularly distinct cancers that are inherently more aggressive. The location of the lesions may contribute to delayed detection or misdiagnosis. The role of UVR in the risk for melanoma in people with darkly pigmented skin is not clear and research is needed. Genetic mutations may be a contributing factor. Educational programs to increase awareness of risk for melanoma among people with darkly pigmented skin, screening, and self-examination can improve outcomes.

Data from Alexandrescu, D. T., Maslin, B., Kauffman, C. L., et al. (2013). *Dermatologic Surgery, 39*(9), 1291–1303; Rouhani, P., Hu, S., & Kirsner, R. S. (2008). *Cancer Control, 15*(3), 248–253; Stubblefield, J., & Kelly, B. (2014). *Surgical Clinics of North America, 94*(5), 1115–1126.

Cutaneous melanomas arise as a result of malignant degeneration of melanocytes located either along the basal layer of the epidermis (see Figure 41.1) or in a benign melanocytic nevus. The clinical varieties of cutaneous melanoma include superficial spreading melanoma, the most common; lentigo malignant melanoma (Figure 41.25), frequently found in older persons and confused with age spots; primary nodular melanoma, an aggressive tumour; and acral lentiginous melanoma, which is rare and aggressive and occurs on non-hair-bearing surfaces (i.e., palms of the hands and soles of the feet) and mucous membranes in people with darker skin.

The pathogenesis of malignant melanoma is complex. Most familial melanomas are associated with cyclin-dependent kinase 4 gene (*CDK4*) and cyclin-dependent kinase inhibitor 2 A gene (*p16/CDKN2A*), located on chromosome 9p21. The *CDKN2A* gene encodes two potent tumour-suppressor proteins (p16 and p14^{ARF}) that are cell-cycle inhibitors. Both *CDKN2A* and *CDK4* are highly penetrant susceptibility genes and result in melanomas. A number of proto-oncogenes have been identified, including *BRAF* point mutations and genes involved in the regulation of mitogen-activated protein kinase (MAPK), and other signalling pathways. Melanomas have a high mutation rate stimulated by UVR, making gene sequencing difficult.[80]

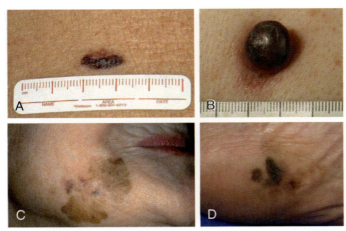

FIGURE 41.25 Lentigo Malignant Melanoma. **A**, Superficial spreading melanoma. **B**, Nodular melanoma. **C**, Lentigo malignant melanoma. **D**, Acral lentiginous melanoma on plantar surface of foot. (From Bolognia, J. L., Schaffer, J., Duncan, K., et al. [2014]. *Dermatology essentials*. Saunders.)

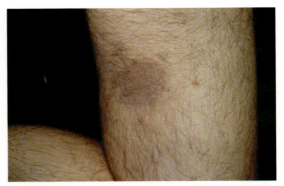

FIGURE 41.26 Kaposi Sarcoma. The purple lesion commonly seen on the skin. (Courtesy Department of Dermatology, School of Medicine, University of Utah, Salt Lake City, UT.)

The relationship between nevi and melanoma makes it important for the clinician to understand the various forms of nevi (see Table 41.7). Most nevi never become suspicious; however, suspicious pigmented nevi need to be evaluated and removed.[71] Indications for biopsy, including sentinel lymph node biopsy, are colour change, size change, irregular notched margin, itching, bleeding or oozing, nodularity, scab formation, and ulceration or an unusual pattern of presentation. The ABCDE rule is used as a guide: *A*symmetry, *B*order irregularity, *C*olour variation, *D*iameter larger than 6 mm, and *E*levation or *E*volving, which includes raised appearance or rapid enlargement. Staging is determined by lesion thickness (presence of *t*umour), lymph *n*ode involvement, and presence of *m*etastasis (TNM staging).[81]

Treatment of melanoma with no evidence of metastatic disease involves a wide surgical excision of the primary lesion site. A lymph node biopsy of the peripherally draining lymph node (sentinel node) is warranted for lesions greater than 1 mm deep. Lesions on the extremities have the best surgical prognosis. Radiation therapy, chemotherapy, and immunotherapy inhibiting the MAPK pathway and *BRAF* mutations are used to treat metastatic disease and have demonstrated long-term improvement in disease outcome.[82] There are some promising new immunotherapies for advanced disease, including checkpoint inhibitors (anti-PD1 antibodies [pembrolizumab (Keytruda), nivolumab (Opdivo)], anti-CTLA4 (cytotoxic T-lymphocyte associated protein 4) antibody [ipilimumab (Yervoy)]), and targeted therapy (*BRAF* or *MEK* inhibition, or both).[83] Vaccines, cell therapy, and biomarkers are under continuing investigation.[84] Early detection is critical to decreasing mortality from metastatic disease.

Kaposi Sarcoma

Kaposi sarcoma (KS) is a vascular malignancy associated with immunodeficiency states and occurs among transplant recipients taking immunosuppressive medications. Genetic and environmental cofactors determine disease progression. Human herpesvirus 8 is found in the lesions of KS. Four forms of the disease have been described: classic (more benign), epidemic (rapidly progressive and associated with acquired immune deficiency syndrome [AIDS]), African endemic, and iatrogenic (associated with immunosuppressant treatment, including organ transplant).[85]

The endothelial cell is thought to be the progenitor of KS. The lesions emerge as purplish-brown macules and develop into plaques and nodules with angioproliferation. They tend to be multifocal rather than spreading by metastasis. The lesions initially appear over the lower extremities in the classic form (Figure 41.26). The rapidly progressive form associated with AIDS tends to spread symmetrically over the upper body, particularly the face and oral mucosa. The lesions are often pruritic and painful. About 75% of individuals with epidemic KS have involvement of lymph nodes, particularly in the gastro-intestinal tract and lungs. Organ involvement is much less common in the classic form. The rapidly progressive form has a poor prognosis and shorter survival rates than the classic form. (See Chapter 8 for a further discussion of AIDS.)

Diagnosis is by medical history, physical examination, and skin biopsy, with a high index of suspicion for those with immunodeficiency. Chest X-ray reveals lesions in the lungs. Local lesions can be excised. Multiple disseminated lesions may be treated with a combination of α-interferon, radiotherapy, and cytotoxic medications. Antiangiogenic agents are being tested. Individuals receiving highly active antiretroviral therapy have a markedly reduced incidence of KS.[86]

Primary Cutaneous Lymphomas

Primary cutaneous lymphomas are cutaneous T-cell and B-cell lymphomas present in the skin without evidence of extracutaneous disease at the time of diagnosis (see Chapter 21 for classification and general pathophysiology of lymphomas). Cutaneous lymphomas are rare but are the second most common site of extranodal non-Hodgkin lymphoma. The incidence rate is about 1 per 100 000, and the cause of these lesions is unknown.[87] Cutaneous lymphomas are more common in men and generally present after age 50.

Cutaneous lymphomas develop from clonal expansion of B cells, T-helper cells, and rarely T-suppressor cells. The most common is cutaneous T-cell lymphoma (66%), and mycosis fungoides is the most prominent subtype. **Mycosis fungoides** can present as focal or widespread erythematous patches or plaques, follicular papules, comedone-like lesions, and tumours. There may be patches of alopecia. The lesions progress over a period of months or years.

The differential diagnosis of the different types of cutaneous lymphomas is based on clinical manifestations, histological appearance, immunological and cytogenetic features, and response to appropriate treatment. Treatment is based on staging of the disease and includes topical and systemic medications and phototherapy.[88,89]

Burns

> **QUICK CHECK 41.8**
> 1. Describe the four degrees of burn injury.
> 2. What dangers accompany frostbite?
> 3. What is alopecia? Compare the different types.
> 4. Describe two disorders of the nail.

In 2018, the World Health Organization estimated that burns cause approximately 180 000 deaths per year (https://www.who.int/newsroom/fact-sheets/detail/burns).[90] Burns may be the result of thermal or nonthermal sources including chemical, electrical, or radioactive sources. Thermal injuries result from thermal contact, scalds, or radiation. Direct contact, inhalation, and ingestion of acids, alkalis, or blistering agents cause chemical burns. Electrical burns occur with the passage of electrical current through the body to the ground or electrical flames or flashes. In addition to cutaneous injury, burns can be associated with smoke inhalation and other traumatic injuries that exacerbate local and systemic responses. There is often a need for ventilatory support with inhalation injury.[91]

Burn Wound Depth

The depth of injury identifies the level of tissue destruction; the extent of injury determines clinical management, healing, and mortality. Table 41.8 summarizes the four categories describing the depth of burns.

First-degree burns require no treatment unless the person is an older person or an infant, in which case severe nausea and vomiting may lead to inadequate fluid intake and dehydration. Fluid therapy may be required in these cases. First-degree burns heal in 3 to 5 days without scarring.

Second-degree burns are either superficial partial-thickness burns or deep partial-thickness burns. Superficial partial-thickness burns are thin-walled, fluid-filled blisters that develop within just a few minutes after injury (Figure 41.27). Tactile and pain sensors remain intact throughout the healing process, and wound care can cause extreme pain. Wounds heal in 3 to 4 weeks with adequate nutrition and no wound complications. Scar formation is unusual and is genetically

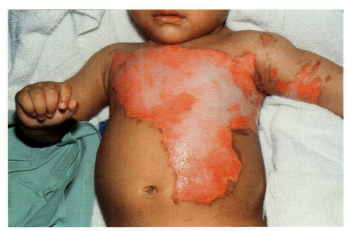

FIGURE 41.27 Superficial Partial-Thickness Burn Vs. Deep Partial-Thickness Burn. Superficial partial-thickness burn around edges (after debridement of blister and nonadherent epithelium), with deep partial-thickness burn in centre (note pale appearance and minimal exudates in the centre). (Courtesy Dr. Rogers.)

TABLE 41.8 Depth of Burn Injury

Characteristic	First Degree	SECOND DEGREE Superficial Partial Thickness	Deep Partial Thickness	THIRD DEGREE Full Thickness	FOURTH DEGREE Full Thickness and Deeper Tissue
Morphology	Destruction of epidermis only; local pain and erythema	Destruction of epidermis and some dermis	Destruction of epidermis and dermis, leaving only skin appendages	Destruction of epidermis, dermis, and underlying subcutaneous tissue	Destruction of epidermis, dermis, and underlying subcutaneous tissue, tendons, muscle, and bone
Skin function	Intact	Absent	Absent	Absent	Absent
Tactile and pain sensors	Intact	Intact	Intact but diminished	Absent	Absent
Blisters	Usually none or present after first 24 hr	Present within minutes; thin walled and fluid filled	May or may not appear as fluid-filled blisters; often is layer of flat, dehydrated tissue paper like skin that lifts off in sheets	Blisters rare; usually is layer of flat, dehydrated tissue paper like skin that lifts off easily	None
Appearance of wound after initial debridement	Skin peels at 24–48 hr; normal or slightly red underneath	Red to pale ivory, moist surface	Mottled with areas of waxy, white, dry surface	White, cherry red, or black; may contain visible thrombosed veins; dry, hard, leathery surface	Black and charred-appearing wound
Healing time	3–5 days	21–28 days	30 days to many months	Will not heal; may close from edges as secondary healing if wound is small	Will not heal; requires skin grafting; may require amputation, reconstructive surgery, or both
Scarring	None	May be present; low incidence influenced by genetic predisposition	Highest incidence because of slow healing rate promoting scar tissue development; also influenced by genetic predisposition	Skin graft; scarring minimized by early excision and grafting; influenced by genetic predisposition	Degree of scarring associated with reconstruction and grafting success

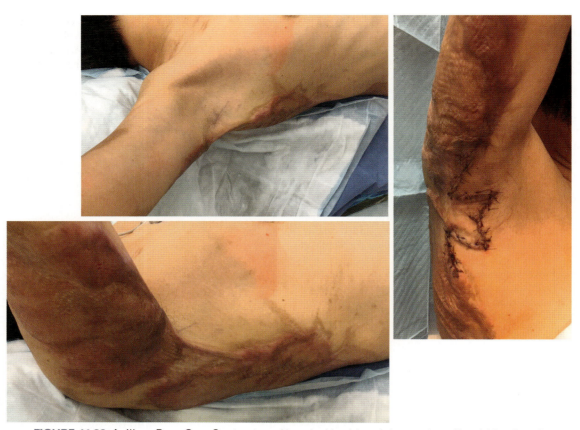

FIGURE 41.28 Axillary Burn Scar Contracture. Note the blanching of the anterior axillary fold and small ulceration from a deep partial-thickness burn, both indicating the diminished range of motion. (Courtesy Dr. Rogers.)

determined. **Deep partial-thickness burns** (Figure 41.27) look waxy white and take weeks to heal. Necrotic tissue is surgically removed followed by an application of the person's own unburned skin from another body area (autograft). Healing commonly results in hypertrophic scarring with poor functional and cosmetic results (Figure 41.28).

Third-degree burns, or **full-thickness burns**, have a dry, leathery appearance from loss of dermal elasticity (Figure 41.29). In areas of circumferential burns, distal circulation may be compromised from pressure caused by edema. **Escharotomies** (tissue decompression by cutting through burned skin) are performed to release pressure and prevent compartment syndrome (the compression of blood vessels, veins, muscles, or abdominal organs resulting in ischemia, necrosis, and irreversible injury).[92] Full-thickness burns are painless because all nerve endings have been destroyed by the injury.

Fourth-degree burns require skin grafting or reconstructive surgery.

The extent of **total body surface area (TBSA)** burned is estimated using either the "rule of nines" (Figure 41.30) or the modified Lund and Browder chart.[93] The severity of burn injury also considers many factors, including age, medical history, extent and depth of injury, and body area involved. Critical Care Services Ontario has defined criteria to assist health care providers in identifying who should be referred to a specialized multidisciplinary burn centre in their Burns Centre Consultation Guidelines (see https://admin.criticall.org/Criticall/media/Resources/BurnCentreConsultationGuidelines_2019-EN.pdf?ext=.pdf).

PATHOPHYSIOLOGY AND CLINICAL MANIFESTATIONS
Burn injury results in dramatic changes in many physiological functions of the body within the first few minutes after the event. Burns exceeding 20%

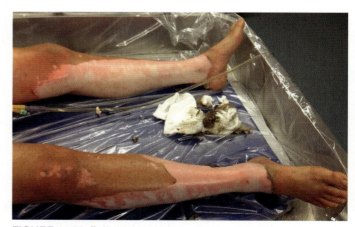

FIGURE 41.29 Full-thickness Burn. The wound is dry and insensate. (Courtesy Dr. M. G. Jeschke.)

of TBSA in most adults are considered to be major burn injuries and are associated with massive evaporative water losses and fluctuations of large amounts of fluids, electrolytes, and plasma proteins into the body tissues, manifested as generalized edema, circulatory hypovolemia, and hypotension.

The immediate (acute) systemic physiological consequences of major burn injury focus on the profound, life-threatening hypovolemic shock that occurs in conjunction with cellular and immunological disruption within a few minutes of injury (Figure 41.31). **Burn shock** is a condition consisting of a hypovolemic cardiovascular component and a cellular component.

CHAPTER 41 Structure, Function, and Disorders of the Integument

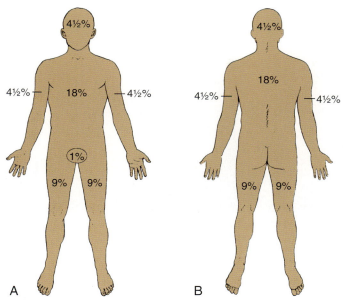

FIGURE 41.30 Estimation of Burn Injury: Rule of Nines. A commonly used assessment tool with estimates of the percentages (in multiples of 9) of the total body surface area burned. **A**, Adults (*anterior view*). **B**, Adults (*posterior view*).

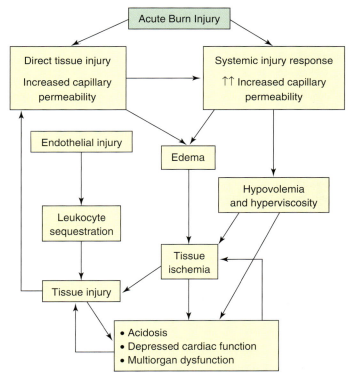

FIGURE 41.31 Immediate Cellular and Immunological Alterations of Burn Shock.

Hypovolemia associated with burn shock results from massive fluid losses and shifts to the interstitial space from the circulating blood volume. The losses are caused by an increase in capillary permeability that persists for approximately 24 hours after burn injury. There is decreased cardiac contractility and decreased blood volume. Blood is shunted away from the liver, kidney, and gut—known as the "ebb phase" of the burn response. This phase lasts during the first 24 hours

after burn injury and most organ systems are affected. Decreased perfusion of the viscera can decrease gut barrier function and result in translocation of bacteria and endotoxemia with sepsis. Intravenous fluid resuscitation is critical to restore the circulating blood volume during this phase, often using lactated Ringer solution. The rate of fluid replacement must be carefully monitored to prevent complications associated with fluid overload. Formulas are available (i.e., Parkland formula or the modified Brooke formula) to guide calculation of fluid volume replacement.[94,95]

Cellular metabolism is disrupted with onset of the burn wound, resulting in altered cell membrane permeability and loss of normal electrolyte allostasis. Many cytokines and inflammatory mediators in burn serum play a role in these cellular processes. The cardiovascular and systemic responses to burn injury are integrated with the cellular response but are described separately for clarification.

Cardiovascular and Systemic Response to Burn Injury

The clinical manifestations of burn shock are the result of multiple physiological alterations related to burn injury and release of inflammatory cytokines, in addition to the loss of fluid. The hallmark of burn shock is decreased cardiac contractility and decreased cardiac output with inadequate capillary perfusion in most tissues. Decreased cardiac output is related to myocardial depressant factor, as well as decreased intravascular volume.

Fluid and protein movement out of the vascular compartment results in an elevated hematocrit level and white blood cell count, and hypoproteinemia. If not treated immediately, profound hypovolemic shock and inadequate perfusion lead to irreversible shock and death within a few hours. Restoration of capillary integrity and renewal of a functional lymphatic system are required for resolution of the edema. Usually this occurs within 24 hours, but in extensive burns, it may take days or weeks. After the individual has reached the endpoint of burn shock, the term used to describe the person's condition is capillary seal.

The liver, with its metabolic, inflammatory, immune, and acute phase functions, plays a pivotal role in burn injury survival and recovery by modulating multiple metabolic pathways. Hepatic changes are common following a major burn, including fatty changes and hepatomegaly, which can influence burn wound recovery.[96] The hepatic response also alters clotting factors, leads to a hypercoagulable state, and can increase the risk for disseminated intravascular coagulation (systemic formation of microthrombi and abnormal bleeding).[97]

Cellular Response to Burn Injury

In addition to capillary endothelial permeability changes resulting in vascular fluid, electrolyte, and protein losses, there are transmembrane potential changes in cells not directly damaged by heat.[98] Cellular dysfunction resulting from burn injury impairs the sodium–potassium pump and results in increased amounts of intracellular sodium and water and decreased potassium level with disruption of the transmembrane potential. Intracellular calcium concentration may also be elevated, thereby influencing myocardial function.[99] Loss of intracellular magnesium and phosphate, hypocalcemia,[100] and elevated serum lactic dehydrogenase level occur.[101]

Metabolic Response to Burn Injury

Major burn injury (greater than 40% of TBSA) initiates a systemic hypermetabolic response with an increase in metabolic rate and a hyperdynamic circulation that begins 24 hours after burn injury—known as the "flow phase."[102] This phase can persist for up to 2 years following a burn.[102] Metabolic responses involve the sympathetic nervous system and other homeostatic regulators. Levels of catecholamines, cortisol, glucagon, are elevated, as is insulin resistance, and there is a corresponding increase in energy expenditure and increased gluconeogenesis, glycogenolysis, lipolysis, proteolysis, and lactic acidosis. Myocardial oxygen consumption increases and there is catabolic loss of muscle mass.[103] Hyperglycemia and insulin resistance can be prolonged in severe burns and require management with intensive insulin therapy to improve postburn morbidity and mortality.[104,105]

Burn injury initiates an inflammatory response with local activation and recruitment of inflammatory cells, such as leukocytes and monocytes, at the site of injury. These cells release inflammatory cytokines that contribute to the hypermetabolic state.[106] The metabolic rate increases in proportion to burn size and compensates for the profound water and heat loss associated with the burn. The inflammatory response and the release of cytokines at the wound level are magnified into a generalized systemic inflammatory response syndrome that can lead to multiple organ dysfunction.[107] Acute kidney injury occurs with hypovolemia, hypervolemia, and the inflammatory response.[108]

Hypermetabolism also increases the thermal regulatory set point and core and skin temperatures. There is persistent tachycardia, hypercapnia, and body wasting. Wound healing may be impaired, contributing to increased risk for infection and sepsis. Increasing the ambient temperature and early excision and grafting can decrease resting energy expenditure and improve mortality after major burns.[109] Inflammatory mediators circulating to the lung result in pulmonary edema that can be life-threatening.[110]

Immunological Response to Burn Injury

The immunological and inflammatory response to burn injury is immediate, prolonged, and severe. The result in individuals surviving burn shock is *immunosuppression* with increased susceptibility to potentially fatal systemic burn wound sepsis. White blood cells are altered at a time when their need to inhibit sepsis is vital.[111] Phagocytosis is impaired, and cellular and humoral immunity is abnormal. Individuals with altered immunocompetence or chronic disease before burn injury are at additional risk for complications, including wound sepsis.[112]

Macrophages, neutrophils, lymphocytes, and platelets release large amounts of inflammatory cytokines and antibodies, with their levels remaining elevated for weeks after burn injury. When combined with bacterial products, they produce peripheral vasodilation, pulmonary vasoconstriction, increased capillary permeability, and local tissue ischemia in the burn wound. There is distant organ dysfunction and multiple organ failure.[113]

Evaporative Water Loss

With major burn injury, there is loss of the skin's barrier function and ability to regulate evaporative water loss. Normally, the skin is the major source of insensible water loss (75%), and the lungs are minor sources (25%), with a total loss of only approximately 600 to 800 mL/day. This changes dramatically with burns because both the skin and the lungs have increased loss of water as a result of hypermetabolism and hyperventilation, especially in an intubated individual. Total evaporative losses exceed many litres per day in an adult with large burn wounds. Replacement of the loss is mandatory to prevent volume deficit and shock.

EVALUATION AND TREATMENT Burn recovery is complex and prolonged, with complications being the rule rather than the exception. Severity of inhalation injury is also a significant morbidity and mortality factor. The goal of burn management is wound debridement and closure in a manner that promotes survival. Scar formation with contractures is often a consequence of healing in deep partial-thickness and third-degree burns (Figure 41.32).

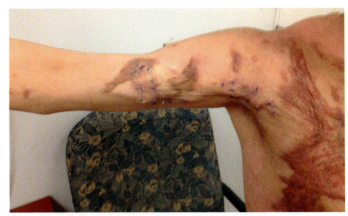

FIGURE 41.32 Hypertrophic Scarring. Deep partial-thickness thermal injury can result in extensive hypertrophic scarring. (Courtesy Dr. M. G. Jeschke.)

The essential elements of survival of major burn injury are (1) provision of adequate fluids and nutrition, (2) meticulous management of wounds with early surgical excision and grafting (Figures. 41.33), (3) aggressive treatment of infection or sepsis, and (4) promotion of thermoregulation.[113] Several medications are used for the management of severe burns, including β-adrenergic antagonists, β-adrenergic agonists, recombinant human growth hormone, insulin, androgenic steroids, and antibiotics.[102] Burn pain is almost always acute and severe, and treatment strategies are aggressive.[114] The risk of developing stress ulcers (Curling ulcers) is reduced with antacids or histamine H2-receptor antagonists.

Nutritional therapy focuses on early enteral therapy to reduce gut-mediated sepsis and to reduce the catabolic state.[115,116] Advancements in skin replacement procedures promote wound closure and healing.[117,118] Reconstructive surgery reduces complications associated with scarring and contractures.[119]

Cold Injury

Exposure to extreme cold includes a spectrum of injuries:[120]

- *Frostnip*—mild and completely reversible injury characterized by skin pallor and numbness
- *Chilblains*—more serious than frostnip; violaceous skin colour with plaques or nodules, pain, and pruritus, but no ice crystal formation; chronic vasculitis can develop and is usually located on the face, anterior lower leg, hands, and feet
- *Frostbite*—tissues freeze and form ice crystals at temperatures less than −2°C (28°F); progresses from distal to proximal and potentially reversible
- *Flash freeze*—rapid cooling with intracellular ice crystals associated with contact with cold metals or volatile liquids

The most common areas affected are fingers, toes, ears, nose, and cheeks. Mild frostbite (frostnip) is cold exposure without tissue freezing. It causes pallor and pain followed by redness and discomfort during rewarming, with no tissue damage. Frostbite occurs when tissues freeze slowly with ice crystal formation. Frozen skin becomes white or yellowish and has a waxy texture. There is numbness and no sensation of pain. Frostbite injury is related to direct cold injury to cells, indirect injury from ice crystal formation, and endothelial cell damage. During rewarming, there is progressive microvascular thrombosis followed by reperfusion injury with release of inflammatory mediators (including thromboxanes, prostaglandins, bradykinins, and histamines) and with impaired circulation and anoxia to the exposed area. Cyanosis and mottling develop, followed by redness, edema, and burning pain on rewarming in more severe cases. Edema can cause capillary compression and vascular stasis. Within 24 to 48 hours, vesicles and bullae appear that resolve into crusts that eventually slough, leaving thin, newly formed skin. Frostbite may be classified by depth of injury: superficial includes partial skin freezing (first degree) and full-thickness skin freezing (second degree); deep includes full-thickness and subcutaneous freezing (third degree) and deep tissue freezing (fourth degree). Third-degree and fourth-degree frostbite result in gangrene with loss of tissue.[121]

Immediate treatment of frostbite is to cover affected areas with other body surfaces and warm clothing. The area should not be rubbed or massaged. Rewarming for severe frostbite should occur after emergency transport. Immersion in a warm water bath (40 to 42°C [104 to 107.6°F) until frozen tissue is thawed is the best treatment. Pain is severe and should be treated with potent analgesics. Antibiotics may be given. Vasodilators, thrombolytics, hyperbaric oxygen, and sympathectomy may improve healing responses. Debridement or amputation of necrotic tissue occurs when there is a clear line of demarcation.[122]

DISORDERS OF THE HAIR

Alopecia

Alopecia means loss of hair from the head or body. Hair loss occurs when there is disruption in the growth phase of the hair follicle. Hair loss can be associated with systemic disorders such as hypothyroidism and iron deficiency, chemotherapy for cancer, malnutrition, compulsive

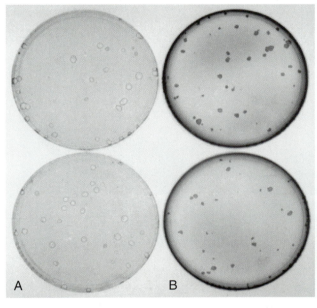
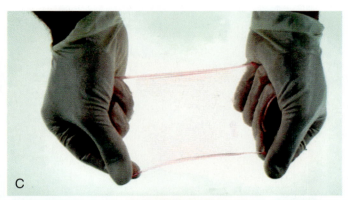
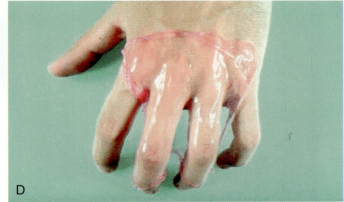
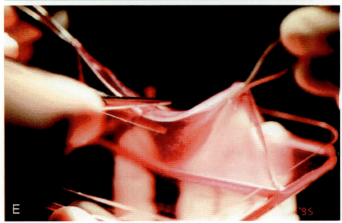

FIGURE 41.33 Cultured Epithelial Autografts. A & B, Keratinocyte culture. Keratinocytes from a severely burnt patient were isolated from a biopsy of unaffected skin and keratinocytes SC colonies, called holoclones, were cultivated in vitro for 2 or 3 weeks to form sheets of epidermal cells. **C–E,** These epidermal sheets were grafted onto the patient's burnt skin following Barrandon and Green's procedure.

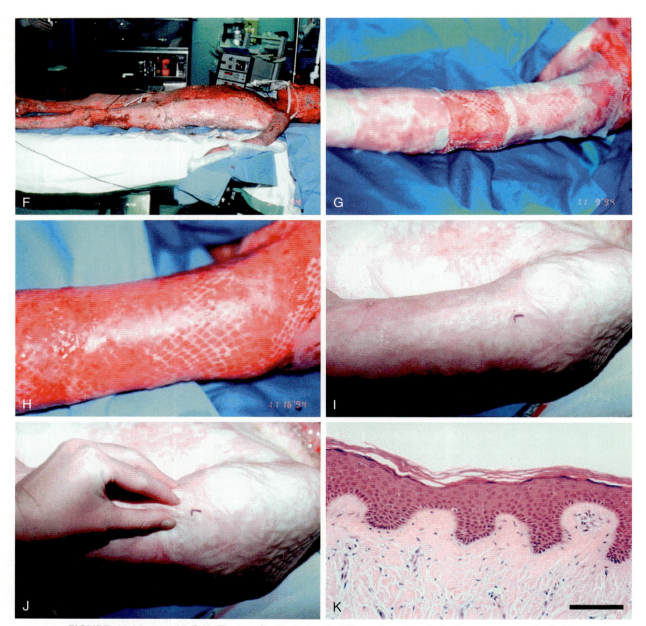

FIGURE 41-33, cont'd F–K, The graft skin is well differentiated and similar to non-grafted skin except the lack of hair follicle and sebaceous gland. (From Ronfard, V., Rives, J. M., Neveux, Y., et al. (2000). Long-term regeneration of human epidermis on third degree burns transplanted with autologous cultured epithelium grown on a fibrin matrix. *Transplantation, 70*, 1588–1598. DOI:10.1097/00007890-200012150-00009. Reprinted with permission.)

hair pulling (trichotillomania), traction on hair from braiding and ponytails, use of hair treatment chemicals, hormonal alterations, and immune reactions.[123]

Androgenic Alopecia

Androgenic alopecia is localized hair loss and occurs in about 80% of men. It is not a disease but a genetically predisposed response to androgens that clusters in families. Within the distribution of hair over the scalp, androgen-sensitive hair follicles are on top and androgen-insensitive follicles are on the sides and back. In genetically predisposed men, the androgen-sensitive follicles are transformed into vellus follicles.

Male-pattern baldness begins with frontotemporal recession and progresses to loss of hair over the top of the scalp. Minoxidil (Loniten) may be used to stimulate hair growth and finasteride (Apo-Finasteride) (a 5α-reductase inhibitor) may decrease the effect of androgens on hair follicles.[124]

Female-Pattern Alopecia

Some genetically susceptible women in their 20s and 30s experience progressive thinning and loss of hair over the central part of the scalp, and prevalence increases with advancing age. Contrary to male-pattern baldness, there is usually no loss of hair along the frontal hairline, but the hairs are shorter and thinner (follicular miniaturization). The mechanism of hair loss is unknown but related to genetic and hormonal changes.[125]

Alopecia Areata

Alopecia areata is an autoimmune T-cell–mediated chronic inflammatory disease directed against hair follicles and results in hair loss. There is rapid onset of hair loss in multiple areas of the scalp, usually in round patches. The eyebrows, eyelashes, beard, and other areas of body hair are rarely involved. Stressful events, cell-mediated immune cytokines, genetic susceptibility, and metabolic disorders, such as Addison's disease, thyroid disease, and lupus erythematosus, are associated with alopecia areata.[126]

The affected areas of skin are smooth or may have short shafts of poorly developed hair that breaks at the surface ("exclamation mark" hair). Regrowth occurs within 1 to 3 months, but hair loss may recur at the same site. Permanent regrowth of hair usually occurs. The pattern of hair loss determines the diagnosis. A biopsy may show a lymphocytic infiltrate around the follicle. There are several treatments for alopecia areata, including corticosteroids and topical immunotherapy, and new treatments are being tested.[127]

Hirsutism

Hirsutism occurs in women and is the abnormal growth and distribution of hair on the face, body, and pubic area in a male pattern. There is also frontotemporal hair recession. These areas of hair growth are androgen sensitive. Variations of hair growth in women are great, and a male pattern may be normal. Women who develop hirsutism may be secreting hormones associated with polycystic ovarian syndrome, adrenal hyperplasia, or adrenal tumours, and these disorders require treatment. If no hormonal pathological conditions exist, treatment may include cosmetic removal of hair, suppression of excessive androgen production, or blockage of peripheral androgen receptors.[128]

DISORDERS OF THE NAIL

Paronychia

Paronychia is an acute or chronic infection of the cuticle. One or more fingers or toes may be involved. Individuals whose hands are frequently exposed to moisture are at greatest risk. The most common causative microorganisms are staphylococci and streptococci. Occasionally *Candida* will be present. Acute paronychia is manifested by the rapid onset of painful inflammation of the cuticle, usually after minor trauma. An abscess may develop, requiring incision and drainage for relief of pain. The skin around the nail becomes more edematous and painful with progressive infection. Pus may be expressed from the proximal nail fold and an abscess may develop. The nail plate is usually not affected, although it can become discoloured with ridges. Chronic paronychia develops slowly, with tenderness and swelling around the proximal or lateral nail folds.[129]

Treatment includes prevention by keeping the hands dry. Oral antifungals are not effective because they do not penetrate the affected tissues. Topical application of thymol is usually effective.[130]

Onychomycosis

Onychomycosis (tinea unguium) is a fungal or dermatophyte infection of the nail unit. The most common pattern is a nail plate that turns yellow or white and becomes elevated with the accumulation of hyperkeratotic debris within the plate. Fungal infections of the nail are differentiated from psoriasis, LP, and trauma by culture and microscopy and the absence of pitting on the nail surface, which is characteristic of psoriasis. Treatment is difficult because topical or systemic antifungal agents do not penetrate the nail plate readily. Systemic antifungal medications are more effective. Surgical excision of the nail may be required. Education is essential to preventing recurrence.[131]

GERIATRIC CONSIDERATIONS
Aging and Changes in Skin Integrity

- Skin becomes thinner, dryer, and more wrinkled.
- DNA repair of damaged skin decreases.
- Epidermal cells contain less moisture and change shape.
- The dermis thins, producing translucent, paper-thin quality that is more susceptible to tearing.
- The dermis becomes more permeable and less able to clear substances, so those substances accumulate and cause irritation.
- There is a loss of epidermal rete pegs, which weakens the connection to the dermis and gives skin a smooth, shiny, and wrinkled appearance with an increased likelihood to tear from shearing forces.
- There is a loss of elastin, contributing to wrinkling.
- There is a loss of flexibility of collagen fibres, so skin cannot stretch and regain shape as readily.
- The barrier function of the stratum corneum is reduced, increasing risk for injury and infection.
- The significantly decreased number of Langerhans cells reduces the skin's immune response.
- The dermoepidermal border flattens, shortening and decreasing the number of capillary loops.

Other Skin Changes With Aging

- Wound healing decreases as a result of decreased estrogen in both men and women, decreased blood flow, and slower rate of basal cell and fibroblast turnover.
- There are fewer melanocytes; pigmentation becomes irregular, giving decreased protection from ultraviolet radiation and leading to greying of hair.
- Atrophy of eccrine, apocrine, and sebaceous glands causes dry skin.
- Pressure and touch receptors and free nerve endings decrease in number, causing reduced sensory perception.
- With compromised temperature regulation, loss of cutaneous vasomotion, and decreased eccrine sweat production, there is an increased risk for heat stroke and hypothermia.
- The nail plate thins, and nails are more brittle.

Data from Amaro-Ortiz, A., Yan, B., & D'Orazio, J. A. (2014). *Molecules, 19*(5), 6202–6219; Chang, A. L., Wong, J. W., Endo, J. O., et al. (2013). *Journal of the American Medical Directors Association, 14*(10), 724–730; Emmerson, E., & Hardman, M. J. (2012). *Biogerontology, 13*(1), 3–20; Kottner, J., Lichterfeld, A., & Blume-Peytavi, U. (2013). *British Journal of Dermatology, 169*(3), 528–542; Ramos-e-Silva, M., Boza, J. C., & Cestari, T. F. (2012). *Clinics in Dermatology, 30*(3), 274–276.

DID YOU UNDERSTAND?

Overview
1. The skin is the largest organ of the body and equals 20% of body weight. The major functions are to provide a protective barrier and to regulate body temperature.

Structure and Function of the Skin
1. The skin has two layers: the dermis and epidermis. The underlying hypodermis contains connective tissue, fat cells, fibroblasts, and macrophages.
2. The epidermis contains basal and spinous layers with melanocytes, Langerhans cells, and Merkel cells.
3. The dermis is composed of connective tissue elements, hair follicles, sweat glands, sebaceous glands, blood vessels, nerves, and lymphatic vessels.
4. The dermal appendages include nails, hair, sebaceous glands, and eccrine and apocrine sweat glands.
5. The papillary capillaries provide the major blood supply to the skin, arising from deeper arterial plexuses.
6. Pressure ulcers develop from pressure and shearing forces that occlude capillary blood flow with resulting ischemia and necrosis. Areas at greatest risk are pressure points over bony prominences, such as the greater trochanters, sacrum, ischia, and heels.
7. Keloids are sharply elevated scars that extend beyond the border of traumatized skin. Hypertrophic scars do not extend beyond the border of injury.
8. Pruritus is itching and is associated with many skin disorders. Small unmyelinated type C nerve fibres transmit itch sensation.

Disorders of the Skin
1. Following is a summary of the various skin disorders discussed in the chapter:

Skin Disorder	Cause/Description	Manifestations
Inflammatory Disorders		
Allergic contact dermatitis	Delayed hypersensitivity reaction	Erythema and swelling with pruritic (itchy) vesicular lesions in areas of contact
Irritant contact dermatitis	Prolonged exposure to chemicals	Erythema and swelling with itchy vesicular lesions in areas of contact
Atopic or allergic dermatitis	Family history of allergic disorder hay fever and increased IgE	Pruritis and thickening of skin over time
Stasis dermatitis	Chronic venous stasis and edema	Development of erythema and pruritis, initially, followed by scaling, petechiae, and hyperpigmentation
Seborrheic dermatitis	*Malassezia* yeasts	Scaly yellowish inflammatory plaques on scalp, eyelids, eyebrows, nasolabial folds, ear canals, axillae, chest and back
Papulosquamous Disorders		
Psoriasis	Chronic inflammatory skin disease associated with a complex inflammatory cascade involving multiple immune cells	Scaly, erythematous, pruritic plaques in epidermis and dermis
Pityriasis rosea	Self-limiting inflammatory disease from herpeslike virus	Oval lesions with scales along the edges along the skin lines of the trunk
Lichen planus	Autoimmune	Papular, violet-coloured inflammatory lesion of unknown origin manifested by severe pruritus
Acne vulgaris	Inflammation of the pilosebaceous follicle	Papules, pustules, and nodules, depending on the severity
Acne rosacea	Altered innate immune responses	On the middle third of the face with hypertrophy and inflammation of the sebaceous glands
Discoid (cutaneous) lupus erythematosus	Autoimmune disease that can affect only the skin	Cutaneous inflammatory lesions in sun-exposed areas with a butterfly distribution over the nose and cheeks
Vesiculobullous Diseases		
Pemphigus	Chronic, autoimmune, blistering disease	Begins in the mouth or on the scalp and spreads to other parts of the body, often with a fatal outcome
Erythema multiforme	T-cell–mediated allergic reactions to medications	Acute inflammation of the skin and mucous membranes (bullous form) with lesions that appear targetlike with alternating rings of edema and inflammation
Bacterial Infections		
Folliculitis	Infection of the hair follicle caused by bacteria, viruses, or fungi, most often by *Staphylococcus aureus*	Erythematous base with small papules and pustules with the hair in the center, though the hair cannot always be seen.
Furuncle	Infection of the hair follicle that extends to the surrounding tissue	A red raised bump on the skin that releases cloudy fluid or pus when ruptured

Skin Disorder	Cause/Description	Manifestations
Carbuncle	Collection of infected hair follicles that forms a draining abscess	Red and painful lump that increases in size over a few days, usually at the nape of the neck, on the back, and the thighs
Cellulitis	Diffuse infection of the dermis and subcutaneous tissue	Redness, warmth, and pain of the skin. Pus can accumulate under the skin and create blisters.
Erysipelas	Acute superficial infection of the skin upper dermis most often caused by *Streptococcus pyogenes*, beta-hemolytic streptococci, and *S. aureus*	Fever, chills, and malaise before the skin lesions that commonly affect the face, ears, and lower legs.
Impetigo	*Staphylococcus* or beta-hemolytic streptococci	Bullous or an ulcerative form. Red sores that rupture and ooze for a few days and then form a yellowish-brown crust. The sores are normally around the nose and mouth but can spread easily with contact.
Lyme disease	Immune response to the spirochete *Borrelia burgdorferi* and transmitted by ticks	Early disease starts with a "bull's eye rash", fever and malaise followed by arthralgias, cardiac conduction irregularities, and neurological symptoms.
Viral Infections		
Herpes simplex virus type 1 (HSV-1)	Cold sores but can infect the cornea, mouth, and labia; it can also cause genital herpes (genital variety more likely due to HSV-2)	Pharyngitis, tonsillitis, fever, malaise, sore throat, and vesicles on tonsils and pharynx that can rupture
Herpes zoster (shingles) and varicella (chickenpox)	Varicella-zoster virus	Headache, malaise, sometimes photophobia. Erythema, vesicles, pain, and lymphadenopathy
Warts	Benign, rough, elevated lesions caused by human papillomavirus; condylomata acuminata, or venereal warts, spread by sexual contact	Small fleshy grainy bumps that are rough to the touch and can become itchy or painful
Fungal infections		
Tinea	Fungal infections classified by location on the body	Lesion with central clearing surrounded by an advancing, red, scaly, elevated border.
Candidiasis	Yeast infections occurring in skin and mucous membranes, GI tract and vagina	White patches on tongue and other affected tissues. Problems swallowing and sore throat when in GI tract.
Vascular Disorders		
Cutaneous vasculitis	Inflammation of skin blood vessels related to immune complex deposition with purpura, ischemia, and necrosis resulting from vessel necrosis	Palpable purpura, petechiae, urticaria, ulcers, livedo reticularis (skin mottling from spasms in blood vessels), and nodules
Urticaria	Hypersensitivity reactions	Lesions appear as wheals, welts, or hives
Scleroderma	Autoimmune-mediated sclerosis of the skin that may also affect systemic organs and cause kidney failure, intestinal obstruction, or cardiac dysrhythmias	Hardening and tightening of skin, Raynaud's disease, and GI symptoms such as heartburn, depending on the tissue affected
Seborrheic keratosis	Proliferation of basal cells that produce elevated, smooth, or warty lesions of varying size, most common in older persons	Waxy, wart-like growth
Keratoacanthoma	Hair follicles on sun-exposed areas	A dome-shaped, crusty lesion filled with keratin that resolves in 3 to 4 months
Actinic keratosis	Pigmented scaly lesion that develops in sun-exposed individuals with fair skin; may become malignant as SCC	Red, scaling papule or plaque on a sun-exposed area, usually 1–3 mm in diameter
Nevi (Moles)	From melanocytes and may be pigmented or fleshy pink; can transition to malignant melanoma	Flattish, pigmented macules or thin papules
Skin Cancer		
Basal cell carcinoma	Most common skin cancer in the world resulting from UVR	Pearly pink or white, dome-shaped papule with prominent telangiectatic surface vessels that develop as the lesion enlarges
Squamous cell carcinoma	Tumour of the epidermis that may be in situ or invasive	Variable presentation that could include a firm red nodule, a flat sore with a scaly crust, a new sore on an old scar, a rough scaly patch on a lip evolving to an open sore, or a red sore inside the mouth
Kaposi sarcoma	Vascular malignancy associated with human herpesvirus 8 and immunodeficiency	Begins as discrete red or purple patches that are bilaterally symmetric and initially tend to involve the lower extremities. Patches become elevated, evolving into nodules and plaques.

Skin Disorder	Cause/Description	Manifestations
Cutaneous melanoma	Malignant tumour that arises from melanocytes with possible metastasis through the lymph nodes	Dark brown-to-black papule or dome-shaped nodule, which may ulcerate and bleed with minor trauma
Primary cutaneous lymphomas	Heterogeneous group of lymphoproliferative neoplasms, with lymphatic proliferation limited to the skin with no involvement of lymph nodes, bone marrow or viscera at the diagnosis	Patches of dry, discoloured (usually red) skin often appear. They can look like more common skin conditions such as dermatitis, eczema, or psoriasis. The patches tend to be dry, sometimes scaly and may be itchy.
BURNS	Thermal injuries: thermal contact, scalds, or radiation Chemical burns: direct contact; inhalation; ingestion of acids, alkalis, or blistering agents Electrical burns: Passage of electrical current through the body to the ground; electrical flames or flashes Burns are classified according to depth and extent of injury as first-, second-, third-, or fourth-degree burns.	Major burn injury causes profound edema and burn shock with severe inflammatory and increased metabolic response, as well as immune suppression and consequent delayed wound healing and risk for infection
COLD INJURY	Exposure to cold; injury usually occurs on the face and digits.	Direct injury to cells and impaired circulation resulting in coagulative necrosis

Disorders of the Hair

1. Alopecia is loss of hair from the head or body.
2. Male-pattern alopecia is an inherited form of irreversible baldness with hair loss in the central scalp and recession of the frontotemporal hairline.
3. Female-pattern alopecia is a thinning of the central hair of the scalp beginning in women at 20 to 30 years of age.
4. Alopecia areata is an autoimmune-mediated loss of hair and may be associated with stress or metabolic diseases; it is usually reversible.
5. Hirsutism is a male pattern of hair growth in women that may be normal or the result of excessive secretion of androgenic hormones.

Disorders of the Nail

1. Paronychia is an inflammation of the cuticle that can be acute or chronic and is usually caused by staphylococci, streptococci, or fungi.
2. Onychomycosis is a fungal or dermatophyte infection of the nail unit.

42

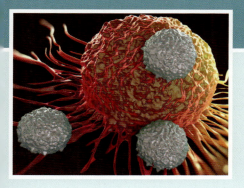

Developmental Alterations of the Integument

Stephanie Zettel, with originating chapter contributions by Noreen Heer Nicol and Sue E. Huether

Additional resources are available online at https://evolve.elsevier.com/Canada/Huether/pathophysiology.

CHAPTER OUTLINE

Acne Vulgaris, 1053
Dermatitis, 1054
   Atopic Dermatitis, 1054
   Diaper Dermatitis, 1055
Infections of the Skin, 1055
   Bacterial Infections, 1055
   Fungal Infections, 1056
   Viral Infections, 1057
Insect Bites and Parasites, 1060
   Scabies, 1060

Pediculosis (Lice Infestation), 1060
Fleas, 1060
Bedbugs, 1061
Cutaneous Hemangiomas and Vascular Malformations, 1061
   Cutaneous Hemangiomas, 1061
   Cutaneous Vascular Malformations, 1061
Other Skin Disorders, 1062
   Miliaria, 1062
   Erythema Toxicum Neonatorum, 1062

LEARNING OBJECTIVES

1. Differentiate between inflammatory and noninflammatory acne vulgaris.
2. Describe the clinical manifestations and treatment of acne conglobata.
3. Describe the clinical manifestations and treatment of atopic and diaper dermatitis.
4. Describe the common skin infections produced by bacteria, fungi, and viruses in children.
5. Compare and contrast the following childhood diseases: rubella, rubeola, roseola, chickenpox, shingles, and smallpox.
6. Describe how scabies and pediculosis are transmitted from one person to another.
7. Discuss the clinical manifestations and treatment of Lyme disease.
8. Compare and contrast the appearance of the various vascular skin disorders seen in children.
9. Define and describe miliaria and erythema toxicum neonatorum.

KEY TERMS

Acne conglobata, 1054
Acne vulgaris, 1053
Atopic dermatitis (AD), 1054
Bedbug, 1061
Chickenpox (varicella), 1059
Cutaneous hemangioma, 1061
Cutaneous vascular malformations, 1061
Diaper dermatitis (diaper rash), 1055
Erythema toxicum neonatorum, 1062
Fleabite, 1060
Herpes zoster (shingles), 1059
Hidradenitis suppurativa (inverse acne), 1054
Impetigo, 1055
Inflammatory (cystic) acne, 1053
Miliaria, 1062
Miliaria crystalline, 1062
Miliaria rubra (prickly heat), 1062
Molluscum contagiosum, 1057
Noninflammatory acne, 1053
Roseola, 1059
Rubella, 1057
Rubeola, 1058
Scabies, 1060
Smallpox (variola), 1059
Staphylococcal scalded-skin syndrome (SSSS), 1056
Strawberry (capillary) hemangioma, 1061
Thrush, 1057
Tinea capitis, 1056
Tinea corporis (ringworm), 1057

ACNE VULGARIS

> **QUICK CHECK 42.1**
> 1. What causes the inflammation of acne vulgaris?
> 2. What lesions are typical of atopic dermatitis in children?
> 3. What causes diaper dermatitis?

Acne vulgaris is the most common skin disease and occurs primarily between the ages of 12 and 25 years. Acne tends to occur in families, and genetic susceptibility may determine the severity of the disease. The incidence of acne is the same in both genders, although severe disease affects males more often.[1] Diets high in simple carbohydrates and dairy products are associated with acne.[2–4]

Acne develops at distinctive pilosebaceous units known as *sebaceous follicles*. Located primarily on the face and upper parts of the chest and

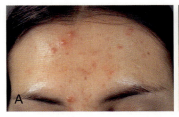
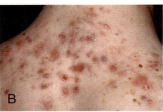

FIGURE 42.1 Acne. **A**, Inflammatory papules and pustules. **B**, Severe nodular cystic acne. (From Kliegman, R. M., Stanton, B. F., St. Geme, J. W., et al. [Eds.]. [2011]. *Nelson textbook of pediatrics* [19th ed.]. Saunders.)

back, these follicles have many large sebaceous glands, a small vellus hair (very short, nonpigmented, and very thin hair), and a dilated follicular canal that is visible as a pore on the skin surface. Acne lesions may be noninflammatory or inflammatory (cystic) (Figure 42.1). In **noninflammatory acne**, the comedones (skin-coloured papules) are open (blackheads) and closed (whiteheads), with distension of the follicle and thinning of follicular canal walls. **Inflammatory (cystic) acne** develops in closed comedones when the follicular wall ruptures, expelling sebum into the surrounding dermis and initiating inflammation. Pustules form when the inflammation is close to the surface; papules and cystic nodules can develop when the inflammation is deeper, causing mild to severe scarring. Both types of lesions may exist in the same individual.

Causes of acne include (1) hyperkeratinization of the follicular epithelium, (2) excessive sebum production, (3) follicular proliferation of anaerobic *Propionibacterium acnes*, and (4) inflammation and rupture of a follicle from accumulated debris and bacteria (see Figure 42.1). *P. acnes* shifts from being symbiotic to pathogenic and from being noninflammatory to inflammatory, and the causal mechanism is unknown.[5] Androgens (dehydroepiandrosterone sulphate and testosterone), synthesized in increasing amounts during puberty, increase the size and productivity of the sebaceous glands, which promotes *P. acnes*. *P. acnes* produces extracellular porphyrins and proinflammatory molecules, including chemotactic factors and lipolytic and proteolytic enzymes. The hydrolytic action of the enzymes converts triglycerides into free fatty acids. Free fatty acids activate Toll-like receptors, T-cell–associated and T-helper 17–associated inflammation, and edema that results in pus formation and breakdown of the follicle wall.[6]

The severity of acne in each individual determines its treatment. Preferred medications include combinations of a topical retinoid [Retin-A], benzoyl peroxide, and antimicrobial agents. Retinoids are *anticomedogenic* (i.e., they do not clog skin pores) and *comedolytic* (i.e., they prevent the formation of blemishes) and have some anti-inflammatory effects. Benzoyl peroxide is antimicrobial with some keratolytic effects. Antibiotics have anti-inflammatory and antimicrobial effects. Use of systemic therapies, including oral antibiotics, sex hormones, corticosteroids, and isotretinoin (Accutane; this medication requires pregnancy prevention), may be limited by side effects.[7] Acne surgery, including comedo extraction, intralesional steroids, and cryosurgery, is useful in selected individuals. Severe scarring may be treated with dermabrasion, lasers, and resurfacing techniques. Diets should avoid high glycemic index foods. Psychological support is important because acne negatively affects quality of life, self-esteem, and mood in adolescents and is associated with an increased risk for anxiety, depression, and suicidal ideation.[8] Special consideration must be given to treatment for those with darker skin because they have greater risk for hyperpigmentation and keloidal scarring.[9] Research is continuing on the development of vaccines to prevent acne.[10]

Acne conglobata is a highly inflammatory form of acne with communicating cysts and abscesses beneath the skin that can cause scarring. Remissions tend to occur during the summer, perhaps from more exposure to sunlight. This type of acne requires the use of systemic and combination therapies to prevent medication resistance.

Hidradenitis suppurativa (inverse acne) is a chronic inflammatory disease characterized by recurrent abscesses, sinus tract formation, and scarring. There is hyperkeratosis and occlusion of the pilosebaceous follicular ducts involving areas of skin where there are folds, hair follicles, and apocrine (sweat) glands (i.e., axillary, inguinal, inframammary, genital, buttocks, and perineal areas of the body). The cause is unknown, but it affects approximately 1 to 4% of the population and is more common in females. Aggravating factors include obesity, stress, and smoking. The lesions present as deep, firm, painful subcutaneous nodules that track and rupture horizontally under the skin. Treatment can include incision and drainage of nodules, culture of exudate, and administration of antibiotics (with concern about the presence of methicillin-resistant *Staphylococcus aureus* [MRSA]), topical or intralesional corticosteroids, and retinoids. The disease can recur for years, with negative effects on quality of life.[11]

DERMATITIS

Atopic Dermatitis

Atopic dermatitis (AD), also known as *atopic eczema*, is the most common cause of eczema in children. Approximately 17% of Canadians experience this at least one point in their lives.[12] More than half of these individuals develop asthma and allergies later in life.[13] Onset is usually from 2 to 6 months of age, and 85% of cases develop within the first 5 years of life.

The cause of this chronic relapsing form of pruritic eczema involves (1) an interplay of genetic predisposition; (2) altered skin barrier function associated with filaggrin gene mutations and filaggrin deficiency (proteins that bind keratin in the epidermis); (3) reduced ceramide (a stratum corneum lipid) levels; (4) decreased antimicrobial peptides; (5) altered innate immunity; and (6) altered immune responses to allergens, irritants, and microbes.[14] Filaggrin gene mutations are also associated with increased risk for asthma in AD and ichthyosis vulgaris (dry, scaly skin)[15] (Figure 42.2). An altered skin microbiome with formation of biofilm by *S. aureus* may cause exacerbations of eczema.[16]

AD has a constellation of clinical features that include severe pruritus and an appearance characteristic of eczema with redness, edema, and scaling. The skin becomes increasingly dry, itchy, sensitive, and easily irritated because the barrier function of the skin is impaired. Itching is the hallmark of AD, and rubbing and scratching to relieve the itch are responsible for many of the clinical skin changes of AD. In young children, a rash appears primarily on the face, scalp, trunk, and extensor surfaces of the arms and legs (see Figure 42.2). In older children and adults, the rash tends to be found on the neck, antecubital and popliteal fossae, and hands and feet. Individuals with AD also tend to develop viral, bacterial, and fungal skin infections in the eczematous areas. There are no specific laboratory features of AD that can be used for diagnostic and treatment purposes.[17] Most affected individuals show increased serum levels of immunoglobulin E (IgE), interleukin-4, and eosinophils (eosinophilia) and positive skin tests to a variety of common food and inhalant allergens.

Management of individuals with AD includes accurate diagnosis and comprehensive evaluation of triggers and response to treatment; management of confounding factors, including sleep disruption; and education of individuals and caregivers. Good therapy includes avoiding triggers and promoting skin hydration, including soaking baths and emollients.[18] Anti-inflammatory agents, such as topical corticosteroids and calcineurin inhibitors, are necessary during active flare-ups of eczema. Immunomodulator therapy and wet wrap therapy[19] are used for severe eczema. Systemic therapy includes the use of sedating

CHAPTER 42 Developmental Alterations of the Integument

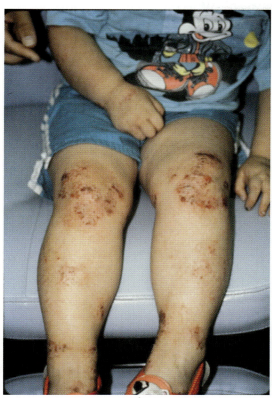

FIGURE 42.2 Atopic Dermatitis. Characteristic lesions with crusting from irritation and scratching over knees and around ankles. (Courtesy Department of Dermatology, School of Medicine, University of Utah, Salt Lake City, UT.)

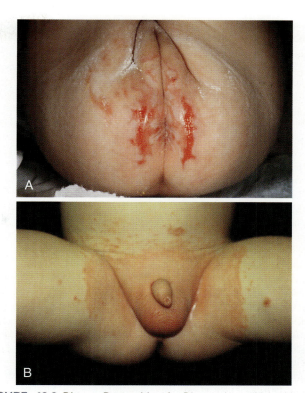

FIGURE 42.3 Diaper Dermatitis. **A,** Diaper dermatitis with erosions. **B,** Diaper dermatitis with *Candida albicans* secondary infection. (Courtesy Department of Dermatology, School of Medicine, University of Utah, Salt Lake City, UT.)

antihistamines and antibiotics. Research is in progress to develop molecule-specific targets to produce long-term disease remission.[20]

Diaper Dermatitis

Diaper dermatitis (diaper rash) is a form of irritant contact dermatitis initiated by a combination of factors, including prolonged exposure to and irritation by urine and feces as well as maceration by wet diapers or airtight plastic diaper covers. Disposable diaper designs have decreased the incidence of diaper dermatitis in infants. Often, diaper dermatitis is secondarily infected with *Candida albicans*. The resulting inflammation affects the lower aspect of the abdomen, genitalia, buttock, and upper portion of the thigh.

The lesions vary from mild erythema to erythematous papular lesions. Candidal (monilial) diaper dermatitis is usually very erythematous, with sharp margination and pustulovesicular satellite lesions (Figure 42.3).

Treatment involves frequent diaper changes to keep the affected area clean and dry or regular exposure of the perineal area to air, use of superabsorbent diapers, and topical protection with a product containing petrolatum or zinc oxide, or both. Topical antifungal medication is used to treat *C. albicans*, when present.[21]

INFECTIONS OF THE SKIN

> **QUICK CHECK 42.2**
> 1. Compare the cause and presentation of impetigo and staphylococcal scalded-skin syndrome.
> 2. Describe rubella and rubeola.
> 3. How are chickenpox and herpes zoster related?

Bacterial Infections

Impetigo Contagiosum

Impetigo is the most common bacterial skin infection in children 2 to 5 years of age. *S. aureus* and, less commonly, *Streptococcus pyogenes* cause impetigo by both direct and indirect contact. The disease is more common in midsummer to late summer, with a higher incidence in hot, humid climates. Impetigo is particularly infectious among people living in crowded conditions with poor sanitary facilities or in settings such as day care facilities. It affects children in good health, but conditions such as anemia and malnutrition are predisposing factors.

Bacterial invasion occurs through minor breaks in the cutaneous surface or as a secondary infection of a pre-existing dermatosis or infestation. The staphylococci produce bacterial toxins called *exfoliative toxins* that cause a disruption in desmosomal adhesion molecules with blister formation. There are two types of impetigo: nonbullous and, more rarely, bullous (caused only by *S. aureus*), where blisters enlarge or coalesce to form bullae (Box 42.1). Both forms of impetigo begin as vesicles with a thin vesicular roof composed of stratum corneum that ruptures to form a honey-coloured crust (Figure 42.4). The lesions are often located on the face, around the nose and mouth, but the hands and other exposed areas also are involved. Impetigo is clinically characterized by crusted erosions or ulcers that may arise as a primary infection or as a secondary infection of a pre-existing dermatosis or infestation.

The treatment of choice for both types of impetigo is topical mupirocin (Bactroban) or fusidic acid (Fucidin) for uncomplicated lesions. For extensive or complicated impetigo, systemic antibiotics may be warranted, but β-lactam antibiotics should be avoided if MRSA is suspected.[22] Prompt treatment prevents complications, such as glomerulonephritis, necrotizing fasciitis, and septic shock syndrome. Lesions

BOX 42.1 Impetigo

Vesicular Impetigo
- Contagious, acute, superficial, vesiculopustular are the most common forms
- Caused by group A Streptococcus pyogenes (alone or with Staphylococcus aureus)
- Spread by direct physical contact with other infected individuals or through insect bites
- Presents as small vesicles with a honey-coloured serum; yellow to white-brown crusts form as vesicles rupture and extend radially
- Untreated lesions last for weeks and cover large area
- Regional lymphadenitis common
- Most significant complication is acute glomerulonephritis
- Treatment is aggressive in light of this complication

Bullous Impetigo
- Caused by *S. aureus*
- Bacterial toxin (exfoliative toxin) produced causes disruption in cellular adhesion with blister formation
- Occurs in neonates
- Highly contagious
- Source is family member with pustule or asymptomatic carrier with pathogen in anterior nares, perineal region, or fingernails
- Transmitted by contact with individual or contaminated equipment
- Presents with vesicles that enlarge or coalesce to form superficial bullae, few localized lesions, or many lesions scattered over the skin surface; as bullae rupture, thin, flat, honey-coloured crust appears (hallmark of impetigo)
- Lesions found on face around the nose and mouth; hands and other exposed areas also susceptible

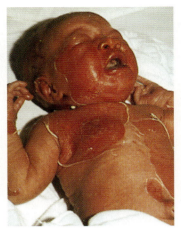

FIGURE 42.5 Staphylococcal Scalded-Skin Syndrome. The skin lesions, showing desquamation and wrinkling of the skin margins, appeared 1 day after drainage of a staphylococcal abscess. (From Kliegman, R. M., Stanton, B. F., St. Geme, J. W., et al. [Eds.]. [2011]. *Nelson textbook of pediatrics* [19th ed.]. Saunders.)

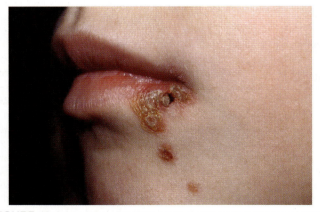

FIGURE 42.4 Impetigo. Multiple crusted and oozing lesions of impetigo. (From Kliegman, R. M., Stanton, B. F., St. Geme, J. W., et al. [Eds.]. [2011]. *Nelson textbook of pediatrics* [19th ed.]. Saunders.)

usually resolve in 2 to 3 weeks without scarring. Using good hand-washing techniques and isolating the infected child's washcloth, towels, drinking glass, and linen are important for prevention.[23]

Staphylococcal Scalded-Skin Syndrome

Staphylococcal scalded-skin syndrome (SSSS) is the most serious staphylococcal infection that affects the skin and is usually seen in infants and children younger than 5 years of age. SSSS is caused by virulent group II strains of staphylococci that produce an exfoliative toxin. The toxin attacks desmoglein and adhesion molecules and causes a separation of the skin just below the granular layer of the epidermis (see Figure 41.1).[24] The toxin is usually produced at body sites other than the skin and arrives at the epidermis through the circulatory system. Staphylococci typically are not found in the skin lesions themselves. Adults have circulating antistaphylococcal antibodies and are better able to metabolize and excrete the toxin. Neonates are at the highest risk because of their lack of immunity with no prior exposure to the toxin.[25] A source of the infection in neonates may be from health care workers who are nasal carriers of the microorganism. This reinforces the need for using good infection control practices with all neonates.[26]

The clinical symptoms begin with fever, malaise, rhinorrhea, and irritability followed by generalized erythema with exquisite tenderness of the skin. There may be associated impetigo, but the infection often begins in the throat or chest. The erythema spreads from the face and trunk to cover the entire body except for the palms, soles, and mucous membranes. Within 48 hours, blisters and bullae may form, giving the child the appearance of being scalded. The pain is severe (Figure 42.5). Fluid loss from ruptured blisters and water evaporation from denuded areas may cause dehydration. Perioral and nasolabial crusting and fissures develop. In severe cases, the skin of the entire body may slough. When secondary infection can be prevented, healing of the involved skin occurs in 10 to 14 days, usually without scarring.

Before medical intervention begins, culture and histological or exfoliative cytological studies must be performed to differentiate SSSS from erythema multiforme and toxic epidermal necrolysis, both of which are usually caused by an immune reaction to medications.[27] When SSSS infection is confirmed, treatment with oral or intravenous antibiotics begins. The skin should be treated in the same manner as a severe burn, with meticulous aseptic technique. Skin substitutes may be used for adjuvant therapy.[28] Special care is required with involvement of the lips and eyelids.

Fungal Infections

Tinea Capitis

Tinea capitis, a fungal infection of the scalp (scalp ringworm), is the most common fungal infection of childhood. It rarely affects infants and is seen in children between 2 and 10 years of age. The primary microorganism responsible for this disease is *Trichophyton tonsurans*.[29] *Microsporum canis* also continues to be a pathogenic micro-organism in this disease and is found on cats, dogs, and certain rodents. Humans appear to be a terminal host for *M. canis*. Children who handle such animals are possible hosts. Direct transmission between humans does not

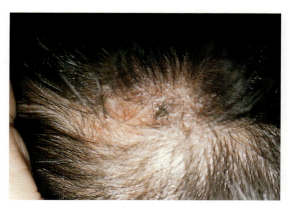

FIGURE 42.6 Tinea Capitis. (Courtesy Department of Dermatology, School of Medicine, University of Utah, Salt Lake City, UT.)

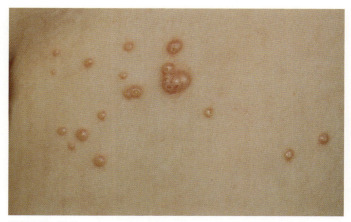

FIGURE 42.7 Molluscum Contagiosum. Waxy pink globules with umbilicated centres. (From Habif, T. P. [2004]. *Clinical dermatology: a color guide to diagnosis and therapy* [4th ed.]. Mosby.)

occur. However, there is direct human transmission of *T. tonsurans* in heavily populated areas, the most prevalent environment of the fungus.[30]

The lesions are often circular and manifested by broken hairs 1 to 3 mm above the scalp, leaving a partial area of alopecia from 1 to 5 cm in diameter (Figure 42.6). A slight erythema and scaling with raised borders can be observed.

Potassium hydroxide (KOH) examination and fungal culture confirm its diagnosis. Tinea capitis always requires systemic treatment because topical antifungal agents do not penetrate the hair follicle. Several oral antifungal agents, particularly griseofulvin (Fulvicin), are available for treatment.[31] Use of Wood's lamp examination has become less popular because there are a number of dermatophytes that fluoresce under an ultraviolet light.

Tinea Corporis

Tinea corporis (ringworm) is a common superficial dermatophyte infection in children. The organisms most commonly responsible for this disease are *M. canis* and *Trichophyton mentagrophytes*. As in tinea capitis, contact with young kittens and puppies is a common source of the disorder. Tinea corporis preferentially affects the nonhairy parts of the face, trunk, and limbs. Lesions are often erythematous, round or oval scaling patches that spread peripherally with clearing in the centre, creating the ring appearance, which is why this disease is commonly referred to as *ringworm*. The lesions are distributed asymmetrically, and multiple lesions, when present, overlap. Transmission occurs by direct contact with an infected lesion and through indirect contact with personal items used by the infected person. KOH examination of the scale from the border of the lesions confirms the diagnosis. Most lesions respond well to applications of appropriate topical antifungal medications.[32]

Thrush

Thrush describes the presence of *C. albicans* in the mucous membranes of the mouths of infants. It occurs less commonly in adults, and infected adults are usually immunocompromised. *C. albicans* penetrates the epidermal barrier more easily than other microorganisms because of its keratolytic proteases and other enzymes. Thrush involves white plaques or spots in the mouth that lead to shallow ulcers caused by keratolytic proteases from the microorganism. The tongue may have a dense, white covering. The underlying mucous membrane is red and tender and may bleed when the plaques are removed. The disease is often accompanied by fever and gastro-intestinal irritation. The infection commonly spreads to the groin, buttocks, and other parts of the body. Treatment may be difficult and includes oral antifungal washes, such as nystatin (Nyaderm) oral suspension. Simultaneous treatment of a *Candida* nipple infection or vaginitis in the mother is helpful in reducing the *C. albicans* surface colonization of the infant. Feeding bottles and nipples should be sterilized to prevent reinfection. The diaper area should be kept clean and dry.

Viral Infections

Viral infections of the skin in children are caused by poxvirus, papovavirus, and herpesvirus.

Molluscum Contagiosum

Molluscum contagiosum is a common, highly contagious viral infection of the skin and, occasionally, conjunctiva that affects school-aged children, sexually active young adults, and immunocompromised individuals. The incidence is higher among children who swim or have eczema; however, the mechanism of disease is not clear.[33] The disease is transmitted by skin-to-skin contact or from autoinoculation.[34]

The poxvirus proliferates within the follicular epithelium and induces epidermal cell proliferation. The epidermis grows down into the dermis to form saccules containing clusters of virus. The characteristic molluscum body is composed of mature, immature, and incomplete viruses and cellular debris.[35]

The lesions of molluscum are discrete, slightly umbilicated, dome-shaped papules 1 to 5 mm in diameter that appear anywhere on the skin or conjunctiva. The lesions are mainly on the trunk, face, and extremities in children (Figure 42.7). There is usually no inflammation surrounding molluscum lesions unless they are traumatized, or secondary infection occurs. Scarring may occur with healing.

The three best diagnostic procedures are (1) staining smears of the expressed molluscum body, (2) examining a biopsy specimen, or (3) inoculating a molluscum suspension into cell cultures to demonstrate the cytotoxic reactions. Most lesions are self-limiting and clear in 6 to 9 months if not manipulated.

Treatment options include immunomodulatory and antiviral therapy and destructive procedures (cryotherapy, curettage, or laser ablation); however, no treatment is universally effective. KOH solution applications can be safe, effective, and inexpensive.[36] Treatment is recommended for genital molluscum to prevent sexual transmission and autoinoculation.[37] Measures to prevent spread of infection must be taken. Recurrences are common.

Rubella (German or 3-Day Measles)

Rubella is a common communicable disease of children and young adults caused by an RNA virus that enters the bloodstream through the respiratory route. This disease is mild in most children. The incubation period ranges from 14 to 21 days. Prodromal symptoms include enlarged cervical and postauricular lymph nodes, low-grade fever, headache, sore throat, rhinorrhea, and cough. A faint pink-to-red coalescing maculopapular rash develops on the face with spread to the trunk and extremities 1 to 4 days after the onset of initial symptoms (Figure 42.8). The rash is thought to be the result of virus dissemination to the skin. The rash subsides after 2 to 3 days, usually without complication. Children are usually not contagious after development of the rash (Table 42.1).

Vaccination for rubella is usually combined with vaccines for measles, mumps, and rubella (MMR). Measles is known to occur in previously immunized children. The *Canadian Immunization Guide* includes vaccine recommendations and is available at https://www.canada.ca/en/public-health/services/canadian-immunization-guide.html (and for measles, specifically, see https://www.canada.ca/en/public-health/services/publications/healthy-living/canadian-immunization-guide-part-4-active-vaccines/page-12-measles-vaccine.html). Rubella has almost been eliminated in North America because of vaccination campaigns. However, challenges to maintaining elimination include large outbreaks of measles in highly travelled developed countries, frequent international travel, and clusters of both Americans and Canadians who remain unvaccinated because of personal belief exemptions.[38] Although MMR vaccine may rarely be associated with adverse neurological events, studies conclude that MMR immunization does not cause autism.[39] Lack of vaccination, however, leads to significant morbidity and mortality, and pneumonia, croup, and encephalitis are causes of death worldwide.

Women of childbearing age are immunized if their rubella hemagglutination-inhibition titre is low. Pregnancy should be avoided for 3 months after vaccination because the attenuated virus in the vaccine may remain viable for this period. Pregnant women who have rubella early in the first trimester may have a fetus who develops congenital defects.

There is no specific treatment for rubella. Recovery is spontaneous, although lymph nodes may remain enlarged for weeks. Supportive therapy includes rest, fluids, and use of a vaporizer. In rare cases, a mild encephalitis or peripheral neuritis may follow rubella.

Rubeola (Red Measles)

Rubeola is a highly contagious, acute viral disease of childhood. Transmitted by direct contact with droplets from infected persons, rubeola is caused by an RNA-containing paramyxovirus with an incubation period of 7 to 12 days, during which there are no symptoms. The virus enters the respiratory tract and attaches to dendritic cells and alveolar macrophages, amplifies in local lymphatic tissue,

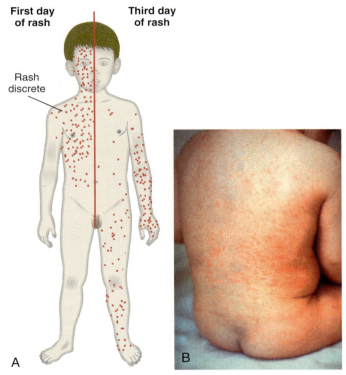

FIGURE 42.8 Rubella (3-Day Measles). **A,** Typical distribution of full-blown maculopapular rash with tendency to coalesce. **B,** Rash of rubella. (From Centers for Disease Control and Prevention Image Bank, Figure #712. https://phil.cdc.gov.)

TABLE 42.1	Differential Presentation of Viral Diseases Producing Rashes			
Viral Disease	**Incubation Period**	**Prodromal Symptoms**	**Duration/Characteristics**	**Clinical Symptoms**
Rubella (German measles)	14–21 days	1–2 days Mild fever Malaise Respiratory symptoms	1–3 days Pink-red maculopapular rash Face and trunk	Enlarged and tender occipital and periauricular lymph nodes
Rubeola (red measles)	7–12 days	2–5 days Fever Cough Respiratory symptoms	3–5 days Purple-red to brown maculopapular rash Face, trunk, extremities	Koplik spots 1–3 days before rash
Roseola (exanthema subitum)	5–15 days	2–5 days High fever	1–3 days Red macular rash Neck and trunk	Rash develops when fever subsides
Varicella (chickenpox)	11–20 days	1–2 days Low-grade fever Cough May be asymptomatic	7–14 days Red papules, vesicles, pustules in clusters	Eruption of new lesions for 4–5 days Occasional ulcerative lesion in mouth
Fifth disease (human parvovirus B19, erythrovirus)	4–28 days	May be asymptomatic Low-grade fever, malaise before rash	7–10 days "Slapped-cheek" rash on face; lacy red rash on trunk and limbs; may itch	Rash develops when fever subsides

and progresses to systemic disease.[40] Prodromal symptoms include high fever (up to 40.5°C [104.9°F]), malaise, enlarged lymph nodes, rhinorrhea, conjunctivitis, and barking cough. Within 3 to 4 days, an erythematous maculopapular rash develops over the head and spreads distally over the trunk, extremities, hands, and feet. Early lesions blanch with pressure, followed by a brownish hue that does not blanch as the rash fades. Characteristic pinpoint white spots surrounded by an erythematous ring develop over the buccal mucosa and are known as *Koplik spots*. These spots precede the rash by 1 to 2 days. The rash then subsides within 3 to 5 days.

Complications associated with measles may be caused by the primary infection or by a secondary bacterial infection. Measles encephalitis occurs in about 1 of 800 cases, and most children recover completely. Only a small minority of children develop permanent brain damage or die. Bacterial complications include otitis media and pneumonia, usually caused by group A hemolytic streptococcus, *Haemophilus influenzae*, or *S. aureus* infection.

Measles is prevented by vaccination. Immunization is key to prevention. There is no specific treatment for measles, and supportive therapy is the same as that recommended for rubella. Antibiotic therapy is initiated if secondary bacterial infections develop.

Roseola (Exanthema Subitum)

Roseola is a presumed viral infection of children between 6 months and 2 years of age and can be seen in children up to 4 years of age. The incubation period is 5 to 15 days, followed by the sudden onset of fever (38.9° to 40.5°C [101.3° to 104.9°F]) that lasts 3 to 5 days. Following the fever, an erythematous macular rash that lasts about 24 hours develops primarily over the trunk and neck. Children usually feel well, eat normally, and have few other symptoms. There is usually no treatment.

Smallpox

Smallpox (variola) was a highly contagious and deadly, but also preventable, disease caused by poxvirus variolae. Smallpox was eradicated worldwide in 1977. Routine immunization programs for infants were discontinued in 1972, in 1977 for health care workers, and in 1988 for Canadian Forces.[41]

Chickenpox and Herpes Zoster

Chickenpox (varicella) and herpes zoster (shingles) are both produced by the varicella-zoster virus (VZV). VZV is a complex deoxyribonucleic acid (DNA) virus of the herpes group. The incubation period is 10 to 27 days, averaging 14 days. Vesicular lesions occur in the epidermis, as infection occurs within keratinocytes. An inflammatory infiltrate is often present. Vesicles eventually rupture, followed by crust formation or the development of transient ulcers on mucous membranes. Varicella occurs in people not previously exposed to VZV, whereas herpes zoster (shingles) occurs in individuals who had varicella in the past. The virus enters the posterior root ganglia and remains latent. Since the introduction of live attenuated VZV vaccine in 1995, there has been a significant reduction in varicella incidence and its associated complications.[42]

Chickenpox. Chickenpox (varicella) is a disease of early childhood, with 90% of children contracting the disease during the first decade of life. Being a highly contagious virus, chickenpox is spread by close person-to-person contact and by airborne droplets. Introduction of an infected person into a household results in a 90% possibility of susceptible persons developing the disease within the incubation period, usually 14 days. Children are contagious for at least 1 day before development of the rash. Transmission of the virus may occur until approximately 5 to 6 days after the onset of the first skin lesions in healthy children. In immunocompromised children, the virus is recoverable for a longer period, but infected children must be considered contagious for at least 7 to 10 days. Transmission occurs more readily in temperate climates than in tropical climates.

Normally, children who develop chickenpox have no prodromal symptoms. The first sign of illness may be pruritus or the appearance of vesicles, usually on the trunk, scalp, or face. The rash later spreads to the extremities. Characteristically, lesions can be seen in various stages of maturation, with macules, papules, and vesicles present in a particular area at the same time (Figure 42.9). The vesicular lesions are superficial and rupture easily. New lesions will erupt for 4 to 5 days, until there are approximately 100 to 300 in different stages of development. The vesicles become crusted, and over time only the crust remains, although there may be an occasional vesicle on the palm later in the disease. Although uncommon, ulcerative lesions are sometimes seen in the mouth and, less commonly, on the conjunctiva and pharynx. Fever usually lasts 2 to 3 days, with body temperature ranging from 38.5 to 40°C (101.3 to 104°F).

Complications are rare in children but more common in adults. They can include transient hematuria (from rupture of vesicles in the bladder), epistaxis, laryngeal edema, and varicella pneumonia. One case of chickenpox produces almost complete immunity against a second attack. Rarely, the fetus may be malformed (congenital varicella syndrome) if chickenpox develops in the first half of pregnancy. Infants whose mothers have chickenpox at any stage of pregnancy have a higher risk of developing herpes zoster during the first few years of life.[43] Varicella-zoster immunoglobulin should be administered to neonates whenever the onset of maternal disease is between 5 days before and 2 days after delivery.[44]

Uncomplicated chickenpox requires no specific therapy. Baths, wet dressings, and oral antihistamines occasionally help to relieve pruritus and to prevent secondary infection from developing as a result of

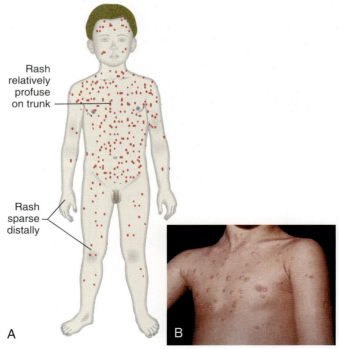

FIGURE 42.9 Chickenpox. **A**, Pattern of generalized, polymorphous eruption. **B**, Chickenpox lesions on fifth day of illness. (From Centers for Disease Control and Prevention Image Bank, Figure #2882. https://phil.cdc.gov.)

scratching. Oral antistaphylococcal medications should be given if secondary bacterial infection is present. Zoster immune globulin may be administered to immunodeficient individuals if given within 72 hours after exposure to chickenpox. Oral acyclovir (Zovirax) may be valuable in immunosuppressed or other select groups of children. The varicella vaccine protects against both varicella and herpes zoster. However, wild-type (vaccine-resistant) viruses are a continuing threat.[45]

INSECT BITES AND PARASITES

QUICK CHECK 42.3
1. Give two examples of insect bites or parasites that affect children. What features are observed in each?
2. Compare a strawberry hemangioma with a cavernous hemangioma.

Scabies

Scabies is a contagious disease caused by the itch mite *Sarcoptes scabiei* (Figure 42.10A), which can colonize the human epidermis. Scabies is a common skin infection in tropical settings, affecting large numbers of people, particularly children. It is transmitted by close personal contact and by infected clothing and bedding. Scabies is often epidemic in areas of overcrowded housing and poor sanitation. Immunocompromised individuals are at greater risk. Scabies can facilitate *S. pyogenes* and *S. aureus* skin co-infections with systemic complications. The scabies mite has adapted mechanisms to overcome host defences, including complement inhibitors.[46] Infestation is initiated by a female mite that tunnels into the stratum corneum, depositing eggs and creating a burrow several millimetres to 1 cm long. Over a 3-week period, the eggs mature into adult mites, which sometimes are recognized as tiny dots at the ends of intact burrows.

Symptoms appear 3 to 5 weeks after infestation. The primary lesions are burrows, papules, and vesicular lesions, with severe pruritus that worsens at night. Pruritus is thought to be related to sensitization to the larval stages of the parasite. In older children and adults, the lesions occur in the webs of fingers; in the axillae; in the creases of the arms and wrists; along the belt line; and around the nipples, genitalia, and lower buttocks. Infants and young children have a different pattern of distribution, with involvement of the palms, soles, head, neck, and face (Figure 42.10B). Secondary infections and crusting develop as a result of scratching and eczematous changes.

Diagnosis of scabies is made by observation of the tunnels and burrows and by microscopic examination of scrapings of the skin to identify the mite or its eggs or feces. Treatment involves the application of a scabicide, which is curative. All clothing and linens should be washed and dried in hot cycles or dry-cleaned.[47]

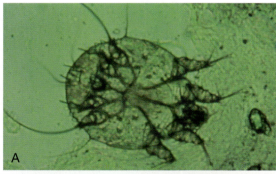

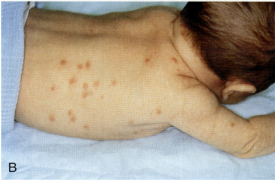

FIGURE 42.10 Scabies. **A**, Scabies mite, as seen clinically when removed from its burrow. **B**, Characteristic scabies bites. (Courtesy Department of Dermatology, School of Medicine, University of Utah, Salt Lake City, UT.)

Pediculosis (Lice Infestation)

The three known types of human lice are (1) the head louse (*Pediculus capitis*), (2) the body louse (*Pediculus corporis*), and (3) the crab or pubic louse (*Phthirus pubis*). They are parasites and survive by sucking blood. The female louse reproduces every 2 weeks, producing hundreds of nits as newly hatched lice mate with older lice. The mouthparts are shaped for piercing and sucking and are attached to the skin of the host while the louse is feeding. When piercing the skin, the louse secretes toxic saliva, and the mechanical trauma and toxin produce a pruritic dermatitis. Head and body lice are acquired directly by personal contact or indirectly by sharing of combs, brushes, or towels or contact with infested clothes, toys, furniture, carpets, or bedding. Crab lice are spread by close body contact, usually with an infected adult. Other common sources of transmission include sharing clothing or headphones.

Pruritus is the major symptom of lice infestation. With head lice, the ova attach to hairs above the ears and in the occipital region. The primary lesion caused by the body louse is a pinpoint red macule, papule, or wheal with a hemorrhagic puncture site. The primary lesion is often not seen, because it is masked by excoriations, wheals, and crusts. The crab louse is found on pubic hairs but also may be found in other body hair, such as eyelashes, mustache, beard, and underarm hair. Young children in particular may become infected with crab lice on their eyebrows or eyelashes.

The live louse, 2 to 3 mm long, is rarely observed. The ova, or nits, can be observed as oval, yellowish, pinpoint specks fastened to a hair shaft. The ova fluoresce under an ultraviolet light (Wood's lamp) and are observed best with a microscope. The Canadian Pediatric Society recommends current treatments: https://www.cps.ca/documents/position/head-lice. Success or failure of therapy for ectoparasitic infestation depends much more on proper use of the topical preparation than on the type of scabicide or pediculicide used.[48]

All clothes, towels, bedding, combs, and brushes should be washed, then dried in hot air or instead be washed in boiling water, or clothes can be ironed to rid them of lice. Individuals who have close personal contact with the infected person should also be treated.

Fleas

Young children are very susceptible to **fleabites**. Bites occur in clusters along the arms and legs or where clothing is tight fitting, such as near elastic bands that circle the thigh or waist. The bite produces an urticarial wheal with a central hemorrhagic puncture (Figure 42.11). Itching can be controlled with antihistamines.[49] Infected animals should be treated, and clothes and bedding should be washed in hot water.

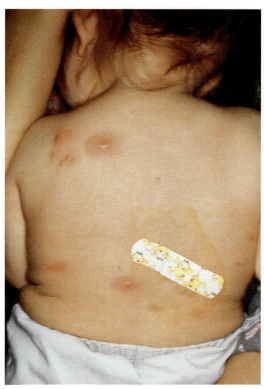

FIGURE 42.11 Fleabites. Fleabite producing an urticarial wheal with central puncture.

Bedbugs

Bedbugs (*Cimex lectularius*) are blood-sucking parasites that live in the crevices and cracks of floors, walls, and furniture and in bedding or furniture stuffing. They are 3 to 5 mm long and reddish brown. Bedbugs are nocturnal, emerging to feed in darkness by attaching to the skin to suck blood, and are attracted by warmth and carbon dioxide. Feeding occurs for 5 to 15 minutes, and the bedbug then leaves. It will move long distances to search for food and can travel from house to house.

Immunological reactions to bedbug saliva vary, but bites typically yield erythematous and pruritic papules. The face and distal extremities, areas uncovered by sleeping clothes or blankets, are preferentially involved. If the host has not been previously sensitized, the only symptom is a red macule that develops into a nodule, lasting up to 14 days. In sensitized children and adults, pruritic wheals, papules, and vesicles may form. Most lesions respond to oral antihistamines or topical corticosteroids, or both. Secondary infections require antibiotic treatment. Bedbugs are eliminated by inspecting and cleaning or disposing of bedding, mattresses, furniture, and other contaminated items and by using applications of approved insecticides, usually by a professional.[50]

CUTANEOUS HEMANGIOMAS AND VASCULAR MALFORMATIONS

Cutaneous vascular anomalies are frequent tumours of early infancy and are categorized as either hemangiomas or vascular malformations.

Cutaneous Hemangiomas

Cutaneous hemangiomas are benign tumours that form from the rapid growth of vascular endothelial cells, which results in formation of extra blood vessels. Hemangiomas can be superficial or deep.[51] *Superficial hemangiomas* are known as infantile (capillary) or **strawberry**

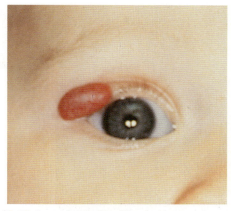

FIGURE 42.12 Superficial (Capillary) Hemangioma. (Courtesy Department of Dermatology, School of Medicine, University of Utah, Salt Lake City, UT.)

hemangiomas. Deep lesions are known as *cavernous or congenital hemangiomas*. The etiology may be related to embolization of fetal placental endothelial cells with placental trauma or loss of placental angiogenic inhibitor of placental and maternal origin. Superficial hemangiomas are associated with endothelial glucose transporter 1 (GLUT1). There is proliferation of mast cells, which are thought to promote the angiogenesis. Infiltration of fat cells, fibrosis, and the rich vascular network give the lesions a firm, rubbery feel. Females are affected more often than males.

About 30% of infantile hemangiomas are apparent at birth, but they usually emerge 3 to 5 weeks after birth. They grow rapidly during the first few years of life and become bright red and elevated with minute capillary projections that give them a strawberry appearance. Only one lesion is usually present and is located on the head and neck area or trunk (Figure 42.12). After the initial growth, the lesion grows at the same rate as the child and then starts to involute at 12 to 16 months of age. Approximately 90% of strawberry hemangiomas involute by 5 to 9 years of age, usually without scarring. Most superficial hemangiomas require no treatment.

Hemangiomas located over the eye, ear, nose, mouth, urethra, or anus may require treatment because they interfere with function and have a higher risk for infection or injury.

Cavernous hemangiomas are a rare variant of superficial hemangiomas and are GLUT1-negative (Figure 42.13). They are present and fully grown at birth and are usually solitary lesions on the head or limbs that appear as a spongy purplish mass of tissue. They have larger and more mature vessels within the lesion. There are two groups of cavernous hemangiomas: rapidly involuting and noninvoluting. Rapidly involuting cavernous hemangiomas disappear by 12 to 14 months of age, leaving an area of thin skin. Noninvoluting cavernous hemangiomas do not undergo involution.

Rapidly progressing hemangiomas are treated with a beta-blocker (e.g., propranolol [Apo-Propranolol]), with regression occurring within 2 weeks and should be considered a first-line agent.[52] Other therapies include systemic or intralesional steroids. Cryosurgery, laser surgery, sclerotherapy, and embolization are alternative treatment options. Interferons, vincristine (Oncovin), cyclophosphamide (Procytox), and radiotherapy can suppress angiogenesis.[53]

Cutaneous Vascular Malformations

Cutaneous vascular malformations are rare congenital anomalies of blood vessels present at birth but may not be apparent for several years.[54] They grow proportionately with the child and never regress. The malformations occur equally among males and females. Occasionally they expand rapidly, particularly during the hormonal changes of puberty

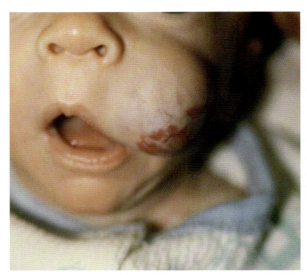

FIGURE 42.13 Cavernous Hemangioma. (Courtesy Department of Dermatology, School of Medicine, University of Utah, Salt Lake City, UT.)

or pregnancy and in association with trauma. Vascular malformations are classified as low flow or high flow. *Low-flow malformations* involve capillaries, veins, and lymphatics. *High-flow malformations* involve arteries. In addition to locations within the skin, they may involve the gastro-intestinal tract, bone (Maffuccis syndrome or Sturge-Weber syndrome),[55] facial capillary malformation, skin, eye, or brain (leptomeningeal hemangioma). *Overgrowth syndromes* can occur with either high-flow or low-flow malformations, with overgrowth of the underlying structures (i.e., legs, arms, facial bones). The most common vascular malformations are nevus flammeus (port-wine stains) and salmon patches (stork bite, angel kiss).

Port-wine (nevus flammeus) stains are congenital malformations of the dermal capillaries. The lesions are flat, and their colour ranges from pink to dark reddish purple. They are present at birth or within a few days after birth and do not fade with age. Involvement of the face and other body surfaces is common, and the lesions may be large (Figure 42.14). Treatments using cryosurgery or tattooing are not satisfactory. The pulsed dye laser is the treatment of choice to successfully lighten the colour and flatten the more nodular and cavernous lesions. Waterproof cosmetics may be used to cover the lesions.

Salmon patches are macular pink lesions present at birth and located on the nape of the neck, forehead, upper eyelids, or nasolabial fold region. They are a variant of nevus flammeus, more superficial, and one of the most common congenital malformations in the skin. The pink colour results from distended dermal capillaries, and 95% of patches fade by 1 year of age. Those located at the nape of the neck may persist for a lifetime. They generally do not present a cosmetic problem.

OTHER SKIN DISORDERS

Miliaria

Miliaria is a dermatosis commonly seen in infants that is characterized by a vesicular eruption after prolonged exposure to perspiration with subsequent obstruction of the eccrine ducts. There are two forms of miliaria: miliaria crystallina and miliaria rubra. In **miliaria crystallina**, ductal rupture occurs within the stratum corneum and appears as 1- to 2 mm clear vesicles without erythema. They rupture within 24 to 48 hours and leave a white scale. In miliaria rubra, the ductal rupture occurs in the lower epidermis, with inflammatory cells attracted to the

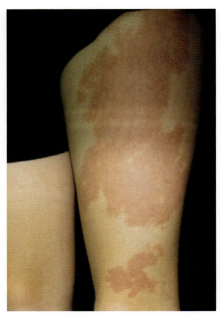

FIGURE 42.14 Port-wine Hemangioma. Port-wine hemangioma in a child. (Courtesy Department of Dermatology, School of Medicine, University of Utah, Salt Lake City, UT.)

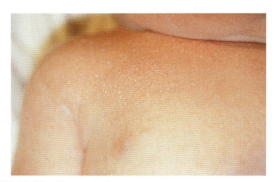

FIGURE 42.15 Miliaria Rubra. Note discrete erythematous papules or papulovesicles. (Courtesy Department of Dermatology, School of Medicine, University of Utah, Salt Lake City, UT.)

site of the rupture. **Miliaria rubra (prickly heat)** is characterized by 2- to 4 mm discrete erythematous papules or papulovesicles (Figure 42.15). Both forms may become secondarily infected, requiring systemic antibiotics. The key to management is avoidance of excessive heat and humidity, which cause sweating. Light clothing, cool baths, and air conditioning assist in keeping the skin surface dry and cool.

Erythema Toxicum Neonatorum

Erythema toxicum neonatorum (toxic erythema of the newborn) is a benign erythematous accumulation of macules, papules, or pustules that appears at birth or 3 to 4 days after birth. The lesions first appear as a blotchy, macular erythematous rash. The macules vary from 1 mm to 1 cm in diameter. When papules or pustules develop, they are light yellow or white and 1 to 3 mm in diameter. There may be a few or several hundred lesions, and any body surface can be affected, with the exception of the palms and soles, where there are no pilosebaceous follicles. The cause of the lesion is unknown but may be related to an innate immune response to the first commensal microflora with release of mast cell mediators. It is self-limiting and resolves spontaneously within a few weeks after birth. No treatment is required.

DID YOU UNDERSTAND?

Acne Vulgaris
1. Acne vulgaris is the most common skin disease and is related to obstruction of pilosebaceous follicles and proliferation of *Propionibacterium acnes*, primarily of the face, neck, and upper trunk. It is characterized by both noninflammatory and inflammatory lesions.
2. Hidradenitis suppurativa is a chronic inflammatory disease with occlusion of the pilosebaceous follicles, primarily where there are folds of skin. The lesions include inflammatory nodules, sinus tracts, fistulae, and scarring.

Dermatitis
1. Atopic dermatitis is an alteration in the skin barrier; occurs as red, scaly lesions on the face, cheeks, and flexor surfaces of the extremities in infants and young children; and is associated with inflammatory cytokines, elevated IgE levels, and a family history of asthma and hay fever.
2. Diaper dermatitis is a type of irritant contact dermatitis that develops from prolonged exposure to urine and feces and often becomes secondarily infected with *Candida albicans*.

Infections of the Skin
1. Impetigo is a contagious bacterial disease occurring in two forms: bullous and vesicular. The toxins from the bacteria produce a weeping lesion with a honey-coloured crust.
2. Staphylococcal scalded-skin syndrome (SSSS) is a staphylococcal skin infection that produces an exfoliative toxin with painful blisters and bullae formation over large areas of the skin, requiring systemic antibiotic treatment.
3. Tinea capitis and tinea corporis are fungal infections of the scalp and body caused by dermatophytes.
4. Thrush is a fungal infection of the mouth caused by *C. albicans*.
5. Molluscum contagiosum is a poxvirus of the skin that produces pale papular lesions filled with viral and cellular debris.
6. Rubella (German or 3-day measles) is a communicable viral disease characterized by fever, sore throat, enlarged cervical and postauricular lymph nodes, and a generalized maculopapular rash that lasts 1 to 4 days.
7. Rubeola is a viral contagious disease with symptoms of high fever, enlarged lymph nodes, conjunctivitis, and a red rash that begins on the head and spreads to the trunk and extremities. The rash subsides within 3 to 5 days. Both bacterial and viral complications may accompany rubeola.
8. Roseola is a benign disease of infants with a sudden onset of fever that lasts 3 to 5 days, followed by a rash that lasts 24 hours.
9. Chickenpox (varicella) is a highly contagious disease caused by the varicella-zoster virus. Vesicular lesions occur on the skin and mucous membranes. Individuals are contagious from 1 day before the development of the rash until about 5 to 6 days after the rash develops.

Insect Bites and Parasites
1. Scabies is a pruritic lesion caused by the itch mite, which burrows into the skin and forms papules and vesicles. The mite is very contagious and is transmitted by direct contact.
2. Pediculosis (lice infestation) is caused by blood-sucking parasites that secrete toxic saliva and damage the skin to produce pruritic dermatitis. Lice are spread by direct contact and are recognized by the ova or nits that attach to the shafts of hairs.
3. Fleabites produce a pruritic wheal with a central puncture site and occur as clusters in areas of tight-fitting clothing.
4. Bedbugs are blood-sucking parasites that live in cracks of floors, furniture, or bedding and feed at night. They produce pruritic wheals and nodules.

Cutaneous Hemangiomas and Vascular Malformations
1. Cutaneous hemangiomas are benign tumours that form from the rapid growth of vascular endothelial cells and result in formation of extra blood vessels.
2. Cutaneous vascular malformations are rare congenital anomalies of blood vessels present at birth.
3. A strawberry hemangioma is a vascular lesion present at birth that proliferates in size and then grows at the same rate as the child. Most lesions resolve spontaneously by 5 years of age.
4. A cavernous hemangioma is present at birth, with larger vessels than a strawberry hemangioma, and is bluish red. Cavernous hemangiomas usually involute by 9 years of age and may require surgical removal if located near the eyes, nares, or genitalia.
5. Port-wine stains are congenital malformations of dermal capillaries that do not fade with age.
6. Salmon patches are macular pink lesions with dilated capillaries that usually resolve by 1 year of age.

Other Skin Disorders
1. Miliaria are small pruritic papules or vesicles that result from obstruction of the sweat duct opening in infants.
2. Erythema toxicum neonatorum is a benign accumulation of macules, papules, and pustules that spontaneously resolves within a few weeks after birth.

APPENDIX

LABORATORY VALUES

The tables in this appendix list some of the most common tests, their normal values, and possible etiologies of abnormal values. Laboratory values are expressed in the Système International d'Unités (SI) units, which are used in Canada. Conventional units, used in the United States, are presented after the SI units in parentheses. ***Laboratory values may vary with different techniques and in different laboratories.*** Possible aetiologies are presented in alphabetical order. SI abbreviations and other symbols appearing in the tables are defined as:

<	=	less than
>	=	greater than
≥	=	greater than or equal to
≤	=	less than or equal to
AU	=	arbitrary unit
cm H_2O	=	centimetres of water
dL	=	decilitre
EU	=	Ehrlich unit
fL	=	femtolitre
g	=	gram
IU	=	international unit
kPa	=	kilopascal
k	=	kilo
L	=	litre
μg	=	microgram (one millionth [10^{-6}] of a gram)
μIU	=	micro–international unit (one millionth [10^{-6}] of an international unit)
μL	=	microlitre
μmol	=	micromole
mEq	=	milliequivalent
mg	=	milligram (one thousandth [10^{-3}] of a gram)
microkat	=	microkatal
microU	=	microunit
mL	=	millilitre
mm	=	millimetre
mm Hg	=	millimetre of mercury
mmol	=	millimole
mOsm	=	milliosmole
mU	=	milliunit (one hundredth [10^{-2}] of a unit)
nmol	=	nanomole (one billionth [10^{-9}] of a mole)
ng	=	nanogram (one billionth [10^{-9}] of a gram)
pg	=	picogram (one trillionth [10^{-12}] of a gram)
pmol	=	picomole (one trillionth [10^{-12}] of a mole)
U	=	unit

TABLE A.1 Serum, Plasma, and Whole Blood Chemistries

	Normal Values (SI Units [Conventional Units])	POSSIBLE ETIOLOGY	
Test		Higher Values	Lower Values
Acetone		Diabetic ketoacidosis, high-fat diet, low-carbohydrate diet, starvation	—
• Quantitative	<200 μmol/L (<1.16 mg/dL)		
• Qualitative	Negative (negative)		
Alanine aminotransferase (ALT; formerly known as serum glutamate pyruvate transferase [SGPT])	5–35 U/L (same as in SI units)	Liver disease, shock	—
Albumin	35–55 g/L (3.5–5.5 g/dL)	Dehydration	Malnutrition, pregnancy, liver disease, protein-losing enteropathies, protein-losing nephropathies, third-space losses, inflammatory disease, familial idiopathic dysproteinemia
α_1-Antitrypsin	0.85–2.13 g/L (85–213 mg/dL)	Acute and chronic inflammatory disorders, infections (i.e., thyroid infections), and stress malignancy, stress, thyroid infections	Chronic lung disease (early onset of emphysema), neonatal respiratory distress syndrome Cirrhosis (in children), end-stage cancer, malnutrition, nephrotic syndrome, protein-losing enteropathy, and hepatic failure

TABLE A.1 Serum, Plasma, and Whole Blood Chemistries—cont'd

Test	Normal Values (SI Units [Conventional Units])	POSSIBLE ETIOLOGY Higher Values	Lower Values
α-Fetoprotein	0–40 µg/L (<40 ng/mL)	Cancers of testes, lymphoma, stomach, colon, breasts, and ovaries; liver cell necrosis (i.e., cirrhosis, hepatitis); carcinoma of liver; fetal death; fetal distress or congenital abnormalities; neural tube defects (i.e., anencephaly, spina bifida) or multiple pregnancies in pregnant women	In pregnant women, fetal trisomy 21 (Down syndrome) or fetal wastage
Ammonia	6–47 µmol/L (10–80 µg/dL)	GI bleeding and obstruction with mild liver disease, genetic metabolic disorder of urea cycle, hemolytic disease of newborn, hepatic encephalopathy and hepatic coma, portal hypertension, Reye syndrome, primary hepatocellular disease, asparagine intoxication, severe heart failure or congestive hepatomegaly	Essential or malignant hypertension, hyperornithinemia
Amylase	25–125 U/L	Acute and chronic pancreatitis, GI disease, acute cholecystitis, mumps (salivary gland disease), perforated ulcers, ruptured ectopic pregnancy, renal failure, diabetic ketoacidosis, pulmonary infarction	Acute alcoholism, cirrhosis of liver, extensive destruction of pancreas
Ascorbic acid	23–85 µmol/L (0.4–1.5 mg/dL)	Excessive ingestion of vitamin C	Connective tissue disorders, hepatic disease, renal disease, rheumatic fever, vitamin C deficiency
Aspartate aminotransferase (AST) (formerly known as serum glutamic oxaloacetic transferase [SGOT])	0–35 U/L (same as SI units)	Acute hepatitis, liver disease, MI, skeletal muscle disease, acute hemolytic anemia, acute pancreatitis	Acute renal disease, chronic renal dialysis, diabetic ketoacidosis, beriberi, pregnancy
B-type (brain-type) natriuretic peptide	<100 µg/L (<100 ng/mL)	Cor pulmonale, heart failure, heart transplant rejection, hypertension, MI	—
Bicarbonate	23–29 mmol/L (23–29 mEq/L)	Use of mercurial diuretics, aldosteronism, compensated respiratory acidosis, metabolic alkalosis	Acute kidney injury, compensated respiratory alkalosis, diarrhea, metabolic acidosis, starvation, chronic use of loop diuretics
Bilirubin • Total • Indirect • Direct	3–22 µmol/L (0.2–1.3 mg/dL) 3.4–12 µmol/L (0.2–0.8 mg/dL) 1.7–5.1 µmol/L (0.1–0.3 mg/dL)	**Direct Bilirubin:** Gallstones, extrahepatic duct obstruction (tumour, inflammation, gallstone, scarring, surgical trauma), extensive liver metastasis, cholestasis from drugs, Dubin-Johnson syndrome, Rotor syndrome **Indirect Bilirubin:** Erythroblastosis fetalis, transfusion reaction, sickle cell anemia, hemolytic jaundice, hemolytic anemia, pernicious anemia, large-volume blood transfusion, resolution of large hematoma, hepatitis, cirrhosis, sepsis, neonatal hyperbilirubinemia, Crigler-Najjar syndrome, Gilbert's syndrome **Increased Urine Levels of Bilirubin:** Gallstones, extrahepatic duct obstruction (tumour, inflammation, gallstone, scarring, surgical trauma), extensive liver metastasis, cholestasis from drugs, Dubin-Johnson syndrome, Rotor syndrome	—
Blood gases* • Arterial pH • Venous pH	7.35–7.45 (same as SI units) 7.35–7.45 (same as SI units)	Alkalosis Alkalosis	Acidosis Acidosis

Continued

TABLE A.1 Serum, Plasma, and Whole Blood Chemistries—cont'd

Test	Normal Values (SI Units [Conventional Units])	POSSIBLE ETIOLOGY Higher Values	Lower Values
• Partial pressure of carbon dioxide in arterial blood (PaCO2)	35–45 mm Hg (same as SI units)	Compensated metabolic alkalosis, respiratory acidosis	Compensated metabolic acidosis, respiratory alkalosis
• Partial pressure of oxygen in arterial blood (PaO2)	80–100 mm Hg (same as SI units)	Administration of high concentration of oxygen	Chronic lung disease, decreased cardiac output
• Partial pressure of oxygen in venous blood (PvO2)	40–50 mm Hg (same as SI units)		
Calcium	Adult: 2.10–2.750 mmol/L (8.4–10.6 mg/dL) Total Calcium: <1.65 mmol/L or >3.25 mmol/L (13 mg/dL)	Hyperparathyroidism, nonparathyroid PTH-producing tumour (e.g., lung or renal carcinoma), metastatic tumour to bone, Paget's disease of bone, prolonged immobilization, milk-alkali syndrome, vitamin D intoxication lymphoma, granulomatous infections such as sarcoidosis and tuberculosis, Addison's disease, acromegaly, hyperthyroidism	Hypoparathyroidism renal failure, hyperphosphatemia secondary to renal failure, rickets, vitamin D deficiency, osteomalacia, hypoalbuminemia, malabsorption, pancreatitis, fat embolism, alkalosis
Calcium, ionized	Adult: 1.15–1.35 mmol/L (4.6–5.1 mg/dL) Ionized calcium: <0.80 mmol/L or >1.58 mmol/L (7 mg/dL)	—	—
Carbon dioxide (CO_2 content)	21–28 mmol/L (21–28 mEq/L)	COPD, metabolic alkalosis, severe vomiting, high volume gastric suction, use of mercurial diuretics	Chronic use of loop diuretics, DKA, metabolic acidosis, renal failure, shock, starvation
Chloride	98–106 mmol/L (98–106 mEq/L)	Dehydration, excessive infusion of normal saline solution, metabolic acidosis, renal tubular acidosis, Cushing's syndrome, kidney dysfunction, hyperparathyroidism, eclampsia, respiratory alkalosis	Overhydration, syndrome of inappropriate secretion of antidiuretic hormone (SIADH), heart failure, vomiting or prolonged gastric suction, chronic diarrhea or high-output GI fistula, chronic respiratory acidosis, metabolic alkalosis, salt-losing nephritis, Addison's disease, diuretic therapy, hypokalemia, aldosteronism, burns
Cholesterol	<5.2 mmol/L (<200 mg/dL) age dependent	Familial hypercholesterolemia, familial hyperlipidemia, hypothyroidism, uncontrolled diabetes mellitus, nephrotic syndrome, pregnancy, high-cholesterol diet, xanthomatosis, hypertension, MI, atherosclerosis, biliary cirrhosis, extrahepatic biliary, stress, and nephrotic syndrome renal disease, uncontrolled diabetes	Malabsorption, malnutrition, advanced cancer, hyperthyroidism, cholesterol-lowering medication, pernicious anemia, hemolytic anemia, sepsis/stress, liver disease, acute MI
• High-density lipoproteins (HDL)	>0.91 mmol/L (>35 mg/dL)		
• Low-density lipoproteins (LDL)	<3.4 mmol/L (<130 mg/dL)		
Cortisol		Adrenal adenoma, Cushing's syndrome, hyperthyroidism, pancreatitis, stress, ectopic ACTH-producing tumours, obesity	Addison's disease, adrenal insufficiency, hypopituitary states, hypothyroidism, liver disease
• 0800 hours	170–635 nmol/L (6–23 µg/dL)		
• 1600 hours	82–413 nmol/L (3–53 µg/dL)		
Creatine		Active rheumatoid arthritis, biliary obstruction, hyperthyroidism, renal disease, severe muscle disease	Diabetes mellitus
• Male	70–120 mmol/L		
• Female	170–635 mmol/L		
Creatine kinase (CK)		Brain damage, exercise, musculoskeletal injury or disease, MI, numerous intramuscular injections, severe myocarditis	—
• Male	20–215 IU/L (same as SI units)		
• Female	20–160 U/L (same as SI units)		
Creatine kinase isozyme of heart (CK-MB [CK-2])		Acute MI	—
• Male	2–6 µg/L (2–6 ng/mL)		
• Female	2–5 µg/L (2–5 ng/mL)		
Creatine kinase mass fraction	<5% fraction of total CK	—	—

TABLE A.1 Serum, Plasma, and Whole Blood Chemistries—cont'd

Test	Normal Values (SI Units [Conventional Units])	POSSIBLE ETIOLOGY Higher Values	Lower Values
Creatinine		Severe renal disease, rhabdomyolysis, acromegaly, gigantism	Diseases with decreased muscle mass (e.g., muscular dystrophy, myasthenia gravis)
• Male	53–106 µmol/L (0.6–1.2 mg/dL)		
• Female	44–97 µmol/L (0.5–1.1 mg/dL)		
Ferritin (serum)		Hemochromatosis, hemosiderosis, megaloblastic anemia, hemolytic anemia, alcoholic/inflammatory hepatocellular disease, inflammatory disease, advanced cancers, chronic illnesses such as leukemias, cirrhosis, chronic hepatitis, or collagen-vascular diseases	Iron-deficiency anemia, severe protein deficiency, hemodialysis
• Male	20–200 µg/L (20–200 ng/mL)		
• Female	20–150 µg/L (20–150 ng/mL)		
Folic acid (folate)	11–57 mmol/L (5–25 ng/mL)	Pernicious anemia, vegetarianism, recent massive blood transfusion	Malnutrition, malabsorption syndrome, pregnancy, folic acid deficiency (megaloblastic) anemia, hemolytic anemia, malignancy, liver disease, chronic renal disease
Gamma-glutamyltranspeptidase (GGT)		Liver diseases (e.g., hepatitis, cirrhosis, hepatic necrosis, hepatic tumour or metastasis, hepatotoxic drugs, cholestasis, jaundice) MI, alcohol ingestion, pancreatic disease, Epstein-Barr virus	—
• Male	8–38 U/L (same as SI units)		
• Female	5–27 U/L (same as SI units)		
Glucose, fasting	3.9–6.1 mmol/L (70–110 mg/dL)	Diabetes mellitus, acute stress response, Cushing's syndrome, pheochromocytoma, chronic renal failure, glucagonoma, acute pancreatitis, diuretic therapy, corticosteroid therapy, acromegaly	Insulinoma, hypothyroidism, hypopituitarism, Addison's disease, extensive liver disease, insulin overdose, starvation
Glucose, 2-h oral glucose tolerance testing (OGTT)		Diabetes mellitus	Hyperinsulinism
• Fasting	4–6 mmol/L (70–110 mg/dL)		
• 1 h	<11.1 mmol/L (<200 mg/dL)		
• 2 h	<7.8 mmol/L (<140 mg/dL)		
Haptoglobin	0.5–2.2 g/L (50–220 mg/dL)	Collagen-rheumatic diseases, infection (e.g., pyelonephritis, urinary tract infection, pneumonia), tissue destruction (e.g., MI), nephritis, ulcerative colitis, neoplasia, biliary obstruction	Hemolytic anemia, transfusion reactions, prosthetic heart valves, primary liver disease, hematoma, tissue hemorrhage
Homocysteine		Cardiovascular disease, cerebrovascular disease, cystinuria, folate deficiency, malnutrition, peripheral vascular disease, vitamin B_6 or B_{12} deficiency, malnutrition	—
• 0–30 years	4.6–8.1 µmol/L (same as SI units)		
• 30–59 years			
• Male	6.13–11.2 µmol/L (same as SI units)		
• Female	4.5–7.9 µmol/L (same as SI units)		
• >59 years	5.8–11.9 µmol/L (same as SI units)		
Insulin	43–186 pmol/L (6–26 microU/mL)	Insulinoma, Cushing's syndrome, acromegaly, obesity, fructose or galactose intolerance	Diabetes mellitus, hypopituitarism
Iron		Hemosiderosis or hemochromatosis, iron poisoning, hemolytic anemia, massive blood transfusions, hepatitis or hepatic necrosis, lead toxicity	Insufficient dietary iron, chronic blood loss (irregular menses, uterine cancer, GI cancer, inflammatory bowel disease, diverticulosis, urologic tract [hematuria] cancer, hemangioma, arteriovenous malformation), inadequate intestinal absorption of iron, pregnancy (late), iron-deficiency anemia, neoplasia
• Male	13–31 µmol/L (75–175 µg/dL)		
• Female	5–29 µmol/L (28–162 µg/dL)		

Continued

TABLE A.1 Serum, Plasma, and Whole Blood Chemistries—cont'd

Test	Normal Values (SI Units [Conventional Units])	POSSIBLE ETIOLOGY Higher Values	Lower Values
Total iron-binding capacity (TIBC)	45–73 µmol/L (250–410 µg/dL)	Estrogen therapy, pregnancy (late), polycythemia vera, iron-deficiency anemia	Malnutrition, hypoproteinemia, inflammatory diseases, cirrhosis, hemolytic anemia, pernicious anemia, sickle cell anemia
Lactic acid (venous blood)	0.6–2.2 mmol/L (5–20 mg/dL)	Shock, tissue ischemia, carbon monoxide poisoning, severe liver disease, genetic errors of metabolism, diabetes mellitus (nonketotic)	—
Lactic dehydrogenase (LDH)	45–90 IU/L (same as SI units)	MI, pulmonary disease (e.g., embolism, infarction, pneumonia, heart failure), hepatic disease (e.g., hepatitis, active cirrhosis, neoplasm), RBC disease, skeletal muscle disease and injury, renal parenchymal disease, intestinal ischemia and infarction, neoplastic states, testicular tumours (seminoma, dysgerminomas), lymphoma and other reticuloendothelial system tumours, advanced solid tumour malignancies, pancreatitis, diffuse disease or injury (e.g., heat stroke, collagen disease, shock, hypotension)	—
Lactic dehydrogenase isoenzymes (LDH)			
• LDH_1	0.17–0.27 (17%–27%)	MI, pernicious anemia, strenuous exercise	—
• LDH_2	0.27–0.37 (27%–37%)	Exercise, pulmonary embolus, sickle cell crisis	—
• LDH_3	0.18–0.25 (18%–25%)	Malignant lymphoma, pulmonary embolus	—
• LDH_4	0.03–0.08 (3%–8%)	Systemic lupus erythematosus (SLE), pancreatitis, pulmonary infarction, renal disease	—
• LDH_5	0.0–0.05 (0%–5%)	Heart failure, hepatitis, pulmonary embolus and infarction, skeletal muscle damage, strenuous exercise	—
Lipase	0–160 U/L (same as SI units)	Pancreatic diseases, biliary diseases, renal failure, intestinal diseases, salivary gland inflammation or tumour, peptic ulcer disease	—
Magnesium	0.65–1.05 mmol/L (1.2–2.1 mEq/L)	Renal insufficiency, ingestion of magnesium-containing antacids or salts, Addison's disease, hypothyroidism	Chronic alcoholism, hyperparathyroidism, hyperthyroidism, hypoparathyroidism, malnutrition, severe malabsorption, chronic renal tubular disease
Myoglobin	1.0–5.3 nmol/L (<90 ng/mL)	MI, myositis, malignant hyperthermia, muscular dystrophy, skeletal muscle ischemia or trauma, rhabdomyolysis, seizures	Polymyositis
Osmolality	285–295 mmol/kg (280–295 mOsm/kg)	Hypernatremia, hyperglycemia, hyperosmolar nonketotic hyperglycemia, ketosis, azotemia, dehydration, mannitol therapy, ingestion of ethanol, methanol, or ethylene glycol, uremia, diabetes insipidus, renal tubular necrosis, severe pyelonephritis	Overhydration, SIADH secretion, paraneoplastic syndromes associated with carcinoma (lung, breast, colon)
Oxygen saturation		Increased inspired oxygen, polycythemia, hyperventilation	Anemia, mucus plug, bronchospasm, atelectasis, pneumothorax, pulmonary edema, acute respiratory distress syndrome, restrictive lung disease, atrial or ventricular cardiac septal defects, emboli, inadequate O_2 in inspired air (suffocation), severe hypoventilation states (such as oversedation or neurological somnolence)
• Arterial	95%–100% (same as SI units)		
• Venous	60%–80% (same as SI units)		

TABLE A.1 Serum, Plasma, and Whole Blood Chemistries—cont'd

Test	Normal Values (SI Units [Conventional Units])	POSSIBLE ETIOLOGY Higher Values	Lower Values
pH	See Blood gases		
Phenylalanine	0–121 µmol/L (0–2 mg/dL)	Phenylketonuria	—
Phosphatase, acid	<30 ng/mL (<3.0 µg/L)	Prostatic carcinoma, benign prostatic hypertrophy, prostatitis, multiple myeloma, Paget's disease, hyperparathyroidism, metastasis to the bone, multiple myeloma, sickle cell crisis, thrombocytosis, lysosomal disorders (e.g., Gaucher's disease), renal diseases, liver diseases (such as cirrhosis), rape or sexual intercourse	—
Phosphatase, alkaline (ALP)	40–160 IU/L (40–160 U/L)	Primary cirrhosis, intrahepatic or extrahepatic biliary obstruction, primary or metastatic liver tumour, metastatic tumour to the bone, healing fracture, hyperparathyroidism, osteomalacia, Paget's disease, rheumatoid arthritis, rickets, intestinal ischemia or infarction, MI, sarcoidosis	Hypophosphatemia, hypophosphatasia, malnutrition, milk-alkali syndrome, pernicious anemia, scurvy (vitamin C deficiency)
Phosphorus, phosphate	1.0–1.5 mmol/L (3.0–4.5 mg/dL) †	Hypoparathyroidism, renal failure, increased dietary or intravenous intake of phosphorus, acromegaly, bone metastasis, sarcoidosis, hypocalcemia, acidosis, rhabdomyolysis, advanced lymphoma or myeloma, hemolytic anemia	Inadequate dietary ingestion of phosphorus, chronic antacid ingestion, hyperparathyroidism, hypercalcemia, chronic alcoholism, vitamin D deficiency (rickets), treatment of hyperglycemia, plasminogen, hyperinsulinism (childhood), malnutrition, alkalosis, Gram-negative sepsis
Potassium	3.5–5.1 mmol/L (3.5–5.1 mEq/L)	Excessive dietary intake, excessive intravenous intake, acute or chronic renal failure, Addison's disease, hypoaldosteronism, aldosterone-inhibiting diuretics (e.g., spironolactone, triamterene), crush injury to tissues, hemolysis, transfusion of hemolyzed blood, infection, acidosis dehydration	Deficient dietary intake, deficient intravenous intake, burns, GI disorders (e.g., diarrhea, vomiting, villous adenomas), diuretics, hyperaldosteronism, Cushing's syndrome, renal tubular acidosis, licorice ingestion, alkalosis, insulin administration, glucose administration, ascites, renal artery stenosis, cystic fibrosis, trauma/surgery/burns
Prostate-specific antigen (PSA)	0–4 µg/L (0–4 ng/mL)	Benign prostatic hypertrophy, prostate cancer, prostatitis	—
Proteins		Burns, cirrhosis (globulin fraction), dehydration	Congenital agammaglobulinemia, increased capillary permeability, inflammatory disease, liver disease, malabsorption, malnutrition
• Total	64–83 g/L (6.4–8.3 g/dL)		
• Albumin	35–50 g/L (3.5–5 g/dL)		
• Globulin	23–34 g/L (2.3–3.4 g/dL)		
• Albumin/globulin ratio	1.5:1–2.5:1 (same as SI units)	Multiple myeloma (globulin fraction), shock, vomiting	Malnutrition, nephrotic syndrome, proteinuria, renal disease, severe burns
Renin		Essential hypertension, malignant hypertension, renovascular hypertension, chronic renal failure, sodium-losing GI disease (vomiting or diarrhea), Addison's disease, renin-producing renal tumour, Bartter syndrome, cirrhosis, hyperkalemia, hemorrhage	Primary hyperaldosteronism, steroid therapy, congenital adrenal hyperplasia
• Upright position, sodium depleted (sodium-restricted diet)	20–39 years: 2.9–24 µg/L/h (2.9–24 ng/mL/h) >40 years: 2.9–10.8 µg/L/h (2.9–10.8 ng/mL/h)		
• Upright position, sodium replaced (normal-sodium diet):	20–39 years: 0.1–4.3 µg/L/h (0.1–4.3 ng/mL/h) >40 years: 0.1–3 µg/L/h (0.1–3 ng/mL/h)		
Sodium	136–145 mmol/L (136–145 mEq/L)	Corticosteroid therapy, dehydration, impaired renal function, increased dietary or IV intake, primary aldosteronism	Addison's disease, decreased dietary or IV intake, diabetic ketoacidosis, diuretic therapy, excessive loss from GI tract, excessive perspiration, water intoxication

Continued

TABLE A.1 Serum, Plasma, and Whole Blood Chemistries—cont'd

Test	Normal Values (SI Units [Conventional Units])	POSSIBLE ETIOLOGY Higher Values	Lower Values
Testosterone			
• Male	9.5–30 nmol/L (275–875 ng/dL)	Idiopathic sexual precocity, pinealoma, encephalitis, congenital adrenal hyperplasia, adrenocortical tumour, testicular or extragonadal tumour, hyperthyroidism, testosterone resistance syndromes	Klinefelter's syndrome, cryptorchidism, primary and secondary hypogonadism, trisomy 21, orchiectomy, hepatic cirrhosis
• Female	0.8–2.6 nmol/L (23–875 ng/dL)	Ovarian tumour, adrenal tumour, congenital adrenocortical hyperplasia, trophoblastic tumour, polycystic ovaries, idiopathic hirsutism	—
Thyroxine (T_4), total	Adult male: 51–154 nmol/L (4–12 µg/dL) Adult female: 64–154 nmol/L (5–12 µg/dL) Adult >60 years: 64–142 nmol/L (5–11 µg/dL)	Primary hyperthyroid states (e.g., Graves' disease, Plummer disease, toxic thyroid adenoma), Acute thyroiditis, familial dysalbuminemic hyperthyroxinemia, factitious hyperthyroidism, Struma ovarii, thyroxine-binding globulin increase (e.g., as occurs in pregnancy, hepatitis, congenital hyperproteinemia)	Hypothyroid states (e.g., cretinism, surgical ablation, myxedema), pituitary insufficiency, hypothalamic failure, protein malnutrition and other protein-depleted states (e.g., nephrotic syndrome), iodine insufficiency, nonthyroid illnesses (e.g., renal failure, Cushing's disease, cirrhosis, surgery, advanced cancer)
Thyroxine (T_4), free	13–27 pmol/L (1.0–2.1 ng/dL)	Primary hyperthyroid states (e.g., Graves' disease, Plummer disease, toxic thyroid adenoma), acute thyroiditis, factitious hyperthyroidism, Struma ovarii	Hypothyroid states (e.g., cretinism, surgical ablation, myxedema), pituitary insufficiency, hypothalamic failure, iodine insufficiency, nonthyroid illnesses (e.g., renal failure, Cushing's disease, cirrhosis, surgery, advanced cancer)
Thyroid-stimulating hormone (TSH)	0.4–4.8 mIU/L (0.4–4.8 mIU/L)	Primary hypothyroidism (thyroid dysfunction), thyroiditis, thyroid agenesis, congenital cretinism, large doses of iodine, radioactive iodine injection, surgical ablation of thyroid, severe and chronic illnesses, pituitary TSH-secreting tumour	Secondary hypothyroidism, hyperthyroidism, suppressive doses of thyroid medication, factitious hyperthyroidism
Triglycerides		Glycogen storage disease (von Gierke disease), familial hypertriglyceridemia, apoprotein C-II deficiency, hyperlipidemias, hypothyroidism, high-carbohydrate diet, poorly controlled diabetes, nephrotic syndrome, chronic renal failure	Hyperthyroidism, malabsorption syndrome, malnutrition, abetalipoproteinemia
• Male	0.45–1.71 mmol/L (40–150 mg/dL)		
• Female	0.40–1.52 mmol/L (35–135 mg/dL)		
Tri-iodothyronine (T_3) uptake	24–34 AU (24%–34%)	Hyperthyroidism, hypoproteinemia (e.g., protein malnutrition, protein-losing enteropathy, nephropathy), familial dysalbuminemic hyperthyroxinemia, nonthyroid conditions (e.g., renal failure, Cushing's disease, cirrhosis, surgery, advanced cancer), factitious hyperthyroidism, Struma ovarii	Hypothyroid states (e.g., cretinism, surgical ablation, pituitary insufficiency, hypothalamic failure, myxedema), hepatitis and cirrhosis, pregnancy, hepatitis, congenital hyperproteinemia
Tri-iodothyronine (T_3)	1.1–2.9 mmol/L (70–190 ng/dL)	Primary hyperthyroid states (e.g., Graves' disease, Plummer disease, toxic thyroid adenoma), acute thyroiditis, factitious hyperthyroidism, Struma ovarii, pregnancy, hepatitis, congenital hyperproteinemia	Hypothyroid states (e.g., cretinism, surgical ablation, myxedema), pituitary insufficiency, hypothalamic failure, protein malnutrition and other protein-depleted states (e.g., nephrotic syndrome), iodine insufficiency, nonthyroid illnesses (e.g., renal failure, Cushing's disease, cirrhosis, surgery, advanced cancer), hepatic diseases
Troponin T (cTnT)	<0.1 µg/L (<0.1 ng/mL)	Cardiac muscle damage (resulting from MI, myocarditis, or pericarditis), chronic renal failure, multiorgan failure, severe heart failure	—
Troponin I (cTnI)	<0.35 µg/L (<0.35 ng/mL)		—

TABLE A.1 Serum, Plasma, and Whole Blood Chemistries—cont'd

Test	Normal Values (SI Units [Conventional Units])	POSSIBLE ETIOLOGY Higher Values	Lower Values
Urea nitrogen, blood (blood urea nitrogen [BUN], serum urea nitrogen)	2.9–8.2 mmol/L (8–23 mg/dL)	Prerenal causes, hypovolemia, shock, burns, dehydration, heart failure, MI, GI bleeding, excessive protein ingestion (alimentary tube feeding), excessive protein catabolism, starvation, sepsis, renal disease (e.g., glomerulonephritis, pyelonephritis, acute tubular necrosis), renal failure, nephrotoxic drugs, ureteral obstruction from stones, tumour, or congenital anomalies, bladder outlet obstruction from prostatic hypertrophy or cancer or bladder/urethral congenital anomalies, postrenal azotemia	Liver failure, overhydration because of fluid overload in SIADH, negative nitrogen balance (e.g., malnutrition, malabsorption), pregnancy, nephrotic syndrome
Uric acid		Increased ingestion of purines, genetic inborn error in purine metabolism, metastatic cancer, multiple myeloma, leukemias, cancer chemotherapy, hemolysis, rhabdomyolysis (e.g., heavy exercise, burns, crush injury, epileptic seizure, MI, gout)	Wilson's disease, Fanconi syndrome, lead poisoning, yellow atrophy of liver
• Male	240–501 µmol/L (4.0–8.5 mg/dL)		
• Female	160–430 µmol/L (2.7–7.3 mg/dL)		
Vitamin A	0.52–2.09 µmol/L (15–60 µg/dL)	Excess ingestion of vitamin A	Vitamin A deficiency
Vitamin B_{12}	118–701 pmol/L (160–950 pg/mL)	Leukemia, polycythemia vera, severe liver dysfunction, myeloproliferative disease	Pernicious anemia, malabsorption syndromes (e.g., inflammatory bowel disease, sprue, Crohn's disease), intestinal worm infestation, atrophic gastritis, Zollinger-Ellison syndrome, large proximal gastrectomy, resection of terminal ileum, achlorhydria, pregnancy, vitamin C deficiency, folic acid deficiency

*Because arterial blood gases are influenced by altitude, the values for $PaCO_2$, PaO_2, and PvO_2 decrease as altitude increases. The lower values are normal for an altitude of 1.6 km (1 mile) above sea level.
†Values for older persons are significantly lower than those for younger adults.
ACTH, Adrenocorticotropic hormone; COPD, chronic obstructive pulmonary disease; DKA, diabetic ketoacidosis; GI, gastro-intestinal; IV, intravenous; MI, myocardial infarction; RBC, red blood cell; SIADH, syndrome of inappropriate antidiuretic hormone.

TABLE A.2 Hematology

Test	Normal Values (SI Units [Conventional Units])	POSSIBLE ETIOLOGY Higher Values	Lower Values
Activated coagulation time or automated clotting time (ACT)	70–120 s (same as SI units)	Heparin administration, clotting factor deficiencies, cirrhosis of the liver, coumadin administration, lupus inhibitor	Thrombosis
Activated partial thromboplastin time (aPTT)	25–40 s* (same as SI units)	Congenital clotting factor deficiencies (e.g., von Willebrand's disease, hemophilia, hypofibrinogenemia), cirrhosis of liver, vitamin K deficiency, disseminated intravascular coagulation (DIC), heparin administration, coumarin administration	Early stages of DIC, extensive cancer (e.g., ovarian, pancreatic, colon)
Bleeding time (Ivy method)	1–9 min	Acetylsalicylic acid (ASA; Aspirin) ingestion, clotting factor deficiency, defective platelet function, thrombocytopenia, vascular disease, von Willebrand's disease	—
D-dimer	<3.0 nmol/L (<0.4 µg/mL)	DIC, primary fibrinolysis, during thrombolytic or defibrination therapy, deep vein thrombosis, pulmonary embolism, arterial thromboembolism, sickle cell anemia with or without vaso-occlusive crisis, pregnancy, malignancy, surgery	—

Continued

TABLE A.2 Hematology—cont'd

Test	Normal Values (SI Units [Conventional Units])	POSSIBLE ETIOLOGY Higher Values	Lower Values
Erythrocyte count† (RBC count [altitude dependent]) • Male • Female	 $4.7–6.2 \times 10^{12}$/L $4.2–5.4 \times 10^{12}$/L	Erythrocytosis, congenital heart disease, severe chronic obstructive pulmonary disease, polycythemia vera, severe dehydration (e.g., severe diarrhea or burns), hemoglobinopathies, thalassemia trait	Anemia, hemoglobinopathy, cirrhosis, hemolytic anemia (as in erythroblastosis fetalis, hemoglobinopathies, drug-induced reactions, transfusion reactions, paroxysmal nocturnal hemoglobinuria), hemorrhage, dietary deficiency, bone marrow failure, prosthetic valves, renal disease, normal pregnancy, rheumatoid/collagen-vascular diseases (e.g., rheumatoid arthritis, lupus, sarcoidosis), lymphoma, multiple myeloma, leukemia, Hodgkin's disease
Erythrocyte sedimentation rate (ESR), Westergren Method • Male • Female	 ≤15 mm/h (same as SI units) ≤20 mm/h (same as SI units)	*Moderate increase:* acute hepatitis, myocardial infarction, rheumatoid arthritis, chronic renal failure (e.g., nephritis, nephrosis), malignant diseases (e.g., multiple myeloma, Hodgkin's disease, advanced carcinomas), bacterial infection, inflammatory diseases, necrotic diseases, diseases associated with increased protein levels, severe anemias (e.g., iron deficiency or vitamin B_{12} deficiency)	Sickle cell disease, spherocytosis, hypofibrinogenemia, polycythemia vera
Fibrin split (degradation) products	<10 mg/L (<10 μg/mL)	Disseminated intravascular coagulation, heart or vascular surgery, thromboembolism, thrombosis, advanced malignancy, severe inflammation, postoperative states, massive trauma, deficiency in protein S and protein C, antithrombin III deficiency	Anticoagulation therapy
Fibrinogen	5.8–11.8 μmol/L (200–400 mg/dL)	Acute inflammatory reactions (e.g., rheumatoid arthritis, glomerulonephritis), trauma, acute infection such as pneumonia, coronary heart disease, stroke, peripheral vascular disease, cigarette smoking, pregnancy	Liver disease (hepatitis, cirrhosis), Disseminated intravascular coagulopathy, fibrinolysins, congenital afibrinogenemia, advanced carcinoma, malnutrition, large-volume blood transfusion
Hematocrit (altitude dependent)† • Male • Female	 0.42–0.52 volume fraction (42%–52%) 0.37–0.47 volume fraction (37%–47%)	Erythrocytosis, congenital heart disease, polycythemia vera, severe dehydration (e.g., severe diarrhea, burns), severe chronic obstructive pulmonary disease	Anemia, hemoglobinopathy, cirrhosis, hemolytic anemia, hemorrhage, dietary deficiency, bone marrow failure, prosthetic valves, renal disease, normal pregnancy, rheumatoid/collagen-vascular diseases, lymphoma, multiple myeloma, leukemia, Hodgkin's disease
Hemoglobin (altitude dependent)† • Male • Female	 140–180 g/L (14–18 g/dL) 120–160 g/L (12–16 g/dL)	Erythrocytosis, congenital heart disease, polycythemia vera, severe dehydration (e.g., severe diarrhea, burns), severe chronic obstructive pulmonary disease	Anemia, hemoglobinopathy, cirrhosis, hemolytic anemia, hemorrhage dietary deficiency, bone marrow failure, prosthetic valves, renal disease, normal pregnancy, rheumatoid/collagen-vascular diseases (e.g., rheumatoid arthritis, lupus), lymphoma, multiple myeloma, leukemia, Hodgkin's disease
Hemoglobin, glycosylated or glycated (hemoglobin A_{1c} [HbA_{1c}])	4–5.9% (adult/child without diabetes)	Newly diagnosed diabetes, poorly controlled diabetes, nondiabetic hyperglycemia, patients with splenectomy, pregnancy	Hemolytic anemia, chronic blood loss, chronic renal failure
International normalized ratio (INR)	0.9–1.1	Same as for PT	—
Mean corpuscular hemoglobin (MCH) [Hb/RBC]	27–31 pg (same as SI units)	Macrocytic anemia	Microcytic anemia, hypochromic anemia
Mean corpuscular hemoglobin concentration (MCHC) [Hb/Hct]	27–31 pg (same as SI units)	Spherocytosis, intravascular hemolysis, cold agglutinins	Iron-deficiency anemia, thalassemia

TABLE A.2 Hematology—cont'd

Test	Normal Values (SI Units [Conventional Units])	POSSIBLE ETIOLOGY Higher Values	Lower Values
Mean corpuscular volume (MCV) [Hct/RBC]	76–100 fL (76–100 mm³)	Pernicious anemia (vitamin B_{12} deficiency), folic acid deficiency, antimetabolite therapy, alcoholism, chronic liver disease	Iron-deficiency anemia, thalassemia, anemia of chronic illness
Partial thromboplastin time (PTT)	60–70 s (same as SI units)	Congenital clotting factor deficiencies, cirrhosis of liver, vitamin K deficiency, disseminated intravascular coagulation (DIC), heparin administration, coumarin administration	Early stages of DIC, extensive cancer (e.g., ovarian, pancreatic, colon)
Platelet count (thrombocytes)	150–400 × 10⁹/L (150 000–400 000/mm³)	Malignant disorders (leukemia, lymphoma, solid tumours such as of the colon), polycythemia vera, rheumatoid arthritis, iron-deficiency anemia or following hemorrhagic anemia	Hypersplenism, hemorrhage, immune thrombocytopenia (e.g., idiopathic thrombocytopenia, neonatal, post-transfusion, or drug-induced thrombocytopenia), leukemia and other myelofibrosis disorders, thrombotic thrombocytopenia, Graves' disease, inherited disorders (e.g., Wiskott-Aldrich, Bernard-Soulier, Zieve syndromes), DIC, SLE, pernicious anemia, hemolytic anemia, cancer chemotherapy, infection
Prothrombin time (PT; Protime)	>20 s	Liver disease (e.g., cirrhosis, hepatitis), hereditary factor deficiency, vitamin K deficiency, bile duct obstruction, coumarin ingestion, disseminated intravascular coagulation, massive blood transfusion, salicylate intoxication	—
Red cell distribution width (RDW)	11%–14.5% (same as SI units)	Iron-deficiency anemia, B_{12} vitamin or folate-deficiency anemia, hemoglobinopathies (e.g., sickle cell disease or protein C disease), hemolytic anemias: fragmentation increases RDW variation, posthemorrhagic anemias	—
Reticulocyte count (manual)	0.5%–2% total number of RBC	Hemolytic anemia (e.g., immune hemolytic anemia, hemoglobinopathies, hypersplenism, trauma from a prosthetic heart valve), hemorrhage (3 to 4 days later), hemolytic disease of the newborn, treatment for deficiency in iron, vitamin B_{12}, or folate	Pernicious anemia and folic acid deficiency, iron-deficiency anemia, aplastic anemia, radiation therapy, malignancy, marrow failure, adrenocortical hypofunction, anterior pituitary hypofunction, chronic diseases
Sickle cell solubility	Negative (negative)	Sickle cell anemia	—
Thrombin time	8–12 s (same as SI units)	DIC, increased tendency to bleed	—
WBC count†	3.5–12.0 × 10⁹/L (3 500–12 000/mm³)	Infection, leukemic neoplasia or other myeloproliferative disorders, other malignancy, trauma, stress, or hemorrhage, tissue necrosis, inflammation, dehydration, thyroid storm, steroid use	Drug toxicity, bone marrow failure, overwhelming infections, dietary deficiency (e.g., vitamin B_{12} deficiency, iron deficiency), congenital bone marrow aplasia, bone marrow infiltration (e.g., myelofibrosis), autoimmune disease, hypersplenism
WBC differential			
• Band neutrophils	0–1 × 10⁹/L (0%–9%)	Acute infections	—
• Basophils	0.01–0.05 × 10⁹/L (15–50/mm³; 0.5%–1%)	Basophilia, myeloproliferative disease (e.g., myelofibrosis, polycythemia rubra vera) leukemia	Basopenia, acute allergic reactions hyperthyroidism stress reactions
• Eosinophils	0.00–0.25 × 10⁹/L (50–250/mm³; 1%–4%)	Eosinophilia, parasitic infections, allergic reactions, eczema, leukemia, autoimmune diseases	Eosinopenia, increased adrenosteroid production
• Lymphocytes	1.5–3.0 × 10⁹/L (1500–3000/mm³; 20%–40%)	Lymphocytosis, chronic bacterial infection, viral infection (e.g., mumps, rubella), lymphocytic leukemia, multiple myeloma, infectious mononucleosis, radiation, infectious hepatitis	Lymphocytopenia, leukemia. sepsis, immunodeficiency diseases, lupus erythematosus, later stages of human immunodeficiency virus infection *Drug therapy:* adrenocorticosteroids, antineoplastics Radiation therapy

Continued

TABLE A.2 Hematology—cont'd

Test	Normal Values (SI Units [Conventional Units])	POSSIBLE ETIOLOGY Higher Values	Lower Values
• Monocytes	0.3–0.5 × 10^9/L (300–500/mm^3; 2%–8%)	Monocytosis, chronic inflammatory disorders, viral infections (e.g., infectious mononucleosis), tuberculosis, chronic ulcerative colitis, parasites (e.g., malaria)	Monocytopenia, aplastic anemia, hairy cell leukemia *Drug therapy:* prednisone
• Neutrophils	3.0–5.8 × 10^9/L (300–5800/mm^3 (55–70%)	Neutrophilia, physical or emotional stress, acute suppurative infection, myelocytic leukemia, trauma, Cushing's syndrome, inflammatory disorders (e.g., rheumatic fever, thyroiditis, rheumatoid arthritis), metabolic disorders (e.g., ketoacidosis, gout, eclampsia)	Neutropenia, aplastic anemia, dietary deficiency overwhelming bacterial infection (especially in older persons), viral infections (e.g., hepatitis, influenza, measles), radiation therapy, Addison's disease *Drug therapy:* myelotoxic drugs (as in chemotherapy)

*For patients receiving anticoagulant therapy, aPTT is 1.5–2.5 times control value in seconds; PT is 1.5–2.0 times control value in seconds.
†Components of complete blood count (CBC).
DIC, Disseminated intravascular coagulation; RBC, red blood cell; WBC, white blood cell.

TABLE A.3 Serology-Immunology

Test	Normal Values (SI Units [Conventional Units])	POSSIBLE ETIOLOGY Higher Values	Lower Values
Antinuclear antibody (ANA)	Negative at 1:40 dilution (same as SI units)	Systemic lupus erythematosus (SLE), rheumatoid arthritis, periarteritis (polyarteritis) nodosa, dermatomyositis, polymyositis, scleroderma, Sjögren's syndrome, Raynaud's phenomenon, other immune diseases, leukemia, infectious mononucleosis, myasthenia gravis, cirrhosis, chronic hepatitis	—
C-reactive protein (CRP)	<10 mg/L (<1.0 mg/dL)	Acute, noninfectious inflammatory reaction, collagen-vascular diseases, tissue infarction or damage, bacterial infections such as postoperative wound infection, urinary tract infection, or tuberculosis, malignant disease, bacterial infection, increased risk for cardiovascular ischemic events	—
Carcinoembryonic antigen (CEA)	<5 μg/L (5 ng/mL)	Cancer (GI, breast, lung, pancreatic, hepatobiliary), inflammation (colitis, cholecystitis, pancreatitis, diverticulitis), cirrhosis, Crohn's disease, peptic ulcer	—
Direct antihuman globulin test (DAT) or direct Coombs' test	Negative (negative) (no agglutination)	Hemolytic disease of the newborn, incompatible blood transfusion reaction, lymphoma, autoimmune hemolytic anemia, mycoplasmal infection, infectious mononucleosis, hemolytic anemia after heart bypass, adult hemolytic anemia (idiopathic)	—
Fluorescent treponemal antibody absorption (FTAAbs)	Negative (nonreactive)	Syphilis	—
Hepatitis A antibody	Negative (negative)	Hepatitis A	—
Hepatitis B surface antigen (HBsAg)	Negative (negative)	Hepatitis B	—
Hepatitis C antibody	Negative (negative)	Hepatitis C	—

TABLE A.3 Serology–Immunology—cont'd

Test	Normal Values (SI Units [Conventional Units])	POSSIBLE ETIOLOGY Higher Values	Lower Values
Immunoglobulins			
• IgA	0.85–3.85 g/L (85–385 mg/dL)	Chronic liver diseases (e.g., primary biliary cirrhosis), chronic infections, inflammatory bowel disease	Ataxia, telangiectasia, congenital isolated deficiency, hypoproteinemia (e.g., nephrotic syndrome, protein-losing enteropathies), drug immunosuppression (steroids, dextran), acquired immune deficiency syndrome (AIDS),
• IgD	Minimal	Chronic infection, connective tissue disease	—
• IgE	Minimal	Anaphylactic shock, atopic disease (allergies), parasite infections	—
• IgG	5.65–17.65 g/L (565–1765 mg/dL)	Chronic granulomatous infections (e.g., tuberculosis, Wegener granulomatosis, sarcoidosis), hyperimmunization reactions, chronic liver disease, multiple myeloma, autoimmune diseases, intrauterine devices	Wiskott-Aldrich syndrome, agammaglobulinemia, AIDS, hypoproteinemia (e.g., nephrotic syndrome, protein-losing enteropathies), medication immunosuppression (steroids, dextran), non-IgG multiple myeloma, leukemia
• IgM	0.55–3.75 g/L (55–375 mg/dL)	Waldenström macroglobulinemia, chronic infections (e.g., hepatitis, mononucleosis, sarcoidosis), autoimmune diseases (e.g., SLE, rheumatoid arthritis), acute infections, chronic liver disorders (e.g., biliary cirrhosis)	Agammaglobulinemia, AIDS, hypoproteinemia (e.g., nephrotic syndrome, protein-losing enteropathies), drug immunosuppression (steroids, dextran), IgG or IgA multiple myeloma, leukemia
Monospot or Mono-Test	Negative (<1:28 titre)	Infectious mononucleosis, chronic Epstein-Barr virus infection, chronic fatigue syndrome, Burkitt lymphoma, some forms of chronic hepatitis	—
Rheumatoid factor (RA factor)	Negative or <60 IU/mL by nephelometric testing	Rheumatoid arthritis, other autoimmune disease (e.g., SLE, Sjögren's syndrome, scleroderma), chronic viral infection, subacute bacterial endocarditis, tuberculosis, chronic active hepatitis, dermatomyositis, infectious mononucleosis, leukemia, biliary cirrhosis, syphilis, renal disease	—
Thyroid antibodies	Titre <1:100 (same as SI units)	Early hypothyroidism, Graves' disease, Hashimoto's thyroiditis, pernicious anemia, SLE, thyroid carcinoma	—

GI, Gastro-intestinal; *IV*, intravenous.

TABLE A.4 Urine Chemistry

Test	Specimen	Normal Values (SI Units [Conventional Units])	POSSIBLE ETIOLOGY Higher Values	Lower Values
Acetone (ketones)	Random	Negative (negative)	Diabetes mellitus, high-fat and low-carbohydrate diets, starvation states	—
Aldosterone	24 h	17–70 nmol/24 h (2–26 µg/24 h)	*Primary aldosteronism:* aldosterone-producing adrenal adenoma (Conn's disease), adrenal cortical nodular hyperplasia, Bartter syndrome *Secondary aldosteronism:* Hyponatremia, hyperkalemia, diuretic ingestion resulting in hypovolemia and hyponatremia, laxative abuse, stress, malignant hypertension, poor perfusion states (e.g., heart failure), decreased intravascular volume (e.g., cirrhosis, nephrotic syndrome), renal arterial stenosis, pregnancy and oral contraceptives, hypovolemia or hemorrhage, Cushing's disease	Renin deficiency, steroid therapy, Addison's disease, patients on a high-sodium diet, hypernatremia, antihypertensive therapy, aldosterone deficiency

Continued

TABLE A.4 Urine Chemistry—cont'd

Test	Specimen	Normal Values (SI Units [Conventional Units])	POSSIBLE ETIOLOGY Higher Values	Lower Values
Amylase	24 h	25–125 IU/L (25–125 U/L)	Acute pancreatitis, chronic relapsing pancreatitis, peptic ulcer penetrating into the pancreas, GI disease, acute cholecystitis, parotiditis (mumps), ruptured ectopic pregnancy, renal failure, diabetic ketoacidosis, pulmonary infarction, after endoscopic retrograde pancreatography	—
Bence-Jones protein	Random	Kappa total light chain: <0.68 mg/dL Lambda total light chain <0.40 mg/dL Kappa/lambda ratio: 0.7–6.2	Multiple myeloma (plasmacytoma), chronic lymphocytic leukemia, lymphoma, metastatic colon, breast, lung, or prostate cancer, amyloidosis, Waldenström macroglobulinemia	—
Bilirubin	Random	3–22 µmol/L (0.2–1.3 mg/dL)	Gallstones, extrahepatic duct obstruction (tumour, inflammation, gallstone, scarring, surgical trauma), extensive liver metastasis, cholestasis from drugs, Dubin-Johnson syndrome, Rotor syndrome	—
Calcium	24 h	2.25–2.75 mmol/day (9.0–10.5 mg/dL)	Bone tumour, hyperparathyroidism, milk-alkali syndrome, lymphoma, Addison's disease	Hypoparathyroidism, malabsorption of calcium and vitamin D, renal failure, pancreatitis
Catecholamines • Epinephrine • Norepinephrine	24 h	<590 mmol/day (<100 µg/24 h) <109 nmol/day (<20 µg/24 h) <590 nmol/day (<100 µg/24 h)	Pheochromocytomas, neuroblastomas, ganglioneuromas, ganglioblastomas, severe stress, strenuous exercise, acute anxiety	—
Chloride	24 h	98–106 mmol/L (98–106 mEq/L)	Dehydration, excessive infusion of normal saline solution, metabolic acidosis, renal tubular acidosis, Cushing's syndrome, kidney dysfunction, hyperparathyroidism, eclampsia, respiratory alkalosis	Overhydration, SIADH, heart failure, vomiting or prolonged gastric suction, chronic diarrhea or high-output GI fistula, chronic respiratory acidosis, metabolic alkalosis, salt-losing nephritis, Addison's disease, diuretic therapy, hypokalemia, aldosteronism
Creatine • Male • Female	24 h	 20–215 IU/L (20–215 U/L) 20–160 IU/L (20–160 U/L)	Diseases or injury affecting the heart muscle, skeletal muscle, and brain	—
Creatinine • Male • Female	24 h	 53–106 µmol/L (0.6–1.2 mg/dL) 44–97 µmol/L (0.5–1.1 mg/dL)	Diseases affecting renal function, such as glomerulonephritis, pyelonephritis, acute tubular necrosis, urinary tract obstruction, reduced renal blood flow (e.g., shock, dehydration, congestive heart failure, atherosclerosis), diabetic nephropathy, nephritis, rhabdomyolysis, acromegaly, gigantism	Debilitation, decreased muscle mass (e.g., muscular dystrophy, myasthenia gravis)
Creatinine clearance		75–125 mL/min	Exercise, pregnancy, high cardiac output syndromes	Impaired kidney function (e.g., renal artery atherosclerosis, glomerulonephritis, acute tubular necrosis), conditions causing decreases in GFR (e.g., heart failure, cirrhosis with ascites, shock, dehydration)
• Male • Female		1.78–2.32 mL/s (107–139 mL/min) 1.45–1.78 mL/s (87–107 mL/min)		

TABLE A.4 Urine Chemistry—cont'd

Test	Specimen	Normal Values (SI Units [Conventional Units])	POSSIBLE ETIOLOGY Higher Values	Lower Values
Estriol	24 h		Feminization syndromes, precocious puberty, ovarian tumour, testicular tumour, adrenal tumour, normal pregnancy, hepatic cirrhosis, liver necrosis, hyperthyroidism	A failing pregnancy, Turner's syndrome, hypopituitarism, primary and secondary hypogonadism, Stein-Leventhal syndrome, menopause, anorexia nervosa
• Female				
• Ovulatory phase		13–54 µg/24 h (104–370 nmol/L)		
• Luteal phase		4–100 µg/24 h (15–37 nmol/L)		
• Pregnancy		*First Trimester:* 0–800 µg/24 h (0–2900 nmol/L) *Second Trimester:* 800–1200 µg/24 h (2900–44000 nmol/L) *Third Trimester:* 5000–12000 µg/24 h (18000–180000 nmol/L)		
• Menopause		1.4–19.6 µg/24 h (5.2–72.5 nmol/L)		
• Male		1–11 µg/24 h (18–67 nmol/L)	—	—
Glucose	Random	Random: negative Fasting: <6.1 mmol/L (70–11 mg/dL)	Diabetes mellitus, acute stress response, Cushing's syndrome, pheochromocytoma, chronic renal failure, glucagonoma, acute pancreatitis, diuretic therapy, corticosteroid therapy, acromegaly	Insulinoma, hypothyroidism, hypopituitarism, Addison's disease, extensive liver disease, insulin overdose, starvation
Hemoglobin	Random		Erythrocytosis, congenital heart disease, severe chronic obstructive pulmonary disease, polycythemia vera, severe dehydration (e.g., severe diarrhea, burns)	—
• Male		140–180 mmol/L (14–18 g/dL)		
• Female		120–160 mmol/L (12–16 g/dL)		
Ketone bodies	Random	Negative (negative)	Poorly controlled diabetes mellitus, starvation, alcoholism, weight-reduction diets, prolonged vomiting, anorexia, fasting, high-protein diets, glycogen storage diseases, febrile illnesses in infants and children, hyperthyroidism, severe stress or illness, excessive aspirin ingestion	—
Lead	24 h	<0.48 µmol/day (<10 µg/day)	Lead exposure	—
Metanephrine	24 h	12–60 pg/mL	Pheochromocytoma	—
Myoglobin	Random	1.0–5.3 nmol/L (<90 ng/mL)	Myocardial infarction, skeletal muscle inflammation (myositis), malignant hyperthermia, muscular dystrophy, skeletal muscle ischemia, skeletal muscle trauma, rhabdomyolysis seizures	Polymyositis
pH	Random	4.6–8.0 (average, 6.0)	Alkalemia, urinary tract infections, gastric suction, vomiting, renal tubular acidosis	Acidemia, diabetes mellitus, starvation, respiratory acidosis
Phosphorus, inorganic	24 h	0.97–1.45 mmol/L (3.0–4.5 mg/dL)	Fever, hypoparathyroidism, nervous exhaustion, rickets, tuberculosis	Acute infections, nephritis
Potassium	24 h	25–100 mmol/day (25–100 mEq/L/day)	Chronic renal failure, renal tubular acidosis, starvation, Cushing's syndrome, hyperaldosteronism, excessive intake of licorice, alkalosis, diuretic therapy	Dehydration, Addison's disease, malnutrition, vomiting, diarrhea, malabsorption, acute renal failure

Continued

TABLE A.4 Urine Chemistry—cont'd

Test	Specimen	Normal Values (SI Units [Conventional Units])	POSSIBLE ETIOLOGY Higher Values	Lower Values
Protein (dipstick)	Random	Negative (negative)	Heart failure, nephritis, nephrosis, physiological stress	—
Protein (qualitative) • At rest • During exercise	24 h	60–80 g/L <50–80 mg/24 h (0.05–0.08 g/day) <250 mg/24 h (<0.25 g/day)	Nephrotic syndrome, glomerulonephritis, malignant hypertension, diabetic glomerulosclerosis, polycystic kidney disease, SLE, Goodpasture's syndrome, heavy-metal poisoning, bacterial pyelonephritis, nephrotoxic drug therapy, trauma, macroglobulinemia, multiple myelomas, pre-eclampsia, heart failure, orthostatic proteinuria, severe muscle exertion, renal vein thrombosis: congestion of the kidneys is associated with proteinuria, bladder tumour, urethritis or prostatitis, amyloidosis	
Sodium, blood	24 h	136–145 mmol/L (136–145 mEq/L)	Increased dietary intake, excessive sodium in intravenous fluids	Cushing's syndrome, hyperaldosteronism
Specific gravity	Random	1.005–1.030 (usually, 1.010–1.025) *	Dehydration, pituitary tumour or trauma, decreased renal blood flow (as in heart failure, renal artery stenosis, or hypotension), glycosuria and proteinuria, water restriction, fever, excessive sweating, vomiting, diarrhea	Overhydration, diabetes insipidus, renal failure, diuresis
Titratable acidity	24 h	20–50 mEq/day (same as SI units)	Metabolic acidosis	Metabolic alkalosis
Uric acid		Male: 240–501 µmol/L (4.0–8.5 mg/dL) Female: 160–430 µmol/L (2.7–7.3 mg/dL)	Increased ingestion of purines, Genetic inborn error in purine metabolism, metastatic cancer, multiple myeloma, leukemias, cancer chemotherapy, hemolysis, rhabdomyolysis, gout	Idiopathic, chronic renal disease, acidosis (ketotic [diabetic or starvation] or lactic), hypothyroidism, toxemia of pregnancy, hyperlipoproteinemia, alcoholism, shock or chronic blood volume depletion states, Wilson's disease, Fanconi's syndrome, lead poisoning, yellow atrophy of liver
Urobilinogen	24 h	0.5–4.0 mg/24 h (0.5–4.0 EU/24 h)	Hemolytic anemia, pernicious anemia, hemolysis because of drugs, hematoma, excessive ecchymosis	Biliary obstruction, cholestasis
Vanillylmandelic acid	24 h	<35 µmol/day (<6.8 mg/24 h)	Pheochromocytomas, neuroblastomas, ganglioneuromas, ganglioblastomas, severe stress, strenuous exercise, acute anxiety	—

*Values decrease with age.
GI, Gastro-intestinal; SIADH, syndrome of inappropriate antidiuretic hormone.

TABLE A.5 Fecal Analysis

Test	Normal Values (SI Units [Conventional Units])	POSSIBLE ETIOLOGY Higher Values	Lower Values
Blood*	Negative (negative)	Anal fissures, hemorrhoids, inflammatory bowel disease, malignant tumour, peptic ulcer	—
Colour			
• Brown		Various shades, depending on diet	—
• Clay		Biliary obstruction or presence of barium sulphate	—
• Tarry		More than 100 mL of blood in GI tract	—
• Red		Blood in large intestine	—
• Black		Blood in upper GI tract or iron medication	—

TABLE A.5 Fecal Analysis—cont'd

Test	Normal Values (SI Units [Conventional Units])	POSSIBLE ETIOLOGY Higher Values	Lower Values
Fecal fat	7–21 mmol/day (2–6 g/24 h)	Cystic fibrosis, malabsorption secondary to sprue, celiac disease, Whipple's disease, Crohn's disease (regional enteritis), or radiation enteritis, maldigestion secondary to obstruction of the pancreatobiliary tree (e.g., cancer, stricture, gallstones), short-gut syndrome secondary to surgical resection, surgical bypass, or congenital anomaly	—
Mucus	Negative (negative)	Mucous colitis, spastic constipation	—
Pus	Negative (negative)	Chronic bacillary dysentery, chronic ulcerative colitis, localized abscesses	—
Urobilinogen	51–372 µmol/100 g of stool (30–220 mg/100 g of stool)	Hemolytic anemias	Complete biliary obstruction

*Ingestion of meat may produce false-positive results. Patient may be placed on a meat-free diet for 3 days before the test.
GI, Gastro-intestinal.

TABLE A.6 Cerebrospinal Fluid Analysis

Test	Normal Values (SI Units [Conventional Units])	POSSIBLE ETIOLOGY Higher Values	Lower Values
Blood	Negative (negative)	Intracranial hemorrhage	—
Chloride	116–122 mmol/L of CSF (116–122 mEq/L of CSF)	Uremia	Bacterial infections of CNS (meningitis, encephalitis)
Glucose	2.8–4.2 mmol/L of CSF (50–75 mg/dL of CSF) or 60–70% of blood glucose level	Diabetes mellitus, viral infections of CNS	Bacterial infections and tuberculosis of CNS
Protein • Lumbar	0.15–0.45 g/L (15–45 mg/dL)	Guillain-Barré syndrome, poliomyelitis, traumatic tap	—
Pressure	100–200 mm Hg H$_2$O	Hemorrhage, intracranial tumour, meningitis	Head injury, spinal tumour, subdural hematoma

CNS, Central nervous system; CSF, cerebrospinal fluid.
Note: The content of this appendix is based on the values presented in Pagana, K. D., Pagana, T. J., & Pike-MacDonald, S. A. (2019). *Mosby's Canadian manual of diagnostic and laboratory tests* (2nd Cdn. ed.). Elsevier.

INDEX

Page numbers followed by "*f*" indicate figures; "*t*" indicate tables; "*b*" indicate boxes. Syndromes and Disorders appear in boldface.

A

A band, 561–562, 562*f*
A beta (Aβ) fibres, 330
A delta (Aδ) fibres, 330
Abbreviations, pulmonary, 664*t*
Abdominal pain, 886
Abducens nerve, 321*t*
Aberrant conduction, 623*t*–624*t*
ABGs. *See* Arterial blood gases
Abnormal uterine bleeding, 790–791, 791*t*
Abscesses, 149
  brain, 401
  cavitation of, 691
  peritonsillar, 703
  respiratory tract, 691
  spinal cord, 401
  tonsillar, 703
Absence seizure, 421*t*
Absolute polycythemia, 508
Absorption atelectasis, 676
Acanthosis nigricans, 256*t*
Accelerated junctional rhythm, 622*t*–623*t*
Accelerated ventricular rhythm, 622*t*–623*t*
Accessory organs of digestion, 873–880. *See also* Exocrine pancreas; Gallbladder; Gastro-intestinal tract; Liver
  anatomy of, 874, 874*f*
  cancer of, 921–924
  disorders of, 906–910
Acetyl coenzyme A, 17, 18*f*
Accidental hyperthermia, 337–338
Accommodation, 340–341
Acetabular dysplasia, 1008
Acetaminophen (Tylenol)
  for osteoarthritis, 984–985
Acetazolamide, 725*t*
Acetylcholine, 305*t*, 866*t*
Acetylcholine receptors (AChRs), 404
Achalasia, 887–888
Achilles tenotomy, 1008
AChRs. *See* Acetylcholine receptors
Acid maltase deficiency, 997
Acid-base balance
  buffer systems in, 124
  CKD progression and, 750*t*
  compensatory changes for, 129*f*
  hydrogen ion in, 124
  pH and, 124
Acid-base imbalances
  ABGs, 130
  compensatory changes for, 129*f*
  metabolic acidosis, 127
  metabolic alkalosis, 128
  respiratory acidosis, 128–129
  respiratory alkalosis, 129–130
Acidemia, 126, 656–657

Acidosis
  ECF hydrogen ions in, 123
  metabolic. *See* Metabolic acidosis
  oxyhemoglobin dissociation curve affected by, 665–666
  respiratory, 128–129
Acids
  bile, 875
  carbonic, 126
  nonvolatile, 124
  renal excretion of, 128*f*
  strong, 124
  titratable, 128*f*
  volatile, 124
  weak, 124
Acinus, 655, 775–776
Acne conglobata, 1054
Acne rosacea, 1033, 1033*f*
Acne vulgaris, 1032, 1053–1054, 1054*f*
Acoustic nerve, 321*t*
ACPA. *See* Anti-citrullinated protein antibody
Acquired heart disease, 647
Acquired hypercoagulability, 533–534
Acquired immune deficiency. *See* Secondary (acquired) immune deficiency
Acquired immunity. *See* Adaptive immunity
Acquired immunodeficiency syndrome (AIDS)
  in children, 297
  lymphocytopenia and, 512
Acquired sideroblastic anemia, 506–507
Acral lentiginous melanoma, 1041
Acrocephaly, 417*f*
Acromegaly, 452–453
ACTH. *See* Adrenocorticotropic hormone
ACTH-independent hypercortisolism, 470
Actin, 561, 958*t*
Actinic keratosis, 1039
Actinin, 958*t*
Action potentials
  cardiac, 556
Activated partial thromboplastin time, 878*t*
Activated platelets, 146
Activator protein-1, 286
Active immunity, 158
Activin, 764*t*, 775, 946*t*
Acute alcoholism, 90
Acute bacterial conjunctivitis, 344
Acute bacterial meningitis, 420
Acute bacterial prostatitis, 842–843, 842*b*
Acute bleeding, 886*t*
Acute bronchitis, 670
Acute colonic pseudo-obstruction, 891
Acute confusional states, 360, 362*b*

Acute coronary syndromes, 601–606
  myocardial infarction. *See* Myocardial infarction
  pathophysiology of, 602–606
  unstable angina, 601–602
Acute cough, 670
Acute cystitis, 737–738
Acute encephalopathies, 419–420
Acute epiglottitis, 702*t*
Acute gastritis, 892
Acute gouty arthritis, 993
Acute hematogenous osteomyelitis, 1010
Acute hydrocephalus, 369
Acute idiopathic TTP, 528
Acute infectious diarrhea, 937
Acute inflammation, 149
Acute inflammatory response, 138*f*
Acute kidney injury (AKI)
  classification of, 744–747
  clinical manifestations of, 746
  definition of, 744
  evaluation of, 746
  intrarenal, 745
  oliguria in, 123, 745*f*, 746
  pathophysiology of, 744–747, 744*t*
  postrenal, 746
  prerenal, 744–745
  RIFLE criteria for, 744*t*
  treatment of, 746
Acute laryngotracheitis, 702
Acute liver failure, 910
Acute lung injury (ALI), 678–682
  in children, 710
Acute lymphocytic leukemia, 296, 514–517
  in children, 547
Acute myeloid leukemia, 513*f*–514*f*
  in children, 547
Acute organic brain syndromes, 360
Acute otitis media, 346
Acute pain, 333
Acute pancreatitis, 915–916, 916*f*
Acute pericarditis, 606–607
Acute poststreptococcal glomerulonephritis, 758–759
Acute pyelonephritis, 738–739, 739*t*, 760
Acute respiratory distress syndrome (ARDS), 678–682
  in children, 710
Acute rheumatic fever, 612–614
Acute toxic inhalation, 677
Acute tubular necrosis (ATN), 744
Acute-phase reactants, 149
Acyanotic heart defects, 667
ADA deficiency. *See* Adenosine deaminase deficiency

1081

INDEX

Adaptation, 73
  cellular. See Cellular adaptation
  diseases of, 216–218
  potassium, 121
Adaptation stage, of general adaptation syndrome, 216–218
Adaptive immunity
  cells of, 135t
  description of, 142
  innate immunity interaction with, 158
Adaptive resizing, 278
ADCC. See Antibody-dependent cellular cytotoxicity
Addison's disease, 123, 472–473
Adenocarcinomas
  characteristics of, 695, 695t, 696f
  definition of, 234–235
  ductal, 922–924
  mammary, 234–235
Adenoid cystic carcinoma, 825t
Adenomas
  pituitary, 451–452
  renal, 736
  toxic, 455
Adenomyosis, 801
Adenosine deaminase deficiency (ADA deficiency), 192–193
Adenosine diphosphate, 16–17, 491, 563
Adenosine monophosphate deaminase deficiency, 997
Adenosine triphosphate (ATP), 15–16, 16b, 335–336, 561
Adenotonsillar hypertrophy, 339
Adenotonsillectomy, 339
ADH. See Antidiuretic hormone
ADHD. See Attention-deficit/hyperactivity disorder
Adipocytes
  cancer-associated, 281f
Adipocytokines, 903–905, 903b
Adipokines, 462
Adiponectin, 823–824, 904–905, 904f
Adipose tissue, 823
Adjuvant chemotherapy, 262
Adolescents, TBW in, 130. See also Children
Adoptive cell therapy, 262
ADP. See Adenosine diphosphate
Adrenal cortex
  aldosterone secretion by, 442
  anatomy of, 441f
  cortisol secretion by, 442
  disorders of, 470–472
    Addison's disease, 123–124, 472–473
    adrenocortical hypofunction, 472–473
    congenital adrenal hyperplasia, 472
    Cushing's syndrome and Cushing's disease, 470–472
    hyperaldosteronism, 472
    hypocortisolism, 472
  glucocorticoids produced by, 440–442
Adrenal glands
  aging and, 444b
  alterations of, 473
  anatomy of, 439, 441f

Adrenal medulla
  catecholamine secretion by, 443
  tumours of, 260, 473–474
Adrenarche, 767
Adrenergic receptors
  α, 221, 322
  β, 221, 322
Adrenergic transmission, 322
Adrenocortical hypofunction, 472–473
Adrenocorticotropic hormone (ACTH), 219, 432
  Cushing's syndrome caused by excessive secretion of, 470
  deficiency of, 451
Adrenomedullin, 573
ADT. See Androgen-deprivation therapy
Advil (ibuprofen), 597
Aerobic glycolysis, 248
Affective-motivational system, 330–331
Afferent arteriole, 736
Afferent loop obstruction, 896
Afferent neuron, 312
Afferent pathways, 301, 330
Afterload, 564, 619
Aganglionic megacolon, 930, 930f
Age-related bone loss, 977
Age-related macular degeneration, 343
Ageusia, 347
Agglutination, 162
Aging, 106–107
  adrenal gland changes and, 444b
  of bone, 961–962
  breast changes secondary to, 818
  cellular, 107–108, 107f
  chest wall and, 666b
  endocrine glands and, 444b
  erythrocytes affected by, 498b
  esophagus by, 880b
  female reproductive system and, 781–782, 781f
  frailty, 108
  gas exchange and, 666b
  gastro-intestinal tract and, 880b
  GH changes and, 444b
  gonads changes and, 444b
  hearing changes with, 344–347
  hematological system affected by, 498b, 498t
  hemoglobin affected by, 498b
  IGF changes and, 444b
  immune response and, 174b
  innate immunity and, 135t
  of joints, 962
  libido and, 781
  liver affected by, 879t
  lungs and, 666b
  male reproductive system and, 782
  menstrual cycle and, 772–775
  of muscles, 962
  olfaction changes with, 348
  pancreas changes and, 444b, 879t
  pituitary gland changes and, 444b
  presbyopia and, 341–343
  prostate cancer risk with, 851–852
  pulmonary system and, 666b
  renal function affected by, 738–739

Aging (Continued)
  reproductive system and, 781–782
  of skeletal muscles, 962
  skin changes in, 1049b
  small intestine affected by, 868–869
  stress-age syndrome and, 230b
  systemic, 108
  taste changes with, 347
  testes and, 777–778
  thyroid gland changes and, 444b
  tissue, 108
  vision changes with, 340–344
Agitated delirium, 362
Agnosia, 360
Agonal rhythm, 622t–623t
Agonist, of muscles, 961
Agranulocytes, 480–482
Agranulocytosis, 510
AIDS. See Acquired immunodeficiency syndrome
Air embolism, 591t
Air pollution
  cancer and, 289
  lung health and, 685b
Air trapping, 683
Airway obstruction, 683, 703f
Airway remodelling, 683
Airway resistance, 661
Airways. See also Pulmonary system
  conducting, 654–655, 656f
  gas-exchange, 655
  lower, 657f
  upper, 656f
Akathisia, 372t
AKI. See Acute kidney injury
Akinesia, 373
Alanine aminotransferase, 878t
Alarm stage, of general adaptation syndrome, 216
Albinism, 98
Albumin, 115, 479, 742–744, 878t, 907–908, 944t
Alcohol
  cancer and, 276–282
  toxic myopathies and, 999
Alcoholic cirrhosis, 911
Alcoholic fatty liver, 910–912
Alcoholic hepatitis, 91f, 911
Alcoholic liver disease, 90
  cirrhosis and, 911
Alcoholic steatohepatitis, 911
Alcoholism, 89
Aldactone, 734t
Aldosterone
  blood pressure affected by, 574
  blood volume regulation and, 720
  nephron function affected by, 725
  potassium regulation by, 116
  secretion of, 442
  sodium balance affected by, 116
  urine regulation and, 720
Alendronate, 1010
Algor mortis, 108
ALI. See Acute lung injury
Alkalemia, 126

Alkaline phosphatase, 878t, 944t
Alkaline reflux gastritis, 896
Alkalosis
   contraction, 128
   metabolic, 128
      hypochloremic, 128
   respiratory, 129–130
Alkylphenols, 823
Allergic alveolitis, 207
Allergic conjunctivitis, 344
Allergic contact dermatitis, 1029–1030, 1030f
Allergy, 199–213
Allodynia, 334
Alloimmune diseases, 199
Allostasis, 218
Allostatic overload, 218
Alnacort, 1016
Alopecia, 258, 1047–1049
Alopecia areata, 1049
Alpha cells, 438
Alpha globulins, 479–480
Alpha rigidity, 370t
α-**Thalassemias**, 543–545
ALS. See Amyotrophic lateral sclerosis
Alternative pathway, of complement system, 140
Alveolar dead space, 672–673
Alveolar ducts, 655, 658f
Alveolar hypoventilation, 128
Alveolar hypoxia, chronic, 656
Alveolar macrophages, 655
Alveolar pressure, 663
Alveolar sac, 658f
Alveolar septum, 655
Alveolar surface tension, 661
Alveolar ventilation, 658
Alveoli, 655
Alveolocapillary membrane
   anatomy of, 655
   oxygen diffusion across, 663, 673
   oxygen toxicity damage to, 677
Alzheimer's disease, 363, 364t, 365b, 365t
Amblyopia, 341, 342t
Ambulatory blood pressure monitoring, 649–650
Amenorrhea, 789–790, 790f
Amiloride, 725t
Amino acid metabolism defects, 419
Ammonia, 624–625
Ammonium, 128f
Amnesia, 358
Amniotic fluid embolism, 591t
Amphiarthrosis, 950
Ampulla, of fallopian tube, 771
Ampulla of Vater, 877
α-Amylase, 862
Amylin, 439, 460
Amyloidosis, 523–524
Amyotrophic lateral sclerosis (ALS), 377–378
Anabolism, 15
Anaphylactic shock, 627
Anaphylatoxins, 139–140
Anaphylaxis, 627

Anaplasia, 234
Androgen insensitivity syndrome, 786
Androgen receptors
   in prostate cancer, 819
   signalling, 848
Androgen-deprivation therapy (ADT), 847
Androgenic alopecia, 1048
Androgens, 443, 772
   in female reproductive system, 783
   hypersecretion of, 452
   in prostate cancer, 844
   testosterone as source of, 844
Andropause, 782
Anemia
   aplastic, 502t
   cancer and, 256t
   in children, 538, 538t
   of chronic disease, 503
   classification of, 501–503
   clinical manifestations of, 501–503
   Cooley's, 544
   Fanconi, 295
   folate deficiency, 504–505
   hemolytic, 502t, 538–540
   hypoplastic, 506–507
   hypoxemia associated with, 503
   iron deficiency, 505–506
      in children, 538–539
      clinical manifestations of, 539
      evaluation and treatment of, 539
      pathophysiology of, 538–539
   leukemia and, 511t
   macrocytic-normochromic, 503–505
   mechanisms of, 258
   megaloblastic, 258, 503
   microcytic-hypochromic, 505–507
   normocytic-normochromic, 507
   pernicious, 503–504
   postgastrectomy, 896–897
   posthemorrhagic, 502t
   progression of, 502f
   sickle cell, 502t, 540–543
   sideroblastic, 506–507
Anencephaly, 413
Aneurysms, 589, 589f
   berry, 397
   fusiform, 397
   giant, 397
   intracranial, 397
   saccular, 397
Angelman syndrome, 65, 65f
Angina pectoris, 598–599
Angioedema, hereditary, 140
Angiogenesis, 152, 555
   cancer cell inducement of, 246–247
   tumour-induced, 247f
Angiogenesis factors, 152
Angiogenic factors, 246
Angiogenic inhibitors, 246
Angiomas, 407t
Angiotensin I, 116
Angiotensin II, 116
Angiotensin receptor blockers, 123, 585, 650, 744

Angular stomatitis, 505
ANH. See Atrial natriuretic hormone
Anhidrotic ectodermal dysplasia, 63
Anion gap, 127
Anisotropic band, 561–562
Ankylosing spondylitis, 989–991, 990f
Anoikis, 253
Anomic aphasia, 360
Anorectal malformations, 931, 931f
Anorexia, 515, 883
Anorgasmia, 811
Anosmia, 347
ANP. See Atrial natriuretic peptide
ANS. See Autonomic nervous system
Antagonist, of muscles, 961
Anterior columns, 311
Anterior fontanelle, 412
Anterior fossa, 313
Anterior horn, 311
Anterior pituitary gland
   anatomy of, 432
   chromophils of, 432
   chromophobes of, 432
   diseases of
      acromegaly, 452–453
      hyperpituitarism, 451–452
      hypopituitarism, 450–451
      prolactinomas, 453
Anterior spinal artery, 318
Anterior spinothalamic tracts, 312
Anterograde amnesia, 358
Antibiotic resistance
   UTI and, 738b
Antibiotics, 137
   broad-spectrum, 137
Antibodies, 158
   antigen binding to, 162
   functions of, 162–164
   heterophilic, 512–513
   immunoglobulins compared to, 161–162
   molecular structure of, 161–162
   monoclonal, 261b, 262
   plasma cells production of, 479
Antibody-dependent cellular cytotoxicity, 205
Antibody screen test, 495t–497t
Antibody-mediated hemorrhagic disease, 546–547
Anticipatory stress responses, 216
Anti-citrullinated protein antibody (ACPA), 988
Anticoagulants, 495t–497t
Antidiuretic hormone (ADH)
   blood volume regulation and, 720, 721f
   diabetes insipidus and, 450
   homeostatic function of, 435
   nephron function affected by, 724–725
   secretion of, 432
   syndrome of inappropriate, 120, 256t, 449–450
   urine regulation and, 720, 721f
   water balance regulated by, 117
Antiemetics, 258
Antigen processing, 167

Antigen receptors
  B cell, 158
  T cell, 158
Antigen-binding fragments, 161
Antigen-binding site, 162
Antigenic determinant, 162
Antigen-presenting cells (APCs), 167, 220
Antigens
  antibodies binding to, 162
  endogenous, 168*f*
  exogenous, 167
  human leukocyte, 167–168
  immunogens compared to, 159–161
  self, 173–174
  superantigens, 171
Antigravity posture, 378
Antimetabolites, 262
Antimicrobial peptides, 136
Antiphospholipid syndrome (APS), 533–534
Antithrombin III (AT-III), 494
Antitoxins, 162
α1-Antitrypsin, 148
Antivascular endothelial growth factor (anti-VEGF), 343
Antrum, 864–865, 865*f*
Anuria, 746
Anus, 862, 872*f*
Aorta, 554
  coarctation of, 639
  semilunar valves, 554
Aortic regurgitation, 610*t*
Aortic stenosis, 610–611, 639–640
APCs. *See* Antigen-presenting cells
Aphasia, 360
Aplastic anemia, 502*t*
Aplastic crisis, 542
Apneusis, 354*f*, 355*t*
Apocrine sweat glands, 1022
Apoferritin, 489–490
Apoptosis, 101, 102*f*, 103–105, 103*t*, 105*f*
  extrinsic pathway of, 248–249
  intrinsic pathway of, 248
Apotransferrin, 490
Appendicitis, 901
  in children, 932
Appendicular skeleton, 948
Apraxia, 378
Aprosody, 378
APS. *See* Antiphospholipid syndrome
Aquaporins, 114
Aquaretics, 725*t*
Aqueduct of Sylvius, 310
Aqueous humor, 340–341
Arachnoid, 314
Arachnoid villi, 315–316
ARBs. *See* Angiotensin receptor blockers
Arcuate arteries, 716
Arcus senilis, of eye, 599–601
ARDS. *See* Acute respiratory distress syndrome
Aredia, 1010
Areflexia, 375
Areola, 777
Arnold-Chiari malformation, 413

Aromatase, 844, 847*f*
Arousal
  alterations in, 352–358
    breathing patterns and, 353, 355*t*
    cerebral death secondary to, 357–358
    clinical manifestations of, 353–357, 353*t*
    infratentorial disorders as cause of, 353
    level of consciousness and, 353
    metabolic disorders as cause of, 353
    motor responses and, 356
    oculomotor responses and, 356
    outcomes of, 357–358
    pathophysiology of, 352–353
    pupillary changes and, 353
    structural, 352–353
    supratentorial disorders as cause of, 352–353
  mediation of, 352
Arrhythmias, 584
Arsenic, inorganic, 290
Arterial aneurysms, 589
Arterial blood gases (ABGs), 130–131
Arterial blood pressure, 571–572
Arterial chemoreceptors, 572
Arterial oxygenation, 664–665
Arterial pressure
  of carbon dioxide, 665*f*
  of oxygen, 665*f*
Arterial thrombi, 533
Arterial thromboembolism, 591*t*
Arterial thrombosis, 590
Arterial vessels, 566
Arteries
  arcuate, 716
  collateral, 555
  elastic, 566
  hypertension. *See* Hypertension
  interlobar, 716
  muscular, 566
  renal, 716–717
  systemic circulation, 566–575
Arteriogenesis, 555
Arteriolar remodelling, angiotensin II mediating, 584
Arterioles, 566
  afferent, 717
  efferent, 717
Arteriosclerosis, 591–592
Arthritis
  gouty, 991, 992*f*
  juvenile idiopathic, 1012
  oligoarthritis, 1012
  osteoarthritis, 982–984, 983*f*
  polyarthritis, 1012
  psoriatic, 1031
  rheumatoid. *See* Rheumatoid arthritis
  septic, 1010–1012
Articular capsule, 950
Articular cartilage, 951–952
  loss of, osteoarthritis and, 984
Asbestos-silicate mineral, 290, 677
Ascending colon, 871
Ascending pathways, 301
Ascites, 116, 906–908, 907*f*

Aseptic meningitis, 400, 420
Ask-Upmark kidney, 758
Aspartate, 305*t*
Aspartate aminotransferase, 878*t*
Asphyxial injuries, 92–95
Aspiration
  foreign body, 702
  pulmonary, 675–676
Aspiration pneumonitis, 708–709
Assessment of SpondyloArthritis International Society, 989–990
Association fibres, 308
Associational neurons, 302
Asterixis, 354*t*
Asthma
  acute responses in, 683
  bronchial, 683, 683*f*
  in children, 709–710
  clinical manifestations of, 683–684
  definition of, 682–683
  evaluation of, 684
  hygiene hypothesis of, 683
  incidence of, 682*b*
  indigenous people in Canada and, 682*b*
  pathophysiology of, 683–684
  risk factors for, 683
  status asthmaticus and, 683–684
  treatment of, 684
Astigmatism, 343
Astrocytes, 302
  swelling of, 388
Astrocytomas, 406, 408*t*, 421
Asymptomatic hyperuricemia, 993
Asystole, 622*t*–623*t*
Ataxia telangiectasia, 514
Ataxic breathing, 355*t*
Ataxic cerebral palsy, 416
Ataxic gait, 378
Atelectasis, 676
Atherogenesis, 592
Atherogenic diet, 597
Atherosclerosis, 591–592
  clinical manifestations of, 592
  diabetes mellitus and, 470*f*
  evaluation and treatment of, 592
  pathophysiology of, 592
Athetosis, 372*t*
AT-III. *See* Antithrombin III
Atmospheric pressure, 662
ATN. *See* Acute tubular necrosis
Atopic dermatitis, 857*t*–859*t*, 1030
  in children, 1054–1055, 1055*f*
ATP. *See* Adenosine triphosphate
Atria, of heart, 554
Atrial fibrillation, 622*t*–623*t*
Atrial flutter, 622*t*–623*t*
Atrial natriuretic hormone (ANH), 116–117
Atrial natriuretic peptide (ANP), 725
Atrial receptors, heart rate and, 566
Atrial tachycardia, 622*t*–623*t*
Atrioventricular bundle (AV bundle), 558
Atrioventricular canal defect, 642–643
Atrioventricular dissociation, 622*t*–623*t*

Atrioventricular node (AV node), 557–558
Atrioventricular septal defect, 642–643
Atrioventricular valves (AV valves), 554
Atrophy, 73–74, 74f
Attention-deficit/hyperactivity disorder (ADHD), 358
Atypical ductal hyperplasia, 814, 815f
Atypical hyperplasia, 814, 815f
Atypical lobular hyperplasia, 814
Atypical pneumonia, 708
Auerbach plexus, 865
Auricle, 345
Autocrine signalling, 14
Autocrine stimulation, 239
Autografts, 1043–1044, 1047f–1048f
Autoimmune diseases
Autoimmune gastritis, 503–504
Autoimmune thyroiditis, 455–456
Autoimmune type 1 diabetes mellitus, 460
Automatic cells, 559
Automaticity, of heart, 559
Autonomic dysfunction, 399
Autonomic hyperreflexia, 389
Autonomic nervous system (ANS)
    neuroreceptors and neurotransmitters of, 322
    parasympathetic nervous system, 223–224, 322
    preganglionic and postganglionic salivation in, 862–864
    sympathetic nervous system, 220–223, 319–322
Autonomic regulation, 575
Autophagy, 105–106, 105b, 106f
Autoregulation, 367–368
    coronary circulation and, 575
Autosomal dominant inheritance, 50–53
    delayed age of onset, 51
    epigenetics and genomic imprinting, 52, 53f
    pedigree chart, 50, 50f, 51f
    pedigrees characteristics, 50–51
    penetrance and expressivity, 51–52, 52f
    recurrence risks, 51
Autosomal recessive inheritance, 53–54
    consanguinity, 54
    pedigrees characteristics, 53–54, 53f
    recurrence risks, 54, 54f
AV bundle. *See* Atrioventricular bundle
AV node. *See* Atrioventricular node
AV valves. *See* Atrioventricular valves
Avanafil, 854
Avastin (bevacizumab), 263t
Avulsions, 969
Awareness
    alterations in, 358–360
        clinical manifestations of, 360
        evaluation and treatment of, 360
        pathophysiology of, 358–360
    definition of, 358
Axial skeleton, 948
Axon hillock, 301
Axons, 301
Azotemia, 744

B

B cell antigen receptor, 164
B cells (B lymphocytes)
    bone marrow as origin of, 158
    class switch in maturation of, 172
    clonal diversity generation and, 158
    clonal selection of, 158
    development of, 164–167
    differentiation sites of, 160f
    in immune response, 158
B lymphocytes. *See* B cells
B vitamins, 276–278
B_{12} vitamin, 504
Bacille Calmette-Guérin (BCG), 691
Bacterial embolism, 591t
Bacterial infections
    in children, 1055–1056, 1056b, 1056f
    of skin, 1035, 1035f
Bacterial meningitis, 400, 420
Bacterial pneumonia, 707
Bacterial tracheitis, 703
Bactrim, 738b
Bainbridge reflex, 566
Balanitis, 835, 835f
Ballism, 372t
Balloon angioplasty, 641
Bare lymphocyte syndrome, 193
Bariatric surgery, 896–897
Barometric pressure, 662
Baroreceptor reflexes, 565
Baroreceptors, 117–118, 565
Barrett esophagus, 918
Bartholinitis, 797, 797f
Basal cell carcinoma, 285–286, 1040, 1040b, 1040f
Basal ganglia, 306–307
Basal ganglia motor syndromes, 378
Basal ganglion gait, 378
Basal ganglion posture, 378
Basal nuclei, 308
Basement membrane, 956
Basic fibroblast growth factor, 246
Basic multicellular units, 949
Basilar skull fractures, 386
Basis pedunculi, 310
Basopenia, 511t
Basophil count, 495t–497t
Basophilia, 511t
Basophils, 144–145, 480t, 511t
BBB. *See* Blood-brain barrier
BCG. *See* Bacille Calmette-Guérin
Bcl-2, 248
BCR-ABL gene, 296, 515f
BCR-ABL protein, 262
Becker muscular dystrophy, 1016
Beckwith-Wiedemann syndrome, 65–66
Bedbugs, 1061
Bell's palsy, 377b
Bence Jones protein, 523
Benign breast disease, 813–814
Benign prostatic hyperplasia, 840–842, 841f
Benign rolandic epilepsy, 421t

Benign tumours
    of adrenal medulla, 260
    description of, 234
    malignant tumours compared to, 234
    of skin, 1039, 1039f, 1039t
Bent nail syndrome, 834
Benuryl (probenecid), 795b
Benzol, 290
Beriberi, 620
Berry aneurysms, 397
Beta cells, 438
Beta globulins, 479–480
Beta-cell dysfunction, 464
β-Thalassemias, 543–545
Bevacizumab (Avastin), 263t
Bicarbonate, 126
Bicornuate uterus, 787f
Bicuspid valve, 554
Bidi smoking, 291
Bile
    acids, 875
    components of, 875
    definition of, 875
Bile acid pool, 875–876
Bile acid-dependent fraction, 875
Bile acid-independent fraction, 875
Bile canaliculi, 874
Bile duct cancer, 288–289
Bile salt deficiency, 897–898
Bile salts, 875, 897
Biliary atresia, 937–938
Biliary cirrhosis, 912
Bilirubin, 99, 489
    conjugated, 876, 908
    definition of, 876
    liver and metabolism of, 876f
    unconjugated, 876
Binding proteins, hormones and, 429t
Bioassays, 430b
Biofeedback, 994
Biphasic effects, of hormones, 429
Bipolar neurons, 301
Birthmarks, 1039
Bisphenol A, 823
Bisphosphonate therapy, 1015–1016
Bladder
    anatomy of, 719f
    cancer of, 736
    exstrophy of, 757–758, 757f
    innervation of, 719
    low bladder wall compliance, 734–735
    neurogenic, 734
    outflow obstruction of, 842
    overactive bladder syndrome, 734
    tumours of, 736
    underactive bladder syndrome, 734
Bladder function tests, 727t–728t
Bladder outlet obstruction, 734
    in children, 758
Blalock-Taussig shunt, 644
Blast cells, 547–548
Blebs, 687–688

Bleeding. *See also* Hemorrhage
  abnormal uterine, 790–791, 791t
  acute, 886t
  gastric, 893
  gastro-intestinal, 886, 886t
  in menstrual cycle, 772–775
  occult, 886, 886t
  types of, 491t
Bleeding time, 495t–497t
Blepharitis, 344
Blindness, 452, 466–467
Blood
  composition of, 478–482
    erythrocytes, 480
    leukocytes. *See* Leukocytes
    plasma, 478–480, 479t
    plasma proteins, 478–480
  oxygen transport in, 663–666
Blood cells, 480t. *See also* Erythrocytes; Hematopoiesis; Leukocytes; Platelets
  components of, 141f
  development of, 485–491
Blood clots
  definition of, 140
  dissolution of, 493f
  lysis of, 495–498
  mechanism of, 494f
  retraction of, 495–498
Blood flow
  in cardiac cycle, 554
  to exocrine pancreas, 877–880
  factors affecting, 568–571
  through heart, 554f
  intrarenal, autoregulation of, 719
  laminar, 570–571
  pulmonary
    congenital heart disease and decreased, 643–644
    congenital heart disease and increased, 641–643
  renal, 719–720, 719f
  splanchnic, 873
  turbulent, 570–571
  in vasa recta, 717
  velocity of, 570
Blood pressure
  aldosterone effects on, 574
  arterial, 571
  baroreceptors effect on, 565
  chemoreceptor reflex control of, 573f
  diastolic, 571
  pericardial sac causing reflex changes in, 553
  regulation of, 572–573
  systolic, 571
  total peripheral resistance effects on, 564
  vasopressin effects on, 574
  venous, 574
Blood supply
  to brain, 316–317
  to CNS, 316–318
  to liver, 872
  to skin, 1022
  to spinal cord, 318
Blood urea nitrogen (BUN), 726–729, 744

Blood velocity, 570
Blood vessel tumours, 407t
Blood vessels. *See also* Arteries; Capillaries
  arterioles, 566
  endothelium of, 566–567
  of kidney, 716–718
  lumen of, 566
  metarterioles, 566
  of nephron, 715–716
  stiffness of, 571
  of stomach, 865f
  vascular compliance of, 571
Blood volume, 478–479
  ADH and aldosterone regulating, 720
  aging effects on, 497b
Blood-brain barrier (BBB), 318
Bloom's syndrome, 244–245, 295, 514
Blowout hemorrhage, 491t
Blue spells, 643–644
BMI. *See* Body mass index
BNP. *See* B-type natriuretic peptide
Body fluids. *See also* Total body water (TBW)
  distribution of, 113–114
  hydrogen ions in, 124
  pH of, 124
Body heat, production and loss of, 335–336
Body of stomach, 865f
Body mass index, 767, 797, 902, 935, 975
Body temperature
  menstrual cycle and, 775
  normal range of, 334–335
  regulation of. *See* Thermoregulation
Body weight, 113t
Bone. *See also* Joints
  age-related loss of, 975
  aging of, 961–962
  anatomy of, 943–950, 944t
  calcification of, 943
  calcium and, 733, 944t, 979b
  cancellous, 947, 947f
  cells of, 943–945, 944f, 944t
  compact, 947, 948f
  cortical, 947
  density, 974–975, 975t
  destruction, bone tumours and, 1001, 1001t
  flat, 948
  formation of, 943
    endochondral, 967–968
  function of, 943–950
  healing, 967–968, 967f
  irregular, 948
  long, 948
  maintenance of, 946t, 949–950
  marrow cavities in, 943
  metastases to, 255
  mineralized, 974
  minerals of, 947
  osteoblasts of, 943–945, 944t
  osteoclasts of, 945, 946t
  osteocytes of, 945, 946t
  phosphate and, 733, 944t
  remodeling of, 946t, 949–950, 951f
  repair of, 950, 990
  short, 949

Bone (Continued)
  spongy, 947, 947f
  tissue, elements of, 943–947
  turnover, biochemical markers of, 979b
  types of, 947–948
  vitamins D and, 979
Bone cancer, 268t–271t
Bone disorders
  metabolic bone diseases, 974–976
  osteomalacia, 979–980
  osteomyelitis, 981–982, 981f
  osteoporosis. *See* Osteoporosis
  Paget's disease, 825t, 980–981
  postgastrectomy, 896–897
Bone fluid, 947
Bone infections
  osteomyelitis, 981–982, 981f, 1010, 1011b, 1012f
  septic arthritis, 1010–1012
Bone marrow
  B cells from, 158
  hematopoiesis in, 485–487
  multiple myeloma and, 523–524
  niches in, 485
Bone matrix, 943
Bone mineral density, 974, 976t
Bone morphogenic proteins, 944t, 946t
Bone tumours
  benign, 1017–1018
  bone destruction patterns of, 1001–1002, 1001t
  classification of, 1000, 1000b
  derivation of, 1001f
  epidemiology of, 1001
  evaluation of, 1001–1002
  malignant, in children, 1018–1019
  osteosarcoma, 1002–1003, 1002f
  staging for, 1002t
  types of, 1002–1004, 1002f
BOOP. *See* Bronchiolitis obliterans organizing pneumonia
Botulinum toxin (Botox), 735
Bowing fractures, 965–966
Bowman capsule, 715
Bowman space, 715
BPD. *See* Bronchopulmonary dysplasia
Brachial plexus, 319
Brachycephaly, 417f
Brachytherapy, 261
Bradykinesia, 373
Bradykinin, 140
Brain. *See also* Hypothalamus
  blood supply to, 316–317
  cerebellum in, 305
  cerebral hemispheres of, 307f
  in children, 412
  CSF flow to, 315–316
  development of, 412
  diencephalon of, 309–310
  divisions of, 306t
  edema of, 368f
  forebrain, 306t
  hindbrain, 306t
  intracerebral hematomas and, 386

Brain (Continued)
   malformations of, 415–416
   metencephalon of, 306t
   midbrain, 306t
   myelencephalon of, 311
   telencephalon of, 306–309
Brain abscesses, 401
Brain cancer, 268t–271t
Brain death, 357
Brain herniation syndromes, 368f
Brain injuries. *See also* Traumatic brain injury
   classification of, 384t
   closed, 383
   diffuse, 386
   focal, 383–386
   open, 386
   secondary, 384t
Brain networks, 305
Brain tumours, 295
   astrocytomas, 406
   in children, 421–422
   of CNS, 405–408
   ependymomas, 406
   glioblastoma multiforme, 406
   gliomas, 405–406
   meningiomas, 407
   metastatic, 408–409
   neurofibromas, 407–408
   oligodendroglioma, 406
   primary intracerebral, 405–407
Brainstem
   anatomy of, 305
   gliomas of, 422
   respiratory centre in, 659
   reticular formation and, 305
   BRCA1, 245–246, 824, 844–847, 855
   BRCA2, 245–246, 824, 844–847, 855
Breast cancer
   clinical manifestations of, 826–830, 829f
   diet and, 822–823
   ductal carcinoma in situ, 235, 816b, 828f
   EMT and, 801–802
   environmental causes of, 821–823
   environmental chemicals and, 823
   estrogen and risk of, 820–821
   evaluation of, 828–830
   genetic heterogeneity and, 823–824
   GH and, 821
   hormonal factors in, 818–820, 819f
   hormone replacement therapy and risk of, 820–821
   IGF and, 821
   incidence of, 817f
   inherited syndromes, 823–825
   insulin and insulin like growth factors, 821
   lobular carcinoma in situ, 825–830, 825t
   lobular involution and, 818
   male, 855
   mammography for, 821
   melatonin and, 821
   menopausal hormone therapy and, 819–820
   obesity and, 823
   oral contraceptives and, 821–822

Breast cancer (Continued)
   pathogenesis of, 824–825, 826f, 827f
   physical activity and, 276–282, 823
   postlactational involution and, 818
   pregnancy and, 814–818
   progesterone and risk of, 820–821
   prolactin and, 821
   radiation exposure causing, 821
   reproductive factors in, 814–818
   risk factors in, 818t
   screening for, 816b
   treatment of, 828–830
   tumour dormancy and, 824
   types of, 825t
   vascular mimicry and, 825–826
Breast disorders
   atypical ductal hyperplasia, 814
   benign breast disease, 813
   galactorrhea, 812–813
   male, 855–856
Breast lesions
   nonproliferative, 813
   proliferative, with atypia, 813–814
   proliferative, without atypia, 813–814
Breasts
   aging effects on, 818
   anatomy of, 776f
   areola, 777
   cysts of, 813
   definition of, 775
   development of, 777, 830
   estrogen effects on, 773t
   lobular involution and, 818
   lymphatic drainage of, 776, 776f
   male, 777
   nipple, 777
   postlactational involution and, 818
   sarcoma of, 825t
   sex hormones and development of, 791
   terminal duct lobular units of, 818
Breathing
   abnormal patterns of, 671
   airway resistance in, 661
   alveolar surface tension and, 661
   elastic properties in, 661
   laboured, 671
   mechanics of, 660–662
   restricted, 671
   work of, 657
Breathing patterns, 355t
Brittle bone disease, 1009
Broad-spectrum antibiotics, 137
Broca area, 307–308
Broca dysphasia, 360
Bromosulfophthalein excretion, 878t
Bronchi, 654–655
Bronchial asthma, 683f
Bronchial circulation, 655
Bronchiectasis, 676–677
Bronchioles, 655
Bronchiolitis, 677
   in children, 706–707

Bronchiolitis obliterans, 677
   in children, 706–707
Bronchiolitis obliterans organizing pneumonia (BOOP), 677
Bronchitis
   acute, 688
   chronic, 686–687
Bronchoconstriction, 661
Bronchodilation, 661
Bronchopulmonary dysplasia (BPD), 705–706, 706t
Brudzinski sign, 398
Brush border, 869
Bruton agammaglobulinemia, 193
B-type natriuretic peptide (BNP), 116–117
   heart failure and, 647
Budesonide, 702
Buerger's disease, 590–591
Buffering
   acid-base balance and, 124
   carbonic acid-bicarbonate, 126
   protein, 124
   renal, 126
Buffers, 124
Bulbar palsy, 377
Bulbourethral glands, 780
Bulla, 1026f
Bullous erythema multiforme, 1034
Bumetanide, 725t
BUN. *See* Blood urea nitrogen
Bundle of His, 558
Burinex, 725t
Burkitt lymphoma, 241–242, 522
   in children, 548
Burn shock, 1044, 1045f
Burning mouth syndrome, 504–505
Burns
   cardiovascular response to, 1045
   cellular response to, 1045
   clinical manifestations of, 1044–1045
   deep partial-thickness, 1043t
   evaluation of, 1046
   evaporative water loss in, 1046
   first-degree, 1043
   fourth-degree, 1044
   full-thickness, 1044, 1044f
   healing, 1027f, 1029
   immunological response to, 1046
   incidence, 1042
   metabolic response to, 1045–1046
   pathophysiology of, 1044–1045, 1045f
   rule of nines in, 1044, 1045f
   second-degree, 1043–1044
   superficial partial-thickness, 1043–1044, 1043f
   third-degree, 1044, 1044f
   total body surface area in, 1044
   treatment of, 1046, 1046f
   wound depth, 1043–1045, 1043f, 1043t, 1044f, 1045f
Bursae, 969, 970f
Bursitis, 969–970, 970f
Butyrate, 276–278
Bystander effects, 284f

C

C cells, of thyroid gland, 436
C fibres, 330
C1, 140
C1 esterase inhibitor, 140
C1 INH deficiency, 140
C3, 140
C5, 140
Cachexia, 255–258, 905
CAD. *See* Coronary artery disease
Calcaneovalgus, 1008*t*
Calcaneovarus, 1008*t*
Calcification, of bone, 943
Calcitonin, 436
Calcitonin gene-related peptide, 225*t*–226*t*
Calcium
    balance, alterations in, 124
    bone and, 733, 944*t*, 979*b*
    formation of, 947*t*
Calcium stones, 733
Calcium-calmodulin complex, 431
Calcium-troponin complex, 563
Calculi, urinary, 732
Caloric ice water test, 356*f*
Calyces, 714, 714*f*
cAMP. *See* Cyclic adenosine monophosphate
CAMs. *See* Cell adhesion molecules
Canadian Cystic Fibrosis Registry, 711
Canadian Nuclear Safety Commission, 282–283
Canaliculi, 947
Cancellous bone, 947, 948*f*
Cancer
    of accessory organs of digestion, 921–924
    adenocarcinomas. *See* Adenocarcinomas
    bladder, 268*t*–271*t*, 736
    bone, 268*t*–271*t*
    brain, 268*t*–271*t*
    breast cancer. *See* Breast cancer
    in Canada, 274*f*
    carcinomas. *See* Carcinomas
    cell surface antigens expressed by, 251
    cellular differentiation during, 234
    cervical. *See* Cervical cancer
    characteristics of, 234–235
    chemotherapy for, 261–262
    childhood. *See* Childhood cancers
    classification of, 268*t*–271*t*
    clinical manifestations of, 255–259
        anemia and, 258
        cachexia and, 255–258, 257*f*
        fatigue associated with, 255
        GI tract and, 258
        hair and, 258
        infection and, 258
        leukopenia and, 258
        pain and, 255
        paraneoplastic syndromes and, 255, 256*t*
        skin and, 258
        thrombocytopenia and, 258
    colorectal, 276, 806–807, 918*t*, 919–921, 920*f*, 921*b*
    definition of, 234
    development of, 272
    diagnosis of, 259–261

Cancer (*Continued*)
    of digestive system, 917
    DNA methylation and, 237–238, 273
    early life conditions, 272–273
    endometrial, 806–807, 806*f*
    environmental-lifestyle factors and, 274–290
        air pollution and, 289
        alcohol and, 279–280
        chemicals and, 293
        diet, 276
        electromagnetic radiation and, 287–288
        ionizing radiation and, 282–285
        nutrition, 276–279
        obesity and, 279
        occupational hazards and, 289–290
        physical activity and, 276–282
        tobacco smoking, 274–276, 275*f*
        ultraviolet radiation and, 285–287
    epigenetics, 69*f*
        DNA demethylating agents, 69
        DNA methylation, 68
        emerging strategies, 69
        epigenetic screening, 68–69
        histone deacetylase inhibitors, 69–70, 70*f*
        microRNA coding, 70
        microRNAs, 68
    epigenetics and, 266–272
    of esophagus, 268*t*–271*t*, 917–919, 918*b*, 918*t*
    familial, 244*t*
    of gallbladder, 268*t*–271*t*, 922
    genes, 242*t*
    genetic lesions in, 261*b*
    genetics of, 261, 266–272
    of GI tract, 883–905, 886*t*
    glucose requirement in, 249*f*
    growth factor signaling pathways in, 241*f*
    hallmarks of, 235
    hereditary nonpolyposis colorectal, 806–807
    heterogeneity of, 238
    immunotherapy for, 251
    laryngeal, 694
    lip, 1041, 1041*f*
    of liver, 921–922, 921*b*
    lung. *See* Lung cancer
    metabolism in, 248*f*
    mortality trends with, 272
    neovascularization of, 246
    ovarian. *See* Ovarian cancer
    pain, 255
    pancreatic, 922–924
    penis, 835–836, 836*b*
    process of, 234*f*
    prostate. *See* Prostate cancer
    radiation therapy for, 261
    skin. *See* Skin cancer
    staging of, 259–261, 260*f*
    stomach, 919
    surgery for, 261
    targeted disruption of, 262–263
    terminology of, 234–235
    testicular, 838
    tissue differentiation during, 236*f*
    TNM staging of, 260*f*, 696–700
    treatment of, 259–263

Cancer (*Continued*)
    tumour markers for, 260*t*
    tumours. *See* Tumours
    vaginal, 805–806
    vulvar, 806
    World Health Organization
    wound healing and, 238
Cancer cells
    anaplasia of, 234
    angiogenesis inducement by, 246–247
    apoptosis resistance by, 240*f*
    dormancy of, 253–255
    EMT and, 253
    energy metabolism reprogramming by, 238–239, 247–248
    genomic instability of, 244–246
    growth suppressor evasion by, 242–244
    heterogeneity of, 252
    metastasis of, 252–255
    proliferative signaling by, 239–242
    in prostate cancer, 848
    tumour-promoting inflammation and, 249–251
    tumour-specific antigens expressed by, 240*f*
Cancer-associated adipocytes, 279
Cancer-associated fibroblasts, 248, 850–852
Candida albicans, 137, 796
Candidiasis, 1037, 1037*t*
Cannabinoids, 333
Cannabis, 92*b*. *See also* Marihuana
Cannon, Walter B., 215–216
Capillaries
    coronary, 555–556
    fenestrations in, 566
    glomerular, 717
    lymphatic, 869
    papillary, 1022
    peritubular, 717
    permeability of, inflammation effects on, 123
Capillary hydrostatic pressure, 114
Capillary oncotic pressure, 114
Capillary pressures, glomerular filtration and, 720
Capillary seal, 1045
Caplan's syndrome, 988
CAR cells. *See* CXCL12-abundant reticular cells
Carbohydrate metabolism, in CKD, 751
Carbohydrates
    liver metabolism of, 876
    small intestine absorption of, 869
Carbon dioxide
    arterial pressure of, 663
    from cellular metabolism, 659*f*
    partial pressure of, 659*f*
Carbon monoxide poisoning, 87–88
Carbonic acid, 126
Carbonic acid–bicarbonate buffering, 126
Carbonic anhydrase, 126
Carbonic anhydrase inhibitors, 725*t*
Carboxypeptidase, 140
Carbuncles, 1035
Carcinogenesis, 286*f*
Carcinogens, 279
Carcinoid syndrome, 256*t*
Carcinoma in situ, 235, 824–825

Carcinomas. *See also* Cancer
  adenocarcinomas, 234–235, 695
  adenoid, 825*t*
  basal cell, 285–286, 1040, 1040*f*
  cholangiocellular, 922
  ductal carcinoma in situ, 235, 816*b*, 825–830, 828*f*
  hepatocellular, 921–922
  infiltrating lobular, 825*t*
  inflammatory, 825*t*
  intraductal, 813
  large cell, 695*t*, 696
  lobular carcinoma in situ, 825*t*, 826
  medullary, 825*t*
  metaplastic, 825*t*
  mucinous, 825*t*
  nipple retraction and, 829*t*
  non-small cell, 695, 695*t*
  oat cell, 696–700
  papillary, 825*t*
  rectal, 921
  renal cell, 736, 736*f*
  renal transitional cell, 736
  small cell, 695*t*, 696–700
  small intestinal, 920
  squamous cell, 285–286, 695, 825*t*, 1040–1041, 1041*f*
  thyroid, 457
  transitional cell, 736
  tubular, 825*t*
Carcinomatous meningitis, 408
Cardiac action potentials, 556, 559–560
Cardiac cycle, 554
Cardiac muscle
  cells of, 561
  skeletal muscle compared to, 560
Cardiac orifice, 864–865
Cardiac output
  afterload, 564
  in elderly, 564*t*
  factors affecting, 563–566
  heart rate effects on, 563
  myocardial contractility and, 564–565
  preload, 564
Cardiac sphincter, 864
Cardiogenic shock, 626
Cardiomyocytes, 553
Cardiomyopathies, 608–609
Cardiopulmonary resuscitation (CPR), 712
Cardiovascular disorders
  acute coronary syndromes. *See* Acute coronary syndromes
  in AIDS patients, 616
  aneurysms. *See* Aneurysms
  arterial thrombosis, 590
  atherosclerosis, 468, 591–592
  cardiomyopathies, 608–609
  chronic venous insufficiency, 580
  congenital heart disease. *See* Congenital heart disease
  coronary artery disease. *See* Coronary artery disease
  deep venous thrombosis, 580–581
  diabetes mellitus complications with, 467*t*

Cardiovascular disorders *(Continued)*
  embolism, 590
  heart failure. *See* Heart failure
  hypertension. *See* Hypertension
  MI. *See* Myocardial ischemia
  MODS. *See* Multiple organ dysfunction syndrome
  Orthostatic hypotension, 589
  peripheral artery disease, 592–595
  PVD, 469
    Raynaud phenomenon, 591
    thromboangiitis obliterans, 590–591
  renin-angiotensin-aldosterone system and, 584–586
  shock. *See* Shock
  superior vena cava syndrome, 581
  varicose veins, 580
Cardiovascular vasomotor control centre, 565
Caretaker genes, 242*t*, 244
Carina, 654–655
Carnitine palmitoyltransferase, 997
Carpopedal spasm, 130
Cartilage
  articular, 951–952
Cartilaginous joints, 950–953
Cascade, 140
Caseous necrosis, 102
Caspases, 249
Catabolism, 15
  protein, 219
Cataracts, 341
Catecholamines
  adrenal medulla secretion of, 443
  physiological effects of, 220*t*
Cathelicidins, 136
Cat's eye reflex, 424
Cauda equina syndrome, 393, 734, 734*t*
Cavernous hemangiomas, 1061, 1062*f*
Cavitation, of abscesses, 691
CD. *See* Crohn's disease
CD3, 166
CD4, 166–167
CD8, 166–167
Cecum, 871, 872*f*
Cefizox (ceftizoxime), 795*b*
Cefoxitin (Mefoxin Pws), 795*b*
Ceftizoxime (Cefizox), 795*b*
Ceftriaxone (Rocephin), 795*b*
Celiac crisis, 934
Celiac disease, 934–935, 934*f*
Cell adhesion molecules, 6, 8, 485–486, 699*b*
Cells. *See also* Blood cells
  of adaptive immunity, 135*t*
  bone, 943–945, 944*f*, 944*t*
  burn response of, 1045
  dendritic, 146
  memory, 158
Cellular accumulations, 95
Cellular adaptation, 73, 74*f*
  atrophy, 73–74, 74*f*
  dysplasia, 76, 77*f*
  hyperplasia, 76, 76*f*
  hypertrophy, 74–76, 75*f*
  metaplasia, 77, 77*f*

Cell cycle, 25–27, 26*f*
Cell surface antigen receptors, 158
Cell-mediated immunity, 172–174
Cell-to-cell adhesions, 11–14
  collagen, 11–12
  elastin, 12
  extracellular matrix, 11–12, 12*f*
  fibronectin, 12
  specialized cell junctions, 12–14, 13*f*
Cellular communication, 14, 14*f*
Cellular components, 3, 4*f*
  cellular receptors, 10–11, 11*f*
  cytoplasmic organelles, 3, 5*t*
  endoplasmic reticulum, 9*b*
  ER stress, 9*b*
  membrane composition, 3–10, 7*f*, 8*f*, 9*f*
  nucleus, 3, 5*f*
  plasma membranes, 3–10, 6*f*, 6*t*
  protein folding, 9*b*
Cellular death, 100–106
  apoptosis, 101, 102*f*, 103–105, 103*t*, 105*f*
  autophagy, 105–106, 105*b*, 106*f*
  necrosis, 101–103, 102*f*, 103*f*, 103*t*
Cellular functions, 2–3
Cellular immunity, 158
Cellular injury, 77–95
  acetaminophen metabolism and toxicity, 89*f*
  alcoholic hepatitis, 91*f*
  asphyxial injuries, 92–95
  cannabis, 92*b*
  carbon monoxide (CO), 87–88
  chronic alcoholism, 90–91
  drugs of abuse, 87*t*
  ethanol, 88–92, 90*f*
  fetal alcohol spectrum disorder, 91*f*
  immunological and inflammatory injury, 95
  infectious injury, 95
  lead exposure, 89*f*, 89*t*
  manifestations, 95–100
    calcium, 99–100, 100*f*, 101*f*
    glycogen, 97
    hemoproteins, 98–99, 99*f*
    intracellular accumulations, 97*f*
    lipids and carbohydrates, 95–97, 98*f*
    melanin, 97–98
    pigments, 97–99
    proteins, 97
    systemic, 101*t*
    urate, 100
    water, 95, 98*f*
  mechanisms, 78–92, 78*t*, 96*t*
    chemical agents, 84–92
    chemical liver injury, 84, 85*f*, 86*f*
    chemical/toxic injury, 83
    human exposure, to pollutants, 83–84, 83*f*
    hypoxic injury, 78–81, 79*f*, 80*f*
    mitochondrial effects, 82–83, 83*b*
    oxidative stress, 81–82, 82*f*, 82*t*, 83*b*, 83*t*
  social/street drugs, 88*t*
  stages, 78*f*
  types, 78*t*
  unintentional and intentional injuries, 92–95, 93*t*–94*t*

Cellular metabolism, 15–18
    adenosine triphosphate, 15–16, 16b
    carbon dioxide from, 658
    food and production, 16–17, 17f
    oxidative phosphorylation, 17–18
Cellular receptors, 10–11, 11f
Cellular reproduction, 25–27, 26f
    cellular division rates, 26–27
    growth factors, 27, 27t
    mitosis and cytokinesis, 26
Cellulitis, 1035
Central chemoreceptors, 660
Central diabetes insipidus, 450
Central fever, 338
Central herniation, 368b
Central line-associated bloodstream infections, 629b
Central nervous system (CNS). See also Brain; Spinal cord; Vertebral column
    deafferentation pain and, 335t
    infections of, 420
    inherited metabolic disorders of, 417–419
    intoxications of, 419
    malformations of, 413–416
        craniostenosis, 414–415
        neural tube defects and, 413–414
    neoplasms of, HIV and, 406f
    tumours of, 405–407
Central nervous system disorders, 383–403.
        See also Spinal cord injuries; Stroke; Traumatic brain injury
    AIDS-related neurologic complications, 383
    brain abscesses, 401
    cerebrovascular accidents, 394
    cerebrovascular disease, 394
    degenerative disorders of spine, 391–394
    low back pain, 391–393
    degenerative joint disease, 393
    encephalitis, 401–402, 401t, 420
    Guillain-Barré syndrome, 377, 403
    headaches, 398–400
    herniated intervertebral disc, 393–394
    infections and, 400–402
    inflammation and, 400–402
    intracranial aneurysms, 397
    meningitis, 400–401
    multiple sclerosis, 402–403
    spinal cord abscesses, 401
    subarachnoid hemorrhage, 397–398
    vascular malformations, 397
    vertebral injuries, 387–394
Central neurogenic hyperventilation, 355t
Central neuropathic pain, 334
Central pontine myelinolysis, 449–450
Central sensitization, 334, 994
Central tolerance, 166
Cerebellar astrocytomas, 421
Cerebellar motor syndromes, 379
Cerebellar tremor, 372t
Cerebral aneurysms, 589
Cerebral artery vasospasm, 398
Cerebral blood flow, 366
Cerebral blood oxygenation, 367b
Cerebral blood volume, 367b

Cerebral death, 357–358
Cerebral edema, 368–369
Cerebral hemodynamics. See also Hydrocephalus
    alterations in, 367–369
    increased intracranial pressure and, 367–368
    terminology associated with, 366t
Cerebral hypoxia, 671
Cerebral infarction, 395–396
Cerebral palsy, 416
    female sexual dysfunction and, 812t
Cerebral peduncles, 310
Cerebral perfusion pressure, 367b
Cerebral thromboses, 395
Cerebral vasoconstriction, 130
Cerebrospinal fluid (CSF), 1079t
    pH of, 656–657
Cerebrovascular accidents, 394. See also Stroke
    female sexual dysfunction and, 812t
Cerebrovascular disease, 394
    in children, 420–421
Cerebrum, 309–310
Ceruloplasmin, 480
Cervical cancer, 251
    classification for precursor lesions to, 805t
    clinical manifestations of, 803–805
    evaluation of, 805
    HPV and development of, 803b, 857t–859t
    incidence of, 802
    pathogenesis of, 803–805, 804f, 805t
    precursor lesions for, 849–850
    prevention of, 805b
    screening for, 803b
    staging of, 805t
    treatment of, 805
Cervical carcinoma in situ, 803, 805t
Cervical intraepithelial neoplasia, 803, 804f, 805t
Cervicitis, 796
Cervix
    anatomy of, 769f
    inflammation of, 796–797
    neoplasm progression in, 237f
Chalazion, 344
Chemical carcinogenesis, 290
Chemical epididymitis, 840
Chemical liver injury, 84, 85f, 86f
Chemicals Management Plan, 823
Chemical signalling modes, 14, 15f
Chemical synapses, 14
Chemokines, 240f
Chemoreceptor trigger zone, 883
Chemoreceptors
    central, 660
    peripheral, 659
Chemotactic factors, 139–140
Chemotaxis, 145
Chemotherapy
    adjuvant, 262
    alopecia caused by, 258
    cancer treatment with, 255
    induction, 248
    neoadjuvant, 262
Chest muscle retraction, 703f

Chest physiotherapy, 677
Chest radiography, 691
Chest wall
    aging and, 657
    disorders of, 673–675
    elastic properties of, 661
    restriction, 673–674
Cheyne-Stokes respiration, 353, 671
Chiari II malformation, 413
Chickenpox, 1036, 1059–1060, 1059f
Chief cells, 867
Childhood cancers
    bone marrow transplants and, 298b
    brain tumours and, 295
    chromosomal abnormalities with, 295
    congenital factors associated with, 296t
    embryonic tumours and, 295
    environmental factors with, 296–297
    Epstein-Barr virus and, 297
    etiology of, 294–297
    genetic and genomic factors in, 295–296
    incidence of, 294–297
    mesodermal germ layer as source of, 295f
    prenatal drug exposures as cause of, 296–297
    types of, 294–297
Children
    AIDS in, 297
    brain growth and development in, 415
    cardiovascular disorders in
        acquired heart disease, 647
        congenital heart disease. See Congenital heart disease
        hypertension, 649–651, 651t
        Kawasaki disease, 648–649, 648b
    coagulation disorders in, 545–547
        hemophilias, 545–546
        ITP, 545–546
    congenital heart disease. See Congenital heart disease
    diarrhea in, 936–937
    erythrocyte disorders in, 537–545
        anemia, 538, 538t
        hemolytic anemia, 539–540
        iron deficiency anemia, 538–539
        sickle cell disease, 540–543
        thalassemias, 543–545
    G6PD deficiency in, 538
    gastro-intestinal tract disorders in
        anorectal malformations, 931
        appendicitis, 932
        celiac disease, 934–935, 934f, 935b
        cleft lip, 928
        cleft palate, 928
        cystic fibrosis, 933–934, 933t
        diarrhea, 936–937
        duodenum obstruction, 929–930
        esophageal atresia, 928–929, 929f
        failure to thrive, 935–936, 936b
        GER, 931–932
        growth faltering, 935–936, 936b
        hepatoblastoma, 940
        Hirschsprung's disease, 930–931, 930f
        idiopathic intestinal pseudo-obstruction, 930

Children (Continued)
    ileum obstruction, 929–930
    infantile hypertrophic pyloric stenosis, 929
    intussusception, 932, 932f
    jejunum obstruction, 929–930
    lactose intolerance, 935
    malignancies, 939–940
    malnutrition, 935
    Meckel diverticulum, 930
    meconium syndromes, 930
    necrotizing enterocolitis, 936
    pancreatic tumours, 940
    tracheoesophageal fistula, 929f
GH deficiency in, 451
hydrocephalus in, 413
leukemia in, 294–295, 547–548
    clinical manifestations of, 547
    evaluation and treatment of, 547–548
    pathophysiology of, 547
liver disorders in
    biliary atresia, 937–938
    cirrhosis, 938–939
    hepatitis, 938
    metabolic disorders, 939
    neonatal jaundice, 540, 937
    portal hypertension, 939
lymphomas in, 295, 548–549
    Burkitt, 548
    Hodgkin's, 548–549
    non-Hodgkin's, 548
metabolic syndrome in, 461–462
musculo-skeletal disorders in
    benign bone tumours, 1017–1018
    clubfoot, 1008, 1008t, 1009f
    developmental dysplasia of hip, 1008–1009, 1009f, 1010f
    Ewing sarcomas, 1018–1019, 1019f
    juvenile idiopathic arthritis, 1012, 1013t
    Legg-Calvé-Perthes disease, 1013–1014, 1014f
    malignant bone tumours, 1018–1019
    muscular dystrophies, 1015–1017, 1015t, 1016f, 1017f
    nonaccidental trauma, 1019–1020, 1019f
    nonossifying fibromas, 1018
    Osgood-Schlatter disease, 1014
    osteochondromas, 1017–1018
    osteochondroses, 1012–1014
    osteogenesis imperfecta, 1009–1010, 1011f
    osteomyelitis, 1010, 1011b, 1012f
    osteosarcomas, 1018
    scoliosis, 1014–1015, 1015f
    septic arthritis, 1010–1012
    Sever disease, 1014
nervous system development in, 412
neurologic disorders in
    amino acid metabolism defects, 419
    anencephaly, 413
    brain malformations, 416
    brain tumours, 421–422
    cerebral palsy, 416
    cerebrovascular disease, 420–421
    Chiari II malformation, 413
    CNS malformations, 413

Children (Continued)
    congenital hydrocephalus, 415
    cortical dysplasias, 415
    craniostenosis, 414–415
    cyclopia, 413
    Dandy-Walker malformation, 416
    encephalocele, 413
    encephalopathies, 416–420
    epilepsy, 420
    inherited metabolic disorders of CNS, 417–419
    meningitis, 420
    meningocele, 413
    microcephaly, 415
    myelomeningocele, 413
    neural tube defects, 413
    neuroblastomas, 422
    perinatal stroke, 420
    phenylketonuria, 419
    retinoblastoma, 423–424
    seizure disorders, 420
    spina bifida, 413
    spina bifida occulta, 414
    storage diseases, 419
    stroke, 420
pain perception in, 330–331
poisoning of, 419
pulmonary diseases and disorders in
acute epiglottitis, 703
    ALI, 710
    ARDS, 710
    aspiration pneumonitis, 708–709
    asthma, 709–710
    atypical pneumonia, 708
    bacterial tracheitis, 707
    BPD, 705–706
    bronchiolitis, 706–707
    croup, 702–703
    cystic fibrosis, 710–711
    foreign body aspiration, 703
    OSAS, 704
    pneumonia, 707–708
    RDS, 704–705
    respiratory tract infections, 706–708
    SUID, 711–712
    tonsillar infections, 703
    upper airways infections, 702t
renal disorders in
    acute poststreptococcal glomerulonephritis, 758–759
    glomerular disorders, 758–760
    hemolytic uremic syndrome, 759–760
    hypoplastic kidneys, 758
    immunoglobulin A nephropathy, 759
    incidence of, 757
    nephroblastoma, 760, 760t
    nephrotic syndrome, 759
    polycystic kidney disease, 758
    renal agenesis, 758
skin disorders in
    acne vulgaris, 1053–1054, 1054f
    atopic dermatitis, 1054–1055, 1055f
    bacterial infections, 1055–1056, 1056b, 1056f

Children (Continued)
    bedbugs, 1061
    chickenpox, 1059–1060, 1059f
    cutaneous hemangiomas, 1061, 1061f, 1062f
    cutaneous vascular malformations, 1061–1062, 1062f
    dermatitis, 1054–1055
    diaper dermatitis, 1055, 1055f
    erythema toxicum neonatorum, 1062
    fleabites, 1060, 1061f
    fungal infections, 1056–1057, 1057f
    herpes zoster, 1059–1060, 1059f
    impetigo, 1055–1056, 1056b, 1056f
    insect bites, 1060–1061
    lice infestation, 1060
    miliaria, 1062, 1062f
    molluscum contagiosum, 1057, 1057f
    parasites, 1060–1061
    pediculosis, 1060
    roseola, 1059
    rubella, 1057–1058, 1058f, 1058t
    rubeola, 1058–1059
    scabies, 1060, 1060f
    smallpox, 1059
    staphylococcal scalded-skin syndrome, 1056, 1056f
    thrush, 1057
    tinea capitis, 1056–1057, 1057f
    tinea corporis, 1057
    viral infections, 1057–1060
strabismus in, 341
urinary system disorders in
    bladder exstrophy, 757, 757f
    bladder outlet obstruction, 758
    epispadias, 757–758
    hypospadias, 757, 757f
    incidence of, 757
    ureteropelvic junction obstruction, 758
    urinary incontinence, 761–763, 762t
    UTI, 760–761
    vesicoureteral reflux, 761, 761f
Chimeric, 517f
Chlamydia, 833, 856
Chlamydia trachomatis, 856t
Chlamydial conjunctivitis, 344
Chlamydial ophthalmia, 857t–859t
Chlamydophila pneumonia, 708
Chloride
    balance, 117
    bicarbonate and, 116
Chloride reabsorption inhibitors, 725t
Choking asphyxiation, 92
Cholangiocellular carcinoma, 922
Cholecystitis, 914
Cholecystokinin, 865, 866t
Cholelithiasis, 914–915
Choleresis, 876
Choleretic agent, 876
Choline deficiency, in pregnancy, 276
Cholinergic crisis, 405
Cholinergic transmission, 322
Chondrocytes, 951–952
Chordae tendineae, 554
Chordee, 757

Chorea, 371–373
Choroid plexuses, 314
Chromaffin cell tumours, 473
Chromophils, 432
Chromophobes, 432
Chromosomes
  abnormalities, 46–49, 49f
  aneuploidy, 43–46, 46f
  characteristics, 47t
  Down syndrome, 48f
  instability of, 246
  polyploidy, 43
  translocations, 49f
    oncogene activation by, 238f
  Turner's syndrome, 48f
Chromosome 5p deletion syndrome, 638t
Chromosome translocations, 237–238
Chronic alcoholism, 90–91
Chronic alveolar hypoxia, 656
Chronic bacterial prostatitis, 842b, 843
Chronic bronchitis, 686–687
Chronic cluster headaches, 399
Chronic conjunctivitis, 344
Chronic cough, 670
Chronic cyanosis, 644
Chronic fatigue syndrome, 996
Chronic gastritis, 892
Chronic hepatitis, in children, 938
Chronic immune gastritis, 893
Chronic inflammation, 149–151, 249–250
Chronic kidney disease (CKD)
  acid-base balance and, 750
  carbohydrate metabolism in, 751
  cardiovascular system and, 751
  clinical manifestations of, 750
  creatinine and urea clearance in, 750
  definition of, 748
  dyslipidemia and, 743t
  endocrine system and, 752
  evaluation of, 752–754
  female sexual dysfunction and, 812t
  fluid and electrolyte balance, 750–751
  gastro-intestinal system and, 752
  hematological system and, 752
  immune system and, 752
  neurological system and, 752
  pathophysiology of, 748–750
  phosphate and calcium balance and, 751
  protein metabolism in, 751
  pulmonary system and, 752
  reproductive system and, 752
  stages of, 748t
  systemic effects of, 749t
  treatment of, 752–754
Chronic Kidney Disease Epidemiology Collaboration, 726
Chronic lymphocytic leukemia, 517–518
Chronic lymphocytic thyroiditis, 455–456
Chronic migraines, 398
Chronic myeloid leukemia, 241, 517–518
  in children, 547
Chronic nonbacterial osteomyelitis, 981
Chronic nonimmune gastritis, 893

Chronic obstructive pulmonary disease (COPD), 684–685
Chronic pancreatitis, 916–917
Chronic pelvic pain syndrome, 842b, 843
Chronic postoperative pain, 335t
Chronic prostatitis, 843
Chronic pyelonephritis, 739, 760
Chronic relapsing TTP, 528
Chronic tension-type headache, 399
Chronic traumatic encephalopathy, 387
Chronic urticaria, 1038
Chronotropic effect, 223
Chylothorax, 675, 675t
Chyme, 864–865
Cialis, 854
Cigar smoking. See Smoking, tobacco
Cigarette smoking. See Smoking, tobacco
Cingulate gyrus herniation, 368b
Circadian rhythm sleep disorders, 339–340
Circle of Willis, 317f
Circulating anticoagulants, 495t–497t
Circulation
  bronchial, 655
  collateral, 555
  coronary, 555
    autonomic regulation and, 575
    autoregulation and, 575
    regulation of, 575
  systemic. See Systemic circulation
Circulatory system. See also Blood; Heart
  anatomy of, 553f
  functions of, 552
Cirrhosis
  alcoholic, 911
  alcoholic liver disease and, 910–912
  ascites caused by, 906–908
  biliary, 912
  causes of, 910b
  in children, 938–939
  clinical manifestations of, 911f
  definition of, 910
  nonalcoholic fatty liver disease and, 912
  nonalcoholic steatohepatitis and, 912
Citrate (Clomid), 792
CKD. See Chronic kidney disease
Clara cell, 657f
Class switch, 172
Clawlike prolongations, 1029, 1029f
Clear cell tumours, 736
Cleft lip, 928, 928f
Cleft palate, 928, 928f
Clinical breast examination, 825–826
Clitoris, 768, 768f
Clomid (citrate), 792
Clonal diversity
  definition of, 158
  generation of, 164
  illustration of, 159f
Clonal expansion, 237–238
Clonal selection
  B cell, 158
  description of, 167–172
  generation of, 166t
  illustration of, 159f

Clonic phase, 366
Closed brain injuries, 383
Closed fractures, 965–968, 966t
Clostridium difficile, 137
  diarrhea and, 885b
Clot retraction test, 495t–497t
Clotting factors
  function of, 480, 494–495
  laboratory tests for, 495t–497t
Clotting system, 494
Clubbing, 671
Clubfoot, 1008, 1008t
Cluster breathing, 355t
Cluster headache, 399
CNS. See Central nervous system
COA. See Coarctation of the aorta
Coagulation disorders. See also Disseminated intravascular coagulation
  in children, 545–547
    hemophilias, 545–546
    ITP, 545–546
  consumptive thrombohemorrhagic disorders, 530–533
  impaired hemostasis, 529–530
  liver disease, 530
  thromboembolic disorders, 533–534
  vitamin K deficiency, 530
Coagulation system. See Clotting system
Coagulative necrosis, 102–103
Coal, 677
Coarctation of the aorta (COA), 639
Cochlea, 345
Cockcroft–Gault formula, 726
Cognitive function. See also Arousal; Awareness; Data-processing deficits; Seizure/seizure disorders
  alterations in, 367–369
  neural systems in, 352
Cognitive-evaluative system, 330–331
Cogwheel rigidity, 370t
Cold injury, 1046–1047
Collagen, 492
Collagen fibres, 945
Collagen zones, 952f
Collateral arteries, 555
Collateral circulation, 555
Collateral ganglia, 319–322
Collecting duct, 714, 716
Collectins, 661
Colon, 871, 872f
  cancer of, 801–802, 885, 919–921
  diverticular disease of, 900–901
Colony-stimulating factor-1, 240f, 250–251
Colony-stimulating factors, 486
Colorado tick fever, 401t
Colorectal cancer, 806–807, 919–921
Colorectal polyps, 920
Colostral antibodies, 164
Colour blindness, 343
Colour vision alterations, 343
Coma
  irreversible, 357–358
  myxedema, 455

Combined oral contraceptive pills, 802
Comminuted fractures, 965–968, 966*t*
Commissural fibres, 308
Common bile duct, 874, 874*f*
Communicating hydrocephalus, 369
Communicating pneumothorax, 674
Community-acquired pneumonia, 688
Compact bone, 947, 947*f*
Compartment I disorders, 789
Compartment II disorders, 789
Compartment III disorders, 789
Compartment syndrome, 972–973, 973*b*
Compensatory hyperplasia, 76, 152
Compensatory hypertrophy, 732
Complement cascade, 139–140
Complement receptors, 142
Complement system, 139–141
Complementarity determining regions, 161–162
Complete fractures, 965–968, 966*t*
Complete precocious puberty, 787, 789*b*
Complex motor performance alterations, 378
Compliance
 lung, 661–662
 vascular, 571
Complicated hypertension, 587–588
Complicated plaque, 592
Compound fractures, 965–968, 1003
Compound skull fractures, 386
Compression atelectasis, 676
Compressive syndrome, 408
Computed tomography (CT) scans
 high-resolution peripheral quantitative, 978
Concentric muscle contraction, 961
Concussions, 383
Conducting airways, 654–655
Conduction system, of heart, 557–560
Conductive hearing loss, 345–346
Condylomata acuminata, 836, 857*t*–859*t*, 1036
Cones, 340
Congenital adrenal hyperplasia, 472
 maternal conditions associated with, 638*t*
Congenital equinovarus, 1008, 1008*t*
Congenital heart disease
 acyanotic heart defects, 638–639
 aortic stenosis, 639–640
 atrial septal defect, 642
 atrioventricular canal defect, 642–643
 COA, 639
 cyanotic heart defects, 638–639
 endocarditis risks and, 641
 heart failure caused by, 646–647, 647*t*
 hypoplastic left heart syndrome, 646
 patent ductus arteriosus, 641–642
 pulmonary stenosis, 640–641
 TAPVC, 645–646
 tetralogy of Fallot, 643–644, 643*f*
 tricuspid atresia, 644
 truncus arteriosus, 646
 ventricular septal defect, 642

Congenital hydrocephalus, 415
Congenital hypothyroidism, 456–457
Congenital nephrotic syndrome, 759
Congenital sideroblastic anemia, 506
Congestive splenomegaly, 524
Conivaptan, 725*t*
Conjugated bilirubin, 876, 908
Conjunctivitis, 344
Connective tissues, 32*t*–34*t*
Conn's syndrome, 472
Consciousness
 definition of, 352. *See also* Arousal; Awareness
Constipation, 884
Constrictive pericarditis, 607–608
Consumptive thrombohemorrhagic disorders, 530–533
Contact activation pathway, of clotting system, 140
Contact-dependent signalling, 14
Contaminated food, 823
Contiguous osteomyelitis, 981
Contractile proteins, of skeletal muscles, 958*t*
Contraction alkalosis, 128
Contractures, 994
Contralateral control, 307–308
Contrecoup injury, 383, 385*f*
Contusions
 description of, 383
Conus medullaris, 311
Convergence, 301
Convulsion, 365
Cooley's anemia, 544
Cooper ligaments, 775–776
COPD. *See* Chronic obstructive pulmonary disease
Coping, with stress, 229–231
Cor pulmonale, 693
Cornea, 340
Cornification, 775
Coronary artery disease (CAD), 595–606
 adipokines and, 597–598
 air pollution and, 509
 atherogenic diet and, 597
 cigarette smoking, 597
 diabetes mellitus, 597
 dyslipidemia and, 595–597
 hypertension and, 597
 infections and, 598
 inflammation markers and, 597
 MI caused by, 598–601
 nontraditional risk factors in, 597–598
 obesity and, 597
 sedentary lifestyle and, 597
 troponin I and, 597
Coronary capillaries, 555–556
Coronary circulation, 555, 558*f*
 autonomic regulation and, 575
 autoregulation and, 575
 regulation of, 575
Coronary heart disease, 222*b*
Coronary ligament, 874
Coronary ostia, 555
Coronary perfusion pressure, 575

Coronary sinus, 555
Coronary veins, 556
Coronary vessels, 555–556
Corpora cavernosa, 779
Corpora quadrigemina, 306*t*
Corpus callosum, 308
Corpus luteum, 771–772, 771*f*
 cysts, 799
Corpus spongiosum, 779
Cortex, of kidney, 714, 714*f*
Cortical bone, 947, 947*f*
Cortical dysplasias, 415
Cortical nephrons, 715
Corticobulbar tract, 307–308
Corticospinal tracts, 307–308
Corticotropin-releasing hormone (CRH), 219, 442
Cortisol, 219
 hypercortisolism and, 470
 secretion of, 442
Cough, 670
Cough reflex, 659
Coup injury, 383
COVID-19, 184*t*
 ACE-2 enzyme, 116
 acute kidney injury, 747–748
 acute respiratory syndrome, 697*b*
 ARDS, 679–681
 chronic obstructive pulmonary disease, 633*b*, 698*b*–699*b*
 coping, 229–230
 cytokine storm syndrome, 142
 digestive symptoms and intestinal inflammation, 917
 immune response, 191
 mass vaccination programs, 190
 mRNA vaccines, 158, 177–178
 multisystem inflammatory syndrome, 648
 obesity, 905
 postinfection, 681
 virus mutations, 185
Cowper glands, 780
Cow's milk allergy, 538
COX. *See* Cyclo-oxygenase
COX-1, 145
"Cracked pot" sign, 416
Cranial nerve palsy, 376
Cranial nerves, 301
Craniopharyngioma, 422
Craniosacral division, 322
Craniostenosis, 414–415
Cranium, 313
C-reactive protein, 982
Creatine kinase, 971, 1016
Creatine phosphokinase-myocardial bound (CPK-MB), 603
Creatinine, CKD progression and clearance of, 750
Creutzfeldt-Jakob disease, 364*t*
CRH. *See* Corticotropin-releasing hormone
Cri du chat syndrome, 638*t*
Crista ampullaris, 345
Critical micelle concentration, 897
Crohn's disease (CD), 898*t*, 899

Cross-bridge theory of muscle contraction, 563, 958–960
Cross-bridges, 561–562
Croup, 702–703, 702f
Crush injury, 971–972
Crush syndrome, 971–972, 974f
Crying, pathological, 378
Cryptorchidism, 837–838
Crypts of Lieberkühn, 869
Crystallizable fragment, 161
CSF. See Cerebrospinal fluid
CT scans. See Computed tomography scans
Cul-de-sac, 768
Curcumin, 845b–846b
Curling ulcers, 895
Cushing's **ulcer**, 895
Cushing's disease, 470–472
Cushing's syndrome, 256t, 470–472
Cushing's-like syndrome, 470
Cutaneous hemangiomas, 1061, 1061f, 1062f
Cutaneous lupus erythematosus, 1033, 1033f
Cutaneous melanoma, 1041–1042, 1042f
Cutaneous vascular malformations, 1061–1062, 1062f
Cutaneous vasculitis, 1038
CXCL12-abundant reticular (CAR) cells, 485
Cyanide, 94
Cyanosis, 638–639, 671
Cyanotic heart defects, 638–639
Cyclic adenosine monophosphate (cAMP), 430, 430t
Cyclic guanosine monophosphate (cGMP), 430, 430t
Cyclin-dependent kinase inhibitor 2A, 286–287
Cyclomen (danazol), 802
Cyclo-oxygenase (COX), 145
Cyclopia, 413
Cystatin C, 726, 746
Cystic duct, 877
Cystic fibrosis
   in children, 710–711, 710f, 711f, 933–934, 933t
   Cystic fibrosis transmembrane conductance regulator (CFTR) proteins, 710–711
Cystinuric stones, 733
Cystitis, 737–738, 760
Cystocele, 797, 798f
Cystometric test, 735
Cystometrogram, 727t–728t
Cystometry, 727t–728t
Cystosarcoma phyllodes, 825t
Cysts, 149
   breast, 813
   corpus luteum, 799
   dermoid, 799
   epididymal, 837
   follicular, 799
   functional, 798
   ovarian, benign, 798–799
Cytokines, 26, 142, 224f. See also Growth factors
   adipocytokines and, 903, 903b
   inflammatory, 460
   proinflammatory, 903b

Cytoplasmic organelles, 3, 5t
Cytotoxic edema, 369
Cytotoxic T cells, 158, 171f

D

D vitamins, 438, 944t
   bone and, 979b
DAF. See Decay accelerating factor
Damage-associated molecular patterns (DAMPs), 141
Danazol (Cyclomen), 802
Dandy-Walker malformation, 416
Dark adaptation, 342t
Data-processing deficits
   acute confusional states, 360
   agnosia, 360
   Alzheimer's disease, 363
   delirium, 360
   dementia, 362
   dysphasia, 329
   frontotemporal dementia, 364t
D-dimer, 495–498
de Quervain's thyroiditis, 456
Deafferentation pain, 335t
Deamination, 876–877
Decay accelerating factor, 143f
Decerebrate posture/response, 357f
Decornification, 775
Decorticate posture/response, 357f
Decubitus ulcer, 152
Deep partial-thickness burns, 1043f, 1043t
Deep venous thrombosis, 529
Defecation reflex, 873
Defence mechanisms, 134–149. See also Immunity
Defensins, 136
Deflazacort, 1016
Degenerative extracellular changes, 107
Degenerative joint disease, 393
Degranulation, 138f
Dehiscence, wound, 153–154
Dehydration
   definition of, 118–119
   isotonic fluid loss as cause of, 118
   signs and symptoms of, 120tb0010
Dehydroepiandrosterone, 764t
Delayed hypersensitivity reactions, 200
Delayed hypersensitivity skin test, 195t
Delayed puberty, 787
Delayed repolarization, 122
Delipidation, 281f
Delirium, 360
Delta cells, 439
Demadex, 725t
Demeclocycline, 450
Dementia, 362
Dementia of Alzheimer's type, 363
Dementia with Lewy body, 364t
Dendrites, 301
Dendritic cells, 142t
Dengue, 401t
Denosumab, 977b

Deoxyhemoglobin, 488
Deoxyribonucleic acid (DNA), 39
   composition and structure, 39
   genetic code, 39–40
   mutation, 40, 42f
   replication, 40, 41f
Depolarization, 559, 622t–623t
Depot medroxyprogesterone acetate, 802
Dermal appendages, 1022
Dermatitis
   allergic contact, 208, 1029–1030
   atopic, 857t–859t, 1030, 1054–1055, 1055f
   in children, 1054–1055
   diaper, 1055
   irritant contact, 1030
   seborrheic, 1030
   stasis, 1030
Dermatomes, 319
Dermatomyositis, 256t, 998–999
Dermatophytes, 185–186
Dermis, 1022
Dermoid cysts, 799
Descending colon, 871–872
Descending facilitatory pathways, 333
Descending inhibitory pathways, 333
Desensitization, to allergens, 208
Detrusor areflexia, 734
Detrusor hyper-reflexia, 734
Detrusor muscle, 718
Developmental basis of health and disease, 272–273
Developmental dysplasia of hip, 1008–1009
Developmental plasticity, 272–273
Diabetes insipidus, 450
Diabetes mellitus
   diagnostic criteria for, 460tb0010
   epidemiology of, 459t
   type 1, 459t
   type 2, 221, 459t
Diabetic glomerulopathy, 743f
Diabetic ketoacidosis (DKA), 461
Diabetic nephropathies, 467t
Diabetic neuropathies, 467t
Diabetic retinopathy, 467t
Diamox, 725t
Diapedesis, 146–148
Diaper dermatitis, 1055
Diaphragm, 660
Diaphysis, 948
Diarrhea
   acute infectious, 937
   clinical manifestations of, 885
   Clostridium difficile and, 885b
   definition of, 884
   evaluation of, 885–886
   motility, 885
   osmotic, 885
   pathophysiology of, 885–886
   secretory, 885
   treatment of, 885–886
Diarthrosis, 950
Diastole, 554
Diastolic dysfunction, 619
Diastolic heart failure, 619

DIC. *See* Disseminated intravascular coagulation
Dichlorodiphenyltrichloroethane, 823
Diencephalon, 305
Diet. *See also* Nutrition
    prostate cancer and, 845b–846b
Dietary acculturation, 583–584
Dietary fat, small intestine and, 869b
Diethylstilbestrol, 273
Diffuse axonal injuries, 384t, 386
Diffuse brain injury, 386
Diffuse papillomatosis, 813
DiGeorge syndrome, 193, 458
Digestive system. *See also* Accessory organs of digestion; Gastro-intestinal tract
    anatomy of, 863f
    cancer of, 917
    mouth, 862–864
Digital rectal examination, 842
Dihydrotestosterone, 849f
1, 25-Dihydroxy-vitamin D_3, 437–438
Dilated cardiomyopathy, 608
Dimorphic fungi, 185
Dioxins, 823
Diplegia, 375b
Diplopia, 341
Dipsogenic polydipsia, 450
Direct antiglobulin test, 495t–497t
Direct effects, of hormones, 429
Discoid lupus erythematosus, 1033
Disease-modifying antirheumatic drugs (DMARDs), 988
Dislocation, 968
Disse space, 875
Disseminated intravascular coagulation (DIC), 530–533
    clinical manifestations of, 531–532
    evaluation of, 532–533
    pathophysiology of, 531–533
    treatment of, 532–533
Distal convoluted tubule, 715
Distal intestinal obstruction syndrome, 930
Disuse atrophy, 994
Diuresis, postoperative, 732
Diverticula, 900
Diverticular disease, 900
Diverticulitis, 900
Diverticulosis, 890t
DKA. *See* Diabetic ketoacidosis
DMARDs. *See* Disease-modifying antirheumatic drugs
DMD. *See* Duchenne muscular dystrophy
DNA. *See* Deoxyribonucleic acid
DNA demethylating agents, 69
DNA methylation
    Alzheimer's disease and, 363
    cancer and, 68, 276
DNA methyltransferase, 276–278
Dolichocephaly, 417f
Doll's eyes phenomenon, 356f
Dopamine
    properties of, 305t
    substantia nigra synthesis of, 310
Dormancy, of cancer cells, 253–255
Dorsal respiratory group, 659

Double uterus, 787f
Double vagina, 787f
Double-helix model, 39
Double-strand break, 283f
Down syndrome, 515, 638t
Downregulation, 429
Down syndrome, 48f
Doxycycline (Teva-Doxycycline), 795b
Driver mutations, 237–238
Droxia, 509
Drugs. *See specific drugs*
Dual X-ray absorptiometry, 978
Duchenne muscular dystrophy (DMD), 1015–1016
Ductal adenocarcinomas, 922
Ductal carcinoma in situ, 235, 825
Ductal intraepithelial neoplasia, 825–826
Duke criteria, 616
Dumping syndrome, 896–897
Duodenum
    anatomy of, 865f
    obstruction of, 929–930
    ulcers of, 893
Dusts, 677
Dutch Famine Birth Cohort, 272–273
Dwarfism, hypopituitary, 451, 451f
Dynorphins, 332
Dysgeusia, 347
Dyskinesia, 371
Dyslipidemia, 595–597
Dysmenorrhea, 788–789
Dyspareunia, 811
Dysphagia, 589, 887
Dysphasia, 360
Dysplasias, 76, 77f
    acetabular, 1008
    cortical, 415
    of hip, developmental, 1008–1009
Dyspnea, 608, 670
Dyspraxia, 364
Dysreflexia, 389
Dysrhythmias, 603
Dyssomnias, 339–340
Dyssynergia, 734
Dystonia, 370t
Dystonic cerebral palsy, 416
Dystonic movements, 378
Dystonic postures, 378
Dystrophic calcification, 99–100
Dystrophin, 1015–1016

E

E vitamins, 845b–846b
Ear
    external, 345
    infections of, 346–347
    inner, 345f
    normal, anatomy of, 345
Eastern equine encephalitis, 401t
EBV. *See* Epstein-Barr virus
Ecchymosis, 491t
Eccrine sweat glands, 1022
ECF. *See* Extracellular fluid

ECF-A. *See* Eosinophil chemotactic factor of anaphylaxis
ECG. *See* Electrocardiogram
ECM. *See* Extracellular matrix
Ectopic kidneys, 760
Ectopic testis, 837–838
Eczema, 1029
Edecrin, 907–908
Edema
    brain, 368f
    cerebral, 368–369
    clinical manifestations of, 116
    cytotoxic, 369
    evaluation of, 116
    formation mechanisms of, 115f
    generalized, 116
    interstitial, 368–369
    localized, 116
    metabolic, 353
    pathophysiology of, 114–116
    pitting, 116f
    treatment of, 116
    vasogenic, 368–369
Effective renal blood flow, 726
Effective renal plasma flow, 726
Efferent arteriole, 716
Efferent lymphatic vessels, 577
EGF. *See* Epidermal growth factor
Ejection fraction, 563
Elastic arteries, 566
Elastic recoil, 661
Elastin, 12
Elderly. *See also* Aging
    age-related macular degeneration and, 343
    hyponatremia in, 120tb0030
    TBW in, 130tb0050
Electrocardiogram (ECG), 588
Electrolytes
    distribution of, 113t
    as solutes, 19–22
Electromagnetic radiation, 287–288
Electromechanical dissociation, 622t–623t
Electromyography, 727t–728t
Electron-transport chain, 17
ELISA. *See* Enzyme-linked immunosorbent assay
Embolic stroke, 395
Embolism
    cardiovascular, 590
    pulmonary, 692
Embolus, 533
Embryonal tumours, 422
Emesis, 883
Emphysema, 686f
Empyema, 675
EMT. *See* Epithelial-mesenchymal transition
Encephalitis, 401–402, 420
Encephalocele, 413
Encephalopathies, 416–420
Endocannabinoids, 333
Endocardial cushion defect, 642–643

Endocardial disorders
   acute rheumatic fever, 612–614
   aortic regurgitation, 611–612
   aortic stenosis, 610–611
   infective endocarditis, 614–615
   mitral regurgitation, 612
   mitral stenosis, 611
   MVPS, 612
   rheumatic heart disease, 612–614
   tricuspid regurgitation, 612
   valvular dysfunction, 609–612
Endocarditis, 641b
Endocardium, 553
Endocervical canal, 769
Endocervical gonorrhea, 857t–859t
Endochondral bone formation, 967–968
Endocrine disorders, 996–997
Endocrine glands. *See also* Adrenal glands; Pancreas; Parathyroid glands; Pituitary gland; Thyroid gland
   aging effects on, 427f
   pineal gland, 436
Endocrine pancreas, 438–439. *See also* Diabetes mellitus
Endocrine system
   female, 819f
   functions of, 427
Endogenous antigens, 167
Endogenous opioids, 331–332
Endogenous pyrogens, 142, 336–337
Endometrial cancer, 806–807, 806f
Endometrial polyps, 800
Endometriosis, 801–802
Endometrium, anatomy of, 769–770
Endomitosis, 491
Endomorphins, 332
Endoplasmic reticulum, 9b
Endorphins
   as endogenous opioids, 331–332
   properties of, 305t
Endothelial cells, 145, 566–567
Endothelial dysfunction, 584
Endothelial injury, 533, 592
Endothelium
   description of, 145
   vascular, 566–567
Endothelium-derived relaxing factor, 574
Endotoxic shock, 183
Endotoxins, 183
End-stage kidney disease, 744
Energy metabolism diseases, 997
Engulfment, 148
Enkephalins
   as endogenous opioids, 332
   properties of, 305t
Enterocytes, 869
Enteroglucagon, 866t
Enterohepatic circulation, 875f
Enthesis, 968–969
Entropion, 344
Environmental tobacco smoke, 274–276
Enzyme-linked immunosorbent assay, 430b, 524
Eosinopenia, 511, 511t

Eosinophil chemotactic factor of anaphylaxis (ECF-A), 163f
Eosinophilia, 510, 511t
Eosinophilic esophagitis, 889, 932
Eosinophils, 141f
Ependymal cells, 302
Epicardium, 553f
Epicondylopathy, 969–970
Epicritic information, 312
Epidermal growth factor (EGF), 239
Epidermis, 1022
Epididymal cysts, 837
Epididymitis, 838
Epidural hematomas, 384
Epigallocatechin gallate, 850–852
Epigenetics, 62
   cancer, 69f
      DNA demethylating agents, 69
      DNA methylation, 68
      emerging strategies, 69
      epigenetic screening, 68–69
      histone deacetylase inhibitors, 69–70, 70f
      microRNA coding, 70
      microRNAs, 68
   ethanol exposure, during gestation, 67–68
      genetic abnormalities, 67–68, 67f
      mental illness, 67
      molecular approaches, 68
      twin studies, 68
   genomic imprinting, 64–66
   human development, 64
   mechanisms, 62–64, 63f
      DNA methylation, 63–64
      histone modifications, 64
      RNA-based mechanisms, 64
   states
      and maternal care, 66–67
      and nutrition, 66
Epilepsy, 365
Epileptogenic focus, 366
Epinephrine, 443, 565
Epithalamus, 309–310
Epithelial cells, 136
Epithelial tissues, 30t–31t
Epithelialization, 151
Epithelial-mesenchymal transition (EMT), 252
   prostate cancer and, 850
Epithelioid cells, 150–151
EPSPs. *See* Excitatory postsynaptic potentials
Epstein-Barr virus (EBV), 251, 512
   Burkitt lymphoma and, 522
   infectious mononucleosis and, 512–513
Equinovalgus, 1008t
Equinovarus, 1008t
Erectile dysfunction treatments, 854
Erectile reflex, of penis, 779
Erlotinib (Tarceva), 263t
Erosion, 1028f
Eryptosis, 503
Erysipelas, 1035
Erythema, 207
Erythema multiforme, 1034
Erythema toxicum neonatorum, 1062
Erythroblasts, 490f

Erythrocyte osmotic fragility test, 495t–497t
Erythrocytes, 480
   aging effects on, 498b
   childhood disorders of, 537–545
      anemia, 538t
      hemolytic anemia, 539–540
      iron deficiency anemia, 538–539
      sickle cell disease, 540–543
      thalassemias, 543–545
   development of
      erythropoiesis, 487
      hemoglobin synthesis and, 487–488
      iron cycle and, 489–490
   disorders involving
      absolute polycythemia, 508
      anemia. *See* Anemia
      familial polycythemia, 508t
      hereditary hemochromatosis, 509–510
      iron overload, 509–510
      myeloproliferative, 507–510
      polycythemia vera, 508–509
      relative polycythemia, 507
      secondary polycythemia, 508
   senescent, normal destruction of, 489–490
   sickled, 542
   in spleen, 482f
Erythrodermic psoriasis, 1031
Erythromelalgia, 529
Erythropoiesis, 487
Erythropoietin, 256t, 488f
Escharotomies, 1044
Escherichia coli, 737f
Esophageal atresia, 928–929
Esophageal varices, 906–908
Esophagitis, 889, 932
Esophagus
   Barrett, 918
   cancer of, 268t–271t
   eosinophilic esophagitis and, 889
   GER, 929
   GERD, 888–889
   GERD and inflammation of, 931
Essential thrombocythemia, 528–529
Estradiol, 429t, 767, 799
Estriol, 772
Estrogen
   adrenal cortex secretion of, 433f
   biological effects of, 772
   biosynthesis of, 820f
   carcinogenicity of, 820
Estrogen receptors, 807
Estrogen receptor-α, 848–849
Estrogen receptor-β, 848–849
Estrone, 772
Ethacrynic acid, 907–908
Ethanol, 88–92, 90f
Ethanol exposure, during gestation, 67–68. *See also* Alcohol
   genetic abnormalities, 67–68, 67f
   mental illness, 67
   molecular approaches, 68
   twin studies, 68
Ethylenediaminetetraacetic acid, 526
Eukaryotes, 2

Ewing sarcoma, 234–235, 1018–1019
Exanthema subitum, 1059
Excess relative risks, with ionizing radiation, 282
Excitatory postsynaptic potentials, 304
Excited delirium syndrome, 362
Excoriation, 1027f
Executive attention deficits, 358
Exocrine pancreas
　anatomy of, 873f
　blood flow to, 873
Exogenous antigens, 134
Exotoxins, 182–183
Expression disorders, 378
Expressive aprosody, 378
Expressive dysphasia, 360
Exstrophy of bladder, 757–758
External anal sphincter, 871–872
External intercostal muscles, 660
External urethral sphincter, 719
Extracellular fluid (ECF)
　in acidosis, 121
　definition of, 113
　hypokalemia in, 121–123
　potassium concentration in, 121
Extracellular matrix, 11–12, 12f
Extradural hematomas, 384t
Extrahepatic portal hypertension, 939
Extramedullary hematopoiesis, 501
Extrinsic allergic alveolitis, 678
Exudate, 149
Eye
　anatomy of, 340–341
　external, structure and disorders of, 343–344
　extrinsic muscles of, 341f
Eyelids, 343

F

F cells, 439
Facioscapulohumeral muscular dystrophy (FSHD), 1017
Factor XII. *See* Hageman factor
FAD. *See* Flavin adenine dinucleotide
Failure to thrive, 935–936
Fallopian tubes, 770f
False vocal cords, 654
Falx cerebri, 314
Familial adenomatous polyposis, 261, 920–921
Familial polycythemia, 508t
Familial tremor, 372t
Fas-associated death domain signaling complex, 248–249
Fas/CD95, 248–249
Fascicles, 318–319
Fasciculus cuneatus, 312
Fasciculus gracilis, 312
Fast-twitch fibres, 955
Fat embolism, 591t
Fatigue, cancer and, 255
Fatigue fractures, 966–967
Fats
　liver metabolism of, 876
　small intestine absorption of, 877t

Fatty liver
　alcoholic, 910–912
　nonalcoholic, 912
Fatty necrosis, 102
Fc receptors, 148
FDPs. *See* Fibrin degradation products
Febrile seizure, 421t
Fecal analysis, 1078t–1079t
Fecal mass, 872, 890t
Female reproductive system
　aging and, 781–782
　breasts. *See* Breasts
　clitoris, 768
　development of, 764–767
　external genitalia of, 767–768, 768f
　fallopian tubes, 771
　internal genitalia of, 768–772
　labia majora, 768
　labia minora, 767
　menopause, 781
　menstrual cycle. *See* Menstrual cycle
　mons pubis, 767–768
　ovaries, 771–772
　perineum in, 768
　sex hormones of, 764t, 772
　uterus. *See* Uterus
　vagina. *See* Vagina
　vestibule in, 768
　vulva, 768
Female reproductive system disorders
　abnormal uterine bleeding, 786, 787f, 791t
　adenomyosis, 801
　amenorrhea, 789–790
　bartholinitis, 797
　breast cancer. *See* Breast cancer
　cervical cancer. *See* Cervical cancer
　cervicitis, 796
　delayed puberty, 787
　dysmenorrhea, 788–789
　endometrial cancer, 806–807
　endometriosis, 801–802
　infections, 793–797
　inflammations, 793–797
　leiomyomas, 800–801
　ovarian cancer. *See* Ovarian cancer
　ovarian cysts, 798–799
　PCOS, 791–792
　pelvic organ prolapse, 797–798
　PID, 793–794
　PMDD, 792–793
　PMS, 792–793
　precocious puberty, 787
　reproductive tract abnormalities, 786
　salpingitis, 794–796
　sexual dysfunction, 811
　sexual maturation alterations, 786–787
　vaginal cancer, 805–806
　vulvodynia, 796–797
　vulvar cancer, 806
Female reproductive tract abnormalities, 786
Female sexual trauma, 739t
Female-pattern alopecia, 1048–1049
Fenestrations, 566
FEP. *See* Free erythrocyte protoporphyrin

Ferritin, 489–490
　serum, determination, 479t
Fetal alcohol spectrum disorder, 91f, 412b
Fetus
　vulnerability of, to environments, 273f
Fever
　benefits of, 337
　in children, 337b
　Colorado tick, 401t
　in elderly, 337b
　pathogenesis of, 336–337, 337f
　of unknown origin, 337
FGF. *See* Fibroblast growth factor
Fibrils, 945
Fibrin degradation products (FDPs), 495–498, 531
Fibrin split products (FSPs), 531
Fibrin-fibrinogen degradation products, 495t–497t
Fibrinogen, 480
Fibrinogen assay, 495t–497t
Fibrinolysis, 530f
Fibrinolytic system, 530f
Fibroblast growth factor, 27t, 807
Fibrocystic disease of pancreas, 933–934
Fibromyalgia, 994–996
Fibronectin, 12
Fibrosarcoma, 1003–1004
Fibrous adhesions, 890t
Fibrous joints, 950
Filtration fraction, 719
Filtration slits, 715–716
Filum terminale, 311
Fimbriae, 771
First messengers, 430
First-degree burns, 1043
Fissure, 1027f
Fissure of Rolando, 306–307
Flagyl (metronidazole), 795b
Flail chest, 674
Flat bones, 949
Flavin adenine dinucleotide, 17
Fleabites, 1060
Fluid resuscitation, 1045
Focal brain injury, 383–386
Focal segmental glomerulosclerosis, 759
Focal seizure, 421t
Folate, 504
Folate deficiency anemia, 504–505
Folic acid, 504
Folic acid deficiency, 89
Follicle cells, of thyroid gland, 436f
Follicle-stimulating hormone (FSH), 432
　functions of, 764t
　in menstrual cycle, 766–767
Follicular cysts, 799
Folliculitis, 1035
Follistatin, 775
Fontan procedure, 646
Fontanelles, 412f
Food additives, 823
Food allergy, 900
Food poisoning, 180t–181t
Foramen of Luschka, 315–316

Foramen of Magendie, 315–316
Foramen of Monro, 315–316
Foramen ovale, 642
Forebrain, 306t
Foreign matter, 591t
Foreskin, 779
Fornix, of vagina, 768
Fosamax, 1010
Fossae, 313
Fourth-degree burns, 1043
Fovea centralis, 340
Fractures
　basilar skull, 386
　bowing, 965–966
　classification of, 965–968
　clinical manifestations of, 967–968
　closed, 965–968
　comminuted, 965–968
　complete, 965–968
　compound, 965–968
　compound skull, 386
　definition of, 965
　delayed union of, 968
　evaluation of, 968
　external fixation of, 968
　fatigue, 966–967
　greenstick, 965–966
　healing, 967–968
　impacted, 966f
　incomplete, 965–968
　insufficiency, 966
　internal fixation of, 968
　linear, 965–968
　malunion of, 968
　nonunion of, 968
　oblique, 965–968
　occult, 966f
　open, 965–968
　open reduction of, 968
　osteoporosis causing, 974–976
　pathological, 966
　pathophysiology of, 967–968
　segmented, 966f
　spiral, 965–968
　stress, 966–967
　torus, 965–966
　traction of, 968
　transchondral, 967
　transverse, 965–968
　treatment of, 968
Fragile sites, 48–49
Fragile X syndrome, 48–49, 67–68
Fragile X tremor ataxia syndrome (FXTAS), 67–68
Fragile X-associated primary ovarian insufficiency, 67–68
Frameshift mutations, 42f
Free erythrocyte protoporphyrin (FEP), 506
Free fatty acids, 462
Freely movable joints, 950
Frontal lobe, 306–307
Frontal lobe ataxic gait, 378
Frontotemporal dementia, 364t
Fructosemia, 939

FSH. See Follicle-stimulating hormone
FSHD. See Facioscapulohumeral muscular dystrophy
FSPs. See Fibrin split products
Full-thickness burns, 1044
Functional constipation, 884
Functional cysts, 798
Functional dysphagia, 887
Functional residual capacity, 661
Fungal diseases, 185–186
Fungal infections, 1036–1038
　in children, 1056–1057
Fungal meningitis, 400
Fungi, 178t, 185
Furosemide, 725t, 907–908
Furuncles, 1035
Fusiform aneurysms, 397
Fusiform muscles, 953
FXTAS. See Fragile X tremor ataxia syndrome

G

G6PD deficiency. See Glucose-6-phosphate dehydrogenase deficiency
GABA. See Gamma-aminobutyric acid
Gait, 1013
Gait disorders, 378
Galactorrhea, 812–813
Galactosemia, 939
Galea aponeurotica, 313
Gallbladder
　aging effects on, 880b
　anatomy of, 853t, 879f
　cancer of, 922
　disorders of, 914–915
Gallstones, 914
Gamma-aminobutyric acid, 92b, 331, 793
Gamma globulins, 479–480
Gamma rigidity, 370t
Gamma-glutamyltranspeptidase, 878t
Ganglia
　basal, 306–307
　collateral, 319–322
　paravertebral, 319–322
　sympathetic, 319–322
Gangrenous cystitis, 737
Gangrenous necrosis, 102–103
Gas-exchange airways, 655
Gas gangrene, 103, 104f
Gasping breathing pattern, 355t
Gastric bleeding, 893
Gastric emptying, 866–867
Gastric glands, 867, 867f
Gastric inflammation, 250
Gastric inhibitory peptide, 866t
Gastric motility, 865–867
Gastric secretion, 867–868
Gastric ulcers, 895t
Gastrin, 439, 865
Gastrin-releasing peptide, 866t
Gastritis, 892–893
Gastrocolic reflex, 872
Gastroduodenal junction, 864–865
Gastroesophageal reflux (GER), 931–932

Gastroesophageal reflux disease (GERD), 888–889, 931
Gastroileal reflex, 870
Gastro-intestinal allergy, 203
Gastro-intestinal bleeding, 886
Gastro-intestinal system. See also specific organs
　CKD and, 752
Gastro-intestinal (GI) tract. See also Accessory organs of digestion
　esophagus. See Esophagus
　immunity and, 873
　microbiome of, 873
　mouth, 862–864
　stomach. See Stomach
Gastro-intestinal tract disorders
　abdominal pain, 886
　anorexia, 515, 883
　appendicitis, 901
　bile salt deficiency, 897–898
　CD, 899
　in children. See Children, gastro-intestinal tract disorders in
　clinical manifestations of, 885
　constipation, 884
　diarrhea. See Diarrhea
　diverticular disease, 900–901
　dysphagia, 887–888
　gastritis, 892–893
　gastro-intestinal bleeding, 886
　GERD, 888–889
　hiatal hernia, 889
　IBD, 898–900
　IBS, 899–900
　intestinal obstruction. See Intestinal obstruction
　lactase deficiency, 897
　malabsorption syndromes, 897–898
　mesenteric vascular insufficiency, 901
　microscopic colitis, 899
　motility disorders, 887–892
　nutrition disorders, 902–905
　pancreatic exocrine insufficiency, 897
　peptic ulcer disease. See Peptic ulcer disease
　pyloric obstruction, 889–890
Gastroparesis, 889
GCT. See Glucose change test
Gegenhalten. See Paratonia
Gene mapping, 56–58, 57f
Genes, 39
　to proteins, 40
General adaptation syndrome, 216
Generalized clonic-tonic seizure, 379
Generalized edema, 116
Generalized lymphadenopathy, 518
Genetic diseases
　autosomal dominant inheritance
　　delayed age of onset, 51
　　epigenetics and genomic imprinting, 52, 53f
　　pedigree chart, 50, 50f, 51f
　　pedigrees characteristics, 50–51
　　penetrance and expressivity, 51–52, 52f
　　recurrence risks, 51

Genetic diseases *(Continued)*
  autosomal recessive inheritance
    consanguinity, 54
    pedigrees characteristics, 53–54, 53f
    recurrence risks, 54, 54f
  mode of inheritance, 50
  X-linked inheritance, 54–56
    pedigrees characteristics, 55
    recurrence risks, 56, 56f
    sex determination, 55, 55f
    sex-limited and sex-influenced traits, 55–56
    X inactivation, 54–55, 54f
Genetic heterogeneity, 823–824
Genetics
  dominance and recessiveness, 50
  elements, 49–50
  phenotype and genotype, 49–50
Genital herpes, 856t
Genomic imprinting, 64–66
GER. *See* Gastroesophageal reflux
GERD. *See* Gastroesophageal reflux disease
Germ cell inheritance, 273t
Germ cell tumours, 407t
German measles, 1058t
Gestational diabetes mellitus, 464–465
GH. *See* Growth hormone
Ghrelin, 439, 464, 866t, 903b
GHRH. *See* Growth hormone-releasing hormone
GI tract. *See* Gastro-intestinal tract
Giant aneurysms, 397
Giant cell tumour, 1004
Giant cells, 150–151
Giantism, pituitary, 451f
Glands of Montgomery, 777
Glans, 779
Glasgow Coma Scale, 384t
Glaucoma, 341
Gleason score, 849b
Gleevec (imatinib), 241, 518
Glioblastoma multiforme, 406
Gliomas, 422
  brainstem, 422
  optic, 422
Glisson capsule, 874
Global dysphasia, 360
Globins, 487
Globulins, 479–480, 876–877
Globus pallidus, 308
Glomerular capillaries, 717
Glomerular disorders, 739–744
  glomerulonephritis. *See* Glomerulonephritis
Glomerular filtration
  capillary pressures and, 720
  definition of, 720
  in distal convoluted tubule, 716
  Loop of Henle and, 716
  in proximal convoluted tubule, 716
  substances transported in, 723b
Glomerular filtration membrane, 715–716
Glomerular filtration rate, 719
  renal clearance and, 726
Glomerular injury, 739
Glomerular lesions, 741t

Glomerulonephritis
  acute, 739
  chronic, 741–742
  clinical manifestations of, 740–741
  evaluation of, 740
  immunological pathogenesis of, 741t
  pathophysiology of, 739–741
  treatment of, 740
  types of, 741t
Glomerulotubular balance, 722
Glomerulus, 715
Glossitis, 506f
Glucagon, 439, 460
Glucocorticoids. *See also* Cortisol
  adrenal cortex producing, 440–443
Gluconeogenesis, 905
Glucophage (metformin), 464
Glucose change test, 465
Glucose transporters (GLUTs), 438
Glucose-6-phosphate dehydrogenase (G6PD) deficiency, 538
Glutathione-S-transferases, 844–847
GLUTs. *See* Glucose transporters
Glycogen storage diseases, 97
Glycogenolysis, 905
Glycolysis, 17, 17f
Glycoprotein hormones, 432, 435t
Glycoprotein PIIb/IIIa (GPIIb/IIIa), 492
Glycoproteins, 944t
Glycosylated hemoglobin, 459
α-Glycoprotein, 947
GM 2 gangliosidosis, 419
GnRH. *See* Gonadotropin-releasing hormone
Goblet cells, 655
Golfer's elbow, 969
Golgi tendon organs, 955
Gomphosis, 950
Gonadarche, 767
Gonadostat, 767
Gonadotropin-releasing hormone (GnRH), 766–767
Gonadotropin-releasing hormone pulse generator, 767
Gonads, 765
Gonococcal infections, 857t–859t
Gonorrhea, 840f, 856t
Gorlin syndrome, 286
Gout, 991–994
Gouty arthritis, 991
GPIIb/IIIa. *See* Glycoprotein PIIb/IIIa
Granulation tissue, 152–153
Granulocytes, 141f
Granulocytopenia, 510
Granulocytosis, 510
Granuloma, 150–151
Granulosa cells, 772
Grasp reflex, 356f
Graves' dermopathy, 455
Graves' disease, 455
Great cardiac vein, 556
Great vessels, of heart, 554
Green tea, 845b–846b
Greenstick fractures, 965–966
Gremlin, 946t

Ground substance, 943
Growth factor-regulated kinases, 244
Growth faltering, 935–936
Growth hormone (GH), 449
Growth hormone-releasing hormone (GHRH), 432
Growth plate, 948–949
Guillain-Barré syndrome, 356f
Guttate psoriasis, 1031
Gynecomastia, 855
Gyri, 306–309

H

H1 receptors, 144–145
H1N1 (swine influenza virus), 185
H2 receptors, 144–145
H5N1 avian influenza virus, 185
Haemophilus influenzae, 420, 981
Hageman factor (factor XII), 140
Hair
  colour of, 1022
Hair cells, 345
Haldane effect, 666–667
Hanging strangulations, 94
Haplotypes, 212
Haptens, 134
Hashimoto's disease, 455–456
Haversian canal, 947
Haversian system, 947
Hayflick limit, 246
HDL. *See* High-density lipoprotein
Headaches, 398–400
Health care-associated pneumonia, 688
Hearing, 344–347. *See also* Ear
Hearing loss, 345–346
Heart
  action potentials of, 556
  ATP for, 561
  automaticity of, 559
  blood flow through, 568–571
  cardiac cycle of, 554
  chambers of, 553–554, 554f
  conduction system of, 557–560
  coronary vessels of, 555
  fibrous skeleton of, 554
  great vessels of, 554
  hypertrophy of, 561
  innervation of, 560
  intracardiac pressures in, 555
  parasympathetic nerves of, 560
  rhythmicity of, 559
  Starling's law of, 564
  structures of, 556–563
  sympathetic nerves of, 560
  valves of, 554
Heart disease
  congenital. *See* Congenital heart disease
  dysrhythmias, 620–621
  rheumatic, 612–614
Heart failure, 646–647
  congenital heart disease causing, 647t
  left, clinical manifestations of, 647b

Heart rate
  atrial receptors and, 566
  cardiac output and, 563–566
  cardiovascular vasomotor control centre and, 565
  pericardial sac causing reflex changes in, 553
Heart rate variability, 229–230
Heart wall
  anatomy of, 553
  disorders of, 606–616
    acute pericarditis, 606–607
    constrictive pericarditis, 607–608
    pericardial effusion, 607–608
Heat cramps, 337–338
Heat exhaustion, 337
Heat stroke, 337
HeLa cells, 246
Helicobacter pylori, 250, 504
Helper T cells, 158
Hemangioblastomas, 407t
Hematemesis, 886t
Hematochezia, 886
Hematocrit determination, 495t–497t
Hematogenous osteomyelitis, 981
Hematological system. *See also* Blood
  aging effects on, 498b, 498t
  blood tests for, 495t–497t
  components of, 478–485
  lymphoid organs
    lymph nodes, 484
    mononuclear phagocyte system, 484–485
    spleen, 483–484
Hematology, 1071t–1074t
Hematomas
  epidural, 384
  extradural, 384
  intracerebral, 386
  subdural, 385
Hematopoiesis
  in bone marrow, 485–486, 486f
  cellular differentiation and, 486–487
  definition of, 485
  extramedullary, 485
Hematopoietic stem cell transplantation, 543
Hematopoietic stem cells (HSCs), 485
Heme, 488
Hemiagnosia, 335t
Hemiparesis, 375b
Hemiplegia, 375b
Hemiplegic posture, 378
Hemochromatosis, 509–510
Hemodynamic stroke, 395
Hemoglobin, 126
  aging effects on, 498b
  glycosylated, 459
  NO binding to, 489f
  oxygen transport by, 663–666
  sickle cell, 540–543
  synthesis of, 487–488
Hemoglobin desaturation, 665–666
Hemoglobin H disease, 542t
Hemoglobin S, 540
Hemolysis, 503
Hemolytic anemia, 554

Hemolytic disease of newborn, 211
  clinical manifestations of, 539–540
  evaluation and treatment of, 540
  incidence of, 539
  pathophysiology of, 539–540
Hemolytic jaundice, 908
Hemophilias, 545–546
Hemoptysis, 670–671
Hemorrhage
  blowout, 491t
  petechial, 491t
  subarachnoid, 396
Hemorrhagic cystitis, 737
Hemorrhagic disorders
  antibody-mediated, 546–547
  classification of, 526–534
  inherited, 545–546
Hemorrhagic exudate, 149
Hemorrhagic infarcts, 400–401
Hemorrhagic stroke, 396–397, 420
Hemosiderin, 98, 489
Hemosiderosis, 99
Hemostasis, 491
  definition of, 491
Hemothorax, 675, 675t
Heparin-induced thrombocytopenia (HIT), 527
Hepatic encephalopathy, 908
Hepatitis, in children, 938
Hepatitis A virus, 913t
Hepatitis B virus, 913t
Hepatitis C virus, 913t
Hepatitis D virus, 913t
Hepatitis E virus, 913t
Hepatoblastoma, 940
Hepatocellular carcinoma, 921–922
Hepatopulmonary syndrome, 906
Hepatorenal syndrome, 908–910
Hepcidin, 258
Herceptin (trastuzumab), 263t
Herd immunity, 190
Hereditary angioedema, 140
Hereditary hemochromatosis, 509–510
Hereditary multiple exostoses, 1017–1018
Hereditary nonpolyposis colorectal cancer (HNPCC), 920–921
Hereditary thrombophilias, 533
Hering-Breuer reflex, 659
Hernia, 890t
  hiatal, 889f
Herniated intervertebral disc, 393–394
Herpes simplex virus, 857t–859t, 1035–1036
Herpes zoster, 1026f
Herpesviruses, 184t
Heterophilic antibodies, 512–513
Heterotopic ossification, 970
Hexose-monophosphate shunt, 148, 193–194
HHS. *See* Hyperosmolar hyperglycemic syndrome
Hiatal hernia, 889f
Hiccups, 356–357
HIF. *See* Hypoxia-inducible transcription factor

High-density lipoprotein, 142, 592, 751, 904
High-output failure, 620
High-resolution peripheral quantitative computed tomography (HRpQCT), 978
High-sensitivity C-reactive protein, 592
Hindbrain, 306t
Hip
  developmental dysplasia of, 1008–1009
  dislocated, 1008
  subluxated, 1008
Hirschsprung's disease, 930–931
Hirsutism, 1049
Histaminase, 140
Histamine, 144–145
Histone acetyl transferase, 276–278
Histone deacetylase inhibitors, 69–70, 70f
HIT. *See* Heparin-induced thrombocytopenia
HIV. *See* Human immunodeficiency virus
HIV-associated neurocognitive disorder, 402
Hives. *See* Urticaria
HLAs. *See* Human leukocyte antigens
HLHS. *See* Hypoplastic left heart syndrome
HNPCC. *See* Hereditary nonpolyposis colorectal cancer
Hodgkin's disease, 262
Hodgkin's lymphoma
  in children, 548–549
Homeostasis, 14, 215
Homunculus, 307–308
Hormonal hyperplasia, 76
Hormonal signalling, 14
Hormone receptors, 429
Hormone replacement therapy, breast cancer risk and, 820–821
Hormones
  adrenal gland, 439–445
  binding proteins and, 429t
  biphasic effects of, 429
  direct effects of, 429
  feedback systems of, 428
  first messengers and, 430
  lipid-soluble, 431
  mechanisms of action of, 427–428
  pineal gland, 436
  pituitary
    regulation of, 437t
  release of, 428
  structural categories of, 427t
  thyroid gland, 436
  water-soluble, 428–429
HPA system. *See* Hypothalamic-pituitary-adrenal system
HPV. *See* Human papillomavirus
HPV DNA test, 803b
HRpQCT. *See* High-resolution peripheral quantitative computed tomography
HSCs. *See* Hematopoietic stem cells
HTLV-1. *See* Human T-cell lymphotropic virus type 1
Human chorionic gonadotropin, 764t
Human epidermal growth factor receptor, 239
Human exposure, to pollutants, 83–84, 83f

Human immunodeficiency virus (HIV)
  antiretroviral therapy for, 196
  genetic map of, 197f
  life cycle and possible sites of, 198f
  neurocognitive disorder associated with, 402
  prevalence of, 199
  viral meningitis and, 400
Human leukocyte antigens (HLAs), 194
Human papillomavirus (HPV), 288
  warts caused by, 1036
Human papillomavirus DNA test, 802
Human T-cell lymphotropic virus type 1 (HTLV-1), 251
Humoral immunity, 158
Hunt and Hess subarachnoid hemorrhage grading system, 397–398
Huntington's disease, 371–373
Huxley, A. F., 958–960
Hyaline membrane disease. See Respiratory distress syndrome of newborn
Hydrea, 529
Hydrocele, 836–837
Hydrocephalus, 310
  clinical manifestations of, 369
  congenital, 415
  definition of, 369
  evaluation and treatment of, 369
  pathophysiology of, 369
Hydrochlorothiazide, 725t
Hydrogen, 722
Hydrogen ions, 124
Hydronephrosis, 731–732
Hydrostatic pressure
  capillary, 114
  interstitial, 114
Hydroureter, 731–732
Hydroxyapatite, 945
11β-Hydroxysteroid dehydrogenase type 1, 221b
Hydroxyurea, 509
  for sickle cell disease, 543
Hyperactive confusional state. See Delirium
Hyperactivity, 358b
Hyperaldosteronism, 128
Hyperbilirubinemia, 539, 908
Hypercalcemia, 457–458, 523–524
Hypercapnia, 128
Hyperchloremia, 119
Hypercoagulability, 526
Hypercyanotic spells, 643–644
Hyperfunction, 732
Hyperglycemia, 458–459
Hypergonadotropic hypogonadism, 788t
Hyperhemolytic crisis, 542
Hyperkalemia
  clinical manifestations of, 123
  evaluation of, 123–124
  pathophysiology of, 123
  treatment of, 123–124
Hyperkinesia, 371
Hypermagnesemia, 125t
Hypermenorrhea, 791t
Hypernatremia, 118–120
Hyperosmolar hyperglycemic syndrome (HHS), 465

Hyperparathyroidism, 457–458
Hyperphosphatemia, 125t
Hyperpituitarism, 451–452
Hyperplasia
  atypical, 814
  atypical ductal, 814
  atypical lobular, 814
  benign prostatic, 840–842
  cellular adaptation, 76, 76f
  mild, 813
  usual ductal, 813–814
Hyperpolarization, 559
Hypersecretion of GH, 452–453
Hypersensitivity, 199–213
Hypersensitivity pneumonitis, 678
Hypersensitivity reactions
  antigenic targets of, 208–213
  delayed, 200
  type 1 (IgE-mediated), 200–204
  type II (tissue-specific), 204–205
  type III (immune complex-mediated), 205–207
  type IV (cell-mediated), 207–208
Hypersomnia, 339
Hypersplenism, 524
Hypertension
  acromegaly-associated, 452
  in children, 649–651
  classification of, 582t
  complicated, 587–588
  incidence of, 582
  primary, 649
    Indigenous people of Canada and, 582–583
    new immigrants and, 583–584
    obesity and, 586
    renin-angiotensin-aldosterone system in, 584–586
  pulmonary artery, 692–693
  secondary, 586–587, 649
  pathophysiology of, 584
Hypertensive crisis, 587
Hypertensive hypertrophic cardiomyopathy, 608–609
Hyperthermia, 337–338
Hyperthyroidism, 453–455
Hypertonia, 370t
Hypertrophic cardiomyopathy, 608–609
Hypertrophic obstructive cardiomyopathy, 608–609
Hypertrophic osteoarthropathy, 256t
Hypertrophic scars, 153, 1029
Hypertrophy
  cellular adaptation, 74–76, 75f
  compensatory, 732
Hyperventilation, 671
Hypervolemic hypernatremia, 119
Hypervolemic hyponatremia, 120
Hypoactive confusional state, 362–363
Hypoactive delirium, 362
Hypoactive sexual desire, 811
Hypoalbuminemia, 743t
Hypocalcemia, 125t, 458
Hypocapnia, 129–130
Hypochloremia, 120

Hypochloremic metabolic alkalosis, 128
Hypodermis, 1022
Hypogeusia, 347
Hypoglossal nerve, 321t
Hypoglycemia, 256t
Hypogonadotropic hypogonadism, 788t
Hypokalemia
  cardiac effects of, 122
  clinical manifestations of, 122
  ECG findings of, 123f
  evaluation of, 122–123
  pathophysiology of, 121–122
  treatment of, 122–123
Hypokinesia, 373
Hypomagnesemia, 458
Hypomimesis, 378
Hyponatremia, 120–121
Hypoparathyroidism, 458
Hypoperfusion, 395
Hypophosphatemia, 125t, 457–458
Hypophysial portal system, 432
Hypopituitarism, 450–451
Hypopituitary dwarfism, 451f
Hypoplastic anemia, 506–507
Hypoplastic left heart syndrome (HLHS), 646
Hypoprothrombinemia, 934
Hyporeflexia, 375
Hypotension, orthostatic, 588–589
Hypothalamic-pituitary-adrenal (HPA) system
  feedback mechanisms of, 219
Hypothalamohypophysial tract, 432
Hypothalamus
  body heat conservation and, 335
  neurosecretory cells of, 432
  sleep and, 338
Hypothermia, 338
Hypothyroidism, 454f
Hypotonia, 369–370
Hypotonic fluid alterations, 120–121
Hypoventilation, 671
Hypovolemia, 1045
Hypovolemic hypernatremia, 119
Hypovolemic hyponatremia, 120
Hypovolemic shock, 626
Hypoxemia, 672–673
Hypoxia, 672
  tissue, 531b
Hypoxia-inducible factor-1α, 246
Hypoxia-inducible transcription factor, 78–79
Hypoxic injury, 78–81, 79f, 80f
Hypoxic pulmonary vasoconstriction, 656

I

I bands, 561–562
IARC. See International Agency for Research on Cancer
IBD. See Inflammatory bowel disease
IBS. See Irritable bowel syndrome
ICF. See Intracellular fluid
Icterus neonatorum, 540
Ictus, 366
Idiojunctional rhythm, 622t–623t
Idiopathic inflammatory myopathies, 998
Idiopathic intestinal pseudo-obstruction, 930

Idiopathic pulmonary arterial hypertension, 693
Idiopathic pulmonary fibrosis (IPF), 677
Idioventricular rhythm, 622t–623t
IFNs. *See* Interferons
IgE-mediated hypersensitivity reactions. *See* Immunoglobulin E-mediated hypersensitivity reactions
IGFs. *See* Insulinlike growth factors
IL-1. *See* Interleukin-1
IL-1β. *See* Interleukin-1β
IL-2. *See* Interleukin-2
IL-4. *See* Interleukin-4
IL-6. *See* Interleukin-6
IL-7. *See* Interleukin-7
IL-10. *See* Interleukin-10
IL-13. *See* Interleukin-13
Ileum, 868
IM. *See* Infectious mononucleosis
Imatinib (Gleevec), 241, 518
Immediate hypersensitivity reactions, 200
Immovable joints, 950
Immune (peripheral) CRH, 224
Immune deficiency. *See also* Acquired immunodeficiency syndrome
   clinical presentation of, 191–194
   combined, 192
   primary (congenital), 191–192, 192t
Immune response, 158, 164–172
Immune system
   burn response of, 1045
   cancer cell evasion from, 252f
Immune thrombocytopenic purpura (ITP), 546–547
Immunity. *See also* Adaptive immunity; Innate immunity
   active, 158
   GI tract and, 873
Immunocompetent cells, 164
Immunocytes, 480–481
Immunoglobulin A pemphigus, 1034
Immunoglobulin E-mediated hypersensitivity reactions, 200–204, 204f
Immunoglobulins
   A, 161
   classes of, 161–162
   D, 161
   E, 161
   G, 161
   M, 161
Immunological and inflammatory injury, 95
Immunotherapy, 251
Impacted fractures, 966f
Impaired hemostasis, 529–530
Impetigo, 1035
Imprinting, genomic. *See* Genomic imprinting
Inclusion body myositis, 998–999
Incomplete fractures, 965–968
Incontinence, 733t
Incretins, 464
Indirect Coombs test, 495t–497t
Indomethacin, 642
Induction chemotherapy, 262
Induration, 207

Infantile hypertrophic pyloric stenosis, 929
Infantile spasms, 415
Infants
   hypothyroidism in, 455–457
   skull of, 412
Infarction, 592
Infections. *See also specific infections*
   active immunization against, 190–191
   antimicrobials treating, 189
   bacterial, 178–183, 1035
   bone
      osteomyelitis, 981–982, 1010
      septic, 1010–1012
   control measures for, 189
   countermeasures against, 188–191
   fungal, 1036–1038
   gastro-intestinal, 180t–181t
   respiratory tract. *See* Respiratory tract infections
   sexually transmitted, 180t–181t
   skin, 179, 1035–1036
   urinary tract. *See* Urinary tract infection
   viral, 1035–1036
Infectious diseases, 177
Infectious injury, 95
Infectious mononucleosis (IM), 512–513
Infectious viral encephalitides, 401
Infective endocarditis, 614–615
Inferior colliculi, 310–311
Inferior vena cava, 554
Infiltrating lobular carcinoma, 825t
Infiltrations. *See* Cellular accumulations
Infiltrative splenomegaly, 525
Inflammasomes, 142
Inflammation
   acute, 138
   acute-phase reactants during, 149
   in cachexia, 255–258
   cellular components of, 141–149
   cellular products of, 142–144
   central nervous system disorders and, 383–403
   chronic, 150–151
   of endothelium, 145
   exudate of, 149
   gastric, 250
   leukocytosis in, 149
   phagocytes in, 138
   plasma protein synthesis and, 149
   plasma protein systems in, 138–139
   type 2 diabetes mellitus and, 221
Inflammatory acne, 1053–1054
Inflammatory bowel disease (IBD), 898–900
Inflammatory carcinoma, 825t
Inflammatory cytokines, 462f
Inflammatory joint disease, 985–994. *See also* Arthritis
   rheumatoid arthritis. *See* Rheumatoid arthritis
Inflammatory response
   acute, 138f
   definition of, 149
Influenza, 183
Infratentorial disorders, 353
Infundibulum, 771

Inguinal canals, 777–778
Inhalation disorders, 677–678
Inheritance
   autosomal dominant
      delayed age of onset, 51
      epigenetics and genomic imprinting, 52, 53f
      pedigree chart, 50, 50f, 51f
      pedigrees characteristics, 50–51
      penetrance and expressivity, 51–52, 52f
      recurrence risks, 51
   autosomal recessive
      consanguinity, 54
      pedigrees characteristics, 53–54, 53f
      recurrence risks, 54, 54f
   X-linked
      pedigrees characteristics, 55
      recurrence risks, 56, 56f
      sex determination, 55, 55f
      sex-limited and sex-influenced traits, 55–56
      X inactivation, 54–55, 54f
Inherited hemorrhagic disease, 545–546
Inherited metabolic disorders of CNS, 417–419
Inhibin, 775
Inhibitory neurotransmitters, 331
Inhibitory postsynaptic potentials (IPSPs), 304
Innate immunity. *See also* Inflammation
   definition of, 134
   description of, 135t
   microbiome and, 136t
Inner dura, 313–314
Inner ear, 345, 346f
Inorganic ions, in plasma, 480
Inositol triphosphate, 431
Inotropic agents, 565
Inotropic effect, 223
Insect bites, 1060–1061
Insomnia, 339
Insufficiency fractures, 966
Insula, 308
Insular lobe, 308
Insulin, 219, 877
Insulin resistance
   diabetes mellitus and, 821
   primary hypertension and, 586
Insulinlike growth factors (IGFs), 444b
Integrin, 945
Integrin αIIbβ3, 492
Integumentary system. *See* Skin
Intercalated cells, 716
Intercalated discs, 561
Intercourse pain, 805
Interferon regulatory factors (IRFs), 141–142
Interferons (IFNs), 144
Interleukin-1 (IL-1), 143, 170f
Interleukin-1β (IL-1β), 630b
Interleukin-2 (IL-2), 170f
Interleukin-4 (IL-4), 173
Interleukin-6 (IL-6), 143, 630b
Interleukin-7 (IL-7), 166
Interleukin-10 (IL-10), 144
Interleukin-13 (IL-13), 173
Interleukins, 143
Interlobar arteries, 716
Internal anal sphincter, 871–872

Internal capsule, 308
Internal carotid arteries, 316–317
Internal fixation, of fractures, 968
Internal hydrocephalus, 369
Internal urethral sphincter, 719
International Agency for Research on Cancer (IARC), 266
International Myeloma Working Group, 524
Interneurons, 302
INTERPHONE study, 287
Interstitial cystitis, 738
Interstitial edema, 369
Interstitial fluid
 definition of, 113
 water movement between plasma and, 114
Interstitial hydrostatic pressure, 114
Interstitial oncotic pressure, 114
Interventricular foramen, 315–316
Intervertebral disc, 316, 316f
Intestinal obstruction
 causes of, 890t
 classification of, 891t
 clinical manifestations of, 891
 evaluation of, 891
 pathophysiology of, 890–892
 treatment of, 891
Intestinointestinal reflex, 870
Intoxications, of CNS, 419
Intracardiac pressures, 555t
Intracellular fluid (ICF)
 definition of, 113
 potassium concentration in, 121
Intracellular overhydration, 120
Intracerebral hematomas, 386
Intracranial aneurysm, 397
Intracranial hemorrhage, 420
Intracranial hypertension, 367
Intracranial pressure, 367–368
Intraductal carcinoma, 825t
Intraductal papillomas, 813
Intrahepatic jaundice, 908
Intrahepatic portal hypertension, 939
Intramural plexus, 862
Intraparenchymal hemorrhagic stroke, 396–397
Intraprostatic conversion, 844
Intrarenal blood flow, autoregulation of, 719
Intravascular fluid, 113
Intraventricular hydrocephalus, 369
Intussusception, 932
Inverse acne, 1054
Inverse psoriasis, 1031
Involucrum, 981, 1010
Iodine deficiency, 823
Ionizing radiation
 acute effects of, 284–285
 definition of, 282
 low-dose, 285, 285b
 microenvironmental effects of, 284–285
 nontargeted effects of, 284
IPF. See Idiopathic pulmonary fibrosis
IPSPs. See Inhibitory postsynaptic potentials
IRFs. See Interferon regulatory factors
Iron, dietary sources of, 538–539

Iron cycle, 489–490
Iron deficiency anemia, 505–506
 in children, 538–539
 clinical manifestations of, 539
 evaluation and treatment of, 539
 pathophysiology of, 538–539
Iron overload, 506
Iron replacement therapy, 506
Irregular bones, 949
Irreversible coma, 357–358
Irritable bowel syndrome (IBS), 899–900
Irritant contact dermatitis, 1030
Irritative syndrome, 408
Ischemia, 591, 672. See also Myocardial ischemia
Ischemia-reperfusion injury, 81f
Ischemic infarcts, 396
Ischemic penumbra, 395–396
Ischemic stroke, 420
Ischemic ulcers, 895
Islets of Langerhans, 438
Isoflavones, 822–823
Isohemagglutinins, 210–211
Isolated cleft palate, 928
Isothiocyanates, 279
Isotonic fluid alterations, 118
Isotonic fluid excess, 118
Isotonic fluid loss, 118
Isotropic bands, 561–562
Isovolemic hypernatremia, 118–119
Isovolemic hyponatremia, 120
Isthmus, 436
ITP. See Immune thrombocytopenic purpura

J

JAK2 gene (Janus kinase gene), 508
Jamestown encephalitis, 401t
Janus family of tyrosine kinases, 431
Janus kinase gene (JAK2 gene), 508
Jaundice
 hemolytic, 908
 intrahepatic, 906
 liver disorders and, 906–910
 neonatal, 540, 937
 in newborns, 908
 obstructive, 908
Jejunum, 868
Jerk nystagmus, 341
Joint capsule, 950
Joint disorders, 982–994
Joint effusion, 983–984
Joint stiffness, 984
Joints. See also Bone
 cartilaginous, 948–949
 fibrous, 950
 freely movable, 950
 immovable, 950
 slightly movable, 950
 synovial, 950
J-receptors, 659
Junctional bradycardia, 622t–623t
Junctional tachycardia, 622t–623t
Juvenile dermatomyositis, 998
Juvenile idiopathic arthritis, 1012

Juvenile myoclonic epilepsy, 421t
Juxtaglomerular apparatus, 716
Juxtamedullary nephrons, 715

K

K vitamins, 944t
 deficiency, 530
Kaposi sarcoma, 268t–271t, 1042
Kawasaki disease, 648–649
Kegel exercises, 797
Keloids, 153, 1029
Keratitis, 344
Keratoacanthoma, 1039
Kernicterus, 539, 937
Kernig sign, 398
Kidney disorders
 acute kidney injury. See Acute kidney injury
 in children. See Children, renal disorders in
 chronic kidney disease. See Chronic kidney disease
 kidney dysfunction, 744
Kidney failure, 744
Kidney stones, 732–733
Kidneys
 anatomy of, 714–718, 714f
 blood vessels of, 716–718
 dysfunction of, 744
 erythropoietin and, 726
 glomerulus. See Glomerulus
 hydronephrosis of, 731–732
 lobes of, 714
 nephron. See Nephron
 substances transported in tubules of, 723b
 vitamin D and, 725–726
Kinin cascade, 140
Kinin system, 138–139
Kissing disease, 512
Klebsiella pneumoniae, 675
Klinefelter's variant, 638t
Knee joints. See Synovial joints
Koilonychia, 505
Kupffer cells, 489, 875
Kussmaul respirations, 671
Kwashiorkor, 935
Kyphosis, 977–978, 979f

L

La Crosse encephalitis, 401t
Labia majora, 767
Labia minora, 768
Lacrimal apparatus, 343
β-Lactamase, 183
Lactase deficiency, 897
Lactate dehydrogenase (LDH), 528, 878t
Lacteal, 869
Lactobacillus sp., 137, 186
Lactose intolerance, 935
Lacuna, 945
Lacunar infarcts, 395
Lacunar strokes, 395
Lamellae, 947
Lamina propria, 869
Laminin, 944t
Laplace's law, 564, 661

Large bowel obstruction, 891
Large cell carcinoma, 695*t*
Large intestine, 871–873
Laryngeal box, 654
Larynx
 anatomy of, 654, 656*f*
 cancer of, 268*t*–271*t*, 694
Latent tuberculosis infection (LTBI), 691
Late-onset Pompe's disease, 997–998
Lateral apertures, 315–316
Lateral columns, 311
Lateral corticospinal tract, 309*f*
Lateral fissure, 306–307
Lateral horn, 311
Lateral spinothalamic tracts, 312
Lateral sulcus, 306–307
LBB. *See* Left bundle branch
LDH. *See* Lactate dehydrogenase
LDL. *See* Low-density lipoprotein
Lead exposure sources of, 89*f*, 89*t*
Lead poisoning, 419
Leak point pressure measurement, 727*t*–728*t*
Lectin pathway, of complement system, 140
Lee-White coagulation time, 495*t*–497*t*
Left bundle branch, 558, 623*t*–624*t*
Left ventricular failure, 605*t*
 in infants, 647
Left ventricular hypertrophy, 74, 587, 609*f*, 619, 639–640, 751
Left-to-right shunting, 642
Legg-Calvé-Perthes disease, 1013–1014
Leiomyomas, 234
Leiomyosarcoma, 1003
Lennox-Gastaut syndrome, 421*t*
Lentiform nucleus, 308
Lentigo malignant melanoma, 1042*f*
Leukemia, 268*t*–271*t*
 acute lymphocytic, 514–517
 acute myeloid, 514–517
 bleeding and, 505
 bone pain and, 516*t*
 chemotherapy for, 517
 in children, 547–548
  clinical manifestations of, 547
  evaluation and treatment of, 547–548
  pathophysiology of, 547
 chronic lymphocytic, 517–518
 chronic myeloid, 241, 517*f*
 clinical manifestations in, 515
 pathophysiology of, 514
 Philadelphia chromosome in, 514
 stem-like cancer cells progressing to, 514
 treatment of, 515–517
Leukemic cells, 547
Leukemoid reaction, 510
Leukocoria, 424
Leukocytes. *See also* Lymphocytes; Phagocytes
 agranulocytes, 480–481
 basophils, 144–145, 482, 511*t*
 disorders involving
  agranulocytosis, 510
  basopenia, 511
  basophilia, 510, 511*t*

Leukocytes *(Continued)*
  eosinopenia, 511
  eosinophilia, 510, 511*t*
  granulocytopenia, 510
  granulocytosis, 510
  infectious mononucleosis, 512–513
  leukemia. *See* Leukemia
  lymphocytosis, 512
  monocytopenia, 511*t*
  monocytosis, 511–512, 511*t*
  neutropenia, 510
  neutrophilia, 511*t*
  quantitative alterations, 510–518
 eosinophils, 146, 480*t*, 683
 granulocytes, 141*f*, 480–481, 510
 immunocytes, 480–481
 lymphocytopenia, 512
 monocytes, 146, 482, 511*t*
 neutrophils, 136, 480*t*, 510
Leukocytosis, 149, 510
Leukopenia, 258
Leukotrienes, 145
Level of consciousness, 353
Levitra, 854
LH. *See* Luteinizing hormone
Libido, 781
 decreased, 811
Lichenification, 1027*f*
Lieberkühn crypts, 869
Life expectancy, 107
Li-Fraumeni syndrome, 244
Ligaments, 961
Ligature strangulation, 94
Limbic system, 308–309
Linear fracture, 965–968
Linkage analysis, 56–58
Linoleic acid, 845*b*–846*b*
Lipids, 595–597
Lipid-soluble hormones, 431
Lipomas, 234
Lipopolysaccharide, 183
Lipoproteins, 480
 low-density, 528
Lips
 cancer of, 268*t*–271*t*, 1041
 cleft, 928
Liver
 bile secretion of, 875–876, 875*f*
 bilirubin metabolism and, 876
 hematological functions of, 876
 lobules, 875*f*
 metabolic detoxification of, 877
 metabolic functions of, 876
 nutrient metabolism of, 876
 vascular functions of, 876
 vitamin storage in, 877
Liver disease, 530, 908
Liver disorders
 acute liver failure, 910
 in children
  biliary atresia, 937–938
  cirrhosis, 938–939
  hepatitis, 938
  metabolic disorders, 939

Liver disorders *(Continued)*
  neonatal jaundice, 937
  portal hypertension, 939
 cirrhosis. *See* Cirrhosis
 complications of
  ascites, 906–908
  hepatic encephalopathy, 908
  hepatorenal syndrome, 908–910
  jaundice, 908
  portal hypertension, 906
 viral hepatitis, 912–914
Lobes, of kidney, 714
Lobular carcinoma in situ, 825–830
Lobular involution, 818
Localized edema, 116
Localized lymphadenopathy, 518
Localized scleroderma, 1038
Locked-in syndrome, 358
Long bones, 948
Longitudinal fissure, 306–307
Long-term starvation, 905
Loop of Henle, 716
Low back pain, 391–393
Low-density lipoprotein (LDL), 528
Low-dose ionizing radiation, 285*b*
Lower airways, 657*f*
Lower esophageal sphincter, 864
Lower gastro-intestinal bleeding, 886
Lower motor neuron syndromes, 374–376
Lower motor neurons, 311
Lower respiratory tract infections, 180*t*–181*t*
Lown-Ganong-Levine syndrome, 623*t*–624*t*
LTBI. *See* Latent tuberculosis infection
Lumbar lordosis, 990
Lumbar plexus, 319
Lumen, 566
Lung cancer
 clinical manifestations of, 696
 definition of, 694
 evaluation of, 696–700
 incidence of, 694
 pathophysiology of, 696
 TNM staging of, 696–700
 tobacco smoking causing, 695
 treatment of, 696–700
Lung receptors, 659–660
Lungs
 acinus of, 655
 aging and, 666*b*
 alveolar pressure in, 663
 alveoli of, 655
 elastic properties of, 661
 epithelial cells of, 655
 hila of, 654–655
Lupus erythematosus, 1033
Lupus nephritis, 741
Luteal phase, 775
Luteinizing hormone (LH), 451
LVH. *See* Left ventricular hypertrophy
Lyme disease, 1035
Lymph, 484, 575–576
Lymph nodes, 484, 576
Lymphadenopathy, 518
Lymphatic capillary, 869

Lymphatic system
    anatomy of, 576f
    definition of, 575–576
    disorders involving
        lymphadenopathy, 517–518
        lymphomas. *See* Lymphomas
    functions of, 576
Lymphatic veins, 576
Lymphatic venules, 576
Lymphatic vessels, 556
Lymphedema, 116
Lymphoblastic lymphoma, 522–523
Lymphoblasts, 547
Lymphocytes, alterations to, 511t
Lymphocytopenia, 511t
Lymphocytosis, 511t
Lymphogranuloma venereum, 857t–859t
Lymphoid organs
    description of, 482–484
    lymph nodes, 484
    mononuclear phagocyte system, 484–485
    primary, 166, 483
    secondary, 159f, 483
    spleen, 483–484
Lymphoid stem cells, 164
Lymphoid tissues, of secretory immune system, 160f
Lymphokines, 142
Lymphomas, 268t–271t
    Burkitt, 241–242
    Hodgkin's
        in children, 548–549
            clinical manifestations of, 519–520
            pathophysiology of, 519–521, 519f
            treatment of, 520–521
    incidence rates of, in Canada, 519
    lymphoblastic, 514–517
    malignant, 518–524
    mucosa-associated lymphoid tissue, 250
    multiple myeloma, 523–524
    non-Hodgkin's
        in children, 548
            clinical manifestations of, 521
            incidence of, 521
            pathophysiology of, 521–522
            treatment of, 521–522
    primary cutaneous, 1042
Lynch syndrome, 920–921
Lysosomal storage diseases, 419
Lysozyme, 136
Lytic lesions, 523–524

M

M line, 561–562
M protein, 523–524
MAC. *See* Membrane attack complex
Macewen sign, 416
Macrocytic-normochromic anemia, 502t
Macrophages
    alveolar, 655
    tissue, 875
    tumour-associated, 250–251
Macrovascular disease, 466
Macula densa, 716

Macula lutea, 340
Maculae, 345
Macular edema, 467
Magnetic resonance imaging (MRI), 970
Major duodenal papilla, 873–874
Major histocompatibility complex (MHC), 193, 211f
Malaria, 188t
Male breast, 777
Male breast cancer, 855
Male breast disorders, 855–856
Male reproductive system
    aging and, 781–782
    andropause and, 782
    bulbourethral glands, 780
    ejaculatory duct, 779–780
    epididymis, 778–779
    external genitalia of, 777–779
    internal genitalia of, 779–780
    penis. *See* Penis
    prostate gland, 780f
    scrotum, 779
    seminal vesicles, 780
    sex hormones of, 780–781
    spermatogenesis, 780
    testes. *See* Testes
    vas deferens, 778–779
Male reproductive system disorders
    benign prostatic hyperplasia, 840–842
    cryptorchidism, 837–838
    delayed puberty, 833
    ectopic testis, 837–838
    epididymitis, 840
    gynecomastia, 855
    hydrocele, 837
    male breast cancer, 855
    male breast disorders, 855–856
    orchitis, 838–839
    penis disorders. *See* Penis disorders
    precocious puberty, 833
    prostate cancer. *See* Prostate cancer
    prostate gland disorders, 840–852
    prostatitis, 842–843
    scrotal disorders, 836–837
    sexual dysfunction, 852–855
    sexual maturation alterations, 833
    sexually transmitted infections, 856–859, 856t
    sperm production impairment, 854–855
    spermatocele, 837
    testicular appendages, 838
    testicular cancer, 838
    testicular torsion, 838
    urethral strictures, 833
    urethritis, 833
Malignant bone tumours, in children, 1018–1019
Malignant hypertension, 587
Malignant hyperthermia, 338, 973
Malleus, 345
Malnutrition, 905
Mammary stem cells, 819–820
Mammographic density, 821
Mammography, 816b, 822
Mannitol, 725t

Mannose-binding lectin (MBL), 136
Manual strangulation, 94
Marasmus, 935
Marfan's syndrome, 611–612
Marginating storage pool, 486
Margination, 146–148
Marihuana, 811
Mast cells, 138f, 141
Mastoid air cells, 345
Mastoid process, 345
Matrix metalloproteinases (MMPs), 152
Maturity-onset diabetes of youth, 464–465
MBL. *See* Mannose-binding lectin
McArdle's disease, 997
Mean arterial pressure, 571
Mean corpuscular hemoglobin, 495t–497t
Mean corpuscular hemoglobin concentration, 495t–497t
Mean corpuscular volume, 495t–497t
Meckel diverticulum, 930
Meconium disease, 930
Meconium ileus, 930
Meconium plug syndrome, 930
Meconium syndromes, 930
Medial epicondylopathy, 969
Mediastinum, 552, 654
Medulla, of kidney, 714
Medulla oblongata, 309f
Medulloblastomas, 421
Megakaryocytes, 146, 482
Megaloblastic anemia, 258, 503
Meissner corpuscles, 347
Meissner plexus, 865
Melanocortin-1, 286–287
Melanocyte-stimulating hormone (MSH), 432
Melanoma, 285–286
Melatonin, 225t–226t
Melena, 886t
Membrane attack complex (MAC), 139–140
Membrane lipid rafts, 6
Membrane potentials, 559
Membrane transport, 18–25, 18f, 19f
    active transport, Na^+ and K^+, 21, 22f, 23t
    caveolae, 22–24
    diffusion, 20, 20f
    electrical impulses, 24–25, 25f
    electrolytes as solutes, 19–22
    endocytic matrix, 24b
    endocytosis and exocytosis, 22, 23f
    filtration, 20, 21f
    osmosis, 20–21
    receptor-mediated endocytosis, 22, 24f
    vesicle formation, 22–24
Memory disorders, 358
Ménière's disease, 346
Meninges, 313–314
Meningiomas, 405
Meningitis, 420
Meningocele, 413
Menometrorrhagia, 791t
Menopausal hormone therapy, 809t
Menopause, 772–773
Menorrhagia, 505, 791t
Menses, 772–773

Menstrual cycle
  bleeding in, 774
  body temperature and, 775
  hormonal control of, 774–775, 774t
  ovarian cycle of, 775
  phases of, 774
  vaginal response in, 775
Menstrual disorders
  abnormal uterine bleeding, 790–791
  amenorrhea, 789–790
  dysmenorrhea, 788–789
  PCOS, 791–792
Menstrual phase, 774
Menstruation, 773–774
Mental stress-induced ischemia, 599
Mercury, thimerosal, 190–191
Merkel discs, 347
Mesangial cells, 715
Mesangial matrix, 715
Mesencephalon. See Midbrain
Mesenchymal stem cells (MSCs), 194
Mesenchymal-epithelial transition (MET), 850
Mesenteric vascular insufficiency, 901
Mesentery, 868
Mesonephric ducts, 765–766
Mesothelium, 268t–271t
Messenger RNA (mRNA), 243f
MET. See Mesenchymal-epithelial transition
Metabolic acidosis, 620
  acid-base imbalances and, 129f
  causes of, 130t
Metabolic alkalosis, 128
Metabolic disorders, 353
Metabolic edema, 369
Metabolic syndrome, 461–462, 597
Metabolically healthy obesity, 905
Metabolism
  amino acid metabolism defects, 419
  muscle, 960
  of myocardium, 553f
Metaphysis, 948
Metaplasia, 77, 77f
Metaplastic carcinoma, 825t
Metastatic brain tumours, 408–409
Metastatic calcification, 100
Metastatic disease, 736
Metencephalon, 310–311
Metformin (Glucophage), 464
Methicillin-resistant *Staphylococcus aureus* (MRSA), 183
Methylenetetrahydrofolate reductase (MTHFR), 533
Methylome, 273
Metronidazole (Flagyl), 795b
Metrorrhagia, 791t
Mexiletine, 996
Mexitil Cap, 996
MGUS. See Monoclonal gammopathy of undetermined significance
MHC. See Major histocompatibility complex
MI. See Myocardial ischemia
Microalbuminuria, 587
Microbiome, 134–137
  GI tract and, 862

Microcephaly, 415
Microcytic-hypochromic anemia, 505–507
Microfilaments, 301
Microglia, 302
β2-Microglobulin, 167–168, 524
Micro-organisms
  antibiotic resistant, 188
  countermeasures against infectious, 188–191
  opportunistic, 137
  parasitic, 186–188
  pathogenic, 178
  tissue damage caused by, 179t
MicroRNA (miRNA), 68, 245
  coding, 70
Microtubules, 301
Microvascular angina, 599b
Microvascular disease, 466
Microvasculature thrombosis, 529
Microvilli, 869
Midbrain, 306t, 310–311
Middle ear, 345
Middle fossa, 313
Migraines, 398–399
Mild concussions, 387
Miliaria, 1062
Miliaria crystallina, 1062
Miliaria rubra, 1062
Mineralization, 947
Mineralocorticoids, 431
Minerals, of bone, 947
Minimal change nephropathy, 741
Minimally conscious state, 357
Minute volume, 658
Mirror focus, 366
Mitochondrial DNA, 90, 108
Mitofusin-2, 256–257
Mitogen-activated protein kinase, 287
Mitosis, 26
Mitotic cells, 234
Mitral regurgitation, 612
Mitral stenosis, 611, 611f
Mitral valve, 554
Mitral valve prolapse syndrome (MVPS), 612
Mixed hearing loss, 346
Mixed incontinence, 733t
Mixed nerves, 319
Mixed precocious puberty, 789b
MLRs. See Membrane lipid rafts
MMPs. See Matrix metalloproteinases
Mobitz I block, 623t–624t
Mobitz II block, 623t–624t
MODS. See Multiple organ dysfunction syndrome
MODY. See Maturity-onset diabetes of youth
Molluscum contagiosum, 1057
Monoclonal antibodies, 163b, 262
Monoclonal gammopathy of undetermined significance (MGUS), 524
Monocytes, 146, 511t
Monocytopenia, 511t
Monocytosis, 511–512

Monokines, 142
Monosodium urate crystals, 985
Motility diarrhea, 885
Motility disorders, 887–892
  acquired, 931–932
  congenital, 928–931
Motor dysphasia, 362t
Motor neuron diseases, 376–377
Motor responses, in arousal alterations, 356
Motor units, of skeletal muscles, 956f
MPNs. See Myeloproliferative neoplasms
MRI. See Magnetic resonance imaging
mRNA. See Messenger RNA
MRSA. See Methicillin-resistant *Staphylococcus aureus*
MSCs. See Mesenchymal stem cells
MSH. See Melanocyte-stimulating hormone
mtDNA. See Mitochondrial DNA
MTHFR. See Methylenetetrahydrofolate reductase
Mucinous carcinoma, 825t
Mucopurulent cervicitis, 796
Mucosa-associated lymphoid tissue lymphoma, 250
Mucoviscidosis, 933–934
Multifactorial inheritance, 58–59, 58f, 59b, 928
Multiple myeloma, 523–524
Multiple organ dysfunction syndrome (MODS), 630–634
Multiple sclerosis, 402–403
Multiple-antibiotic resistance, 189
Multipolar neurons, 301
Muscle cells, 956–957
Muscle contraction
  calcium-troponin complex in, 562
  concentric, 947
  cross-bridge theory of, 563, 958–960
  dynamic, 961
  eccentric, 961
  excitation-contraction coupling in, 563
  isometric, 961
  static, 961
Muscle fibre action potential, 958
Muscle fibres, 955–957
Muscle membrane, 956
Muscle movement alterations
  akinesia, 371
  bradykinesia, 373
  dopamine and, 373
  Huntington's disease, 371–373
  hyperkinesia, 372t
  hypokinesia, 373
  Parkinson's disease, 373
  paroxysmal dyskinesia, 371
  tardive dyskinesia, 371
  Tourette syndrome, 371
Muscle pumps, 567
Muscle strain, 970
Muscle tissues, 34t–35t
Muscle tone alterations, 369–371
Muscle tumours, 1004–1005
Muscle wasting, in cachexia, 255–258

Muscles
  aging of, 962
  agonist of, 961
  antagonist of, 961
  cardiac. *See* Cardiac muscle
  metabolism of, 960
  movement of, 958
  skeletal. *See* Skeletal muscles
  strains of, 968–969
Muscular arteries, 566
Muscular dystrophies, 1015–1017
Musculo-skeletal disorders
  bone tumours. *See* Bone tumours
  bursitis, 969–970
  in children. *See* Children, musculo-skeletal disorders in
  compartment syndrome, 972–973
  dislocation, 968
  epicondylopathy, 969–970
  fractures. *See* Fractures
  joint disorders. *See* Joint disorders
  ligament sprains and strains, 969
  malignant hyperthermia, 973
  muscle strain, 970
  muscle tumours, 1004–1005
  rhabdomyolysis, 970–972
  skeletal trauma, 965–968
  subluxation, 968
  tendinopathy, 969–970
Mutualistic relationship, 137
MVPS. *See* Mitral valve prolapse syndrome
Myalgic encephalomyelitis, 996
Myasthenia gravis, 404–405
Myasthenic crisis, 404–405
MYC proto-oncogene, 241–242
Myelencephalon, 311
Myelin, 301
Myelin sheath, 301
Myelodysplasia, 415t
Myelodysplastic syndrome, 506
Myelogenic tumours, 1004
Myeloma cells, 523
Myelomeningocele, 413
Myeloproliferative disorders, 517
Myeloproliferative neoplasms (MPNs), 508
Myenteric plexus, 865
Myoadenylate deaminase deficiency, 997
Myoblasts, 955–957
Myocardial hypertrophy, 74–76, 75f
Myocardial infarction, 601–606, 601f
  complications with, 605t
  definition of, 606b
Myocardial ischemia (MI), 598–601
Myocardial oxygen consumption, 562
Myocardial stunning, 603
Myocardium, 553f
Myoclonic seizure, 421t
Myoclonus tremor, 354t
Myofascial pain, 335t
Myofibrils, 560–561, 955–957
Myofibroblasts, 153
Myoglobin, 575, 956
Myoglobinuria, 970–971
Myomas, 800

Myoneural junction. *See* Neuromuscular junction
Myophosphorylase deficiency, 997
Myopia, 343
Myosin, 561–562, 957f
Myositis, 970
Myositis ossificans, 970
Myotonia, 996
Myotonic muscular dystrophy, 1017
Myxedema, 455
Myxedema coma, 456

N

NAD. *See* Nicotinamide adenine dinucleotide
Nails, 1022
Naloxone (Narcon), 332–333
Narcolepsy, 339
Nasal cavity cancer, 268t–271t
Nasopharynx
  anatomy of, 654
  cancer of, 268t–271t
National Council on Radiation Protection and Measurements, 282–283
Natriuretic peptides, 566
Natural immunity. *See* Innate immunity
Natural killer (NK) cells, 227, 875
Nausea, 883
NAUTICA. *See* North American Urinary Tract Infection Collaborative Alliance
NCF. *See* Neutrophil chemotactic factor
ncRNA. *See* Noncoding RNA
Nebulin, 958t
Necrosis, 101–103, 102f, 103f, 103t
Necrotizing enterocolitis, 936
Necrotizing fasciitis, 1035
Negative feedback, 428
Neglect syndrome, 358–360
Neisseria gonorrhoeae, 162
Neisseria meningitidis, 420
Neoadjuvant chemotherapy, 262
Neonatal jaundice, 540, 937
Neoplasms
  clonal proliferation model of, 237–238
  infectious agents associated with, 250t
  inflammatory conditions associated with, 250t
  myeloproliferative, 508
Neoplastic polyps, 920
Neovascularization, 246
Nephritic syndrome
  clinical manifestations of, 743
  definition of, 742
  evaluation of, 744
  pathophysiology of, 742–744
  treatment of, 744
Nephroblastoma, 760
Nephron
  blood vessels of, 716–718
  components of, 715f
  cortical, 715
  definition of, 715
  distal convoluted tubule, 716

Nephron (*Continued*)
  functions of, 720–726
  juxtamedullary, 715
  loop of Henle of, 716
  midcortical, 715
  proximal convoluted tubule of, 716
Nephropathy, 466
Nephrotic syndrome, 256t
  clinical manifestations of, 743
  definition of, 742
  evaluation of, 744
  pathophysiology of, 742–744
  treatment of, 744
Nerve growth factor, 27t
Nerve impulse, 304–305
Nerve sheath tumours, 407–408
Nervous system. *See* Autonomic nervous system; Central nervous system; Peripheral nervous system; Somatic nervous system
Neural lobe, 433
Neural reflexes, heart rate and, 565
Neural tube defects, 413–414
Neurilemma cells. *See* Schwann cells
Neurilemmoma, 407t
Neuritic plaques, 363–364
Neuroblastomas, 422–424
Neuroendocrine hormones, 227
Neuroendocrine tumours, 694–700
Neurofibrillary tangles, 363–364
Neurofibrils, 301
Neurofibromas, 407–408
Neurofibromatosis type 1, 407–408
Neurofibromatosis type 2, 407–408
Neurogenic bladder, 734
Neurogenic diabetes insipidus, 450
Neurogenic shock, 389
Neuroglia, 302
Neuroglial cells, 301
Neurohormonal signalling, 14
Neuromotor function alterations
  ALS, 377–378
  hypertonia, 370–371
  hypotonia, 369–370
  lower motor neuron syndromes, 375–376, 376f
  motor neuron diseases, 376–377
  muscle movement
    akinesia, 371
    bradykinesia, 373
    Huntington's disease, 371–373
    hyperkinesia, 372t
    hypokinesia, 373
    Parkinson's disease, 373
    paroxysmal dyskinesia, 371
    tardive dyskinesia, 371
    Tourette syndrome, 371
  muscle tone, 369–371, 370t
  upper motor neuron syndromes, 374–375, 375b, 375f, 376f
Neuromuscular junction, 314f
Neuromuscular junction disorders, 403–405

Neurons
  afferent, 312
  associational, 302
  bipolar, 301
  components of, 301, 301f
  definition of, 301
  efferent, 322
  interneurons, 302
  motor, 311
    lower, 311
    upper, 311
  multipolar, 301
  postganglionic, 319
  postsynaptic, 304
  preganglionic, 319
  presynaptic, 304
  pseudounipolar, 301
  sensory, 302
  third order, 312
  unipolar, 301
Neuropathic pain, 334
Neuropathies, 404t
Neuropeptides
  properties of, 305t
  Y, 224
Neuroplasticity, 304
Neuroreceptors, 322
Neurotransmitters
  of ANS, 322
  chemical signaling through, 14
  excitatory, 331
  inhibitory, 331
  of pain modulation, 331–333
Neutropenia, 510
Neutrophil chemotactic factor (NCF), 145
Neutrophil count, 495t–497t
Neutrophilia, 510
Neutrophils, 480t, 511t
Newborns
  hemolytic disease of
    clinical manifestations of, 539–540
    evaluation and treatment of, 540
    incidence of, 539
    pathophysiology of, 539–540
NGF. See Nerve growth factor
Niches, in bone marrow, 485
Nicotinamide adenine dinucleotide, 17
Night terrors, 340
Nipple, 777
NIPPV. See Noninvasive positive-pressure ventilation
Nitric oxide (NO), 488
  hemoglobin binding to, 489f
NK cells. See Natural killer cells
NLRs. See NOD-like receptors
NO. See Nitric oxide
Nociceptin/orphanin FQ, 332
Nociception, 330
Nociceptive pain, 330
Nociceptive transmission, 330
Nodes of Ranvier, 301
NOD-like receptors (NLRs), 142
Nodular thyroid disease, 455
Noggin, 946t

Nonaccidental trauma, 1019–1020, 1019f
Nonalcoholic fatty liver disease, 912
Nonalcoholic steatohepatitis, 912
Nonbacterial prostatitis, 843
Nonbacterial thrombotic endocarditis, 615
Nonceliac gluten sensitivity, 934
Noncoding RNA (ncRNA), 237–238
Nondividing support cells, 780
Nonerosive reflux disease, 888
Non-Hodgkin's lymphomas
  in children, 548
  clinical manifestations of, 521
  incidence of, 521
  pathophysiology of, 521–522
  treatment of, 521–522
Nonhomologous end joining pathway, 283–284
Nonimmunologic urticaria, 203–204
Noninfectious cystitis, 738
Noninflammatory acne, 1053–1054
Noninvasive positive-pressure ventilation (NIPPV), 676
Nonossifying fibromas, 1018
Nonpuerperal hyperprolactinemia, 812–813
Nonpurulent meningitis, 400, 420
Non-REM (NREM) sleep, 338
Nonspastic cerebral palsy, 416
Non-ST elevation myocardial infarction, 601
Nonsteroidal anti-inflammatory drugs (NSAIDs)
  gastritis caused by, 892
  peptic ulcer disease caused by, 893
Nonstructural scoliosis, 1014–1015
Nontargeted effects, 284
Nonvolatile acid, 124
Norepinephrine, 322
  properties of, 305t
Normal transit constipation, 884
Normal weight obesity, 905
Normoblasts, 487
Normocytic-normochromic anemia, 502t
North American Urinary Tract Infection Collaborative Alliance (NAUTICA), 738b
NREM. See Non-REM sleep
NS1 protein, 185
NSAIDs. See Nonsteroidal anti-inflammatory drugs
Nuclear factor of activated B cells, 946t
5′-Nucleotidase, 878t
Nucleus accumbens, 308
Nucleus pulposus, 316
Nutrigenomics, 276
Nutrition, 66, 73–74, 153, 276–279, 291, 387, 488, 489t, 793b, 902–905, 932–936
  erythropoiesis requirements with, 487
Nutrition disorders, 902–905
  malnutrition, 905
  obesity. See Obesity
  starvation, 905
Nystagmus, 341

O

Oat cell carcinoma, 696–700
Obesity
  adipocytokines and, 903b
  in children with cardiovascular

Obesity (Continued)
  clinical manifestations of, 904–905
  definition of, 902
  evaluation of, 905
  incidence of, 902–903
  insulin resistance from, 459t
  metabolically healthy, 905
  normal weight, 905
  overweight compared to, 905
  pathophysiology of, 903–905
  treatment of, 905
Obesity hypoventilation syndrome, 339
Oblique fractures, 965–968
Obscurin, 958t
Obstructive jaundice, 908
Obstructive lung diseases
  asthma. See Asthma
  chronic bronchitis, 686–687
  COPD, 684–685
  emphysema, 687–688
Obstructive sleep apnea syndrome (OSAS), 339
  in children, 704
Obstructive uropathy, 731
Occipital lobe, 308
Occlusive stroke, 420
Occult bleeding, 886
Occult fractures, 966f
Occupational hazards, as carcinogens, 289–290
Ocular movement alterations, 341
Oculomotor nerve, 321t
Olfaction, 347–348
Olfactory hallucinations, 347
Olfactory nerve, 321t
Oligoarthritis, 1012
Oligodendrocytes, 302
Oligodendroglia, 302
Oligodendroglioma, 406
Oligomenorrhea, 792b
Oliguria, 123, 745f
Omalizumab (Xolair), 684
Oncogenes, 239, 242–244, 242t, 248
Oncomirs, 245
Oncotic pressure
  capillary, 114
  interstitial, 114
Onychomycosis, 1049–1050
Open fractures, 965–968
Open pneumothorax, 674
Open reduction, of fractures, 968
Open wounds, 152
OPG. See Osteoprotegerin
Opioids, endogenous, 331–332
Optic chiasm, 340–341
Optic disc, 340
Optic glioma, 422
Optic nerves, 321t, 340–341
Oral cavity, cancer of, 268t–271t
Oral contraceptives, breast cancer and, 821
Orchitis, 838–839
Organ of Corti, 345
Orgasmic dysfunction, 811
Oropharyngeal phase of swallowing, 864
Oropharynx, 654

Orthopnea, 670
Orthostatic hypotension, 588–589
OSAS. *See* Obstructive sleep apnea syndrome
Osgood-Schlatter disease, 1014
Osmitrol, 725*t*
Osmolality, plasma, 117
Osmoreceptors, 117
Osmosis, 20–21
Osmotic diarrhea, 885
Osmotic diuretics, 725*t*
Osseous labyrinths, 345
Osteoarthritis, 982–984
Osteoblastic niche, 485
Osteoblasts, 943–945, 967
Osteocalcin, 943–945
Osteochondromas, 1017–1018
Osteochondroses, 1012–1014
Osteoclasts, 944*t*
Osteocytes, 945
Osteogenesis imperfecta, 1009–1010
Osteogenic tumours, 1002–1003
Osteoid, 943–945
Osteomalacia, 979–980
Osteomyelitis, 981–982
  in children, 1010
Osteophytes, 982
Osteoporosis, 974–976
  clinical manifestations of, 977–978
  definition of, 974
  electron microscopic image of, 975*f*
  evaluation of, 978–979
  pathophysiology of, 976
  postmenopausal, 976
  regional, 976
  risk factors of, 977*b*
  secondary, 976
  treatment of, 978–979
  in vertebral body, 975*f*
Osteoprotegerin (OPG), 945, 976–978
Osteosarcoma, 1002–1003
Ostium primum atrial septal defect, 642–643
Ostium secundum atrial septal defect, 642–643
Otitis externa, 346
Otitis media infections, 180*t*–181*t*
Outlet dysfunction, 884
Ovarian cancer
  clinical manifestations of, 810
  evaluation of, 811
  global incidence of, 807
  metastasis of, 811*f*
  pathogenesis of, 808–811
  risk factors of, 809*t*
  staging of, 811*t*
  treatment of, 811
Ovarian cycle, 771–772
Ovarian cysts, 798–799
Ovarian follicles, 771*f*
Ovarian tumours, 808*f*
Ovaries
  anatomy of, 771–772
  PCOS, 791
  torsion of, 799
Overactive bladder syndrome, 734
Overflow incontinence, 733*t*

Overweight, obesity compared to, 905
Oviducts, 765
Ovulation, 773–774, 773*f*
Ovum, 764
Oxidative phosphorylation, 17–18, 247–248
Oxidative stress, 81–82, 82*f*, 82*t*, 83*b*, 83*t*
Oximeter, 664
Oxycephaly, 417*f*
Oxygen
  arterial pressure of, 663
  diffusion of, across alveolocapillary membrane, 655
  partial pressure of, 660
Oxygen debt, 960
Oxygen saturation, 664
Oxygen toxicity, 677
Oxygenation, arterial, 664–665
Oxygen-dependent killing mechanisms, 148
Oxyhemoglobin, 488, 665–666
Oxyhemoglobin dissociation curve, 665*f*
Oxytocin, 773*t*
  function of, 432
  in stress response, 225*t*–226*t*
  synthesis of, 435–436

P

Para-aminohippuric acid, 726
P wave, 559
Pacinian corpuscles, 347
PAF. *See* Platelet-activating factor
Paget's disease, 825*t*, 980–981
PAH. *See* Para-aminohippuric acid
Pain
  abdominal, 886
  acute, 333
  central neuropathic, 334
  chronic postoperative, 335*t*
  clinical descriptions of, 333–334
  deafferentation, 335*t*
  heterosegmental inhibition of, 333
  intractable, 334
  modulation of, 331–333
    neurotransmitters of, 331–333, 332*f*
    pathways of, 333
  myofascial, 335*t*
  neuroanatomy of, 330–331
  neuropathic, 334
  nociceptive, 330
  parietal, 886
  perception of, 330–331
  peripheral neuropathic, 334
  persistent, 334
  phantom limb, 335*t*
  referred, 333–334, 886
  somatic, 333–334
  theories of, 329–330
  threshold for, 331
  tolerance for, 331
  transduction of, 330
  transmission of, 330
  visceral, 333–334, 886
Painful bladder syndrome/interstitial cystitis (PBS/IC), 738
Painless thyroiditis, 456

Palate, cleft, 928
Palmomental reflex, 356*f*
Pamidronate, 1010
PAMPs. *See* Pathogen-associated molecular patterns
Pancreas. *See also* Diabetes mellitus
  anatomy of, 427*f*
  exocrine, 877–880
  fibrocystic disease of, 933–934
  tumours of, in children, 940
Pancreatic duct, 877
Pancreatic exocrine insufficiency, 897
Pancreatic polypeptide, 439, 877
Pancreatitis
  acute, 915–916
  chronic, 916–917
Paneth cells, 873
Panhypopituitarism, 451
Pannus, 986
Papanicolaou (Pap) test, 803*b*
Papillary apocrine change, 813
Papillary carcinoma, 825*t*
Papilledema, 342*t*
Papulosquamous disorders, 1030–1033
Parabens, 823
Paracentesis, 907–908
Paracetamol. *See* Acetaminophen
Paracrine signalling, 14
Paraesophageal hiatal hernia, 889
Parafollicular cells, 436
Paralysis, 374
  periodic, 996
  thyrotoxic periodic, 996
Paralysis agitans, 373
Paralytic ileus, 890–892
Paramesonephric ducts, 765–766
Paranasal sinus cancer, 268*t*–271*t*
Paraneoplastic pemphigus, 1034
Paraneoplastic syndromes, 255
Paraparesis, 375*b*
Paraplegia, 375*b*
Paraprotein, 523
Parasites, 1060–1061
Parasitic diseases, 186–188
Parasitic micro-organisms, 186
Parasomnias, 340
Parasympathetic nervous system, 319
  anatomy of, 322, 323*f*
Parathyroid glands
  disorders of
    hyperparathyroidism, 457–458
    hypoparathyroidism, 458
Paratonia, 356
Paravertebral ganglia, 319–322
Paresthesias, 461*t*
Parietal cells, 867
Parietal lobe, 308
Parietal lobe disease, 358–360
Parietal pain, 886
Parietal peritoneum, 769–770
Parietooccipital sulcus, 308
Parkinsonian syndrome, 373
Parkinsonian tremor, 372*t*
Parkinsonism, 373

Parkinson's disease, 373
Parkinson's syndrome, 373
Paronychia, 1049
Paroxysmal dyskinesia, 371
Paroxysmal nocturnal dyspnea, 670
Pars distalis, 432
Pars intermedia, 432
Pars nervosa, 433
Pars tuberalis, 432
Partial seizure, 421t
Partial thromboplastin time, 495t–497t
Passenger mutations, 237–238
Passive immunity, 158–159
Pasteurella multocida, 981
Patch (skin lesion), 1037t
Pathogen-associated molecular patterns (PAMPs), 141
Pathogenic micro-organisms, 191
Pathological atrophy, 73–74
Pathological crying, 378
Pathological fractures, 967–968
Pathological fungi, 186
Pathological hyperplasia, 76
Pattern recognition receptors (PRRs), 141
Pavementing, 146–148
Pavlik harness, 1008–1009, 1010f
PBS/IC. *See* Painful bladder syndrome/interstitial cystitis
PCI. *See* Percutaneous coronary intervention
PCOS. *See* Polycystic ovary syndrome
PDE5i. *See* Phosphodiesterase type 5 inhibitors
PDGF. *See* Platelet-derived growth factor
Peak bone mass, 975
Pediculosis, 856t, 1060
Pedigrees analysis of, 56, 57f
Pelvic floor dysfunction, 884
Pelvic inflammatory disease (PID), 793–794, 795b, 856
Pelvic organ prolapse, 734, 797–798, 799b
Pemphigus, 1033–1034
Pemphigus erythematosus, 1034
Pemphigus foliaceus, 1034
Pemphigus herpetiformis, 1034
Pemphigus vegetans, 1034
Pemphigus vulgaris, 1034
Pendular nystagmus, 341
Penetrating trauma, 383–386
Penis
　anatomy of, 779, 779f
　cancer of, 268t–271t
　ejaculation of, 780
　erectile reflex of, 779
　sexual excitement of, 768
　tumours of, 835
Penis disorders
　balanitis, 835, 835f
　cancer, 268t–271t, 835–836
　paraphimosis, 833–834
　Peyronie disease, 834–835
　phimosis, 833–834
　priapism, 835
　tumours, 835
Pennate muscles, 953
Pepsin, 867

Peptic ulcer disease
　definition of, 893
　duodenal ulcers, 894–895
　gastric ulcers, 895
　Helicobacter pylori causing, 892
　lesions caused by, 893f
　postgastrectomy syndromes, 896–897
　risk factors of, 893b
　stress ulcers, 895
　surgical treatment of, 895–896
　Zollinger-Ellison syndrome and, 893–897
Percutaneous coronary intervention, 81
Pericardial cavity, 553
Pericardial effusion, 607–608
Pericardial fluid, 553
Pericardial sac, 553
Pericarditis
　acute, 606–607
　constrictive, 607–608
Pericardium, 553
Perimysium, 953
Perinatal stroke, 420
Periodic paralysis, 996
Periosteal reaction, 1003
Periosteum, 947–948
Peripheral artery disease, 592–595
Peripheral (immune) CRH, 224
Peripheral cyanosis, 671
Peripheral nervous system (PNS), 318–319
Peripheral vascular disease (PVD), 590–591
Peripheral vascular resistance-mediated ischemic cellular injury, 618
Peripheral vascular system, 566
Peristalsis, 862
Peritoneal cavity, 868
Peritoneum, 868
Peritubular capillaries, 717
Permissive effects, of hormones, 429
Pernicious anemia, 503–504
Persistent pain, 334
Pertussis vaccine, 190
Petechial hemorrhage, 491t
Peyronie disease, 834–835
PGI 2. *See* Prostacyclin
pH
　hydrogen ion, 124
Phagocytes, 138, 480–481. *See also* Macrophages
　basophils, 144–145
　dendritic cells, 142t
　eosinophils, 146
　monocytes, 146
Phagocytosis, 146
Phagolysosomes, 146
Phantom limb pain, 335t
Pharyngeal cancer, 268t–271t
Pharyngotympanic tube, 345
Phase I activation enzymes, 278
Phase II detoxification enzymes, 278
PHDs. *See* Prolyl hydroxylases
Phenylalanine hydroxylase, 419
Phenylketonuria (PKU), 419
Pheochromocytomas, 473
Philadelphia chromosome, 241, 514
Phimosis, 833–834

Phlebotomy, 506
Phosphate
　bone and, 733
Phosphatidylserine, 142
Phosphodiesterase type 5 inhibitors (PDE5i), 854
Phthalates, 823
Physical activity
　breast cancer and, 823
　cancer and, 276–282
Physical barriers, 134–136
Physiological atrophy, 73–74
Physiological jaundice of newborn, 937
Physiological stress, 216
Physiological tetanus, 960
Pia mater, 314
Pick disease, 365
PID. *See* Pelvic inflammatory disease
PIF. *See* Prolactin-inhibiting factor
PIN. *See* Prostatic intraepithelial neoplasia
Pineal gland, 436
Pinkeye, 344
Pipe smoking. *See* Smoking, tobacco
Pitting edema, 116f
Pituitary adenomas, 451–452
Pituitary giantism, 451f
Pituitary gland
　anatomy of, 428f
　anterior
　　anatomy of, 432
　　chromophils of, 432
　　chromophobes of, 432
　　hyperpituitarism and, 451–452
　　hypopituitarism and, 450–451
　　prolactinomas and, 453
　posterior
　　anatomy of, 434f
　　diabetes insipidus and, 450
　　SIADH and, 449
Pituitary stalk, 432
PKU. *See* Phenylketonuria
Plagiocephaly, 417f
Plaque, 591–592
Plaque (skin lesion), 1025f
Plaque psoriasis, 1031
Plasma, 1064t–1071t
　composition of, 478–480, 478f
　inorganic ions in, 480
　osmolality, 118f
Plasma cell count, 495t–497t
Plasma cells
　antibody production by, 495t–497t
　in asthma, 683
Plasma creatinine concentration, 726
Plasma protein systems, 138–139
Plasma proteins
　albumin, 479
　composition of, 479t
　globulins, 479–480
Plasmin, 140, 495
Plasminogen, 140
Plasmodium, 186
Plastic rigidity, 379t
Plasticity, developmental, 272–273

Platelet count, 495t–497t
Platelet-activating factor (PAF), 145
Platelet-derived growth factor (PDGF), 946t
Platelets
    activated, 146
    disorders of, 526–529
        thrombocythemia, 528–529
        thrombocytopenia, 526–528
    hemostasis function of, 529–530
Pleomorphic liposarcoma, 1003
Pleura
    abnormalities of, 674–675
    anatomy of, 658f
Pleural cavity, 657
Pleural effusion, 675
Pleural space, 657
Plexus injuries, 404t
Plexuses, 301
    brachial, 312f
    lumbar, 319
    sacral, 319
PMDD. *See* Premenstrual dysphoric disorder
PMS. *See* Premenstrual syndrome
Pneumococcal pneumonia, 690f
Pneumococcus, 689
Pneumoconiosis, 677
Pneumonia
    clinical manifestations of, 690
    community-acquired, 682
    evaluation of, 690
    hospital-acquired, 688
    pathophysiology of, 689–691
    pneumococcal, 690f
    treatment of, 690
    urine antigen testing of, 690
    ventilator-associated, 688
    viral, 690
Pneumothorax, 674
PNS. *See* Peripheral nervous system
Podocytes, 715–716
Podosomes, 945
Poiseuille's law, 568–570
Poison ivy, 209f, 1030f
Poisoning
    lead, 419
Poliovirus, 190
Polyarthritis, 1012
Polycystic kidney disease, 758
Polycystic ovary syndrome (PCOS), 791–792
Polycythemia, 256t
    absolute, 508
    familial, 508t
    relative, 507
    secondary, 508
Polycythemia vera, 508–509
Polydipsia, 450
Polymenorrhea, 791t
Polymorphonuclear neutrophil, 146. *See also* Neutrophils
Polymyositis, 998–999
Polyphagia, 461
Polyphenols, 276–278
Polyploidy, 43

Polyps
    colorectal, 920
    neoplastic, 920
Polysomnography, 339
Polyuria, 461t
Pompe's disease, 997
Pons, 305
Pores of Kohn, 655, 676f
Porphyrin analysis, 495t–497t
Portal hypertension, 906
Portopulmonary hypertension, 906
Port-wine stains, 1061–1062
Postcentral gyrus, 308
Postconcussion syndrome, 387
Posterior columns, 312
Posterior fontanelle, 412
Posterior fossa, 313
Posterior horn, 311
Posterior pituitary gland
    anatomy of, 434f
    diseases of
        diabetes insipidus and, 450
        SIADH, 256t, 449
Posterior spinal artery, 318
Postganglionic neurons, 319
Postgastrectomy syndromes, 896
Posthemorrhagic anemia, 502t
Posthyperventilation apnea, 355t
Postictal phase, 366
Postinflammatory IBS, 900
Postlactational involution, 818
Postmenopausal osteoporosis, 976
Postpartum thyroiditis, 456
Postrenal acute kidney injury, 746
Postsynaptic neurons, 304
Post-translational modifications, 6–9
Post-traumatic seizures, 387
Post-traumatic stress disorder (PTSD), 216
Postural abnormalities, 374
Posture disorders, 378
Postvoid residual urine, 727t–728t
Postvoid urine, 735
Potassium, 121–124. *See also* Hyperkalemia; Hypokalemia
Potassium-sparing diuretics, 725t
Pouchitis, 899
Powassan encephalitis, 401t
PP cells, 438
PR interval, 559
Prader-Willi syndrome, 65, 65f, 66f
Precapillary sphincter, 566
Precentral gyrus, 307–308
Preclinical diastolic dysfunction, 619
Precocious puberty, 787, 833
Predominantly antibody deficiencies, 192t
Pre-excitation syndromes, 623t–624t
Preganglionic neurons, 319
Pregnancy
    choline deficiency in, 276–278
    pyelonephritis and, 738
    sickle cell test and, 544f
Preictal phase, 366
Prekallikrein, 140
Preload, 564

Premature atrial contractions, 622t–623t
Premature junctional contractions, 622t–623t
Premature ventricular contractions, 622t–623t
Premenstrual dysphoric disorder (PMDD), 792–793
Premenstrual syndrome (PMS), 792–793
Premotor area, 306–307
Prepuce, 779
Prerenal acute kidney injury, 744–745
Presbycusis, 346
Presbyopia, 341–343
Pressure flow study, 727t–728t
Pressure ulcers, 1024–1029
Presynaptic neurons, 302f
Pretibial myxedema, 455
PRF. *See* Prolactin-releasing factor
Priapism, 835, 835f
Primary adrenal insufficiency, 472–473
Primary aldosteronism, 472
Primary biliary cirrhosis, 912
Primary cutaneous lymphomas, 1042
Primary emphysema, 687
Primary glomerular injury, 739
Primary hyperaldosteronism, 122
Primary hyperparathyroidism, 457–458
Primary hypertension, 649
Primary hypothyroidism, 453
Primary (congenital) immune deficiency, 191–192
Primary intention wound healing, 151
Primary nodular melanoma, 1041
Primary particles, 289
Primary polycythemia. *See* Polycythemia vera
Primary polydipsia, 450
Primary spermatocytes, 780
Primary spinal cord injury, 387–394
Primary thyroid disorders, 453
Prinzmetal angina, 599
Prodroma, 366
Proerythroblasts, 487
Progesterone, 773t
    biological effects of, 772
Progesterone receptor, 807
Progressive relaxation training, 994
Prokaryotes, 2, 178
Prolactin
    secretion of, 452
    in stress response, 225t–226t
Prolactin-inhibiting factor (PIF), 435t, 812–813
Prolactinomas, 453
Prolactin-releasing factor (PRF), 435t
Proliferative inflammatory atrophy, 844
Proliferative phase, of wound healing, 152
Prolyl hydroxylases, 78–79
Propionibacterium acnes, 1054
Proprioception, 347–348
Prostacyclin, 574
Prostacyclin (PGI 2), 145, 491
Prostaglandins, 145
Prostate cancer
    aging and risk of, 843f
    cancer cells in, 844
    chronic inflammation and, 844
    clinical manifestations of, 851–852

Prostate cancer (Continued)
  diet and, 845b–846b
  epigenetic factors in, 844–847
  evaluation of, 851–852
  genetic factors in, 844–847
  Gleason score for, 849b
  hormones involved in, 844
  incidence of, 843–844
  pathogenesis of, 847
  prostate epithelial neoplasia and, 849–850
  stromal environment in, 850–852
  treatment of, 851–852
  vasectomy and risk of, 844
Prostate epithelial neoplasia, 849–850
Prostate gland
  anatomy of, 780f
  disorders of, 840–852
Prostate-specific antigen (PSA), 852f
Prostatic hyperplasia, 841f
Prostatic intraepithelial neoplasia (PIN), 849–850
Prostatitis, 842–843
Proteases, 223
Protein C, 495
Protein kinases, 431
Protein S, 495
Protein-energy malnutrition, 935
Protein-free fluid, 720
Proteins
  catabolism of, 219
  contractile, of skeletal muscles, 958t
  synthesis, 44f
Proteinuria
  CKD progression and, 743t
  in multiple myeloma, 524
Proteoglycans, 945–947
Prothrombin time, 495t–497t, 878t
Prothrombinase complex, 494
Prothrombotic state, 527
Proton pump inhibitors, 889
Protoporphyrin, 488
Protoporphyrin analysis, 495t–497t
Protozoan parasites, 188
PRRs. See Pattern recognition receptors
Pruritus, 1029, 1059
PSA. See Prostate-specific antigen
Pseudohypoparathyroidism, 448
Pseudomonas aeruginosa, 137
Pseudounipolar neurons, 301
Psoriasis, 1030
Psoriatic arthritis, 1031
Psoriatic nail disease, 1031
Psychological stressors, 216
Psychoneuroimmunology, 216–218
Psychosocial distress, 227
Psychosocial stress, 219
PTMs. See Post-translational modifications
PTSD. See Post-traumatic stress disorder
Puberty
  definition of, 767
  delayed, 787
  precocious, 787
  reproductive system and, 767
Puerperal infections, 793–794

Pulmonary artery, 656–657
Pulmonary artery hypertension, 692–693
Pulmonary atresia, 640–641
Pulmonary blood flow
  congenital heart defects with decreased, 643–644
  congenital heart defects with increased, 641–643
Pulmonary circulation, 663. *See also* Heart
  control of, 656–657
Pulmonary diseases and disorders
  acute bronchitis, 688
  ALI, 678–682
  ARDS, 678–682
  aspiration, 675–676
  asthma. *See* Asthma
  atelectasis, 676
  bronchiectasis, 676–677
  bronchiolitis, 677
  in children. *See* Children, pulmonary diseases and disorders in
  chronic bronchitis, 686–687
  conditions caused by
    hypercapnia, 672
    hypoxemia, 672–673
    respiratory failure, 673
  COPD, 684–685
  cor pulmonale, 693
  emphysema, 687–688
  inhalation disorders, 677–678
  obstructive lung diseases, 682–688
  pneumonia. *See* Pneumonia
  pulmonary artery hypertension, 692–693
  pulmonary edema, 678
  pulmonary embolism, 692
  pulmonary fibrosis, 677
  respiratory tract infections. *See* Respiratory tract infections
  restrictive lung diseases, 675–682
  signs and symptoms of
    breathing pattern abnormalities, 671
    clubbing, 671
    cough, 670
    cyanosis, 671
    dyspnea, 670
    hemoptysis, 670–671
    hyperventilation, 671
    hypoventilation, 671
    pain, 671–672
    sputum abnormalities, 670
  tuberculosis. *See* Tuberculosis
Pulmonary edema, 678
Pulmonary embolism, 692
Pulmonary fibrosis, 677
Pulmonary function tests, 661
Pulmonary stenosis, 663
Pulmonary system
  abbreviations for, 664t
  bronchial circulation in, 655
  chest wall in, 657
  conducting airways of, 654–655
  defense mechanisms of, 655t
  functions of, 657–667
  gas-exchange airways of, 655

Pulmonary system (Continued)
  larynx. *See* Larynx
  lungs. *See* Lungs
  pleura in, 657
  trachea. *See* Trachea
Pulmonary vascular resistance (PVR), 642
Pulmonary veins, 554, 655
Pulmonic semilunar valves, 554
Pulse pressure, 571–572
Pulsus paradoxus, 683–684
Purified protein derivative, 691
Purkinje fibres, 558–559
Purpura fulminans, 400–401
Purulent exudate, 146
Pustular psoriasis, 1031
Pustule, 1035
Putamen, 308
PVD. See Peripheral vascular disease
PVR. See Pulmonary vascular resistance
Pyelonephritis, 738
Pyloric obstruction, 889–890
Pyloric sphincter, 864–865
Pylorus, 864–865
Pyramidal motor syndrome, 379t
Pyramidal system, 307–308
Pyramids, of kidney, 714
Pyrogenic bacteria, 183

Q

QRS complex, 559, 560f
QT interval, 559, 560f
Quadriparesis, 375b
Quadriplegia, 375b
Quality-adjusted life year (QALY), 107

R

RAAS. See Renin-angiotensin-aldosterone system
Rabies vaccine, 198
Radial scar, 813–814
Radiation therapy
  for cancer, 261
  secondary malignancies caused by, 822
Radicular pain, 393
Radicular syndrome, 408
Radiculopathy, 393–394, 404t
Radiofrequency electromagnetic radiation, 287
Radioimmunoassay (RIA), 430b
Radiolysis, 283–284
Radon, 289
Raloxifene, 977b, 978–979
RANKL. See Receptor activator nuclear factor kappa-B ligand
RANK. See Receptor activator nuclear factor kappa-B
Rapid eye movement (REM) sleep, 338
RAS (rat sarcoma), 239–242
Raynaud phenomenon, 207, 591
RBB. See Right bundle branch
RDS. See Respiratory distress syndrome of newborn
Reactive oxygen species (ROS)
  sun exposure as cause of, 286
Reactive stress response, 216

Rebound headaches, 399
Receptive aprosody, 378
Receptive dysphasia, 360, 362t
Receptor activator nuclear factor kappa-B (RANK), 945, 946t, 976–978, 978f
Receptor activator nuclear factor kappa-B ligand (RANKL), 945, 946t, 976–978, 978f
Recombinant human erythropoietin (r-HuEPO), 487
Recombinant human granulocyte colony-stimulating factor, 258
Recombination activating genes, 164
Rectal carcinomas, 921
Rectocele, 798, 798f
Rectosigmoid sphincter, 871–872
Rectosphincteric reflex, 873
Rectum, 873
   cancer of, 268t–271t, 806, 917–921, 918t, 919b, 920f, 921b
Red cell count, 495t–497t
Red measles, 1058–1059, 1058t
Red muscle, 955, 957t
Red nucleus, 310
Reed-Sternberg (RS) cells, 519, 519f, 548, 549f
Refeeding syndrome, 905
Referred pain, 333–334, 334f, 886
Reflex arcs, 311, 314f
Reflexes, in infants, 412, 413t
Refraction alterations, 343, 343f
Refractory period, 559
Regeneration, tissue, 151
Regional osteoporosis, 976
Regulatory T cells, 158, 173–174
Regurgitation
   aortic, 611–612
   mitral, 612
   tricuspid, 612
   valvular, 609–612, 610t, 611f
Relative polycythemia, 507
Relaxin, 764t
Remitting-relapsing multiple sclerosis, 403
REM. See Rapid eye movement sleep
Renal adenomas, 736
Renal agenesis, 758
Renal aplasia, 758
Renal arteries, 716–717
Renalase, 720
Renal autoregulation, 719, 719f
Renal blood flow, 719–720, 719f, 726
Renal cancer, 268t–271t
Renal capsule, 714, 714f
Renal cell carcinoma, 736, 736f
Renal clearance
   BUN and, 726–729
   glomerular filtration rate and, 726
   plasma creatinine concentration and, 726
   renal blood flow and, 726
Renal colic, 733
Renal columns, 714, 714f
Renal corpuscle, 715, 715f
Renal disorders. See Children, renal disorders in
Renal fascia, 714

Renal function
   aging effects on, 728b
   elderly and, 728b
   infants and, 728b
   tests of, 726–729, 727t, 727t–728t
Renal insufficiency, 744
Renal papillae, 718
Renal plasma flow, 719
Renal system, 714–718. See also Kidneys
Renal transitional cell carcinoma, 736
Renal tumours, 736, 736f
Renal veins, 717
Renin, 116
Renin-angiotensin-aldosterone system (RAAS), 116, 117f, 584–586
   renal blood flow regulation by, 720
Repair, of scar tissue, 151
Reperfusion injury, 81
Repetitive discharge, 960
Repolarization, 559–560
   delayed, 122
Reproductive system
   aging and, 781–782
   CKD effects on, 749t, 752
   development of, 764–767
   female. See Female reproductive system
   male. See Male reproductive system
   maturation and, 767
   puberty and, 767
   sexual differentiation in utero, 765–767
Resistance, blood flow affected by, 570
Resistance stage, of general adaptation syndrome, 216–218
Resistin, 903b
Resolution, of inflammation, 151
Respiration. See also Breathing; Ventilation
   brainstem control of, 659, 659f
   Cheyne-Stokes, 353, 355t, 671
   Kussmaul, 127, 671
   neurochemical control of, 659–660, 659f
   physiology of, 674f
Respiratory acidosis, 128–129, 129f
Respiratory alkalosis, 129–130, 129f
Respiratory bronchioles, 655, 657f, 658f
Respiratory burst, 148
Respiratory distress syndrome of newborn (RDS), 704–705, 704b, 705f
Respiratory failure, 673
Respiratory rate, 658
Respiratory tract
   laryngeal cancer of, 268t–271t, 694, 694f
   lung cancer. See Lung cancer
   malignancies of, 268t–271t, 693–700
Respiratory tract infections, 180t–181t
   abscesses, 691
   acute bronchitis, 688
   in children, 706–708
   pneumonia. See Pneumonia
   tuberculosis. See Tuberculosis
Rest legs syndrome, 340
Restricted breathing, 671
Restrictive cardiomyopathy, 608–609, 608f

Restrictive lung diseases, 675–682
   ALI, 678–682
   ARDS, 678–682, 680f
   aspiration, 675–676
   atelectasis, 676, 676f
   bronchiectasis, 676–677
   bronchiolitis, 677, 706–707
   inhalation disorders, 677–678
   pulmonary edema, 678
   pulmonary fibrosis, 677
Resveratrol, 278–279
Retching, 883
Rete testis, 778, 778f
Reticular activating system, 305, 306f
Reticular formation, 305, 306f
Reticulocyte, 487
Reticulocyte count, 495t–497t
Reticuloendothelial system, 876
Retina, 340, 340f
Retinal detachment, 340–341
Retinoblastoma, 295
   in children, 423–424, 423f
   familial, 244
   gene for, 244
Retinoids, 1054
Retractile testis, 838
Retrograde amnesia, 358, 359t
Retrograde menstruation, 801
Retropulsion, 866
Reverse transcriptase, 196
Reverse transcriptase inhibitors, 197–198
Reverse Warburg effect, 248
Reversible sideroblastic anemia, 506–507
Rhabdomyolysis, 746, 970–972, 972b
Rhabdomyomas, 1004
Rhabdomyosarcomas, 234–235, 295, 1003–1004
Rh blood group, 211
Rheumatic heart disease, 612–614, 614f
Rheumatoid arthritis
   ankylosing spondylitis compared to, 989–990
   cause of, 985–986
   classification criteria for, 989t
   clinical manifestations of, 987–988
   evaluation of, 990–991
   female sexual dysfunction and, 812t
   of hand, 986f
   HLAs and, 985–986
   incidence of, 985
   mechanisms of, 985
   molecular imaging of, 988b
   pathophysiology of, 986–989, 986f, 987f
   treatment of, 988
Rheumatoid factors, 985–986
Rheumatoid nodules, 988
Rh incompatibility, 539
Rhinovirus, 183
r-HuEPO. See Recombinant human erythropoietin
Rhythmicity, of heart, 559
RIA. See Radioimmunoassay

Ribonucleic acid (RNA)
　gene splicing, 41
　messenger, 245
　micro, 245
　noncoding, 237–238, 244
　transcription, 40, 42f, 43f
　translation, 41
Ribosomal RNA, 3, 41, 64, 487
Rickets, 979
RIFLE criteria, 744–747, 744t
Right atrium, 553, 554f
Right bundle branch (RBB), 558
Right coronary artery, 555, 556t, 558f
Right lymphatic duct, 576, 576f
Right-to-left shunting, 638–639, 639f
Right ventricle, 553, 554f
Right ventricular failure, 620, 620f
Rigidity, 370, 370t
Rilutek (riluzole), 377
Riluzole (Rilutek), 377
Ringed sideroblasts, 506
Rituximab (Rituxan), 263t, 528
RNA. See Ribonucleic acid
Rocephin (ceftriaxone), 795b
Rods, 340
ROS. See Reactive oxygen species
Roseola, 1058t, 1059
Rotavirus, 937
rRNA. See Ribosomal RNA
RS cells. See Reed-Sternberg cells
Rubella, 1057–1058, 1058f, 1058t
Rubeola, 1058–1059, 1058t
Rubral tremor, 372t
Rubrospinal tract, 311
Ruffini endings, 347
Rugae, 768
Rule of nines, in burns, 1044, 1045f
Russell-Silver syndrome, 66

S

Sabin vaccine, 164, 190
Saccular aneurysms, 397, 589
Sacral plexus, 319
SAGs. See Superantigens
Saliva, 862–864, 864f
Salivary α-amylase, 862
Salivary glands, cancer of, 268t–271t
Salivation, 862–864, 864f
Salivatory glands, 862–864, 864f
Salk vaccine, 164, 190
Salmonella, 981
Salpingitis, 794–796, 794f
Saltatory conduction, 301
SA node. See Sinoatrial node
Saphenous veins, 580
Sarcolemma, 956
Sarcomas, 234–235
　of breast, 825t
　Ewing, 234–235, 295, 1003, 1018–1019, 1019f
　fibrosarcoma, 1003–1004
　Kaposi, 251, 268t–271t, 297, 1042, 1042f
　leiomyosarcoma, 1003
　osteosarcomas, 1002–1003, 1002f, 1002t, 1018
　pleomorphic liposarcoma, 1003

Sarcomas *(Continued)*
　rhabdomyosarcomas, 234–235, 295, 1003
　synovial, 1003
Sarcomeres, 560–561, 561f, 562f, 956–957
Sarcopenia, 962
Sarcoplasm, 956–957
Sarcoplasmic reticulum, 956–957
Sarcotubular system, 956–957
Sarcotubules, 956–957
SARS-CoV-2, 184t, 697b
　ACE-2 receptor, 183
　acute kidney injury, 747
　antigenic drift, 185
　ARDS, 679–681
　chronic obstructive pulmonary disease, 633b, 698b–699b
　cytokine storm, 142
　digestive symptoms and intestinal inflammation, 917
　human ACE2 receptor, 680–681
　mRNA vaccines, 158
　multisystem inflammatory syndrome, 648
　obesity, 905
　vaccines and therapeutic antibodies, 191
Satellite cells, 301, 955–957
Saturated fatty acids, 869b
Scabies, 856t, 857t–859t, 1060, 1060f
Scale (skin lesion), 1028t
Scaphocephaly, 417f
Scars
　hypertrophic, 153, 154f, 1029, 1029f, 1046f
　keloids, 153, 154f, 1028f, 1029
　radial, 813–814
Scar tissue
　contracture of, 154
　definition of, 151
　repair of, 151
Schwann cells, 301–302, 303f
Sciatica, 393
SCIDs. See Severe combined immunodeficiencies
Sclera, 340, 340f
Scleroderma, 1038, 1038f
Sclerosing adenosis, 813
Scoliosis, 1014–1015, 1015f
Scotoma, 342t
Scrotum, 778f, 779
　disorders of, 836–840, 837f
Sebaceous glands, 1022
Seborrheic dermatitis, 1030, 1031f
Seborrheic keratosis, 1039, 1039f
Secondary amenorrhea, 789–790, 810f
Secondary bile acids, 875–876
Secondary biliary cirrhosis, 912
Secondary brain injury, 384t, 387
Secondary dysmenorrhea, 788–789
Secondary glomerular injury, 739
Secondary hyperaldosteronism, 472
Secondary hyperparathyroidism, 457
Secondary hypertension, 582, 586–587, 649, 650b
Secondary hypocortisolism, 473
Secondary hypothyroidism, 455, 456f

Secondary (acquired) immune deficiency, 191, 194, 195b
Secondary immune response, 167
Secondary incontinence, 761
Secondary intention wound healing, 151f, 152
Secondary lymphoid organs, 158, 160f, 483
Secondary osteoporosis, 976
Secondary Parkinsonism, 373
Secondary particles, 289
Secondary peristalsis, 864
Secondary pneumothorax, 674
Secondary polycythemia, 508, 508t
Secondary-progressive multiple sclerosis, 403
Secondary spermatocytes, 780, 780f
Secondary spinal cord injury, 388
Secondary thrombocythemia, 528
Secondary thyroid disorders, 453
Secondary ureteropelvic junction obstruction, 758
Second-degree block, 623t–624t
Second-degree burns, 1043–1044, 1043f, 1043t
Secondhand smoke, 274–276, 685b
Second messengers, 430–431, 430f, 448
Secretin, 865–866, 866t
Secretory diarrhea, 885
Secretory IgA, 193
Secretory immune system, 164, 165f
Secretory immunoglobulin, 164
Secretory phase, 771f, 774
Sedentary lifestyle, 597
Segmental pain inhibition, 333
Segmented fractures, 966f
Seizure/seizure disorders
　absence, 421t
　atonic, 421t
　in children, 420, 421t
　clinical manifestations of, 366
　conditions associated with, 365–366, 366t
　definition of, 365
　evaluation and treatment of, 366
　febrile, 421t
　focal, 421t
　generalized clonic-tonic, 366, 421t
　myoclonic, 421t
　partial, 421t
　post-traumatic, 387
　types of, 366, 366t
Selective attention, 358, 359t
Selective attention deficits, 358
Selective auditory attention, 358
Selective estrogen receptor modulator, 977b
Selective IgA deficiency, 192t, 193
Selective visual attention, 358
Selenium, 845b–846b
Self-antigens, 166
Selye, Hans, 216
Semen, 779
Semicircular canals, 345, 345f, 346f
Semilunar valves, 554, 554f, 555f
Seminal vesicles, 779–780, 780f
Seminiferous tubules, 778, 778f
Senile disease complex, 363
Sensorimotor syndrome, 408
Sensorineural hearing loss, 346

Sensory-discriminative system, 330–331
Sensory dysphasia, 360, 362t
Sensory inattentiveness, 358–360
Sensory neurons, 302
Sensory pathways, 312
Sensory speech area, 307f, 308
Sepsis
   central line-associated bloodstream infections as cause of, 629b
   deaths involving, 627–630
   description of, 183
   guidelines for surviving, 630, 630b
Septic arthritis, 1010–1012
Septicemia, 183, 620
Septic shock, 627–630, 628t, 629b, 629f
Sequestosome-1, 980
Sequestrum, 981–982
Serology–immunology, 1074t–1075t
Serotonin, 866t
   properties of, 305t
Serous cell, 657f
Serous exudate, 149
Sertoli cells, 780, 780f
Serum, 478–479, 1064t–1071t
Serum electrolytes, 907–908
Serum electrophoresis, 479–480
Serum enzymes, 878t
Serum ferritin determination, 495t–497t
Serum proteins, 878t
Serum sickness, 205–207
Sever disease, 1014
Severe combined immunodeficiencies (SCIDs), 192–194, 192t
Severe congenital neutropenia, 192t, 193–194
Sex hormones
   breast development and, 818–819
   definition of, 764–765
   female, 764t, 772, 772b, 773t
   male, 764t, 780–781
Sexual differentiation, 765–767
Sexual dysfunction
   female, 811, 812t
   male, 852–855
Sexually transmitted infections/diseases, 180t–181t, 856–859, 856t, 857t–859t
   cancer and, 288, 288t
Sexual maturation alterations, 786–787, 788b, 788t, 789b, 833
Sexual trauma, female, 739t
SGLT2. See Sodium-glucose cotransporter 2
Shear stress, 555
Sheehan's syndrome, 450–451
Shift to the left, 510
Shift to the right, 510
Shift work sleep disorder, 339–340
Shingles, 1036, 1059
Shock, 671
   anaphylactic, 627, 628f
   cardiogenic, 626, 626f
   cellular metabolism impairment in, 621, 625f
   clinical manifestations of, 625
   compensatory mechanisms for, 621
   description of, 621
   glucose impairment in, 621–625, 625f

Shock (Continued)
   hypovolemic, 626, 627f
   neurogenic, 626–627, 628f
   oxygen use impairment in, 621–625
   septic, 627–630, 628t, 629b, 629f
   treatment for, 625
   types of, 625–630
   vasogenic, 626–627
Short bones, 949
Short-term starvation, 905
Shunt, 638–639, 639f, 643
Shunting
   left-to-right, 638–639, 639f
   right-to-left, 638–639, 639f
   ventilation-perfusion mismatch caused by, 672–673, 673f
Shwachman syndrome, 514
SIADH. See Syndrome of inappropriate antidiuretic hormone
Sialoprotein, 944t, 947
Sickle cell anemia, 502t, 541
Sickle cell disease, 540–543, 541f, 542f, 542t, 543f, 544f
Sickle cell-hemoglobin C disease, 541–542
Sickle cell test, 495t–497t, 544f
Sickle cell-thalassemia disease, 541–542
Sickle cell trait, 541
Sickled erythrocytes, 542, 542f, 543f
Sideroblastic anemia, 502t, 506–507
Sigmoid colon, 871–872, 872f
Sildenafil, 854
Silent ischemia, 599, 599f, 600f
Silent thyroiditis, 456
Simple fibroadenomas, 814
Simple sinus tachycardia, 622t–623t
Single gene defects, 191–199
Single nucleotide polymorphisms, 276
Single-photon emission computed tomography (SPECT), 600
Signal transduction pathway, 14, 16f
Sinoatrial node (SA node), 557–558, 559f
Sinus block, 623t–624t
Sinus bradycardia, 622t–623t
Sinus dysrhythmias, 622t–623t
Sinusoids, 874, 875f
SIRS. See Systemic inflammatory response syndrome
Skeletal muscle disorders
   acid maltase deficiency, 997
   chronic fatigue syndrome, 994
   contractures, 994
   dermatomyositis, 998–999, 998f
   disuse atrophy, 994
   endocrine disorders, 996–997
   energy metabolism diseases, 997
   fibromyalgia, 994–996, 995b, 995f
   idiopathic inflammatory myopathies, 998, 998f
   inclusion body myositis, 998–999
   lipid deficiency, 997
   McArdle's disease, 997
   myoadenylate deaminase deficiency, 997
   myositis, 997–998
   myotonia, 996

Skeletal muscle disorders (Continued)
   periodic paralysis, 996
   polymyositis, 998–999
   stress-induced muscle tension, 994
   toxic myopathies, 999, 999b
Skeletal muscles
   cardiac muscle compared to, 561
   contractile proteins of, 957, 958t
   extrafusal, 954
   fast-twitch, 955
   fibres, 955–957, 957f, 957t
   function of, 953
   fusiform, 953
   motor units of, 954–958, 956f
   myofibrils of, 957, 957f, 958t
   nonprotein constituents of, 958
   pennate, 953
   sensory receptors of, 955
   slow-twitch, 955
   striated, 954
   structure of, 953–961, 955f, 956f, 957t
   voluntary, 954
Skeletal muscles, aging of, 962
Skeletal system, CKD and, 749t
Skeletal trauma, 965–968
Skeleton, 948, 949f
Skin
   aging changes to, 1022
   anatomy of, 1023f, 1023t, 1024f
   apocrine sweat glands of, 1022
   blood supply to, 1022
   cancer manifestations of, 258
   CKD effects on, 749t, 752
   cysts, 1025f
   dermal appendages, 1022, 1024f
   dermis, 1022, 1023f, 1023t
   eccrine sweat glands of, 1022
   epidermis, 1022, 1023f, 1023t
   layers of, 1022–1024, 1023f, 1023t
   sebaceous glands of, 1022
   subcutaneous layer of, 1022, 1023f
   tumours of, 1025f
   ulcers, 1027f
Skin cancer, 258
   basal cell carcinoma, 286, 1040, 1040f
   cutaneous melanoma, 1041–1042, 1042f
   description of, 268t–271t
   Kaposi sarcoma, 251, 268t–271t, 297, 1042, 1042f
   melanoma, 285–286
   multistep, theoretical scheme of, 286, 286f
   primary cutaneous lymphomas, 1042
   squamous cell carcinoma, 286, 1040–1041, 1040f
   sun exposure and, 286
   trends for, 1040b
   types of, 285–286
   ultraviolet radiation as cause of, 1022
Skin disorders
   acne rosacea, 1033, 1033f
   acne vulgaris, 1032
   actinic keratosis, 1039
   allergic contact dermatitis, 209f, 1029–1030, 1030f

Skin disorders *(Continued)*
    atopic dermatitis, 857t–859t, 1030
    bacterial infections, 1035, 1035f
    benign tumours, 1039, 1039f, 1039t
    burns. *See* Burns
    candidiasis, 1037, 1037t
    carbuncles, 1035
    cellulitis, 1035
    chickenpox, 1036
    in children. *See* Children, skin disorders in
    cold injury, 1046–1047
    cutaneous vasculitis, 1038
    eczema, 1029–1030
    erysipelas, 1035
    erythema multiforme, 1034
    folliculitis, 1035
    fungal infections, 1036–1038, 1037f, 1037t
    furuncles, 1035, 1035f
    herpes simplex virus, 856t, 857t–859t, 1035–1036, 1036f
    herpes zoster, 1036, 1036f
    hypertrophic scars, 153, 154f, 1029, 1029f
    impetigo, 1035
    infections, 180t–181t, 1034–1038, 1035f, 1036f, 1037t
    inflammatory, 1029–1030
    irritant contact dermatitis, 1030
    keloids, 153, 154f, 1027f, 1029, 1029f
    keratoacanthoma, 1039
    lesions, 1024–1029, 1025f, 1027f
    lupus erythematosus, 1033, 1033f
    Lyme disease, 1035
    necrotizing fasciitis, 1035
    papulosquamous, 1030–1033, 1031b, 1031f, 1032f
    pemphigus, 1033–1034, 1034f
    pressure ulcers, 1024–1029, 1024b, 1028f
    pruritus, 1029, 1032
    psoriasis, 1031–1032, 1031b, 1031f
    scleroderma, 1038, 1038f
    seborrheic dermatitis, 1030, 1031f
    shingles, 1036
    stasis dermatitis, 1030, 1030f
    tinea infections, 1037, 1037f, 1037t
    urticaria, 203–204, 204f
    varicella, 1036
    vascular, 1038–1039
    vesiculobullous diseases, 1033–1034, 1034f
    viral infections, 1035–1036, 1036f
    warts, 1036, 1036f
Skin lesions, 1024–1029, 1025f
Skull
    fontanelles of, 412, 412f
    of infants, 412
    malformations of, 415–416, 417f
    periosteum of, 313–314
    sutures of, 412, 412f
Sleep
    definition of, 338
    deprivation, 218, 339
    disorders of, 339–340
    elderly characteristics of, 339b
    hypothalamus and, 338
    infant characteristics of, 338b

Sleep *(Continued)*
    non-REM, 339
    REM, 338–339
Sleepwalking, 340
Sliding hiatal hernia, 889, 889f
Slightly movable joints, 950
Slit membranes, 715–716
Slow-reacting substances of anaphylaxis (SRS-A), 145
Slow-transit constipation, 884
Slow-twitch fibres, 955
Small bowel obstruction, 890–892, 890t
Small cell carcinoma, 695t, 696–700
Small intestinal carcinoma, 920
Small intestine
    aging effects on, 880
    anatomy of, 868–869, 868f
    dietary fat and, 869b
    digestion and absorption in, 869, 869b, 870f, 871b, 871f
    duodenum, 868, 868f
    ileum, 868, 868f
    jejunum, 868, 868f
    motility in, 869–871
    mucosa of, 866t
    nutrients absorbed in, 871b
    obstruction of, 891
    villi, 868f, 869
Small lymphocytic lymphoma, 517–518
Small vessel disease, 395
Smallpox, 1059
Smoking, tobacco, 823
    CAD and, 597
    cancer and, 274–276, 274f
    environmental tobacco smoke, 274–276
    facts on, 695b
    health consequences of, 275f
    lung cancer and, 694–700
    lung health and, 685b
    prevalence of, in Canada, 274f
    secondhand, 274–276
Snout reflex, 356f
Social support, 230
Sodium
    balance
        aldosterone effects on, 116
        alterations in, 118–121, 118t, 119f
        hypertonic alterations to, 118–120, 119f
        hypotonic alterations to, 119f, 120–121
        isotonic alterations to, 118, 119f
        maintenance of, 116–118
    CKD progression and water balance with, 750t
    in ECF, 116
    functions of, 116
Sodium bicarbonate, 124
Sodium-glucose cotransporter 2 (SGLT2), 464
Sodium reabsorption inhibitors, 725t
Soluble immune-complex glomerulonephritis, 741t
Somatic cell inheritance, 273t
Somatic cell mutation, 242

Somatic death, 108–109
Somatic nervous system, components of, 301
Somatic pain, 333–334
Somatic recombination, 164–166
Somatosensory function, 347–348
Somatostatin, 225t–226t, 435t, 439, 866t
Somatotropic hormones, 432, 435t
Somnambulism (sleepwalking), 340
Somogyi effect, 465
Spasmodic croup, 702–703
Spastic cerebral palsy, 416
Spasticity, 370, 370t, 371f, 375
Spatial summation, 304
Specific immunity. *See* Adaptive immunity
Specificity theory, 329
SPECT. *See* Single-photon emission computed tomography
Spermatids, 780
Spermatocele, 837, 837f
Spermatocytes, 780, 780f
Spermatogenesis, 780, 780f, 854
Spermatogonia, 780
Spermatozoon, 764
Sperm cells, 764, 778–779, 781f
    production impairment, 854–855
Sperm motility, 855
Sphincter of Oddi, 873–874, 877
Spina bifida, 413, 415f
Spina bifida occulta, 414
Spinal accessory nerve, 321t
Spinal cord
    anatomy of, 311, 312f, 313f, 314f
    blood supply to, 318, 320f
    central canal of, 311
    coverings of, 311, 313f
    cross section of, 311, 314f
    description of, 306t
    reflex arcs of, 311, 314f
    tracts of, 313f
    tumours of, 408–409
    in vertebral column, 311, 312f
Spinal cord abscesses, 401
Spinal cord injuries
    clinical manifestations of, 389–391, 390t
    evaluation and treatment of, 391
    female sexual dysfunction and, 812t
    pathophysiology of, 387–394
    primary, 387–394
    secondary, 387–394
    types of, 388t
Spinal multiple sclerosis, 402–403
Spinal nerves, 312f, 318–319
Spinal shock, 374–375, 390t
Spinal stenosis, 393
Spinal tracts, 311
Spindles, 955
Spine
    axial compression injuries of, 389f, 389t
    degenerative disorders of, 391–394
        low back pain, 391–393
    flexion injuries of, 388f, 389t
    flexion-rotation injuries of, 389f, 389t
    hyperextension injuries of, 388f, 389t

Spinnbarkeit mucus, 770–771
Spinothalamic tract, 311, 313f
  anterior, 311
  lateral, 311
Spiral fractures, 965–968, 966f, 966t
Spirochetes, 178
Spironolactone, 725t
Splanchnic blood flow, 873
Splanchnic nerves, 319–322
Spleen
  absence of, 484
  anatomy of, 483–484, 483f
  disorders involving, 524–526, 525b
  erythrocytes in, 482f
  functions of, 483–484
Splenectomy, 526
Splenic pulp, 483–484
Splenomegaly, 512, 517–518, 906
  congestive, 524
  diseases related to, 524–526, 525b
  infiltrative, 525
Spondyloarthropathies, 989–990
Spondylolisthesis, 393
Spondylolysis, 393
Spongy bone, 947, 947f
Spousal death, 228b
Sputum abnormalities, 670
Squamocolumnar junction, 770
Squamous cell carcinoma, 285–286, 695, 695t, 696f, 825t, 1040–1041, 1040f, 1041f
SRS-A. *See* Slow-reacting substances of anaphylaxis
SRY gene, 765
Stable angina pectoris, 598–599
Staghorn calculus, 733
Stance disorders, 378
Stapes, 345, 346f
Staphylococcal pneumonia, 707, 708t
Staphylococcal scalded-skin syndrome, 1056, 1056f
Staphylococcus aureus, 171, 178, 182f, 675
  methicillin-resistant, 183
  osteomyelitis and, 981
Strangulation, 92–94
Starling forces, 114
Starling's law of the heart, 563f, 564
Starvation, 905
Stasis dermatitis, 1030, 1030f
Static encephalopathies, 416–417
Static muscle contraction, 961
Status asthmaticus, 683–684
Status epilepticus, 366, 421t
Steatorrhea, 885
ST elevation myocardial infarction, 601, 601f
Stellate cells, 875
Stem cells, 278
  hematopoietic, 485, 486f
  mammary, 819–820
  mesenchymal, 194, 485, 486f
Stem-like cancer cells, 514, 516f
Stendra, 854

Stenosis, 555
  aortic, 610–611, 611f, 639–640, 640f
  mitral, 611, 611f
  pulmonary, 640–641, 641f
  valvular, 609, 610t, 611f
Steroid hormones, 427, 480
Stevens-Johnson syndrome, 1034
Sticky platelets, 492b
Still disease, 1012
ST interval, 559, 560f
St. Louis encephalitis, 401t
Stomach
  aging effects on, 880
  anatomy of, 864–871, 865f
  blood vessels of, 865, 865f
  cancer of, 268t–271t, 918t, 919
  gastric motility in, 865–867, 866t
  gastric secretion in, 867–868, 867f
  mucosa of, 866t
Storage diseases
  in children, 419
Strabismus, 341
Strains
  muscle, 970, 971t
  stress and, 216
Strawberry hemangiomas, 1061
Streptococcal pneumonia, 707, 708t
Streptococcus pneumoniae, 193, 420
Streptococcus pyogenes, 171
Stress
  acute, 218
  adverse heart effects of, 228b
  anti-inflammatory effects of, 223–224
  behavioral, 216f
  chronic, 227
  coping with, 229–231, 229f
  coronary heart disease and, 222b
  cortisol secretion during, 219, 220t
  cytokine secretion affected by, 223
  definition of, 215
  diseases and conditions associated with, 218t
  exogenous glucocorticoids effect on, 220
  good types of, 229f
  health outcome determination in, 227, 228f
  historical background on, 216–219
  HPA system and, 222b
  immune system in, 224–227, 227f
  nonlinear and complex interactions of, 222f
  overview of, 218
  physiological, 216, 216f
  proinflammatory effects of, 223
  psychosocial, 222b
  shear, 555
  sleep deprivation caused by, 218
  strain and, 216
  type 2 diabetes mellitus and, 221b
Stress-age syndrome, 219, 230b
Stress echocardiography, 600
Stress fractures, 966–967, 966t
Stress incontinence, 733–736, 733t
Stress-induced muscle tension, 994

Stressors
  definition of, 215
  personality characteristics and, 228
  psychological, 216
  repetitive exposure to, 227
Stress-related mucosal disease, 895
Stress response
  anticipatory, 216
  definition of, 215
  hormones influencing, 224, 225t–226t
  HPA system regulation and, 219–220
  mechanisms of, 219–227
  neuroendocrine regulation of, 220–224
  parasympathetic nervous system in, 223–224
  reactive, 216
  schematic diagram of, 217f
  sympathetic nervous system in, 220–223
Stress ulcers, 895
Stretch receptors, 659
Striated muscles, 954. *See also* Skeletal muscle
Striatum, 308, 310f
Stroke
  childhood, 420
  diabetes mellitus complications with, 467t, 468
  dietary potassium and lower risk of, 122
  embolic, 395
  heat, 337
  hemodynamic, 395
  hemorrhagic, 396–397, 420
  ischemic, 395–396, 420
  lacunar, 395
  occlusive, 420
  perinatal, 420
  prevention of, in women, 395b
  signs of, 389
  thrombotic, 395
Stroke volume, 563
Stroma, 234, 235f, 850–852
Stromal cells, 239, 485
Strong acid, 124
Structural scoliosis, 1014–1015
Struvite stones, 733
Stye, 344
Subacute thyroiditis, 456
Subarachnoid hemorrhage, 397–398, 398t
Subarachnoid space, 314, 315f
Subclinical hypothyroidism, 456–457
Subclinical thyroid disease, 453
Subcutaneous layer of skin, 1022–1024, 1023f, 1023t
Subdural hematomas, 384t, 385
Subdural space, 314, 315f
Subluxation, 968
Submucosal plexus, 865, 869
Substance P, 435t
  properties of, 305t
  in stress response, 225t–226t
Substantia gelatinosa, 311
Substantia nigra, 308, 310, 310f
Subthalamic nucleus, 308, 310f
Subthalamus, 309–310
Subvalvular aortic stenosis, 640
Succussion splash, 889

Suck reflex, 356f
Sudden cardiac death, 604, 605f
Sudden unexpected infant death (SUID), 711–712, 712b
Suffocation, 92
SUID. See Sudden unexpected infant death
Sulci, 306–307, 307f
Summation, 304
Sun burn, 286
Sun exposure, 286
Superantigens (SAGs), 171
Superficial hemangiomas, 1061, 1061f
Superficial mycoses, 185–186
Superficial partial-thickness burns, 1043–1044, 1043f, 1043t
Superficial spreading melanoma, 1041
Superior colliculi, 310
Superior vena cava, 554, 554f
Superior vena cava syndrome, 581
Supply-dependent oxygen consumption, 632
Suppurative cystitis, 737
Suppurative exudate, 149
Suprachiasmatic nucleus, 340–341
Supratentorial disorders, 352–353, 353t
Supratentorial herniation, 368b, 368f
Supravalvular aortic stenosis, 640
Surface tension, 661
Surfactant, 655, 657f, 661
  deficiency, RDS from, 704–705
  impairment of, 676
Surgery, for cancer, 261
Sustained attention deficits, 358
Sutures, 950
  cranial, 412, 412f
Swallowing, 863f, 864
  dysphagia and, 589, 887–888, 888f
Sweat glands, 1022
Swine influenza virus (H1N1), 185
Sylvian fissure, 306–307, 307f
Sympathetic ganglia, 319–322
Sympathetic nervous system
  anatomy of, 319–322, 323f
  myocardial performance affected by, 560
  primary hypertension and, 582–584, 612
  in stress response, 220–223
Symphysis, 950
Synapses, 302f, 304
Synaptic bouton, 304
Synaptic cleft, 302f, 304
Synarthrosis, 950
Synchondrosis, 950
Syndesmophyte, 990
Syndesmosis, 950
Syndrome of inappropriate antidiuretic hormone (SIADH), 120, 256t, 449–450, 450t
Syndromic cleft palate, 928
Synovial cavity, 950
Synovial fluid, 951
Synovial joints, 952f, 953, 953f, 954f
Synovial membrane, 950
Synovial sarcoma, 1003
Synovitis, 986f
Syphilis, 856t, 857t–859t

Systemic circulation
  anatomy of, 553f, 566, 567f
  arterioles of, 566, 567f
  blood vessel structure in, 566–568
  bronchial circulation, 655
  capillaries, 566, 567f
  function of, 552
Systemic exertional intolerance disease, 996
Systemic immune system, 164
Systemic inflammatory response syndrome (SIRS), 628–629
Systemic lupus erythematosus, 209–210
Systemic scleroderma, 1038
Systemic vascular resistance, 564
Systole, 554
Systolic blood pressure, 571
Systolic compressive effect, 575
Systolic heart failure, 616

T

Tadalafil, 854
Talipes, 1008t
Tamm-Horsfall protein, 724
Tamponade, 607
TAPVC. See Total anomalous pulmonary venous connection
Tarceva (erlotinib), 263t
Tardive dyskinesia, 371
Target cells, for hormones, 429–431, 430f, 448–449
Taste, 347, 347f, 348b
Tay-Sachs disease, 419
TBI. See Traumatic brain injury
TBW. See Total body water
T-cell-independent antigens, 172, 172f
T-cell receptors, 141
T cells (T lymphocytes), 146
  autoreactive, 199
  CD4+, 195–196
  clonal diversity generation and, 164, 166t
  cytotoxic, 158, 171, 171f, 220
  description of, 158
  development of, 166–167
  differentiation sites of, 160f
  functions of, 172–174
  helper, 158, 168–170, 170f, 220
  in immune response, 164–172
  lymphokine-secreting, 173
  regulatory, 158, 173–174
  subsets of, 170, 170f
  thymus as origin of, 164–172
Tears, 343, 344f
Tegmentum, 310–311
TEL-AML1 gene, 296
Telangiectasia, 1025f
Telencephalon (cerebral hemispheres), 306–307, 307f
Telomerase, 246, 246f
Telomeres, 246, 246f
Temporal fossa, 313
Temporal lobe, 307f, 308
Temporal summation, 304
Tenase complex, 494
Tendinopathy, 969–970, 970f

Tendons, 961, 962f
Teniae coli, 872, 872f
Tension pneumothorax, 674
Tension-type headache, 399, 399t
Tentorium cerebelli, 314
Terminal duct lobular units, 818
Tertiary hyperparathyroidism, 457
Testes
  aging and, 782
  anatomy of, 777–778, 777f, 778f
  cancer of, 268t–271t, 839–840, 839b, 839f
  development of, 787
  ectopic, 837–838
  function of, 777
  torsion of, 838, 838f
  tumours of, 839, 839f
Testes-determining factor, 765
Testicular appendages, 838
Testosterone
  androgens and, 844, 849
  functions of, 764t, 781
  libido and, 781
  in sexual differentiation, 766
  in stress response, 225t–226t
Tetralogy of Fallot, 638–639, 639f, 643–644, 643f
Tet spells, 643–644
Teva-Doxycycline (doxycycline), 795b
TFPI. See Tissue factor pathway inhibitor
TF. See Tissue factor
TGA. See Transposition of great arteries
TGF-β. See Transforming growth factor-beta
TGV. See Transposition of great vessels
Thalamus, 309–310
Thalassemias, 502t, 507
  α-, 543–545
  β-, 543–545, 545f
  in children, 543–545
  discovery of, 543–545
  sickle cell, 540–543
Th1 cells, 170, 220
Th2 cells, 170, 220
Th17 cells, 170
Theca cells, 772
Thelarche, 767, 787
T-helper cells, 683
Therapeutic hyperthermia, 337
Thermoregulation. See also Fever
  disorders of, 337–338
  in elderly, 336
  in infants, 336
  mechanisms of, 335, 336t
  trauma and, 338
Thiamine deficiency, 620
Thiazides, 725t
Thimerosal, 190–191
Third-degree block, 623t–624t
Third-degree burns, 1043t, 1044, 1044f
Third order neurons, 312
Thoracic aortic aneurysms, 589
Thoracic cavity, 657, 658f
Thoracic duct, 576, 576f
Thoracolumbar division, 319–322
3-Day Measles, 1057–1058, 1058f, 1058t

Thrombin time, 495t–497t
Thromboangiitis obliterans, 590–591
Thrombocytes. *See* Platelets
Thrombocythemia, 528–529
Thrombocytopenia, 258
Thrombocytopenia, 526–528
Thrombocytosis, 528–529
Thromboembolic disease, 526
Thromboembolic disorders, 533–534, 533f
Thromboembolus, 580–581
Thrombolysis, 396
Thrombomodulin, 495
Thrombophilia, 533
Thrombopoietin, 491
Thrombosis, 526. *See also* Deep venous thrombosis
  arterial, 590
  microvasculature, 529
Thrombospondin-1, 247
Thrombotic crisis, 542
Thrombotic strokes, 395
Thrombotic thrombocytopenic purpura (TTP), 528
Thromboxane A_2 (TXA_2), 146
Thrombus, 533–534, 533f
  venous, 580–581
Thrush, 1057
Th1 to Th2 shift, 220
Thymus, T cells from, 164–172
Thyroid carcinoma, 457
Thyroid gland
  aging and, 444b
  anatomy of, 436, 436f
  C cells of, 436, 436f
  disorders of, 453–455
    carcinoma, 457
    central, 453
    Graves' disease, 455, 455f
    hyperthyroidism, 453–455, 454f, 455f
    hypothyroidism, 455–457, 456f, 457f
    nodular thyroid disease, 455
    primary, 453
    secondary, 453
    subclinical thyroid disease, 453
    thyrotoxic crisis, 455
    thyrotoxicosis, 453–455, 454f, 455f
  follicle cells of, 436, 436f
  hormones of
    actions of, 437, 437t
    creation of, 437
    regulation of, 436–437, 437t
Thyroid-stimulating hormone (TSH), 335, 428, 432, 433f, 435t
  deficiency of, 451
  regulation of, 436–437, 437t
Thyroid storm, 455
Thyrotoxic crisis, 455
Thyrotoxicosis, 453–455, 454f, 455f
Thyrotoxic periodic paralysis, 996
Thyrotropin-releasing hormone (TRH), 428, 435t
  regulation of, 436–437, 437t

Thyrotropin-stimulating hormonereleasing hormone, 335–336
Thyroxine, 428
Thyroxine-binding globulin, 437
Tidemark, 952
Tight junctions, 13–14, 561
Tinea capitis, 1056–1057, 1057f
Tinea corporis, 1057
Tinea unguium, 1049
Tinnitus, 346
TIPS. *See* Transjugular intrahepatic portosystemic shunts
Tissue factor (TF), 140
Tissue factor pathway inhibitor (TFPI), 494
Tissue factor pathway, of clotting system, 140
Tissue hypoxia, 503
Tissue inhibitors of metalloproteinases, 946t
Tissue macrophages, 875
Tissue plasminogen activator, 495
Tissues
  connective tissues, 32t–34t
  epithelial tissues, 30t–31t
  formation, 28, 29f
  granulation, 152–153
  micro-organisms causing damage to, 178, 179t
  muscle tissues, 34t–35t
  regeneration of, 151
  types, 28
  wound healing formation of, 152–155
Tissue-specific antigens, 204–205
Tissue-specific hypersensitivity reactions, 202t, 204–205, 206f
Tissue thromboplastin, 494
Titin, 562, 958t
Titratable acid, 128f
TLRs. *See* Toll-like receptors
T lymphocytes. *See* T cells
Tonicity, 21, 21f
TNF-α. *See* Tumour necrosis factor-alpha
TNM staging, 259–260, 260f, 696–700
Tobacco. *See* Smoking, tobacco
Tolerance, 209
Toll-like receptors (TLRs), 141–142, 142t
Toloxin (digoxin), 619
Tongue, glossitis and, 506f
Tonic phase, 366
Tonsil cancer, 268t–271t
Tonsillar abscesses, 703
Tonsillar infections, 703
Tophaceous gout, 993
Tophi, 991
Torsemide, 725t
Torsion
  intestinal obstruction from, 890t
  of ovaries, 799
  of penis, 757
  of testes, 838, 838f
Torus fractures, 965–966, 966t
Total anomalous pulmonary venous connection (TAPVC), 645–646, 645f
Total body surface area, in burns, 1042–1046, 1043f

Total body water (TBW)
  in adolescents, 130tb0050
  age-related changes in, 113, 113t
  body weight in relation to, 113, 113t
  in children, 130tb0050
  distribution of, 113–114, 113t
  in elderly, 130tb0050
  in infants, 130tb0050
Total iron-binding capacity, 495t–497t
Total peripheral resistance, 564, 572
Total resistance, 570
Touch, 347
Tourette syndrome, 371, 371b
Toxic adenoma, 455
Toxic epidermal necrolysis, 1034
Toxic gas exposure, 677
Toxic multinodular goitre, 455
Toxic myopathies, 999, 999b
Toxins, bacteria secreting, 162
Toxoids, 190
TP53 (tumour protein p53), 244, 245f, 248
Trabeculae, 947, 947f
Trabecular bone score, 978
Trachea, anatomy of, 654–655, 654f, 656f
Tracheitis, 703, 706t
Tracheoesophageal fistula, 928–929, 929f
Trachoma, 344
Traction, of fractures, 968
Trait anger, 222b
Transcalvarial herniation, 368b, 368f
Transchondral fractures, 966t, 967
Transcortical dysphasia, 360
Transferrin, 480, 490, 878t
Transferrin saturation, 495t–497t
Transfer RNA (tRNA), 41
Transformation, of cancer cells, 237–238
Transformation zone, 770
Transforming growth factor-beta (TGF-β), 144, 153, 946t
Transforming growth factors, 144
Transfusion reactions, 210–211
Transgenerational phenotypes, 273t
Transient ischemic attacks, 395
Transient regional osteoporosis, 976
Transitional cell carcinoma, 736
Transjugular intrahepatic portosystemic shunts (TIPS), 906
Translocations, chromosome
  oncogene activation by, 239, 241f
Transmural myocardial infarction, 602, 603f
Transplant rejection, 211–213
Transport maximum, 721–722
Transposition of great arteries (TGA), 644–645
Transposition of great vessels (TGV), 644–645, 645f
Transthoracic echocardiography (TTE), 610
Transudative pleural effusion, 675, 675t
Transverse colon, 871–872, 872f
Transverse fibres, 308
Transverse fractures, 965–968, 966f, 966t
Transverse tubules, 956–957
Trastuzumab (Herceptin), 263t

Trauma
  skeletal, 965–968
  thermoregulation and, 338
Traumatic brain injury (TBI)
  closed, 383–386, 384t
  complications of, 387
  definition of, 383
  diffuse axonal injuries and, 384t, 386
  focal brain injury, 383–386, 384t, 385f
  open, 384t, 386
  primary, 383–387
  secondary, 384t, 387
Treitz ligament, 868, 868f
Tremors, 372t
Trendelenburg gait, 1013
TRH. See Thyrotropin-releasing hormone
Triamterene, 725t
Trichinella larvae, 997
Trichomoniasis, 856t, 857t–859t
Tricuspid regurgitation, 612
Tricuspid valve, 554, 554f, 555f
  atresia of, 644, 644f
Trigeminal autonomic cephalalgias, 399
Trigeminal nerve, 321t
Trigone, 718, 719f
Triiodothyronine, 428, 437t
Trimethoprim-sulfamethoxazole, 738b
Trisomy 21. See Down syndrome
Trisomy 13 syndrome, 638t
Trisomy 18 syndrome, 638t
Trisomy 21 syndrome, 638t
Trochlear nerve, 321t
Tropism, 183
Tropomyosin, 562, 562f
Troponin C, 562
Troponin I, 562, 604
  CAD and, 597
Troponin T, 562
Troponin-tropomyosin complex, 562, 562f, 563f
Trousseau phenomenon, 256t
True aneurysms, 589, 589f
True vocal cords, 654
Truncus arteriosus, 646, 646f
Trypanosoma brucei, 188
Trypanosoma cruzi, 188
TSH. See Thyroid-stimulating hormone
TTE. See Transthoracic echocardiography
TTP. See Thrombotic thrombocytopenic purpura
Tuberculin skin test, 691
Tuberculosis
  clinical manifestations of, 691
  definition of, 691
  evaluation of, 691
  granuloma with, 150f, 151
  Indigenous people in Canada and, 195b
  latent infection of, 691
  pathophysiology of, 691
  risk factors of, 691
  treatment of, 691
Tubular carcinoma, 825t
Tubular reabsorption, 720, 723f
Tubular secretion, 720, 723f

Tubuloglomerular feedback, 719
Tubulointerstitial fibrosis, 731–732
Tubulus rectus, 778, 778f
Tumour-associated macrophage, 250–251, 253
Tumour-infiltrating lymphocytes, 252
Tumour markers, 260–261, 260t
Tumour necrosis factor-alpha (TNF- α), 630b
Tumour necrosis factor-alpha (TNF-α), 142, 221b
Tumour protein p53 (TP53), 244, 245f, 248
Tumours
  of adrenal medulla, 260, 473–474
  angiogenesis induced by, 247f
  benign. See Benign tumours
  bladder, 736
  bone tumours. See Bone tumours
  chondrogenic, 1003
  chromaffin cell, 473
  classification of, 234–235, 261
  clear cell, 736
  of CNS, 405–407
    brain, 405–408, 405f, 407t, 408t
  collagenic, 1003–1004
  dormancy of, 824–825
  embryonal, 422–424
  estrogen-secreting, 472
  giant cell, 1003
  inflammation promotion by, 249–251, 250t
  initiation of, 235–237
  intestinal obstruction from, 890t
  malignant, 234–235, 235f
  muscle, 1004–1005
  myelogenic, 1004
  neuroendocrine, 695t, 696–700
  nomenclature for, 234–235
  osteogenic, 1002–1003
  ovarian, 810f
  pancreatic, in children, 940
  of penis, 835
  of pituitary gland, 453
  progression of, 235–237
  promotion of, 235–237
  renal, 736, 736f
  skin, 1025f
  spinal cord, 408–409
  testicular, 839, 839f
  Wilms, 296, 760, 760t
Tumour-suppressor genes
  childhood cancers associated with, 295, 296t
  deactivation of, 243f
  familial cancer caused by function loss of, 244t
  functions of, 242, 242t
  retinoblastoma gene and, 244
  silencing, 243f
  TP53, 244, 245f
Tunica albuginea, 778, 778f
Tunica externa, 566, 569f
Tunica intima, 566, 569f
Tunica media, 566, 569f
Tunica vaginalis, 777–778, 778f
Turbulent blood flow, 570–571, 571f

Turner's syndrome, 638t
T wave, 559, 560f
TXA$_2$. See Thromboxane A$_2$
Turner's syndrome, 48f
Tylenol. See Acetaminophen
Tympanic cavity, 345
Tympanic membrane, 345, 345f
Tyrosine kinase inhibitors, 241
Tyrosine kinases, 430, 430t

U

Ubiquitin–proteasome system, 9–10, 74
Ulcerative colitis (UC), 898t, 899
Ulcerative cystitis, 737
Ulcers
  duodenal, 894–895, 894f
Ulcers
  curling, 895
  Cushing, 895
  duodenal, 895t
  gastric, 895, 895t
  ischemic, 895
  peptic. See Peptic ulcer disease
  pressure, 1024–1029, 1024b, 1024f
  skin, 1027f
  stress, 895
  surgical treatment of, 895–896
  venous stasis, 580, 581f
Ultraviolet radiation, 285–287, 1022
Umbilical cord blood, antibodies in, 174b
Uncal herniation, 368b, 368f
Unconjugated bilirubin, 876
Underactive bladder syndrome, 734
Unicornuate uterus, 787f
Unilateral neglect syndrome, 358–360
Unintentional and intentional injuries, 92–95, 93t–94t
Unipolar neurons, 301
Universal donors, 211
Unsaturated fatty acids, 869b
Unstable angina, 601–602, 602b, 603f
Upper airway
  anatomy of, 654, 656f
  infections of, in children, 702–703, 702t
Upper esophageal sphincter, 864
Upper gastro-intestinal bleeding, 886
Upper motor neuron gait, 378–379
Upper motor neuron paresis/paralysis, 374–375, 375b
Upper motor neurons, 311
Upper motor neuron syndromes, 374–376, 374t, 375b, 375f, 376f
Upper respiratory tract infections, 180t–181t
Upregulation, 429
UPR. See Unfolded-protein response
UPS. See Ubiquitin–proteasome system
Urate, 991, 991t
Urea, 724, 725t
  CKD progression and clearance of, 750, 750t
Ureaphil, 725t
Uremia, 744
Uremic syndrome, 744
Ureterocele, 757

Ureterohydronephrosis, 731–732, 732f
Ureteropelvic junction obstruction, 758
Ureterovesical junction obstruction, 758
Ureters, anatomy of, 718–719
Urethra
    anatomy of, 718–719, 719f
    partial obstruction of, 734–735
Urethral strictures, 734, 833
Urethritis, 833
Urge incontinence, 733t
Uric acid, 991, 991f
Uric acid stones, 733
Urinalysis, 727–729, 727t, 727t–728t
Urinary bladder. *See* Bladder
Urinary calculi, 732
Urinary incontinence, 733t, 761–763, 762t
Urinary system
    disorders, in children. *See* Children, urinary system disorders in
    structures, 718–719
Urinary tract infection (UTI)
    acute cystitis, 737–738
    antibiotic resistance and, 738b
    causes of, 737
    in children, 760–761, 760b
    complicated, 737
    mechanisms of, 743f
    uncomplicated, 737
Urinary tract obstruction
    anatomical obstructions in, 734–736
    definition of, 731
    kidney stones, 732–733, 739t
    lower, 733–736, 733t
    major sites of, 731f
    neurogenic bladder, 734, 734t, 739t
    overactive bladder syndrome, 734
    upper, 731–733, 731f, 732f
Urination (micturition), 718
Urine
    ADH and aldosterone regulating, 720, 721f
    chemistry, 1075t–1078t
    composition of, 724
    concentration of
        countercurrent exchange system and, 723–724, 724f
        in Loop of Henle, 722–724
    diuretics and flow of, 725, 725t
    flow, anatomical obstructions to, 734–736
    glomerular filtration and, 720–724, 723f
    myoglobin in, 970–972
    postvoid, 735
    properties of, 727t
    tubular reabsorption and, 720, 723f
    tubular secretion and, 720, 723f
Urine antigen testing, 690
Urobilinogen, 876
Urodilatin, 116–117, 720
Urodynamic tests, 727t–728t
Uroflowmetry, 727t–728t, 735
Urokinaselike plasminogen activator, 495
Uromodulin, 724
Urticaria (hives), 203–204, 204f, 1038
Urticarial lesions, 1038
Urushiol, 159–161

Usual ductal hyperplasia, 813–814
Uterine cancer, 268t–271t
Uterine fibroids, 800–801, 800f
Uterine phases, of menstrual cycle, 774
Uterine tubes, 771
Uterus
    abnormal bleeding of, 790–791, 791t
    abnormalities of, 786, 787f
    anatomy of, 769–771, 769f, 770f
    bicornuate, 787f
    corpus of, 769, 770f
    double, 787f
    fundus of, 769
    isthmus of, 769, 770f
    positions of, 769, 770f
    prolapse of, 797, 797f
    unicornuate, 787f
    wall of, 769–770, 770f
UTI. *See* Urinary tract infection

V

Vaccinations
    fears with, 190–191
    in HIV, 199
    immune response from, 190
    mass, 190
    purpose of, 190
    rabies, 198
Vaccines, 190
Vagina
    anatomy of, 767–768, 768f
    cancer of, 268t–271t, 805–806
    double, 787f
    fornix of, 768
    menstrual cycle response by, 775
    pH of, 769, 796
    prolapse of, 799b
    self-cleansing action of, 769
    wall of, 768
Vaginismus, 811
Vaginitis, 796
Vaginosis, 796, 856t, 857t–859t
Vagus nerve, 321t
Valsalva manoeuvre, 873
Valvular aortic stenosis, 639–640
Valvular dysfunction, 609–612, 610t, 611f
Valvular hypertrophic cardiomyopathy, 608–609
Valvular regurgitation, 609–612, 610t, 611f
Valvular stenosis, 609, 610t, 611f
Vaprisol, 725t
Vaptans, 449–450
Vardenafil, 854
Varicella, 1036, 1058t, 1059, 1059f
Varices, 906, 906f
Varicose veins, 580, 581f
Variocele, 836–837, 837f
Variola, 1059
Vasa recta, 717, 724
Vasa vasorum, 566
Vascular compliance, of blood vessels, 571
Vascular dementia, 364t
Vascular endothelial growth factor (VEGF), 152, 246

Vascular endothelium, 552, 566–567, 569f, 570t
Vascular malformations, 397
Vascular mimicry, 824–825
Vascular niche, 485, 486f
Vascular permeability, 137
Vas deferens, 780f
Vasectomy, prostate cancer risk and, 844
Vasoactive intestinal peptide, 225t–226t, 866t
Vasoactive intestinal polypeptide, 423
Vasoconstriction, 566
    hypoxic pulmonary, 656
Vasoconstrictor hormones, 573–574
Vasodilation, 137–138, 566
Vasodilator hormones, 574
Vasogenic edema, 368–369
Vasogenic shock, 389, 626–627
Vasomotor flushes, 782
Vaso-occlusive crisis, 542
Vasopressin, 449–450
    blood pressure affected by, 557f, 574
Vasopressin blockers, 725t
VDLs. *See* Very-low-density lipoproteins
VEDP. *See* Ventricular end-diastolic pressure
VEDV. *See* Ventricular end-diastolic volume
Vegetables, 845b–846b
Vegetative state, 357–358
VEGF. *See* Vascular endothelial growth factor
Veins
    anatomy of, 567, 569f
    blood pressure in, 574
    chronic venous insufficiency of, 580
    coronary, 556, 558f
    distension of, 580
    lymphatic, 577
    renal, 717
    saphenous, 580
    valves in, 564, 570f
    varicose, 580, 581f
Venereal warts, 1036
Venezuelan encephalitis, 401t
Venous sinuses, 484
Venous stasis ulcers, 580, 581f
Venous thrombi, 533
Venous thromboembolism, 591t
Venous thrombosis, 256t
Ventilation. *See also* Breathing
    alveolar, 658
    alveolar surface tension and, 661
    chemoreceptors in, 660
    definition of, 658
    distribution of, 663, 664f
    lung receptors in, 659–660
    maintaining adequate, 661–662, 663f
    muscles of, 660–661, 660f
    neurochemical control of, 659–660, 659f
    noninvasive positive-pressure, 676
Ventilation-perfusion mismatch, 672–673, 673f
Ventilation-perfusion ratio, 663, 672–673, 673f
Ventilator-associated pneumonia, 688, 689b
Ventral horn, 311
Ventral respiratory group, 659
Ventricles, 314
    of heart, 554, 554f
Ventricular block, 623t–624t

Ventricular bradycardia, 622t–623t
Ventricular end-diastolic pressure (VEDP), 564
Ventricular end-diastolic volume (VEDV), 564, 564f
  myocardial infarction effects on, 616–617
Ventricular fibrillation, 622t–623t
Ventricular remodelling, 616
Ventricular septal defect, 642
Ventricular standstill, 622t–623t
Ventricular system, 314–316
Ventricular tachycardia, 622t–623t
Venules
  functions of, 552
  lymphatic, 576
  systemic circulation, 566
Vermiform appendix, 871–872, 872f
Vermis, 310–311
Vertebral arteries, 316–317, 317f
Vertebral body osteoporosis, 975f
Vertebral column
  anatomy of, 316, 316f
  spinal cord in, 311, 312f
Vertebral fractures, 389t, 397
Vertebral injuries, 387–394, 389f, 389t
Vertigo, 347
Very-low-density lipoproteins (VLDLs), 595
Vesicle, 1025f
Vesico-sphincter dyssynergia, 734
Vesicoureteral reflux, 739t
  in children, 761, 761f
Vesiculobullous diseases, 1033–1034, 1034f
Vestibular nystagmus, 347
Vestibule, 345, 345f, 346f
  in female reproductive system, 768, 768f
Vestibulitis, 796–797
Vestibulocochlear nerve, 321t
Vestibulospinal tract, 311
Viagra, 854
Video urodynamics, 727t–728t, 735
Villi, 868f, 869
Viral conjunctivitis, 344
Viral diseases
  description of, 183–185
  examples of, 184t
  opportunistic, 199b
  stages of, 185f
Viral encephalitis, 420
Viral hepatitis, 912, 913t
Viral infections, 1035–1036
  in children, 1054–1057, 1054f, 1055f, 1059–1060
Viral meningitis, 400, 420
Viral pneumonia, 690, 707–708, 708t
Virchow triad, 533, 580–581
Virilization, 472, 473f
Viruses
  attenuated, 190
  cancer associated with, 251
  cellular effects of, 183–185
  life cycle of, 185f
  pathogenicity of, 183
  poliovirus, 190
Visceral pain, 333–334, 886
Visceral pleura, 657, 658f

Visfatin, 903b
Vision. See also Eye
  aging changes in, 348b
  colour, alterations in, 343
  diabetic retinopathy impact on, 467–468, 467t, 468f
  dysfunctions of, 341–343
    neurological disorders causing, 343, 344f
  elderly changes in, 348
  overview of, 340–344
Visual acuity alterations, 341–343, 342f, 342t
Vitamins
  B, 276–278
  B_{12}
    deficiency of, 503–504
    oral replacement of, 504
  D, 437–438, 944t
    bone and, 979b
    deficiency, 743
    kidneys and, 725–726
    supplementation of, 751
  E, 845b–846b
  K, 944t
    deficiency, 530
    liver storage of, 877
    small intestine absorption of, 871b
Vitreous humour, 340–341, 342t
Vocal cords
  false, 654, 656f
  true, 654
Volatile acid, 124
Volkmann canals, 947–948, 948f
Volkmann ischemic contracture, 973
Volume-sensitive receptors, 117–118
Voluntary muscles, 954
Voluntary phase of swallowing, 864
Vomiting, 356–357, 883–884, 889
von Willebrand factor (vWF), 492
Vulva, 767–768, 768f
Vulvar cancer, 806
Vulvar cancer, 268t–271t
Vulvitis, 796–797
Vulvodynia, 796–797
Vulvovestibulitis, 796–797
Vulvovestibulitisdynia, 796–797
vWF. See von Willebrand factor

W

Waist-hip ratio, 823
Wallerian degeneration, 302
Wandering, 372t
Warts, 1036, 1036f
Water. See also Total body water
  balance
    ADH regulating, 116–118, 117f
    alterations in, 118–121, 118t, 119f
    hypertonic alterations to, 118–120, 119f
    hypotonic alterations to, 119f, 120–121
    isotonic alterations to, 118, 119f
    maintenance of, 116–118
  burns and evaporative loss of, 1042–1046
  CKD progression and sodium balance with, 750t

Water (Continued)
  gaining of, 114t
  intoxication with, 120
  loss of, 114t
  movement of
    alterations in, 114–116
    between ECF and ICF, 114
    between plasma and interstitial fluid, 114, 115f
  small intestine absorption of, 871b
Water-soluble hormones, 428–429, 429t
Watson–Crick model, 40f
Weak acid, 124
Weight gain, in Cushing's syndrome, 470–471, 471f
Weight loss
  in cachexia, 255–258
  leukemia and, 516t
  postgastrectomy, 896–897
Weight loss surgery, 905
Wenckebach block, 623t–624t
Wernicke area, 307f, 308
Wernicke dysphasia, 360, 362t
Western equine encephalitis, 401t
West Nile virus, 401–402, 401t
West's syndrome, 421t
Wheal, 1025f
Wheal and flare reaction, 203–204, 204f
White adipose tissue, 256–257
White graft, 212
White matter, 306–307
White muscle, 955, 957t
White reflex, 424
Whole blood clotting time, 495t–497t
Wilms tumour, 296, 760, 760t
Wilson's disease, 939, 939t
Wirsung duct, 877
Wiskott-Aldrich syndrome, 192t, 193
Wolffian ducts, 765, 765f
Wolff-Parkinson-White syndrome, 623t–624t
Women. See also Female reproductive system
  microvascular angina and, 599b
  stroke prevention in, 395b
Work of breathing, 661–662, 663f
World Health Organization, cancer prevention strategy of, 272b
Wound healing
  cancer and, 238
  diabetes mellitus and, 153
  drug effects on, 153
  dysfunctional, 153
  fibrin deposition in, 153
  fibroblasts in, 153
  inflammation phase of, 152, 152f
  macrophages in, 146, 152
  maturation phase of, 153
  new tissue formation phase of, 152–155
  nutrition and, 153
  obesity delaying, 153
  open, 152
  primary intention, 151, 151f
  proliferative phase of, 152–155
  remodeling phase of, 153
  secondary intention, 151f, 152

Wounds. *See also specific wounds*
  contraction of, 154–155
  dehiscence and, 153–154
  disruption of, 153–154
  infections of, 180t–181t

X

Xanthelasmas, 599–601
Xanthine stones, 733
Xenobiotics, 278
Xenoestrogen, 823
Xeroderma pigmentosum, 244–245

X-linked inheritance, 54–56
  pedigrees characteristics, 55
  recurrence risks, 56, 56f
  sex determination, 55, 55f
  sex-limited and sex-influenced traits, 55–56
  X inactivation, 54–55, 54f
X-linked SCID, 192–193, 192t
Xolair (omalizumab), 684
X-ray absorptiometry, 975

Y

Yawning, 356–357

Z

Zeranol, 823
Z line, 561–562, 562f
Zoledronic acid, 980–981
Zollinger-Ellison syndrome, 893–897
Zona fasciculata, 440, 441f
Zona glomerulosa, 440, 441f
Zona reticularis, 440, 441f
Zoonotic infections, 180t–181t, 183

PREFIXES AND SUFFIXES USED IN MEDICAL TERMINOLOGY

Prefix	Meaning	Suffix	Meaning
a-	Without, not	-al, -ac	Pertaining to
acantho-	Spiny, thorny	-algia	Pain
af-	Toward	-aps, -apt	Fit; fasten
an-	Without, not	-arche	Beginning; origin
ante-	Before	-ase	Signifies an enzyme
anti-	Against; resisting	-blast	Sprout; make
auto-	Self	-centesis	A piercing
bi-	Two; double	-cide	To kill
blast-	Immature cell, embryonic	-clast	Break; destroy
circum-	Around	-crine	Release; secrete
co-, con-	With; together	-cytosis	Increase in number
contra-	Against	-ectomy	A cutting out
crine-	Secrete, separate	-emesis	Vomiting
de-	Down from, undoing	-emia	Refers to blood condition
dia-	Across; through	-flux	Flow
dipl-	Twofold, double	-gen	Creates; forms
dys-	Bad; disordered; difficult	-genesis	Creation, production
ecto-	Displaced, outside	-gram	Something written
ef-	Away from	-graph(y)	To write, draw
em-, en-	In, into	-hydrate	Containing H_2O (water)
endo-	Within	-ia, -sia	Condition; process
epi-	Upon, above	-iasis	Abnormal condition
eu-	Good	-ic, -ac	Pertaining to
ex-, exo-	Out of, out from	-in	Signifies a protein
extra-	Outside of	-ism	Signifies "condition of"
hapl-	Single	-itis	Signifies "inflammation of"
hem-, hemat-	Blood	-lemma	Sheath, covering
hemi-	Half	-lepsy	Seizure
hom(e)o-	Same; equal	-lith	Stone; rock
hyper-	Over; above	-logy	Study of
hypo-	Under; below	-lunar	Moon; moonlike
infra-	Below, beneath	-malacia	Softening
inter-	Between	-megaly	Enlargement
intra-	Within	-metric, -metry	Measurement, length
iso-	Same, equal	-oid	Like; in the shape of
juxta-	Near	-oma	Tumour
macro-	Large	-opia	Vision, vision condition
mega-	Large; million(th)	-oscopy	Viewing
mes-	Middle	-ose	Pertaining to, sugar
meta-	Beyond, change, after	-osis	Condition, process
micro-	Small; millionth	-ostomy	Formation of an opening
milli-	Thousandth	-otomy	Cut
mono-	One (single)	-penia	Lack
necro-	Death	-philic	Loving
neo-	New	-phobic	Fearing
non-	Not	-phragm	Partition
oligo-	Few, scanty	-plasia	Growth, formation
ortho-	Straight; correct, normal	-plasm	Substance, matter
para-	By the side of; near	-plasty	Shape; make
per-	Through	-plegia	Paralysis
peri-	Around; surrounding	-pnea	Breath, breathing
poly-	Many	-(r)rhage, -(r)rhagia	Breaking out, discharge
post-	After	-(r)rhaphy	Sew, suture
pre-	Before	-(r)rhea	Flow
pro-	First; promoting	-some	Body
quadri-	Four	-tensin, -tension	Pressure
re-	Back again	-tonic	Pressure, tension
retro-	Behind	-tripsy	Crushing
semi-	Half	-ule	Small, little
sub-	Under	-uria	Refers to urine condition
super-, supra-	Over, above, excessive		
trans-	Across; through		
tri-	Three; triple		